For Reference

Not to be taken from this room

W9-AEM-570

GRACE LIBRARY CARLOW UNIVERSITY
PITTSBURGH PA 15213

PHARMACOTHERAPEUTICS
for Nurse Practitioner Prescribers

Anita Lee Wynne, PhD, FNP-C
Associate Professor of Nursing
School of Nursing
University of Portland
Portland, Oregon
and
Family Nurse Practitioner
Urgency Care
Kaiser-Permanente HMO
Portland, Oregon

Teri Moser Woo, RN, MS, CPNP
Pediatric Nurse Practitioner
Kaiser Permanente Northwest Region
and
Adjunct Clinical Faculty
Oregon Health Sciences University
School of Nursing
Portland, Oregon

Michael Millard, MS, RPh
Director of Pharmacy
Sacred Heart Medical Center
Eugene, Oregon
and
Assistant Professor of Pharmacy Practice
Oregon State University
Corvallis, Oregon

Ref.
RM
300
W96
2002

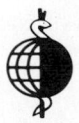 **F. A. DAVIS COMPANY** • Philadelphia

CATALOGUED

GRACE LIBRARY CARLOW UNIVERSITY
PITTSBURGH PA 15213

F. A. Davis Company
1915 Arch Street
Philadelphia, PA 19103
www.fadavis.com

Copyright © 2002 by F. A. Davis Company

All rights reserved. This book is protected by copyright. No part of it may be reproduced, stored in a retrieval system, or transmitted in any form or by any means, electronic, mechanical, photocopying, recording, or otherwise, without written permission from the publisher.

Printed in the United States of America

Last digit indicates print number: 10 9 8 7 6 5 4 3 2

Acquisitions Editor, Nursing: Joanne Patzek DaCunha, RN, MSN
Developmental Editor: Diane Schweisguth, RN, BSN
Production Editor: Stephen D. Johnson
Cover Designer: Louis J. Forgione

As new scientific information becomes available through basic and clinical research, recommended treatments and drug therapies undergo changes. The authors and publisher have done everything possible to make this book accurate, up to date, and in accord with accepted standards at the time of publication. The authors, editors, and publisher are not responsible for errors or omissions or for consequences from application of the book, and make no warranty, expressed or implied, in regard to the contents of the book. Any practice described in this book should be applied by the reader in accordance with professional standards of care used in regard to the unique circumstances that may apply in each situation. The reader is advised always to check product information (package inserts) for changes and new information regarding dose and contraindications before administering any drug. Caution is especially urged when using new or infrequently ordered drugs.

Library of Congress Cataloging-in-Publication Data
Wynne, Anita Lee, 1941–
    Pharmacotherapeutics for nurse practitioner prescribers / Anita Lee Wynne, Teri Moser Woo, Michael Millard.
       p. cm.
    Includes bibliographical references and index.
    ISBN 0-8036-0535-8 (alk. paper)
    1. Pharmacology. 2. Therapeutics. 3. Nurse practitioners. I. Woo, Teri Moser, 1962– . II. Millard, Michael, |
1949– . III. Title.
    RM300 .W96 2001
    615'.1—dc21
                                                                                              00-060152

Authorization to photocopy items for internal or personal use, or the internal or personal use of specific clients, is granted by F. A. Davis Company for users registered with the Copyright Clearance Center (CCC) Transactional Reporting Service, provided that the fee of $.10 per copy is paid directly to CCC, 222 Rosewood Drive, Danvers, MA 01923. For those organizations that have been granted a photocopy license by CCC, a separate system of payment has been arranged. The fee code for users of the Transactional Reporting Service is: 8036-0535/02 0 + $.10.

To my loving husband and my esteemed colleagues at the University of Portland, without whose patience and support this book never would have been completed; to my parents, who consistently taught me to shoot for the stars; and to my children and grandchildren, who daily make my life complete.

ALW

I would like to dedicate this book to my family. My husband, John, and my three sons, Michael, Patrick, and Nicholas, have been wonderfully supportive as I have completed this project.

TMW

To my wife and children, who really wanted me to do this and did everything in their power to make it easy for me. To all the pharmacists and nurses who are trying to make the lives of their patients better.

MM

RIT $ 105.00 HF-05 Credits

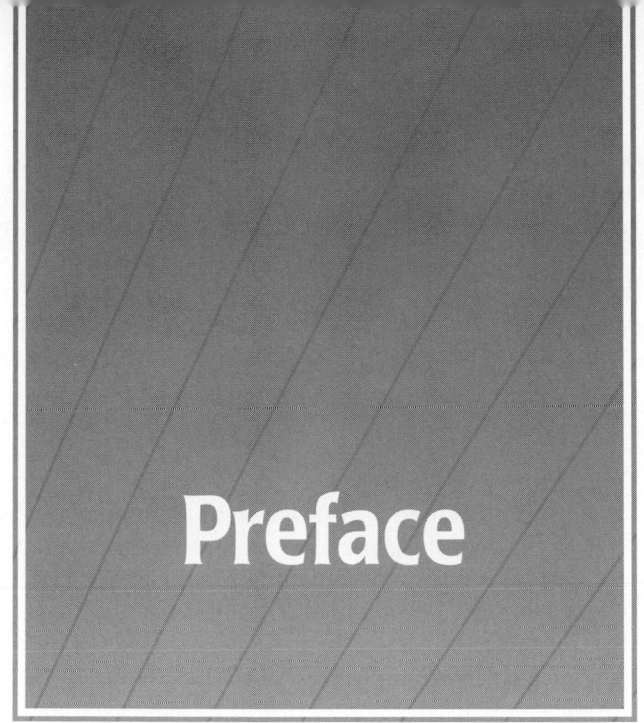

Preface

*T*he increasing volume of pharmacology-related information presents a challenge to acquire and maintain current knowledge in the area of pharmacotherapeutics. The number of new drugs coming on the market each year, the changes in "the best" drugs to use for any given disease state based on the latest research, the influence on patient and practitioner alike of advertising and promotion, and the increasing incursion of managed care and restricted formularies into practice decisions about drug selection is phenomenal. This book is designed to provide nurse practitioner students and the nurse practitioner in the primary care setting with a thorough, current, and usable pharmacology text and reference to address this challenge.

The design of this book assumes knowledge of basic pharmacology from one's undergraduate education in nursing. Although a brief review of basic pharmacology is presented in **Chapter 2,** the focus of the book is on advanced pharmacology and the role of the advanced practice nurse in pharmacotherapeutics. The authors of the text are practicing nurse practitioners or selected specialists in a field. The book is by nurse practitioners, for nurse practitioners.

Organization

This book is organized around four distinct content areas: The Foundation, Pharmacotherapeutics with Single Drugs, Pharmacotherapeutics with Multiple Drugs, and Special Drug Treatment Considerations.

The Foundation

The 11 chapters in **Unit I** provide the foundation of advanced pharmacology and the link between this knowledge and professional practice. **Chapter 1** discusses the role of the nurse practitioner as prescriber and the knowledge needed to actualize this role. Factors involved in clinical judgment related to prescribing are a central focus, and collaboration with other health care providers is also presented.

The pharmacology knowledge required for rational drug selection requires more depth than that given in undergraduate pharmacology, where the focus is on safe administration of drugs prescribed by someone else. Advanced pharmacology information on receptor reserve and regulation, bioavailability and bioequivalence, metabolism of drugs including a focus on the cytochrome P450 microsomal enzyme system, half-life, and steady state are provided in **Chapters 3 and 5.** New information not normally covered in undergraduate nursing courses but central to the prescribing role includes an in-depth discussion of volume of distribution and therapeutic drug monitoring. Volume of distribution is important in prescribing drugs with very large or very small volumes of distribution and for selecting drugs for patients with cardiac or renal failure, during pregnancy, or when a patient is underweight or obese. Knowing what tests to order and when to order them to assess plasma drug levels by bioassay and to monitor for adverse drug reactions are necessary to make choices about when or if dosage alterations are required or drugs need to be stopped. These are also covered in **Unit I.**

Legal aspects of the prescriber role are presented in **Chapter 4.** Issues surrounding the legal authority of a nurse practitioner to prescribe a drug, the conditions under which the prescription may be written, and how to write the prescription are presented. Risk management issues are also discussed including informed consent, dealing with multiple providers, and substance abuse and drug-seeking behaviors.

Nurse practitioners have a history of high levels of patient satisfaction with the care provided. This is related, in part, to their holistic approach to each patient. Several chapters are devoted to information that reflects this approach. Cost, knowledge deficits, dealing with complex treatment regimens, and negotiating a shared responsibility for drug management are discussed in **Chapter 6.** Many patients choose to use complementary therapies such as herbal remedies. **Chapter 9** discusses these complementary therapies and provides a list of resources in this area.

A relatively new area in pharmacotherapeutics is ethnopharmacology. As more research is occurring in this area, treatment guidelines are beginning to include which drugs are best for different racial groups. Cultural considerations in prescribing drugs as well as racial differences in patient responses to drugs are the subject of **Chapter 7.**

Consideration of drug and food interactions has long been a part of nursing knowledge, but the interrelationship between nutrition and drug therapy beyond these interactions has been largely missed. **Chapter 8** provides an in-depth discussion of this interrelationship including nutritional supplementation and nutrition as therapy.

In an age of increasing use of technology, the nurse practitioner must be able to acquire information about drugs and to deliver care to patients using this technology. **Chapter 10** focuses on computers and the Internet as sources of information and for care delivery. Especially helpful is a large table that presents up-to-date sites for drug information from government, commercial, organizational, and other sources. Where it is possible to determine, each site has a discussion of its content, reliability, frequency of update, link to other sites, charges or fees, and who is the "owner or operator" of the site. If the site is supported by advertising, this is also mentioned. Telehealth, the use of telecommunications technology to provide health care services, as well as the future use of information technology in obtaining drug-related information and the delivery of health care services, is also included.

Over-the-counter drugs may be prescribed by the practitioner or chosen by patients on their own. These drugs are often erroneously perceived to be less powerful and having fewer adverse reactions than prescription drugs. Understanding their role in pharmacotherapeutics is the focus of **Chapter 11.**

Pharmacotherapeutics With Single Drugs

The next two units are organized around specific drugs and the diseases they are used to treat. The chapters in **Unit II** are organized to provide easy access to information based on specific drug classes. Many practitioners have a personal formulary of drugs they use for disease processes that they commonly see. When presented with a patient requiring drug therapy, they know the class of drug from which they will make a rational drug choice. The information they seek is about drugs within that class that would be most appropriate for this patient.

Pharmacokinetics, pharmacodynamics, and pharmacotherapeutics for each drug class are discussed. Tables with easy-to-access information on pharmacokinetic properties of each drug, drug interactions, clinical use and dosing, and available dosing forms are presented. There is a major focus on rational drug selection and on monitoring parameters. Patient education specific to each drug class is provided—designed around administration of the drug, adverse drug reactions to monitor for and what to do if they occur, and lifestyle modifications that complement the drug therapy.

To provide the most up-to-date, accurate, and relevant information possible, contributors to this unit are practicing clinicians. Clinical pearls drawn from the daily practice world of these contributors are incorporated throughout the text. Drugs currently in development that may influence drug choices in the near future are also included in the "On the Horizon" feature.

Pharmacotherapeutics With Multiple Drugs

Unit III chapters provide access to drug information from the viewpoint of the disease processes they are commonly used to treat. Patients often have complex health and illness issues and treatment needs. Nurse practitioner students find these especially perplexing, and these patients may have disease processes that extend beyond those a given nurse practitioner commonly sees. The knowledge the student or practitioner needs to select the appropriate drug to treat a given disease may be limited. Unit III facilitates acquisition of this knowledge by providing access to information from a disease process format. The diseases in this unit are those commonly seen in primary care and for which multidrug therapy from more than one drug class may be recommended.

Pharmacotherapeutics is discussed in relation to the pathophysiology of the disease and the goals of treatment. Each chapter explores how patient variables, economic considerations, concurrent diseases, and drug characteristics influence rational drug selection. Outcome evaluation is presented with guidelines for consultation and referral. Where relevant professional guidelines exist, they are incorporated. Each patient is unique and no set of guidelines or treatment algorithm applies to each patient. However, these tools, drawn from the clinical knowledge and experience of experts in a given specialty, are helpful in rational drug selection, especially for the student and novice practitioner. Clinically based case studies in each chapter also provide a framework for application of pharmacotherapeutic knowledge.

Special Drug Treatment Considerations

Unit IV focuses on special populations. Age-related variables are explored in the chapters on pediatric and geriatric patients, and variables specific to women are discussed in the women-as-patients chapters. Information on safe prescription of drugs for lactating patients is often difficult to find, and tables with the most current information on the effect of drugs on the nursing infant are found in the pediatric chapter. The prevalence of chronic illness is increasing as acute illnesses that formerly accounted for most of the morbidity and mortality in developed countries have been eradicated or come under control. The last chapter in the text discusses the modification of pharmacotherapeutics in patient populations with chronic illness or in long-term care facilities.

Features

Throughout the text, care has been taken to provide the reader with a consistent and logical presentation of material. Visual appeal is provided through the generous use of tables, illustrations, and flowcharts. Other features are unique to the specific units:

Unit I chapters

In-depth pharmacology base for advanced pharmacotherapeutics
Herbal therapies
Ethnopharmacology
Nutrition as therapy
Information technology and telehealth

Unit II chapters

Tables for ease of access to information
    Pharmacokinetics tables
    Drug Interactions tables
    Dosage Schedule tables
    Available Drug Dosage Forms tables
Rational drug selection and monitoring parameters
Patient Education
Clinical Pearls
On-the-Horizon feature

Unit III chapters

Integration of pathophysiology and pharmacotherapeutics
Integration of professional treatment guidelines
Drugs Commonly Used tables
Patient Education displays
Case Study displays

Unit IV chapters

Variables related to special populations

Summary

Every effort has been made to make this text as comprehensive, accurate, and user friendly as possible. The generous use of tables for ease of access to information, the focus on rational drug selection, the inclusion of often hard to find monitoring parameters, and the integration of patient education throughout the text are examples of this user-friendly approach. The authors hope that you will find this a valuable resource both as a student and in your practice.

ALW

TMW

MM

Acknowledgments

I would like to acknowledge my mentors at the OHSU School of Nursing who have supported me throughout my nursing career. They include Dr. Sheila Kodadek, Dr. Pam Hellings, and Dr. Cathy Burns, as well as many other fine faculty mentors.

TMW

About The Authors

Anita Lee Wynne, PhD, FNP-C

Anita Lee received her Bachelor of Science in nursing from San Diego State University, a Master of Science in Nursing with a focus in Adult Health from the University of Colorado Health Science Center, and a Master of Public Health and PhD with a focus in Health Behavior from the University of Oklahoma College of Health. She received her Family Nurse Practitioner preparation at Gonzaga University in the Post Master's Certificate Option program. Her 25 years of teaching experience include baccalaureate and master's degree programs in Oklahoma and Oregon, and her favorite teaching areas are pathophysiology, pharmacotherapeutics, and health assessment. She is currently teaching in the Family Nurse Practitioner graduate program at the University of Portland and practicing in Urgency Care for Kaiser Permanente in Portland, Oregon.

Teri Moser Woo, RN, MS, CPNP

Teri has been a pediatric health care provider for 15 years. She received her MSN in Childrearing Family Nursing in 1989 and a Post-Masters Pediatric Nurse Practitioner Certificate in 1993. She has taught undergraduate nursing students, precepted nurse practitioner students, and lectured in nurse practitioner courses. Teri was president of the Oregon Pediatric Nurse Practitioner Association from 1998–2000.

Michael Millard, MS, RPh

Mike has had a wide variety of experiences in many various types of health systems, from 80-bed inpatient psychiatric hospitals to large HMO medical centers. He achieved his master's degree in clinical pharmacokinetics and has been on the faculty of OSU College of Pharmacy, as a preceptor for clinical and administrative clerkships. Mike has been a nurse educator since 1975 at both the community college and university level. He has been involved with the education of nurse practitioners since 1985 and is committed to the success of these critical health care providers

Contributors

Danita Lee Ewing, RN, MS
Doctoral Student and Graduate Research Assistant
Oregon Health Sciences University
Portland, Oregon
Adjunct Faculty
University of Portland
Portland, Oregon

Karen Groth, MN, RN, CS, FNP
Assistant Professor
Department of Nursing
Gonzaga University
Spokane, Washington

Barbara J. Limandri, DNSc, RN, CS, PMHNP
Associate Professor
Oregon Health Sciences University
School of Nursing
Department of Primary Care, Mental Health Nursing Division
and
Private Practice
Hamilton House
Portland, Oregon

Karen W. Loveless, RN, MSN, ANP
Nurse Investigator
The Research and Education Group
Portland, Oregon

Patricia M. McChesney, MN, RN, PMHNP
Private Practice
Lincoln City, Oregon

Mary K. Miller, MS, ANP-C
Certified Nurse Practitioner
Willamette View Outpatient Clinic
Portland, Oregon

Kay E. Ortman, RN, MN, FNP-C
FNP Preceptor Liaison
Teaching Associate
University of Portland
Portland, Oregon
and
Private Practice
Maple Street Clinic
Forest Grove, Oregon

Ginette A. Pepper, PhD, RN, FAAN
Assistant Professor
University of Colorado Health Sciences Center
School of Nursing
Denver, Colorado

Reviewers

Tom G. Bartol, RN, MN
Family Nurse Practitioner
Richmond Area Health Center
Richmond, Maine
and
Adjunct Faculty
Husson College School of Nursing
Orono, Maine

Karen Griffith, RN, MN, ANP
Adult Nurse Practitioner
Division of Cardiology
Oregon Health Sciences University
Portland, Oregon

Toni Karle, RN, MN, CNS, C-FNP
Chesapeake Family Medical Center
Chesapeake, Ohio

Dawn McElhaney, RN, MSN, CS-ANP, CS-FNP
Family and Adult Nurse Practitioner
Lake County Medical Center
Lakeview, Oregon

Renee McLeod, DNSc(c), RN, CS, CPNP
Pediatric Clinical Faculty
Scripps Mercy Hospital and Clinic
and
Faculty, School of Medicine
University of California, San Diego
San Diego, California

Linda E. Moody, RN, PhD, MPh, FAAN
Professor
College of Nursing
University of South Florida
Tampa, Florida

Mary Ann Notarianni, DNSc, CRNP
Associate Professor
Coordinator, Family Nurse Practitioner Program
College Misericordia
Dallas, Pennsylvania

Stephanie Oetting, RN, MSN
Associate Professor
Director, Generic BSN Program
University of Saint Francis
Fort Wayne, Indiana

Lori Martin Plank, RN, MSPH, MSN, CS, FNP, GNP
Nurse Practitioner, Community Health
St. Luke's Hospital and Health Network
Bethlehem, Pennsylvania
VNA Community Services, Inc.
Abington, Pennsylvania
Adjunct Faculty
The College of New Jersey
Ewing, New Jersey
Doctoral Student
Duquesne University
Pittsburgh, Pennsylvania

Jacqueline Rhoads, RN, PhD, CCRN, ACNP-CS
Professor, Family Nurse Practitioner Program
Louisiana State University Health Sciences Center
School of Nursing
New Orleans, Louisiana

Nancy Ridenour, RN, CS, PhD, FNC, FAAN
Dean and Professor
Illinois State University
Mennonite College of Nursing
Normal, Illinois

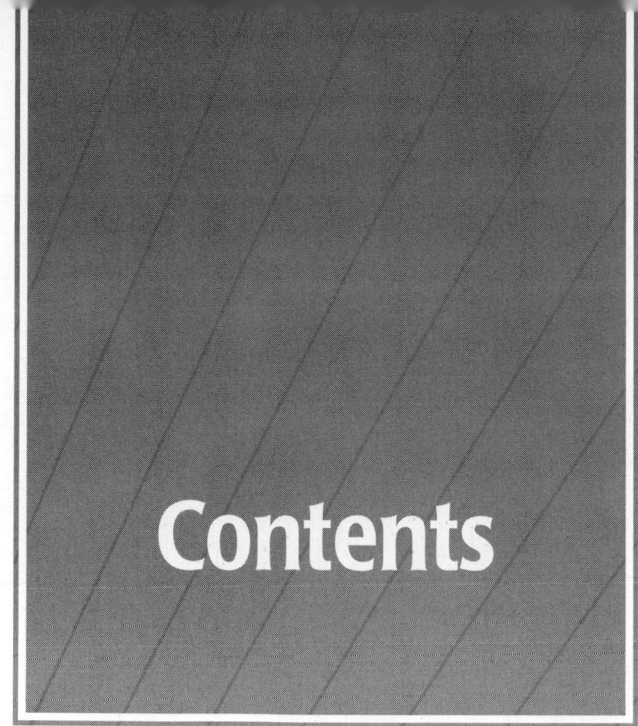

Contents

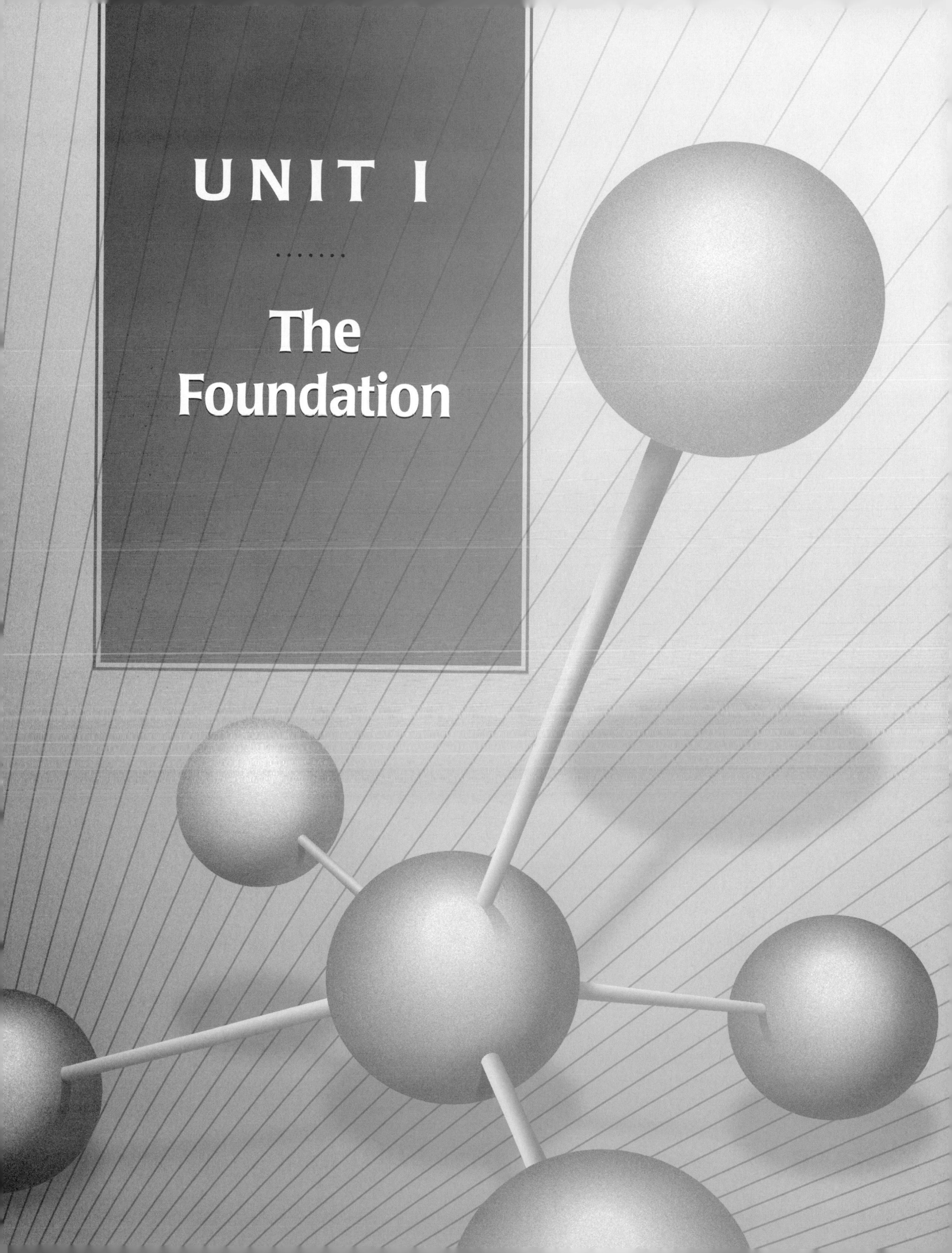

UNIT I

·······

The
Foundation

CHAPTER 1

· · · · · · ·

The Role of the Nurse Practitioner as Prescriber

CHAPTER OUTLINE

Nurses have been administering medications prescribed by another provider for many years. The knowledge base to safely perform this activity has been an integral part of basic nursing programs. With the advent of the advanced practice nurse (APN), especially the nurse practitioner (NP), the role of the nurse in relation to medications evolved to include prescribing the medications as well as administering them. This new role requires additional knowledge beyond that taught in undergraduate nursing programs. More than that, it requires the willingness and ability to assume a different kind of responsibility for this activity.

Roles of Registered Nurses and Advanced Practice Nurses Who Are Not Nurse Practitioners

Registered Nurses Who Are Not Nurse Practitioners

Experienced registered nurses often find themselves in the position of discussing with a physician or other provider which drug a patient should receive. Their input is sought and highly valued. Collaboration of this nature increases the nurse's self-esteem and results in improved patient care as the disciplines of medicine and nursing work together. The responsibility for the final decision, however, remains with the physician or other provider in this case. The role of the registered nurse is advisory only.

Advanced Practice Nurses Who Are Not Nurse Practitioners

Nurses in advanced practice (APNs) have a higher level of responsibility related to pharmacotherapeutics. The nature of this responsibility depends on whether the nurse can prescribe drugs. Often, APNs who are not NPs do not have prescriptive authority. Because they have in-depth knowledge of the drugs used in their specialty area, their collaboration with the health care provider who is prescribing is at a different level than that of the registered nurse. They may assist in determining the pharmacotherapeutic protocols for their patients and select drugs within those protocols to be administered to their patients. These roles related to pharmacotherapeutics represent an intermediate level of responsibility between the registered nurse who administers drugs chosen by another provider and the NP who prescribes a drug without the need for a protocol. APNs also often collaborate with other providers in designing and implementing research protocols to test the efficacy of a new drug. They also have a central role in educating nurses and other providers in the appropriate use of these new drugs.

Roles and Responsibilities of Nurse Practitioners

NPs differ from other APNs in that they have prescriptive authority. The role of the NP as prescriber places in the hands of the NP the responsibility for the final decision of which drug to use and how to use it. The degree of autonomy in this role and the breadth of drugs that can be prescribed vary from state to state, based on the nurse practice act of each state. As of January 1999, 11 states permitted NPs to prescribe, including controlled substances, independent of any required physician involvement in prescriptive authority. All states have some statutory prescribing authority for NPs. Each year the January issue of *The Nurse Practitioner* journal presents a summary of each state's practice acts as they relate to titling, roles, and prescriptive authority.

Knowledge about the pharmacokinetics and pharmacodynamics of drugs, how to safely administer them, and what to teach the patient are learned in undergraduate nursing courses and refined in practice. This knowledge is critical to the decision the NP is about to make, but additional knowledge and responsibility now come into play. The advanced practice role of the NP, while clearly an example of expanded nursing role functions and not "junior doctoring," is, nonetheless, a blending of the disciplines of medicine and nursing. Medical, pharmacological, and nursing kinds of knowledge intertwine in the NP role. It now becomes the role and responsibility of the NP to determine the diagnosis for which the drug will be prescribed and to prescribe the appropriate drug.

Advanced Knowledge

This new role requires advanced knowledge about pathophysiology and medical diagnoses and their relationship to choosing an appropriate drug. Determining the medical diagnosis is not within the scope of this book, but rational drug selection requires knowledge of the disease processes (medical diagnoses) for which a drug may be prescribed and the mechanism of action of a specific drug and how it affects this disease process. Rational drug selection is discussed throughout the book.

This new role also requires advanced pharmacology knowledge beyond that taught in undergraduate education. Knowledge required for rational drug selection includes bioequivalence and cost for deciding whether to use a generic form of a given drug, the enzyme systems used to metabolize a drug for deciding about potential drug interactions, and the pharmacokinetics of a drug for determining the loading, maintenance, and tapering doses. The terms may sound familiar, but the underlying depth of information and the role of this information in determining the best drug to prescribe are beyond basic knowledge. Volume of distribution, for example, receives little discussion in undergraduate pharmacology texts, but it is often critical in determining dosage for drugs with very large or small volumes of distribution and in selecting drugs for patients with cardiac or renal failure, pregnant patients, or patients who are underweight or obese. Assessment of plasma drug levels by bioassay may be familiar, but the use of this knowledge to determine whether a drug should be prescribed or the prescription altered will be new. The registered nurse may know a given drug's effect on renal functioning, but the prescribing NP needs to know what tests to order and when to order them to appropriately monitor that functioning, as well as when or if to alter the dosage or stop the drug. Diagnostic tests and their role in drug monitoring will be new. Additional knowledge is also needed about prescriptive authority. Does the chosen drug fit within the legal authority of an NP to prescribe in this state? What are the conditions under which the prescription may be written, and how does one correctly write it? What constraints may be in place because of the patient's health insurer or lack of health insurance?

Benefits of a Nurse Practitioner as Prescriber

Although the focus of this book is on pharmacotherapeutic intervention, other treatment options are also part of the NP armamentarium to treat a given disorder and often interact with the pharmacotherapeutic intervention to provide the desired outcome. Common therapies that may be chosen as treatment options or that are integral to drug therapy are integrated throughout the drug-specific and disease-specific chapters. Some of them have traditionally been part of what all nurses teach, and they remain central to the role of the NP: for example, lifestyle management issues for a cardiac patient, relaxation techniques for a patient experiencing stress, and appropriate exercise for a patient with low back pain or arthritis. Herbal therapies have been part of the health practices of people for a long time, but only recently have health care providers acknowledged them and considered them in planning treatment. If the NP chooses to use herbal therapy or the patient is using this therapy from another provider, the NP must have reliable information sources about this therapy. Nutrition is also a common issue in nursing, but often the nurse's knowledge of nutrition related to pharmacology is limited to food-drug interactions or the low-sodium diet for a patient with hypertension. The NP uses more in-depth knowledge about nutrition as therapy.

Choosing among pharmacological and other treatment options also involves advanced knowledge. The right choice depends on accurate information about the patient and his or her situation and about the effects of the alternative treatment options on health outcomes. Choices also depend on the patient's culture, preferences for different health outcomes, attitudes toward taking risks, and willingness to endure morbidity now for some possible future benefit. Characteristic of NPs and their practice are consideration of the whole patient, the joint setting of therapeutic goals, and the inclusion of the patient in each decision about care. This remains a central element in NP practice and is often cited by patients and other providers as a hallmark and distinguishing feature of NP practice. Adherence to a drug treatment regimen has traditionally not been good. Statistics cited often place patient adherence (taking the drugs as prescribed) at less than 50 percent. Research shows that adherence is better for prescriptions given by NPs, and the proposed reasons for the difference are these very issues of consideration of the whole patient and inclusion of the patient in decision making. Another factor in improved adherence is patient education; NPs spend more time than other providers in teaching their patients about their disease process and the relationship of the treatment regimen to it.

Clinical Judgment in Prescribing

Prescribing a drug results from clinical judgment based on a thorough assessment of the patient and the patient's environment, the determination of medical and nursing diagnoses, a review of potential alternative therapies, and specific knowledge about the drug chosen and the disease process it is designed to treat. In general, the best therapy is the least invasive, least expensive, and least likely to cause adverse reactions. Frequently, the choice is nonpharmacological and pharmacological therapies working together. When the choice of treatment options is a drug, several questions arise.

IS THERE A CLEAR INDICATION FOR DRUG THERAPY? In the age of managed care and increased awareness of the limitations of drugs, this has become an important question. For example, in treating otitis media there is controversy about the use of antibiotics. A high percentage of otitis media infections resolve on their own, so how do we know that the antibiotic was the cause of the cure? Antibiotic resistance of organisms is on the rise. Is overtreatment with antibiotics a contributing factor? Before drug therapy is chosen, the indication for using a drug should be thought through carefully.

WHAT DRUGS ARE EFFECTIVE IN TREATING THIS DISORDER? Several drugs are often effective; which is the best one for this unique patient? Even if only the best class of drug is considered, few classes of drugs have only one drug in them. How does one determine "best"; what are the criteria? Are there nationally recognized guidelines that can be used as criteria? The Agency for Health Care Policy and Research (AHCPR), the National Institutes of Health (NIH), and many specialty organizations publish disease-specific treatment guidelines that include both pharmacological and nonpharmacological therapies.

WHAT IS THE GOAL OF THERAPY WITH THIS DRUG? Is it the best drug to achieve that goal? A variety of goals are possible in the choice of any therapy. The goal may be cure of the disease and short-term in nature. If this is the goal, troublesome adverse effects may be better tolerated, and cost may be less of an issue. If the goal is long-term treatment for a chronic condition, adverse effects and cost take on a different level of importance, and how well the drug fits into the lifestyle of the patient can be a critical issue.

UNDER WHAT CONDITIONS IS IT DETERMINED THAT A DRUG IS NOT MEETING THE GOAL AND A DIFFERENT THERAPY OR DRUG SHOULD BE TRIED? At the onset of therapy, monitoring times are established to see how well the drug is meeting the goal. Monitoring parameters are often published for the drug, but they may need to be adjusted, based on the age or concurrent disease processes of the patient. Part of this decision making may include questions about when to consult or refer the patient.

ARE THERE UNNECESSARY DUPLICATIONS WITH OTHER DRUGS THE PATIENT IS ALREADY TAKING? Sometimes drugs from different classes are given together to achieve a desired effect, and this is a therapeutic choice. It may also be that the provider did not notice the overlap, especially if the patient is seeing several different providers. For example, a patient who is on a diuretic to treat hypertension may have potassium supplementation. Another provider may decide to use an angiotensin-converting enzyme (ACE) inhibitor to treat heart failure. An ACE inhibitor can also be used to treat hypertension. Rather than a treatment regimen with three drugs, it may be possible to use a combination of an ACE inhibitor with a diuretic in one tablet and, because ACE inhibitors cause potassium retention, no supplemental potassium would be needed. Any time a regimen can be simplified, adherence is more likely.

WOULD AN OVER-THE-COUNTER DRUG BE JUST AS USEFUL AS A PRESCRIPTION DRUG? Increasing numbers of drugs are being moved from prescription-only to over-the-counter (OTC) status. Often, this results in a significant reduction in cost for the patient. It also can create problems, however, unless the provider takes a good drug history because many patients do not consider these as "drugs" once they are not prescribed.

WHAT ABOUT COST? Who will pay for this drug? Can the patient afford it? What patient advocacy issues does this raise? Will these issues affect adherence to the treatment regimen? Cost is an issue for several reasons. Many insurance policies do not cover the cost of drugs so the patient must pay "out of pocket." The newer the drug, the more likely the cost is to be high, based on the drug manufacturer's need to reclaim research and development costs while the corporation still holds the patent on that drug. Newest is not always best, and consideration of cost may be a major factor in choosing between newer drugs and ones that have been available long enough to be available in generic form. Factors that are likely to lead to poor adherence include a drug that is expensive in relation to a patient's finances, a drug that must be taken daily as part of a complex regimen, and a drug that is not covered by insurance.

WHERE IS THE INFORMATION TO ANSWER THESE QUESTIONS? Nurses have always evaluated sources of drug information and learned which ones to trust. For an NP, the sources of drug information expand to include the drug company representative who visits the clinic, the medical literature that ranges from the well-reputed *New England Journal of Medicine* to what some NPs refer to as "throw-away" literature that can fill the NP's mailbox, the multitude of computerized drug databases, information from the Food and Drug Administration, and the Internet. How reliable is that information, and how can reliability be determined? Is the information source written by someone who may benefit from presenting biased information? Is the information source up to date? Today's "wonder drug" may be removed from the market tomorrow. Is the information relevant to the specific patient for whom the drug will be prescribed? If the information is a research report, what type of research design was used? Are there questions about the validity and reliability of the data? To prescribe drugs appropriately, NPs must be able to answer these questions, and to answer them, they must master sources of information and use them on a regular basis.

Collaboration with Other Providers

No one member of the health care team can provide high-quality care without the collaboration of other team members. The NP most often collaborates with physicians, pharmacists, and other nurses.

Physicians

Collaboration with physicians has been something of a roller-coaster ride for NPs. Early in NP role development, physicians were the teachers in the NP programs and accepted NPs as physician-extenders. As the role of the NP evolved to clearly indicate that it was advanced nursing practice and as legislation made autonomy of practice possible, the role became more adversarial, often for economic reasons. While this struggle still continues at the national level, NPs and physicians must work together on an individual basis. Especially in an era of managed care, our joint concerns about patient care decisions require us to be allies. Physicians have a history as prescribers and can offer suggestions born of experience. Their focus related to pharmacology is on understanding biochemistry and prescribing for a given pathophysiology. Their emphasis is on the disease and the drug, with less emphasis on the impact on the patient. Patient education is limited or left to the nurse or pharmacist. NPs will always approach prescribing drugs in a slightly different manner than physicians. As they prescribe a drug for a given pathophysiology, their nursing background leads them to place equal emphasis on understanding the impact the drug will have on the patient. Patient education is a central focus. Knowledge and clinical experience shared from these two perspectives are mutually beneficial to the providers and the patient. The NP can benefit from the in-depth knowledge about the drugs in the physician's specialty area and from the power base physicians have established in dealing with drug companies. The physician can benefit from NPs' focus on the impact of the drug on the patient and from their patient education skills. In the age of managed care, increasing emphasis is being placed on these latter issues.

Pharmacists

Collaboration with pharmacists requires an understanding of the slightly different preparation and focus of retail pharmacists and clinical pharmacists. Both have basic pharmacological science preparation, but the retail pharmacist, often prepared at the undergraduate level, focuses on securing and dispensing drugs prescribed by health care providers. Patient education about these drugs is also a major emphasis. Clinical pharmacists, often with graduate-level education including the doctorate in pharmacy (PharmD), have more knowledge about pathophysiology and take a more active role in determining the best drug to prescribe. Both can provide the information necessary, such as available dosage forms, potential adverse reactions, and drug interactions, for the NP to choose a drug and write a valid prescription. The clinical pharmacist, like the physician, can add clinical knowledge to the drug choice. Both physicians and nurse practitioners increasingly consult clinical pharmacists for this knowledge. As both retail and clinical pharmacists take on the relatively new role of patient educator, they can benefit from the expertise in this area that NPs bring.

Other Nurse Practitioner Prescribers

Collaboration with other NPs who have prescriptive privileges has two major advantages. On a one-to-one basis dealing with individual patient issues, NPs can share "clinical pearls" from their knowledge base and practice experience to improve the care of the patient and expand the knowledge of the two NPs. On a bigger scale, there is power in numbers. Collaboration on issues related to scope of practice and prescriptive privilege at the state and national level is critical to obtaining and maintaining the autonomy of practice needed to provide optimal patient care.

Advanced Practice Nurses Who Are Not Prescribers

Because they cannot prescribe drugs, these APNs have often had to develop creative nonpharmacological strategies to deal with patient problems. Prescribing a drug is not the only or even always the best therapy. Collaboration at this level can increase the expertise of NPs in a wide range of therapies and make these therapies available to our patients. Those APNs who currently cannot prescribe may want to add prescriptive privilege to their practice. The same power of numbers related to scope of practice and prescriptive privilege issues applies here. It is in the interest of all APNs to work together to foster the optimal scope of practice for both prescribing APNs and nonprescribing APNs.

Other Health Team Members

NPs also regularly collaborate with other nurse colleagues who are not in advanced practice roles. These nurses and their assistants carry out the prescriptive orders of the NP. For each of these care providers, it is important to remember their preparation and knowledge level and their legal responsibility in carrying out the NP's orders. Registered nurses and licensed practical/vocational nurses function under their own licenses. Their preparation and responsibility are defined by the nurse practice act in each state. Whether they can legally take orders from an NP is also delineated in these statutes. When prescribing drugs that others will administer, NPs must know these parameters. Medical assistants, who often have a role in clinics, may have certification in the state that delineates their preparation, but generally they are not licensed. Their knowledge of drugs is very limited, if they have had any formal education in the area of pharmacology at all. When prescribing drugs to be administered by medical assistants, NPs must take care to assure that they clearly understand what they are to do; careful supervision is critical.

Current Issues and Trends in Health Care and Their Effect on Prescriptive Authority

The growth in autonomy and prescriptive authority for NPs is a source of pride. NPs have now successfully overcome the "cannot prescribe," "cannot diagnose and treat," and "cannot admit" prohibitions to practice that have required so much of our time and energy in the past. These gains are not written in stone, however, and can be reversed. Major concerns related to prescriptive authority must continue to be addressed. Turf battles between NPs and physicians at national and many state levels over physician supervision requirements and cosignatures on prescriptions continue. A recent example was the "invitation" by the California Medical Association (CMA) to allow NPs to join as equal dues-paying members. Although it seemed favorable at the outset, the CMA invitation was based on the claim that physicians and NPs share the common goal of "practicing medicine" and that patients accept NPs as legitimate providers because NPs have adopted the medical knowledge base and the medical ethic. Bringing NPs into the CMA would assure an appropriate supervisory arrangement and prevent unsupervised nonphysicians from "pursuing independent and perhaps competitive or adversarial roles with physicians" (Johnson, 1996). The potential transfer of accountability for Medicaid from the federal government to the states also has the potential to jeopardize implementation of federal mandates for services and access to NPs as providers, especially if NPs are seen as primary care providers only to underserved populations that are undesirable for physicians. NPs must be careful that they are not seen as physician-substitutes or physician-extenders, but rather as APNs; otherwise, the current autonomy we enjoy and the level of autonomy we hope to attain may disappear as the number of family practice and other primary care physicians increases.

Private-sector restructuring of health care with a focus on cost control and for-profit groups has both positive and negative potential for the autonomy of the NP. Negatively, this means treatment options and decision making about their use are often transferred to the corporation. This can limit the NP's ability to determine treatment options, and the extra time the NP takes to educate and counsel patients may be seen as a liability rather than an asset. Positively, NPs have demonstrated their ability to control costs and improve patient outcomes. We must continue to conduct research on the ability of NPs to provide competent, cost-effective, high-quality services to improve the health of our patients, whether in NP-only practices or in collaborative practices, and to share the findings of that research with the decision makers in the changing world of health care. Better yet, we must become decision makers.

To do this requires a commitment of time and energy from each NP to work together with other nurses to deal with these issues at local, state, and national levels. Keeping current on new knowledge in pharmacology and on the latest drugs and their clinical applications is only part of the role of nurse practitioner as prescriber. NPs should join and support their professional organizations and engage in positive political activity to maintain the prescriptive authority already gained in each state and to extend autonomous prescriptive authority to all states.

REFERENCES

Brush, B., & Capezuti, E. (1997). Professional autonomy: Essential for nurse practitioner survival in the 21st century. *Journal of the American Academy of Nurse Practitioners, 9*(6), 265–270.

Coeling, H., & Cukr, P. (1997). Don't underestimate your collaboration skills. *Journal of the American Academy of Nurse Practitioners, 9*(11), 515–519.

Ford, V., & Kish, C. (1998). Family physician perceptions of nurse practitioners and physician assistants in a family practice setting. *Journal of the American Academy of Nurse Practitioners, 10*(4), 167–171.

Goroll, A., May, L., & Mulley, A., Jr. (1995). *Primary care medicine* (3rd ed.). Philadelphia: Lippincott.

Hamric, A., Lindebak, S., Worley, D., & Jaubert, S. (1998). Outcomes associated with advanced nursing practice prescriptive authority. *Journal of the American Academy of Nurse Practitioners, 10*(3), 113–118.

Hawkins, J., & Thibodeau, J. (1993). *The advanced practitioner* (3rd ed.). New York: Tiresias Press.

Johnson, B. (1996). Should the CMA allow PAs and NPs to join? *Clinician Reviews, 6*(7), 29–30.

Pearson, L. (1996). Annual update of how each state stands on legislative issues affecting advanced nursing practice. *Nurse Practitioner, 21*(1), 10–22.

Pearson, L. (1999). Annual update of how each state stands on legislative issues affecting advanced practice. *Nurse Practitioner, 24*(1), 16–24.

Walker, P., Baldwin, D., Fitzpatrick, J., Ryna, S., Bulger, R., DeBasio, N., Hanson, C., Haravan, R., Johnson-Pawlson, J., Kelly, M., Lacey, B., Ladden, M., McLaughlin, C., Selker, L., Sluyterm, D., & Vanselow, N. (1997). Building community: Developing skills for interprofessional health professions education and relationship-centered care. *Journal of the American Academy of Nurse Practitioners, 9*(9), 413–418.

CHAPTER 2

· · · · · · ·

Review of Basic Principles of Pharmacology

As recently as the 1920s, most drugs were impure mixtures of only vaguely known composition and primarily of plant and animal origin. A prescriber was required to know only what happened when the drug was administered. How the product produced such effects was beyond the knowledge of the day. Today, a prescriber is required to know the expected benefits, contraindications, likely adverse effects, drug interactions, and the precise mechanism by which the beneficial effects are brought about. Rational drug selection may require choosing among several similar drugs with similar effects and different mechanisms of action.

Rational drug therapy of any patient requires adequate knowledge of the disease, the pharmacodynamic properties of the drug selected, and the pharmacokinetics of the drug (the individual patient's ability to absorb, distribute, metabolize, and eliminate the drug). Basic principles in drug therapy are based on the concept that drugs are molecules with specific characteristic chemical and pharmacokinetic properties, based on basic scientific principles of biochemistry, physiology, organic chemistry, and biochemistry.

The aim of drug therapy is to rapidly deliver and maintain therapeutic, yet nontoxic, levels of drug in the target tissues. To achieve this goal, the clinician must have basic knowledge of onset of action, intensity of drug effect, and duration of drug effect. These factors are controlled by absorption, distribution, and excretion of the drug. First, drug absorption permits entry of the drug into plasma. Second, the drug may then leave the bloodstream and distribute into the interstitial and intracellular fluids. Third, a process consisting primarily of urinary excretion and/or hepatic metabolism causes the drug and its metabolites to be eliminated from the body.

Understanding the time course of drug effects is based on knowledge of the relationship between drug concentration and effect. Drugs act by affecting biochemical and physiological processes in the body. Most drugs act at specific receptors but may produce multiple effects because of the location of the receptor in various organs. Knowledge of these properties helps to predict the behavior of a drug in the body and is an important guide in the selection of appropriate doses and dosage intervals.

A complete presentation of these basic pharmacological principles is beyond the scope of this book. This chapter briefly reviews basic principles for quick reference.

Pharmacodynamics

The pharmacodynamic phase studies the effects of the drugs on the body. This effect is the result of an interaction between the drug and a target cell to produce a therapeutic effect. Most medications are thought to work with a receptor at the site of action. These receptors are found in cell membranes, enzymes, cellular proteins, and constituents of the cells, such as nucleic acids. The combination of the receptor and the drug is the action, and the results are considered the effect of the drug. These effects can be momentary or last for days.

Drug-Receptor Interaction

There is a fundamental hypothesis of pharmacology that a relationship exists between a beneficial or toxic effect of a drug and the concentration of the drug at the site of actions as measured by the concentration in the blood.

This hypothesis has been confirmed for many drugs and is the basis for the determination of effective or toxic concentrations reported in the literature and followed clinically by serum drug level testing. Knowing the relationship between drug concentration and effects allows the clinician to take into account the various pathological and physiological features of a particular patient that make that patient different from the "average" individual, based on clinical trials and mean statistical data.

Drug Receptor Activity

Drugs have an affinity for certain portions of a cell or tissue that can be occupied to cause a certain effect. If the drug is an **agonist,** the drug combines with the receptor that stimulates the target organ. If the drug is an **antagonist,** the drug combines with the receptor but interferes with the naturally occurring agonist or other drug agonists that may be present. The antagonist is not capable of producing a biologic effect (Fig. 2–1).

Through the years, a variety of natural agonists of many different receptors have been identified. These **receptor subtypes** have been noted for a number of therapeutic agents that have selectivity for subtype receptors so that effects can be specific and adverse reactions minimized. For example, several histamine receptors, H_1 and H_2, and catecholamine receptors, alpha$_1$, alpha$_2$, beta$_1$, and beta$_2$, have been identified.

Receptors interact with natural agonists to regulate the functioning of the body. If receptors are continually stimulated by drugs, their responsiveness may be decreased, which is referred to as **down-regulation,** or **desensitization.** This can be due to a decrease in the number of receptors or a change in the existing receptors. Severe down-regulation may result in **refractoriness,** or a lack of response to the drug.

If a receptor's activity is chronically reduced by antagonists, a state of **up-regulation,** or **hypersensitization,** may occur. If the drug is rapidly withdrawn, the receptors react strongly to the natural agonists, resulting in exaggerated response because of the exaggerated response of the supersensitive receptors to the normal amounts of natural agonist. For example, rapid withdrawal of antihypertensives may result in hypertensive episodes.

In most cases, the interaction between a drug and a receptor is temporary, with the drug action ending when the drug leaves the receptor site. This drug-receptor relationship is termed a **reversible agonist.** This principle provides for the relationship between drug concentration and drug effect. When there is a high concentration of drug present, the receptors are frequently stimulated, and as the concentration goes down, fewer receptors are filled, and the drug effect dissipates with time. If a drug occupies a receptor permanently, the interaction is termed **irreversible.**

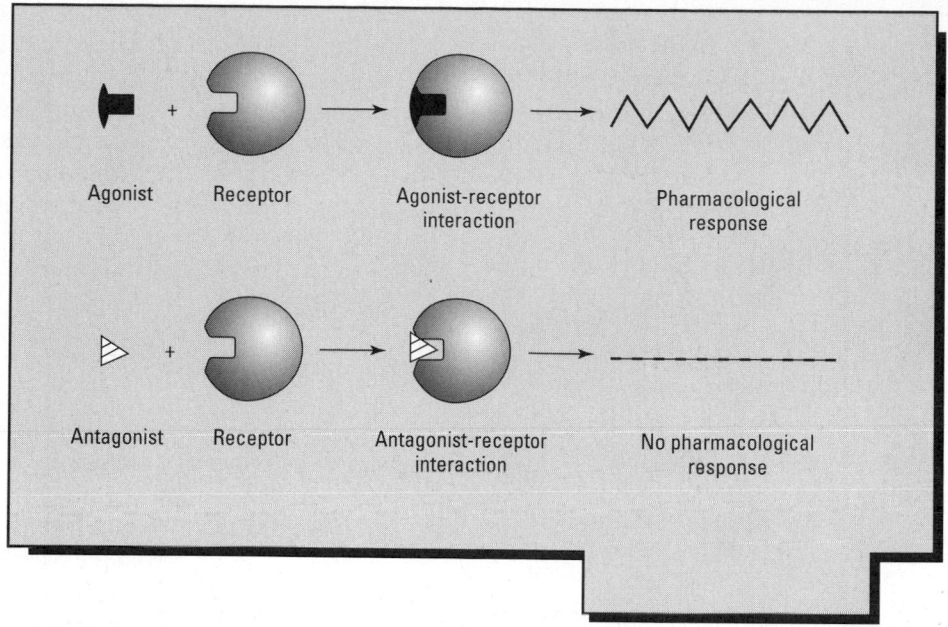

Figure 2–1. Drug receptor activity. (From Kuhn, M. A.: *Pharmacotherapeutics: A Nursing Process Approach*, 4th ed. F. A. Davis, Philadelphia, 1998, p. 46, with permission.)

The same is true if the drug acts as an antagonist; if the binding of drug and antagonist is reversible, the antagonist is called a **competitive antagonist.** This refers to the fact that the effect of the antagonist can be overcome by higher doses of the agonist competing for the receptor site with the antagonist, with the blocking of the receptor overcome by higher concentrations of the drug. If the receptor is irreversibly blocked by the antagonist, then the effect of the antagonist cannot be overwhelmed by the agonist, and the antagonist is a **noncompetitive inhibitor** of the receptor.

The Dose-Response Relationship

In general, the larger the drug dose, the higher the drug concentration at the site of action and the greater the effect of the drug, up to a maximum effect. Further increases in drug dose will not cause further effects because all possible receptor sites are being stimulated by the drug. At this point, a further increase in dose will not increase response; the maximal response has been attained (Fig. 2–2). Once the drug is administered and absorption begins, blood levels start to rise. However, there will be no measurable response until a **minimum effective concentration** of free drug molecules in the blood is reached. The **onset of action** is the time needed for the drug concentration to reach this minimum level. While blood concentration and the intensity of the response are rising toward the peak, absorption rates are greater than elimination rates. The **time to peak** is the

time required for the maximum effect to occur after administration. The fall of blood levels and decreased response reflect metabolism, excretion, and distribution at rates faster than absorption. The **duration of action** is the time during which the blood levels are above the minimum effective concentration.

Therapeutic Index

All drugs elicit more than one response. Some adverse reactions occur at the same doses used to elicit therapeutic responses. On a dose-response curve, the curve representing adverse reactions would overlap the drug-response curve for desirable responses. Ideally, a drug-response curve for desired outcomes does not overlap the curve for undesirable outcomes. This would reduce the patient's risk of an adverse reaction at therapeutic doses. However, this is not the case for most drugs in clinical use. The relationship between a drug's desired therapeutic effects and its adverse effects is called its **therapeutic index** (Fig. 2–3). The therapeutic index is the ratio of the doses required to produce death or serious toxicity in 50 percent of subjects compared with the doses required for effective treatment of 50 percent of subjects. If the difference is wide, several orders of magnitude, then the therapeutic index is wide, the drug is safe, and close therapeutic monitoring is not usually required. If the difference is small, less than 10-fold, then the index is narrow, and close monitoring of doses is needed to prevent adverse reactions in the patient.

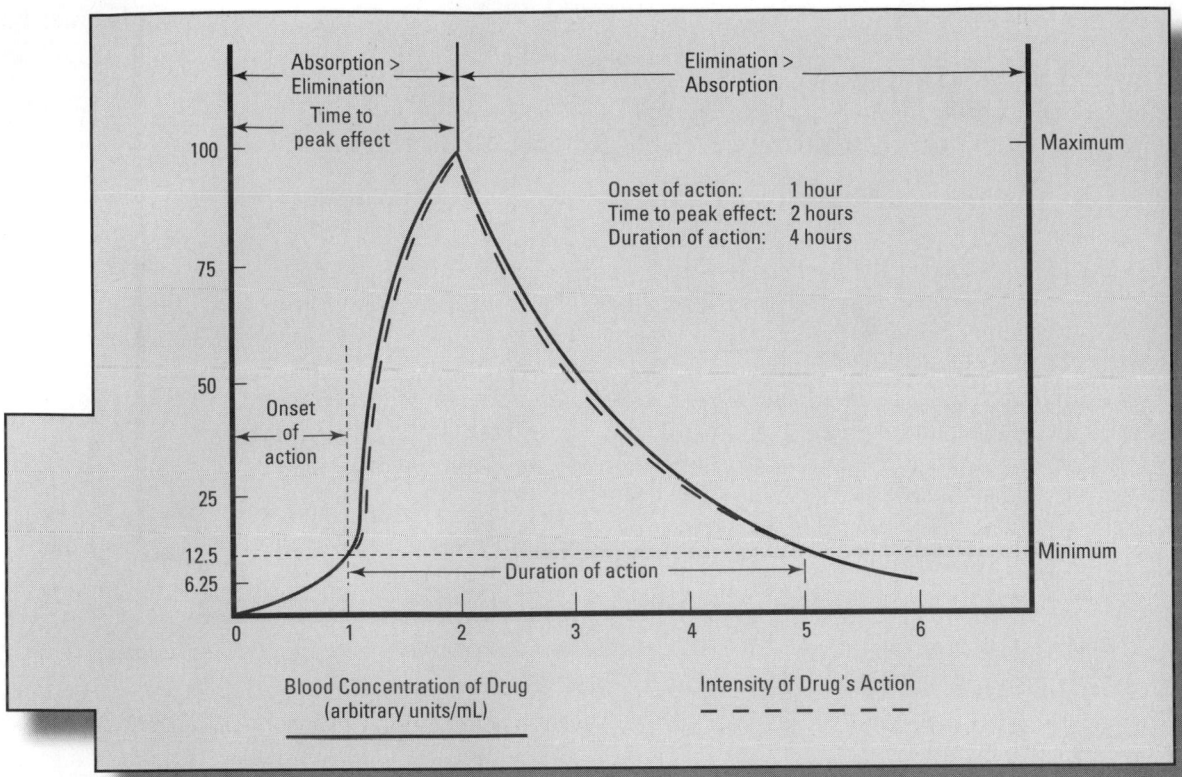

Figure 2–2. The dose-response relationship. (From Shlafer, M.: *The Nurse, Pharmacology, and Drug Therapy: A Prototype Approach,* 2nd ed. Addison-Wesley Nursing, Redwood City, CA, 1993, p. 68, with permission.)

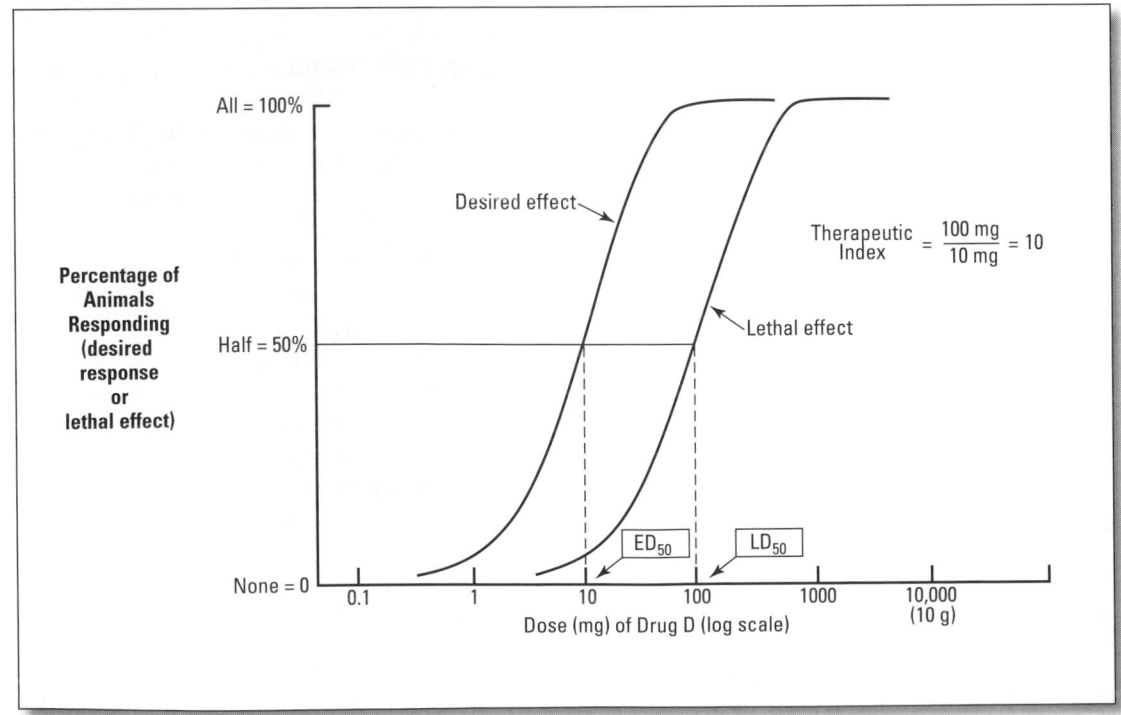

Figure 2–3. The therapeutic index. (From Shlafer, M.: *The Nurse, Pharmacology, and Drug Therapy: A Prototype Approach,* 2nd ed. Addison-Wesley Nursing, Redwood City, CA 1993, p. 82, with permission.)

Drug Potency and Efficacy

The dose response of a drug has two important properties, efficacy and potency. **Efficacy** is measured by the maximum effect that the drug can achieve. **Potency** of a drug is a relative measure that compares the doses of two different drugs that are required to achieve the same effect. A drug is said to be potent when it possesses a high intrinsic activity at low unit doses. Potency is influenced by absorption, distribution, biotransformation, and excretion. When similar drugs with different potencies are switched, the ratio of equi-effective doses needs to be considered.

For clinical use, it is helpful to distinguish between a drug's potency and its maximum effect (Fig. 2–4). The clinical effectiveness of a drug depends not on its potency but on its maximal efficacy and its ability to reach relevant receptors. In deciding which of two drugs to prescribe, the provider must consider their relative maximum effectiveness rather than their relative potency.

Pharmacokinetics

Pharmacokinetics is the study and analysis of the time course of the drug in the body. The ease with which drugs pass through membranes is the key to assess the rates of absorption and extent of distribution throughout the many body compartments. Drugs are transported throughout the circulatory system and end up at tissues and organs where their presence is beneficial and also at some areas where their presence may be detrimental. The principal reasons drugs disappear from the body are (1) elimination of unchanged drug and (2) metabolism to pharmacologically active or inactive chemicals that may be subject, in turn, to further metabolism and elimination.

Drug Absorption

The first stage of pharmacokinetics is drug absorption. Drug absorption includes all the chemical and biologic processes during a drug molecule's progress from the pharmaceutical dosage form to the systemic circulation. To reach the site of action, the drug must be absorbed from the dosage form into the body. There are many important basic pharmacological principles pertaining to drug absorption. The mechanisms of drug absorption are shown in Figure 2–5.

Parenteral Drug Absorption

Parenteral drug formulations are commonly clear solutions of a drug, designed for direct injection. These drug solutions have few absorption problems because they are in solution when given. Drugs injected directly into the venous circulation (intravenous [IV]) begin distribution throughout the body immediately. This is the unique property and advantage of IV administration.

However, drugs for intramuscular (IM) or subcutaneous (SC) administration do undergo absorption from the injection site and are subject to some of the factors affecting oral drug absorption. Although they do not have to dissolve and diffuse through the gastrointestinal (GI) membrane and are not affected by the first-pass effect, they are affected by blood flow to the site of injections. Some IM preparations are formulated in oil or as a suspension to prolong absorption and provide a pro-

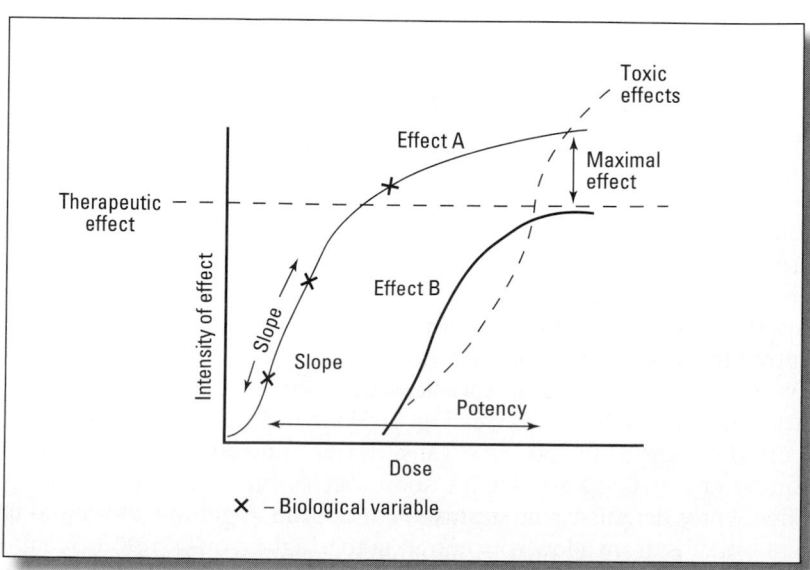

Figure 2–4. Drug potency and maximal effect. (From Kuhn, M. A.: *Pharmacotherapeutics: A Nursing Process Approach,* 4th ed. F. A. Davis, Philadelphia, 1998, p. 48, with permission.)

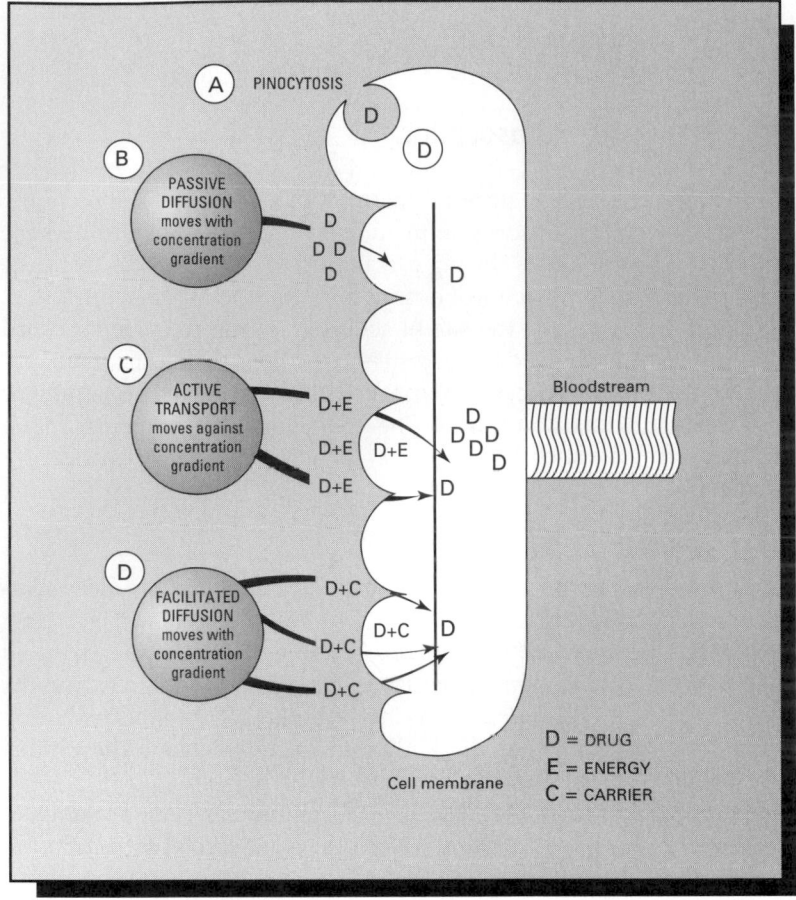

Figure 2–5. Mechanisms of drug absorption. (From Kuhn, M. A.: *Pharmacotherapeutics: A Nursing Process Approach,* 4th ed. F. A. Davis, Philadelphia, 1998, p. 39, with permission.)

longed drug effect. These preparations cannot be given IV because of the risk of pulmonary emboli with the insoluble drugs and ingredients.

Oral Drug Absorption

The active drugs must dissolve in liquid and be available in solution because the body cannot absorb solids. Oral drug absorption is the most common type of drug absorption, and oral dosage forms comprise most of the medications given to patients. In most cases, drug absorption across membranes occurs in the same manner as nutrient absorption from foods. **Passive diffusion** includes simple diffusion, convective absorption, and carrier-mediated diffusion; requires no energy expenditure; and can be described as drug movement from an area of high concentration to an area of lower drug concentration. Most drugs are absorbed by passive diffusion. Only un-ionized lipid-soluble drugs diffuse well. Other absorption processes (see Fig. 2–5) are important to certain drugs or in specific organs. **Active transport** requires energy and an active transport mechanism and is frequently demonstrated against a concentration gradient—that is, from a low concentration to a higher concentration of drug molecules. Active transport is used in

the absorption of electrolytes and some drugs such as levodopa. **Pinocytosis** is a form of active transport in which the cell engulfs the drug particle in a lipid vacuole and transports it across the cell membrane. Pinocytosis is commonly used to transport fat-soluble vitamins across the cell membrane.

EFFECT OF pH ON ORAL ABSORPTION. Drug molecules can pass through the cell membrane if they are un-ionized; that is, they do not have an electrical charge. The local pH of the GI tract and the chemical nature of the drug (pK_a) will determine how much of the total drug concentration is un-ionized (Fig. 2–6). For example, theophylline and phenytoin are weak acids and are mostly un-ionized in an acid environment such as the stomach. Therefore, absorption occurs mostly in the stomach. Conversely, quinidine is a weak base and is un-ionized in a basic environment such as the intestine, where most of its absorption occurs. For example, a weak base ($pK_a = 7$) in the low-pH environment of the stomach is highly ionized, with a ratio of ionized to un-ionized of 5000:1. Most of the drug cannot be absorbed. In the higher-pH environment of the intestine, the ratio of ionized to un-ionized changes to 1:10. In this situation, 90 percent of the drug is available for absorption in the intestine. The site of absorption determines which fac-

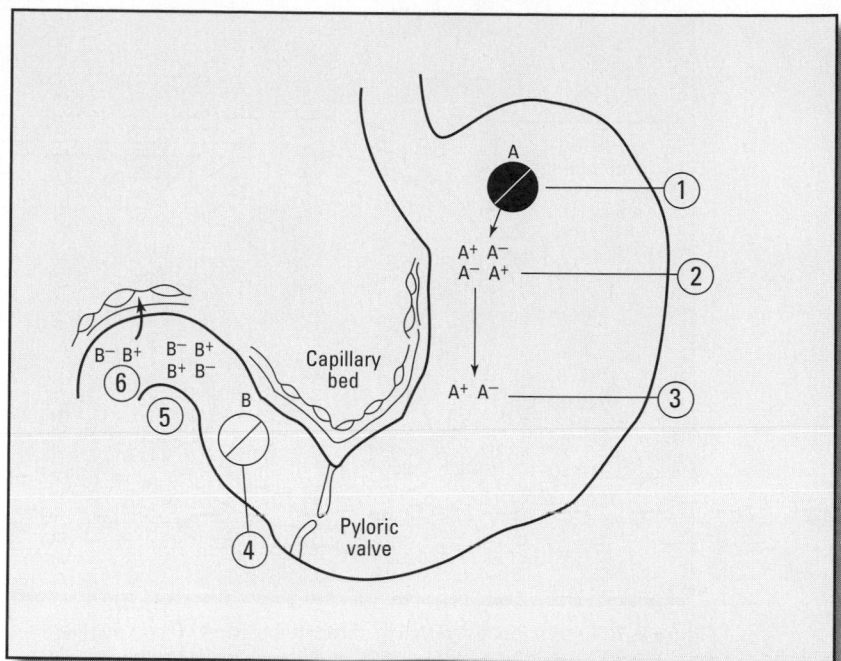

Figure 2–6. Effect of pH on oral absorption. (From Kuhn, M. A.: *Pharmacotherapeutics: A Nursing Process Approach,* 4th ed. F. A. Davis, Philadelphia, 1998, p. 39, with permission.)

tors, such as gastric emptying time and intestinal motility, will have an effect on a specific drug's absorption.

MOTILITY OF THE GUT. Most absorption of orally administered drugs occurs in the small intestine, where the mucosal villi provide the largest surface area in the GI tract. If the intestinal transit time is reduced or sections of the intestine have been removed, drug absorption is significantly reduced. The gastric emptying time and the intestinal transit time affect the total drug absorption by changing the drug contact time with the intestinal mucosa. Rapid transit through the part of the GI tract most favorable for drug absorption reduces absorption, and prolonged contact through slowing transit increases absorption. Solid, high-fat foods prolong gastric emptying and delay drug delivery to the intestine for absorption. Anticholinergics prolong intestinal transit time and may increase total drug absorption. Laxatives decrease intestinal transit time, thereby decreasing drug absorption.

Blood Flow

Drug absorption depends on normal blood flow past the absorptive surface. For oral administration, food stimulates gastric blood flow and absorption, and physical exercise, by diverting blood to the muscles, decreases GI blood flow and lowers absorption. If blood flow is reduced by cardiac disease, then IM medications are absorbed more slowly from the injection site.

First-Pass Metabolism

The metabolism of a part of the administered dose of a drug before it reaches the systemic circulation is referred to as the *first-pass metabolism.* Orally administered drugs move through the portal vein into the liver before passing into the general circulation. For some drugs, a clinically significant portion of the drug taken is destroyed by this method, so that the oral dose required for a given effect is much higher than for other routes that do not use the portal circulation (parenteral or sublingual). For example, propranolol has a recommended oral dose of 40 to 120 mg and an equivalent intravenous dose of 1 to 3 mg because of the first pass metabolism of portal circulation. Drugs with clinically significant first-pass metabolism include dopamine, lidocaine, propranolol, imipramine, morphine, reserpine, nitroglycerin, isoproterenol, and warfarin.

Enterohepatic Recycling

After being absorbed, drugs move through the bloodstream and return to the liver for metabolism. Some drugs leave the liver circulation and enter the biliary tract to be excreted in bile, eventually returning to the intestine and becoming available for reabsorption through the intestinal wall back into the bloodstream. Each day, 80 percent of bile is reabsorbed, so the active drug or metabolites recirculate for a long time. Some of the drug may go to the kidney for renal elimination. This process is defined as *enterohepatic recycling* (Fig. 2–7).

Bioavailability

The combination of inert ingredients determines the disintegration, dissolution, and drug availability in the body, and different combinations can result in different

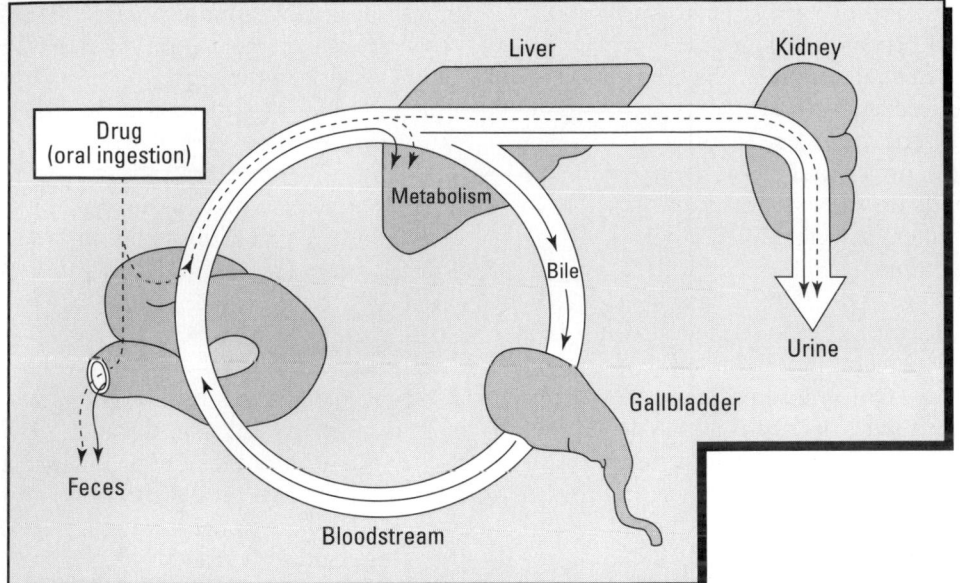

Figure 2–7. Enterohepatic recycling. (From Kuhn, M. A.: *Pharmacotherapeutics: A Nursing Process Approach,* 4th ed. F. A. Davis, Philadelphia, 1998, p. 45, with permission.)

clinical effects among products of the same labeled potency. The amount of the drug dose that reaches the systemic circulation determines its bioavailability. A product that is not completely absorbed or is eliminated by the liver in its first pass has low bioavailability. Differences in bioavailability may be evident between two products that contain the same amount of drug but result in two different plasma concentrations. The total amount of drug reaching the systemic circulation is reflected by the area under the curve (AUC) of a plasma concentration versus the time curve. Comparisons of the AUCs of various dosage forms of a drug compare their bioavailabilities. It should be emphasized that bioavailability does not take into account the rate of absorption; it only estimates the extent of absorption. Although rate of absorption can be important when rapid effects are required, it is usually not important when a drug is administered chronically.

Drug Distribution

After a drug reaches the bloodstream or is absorbed into the body, the drug molecules are distributed throughout the body in several phases. The initial phase distributes medication to high-flow areas such as the heart, liver, kidney, and brain. The second phase occurs to areas of slower blood flow such as fat, bone, and skin. The rate and extent of distribution of a drug throughout the body determine how much of the drug will be available to exert the pharmacological actions in the body and how soon the drug will be eliminated. Drug distribution to various body tissues and compartments is affected by many factors,

such as body composition, cardiac output, regional blood flow, and binding propensities. Drug diffusion is also dependent on protein binding and lipid solubility.

Plasma Protein Binding

The drug's affinity for aqueous or lipid tissue and its degree of binding to proteins determine where the drug goes and whether it reaches a therapeutic drug level at the site of desired action. During distribution throughout the body, the drug comes in contact with plasma carrier proteins, storage tissue, or receptor protein. Drug molecules that attach to the plasma proteins cannot leave the vascular space. The amount of drug that remains free of binding circulates to the receptor sites and stimulates the drug's effects. The drug that is bound to protein becomes inactive and is unavailable for binding to receptor sites and exerting therapeutic activity. Because most medications are bound to serum albumin, the patient with hypoalbuminemia may demonstrate exaggerated pharmacological response because of excess free drug. Equilibrium is achieved when a stable ratio of drug is found within all body compartments. However, a bound drug can rapidly free itself from binding to restore the equilibrium between bound and free drug in the body.

The percentage of free drug is constant for a single drug but differs between drugs. For example, about 90 percent of the total gentamicin in the plasma is free, whereas only about 1 percent of the total warfarin in the plasma remains unbound. Administering a single dose of aspirin to a patient on warfarin therapy causes competition for protein binding between the two drugs. As a result, the amount of free warfarin in the plasma is increased from 1 to 2 percent, as some of the warfarin is replaced by aspirin on the plasma protein and becomes unbound. Although the 1 percent increase seems unimportant, the amount of free warfarin available to exert anticoagulant effects is doubled, with possible serious consequences.

The percentage of drug that remains free and available for binding depends on the amount of plasma protein available, which differs among patients, depending on their medical condition. The affinity of a drug for protein and the percentage of bound plasma protein and tissue are usually constant for an individual drug. This is usually called the percent protein bound or protein binding of the drug. Only free drug can cross membranes to enter body tissues or to be eliminated, and only free drug can interact with receptors to produce therapeutic effects. Clinical laboratories usually report the total serum concentration, which includes both free and bound drug. For most patients, this is a good indicator of drug effect; in some circumstances, however, free drug concentration must be obtained.

Volume of Distribution

Volume of distribution (V_d) is a mathematically determined measure of the size of a compartment that would be filled by the amount of a drug in the same concentration as that found in the blood or plasma. In reality, the amount of drug in the body is constantly changing because of elimination, making it difficult to calculate the volume in which a drug distributes. One way to calculate the apparent volume distribution is to administer an IV dose and measure the serum concentration right away, before elimination has had much of an effect. The concentration just after IV administration is known as C_0, and the amount of drug given is X_0 or $V_d = X_0/C_0$ (Table 2–1). This volume is not real, but it is useful in expressing the affinity of a drug to tissue and storage sites and in calculating a drug's clearance from the body. A larger volume of distribution indicates that a larger dose should be administered to achieve a target concentration. It is not useful in determining the drug's effectiveness or duration of action.

In the example in Table 2–1, it can be seen that water-soluble drugs (hydrophilic) have a smaller volume of distribution than more lipid-soluble drugs. If a drug's volume of distribution approximates physiological fluid volumes, some assumptions about the distribution of that drug in the body can be made. If a drug has a volume of distribution of 0.2 to 0.25 L/kg (15 to 18 L in a 70-kg person), we might assume that its distribution is limited to the extracellular fluid. If a drug has a volume of distribution of 0.5 to 0.6 L/kg (40 L in a 70-kg person), it may be distributing into all body water.

A highly water-soluble drug has a small volume of distribution and a high plasma concentration. A highly fat-soluble drug possesses a large volume of distribution and has a low plasma concentration (Table 2–2). Variable drug concentrations among different organs and tissues can complicate drug distribution. For example, antibiotics do not distribute to abscesses and exudates. The distribution of a drug can also be affected by the drug's ability to cross various barriers like the blood-brain barrier or placental barrier.

Blood-Brain Barrier

The *blood-brain barrier* refers to a network of capillary endothelial cells in the brain. These cells have no pores and are surrounded by a sheath of glial connective tissue that makes them impermeable to water-soluble drugs. This barrier excludes ionized drug molecules like dopamine from the brain and allows un-ionized drug molecules, such as **barbiturates,** to pass readily and enter the brain. Usually only medications that are lipid soluble, such as atropine, general anesthetics, and psychotropics, cross this barrier.

The Placental Barrier

The placental barrier is a lipid membrane that allows passage of drugs by simple diffusion. The fetus is generally exposed to the same drug concentrations as the mother. Placental transfer is responsible for many of the untoward effects of alcohol, cigarettes, narcotics, and other drugs. Some drugs may have teratogenic effects, causing physical defects in the developing fetus.

Table 2–1. Example of Volume of Distribution Calculation

Type of Drug	Water Soluble	Fat Soluble
Percent in tissue (30% of body)	10%	90%
Percent in fluids (70% of body)	90%	10%
Dose given	100 mg	100 mg
Amount found in fluids (blood)	90 mg	10 mg
Serum concentration	1.29 mg/mL	0.14 mg/mL
V_d calculation	100 mg	100 mg
	1.29 mg/mL	0.14 mg/mL
Volume of distribution	78 mL	714 mL

Table 2–2. Examples of Physiological Tissues and
Approximate Volumes of Distributions of Various Drugs

Compartment	Volume	Type of Drug	Example
Total body water	0.6 L/kg	Water soluble	Ethanol
Extracellular water	0.2 L/kg	Higher molecular weight, water soluble	Mannitol
Plasma	0.04 L/kg	Highly protein bound	Heparin
Fat	0.2–0.35 L/kg	Highly fat soluble	Chlorpromazine
			Imipramine
Bone	0.07 L/kg	Some ions	Fluoride
			Calcium

Drug Metabolism

Drug metabolism refers to the process of chemical change to a different compound called a **metabolite.** When drugs are metabolized, the change is usually an increase in water solubility, often accompanied by a decrease in lipid solubility. The resulting compounds can be more readily excreted in the urine. The metabolites formed are usually less active than the parent compound. Many other drugs are active per se but also have active metabolites whose pharmacokinetic and pharmacological profiles differ from that of the parent drug. The pharmacological effects seen in the patient are the result of the parent compound and all of its metabolites. Some drugs, such as ACE inhibitors, are administered as an inactive **prodrug** that must be metabolized to an active metabolite to have any effect. Drug metabolism occurs mainly in the liver (see the discussion of the first-pass effect), but other tissues such as lungs, kidneys, and the gut wall may also metabolize drugs.

Although many different types of chemical reactions are seen in drug metabolism, the most important are the **phase one** reactions such as oxidation, reduction, and hydrolysis. **Oxidation** reactions typically insert an oxygen atom into the drug molecule. The most clinically significant oxidation enzymes include **cytochrome P-450. Phase two** reactions, called synthetic or **conjugation** reactions, involve the attachment of another chemical group to the drug, resulting in a chemical with greater water solubility and renal elimination. Drugs may undergo one or both of the phases during their metabolism to produce a metabolite that will be easily excreted in the urine.

Drug Interactions Due to Changes in Metabolism

Alcohol, a variety of drugs, and cigarette smoke stimulate the synthesis of drug-metabolizing enzymes. This process is called **enzyme induction** and is clinically significant for many drug products. Other drugs inhibit the metabolism of another drug and are called **enzyme inhibitors.** These changes in drug metabolism can result in drug interactions, clinically significant changes in drug dose, and adverse effects. Common drugs that cause drug interactions through their effect on metabolism are listed in Table 2–3.

Table 2–3. Common Drugs That Cause Drug Interactions through the Effect on Metabolism

Drugs that inhibit enzymes	*Drugs that have metabolism inhibited*
erythromycin	amphetamines
cimetidine	ephedrine
sodium valproate	phenylephrine
oral contraceptives	digoxin
propranolol	warfarin
some sulfonamides	theophylline
	carbamazepine
	propranolol

Drugs that induce enzymes	*Drugs that have metabolism accelerated*
rifampin	theophylline
phenytoin	imipramine
carbamazepine	pentazocine
primidone	chlorpromazine
griseofulvin	diazepam
cigarette smoke	dexamethasone
	prednisone
	methadone

Patient Variation in Drug Metabolism

Much of the observed difference in drug effects from one patient to the other is due to differences in drug metabolism caused by a variety of factors that determine the ability of a specific patient to metabolize a specific drug at a specific time:

1. Genetic influences: Some acetylation and oxidative reactions have ethnic and familial patterns.
2. Age: Neonates and older adults may have reduced drug metabolism.
3. Pregnancy: Drug metabolism may be increased or decreased during pregnancy.
4. Liver disease: The rate of elimination of high-clearance drugs may be reduced.
5. Time of day: Circadian rhythm has some effect on drug metabolism.
6. Environment: Smoking, air pollution, and exposure to industrial chemicals may affect drug metabolism.
7. Diet: Drug metabolism may be affected by food-drug interactions or by malnutrition.
8. Alcohol: Alcohol may cause induction of drug metabolism.
9. Drug interactions: The concentration or function of various hepatic enzymes may change.

Drug Elimination

Drug elimination refers to the metabolism and excretion of drugs and their transport outside the body. Some drugs are excreted unchanged, and others are metabolized by the body. In excretion, a drug is removed from tissues and circulation. Most drugs and drug metabolites are excreted by the kidney through active and passive mechanisms. The biliary route of excretion is important for some drugs, such as ampicillin and rifampin, and is the beginning of enterohepatic recirculation, which is important for a few drugs, such as digoxin and the estrogens. Drugs can also be excreted by the lungs, skin, breast milk, and sweat.

Renal Excretion

Renal excretion is by far the most common method of excretion from the body. The kidney usually removes drug that is unbound and free in the plasma. Renal excretion is the net effect of three different mechanisms within the kidney: (1) glomerular filtration, (2) tubular secretion, and (3) tubular reabsorption.

GLOMERULAR FILTRATION. With **glomerular filtration,** blood flows into the glomeruli in the kidney, and there is passive diffusion of fluids and solutes across the glomerular membrane. In a healthy adult, up to 130 mL/min of fluid crosses this membrane. Three factors determine whether a drug will be filtered: molecular size, protein binding, and glomerular integrity and function. Drugs dissolved in plasma can cross the membrane, whereas drugs that are protein bound or have a molecular weight higher than 60,000 are not filtered. Renal disease alters glomerular function and drug excretion.

TUBULAR SECRETION. Some drugs undergo **tubular secretion,** during which they are actively secreted from the proximal tubule into the urine. These drugs (primarily weak acids) are secreted by processes that may be subject to competition from other drugs or chemicals in the body that are also actively secreted. For example, probenecid and penicillin are both secreted from the tubule; if given together, they compete, and penicillin is secreted more slowly in the presence of probenecid. In this particular case, the drug interaction can be used to prolong the effect of penicillin.

TUBULAR REABSORPTION. Most drugs undergo **tubular reabsorption** passively in the distal tubules for drugs that are lipid soluble or not highly ionized. Tubular reabsorption is dependent on the physical and chemical properties of the drug and the pH of the urine. Drugs that are ionized at urine pH have less tubular reabsorption and tend to be excreted. Any change in the pH of the urine influences the excretion process. It is the ionized portion of the drug molecule that is water soluble and can be excreted by the kidney. Weak acids are excreted more rapidly in alkaline urine; weak bases are excreted more rapidly in acid urine. The rate of excretion can be changed for these drugs by changing the pH of the urine with other drugs. For example, an overdose of a weak base like amphetamine can be eliminated from the body more quickly by acidifying the urine with ammonium chloride.

Biliary Excretion

Many drugs are actively transported by the liver cells from blood to bile. These drugs or a conjugated metabolite of a drug is excreted in the bile and enters the GI tract, where it is excreted in the feces. Some of these conjugates can be broken down by enzymes in the gut bacteria to liberate the original drug, which may be reabsorbed into the body through oral absorption. This enterohepatic reabsorption may be interfered with by oral antibiotics that remove the gut bacteria; this is the mechanism of the interaction between oral contraceptives and antibiotics. Biliary excretion may serve as an alternative route of elimination of some drugs, such as digoxin and oxazepam, in patients with renal impairment.

Other Excretion

Pulmonary excretion occurs commonly with drugs administered by inhalation or drugs in a vapor state. The pulmonary excretion of alcohol, for example, is the basis of the alcohol breath test that is correlated to blood alcohol levels. Drugs can be excreted by the skin, sweat, saliva, and tears. Although routes seldom result in significant loss of drug concentration, they may be important to some patients if an adverse drug reaction occurs or if these functions play a role in the disorder being treated.

Biologic Half-Life

The half-life of a drug (Fig. 2–8) ultimately determines how often a drug is administered. The half-life is usually not dose dependent; therefore, doubling the dose does not double the half-life. The half-life for a given drug generally remains the same for a given patient, but a patient with renal or hepatic disease may have increased drug half-life. Half-life is an important variable to consider for solving problems concerning time:

1. Estimating the time needed to reach steady-state plasma concentration after the change of a maintenance dose
2. Estimating the time required to eliminate all or a portion of a discontinued drug from the body
3. Predicting the plasma levels following the initiation of therapy
4. Determining the dose interval needed to provide a desired fluctuation in plasma concentration during that interval

5. Determining the fluctuation in plasma concentrations, given a specific dosing interval

Drug Response versus Time Curve (Single Dose)

The effect of the drug absorbed is concentration related and also related to the action of the target organ and the number of receptors occupied by drug. The drug concentration–time curve represents the plasma concentration of drug as plotted against time (see Fig. 2–2). A single dose of a drug results in a single peak in plasma concentration, followed by a continuous decline in drug levels. Immediately after administration, the absorption phase results in a rapid rise in plasma concentration. When the plasma concentration reaches a minimum effective level, the drug's effects can be seen, and the **onset of action** is noted. As the body absorbs more drug, the blood concentration rises, more drug reaches the site of action, and the response increases. As the amount absorbed equals the amount being eliminated, the plasma concentration reaches the peak level or maximum level achieved during that dose interval. As elimination continues, the plasma level declines until it drops below the minimum effective level. The time between onset and termination of effect is the **duration of action** of the drug. Any time after the peak plasma concentration, an elimination **half-life** can be calculated by measuring the time it takes to reduce the plasma level to half a previous level on this drug concentration–time curve.

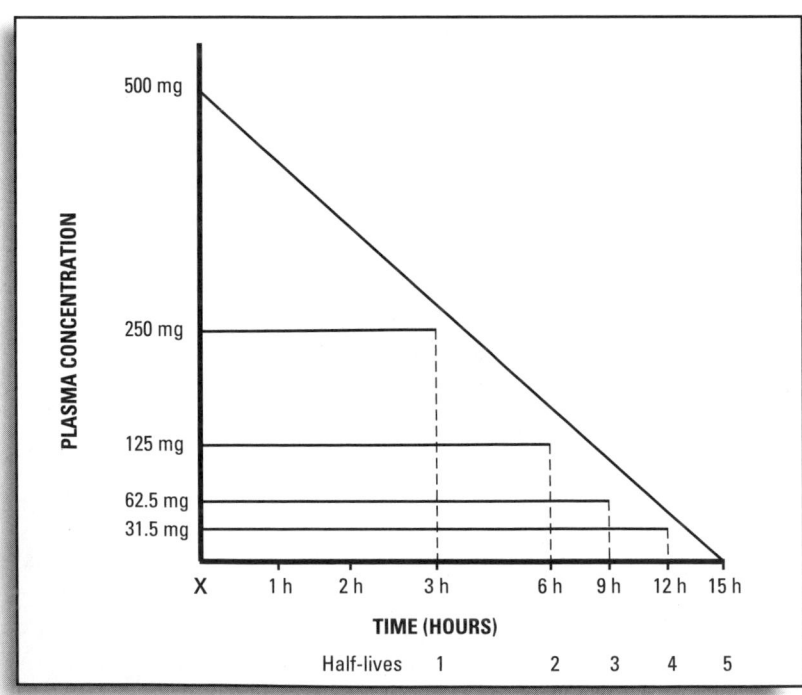

Figure 2–8. Elimination half-life determination. (From Kuhn, M. A.: *Pharmacotherapeutics: A Nursing Approach,* 4th ed. F. A. Davis, Philadelphia, 1998, p. 43, with permission.)

Multiple Dosing

Most clinical situations require a therapeutic effect for longer than one dose, and multiple doses are given to maintain a therapeutic plasma concentration within a constant range. Repeated administration of a drug results in oscillations in plasma concentrations that are influenced by both the rate of drug absorption and rate of drug elimination (Fig. 2–9). If the second dose is administered before the first dose is completely eliminated, the peak concentration is higher for the second dose than for the first dose. The curves are very similar, but the second dose is higher because some drug remains from the first dose. The time elapsing between the first and second doses is the **dosing interval (τ)**, which is generally determined by the drug half-life. Rapidly eliminated drugs have to be given more frequently to maintain a therapeutic plasma level. Drugs that are given chronically accumulate in the body until the amount given in the maintenance dose is the same as the amount eliminated in the dosage interval. When this occurs, the plasma concentrations have reached a steady state. The time required for a drug to reach steady state is determined by its half-life. The number of half-lives needed to achieve a certain percentage of the steady state is shown in Table 2–4.

Steady-State Plasma Concentrations

As successive doses of a drug are administered, the drug begins to accumulate in the body. Accumulation continues until the rate of elimination approaches the rate of administration. After that point, there is no further accumulation; each dose has a constant maximum and minimum concentration, and the amount of drug eliminated equals the amount of drug being administered. When the maximum and minimum drug concentrations are the same for two successive doses, steady state (C_{ss}) is reached. The time needed to reach steady state varies from drug to drug and is dependent on the drug half-life. For all practical purposes, steady state is reached in five half-lives (see Table 2–4). Each time a dose or dosing interval is changed, the time needed to reach a new steady state is five half-lives. The concentration achieved at steady state depends on the drug clearance, volume of distribution, dose, and dosing interval:

$$C_{ss} = \frac{Dose}{Clearance \times Interval}$$

Drug Clearance

Clearance refers to the removal of drug from plasma and relates the rate at which a drug is eliminated to the resulting plasma concentration. A drug's clearance and volume of distribution determine its half-life. Clearance is expressed as a volume of plasma from which drug is completely removed in a given time period (mL/min, L/h). Clearance is the proportionality constant that relates the average steady-state concentration (C_{ss}) and the dose administered:

$$(Fraction\ of\ dose\ absorbed) \times (Dose/Dose\ interval) = (\textbf{Clearance}) \times (C_{ss})$$

If the steady-state plasma concentration and the rate of drug administration are known, then clearance can be calculated by the equation:

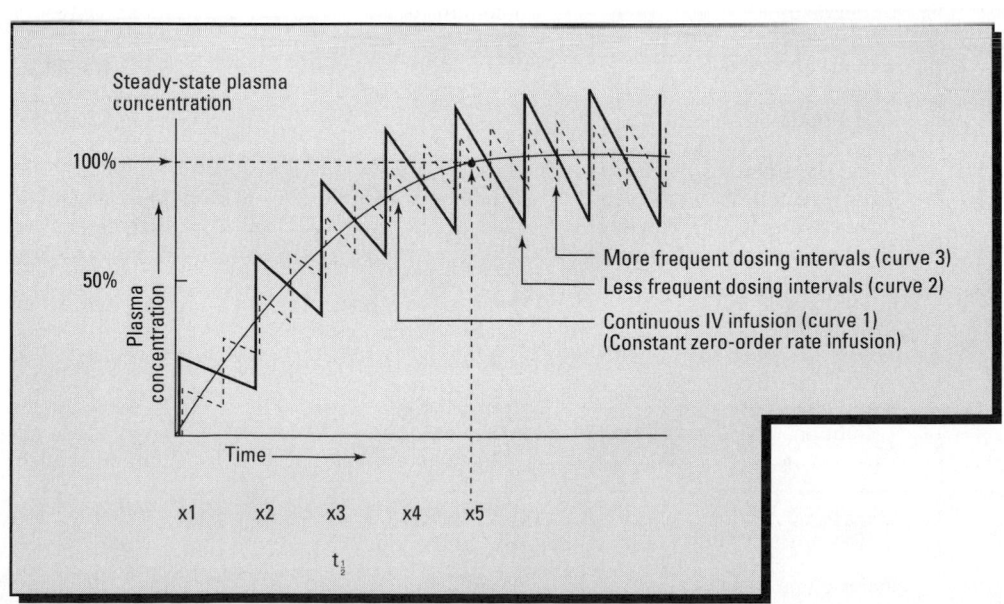

Figure 2–9. Multiple dosing curve. (From Kuhn, M. A.: *Pharmacotherapeutics: A Nursing Process Approach*, 4th ed. F. A. Davis, Philadelphia, 1998, p. 44, with permission.)

Table 2–4. Relationship between Drug Half-Life
and Percent of Steady-State Plasma Levels

	HALF-LIVES					
	1	2	3	4	5	Infinity
% Accumulation or % steady state	50%	75%	87.5%	93.75%	96.875%	100%
% Elimination if drug is discontinued	50%	75%	87.5%	93.75%	96.875%	100%

Clearance =

$$\frac{(\text{Fraction of dose absorbed}) \times (\text{Dose/Dose interval})}{C_{ss}}$$

For example, if lidocaine is infusing IV at 2 mg/min and the concentration is 3 mg/L, then the clearance would be 0.667 L/min.

$$\text{Clearance} = \frac{(1)(2 \text{ mg/min})}{3 \text{ mg/L}} = 0.667 \text{ L/min}$$

Abnormal clearance may be anticipated when there is major impairment of the function of the kidney, liver, or heart. Creatinine clearance is a useful quantitative indicator of renal function. Hepatic disease has been shown to reduce the clearance and prolong the half-life of many drugs. However, from other drugs eliminated by the liver, no changes in half-life have been noted with similar levels of hepatic dysfunction. At present, there is not a predictor of liver clearance that is as predictable as creatinine clearance for renal clearance.

Routes of Administration

The three general routes of administration used for most drugs are enteral, parenteral, and topical (Table 2–5). The enteral route is used when the drug is introduced into the intestinal system and is absorbed through similar mechanisms such as nutrients and vitamins. The parenteral (or "not enteral") route includes all the various injection routes by which a drug is introduced to tissue and absorbed into the bloodstream without the barriers that are present in the enteral route. The topical route

Table 2–5. Selected Routes of Administration and Their Characteristics

Route of Administration	Absorption Characteristics	Advantages	Disadvantages
Oral	Variable Depends on: • Drug solubility • GI pH and motility • Food • GI blood flow	Convenient Economical Best for self-administration	Unsuitable for: • Poorly adsorbed drugs • Infants • Dysphagia • Vomiting
Intramuscular	Rapid if solutions are used Slow if suspensions are used Speed depends on blood flow	Requires training for self-administration Suitable for small volumes	Painful Muscle damage Bleeding risk with anticoagulants
Intravenous	Immediate effect	Ideal for emergency use Large volumes of drug	Frequent administration Infection risk Vasculitis
Inhalation	Rapid absorption if in solution	Bronchodilators directly to site of action General anesthetics	Special equipment and technique needed for optimal effect
Transdermal	Incomplete unless specially formulated	Convenient Constant drug levels	Limited number of drugs can be absorbed
Topical	Incomplete, poor systemic absorption	Useful in dermatological, ophthalmic, nasal, and otic drugs	Drug may damage skin Allergic reactions to drugs Dose not precise

applies a drug directly to skin or other organs and is useful when the target organ can be reached externally or local effects from the drug are needed.

The Enteral Route

The enteral route includes buccal, sublingual, oral, and rectal administration. For the buccal and sublingual methods, only a small quantity of the drug can be used, the drug must be water soluble, the drug can have little flavor, and a rapid onset of action must be desired. Oral administration predominantly results in the dissolution and disintegration of the dose in the stomach and the absorption of the drug in the small intestine; the large surface area and rapid blood flow facilitate the rapid and complete absorption of drug into the systemic circulation. Rectal administration is poor because the large intestine absorbs mostly water and electrolytes rather than drugs.

ORAL ROUTE FORMULATIONS. The physical characteristics of a dosage form, such as shape, size, color, inert ingredients, dissolution, stability, and disintegration rate, make up the formulation or formula of the dosage form. **Compressed tablets** and **capsules** are the most frequently prescribed dosage forms. They provide a standard dose that is readily administered, easily recognized and identified, and safe to store for long periods of time without losing potency. **Tablet disintegration** must occur to allow the solid drug to dissolve in the liquid of the GI tract and be absorbed through the intestinal mucosa. **Sustained-release formulations** control the disintegration and solution of drugs in a predictable manner to provide drug absorption throughout the entire GI tract. Enteric coatings, protective coatings, wax matrices, osmotic pumps, and repeat action are some of the processes used to prolong the absorption of a dosage form. **Inert ingredients**, including diluents, lubricants, disintegrating agents, binders, and coloring agents, allow the drug powder to flow through the manufacturing equipment, provide a finished product of a manageable size that does not crumble in shipment (binders), enhance the disintegration of the tablet in the GI tract, and provide an aesthetically pleasing product that the patient can distinguish from other medications. Some patients are allergic to various inert ingredients, which cause adverse reactions unrelated to the active ingredient. An example is tartrazine (FDC yellow #5), a well-known causative agent of asthma attacks in sensitive, asthmatic patients. Many manufacturers have removed tartrazine from their products for this reason.

The Parenteral Route

The parenteral route includes SC, IM, and IV administration. The SC route involves administering the drug below the epidermis to the capillary vascular system, where the drug can diffuse into the bloodstream. Adding vasoconstrictors slows the uptake of the drug by reducing blood flow. Drug absorption from the IM site depends on whether a solution or suspension is used. Solutions, which are clear liquids, provide rapid absorption from the injection site. Suspensions, which contain drug particles that give the preparation a cloudy appearance, slow the absorption of the drug and prolong the drug's effects. The volume of blood flow in the muscle also affects the rate of absorption of IM-administered drugs.

Administering the drug by the IV route provides immediate systemic response. The injection of drug into the bloodstream eliminates absorptive barriers and the time needed for absorption. The IV route is preferred when rapid response is needed or the drug cannot be tolerated or absorbed by the other administration routes.

The Topical Route

The topical route requires application of the drug to a body surface. Topical routes include ointments and creams, ophthalmic and otic preparations, nasal instillation, and inhalation. These topical preparations are usually meant to provide effects locally at the site of administration, and they minimize systemic absorption and adverse effects. Drug administration by inhalation uses small particle sizes to navigate the bronchioles and reach the affected portions of the lung. This route provides a local effect in the bronchial tubes and a systemic effect from the absorption of drug by the pulmonary capillaries.

The transdermal delivery system has been used more frequently in recent years to provide a constant systemic effect through the absorption of a drug through the skin. The advantages of transdermal drug administration are steady-state levels that do not vary over the day, reduction of adverse reactions, and ease of administration. The disadvantage is the slow onset of action and the lack of dose flexibility. The rate and predictability of the drug absorption are dependent on intact, healthy skin and the surface area of the skin that is absorbing the drug.

REFERENCES

DiPiro, J. T., Blouin, R. A., Pruemer, J. M., and Spruill, W. J. (1996). *Concepts in clinical pharmacokinetics* (2nd ed.). Bethesda, MD: American Society of Health-Systems Pharmacists.

Katzung, B. G. (1998). *Basic and clinical pharmacology* (7th ed.). Stamford, CT: Appleton & Lange.

MacDermott, B. L., and Deglin, J. H. (1994). *Understanding basic pharmacology: Practical approaches for effective application.* Philadelphia: F. A. Davis.

CHAPTER 3

. . . .

Rational Drug Selection

CHAPTER OUTLINE

A t the start of clinical training, most nurse practitioners (NPs) find that they do not have a very clear idea of how to prescribe a drug for their patients or what information they need to provide. This is usually because their earlier pharmacology training was "drug-centered" and focused on the indications and adverse effects of different drugs. But in this book the reverse

approach has been taken, from the diagnosis to the drug. Moreover, patients vary in age, gender, size, and many other ways, all of which may affect treatment choices. All this is not always taught in school, and the number of hours spent on therapeutics may be low, compared with traditional pharmacology teaching.

Clinical training for NPs often focuses on diagnostic

rather than therapeutic skills. Sometimes practitioners are expected only to copy the prescribing behavior of physicians or the existing standard treatment guidelines, without explanation as to why certain treatments are chosen. Books may not be much help either. Pharmacology reference works and formularies are drug-centered, and although clinical textbooks and treatment guidelines are disease-centered and provide treatment recommendations, they rarely discuss why these therapies are chosen. Different sources may give contradictory advice.

Bad prescribing leads to ineffective and unsafe treatment, exacerbation or prolongation of illness, distress and harm to the patient, and higher costs. It also makes the prescriber vulnerable to influences that can cause irrational prescribing, such as patient pressure, bad examples by colleagues, and high-powered salesmanship. This chapter is primarily intended for NPs who are about to enter the clinical phase of their studies. It provides step-by-step guidance to the process of rational prescribing. It teaches skills that are necessary throughout a clinical career. Postgraduate students and practicing physicians may also find it a source of new ideas and perhaps an incentive for change. In this chapter, you will find a process for selecting a small group of drugs for your personal formulary, as well as information on the process of prescribing. It gives you the tools to think for yourself and not blindly follow what other clinicians think and do. It also helps you understand why standard treatment guidelines have been chosen and teaches you how to make the best use of such guidelines. Target drug concentration and monitoring plasma drug concentrations are discussed.

Your Personal Formulary

As a clinician, you may see dozens of patients per day, many of whom need treatment with a drug. How do you manage to choose the right drug for each patient in a relatively short time? You must preselect drugs, doses, and regimens for commonly encountered diagnoses and make a personal formulary. Your personal formulary is a compilation of the drugs you have chosen to prescribe regularly and with which you have become familiar. They are your priority choice for given indications. Your formulary is more than just the name of a drug. It also includes the dosage form, dosage schedule, and duration of treatment. And, as you use your formulary drugs regularly, you will get to know their effects and adverse effects thoroughly, with obvious benefits to your patients.

Most clinicians use only 40 to 60 drugs routinely. It is therefore useful to make your own selection from the various chapters of this book and to make this selection in a rational way. The next section of this chapter contains detailed information on the process of selection. It is important to compile your own formulary rather than copy your clinical teacher's or physician's practice patterns. There are four good reasons to do this:

1. You have final responsibility for your patient's well-being, and you cannot pass this on to others. Although you can and should draw on expert opinion and consensus guidelines, you should always think for yourself.

2. Through developing your own formulary, you will learn how to handle pharmacological concepts and data. This will enable you to discriminate between major and minor pharmacological features of a drug, making it much easier for you to determine its therapeutic value. It will also enable you to evaluate conflicting information from various sources.

3. Through compiling your formulary, you will know the alternatives when your preferred drug cannot be used, for example, because of serious adverse effects or contraindications. The same applies when a recommended standard treatment cannot be used. With the experience gained in choosing your formulary drugs, you will more easily be able to select an alternative drug.

4. You will regularly receive information on new drugs, new adverse effects, and new indications. Remember, however, that the latest and most expensive drug is not necessarily the best, the safest, or the most cost-effective. If you cannot effectively evaluate such information, you will not be able to update your formulary, and you will end up prescribing drugs that are dictated to you by your colleagues or sales representatives.

Choosing a Personal Formulary

Choosing a personal formulary drug is a process that can be divided into five steps (Table 3–1). You will choose a drug of first choice for a common condition, without a specific patient in mind.

Define the Indication

In selecting a drug, it is important to remember that you are choosing a drug of first choice for a common condition. You are not choosing a drug for an individual patient. (When actually treating a patient, you will verify whether your formulary drug is suitable for that particular patient.)

To be able to select the best drug for a given condition, you should study the pathophysiology of the disease. The more you know about this, the easier it is to choose a personal drug of choice. Sometimes the physiology of the disease is unknown, yet treatment is possible and neces-

Table 3–1. Steps in Choosing a Personal Formulary Drug

1 Define the indication.

2 Define the therapeutic objective.

3 Prepare an inventory of possible therapeutic classes.

4 Choose an effective group(s) according to criteria:

  Efficacy

  Safety

  Suitability

  Cost

5 Choose a drug from the group(s) for your personal formulary:

  Efficacy

  Safety

  Suitability

  Cost

6 Verify the suitability of your personal formulary drug:

  Drug and dosage form

  Standard dosage schedule

  Standard duration of treatment

  (For each of these, check effectiveness [indication, convenience] and safety [contraindications, interactions, high-risk groups].)

sary. Treating symptoms without really treating the underlying disease is called symptomatic treatment.

Define the Therapeutic Objective

It is very useful to define exactly what you want to achieve with a drug, for example, to decrease the diastolic blood pressure to a certain level, to cure an infectious disease, or to suppress feelings of anxiety. Always remember that the pathophysiology determines the possible site of action of your drug and the maximum therapeutic effect that you can achieve. The better you define your therapeutic objective, the easier it is to select the best drug.

Prepare an Inventory of Possible Therapeutic Classes

In this step, you link the therapeutic objective to various drugs. Drugs that are not effective are not worth examining any further, so efficacy is the first criterion for se-

lection. Initially, look at groups of drugs rather than individual drugs. There are tens of thousands of different drugs, but only about 70 pharmacological groups. All drugs with the same working mechanism (pharmacodynamics) and a similar molecular structure belong to one group. As the active substances in a drug group have the same working mechanism, their effects, adverse effects, contraindications, and interactions are also similar. The benzodiazepines, beta blockers, and penicillins are examples of drug groups. Most active substances in a group share a common stem in their generic name, such as diazepam, lorazepam, and temazepam for benzodiazepines and propranolol and atenolol for beta blockers.

There are two ways to identify effective groups of drugs. The first is to look at guidelines in your hospital or health system or at national guidelines. Another way is to review material in Unit II of this book and determine which groups are listed for your diagnosis or therapeutic objective. In most cases, you will find only two to four groups of drugs that are effective.

Choose an Effective Group According to Criteria

To choose a group of effective drugs, you need information on efficacy, safety, appropriateness, and cost.

EFFICACY. Most prescribers choose drugs on the grounds of efficacy, and adverse effects are taken into consideration only after they have been encountered. This means that too many patients are often treated with a drug that is stronger or more sophisticated than necessary (e.g., the use of wide-spectrum antibiotics for simple infections). In addition, some drugs may score favorably on an aspect that is of little clinical relevance. Sometimes kinetic characteristics that are clinically of little importance are stressed to promote an expensive drug, although many cheaper alternatives are available. To be effective, the drug has to reach a minimum plasma concentration, and the kinetic profile of the drug must allow this with an easy dosage schedule. Kinetic data on the drug group as a whole may not be available because they are related to dosage form and product formulation, but in most cases general features can be listed. Kinetics should be compared on the grounds of absorption, distribution, metabolism, and excretion.

SAFETY. Possible adverse effects and toxic effects must be listed and considered. If possible, the incidence of frequent adverse effects and the safety margins should be known. Almost all adverse effects are directly linked to the working mechanism of the drug, with the exception of allergic reactions.

Each drug has adverse effects, even your drugs of choice. Adverse effects are a major hazard in the industrialized world. It is estimated that up to 10 percent of hospital admissions are due to adverse drug reactions. Not all drug-induced injury can be prevented, but much of it is caused in high-risk groups that can be distinguished. Often these are exactly the groups of patients with whom you should always be very careful: elderly people, children, pregnant women, and those with kidney or liver disease.

APPROPRIATENESS. Although the final check will be made with only the individual patient, some general aspects of appropriateness can be considered in selecting drug groups. Contraindications are related to patient conditions, such as other illnesses that make it impossible to use a personal formulary drug that is otherwise effective and safe. You may eliminate or favor a group of drugs depending on your practice. For example, if you see primarily elderly or pediatric patients, you may choose different drug groups for your personal formulary. A change in the physiology of your patient may influence the dynamics or kinetics of your first choice: The required plasma levels may not be reached, or toxic adverse effects may occur at normal plasma concentrations. In pregnancy or lactation, the well-being of the child has to be considered. Interactions with food or other drugs can also strengthen or diminish the effect of a drug. A convenient dosage form or dosage schedule can have a strong impact on patient adherence to the treatment. All these aspects should be taken into account when choosing your drug of choice. For example, in the elderly and children, drugs should be in convenient dosage forms, such as tablets or liquid formulations that are easy to handle.

COST OF TREATMENT. The cost of the treatment is always an important criterion, whether it is paid by the state, by an insurance company, or directly by the patient. Cost is sometimes difficult to determine for a group of drugs, but you should always keep it in mind. Certain groups are definitely more expensive than others. Always look at the total cost of treatment rather than the cost per unit. The cost arguments really start counting when you choose between individual drugs. The final choice between drug groups is your own. It needs practice, but making this choice on the basis of efficacy, safety, appropriateness, and cost of treatment makes it easier. Sometimes you will not be able to select only one group and will have to take two or three groups on to the next step.

The conditions of health insurance and reimbursement schemes may also have to be considered. The best drug in terms of efficacy and safety may not (or only partially) be reimbursed; patients may request you to prescribe the reimbursed drug rather than the best one. When too many drugs are prescribed, the patient may buy only some of them, or insufficient quantities. In these circumstances, you should make sure that you prescribe only drugs that are really necessary, available, and affordable. As the prescriber, you should decide which drugs are the most important, not the patient or the pharmacist.

Choose a Drug from the Group for Your Personal Formulary

There are several steps to the process of choosing a drug of choice for your personal formulary. Using this reference is very helpful and will make it much easier to begin, but do not forget to collect and consider all essential information, including existing treatment guidelines. The choice of a drug includes the active drug, dosage form, dosage schedule, and duration of the drug therapy.

CHOOSE AN ACTIVE SUBSTANCE AND A DOSAGE FORM. Choosing an active substance is like choosing a drug group, and the information can be listed in a similar way. In practice, it is almost impossible to choose an active substance without considering the dosage form as well, so consider them together. First, the active substance and its dosage form have to be effective. This is mostly a matter of kinetics.

Although active substances within one drug group share the same mechanism of action, differences may exist in safety and suitability because of differences in kinetics. There may be large differences in convenience to the patient, which will have a strong influence on adherence to treatment. Different dosage forms usually lead to different dosage schedules, and this should be taken into account when choosing your drug of choice. Last but not least, cost of treatment should always be considered.

Keep in mind that drugs sold under generic names are usually cheaper than patented brand-name products. If two drugs from the same group appear equal, you could consider which drug has been on the market longer (indicating wide experience and probably safety). When two drugs from two different groups appear equal, you can choose both. This will give you an alternative if one is not suitable for a particular patient. As a final check, you should always compare your selection with existing treatment guidelines.

CHOOSE A STANDARD DOSAGE SCHEDULE. A recommended dosage schedule is based on clinical investigations in a group of patients. However, this statistical average is not necessarily the optimal schedule for your individual patient. If age, metabolism, absorption, and excretion in your patient are all average, and if no other diseases or other drugs are involved, the average dosage is probably adequate. The more your patient varies from this average, the more likely the need for an individualized dosage schedule. Recommended dosage schedules for drugs can be found in formularies, desk references, or this textbook.

DURATION OF TREATMENT. When you prescribe your drug of choice to a patient, you need to decide the duration of the treatment. By knowing the pathophysiology and the prognosis of the disease, you will usually have a good idea of how long the treatment should be continued. Some diseases require lifelong treatment (e.g., diabetes mellitus, heart failure, and Parkinson's disease).

The total amount of a drug to be prescribed depends on the dosage schedule and the duration of the treatment. It can easily be calculated. For example, for a patient with bronchitis, you may prescribe penicillin for 7 days. You will need to see the patient again only if there is no improvement, and so you can prescribe the total amount at once.

If the duration of treatment is not known, the monitoring interval becomes important. For example, you may request a patient with newly diagnosed hypertension to come back in 2 weeks so that you can monitor blood pressure and any adverse reactions to the treatment. In this case, you would prescribe for only the 2-week period. As you get to know the patient better, you could extend the monitoring interval, perhaps to 1 month. Three months should be about the maximum monitoring interval for drug treatment of a chronic disease.

The Process of Rational Treatment

Rational treatment requires a logical approach and common sense. After reading this chapter, you will know that prescribing a drug is part of a process that includes many other components, such as specifying your therapeutic objective and informing the patient. The process of rational treatment includes six steps:

1. Define the patient's problem.
2. Specify the therapeutic objective.
3. Verify the suitability of your selected treatment.
4. Initiate the selected treatment.
5. Discuss the treatment with the patient.
6. Monitor the treatment.

This chapter presents a first overview of the process of choosing a drug treatment. The process is illustrated with the example of a patient with a dry cough (Table 3–2). The chapter focuses on the principles of a stepwise approach to choosing a drug, and is not intended as a guideline for the treatment of dry cough. In fact, some prescribers would dispute the need for any drug at all.

A good scientific experiment follows a rather rigid methodology, with a definition of the problem, a hypothesis, an experiment, an outcome, and a process of verification. This process, especially the verification step,

Table 3–2. The Process of Rational Treatment

1 Define the patient's problem.
2 Specify the therapeutic objective.
3 Verify the suitability of your selected treatment.
4 Initiate the selected treatment.
5 Discuss the treatment with the patient.
6 Monitor the treatment.

ensures that the outcome is reliable. The same principles apply when you treat a patient. First you need to carefully define the patient's problem (the diagnosis). After that, you have to specify the therapeutic objective and choose a treatment of proven efficacy and safety from different alternatives. You then start the treatment, for example, by writing an accurate prescription and providing the patient with clear information and instructions. After some time, you monitor the results of the treatment; only then will you know if it has been successful. If the problem has been solved, the treatment can be stopped.

When you observe experienced clinicians, the process of choosing a treatment and writing a prescription seems easy. They reflect for a short time and usually decide quickly what to do. Choosing a treatment is more difficult than it seems, and to gain experience you need to work very systematically. The patient's problem can be described as a persistent dry cough and a sore throat. These are the symptoms that matter to the patient, but from the clinician's viewpoint there might be other dangers and concerns. The patient's problem could be translated into a working diagnosis of persistent dry cough for 2 weeks after a cold. There are at least three possible causes. The most likely is that the mucous membrane of the bronchial tubes is affected by the cold and therefore easily irritated. A secondary bacterial infection is possible but unlikely (no fever, no green or yellowish sputum). It is even less probable that the cough is caused by a lung tumor, although that possibility should be considered if the cough persists.

Define the Patient's Problem

A patient usually presents with a complaint or a problem. It is obvious that making the right diagnosis is a crucial step in starting the correct treatment. Making the right diagnosis is based on integrating many pieces of information: the complaint as described by the patient, a detailed history, physical examination, laboratory tests, x-rays, and other investigations. In the next sections on treatment, we therefore assume that the diagnosis has been made correctly.

Patient complaints are mostly linked to symptoms. A symptom is not a diagnosis, although it will usually lead to it. Patients may come to you with a request, a complaint, or a question. All may be related to different problems: a need for reassurance, a sign of underlying disease, a hidden request for assistance in solving another problem, an adverse effect of drug treatment, nonadherence to treatment, or psychological dependence on drugs. Take a look at five complaints of "sore throat":

1. Cause: minor viral infection; needs reassurance.
2. Cause: AIDS; needs treatment of underlying disease.

3. Cause: none, patient is 3 months pregnant; needs assistance with another problem.
4. Cause: bacterial infection treated with penicillin; needs counseling on lack of compliance or treatment failure and/or new treatment regimen.
5. Cause: dry mouth due to drug therapy with antidiarrhea medication; needs treatment of the cause of the diarrhea and/or new treatment regimen.

As you can see in these examples, the same complaint can come from very different patient problems. Through careful observation, structured history taking, physical examination, and other examinations, you should try to define the patient's real problem. Your definition (working diagnosis) may differ from how the patient perceives the problem. Choosing the appropriate treatment will depend on this critical step. In many cases, you will not need to prescribe a drug at all.

Specify the Therapeutic Objective

Before choosing a treatment, it is essential to specify your therapeutic objective. What do you want to achieve with the treatment? The following examples illustrate this crucial step:

1. A 4-year-old girl, slightly undernourished, has had watery diarrhea without vomiting for 3 days. She has not urinated for 24 hours. On examination, she has no fever but does have a rapid pulse and low elasticity of the skin. With this patient, the diarrhea is probably caused by a viral infection because it is watery (not slimy or bloody) and there is no fever. She has signs of dehydration (listlessness, little urine, and decreased skin turgor). This dehydration is the most worrying problem in that she is already slightly undernourished. The therapeutic objective in this case is therefore (1) to prevent further dehydration and (2) to rehydrate, not to cure the infection. Antibiotics would be ineffective anyway.
2. A 44-year-old man has had insomnia for the last 6 months and comes for a refill of diazepam tablets, 5 mg, 1 tablet before sleeping. He wants 60 tablets. The problem with this patient is not which drugs to prescribe but how to stop prescribing them. Diazepam is not indicated for long-term treatment of insomnia because tolerance quickly develops. It should be used only for short periods, when strictly necessary. The therapeutic objective in this case is not to treat the patient's sleeplessness but to avoid a possible dependence on diazepam. This objective could be achieved through a gradual and carefully monitored lowering of the dose to diminish withdrawal symptoms, coupled with more

appropriate behavioral techniques for insomnia, which should lead to eventual cessation of the drug.

As these examples show, in some cases the therapeutic objective is straightforward: the treatment of an infection or a condition. Sometimes the picture is less clear, such as the patient with insomnia. You will have noticed that specifying the therapeutic objective is a good way to structure your thinking. It forces you to concentrate on the real problem, which limits the number of treatment possibilities and so makes your final choice much easier.

Specifying your therapeutic objective will prevent a lot of unnecessary drug use. It should stop you from treating two diseases at the same time if you cannot choose between them, for example, prescribing antifungal and corticosteroid skin ointments when you cannot choose between a fungus and eczema.

It is a good idea to discuss your therapeutic objective with the patient before you start the treatment. This step may reveal that the patient has quite different views about illness causation, diagnosis, and treatment. It also makes the patient an informed partner in the therapy and improves adherence to treatment.

Verify Whether Your Usual Treatment Is Suitable for This Patient

You have already determined your personal formulary, the most effective, safe, suitable, and least expensive treatment for dry cough in general. Now you have to verify whether your usual treatment is also suitable for this particular patient: Is the treatment also effective and safe in this case?

The starting point for this step is to look up your personal formulary, or the treatment guideline that is available to you. In all cases, you will need to check three aspects:

1. Are the active substance and the dosage form effective or suitable for this patient?
2. Is the standard dosage schedule suitable?
3. Is the standard duration of treatment suitable?

For each aspect, you have to check whether the proposed treatment is effective and safe. A check on effectiveness includes a review of the drug indication and the convenience of the dosage form. Safety relates to contraindications and possible interactions. Be careful with certain high-risk groups.

Drug and Dosage Form Effectiveness

We assume that all your personal formulary drugs of choice have already been selected on the basis of efficacy. However, you should now verify that the drug will also be effective in this individual patient. For this purpose, you have to review whether the active substance is likely

to achieve the therapeutic objective and whether the dosage form is convenient for the patient. Convenience contributes to patient adherence to the treatment and therefore to effectiveness. Complicated dosage forms or packages and special storage requirements can be major obstacles for some patients.

Drug and Dosage Form Safety

The safety of a drug for the individual patient depends on contraindications and interactions; these may occur more frequently in certain high-risk groups. Contraindications are determined by the mechanism of action of the drug and the characteristics of the individual patient. Drugs in the same group usually have the same contraindications. Some patients fall into certain high-risk groups, and any other illnesses should also be considered. Some adverse effects are serious only for categories of patients, such as drowsiness for drivers. Interactions can occur between the drug and nearly every other substance taken by the patient. The best-known interactions are with other prescribed drugs, but you must also think of over-the-counter (OTC) drugs the patient might be taking. Interactions may also occur with food or drinks (especially alcohol). Some drugs interact chemically with other substances and become ineffective (e.g., tetracycline and milk). Fortunately, in practice only a few interactions are clinically relevant. Take a look at this example:

PATIENT EXAMPLE. A 45-year-old man with a history of asthma uses an albuterol (Ventolin) inhaler. A few weeks ago, you diagnosed essential hypertension (145/100 mm Hg on various occasions). You advised a low-salt diet, but his blood pressure remains high. You decide to add a drug to your treatment. Your drug of choice for hypertension in patients under age 50 is atenolol tablets, 50 mg a day. Atenolol is a good drug for the treatment of essential hypertension in patients younger than 50, and it is very convenient. However, like all beta blockers, it is relatively contraindicated in asthma. Despite the fact that it is a selective beta blocker, it can induce asthmatic problems, especially in higher doses because selectivity then diminishes. If the asthma is not very severe, atenolol can be prescribed in a low dose. In severe asthma, you should probably switch to diuretics; almost any thiazide is a good choice.

Dosage Schedule

The aim of a dosage schedule is to maintain the plasma level of the drug within the therapeutic window. As in the previous step, the dosage schedule should be effective and safe for the individual patient. There are two main reasons to adapt a standard dosage schedule: The window and/or plasma curve may have changed, or the dosage schedule is inconvenient to the patient.

For a variety of reasons (e.g., age, pregnancy, disturbed organ functions), individual patients may differ from the standard. These differences may influence the pharmacodynamics or pharmacokinetics of your drug of choice. A change in pharmacodynamics may affect the level (position) or width of the therapeutic window. The therapeutic window reflects the sensitivity of the patient to the action of the drug. Changes in the therapeutic window are sometimes expressed as the patient's being "resistant" or "hypersensitive." The only way to determine the therapeutic window in the individual patient is by trial, careful monitoring, and logical thinking.

Four factors determine the course of the concentration curve, usually called ADME (absorption, distribution, metabolism, and excretion) factors. You always have to check whether ADME factors in your patient are different from those in average patients. If so, you have to determine what this difference will do to the plasma curve. Any change in ADME factors influences plasma concentration.

The plasma concentration curve will *drop* in the following cases:

1. Absorption is low.
2. Distribution is high.
3. Metabolism is high.
4. Excretion is high.

The plasma concentration curve will *rise* in the following cases:

1. Absorption is high.
2. Distribution is low.
3. Metabolism is low.
4. Excretion is low.

How can you define the position of the plasma curve in an individual patient? The plasma concentration can be measured by laboratory investigations, but in many settings this is not possible and it may be expensive. More important, each measurement represents only one point of the curve and is difficult to interpret without special training and experience. More measurements are expensive and may be stressful to the patient, especially in an outpatient setting. It is simpler to look for clinical signs of toxic effects. These are often easy to detect by history taking and clinical investigation.

CHANGES IN WINDOW AND CURVE. Elderly people are one of several categories of high-risk patients. Dosage schedules for antidepressant drugs in the elderly usually recommend that the dose be reduced to half the adult dose, for two reasons: First, in the elderly the therapeutic window of antidepressant drugs shifts down (a lower plasma concentration will suffice). At a full adult dose, the plasma curve may rise above the therapeutic window, leading to adverse effects, especially anticholinergic and cardiac effects. Second, metabolism and renal clearance of the drug and its active metabolites may be reduced in the elderly, also increasing the plasma curve. Thus, if you prescribe the normal adult dosage, your patient will be exposed to unnecessary and possibly harmful adverse effects.

CONVENIENCE. A dosage schedule should be convenient. The more complex the schedule, the less convenient it is. For example, 2 tablets taken once daily are much more convenient than ½ tablet four times daily. Complex dosage schedules decrease patient adherence to treatment, especially when more than one drug is used, and thus decrease effectiveness. Try to adjust a dosage schedule to the patient's other schedules.

DURATION OF THERAPY. Many clinicians prescribe not only too much of a drug for too long but also frequently too little of a drug for too short a period. In one study, about 10 percent of patients on benzodiazepines received them for a year or longer. Another study showed that 16 percent of outpatients with cancer still suffered from pain because clinicians were afraid to prescribe morphine for a long period. They mistook tolerance for addiction. The duration of the treatment and the quantity of drugs prescribed should also be effective and safe for the individual patient.

Overprescribing leads to many undesired effects. The patient receives unnecessary treatment, or drugs may lose some of their potency. Unnecessary adverse effects may occur. The quantity available may enable the patient to overdose. Drug dependence and addiction may develop. Some reconstituted drugs, such as eyedrops and antibiotic syrups, may become contaminated. It may be very inconvenient for the patient to take so many drugs. Last but not least, valuable and often scarce resources are wasted.

Underprescribing is also serious. The treatment is not effective, and more aggressive or expensive treatment may be needed later. Prophylaxis may be ineffective, resulting in serious disease. Most patients find it inconvenient to return for further treatment. Money spent on ineffective treatment is money wasted.

In long-term treatment, patient compliance can be a problem. Often the patient stops taking the drug when the symptoms have disappeared or if adverse effects occur. For patients with chronic conditions, repeat prescriptions are often prepared by the receptionist or assistant and just signed by the NP. This practice may be convenient for the clinician and the patient, but it has certain risks because the process of renewal becomes a routine rather than a conscious act. Automatic refills are one of the main reasons for overprescribing in industrialized countries, especially in chronic conditions. When patients live far away, convenience may lead to prescriptions for longer periods, which may also result in overprescribing.

Initiate Selected Treatment

The advice should be given first, with an explanation of why it is important. Be brief and use words the patient can understand.

The basic elements of a legal prescription are as follows:

1. *Name, address, and telephone number of the prescriber.* This is usually preprinted on the prescription form. If the pharmacist has any questions about the prescription, the pharmacist can easily contact the prescriber.
2. *Date.* The date of the prescription is needed because prescriptions for controlled substances are good for only 6 months, and many states limit the validity of a prescription to 1 year from the time it was written.
3. *Generic name of the drug and strength of the drug.* Rx is derived from *recipe* (Latin for "take"). After Rx, you should write the name of the drug and the strength. It is strongly recommended to use the generic (nonproprietary) name. This facilitates education and information. It means that you do not express an opinion about a particular brand of the drug, which may be unnecessarily expensive for the patient. It also enables the pharmacist to maintain a more limited stock of drugs or to dispense the cheapest drug. However, if there is a particular reason to prescribe a special brand, the trade name can be added. Many states allow generic substitution by the pharmacist and require the addition "Do not substitute" or "Dispense as written" if that brand, and no other, is to be dispensed. The strength of the drug indicates how many milligrams each tablet, suppository, or milliliter of fluid should contain. Internationally accepted abbreviations should be used: *g* for gram, *mL* for milliliter. Try to avoid decimals and, where necessary, write words in full to avoid misunderstanding. For example, write levothyroxine 50 micrograms, not 0.050 milligrams or 50 μg. Badly handwritten prescriptions can lead to mistakes, and it is the legal duty of the prescriber to write legibly. In prescriptions for controlled drugs or those with a potential for abuse, it is safer to write the strength and total amount in words to prevent tampering. Instructions for use must be clear, and the maximum daily dose mentioned. Use indelible ink.
4. *Dosage form and total amount.* Use only standard abbreviations that will be known to the pharmacist.
5. *Information for the package label (e.g.,instructions, warnings).* S stands for *signa* (Latin for "write"). All information following the *S* or the word *Label* should be copied by the pharmacist onto the label of the package. This includes how much of the drug is to be taken, how often, and any specific instructions and warnings. These should be given in lay language. Do not use abbreviations or statements like "as before" or "as directed." When stating "as required," the maximum dose and minimum dose interval should be indicated. Certain instructions for the pharmacist, such as "Add 5-mL measuring spoon," are written here but, of course, are not copied onto the label.
6. *Name and address of the patient and, if the patient is a child or older adult, age.*
7. *Prescriber's initials or signature.*

Discuss Treatment with the Patient

On average, 50 percent of patients do not take prescribed drugs correctly, take them irregularly, or do not take them at all. The most common reasons are that symptoms have ceased, adverse effects have occurred, the drug is not perceived as effective, or the dosage schedule is complicated for patients, particularly the elderly. Nonadherence to treatment may have no serious consequences. For example, irregular doses of a thiazide still give the same result because the drug has a long half-life and a flat dose-response curve. But drugs with a short half-life (e.g., phenytoin) or a narrow therapeutic margin (e.g., theophylline) may become ineffective or toxic if taken irregularly.

Patient adherence to treatment can be improved in three ways.

1. Prescribe a well-chosen drug treatment.
2. Create a good practitioner-patient relationship.
3. Take the time to give the necessary information, instructions, and warnings.

A well-chosen drug treatment consists of as few drugs as possible (preferably only one), with rapid action, with as few adverse effects as possible, in an appropriate dosage form, with a simple dosage schedule (once or twice daily), and for the shortest possible duration.

A good patient relationship is established through respect for the patient's feelings and viewpoint, understanding, and willingness to enter into a dialogue that empowers the patient as a partner in therapy. Patients need information, instructions, and warnings to provide them with the knowledge to accept and follow the treatment and to acquire the necessary skills to take the drugs appropriately. In some studies, fewer than 60 percent of patients had understood how to take the drugs they had received. Information should be given in clear, common language, and it is helpful to ask patients to repeat in their own words some of the core information to be sure that it has been understood. A functional name, such as a "heart pill," is often easier for the patient to remember and clearer in terms of indication. Table 3–3 presents the minimum information that should be given to a patient.

You may think that there is not enough time, that the pharmacist or dispenser should give this information, or that too much information on adverse effects could even decrease adherence to treatment. Yet it is the prime responsibility of the clinician to ensure that the patient understands the treatment, and this responsibility cannot be shifted to the pharmacist or written material. Maybe not

Table 3–3. Patient Teaching: The Minimum

The six points listed below summarize the minimum information that should be given to the patient.

Effects of the Drug

Why the drug is needed.

Which symptoms will disappear, and which will not.

When the effect is expected to start.

What will happen if the drug is taken incorrectly or not at all.

Adverse Effects

The adverse effects that may occur.

How to recognize them, how long they may continue, and how serious they are.

The action to take.

Instructions

How the drug should be taken.

When it should be taken.

How long the treatment should continue.

How the drug should be stored.

What to do with leftover drugs.

Warnings

When the drug should not be taken.

The maximum dose.

Why the full treatment course should be taken.

Future Consultations

When to come back (or not).

In what circumstances to come back earlier.

What information you will need at the next appointment.

Everything Clear

Ask the patient whether everything is understood.

Ask the patient to repeat the most important information.

Ask whether the patient has any more questions.

all adverse effects have to be mentioned, but you should at least warn your patients of the most dangerous or inconvenient adverse effects. Having too many patients is never accepted by a court of law as a valid excuse for not informing and instructing a patient correctly.

Monitor the Treatment

If the patient's symptoms continue, you will need to consider whether the diagnosis, treatment, adherence to treatment and the monitoring procedure were all correct. You may wish to obtain a plasma drug concentration. In fact, the whole process starts again. Sometimes there may be no end solution to the problem. For example, in chronic diseases such as hypertension, careful monitoring and improved patient adherence to the treatment may be all that you can do. In some cases, you will change a treatment because the therapeutic focus switches from curative to palliative care, as in terminal cancer or AIDS.

Making a Rational Drug Selection

So, what at first seems just a simple consultation of only a few minutes in fact requires a quite complex process of professional analysis. What you should not do is copy the doctor and memorize that dry cough should be treated with 15 mg codeine three times daily for 3 days—which is not always true. Instead, build your clinical practice on the core principles of choosing and giving a treatment, which have been outlined.

In fact, there are two important stages in choosing a treatment. You start by considering your "first choice" treatment, which is the result of a selection process done earlier. The second stage is to verify that your first-choice treatment is suitable for this particular patient.

Take a look at this example: You sit in with an NP and observe the following case. A 52-year-old taxi driver complains of a sore throat and cough that started 2 weeks earlier with a cold. He has stopped sneezing but still has a cough, especially at night. The patient is a heavy smoker who has often been advised to stop. Further history and examination reveal nothing special, apart from a throat inflammation. The NP again advises the patient to stop smoking and writes a prescription for codeine tablets, 15 mg, 1 tablet three times daily for 3 days.

Now that we have defined our drug of choice for dry cough, we can review the process of rational prescribing as a whole. This process consists of six steps, using the example of our patient with a dry cough.

1. Define the patient's problem. The patient's problem can be described as a persistent dry cough and a sore throat. These are the symptoms that matter to the patient, but from the practitioner's viewpoint there might be other dangers and concerns. The patient's problem could be translated into a working diagnosis of persistent dry cough for 2 weeks after a cold. There are at least three possible causes. The most likely is that the mucous membrane of the bronchial tubes is affected by the cold and therefore easily irritated. A secondary bacterial infection is possible but unlikely (no fever, no green or yellowish sputum). It is even less probable that the cough is caused by a lung tumor, although that should be considered if the cough persists.

2. Specify the therapeutic objective. Continuous irritation of the mucous membranes is the most likely cause of the cough. The first therapeutic objective is therefore to stop this irritation by suppressing the cough, to enable the membranes to recover.

3. Verify the suitability of your selected treatment (e.g., your personal formulary drug). You have already determined your personal formulary, the most effective, safe, suitable, and least expensive treatment for dry cough in general. Now you have to verify whether your drug of choice is also suitable for this particular patient: Is the treatment also effective and safe in this case? In this example, there may be reasons why this advice is unlikely to be followed. The patient will probably not stop smoking. Even more important, he is a taxi driver who cannot avoid traffic fumes in the course of his work. So although advice should still be given, your drug of choice should also be considered and checked for suitability. Is it effective, and is it safe? Codeine is effective, and it is not inconvenient to take a few tablets every day. However, there is a problem with safety because the patient is a taxi driver and codeine has a sedative effect. For this reason, it would be preferable to look for a cough depressant that is not sedative. Other opiates share the same adverse effects; this is often the case. The antihistamines are even more sedative and probably not effective. We must therefore conclude that it is probably better not to prescribe any drug at all. If we still consider that a drug is needed, codeine remains the best choice but in as low a dosage as possible and for a few days only.

4. Initiate the selected treatment. The advice should be given first, with an explanation of why it is important. Be brief and use words the patient can understand. Then codeine can be prescribed: Rx codeine 15 mg; 10 tablets; 1 tablet three times daily; date; signature; name, address, and age of the patient. Write clearly!

5. Discuss the treatment with the patient. Give information, instructions, and warnings. The patient should be informed that codeine will suppress the cough, that it works within 2 to 3 hours, that it may cause constipation, and that it will make him

sleepy if he takes too much of it or drinks any alcohol. He should be advised to come back if the cough does not go away within 1 week or if unacceptable adverse effects occur. Finally, he should be advised to follow the dosage schedule and warned not to take alcohol. A good idea is to ask him to summarize in his own words the key information to be sure that it is clearly understood.

6. Monitor the treatment. If the patient does not return, he is probably better. If there is no improvement and the patient does come back, there are three possible reasons: The treatment was not effective, the treatment was not safe (e.g., because of unacceptable adverse effects), or the treatment was not convenient (e.g., the dosage schedule was hard to follow or the taste of the tablets was unpleasant). Combinations are also possible.

Individualizing Drug Therapy

Occasionally, it is necessary to closely monitor the drug dosage and regimen to ensure that the therapeutic objectives are met. This monitoring is usually accomplished by closely monitoring the serum drug levels and making careful adjustments in the drug treatment regimen. Pharmacokinetic concepts, as discussed in Chapter 2, have been used successfully to individualize patient drug therapy.

Target Drug Concentrations

Laboratories routinely measure patient serum for many drugs, including antibiotics, theophylline, phenytoin, lithium, and antiarrhythmics. Combined with knowledge of the disease states and conditions that influence the disposition of a particular drug, kinetic concepts can be used to modify doses to produce desirable pharmacological effects without unwanted adverse effects. This narrow range of drug concentrations is called the *target concentration*. A rational series of steps useful to achieve a target concentration in an individual patient are as follows:

1. Select a target concentration from the literature.
2. Predict clearance and volume of distribution values for the patient from the population-based estimates in the literature.
3. Calculate a loading dose and maintenance dose to achieve the target concentration.
4. Prescribe the doses and measure the plasma concentration.
5. Use the measured values to predict the individual's values for clearance and volume of distribution.
6. Revise the target concentration based on clinical assessment, if needed.
7. Go back to step 3.

The target concentration is a substitute for the desired therapeutic outcome, similar to a target blood pressure or serum cholesterol. In many situations, the therapeutic benefit is difficult to assess, in which case step 6 is not feasible. The target concentration can provide some assurance that treatment is adequate, even if the therapeutic benefit cannot be observed. Given an accurate dose history and one or more serum concentrations, the prediction of concentrations at future points in time will be much more precise. This process allows the clinician to tailor the dosage for the individual patient with confidence and provides the full benefit of the drug to the patient.

As an example, consider how a target concentration for theophylline might be defined. Theophylline is a bronchodilator that might be used in the acute management of severe bronchospasm due to asthma. Studies have been done in asthmatics and examined the increase in forced expiratory volume in 1 second (FEV_1) and theophylline concentration. The relationship between theophylline concentration and change in FEV_1 is not a straight line. As concentrations increase, the increase in FEV_1 is less and approaches a maximum response (Emax—the largest effect that can be expected from the drug). Half the improvement is achieved at 10 mg/L (EC_{50}—the concentration where 50 percent of the maximum effect is seen). It can be predicted that concentrations of 40 mg/L are required to obtain 80 percent response. However, this calculation does not consider adverse effects. Although FEV_1 changes little between 10 and 20 mg/L, the incidence of vomiting increases fivefold to 12 percent. Selection of the target concentration, then, is dependent on whether a 20 percent improvement in FEV_1 justifies a fivefold risk in vomiting.

Note that 30 percent of the maximal benefit is expected at concentrations of 5 mg/L, and almost no adverse effects are likely at this level. In contrast, there is additional benefit to the occasional patient who can tolerate higher levels without adverse reactions. Sixteen percent of patients with theophylline levels above 20 mg/L have no signs of toxicity. For an individual patient, target concentrations may be chosen outside the normal range: lower concentrations for patients who are responding to even low levels of the drug and higher concentrations for patients who are receiving continued improvement in effect without adverse effects.

Some drugs, such as antiarrhythmics, have effects that are all or none. The patient either has an arrhythmia or not. The target drug concentration here is the concentration that exceeds the threshold at which the arrhythmia is suppressed. Higher concentrations offer no benefit, and the risk of toxicity increases. When a sample of patients is studied, a target can be defined at which the benefit is reasonably high and toxicity is relatively low. For example, the chance of an arrhythmia decreases with concentration, but the chance of toxicity increases. Between 1 and 2 mg/L, the benefits appear to be about 80 percent responding, with the toxicity at 40 percent. Any higher concentrations do not significantly increase the percentage responding but significantly increase the percentage with adverse effects. From these data, a target concentration of 1.5mg/L for amiodarone would be reasonable.

Establishing a target concentration is based on a knowledge of Emax and EC_{50}, which define the extent of the therapeutic response and the steepest part of the response curve, where the most gain can be expected for the smallest increase in concentration.

The selection of dose needed to achieve the target concentration selected rests on the pharmacokinetic parameters of the drug. The volume of distribution determines loading dose:

$$\text{Loading Dose} = \text{Volume of Distribution} \times \text{Target Concentration}$$

Using theophylline as an example, the loading dose would be 350 mg (35 L for a 70-kg patient $\times$ 10 mg/L).

The maintenance dose rate is calculated from the clearance:

$$\text{Maintenance Dose Rate} = \text{Clearance} \times \text{Target Concentration}$$

Using theophylline as an example, the maintenance dose rate would be 720 mg/day (3 L/h for a 70-kg patient $\times$ 10 mg/L).

This example shows the importance of estimating the volume of distribution and clearance in each individual patient. Once this has been done, other useful parameters can be derived to assist in determining the appropriate dosage interval, time needed to reach steady state, and half-life.

Half-life is calculated by using the following formula:

$$0.7 \times \text{Volume of Distribution} \div \text{Clearance}$$

Using the theophylline as an example, the half-life would be 8 hours (0.7 $\times$ 35 L $\div$ 3 L/h).

Thus, the expected dosage interval is 8 hours, and the time to achieve about 90 percent of steady-state theophylline concentrations is 32 hours (about 4 half-lives).

Factors Affecting Interpretation of Plasma Drug Concentration

A key piece of information is the recent dose history. All doses within 4 half-lives must be known to determine if the drug is at steady-state concentrations. The interpretation of a target concentration of a long-lived drug such as digoxin will focus on volume of distribution in determining the measured value within the first 24 hours of therapy. After 4 half-lives (steady state), the dose will be determined by clearance. It is most useful to adjust doses based on plasma concentrations obtained after steady state is reached and total clearance can be determined.

Nothing is more confusing than the effects of altered plasma protein binding on the interpretation of plasma drug concentrations. For reasons of convenience and expense, routine drug concentration measurement is expressed as total concentration of drug in plasma. The drug effects are due to the amount of unbound drug. The relevance of the percent of drug bound to plasma versus the percent unbound is in the interpretation of the reported value. A hypothetical example of phenytoin protein binding can demonstrate this principle.

With normal plasma concentrations and affinity, the bound concentration of phenytoin is 90 percent of the total plasma concentration. So if a normal patient has a reported value of 10 mg/L, then 9 mg/L is bound and 1 mg/L is free to provide the antiepileptic effects. In renal failure, because of decreased albumin and plasma protein affinity, the bound concentration is about 80 percent of total plasma concentration. In this case, the reported value of 10 mg/L will be the result of 8 mg/L of bound drug and 2 mg/L of free drug. Patients with and without renal failure may have identical total drug concentrations and a twofold difference in free (active) drug concentration.

Because only the unbound drug is active, the patient with normal renal function with a total drug concentration of 10 mg/L is considered "in the therapeutic range," and no change in dose would be considered unless the patient is having seizures. A patient with renal failure with a total concentration of 5 mg/L might be considered "subtherapeutic" and a candidate for a dosage increase. However, as in the following example, this patient would have the same unbound drug concentration as the normal patient. So the total drug concentration of 5 mg/L will probably be effective in controlling seizures.

An example is altered protein binding. In the normal patient, there is 90 percent protein binding.

$$10 \text{ mg/L} = 9 \text{ mg/L bound} + 1 \text{ mg/L free}$$

A patient with renal failure has 80 percent protein binding.

$$5 \text{ mg/L} = 4 \text{ mg/L bound} + 1 \text{ mg/L free}$$

This example highlights the effect of altered protein binding on the free drug concentrations with drugs that are 90 percent protein bound or greater. In these drugs, the practitioner must take into account changes in protein binding in evaluating target drug concentrations and dosage adjustments to achieve these total drug concentrations. Special care must be taken in interpreting concentrations of highly protein bound drugs in patients who have low albumin concentrations from severe liver disease, malabsorption, or renal failure.

Using Plasma Drug Concentrations in Clinical Practice

The primary reasons for target concentration intervention are that the desired therapeutic effect is itself difficult to monitor and that the drug has a relatively narrow therapeutic index. For instance, with an antiepileptic drug, it is not sufficient to know that the patient is not actually having a seizure at the time of review. Seizures may be quite infrequent yet devastating when they occur. The absence of seizures is not an adequate measure of efficacy until a sufficiently long interval, such as a year without a seizure, has elapsed. In the meantime, the patient and practitioner would like some reassurance of a reasonable chance that therapeutic effectiveness is likely to be achieved. If antiepileptic drugs, like most antibiotics, had a wide therapeutic index, it would be sufficient to give large doses to all patients in the knowledge that the concentrations would always be sufficient to suppress seizure activity, irrespective of the interpatient variability in pharmacokinetics. However, this is not the case. Target concentrations for most antiepileptic drugs are frequently close to those producing significant adverse effects.

For similar reasons, the absence of an arrhythmia in a patient using an antiarrhythmic drug, the absence of mania or depression in a patient using lithium, or the absence of signs of transplant rejection in a patient using cyclosporine, coupled with the significant risk of toxicity for patients using these drugs in effective doses, makes them prime candidates for target concentration intervention.

The indications for other drugs rely on softer criteria. The bronchodilator response to theophylline is readily measurable, but the flat concentration-response curve above 10 mg/L and the real risk of serious toxicity at concentrations only twice this value make the measurement of concentrations valuable in assessing whether a further increase in dose, and by how much, is likely to bring therapeutic reward.

The effectiveness of digoxin in controlling atrial fibrillation is simply assessed by taking the pulse and cardiac auscultation. Like theophylline, however, if the response is inadequate, a decision to increase the dose, and to what extent, is made easier if the current concentration is known.

If a patient reports a symptom or exhibits a sign that may be due to a drug effect, whether therapeutic or toxic, then obtaining a sample for measurement of the drug concentration at that time can be quite useful. By considering the concentration along with the patient's clinical picture, it is possible to make a more reasonable judgment as to whether the drug is contributing to the signs and symptoms. For example, if a patient who is taking theophylline complains of not feeling well and has a headache, it is possible that the drug is the cause of the problems or, alternatively, that some illness is responsible. If, on one hand, the theophylline concentration is less than 5 mg/L, the clinician can be reasonably confident that the drug is not causing the problems. On the other hand, if the concentration is over 15 mg/L, there is a very good chance that theophylline is the culprit. In between these concentrations, the situation is not well resolved, but a drug cause is more likely at a higher drug concentration.

The most widespread use of drug concentration measurements is to find out its relationship to the therapeutic range. Some clinicians interpret drug concentration in one of three ways:

1. If the concentration is within the therapeutic range, they do nothing further.
2. If it is above the range, they reduce the dose in proportion to the degree that the measured concentration exceeds that desired.
3. If it is below the range, they increase the dose along similar lines.

If the previous dosage has been constant long enough to achieve steady state or if the drug has a long half-life in relation to the dosage interval (e.g., digoxin), this course of action is likely to be effective (as long as it is consistent with clinical assessment of the patient), and the procedure is simple to follow and apply.

The ideal times for plasma drug determination depend on the usual pattern of dose administration and the expected half-life of the drug.

REFERENCES

Avery, G. S. (1997). *Avery's drug treatment*. Auckland, New Zealand: Adis International.

DiPiro, J., Talbert, R. L., Yee, G. C., & Posey, L. M. (1996). *Pharmacotherapy: A pathophysiologic approach*. Stamford, CT: Appleton & Lange.

Katzung, B. G. (Ed.). (1995). *Basic and clinical pharmacology*. Norwalk, CT: Appleton & Lange.

World Health Organization. (1995). *WHO guide to good prescribing*. Geneva: WHO.

CHAPTER 4

. . . .

Legal and Professional Issues in Prescribing

CHAPTER OUTLINE

The Prescription

Writing the Prescription

A number of decisions need to be communicated in writing or verbally to the dispensing pharmacist to complete a prescription properly. The following are the most important of these issues. Based on reports re-ceived through the USP Medication Errors Reporting Program, the following practices reduce medication errors:

1. Use preprinted prescription pads that contain the name, address, and telephone number of the prescriber. This will allow the pharmacist to contact the prescriber if there are any questions about the prescription.
2. Write the complete drug name, strength, dosage, and form.
3. Write the date of the prescription.

4. Use metric units of measure such as milligrams and milliliters; avoid apothecary units of measure.
5. Avoid abbreviations.
6. Avoid the use of "as directed" or "as needed."
7. Include the general indication, such as "for infection."
8. Write "Dispense as Written" if generic substitution is not desired.

Positive Outcomes

Including the name of the drug and its strength on the patient label has numerous positive outcomes for the patient. It fulfills the right of the patient to be informed about the medications prescribed. It minimizes mistaken ingestion and is helpful in accidental overdose. It is useful to other providers prescribing for the patient. It enables the pharmacist and patient to verify that the prescribed drug is being dispensed. Finally, it helps patients when subsequent directions or warnings are given for the specific drug.

The appropriate amount of drug and the refill authorization benefit the patient in convenience and may reduce the cost of therapy. For acute therapies, the amount prescribed should be enough to cure the illness or maintain therapy until the next patient visit. Overprescribing is costly, permits inappropriate self-treatment with leftover doses, and contributes to the risk of accidental overdose. Patients cannot return unused drugs to the pharmacy for credit. Conversely, for the treatment of chronic illness, it is more economical to obtain a supply of medication for 1 to 3 months instead of repeated refills of smaller quantities. It is judicious to prescribe small initial trial supplies until patient dosage and compliance can be determined, followed by larger refill quantities for chronic therapy.

Federal Drug Legislation

History

The Food, Drug, and Cosmetic Act of 1906 was the first federal law designed to protect the public by restricting the manufacture and distribution of drugs. The law designated that drugs must meet official standards for strength and purity. The law prohibited "the manufacture of adulterated or misbranded or poisonous or deleterious foods, drugs, medicines, and liquors."

In 1937, a manufacturer marketed an elixir of sulfanilamide that used ethylene glycol as a solvent for the new antibiotic. Because its pharmacological effects were not tested, its toxicity went unnoticed until reports of more than 100 patient deaths were collected. The public outcry for new laws resulted in the federal Food, Drug, and Cosmetic Act of 1938. This act created the

Food and Drug Administration (FDA) to order drug recalls if a drug was determined to be unsafe.

From 1938 to 1962, the approval of new drugs was based on safety. In the early 1960s, the use of thalidomide by women in the early stages of pregnancy resulted in the birth of hundreds of deformed babies in Europe. A tragedy of this scale was avoided in the United States because the drug was not marketed here. This situation spurred the passage of the Kefauver-Harris amendments in 1962. These amendments required that both safety and efficacy of a drug be proven before it is marketed. In addition, the act required that all drugs marketed from 1938 to 1962 be evaluated for efficacy. This study was performed by the National Academy of Sciences and called the Drug Efficacy Study Implementation (DESI). Thousands of drugs were studied, and ineffective drugs were withdrawn from the market.

Two additional acts have had considerable influence on improving drug availability and benefiting patients with rare diseases. The Orphan Drug Act of 1983 fosters orphan drug development, for diseases so rare that the usual approval process would take decades to complete. The Drug Price Competition and Patent Term Restoration Act of 1984 expanded the number of generic drugs suitable for an abbreviated new drug application (ANDA). This makes it possible for generic drug companies to market generic versions of drugs by proving bioequivalence rather than duplicating the clinical trials needed for initial drug approval.

Food and Drug Administration Regulatory Jurisdiction

The FDA regulatory jurisdiction over drugs encompasses the standardization of nomenclature, the approval process for new drugs and new indications, official labeling, surveillance of adverse drug events, and methods of manufacture and distribution. The classification of a drug as a prescription or nonprescription medication is a matter of federal law. Products labeled with the legend "Caution: Federal law prohibits dispensing without a prescription" are regulated by the FDA and are referred to as *legend drugs*.

The FDA also regulates advertisements but only for prescription drugs and biologics. This role of the FDA was created by the Durham-Humphrey amendment of 1951, which provided that drug products labeled with the legend did not need to contain detailed instructions and that, when dispensed, the inclusion of directions from the prescriber on the label fulfilled the labeling requirement.

Controlled Substance Laws

The most significant drug legislation of recent years is the Controlled Substances Act of 1970. This law was designed to improve regulation of the manufacturing, distribution, and dispensing of certain controlled drugs by providing a closed system for legitimate providers of these substances. Every person who manufactures, distributes, prescribes, administers, or dispenses any controlled substance must register annually with the Drug Enforcement Administration (DEA). A pamphlet written for the physician that outlines regulations and requirements for controlled drug prescribing is available from the DEA. All those who regularly dispense and administer controlled substances during the course of their practice must maintain and keep on file for 2 years accurate records of drugs they purchase, distribute, and dispense.

In an effort to control drug distribution, a classification system was developed to categorize drugs according to their abuse and diversion potential. Nurse practitioners (NPs) have to know the different classifications and schedules of controlled drugs as well as the associated prescribing rules and regulations. Controlled drugs are placed into different schedules to which different regulations apply. There are five different schedules: I, II, III, IV, and V.

Table 4–1 presents the schedules, controls required, and examples of drugs.

Many states have controlled substance acts patterned after federal law. Because differences are allowed in the scheduling of drugs among states (a state may be more restrictive but not less restrictive), NPs must become acquainted with the provisions of the regulations in the state in which they are licensed. NPs wanting authority to prescribe controlled substances must apply for state authority prior to application for a federal DEA number.

Applications for a DEA number may be obtained from the state DEA office in your local jurisdiction.

Controlled Substance Prescribing Precautions

The practitioner should take precautions with controlled drug prescription pads and information included on the controlled substance prescription to minimize the chance for fraud and diversion of these drugs.

The prescription pad (or blanks) should be stored in a locked area, and supplies in use should be kept in sight of the practitioner. Prescriptions should never be signed in advance or used as notepads. The prescriber's name, address, and telephone number should be printed on the pads to allow verification by the dispensing pharmacist. The DEA registration number should appear on all controlled substance prescriptions. The prescription should be dated and legible and indicate any authorized refills. It is helpful to spell out the quantity dispensed as well giving an arabic number (e.g., "forty [40]") to discourage alterations in the intended quantity.

A few medications have such high abuse potential or potential for serious adverse effects, without clear therapeutic benefit, that they should be prescribed sparingly, if at all. The medications with high abuse potential that fall into this category include methadone, ethchlorvynol, amphetamine, and scheduled diet pills. Medications with especially problematic adverse-effect profiles include propoxyphene, meperidine, and butalbital. Med-

Table 4–1. Controlled Drug Schedules

Schedule	Controls Required	Drug Examples
I	No accepted medical use No legal use permitted For registered research facilities only	Heroin, LSD, mescaline, peyote, marijuana
II	No refills permitted Written prescriptions only (no telephone orders) Prescription expires in 72 h if not filled	Narcotics (morphine, codeine, meperidine, opium, hydromorphone, oxycodone, oxymorphone, methadone) Stimulants (cocaine, amphetamine, methylphenidate) Depressants (pentobarbital, secobarbital)
III	Prescription must be rewritten after 6 mo or 5 refills Telephone prescriptions okay	Narcotics (codeine in combination with nonnarcotic ingredients not to exceed 90 mg/tab; hydrocodone not to exceed 50 mg/tab) Stimulants (benzphetamine, chlorpheniramine, diethylpropion) Depressants (butabarbital)
IV	Same as schedule III Penalties for illegal possession are different	Pentazocine, propoxyphene, phentermine, benzodiazepines, meprobamate
V	Same as all prescription drugs May be dispensed without a prescription unless regulated by the state	Loperamide, diphenoxylate

ications with exceptionally narrow safety margins include secobarbital, pentobarbital, meprobamate, and ethchlorvynol. Medications with little established efficacy include propoxyphene, carisoprodol, butalbital, and scheduled diet pills.

Prescribing two or more controlled drugs from the same or different classes for one patient is to be done with extreme caution. Rarely does one patient meet diagnostic and symptomatic criteria to require the concomitant prescribing of two or more controlled drugs, whereas the natural history of chemical dependence frequently involves polysubstance abuse. Avoidance of polypharmacy when prescribing controlled drugs is therefore an important clinical, pharmacological, and medical-legal safeguard.

Opioids such as morphine have legitimate clinical usefulness, and the practitioner should not hesitate to prescribe them when indicated for patients who require analgesia or symptomatic relief not provided by other analgesics.

The most difficult clinical issues regarding controlled drug prescribing are with patients who have histories of drug or alcohol abuse or dependence and who need management of pain, anxiety, and insomnia. Special attention should be given to patients with current dependence on opioids or other central nervous system depressants. If a genuine symptomatic need is confirmed by adequate diagnostic evaluation and other analgesics or nondrug treatments are ineffective, it is the practitioner's responsibility to prescribe opioids. In this situation consider: (1) the patient may be simulating a disease to obtain the drug, (2) the effective dose will vary according to the degree of tolerance that the patient has developed, and (3) abrupt discontinuation can precipitate a withdrawal syndrome if the patient undergoes major surgical or medical trauma while dependent on the drug. Drug dependence can be maintained until the patient begins to recover from the intervening illness.

The practitioner must caution any patient for whom an antianxiety or hypnotic is prescribed about the potentiating effects of alcohol. Patients with a history of alcohol abuse or alcoholism should seldom receive these drugs.

Drug-Seeking Behavior

Within standard medical practice, there are many opportunities for individuals to obtain excessive quantities of controlled drugs, either intentionally or as a result of duplicate prescribing, often by different prescribers. The problems and costs associated with excessive use of controlled prescription drugs may have an impact on patients and their prescribers.

Drug-seeking behavior is a widely used, yet poorly defined term. For the purposes of this chapter, drug-seeking behavior describes the overreporting or manufacturing of symptoms to obtain prescriptions for controlled substances. Typical behaviors include multiple somatic complaints; vague symptom complexes of unclear origin involving pain, anxiety, or insomnia; insistence that no other medications work; multiple medication allergies; remarks about having a high tolerance; insistence on controlled drug prescriptions on the first visit; symptom complexes that seem to indicate a need for multiple controlled drugs or classes of drugs; arguing about pharmacology;

Table 4–2. Drug-Seeking Behaviors

Overreporting symptoms
Multiple somatic complaints
Vague symptom complexes
Insistence on specific medications
Refusal of generic equivalent
Self-asserted high tolerance
First-visit insistence on controlled prescriptions
Veiled threats
Flattery followed by prescription request
Demands for polypharmacy
More than two pharmacies
More than two prescribers of controlled drugs

veiled threats; and comments that "you are the only person who understands me." Table 4–2 lists common drug-seeking behaviors.

Although not diagnostic of drug-seeking behavior, many of these types of comments indicate the basic pathological state involved in drug-seeking behavior—a progressive preoccupation with obtaining, using, and recovering from the use of mood-altering drugs at the expense of other relationships. In the instance of prescription drug abuse, the provider-patient relationship becomes increasingly strained.

Generally, if the NP has a vague sense of uneasiness about a diagnosis and controlled drug prescription, caution is indicated. If the practitioner experiences a feeling of being pressured by the patient about a symptom and controlled drug prescription, drug-seeking behavior is present until proved otherwise.

Strategies to combat drug-seeking behavior include the following:

1. Acquisition and wide use of chemical dependence screening skills
2. Early and firm limit setting regarding indications for controlled drug prescribing
3. Careful documentation of a firm diagnosis and the ruling out of chemical dependence before initiating a controlled prescription
4. Practice in "just saying no" and feeling comfortable in being firm without escalating into an argument with the patient

A practitioner must not take drug-seeking behavior personally. The behavior has little if anything to do with the practitioner, but rather it indicates the patient's underlying pathology of chemical dependence. As such, it is a patient symptom that can be assessed and addressed objectively and compassionately (but without prescribing) rather than angrily and personally.

Scams

Scams are common ruses that chemically dependent patients use to obtain increasing supplies of controlled prescriptions. Once a scam has worked in a given practice, that scam will continue to surface periodically in that office practice until the provider ceases to reinforce the scam. Drug enforcement investigators and prescription drug–abusing patients commonly observe that the greater the ease patients find when practicing scams and drug-seeking behavior in a provider's practice, the higher the prevalence of prescription drug–abusing patients there will be in that practice. Dealing with scams consists of the following steps:

1. Learning to recognize the common ones
2. Refusing to give in to them
3. Practicing the skill of turning the tables on the scammer

Scams are generally reasons for more medications, indications for more potent or higher dosage formulations, indications for higher street value brands of drugs, ways to obtain a controlled drug without a chart or visit note, or reasons to avoid noncontrolled alternatives. Most scams produce discomfort in providers, and patients using scams are often willing to push the practitioner if they encounter resistance to the scam. Patient-generated pressure to prescribe in the face of clinician hesitancy is one classic sign of a scam. Patients rarely argue pharmacology with providers unless the issue of prescribing controlled drugs is being contested. The clinical phenomenon of an initial "no" (refusal to prescribe by the practitioner) becoming a "yes" (eventual willingness to prescribe) if the patient brings the right pressure to bear on the practitioner is pathognomonic of prescription drug abuse.

Prescription altering and forging is a frequently encountered scam. Variations include stealing prescriptions, forging blank prescriptions, photocopying prescriptions, and rewriting prescriptions. Additional prescription alteration strategies that are more common include changing the strength of drug prescribed, the number of pills prescribed, the number of refills indicated, or the date of the prescription.

Pressure to Prescribe

Another factor that increases the demand for controlled substances is the pressure to prescribe at every visit and the expectation that patients deserve a prescription for something at each visit or for each symptom offered. This process results in two well-known adverse situations: (1) overprescribing of antibiotics and resulting antibiotic resistance and (2) polypharmacy, especially of the elderly. It also may result in a tendency on the part of practitioners to prescribe higher-potency noncontrolled substances and then ultimately controlled drugs when patients persist with vague somatic complaints.

Enabling

Enabling refers to the powerful instinct in practitioners to do anything medically possible to enable patients with present or potential disability to live at a higher level of function. Unfortunately, the disease of chemical dependence has a bottomless appetite for enabling, also defined as behaviors on the part of a friend, family member, or health care provider that shelter the chemically dependent individual from the adverse consequences of the disease. When the practitioners' overdeveloped enabling instincts interact with chemically dependent patients, the patients are often able to manipulate the practitioners to avoid the consequences of their disease process, thus permitting that disease to progress to further, more pathological levels. This is especially true when controlled drug prescribing is involved. A common statement from practitioners who have been manipulated into enabling and overprescribing to patients is "I was only trying to help." Chemical dependence is one disease process in which practitioners must strive against their natural enabling tendencies, especially when prescribing controlled drugs.

Confrontation Phobia

Finally, there is confrontation phobia. Newer curricula in training programs over the past two or three decades have led to an emphasis on the clinical interview and practitioner-patient relationship-building skills. Skill building involves active learning strategies in the areas of verbal and nonverbal communication, empathy, and rapport building. Rarely, if ever, are NPs coached on how to say no. This emphasis on rapport-building techniques to the virtual exclusion of limit-setting skills helps to create the current clinical reality in which NPs feel acutely uncomfortable with conflict and interpersonal confrontation. It is obvious how the practitioner's fear and avoidance of confrontation plays into the hands of chemically dependent patients, who have a stronger relationship with the prescription than they do with the practitioner.

Solutions to Problems of Controlled Substance Prescribing

Law enforcement and legislative efforts have produced few solutions to the problem of imbalance in controlled drug prescribing. Until recently, these approaches have targeted diversion of drugs and overprescribing. Results of duplicate and triplicate prescription policies, as well as stricter investigation and enforcement, have led to physicians' decreased prescribing of controlled drugs across the board. The outcome has not been the optimal practice of more prescribing to the many patients who are currently undertreated and little or no prescribing to those with chemical dependence and other contraindications.

Practitioners must be able to identify common scams and defuse them efficiently and effectively. One strategy is to just say no and mean it. Chemically dependent patients have learned that the practitioners' enabling instincts and confrontation discomfort are so great that when NPs initially say no, it usually ultimately can be turned into a yes if enough pressure is applied. Thus, it is important to be able to mean no and to stick with it. A higher-level clinical skill is initially to say no and then to turn the tables on a patient who demands the prescription. This strategy is based on the clinical fact that patients who demand controlled drugs generally have a

pathological relationship with that prescription because of underlying chemical dependence. By making the statement "I am feeling pressured by you to write a prescription today that is not clinically indicated. Because of this I am really concerned about you, and we need to talk about your use of alcohol or other substances," the NP can often effectively turn the tables and shift the discomfort to the patient while still refusing to prescribe.

Careful charting and documentation habits are essential for prescribing controlled drugs. Document clearly in a progress note (1) the diagnosis, (2) the clinical indications, (3) the expected symptom end point, and (4) the treatment time course whenever prescribing controlled drugs.

These strategies reduce the risk of significant controlled drug diversion from one's practice. Therefore, controlled medications can be much more comfortably and safely prescribed, with the overall effect of increasing appropriate prescribing.

State Practice Acts

Federal law establishes whether a drug requires a prescription but does not dictate who may prescribe. The authority to prescribe is a function of state law. Unlike the uniform nature of federal law, prescriptive authority varies from state to state. The states have the authority to license health care professionals, and NPs are well aware that they possess a state license and not a federal license to practice nursing.

The idea of regulation of medical and nursing education and practice is relatively recent, beginning with the licensing of NPs in the 1970s. States have this authority under the states' "police power" to take regulatory action to protect public health, welfare, and safety. The courts have consistently upheld professional licensing laws as legitimate use of this power. The purpose of these laws is to ensure that those who provide health care services for a fee have demonstrated a minimum level of competency.

Each state therefore has practice acts that set forth licensing requirements for health professionals, define the scope of practice, and prohibit unauthorized practice. These laws usually provide for a state board that governs each profession and establishes administrative rules of conduct for each profession. Usually, prescriptive authority is given expressly to NPs; however, prescribing authority need not be restricted to NPs. For example, Connecticut defines a "prescribing practitioner" as an NP, dentist, podiatrist, optometrist, osteopath, nurse practitioner assistant, advanced practice registered nurse, nurse-midwife, or veterinarian licensed by the state. Similar definitions appear in other state statutes. Most states permit advanced practice nurses, NPs, or clinical nurses to have some degree of prescriptive authority.

Prescriptive authority exists as dependent and independent authority. Independent authority, as granted NPs, permits the prescriber to exert autonomous judgment. Dependent authority exists when the primary prescriber delegates the authority to another through a collaborative agreement. These agreements usually involve written guidelines and/or a protocol for treatment. Some states limit authority by restricting prescribing to a written formulary. Other restrictions may apply, including limits on the geographic locations of the clinical site, limits on the number of doses or refills that may be authorized, or requiring written agreements with a practicing NP that spell out the scope of the prescribing authority.

Fifteen states permit NPs to function independently of physicians. Washington, for example, requires no collaborative or supervising agreements with a physician for nonschedule drugs and does not require a formulary. The Nursing Board has the power to establish the conditions of the prescribing authority. The only restriction on prescribing is that the drug must relate to the nurse's scope of practice. Nurse prescribers must complete 30 contact hours of pharmacotherapeutics and provide evidence of an additional 15 hours every 2 years.

Each year, the January issue of the journal *Nurse Practitioner* contains a review of the current state laws regarding prescriptive authority for advanced practice nurses. This review is useful in determining the current status of prescribing in each state.

The New Drug Approval Process

The U.S. system of new drug approvals is perhaps the most rigorous in the world. On average, it costs a company $359 million to get one new medicine from the laboratory to the pharmacist's shelf, according to a February 1993 report by the Congressional Office of Technology Assessment (Congressional Office of Technology Assessment, 1993). It takes 12 years on average for an experimental drug to travel from lab to medicine chest. Only 5 in 5000 compounds that enter preclinical testing make it to human testing. One of these five that are tested on people is approved.

Preclinical Research

The process of synthesis and extraction identifies new molecules with the potential to produce a desired change in a biologic system (e.g., to inhibit or stimulate an important enzyme, to alter a metabolic pathway, or to change cellular structure). The process may require research on the fundamental mechanisms of disease or biologic processes, research on the action of known therapeutic agents, or random selection and broad biologic

screening. New molecules can be produced through artificial synthesis or extracted from natural sources (plant, mineral, or animal). The number of compounds that can be produced based on the same general chemical structure runs into the hundreds of millions.

Biologic screening and pharmacological testing use nonhuman studies to explore the pharmacological activity and therapeutic potential of compounds. These tests involve the use of animals, isolated cell cultures and tissues, enzymes, and cloned receptor sites, as well as computer models. If the results of the tests suggest potential beneficial activity, related compounds are tested to see which version of the molecule produces the highest level of pharmacological activity and demonstrates the most therapeutic promise, with the smallest number of potentially harmful biologic properties.

Pharmaceutical dosage formulation and stability testing is the process of turning an active compound into a form and strength suitable for human use. A pharmaceutical product can take any one of a number of dosage forms (e.g., liquid, tablets, capsules, ointments, sprays, patches) and dosage strengths.

Toxicology and safety testing determines the potential risk a compound poses to people and the environment. These studies use animals, tissue cultures, and other test systems to examine the relationship between factors such as dose level, frequency of administration, and duration of exposure to both the short- and long-term survival of living organisms. Tests provide information on the dose-response pattern of the compound and its toxic effects. Most toxicology and safety testing is conducted on new molecular entities prior to their human introduction, but companies can choose to delay long-term toxicity testing until after the therapeutic potential of the product is established.

Clinical Studies

Investigational New Drug Application

An investigational new drug (IND) application is filed with the FDA prior to human testing. The IND application is a compilation of all known information about the compound. It also includes a description of the clinical research plan for the product and the specific protocol for phase I study. Unless the FDA says no, the IND is automatically approved after 30 days, and clinical tests can begin. The FDA has formulated IND regulations for the clinical study of a new drug's safety and efficacy and has divided this evaluation into three phases:

1. Phase I clinical evaluation is the first testing of a new compound in subjects, for the purpose of establishing the tolerance of healthy human subjects at different doses, defining its pharmacological effects at anticipated therapeutic levels, and study-

ing its absorption, distribution, metabolism, and excretion patterns in humans.

2. Phase II clinical evaluation is controlled studies performed on patients with the target disease or disorder to determine a compound's potential usefulness and short-term risks. A relatively small number of patients, usually no more than several hundred subjects, are enrolled in phase II studies.

3. Phase III trials are controlled and uncontrolled clinical trials of a drug's safety and effectiveness in hospital and outpatient settings. Phase III studies gather precise information on the drug's effectiveness for specific indications, determine whether the drug produces a broader range of adverse effects than those exhibited in the small study populations of phase I and II studies, and identify the best way of administering and using the drug for the purpose intended. If the drug is approved, this information forms the basis for deciding the content of the product label. Phase III trials verify that the acceptable benefit-to-risk ratio seen in phase II persists under conditions of anticipated usage and in groups of patients large enough to identify statistically and clinically significant responses.

Conferences between the sponsor and the FDA are held during all three phases of development. While an IND is in effect, the sponsor must report in writing to the FDA within 10 working days any serious and unexpected adverse reactions that may be drug related.

The treatment IND program is part of the FDA's efforts to facilitate the development of significant new therapies. Under this program, treatment protocols using an investigational drug can be approved for life-threatening illnesses for which there is no comparable alternative therapy. Information on the availability of an investigational drug under a treatment IND is published in the *Journal of the American Medical Association* and other public means.

Bioavailability Studies

Healthy volunteers are used to document the rate of absorption and excretion from the body of a compound's active ingredients. Companies conduct bioavailability studies both at the beginning of human testing and just prior to marketing to show that the formulation used to demonstrate safety and efficacy in clinical trials is equivalent to the product that will be distributed for sale. Companies also conduct bioavailability studies on marketed products whenever they change the method used to administer the drug (e.g., from injection or oral dose form), the composition of the drug, the concentration of the active ingredient, or the manufacturing process used to produce the drug.

Regulatory Review: New Drug Application

To market a new drug for human use, a manufacturer must have a new drug application (NDA) approved by the FDA. All information about the drug gathered during the drug discovery and development process is assembled in the NDA. During the review period, the FDA may ask the company for additional information about the product or seek clarification of the data contained in the application. The FDA must review the NDA within 180 days. Usually, the FDA requests additional information, and the manufacturer needs from 1 to 5 years to complete any additional well-controlled trials necessary to support the claimed indications or prove the drug's safety.

Accelerated Approval of a New Drug Application

The timely availability of new drugs remains the subject of considerable debate. In December 1992, the FDA published new regulations to accelerate approval of certain new drugs that provide therapeutic benefit to patients with serious or life-threatening illnesses. The FDA can approve these drugs based on well-controlled clinical trials establishing that the product has an effect on a therapeutic end point that is likely to predict clinical benefit. The applicant is required to conduct postmarketing studies.

Postapproval Research

Clinical experience with a new drug may include no more than 1000 to 2000 patients. The detection of rare (less than 1:1000) adverse drug reactions is not reliable until hundreds of thousands of patients have taken the drug. Clinical trials conducted after a drug is marketed (referred to as phase IV studies in the United States) are an important source of information on as-yet undetected adverse outcomes, especially in populations not included in the premarketing trials (e.g., children, the elderly, pregnant women), and the drug's long-term morbidity and mortality profile. Regulatory authorities can require companies to conduct phase IV studies as a condition of market approval. Companies often conduct postmarketing studies in the absence of a regulatory mandate.

Official Labeling

The legal distinction between a prescription drug and an over-the-counter (OTC) drug is not founded on relative safety per se but rather involves a regulatory decision on whether adequate directions for the drug's proper use can be written for the layperson. If the FDA determines that adequate directions can be written, the manufacturer is not allowed to identify the drug with a prescription legend.

Conversely, for a prescription drug, the manufacturer's directions or FDA-approved labeling (the package insert) is intended for the prescriber, pharmacist, or nurse and provides a summary of information about the chemical and physical nature of the product, pharmacological indications and contraindications, means of administration, dosages, side effects and adverse reactions, how the drug is supplied, and any other information pertinent to safe and effective use. This summary, or official labeling, is developed by discussion between the FDA and the drug manufacturer. The material in the *Physician's Desk Reference* (PDR) is a verbatim presentation of the official labeling.

The FDA's jurisdiction over the uses of marketed drugs and doses extends only to what the manufacturer may recommend and must disclose in its labeling. The FDA is not charged with dictating how a prescriber should practice. The FDA is concerned with the marketing and availability of drugs that have demonstrated substantial evidence of an acceptable benefit-to-risk ratio for labeled indications. The proper and successful therapeutic use of these drugs is the responsibility of the prescriber.

Off-Label Use

The prescription of a drug for an off-label (unlabeled) indication is entirely proper if the proposed use is based on rational scientific theory or controlled clinical studies. The FDA has made it clear that it neither has nor wants the authority to compel prescribers to adhere to official uses.

NPs are well advised to be aware of the package insert and give it due weight. However, a decision on how to use a drug must be based on what is best for the patient. In professional liability suits, such drug labeling may have evidentiary weight, but drug labeling is not intended to set the standard for what is good medical practice.

Direct to Consumer Advertising

The federal Food, Drug, and Cosmetic Act provides that the advertising of prescription drugs must conform to the labeling. Any advertisement that describes a drug's use must contain the generic name and amount of active ingredient, the name and address of the manufacturer, and a brief summary of the prescribing information. A prescription drug advertisement that implies incorrectly that a drug is the treatment of choice or is useful for an unlabeled indication is unlawful. Drug manufacturers are increasingly marketing prescription drugs to patients through print and electronic media, which has increased the demand on practitioners to prescribe advertised drug products.

Informed Consent

The notion of informed consent is shorthand for the doctrine of informed decision making, which proposes that each patient has the right to make informed decisions about those things that will have an impact on himself or herself. Although some question whether consent to medical procedures can ever be truly informed, the doctrine has been assimilated into American society's concept of what medical practice should include. Informed consent should be obtained from a patient before all medical interventions, diagnostic as well as therapeutic. A patient may either agree to or refuse a proposed intervention; in both situations, the patient is making her or his own informed decision.

The provider who performs a specific service is responsible for obtaining consent to that specific service. The consent usually is given to the identified individual and others working with him or her to perform the specific procedure and other procedures within the scope of the consented-to procedure. In general, a referring provider is not responsible for getting consent for a procedure performed by another provider. Some exceptions may apply, however, and practitioners who send patients for tests or consultations should inform them generally about the procedures.

There are four critical features of informed consent: (1) a competent patient (2) who is provided adequate information with which to make a decision (3) and who voluntarily (4) consents to a proposed intervention. Although legal opinions tend to merge the concepts, it is helpful to consider competence as two related but distinct areas: legal competence and clinical competence. A patient must be both legally and clinically competent to give informed consent. In general, an adult is presumed to be legally competent unless declared incompetent in formal legal proceedings. To be clinically competent for medical decision making, a patient must be able to comprehend information that is provided, formulate a decision about a proposed intervention, and communicate that decision to the health care team.

Clinical competence is not an all-or-none phenomenon. A patient may be competent to make some choices but not others. Clinical competence may vary over time and is affected by the vagaries of the individual's illness and therapies currently in use. Assistive devices and environmental modification may be important to maintaining and enhancing clinical competence. Hearing aids, interpreters, and communication boards may be important assistive devices to certain patients. Examples of environmental factors that affect clinical competence include sedative medications, presence of background noise for a patient with a hearing disability, and the side of approach to a patient with a visual field loss.

REFERENCES

AMA. (1993). *AMA drug evaluations* (pp.1–16). Chicago: American Medical Association.

Congressional Office of Technology Assessment. (1993). *Pharmaceutical R&D costs, risks, and rewards*. Washington, D.C., U.S. Government Printing Office (stock #052-003-01315-1).

Drug Enforcement Administration. (1990). *Guidelines for prescription of narcotics for physicians*. Washington, D.C.: U.S. Government Printing Office.

Parran, T. (1997). Alcohol and other substance abuse. *Medical Clinics of North America, 81*.

CHAPTER 5

Adverse Drug Reactions

CHAPTER OUTLINE

In general, when drug products are administered, the benefit should outweigh the risk. However, all use of drug products has certain risks. An adverse drug reaction (ADR) is an unintended and undesired response to an appropriate drug administered for diagnostic, therapeutic, or prophylactic purposes. This chapter describes the various types of adverse reactions to drugs.

The terms *adverse drug event* and *side effect* describe the potential unwanted effects that patients experience as a result of medication therapy. Adverse events include symptoms that are uncomfortable for the patient but may be tolerable, such as nausea, vomiting, fatigue, dizziness, and hypotension. Adverse events may also include syndromes that require immediate termination of therapy, such as anaphylaxis, thrombocytopenia, and lupus.

Adverse drug events may occur within minutes of drug exposure (e.g., anaphylaxis), days (e.g., gastrointestinal [GI] bleeding), or weeks (e.g., renal failure). Alternatively, important reactions can develop insidiously over a prolonged period (e.g., corticosteroid-induced cataracts). Other reactions may be apparent only after the drug has been discontinued (e.g., cancer related to immunosuppressants). It is even possible that the adverse effect will affect the offspring of the patient, without affecting the patient at all (e.g., congenital abnormalities caused by drug therapy).

Numerous studies have been done to determine the actual incidence of adverse drug events, and they range from 10 to 30 percent of hospitalized patients, with a mortality of 0.1 to 0.5 percent. It has been estimated that 2 to 6 percent of hospital admissions are due to adverse drug events. Adverse drug events are more likely to occur in females, the elderly, patients with renal impairment, and patients taking many medications.

The incidence of adverse drug reaction increases with the number of drugs a patient takes. A study showed that in patients receiving no to five drugs, the incidence of adverse drug reactions was 4.2 percent; however, the incidence rose to 24.2 percent when 11 to 15 drugs were administered and to 45 percent when 21 or more drugs were given.

There is some temptation to add drugs to existing treatments, especially if the current regimen was prescribed by someone else. The nurse practitioner (NP) may feel that the earlier prescriber knew more about the clinical situation. Even if this is true, it is important to review all of the patient's medications, including over-the-counter (OTC) medications and herbal remedies, before adding to them.

Some drug effects are dose related. Because of individual differences in pharmacokinetics, a dose tolerated by one patient may cause adverse effects in another. Medication errors may lead to an excessive amount of the drug being given or taken, as may a change of products of the same drug entity (changing from depot or sustained-release forms to regular forms of the same drug product). It is possible to overdose a patient on a newly developed drug because the dose is usually determined in a very small group of patients. Many drugs are found to be effective at a lower dose than that initially suggested.

The presence of disease can markedly influence the incidence and occurrence of adverse drug reactions. Diseases of the kidney and liver increase the risk of adverse drug reaction. Table 5–1 presents examples of adverse drug reactions associated with diseases.

Categories of Adverse Drug Reactions

Adverse drug reactions are classified into three categories. Type A adverse drug reactions, which produce 70 to 80 percent of all adverse events, are dose-dependent and related to the pharmacological effects of the drug. These reactions, which are often predictable and preventable, are the ones frequently listed in the product information and in textbooks. They are important factors in drug selection, and the practitioner must be familiar with them to safely prescribe drugs.

Type B reactions are allergic or idiosyncratic reactions. They are not dose-dependent or an extension of the pharmacology of the drug. Most adverse drug reactions are not allergic; only about 6 to 10 percent are true allergic reactions. The risk of an allergic reaction is 1 to 3 percent for most drugs. Type B reactions are usually not predictable or preventable.

The third type of adverse drug reaction is a delayed form of type A reaction, such as carcinogenesis or teratogenesis. These reactions must be prevented by not administering the drug unless the benefits exceed the potential risk of these long-term and irreversible effects on the patient or fetus.

Table 5–2 presents the categories of adverse drug reactions.

Type A Adverse Drug Reactions

Type A adverse drug reactions are the result of an unwanted but otherwise normal pharmacological action of a drug given in the usual therapeutic doses. Type A reactions are predictable from a drug's known pharmacological properties. They are usually dose-dependent, and their incidence and morbidity are generally well known. Their mortality is usually low. When a group of individuals receives a drug, a spectrum of response is observed. This variability manifests itself as different doses to achieve the desired therapeutic effects, or differing responses to the same dose. Type A reactions are likely to occur when the therapeutic index is low. In some instances, the type A reaction occurs as an exaggeration of the primary pharmacological effect. Examples include bleeding with anticoagulants, hypoglycemia with insulin, and hypotension with antihypertensives. In other circumstances, the type A reaction is the result of the

Table 5–1. Examples of Adverse Drug Reactions Associated with Disease

Disease	Drug	Possible Adverse Drug Reaction
Renal failure	Aminoglycosides Digoxin Furosemide	Nephrotoxicity, ototoxicity Digitalis toxicity Ototoxicity
Hepatic precoma	Morphine	Precipitate encephalopathy
Ascites	Diuretics	Precipitate encephalopathy
Peptic ulcer disease	Corticosteroids, nonsteroidal anti-inflammatory drugs (NSAIDs)	Increased risk of GI bleeding
Heart failure	Beta blockers, NSAIDs	Aggravate or precipitate heart failure
Epilepsy	Phenothiazines, tricyclic antidepressants	May aggravate seizures
Hyperthyroidism	Digoxin	Digitalis toxicity

Table 5–2. Categories of Adverse Drug Reactions

Type A (Predictable)	Type B (Unpredictable)	Delayed
Side effects	Allergy	Teratogenesis
Secondary effects	Idiosyncrasy	Carcinogenesis
Drug interactions	Intolerance	

drug's secondary reactions. Examples include tricyclic antidepressants' anticholinergic properties or the action of terfenadine (Seldane) on myocardial potassium channels, which are unrelated to the effects that mediate the drug's therapeutic action. At times, reduction of the dose may be sufficient to lessen or stop these reactions; otherwise, the drug has to be discontinued.

Causes

Type A reactions develop in individuals who are at the extremes of the dose-response curves for pharmacological and secondary drug effects. There are three basic reasons for unexpected type A reactions: (1) defects in drug quality, (2) abnormal pharmacokinetics, and (3) altered sensitivity of the target receptors because of disease or individual genetics. If the drug product is of poor quality, then there can be more actual drug than the amount stated, or the release of the drug from the dosage form can be much faster than desired, which will result in a adverse reaction. Changes in the individual pharmacokinetic parameters of adsorption, distribution, or elimination may result in high concentrations of the drug in the body and an exaggerated effect in the body. Many adverse drug reactions result from abnormal pharmacokinetic handling of the drug in an individual patient. Adverse reactions may also be due to differences in target

organ sensitivity to the drug. These differences may be due to genetic differences in the number of receptors among individuals, the presence of other drugs in the body, or the effect of diseases on various physiological systems in the body. Any or all of these factors may result in unwanted adverse effects on the administration of a drug. Table 5–3 presents the causes of type A adverse drug reactions.

Type B Adverse Drug Reactions

Type B adverse drug reactions are allergic or idiosyncratic effects that are not dose-dependent or expected from the pharmacological actions of the drugs. They are usually unpredictable and unavoidable. Examples include anaphylactic reactions, serum sickness, lupus erythematosus, urticaria, hemolytic anemia, and photosensitivity. The development of type B adverse reactions usually requires discontinuation of the therapy.

Allergic Causes

Drug allergies range from very mild (e.g., urticaria) to very severe (e.g., anaphylactic shock) reactions. Patients who report drug allergies need to be evaluated carefully, even though often the events reported are type A reac-

Table 5–3. Causes of Type A Adverse Drug Reactions

Cause of Reaction	Mechanism of Reaction	Examples
Drug quality	Drug overdose	Mislabeled drug has more active ingredient than shown on the label.
	Release rate too fast	Long-acting dosage form releases all of the drug at once instead of over several hours.
Pharmacokinetics	Unexpectedly high drug levels cause an enhanced pharmacological response	Reduced elimination in renal disease causes drug to accumulate and cause toxicity. Reduced protein binding causes more free drug to be available.
Receptor sensitivity	Exaggerated or secondary pharmacological effects of a drug	Anticholinergic effects in some patients at very low doses. Cardiac failure may be unmasked in some patients by beta blockers.

tions such as nausea and vomiting rather than true allergic reactions.

Drugs are usually extremely small molecules and have no antigenic activity. The drug combines with a carrier molecule or protein and forms a drug-protein complex. It is this drug-protein complex that possesses antigenic activity and invokes specific antibody formation, thereby sensitizing the body to the drug. This synthesis of antibodies usually occurs after a period of 1 to 2 weeks. When subsequent exposure to the drug occurs, an antigen-antibody interaction results in the typical allergic manifestations. Extremely small quantities of antigen are required to provoke an allergic reaction. Drug allergies may manifest themselves over a full spectrum of immediate and delayed reactions. As an example, skin reactions may extend from mild rash to severe exfoliative dermatitis.

Drug allergies are classified into five types of reactions:

1. In type I reactions, called *immediate hypersensitivity reactions,* the drug-protein complex binds with IgE on the surface of basophils and mast cells, which causes the release of mediators such as histamine, prostaglandins, and leukotrienes. These substances cause the clinically apparent symptoms of urticaria, bronchospasm, or anaphylactic shock. Drug-induced skin reactions such as urticaria or angioedema can occur as isolated reactions or can be accompanied by other types of allergic reactions.

2. In type II reactions, called *cytotoxic hypersensitivity reactions,* the IgG or IgM antibody reacts with the drug-protein complex on the wall of blood cells. This destruction of the formed elements of the blood results in drug-induced thrombocytopenia, neutropenia, hemoloysis, or anemia.

3. In type III allergic reactions, called *immune complex hypersensitivity,* the drug-protein complex combines with IgG and IgM to trigger the release of complement and cause local vascular damage. This is seen clinically as serum sickness, fever, joint and muscle pain, and lymphadenopathy. Such reactions may take the form of fever only or involve generalized lymphadenopathy and joint swellings accompanied by urticaria and angioedema. Serum sickness may also be due to the injection of contaminant foreign proteins, for example, the egg protein in influenza vaccine. In the initial exposure to the drug, the symptoms develop after significant amounts of antibody are synthesized by the body, usually about a week. Symptoms may appear 3 weeks after the drug has been discontinued. Penicillin and sulfa drugs have been associated with these adverse reactions.

4. Type IV allergic reactions, called *delayed hypersensitivity reactions,* occur if the drug-protein complex is recognized by T lymphocytes, which causes a direct cytotoxicity and activation of macrophages to the cell. Clinically, this is seen as fixed drug eruptions or topical contact dermatitis to topical drug preparations.

5. Another type of allergic reaction is the autoimmune reaction. In this case, the drug-protein complex puts into effect changes in the immune system that result in increased cytotoxic T-cell proliferation and formations of immunoglobulins that produce such conditions as systemic lupus erythematosus, glomerulonephritis, and certain types of granulocytopenia.

Idiosyncratic Causes

Individual patients vary widely in their reactions to drugs. Some patients have reactions that are not expected from the known pharmacological actions of a drug. The patient's unique genetic makeup contributes to the variability. When given an average and safe dose of a drug, some patients experience no effects, and others have severe adverse reactions. The cause of these bizarre effects may be pharmaceutical, pharmacokinetic, or genetic in origin.

Three potential sources of idiosyncratic type B adverse reactions are due to problems with the drugs themselves: (1) decomposition of the active ingredients, (2) effects of additives placed in the dosage form for pharmaceutical reasons, and (3) effects from the by-products of the manufacturing of the drug.

The administration of decomposed product is most likely to produce a therapeutic failure; however, the decomposed compounds may be toxic. An example is tetracycline, which can degrade into compounds that can cause renal failure (Fanconi's syndrome). It is well known that tartrazine dye in some products causes allergic reactions and bronchospasm. Recently, L-tryptophan was withdrawn from the market when certain brands contained a manufacturing by-product that caused eosinophilia and myalgia. When patients exhibit bizarre adverse reactions to common drugs, it is useful to keep drug product problems in mind as a possible cause.

Patients can also react to drugs in an unexpected way if they have an abnormality of metabolism of the drug that creates a toxic substance that causes direct organ damage. Examples of these reactions are hepatotoxicity with tacrine and halothane, agranulocytosis with clozapine, and hypersensitivity with carbamazepine. Why a very few individuals develop these reactions is unknown. These patients may have overactive activation pathways, underactive protective pathways, or immunologic systems that are more responsive to allergic stimuli.

The final source of idiosyncratic reactions is some qualitative or quantitative abnormal response by the patient. Many of these abnormal responses are genetic in origin. For example, the patient with hemophilia may bleed excessively if given aspirin, the patient with G6PD deficiency may develop hemolytic anemia if given primaquine, or the patient with excess aminolevulinic acid may develop porphyria if given drugs such as barbiturates or estrogens.

Delayed Adverse Drug Reactions

Delayed adverse drug reactions, a form of a type A reaction, results from teratogenesis (congenital malformation) or carcinogenesis.

Teratogenesis (Congenital Malformation)

The possibility that a drug may cause teratologic changes is well known. These adverse reactions are type A, being dose related and predictable. Congenital malformations are defined as irreversible functional or morphologic defects present at birth and can be caused by genetic or environmental (including drug) factors. A *teratogen* is generally defined as an exogenous agent that has the ability to produce congenital malformations during fetal development. Major congenital malformations occur in 2 to 4 percent of all live births, and up to 15 percent of all diagnosed pregnancies result in fetal loss. The cause of these adverse outcomes is poorly understood, but it is important to understand this background risk in evaluating the prevalence of drug-induced malformations. Associations of congenital malformations with drugs have been described in case reports and case series. Although

these are important in drawing attention to a suspected teratogen, they do not prove teratogenicity. Epidemiological studies, which correct for confounding factors and have appropriate statistical analyses, are needed to detect associations between drug therapy and adverse outcomes.

The FDA's use-in-pregnancy rating system (Table 5–4) weighs the degree to which available information has ruled out risk to the fetus against the drug's potential benefit to the patient. All drugs available are not rated, and the list is not inclusive. If a drug is not rated, there may be pregnancy precautions listed in the prescribing information.

In general, the decision to use a drug for therapy in any patient is made by evaluating the benefits versus the risks to the patient. The situation is more complex in treating the pregnant patient because this evaluation must be made for two patients, the mother and the unborn child, and the adverse reactions in the fetus are usually irreversible. Unfortunately, many new drugs' risks to the fetus are unknown. Table 5–5 lists drugs identified with FDA ratings of X and D. Because a number of drugs have never been rated, the lists are not all inclusive; precautions do need to be taken with many of the drugs that are not rated.

The identification of a drug or chemical as a teratogen is hampered by the fact that all exposed fetuses do not show congenital malformations. Even with drugs such as thalidomide and retinoids, the occurrence is 20 to 40 percent. Other substances, such as carbamazepine and valproic acid, cause malformations in only 1 to 2 percent of prenatal exposures. In addition, the use of animal models is not very helpful. There are known teratogens

Table 5–4. FDA Use-in-Pregnancy Ratings

FDA Rating (category)	Criteria for Rating
X	*Contraindicated in Pregnancy* Studies in animals or humans have demonstrated fetal risk that clearly outweighs any possible benefit to the patient.
D	*Positive Evidence of Risk* Investigational or postmarketing data show risk to the fetus. Nevertheless, potential benefits may outweigh the potential risk.
C	*Risk Cannot Be Ruled Out* Human studies are lacking, and animal studies are either positive for risk or are lacking as well. However, potential benefits may outweigh the potential risk.
B	*No Evidence of Risk in Humans* Either animal findings show risk while human findings do not, or, if no adequate human studies have been done, animal findings are negative.
A	*Controlled Studies Show No Risk* Adequate, well-controlled studies in pregnant women have failed to demonstrate risk to the fetus.

Table 5–5. Drugs Listed as Pregnancy Risk Rating X and D

FDA Rating	Drugs
X Contraindicated in Pregnancy	Acetohydroxamic acid, anisindione, belladonna/ergot/phenobarbital, benzphetamine, chlorotrianisene, clomiphene, danazol, demecarium, desogestrel, dienestrol, diethylstilbestrol, dihydroergotamine, ergotamine, estazolam, estradiol, estramustine, estrogens (conjugated), estrone, estropipate, ethinyl estradiol, etretinate, finasteride, fluoxymesterone, fluvastatin, goserelin, histrelin, isoflurophate, isotretinoln, leuprolide, levonorgestrel, lovastatin, medroxyprogesterone, misoprostol, nafarelin, nandrolone, norethindrone, norgestrel, oxandrolone, oxymetholone, oxytocin, plicamycin, pravastatin, quazepam, quinestrol, quinine, ribavirin, simvastatin, stanozolol, temazepam, testosterone, triazolam, urofollitropin, vitamin A, warfarin
D Positive Evidence of Risk	Alprazolam, altretamine, amikacin, aminoglutethimide, amiodarone, amitriptyline, amobarbital, aspirin, atenolol, azathioprine, benazepril, busulfan, butabarbital, calcium iodide, captopril, carboplatin, carmustine, chlorambucil, chlordiazepoxide, cisplatin, cladribine, colchicine, cortisone, cyclophosphamide, cytarabine, daunorubicin, dicumarol, divalproex, doxorubicin, doxycycline, enalapril, etoposide, floxuridine, fludarabine, fluorouracil, flutamide, fosinopril, halazepam, hydroxyprogesterone, idarubicin, ifosfamide, kanamycin, lisinopril, lithium, lomustine, lorazepam, mechlorethamine, melphalan, mephobarbital, meprobamate, mercaptopurine, metaraminol, methimazole. midazolam, minocycline, mitoxantrone, nalbuphine, neomycin, netilmicin, nicotine, nortriptyline, oxazepam, oxytetracycline, paclitaxel, paramethadione, pentobarbital, pentostatin, phenacemide, phenobarbital, phensuximide, pipobroman, polythiazide, potassium iodide, primidone, procarbazine, progesterone, propylthiouracil, quinapril, quinethazone, ramipril, reserpine, secobarbital, streptomycin, strontium-89, tamoxifen, teniposide, thioguanine, tobramycin, trimethaphan, trimetrexate, valproic acid, vinblastine, vincristine

that do not cause malformations in some animals, and some substances that cause malformations in animals are not teratogens for people. Given that the expected rate of malformation is 2 to 4 percent, an agent that is given frequently during pregnancy will be associated with some malformations. Rational drug selection for pregnant patients depends on careful examination of available information on the drugs being used and of the risks of withholding treatment to both mother and child.

PRINCIPLES OF TERATOGENICITY. No teratogenic drug compound causes malformations with every exposure. Some patients can take drugs without any apparent ill effects on the fetus. The specific malformations induced by a given drug are often similar but may be seen with a spectrum of severity. The presence and severity of malformations depend on three main factors: genetic susceptibility, developmental stage during the exposure, and dose of the drug.

A complicating factor in teratogenicity is the large differences between species in the adverse effects of drugs on the fetus. All human teratogens have been found to cause malformations in at least one animal; however, some drugs (e.g., aspirin) can induce malformations in animals but do not produce them in humans. Interpatient variation in susceptibility is found in humans as well. Only a small percentage of exposed fetuses demonstrate malformations, and some of this resistance is due to resistance to the effects of the drug.

The damage drugs cause is highly dependent on the time of exposure. The fetus's stage of development at the time of exposure—blastogenesis (2 weeks), embryogenesis (2–8 weeks), or fetogenesis (8–32 weeks)—determines whether the malformation will be seen. Malformations are not induced during the first 2 weeks after conception. Embryogenesis is the period of greatest susceptibility to malformations, a period when some women do not know they are pregnant.

During fetogenesis, the major risk is to the development of the central nervous system. Functional and behavioral defects have been associated with exposure while the brain is still growing and developing. Knowledge of fetal milestones and specific drug exposure is clinically important for making treatment decision in pregnant patients. Most drugs have a window of opportunity for malformations, which may allow their use outside these periods if drug therapy is essential. For example, carbamazepine causes neural tube defects only during the blastogenesis stage, the first 2 weeks after conception.

Teratogenic effects depend on the dose of the teratogen. This dose dependency may have a steep dose-response curve, giving a clear threshold of teratogenicity. Because of wide differences between patients in placental function and fetal and maternal metabolism of drugs, there is wide variability in toxic doses from one patient to another. This makes identification of a safe dose of a teratogen impossible. Teratogens may cause spontaneous abortion, fetal malformations, growth retardation, mental retardation, carcinogenesis, and mutagenesis. Factors that influence the teratogenicity of a drug include the fetus's gestational age, the type of malformation induced, and simultaneous exposure to other drugs or environmental agents.

Often a patient has already taken a drug before seeking advice about the teratogenic risk. In this situation, it is important to accurately determine the drug(s), dose, route of administration, exact gestational age at exposure, and other drugs taken concurrently. The patient's general health and previous obstetric history may be helpful. The practitioner can then provide all the information available about the teratogenic risk.

Mechanisms of teratogenicity are poorly understood, and drug therapy is to be avoided if at all possible in pregnant patients. Occasionally, however, the mother's treatment is essential for both mother and child. Rational drug selection is then determined by carefully examining the dose, timing, and functional effects of the drug on both patients.

Carcinogenesis

Today, we know that certain drugs and environmental agents are capable of inducing cancer. Carcinogenesis may arise from genetic damage that is dose related; this may be due to activation of oncogenes or inactivation of suppresser genes. It may also occur as the result of some potentially neoplastic tissue in the patient; a preneoplastic cell may be transformed into cancer by the administration of a drug, such as an estrogen or androgen, given for an unrelated condition.

Drugs that are potentially carcinogenic include androgens, antineoplastics, busulfan, clofibrate, corticosteroids, cyclamates, estrogens, griseofulvin, metronidazole, nitrites, nitrofurans, oral contraceptives, and progestins.

Chemicals and other substances that are potentially carcinogenic include asbestos, benzene, carbon tetrachloride, chloroform, dioxin, herbicides, nitrosamines, pesticides, tobacco smoke, and TRIS (a flame retardant).

Conclusion

Recent evidence suggests that adverse drug events are a significant and growing problem in health care. The risk-to-benefit ratio of each drug therapy decision must be carefully weighed, and the why, how, and when of therapy, including the risks, must be explained to the patient.

REFERENCE

Freidman, J. M., & Polifka, J. E. (1996). *The effects of drugs on the fetus and nursing infant.* Baltimore: Johns Hopkins Press.

CHAPTER 6

·······

Factors That Foster Positive Outcomes

CHAPTER OUTLINE

H ealth care providers work in this field because they have an altruistic motivation to help people become healthier. When the patient does not or cannot follow recommendations or instructions, the provider may become very frustrated. Nurse practitioners (NPs) may experience a higher degree of frustration because we expect of ourselves a better job of teaching. Multiple clinical studies have revealed that even though providers expect positive outcomes, in reality it often does not happen.

No longer is the health care provider–patient relationship viewed as a parent-child relationship; now it is one of setting and working toward realistic mutual goals (Stone et al., 1998). No longer are providers expecting compliance. Compliance implies an involuntary act of submission. What is expected is adherence or positive outcomes, which imply a voluntary act of accepting a point of view. Because of this change in attitude between provider and patients, the provider now has an increased responsibility to educate patients about their diseases and medications.

Nonadherence to pharmacological regimens can com-

promise the efficacy of a medicine, which may lead to failure of the desired treatment goal. The provider then may make changes in the medication regimen because the provider believes the medicine failed. If patients then realize they must adhere to the regimen more closely, the likelihood of toxicity may increase, creating a possible increase in morbidity and wasted resources (Matsui, 1997).

Why does a patient not follow our directions? What occurs outside the office setting to sabotage the best of intentions? What is the patient's responsibility, and what is the provider's? This chapter will guide the novice and the experienced NP toward fostering positive outcomes.

Adverse Drug Reactions

Adverse drug reactions can take many forms. Some of them are real; some are the patient's perceptions about a medication learned from well-meaning friends. A telephone survey (Wysocke & Davis, 1999) contacted approximately 700 women regarding their use of oral contraceptives. Half of those women surveyed thought that oral contraceptives caused most women to gain weight, and about one-fourth of those women reported never using oral contraceptives because of the fear of gaining weight. Studies comparing oral contraceptive use and weight gain revealed that weight gain could not be attributed to oral contraceptive use. More often, the weight gain is attributed to interpersonal relations and the subsequent increase in frequenting restaurants. The providers' education regarding the real side effects of oral contraceptives provided women with greater choices.

Intermittent adherence to antihypertension medications is one of the major reasons for uncontrolled hypertension and presumably persistent left ventricular hypertrophy (Leenen, 1999). Patients may realize through education that control of hypertension is very important to their morbidity but may not adhere to the regimen secondary to the adverse reactions they experience, either by continuous doses or by missed doses. Antihypertensive medications that have a rapid onset and short duration of action are not very desirable in long-term therapy secondary to possible large variations in blood pressure. These particular medications have rapid onset, lowering the blood pressure quickly. If the patient misses one dose, the antihypertensive effect disappears, creating a possible rebound or adverse reaction. Antihypertensives that require several dose titrations (e.g., alpha-1 blockers) can be particularly troublesome if the patient misses some doses and then restarts at the full dose. Excessive drug action and symptomatic hypotension may result.

Short-acting antihypertensives (e.g., short-acting beta blockers of clonidine-like medications) may lead to rebound sympathetic responses if the doses are missed after 1 or 2 days. This sequence may lead not only to adverse reactions but also to adverse events, particularly in patients with silent coronary artery disease.

Obviously, intermittent hypertension control is not an appropriate approach to the management of hypertension. This type of adherence may cause additional risks, depending on the type of antihypertensive medication. The savvy provider, without judgment, must explore with the patient how and when the patient is taking the medication. Some patients are very exacting and precise, never missing a dosage; others may be more relaxed in their adherence. In the patient on hypertensives discussed previously, medications with slow onset and long duration of action will provide better outcomes when the patient does not take the medication.

Erectile dysfunction is a highly publicized and actual medical problem affecting a significant number of men. The cause of erectile dysfunction may be a significant adverse reaction secondary to medication therapy (Keene & Davies, 1999). Antihypertensives and psychotherapeutic medications have been commonly implicated as the cause of this particular adverse reaction because of the predi-

cated pharmacological action. The savvy provider must explore possible drug action first, before other specific investigations and therapy related to erectile dysfunction.

Drug holidays to help with erectile dysfunction give the patient the wrong message. The patient may hear that it is okay not to consistently take their medications (Weber, 1999). This misunderstanding would be a particular problem with control of hypertension or psychological problems. The provider must be open and willing to help explore all options for the patient.

Several medications are now available for control of hypertension and psychological problems. We know that these medications have several possible adverse reactions, so the tolerability profile must be discussed in selecting medications for a particular patient (Roose, 1999). Tolerability is directly linked to patient adherence for both short- and long-term therapy and ultimately to the overall success of treatment. Knowledge of a medication's possible interactions and adverse reactions is a must for assessing tolerability and adherence to the regimen for each individual patient.

Real or perceived adverse reactions directly affect the outcome of a prescribed medication regimen. If patients perceive that a prescribed medication is causing a reaction, the NP must explore alternative options to treating the problem. This response assures patients that the provider is willing to listen and work with them until the right medication or right dosage is prescribed.

Knowledge Deficit

Providing educational material, written or oral, cannot ensure that the patient will not have a knowledge deficit regarding their medication regimen (Demi, Brown, & Jones, 1998; Thiel & McDonnell, 1999; Wiecker, 1999). In this era of managed care, the NP may well feel pressured into shorter visits with the patient. The practitioner, then, must become an excellent communicator. A greater length of time spent with a patient is not related to increased patient satisfaction but rather to the quality of the communication and interaction (Halperin, 1998). Patients report greater satisfaction and adherence to a medication regimen if they feel that their concerns, rather than the provider's concerns, are addressed. They feel that their specific points of knowledge deficit are being addressed. The right amount of information is elegant, just enough to be read, understood, and acted on by the patient (Halperin, 1998), which fosters greater positive outcomes.

Other influences regarding a patient's knowledge deficit include health beliefs the patient holds, cultural beliefs, literacy, characteristics of the site in which treatment occurs, life circumstances, and the relationship between the patient and the provider (Ailinger & Dear, 1998; Ladebauche, 1997; Thiel & McDonnell, 1999).

Some patients do not want to share in the decision-making process. Because of health beliefs or cultural beliefs, they perceive that they need to do what the health care provider tells them to do. The idea of having to share the control of taking care of themselves is very foreign, and the patient may not return to the provider. Patients who expect the provider to tell them what to do perceive that the decision-sharing provider does not know what he or she is doing. Conversely, the patient who wants to be in control and the provider who presents information in an authoritarian manner together can also create a lose-lose situation.

NPs must educate themselves to be sensitive to the patient's particular beliefs. In an atmosphere of shared values, shared language, and mutual respect, positive patient outcomes occur.

Using language that the patient understands increases the chances of reversing knowledge deficit. Listen actively to patients' terminology when they refer to their body parts or disease processes. When a provider refers to "cystitis," the patient may not understand; if the provider says, instead, "urinary tract infection," usually the patient understands. By using biomedical terminology, the provider is putting up a barrier that may unintentionally create a greater knowledge deficit. Using the patient's terminology can reduce the possible trial-and-error period that may result when the provider attempts to communicate the physiological findings. Finding common terminology with the patient will increase the patient's confidence in the provider's desire to help.

Research by Fisch and O'Connell (1998) posed this question of finding common terminology. Through their work, they composed a dictionary for the provider that defines common terminology. Their work was based on the fact that patients are encouraged to play a more active role in their health care. The drug information sheets that are included with prescription and over-the-counter (OTC) medications may include terminology that is confusing. By defining terms and cross-referencing these terms between lay and professional language, they believe they have increased patient satisfaction and fostered positive outcomes. For any provider who has difficulty in the communication process, certainly this would be an excellent resource.

The inclusion of a drug insert may make patients anxious as they read how many adverse reactions may occur. Certainly, the information about interactions has prevented serious complications, but what about patients who are sure they have every possible complication that might develop from any medication? In this situation, the provider and pharmacist must work closely together to provide the patient with correct information. Having open communication with patients and using their terminology can enhance the positive outcomes from the medication regimen. Enhanced, clear communication then forms a positive relationship between patient and provider.

Complexity of Medicinal Regimen and Polypharmacy

An increased number of medications used to manage multiple complex disease processes increases the possibility of a decreased ability to follow multiple medication regimens. This decreased ability, in turn, increases the chances of a decreased positive outcome for the patient. Deciding what to do and when to do it can be complex and frustrating for all involved, patient and provider alike.

Education for the patient, written and oral, regarding the importance of following a daily schedule is the gold standard (Czenis, 1999). However, this is only one of the components in solving the dilemma of complex medicinal regimens or polypharmacy.

Helping patients set up a personalized medication schedule devised only for them (Martens, 1998) is one possible solution. In the era of managed care, the provider does not have the time to do this. Designating this important task to the nursing staff can help the provider and the patient. The provider may oversee the process, but nurses are certainly appropriate people to help the patient set up a medication regimen that works.

At the time of the visit, making follow-up appointments is extremely important. Saying to the patient, "I want to see you in x amount of time" stresses that the patient is important and may enhance the likelihood of adherence. It also gives the provider the opportunity to assess for adverse reactions in the medication regimen (Ladebauche, 1997).

Another method that fosters positive outcomes with complex medication regimens or polypharmacy is the anticipatory guidance framework. This method anticipates what education and guidance will be needed at different intervals of the patient's learning process (Ladebauche, 1997).

The provider who chooses to utilize this method must have knowledge of the physiological, psychological, and developmental concerns of the individual patient. A child, teenager, young adult, and older adult are in definite stages of development. Interventions designed for a child certainly are not appropriate for other age levels unless a cognitive deficiency is present. The theme of individualized assessment and education is repeated, but its importance cannot be stressed enough. A practitioner who is pressed for time management can utilize the multidisciplinary format to help achieve the most positive outcomes.

Another way to help patients with the complexity of medications and polypharmacy is psychoeducational intervention (Peyrot & Rubin, 1999). This technique has been shown to enhance positive outcomes in the coping ability of diabetic patients who are clinically depressed.

Certainly, this technique could be utilized for patients with multiple medical diagnoses. Coping with one chronic disease is, at best, difficult. The patient with several chronic diseases must be provided with whatever educational technique may work for them. The provider can be challenged and rewarded with successful interventions. Several techniques might enhance a patient's ability to adhere to polypharmacy. Finding the correct technique takes patience and humor on the part of the provider.

Patient's Responsibilities

Forgetting to take the medication or forgetting to take the medication on time is a common form of nonadherence to medication regimens. Failure to fill the prescription, incorrect dosage, improper dose intervals, and premature discontinuation of the medication are other forms of omission of adherence (Heymann, Sell, & Brewer, 1998; Matsui, 1997; Starr, 1999).

Over the last few years, antibiotic resistance has become a great concern for health care providers. The responsibility for overuse and misuse of antibiotics lies with the public, which is uneducated about the appropriate use of antibiotics (Pinkowish, 1999). A patient who presents with a cold may demand an instant fix to the situation. Most health care consumers do not know the difference between viruses and bacteria. Explaining why an antibiotic does not work on a viral infection must be done in terminology the patient understands. Taking the time to explain can be time-consuming and tiring, but as a health care provider, the NP has the responsibility to protect patients from resistant organisms.

It becomes clear through literature reviews that chronic illness, such as tuberculosis, asthma, or diabetes, creates some of the greatest problems for the patient who has to adhere to ongoing therapy. Time, finances, and a desire to be perceived as healthy appear to have the greatest impact.

In the recent past, public health departments attempted to control the increasing epidemic of tuberculosis. This was attempted in several ways, one of which was creating directly observed therapy programs. Directly observed programs were more effective than self-administration programs; however, many patients delayed treatment to avoid mandatory therapy or detainment (Heyman, Sell, & Brewer, 1998). The patients who had positive adherence to the medication regimen were those who had a personal desire to be free of the symptoms associated with tuberculosis. This personal investment is one of the keys to successful long-term management of any chronic disease.

Improved adherence to long-term medication use should include education regarding acute and symptomatic therapy. The patient must accept the responsibility of adhering to a long-term management plan, or all the education provided by the NP will be of no use. Written treatment plans, reviews of treatment recommendations that help correct misinformation, and improved communication between patient, provider, and family members are some of the suggestions for fostering positive outcomes.

Self-monitoring has been shown to have positive effects on outcomes of medication regimens. For the patient with asthma, self-monitoring of peak expiratory flow rates can improve disease awareness and predict asthma flareups (Ladebauche, 1997; Simmons et al., 1996; Wiecker, 1999). Patients demonstrated better adherence after the first follow-up visits but gradually tapered off unless the use of the medications was reiterated in follow-up visits. This technique can be utilized with other chronic diseases (e.g., diabetes, chronic obstructive pulmonary disease, cardiac disease, hypertension, depression) by reviewing whatever device is utilized for home management.

The social stigma of a chronic disease process has a definite impact on the patient's adherence to chronic pharmacological regimens (Ailinger & Dear, 1998). Patients with a long-term or chronic disease process may have difficulty pursuing a work schedule that is conducive to their pharmacological regimens. The stigma of the disease may cause the patient to attempt to deny the disease, leading to denial of the need for the pharmacological interventions (e.g., stopping diuretics so that frequent urination does not occur). Certainly, in these situations the provider needs to explore possible changes in the medication, but patients also have the responsibility to inform the provider of the impact the disease has made on their lives. The provider then can possibly modify the medication regimen to enhance positive outcomes.

Do not assume that patients with a history of homelessness or substance abuse will not follow a treatment plan or that the well-educated, affluent patient will. The NP must find out if the patient actually wants to take the medication and is committed to adhere to a strict schedule. Patients have the responsibility to try to adhere to pharmacotherapeutics, but it is also the provider's responsibility to attempt to discover the barriers that are impeding a positive outcome.

Financial Impacts

Pharmacological interventions cost money. This cost can have a huge impact on the ability and willingness of the patient to adhere to medication regimens. Even if the patient has access to financial assistance (e.g., Medicaid, insurance coverage for drugs), this does not ensure that the patient will view medications as a primary financial need (Avorn et al., 1998). Basic needs (e.g., food, housing) may take precedence over medication in dividing a monthly budget.

Having an adequate payment system to cover the cost of medications does not in itself guarantee appropriate utilization of this benefit. Certainly, those who have to cover the cost of medications out of pocket are at greater risk for inadequate adherence to costly pharmacological interventions.

Patients who have several family members to support may view pharmacological interventions for themselves as selfish. The child who has a chronic disease also affects the financial stability of the family, which may cause resentment from parents or siblings.

This whole issue is certainly complex and difficult. The provider must be aware of the psychological impact a disease is making financially. Having an awareness of possible public programs available to assist financially is only a part of the whole picture. The provider also has to have knowledge of the patient and whether that patient will accept public assistance. The patient's acceptability must also be considered prior to selecting a public health intervention (Heymann, Sell, & Brewer, 1998). All the public assistance in the world will not work if the patient or family views it as a social or cultural stigma that is unacceptable. By considering the potential financial impact polypharmacy or the use of expensive medications has on the patient, the provider can avoid nonadherence by the patient. Financial concerns for the patient and family can have a huge effect in fostering positive outcomes.

Caregiver's Roles

When the patient an NP sees is a child, an older adult, or a person with mental disabilities, the patient's caregiver must be involved in the educational process. The caregiver can provide valuable information regarding the patient's responses to medication or difficulties in adhering to the prescribed medication regimen.

If the provider detects that the caregiver may be having difficulty in adhering to the pharmacological interventions, it is possible that the caregiver may need to be provided one-on-one interventions to help foster positive outcomes for the patient.

Certainly, the impact on the caregiver's quality of life has a huge impact on the patient's quality of life (Demi, Brown, & Jones, 1998). By exploring the psychological, physical, and social impact with the caregiver, the provider is acknowledging the difficulties the caregiver must face every day. This, in turn, will foster a positive relation with the provider. By being open to the impact the caregiver has on the patient, greater adherence and positive outcomes can occur.

Behavioral changes may have to be explored. This type of intervention can empower the caregiver to provide appropriate interventions (Helliwell et al., 1999). Behavioral changes that may be needed must be identified early in the disease process for the caregiver and patient. It may be that an interdisciplinary approach is the best intervention for caregivers and patients with a multitude of complicating factors. Caregivers have a huge role in communicating to the provider and patient the possibility of adverse reactions. Always include the caregiver, if there is one, when providing education to the patient. Acknowledgment of the caregiver's roles in the patient's outcome is a powerful topic. The thoughtful provider realizes this impact and considers its potential outcome in every encounter.

Communication Difficulties

Communication difficulties exist not only in finding common terminology but also in speech and hearing difficulties or in language barriers. Such difficulties can cause considerable frustration for the provider and patient. Cooperation between the provider and patient is a must for any positive outcome, but this becomes a very clear problem with those patients who cannot hear, cannot read, or do not understand the language that is predominantly spoken.

Most health care clinics advise patients that they must provide an interpreter if their primary language is different from the provider's. Some clinics are able to contact interpreters for a number of different languages. The difficulty that arises is whether the interpreter is repeating exactly what the provider is saying and in return whether the interpreter is saying exactly what the patient is saying. A certain amount of trust must be exhibited between the interpreter and provider. Certainly, language barriers are a difficulty in adhering to a medication regimen.

Professional interpreters are preferable but not always accessible. The provider who is unsure that correct information is being translated can refuse to treat the patient. However, in a medical emergency, every effort must be made to find an alternative provider. The referring provider can be held liable for poor outcomes. Legal and personal liability must be taken into account and considered before refusing to treat a patient.

Patients with hearing, speech, or sight difficulties are usually easier to work with than patients with language barriers. Patients with hearing difficulties may have learned to compensate by reading lips. With partial hearing loss, such as from the aging process, if the provider speaks in low tones, the patient usually has greater hearing ability. The patient with speech difficulties usually has learned coping mechanisms, but the provider must recognize that these complicating factors may have a huge impact on the outcomes of pharmacological interventions. The provider cannot assume, just because the patient says, "Yes," that the patient really heard or understood what was said. Communication barriers between patients and providers can take many forms. Speech, hearing, and language barriers can be devastating complications. Ability to access barrier breakers is a must in providing appropriate care.

Communication Between Providers

Nothing can be more disconcerting and exasperating than attempting to coordinate health care for a patient who sees several different providers. Not much research has been done in this area to help the provider decide how to best improve communication between providers. Common sense and open lines of communication are a must between the patient and providers and among health care providers. If a patient sees a specialist for whatever reason, ask the patient to request that the records of each visit be sent to the coordinating primary care provider. However, either the patient or the specialist's staff does not always follow through on this request.

A congenial call by the primary care provider will do much toward receiving the reports; coordinating care, regimens, and appointments; letting patients know you think they are important; and reminding the specialists that you are a primary care provider, thus also enhancing the visibility and credibility of the practice.

Patients who see several health care providers or who do not consistently have the same provider show greater problems with adherence to treatment therapy (Matsui, 1997). Encouraging repeat visits to the same provider increases communication and knowledge between the patient and the provider.

Coordination by one primary health care provider alleviates part of the problem between multiple providers. Communication in identifying the patient's major concerns and meeting expectations is extremely important. If the patient must be referred to a specialist, making a follow-up appointment that does not interfere with the specialist's appointments informs the patient that you believe the patient and specialist are important. Patients may feel abandoned if follow-up appointments are not made or at least suggested when the patient must be turned over to a specialist. The primary care provider can enable a positive outcome by creating open communication between providers.

Summary

Patient education, enhanced communication, and consideration of multiple complicating social factors all contribute to fostering positive pharmacological interventions and positive outcomes. These complicating factors can create a huge burden for the provider and patient. NPs have the educational background to promote positive outcomes and provide a positive force in creating a healthier world.

REFERENCES

Ailinger, R. L., & Dear, M. R. (1998). Adherence to tuberculosis preventative therapy among Latino immigrants. *Public Health Nursing, 15*(1), 19–24.

Avorn, J., Monette, J., Lacour, A., Bohn, R., Monane, M., Mogun, H., & LeLorier, J. (1998). Persistence of use of lipid-lowering medications: A cross-national study. *Journal of American Medical Association, 279*(18), 1458–1462.

Czenis, A. L. (1999). Thyroid disease in the elderly: Not a typical presentation. *Advance for Nurse Practitioners, 7*(9), 38–44.

Demi, A. S., Brown, J. V., & Jones, K. D. (1998). Promoting asthma self-management skills in young children through a home based nursing intervention: A pilot study. *The American Journal of Nurse Practitioners, 2*(10), 15–30.

Fisch, M. K., & O'Connell, C. A. (1998). Creation of a dictionary of medical and lay terms for use in the preparation of patient information leaflets. *Drug Information Journal, 32,* 533–538.

Halperin, J. A. (1998). Useful patient information on prescription drugs. *Annals of Pharmacotherapy, 32*(5), 612.

Helliwell, P. S., O'Hara, M., Holdsworth, J., Hesselden, A., King, T., & Evans, P. (1999). A 12-month randomized controlled trial of patient education on radiographic changes and quality of life in early rheumatoid arthritis. *Rheumatology, (Oxford) 38* (4), 303–308.

Heymann, S. J., Sell, R., & Brewer, T. F. (1998). The influence of program acceptability on the effectiveness of public health policy: A study of directly observed therapy for tuberculosis. *American Journal of Public Health, 88*(3), 442–444.

Keene, L. C., & Davies, P. H. (1999). Drug-related erectile dysfunction. *Adverse Drug Reactions Toxicology Review, 18*(1), 5–24.

Ladebauche, P. (1997). Managing asthma: A growth and development approach. *Pediatric Nursing, 23*(1), 37–44.

Leenen, F. H. (1999). Intermittent blood pressure control: Potential consequences for outcome. *Canadian Journal of Cardiology, May: 15,* Supplement C: 13–18.

Martens, K. H. (1998). An ethnographic study of the process of medication discharge education (MDE). *Journal of Advanced Nursing, 27,* 341–348.

Matsui, D. M. (1997). Drug compliance in pediatrics: Clinical research issues. *Pediatric Clinics of North America, 44*(1), 1–13.

Peyrot, M., & Rubin, R. R. (1999). Persistence of depressive symptoms in diabetic adults. *Diabetes Care, 22,* 448–452.

Pinkowish, M. D. (1999). Infectious diseases: Still emerging. *Patient Care for the Nurse Practitioner,* (Special Reports, Infectious Diseases) March, 1999.

Roose, S. P. (1999). Tolerability and patient compliance. *Journal of Clinical Psychiatry, Supplement 17,* 14–17.

Simmons, M. S., Nides, M. A., Rand, C. S., Wise, R. A., & Tashkin, D. P. (1996). Trends in compliance with bronchodilator inhaler use between follow up visits in a clinical trial. *Chest, 109*(4), 963–968.

Starr, C. (1999). The latest recommendations for antiretroviral therapy. *Patient Care of the Nurse Practitioner,* (Special Reports, Infectious Diseases) March, 1999.

Stone, M. S., Bronkesh, S. S., Gerbarg, Z. B., & Wood, S. D. (1998). *Improving patient compliance: Strategic medicine.* Scottsdale, AZ: HSM Group.

Thiel, J., & McDonnell, M. (1999). Tuberculosis in children. *American Journal for Nurse Practitioners, 3*(4), 23–29.

Weber, S. S. (1999). *Psychiatric pharmacotherapy update.* Lecture at Oregon Nurse Practitioner Conference, Wilsonville, OR, August, 1999.

Wiecker, T. L. (1999). Managing asthma with behavior modification: Putting ideas into practice. *Clinical Reviews, 9*(3), 65–82.

Wysocke, S., & Davis, A. J. (1999). *Clinical challenges in women's health: A handbook for nurse practitioners.* Jamesburg, NJ: NP Communications.

CHAPTER 7

....

Cultural and Ethnic Influences in Pharmacotherapeutics

CHAPTER OUTLINE

In prescribing drugs, a wide variety of factors come into play. The practitioner must consider the pharmacodynamics and pharmacokinetics of the drugs themselves, potential adverse drug reactions, the potential drug interactions with any other drugs the patient may be taking, and economic factors such as drug cost and whether the drug will be covered by insurance.

Equally important is consideration of cultural factors. Who makes the decisions in the family about health care? Does this person support the use of the prescribed drug? How well does the patient's view of health and illness and the way it should be managed match the provider's view? Will this attitude create problems with adherence? Although each person with a specific cultural heritage is a unique individual who may not subscribe to all or even most of the health beliefs and health practices of that cultural group, it is important to know what is common among members of the group. Cultural heritage plays an important role in helping to explain attitudes, beliefs, and health practices.

Another factor only recently being incorporated into pharmacotherapeutic decision making is that of ethnopharmacology, a study of racial differences in drug metabolism and response. Practitioners may know and guidelines may sometimes specify that certain drugs are less efficacious with certain racial groups. Research is increasingly demonstrating the underlying genetic reasons for these differences in efficacy. Research with the cytochrome P-450 (CYP-450) enzyme system has been especially fruitful in this area, but it is not the only source of racial differences. Review of current literature on racial differences in pharmacokinetics of drugs supports the premise that only pharmacokinetic processes that are biologically or biochemically mediated have the potential to exhibit differences between racial or ethnic groups (Johnson, 1997). The pharmacokinetic factors that can be expected to potentially exhibit these differences are (1) bioavailability for drugs that undergo gut or hepatic first-pass metabolism, (2) protein binding, (3) volume of distribution, (4) hepatic metabolism, and (5) renal tubular secretion. Absorption, filtration at the glomerulus, and passive tubular reabsorption would not be expected to exhibit racial differences. Because there are relatively few drugs that have research evidence of racial differences, it is often necessary to predict whether these differences might exist. For example, a drug that is eliminated entirely by the kidney through filtration and reabsorption and is not highly protein bound is highly unlikely to exhibit racial differences. Conversely, a drug that undergoes significant hepatic first-pass metabolism and is highly protein bound is more likely to exhibit pharmacokinetic differences between racial groups.

This chapter focuses on both cultural and ethnopharmacological factors that influence the choice of drugs that practitioners prescribe. The data provided are based both on evidence derived from drug research and on identifying those drugs most likely to exhibit differences in their pharmacokinetics. In using this information, it is important to keep in mind that most Americans are not of any "pure" cultural or racial background and that patients must be treated as unique individuals.

The American Anthropological Society (AAS) has raised several pertinent issues related to both racial and cultural heritage in the United States. Although the U S. Census collects data based on five distinct groupings, the AAS states that the United States is home to at least 26 different and distinct racial and cultural groupings. It is not possible within this chapter to delineate all of these groupings, so the five groups delineated by the census are used. It is important, however, to remember that these are artificial groupings and that people listed within a specific group may be very divergent from each other.

Socioeconomic factors also influence prescription choices and may supersede cultural and racial differences. For this reason, discussion of cultural factors includes such socioeconomic data as demographics, education and employment (most patients obtain health insurance through their employment), and health care utilization. This information is based on data from the 1990 U.S. Census.

African-Americans

Cultural Factors

Demographics

African-Americans make up about 12 percent of the population, and their numbers are increasing 1.5 times faster than the overall population. As a group, they are younger (35% under age 20) and more likely to be unmarried (61%), urban (81%), and female (53%). The proportion below the poverty line is 29 percent, compared with 13 percent for all races and 10 percent for white Americans. The mean household income in 1990 was $19,758.

Education and Employment

Fewer African-Americans complete high school (63%) and college (11.4%) than do white Americans. The unemployment rate is 13.7 percent, more than twice that of white Americans and higher than that of any other ethnic group except American Indian–Alaska Natives.

Family Relationships

Although over half are raised in single-parent homes, there is still a strong kinship bond between family members. Ever alert for signs of discrimination, they may see health care providers as "outsiders" in health decisions. The female is the dominant family force, and the grandmother is often the major decision maker.

Health Care Utilization

More African-Americans than whites have no usual source of health care and no health insurance, and cost considerations for prescribing drugs are especially important. They use hospital clinics and emergency rooms as their care providers more than any other ethnic group, perhaps in part because of their urban residence.

Health Status

Life expectancy for males is lowest of all ethnic groups. African-American females, however, have life expectancies only slightly shorter than those of white females. Maternal mortality rates are almost three times higher than other ethnic groups or whites. Their patterns of illness include a higher prevalence of coronary heart disease and stroke. The prevalence and age-adjusted mortality rate for diabetes is twice that of whites, and prevalence of hypertension is more than twice that of whites. Cigarette smoking is more prevalent.

Health Beliefs and Practices

For a significant portion of the African-American population, health is a gift from God, and illness and suffering are God's will or are caused by evil influences. Because God's will is the source of the illness, they rely heavily on the healing powers of religious ritual and the advice of their minister. Folk healers and folk medicine, such as cod liver oil to prevent colds, sulfur and molasses in the spring to promote health, and copper or silver bracelets to protect from harm, are often used. Herbal remedies are also used. Allopathic health care is not considered for prevention.

Regional differences are as often a factor as ethnic differences for all ethnic groups, including African-Americans. Those who were raised in the southeastern part of the United States are more likely to subscribe to health beliefs and practices common to that region than are African-Americans raised elsewhere, for example.

Racial Differences in Drug Pharmacokinetics and Response

African-Americans have been studied more than other ethnic groups in relation to ethnopharmacology, which has resulted in a larger body of knowledge about racial differences in pharmacokinetics.

Using **metoprolol** as a prototype drug, Johnson and

Burlew (1996) looked at metabolism of drugs by the CYP-450 2D6 isoenzyme group. This particular isoenzyme group is responsible for several important drug groups, including **antiarrhythmics, antidepressants,** and **neuroleptics**. They concluded that drugs primarily metabolized by this isoenzyme system will not exhibit racial differences between African-Americans and whites.

Bertilsson (1995) studied CYP-450 2C19 in relation to the difference between Asian-Americans and whites (see discussion later). Because the separation of whites from Asians is fairly recent in the evolutionary process and the separation of Africans from whites and Asians occurred much earlier, it might be expected that African-Americans will show even greater differences in drugs metabolized by CYP-450 2C19 than do Asian-Americans.

Differences have also been demonstrated between African-Americans and whites in plasma protein binding (Johnson & Livingston, 1997). The study found increased unbound fractions of drugs bound to albumin, a common binding site for many drugs. The researchers were careful to point out, however, that differences in protein concentrations might also explain the racial differences. Further study is needed in this area, because a large number of drugs could be affected by this racial difference if it can be replicated.

Hypertension has a high prevalence in African-Americans. One reason behind this phenomenon appears to be salt sensitivity (Weinberger, 1993), which is often cited as the reason to use **diuretics** as first-line therapy for this ethnic group. In a study looking at the use of **beta-adrenergic blockers** to treat hypertension in African-Americans, a practice that is not usually recommended, Prisant and Mensah (1996) found that not all African-Americans are salt-sensitive. When salt sensitivity was controlled for, there was no racial difference in efficacy when **beta-adrenergic blockers** were used with **diuretics** as combination therapy for hypertension. This study suggests that **beta-adrenergic blockers** should be given to some African-Americans for certain indications, such as myocardial infarction prophylaxis.

A study by Weir et al. (1998) also demonstrated that controlling for salt sensitivity affected response to two other classes of drugs (**angiotensin-converting enzyme inhibitors** and **calcium channel blockers**). **Calcium channel blockers** are recommended second-line therapy for African-Americans. African-Americans who were salt-sensitive had more blood pressure lowering with **isradipine** (a **calcium channel blocker**) than with **enalapril** (also a **calcium channel blocker**). The differences appear to be not only between drug classes but also within them.

To further confuse the issue of **beta-adrenergic blockers,** studies have been done related to racial differences in nucleotide-mediated smooth muscle relaxation (vasodilation) in response to nitric oxide. Studies by Cardillo et al. (1998; 1999) support a difference between African-Americans and whites in vasodilation response. The vasodilation effect of **beta-adrenergic blockers** stems from the combination of direct smooth muscle stimulation and endothelial nitric oxide release.

Other drugs dependent on nitric oxide for their action include the **nitrates**. Both drug classes may not be efficacious or may require dosage alterations to achieve efficacy in African-Americans.

Angiotensin-converting enzyme (ACE) inhibitors are also useful in treating hypertension, but African-Americans appear to have less renin-dependent hypertension, and these drugs are less useful with that group. A study by Mitchell et al. (1997) confirmed racial differences in the renal hemodynamic response to chronic use of ACE inhibition that was independent of **diuretic** use and the magnitude of blood pressure lowering.

A serious adverse reaction to **ACE inhibitors** that contraindicates their use is angioedema. It is thought to be related to the reduced breakdown of bradykinin in patients taking this class of drugs. A study by Gainer et al. (1996) concluded that African-Americans show racial differences in the kallikrein-kinin system and are more sensitive to bradykinin, placing them at increased risk of **ACE inhibitor**–associated angioedema, independent of dose or concurrent drugs.

Diabetes mellitus has a higher prevalence in African-Americans. The Bogalusa Heart Study (1995) suggested that elevated insulin levels observed in African-American adolescents, especially girls, may be attributed to their decreased hepatic insulin clearance. This suggests consideration of drugs that affect hepatic insulin clearance (e.g., **metformin [Glucophage]**) for treating African-Americans with type 2 diabetes. Stephens et al. (1990) also found racial differences in the incidence of end-stage renal disease associated with diabetes, which suggests that more aggressive management may be needed to prevent this complication.

Cryer and Feldman (1996) studied racial differences in gastric function among African-Americans and whites. Gastric bicarbonate secretion was significantly higher in African-Americans, making their gastric pH also higher. This might be a factor in the absorption of drugs that require highly acid media for absorption. Mucosal biopsies demonstrated a much higher prevalence of *Helicobacter pylori* infection and chronic active superficial gastritis in African-Americans. Even those who were negative for this infection had differences in gastric bicarbonate secretion. Drug combinations used to treat *H. pylori* infection include those that have pH-raising drugs. Are these the best ones for African-Americans?

Finally, a study by Carmel (1999) looks at racial differences in cobalamin and homocysteine levels among African-Americans and whites. Concern was raised about potential underreporting and undertreatment of pernicious anemia because African-Americans have significantly higher serum cobalamin levels than whites. They also have significantly lower homocysteine levels, metabolize homocysteine more efficiently, and do not show the same benefit from **vitamin** therapy in treating this anemia. A further question raised related to the prescription of **folate**: "Given their lower rate of neural tube defects, possibly lower homocysteine levels, more efficient homocysteine metabolism and lesser impact of **vitamin** therapy on it, does the untargeted promotion of high **folate** intake provide less benefit to blacks than to whites while exposing them to an equal risk for adverse effects because of unrecognized pernicious anemia?"

American Indian–Alaska Native Group

Cultural Factors

Demographics

American Indian (Native American) and Alaska Native people are a diverse group with more than 500 different tribes recognized by the federal government and others not so recognized. The census records that this group represents 0.8 percent of the population and that their numbers are increasing 1.5 times faster than the overall population. As a group, they are young (30% under the age of 15), less educated, and poorer than the rest of the United States. The median household income, according to the 1990 Census, is $19,886, and 32 percent live below the poverty level. They are divided in residence, with 50 percent living in urban areas.

One problem in reporting the actual numbers of American Indians is the tendency of this population group to avoid being counted as American Indians and the requirement by many tribal groups that an individual be at least one-quarter American Indian to be recorded as a member of that tribe. Interracial marriages are also common, and the children are often documented as being of the race of the non-Indian parent. A recent shift to recognition and pride in American Indian heritage has occurred. If the 2000 Census permits individuals to write in percentages of more than one race or even to list more than one race, the percentages of several minority groups, including American Indians, may change.

Education and Employment

The proportion completing college is less than half that of all races in the United States, and the unemployment rate is twice as high as all other races combined. The unemployment rate for American Indian men is approximately 16 percent.

Family Relationships

The average family household has four to five members, making it the largest family size of any of the ethnic minority groups. Women head 25 percent of the households. The family is extended, including relatives from both sides. Elder members assume leadership roles. Some tribal groups are matriarchal and some are patriarchal, with the leadership and the health decision making coming from the sex that matches this orientation.

Health Care Utilization

Since 1995, the U.S. Public Health Service has provided no-cost comprehensive health care to American Indians and Alaska Natives, and approximately 70 percent of all members of this group who claim American Indian heritage receive that care. Many people live in remote areas, however, where the ratio of providers to patients is half the national average. The main reason for utilization of health care services is obstetrical care.

Health Status

Life expectancy is 73.2 years, compared with about 79 years for white females. The four top causes of mortality are not that different from the general population: heart disease, injury, cancer, and diabetes. Other causes, in descending order, are chronic liver disease (associated with high rates of alcohol abuse), cerebrovascular disease, pneumonia and influenza, and suicide.

The higher the percentage of American Indian or Alaska Native genetic heritage, the more likely the individual is to manifest diabetes, and this diabetes is almost exclusively type 2. This may be correlated with the increased obesity found in this group.

Health Beliefs and Practices

Health is harmony with nature and oneself. Illness is disharmony and may be caused by a supernatural force or by violation of a restriction or prohibition. Because the cause of the illness is external, illness prevention practices that relate the cause of illness to the behavior of the patient are questioned. This is an interesting conflict, because self-control is considered to be a central attribute to maintaining harmony.

Theology and medicine are strongly interwoven. Witchcraft is feared, and medicine bags may be worn or carried to protect a person from witchcraft or to promote wellness and harmony. "Medical" care is often sought from a member of the family or tribe who has the ability to use his or her powers of healing in conjunction with herbs and rituals in a purely positive way to heal. The medicine person may use negative force powers, but only against the sick person's enemies. Singing is often part of the healing ritual.

Allopathic medicine is accepted but not seen as able to heal except when used with native healing practices. Because the hospital is considered the place to die, the patient may resist hospitalization.

Racial Differences in Drug Pharmacokinetics and Response

Although a large portion of this ethnic group has health care provided by the U.S. Public Health Service, little research has been done related to racial considerations in pharmacokinetics or other therapies. The few studies in the literature were related to metabolism of alcohol, which were contradictory (Bennion & Li, 1976; Chan, 1986), and to lipoprotein levels. A study related to lipoproteins (Harris-Hooker & Sanford, 1994) reported that American Indians have a lower prevalence of coronary heart disease related to lower LDL-cholesterol and higher HDL-cholesterol levels. Few studies were found related to diabetes and its treatment, despite a prevalence of 50 percent in Pima Indians and a lower but still elevated prevalence in other American Indian groups. Clearly, this ethnic group requires more study.

Asian-Americans/Pacific Islanders

Cultural Factors

Demographics

Asian-Americans and Pacific Islanders made up 3 percent of the population in the 1990 Census. Because they are the fastest-growing segment of the population, their percentage will probably be higher in the 2000 Census. Like the American Indian–Alaska Native group, they are extremely diverse, with more than 20 different subgroupings. Most of them (92%) live in urban areas, and the majority live in California. Their mean household income in 1990 was $36,784, higher than the average for all races, which was $30,056.

Education and Employment

Asian-Americans are better educated and better paid than the general U.S. population. The unemployment rate is lower than that of the general population.

Family Relationships

Family relationships are strong, with extended (multigenerational) families and an expectation of family loyalty from all members. Respect for elders is taught at an early age. Males are more "valued" than females, and they are the decision makers in the family. Females are submissive to males. Individuals' wishes and needs are subordinated to the needs of the group.

Health Care Utilization

Visits to health care providers are less frequent, with Asian-Americans over age 65 making about half as many visits to health care providers as their white counterparts.

Health Status

The health status of this group as a whole is excellent. They have a longer life expectancy and lower death rates from all causes than the general population. The illnesses that are higher than those in the general population include stomach cancer (among Japanese) and suicide (among elderly Chinese women). Southeast Asian refugees have a higher incidence of intestinal parasites, positive tuberculin tests, and presence of hepatitis B antigen and more anemia than other Asian-Americans or the general population.

Health Beliefs and Practices

Health beliefs and practices vary among different Asian-American subgroups.

Chinese and Vietnamese people believe that health is a result of forces that rule the world: yin (cold) and yang (hot). Illness results when there is an imbalance in these forces. Illness is diagnosed by pulses (there are seven different ones), color and texture of the tongue, and other means not commonly used by allopathic medicine. Treatment is provided with the opposing force to achieve balance. For example, a "cold" illness (e.g., colic, diarrhea, or edema) is treated with "hot" herbs and foods. "Hot" illnesses (e.g., hypertension, blood diseases, or a cough) are treated with "cold" herbs and foods. Healers within the group are skilled at diagnosis and prescription of therapy. Such therapy may include acupuncture, acupressure, tai chi, moxibustion, or medicinal herbs. Chapter 9 discusses herbal therapy, with the important caveat that one must understand and subscribe to a totally different view of health and illness to prescribe these herbs appropriately. "Chi" is innate energy, and lack of it results in fatigue and long illnesses.

Japanese beliefs are influenced by Shinto, a religious orientation. They believe that humans are inherently good, and that evil is caused by outside spirits. Both Japanese and Vietnamese people believe that pleasing good spirits and avoiding evil ones help to maintain harmony and health. Evil is removed by purification, and there are rituals for this purpose.

Filipinos also subscribe to the concept of yin and yang, but believe that God's will and supernatural forces govern the universe and determine health and illness. Illness is punishment for violations of God's will. Amulets and religious medals may be worn as a shield from witchcraft or as a good-luck charm.

All of these groups use combinations of allopathic and ethnically defined health and illness care. The allopathic approach, however, is often chosen last or to supplement ethnically defined care.

Racial Differences in Drug Pharmacokinetics and Response

Bertilsson (1995) compared Asian-Americans and whites on the basis of drug metabolism by the CYP-450 2D6 and 2C19 isoenzyme systems. The 2D6 isoenzyme system is responsible for metabolism of **antiarrhythmics, antidepressants,** and **neuroleptics,** among others. The mean activity of 2D6 extensive metabolizers is lower in Asian-Americans and is the molecular genetic basis for slower metabolism of **antidepressants** and **neuroleptics** in Asian-Americans. This difference in metabolism requires lower doses of these drugs. The 2C19 system is involved in the metabolism of acids (e.g., **mephenytoin**), bases (e.g., **imipramine** and **omeprazole**), and neutral drugs (e.g., **diazepam**). **Diazepam (Valium)** is partially demethylated by 2C19, and the high frequency of mutated alleles in Asian-Americans is probably the reason that such populations have slower metabolism and are treated with lower doses of **diazepam** than whites. Although other drugs in this same class have not been studied, it is likely that they have similar metabolic fates as **diazepam**. **Omeprazole (Prilosec)** is hydroxylated to a major extent by 2C19, and there is an approximately tenfold difference in oral clearance between Asian-Americans and whites. Hence, a lower dose is required among Asian-Americans for this drug.

McSweeney and Zhan (1994) state that many Asians have a deficiency of the active form of dehydrogenase, an enzyme used in the metabolism of alcohol. In these people, a "flushing" may appear after they ingest only a small amount of alcohol. Chan (1986) also reports this "atypical" dehydrogenase, which he states is present in 85 to 90 percent of Asian-Americans.

Asians have also been described as "fast acetylators" (Katsung, 1998). Hepatic acetylation is responsible for metabolism of many drugs, including cardiac and psychotropic drugs, and 78 to 93 percent of Asians are "fast acetylators" (Lin et al., 1991). This faster metabolism may require a more frequent or higher dose of drugs metabolized by acetylation to achieve efficacy.

Frackiewicz et al. (1997) did a MEDLINE search of articles from 1966 to 1996 that identified racial differences in response to **antipsychotic** drugs. Their studies suggest that Asians may respond to lower doses of **antipsychotics** because of pharmacokinetic and pharmacodynamic differences. Confounding the issue, however, Lee, Yang, and Hu (1998) found lack of racial differences in **lithium** pharmacokinetics between Taiwanese Chinese bipolar patients and whites.

A class of drugs used to treat Parkinson's disease is **dopaminergics.** Filipinos require lower doses of **levodopa** than whites, and they develop dyskinesia more readily at comparable doses. This difference appears to be related to racial differences in erythrocyte catechol-O-methyltransferase (Rivera-Calimlim & Reilly, 1984).

In comparing Asian-American children with African-Americans, Hispanics, and whites, Liu and Levinson (1996) found a higher prevalence of elevated blood pressure in Asian-Americans. This suggests a need to consider any racial differences in antihypertensive drug metabolism and responses. Studies do appear to support such differences, including the need for lower doses of **beta-adrenergic blockers** (Hui & Pasic, 1997; Matthews, 1995), and **ACE inhibitors** and **calcium channel blockers** (Hui & Pasic, 1997), based in part on increased adverse drug reactions at doses used for whites.

Recently, the National Academy of Sciences released **calcium** requirements for North Americans. Adequate intake for individuals over age 50 was set at 1200 mg/day. This amount appears necessary to eliminate dietary **calcium** as the limiting factor in age-related bone loss. The evidence to determine the amount required was accumulated primarily in whites. Weaver (1998) reports a fractional **calcium** absorption rate that is much higher in Chinese women than values reported for whites. If **calcium** is generally better absorbed from the Chinese diet and if Chinese individuals absorb **calcium** more efficiently than do whites, as the Weaver-reported studies have found, **calcium** requirements may be lower for this population. No specific amount of supplementation was given in this article, and the number remains to be determined by research.

Hispanics/Mexicans

Cultural Factors

Demographics

Individuals of Hispanic descent include Mexicans, Puerto Ricans, Cubans, and people from Central and South America. They make up 9 percent of the U.S. population and are the second largest minority group. This group is young, with 33 percent under age 18. Most live in urban areas, with the highest percentage living in southwestern states (Arizona, California, Colorado, New Mexico, and Texas). The mean household income in 1990 was $24,156, and the percentage of families below the poverty line was 25.3 percent.

Education and Employment

Thirty-one percent of Hispanics have less than a ninth-grade education, 50 percent have a high school education, and 9.2 percent have a college education. The unemployment rate for Hispanic men is 9.8 percent, but this may not accurately reflect the migrant farm worker population.

Family Relationships

The family is the center of the person's life, and strong kinship bonds include godparents, who are established by ritual kinship. The family is usually large and home-centered. Respect for parents and elders is taught early. There are clearly differentiated roles for males and females. The father is the main decision maker in the family, but women, who are considered the primary healers in the group, decide health-related issues. Native healers (*curanderas*) are usually women.

Health Care Utilization

The combination of unemployment and lack of documentation of farm workers means that this group has the highest percentage of people without health insurance. Public health clinics and emergency departments are often the sites for health care.

Health Status

Obtaining accurate health statistics on Hispanics is difficult because their data are often included with those of whites. In addition, this group is more likely than others to have "undocumented aliens" who actively seek not to have their status reported, including health status. What is known is that the prevalence of type 2 diabetes is nearly twice that of whites. Their strong religious traditions and connection with the Roman Catholic church mean that they are the least likely minority group to use contraception, which increases their risk for pregnancy and sexually transmitted infections. The leading causes of mortality are cardiovascular disease, diabetes, cancer, and homicide. The suicide rate is the lowest among the ethnic groups.

Health Beliefs and Practices

Similar to the Asian concept of yin and yang, Hispanic peoples subscribe to the concept of hot and cold but also consider wet and dry. Illness results from an imbalance of these forces. Illness may also be caused by *mal ojo* (evil eye) that results from the look or gaze of an individual thought to possess evil intention and evil powers. Health care providers can inadvertently give this look. Health beliefs often have a strong religious association, with health a gift from God as a reward for good behavior. Eating proper foods, working the proper amount of time, wearing religious medals, and sleeping with relics in the home are thought to prevent illness. *Curanderas* treat illness with a variety of herbs, teas, visits to shrines, medals, candles, and promises to God to change behavior. Understanding the herbs used and considering them when prescribing other drugs will reduce the risk for drug interactions. Like Asian medicinal therapies, it is important to understand that illness conditions are defined differently and that there are illnesses that have no correlate in allopathic medicine. Having worked in a clinic where a *curandera* was an integral part of the health care team, the author can state that referral to the *curandera* for these illnesses can result in referral from the *curandera* for illnesses that she recognizes as treatable by allopathic medicine. This practice also increases the willingness of the Hispanic population to accept allopathic care and to adhere to allopathic prescriptions.

Racial Differences in Drug Pharmacokinetics and Response

An interracial comparison of the pharmacokinetics of **HMG-CoA reductase inhibitors** (Muck et al.,1998) was undertaken because these drugs are extensively metabolized by the liver and therefore are in a class at risk for racial differences. The results of this study showed no evidence of any clinically relevant interethnic difference in their metabolism among white, African-American, Hispanic, and Japanese subjects. Studies of other drugs in a class at risk for racial differences that included Hispanic patients (Jamerson & DeQuattro, 1996) reported a similar lack of difference between Hispanic Americans and whites.

Despite preliminary evidence of racial differences in insulin secretion and glucose metabolism and in factors associated with cardiovascular risk, evidence of differences in drug pharmacokinetics and response to drugs is lacking. This may be related to the genetic variability among persons classified as Hispanic.

Non-Hispanic Whites

Limited discussion is required about this segment of the population because most allopathic health care is currently directed at this group. There are within this group, however, some subgroups that bear a short discussion.

Whites of various ethnic backgrounds may hold to beliefs in the "evil eye" and to the curative powers of folk medicine. **German-, Polish-,** and **Italian-**Americans also see stress and environmental changes as sources of illness. Along with **Irish-**Americans, they have strong family ties, with the male as the dominant force and de-

cision maker. **Polish-** and **Italian-**Americans may use folk remedies and native healers. All four groups have strong religious ties, with **Polish-, Irish-,** and **Italian-**Americans having Roman Catholicism as their main religion. Religious medals and rituals are often used to promote health, prevent illness, and heal.

Summary

Consideration of demographic, socioeconomic, and cultural factors is important in prescribing appropriate drugs for patients and in recognizing the potential for drug interactions with herbs or foods that may be used in culture-specific healing practices. Becoming culturally sensitive requires recognizing that cultural diversity exists, identifying and exploring one's own cultural beliefs, and being willing to modify health care delivery to be more congruent with the patient's cultural background.

As can be seen from the research and other articles discussed, the study of ethnopharmacology often presents conflicting data. It is incumbent upon prescribers to keep current in the literature and to take the time to review research studies for the validity and reliability of the methods and statistics used in the research and for the appropriateness of application to their patients. Studies that report differences without stating a specific metabolic or biochemical relationship should be especially suspect. It is also important to look at articles in journals with reputations for peer review and careful selection of their research reports. Just because an article is published does not mean it is "good" research.

Many racial differences in drugs relate to their metabolism by the CYP-450 enzyme system. One quick way to review the literature in ethnopharmacology related to this system is a relatively new Website that is devoted exclusively to CYP-450 drug interactions. It includes a full discussion of the cytochrome enzymes and gives clinically relevant information and recommendations (including racial differences) in one window while showing the data used to arrive at these conclusions in another window. The site, maintained by two physicians and updated on a regular basis, can be found at *http://www.mhc.com*.

REFERENCES

Afzal, A., Brar, J., Ali, A., Jafri, S., Goldstein, A., & Khaja, F. (1997). Racial difference in patients with chest pain syndrome and abnormal coronary angiography. *Chest, 112*(3S), 24.

Aronoff, S., Bennett, P., Rushforth, N., Miller, M., & Unger, R. (1976). Arginine-stimulated hyperglucagonemia in diabetic Pima Indians. *Diabetes, 25*(5), 404–407.

Bell, R. (1994). Prominence of women in Navajo healing beliefs and values. *Nursing and Health Care, 15*(5), 232–240.

Bennion, L., & Li, T. (1976). Alcohol metabolism in American Indians and whites: Lack of difference in metabolic rate and liver alcohol dehydrogenase. *New England Journal of Medicine, 294*(1), 9–13.

Bertilsson, L. (1995). Geographic and interracial differences in polymorphic drug oxidation: Current state of knowledge of cytochromes P450 (CYP) 2D6 and 2C19. *Clinical Pharmacokinetics, 29*(3), 192–209.

Bogalusa Heart Study Twentieth Anniversary Symposium. (1995). *American Journal of Medical Science, 310,* S1–S138.

Cardillo, C., Kilcoyne, C., Cannon III, R., & Panza, J. (1998). Racial differences in nitric oxide-mediated vasodilator response to mental stress in forearm circulation. *Hypertension, 31*(6), 1235–1239.

Cardillo, C., Kilcoyne, C., Cannon III, R., & Panza, J. (1999). Attenuation of cyclic nucleotide-mediated smooth muscle contraction in blacks as a cause of racial differences in vasodilator function. *Circulation, 99*(1), 90–95.

Carmel, R. (1999). Ethnic and racial factors in cobalamin metabolism and its disorders. *Seminars in Hematology, 36*(1), 88–100.

Chan, A. (1986). Racial differences in alcohol sensitivity. *Alcohol, 21*(1), 93–104.

Cryer, B., & Feldman, M. (1996). Racial differences in gastric function among African-Americans and Caucasian Americans: Secretion, serum gastrin and histology. *Professional Association of American Physicians, 108*(6), 481–489

Cubeddu, L., Arnada, J., Singh, B., Klein, M., Brachfeld, J., Freis, E., & Roman, J. (1986). A comparison of verapamil and propranolol for the initial treatment of hypertension: Racial differences in response. *Journal of the American Medical Association, 256*(16), 2214–2221.

Dries, D., Exner, D., Gersh, B., Cooper, H., Carson, P, & Domanski, M. (1999). Racial difference in the outcome of left ventricular dysfunction. *New England Journal of Medicaine, 340*(8), 609–616.

Flaws, J., & Bush, T. (1998). Racial differences in drug metabolism: An explanation for higher breast cancer mortality in blacks? *Medical Hypotheses, 50*(4), 327–329.

Frackiewicz, E., Srmek, J., Herrera, J., Kurtz, N., & Culter, N. (1997). Ethnicity and antipsychotic response. *Annals of Pharmacotherapeutics, 31*(11), 1360–1369.

Friday, K., Srinivasan, S., Elkasabany, A., Dong, C., Wattigney, W., Dalferes Jr, E., & Berenson, G. (1999). Black-white differences in postprandial triglyceride response and postheparin lipoprotein lipase and hepatic triglyceride lipase among young men. *Metabolism, 48*(6), 749–754.

Gainer, J., Nadeau, J., Ryder, D., & Brown, N. (1996). Increased sensitivity to bradykinin among African-Americans. *Journal of Allergy and Clinical Immunology, 98*(2), 283–287.

Harris-Hooker, S., & Sanford, G. (1994). Lipid, lipoproteins and coronary heart disease in minority populations. *Atherosclerosis, 108* (suppl), S03–104.

Hui, K., & Pasic, J. (1997). Outcome of hypertension management in Asian Americans. *Archives of Internal Medicine, 157*(12), 1345–1348.

Jamerson, K., & DeQuattro, V. (1996). The impact of ethnicity on response to antihypertensive therapy. *American Journal of Medicine, 101*(3A), 22S–32S.

Johnson, J. (1997). Influence of race or ethnicity on pharmacokinetics of drugs. *Journal of Pharmacology Science, 86*(12), 1328–1333.

Johnson,J., & Burlew, D. (1996). Metoprolol metabolism via cytochrome P450 2D6 in ethnic populations. *Drug Metabolism Disposition, 24*(3), 350–355.

Johnson, J., & Livingston, T. (1997). Differences between blacks and whites in plasma binding of drugs. *European Journal of Clinical Pharmacology, 51*(96), 485–488.

Katsung, B. (1998). *Basic and clinical pharmacology* (7th ed.). Stamford, CT.: Appleton & Lange.

Koup, J., Abel, R., Smithers, J., Eldon, M., & de Vries, T. (1998). Effect of age, gender, and race on steady state procainamide pharmacokinetics after administration of Procanbid sustained-release tablets. *Therapeutic Drug Monitoring, 20*(91), 733–737.

Lannin, D., Mathews, H., Mitchell, J., Swanson, M., Swanson, F., & Edwards, M. (1998). Influences of socioeconomic and cultural factors on racial differences in late-stage presentation of breast cancer. *Journal of the American Medical Association, 279,* 1801–1807.

Lee, C., Yang, Y., & Hu, O. (1998). Single-dose pharmacokinetic study of lithium in Taiwanese/Chinese bipolar patients. *Australia and New Zealand Journal of Psychiatry, 32*(1), 133–136.

Lin, K., Poland, R., Smith, M., Strickland, T., & Mendoza, R. (1991). Pharmacokinetic and other related factors affecting psychotropic responses in Asians. *Psychopharmacology Bulletin, 27*(4), 427–437.

Liu, K., & Levinson, S. (1996). Comparisons of blood pressure between Asian-American children and children from other racial groups in Chicago. *Public Health Reports. 111*(Suppl 2), 65–67.

Liu, K., Ruth, K., Flack, J., Jones-Webb, R., Burke, G., Savage, P., & Hulley, S. (1996). Blood pressure in young blacks and whites: Relevance of obesity and lifestyle factors in determining differences: The CARDIA study. *Circulation, 93,* 60–66.

Matthews, H. (1995). Racial, ethnic and gender difference in response to medicines. *Drug Metabolism and Drug Interaction, 12*(2), 77–91.

McSweeney, E., & Zhan, L. (1994). Cultural and pharmacologic considerations when caring for Chinese elders. *Journal of Gerontological Nursing,* (October), 11–16.

Mitchell, H., Smith, R., Cutler, R., Sica, D., Videen, J., Thompsen-Bell, S., Jones, K., Bradley-Guidry, C., & Toto, R. (1997). Racial differences in the renal response to blood pressure lowering during chronic angiotensin-converting enzyme inhibition: A prospective double-blind randomized comparison of fosinopril and lisinopril in older hypertensive patients with chronic renal insufficiency. *American Journal of Kidney Diseases, 29*(6), 897–906.

Moskowitz, W., Schwartz, P., & Schieken, R. (1999). Childhood passive smoking, race, and coronary artery disease risk: The Medical College of Virginia Twin study. *Archives of Pediatric Adolescent Medicine, 153*(5), 446–453.

Muck, W., Unger, S., Kawano, K., & Ahr, G. (1998). Inter-racial comparisons of the pharmacokinetics of the HMG-CoA reductase inhibitor cervistatin. *British Journal of Clinical Pharmacology, 45*(6), 583–590.

O'Hara, E., & Zhan, L. (1994). Cultural and pharmacologic considerations when caring for Chinese elders: Knowledge of traditional Chinese medicine is necessary. *Journal of Gerontological Nursing,* (October), 11–16.

Osterheld, J., & Osser, D. (1999). The P450 drug interactions home page. *http://www.mhc.com/cytochromes*

Prisant, L., & Mensah, G. (1996). Use of beta-adrenergic receptor blockers in blacks. *Journal of Clinical Pharmacology, 36*(10), 867–873.

Rivera Calimlim, L., & Reilly, D. (1984). Difference in erythrocyte catechol-o-methyltransferase activity between Orientals and Caucasians: Difference in levodopa tolerance. *Clinical Pharmacology and Therapeutics, 35*(6), 804–809.

Stephens, G., Gillaspy, J., Clyne, D., Mejia, A., & Pollack, V. (1990). Racial differences in the incidence of end-stage renal disease in types I and II diabetes mellitus. *American Journal of Kidney Diseases, 15*(6), 562–567.

Summerson, J., Bell, R., & Konen, J. (1995). Racial differences in the prevalence of microalbuminuria in hypertension. *American Journal of Kidney Diseases, 26*(4), 577–579.

Thompson, J., & Wilson, S. (1996). *Health assessment for nursing practice.* St. Louis: Mosby.

Tortolero, S., Goff Jr, D., Nichaman, M., Labarthe, D., Grunbaum, J., & Harris, C. (1997). Cardiovascular risk factors in Mexican-American and non-Hispanic white children: The Corpus Christi heart study. *Circulation, 96,* 418–423.

Weaver, C. (1998). Calcium requirements: The need to understand racial differences. *American Journal of Clinical Nutrition, 68,* 1153–1154.

Weinberger, M. (1993). Racial differences in renal sodium excretion: Relationship to hypertension. *American Journal of Kidney Diseases, 21*(4), 41–45.

Weir, M., Chrysant, S., McCarron, D., Canossa-Terris, M., Cohen, J., Gunter, P., Lewin, A., Mannella, R., Kirkegaard, L., Hamilton, J.,

Weinberger, M., & Weder, A. (1998) Influence of race and dietary salt on the antihypertensive efficacy of an angiotensin-converting enzyme inhibitor or a calcium channel antagonist in salt-sensitive hypertensives. *Hypertension, 31*(5), 1088–1096.

Winkleby, M., Kraemer, H., Ahn, D., & Varady, A. (1998). Ethnic and socioeconomic differences in cardiovascular disease risk factors: Findings for women from the Third National Health and Nutrition Examination Survey, 1988–1994. *Journal of the American Medical Association, 280,* 356–362.

Winkleby, M., Robinson, T., Sundquist, J., & Kraemer, H. (1999). Ethnic variations in cardiovascular disease risk factors among children and young adults. *Journal of the American Medical Association, 281*(11), 1006–1013.

Wood, A. (1998). Ethnic differences in drug disposition and response. *Therapeutic Drug Monitoring, 20*(5), 525–526.

Youngkin, E., Sawin, K., Kissinger, J., & Israel, D. (1999). *Pharmacotherapeutics: A primary care clinical guide.* Stamford, CT: Appleton & Lange.

CHAPTER 8

·······

Nutrition and Drug Therapy

CHAPTER OUTLINE

The role of nutrition in drug pharmacokinetics has great clinical importance and growing public interest. This chapter examines the significant role that nutrition plays in pharmacotherapy. The use of nutrition as therapy is beginning to take its rightful place in health promotion, disease prevention, and disease treatment. This is partly due to the fact that nutrition is often associated with the consumer trend to seek broader, preventive, more holistic approaches in health care, often referred to as *alternative* or *complementary* medicine. It should be argued, however, that nutritional concepts should be and sometimes are part of traditional health care. We have significant knowledge about the importance of nutrition as a key factor in health promotion, disease prevention, and treatment. We know that nutrition therapy can provide effective and efficient treatment when the medical condition affects nutritional needs or the diet affects the medical condition. Nutrition impacts disease progression. When nutritional considerations are part of the plan of care, the nurse practitioner (NP) helps patients feel better, improves management of their health care problems, and avoids complications that affect quality of life, productivity, and health care costs. There has been a deluge of both lay and professional resources on the topic of nutrition in health and disease. This chapter focuses on the role nutrition plays in the pharmacological management of patients.

Nutrient-Drug Interactions

Drugs do not create new bodily functions but rather interact with cellular function. Key to adequate cell function is the supply of needed nutrients. Because drugs are designed to improve altered cell function, it seems logical to conclude that nutritional factors can, in turn, affect pharmacological therapy. Clinically, the NP is concerned about the effect of drugs on the absorption, transport, metabolism, cellular uptake, and excretion of nutrients and the effect of nutrients on the pharmacokinetics of drugs. Therefore, drug-nutrient interactions must be considered for the NP to effectively utilize drugs in the prevention and treatment of disease. The relationship of nutrients and drugs is one of interaction or modification of cellular activity. The gap that once separated nutrition and pharmacology is closing, as research emerges that clearly demonstrates this relationship.

The ability of drug-nutrient interactions to alter the patient outcome has been established. Consumer education about drug therapy has become an expectation. Health care accrediting agencies such as the Joint Commission on Accreditation of Healthcare Organizations (JCAHO) and the National Committee on Quality Assurance (NCQA) require that patients be counseled and provided instruction about their care, including the pharmacological therapy that is prescribed. An important aspect of the patient education provided is information about drug-nutrient interactions, especially if there is a potential for adverse patient outcomes.

Consumers have shown increased interest and awareness of the importance of nutrition and nutrients in staying healthy. An outcome of this knowledge is increased use of nutrient supplementation. There are approximately 50 essential nutrients that must be acquired in the diet to maximize health. Although all nutritionists will tell you that the interplay of these nutrients is significant to their role in the body, many still will recommend supplementation of specific nutrients or combinations of nutrients for individuals at risk. It is vital that all practitioners engage in recommendations about how to utilize diet as part of the plan of care, but it is not uncommon that the ability to accomplish the recommendation by diet alone is difficult for given individuals. Additionally, recommended diet alterations might not be best, in consideration of other health problems. Therefore, the NP must become skilled in accurately advising patients about the benefits of nutrient supplementation in maintaining health, preventing disease, and treating disease. This advice must be based on the best scientific knowledge available, given that our knowledge about the nutritional implications in health and disease is moving forward at a very fast pace. All of these products can be purchased over the counter, and the NP must assist the patient with making the best decision possible about nutrient supplementation. Those individuals who might be on drug therapy that can induce nutrient deficiencies need specific recommendations about diet and nutrient supplementation to avoid additional drug adverse reactions. Patients at high risk for drug-food interactions include those who are elderly, have a multidrug regimen, require long-term therapy, or have marginal nutritional status.

Health care providers are often viewed as a reliable resource for pharmacological and nutritional information.

Yet, the knowledge base needed to accompany this responsibility is often deficient. This is demonstrated when the drug effect of nutrients or nutrient effects on a drug are not included in patient education. The lack of thorough patient education and of a holistic approach in health care is often attributed to the medical model of health care delivery. A holistic health care delivery model that includes prevention is within the grasp of NPs. Nurses are in a key position to facilitate that change and to make a difference. Holistic care and patient education have always been an essential component of nursing. The challenge for NPs is to enhance their knowledge base about the cellular action and interaction of drugs and nutrients to maximize the effectiveness of pharmacological therapy.

A complete or focused nutritional assessment should be part of the information gathered during the patient interaction. Data from the diet history, anthropometric measurement, physical examination, and laboratory findings are useful for pharmacological decision making. Team members such as a pharmacist and a registered dietitian are especially important in the care of patients with complex medical problems or pharmacological treatment plans. Although disease-specific nutritional therapy is beyond the scope of this chapter, recommendations about nutrient intake can promote health and prevent disease. The level, content, and frequency of nutrition care that are appropriate, as based on the patient's diagnosis, are clearly defined in available protocols. The American Dietetic Association (ADA) has developed medical nutrition therapy protocols for a variety of diagnoses.

Influence of Diet on the Pharmacokinetics of Drugs

Drug Absorption

The most frequent type of drug-food interaction is the effect that food has on the gastrointestinal (GI) absorption of drugs. The common result of this interaction is a change in the rate or amount of drug absorption. Drug absorption takes place across the mucosa of the GI tract. The proximal part of the small intestine plays a significant role in drug and nutrient absorption, secondary to its large surface area. Drugs utilize the same transport mechanisms as nutrients: passive and facilitated diffusion, endocytosis, and active transport. Several physiological factors affect drug absorption during the transport process: bioavailability, presystemic metabolism, gastric emptying time, concentration gradient, and absorptive surface area. Food in the GI tract at the time of drug administration affects absorption and bioavailability of the drug by changing the gastric emptying time, through interaction within the GI lumen, and by competitive inhibition.

Bioavailability—the percentage of drug available to produce a pharmacological effect—is influenced by the presence of food within the GI tract. Therefore, absorption of drugs can be increased or decreased, depending of the presence of food. Food decreases the amount of fluid in the GI tract, thus slowing down drug dissolution. Lack of food for an extended period—fasting for a day, for example—can decrease absorption secondary to vasoconstriction. Gastric emptying time also can influence drug absorption. However, the effect varies, depending on the type of drug preparation and the need for presystemic metabolism or dissolution. A drug that requires interaction in the stomach for disintegration and dissolution would have reduced absorption on account of the rapid gastric emptying time that might accompany a fasting state. Delayed gastric emptying that might occur with a meal high in fat would facilitate drug absorption because the drug is given more time for maximal disintegration and dissolution. Clearly, a change in gastric emptying can affect drug absorption, but the impact of the change is related to the dosage form and dissolution characteristics of the drug. A change in the drug form or time of administration can potentially affect bioavailability. Questioning the food intake of a patient who has had a change in the effectiveness of a pharmacological therapy can be an important part of the clinical decision-making process.

Additionally, the effect of food on the pH of the stomach can change bioavailability. The degree of ionization that occurs when a drug is taken into the stomach is a function of GI pH. If a drug that is a weak acid with best absorption in the nonprotonated (un-ionized) state, then the low pH of the stomach is essential to drug absorption to allow the acid to remain un-ionized and absorbable.

Chemical and physical changes in the drug can also occur as a result of interaction with food. These changes affect the absorption of the drug. Every nurse is aware of the need to advise patients to take **tetracycline** on an empty stomach or with foods that are not high in calcium, aluminum, iron, and magnesium because of decreased absorption as the drug chelates with these minerals. The binding of **phenytoin** with enteral nutrition products that results in fluctuation of phenytoin levels has provided impetus to the development of protocols that stop enteral nutrition before, during, and after delivery of this medication when the patient is tube-fed.

Additional physiological factors that may change a drug's absorption from the GI tract include food-induced changes in splanchnic blood flow, resulting in variation of drug absorption. As pointed out earlier, use of the same cellular transport proteins could result in competition for transport systems. **Levodopa** absorption is thought to be reduced with high-protein diets because of competition for the same transport system. The potential for change in drug absorption by food or nutrients in the GI system is quite high. In reality, we know of relatively few interactions that are clinically significant. Much of what we know is learned through clinical trials during drug approval or in specific research designed to investigate reports of clinically relevant, food-related variation in drug bioavailability. Further exploration of food effects on drug absorption would enhance our ability to predict and prevent drug-food interactions of this type.

Drug Metabolism

The rate of drug metabolism in both the GI tract and the liver is affected by nutrient intake. One of the impacts of the high-protein weight-loss diet that many people are now utilizing is an increase in drug-metabolizing enzymes. As individuals increase their intake of antioxidant cruciferous vegetables, one outcome could also be increased activity of drug-metabolizing enzymes. Most of the information about diet or nutrient interaction on drugs is obtained from animal studies. Yet, clinically we see examples of the effect daily, as unexplained variability in drug response or therapeutic drug levels is common. Even the lay press picks up some of the professional discussion about diet or nutrient interactions with drugs—for example, the interaction between grapefruit juice and **calcium channel blockers** that produces significant increases in area under the curve (AUC) and untoward adverse reactions.

The cytochrome P450 system is the major enzyme group responsible for the metabolism of foreign chemicals that come into the body. It is important to remember, however, that numerous other enzymes can be affected by drugs. Information is expanding about the clinically significant interactions between nutrients and drugs utilizing the cytochrome P450 enzyme system. Interestingly, as we get more sophisticated about the specificity of drug action, it is not uncommon to see adverse reactions related to cytochrome P450 interactions.

The cytochrome P450 proteins are found in the endoplasmic reticulum of the liver, intestine, lung, kidney, and brain. These proteins catalyze oxidative reactions and are not highly specific. The classification of these enzymes is based on similarity in amino acid structure. CYP is the superfamily name for this entire group of heme-containing enzymes. The next Arabic number indicates the family, the next letter indicates the subfamily, and the last Arabic number indicates the gene. Interestingly, the enzyme action associated with the cytochrome P450 system often results in metabolic products that are detrimental to the human body. It is thought that the nutrient inducers of these enzymes potentially increase carcinogen formation and that nutrient inhibitors offer cancer protection. Additionally, the cytochrome P450 system has a significant amount of polymorphism associated with it; that is, there are between-individuals differences in the presence and/or function of a particular enzyme group. This is one area where race is known to be a factor in physiological differences.

Asians are more likely to have a deficit in CYP2C19, whereas whites are more likely to have an inactive CYP2D6 enzyme. There are also differences in the function of particular enzymes between individuals, with some exhibiting slow metabolism and others exhibiting rapid metabolism. This difference is one of the factors involved in the individual differences seen clinically in drug effect and serum blood levels for the same dose of drug. A patient with deficient CYP2D6 does not convert codeine to morphine and thus gets little analgesic effect, whereas a rapid metabolizer of codeine has significant adverse reactions, such as GI pain and dizziness, due to fast conversion of codeine to morphine. This difference reinforces the need to understand the nutrient effect on metabolizing enzymes. Those who are slow metabolizers will have high concentrations of parent drug and low concentrations of metabolites, and they will be less influenced by cytochrome P450 system induction or inhibition. The high metabolizers will have low concentrations of parent drug, high concentrations of metabolites, and more susceptibility to the effects of enzyme inhibition or induction (Jefferson, 1999).

Currently, we know that the dietary factors that influence drug oxidation or conjugation reactions include protein quality, indolic compounds in vegetables (cruciferous), methylxanthine-containing beverages (caffeine), dietary fiber, and charcoal broiling. Much of our understanding about the effect of nutrients on the cytochrome P450 system has been obtained in animal research. There is a need to expand the research to epidemiological and metabolic studies in humans so that we can better predict potential interactions. Could part of the reason for the high number of adverse drug reactions in certain populations, such as older adults and the chronically ill, be related to nutrient-drug interactions?

Drug Excretion

A change in renal blood flow and thus clearance can affect drug excretion. A significant change in food and fluid intake could reduce renal blood flow and thus reduce renal drug clearance. Similarly, a low-protein diet can result in reduced renal clearance of drugs. The elderly are very susceptible to changes in renal elimination of drug that are due to dietary changes, particularly fluid intake.

The ionization of drug or drug metabolites that is important in GI pH also comes into play in the urine. Certain foods can change the urinary pH, which then increases or decreases the amount of the ionized form of a drug or metabolite. Higher ionization is associated with less tubular reabsorption and higher excretion. For example, **gentamicin** as a basic drug would be more likely to be reabsorbed in the renal tubule when there is an alkaline pH. This is one of the factors involved in the high variability in dose requirements to maintain **gentamicin** therapeutic serum levels. Competition between drugs and nutrients for tubular secretion sites and thus elimination of drug could be another mechanism for drug-nutrient interaction on drug excretion.

Drug-Food Incompatibilities

The level of nutrient intake can also affect a drug's activity in the body. The variability of vitamin K and fat intake while a patient is on **warfarin (Coumadin)** therapy can cause variation in anticoagulant effect and stability of INR measurements. A high intake of food containing tyramine can result in enhanced **norepinephrine** synthesis—problematic if the same patient is taking drugs that increase **norepinephrine** availability at the neurological synapse. For example, the adverse effect of acute hypertension associated with the use of **monoamine oxidase inhibitors (MAOIs)** is enhanced by intake of foods high in tyramine. The inhibition of aldehyde dehydrogenase by **metronidazole** results in a **disulfiram** reaction—flushing, headache, nausea, and abdominal or chest pain—when it is taken with alcohol or alcohol-containing products because of alteration in the alcohol metabolism.

Food contains many highly interactive ingredients that can have an impact on drug therapy. For example, the use of caffeine with known central nervous system (CNS) effects is problematic for patients utilizing psychotropic medications. The ability to manage the mental health problem becomes a challenge when high or variable levels of caffeine are consumed. For example, sorbitol, a common ingredient in sugar-free foods, has a significant effect on GI transit time and thus can influence the absorption of both drugs and nutrients.

Alcohol consumption is also associated with significant drug interaction problems. Alcohol can either induce or inhibit the cytochrome P450 system enzymes, depending on the ingestion pattern. Chronic low levels cause enzymatic induction, whereas high binge intake or high chronic use, resulting in hepatic failure, inhibits the metabolizing enzymes. Therefore, the practitioner needs to know the patient's specific level of alcohol consumption to better understand the potential for interaction with drugs.

Influence of Drugs on Nutrients

Drug-Induced Nutrient Depletion

Another mechanism of interaction between drugs and nutrients is the impact drugs can have on nutrient absorption, synthesis, transport, storage, metabolism, and excretion. The side effect profile of a drug taken over a period of time can be related to the effect of that drug on nutrient depletion. The number of potential drug-induced nutrient deficiencies is large and growing, as research in this area continues. A summary of those data in this text would be impossible. However, an excellent handbook listing the known interactions is available and would be a valuable tool in the clinical setting (Pelton, LaValle, Hawkins, & Krinsky, 1999). Often the clinician is faced with a patient on a long-term drug regimen who presents with a new set of complaints that do not fit into the current diagnostic picture and yet do not clearly suggest a new diagnosis. The differential diagnosis should include the potential for drug-induced nutrient depletion.

The mechanisms of action for drug-induced nutrient deficiencies are varied. As discussed previously, the gastrointestinal changes due to dietary factors that affect drug absorption can also be induced by drugs and thus affect nutrient absorption. The alterations in gastric emptying time, changes in pH, mucosal irritation (enteropathy), and formation of complexes that can be the result of drug therapy often have an impact on nutrient absorption. For example, changes in the pH from antacid therapy or potassium therapy can reduce absorption of folic acid, iron, and vitamin B_{12}. Drugs can induce or inhibit metabolic processes and, as a result, impact nutrient metabolism and bioavailability. For example, **phenytoin** reduces the level of folic acid by inhibition of intestinal enzymes needed for folic acid absorption. Many metabolic pathways rely on specific nutrient availability, so a deficiency results in cellular dysfunction. For example, the synthesis of vitamins, coagulation factors, and neurotransmitters can be affected by reduction in nutrient substrates. Just as the nutrient can affect excretion of drugs, drugs can affect urinary secretion, reabsorption, and elimination of nutrients. For example, the commonly seen depletion of sodium, calcium, and potassium with **loop diuretic** use is the result of interference with renal reabsorption. Thus, drug-induced nutrient malabsorption, maldigestion, and vitamin antagonism are potential adverse reactions of commonly prescribed drugs.

Outcomes of Nutrient-Drug Interactions

The physiological and cellular basis for drug-nutrient interactions is strong. However, it is the outcome of the interaction that takes the spotlight. Does the interaction cause a change in the expected outcome of drug therapy or a nutrient deficiency that enhances the potential for adverse reactions or disease progression? Clinically, practitioners often overlook this area. In the past, the availability of this information has not been good, and the research has been lacking. The increased interest in nutrition's role in health and disease has fueled experts to provide resources for current knowledge and to increase investigation in this area. When the availability of solid scientific information is limited, the NP is the most important tool in ensuring effective and efficient pharmacological treatment. If the expected outcome is not occurring or the adverse reaction profile is enhanced, the practitioner must know the key questions to ask to determine what is happening. It should be clear that a piece of the data needed is related to food and nutrient intake. Could the patient who became pregnant on the low-**estrogen** birth control pill have a reduction in drug bioavailability due to food intake? Is the **antidepressant** not working secondary to high caffeine intake? Is the **digoxin** (**Lanoxin**) serum level low because of an aggressive bowel care program with high fiber intake? And even more important, did the change in dietary fiber intake during a recent trip contribute to the **digoxin** toxicity the patient is experiencing?

Nutrient-Drug Interactions and the Nurse Practitioner

What can practitioners do to improve their skill in recognizing nutrient-drug interactions? The need to keep up to date about current and new drugs is vital in health care today. Journals, peer communication, the Internet, conferences, and improved references are available to the practitioner. It is not easy. Time is a precious commodity that few of us have in excess. Keep requesting that drug information be made available in an efficient and effective format. Seek out educational materials that can provide accurate and appropriate drug information to patients who must assume responsibility for their health. Have tools available in the office to allow you to quickly get information about drug-nutrient interactions. Utilize the Internet in your data search. Understand that you are not alone in providing care to the patient; consult with other practitioners, pharmacists, and registered dietitians. This provides a combined effort in pharmacological and nutritional knowledge to enhance identification of drug-nutrient interactions. Get a complete patient profile in terms of drug, herb, and nutrient intake. Knowing all of the medications taken—prescribed, over-the-counter, herbs, vitamins, alcohol, nutrient supplements—is key to identification of interaction potential. The NP must understand how the medication is taken in relation to food and fluids. How stable is food intake in terms of the substances known to impact drug absorption, like fiber, protein, and fat? Clearly communicate to the patient the best routine for medication administration. Ensure that you and the patient read warning labels for instructions about mixing with food, using with nutritional supplements, and taking with fluid. As clinicians, we have the advantage of knowing specific cellular function of the pharmacological therapy we prescribe. As a result, there has been significant improvement in our knowledge about drug-nutrient interactions. As professionals, we must utilize this information to maximize the intended pharmacological outcome for the patient, while minimizing the adverse reactions.

Nutritional Supplementation

Nutritional supplementation is the use of vitamins, minerals, or other food factors to support health and prevent or treat disease. In the last few years, increasing numbers of people are buying and taking nutritional supplements. Although much of the research surrounding use of supplements is not conclusive in terms of randomized clinical trials and is even sometimes contradictory, patients' use of nutritional supplementation is not waiting for conclusive outcomes. To partner with the patient who is interested in nutritional supplementation, NPs must have a clear understanding of the patient's philosophy surrounding nutritional supplementation and the recommendations of experts in the area. We must remind ourselves that nutritional supplementation does not replace a healthy diet but rather complements the two important basics of good health: nutrition and exercise.

To supplement or not to supplement, that is the question. The ADA has developed a position statement about vitamin and mineral supplementation. This statement provides a solid foundation for assisting patients with their nutriment supplementation decisions. It supports obtaining nutrients through a wide variety of foods as the best way to promote health and reduce risk of disease. The one thing that is clear in nutritional research is that the more evidence mounts about the role of nutrients in health, the fuzzier the picture gets. It seems that nutrient interplay within foods is critical in order to realize the health benefit. As single nutrients are studied for their effect on health or disease progression, often the same beneficial outcome is not available. For example, the results of beta carotene trials in cancer prevention demonstrated the problem of extrapolating strong epidemiological research on food consumption to single nutrients. The ADA recognizes the need for strong scientific evidence based on controlled clinical trials.

However, the ADA also defines clearly in the position statement the circumstances in which supplementation is indicated. Nutritional supplementation for vulnerable or at-risk populations has been recently advocated in the development of a food pyramid for older adults. A less wide variation in the number of servings within each group, a suggestion to increase the use of nutrient-dense food, and the addition of nutritional supplementation differentiate the food pyramid for older adults. Patients frequently ask for advice from nurse practitioners about nutritional supplementation. Often, they need an interpretation of what they read or hear about nutritional supplementation. It is best to assist the patient in this decision by reviewing the patient's

1. Current intake (assessing for potential areas of deficiency)
2. Daily requirements of the nutrient for health
3. Health problems currently present
4. Disease risk profile, if there is increased loss of nutrients
5. Drug-nutrient interaction potential

Obviously, the need to utilize nutritional supplementation is highly individual. The NP must guide patients to understand their particular situation and need. Most important in this interaction between patient and practitioner is an open, honest discussion of the nutritional supplementation decision. This is critical to assessing the potential for impact on therapy that the practitioner might prescribe for the patient. Although vitamin supplementation is often inexpensive and unlikely to cause harm, the same cannot be said for many other nutrients for which there is no recommended daily allowance (RDA) and no established standard for supplementation. If you do recommend or prescribe a multiple vitamin and mineral supplement for an at-risk individual, it is important to frame the dosage needed around the RDA and recommended vitamin and mineral intake ranges.

REFERENCES

Jefferson, J. (1999). Drug and diet interactions: Avoiding therapeutic paralysis. *Journal of Clinical Psychiatry, 59*(Suppl 16), 31–39.

Jones, M., & Tracy, T. (1998). Cytochrome P450: New nomenclature and clinical implications. *American Family Physician, 57*(1), 107–116.

Pelton, R., LaValle, J., Hawkins, E., & Krinsky, D. (1999). *Drug-induced nutrient depletion handbook.* Hudson, OH: Lexi-Comp.

Pronsky, Z. (1997). *Food medication interactions* (10th ed.). Pottstown, PA: Food Medication Interactions.

RESOURCES

American Dietetic Association
http://www.eatright.org
Food and Drug Interactions
http://vm.cfsan.fda.gov/~lrd/fdinter.html
Food and Drug Interactions Patient Brochure
http://www.natlconsumersleague.org/fooddruord.html
Food and Medication Interactions
http://www.foodmedinteractions.com

CHAPTER 9

....

Pharmacology in Complementary Medicine

CHAPTER OUTLINE

T he pharmacopeia in primary care is vast and to the novice may seem overwhelmingly so. In addition, medicinal remedies available through naturopathic medicine broaden the possibilities for relieving the symptoms of patients who are seeking primary care. All these medicines by definition are available through the various plants and plant products and therefore have been around since the beginning of time. Early practitioners of the healing arts had only these medicines, which they discovered through trial and error, and eventually these medicines were passed on to their students. This chapter serves as an introduction to phytomedicine—"the practice of using plants or plant parts to achieve a therapeutic cure" (Fetrow & Avila, 1999, p. 1)—which is a large part of the field of complementary medicine. Because this is a relatively new area of study for Western health practitioners, definitions of terms are necessary, as is knowledge of the variables involved in producing and distributing these medicines in North America. This chapter also addresses herbal remedies for common health conditions. A cautionary note, however, is that this chapter is meant to be used in an informative way rather than in a prescriptive sense. With a basic understanding of these treatments, the primary care practitioner can better understand what patients may be using along with medicines they are prescribed by Western practitioners and collaborate with naturopathic practitioners in providing complete care for patients.

Basic Assumptions

Chinese herbalists and naturopathic physicians train for many years to learn to prescribe herbal medicines appropriately. The conceptual base by which they make clinical decisions is remarkably different from Western allopathic medicine. Allopathic and naturopathic medicines can be used together by the primary care practitioner who has this full range of knowledge; but without that background the practitioner is likely to be practicing outside the scope of advanced primary care nursing practice. This chapter is based on the following three basic assumptions:

1. A role of advanced practice primary care nurses is to learn from patients, teach and inform patients, and clarify the theoretical perspectives and biases of their practice.
2. Prescribing nonallopathic medicines requires further individual study of both the medicines and the conceptual foundation of the practice.
3. Using this information within an allopathic framework requires additional research in naturopathic medicines' mechanisms of action, pharmacokinetics, pharmacodynamics, effects, and interactions with other medicines.

Definition of Terms

This chapter deliberately avoids the terms *complementary*, *alternative,* and *traditional medicine* because of their vague and misunderstood reference points. The implied assumption of alternative medicine is that the preferred approach is Western allopathic medicine. Similarly, complementary medicine refers to using these approaches to complement allopathic medicine. If the term *traditional medicine* is used, confusion arises concerning on what traditions it is based and over what period of time. Historically, herbal medicines have been used at least as early as the Egyptian and Greek cultures of the Old World and the Anasazi and Hohokam cultures of the Americas. Currently, the terms *complementary* and *alternative medicine* refer to the broad approach of using a variety of healing strategies, including massage, acupuncture, chiropractic, biofeedback, ayurvedic, and others; a more appropriate overarching term for the medicines they use would be *phytomedicine.*

Phytomedicine refers to using plant derivatives for their medicinal value as determined by early use among folk healers. Actually, many of the drugs used in allopathic medicine were derived from plants, including foxglove for digitalis, *Ephedra* for ephedrine, and *Claviceps purpurea* for ergotamine. *Naturopathic medicine* refers to the practice of using only natural remedies for the treatment of illnesses. Remedies include not just plant derivatives but also massage, exercise, and nutrition. *Allopathic medicine* refers to the use of medicines that are unrelated to the illness to be cured, whereas *homeopathic medicine* refers to the use of minute quantities of substances that in much larger quantities would produce effects similar to the illness to be cured (*American Heritage Dictionary,* 1976). Like naturopathy, allopathic practices include more than administering drugs, such as physical therapy, nutrition, and surgery.

Pharmacognosy is the branch of pharmacology that uses the chemicals from plants, molds, fungi, insects, and marine animals for their medicinal value. Development and preparation of medicines from these plant and animal products can introduce wide variations, based on the conditions of their growth, harvesting, processing, storing, and shipping. Plants grown in the wild may be quite different from the same plants grown agriculturally. When harvested in the wild, they contain the inevitable uncontrollable contaminants, including insects and plant diseases. If the weather is particularly warm, the plants that are harvested may be quite different from the ones harvested in a wet and cool season. After harvest, the processing also introduces variations based on the drying and sterilizing techniques that are used. If products are not stored carefully, contaminants and moisture may again influence the character of the herbs.

In the United States, pharmaceuticals must meet a strict standard established by the Food and Drug Administration (FDA) not only in the research and development stages but also in the processing to maintain consistent standards of quality. Herbs, however, are not considered drugs but rather food products and do not have to meet FDA standards. The government agency in Germany that is similar to the FDA, Commission E, maintains a compendium of more than 300 herbal medicines and their safety and efficacy. The European Scientific Cooperative for Phytotherapy is a committee of herbal manufacturers, herbal associations, and European researchers that seeks to establish standards for herbal medicines put on the market. However, there is still a large gap between the rigorous studies required by the FDA and the experiential history of countries that have been using herbs for medicines for a very long time. Furthermore, the efficacy of the medicine does not come from just the herb but also the philosophical foundation of the prescriber, the assessment and diagnosis of the provider, and the specific manner of the prescription.

Herbal medicine refers to the use of plants, not limited to herbs, that are edible and useful to humans and other mammals (e.g., dogs and cats). Chinese medicine includes herbal medicine based on the notion of health as a state of balance and harmony of physical, emotional, and environmental influences. Chinese herbal medicine uses herbs to promote balance. The herbs are organized around the effects on body energies on a continuum: warm and cool, dispersion and concentration, strengthening and draining, dry and moist, calm and active, lubricate and bind. The overriding principle of two opposing forces—yin and yang—serves as the organizing element according to which the internal and external environments interact. Yin and yang are not really in opposition but rather are in confrontation and interaction. There are five elements of various processes in the body that interact with the environment (Table 9–1); however, the interaction is one of confluence and divergence not easily depicted in two linear dimensions. Herbs are used to restore harmony and

Table 9–1. Interaction of Elements and Internal and External Environments Used in Assessing and Prescribing within Chinese Herbal Medicine Tradition

Element	Organ	Emotion	Taste	Climate
Wood (straight)	Liver	Anger	Acid	Windy
Fire (rises)	Heart	Joy	Bitter	Hot
Earth (quiet and solid)	Spleen	Melancholy	Sweet	Damp
Metal (luminous and firm)	Lung	Grief	Acrid	Dry
Water (fluid and descendent)	Kidney	Fear	Salty	Cold

exhibit two properties: *Qi* or "nature" can be hot, warm, cool, or cold; *wei* or "taste" can be acid, bitter, sweet, acrid, or salty. Yang is the confluence of hot and warm and acrid and sweet. Yin is the confluence of cool and cold and acid, bitter, and salty. Each drug has a nature and one or more tastes. The herbalist assesses the patient by asking many questions about the sensations of the symptoms, as well as emotions and environmental influences. Physical assessment includes looking at the tongue, feeling the pulses on both sides of the body, and looking at the color of the patient. The herbalist arrives at a very individual determination of the disharmony and blends herbs together based on that particular assessment. The diagnoses that develop from this theoretical base and assessment sound very foreign to the Western ear and, without an understanding of the medical art, may even seem silly; for example, a diagnosis may be dampness in the lower burner or exogenous wind cold. Although the herbs that are prescribed may be the same or similar to herbs in the general pharmacognosy, their blend and preparation are highly individual. Clearly, these are not prescriptions that can be easily emulated without full immersion in the philosophy and practice of Chinese herbology.

Alternative or complementary medicine as a field also includes practices that may not use medicines at all: many different kinds of massage therapies (e.g., myofascial release, rolfing, shiatsu), movement therapy, combinations of massage and movement (e.g., Feldenkrais, Trager, Pilates), chiropractic or adjusting and releasing spinal fixations, and osteopathy or manipulation of bone articulations. Incorporation of these therapeutic methods in practice requires additional training and experience. Unless the practitioner has a strong background in these therapies, it is best to refer the patient to a skilled practitioner if the patient wishes to try them as part of an overall treatment.

Common Herbs Used for Medicine

Today it is possible to go to the grocery store in most communities in the United States and find a health section that sells various herbal remedies. They are available without

prescription or even any particular guidance except what the consumer may gather from sources that may or may not be reliable. The FDA does not permit the marketing and labeling of these products to make any therapeutic claims or to use terms such as *diagnose, treat, prevent,* or *cure.* In fact, the Dietary Supplement Health and Education Act (DSHEA) requires dietary supplements to carry on the label this statement: "This product has not been evaluated by the FDA. This product is not intended to diagnose, treat, cure, or prevent any disease."

Popular media now advertise herbal products with celebrities' endorsements of how the products have affected them. Consumers, therefore, may have a great deal of knowledge and may even consult an herbalist, or they may have only the testimonials of advertising to suggest particular herbal preparations for different symptoms or desired health states. This section discusses some common herbs used for different symptom constellations and what research literature there is about the herb. The purpose is simply to inform the advanced practice nurse (APN) of what herbal remedies patients may be using and how they can or should be used. Herbal and botanical products are not easily categorized, and many have multiple uses. In keeping with the organization of this book, these products are listed by the target symptoms for which they have some effect. Included are the common names and botanical names, the forms that are available, the putative mechanism of action, dosage as available, adverse effects, and some cautionary comments if necessary. This section is not meant as a recommendation for prescribing to clients. Instead, the APN needs to talk with patients about these medicines and take them into consideration when prescribing pharmaceutical medicines. Following this section are some resources available to provide greater depth of knowledge about herbal medicines; the APN should consult these references when working with a patient who is using them.

Mental Health Symptoms

The most common symptoms for which people use herbs are anxiety, difficulty in sleeping, depression or dysphoria, and forgetfulness and confusion. Like pharmaceutical drugs, some herbs may be beneficial for multiple similar symptoms.

Anxiety

Kava, pill-bearing spurge, mugwort, wormwood, and passion flower are commonly used for relief of anxiety. Kava and wormwood are presented here as exemplars in this category. Kava, also known as *ava, awa, kava-kava, kawa, kew,* or *tonga,* comes from the dried root of the *Piper methysticum,* which is a member of the black pepper family. This shrub is native to the Pacific Islands and kava-kava is a common substance Hawaiians use. It can be prepared as a drink from the pulverized root and also comes in tablet, capsule, and extract forms. This herb has been studied with humans and appears to have more than one active component to produce the effects. One component acts as a local anesthetic when chewed, and it produces intense muscle relaxation. It appears to act on the limbic system to suppress emotional excitability and produce mild euphoria without affecting memory or cognition. In therapeutic drug trials, kava seems to act on the gamma-amino butyric acid (GABA) receptor, like the benzodiazepines. Like the benzodiazepines, kava can reduce seizure activity and can be used for sedation. Dose varies, depending on the form and the amount of active components retained in the preparation, and studies indicate 70 to 240 mg daily as the adult dose. Pharmacokinetics are unavailable for kava, but it seems to be preferred in divided doses, usually three times a day. Unlike the benzodiazepines, it does not seem to produce dependence, but the studies are very limited. When used short term, it seems to have few adverse reactions, including decreased motor reflexes, diminished judgment, and visual disturbances. Chronic use may decrease platelet count and cause dry, flaky skin, reddened eyes, shortness of breath, pulmonary hypertension, and weight loss. Because it seems to act like the benzodiazepines, it may potentiate alcohol, other sedatives, and GABA-ergic drugs such as phenobarbital and benzodiazepines. At higher doses, kava seems to block dopamine receptors and therefore to improve psychotic levels of anxiety as well as interact with antipsychotic drugs. It should not be used in pregnancy or when breastfeeding because its safety is uncertain during pregnancy (Volz, 1997).

Mugwort, also know as *felon herb, wild wormwood,* and *St. John's plant,* comes from the roots of the *Artemisia vulgaris* plant. It should not be confused with wormwood or St. John's wort, which come from different plants. Mugwort is available as dried leaves and roots, fluid extract, tincture, or a tea infusion. It is a very versatile herb that is reported to be useful as an analgesic, anthelmintic, antibacterial, antifungal, aphrodisiac, appetite stimulant, central nervous system (CNS) depressant, diuretic, emetic, expectorant, hemostatic, laxative, sedative, uterine stimulant, and uterine vasodilator. It is also a primary ingredient in moxa sticks, used in Chinese medicine by burning the stick and holding it over acupuncture points with or without needles. In addition to relieving anxiety and causing sedation, mugwort is also used for gastrointestinal problems, menstrual cramps, anorexia, gout, headache, epilepsy, and circulatory problems. When taken for anxiety and sedation, the usual dose is 5 mL of tincture 30 minutes before bedtime. For use as an appetite stimulant, 150 mL of boiling water is poured over 1 or 2 teaspoons of the dried leaves, allowed to steep for 5 to 10 minutes, and drunk before meals as two or three cups of tea. Adverse reactions of mugwort include anaphylaxis, contact dermatitis, and induction of premature birth or miscarriage. It should not be used during pregnancy or breastfeeding or by people who have clotting abnormalities or allergies to hazelnuts. Because there are no controlled studies on mugwort, no therapeutic claims can be made.

Difficulty in Sleeping

In addition to mugwort, passion flower, melatonin, valerian, and chamomile are used for sedation. Melatonin and valerian are used here as exemplars. Melatonin is not an herb but a hormone produced by the pineal gland. Because it is a hormone, exogenous consumption over extended periods of time may act as negative feedback and suppress normally secreted melatonin. Melatonin is produced when serotonin is broken down in the pineal gland. Under physiological conditions, melatonin is released during the fourth stage of sleep, along with prolactin and growth hormone. It is used to induce sleep via the same GABA-ergic mechanism as benzodiazepine sedatives and is widely used to prevent and treat jet lag. A single study identified the utility of melatonin in elderly people to help induce and maintain sleep, probably because the elderly usually have some degree of melatonin deficiency under normal circumstances. Used long term, it can increase prolactin secretion, which can decrease luteinizing hormone, progesterone, and estradiol levels. Long-term use can also reset the sleep-wake cycle and contribute to disturbed sleep cycling. Melatonin is available in tablets, capsules and extended-release capsules, and liquid forms. For difficulty in getting to sleep, 1 to 5 mg taken at bedtime is the usual dosage, but it should not be used more than three nights a week. In the elderly, the dosage is usually 1 to 2 mg taken 2 hours before bedtime. Adverse reactions include altered sleep patterns, confusion, headache, tachycardia, and hypothermia. Melatonin potentiates benzodiazepines. It also potentiates succinylcholine, thereby increasing the blocking action, which can be dangerous. Its content of active drug may vary widely in commercial melatonin, making it difficult to determine correct dosages (Brzezinski, 1997; Fetrow & Avila, 1999).

Valerian is derived from the roots of *Valeriana officinalis* and is known also as *all heal, amantilla, setewale capon's tail,* and *herba benedicta.* It seems to inhibit uptake and increase presynaptic release of GABA; however, it is not readily absorbed, is highly unstable, and readily decomposes. Therefore, availability of the active drug is minimal when it is taken orally. German Commission E suggests valerian root for anxiety, restlessness, and difficulty in getting to sleep. Because of the instability, dosages are difficult to determine, especially between different brands. Usually 400 to 900 mg of extract at bedtime or 1 teaspoon of dried herb in tea several times a day is useful in inducing sleep. Commercial valerian tea at bedtime acts more as a relaxant and permits the person to fall asleep spontaneously. Valerian has no adverse reactions when used at the recommended level; however, overdosage at 2.5 g or more can cause cardiac disturbance, excitability, headache, insomnia, and nausea. It can potentiate alcohol and other CNS depressants if taken in large amounts. Because clinical trial studies are very limited, it should not be used by pregnant or breastfeeding women, children, or patients with impaired liver function.

Depression

The popular media have touted the benefits of St. John's wort for depression, contributing to its great popularity. Additionally, kava, mugwort, and DHEA have been used to treat mild depression. Because kava and mugwort have already been described, St. John's wort and DHEA are used as exemplars here.

St. John's wort is obtained from the tops and flowers of the *Hypericum perforatum* plant, which is common all over Europe, Asia, and the United States. The exact mechanism of action is still unknown but assumed to be related to inhibition of serotonin presynaptic uptake. Early studies showed inhibition of monamine oxidase (MAO) type A and minimally type B; however, this was later attributed to contaminants. In studies to determine effective dosages, St. John's wort was effective at blocking serotonin reuptake at much higher doses than could be achieved. St. John's wort also seems to act on the benzodiazepine receptor of GABA, norepinephrine reuptake inhibition, and acetylcholine blocking, as well as inhibiting stress-induced corticotropin-releasing hormone, adrenocorticotropic hormone (ACTH), and cortisol and increasing nighttime release of melatonin. Some reports have also indicated antiviral activity, including retroviruses (Chavez, 1997). With such a wide range of receptor activity, it is not surprising that it is used to treat depression, enuresis, gastritis, hypothyroidism, insomnia, kidney disorders, scabies, hemorrhoids, wound healing, HIV infection, and Kaposi's sarcoma.

Most commonly, St. John's wort is used to relieve mild to moderate depression, less than would meet the criteria for major depressive episode or dysthymia. Therefore, it seems most effective for those who have sadness and lesser degrees of depression. When used for clinically diagnosed depression, St. John's wort is relatively ineffective and may dishearten or demoralize the person who is trying to avoid using more potent antidepressants. For standardized, commercially prepared St. John's wort, the usual dosage is 300 mg taken three times daily; because of the delayed neuroreceptor response, it may take 4 to 6 weeks to determine effectiveness. When St. John's wort is used as a tea, it requires 2 to 4 g of tea steeped in 1 to 2 cups of boiling water for 10 minutes and taken daily to be effective within 4 to 6 weeks. There are a few adverse reactions, attributable to the anticholinergic blockade, including constipation, dry mouth, dizziness, gastrointestinal (GI) upset, restlessness, and insomnia. St. John's wort interacts with MAO inhibitors (MAOIs), tricyclic antidepressants, serotonin reuptake inhibitors, over-the-counter (OTC) cold and flu medications, narcotics, and sympathomimetics. Because there are inadequate studies available, St. John's wort should not be taken by children or pregnant or breastfeeding women. The primary care provider who determines that the patient meets the *Diagnostic and Statistical Manual of Mental Disorders, Fourth Edition* (1994) criteria for depression might advise the client to consider taking another kind of antidepressant if there are minimal results in 3 to 4 weeks.

Dehydroepiandrosterone (DHEA) is a steroid precursor found in plants from the yam family and secreted by primate adrenal glands. Physiologically, DHEA is converted into androgens and estrogens (depending on the person's gender) and may raise the blood level of a precursor of the human growth hormone. There are many benefits attributed to DHEA including immune enhancement, prevention of osteoporosis, antineoplastic, and antiaging, as well as antidepressant. Because few studies on humans are available, exact pharmacokinetics and pharmacodynamics are not known, but it does not seem to be readily absorbed through the GI tract. Similarly, it is difficult to determine dosage for the particular effect that is desired. At present, 50 mg daily is commonly used, but serum levels should be checked, with an expected level of 3600 ng/mL for men and 3000 ng/mL for women. Because DHEA is a hormonelike drug, it may cause negative feedback to the adrenal glands, thereby reducing production of endogenous hormones. Adverse reactions to be expected with an androsteroid include aggressiveness, hirsutism, insomnia, and irritability. Patients with hormone-sensitive cancers should be discouraged from using DHEA, as should pregnant and breastfeeding women. DHEA is likely to interact with other hormone therapy, such as estrogen replacement therapy. When it is used for depression, there may be a 4-week lag time before seeing an effect on depression (Wolkowitz, 1997).

Confusion and Forgetfulness

Confusion and forgetfulness, along with other cognitive impairments, are often seen in dementia, depending on the root cause of the dementia. Additionally, people who are concerned about benign forgetfulness are taking herbs both to improve their cognitive abilities and to prevent memory problems. Common herbs used include chaparral, ginkgo, ginseng, and galanthamine. This chapter uses ginkgo and ginseng as exemplars, and often they are taken together or combined in a single preparation.

Ginseng (American ginseng, Asian ginseng, Chinese ginseng, five-fingers, Japanese ginseng, Jintsam, Korean ginseng, ninjin, seng and sang, or schinsent) should not be confused with Siberian ginseng, which seems to bind with estrogen receptors. It is from the *Panax quinquefolius* plant, especially the root. The Asian ginseng is usually dried or cured and is highly valued, whereas the American ginseng has less processing but is not as widely sought. Several compounds have biological activity, producing different effects. The mechanisms of action are not understood, but ginseng is said to have differing effects depending on the involved active component: anticonvulsant, analgesic, and antipsychotic effects; CNS-stimulating, antifatigue, hypertensive, and stress ulcer exacerbation; improvement of cardiac function; depression of cardiac function; antiarrhythmic activity; reduction of cholesterol and triglycerides; decrease in platelet adhesiveness; impaired coagulation; and increased fibrinolysis. The presumed focus of action is in the adrenal gland, although there are claims in popular literature that it decreases thymus gland activity. Consequently, it is used as a sedative, aphrodisiac, antidepressant, hypnotic, and diuretic. It is also used to improve stress resistance, stamina, work efficiency, concentration, mental performance, and general feelings of well-being. Some studies found it decreased fasting blood sugar and hemoglobin to such a degree that some diabetics no longer needed insulin. Ginseng comes in capsules, tea bags, and extract, and in some places ginseng root can be bought in bulk in Asian markets. In processed form, however, it is difficult to standardize. Used for illness, it is usually taken at 0.5 to 2 g a day of dry root or 200 to 600 mg of extract daily in divided doses. For dementia in frail elderly, it is usually taken at 0.4 to 0.8 g of dry root daily. There seems to be a lag time in achieving maximum effectiveness—up to 90 days to see full results. It seems to have minimal and mild adverse reactions, including dizziness, drowsiness, headache, and insomnia, although chest pain, diarrhea, hypertension, impotence, nervousness, agitation, palpitations, nausea, and vomiting have also been reported. It may potentiate insulin and oral hypoglycemics, and it interacts with MAOIs to cause headaches, tremors, and mania. There are more studies on ginseng to identify its effectiveness, yet the pharmacodynamics are elusive. The German Commission E considers ginseng to be an effective drug (Sorensen, & Sonne, 1996; Wesnes et al., 1997).

Ginkgo, also known as *ginkgo biloba* or *ginkogink,* is an extract from the leaves of the ginkgo tree, with the toxic ginkgolic acid removed. It is available in many forms, including tablets, capsules, sublingual sprays, and even included in juices and foods. It is believed to stimulate prostaglandin synthesis and thereby cause vasodilation, increasing tissue perfusion and cerebral blood flow. Ginkgo has been used for centuries in Asian countries to improve mental alertness and today is used in the treatment of cerebrovascular disease and peripheral vascular disease. Additionally, it is popularly taken to improve thinking abilities, concentration, and memory. Dosage for confusion and dementia symptoms is 120 to 240 mg daily in two or three divided doses. For vascular disease, 120 to 320 mg daily has been used, but there is a 4- to 6-week lag time before maximum effect is obtained. Adverse reactions include diarrhea, headache, nausea, vomiting, bruising, excessive bleeding, and seizures in overdose. Trying to use ginkgo leaves to make a home remedy is potentially dangerous because of the ginkgolic acid and the difficulty in determining the quantity of active ingredients. Because it reduces platelet-activating factor and erythrocyte aggregation, it should not be taken with anticoagulants or antiplatelet medications. The German Commission E approved ginkgo for the treatment of dementia and peripheral arterial occlusive disease (Fetrow & Avila, 1999).

Gastrointestinal Problems

Probably the most common use of home remedies is for GI upset, such as constipation, diarrhea, indigestion, and nausea. Because the underlying cause of these complaints is also common, the herbal medications used for them overlap. The herbs most often used for constipation are also incorporated into commercial OTC medications: cascara, castor bean, and senna. Cascara sagrada is dried bark from the *Rhamnus purshiana* tree (found primarily in the Pacific Northwest and from Canada to California) that has been dried and aged for at least a year and up to 3 years. Cascara acts by increasing the smooth muscle tone of the large intestine and thus peristalsis. The FDA approved cascara as a safe and effective laxative to be sold OTC. It is available in an extract or extract capsules. Although it is very safe, it may produce such adverse reactions as abdominal cramping, diarrhea, fluid and electrolyte imbalance, steatorrhea, vomiting, and vitamin and mineral deficiencies in long-term use. Cascara can be used in pregnancy but should not be used by breastfeeding women because it is excreted in milk and may cause serious diarrhea in the infant. Because a person can become dependent on cascara, it should be limited to short-term use.

Senna comes from the leaves and pods of the *Cassia* tree. It is the active ingredient in OTC medications such as Senokot, Senokot-S, and Senolax and comes in capsules, tablets, and syrup. Dried senna leaves can also be made into a tea by adding 100 g of leaves to a liter of boiling water to steep for 10 minutes. Sliced ginger or crushed coriander leaves make the tea more palatable. When it enters the intestinal tract, bacteria convert it into a biologic active agent. Senna increases peristaltic action in the lower bowel. It is excreted in breast milk and should not be taken by the breastfeeding woman. The usual adult dosage is about 340 mg taken at bedtime or 0.5 to 1 dram of syrup. Adverse reactions are similar to those of cascara: abdominal cramping, diarrhea, hypokalemia, and clubbing of the fingers with chronic use. Calcium channel blockers or indomethacin blocks the diarrheal effects. A patient with irritable bowel, hemorrhoids, GI inflammatory conditions, or prolapsed rectum should not use senna. Again, it can be overused and create a laxative dependency.

Indigestion and heartburn plague Americans, as evidenced by the large amounts of antacids sold. In addition to these antacids, common household herbs can be used effectively and safely. Caraway oil distilled from dried seeds of the *Carum carvi* herb or caraway water made from soaking 1 oz of crushed caraway seeds in a pint of cold water for 6 hours can be used for indigestion, flatulence, constipation, and menstrual cramps. Because of its mild action, it can be given to infants for colic. The usual dosage for adults is 1 to 4 drops of oil in a teaspoon of sweetened water; and for infants 1 to 3 tsp of caraway water. The only adverse reactions reported are diarrhea and mucous membrane irritation.

Licorice root has also been used for gastric irritation and dyspepsia. Licorice comes from the dried roots of the *Glycyrrhiza glabra* shrub and is available in capsules, tablets, liquid extracts, chewing gum, tea, and candy. Studies indicate that glycyrrhetic acid is the active element that potentiates endogenous steroids and stimulates gastric mucus synthesis. It is a soothing and mild expectorant, mild laxative, and antispasmodic. Additionally, licorice has antiarrhythmic effects, lowers cholesterol and triglyceride levels, and may even cause immunosuppression. The usual dose is 200 to 600 mg tablets taken daily for 4 to 6 weeks or licorice tea simmered for 5 minutes and taken three times a day after eating. Reported adverse reactions include mineralocorticoid effects of headache, lethargy, sodium and water retention, hypokalemia, and hypertension, as well as, in overdose, muscle weakness, heart failure, and cardiac arrest. Licorice interacts with many medications such as antihypertensives, diuretics, corticosteroids, digoxin, loratadine, procainamide, quinidine, and spironolactone. A patient who is taking licorice regularly should be warned against excessive and chronic use, especially when it is combined with diuretics. Licorice candy does not actually contain the herb but rather licorice flavoring, usually from anise oil.

Papaya enzymes, available in tablets and chewable tablets, are frequently used to prevent or treat common heartburn, although it is not effective with gastro-esophageal reflux. Papaya is a proteolytic enzyme in the leaves, seeds, pulp, and latex of the *Carica papaya* tree. The clinical trials with humans have mostly focused treating inflammation from trauma and surgery. It also has been used effectively as a debriding agent and for intradiskal injections in patients with herniated disks. The dosage for inflammation is 10 mg four times a day for a week. Dosage for dyspepsia is variable and not standardized, but usually 4 to 5 tablets are taken immediately after eating. Adverse reactions are uncommon and limited to dermatitis, hypersenstivity, decreased heart rate and CNS activity, and perforation of the esophagus with excessive ingestion. No drug interactions have been reported. There have been no studies with pregnant and breastfeeding women, so it is safest to avoid use during pregnancy and breastfeeding.

Pain

Joint pain, soft tissue pain, and headache are frequent problems that people often treat with herbal and home remedies. There is little overlap in medications to treat each of these kinds of pain. Two products currently in health food stores are glucosamine and chondroitin, both of which are not herbal. Glucosamine, sold under such names as Arth-X Plus, Glucosamine Mega, Joint Factors, and Nutri-Joint, is a natural substance found in mucopolysaccharides and chitin. Most of what is sold in stores in the United States, however, is synthetically made. It is usually in capsules or tablets of a wide range of dosages. Glucosamine is thought to stimulate cartilage production and enhance rebuilding of damaged cartilage. Some studies done in Europe demonstrated good relief of pain and rapid restoration of mobility and range of motion in people with osteoarthritis. The dose used was 500 mg three times a day. Adverse reactions were benign, with constipation, diarrhea, drowsiness, headache, heartburn, nausea, and rash the most common. There were no drug interactions reported. Frequently, glucosamine is combined with chondroitin for greater efficacy.

Chondroitin is extracted from the cartilage of cow trachea and is available in 200- and 400-mg capsules. It seems to stimulate chondrocyte metabolism and synthesis of collagen, improving the formation of cartilage. Other studies identified stimulation of hyaluronic acid in synovial cells in patients with rheumatic disease, resulting in increased viscosity and amount of synovial fluid. When it was used for up to 4 months, patients used much less pain medication and were doing weight-bearing exercises comfortably. The dosage depends on the patient's weight: for patients under 120 lb, the dosage was 1000 mg of glucosamine and 800 mg of chondroitin; for patients 120 to 200 lb, the dosage was 1500 mg of glucosamine and 1200 mg of chondroitin. Used alone, the usual dose was 800 to 1200 mg daily, taken in either divided doses or a single dose. Adverse reactions include dyspepsia, headache, motor restlessness, euphoria, nausea, and risk of internal bleeding. Chondroitin may potentiate anticoagulants. Because there have been no studies with pregnant or breastfeeding women, glucosamine and chondroitin should not be used by this population.

Wintergreen oil and liniments have been deemed effective in relieving pain from muscle strains, inflamed muscles, ligaments, and joints. Usually the oil is a combination of oil extracted from the leaves and bark of *Gaultheria procumbens* and methyl salicylate. Although there have been no studies of the efficacy of wintergreen, it is assumed to act through counterirritation, which masks pain, or through the analgesic and anti-inflammatory effects of the salicylate. The 10 percent wintergreen oil is applied to the skin no more often than three to four times a day. Overgenerous application can result in salicylate poisoning from absorption into the bloodstream. People who are allergic to aspirin or who are taking oral anticoagulants should not use it.

Feverfew is an interesting herb used most often to treat headache and migraines. It has also been used for toothache, joint pain, asthma, stomachache, menstrual problems, and threatening miscarriage. It is extracted from the leaves of the feverfew plant, also called bachelors' buttons, featherfoil, Santa Maria, midsummer daisy, or its botanical name, *Chrysanthemum parthenium*. The assumed mechanism of action is the inhibition of serotonin release from platelets. It is available in capsules, liquid, tablets, and dried leaves for tea. The research with feverfew showed improvement in the number, duration, and severity of migraines in a double-blind, crossover study (Murphy et al., 1988). The average dose for the treatment of migraines was 543 μg of parthenolide (the active component of feverfew) daily; for migraine prevention, the dose was 25 mg daily of freeze-dried leaf extract. The most common adverse reactions were mouth ulcerations, hypersensitivity, and a withdrawal syndrome characterized by moderate to severe pain and joint and muscle stiffness.

Other Disorders

Table 9–2 presents additional information on herbal medicines for common health problems. Although many other herbs may be used for these disorders, the ones listed have all been studied in some kind of human trial. Those not listed have been used but reported in case or anecdotal reports.

Considerations for the Advanced Practice Nurse Prescriber

There are many reasons for people to use herbal remedies instead of conventional medicines. Sometimes these reasons may not be rational or supported by studies; however, we must respect the consumer's autonomy and free choice. Twenty-five percent of current pharmaceuticals originated in part or entirely from some naturally occurring plant or plant product. Herbal medicines have been around for centuries, and the practice of herbal medicine continues now and into the twenty-first century. The *Materia Medica,* the first known pharmacopeia, provided rigorous documentation of plants for the treatment of disease by early people of the Middle East.

Just because a product is natural, however, does not mean it is risk-free. Some plants can cause serious illness or death in even minute amounts; some in minute amounts treat diseases but in larger amounts can cause death (e.g., digitalis from foxglove). Adverse responses from herbs may be related to the herb itself, a specific chemical component of the herb, or mishandling during processing or packaging. Because these remedies are classified as dietary supplements rather than drugs, there are no requirements to report adverse effects. Yet, in the late 1980s a particular brand of L-tryptophan tablets resulted in several cases of fatal eosinophilia myalgia, and from 1993 to 1997 several hundred cases of serious adverse effects were documented from ephedra in diet and weight loss supplements, resulting in severe hypertension, tremors, arrhythmias, seizures, strokes, heart attack, and death. Table 9–3 presents selected herbal product and drug interactions.

These medicines can be purchased and consumed freely by anyone. With many, the doses are not certain; because a little helps, some consumers take many more because they assume they are safe. They can be abused and misused. High school athletes have used the glucosamine-chondroitin combination to reduce pain, swelling, and inflammation from sport injuries and permit them to continue playing at the risk of more serious injury. Some remedies may have widely accepted beneficial effects yet also have rare but serious adverse reactions. For example, pennyroyal is an effective insect and flea repellent that may also cause miscarriage in pregnant women. Many seriously depressed people are using St. John's wort to treat their depression and forestalling more effective treatments such as psychotherapy and antidepressants. An often-overlooked result of untreated or inadequately treated depression is suicide.

Health care professionals need to keep an open mind to all the possible ways to treat physical and mental health problems, and they must remember that open-mindedness also needs to extend to the negative effects of natural products as well as the positive. It is important to advocate for patients' rights to choose and to provide sufficient accurate information for their informed decisions. Primary care providers may need to explore the resources that are available to the public at large, critique the information, and assist the patient in finding practitioners that can meet their needs for non–Western-based treatments.

Table 9–2. Selective Herbal Agents Used for Common Disorders

Disorder	Herbal Agent	Dosage Range
Arthritis	Borage	1.1–1.4 g PO qd
	Capsicum	0.025–0.25% topically tid
	Chondroitin	800–1200 mg PO qd
	Evening primrose oil	No consensus
	Ginger	No consensus
	Glucosamine	500 mg PO tid
	Turmeric	8–60 g PO tid (on empty stomach)
Benign prostatic hypertrophy	Nettle	1–2 tsp/1 cup water PO bid
	Pumpkin seed	60–500 g PO qd
	Saw palmetto	160 mg PO bid
Cancer	Green tea	6–10 cups qd
	Lavender	1–2 tsp/150 mL of water qd
	Mayapple	Root: 6 g PO qd
		Leaf: 5 g PO qd
	Melatonin	20 mg IM × 2 mo, then 10 mg PO qd
	Mistletoe	Dried leaves: 2–6 g PO tid
		Extract: 1–3 mL PO tid (1:1 solution in 25% alcohol)
	Shark cartilage	Depending on type of preparation and amount of pure shark cartilage contained
		500–4500 mg PO qd
	Skull cap	Dried herb: 1–2 g/1 cup water PO tid
		Extract: 2–4 mL PO tid (1:1 in 45% alcohol)
Diabetes	Basil	2.5 g/half cup water qd–bid
	Ginseng	0.5–5 g dry gingerroot qd
Eczema	Evening primrose oil	Adults: 320 mg–8 g PO qd
		Children: 160 mg–4 g PO qd
Edema	Tonka bean	60 mg PO qd
Hyperlipidemia	Fenugreek	Seeds: 1–6 g PO tid
	Flax	1–2 Tbsp oil PO qd
	Garlic	Powder: 600–900 mg PO qd
		Fresh: 4 g qd; oil 8 mg qd
	Safflower	Powder: 2–3 g PO tid
		Extract: 3 g:15 mL alcohol & 15 mL water PO tid
Impotence	Yohimbe	5.4 mg PO tid
	Tonka bean	60 mg PO qd
Infection	Cranberry	10–16 oz juice PO qd
	Echinacea	Capsules: 900 mg–1 g PO tid
		Tincture: 0.75–1.5 mL (15–30 gtt) PO 2–5 times/day
Liver disorders	Dandelion	Dried root: 2–8 g PO tid
		Dried leaf: 4–10 g PO tid
		Extract: 4–8 mL PO tid (1:1 in 25% alcohol)
	Milk thistle	420–800 mg PO qd
Menopause	Black cohosh	Not standardized
		8–2400 mg qd

Continued on next page

Table 9–2. Selective Herbal Agents Used for Common Disorders *(continued)*

Disorder	Herbal Agent	Dosage Range
Premenstrual syndrome	Evening primrose oil	3–4 g PO qd
Warts	Mayapple	1–10 gtt qd or bid (5–25% solution in alcohol)
Wound healing	Aloe Echinacea Gotu kola	Apply liberally as needed Capsules: 900 mg–1 g PO tid Tincture: 15–60 gtt PO 2–5 times/day Dried leaf: 0.6 g PO tid Capsule: 450 mg PO qd

Adapted from: Fetrow, C. W., & Avila, J. R. (1999). *Professional's handbook of complementary & alternative medicines.* Springhouse, PA: Springhouse Corp.

Table 9–3. Herbal Product and Drug Interactions

Herbal Product	Indication for Herb	Interacting Drug and Consequence
Broom	Tooth decay, toothache	**Lithium:** Potentiates, possible toxicity
Danshen	Cardiovascular disorders	**Warfarin** (Coumadin): Increases the anticoagulating effect
Ephedra (ma huang)	Bronchodilation, breathing problems, urinary problems	**Theophylline:** Increased theophylline toxicity
Feverfew	Promote menstruation, induce miscarriage	**Warfarin:** Decreased platelet aggregation, bruising and increased bleeding
Ginkgo biloba	Cerebral insufficiency, dementia, circulatory problems	**Warfarin:** Increased risk for bleeding because of the antiplatelet activity of ginkgo
Ginseng	Reduce stress, lower cholesterol and blood sugar, increase estrogen effect	**Digoxin** (Lanoxin): Elevated levels of digoxin **Hypoglycemic agents:** May antagonize or potentiate hypoglycemic effect **Phenelzine** (Parnate): headache, irritability, visual hallucinations, tremor **Warfarin:** decreased anticoagulating effect
Hawthorn	Hypertension	**Digoxin:** Increased cardiac toxicity
Kava	Decrease anxiety, promote sleep	**Alprazolam** (Xanax): Potentiates effect of both, which can lead to coma
Khat	Mood elevation, euphoria	**Penicillins:** Delayed or reduced absorption if taken at the same time; allow 2 h between each
Licorice	Indigestion, gastritis	**Spironolactone** (Aldactone): Interferes with mineralocorticoid activity
St. John's wort	Anxiety and depression	**Paroxetine** (Paxil): Potentiation contributing to cognitive impairment and slowing, nausea, weakness, fatigue

However, professionals must also recognize their scope of practice and not venture into prescribing or recommending without adequate knowledge and training in the area. Instead, they can become familiar with those in the community who provide non-Western care and develop a collaborative and consultative role with them. In this way, health care becomes truly complementary.

REFERENCES

Brzezinski, A. (1997). Melatonin in humans. *New England Journal of Medicine, 336,* 186–195.

Chavez, M. L. (1997). Saint John's Wort. *Hospital Pharmacy, 32,* 1621–1632.

Fetrow, C. W., & Avila, J. R. (1999). *Professional's handbook of complementary & alternative medicines.* Springhouse, PA: Springhouse Corp.

Murphy, J. J., Heptinstall, S., & Mitchell, J. R. (1988). Randomised, double-blind, placebo-controlled trial of feverfew in migraine prevention. *Lancet, 2,* 189–192.

Sorensen, H., & Sonne, J. (1996). A double-masked study of the effects of ginseng on cognitive function. *Current Therapy Research, 57,* 959–968.

Volz, H. P. (1997). Kava-kava extract WS-1490 versus placebo in anxiety disorders: A randomized placebo-controlled 25-week outpatient trial. *Pharmacopsychiatry, 30,* 1–5.

Wesnes, K. A., Faleni, R. A., Hefting, N. R., Hoogsteen, G., Houben, J. J., Jenkins, E., Jonkman, J. H., Leonard, J., Petrini, O., & van Lier, J. J. (1997). The cognitive, subjective, and physical effects of a ginkgo biloba/panax ginseng combination in health volunteers with neurasthenic complaints. *Psychopharmacology Bulletin, 33*(4), 677–683.

Wolkowitz, O. M. (1997). Dehydroepiandrosterone treatment of depression. *Biological Psychiatry, 41,* 311–318.

CHAPTER 10

....

Information Technology and Pharmacology

CHAPTER OUTLINE

he explosion in the volume of health-related information, combined with pressures from the government and third-party payers to increase clinical productivity, has resulted in dramatic changes in the way information is managed in health care. The challenge to maintain current knowledge in the area of pharmacotherapeutics is daunting. The number of new drugs coming on the market each year, the withdrawal of some of them almost as fast as they were introduced, and the changes in the "best" drugs for any given disease state based on the latest research are phenomenal.

Added to this volume of new information are the changes in how we use and document the use of these drugs. It has become inefficient if not impractical to maintain the typical paper-charting system. Communications between providers and between the direct provider of care and the providers of the services that support that care are also increasingly complex. Third-party payers and government regulatory bodies require "written" documentation, but documenting on paper takes an inordinate amount of time and lengthens the time between patient contact with the provider and the provision of other services. Computer networks to call up specific patient information such as the latest medication list can save time and keep track of patient medications more accurately, especially if the patient has multiple providers.

Multiple providers and changes in drug information also increase the risk for drug reactions and interactions. Technology-based systems in many hospitals and pharmacies identify these potential drug problems, and primary care providers need to develop similar systems. If such systems were integrated with clinical data that contain all the drugs and disease states for each patient, drug reactions and iatrogenic morbidity could decline markedly.

Not just the government and third-party payers want speed and accuracy in care delivery. Patients who are used to shopping in a supermarket that scans their groceries for payment and simultaneously orders new stock for the shelves find it hard to accept an expensive health care delivery system that cannot perform at a similar level. These patients also have not escaped the impact of the Internet and other health information sources such as the media, and an increasing number of patients own and regularly use a computer, either at home or at work. They have access to and use information obtained via that computer and other technology to determine the "state of the art" in health care from their viewpoint, and they demand that level of care for themselves. Of the approximately 357 million users of the World Wide Web, retrieval of health-related material now may be up to 49 percent of U.S. Internet use (Glascow et al., 1999). To provide state-of-the-art care, providers need to be able to access and use the latest health-related information. At the very least, providers need to know as much as their patients!

The prevalence of chronic illnesses is on the rise. Patients with chronic conditions are often the "experts" in the lived experience of that illness. These patients are increasingly dissatisfied by traditional care with the provider as "expert in control" and the patient as "compliant" to the "orders" of the provider. Technology that accesses information gives them a more equal footing in the patient-provider relationship. Patients want joint decision making in setting health-related goals, in diagnosing health problems, and in determining appropriate interventions to deal with these issues. Helping the patient access reliable information and accepting their input as central to the process of providing care can empower patients and increase clinicians' ability to individualize care.

On the other end of the disease spectrum, health promotion and preventive services are an important focus for primary care. The U.S. Preventive Services Task Force (1996) has developed recommendations for providers to follow, and the Health Plan Employer Data and Information Set (HEDIS) and many government and specialty organizations have generated guidelines. With shorter patient-provider interactions and increased demand for evidence-based care according to outcome criteria, the health care provider needs ready access to these recommendations and guidelines. Technology can improve this access and even ensure timely, individualized prompts and reminders to both patients and providers that are integrated into patients' health records.

To manage their own practices and steer patients to reputable sources of consumer health information, providers also need to be knowledgeable about the advantages and disadvantages of different information systems. This chapter focuses on the use of technology, especially computers and the Internet, both in obtaining pharmacotherapeutic knowledge and in providing care. Other forms of electronic information technology, such as the telephone and fax, are more familiar tools. They are important, but they are discussed minimally here because providers already use them regularly.

Although specific computer programs and Internet sites are mentioned, and their pros and cons discussed, the authors offer no endorsement of any product or Internet site. Like any other source of drug information, each site must be evaluated for its quality and application to the needs of the nurse practitioner (NP). The criteria for evaluation of Internet sources of drug information are covered in Chapter 3.

This chapter is not a primer for computer and Internet use. To maximize the information in this chapter, the reader needs at least minimal skill in using a computer and accessing the Internet. If the terminology and directions given here do not sound familiar, the reader would do well to seek out courses or books to acquire that knowledge and then return to read this chapter. Recent books include *Internet for Physicians* (1999) and *Nurse's Guide to the Internet* (1998). One Website that teaches Internet use is *www.ohsu.edu/son/ed-tools;* although not specifically a health-related site, *http://library.berkeley. edu/help/search.html* has instructions for searching online and using Internet directories. Professional organizations, workshops, and medical and public libraries are other sources of information about computers and how to use them. Journals such as *Computers in Nursing, MD Computing,* and *Journal of the American Medical Informatics Association* are other sources of information about computers and information systems.

The Computer

Desktop personal computers, laptops, and handheld digital devices are proliferating rapidly in both personal and professional settings. Patients and providers are increasingly using computers to obtain information, manage information, or do a host of other activities such as word processing. Children are introduced to computers in elementary school and learn to access information and use computer applications in their schoolwork. Each succeeding generation is likely to be more comfortable than the former one. Even older adults are logging on and using the Internet to obtain health information and maintain contact with their families and their health care providers. Senior citizens even have a national organization, Senior Net, to teach their peers about computers (Glascow et al., 1999) Homebound patients may find the Internet an important way to contact their provider and a source of health-related information, support, and social contact.

A number of factors are driving the increased use of computers and computer networks in practice. Computer technology has become both more user-friendly and less expensive. The ability to link computers together to form networks can provide increased access to fellow providers and other information resources. With computer linkage, one command can result in information transfer to multiple services for patients and providers, increasing the efficiency of health care delivery. The computer as the tool to access the Internet and other online information sources is a major factor. Even if not connected to the Internet, the computer may serve as a source of information for patients and providers through CD-ROM and interactive educational materials.

Computers and computer systems are increasingly an integral part of prescribing and monitoring drug therapy Although they can increase the speed and safety with which drugs are prescribed and delivered to patients, their use has both advantages and disadvantages. Like any resource, there are trade-offs.

Use of Computer Technology to Obtain Information

Many forms of information technology, including databases, CD-ROM, and computer-assisted instruction, are computer-based. Use of computer technology to obtain information has both advantages and disadvantages that must be weighed in choosing to use the technology and in choosing which technology to use (Table 10–1).

From the Patient's View

From the patient's standpoint, the use of computers to obtain information has several advantages. Computers are *convenient* for accessing reliable health care information on demand from home or workplace at any time during the day. This information can be *individualized* to the specific needs or characteristics of the individual patient or group. For example, educational simulators and computerized diabetes self-management education modules facilitate teaching the program recommended by the American Diabetes Association (Lehman, 1998; Tomky, 1999). This education is accurate, reliable, and convenient and can be individualized. In addition, the educational simulator (Lehman, 1998) offers a method of teaching patients with type 1 diabetes how to modify their therapy based on self-monitored blood glucose data; they can experiment with various therapeutic options without the personal risks of hypoglycemia. *Distance learning* is possible in isolated rural communities and for patients with disabilities who cannot readily leave their homes. Chat groups can provide *emotional support* without the cost, inconvenience, and transportation and scheduling challenges associated with traditional group participation. Computers provide *anonymity and perceived objectivity* when patients are disclosing sensitive in-

Table 10–1. Advantages and Disadvantages of Computers as Information Sources

	Advantages	Disadvantages
From the patient's view	• Convenience of access to information on demand • Ability to individualize the information search • Access at distant sites, in rural areas, and to patients with mobility issues • Provision of emotional support, especially from peers • Anonymity and perceived objectivity of information	• Cost, especially of initial investment • Potential for misinformation • Confidentiality risks • Lack of access to the technology • Lack of access to information on how to use the technology
From the provider's view	• Convenience of access to information on demand • Access to highly skilled experts • Access at distant sites and in rural areas • Access to evidence-based guidelines and recommendations	• Cost, especially of initial investment • Compatibility between systems • Frequent system updates required • Patient confidentiality risks • Time needed to learn to use vs. time it saves

formation. Taken together, these factors increase patients' feelings of *personal control.*

The disadvantages of computers include *cost* (especially the initial investment), the *complexity* of some applications, *confidentiality* risks, and the *potential for misinformation* without an expert to filter or validate the data. Misinformation can result in inappropriate treatment, delay necessary health care, and damage people's trust in their health care providers and prescribed treatments. Within a few hours, the Federal Trade Commission, for example, found more than 400 Websites and Usenet news groups that contained false or deceptive advertising claims for products or services for six diseases (Robinson et al., 1998). Many interactive health communication applications do not have consistent standards of evaluation that enable users to compare or assess data for accuracy and reliability. The Scientific Panel on Interactive Communication and Health has proposed the Evaluation Reporting Template for Interactive Health Communication Applications (Robinson et al., 1998). Table 10–2 summarizes the items in the template. This template has yet to be widely disseminated and used. The Health on the Net (HON) Foundation, based in Geneva, has developed a code of conduct for medical and health Websites that addresses many of the same issues; it is discussed in the Internet section. To ad-

dress these issues, the cooperation of providers, patients, and the developers of technology is critical.

From the Provider's View

The advantages for the provider are similar. Computers provide *convenient* access to information on demand, including access to input and advice from *highly skilled experts* in pharmacy and health care for less experienced providers and for those in *remote locations.* Computers can also provide access to *evidence-based care guidelines* to facilitate choosing the "best" drug or the most appropriate intervention for each patient.

The disadvantages include the *cost* of the initial equipment, the rapid changes in technology that require frequent system *updates,* and the *time* required to learn to use it against the time that its use can save. *Compatibility* between systems, so that information in one system may not be easily shared with another system, can also be a problem.

From Both Points of View

For both obtaining information and providing care, another concern is *lack of access* to the technology, with a gap between more and less affluent users. Glascow et al.

Table 10–2. Evaluation Reporting Template for Interactive Health Communications Applications

Description of application	1. Title of product or application 2. Name(s) of developers with their relevant qualifications 3. Contact(s) for additional information 4. Funding sources for development 5. Category of application (e.g., health information, clinical decision support, risk assessment) 6. What the application is intended to do and for what target audience 7. Technical and resource requirements 8. How confidentiality or anonymity will be protected 9. Who will be able to access and use the information
Formative and process evaluation	1. Processes and information source(s) to ensure validity of content 2. Citation of these sources within the document 3. Methods of instruction and/or communication used 4. Media formats used 5. Reading level or understandability tested? 6. Length of time to train beginner to use 7. How application was beta tested or debugged
Outcome evaluation	1. How much did users like the application? 2. How useful did the users find it? 3. Did it increase their knowledge; change their behavior, beliefs, or attitudes? 4. Are changes seen in morbidity or mortality, cost or resources allocation?
Evaluators	1. Name(s) and contact information for evaluator(s) who determined the above 2. Do they have any financial interest in the application they evaluated? 3. Funding sources for the evaluation 4. Copy of evaluation report available on request

(1999) discuss this "socioeconomic paradox": The current users of computer technology are typically educated and affluent, whereas the greatest potential for technology may lie in extending high-quality services to underserved and disenfranchised populations, those traditionally advocated for by nurse practitioners. Community outreach efforts are needed to ensure that computers and other information technologies narrow rather than widen disparities between the haves and the have-nots. The 1996 Telecommunications Act put Internet capabilities in more accessible places: "Congress was especially concerned that health care providers, schools, and libraries have early access to the benefit of advanced telecommunications services" (Jones, 1997, p. 405). Unfortunately, only health care providers in rural areas qualify for universal service support, and that is to subsidize the cost of services compared with urban rates.

On June 22, 1998, the Health Care Financing Administration (HCFA) published a regulation in the *Federal Register* (63 [119]), "Payment for Teleconsultations in Rural Health Professional Shortage Areas (HPSA)," that would pay for professional consultation by providers, including NPs, via interactive telecommunications for Medicare beneficiaries residing in a rural

HPSA. Once again, however, the technology is limited to rural areas.

Sources of Information

DATABASES. Databases are collections of documents that can be accessed by a computer system. Databases can be on a computer's hard drive or CD-ROM, part of a computer network, or available via the Internet. There are several types of databases. Bibliographic databases contain references to literature (Hersh, 1996). Databases increasingly include full text; the searcher can not only find the citation but also has the option of downloading the full-text of the document, including graphs and photographs. These documents may or may not be free. The National Library of Medicine listing is available at *www. ncbi.nlm. nih.gov/PubMed/fulltext.html.* Documents from this database are usually free.

Several databases are specifically related to pharmacotherapeutics, including eight major databases using the National Drug Code (NDC). Table 10–3 lists these databases. The NDC system was created by the Food and Drug Administration and is currently widely used in provider drug order entry and clinical patient profiling.

Table 10–3. National Drug Code Database

Database Name	Organization	Description
NDC Directory	Food and Drug Administration, Rockville, MD	Entire current prescription drugs and partial OTC drugs.
Rebate Drug Product Data	Health Care Financing Administration, Baltimore	Entire formulary of drugs that are used in Medicaid and Medicare drug rebate programs. Includes prescription and OTC drugs.
Veterans Affairs Drug File	Department of Veterans Affairs, Washington, DC	Entire formulary of drug products used in VA hospitals.
Redbook	Medical Economics Data, Inc., Montvale, NJ	Entire drug products from major drug companies. Includes all active and obsolete prescription and OTC drugs.
National Drug Data File	Hearst Corporation, First Data Bank, San Bruno, CA	Entire drug products from major drug companies. Includes all active and obsolete prescription and OTC drugs.
Medi-Span Electronic Drug File	Medi-Span Inc., Indianapolis	Entire drug products from major drug companies. Includes all active and obsolete prescription and OTC drugs.
Bergen, Durr-Fillauer Drug File	Bergen Brunswig, Durr-Fillauer Medical Inc., Montgomery, AL	Entire drug products from major drug companies in a regional wholesaler. Includes all active prescription and OTC drugs.
Medicaid Drug File	Alabama Medicaid Agency, Montgomery, AL	Entire drug products in Medicaid drug formulary. Includes all active prescription and OTC drugs.

Unfortunately, the product codes and package size codes are not standardized, so any two labelers may use completely different codes to indicate the same generic drug or the same package size. With the development of computerized information systems, the NDC database system has become increasingly important for accessing specific drug information. There is no gold standard NDC information database in the market, and Guo et al. (1998) call for a public central repository of a complete standard NDC reference for the health care industry in order to improve the comparability, accessibility, and quality of drug information.

One advantage of databases is the amount of information available. Two search systems, Internet Grateful Med and PubMed, can be used to search through the National Library of Medicine (NLM) site. MEDLINE, which is free, can also be accessed through the NLM site. Databases can contain best evidence for clinical practice, for example, Cochrane Collaboration (*http://hiru.mcmaster. ca/COCHRANE/*) or the Agency for Health Care Policy and Research clinical practice guidelines (*http://www. guidelines.gov*). It is also possible to do a quick, focused search. Graber, Bergus, and York (1999) report, however, that most medicine-specific search engines on the Web, compared with general search engines, fare poorly in answering clinical questions. In a study reported in the *Journal of Family Practice,* the search engines MD Consult, Excite, HotBot, and Hardin MD found the greatest number of answers to 10 specific clinically based questions. (Search engines are discussed again in the Internet section.) A practitioner can also conduct a search and find information to read later by saving the search results on a disk or hard drive or can conduct more thorough searches for research or an in-depth review of a topic of interest. There are also services that search for information for the provider or send the provider information about a particular topic on a regularly scheduled basis.

Databases are indexed to "represent the content of individual documents for searchers to retrieve them, and . . . to organize the content so that computer programs may determine rapidly which documents contain content about the concepts" (Hersh, 1996, p. 75). Documents can be indexed by using controlled vocabularies such as the MEDLINE system. Human indexers assign vocabulary terms, usually from a standardized list. A major problem is that the searcher may not be using the same term to search the database as the indexer used, and the searcher may therefore be unable to find the information desired. Human indexing can also be time-consuming and expensive, given the large volume of information that must be indexed to keep the database current. Human indexers, however, have an understanding of language that word indexing lacks. In word indexing, computers use a preprogrammed process to break words into root parts and match that part to the search term (Hersh, 1996).

Internet-based search engines can use word indexing, although human-indexed databases can also be searched via the Internet. The advantages of word indexing are the more natural search terms, less time, and less expense. The word-indexing program must not break down the words so far that compound words lose the meaning the searcher intends or that important meaning cues from the words' context is lost.

Databases search problems include retrieving too many documents, too few, or the wrong type of document. All three can be frustrating. Some search systems do have help or coaching components for conducting more skillful searches (Hersh, 1996). Unfortunately, searching one or more databases can be time-consuming and frustrating if the desired information is not retrieved. Search engines, whether searching a database or the Internet, retrieve only a portion of the relevant documents. Graber et al. (1999) discuss the efficiency of selected search engines for answering clinical questions. Modem and connection speeds can also determine how long retrieving the desired documents takes, especially if the searcher is downloading full-text articles with graphics or photographs. Search engines do not search limited-access databases, such as Micromedix and CINAHL, unless you have subscribed to (paid for) the service. Micromedix requires a subscription from the user for products such as Poisindex, Drugdex, Emergindex, and Aftercare Illness and Injury (Baker, Smith, & Abate, 1994), either singly or in various combinations. The OVID combination of databases, including MEDLINE, CINAHL, and Best Evidence, can also be purchased.

CD-ROM.   Various drug references are available on CD-ROM. Mercado (1997) discusses *Mosby's Complete Drug Reference: Physicians GenRX.* Another excellent CD-ROM program is *CliniSphere,* produced by Facts and Comparisons, which contains drug information that is updated monthly, patient education materials for selected drugs, a natural and herbal products section, and detailed discussion of commonly used products, including drug interactions.

A CD-ROM can be used as a database, for patient education, or for patient records. Hersh (1996, p. 62) lists the advantages of this technology, including "increased durability over magnetic disks, relatively cheap cost to reproduce, and a common file format (ISO9660) that can be read by virtually all computers." Hersh (1996) also points to another advantage, that the data on the CD-ROM can be on put on the computer itself, which enables the user to print or store on a floppy disk information retrieved in a search. CD-ROMs do not depend on a modem or online connection that can be lost and requires additional equipment. Most computer systems now sold have a CD-ROM drive as a standard feature. CD-ROMs also have the advantage of being easily portable, and the same CD-ROM can be used to put the desired information on multiple computers in a practice or health care system once the licensing fees per use are paid.

The CD-ROM also can take advantage of multimedia technology. Castalsini et al. (1998) pilot-tested a multimedia CD-ROM for diabetic education. Participants found the program easy and fun to use and reported that the program increased their knowledge about diabetes. Animated cartoons and audio were found particularly helpful. Individualization of learning, interactivity, and an interesting presentation of information were noted as advantages. Quiz sections that tested knowledge gave users immediate feedback for correct answers and positive reinforcement to increase their confidence and self-esteem. The Internet and other computer-based instruction formats can also take advantage of multimedia capability.

A disadvantage of CD-ROM is that most databases, especially those with such a large topic area as pharmacology information, require more than one CD-ROM. The disks can also become rapidly obsolete in an area with as much change as pharmacotherapeutics. It is important to purchase CD-ROM products that include regular updates to keep them current. These products usually require an annual subscription, which is often expensive, to obtain the updates.

MEDICAL BOOK SYSTEMS. Handheld computers with books on disklike inserts are called *medical book systems*. Several are available, including *Drug Facts and Comparisons*. They provide instant access to critical information that is retrieved by keyboard entry This electronic application contains thousands of abridged drug monographs that include drug actions, indications, interactions, adverse reactions, warnings, and brief patient education notes. Tables present details on dosing, dosage forms, and product identification codes. Because the printed book is definitely too large to be portable, this electronic book is wonderful in the clinical setting.

COMPUTER-ASSISTED INSTRUCTION. Computer-assisted instruction (CAI) is increasingly common as an information source. Huss, Salerno, and Huss (1991) studied the effects of CAI that was used to reinforce adult asthmatics' education and promote adherence to implementing an environmental control program. The CAI group had significantly higher adherence scores and increases between pretest and posttest scores than the control group. The CAI group was also more likely to report changes in behaviors on a self-report measure of implementing allergen-avoidance behaviors.

Krishna et al. (1997), studying CAI use in diabetic education, saw a 10 to 20 percent reduction in blood glucose. No significant difference between controls and experimental subjects on knowledge scores was noted, but 40 percent of those using CAI reported more involvement in their disease management. Another study found that the CAI users spent 39 percent more time with their physicians. Diabetes and nutrition knowledge levels did increase. Tomky's (1999) and Lehman's (1998) studies of CAI for patients with diabetes have already been mentioned.

Scores also increased in one study that used instructional computer feedback instead of right-or-wrong feedback. CAI users reported higher levels of satisfaction with their care and a more positive attitude toward their blood glucose monitoring. Patients with asthma, rheumatoid arthritis, and hypertension who were CAI users showed significant knowledge gains over controls. Clean-catch urine specimen collections were performed with fewer errors when instructions were given with CAI. Medication recall with CAI had 20 percent less total nonadherence than the control group. The authors also noted that some studies found that patients seemed more willing to confide in computers than in human interviewers, possibly because the computers were perceived as nonjudgmental or evoked less embarrassment on sensitive subjects (Krishna et al., 1997, p. 32). Across the studies, age did not affect CAI acceptance; positive results were shown in ages from children to elders. The authors point out that the benefits of CAI for those with lower literacy and education levels have not been established.

Use of Computer Technology to Deliver Care

Telephone Messages

The telephone is the oldest communications technology used to deliver care (Friedman et al., 1997). Recent innovations include automated voice messaging systems that deliver information and reminders to patients and/or obtain information from them about their health status. Friedman et al. (1997) describe a telephone-linked care (TLC) system that conducts virtual telephone visits with patients with chronic illnesses and patients who need to change health behaviors. The system also provides emotional support and information to users and has caregiver support applications as well. The calls may be initiated by the patient, the caregiver, or the system, and thus the frequency of calls and their duration vary. Reports of the calls are available to health care providers, and alerts are issued if any problems require immediate provider action. So far, the authors have evaluated patients with hypertension, medication adherence, cholesterol, and exercise. The medication adherence group improved 18 percent compared with the control group's 12 percent. The TLC groups showed decreased diastolic blood pressure. Patients reported satisfaction with the system and ease in using it, and providers found the reports generated by TLC useful. In a randomized pilot study conducted over 3 months, total cholesterol levels were lower in the TLC group (by 21.3 mg/dL) than in the control group (by 1.3 mg/dL).

In a randomized trial of an exercise program for sedentary seniors, TLC users walked more (mean 120 min per week) than nonusers (mean 40 min per week). The authors state that the system was effective with diverse age, socioeconomic, and ethnic groups.

Grymonpre and Steele (1998) describe a telephone-based medication information line (MILE) directed at older adults. An 8-year cumulative analysis of MILE found that it reduced calls to providers and possibly prevented drug reactions in users. A few of the calls (0.3%) were for severe problems that could have resulted in injury or death. Follow-up findings indicated that 90 percent of those contacted had a positive outcome from the information MILE provided.

Meneghini et al. (1998) used an electronic case manager for diabetes control. Their feasibility study found that this automated voice messaging system was an effective, cost-efficient way to help manage diabetic care, with significant reductions in hypoglycemia and improvement in other clinical indicators. Utilization of clinic services decreased by half over the year during which the study was conducted.

Electronic Medical Records and "Smart Cards"

Electronic medical records for all patients in the United States has been set as a goal, despite large potential capital outlays, because of the anticipated benefits to the public health sector, patient care, and health research (Cushman, 1997). Health care computer systems are rich with patient data, but rather than a seamless web, the data often come from a diverse group of individual computer systems. For example, word processing systems hold discharge summaries and operative reports, laboratory systems produce laboratory results, pharmacy systems organize prescription records, and radiology systems produce images and their interpretations. Consequently, even at a single patient encounter, one patient's data are scattered over multiple separate systems. If the patient has multiple providers, the number of systems may increase exponentially.

The benefits of electronic medical record (EMR) systems include unification of data from many different information sources, ready access to relevant and current patient information, portability (e.g., the information can go to the point of care), and some of the previously mentioned general benefits of electronic systems. With "smart cards," patients could carry their health information with them to appointments or when traveling. For the prescribing NP, there would be no more patients or family members trying to recall drugs, dosages, and frequencies. The EMR could be updated as changes in drugs are made, organize diverse clinical information, and eliminate filing costs, illegible notes, and lost charts. They can also improve care by detecting dangerous trends, drug interactions, and possible oversights and provide a system for outcomes management. Research, especially public health and outcomes research, could benefit by having access to a large volume of data, stripped of identifiers to protect patient anonymity, available for analysis (Cushman, 1997). National databases could be available to providers and researchers.

The World Wide Web offers most of the tools necessary to build an effective and efficient EMR. Almost every large system vendor now offers Web-based medical record systems. These systems make it possible for the provider to access current data on each patient at the time of the visit, even if the chart was last in x-ray or the laboratory or with a different provider at a different site. In some cases, systems allow the provider to check on results of laboratory tests and other patient data from home via secure access lines. With a comprehensive, Web-based system, the provider can also check the Web for relevant clinical practice guidelines or other data to make clinical decisions while the patient is still in the office.

Equally important are time-saving features. Orders and prescriptions can be generated at the computer and simultaneously printed out in the location where the order is to be carried out or the prescription filled. By the time patients reach the site where the order or prescription is to be completed, the distant site is ready for them. Orders or prescriptions generated by computer can also have prompts to remind the provider about required data to facilitate the best application of the order. These orders or prescriptions are also legible, reducing the chance of errors.

The provider can create charting macros or templates for common problems that can then be individualized for each patient. Documents can include specific reminders of areas to assess or treatments commonly done, as well as links to patient education documents that can be individualized. Finally, the EMR facilitates giving the patient an after-visit summary detailing the name of the provider seen, patient vital signs, diagnosis determined, orders or prescriptions written, patient education in language they can understand, and time and place of any follow-up visits. Some programs can translate the summary into several languages.

Like all systems, EMR has disadvantages, too. The top of the list is the time it takes to learn the system with enough proficiency to actually save time and effort. If macros and templates are to be used, they must be created, often by the providers because they determine the information they want documented and the orders or patient education they want for their patients. Providers are not always skillful in computer applications, and a common caveat among computer users is "garbage in, garbage out." Providers may need assistance from computer experts to learn the system and design their individual macros.

Macros and templates can also have an unwanted side effect. In the process of "saving time," using the macro may become more convenient than individualizing the charting. Working in a system that has extensive EMRs, the author has seen several such instances that might have been humorous if a patient's legal medical record had not been involved.

Practical issues also abound. Cost is a major issue, and the capital outlay is large (Institute of Medicine, 1994). How will the cost be borne? Will patients, providers, or the federal government be responsible for paying for the infrastructure and computer systems necessary, especially if the goal is a national EMR? In primary care, an informatics-based practice such as that described by Nordyke and Kulikowski (1998) provides an example of what is possible and some of the implications for research and clinical practitioners. For 35 years, the chronic thyroid disease clinic they describe used informatics to improve practice. Worksheets that featured flexibility, fit with the patient population, completeness, and the ability of the provider to use quick shorthand notes facilitated patient care and tracking of information. A computer report from the worksheet was immediately generated and stored for future use in research, administration, and practice. Other providers in the practice had ready access to the information when it was needed. The authors report major benefits in research and patient care and management. Other chronic disease clinics have been able to adapt the same techniques to generate their own informatics systems that fit their patient care and research needs.

Another important practical issue is determining what information multidisciplinary users of such a record would need. Can a system meet the needs and wants of multiple users and enable multiple providers to access the same patient record simultaneously and enter data into it? The latter is most problematic in areas such as urgency care and emergency departments. Moran et al. (1994) describe creating such a system to facilitate care of primary care patients in a particular area. The problem addressed was fragmentation of care among multiple providers and agencies for patients with chronic illness. Data included patient functional status, mental status, caregiver and home information, and information about the community health and social services the patient received. Standardized instruments with known reliability and validity, such as the Mini-Mental Status Exam and Center for Epidemiologic Studies Depression Scale, were used whenever possible.

For maximum utility of an EMR system purchased for a practice setting, products must be Web-enabled, use standard coding systems, and communicate with other computer systems via broadly accepted protocols (McDonald et al., 1998).

Ethical and legal issues must be considered as well. Crucial ethical issues are patient privacy and confidentiality and informed consent. Current computer security systems in health care are rarely adequate to ensure privacy and confidentiality of patients' health information, and in some incidents sensitive information has been made pub-

lic (Cushman, 1997). Adequate security systems must be developed or purchased for the information system, and security procedures must be followed consistently to protect patient privacy and the confidentiality of their health information. Some of those procedures can be time-consuming. For example, logging off each time a practitioner steps away from the computer and then logging back on to use the computer again when the next patient is in the examination room takes time but helps keep those with unauthorized access out of the patient record. Such steps may actually make electronic records more secure than paper.

A proposed use for a nationally standardized EMR is the creation of national databases for monitoring public health, tracking trends and outcomes, assessing the efficacy of interventions, and providing an incredibly rich data source for research. Ensuring anonymity and limiting access to the database would be difficult, however. The issue of patient consent also arises. Would patients have to go through an informed consent procedure each time they went to a provider's office? What data would be collected and on whom? How would the data be used? Health research has been used in very unethical ways, and some ethnic or racial groups justifiably view such research with mistrust. The Tuskegee syphilis study is just one example of how the poor or those belonging to a specific racial group can be exploited by health research. Some of these groups do not participate in research at representative rates, and data on them are lacking. A national database could capture this missing information but only if they agree to participate. Because the data would theoretically be stripped of identifying information, does anyone have the right to refuse? Who owns the health care data? Who has access to it? Who benefits from it?

Legal issues are related to some of the ethical concerns. Ownership of health information is a critical question from a legal standpoint. Does the health care provider who generates the data own it? Do the patients own it because the information is about them? Does the health care institution or insurer own the data? What about the government? Who is responsible for maintaining the data—the patient, the provider or the health system? Usually, the owner gets to specify how the information is used, but many individuals and groups can claim ownership of the data. The advantage of portability of the data and easier access to an electronic record is a double-edged sword.

All of these ethical and legal issues relate to the microsystem of the provider's office and the macrosystem of a potential national EMR. In addition, there are comparability and compatibility issues. For an EMR to be put into use, standards and cross-platform compatibility are necessary. In short, providers need to be entering similar data, using the same language, into a computer system that can "talk" with other computer systems. Standardized taxonomies and classification systems are critical for such a system to function. Efforts are currently under way to develop standardized language, classification systems, and taxonomies. How the implementation of nursing informatics on a wide scale will affect nursing education, practice, and research is currently unknown. The questions outlined here are only a brief overview of issues that must be addressed before the full benefits of an EMR can be realized and some of the disadvantages of such a system can be prevented or mitigated.

Computerized Drug Systems

Computerized drug systems can link the prescriber directly to the pharmacist so that the prescription may be filled more expediently and the prescription is not misplaced. They also reduce the risk for misinterpretation of the prescription because of misspelling or illegible handwriting.

Drug alerts can also be programmed into the computer to reduce the risk of allergic reactions, drug interactions, and inappropriate dosing. This feature is especially important for older adults, who are often on many different medications and may have multiple providers. Some programs include cost variables in choosing among drug alternatives and links to national guidelines that suggest the latest research findings for drug therapy in a particular disease state (Glascow et al., 1999, p. 467).

Prompting systems can integrate information on risk, morbidity, medication use, laboratory data, and needed preventive services for each patient. As a time-saver for obtaining patient information, handheld or touch-screen computers in waiting rooms can be used to collect patients' history information, which can be uploaded immediately into their records.

The system can also be programmed with prompts so that when a particular drug is ordered, a prompt appears on the screen to allow the provider the option of automatically ordering the recommended treatment or a related drug. A randomized trial of such a system detected significant differences in the use of corollary orders between physicians who received such computer prompts and those who did not. The system was set up to allow physicians to decide which order prompts would be used and which would not (Overhage et al., 1997). Errors of omission as well as errors of commission can be detected. For example, the pharmacy where a patient fills prescriptions can keep track of medications the patient is taking and detect allergies or a drug prescribed by one provider that could interact with a drug prescribed by another.

The Internet

The Internet and its most successful application, the World Wide Web, have penetrated into the homes of pa-

tients and providers, schools, and workplaces at a more rapid rate than almost any other technology, including television and videocassette recorders. Although accurate estimates of Internet use are difficult to obtain, more than 9 million users are online daily with 60 million Internet users in the United States and Canada alone (Izenberg & Lieberman, 1998). Estimates are that anywhere from 25 to 49 percent (Glascow et al., 1999) of Internet use is related to health information and that there are approximately 10,000 health-related sites. That represents a significant population already using the Internet as a source of health information. Before the advent of Internet Grateful Med, the National Library of Medicine (NLM) conducted a user survey that found that approximately 15 percent of users were lay consumers (journalists, patients, or students) rather than health professionals (Wood, Wallingford, & Siegel, 1997). When free Web access via Internet Grateful Med or PubMed was introduced in June 1997, usage jumped tenfold to a rate of 75 million searches annually (Lindberg & Humphreys, 1998). Efforts to link lay consumers to online databases and other information resources are already occurring (Kantz et al., 1998; Tarby & Hogan, 1997). These figures for only one type of technology demonstrate that people are searching for health information with information technology and doing it independently of the formal health care system. The fact that consumers are searching for health information so often may indicate that they are empowered; it may indicate that they are not receiving the type, quality, or quantity of information they need; or other unknown factors may be at work.

The World Wide Web uses text, animation, sound, and graphics via a hypertext transfer protocol. Thus, World Wide Web sites are *http://www,* followed by the remainder of the site address. This makes up the uniform resource locator (URL). Telnet allows keyboard-shortcut commands to access and use another computer remotely. A browser is the software on a computer that allows the user to view the Internet.

New applications of Internet technology that are useful for nurse practitioners, including both care delivery and information-based applications, are occurring almost daily. Computer-based medical information systems, including patient data, ordering of therapies, referral mechanisms, and documentation of patient-provider interactions, are being tied to the Internet so that providers can access these data from sites other than the hospital or clinic. By using a modem and a telephone, patients can have a disease process and the therapies to treat it monitored on the Internet. Biomedical information and research reports are being distributed through the Internet. Drug companies have found the Web to be an inexpensive and useful way to distribute information on new drugs. It is more readily available to providers and less intrusive than the "drug rep," who must travel to providers' offices and try to fit into their busy schedules. Martin

(1998) proposes that the most practical method of drug information dissemination is electronically via the Internet. The Food and Drug Administration Center for Drug Evaluation and Review (CDER) is currently moving ahead with making 8.5- × 11-inch, 12-point versions of approved drug labeling available on the Internet to all CDER reviewers. If this information were available to all providers, it would (1) enable instant access to the latest prescribing information, (2) ensure that all referenced labeling is the most current, (3) virtually eliminate product misbranding due to package insert errors, (4) save the pharmaceutical industry the significant cost of producing package inserts, and (5) allow products to reach the market almost immediately upon regulatory approval.

Drug information sources are also accessed by patients, who then ask their providers about the new drug. E-mail, chat rooms, and "listservs" offer networking and consultation opportunities among NPs, between NPs and other providers, and between NPs and their patients. These opportunities are especially important for NPs in rural settings or small towns, where access to major medical center libraries is limited. Major medical centers are also going online to providers with services such as remote access to library resources and consultation.

Despite the great amount of information available via the Internet, like all resources, it has both advantages and disadvantages. By recognizing these strengths and drawbacks, providers can use this resource judiciously to improve the care they give.

Use of the Internet to Obtain Information about Pharmacotherapeutics

The volume of information on drugs and prevention or treatment of disease with drugs is large, and it changes almost daily. Books provide data that are, at best, 2 years old. Martin (1998) states that third-party publications can be as much as a year out of date for new products. Company-produced materials are more current but also may contain prescribing information that has been changed since they were printed. He laments that, even with a streamlined process for generating package inserts for new products, the best-case time frame is several weeks to print a package insert. Drug companies also have a "use up and replace" policy for minor labeling changes. Journals provide more up-to-date information, but the cost and time required to read widely in the medical literature are prohibitive, especially for providers in rural settings. Although some of the information available in books and journals will never be available on the Internet, using the Internet can help the provider overcome some of the problems of accessing extensive up-to-date information about drugs. The provider who develops Internet searching skills can find this information quickly when it is needed, often while the patient is still in the ex-amining room. This speed improves quality of care and may sometimes eliminate the need for a return visit.

Searching

As mentioned earlier, searching can be frustrating and time-consuming unless the provider knows how to search effectively. Keys to effectiveness and efficiency include the following:

1. Using the fastest modem and connection possible. This makes connecting with information faster and avoids lengthy delays in downloading information, especially if it has multimedia components such as graphics.
2. Deciding what you need to know, how much time you have to search, and where you want to go to find it, ahead of time if possible.
3. Practicing searching during less hurried times.
4. Trying out different search engines. Some, such as *hotbot.com, dogpile.com,* or *metacrawler.com,* search multiple engines. Other search engines are *lycos.com, excite.com, infoseek.com,* and *altavista.com.* Graber et al. (1999) recommend MDConsult.com for clinical questions. This familiarity allows the provider to determine which sites tend to return which kinds of information. Trying out advanced search features, such as limitations to a particular language, site type, or time frame, can shorten the time it takes to focus a search and obtain only the relevant information.
5. Bookmarking "favorite places" facilitates faster acquisition of useful sites and organizes information.

Accessing the Internet can also enable the provider to evaluate some of the material about drugs and drug therapies that patients are reading. Evaluating the information for accuracy and reliability is essential to answering patients' questions and directing them to reliable sites for obtaining future information. Health care providers have lamented the lack of patient involvement in their own care. With the advent of the Internet, that involvement is increasing. More patients are seeking out information about their drugs and their diseases and coming to the provider's office with questions and suggestions. Providers need to be ready to encourage appropriate patient-centered decision making. This includes helping them search for and find reliable information. To highlight reliable content, health science libraries and other organizations are producing *directories* of Internet-accessible health information sites from sources they consider dependable and useful. Examples of such directories include HealthWeb (*http://healthweb.org*) and New York Online Access to Health (*http://www.noah.cuny.edu*). Healthfinder (*http://www.healthfinder.gov*) also is a site for highly filtered information for consumers. These sites should be reviewed to increase the likelihood of accurate, reliable data.

The Health on the Net (HON) Foundation, based in

Table 10–4. Health on the Net: Statement of Principles

- Information must come from medically/health trained professionals or state that it does not.
- The information is supplemental to the patient-provider relationship.
- Confidentiality of data related to individual patients and visitors to the site is respected.
- Wherever possible, source of the information is supported by clear references and HTML links to the data. The date the site was last updated is displayed.
- Balanced evidence—pro and con statements—is provided.
- Information is provided in the clearest possible manner and the Webmaster displays his or her e-mail address throughout the site.
- Support for any advice or data given (e.g., financial, commercial) is identified.
- If advertising is a source of funding, it is clearly stated. Advertising is presented in a manner and context so that the viewer can clearly differentiate it from the original material created by the operator of the site.

Geneva, has developed a code of conduct for medical and health Websites. Sites that subscribe to this code agree to eight principles (Table 10–4).

Any blatant violation of these principles on a Website displaying the HON Code logo will result in a request for appropriate modifications to the site. If the modifications are not made in a timely manner, the logo is withdrawn from the site. Although the foundation does not suggest using the HON Code logo as a rating service, it is valuable in determining certain data about the reliability and potential biases of a site.

Types of Sites

A variety of Websites are available:

1. *.gov* sites: government sites
2. *.com* sites: commercial sites
3. *.edu* sites: school/education sites
4. *.org* sites: nonprofit organization sites
5. *.net* sites: network infrastructure sites
6. *.mil* sites: military sites

These are all United States or Canadian site domain names. Other countries such as the United Kingdom (*.uk*), Australia (*.au*), Israel (*.il*), and Moldova (*.md*) have their own suffixes. Table 10–5 provides general information on different types of sites, including the type of information they provide, the reliability of their information, who maintains the site, if it has links to other related sites, and if there are any charges or fees for using the site.

Table 10–6 describes selected Internet-accessible drug-related sites. It is certainly not an exhaustive list, but the goal is to provide information on some sites with

Table 10–5. Types of Internet Sites

Site Type	Type of Information	Reliability	Who Maintains	Links to Other Sites	Charges or Fees for Use
.gov	Government reports/ information available to the public.	Excellent	Federal, state, local governments	Available on many pages	Almost always free.
.com	Information from for-profit organizations and those selling products or services. Some patient-support groups also use *.com* sites or *.net* sites.	Variable	Variable, sometimes by individuals who are selling a product or service	Available on many pages	Charges for services or products. Some things may be free.
.edu	Information from educational institutions, including current research, online or other educational offerings.	Excellent	Educational institution	Available on many pages	Information is usually free unless associated with a course.
.org	Information from not-for-profit organizations.	Very good to excellent	Not-for-profit organization	Available on many pages	Some is free but not always.

Table 10–6. Selected Drug-Related Internet Sites

Site	Address	Comments
.gov sites		
Agency for Health Care Policy and Research	www.ahcpr.gov	Access to AHCPR clinical guidelines, including those that have drug treatment protocols. Information is as current as latest guidelines, but some guidelines are several years old, and there are a limited number of guidelines. Maintained by AHCPR. No charges or fees.
Centers for Disease Control and Prevention	www.cdc.gov/travel/html	Current CDC recommendations for screening and treatment of communicable disease and immunizations for travel. Updated frequently with new guidelines, often before they appear in written publications. Maintained by CDC. No charges or fees.
Food and Drug Administration	www.fda.gov/	Access to information about drugs, foods, and devices regulated by FDA.
	www.fda.gov/medbull/contents.html	Medical bulletin with information on drugs, foods, and devices and the MedWatch program.
National Institutes of Health	www.nih.gov	NIH guidelines for treatment of specific diseases, including drug therapies for these diseases. Current research on drugs and drug therapies. Site has search engine to help locate information. Each institute has a separate address that includes the NIH link. Some of these documents require an Adobe Acrobat Reader to print and read. The reader is available via free download from most large servers. Updated frequently. No charges or fees. Highly recommended site.
	www.nih.gov/database/alerts/clinical_alerts.html	Clinical alerts provide latest results of clinical trials on a variety of therapies, including drugs. Includes information on upcoming information releases, making it extremely current. Links to other sites. Maintained by NIH. No charges or fees. Highly recommended site.
	www.nlm.nih.gov	Access to data from National Library of Medicine. Provides access to premier databases and search engines, including MEDLINE, that can be searched at no cost. Excellent site.
.com sites		
American Academy of Neurology	www.aan.com/	Patient and provider information on neurological diseases, with links to other sites and Internet search engine. Includes data on drug therapies. Maintained by AAN. Cocharges or fees. Excellent site.
Drug Info Net	www.druginfonet.com/	Patient- and provider-oriented information. Information comes from "medically/health trained professionals" unless otherwise stated. Has search engine and links to .gov, .org, and drug manufacturer sites. Frequent updates. Subscribes to HON code. Excellent site.
Internet Mental Health	www.mentalhealth.com/	Primary care provider–and patient-oriented information regarding 52 of the most common psychiatric disorders, with guidelines for treatment and diagnosis. Comprehensive information on 65 of the most frequently used psychiatric drugs. Includes both American and European information. Extensive links to other mental health–related Internet sites. Highly recommended site.
Medicinenet	http://medicinenet.com/	Patient- and provider-oriented information regarding drugs, side effects, and related material. Drugs listed in alphabetical order by brand and generic name. Listing of

Continued on next page

Table 10–6. Selected Drug-Related Internet Sites (*continued*)

Site	Address	Comments
		clinical trials and poison control centers. Source is network of physician educators. Links to other sites. Adding chat feature. Limited depth of information. No charges or fees.
MDConsult	*www.MDConsult.com*	Reliable, comprehensive medical information service. Integrated collection of trusted resources: 35 medical texts, 48 medical journals, and more than 600 peer-reviewed clinical practice guidelines searched. Simplifies searches to answer clinically based questions quickly. Uses common terms, so no need to learn search language. Has 2500 patient education handouts that can be individualized with practitioners' own special instructions. Regularly updated prescribing information on more than 300,000 drugs. Has fee for use, but allows 10-day free trial before subscribing.
RXList: The Internet Drug Index	*www.rxlist.com/*	Full package-insert information for more than 4000 prescription products and simplified listing for OTC drugs. Can be searched by entering brand or generic names or therapeutic category. Also can search by imprint codes, important to identification of generic drugs. Information similar to PDR. Checked by PharmD who works for major pharmaceutical distributor. Lists top 200 prescribed drugs. No charges or fees.
Pharmaceutical Information Network	*http://pharminfo.com*	Drug information available by brand and generic names, with limited information at the site itself. Has search engine and links to other sites with more detailed information. Has received Internet awards. Latest information on this site was almost 1 year old. Supported by advertising.
.edu sites HIV Insite Home Page	*http://hivinsite.ucsf.edu/*	Up-to-date research findings and clinical information regarding effectiveness of treatment strategies, risk analysis, and prognoses. Latest treatment protocols and guidelines. Source is University of California San Francisco AIDS Research Institute, University of California San Francisco AIDS project at San Francisco General Hospital, and the Center for AIDS Prevention Studies. Links to other sites. Excellent site.
Oncolink: University of Pennsylvania	*http://cancer.med.upenn.edu*	Disease-specific therapies including drug therapies. Clinical trials in progress and results of completed trials.
Oregon Health Science University Cliniweb	*www.ohsu.edu/cliniweb/wwwvl*	Includes pharmacy site with multiple links to other Web sites. Up-to-date information on drug therapy. Has disease-specific and drug-specific search engines. Source is Oregon Health Science University. Originally designed to provide access to the expertise available on that campus for providers in rural areas. No charges or fees. Excellent site.
Virtual Pharmacy Center	*www.sci.lib.uci.edu/~martindale/ Pharmacy.html*	According to Korn, this site provides a "listing of sites that is second to none." "Links to sites concerning virtually every conceivable aspect regarding pharmacy and pharmacology." Links major drug databases and drugs currently in development. Source is University of California—Irvine. Not easy to access.

Continued on next page

Table 10–6. Selected Drug-Related Internet Sites (*continued*)

Site	Address	Comments
.org sites American Academy of Allergy, Asthma and Immunology	*www.aaaai.org*	Patient- and provider-oriented information on allergic disorders, asthma, and immunologic disorders, including drug therapies. Includes frequently asked questions (FAQ). Sponsored by unrestricted grant from Schering/Key Pharmaceuticals.
American Cancer Society	*www.cancer.org*	Information on all aspects of cancer, with links to other sites. Cancer treatment guidelines, including drug therapies. Patient and family information, including alternative treatments. Highly recommended site for cancer information.
American Heart Association	*www.amhrt.org/*	One of the most comprehensive reference sources on Internet. Patient- and provider-oriented information, including prevention and treatment protocols. Visit home page to see all that is available. Excellent site.
United States Pharmacopeia	*www.usp.org*	Different subsites for health care providers, pharmaceutical manufacturers, patients, and distributors of book form of USPDI. Information on drugs and botanicals, anonymous medication error reporting (MER) program (MedMARx), and drug products problem reporting (DPPR) program. Has search engine and links to many other sites. Data on current MedWatch alerts. Updated frequently. Subscribes to HON code. Highly recommended site.
Listservs Maelstrom	*Listserv@maelstrom.etjohns.edu*	Has a link to an online catalog of all public listservs. Few are drug-related, but some interesting sites include CHILD-PHARM for professionals interested in child and adolescent psychopharmacolgy; CIMH with discussions of the use of computers in mental health; PROZAC, a discussion group on the use of this drug, and TELEHEALTH, a professional forum for all aspects of telehealth, which had 476 subscribers in the fall of 1999. Some of these listservs are free, but many require subscription.

Many of these sites are reviewed by Ken Korn in the *Journal of the American Academy of Nurse Practitioners*. Only the drug-related information at each site is discussed. Other information may be available at each site.

information across specialty and disease processes and some that provide entry information with links to other sites. The articles by Korn cited in the references give other sites that he has reviewed and finds helpful for specific disease states.

The general information presented previously about specific types of sites applies in this table and is not repeated. Where it is possible to determine, each site's content, reliability, frequency of update, links to other sites, charges or fees, advertising support, and "owner or operator" are discussed. Of interest, some Internet sites "hide" the identity of the owner or operator of the site behind site-specific names. In these cases, it is not possible to determine if the site is sponsored by a drug company or other organization or business that might have

a vested interest in slanting the data in the site. Sites that claim to subscribe to the HON code have this information stated.

Listservs

Listservs automatically deliver e-mail directly to a subscriber's e-mail account. Listservs have abbreviations such as *.majordomo, .listserv,* or *.listproc* in the URL. They are either one-way listservs, in which the editor or person who controls the list is the one who posts to members, or two-way listservs, in which members can communicate with each other. Listservs are often used for discussion groups and as a teaching strategy for courses, such as those provided by universities. NP groups have formed listservs for discussion of clinical problems.

News Groups

News groups also post sites on the Web. They are unmoderated forums for discussion. Although they may provide useful information, they must be used cautiously because material presented is not routinely monitored for accuracy except by those involved in the group. News groups differ from listservs in that the news group site has to be visited periodically to see new postings. Information is not automatically delivered.

Resources

Even the most skillful users of information technology need assistance from time to time. There are two excellent resources for that assistance related to nursing and pharmacotherapeutics information.

Informaticists

Informaticists are experts in organizing and synthesizing information, as well as in using or creating systems to make information as accessible and comprehensible as possible. Nursing informatics draws on nursing, informatics, and computer science to manage and process information of interest to nursing. This is an emerging science in nursing, but more educational programs are offering preparation in informatics. As information becomes both more plentiful and complex and as evidence-based practice evolves, NPs need to be more sophisticated users of information and information technologies. Knowledge and experience are related to the quality of assessment, diagnosis or clinical inference, and planning of care. Information technology can provide access to a variety of information resources, such as knowledge bases and decision support systems, to increase the NP's level of knowledge. Structured patient assessment forms with linkages to knowledge bases have the potential to improve the quality of patient assessment and the accuracy of the diagnosis or clinical inference. NPs often deal with complex tasks in which a number of options are potentially appropriate. Model-based decision-support applications, such as decision analysis and multiattribute utility theory, can assist them and patients to analyze and compare the treatment alternatives in a systematic manner. Informaticists are an excellent resource for practice, research, and education information needs.

Technical Support

Determining what technical support is available from the technology provider or vendor, the practitioner's own system or network, and other sources such as online help or help applications within the program is important. The user needs to know ahead of time—ideally, in advance of the information technology purchase—where to find assistance and the costs and limitations of that assistance. Experiment with your computer program's tutorial and help functions before trying to use it with patients. In case of a problem, have a backup plan when using information or "telehealth" technologies. Keeping current with the latest software or system can be difficult. It is rarely necessary or cost-effective to update a system with each new version.

Like the other technologies, there are advantages and disadvantages to using the Internet as an information source. Issues such as confidentiality and privacy, the time it takes to learn and use the technology effectively and efficiently, and initial costs and upgrading are similar to those for computers.

Use of the Internet to Deliver Care

Brennan et al. (Brennan, Moore, & Smyth, 1991, 1992; Brennan & Ripich, 1994; Brennan, Ripich, & Moore, 1991) were innovators in the use of a computer system (ComputerLink) to deliver nursing care via the Internet. ComputerLink is a system with three components: an electronic encyclopedia with information tailored to the needs of the user, a decision support system that helps the user through the decision-making process, and a communications system. The communications system includes e-mail and a bulletin board for patients or caregivers to communicate with nurses or each other. The communications system operates via a free net site, and access to the site was limited for confidentiality reasons.

The system has been tested with caregivers of patients with Alzheimer's disease and with persons living with AIDS. Content analysis of caregiver messages showed that caregivers used the forum function to communicate information about Alzheimer's disease and available community resources, behavior management, and ways for the caregiver to cope (Brennan, Moore, & Smyth, 1991). Although individual use and use patterns varied widely, caregivers most often used ComputerLink to communicate with other caregivers or the nurses and for social support (Brennan, Moore, & Smyth, 1992). The authors found that patients were more empowered, information-seeking patterns and preferences changed, patients felt more competent in self-care, and sensitive issues could be discussed with others going through similar situations as they felt safe and supported enough in the online system to share issues (Brennan, Ripich, &

Moore, 1991). Further, Brennan, Ripich, and Moore (1991) noted that the convenience of accessing the system at patients' own time and pace had positive benefits and that patients tended to reach out more to others while using the system than in face-to-face encounters.

Fitting Information Technology into a Busy Practice

Every NP feels pressure to shorten the time spent with the patient. It is not the style or desire of nurse practitioners to reduce this time, so time cuts that can be made in other areas are welcome. Information technology can provide those time cuts if it is used appropriately. Following are some suggestions for making information technology a help rather than a hindrance:

1. Use the search strategies outlined previously.
2. Separate professional and personal searching. Personal searching, even for material that might be useful to patient care in general, must take place outside office hours.
3. Prioritize *needed information* according to how much time you have, and be systematic. It is easy to begin searching a subject and find "interesting" information that is not central to the problem at hand. Looking something up in a journal can lead you astray as well. Quickly determine whether information is relevant and needed, nice to know but not immediately relevant, or marginally relevant. Move past the last two categories unless you have a lot of time.
4. Automate computer tasks such as virus scanning and file backup.
5. Do not check e-mail frequently. Establish a routine such as a check first thing in the morning and another in midafternoon. Set aside time to deal with e-mail. Many practitioners already do this for telephone messages. Use a similar strategy with information technology.
6. Use separate accounts for personal and professional e-mail. Give out your professional e-mail address only to professional or close personal contacts, and check it more frequently than your personal account. You can also use your personal account address for trying out new sites or listservs from which you might later want to unsubscribe or to avoid spending a lot of work time going through "spam."
7. If you have a slow modem or connection or are just not interested in graphics, you can turn off the default browser setting to download graphics.
8. Set your default browser home page to a blank page or set it to your most frequently used site, such as a favorite search engine or a page of links to drug sites.

Telehealth

Telehealth is the use of telecommunications technology to provide health care services. Although *telehealth* is the broader term, some people use *telemedicine* interchangeably with *telehealth,* which involves clinical care, health care professional education and consultation, consumer health education, research, administration, and public health applications such as community health information networks (CHINs). (Puskin, Mintzer, & Wasem, 1998). Examples of telemedicine are provider consultation via phone, fax, or Internet connection and the transmission of radiologic or dermatologic information over a telecommunications system (Viegas & Dunn, 1998). Telenursing includes services such as telephone advice nursing, the fastest-growing area of nursing practice. Telehealth uses a combination of technologies from the telephone and fax to virtual visiting in real time via high-speed computer.

Management of common acute illnesses; when to get a tetanus booster, screening tests, or immunizations; reminders for monitoring tests related to drug therapy such as PT/INR tests for patients on warfarin; and when or if to refill a drug can all be handled via telehealth. Patients are becoming more knowledgeable about their health and more capable of providing accurate history and physical data. Home monitoring devices that provide reliable laboratory data are available for many tests.

The possible benefits of telehealth applications include increasing access to health care for rural and underserved populations, decreasing the isolation of rural providers (McGhee & Tangalos, 1994), and decreasing or eliminating travel time. A major advantage of telehealth is that providers and patients do not have to be in the same place at the same time for care to occur (Puskin, Mintzer, & Wasem, 1998; Stoeckle & Lorch, 1997). Patients can collect relevant health information and transmit it to the provider, who can then make decisions and relay them to the patient, all without face-to-face contact (Friedman et al., 1997; Meneghini et al., 1998). This application is especially helpful for patients and providers in rural sites, where the provider-to-patient ratio is high and where distances between the clinic and the patient are often vast.

Patients may also be able to use systems to diagnose and treat themselves at home (Stoeckle & Lorch, 1997). These trends will affect how primary care is practiced and how patients and providers relate to each other. Telehealth systems are generally well accepted by patients and providers (Allen et al., 1997; Whitten & Collins, 1998; Whitten, Mair, & Collins, 1997) and can be used to provide an array of services that better manage care (Warner, 1997). Patients learn to use a telehealth system with minimal difficulty (Mahmud & Lenz, 1995).

One example of a telehealth system in primary care uses a home monitoring system to improve outcomes for patients with congestive heart failure. For the initial 8 weeks of the year-long program, patients received weekly mailings of educational materials covering topics such as commonly used drugs. Patients were given equipment such as an electronic blood pressure cuff, scale, and pager and taught how to use them. They were contacted weekly by telephone to collect physiological data and monitor their clinical status. A 24-hour telephone number was also available to call the nurse in the event of emergent changes in health status. Providers were notified immediately by fax if there were significant changes and also received printouts of current medications, daily weight, and daily blood pressure. Patients and providers were contacted to find out what actions were taken after providers received notification of problems. There were significant declines in the number of hospital admissions from all causes as well as cardiovascular causes, and hospital stays were shorter. Patient acceptance of the intervention was high, with 82 percent reporting the program useful or very useful. The patients with New York class III or IV disease were very enthusiastic, with 88 percent rating the program as very useful. All the patients were pleased with the 24-hour access to a nurse. "More than 90 percent of patients found the educational material very useful and thought it increased their understanding of the disease, their medications, and the importance of dietary discretion" (p. 376). Increased adherence to drug taking because of the computer-generated drug reminders was reported by 80 percent of the patients. Providers found the physiological data reports helpful adjuncts in managing patient health status.

Another example used an automated telephone system to provide a variety of services to pregnant, substance-abusing women (Alemi & Stephens, 1996). The authors found minimal if any effect on patient health status, but service utilization patterns changed. Computer-generated reminder calls increased patient visits to the clinic; other computer services such as the computer bulletin board reduced clinic visits because questions could be left for the provider to call back with an answer and an appointment was unnecessary.

Recognizing the value of telehealth, the Health Resources and Services Administration (HRSA) has established an Office for Advancement of Telehealth to support telecommunications for technical assistance, training, and knowledge exchange. Later developments will also focus on delivery of patient care. The focus to date is on rural and underserved populations, but this technology does not need to be limited to that population.

There are barriers to successful implementation of telehealth, however. Legal issues such as cross-state licensure are complex and currently the subject of much discussion at the national level, with the state boards of nursing desirous of pushing ahead with multistate licensure and nursing professional organizations raising serious concerns. Some of the licensure issues include which state's practice acts should be followed if the patient is in one state and the provider in another and who is accountable for what outcomes if there is a consultant in another state and a primary care provider in the patient's home state (Kovner & Hardy Havens, 1996). For registered nurses, the nurse practice acts in most states are similar, making some of these issues less dramatic. For advanced practice nurses, this is not the case. As can be seen in the January issue each year of *Nurse Practitioner*, the scope of practice, who is able to use the title "nurse practitioner" or "advanced practice nurse" and how they are educated, and the ability to prescribe drugs and which ones are all different across states. A very real concern for NPs in states with broad scopes of practice, prescriptive authority, and autonomy is the possibility that they might lose some hard-won privileges in the push to incorporate information technology into the practice arena.

Other challenges are technological (namely, bandwidth and data transmission speed), assurance of patient confidentiality, documentation standards, and reimbursement for telehealth services (Burdick, Mahmud, & Jenkins, 1996). They have to be solved before telehealth can be widespread.

The Future in Information Technology

Clear, full-motion video images with high-fidelity audio links will permit physical assessment at a distance with less choppy motion. Imagine how this would affect a clinic nurse practitioner's practice. NPs could make some virtual "home visits" to replace some office visits, and these visits might be made from the nurse practitioner's home. Although virtual visits are not appropriate for every situation and cannot always be an adequate substitute for in-person visits, they can replace office visits for many patients. NPs could check e-mail from patients and others while still at home and address problems before coming to the office. For example, e-mail may include patients' requests for prescription refills or laboratory results or messages about a call from one of the patients to the telephone advice nurse. Once at the office, the day might include a combination of real and virtual visits at prescheduled times. Patients could have already filled out their current medical history, drug and treatment list, and presenting problem on a computer for the practitioner's review before the patient is seen, either ahead of time at home or in the office right before the visit. Patients can also swipe their "smart cards" through a reader to get information from other providers they have seen into the electronic record system. Times for appointments can be prescheduled on an Internet electronic calendar so that the nurse practitioner can download the schedule to the personal electronic calendar. The office secretary or manager who schedules the appointments can determine when the nurse practitioner has an opening without face-to-face contact with the provider.

Conclusion

This chapter provides a general overview of some information technologies that an NP may find useful in practice and a specific overview of their use in pharmacotherapeutics. Possible strengths and weaknesses are discussed to assist in determining which technology will best fit the practice's information management needs.

Caring for informed patients means relating to them in new ways, and new practice patterns become possible. More patients are becoming proactive and empowered in using information technologies. Many are interested in health promotion or self-care activities. The population is aging, and patients are more likely to have chronic conditions for which empowerment and self-care are central to disease management. The NP can play an important role as information facilitator or guide rather than as the sole or main source of health or illness-related information. Maintaining a list of Websites or having a CD-ROM library and computer at the practice site may become commonplace. Patients would be able to borrow these resources or use them in the office. Both the quality and quantity of patient education can be improved by the judicious use of information technology.

How NPs manage their time in relation to pharmacotherapeutics is changing. Information technologies can save time by catching potential problems such as drug interactions before they happen, by providing rapid access to the latest information on specific drugs and practice guidelines, and by enabling the practitioner to access the current medication record of the patients.

In the information age, particularly in health care, there is an abundance of information to sift through. Determining what is relevant and useful and what is extraneous can be challenging. The time and expense of acquiring and learning new systems or system upgrades and the potential for "information overload" are all very real. Careful selection of information technologies that "fit" the NP's practice can address these issues. It is important to stress, however, that no information technology alone can replace the judgment and skill of the NP. These technologies are intended to supplement rather than supplant the NP's knowledge and patient contact.

REFERENCES

Abbott, R. (1998). An overview of knowledge integration for innovation in health care and pharmaceuticals. *Drug Information Journal, 32,* 905–915.

Alemi, F., & Stephens, R. C. (1996). Computer services for patients: Description of systems and summary of findings. *Medical Care, 34*(10 Suppl), OS1–OS9.

Allen, A., Roman, L., Cox, R., & Cardwell, B. (1997). Home health visits using a cable television network: User satisfaction. *Journal of Telemedicine and Telecare, 2*(1), 92–94.

Baker, D., Smith, G., & Abate, M. (1994). Selected topics in drug information access and practice: An update. *Annals of Pharmacotherapy, 28*(12), 1389–1394.

Becker, L. (1997a). Handheld computers in clinical practice. *Primary Care, 9*(9), 190–192.

Becker, L. (1997b). How to manage the medical literature. *Primary Care, 9*(9), 184–185.

Becker, L. (1997c). Using your computer to keep up to date. *Primary Care, 9*(9), 186–190.

Bergeron, B. (1997a). The electronic medical record: A benefit-based analysis. *Primary Care, 9*(9), 192–193.

Bergeron, B. (1997b). Understanding the Internet and World Wide Web. *Primary Care, 9*(9), 182–184.

Biermann, J., Golladay, G., & Baker, L. (1999). Evaluation of cancer information on the Internet. *Cancer, 86*(3), 381.

Brennan, P. F., Moore, S. M., & Smyth, K. A. (1991). ComputerLink: Electronic support for the home caregiver. *Advances in Nursing Science, 13*(4), 14–27.

Brennan, P. F., Moore, S. M., & Smyth, K. A. (1992). Alzheimer's disease caregivers' uses of a computer network. *Western Journal of Nursing Research, 14*(5), 662–673.

Brennan, P. F., & Ripich, S. (1994). Use of a home-care computer network by persons with AIDS. *International Journal of Technology Assessment in Health Care, 10*(2), 258–272.

Brennan, P. F., Ripich, S., & Moore, S. M. (1991). The use of home-based computers to support persons living with AIDS/ARC. *Journal of Community Health Nursing, 8*(1), 3–14.

Burdick, A. E., Mahmud, K., & Jenkins, D. P. (1996). Telemedicine: Caring for patients across boundaries. *Ostomy/Wound Management, 42*(9), 26–37.

Buswell, L., & Kunsmand, J. (1997a). Computer links clinical trials registration and patient information. *Oncology Nurse Forum, 24*(9), 1500.

Buswell, L., & Kunsmand, J. (1997b). Computerized system streamlines chemotherapy order process. *Oncology Nurse Forum, 24*(9), 1499–1500.

Castalsini, M., Saltmarch, M., Luck, S., & Sucher, K. (1998). The development and pilot testing of a multimedia CD-ROM for diabetes education. *Diabetes Educator, 24*(3), 285–296.

Chatterton, H. (1999). Efficacy, risk, and the determination of value: Shared medical decision making in the age of information. *Journal of Family Practice, 48*(7), 505–507.

Christensen, D., Williams, B., Goldberg, H., Martin, D., Engelberg, R., & LoGerfo, J. (1997). Assessing compliance to antihypertensive medications using computer-based pharmacy records. *Medical Care, 35*(11), 1164–1170.

Cushman, R. (1997). Serious technology assessment for health care information technology. *Journal of the American Medical Informatics Association, 4*(4), 259–265.

Ferguson, T. (1997). Health online and the empowered medical consumer. *Journal on Quality Improvement, 23*(5), 251–257.

Ferrill, M. (1998). The national library of medicine on the Internet: Part I. *Drug Facts and Comparisons News* (December), 50–54.

Foisy, M., & Tseng, A. (1998). Development of an interactive computer-assisted program to manage medication therapy in HIV infected patients. *Drug Information Journal, 32,* 649–656.

Friedman, R. H., Stollerman, J. E., Mahoney, D. M., & Rozenblyum, L. (1997). The virtual visit: Using telecommunications technology to take care of patients. *Journal of the American Medical Informatics Association, 4*(6), 413–425.

Gallagher, S., & Zeind, A. (1998). Bridging patient education and care. *American Journal of Nursing, 98*(8), 16AAA–16DDD.

Glascow, R., McKay, G., Boles, S., & Vogt, T. (1999). Interactive computer technology, behavioral science and family practice. *Journal of Family Practice, 48*(9), 464–470.

Graber, M., Bergus, G., & York, C. (1999). Using the world wide web to answer clinical questions: How efficient are different methods of information retrieval? *Journal of Family Practice, 49*(7), 520–524.

Grymonpre, R. E., & Steele, J. W. (1998). The medication information line for the elderly: An 8-year cumulative analysis. *Annals of Pharmacotherapy, 32,* 743–748.

Guo, J., Diehl, M., Felkey, B., Gibson, J., & Barker, K. (1998). Comparison and analysis of the national drug code system among data information databases. *Drug Information Journal, 32,* 769–775.

Henry, S. B. (1993). Nursing informatics: State of the science. *Journal of Advanced Nursing, 22,* 1182–1192.

Henson, D. (1999). Cancer and the Internet. *Cancer, 86*(3), 373.

Hersh, W. R. (1996). *Information retrieval: A health care perspective.* New York: Springer.

Huss, K. Salerno, M., & Huss, R. W. (1991). Computer-assisted reinforcement of instruction: Effects on adherence in adult atopic asthmatics. *Research in Nursing and Health, 14,* 259–267.

Institute of Medicine (1994). *Health data in the information age: Use, disclosure and privacy.* Washington, DC: National Academy Press.

Isaksen, S., Jonassen, J., Malone, D., Billups, S., Carter, B., & Sintek C. for the IMPROVE investigators. (1999). Estimating risk factors for patients with potential drug-related problems using electronic pharmacy data. *Annals of Pharmacology, 33*(4), 406–412.

Izenberg, N., & Lieberman, D. A. (1998). The Web, communication trends and children's health, part 3: The Web and health consumers. *Clinical Pediatrics, 37,* 275–285.

Johnson, S., & Wordell, C. (1998). Internet utilization among medical information specialists in the pharmaceutical industry and academia. *Drug Information Journal, 32,* 547–554.

Jones, M. G. (1997). Telemedicine and the National Information Infrastructure: Are the realities of health care being ignored? *Journal of the American Medical Informatics Association, 4*(6), 399–412.

Kantz, B., Wandel, J., Fladger, A., Folcarelli, P., Burger, S., & Clifford, J. C. (1998). Developing patient and family education services. *Journal of Nursing Administration, 28*(2), 11–18.

Keockeritz, J., & Wood, D. (July 1998). Internet for advanced practice nurses. Presentation at the 23rd National Primary Care Nurse Practitioner Symposium, Keystone, CO.

Korn, K. (1997a). Cancer information on the Internet. *Journal of the American Academy of Nurse Practitioners, 9*(8), 385–386.

Korn, K. (1997b). Dermatology on the Internet. *Journal of the American Academy of Nurse Practitioners, 9*(10), 487–488.

Korn, K. (1997c). Health care for travelers: Internet sites of interest. *Journal of the American Academy of Nurse Practitioners, 9*(6), 277–278.

Korn, K. (1997d). Reference books for professional use of the "information superhighway." *Journal of the American Academy of Nurse Practitioners, 9*(5), 225–226.

Korn, K. (1998a). Allergy information on the Internet. *Journal of the American Academy of Nurse Practitioners, 10*(7), 321–322.

Korn, K. (1998b). Cardiac information on the Internet. *Journal of the American Academy of Nurse Practitioners, 10*(3), 127–128.

Korn, K. (1998c). Diabetes mellitus information on the Internet. *Journal of the American Academy of Nurse Practitioner, 10*(2), 61–63.

Korn, K. (1998d). HIV and AIDS information on the Internet. *Journal of the American Academy of Nurse Practitioners, 10*(4), 173–174.

Korn, K. (1998e). Mental health information on the Internet. *Journal of the American Academy of Nurse Practitioners, 10*(6), 267–268.

Korn, K. (1998f). Neurology resources on the Internet. *Journal of the American Academy of Nurse Practitioners, 10*(5), 219–220.

Korn, K. (1998g). Pharmacology resources on the Internet. *Journal of the American Academy of Nurse Practitioners, 10*(1), 29–30.

Korn, K. (1999). Hepatitis information on the Internet. *Journal of the American Academy of Nurse Practitioners, 11*(1), 21–22.

Kovner, R. & Hardy Havens, D. M. (1996). Telemedicine: Potential applications and barriers to continued expansion. *Journal of Pediatric Health Care, 10*(4), 184–186.

Krishna, S., Balas, A., Spencer, D. C., Griffin, J. Z., & Boren, S. A. (1997). Clinical trials of interactive computerized patient education: Implications for family practice. *Journal of Family Practice, 45*(1), 25–33.

Lehman, E. (1998). AIDA: A computer-based interactive educational diabetes simulator. *Diabetes Educator, 24*(3), 341–348.

Lindberg, D., & Humphreys, B. (1998). Medicine and health on the Internet: The good, the bad and the ugly. *Journal of the American Medical Association, 280*(15), 1303–1304.

Lybecker, C. (1997). A nurse explores the Internet. *American Journal of Nursing, 97*(6), 42–51.

Mahmud, K., & Lenz, J. (1995) The personal telemedicine system: A new tool for the delivery of health care. *Journal of Telemedicine and Telecare, 1*(3), 173–177.

Marousky, R. (1996). Nurses' guide to the Internet—Professional and personal benefits. *AORN Journal, 64*(3), 463–469.

Martin, I. (1998). Electronic labeling: A paperless future? *Drug Information Journal, 32*(4), 917–919.

McDonald, C., Overhage,. J., Dexter, P., Blevins, L., Meeks-Johnson, J., Suico, J., Tucker, M., & Schadow, G. (1998). Canopy computing: Using the web in clinical practice. *Journal of the American Medical Association, 280*(15), 1325–1329.

McGhee, R., & Tangalos, E. G. (1994). Delivery of health care to the underserved: Potential contributions of telecommunications technology. *Mayo Clinic Proceedings, 69,* 1131–1136.

Meneghini, L. F., Albisser, A. M., Goldberg, R. B., & Mintz, D. H. (1998). An electronic case manager for diabetes control. *Diabetes Care, 21*(4), 591–596.

Mercado, A. D. (1997). Drug reference software on CD-ROM. Part 1. *Pacing and Clinical Electrophysiology, 20,* 976–979.

Monane, M., Matathias, D., Nagle, B., & Kelly, M. (1998). Improving prescribing patterns for the elderly through an online drug utilization review intervention. *Journal of the American Medical Association, 280* (14), 1249–1252.

Moran, W. P., Messick, C., Guerette, P., Anderson, R., Bradham, D., Wofford, J. L., Velez, R., & The Community Care Coordination Network Database Group (1994). A practice-based information system for multi-disciplinary care of chronically ill patients: What information do we need? *Proceedings of the American Medical Informatics Association Annual Symposium on Computer Applications in Medical Care,* 585–589. Bethesda, MD: AMIA, Inc.

Nicole, L. (1998). *Nurse's guide to the internet.* Philadelphia: Lippincott.

Nordyke, R. A., & Kulikowski, C. A. (1998). An informatics-based chronic disease practice: Case study of a 35-year computer-based longitudinal record system. *Journal of the American Medical Informatics Association, 5,* 88–103.

Overhage, J. M., Tierney, W. M., Zhou, X., & McDonald, C. J. (1997). A randomized trial of corollary orders to prevent errors of omission. *Journal of the American Medical Association, 4*(5), 364–375.

Pucket, F. (1995). Medication-management component of a point-of-care information system. *American Journal of Health-System Pharmacists, 52,* 1305–1309.

Puskin, D. S., Mintzer, C. L., & Wasem, C. (1998). Telemedicine: Building rural systems for today and tomorrow. *www/nal.usda.gov/ric/richs/chapter.htm.*

Raw, A., & White, K. (1996). Nurses' guide to the internet: AORN online. *AORN Journal, 64*(3), 286–289.

Robinson, T., Patrick, K., End, T., & Gustafson, D., for the Science Panel on Interactive Communication and Health. (1998). An evidence-based approach to interactive health communication. *Journal of the American Medical Association, 280*(14), 1264–1269.

Sharp, N. (1998). Teleconsultation: The death of distance. *Nurse Practitioner, 23*(10), 84–88.

Shortliffe, D. (1998). Health care and the next generation Internet. *Annuals of Internal Medicine, 129*(2), 138–140.

Smith, R. (1999). *Internet for physicians.* New York: Springer-Verlag.

Stoeckle, J., & Lorch, S. (1997). Why go see the doctor? Care goes from office to home as technology divorces function from geography. *International Journal of Technology Assessment in Health Care, 13*(4), 537–546

Tarby, W., & Hogan, K. (1997). Hospital-based patient information services: A model for collaboration. *Bulletin of the Medical Library Association, 85*(2), 158–166.

Tomky, D. (1999). Developing a computerized diabetes self-management education module for documenting outcomes. *Diabetes Educator, 25*(2), 197–208.

Tribble, D. (1996). How automated systems can (and do) fail. *American Journal of Health-System Pharmacists, 53,* 2622–2627.

U. S. Preventive Services Task Force. (1996). *Guide to clinical and preventive services* (2nd ed.). Baltimore: Williams & Wilkins.

Viegas, S. F., & Dunn, K. (Eds.). (1998). *Telemedicine: Practicing in the information age.* Philadelphia: Lippincott-Raven.

Warner, I. (1997). Telemedicine applications for home health care. *Journal of Telemedicine and Telecare, 2*(1), 65–66.

Whitten, P., & Collins, B. (1998). Nurse reactions to a prototype telemedicine system. *Journal of Telemedicine and Telecare, 4*(1), 50–52.

Whitten, P., Mair, F., & Collins, B. (1997). Home telenursing in Kansas: Patients' perceptions of uses and benefits. *Journal of Telemedicine and Telecare, 3*(1), 67–69.

Wood, F. B., Wallingford, K. T., & Siegel, E. R. (1997). Transitioning to the Internet: Results of a National Library of Medicine user survey. *Bulletin of the Medical Library Association, 85,* 331–340.

CHAPTER 11

·······

Over-the-Counter Medications

CHAPTER OUTLINE

Nonprescription Drug Use

P atients are now taking a more active and informed role in their own health care. Thousands of self-help books, articles, Websites, and television commercials demonstrate the rapidly growing trend for self-care. Surveys consistently show that consumers are increasingly self-medicating with nonprescription drugs. This trend must be taken into account by the nurse practitioner (NP). In a 1992 survey conducted by the Nonprescription Drug Manufacturers Association, the following results were reported:

1. Almost 70 percent of consumers prefer to fight symptoms without taking any medication if possible.
2. Eighty-five percent of consumers believe it is important to have access to nonprescription medications.
3. Fifty-four percent of consumers believe that the over-the-counter (OTC) availability of former prescription drugs has made it possible to save the time and expense of going to a physician or other provider.

4. Ninety percent of consumers discontinue their nonprescription medication because their problem was resolved.

The problems most likely to be treated with nonprescription, or OTC, medications in order of frequency follow:

1. Headache
2. The common cold
3. Muscle aches (e.g., sprains, strains)
4. Dermatologic conditions (e.g., acne, cold sores, dandruff, dry skin, athlete's foot)
5. Minor wounds
6. Premenstrual and menstrual symptoms
7. Upset stomach
8. Sleeping problems

Because patients are likely to treat many symptoms and conditions first with nonprescription drugs, the practitioner should assume that some therapy has been started when patients present for care and therefore should ask about OTC medication use. Patients are more likely to self-treat themselves or their children when they feel their illnesses are not serious enough to require medical care. There are more than 300,000 nonprescription products, some of them available only on a local basis, making the situation confusing for both patient and practitioner. Table 11–1 presents conditions for which OTC drugs are marketed.

Nonprescription drug therapy should not be undervalued or underestimated in the current health care environment. OTC drugs are powerful drugs that should be considered just like prescription drugs with respect to their pharmacology, toxicology, contraindications, precautions, adverse effects, and drug interactions. In fact, many former prescription drugs have recently been converted to nonprescription status (Table 11–2). All the care and thought needed to monitor prescription drug use are necessary for nonprescription drugs as well.

This chapter discusses OTC drugs patients commonly use. For more specific information on these drugs, see the appropriate chapter in this book.

Analgesics and Antipyretics

The OTC **analgesics** and **antipyretics** available in the United States are aspirin and other **salicylates, acetaminophen, ibuprofen, naproxen,** and **ketoprofen.**

Aspirin and Other Salicylates

Chemically, **aspirin** is acetylsalicylic acid (ASA). The acetyl group acetylates platelets, causing irreversible inhibition of platelet aggregation. This effect provides a unique advantage in preventing thrombus, but it increases the risk of bleeding. A single 650-mg dose can double bleeding times. **Aspirin** is contraindicated in those with hemophilia, vitamin K deficiency, or a history of peptic ulcer disease. Patients with these conditions should avoid **aspirin** and be aware that it is an ingredient in many products.

Aspirin and other **salicylates** can affect uric acid secretion and reabsorption. Doses of 1 to 2 g per day increase plasma uric acid levels. All **salicylates** should be avoided in patients with a history of gout or hyperuricemia.

Aspirin produces local gastrointestinal (GI) damage by penetrating the gastric mucosa and leading to cellular and vascular erosion by the stomach acid. There are two different ways that this can happen: a local effect from the drug coming in contact with the stomach lining and a systemic effect of prostaglandin inhibition. Ulceration can be asymptomatic until it is advanced. Moderate **aspirin** intake increases the daily GI blood loss to 6 to 10 mL a day, with 15 percent of patients losing in excess of 10 mL a day. This level of blood loss can produce iron-deficiency anemia. In a small number of patients, **aspirin** can produce GI bleeding, resulting in hematemesis or melena. Acute **aspirin** ingestion is associated with about half of the cases of acute hemorrhagic gastritis. Older patients, patients with a history of gastric ulceration or bleeding, and those with alcoholic liver disease are at increased risk for gastric bleeding and should avoid **aspirin.**

Table 11–1. Conditions for Which OTC Drugs Are Marketed

Most frequently treated conditions	Acne, athlete's foot, cold sores, colds, cough, cuts, dandruff, headache, heartburn, indigestion, insomnia, premenstrual, sinusitis, sprains
Other conditions	Abrasions, aches and pains, allergic rhinitis, anemia, arthralgia, asthma, bacterial infection (superficial), boils, burns, candidal vaginitis, canker sores, chapped skin, congestion, conjunctivitis, constipation, contact lens care, contraception, corns, dental care, dermatitis (contact), diaper rash, diarrhea, dysmenorrhea, dyspepsia, feminine hygiene, fever, gastritis, gingivitis, hair loss, halitosis, head lice, impetigo, insect bites, jet lag, motion sickness, nausea, obesity, otitis (external), periodontal disease, pharyngitis, pinworms, prickly heat, psoriasis, ringworm, seborrhea, smoking cessation, stye, sunburn, swimmer's ear, teething, toothache, vomiting, warts, xerostomia

Table 11–2. Selected Drugs Converted to Nonprescription Status

Drug	Indication
Brompheniramine (Dimetapp)	Antihistamine
Butoconazole (Femstat, Mycelex-3)	Antifungal
Chlorpheniramine (Chlor-Trimeton)	Antihistamine
Cimetidine (Tagamet)	Heartburn/acid peptic
Clemastine (Tavist)	Antihistamine
Clotrimazole (Mycelex-7)	Antifungal
Diphenhydramine (Benadryl)	Antihistamine/sleep aid
Doxylamine (Unisom)	Sleep aid
Famotidine (Pepcid)	Heartburn/acid peptic
Haloprogin (Halotex)	Antifungal
Hydrocortisone (Cortatid)	Antipruritic, anti-inflammatory
Ibuprofen (Motrin IB, Advil, Nuprin)	Analgesic, antipyretic
Ketoprofen (Orudis)	Analgesic
Loperamide (Imodium)	Antidiarrheal
Minoxidil (Rogaine)	Baldness
Naproxen (Aleve)	Analgesic, anti-inflammatory
Nicotine (Nicorette, Nicotrol)	Smoking cessation
Permethrin (Nix)	Pediculicide
Pyrantel pamoate (Antiminth)	Pinworm treatment
Sodium fluoride (ACT, Fluorogard)	Dental rinse
Stannous fluoride	Dental rinse/gel
Tolnaftate (Tinactin)	Antifungal
Triprolidine (Actifed, Allerfrin)	Antihistamine

Aspirin allergy is uncommon, occurring in less than 1 percent of patients. Many patients report **aspirin** allergy based on heartburn or gastric pain, which are common side effects, but not allergy. Symptoms of **aspirin** allergy include hives, edema, shortness of breath, bronchospasm, rhinitis, or shock. The allergic symptoms are usually due to the acetyl group, so that patients allergic to **aspirin** may use nonacetylated salicylates. **Aspirin** allergy occurs commonly (10 to 30%) in patients with chronic urticaria, asthma, and nasal polyps; these patients should avoid **aspirin**. Patients allergic to **aspirin** may cross-react with other drugs. The cross-reaction rate for **ibuprofen** is 97 percent, for **tartrazine #5** dye 15 percent, and for **acetaminophen** 6 percent; therefore, patients with these allergies should also avoid all **nonsteroidal anti-inflammatory drugs (NSAIDs)** as well.

Reye's syndrome is a potentially fatal illness characterized by vomiting, liver damage, encephalopathy, and hypoglycemia. The syndrome usually follows a viral infection with influenza or chickenpox. The mortality rate can be as high as 50 percent. The Centers for Disease Control and Prevention (CDC) and the American Academy of Pediatrics have confirmed an association between these viral infections, **aspirin** ingestion, and Reye's syndrome. More than 90 percent of patients with Reye's syndrome had taken **salicylates**. Since 1988, the Food and Drug Administration (FDA) has required that labels of nonprescription drugs containing **aspirin** warn that children and teenagers with flu or chickenpox should not use the medication. A common cold is not a contraindication to **aspirin** use; because symptoms of flu and chickenpox can be similar, however, most clinicians avoid **aspirin** altogether in this age group. The use of **aspirin** as a pediatric antipyretic has all but ceased in the United States, as have reports of Reye's syndrome. The CDC has been monitoring the safety of **ibuprofen** in these patients and an association with Reye's syndrome, and it appears to be a safe alternative to **aspirin**.

Acetaminophen

Acetaminophen is sometimes underdosed, especially when growing infants outgrow previous dose recommendations or when the parents use the infant dropper (0.8 cc) to dose the junior elixir (160 mg/5 cc), assuming they are the same strength.

Acetaminophen does not have any of the clinical problems noted for the **NSAIDs** (listed later). It has no effect on platelets, urinary excretion of uric acid, bleeding time, GI mucosa, renal function, or **aspirin**-allergic patients.

Acetaminophen is toxic to the liver in doses higher than 12 tablets per day (about 4 g). Patients taking large doses of **acetaminophen** should be monitored for liver function. Patients with preexisting liver disease are at increased risk for toxicity.

Acetaminophen produces no clinically significant drug interactions. Chronic **acetaminophen** therapy has been shown to elevate zidovudine levels and perhaps increase the bone marrow depression seen with this drug. Short-term or intermittent use of **acetaminophen** appears to be safe.

Ibuprofen, Ketoprofen, and Naproxen

Ibuprofen, **ketoprofen**, and **naproxen** are very similar and share the properties for **ibuprofen** listed later. The most frequent adverse effects of **ibuprofen** affect the GI tract. Heartburn, nausea, and epigastric pain are common complaints. **Ibuprofen** produces less GI bleeding than **aspirin** and less gastric erosion with chronic therapy. Although **ibuprofen** inhibits platelet aggregation, the effect is reversible, lasting about 24 hours. **Ibuprofen** has been shown to be as safe as **acetaminophen** for children under age 12, at a dose of 7.5 mg/kg.

Ibuprofen may decrease renal blood flow as a result of inhibiting prostaglandin synthesis. This effect is important in patients with congestive heart failure or chronic renal impairment. Patients with these conditions should not take **ibuprofen**.

Ibuprofen is contraindicated for patients with **aspirin** allergy because of the 97 percent cross-reactivity with **aspirin**. Patients with asthma may experience bronchospastic symptoms with **ibuprofen**.

Antihistamines and Decongestants

Antihistamines

Antihistamines are first-line agents for the prophylaxis and treatment of allergic rhinitis. However, **antihistamines** can reduce symptoms by only 50 percent. They competitively compete with only one of the mediators of allergic reaction (histamine), and their effectiveness depends on the timing and dosage of the drug. Histamine is the primary mediator for sneezing and itching, and **antihistamines** are very effective with these symptoms, but much less effective for rhinorrhea and congestion.

Antihistamines are highly lipophilic and cross the blood-brain barrier to cause significant sedation. **Chlorpheniramine** and **brompheniramine** are the least sedating OTC **antihistamines**. They are anticholinergic (dry mouth, eyes, and nose; urinary retention; blurred vision) and have quinidine-like effects on the heart. Second-generation (nonsedating) **antihistamines** are currently prescription only.

Decongestants

Decongestants are vasoconstrictive drugs that reduce nasal congestion; however, they have no effect on histamine or other mediators of allergy. They are frequently given in combination with **antihistamines**.

Decongestants are available for either oral or nasal administration. **Topical decongestants** are minimally absorbed, and their side effects tend to be minimal. Rebound congestion is a common problem when nasal preparations are administered for more than 5 days. It is more common with the short-acting preparations like **naphazoline** and **phenylephrine**. Treatment of rebound congestion consists of slow withdrawal—one nostril at a time—and replacement with topical normal saline. Resolving the condition takes 1 to 2 weeks after the **topical decongestant** is discontinued.

Systemic decongestants constrict vascular beds and stimulate the central nervous system (CNS). This causes increased blood pressure, insomnia, and increased heart rate. Stimulation of alpha-adrenergic receptors may cause urinary sphincter constriction in men with benign prostatic hyperplasia (BPH) and increase intraocular pressure in patients with glaucoma.

Table 11–3. Common Antihistamines, Decongestants, and Combination OTC Products

Brand Name Product	Generic Name/Contents	Dosage Forms
ANTIHISTAMINES		
Benadryl, Benadryl 25, Benadryl Dye Free	Diphenhydramine HCl	Elixir, tablet, capsule, liquid
Chlor-Trimeton 4-Hour Allergy	Chlorpheniramine maleate	Tablet
Contac 12-Hour Allergy	Clemastine fumarate	Tablet
Dimetapp Allergy, Dimetapp Allergy Extentabs	Brompheniramine maleate	Tablet, elixir, liqui-gel, time-release tablet
Tavist-1	Clemastine fumarate	Tablet
DECONGESTANTS		
Afrin 12-Hour, Afrin 12-Hour Pediatric, Afrin Extra Moisturizing, Afrin Sinus	Oxymetazoline HCl	Nasal spray, drops, pump, nasal drops
Allerest	Oxymetazoline HCl	Nasal spray
Benzedrex 12-Hour	Oxymetazoline HCl	Nasal spray
Benzedrex (Menthol)	Propylhexedrine	Nasal inhaler
Chlor-trimeton Non-Drowsy 4-Hour	Pseudoephedrine HCl	Tablet
Decongestant Inhaler	Levmetamfetamine	Nasal inhaler
Dimetapp Decongestant NonDrowsy, Dimetapp Decongestant Pediatric	Pseudoephedrine HCl	Liqui-gel, drops
Dristan	Phenylephrine HCl	Nasal spray
Dristan 12-Hour	Oxymetazoline HCl	Nasal spray
Drixoral Non Drowsy Formula	Pseudoephedrine HCl	Time-release tablet
Duration	Oxymetazoline HCl	Nasal spray, pump
4-Way Fast Acting	Phenylephrine HCl and Naphazoline HCl	Nasal spray
4-Way Long Lasting	Oxymetazoline HCl	Nasal spray
Neo-Synephrine Extra, Neo-Synephrine Mild, Neo-Synephrine Pediatric, Neo-Synephrine Regular	Phenylephrine HCl	Nasal spray, drops, pump
Neo-Synephrine Maximum 12-Hour	Oxymetazoline HCl	Nasal spray
Pediacare Infants' Decongestant	Pseudoephedrine HCl	Drops
Sinex Long Acting	Oxymetazoline HCl	Nasal spray
Sinex Regular	Phenylephrine HCl	Nasal spray

Continued on next page

Table 11–3. Common Antihistamines, Decongestants, and Combination OTC Products (*continued*)

Brand Name Product	Generic Name/Contents	Dosage Forms
Sudafed, Sudafed 12-Hour, Sudafed 12-Hour Caplet, Sudafed Children's, Non-Drowsy Sudafed Decongestant (Children & Infant)	Pseudoephedrine HCl	Tablet, time-release tablet, time-release caplet, liquid, chewable tablet
Triaminic AM Decongestant Formula, Triaminic Infant's Oral Decongestant	Pseudoephedrine HCl	Liquid drops
Vicks Sinus	Phenylephrine HCl	Nasal spray
Vicks Sinex 12-Hour	Oxymetazoline HCl	Nasal spray
COMBINATION PRODUCTS	**DECONGESTANT/ANTIHISTAMINE**	
Actifed	Pseudoephedrine/triprolidine	Tablet, syrup
Actifed Allergy Daytime/Nighttime	Pseudoephedrine/ nighttime only: Diphen- hydramine	Caplet
Allerest Maximum Strength	Pseudoephedrine/ chlorpheniramine	Tablet
Benadryl Allergy Decongestant Medication, Benadryl D	Pseudoephedrine/diphen- hydramine	Liquid, tablet, capsule
Chlor-Trimeton 12-Hour Allergy Decongestant, Chlor-Trimeton 4-Hour Allergy Decongestant	Pseudoephedrine/ chlorpheniramine	Tablet
Contac 12-Hour Cold	Phenylpropanolamine/ chlorpheniramine	Capsule, time-release
Dimetapp, Dimetapp Cold & Allergy, Dimetapp Maximum Strength 12-Hour Extentabs, Dimetapp Maximum Strength 4-Hour	Phenylpropanolamine/ brompheniramine	Chewable tablet, quick-dissolve tablets, time-release tablets, liqui-gel
Drixoral Cold & Allergy Sustained-Release	Pseudoephedrine/ dexbrompheniramine	Time-release tablets
Pediacare Cold Allergy for ages 6 to 12	Pseudoephedrine/ chlorpheniramine	Chewable tablet
Sudafed Cold and Allergy	Pseudoephedrine/ chlorpheniramine	Tablet
Tavist-D	Phenylpropanolamine/ clemastine fumarate	Tablet
Triaminic Cold & Allergy	Phenylpropanolamine/ chlorpheniramine	Syrup

Monoamine oxidase (MAO) inhibition intensifies the sympathomimetic effects of the **decongestants,** and oral agents are contraindicated in patients who are taking **MAO inhibitors (MAOIs).**

There are hundreds of combinations of **antihistamines, decongestants,** and **analgesics** cobined in products available for patients to select for self-medication. Table 11–3 lists the most commonly available national brand names.

Antacids and Histamine₂ Antagonists

Antacids

Antacids neutralize gastric acid secreted by the parietal cells of the stomach. **Antacids** neutralize the existing acid; they do not affect the amount of acid being secreted. **Antacids** do not neutralize the gastric pH but do raise it to about 4 to 5. At this level, gastric pepsin is inhibited.

Antacid potency is expressed as acid-neutralizing capacity (ANC), the amount of acid buffered per dose. The FDA requires that an **antacid** neutralize at least 5 mEq per dose and act for at least 10 minutes. The ANC is highly variable, so dosing should be determined by the amount needed to neutralize a standard amount of acid.

Table 11–4 presents the potency of selected **antacids** needed to provide 80 mEq of ANC.

The formulation of an **antacid** is important for neutralizing capacity, as well as for patient acceptance and compliance. Only dissolved antacid can react with stomach acid, and the size of **antacid** particle is the determinant of neutralizing capacity. **Antacid** suspensions are already in a form to react with acid, whereas tablets must be chewed so they will dissolve and react with the acid. Because of this difference, suspensions are more potent than tablets of the same milligram strength. Many patients prefer tablets, but they should be instructed to chew them well and take them with a glass of water.

Antacids must be taken in large doses, so their palatability is very important. One of the reasons there are so many products is the difference in patient preference. In one study, 14 aluminum and/or magnesium suspensions were tested. Overall, **Mylanta Cherry Creme** and **Mylanta Double Strength Cool Mint Creme** were selected as the most palatable, with **Di-Gel** lemon/orange and **Riopan 2** the least palatable.

All **antacids** are basic compounds that react with gastric acid to form a salt and water. Four primary compounds are found in today's products: sodium bicarbonate, calcium carbonate, aluminum hydroxide, and magnesium hydroxide. Most commercially available products contain a mixture of aluminum and magnesium hydroxide (Table 11–5). Because constipation from aluminum and diarrhea from magnesium are dose-related, combining these two agents allows potent ANC with lower doses of each agent. Theoretically, the two effects would balance out, but diarrhea appears to be the predominant effect. Up to 75 percent of patients taking combination products experience diarrhea, whereas constipation is rarely encountered. Patients with poor renal function may experience hypermagnesemia, hyperaluminumemia, or metabolic alkalosis.

Antacid drug interactions, most of which are not clinically significant, have been reported with more than 30 classes of drugs. Most interactions can be avoided by sep-

arating the **antacids** by at least 2 hours from the dosing of the other oral medications. Intraluminal interactions occur in the stomach when an **antacid** chelates another drug or adsorbs another drug onto its surface. **Antacids** can interfere with another drug's adsorption and elimination by changing the pH of the stomach or urine.

The best-known interaction is with **tetracycline**. Aluminum hydroxide and magnesium hydroxide have a strong affinity for **tetracycline** and form an insoluble and inactive chelate. This interaction can reduce bioavailability by 90 percent and result in clinical failures. This chelation occurs with all other forms of **tetracycline**, such as **doxycycline** and **minocycline**. Patients should not take any **antacid** until at least 2 hours after **tetracycline** administration. A similar interaction exists with the **quinolone antibiotics**, such as **ciprofloxacin** and **ofloxacin**.

Histamine₂ Receptor Antagonists

The introduction of **histamine₂ (H₂) receptor antagonists** in 1977 completely changed the treatment of acid peptic disorders. Today all of these products are now available in OTC tablet formulations: **cimetidine (Tagamet HB)**, **ranitidine (Zantac 75)**, **nizatidine (Axid AR)**, and **famotidine (Pepcid AC** and **Mylanta AR)**.

The **H₂ antagonists** inhibit gastric acid secretion by blocking the histamine₂ receptors. Although all phases of acid production are inhibited, baseline and nocturnal acid secretion are inhibited to a greater extent. An effect begins within 1 hour and continues for 6 to 12 hours. Both the degree and the duration of acid suppression are dose-dependent, so the reduction in acid and duration of effect are significantly lower with nonprescription-strength products.

As a class, the **H₂ antagonists** are among the most studied drugs. More than 60 million patients have taken these agents, which have rarely caused severe side effects. This safety profile suggests that the lower OTC doses are safe. The most common side effects are headache, nausea, and diarrhea, at rates (less than 10%) that are usually the same as the placebo.

Cimetidine has the greatest potential to interact with other drugs because it binds to cytochrome P-450 enzymes to impair hepatic metabolism of drugs that are normally cleared by the liver. The inhibition is dose-dependent, with very little effect at doses lower than 400 mg a day. However, the potential for adverse clinical consequences exists, particularly in older patients with declining renal function and multiple medications. **Famotidine** and **nizatidine** do not bind appreciably to the system and therefore do not inhibit the metabolism of other drugs.

A major concern with OTC **H₂ antagonists** is that patients with angina, cancer, or gastroesophageal reflux disease (GERD) will self-medicate and delay appropriate treatment. The potential for undertreatment of peptic ul-

Table 11–4. Potency of Selected Antacids

Antacid Tablet	Equivalent Volume*
Riopan Extra Strength	13.3 mL
Extra Strength Maalox	13.8 mL
Maalox TC	15 mL
Mylanta II	16 mL
Gelusil Ii	17 mL
Alternagel	25 mL
Milk of Magnesia	29 mL
Maalox	30 mL
Mylanta	32 mL
Di-Gel	33 mL
Titralac Plus	37 mL
Amphojel	40 mL
Gaviscon	100 mL

Antacid Tablet	Equivalent Number of Tablets*
Maalox TC	3
Riopan Plus 2	3
Extra Strength Maalox	4
Mylanta II	4
Gelusil II	4
Amphojel (600 mg)	5
Tums EX	6
Mylanta	7
Maalox Plus	7
Tums	8
Maalox	9
Rolaids	10
Gaviscon	160

*Number of milliliters or tablets needed to provide 80 mEq of acid-neutralizing capacity.

cer disease (PUD) also exists because the H_2 antagonist treats pain without healing the ulcer. On account of these concerns, these OTC products are not recommended to be taken for longer than 2 weeks.

Despite the fact that these drugs may cause problems for certain patients and have the possibility of interacting with prescription drugs, the nonprescription strengths of H_2 antagonists offer convenient self-care for patients. The overall safety record of these drugs supports their OTC availability. NPs can minimize the risks by recognizing and triaging patients who are at risk for serious GI disorders, by recognizing patients at risk for **cimetidine** drug interactions, and by taking a careful history for their OTC use.

Laxatives

Extensive advertising suggests that bowel movements somehow enhance physical well-being and mood. **Laxatives** are widely used and are a common part of a nonprescription medication history. By definition, a **laxative** facilitates the passage and elimination of feces from the colon and rectum. **Laxative** drugs have been classified by their mechanism of action.

Bulk-Forming Laxatives

Bulk-forming laxatives cause water to be retained in the small and large intestines. This water helps to produce formed stools. **Bulk-forming laxatives** are the best choice for the initial treatment of constipation. They are made from natural sources such as semisynthetic hydrophilic polysaccharides and cellulose derivatives, most of which are not absorbed by the body. They produce bulk in the form of a gel that passes easily through the intestines. **Bulk-forming laxatives** generally take 12 to 24 hours to work, but they can take as long as 72 hours. It is very important that patients drink a large glass of water (8 oz) when taking these **laxatives.** Not only does the water promote stool formation but also it prevents obstruction in the intestines or esophagus. **Bulk-forming laxatives** are the safest form of **laxatives** for long-term use.

The main ingredients in **bulk-forming laxatives** are methylcellulose, polycarbophil, tragacanth, and psyllium. Polycarbophil is the calcium salt of a polyacrylic resin and has a large capacity for binding water. The calcium content of this product is approximately 150 mg per tablet, which may increase the risk of hypercalcemia in susceptible patients.

If **bulk-forming laxatives** are taken in dry form or the tablets are chewed and swallowed, esophageal obstruction may occur. It is essential that all forms of **bulk laxatives** be taken with at least 8 oz of water to ensure that they are cleared of the upper GI tract. **Psyllium** products are not absorbed and do not seem to interfere with nutrient absorption. The dose can be titrated up to effect, and they are appropriate for long-term therapy.

Table 11–5. Combination Antacids

Combinations of Antacids	Brand Name Product	Dosage Forms	Other Compounds
Aluminum hydroxide and magnesium hydroxide	Gelusil	Tablet	Simethicone
	Maalox	Suspension, tablet	
	Maalox Antacid Plus AntiGas	Tablet	Simethicone
	Maalox Extra Strength Plus	Suspension	Simethicone
	Mylanta (Regular & Double Strength)	Gelcap, chewable tablet, suspension	Simethicone
Aluminum hydroxide and magnesium carbonate	Gaviscon ESR, Gaviscon ESRF	Chewable tablet, suspension	Alginic acid (ESR)
Aluminum hydroxide, magnesium trisilicate, and sodium bicarbonate	Gaviscon, Gaviscon-2	Chewable tablet	Alginic acid
Calcium carbonate and magnesium hydroxide	Di-Gel	Chewable tablet, liquid	Simethicone
	Rolaids Calcium & Magnesium	Tablet	

Stimulant Laxatives

Stimulant laxatives are conveniently classified according to their chemical structure and pharmacological activity. It has been suggested that these **laxative** products stimulate secretion of water and electrolytes in either the small or large intestine, or both, depending on the specific **laxative**. Intensity of action is proportional to dosage, but individually, effective doses vary. All **stimulant laxatives** may produce gripping, colic, increased mucus secretion, and, in some people, excessive evacuation of fluid. **Stimulant laxatives** are most commonly used to empty the colon prior to rectal and bowel examinations and before surgical procedures involving the GI tract. They should never be used routinely. Because they act fairly quickly, they are often abused. Abuse can lead to dehydration, loss of protein, loss of potassium, severe cramping, or a dysfunctional colon. Because these products do have a quick onset of action, it is best not to use them at certain times (e.g., at bedtime).

The most commonly used **stimulant laxatives** are bisacodyl and phenolphthalein.

Bisacodyl, administered in a combination of tablets and suppositories or tablets and enemas, has been recommended for cleaning the colon before GI surgery, endoscopy, or radiography. **Bisacodyl** is effective in patients with colostomies, and it may reduce or eliminate the need for irrigation. **Bisacodyl** acts in the colon on contact with the mucosal nerve plexus. Its action is independent of intestinal tone, and the drug is minimally absorbed systemically (approximately 5%). Action on the small intestine is negligible. A soft, formed stool is usually produced 6 to 10 hours after oral administration and 15 to 60 minutes after rectal administration. Adverse effects, which come with chronic, regular use (abuse), include metabolic acidosis or alkalosis, hypocalcemia, tetany, loss of enteric protein, and malabsorption. The suppository form may produce a burning sensation in the rectum. No adverse effects on the liver, kidney, or hematopoietic system have been observed after administration. Enteric-coated **bisacodyl** tablets prevent irritation of the gastric mucosa and therefore should not be broken, crushed, chewed, or administered with agents that increase gastric pH, such as **antacids, histamine-receptor antagonists,** or **proton pump inhibitors.**

Phenolphthalein is effective in small doses and is tasteless, making it desirable for use in candy, wafer, and chewing gum dosage forms. When ingested, it passes through the stomach unchanged and is dissolved in the intestine by bile salts and the alkaline intestinal secretions. As much as 15 percent of the dose is absorbed; the rest is excreted unchanged in the feces. This drug exerts its stimulating effect primarily on the colon. It is usually active 6 to 8 hours after administration. Part of the absorbed **phenolphthalein** is secreted into the intestinal tract along with bile. Enterohepatic recycling may prolong the action of **phenolphthalein** for 3 or 4 days. Because bile must be present for **phenolphthalein** to be effective, the drug does not relieve constipation for patients who have obstructive jaundice.

Phenolphthalein is usually nontoxic. However, at least two types of allergic reactions may follow its use. In susceptible individuals, a large dose may cause diarrhea, colic, cardiac and respiratory distress, or circulatory collapse. The other reaction is a polychromatic rash that ranges from pink to deep purple. The eruptions may be as small as a pinhead or as large as the palm of the hand. Itching and burning may be moderate or severe. If the rash is severe, it may lead to vesication and erosion, especially around the mouth and genital areas. Patients should be advised to report any rash immediately. Some of the absorbed drug appears in the urine, which is colored pink to red if it is sufficiently alkaline. Similarly, the drug excreted in the feces causes a red coloration if the feces are sufficiently alkaline. This effect may be alarming, so the patient should be forewarned.

Anthraquinone Stimulant Laxatives

Anthraquinone stimulant laxatives include **aloe, cascara sagrada, casanthranol, senna, aloin, danthron, rhubarb,** and **frangula.** The drugs of choice in this group are the **cascara, casanthranol,** and **senna** compounds. The precise mechanism by which peristalsis is increased is unknown. The cathartic activity of **anthraquinones** is limited primarily to the colon. **Anthraquinones** usually produce their action 8 to 12 hours after administration but may require up to 24 hours. The active principles of **anthraquinones** are absorbed from the GI tract and subsequently appear in body secretions, including human milk. After taking a **senna-containing laxative,** postpartum patients have reported a brown discoloration of breast milk and subsequent catharsis by their nursing infants. A study with constipated postpartum breastfeeding women receiving a **senna laxative** reported that 17 percent of their infants experienced diarrhea. Preparations of **senna** are more potent than those of **cascara** and can produce considerably more abdominal cramping. Chrysophanic acid, a component of **senna** that is excreted in urine, colors acidic urine yellowish brown and colors alkaline urine reddish violet. The prolonged use of **anthraquinone laxatives,** especially **cascara sagrada,** can result in a harmless, reversible melanotic pigmentation of the colonic mucosa (melanosis coli), which is usually found on sigmoidoscopy, colonoscopy, or rectal biopsy.

Surfactant Laxatives

Surfactant laxatives are anionic surfactants that, when taken orally, increase the wetting efficiency of intestinal fluid and soften fecal mass. **Laxatives** that contain only surfactants should not be used to relieve long-term constipation. These **laxatives** are considered "stool softeners." They work best to prevent rather than cure constipation. They are best for people who should not strain while having a bowel movement, such as new mothers, patients who have had rectal or vaginal surgery, and those with heart disease or high blood pressure. **Surfactant laxatives** do not stimulate bowel movements when used alone and are usually effective after 1 to 2 days. These **laxatives** are nonabsorbable, nontoxic, and inert; however, their detergent properties may facilitate the ab-

sorption of other substances in the GI tract, including prescription drugs.

Table 11–6 presents common OTC **laxatives.**

Geriatric Laxative Use

Constipation is a common complaint of many older patients. It may progress with age, and prolonged and excessive **laxative** use is not uncommon in this population. Because of the physiological effects of chronic **laxative** use on the intestine, **laxative** dependency is often difficult to manage. Thus, proper education about **laxative** products and advice on product selection and use are particularly crucial for the older patient.

For geriatric patients without a history of constipation, a thorough investigation should be conducted to determine whether acute cases of constipation have resulted from new or old diseases or from the use of medications. The colon in the older adult can lack normal tone, resulting in an overreliance on oral **laxatives** or rectal enemas. A low-residue diet, a diet consisting mainly of soft foods, or inadequate chewing of food may be associated with the development of constipation in this age group.

Constipation in older people can result from a number of factors, including failure to establish a time habit, insufficient fluid and/or bulk intake, abuse of **stimulant laxatives,** and immobility. Constipation in this population is often associated with a prolonged transit time through the colon and a decreased perception of the need to defecate, which is often precipitated by conditions such as neuromuscular disorders, confusion, and depression. Older patients often strain to pass hard stools, which may predispose them to serious complications, including cardiovascular problems and hemorrhoids. In addition, geriatric patients tend to have multiple diseases and take multiple medications, some of which may contribute to the development of constipation. Such agents include **sedatives; hypnotics; antispasmodics; antidepressants; antipsychotics; calcium-, aluminum-,** and **iron-containing products;** and **calcium channel blockers. Laxative** preparations can increase the rate at which other drugs pass through the GI tract by increasing GI motility, which then decreases the absorption and effectiveness of concurrently administered medications.

For older patients requiring **laxatives, bulk-forming agents** are generally preferred; onset is usually in 2 to 3 days. Sugar-free products (e.g., **Konsyl, Serutan,** and various **Metamucil** products) are recommended for diabetic patients.

Antidiarrheal Products

In the United States, most acute nonspecific diarrhea is self-limiting in nature. Some health care providers rec-

Table 11–6. Common OTC Laxatives

Brand Name Product	Active Ingredient	Dosage Forms
Bulk-Forming Laxatives		
Citrucel (Regular and Sugar Free)	Methylcellulose	Powder
Equalactin	Polycarbophil	Chewable tablet
Fibercon	Polycarbophil	Tablet
Fiberall	Polycarbophil	Tablet
Fiberall (Oatmeal Raisin)	Psyllium	Wafer
Fiberall (Orange)	Psyllium	Powder
Konsyl	Psyllium	Powder
Konsyl Fiber	Polycarbophil	Tablet
Metamucil Fiber (Apple Crisp)	Psyllium	Wafer
Metamucil (Original and Sugar Free)	Psyllium	Packet
Metamucil (Original Texture; Smooth Texture-Orange, Regular; Smooth Texture-Sugar Free, Citrus)	Psyllium	Powder
Perdiem Fiber	Psyllium	Granule
Stimulant Laxatives		
Alophen	Phenolphthalein	Tablet
Dulcolax	Bisacodyl	Suppository, tablet
Evac-U-Gen	Phenolphthalein	Chewable tablet
Ex-Lax Chocolate, Regular, or Maximum	Phenolphthalein	Tablet
Ex-Lax Gentle Nature	Sennosides	Tablet
Fleet	Bisacodyl	Suppository, tablet, enema
Fletcher's Castoria	Senna	Liquid
Fletcher's, Fletcher's Children's Cherry	Phenolphthalein	Liquid
Kellogg's Tasteless Castor Oil	Castor oil	Liquid
Milk of Magnesia Cascara	Cascara sagrada	Suspension
Modane	Phenolphthalein	Tablet
Nature's Remedy	Cascara sagrada, aloe	Tablet
Senokot	Senna	Tablet
Surfactant Laxatives		
Colace	Docusate sodium	Capsule, liquid, syrup
Correctol Stool Softener Laxative	Docusate sodium	Softgel

Continued on next page

Table 11–6. Common OTC Laxatives (*continued*)

Brand Name Product	Active Ingredient	Dosage Forms
Ex-Lax Stool Softener	Docusate sodium	Caplet
Surfak	Docusate sodium	Liqui-gel
Combination Laxative Products Correctol	Stimulant: Phenolphthalein Stool softener: Docusate sodium	Caplet, tablet
Doxidan	Stimulant: Phenolphthalein Stool softener: Docusate sodium	Liqui-gel
Ex-Lax Extra Gentle	Stimulant: Phenolphthalein Stool softener: Docusate sodium	Tablet
Feen-A-Mint Pills	Stimulant: Phenolphthalein Stool softener: Docusate sodium	Tablet
Perdiem	Bulk former: Psyllium Stimulant: Senna	Granule
Peri-Colace	Stimulant: Casanthranol Stool softener: Docusate sodium	Tablet
Senokot-S	Stimulant: Senna Stool softener: Docusate sodium	Tablet

ommend **loperamide** or adsorbents in acute diarrhea. With the exception of **loperamide** and **bismuth subsalicylate** in traveler's diarrhea, however, scientific evidence is lacking to prove that pharmacological agents reduce stool frequency or duration of disease. Nevertheless, when used according to labeling, nonprescription **antidiarrheals** may provide relief.

Antiperistaltics

The most commonly used nonprescription **antidiarrheal** medication currently available is **loperamide.** It is the drug of choice for treating uncomplicated diarrhea. It is used for traveler's diarrhea, nonspecific acute diarrhea, and chronic diarrhea associated with inflammatory bowel disease, and it possesses a more favorable side effect profile than **opiate** and **opiate-like agents.** It not only reduces the frequency of stool loss but also helps relieve the cramping that often accompanies diarrhea. It slows intestinal motility and produces a positive movement of electrolytes and water through the gut. Like other **antiperistaltic drugs,** it should be used for no more than 48 hours in acute diarrhea. The usual nonprescription adult dosage is 4 mg initially and then 2 mg after each loose bowel movement, not to exceed 8 mg per day.

Loperamide is also effective in treating traveler's diarrhea. Traveler's diarrhea is caused by eating or drinking fecally contaminated food or water that is not inacti-

vated by cooking or processing. Typically, symptoms occur within 24 to 48 hours of exposure and include diarrhea, nausea, fever, chills, and muscle pain.

Adsorbents

Many **antidiarrheal** products contain **adsorbents** that both help to alleviate the symptoms, such as gastric pain, that accompany diarrhea and absorb the excessive fluid that is present with diarrhea. Often large quantities of **adsorbents** are necessary to accomplish an antidiarrheal effect. Most commercially available products are formulated as flavored liquid suspensions to improve palatability. Constipation may result if **adsorbents** are taken in excess. Adsorption is not selective, and when **adsorbents** are given orally, they may adsorb nutrients and digestive enzymes as well as toxins, bacteria, and various noxious materials in the GI tract. They may also have the undesirable effect of adsorbing drugs in the GI tract. Although the systemic absorption of an orally administered drug from the GI tract is compromised during a diarrheal episode, absorption may be further hampered by the concomitant administration of an antidiarrheal **adsorbent.** Thus, a clinical judgment must be made regarding when the patient will take medications other than the **antidiarrheal** preparations.

Following initial treatment, most **antidiarrheal** preparations containing **adsorbents** are taken after each loose bowel movement until the diarrhea is controlled or the maximum daily dosage is reached. The total amount of **adsorbent** taken may be quite large if the diarrhea episodes recur in rapid succession over several hours. Because there is negligible systemic absorption of the adsorbent drug, the most common side effects associated with adsorbents include constipation, bloating, and fullness.

Bismuth Subsalicylate

Bismuth subsalicylate (Pepto-Bismol) is available as 262.5 mg per tablet (original and cherry-flavored), 262.5 mg per swallowable caplet, 262.5 mg per 15 mL, or 525 mg per 15 mL (maximum strength). The usual adult dosage is 30 mL every 30 to 60 minutes as needed, to a maximum of eight doses in a 24-hour period. **Bismuth subsalicylate** dosage forms contain various amounts of **salicylate**. Methylsalicylate (oil of wintergreen) is used as a flavoring agent in the suspension dosage form and the original tablets. The suspension dosage form (262.5 mg/15 mL) contains 130 mg of **salicylate**, whereas the original tablets (262.5 mg) contain 102 mg of **salicylate**. Further, the caplets (262.5 mg) and cherry-flavored tablets (262.5 mg) contain 99 mg of **salicylate**.

The **salicylate** may be a problem if the patient is taking **aspirin** or other **salicylate**-containing drugs. Toxic levels of **salicylate** may be reached even if the patient follows dosing directions on the label for each drug. Thus, patients who are sensitive to **aspirin** should not use **bismuth subsalicylate**. Children and teenagers who have or are recovering from chickenpox or flu are at risk of **salicylate**-induced Reye's syndrome. This product may also interact adversely with **oral anticoagulants, methotrexate, probenecid,** and any other drug that potentially interacts with **aspirin**. Also, **serum salicylate** concentrations may exert an antiplatelet effect. Harmless black-stained stool may occur, which should not be confused with melena; harmless darkening of the tongue may occur as well. Mild tinnitus is a side effect that may be associated with moderate to severe **salicylate** toxicity. If diarrhea is seen with high fever or continues beyond 24 hours, the patient should seek medical care. **Bismuth** is radiopaque and may interfere with radiographic intestinal studies.

Table 11–7 presents common OTC **antidiarrheal** products.

Antifungal Preparations

The most common types of fungal infections that affect the skin are tinea pedis (athlete's foot), tinea cruris (jock itch), tinea capitis (scalp itch), tinea corporis (ringworm), tinea versicolor, and candidiasis (vaginal yeast

Table 11–7. Common OTC Antidiarrheal Products

Brand Name Product	Dosage Forms
Products Containing Loperamide	
Diar Aid	Tablets
Imodium A-D	Liquid, caplet
Kaopectate 1-D	Caplet
Maalox AntiDiarrheal	Caplet
Pepto Diarrhea Control	Liquid
Products Containing Adsorbents	
Charco-Caps	Caplet, capsule, tablet
Diasorb	Liquid, tablet
Donnagel	Chewable tablet, suspension
Kaopectate	Liquid
Kaopectate Children's	Chewable tablet, liquid
Parapectolin	Suspension
Rheaban	Caplet

infection and thrush). These infections respond well to topical OTC antifungal medications.

Tinea pedis, or athlete's foot, is the most commonly encountered type of fungal infection involving the skin. Symptoms may include itching, burning, stinging, odor, scaliness, and dryness. In severe conditions, inflammation, oozing, weeping, and pain may be present.

Currently, recommended initial therapy for candidal vulvovaginitis is with an **imidazole** product. There are currently four topical **imidazole** derivatives available in the United States for treating candidal vulvovaginitis: **butoconazole, clotrimazole, miconazole,** and **tioconazole**. These products are available as vaginal creams, suppositories, and tablets. Studies have shown the **imidazole** to be equally effective and without major toxicities; effectiveness rates are approximately 85 to 90 percent.

Side effects from topical therapy are minimal. **Topical imidazoles** are associated with vulvovaginal burning, itching, and irritation in about 7 percent of patients. These side effects are more likely to occur with the initial application of the vaginal preparation and are similar to symptoms of the vaginal infection. Abdominal cramps, headache, penile irritation, and allergic reactions are rare. Different treatment durations have been studied. Initially, **antifungal** treatment regimens of 14 days were used. Currently, the 7-day regimens of **clotri-**

mazole and **miconazole** and the 3-day regimen of **butoconazole** are available without a prescription.

Adverse effects include abdominal cramping, headache, urticaria, hives, and skin rash. The vaginal **antifungals** can be used during menses, and women should be instructed to continue therapy if menses begin during the course of therapy. However, some patients object to using the vaginal **antifungals** during menses; postponement of treatment may be reasonable. The practitioner should also emphasize the importance of continuing therapy despite early symptomatic relief. Relief of symptoms can occur as early as several hours after initiation of therapy, but relief of symptoms is not synonymous with cure.

Table 11–8 presents common topical OTC **antifungal** products.

Sleep Aids

Insomnia is one of patients' most common complaints, listed third after the common cold and headache. More than 2.5 percent of Americans use a prescription **hypnotic**, and 3 percent buy nonprescription **sleep aids**. It is very common for these drugs to appear in a patient's OTC drug history. Only a small percentage of patients with a sleep disorder verbalize their complaints to the practitioner. Insomnia is a symptom for which there is no definitive definition. Some patients who complain of insomnia sleep the same length of time as others who say they sleep well. Patients may complain of sleep latency, nocturnal awakening, early morning awakening, or poor quality of sleep. Patients feel that they sleep poorly at night and function poorly during the day.

Table 11–8. Common Topical OTC Antifungal Products

Brand Name Product	Active Ingredient	Dosage Forms	Use
Betadine First Aid	Povidone-iodine	Cream, spray	
Betadine	Povidone-iodine	Gel, douche, ointment	
Cruex Antifungal	Undecylenate	Spray-powder, cream	Tinea cruris, pedis
Desenex Antifungal	Tolnaftate	Spray-liquid	Tinea pedis, cruris, corporis, versicolor
Desenex Antifungal Aerosol	Undecylenate	Spray-powder	Tinea pedis, cruris
Desenex Antifungal	Undecylenate	Cream, ointment, powder	Tinea pedis, cruris
Desenex Foot & Sneaker Deodorant Powder Plus	Undecylenate	Powder	Tinea pedis
Femstat-3	Butoconazole	Cream, prefilled applicators	Candidiasis
Gyne-Lotrimin (Vaginal)	Clotrimazole	Vaginal inserts, cream	Candidiasis
Lotrimin AF	Clotrimazole	Cream	Tinea pedis, cruris, corporis, versicolor
Lotrimin AF Jock Itch	Clotrimazole	Spray-powder, lotion	Tinea cruris
Micatin Athlete's Foot	Miconazole nitrate	Cream	Tinea pedis
Monistat 7 (Vaginal)	Miconazole nitrate	Vaginal inserts, cream	Candidiasis
Monistat 3 (Vaginal)	Miconazole nitrate	Vaginal cream	Candidiasis
Tinactin Cream	Tolnaftate	Cream	Tinea pedis
Tinactin Powder	Tolnaftate	Powder	Tinea pedis
Vagistat-1	Tioconazole	Ointment	Candidiasis
Zeasorb-AF	Miconazole nitrate	Powder	Tinea pedis, cruris, corporis, versicolor

Table 11–9. Common OTC Sleep Aids

Brand Name Product	Antihistamine	Analgesic	Dosage Form
Doan's P.M.	Diphenhydramine	Magnesium salicylate	Tablet
Excedrin P.M.	Diphenhydramine	Acetaminophen	Caplet, tablet, softgel
Nytol (Regular & Extra Strength)	Diphenhydramine		Caplet, tablet
Sleepinal (Regular & Maximum Strength)	Diphenhydramine		Capsule
Sominex	Diphenhydramine		Caplet, tablet
Sominex Pain Relief	Diphenhydramine	Acetaminophen	Caplet, tablet, gelcap
Tylenol P.M. (Regular & Extra Strength)	Diphenhydramine	Acetaminophen	Caplet, tablet, gelcap
Unisom	Doxylamine		Tablet
Unisom Sleepgels (Maximum Strength)	Diphenhydramine		Softgel

Currently, there are only two active ingredients available in OTC **sleep-aid** medications. These ingredients are the **antihistamines diphenhydramine** and **doxylamine.**

Many OTC **analgesic** or **antifever products** are also marketed as products that promote sleep. These products contain **aspirin** or **acetaminophen** and have a **sleep aid** added to enhance their appeal. If mild pain symptoms are present or more pronounced at bedtime, these combination medications can be quite effective.

The primary adverse effects of **diphenhydramine** and **doxylamine** are anticholinergic, such as dry mouth, constipation, blurred vision, and tinnitus. Older male patients may have difficulty in urinating. These effects may be additive with the anticholinergic effects of other drugs that are being taken. Older patients may develop delirium from modest doses of **diphenhydramine.** All of these issues must be considered if a patient is taking these OTC drugs.

Table 11–9 presents common OTC **sleep aids.**

Summary

The practitioner must keep in mind that the prescription drug history, although very important, is usually not the only story of a patient's drug use. A careful OTC and herbal drug history is needed to avoid overlooking important aspects, such as adverse drug effects and drug interactions, caused by the OTC drugs that the patient is taking.

Many people diagnose their own symptoms, select a nonprescription drug product, and monitor their own therapeutic response. This process is not often reliably reported when, during a routine health history, a patient is asked, "Do you take any medications?" Specific questions need to be asked.

Properly used, OTC medications are useful in self-care to relieve minor complaints and transient conditions. If used improperly or in combination with other medications, these medications can cause a multitude of problems, adverse drug events, and drug interactions.

REFERENCES

Nonprescription Drug Manufacturers Association. (1992). Self-medication in the '90s: Practices and perceptions. Washington, DC: Author.

Rosefsky, J. B. (1992). Ibuprofen safety (letter). *Pediatrics, 89,* 166–167.

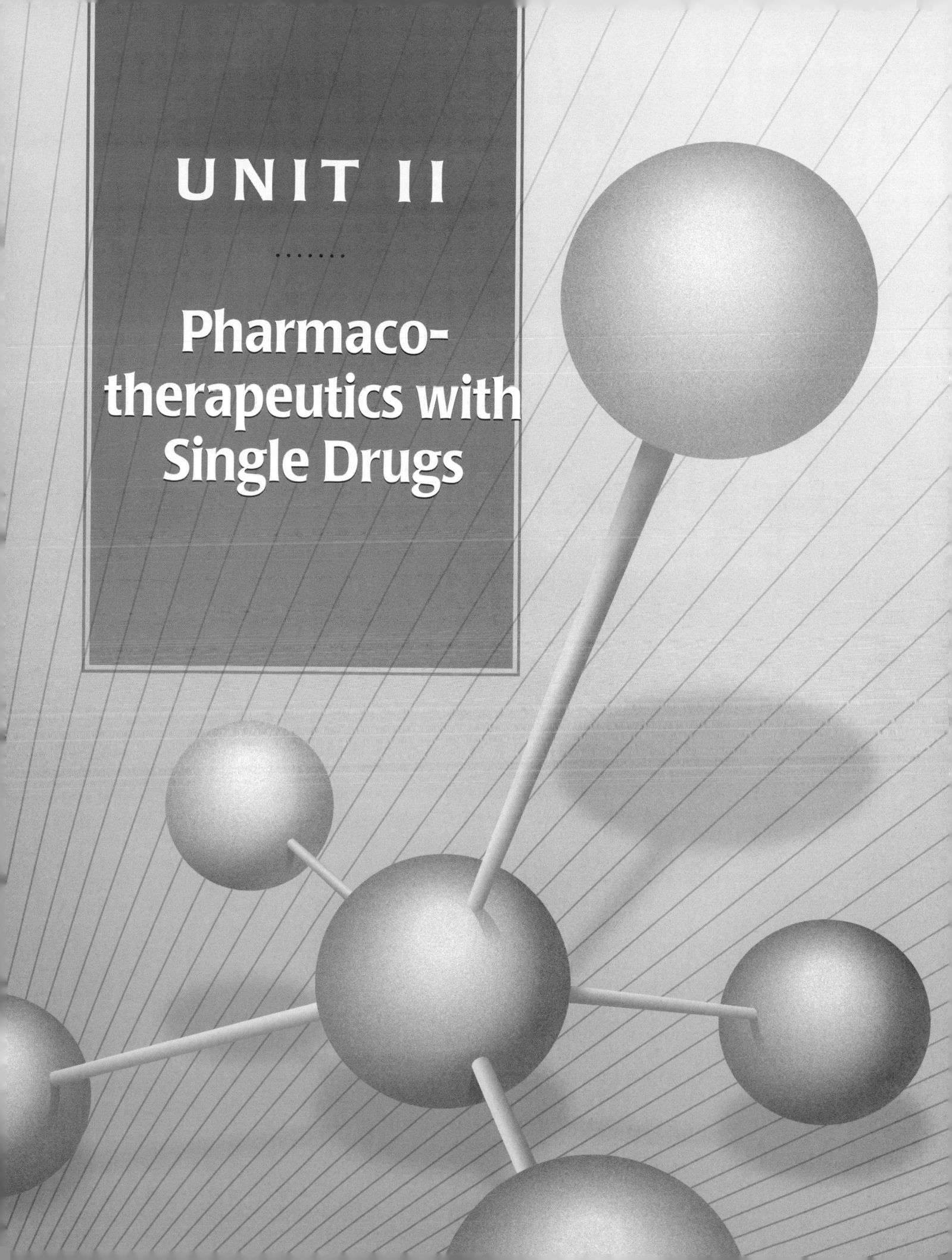

UNIT II

. . . .

Pharmaco-
therapeutics with
Single Drugs

CHAPTER 12

·······

Drugs Affecting the Autonomic Nervous System

*Reversal of nonpolarizing neuromuscular
    blockade*
Alzheimer's disease
Rational drug selection
Formulation
Cost
Dosing schedule
Adverse reactions profile
Time to recurrence of disease progression
Monitoring
Patient education
Administration
Adverse reactions
Lifestyle management

NICOTINE
Pharmacodynamics
    Cardiovascular effects
    Gastrointestinal effects
    Central nervous system effects
Pharmacokinetics
    Absorption and distribution
    Metabolism and excretion
Pharmacotherapeutics
    Precautions and contraindications
    Adverse drug reactions
    Drug interactions
    Clinical use and dosing
    Rational drug selection
    Cost
    Convenience
    Success rates
    Concomitant diseases
    Monitoring
    Patient education
    Administration
    Adverse reactions
    Lifestyle management

CHOLINERGIC BLOCKERS
Pharmacodynamics
    Cardiovascular effects
    Respiratory effects
    Exocrine gland effects
    Urinary and gastrointestinal effects
    Central nervous systems effects
    Optic effects
Pharmacokinetics
    Absorption and distribution
    Metabolism and excretion
Pharmacotherapeutics
    Precautions and contraindications
    Adverse drug reactions
    Cardiovascular
    Respiratory
    Exocrine glands
    Gastrointestinal and urinary
    Eye
    Central nervous system
    Drug interactions
    Clinical use and dosing
    Parkinson's disease
    *Management of extrapyramidal symptoms
        (EPS) secondary to drug therapy*
    Antispasmodic for bladder instability
    *Prevention of nausea and vomiting associated
        with motion sickness*
    *Adjunct therapy in management of irritable
        bowel syndrome and peptic ulcer disease*
    Rational drug selection
    Cost
    Formulation
    Monitoring
    Patient education
    Administration
    Adverse reactions
    Lifestyle management

he resting activity of most organs is maintained by opposing influences from the parasympathetic nervous system (PNS) and its neurotransmitter, acetylcholine (ACh), and the sympathetic nervous system (SNS) and its neurotransmitters, epinephrine, norepinephrine, and dopamine. Changes in resting activity can occur by increasing the activity of either the PNS or the SNS or by decreasing the activity of the opposing system (see Fig. 12–1).

Because these drugs are not organ-specific, when one organ is targeted for therapeutic reasons, the drug simultaneously produces effects in other organs. The targeted organ effects become the desired drug action and the other organ effects become the adverse drug effects.

Drugs that produce these effects are used for a wide variety of diseases and in settings from intensive care to primary care. This chapter focuses on the drugs used in primary care to treat conditions usually managed by nurse practitioners (NPs). Intravenous (IV) forms of the drugs are generally not used in primary care and are not discussed. **Dopamine** and drugs affecting dopamine are discussed in Chapter 13. **Alpha₁** and **alpha₂ agonists** acting peripherally are used mainly as **decongestants,**

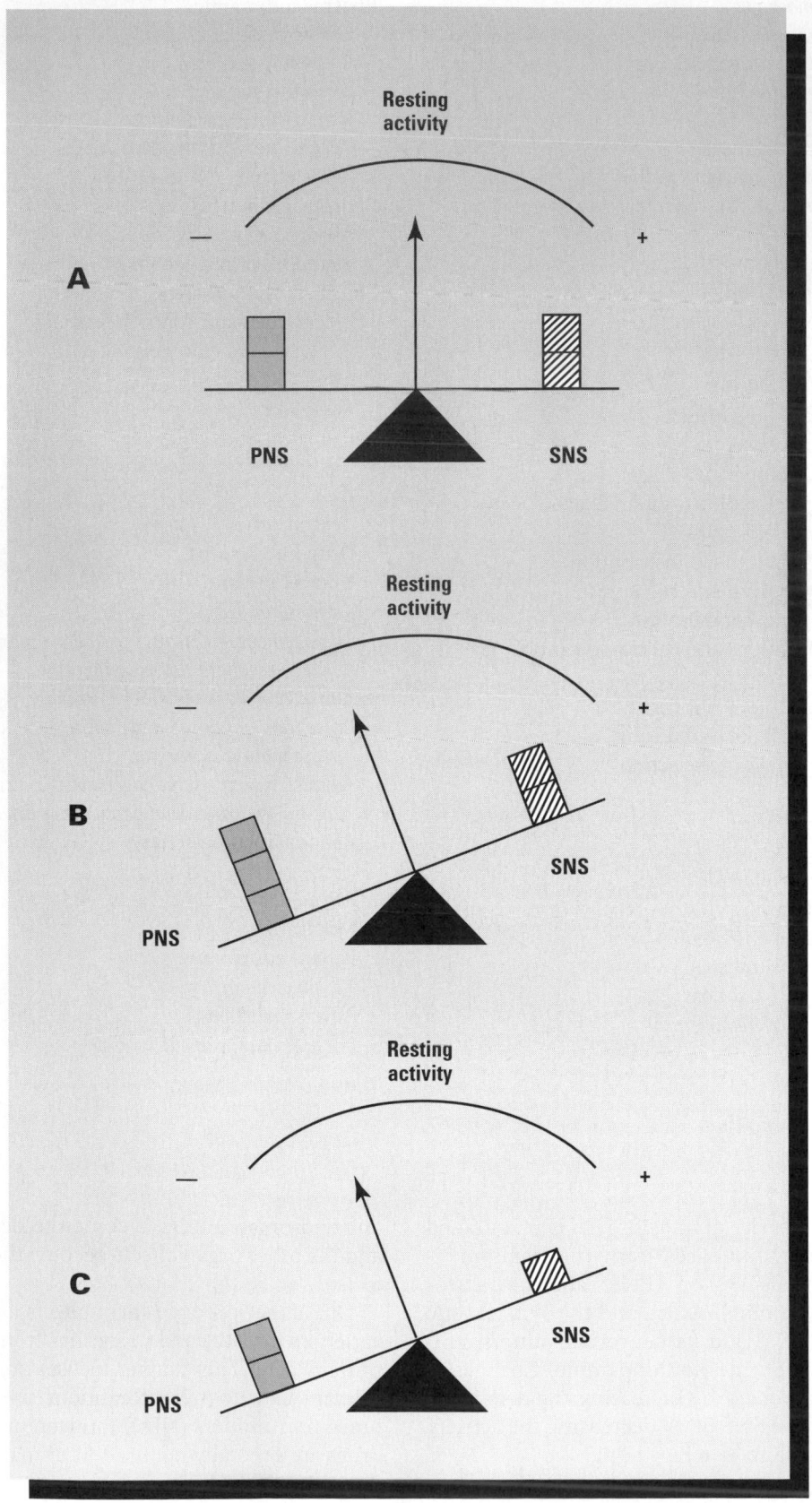

Figure 12–1. Resting activity and the autonomic nervous system.

and **beta agonists** are used mainly for their bronchodilating effects. These drugs are discussed in Chapter 15.

Adrenergic Agonists

Adrenergic agonists act directly on the SNS by: direct receptor binding to organs or tissues, promotion of norepinephrine release, or mimicking the action of norepinephrine or epinephrine. Four receptor types are involved: alpha$_1$, alpha$_2$, beta$_1$, and beta$_2$. Alpha$_1$ receptors are mostly associated with excitation or stimulation and are found mainly in the eye, salivary glands, arterioles, postcapillary venules, and gastrointestinal (GI) and genitourinary (GU) sphincters. Alpha$_2$ receptors are mostly associated with relaxation or inhibition and are located mainly in the nerve terminals of smooth muscle. Beta$_1$ receptors, found mostly in the heart and kidney, are associated with stimulation. Beta$_2$ receptors are located in the eye, arterioles, venules, lungs, liver, pancreas, and GI track. Norepinephrine stimulates all alpha and beta$_1$ receptors. Epinephrine stimulates all four types of receptors. Centrally acting **alpha$_2$ agonists** are the relevant agonist drugs, and they are discussed here (see Table 12–1).

Alpha$_2$ Agonists: Central

Pharmacodynamics

Activation of central alpha$_2$ receptors results in inhibition of cardioacceleration and vasoconstriction centers in the brain. This action causes a decrease in peripheral outflow of norepinephrine, leading to decreases in peripheral resistance, renal vascular resistance, heart rate, and blood pressure. Because they lower blood pressure by altering sympathetic function, they can produce compensatory effects on blood pressure, resulting in retention of sodium and expansion of blood volume through mechanisms that are not dependent on adrenergic nerves. For this reason, they are usually given in combination with a **diuretic**. The drugs in this class, commonly used to treat hypertension, are **clonidine (Catapres), guanabenz (Wytensin), guanfacine (Tenex),** and **methyldopa (Aldomet).** Centrally activating **alpha$_2$ agonists** are used largely as second-line drugs in the treatment of mild to moderate hypertension. **Clonidine** is also used to treat withdrawal symptoms from **heroin, alcohol,** and **nicotine,** based on its ability to lower the adrenergic stimulation that is associated with this withdrawal.

Clonidine activates alpha$_2$ receptors in the medulla of the brain, reducing sympathetic tone and increasing parasympathetic tone, which results in lower blood pressure and bradycardia, particularly when patients are upright. It also directly stimulates peripheral alpha$_2$ receptors in arterioles, resulting in vasodilation and decreased renal vascular resistance with maintenance of renal blood flow. This combination of actions rarely results in postural hypotension. **Clonidine** also binds to a nonadrenergic receptor, the imidazoline receptor, which is considered to be part of the final common pathway for sympathetic vasomotor outflow.

Guanabenz and **guanfacine** also reduce sympathetic outflow by activating alpha$_2$ receptors in the brain but do not directly stimulate peripheral receptors, so that blood pressure is reduced in both the supine and standing positions without alterations in normal postural mechanisms. Postural hypotension has not been observed. Pulse rates are reduced by about 5 beats per minute (bpm).

Methyldopa is an analogue of **L-dopa.** Stimulation of central alpha$_2$ receptors by its active metabolites produces a decrease in sympathetic outflow to the heart, kidney, and blood vessels. The end result is a decrease in blood pressure and peripheral resistance, a slight decrease in heart rate, but no change in cardiac output.

Pharmacokinetics

Absorption and Distribution

Absorption following oral administration varies among the drugs. **Clonidine, guanabenz,** and **guanfacine** are well absorbed (70 to 80%), but **methyldopa** is incompletely absorbed (50%). All of the drugs are widely distributed in body tissues. Both **Clonidine** and **methyldopa** cross the blood-brain barrier and the placenta and are found in breast milk.

Metabolism and Excretion

The liver in varying degrees metabolizes each of these drugs. **Guanfacine** has a significant first-pass effect, with more than 95 percent of the oral dose metabolized to inactive metabolites by the liver. **Methyldopa** is also extensively metabolized to inactive metabolites, with only approximately 17 percent of the active drug appearing in the plasma. The kidney is the organ of excretion for each of these drugs. Table 12–2 shows the pharmacokinetics of these drugs.

Pharmacotherapeutics

Precautions and Contraindications

Cautious use is recommended in the presence of severe coronary insufficiency, recent myocardial infarction (MI), and renal function impairment. Because they cross the blood-brain barrier, **methyldopa** and **clonidine** are used cautiously in the presence of cerebrovascular disease. **Clo-**

Table 12–1. Actions of Autonomic Nervous System Based on Receptor

Organ or Tissue	Receptor	Adrenergic Effect	Cholinergic Effect
Eye (radial muscle)	Alpha$_1$	Contraction (mydriasis)	None
Eye (ciliary muscle)	Beta$_2$	Relaxation for far vision	Contraction for near vision
Eye (sphincter muscle)		None	Contraction (miosis)
Lacrimal glands		None	Secretion
Nasopharyngeal glands		None	Secretion
Salivary glands	Alpha$_1$	Secretion of potassium and water	Secretion of potassium and water
Heart (SA node)	Beta$_1$	Increases heart rate	Decreases heart rate; vagus arrest
Heart (atria)	Beta$_1$	Increases contractility and conduction velocity	Decreases contractility; shortens action potential duration
Heart (AV junction)	Beta$_1$	Increases automaticity and propagation velocity	Decreases automaticity and propagation velocity
Heart (ventricles)	Beta$_1$	Increases contractility	None
Arterioles (coronary)	Alpha$_1$ Beta$_2$	Constriction Dilation	Dilation
Arterioles (skin and mucosa)	Alpha$_1$ and alpha$_2$	Constriction	Dilation
Arterioles (skeletal muscle)	Alpha$_1$ Beta$_2$	Constriction Dilation	Dilation
Arterioles (cerebral)	Alpha$_1$	Constriction (slight)	None
Arterioles (pulmonary)	Alpha$_1$ Beta$_2$	Constriction Dilation	None
Arterioles (renal)	Alpha$_1$ Beta$_1$ and beta$_2$	Constriction Dilation	None
Veins (systemic)	Alpha$_1$ Beta$_2$	Constriction Dilation	None
Platelets	Alpha$_2$	Aggregation	None
Lungs (bronchial muscle)	Beta$_2$	Relaxation	Contraction
Lungs (bronchial glands)	Alpha$_1$ Beta$_2$	Decreases secretion Increases secretion	Stimulation
GI (motility)	Alpha$_1$ and beta$_2$	Decrease	Increase
GI (sphincters)	Alpha$_1$	Contraction	Relaxation
GI (secretion)			Stimulation
Liver	Alpha$_1$, alpha$_2$, and beta$_2$	Glycogenolysis and gluconeogenesis	Glycogen synthesis
Pancreas (islet cells)	Alpha$_2$ Beta$_2$	Decreases secretion Increases secretion	None
Adrenal medulla			Secretion of epinephrine and norepinephrine (nicotinic effect)
Kidney	Alpha$_1$ Beta$_1$	Decreases renin secretion Increases renin secretion	None
Ureter (motility and tone)	Alpha$_1$	Increases	Increases
Urinary bladder (detrusor)	Beta$_2$	Relaxation	Contraction
Urinary bladder (trigone and sphincter)	Alpha$_1$	Contraction	None
Uterus	Beta$_2$	Promotes smooth muscle relaxation	None
Male sex organs	Alpha$_1$	Ejaculation	Erection
Fat cells	Alpha$_2$ Beta$_1$	Inhibition of lipolysis Stimulation of lipolysis	

nidine should not be given to patients who are at risk for mental depression, and it should be discontinued if depression occurs. Because they affect cognitive function, **centrally acting alpha$_2$ agonists** should be avoided or used with extreme caution with older adults and others for whom this adverse response creates a significant problem.

Pregnancy categories vary greatly among these drugs. *Guanabenz* may have adverse fetal effects when given to pregnant women. Skeletal anomalies were found in the offspring of mice that were given this drug. *Clonidine* crosses the placenta with a cord:maternal ratio of 0.89. It is listed as Pregnancy Category

Table 12–2. Pharmacokinetics: Selected Centrally Acting Alpha$_2$ Agonists

Drug	Onset	Peak	Duration	Protein Binding	Bioavail-ability	Half-Life	Elimination
Clonidine	Oral: 30–60 min	Oral: 3–5 h	Oral: 8 h	20–40%		12–16 h; up to 41 h in impaired renal function	40–60% unchanged in urine
	Transdermal: 2–3 d	Transdermal: unknown	Transdermal: 7 d (8 h of effect after patch is removed)				
Guanabenz	60 min	2–5 h	12 h	90%		6 h; prolonged in renal impairment	<1% unchanged in urine
Guanfacine	1 h	1–4 h	24 h	70%	80%	Adults: 17 h Younger adults: 13–14 h Older adults: 17–18 h	50% unchanged in urine 70% in urine unchanged or as metabolites
Methyldopa	2–3 h	2–6 h	12–24 h	8%	50%	1.8 h; blood pressure reduction is pronounced and prolonged in renal failure	

C, and there are no well-controlled studies in pregnant women. *Clonidine* should be used only if clearly needed. *Guanfacine* is listed as Pregnancy Category B but should be used only when clearly needed because of the lack of adequate, well-controlled studies in pregnant women. *Methyldopa* crosses the placenta and achieves fetal concentrations approximately equal to maternal levels; however, no adverse reactions or teratogenic effects have been observed. It is recommended for use with pregnant women.

The American Academy of Pediatrics considers **methyldopa** compatible with breastfeeding. All of the other drugs are not recommended for nursing mothers. **Methyldopa** and **clonidine** have pediatric doses and can be safely used in children younger than 12.

Adverse Drug Reactions

The major adverse reactions are related to the action of the drug on organs other than the targeted organ. They include drowsiness, dry mouth, constipation, and impotence. Cardiac symptoms include hypotension, chest pain, and bradycardia. GI symptoms are more commonly associated with **guanabenz** and additionally include abdominal pain, vomiting, anorexia, and altered taste. Gynecomastia has also been associated with **guanabenz** and **clonidine**. All drugs in this class have also been associated with life-threatening rebound hypertension mediated by increased SNS activity after sudden withdrawal of these drugs. **Clonidine** and **methyldopa** have especially been noted to have this adverse reaction, which is exacerbated if the patient is also taking **beta-adrenergic blockers** (Table 12–3). All patients given these drugs should be warned about this possibility. If the drug must be withdrawn, it should be done gradually. All of the drugs in this class may result in pruritic rashes.

Methyldopa has been associated with development of a positive Coombs' test, usually between 6 and 12 months after initiation of therapy. Rarely, this is associated with hemolytic anemia. The lowest incidence of this problem is reported with doses of less than 1 g. Perform baseline hemoglobin and hematocrit levels, and repeat them at 6 and 12 months after initiation of therapy.

Drug Interactions

All **centrally acting alpha$_2$ agonists** have additive sedation with central nervous sytem (CNS) depressants and additive hypotension with other drugs that also reduce blood pressure. Table 12–3 gives the specific drugs. **Tricyclic antidepressant (TCA) agents** decrease the antihypertensive effects of all **centrally acting alpha$_2$ agonists**. Several other drugs used to treat psychoses interact with **centrally acting alpha$_2$ agonists**, resulting in toxic-

Table 12–3. Drug Interactions: Centrally Acting Alpha₂ Agonists

Drug	Interacting Drug	Possible Effect	Implications
Clonidine	Alcohol, antihistamines, phenothiazines, barbiturates, benzodiazepines	Additive sedation	Avoid concurrent use
	Beta-adrenergic blockers	Attenuation or reversal of antihypertensive effect of clonidine; may result in life-threatening hypertension (HTN)	Avoid concurrent use; if patient is taking both drugs and withdrawal is required, withdraw beta-adrenergic blocker first to prevent excessive unopposed alpha stimulation that may lead to malignant HTN within 12 h
	Nitrates, other antihypertensives	Additive hypotensive effects	Avoid concurrent use
	Prazosin	Decreased antihypertensive effect of clonidine	Choose alternative drug
	TCAs	Block antihypertensive effects of clonidine and may result in life-threatening HTN	Choose alternative antidepressant
	Verapamil	Synergistic pharmacological and toxic effects; may result in atrioventricular block and severe hypotension	Choose alternative calcium channel blocker or antihypertensive
Guanabenz, guanfacine	Alcohol, antihistamines, phenothiazines, barbiturates, benzodiazepines	Additive sedative effects	Avoid concurrent use or choose alternate antihypertensive
	TCAs, NSAIDs	Decrease antihypertensive effects of guanabenz or guanfacine	Choose alternative antihypertensive
	Alcohol, nitrates, other antihypertensives	Additive hypotension	Avoid concurrent use or monitor blood pressure closely
Methyldopa	Alcohol, antihistamines, phenothiazines, barbiturates, benzodiazepines	Additive sedation	Avoid concurrent use
	Beta-adrenergic blockers	May result in life-threatening HTN	Less likely with beta₁ selective agents; see clonidine above for implications
	Haloperidol	Potentiate antipsychotic effects or may produce psychosis	Choose different antipsychotic
	Levodopa	Potentiate antihypertensive effects of methyldopa and central effects of levodopa in Parkinson's disease	Avoid concurrent use; choose alternative antihypertensive
	Lithium	Increased risk for lithium toxicity	Choose alternative antihypertensive
	Monoamine oxidase inhibitors (MAOIs)	Metabolites of methyldopa stimulate release of endogenous catecholamines that are usually metabolized by MAOIs; result is excessive SNS stimulation	Avoid concurrent use
	Nitrates, other antihypertensives	Additive hypotension	Avoid concurrent use
	Phenothiazines, sympathomimetics	May result in serious elevations of blood pressure	Avoid concurrent use

Continued on next page

Table 12–3. Drug Interactions: Centrally Acting Alpha$_2$ Agonists (*continued*)

Drug	Interacting Drug	Possible Effect	Implications
	Tolbutamide	Tolbutamide metabolism may be impaired, resulting in enhanced hypoglycemic effects	Choose alternative hypoglycemic
	TCAs	Attenuation or reversal of antihypertensive effect of methyldopa	Avoid concurrent use; choose alternative drugs for depression or hypertension

ity, psychoses, or excessive SNS stimulation. Careful selection of the drugs to treat each condition is required. **Beta-adrenergic blockers** interact with **clonidine** and **methyldopa** to produce potentially life-threatening hypertension. They should not normally be used concurrently, but there are occasions, such as when **beta-adrenergic blockers** are used for MI prophylaxis, when use of both drugs is necessary. If withdrawal of one or both of these drugs is required because of adverse effects, the **beta-adrenergic blocker** is always withdrawn first to prevent excessive unopposed stimulation of alpha$_2$ receptors that can result in a hypertensive crisis in as little as 12 hours. **Methyldopa** enhances the hypoglycemic effects of **tolbutamide (Orinase)**, which may result in serious hypoglycemia. There are a variety of **oral hypoglycemics** so that an alternative **oral hypoglycemic** can be chosen.

Clinical Use and Dosing

HYPERTENSION. Centrally acting alpha$_2$ agonists are used to treat mild to moderate hypertension and are second-line drugs usually chosen when other drugs are not effective in achieving blood pressure control. The exception is **methyldopa**, which is first-line therapy for pregnant patients. These drugs are not well suited for monotherapy because they produce troublesome adverse reactions in almost all patients who take them. They can be used effectively when combined with a diuretic to address the problems with sodium and water retention.

Doses vary with each drug, but adverse reactions occur at higher doses and with older adults. Beginning with the lowest dose recommended for each drug, the dose is increased at weekly intervals until blood pressure control or the maximum dose is reached. To minimize the sedation, which is more common with **clonidine** and **methyldopa**, the dose may be divided, with a higher dose in the evening than in the morning. Smaller doses are required in renal impairment. Use of the low end of the dose range of **guanfacine** produces the least problems for patients with renal insufficiency.

UNLABELED USES OF CLONIDINE. **Clonidine** has been evaluated for many unlabeled uses. It lowers the adrenergic stimulation associated with **alcohol** and **nicotine** withdrawal and lessens the unpleasant symptoms of withdrawal. Attention-deficit hyperactivity disorder is associated with decreased stimulation of certain centers in the brain, and the stimulation of central alpha$_2$ receptors by **clonidine** has resulted in improved concentration and reduced behavioral symptoms in some children. Dosage schedules for these and other unlabeled uses are presented in Table 12–4.

Rational Drug Selection

AGE. Only **clonidine** and **methyldopa** have pediatric doses and are approved for use with children. **Clonidine** works better in older adults. Dosage reductions may be required for all drugs in this class when prescribed for older adults because of the risk for fluid retention and orthostatic hypotension.

CONCOMITANT DISEASE PROCESSES. Because it does not affect the renin-angiotensin-aldosterone (RAA) axis, **clonidine** works well for patients with decreased renal function. It also does not affect glucose metabolism and is useful for patients with diabetes. **Guanabenz** is not associated with as much fluid retention as **clonidine** and **methyldopa**, making a concurrent **diuretic** less necessary, and it would be preferred in conditions that would be worsened with fluid retention (e.g., congestive heart failure).

PREGNANCY. The Sixth Report of the Joint National Committee on Prevention, Detection, Evaluation, and Treatment of High Blood Pressure (1997) recommends **methyldopa** as the drug of choice for pregnant women. **All other drugs in this class are associated with varying degrees with teratogenesis.**

ROUTE OF ADMINISTRATION. Patients who have difficulty taking pills, who have trouble remembering more frequent doses, or who for other reasons would have better adherence to the treatment regimen with a transdermal system can be given **clonidine**. This drug is the only **antihypertensive** currently available in a transdermal formulation (see Table 12–5).

Table 12–4. Schedule: Centrally Acting Alpha$_2$ Agonists

Drug	Indication	Initial Dose	Maintenance Dose
Clonidine	Hypertension	Adults: 0.1 mg bid PO (older adults may need lower dose)	Adults: Increase in increments of 0.1 mg PO in weekly intervals; maintenance dose 0.1–0.3 mg bid; max dose: 1.2 mg bid
		Transdermal: Catapres-TTS 1 (0.1 mg)	After 1–2 wk, if desired blood pressure (BP) is not achieved, increase in increments of 0.1 mg/wk (Catapres-TTS comes in 2 (0.2 mg) and 3 (0.3 mg) patches)
		Children: 0.05 mg bid	Children: Increase in 0.05-mg increments at weekly intervals; maintenance dose 0.05–0.2 mg bid

	Unlabeled uses:
	  Alcohol withdrawal
	  ADHD
	  Nicotine withdrawal
	  Postherpetic neuralgia
	  Restless leg syndrome
	  Ulcerative colitis
			0.3–0.6 mg q6h
			
			0.005 mg/kg/d for 8 wk
			0.15–0.4 mg/d or 0.2 mg/24 h patch
			0.2 mg/d
			0.1–0.3 mg/d; up to 0.9 mg/d
			0.3 mg tid

Guanabenz	Hypertension	4 mg bid	Increase in increments of 4–8 mg/d every 1–2 wk until target BP achieved; max dose 32 mg bid
Guanfacine	Hypertension	1 mg qd at bedtime	May increase to 2 mg qd after 3–4 wk if target BP not achieved; 2-mg dose may be given as 1 mg bid; max dose 3 mg qd
Methyldopa	Hypertension	Adults: 250 mg bid or tid for first 48 h	Increase in increments of 250 mg every 2 d until target BP is achieved; to minimize sedation, increase dose in evening; smaller doses should be used in renal impairment; maintenance dose 500–2000 mg/d in 2–4 divided doses
		Children: 10 mg/kg/d in 2–4 divided doses	Children: max dose is 65 mg/kg or 3000 mg, whichever is less

Monitoring

Clinical monitoring of blood pressure is appropriate for all drugs in this class as with any other **antihypertensive** drug. Baseline blood pressure should be taken before initiating therapy and with each change in dosage. Weight and other indicators of fluid status should also be monitored. See Chapter 38 for further discussion of blood pressure monitoring.

For patients who have or are at risk for renal impairment, dosage alterations are required. Assess serum creatinine prior to initiation of therapy and regularly thereafter for up to 1 year.

Methyldopa is associated with a risk for development of hemolytic anemia. A forewarning of this development is a positive Coombs' test between 6 and 12 months after initiation of therapy. Patients receiving this drug should have a baseline Coombs' test and complete blood count (CBC) done prior to initiation of therapy and at 6

and 12 months of therapy. Although only about 5 percent of patients who develop the positive Coombs' test go on to develop hemolytic anemia, the drug is withdrawn in the presence of a positive test. Hemolytic anemia resolves soon after the withdrawal, even though the Coombs' test may remain positive for several months.

Liver function studies are also done prior to therapy and at 6 and 12 months. **Methyldopa** has been associated with hepatotoxicity. Liver function usually returns to normal after withdrawal of the drug.

Patient Education

ADMINISTRATION. The drug should be taken exactly as prescribed, at the same time each day, even if the patient is feeling well. Missed doses are taken as soon as they are remembered unless it is almost time for the next dose. Doses are not doubled. If more than one oral dose of any of these drugs is late or if the **clonidine** transdermal sys-

Table 12–5. Available Dosage Forms: Selected Centrally Acting Alpha$_2$ Agonists

Drug	Dosage Form	Package
Clonidine (Catapres)	Tablets: 0.1 mg (scored) 0.2 mg (scored) 0.3 mg (scored)	In bottles of 100, 500, 1000 tablets and in unit dose In bottles of 100, 500, 1000 tablets and in unit dose In bottles of 100 tablets and in unit dose
Clonidine (Catapres-TTS)	Transdermal: Catapres-TTS 1: 0.1 mg/24 h Catapres-TTS 2: 0.2 mg/24 h Catapres-TTS 3: 0.3 mg/24 h	In packages of 12 In packages of 12 In packages of 4
Guanabenz (Wytensin)	Tablets: 4 mg 8 mg	In bottles of 100, 500 tablets (Wytensin in Redipak 100s) In bottles of 100, 500 tablets
Guanfacine (Tenex)	Tablets: 1 mg 2 mg	In bottles of 100, 500 tablets In bottles of 100 tablets
Methyldopa (Aldomet)	Tablets: 125 mg 250 mg 500 mg Oral suspension: 50 mg/cc	In bottles of 100 tablets In bottles of 100, 500, 1000 tablets and in unit dose In bottles of 100, 500 tablets and in unit dose In 473 cc orange-pineapple flavor

tem is changed 3 or more days late, report this to the health care provider. These drugs must be withdrawn slowly over 2 to 3 days to prevent rebound hypertension, and missed doses increase the risk for the occurrence of rebound hypertension. To prevent missing doses, patients should make certain they have enough medication available for weekends, holidays, and vacations.

Nonsteroidal anti-inflammatory drugs (NSAIDs) decrease the antihypertensive effects of **guanabenz** and **guanfacine.** Over-the-counter (OTC) medications that contain NSAIDs should be avoided. Advise patients to consult their health care provider before taking any OTC drug, especially cough, cold, and allergy remedies.

Instruct patients who are on the transdermal **clonidine** system in proper application of the patch. They should not cut or trim the patch. It can remain in place during bathing and swimming.

ADVERSE REACTIONS. Hypotension is the most common adverse reaction. Changing positions slowly, not exercising in hot weather, avoiding alcohol, and drinking more than 2 L of noncaffeinated fluid per day will decrease these reactions.

Drowsiness and dry mouth are also common. Avoid activities requiring mental alertness until the patient's individual response to the drug is known. Drowsiness frequently subsides after 7 to 10 days of continuous therapy. Dry mouth can be minimized by good oral hygiene, chewing sugarless gum, or sucking on hard candy.

Concurrent use of **alcohol** or other **CNS depressants** should also be avoided. **Centrally acting alpha$_2$ agonists** can produce additive sedation with these drugs.

Fluid retention is indicated by weight gain and swelling in the feet and ankles. Report any weight gain of more than 2 lb in 1 day to the health care provider. Fluid retention may be treated by the addition of a **diuretic** to the treatment regimen.

Methyldopa has some unique adverse reactions. Jaundice may indicate hepatotoxicity and should be reported to the health care provider. Decreased energy levels may indicate anemia. In the absence of another explanation for decreased energy, this symptom should also be reported to the health care provider. Warn the patient that urine left standing may darken or turn red-black. This does not indicated hematuria.

LIFESTYLE MANAGEMENT. Drugs control hypertension, but they do not cure it. Encourage patients to adhere to other interventions for management of hypertension such as weight loss, aerobic exercise, a low-sodium diet, smoking cessation, and stress management.

Adrenergic Antagonists

Adrenergic antagonists act directly by blockade of adrenergic receptors or indirectly by decreasing norepinephrine release within SNS terminals. Most of the clinically useful actions of these drugs result from blockade of alpha$_1$ receptors in blood vessels, beta$_1$ receptors in the heart, and alpha$_1$ receptors in the bladder neck and prostate gland. **Adrenergic antagonists** are categorized on the basis of receptors that are blocked and include drugs that block only one receptor and those that block more than one receptor. This section discusses **antagonist drugs** whose major effect is on alpha$_1$ and beta receptors outside the CNS (peripherally acting).

Alpha₁ Antagonists

Although they are capable of blocking the vasoconstricting effects of catecholamines and of lowering blood pressure, the tendency of **alpha₁ antagonists** to produce orthostatic hypotension has limited their use in treating essential hypertension. **Alpha₁ antagonists** are also used clinically for treatment of pheochromocytoma and in the symptomatic management of benign prostatic hyperplasia (BPH). Six drugs in this class are used clinically: **doxazosin (Cardura), prazosin (Minipress), terazosin (Hytrin), tamsulosin (Flomax), phentolamine (Regitine),** and **phenoxybenzamine (Dibenzyline).** The first four drugs selectively block alpha₁ receptors in a reversible manner. **Doxazosin, prazosin,** and **terazosin** are used to treat hypertension and in the management of outflow obstruction secondary to BPH. **Tamsulosin** is used only to manage outflow obstruction secondary to BPH. **Phentolamine** reversibly blocks both alpha₁ and alpha₂ receptors, and its use is limited to treatment of pheochromocytoma and prevention of tissue necrosis following extravasation of drugs that produce alpha₁-mediated vasoconstriction. **Phenoxybenzamine** irreversibly blocks both alpha₁ and alpha₂ receptors. It is approved only for the treatment of pheochromocytoma. Because the latter two drugs are used almost exclusively by specialists and not in a primary care setting, they are not discussed here.

Pharmacodynamics

Reversible **alpha₁ antagonists** block postsynaptic alpha₁ receptors in the vasculature, resulting in a decrease in both arterial and venous vasoconstriction. Because arteriole and venous tone are determined largely by the stimulation of alpha₁ receptors in vascular smooth muscle, the result is a decrease in peripheral vascular resistance and lowered blood pressure. Both supine and standing blood pressures are lowered, with the most pronounced effect on diastolic blood pressure. Orthostatic hypotension may result from their action on receptors in venous smooth muscle. Reflex tachycardia may result from compensatory mechanisms but is minimal. **Prazosin** and **terazosin** rarely produce reflex tachycardia. Chronic use of **alpha₁ antagonists** may result in compensatory increases in blood volume through sodium and water retention. **Tamsulosin** has not been approved for treatment of hypertension.

The reduction in symptoms and improved urine flow rates in patients with BPH is related to relaxation of smooth muscle produced by blockade of the alpha₁ receptors in the bladder neck and prostate gland. Because there are few alpha₁ receptors in the body of the bladder, these drugs are able to reduce bladder outflow obstruction without affecting bladder contractility. **Tamsulosin** is a competitive alpha₁ receptor antagonist with a structure very different from other **alpha₁ antagonists,** but it also acts by preventing contraction of prostate gland smooth muscle.

Pharmacokinetics

Absorption and Distribution

All four drugs are well absorbed after oral administration (Table 12–6), although **tamsulosin** is more slowly absorbed. All are widely distributed in the body. **Doxazosin** accumulates in breast milk with a concentration 20 times that in maternal plasma. **Prazosin** is found in small amounts in breast milk, and it is not known if **terazosin** is excreted in breast milk. No information about breast milk concentration is provided for **tamsulosin,** which would not be given to female patients.

Metabolism and Excretion

Extensively metabolized by the liver, reversible **alpha₁ antagonists** are excreted in both feces and urine. Elimination of **prazosin** is slower in patients with congestive heart failure (CHF) than in normal individuals. In the presence of renal failure, elimination half-life of this drug

Table 12–6. Selected Alpha₁-Adrenergic Antagonists

Drug	Onset	Peak	Duration	Protein Binding	Bioavailability	Half-Life	Elimination
Doxazosin	60–120 min	2–3 h	24 h	98%	65%	22 h	63% in bile/feces; 9% in urine
Prazosin	120–130 min	1–3 h	6–12 h	92–97%	48–68%	2–3 h	90% in bile/feces; 10% in urine
Tamsulosin	Unknown	5 d	Unknown	94–99%	>90%	9–15 h	<10% unchanged in urine
Terazosin	15 min	1–2 h	12–24 h	90–94%	90%	9–12 h	60% in bile/feces; 40% in urine

may be prolonged, protein binding decreased, and peak plasma levels increased.

Pharmacotherapeutics

Precautions and Contraindications

All the "**azosin**" drugs are contraindicated in the presence of volume depletion and CHF. Peripheral vasodilation caused by these drugs decreases venous return to the heart and may precipitate significant heart failure. All four drugs are associated with fluid retention that may exacerbate CHF.

Administer all four drugs with caution to patients with hepatic impairment or on other drugs known to influence hepatic metabolism. They are all extensively metabolized by the liver.

Doxazosin, prazosin, and *terazosin* **are Pregnancy Category C. Teratogenicity and reduced fertility have been demonstrated in animal studies. There are no adequate and well-controlled studies in pregnant women. Because of its high concentration in breast milk,** *doxazosin* **should not be given to nursing mothers.** *Prazosin* **has also been found in breast milk. Exercise caution when administering** *prazosin* **or** *terazosin* **to nursing mothers, and do so only when benefits clearly outweigh risks to the baby.** *Tamsulosin* **is not prescribed to female patients.**

Safety and efficacy for use with children have not been established. *Drug Facts and Comparisons* (1998) provides a suggested dose of **prazosin** that can be used to treat hypertension in children.

Adverse Drug Reactions

Each of these drugs carries a risk for significant first-dose orthostatic hypotension that may result in syncope and tends to occur within 30 to 90 minutes of drug administration. This adverse reaction is decreased with continued doses, but returns if therapy is interrupted for even a few doses, if the dosage is increased, or if another **antihypertensive** is added to the treatment regimen. The first dose should be given in the clinic or taken at bedtime. The "first-dose" reaction may be minimized by starting with a 1-mg dose and slowly increasing the dosage at 2-week intervals (see Table 12–8). **Terazosin** exhibits this reaction most often, **prazosin** is average, and it occurs least with **doxazosin.**

Fluid retention that results in peripheral edema is also common to all these drugs. Close monitoring of weight changes may be needed, especially early in therapy, and the addition of a diuretic to the therapy regimen is often required.

Other adverse reactions are associated with alpha$_1$ adrenergic blockade (nasal congestion, blurred vision, dry mouth, constipation, impotence, and urinary frequency) or with hypotension (dizziness, headache, fatigue, tachycardia, and nausea).

Drug Interactions

The major drug interactions result in decreased antihypertensive effects with the interacting drug or in additive hypotension, with increased risk for postural hypotension. All four drugs have increased risk for postural hypotension when administered with acute **alcohol** ingestion, other **antihypertensives,** or **nitrates.** **Doxazosin** has the fewest published drug interactions and **prazosin** has the most. **Cimetidine** interacts with **tamsulosin** to decrease **tamsulosin's** effects. Table 12–7 depicts the common drug interactions.

Clinical Use and Dosing

HYPERTENSION. **Alpha$_1$-adrenergic antagonists** are the drugs of choice for treating hypertension in older men with concomitant BPH. Their actions simultaneously improve both conditions. They are also effective for African Americans, although not the first-line drugs. All drugs in this class reduce total cholesterol and triglycerides and raise high-density lipoprotein levels. **Doxazosin** and **terazosin** also lower low-density lipoprotein levels. This class of drugs is useful for patients with hypertension who also have altered lipoprotein levels. They also enhance insulin sensitivity, cause regression of left ventricular hypertrophy, and improve the activity of the fibrinolytic system, making them useful for patients with diabetes and heart failure. Because they do not aggravate bronchospastic disease, they are useful for patients with asthma. **Alpha$_1$-adrenergic antagonists** are usually not used for monotherapy because they cause troublesome adverse reactions in almost all patients who take them. They can be use effectively in combination with other drugs that address these adverse reactions.

To reduce "first-dose" postural hypotension, the adult dose is begun at 1 mg qd to bid, depending on the drug (Table 12–8). **Prazosin** has a suggested starting dose of 0.5 mg tid (*Drug Facts and Comparisons,* 1998) for children. No other drug in this class is suggested for children.

The dose is then gradually increased until target blood pressure is achieved or the maximum dose reached. When the dose is increased, the first larger dose is always given at bedtime. **Doxazosin** has once-daily dosing. Postural hypotension effects are most commonly seen 2 to 6 hours after taking a dose. Measure the blood pressure at this time interval for the first dose and when increasing the dose to determine if the target blood pressure is being reached. **Prazosin** has a bid or tid dosing schedule. Measure blood pressure 2 to 3 hours after dosing to see when maximum and minimum benefits in blood pressure lowering result. If the response is substantially diminished at 24 hours on

Table 12–7. Drug Interactions: Selected Alpha$_1$-Adrenergic Antagonists

Drug	Interacting Drug	Possible Effect	Implications
Doxazosin	Clonidine	May decrease antihypertensive effect of clonidine	Avoid concurrent use.
Prazosin	Beta-adrenergic blockers	May enhance acute postural hypotension following first dose of alpha$_1$-adrenergic blocker	Select different alpha$_1$-adrenergic blocker. No adverse reaction seen with doxazosin or terazosin.
	Indomethacin	Antihypertensive action of prazosin may be decreased	Select different alpha$_1$-adrenergic blocker or different NSAID. No adverse reaction with doxazosin or other NSAIDs.
	Verapamil	Increases serum prazosin levels and may increase sensitivity to prazosin-induced postural hypotension	Avoid concurrent use.
Tamsulosin	Cimetidine	May increase blood levels of tamsulosin, with increased risk for hypotension and toxicity	Select different histamine$_2$ blocker if one must be used.
Terazosin	NSAIDs, sympatho-mimetics, estrogens	May decrease antihypertensive effects of terazosin	Avoid concurrent use or select doxazosin or another drug class for antihypertensive therapy.
	Finasteride	Increase in peak plasma concentration and AUC of finasteride	Clinical significance unknown; monitor for adverse effects of finasteride.
Doxazosin, prazosin, tamsulosin, terazosin	Alcohol, antihyper-tensives, nitrates	Additive hypotension	Avoid concurrent use or administer first dose in the office and monitor blood pressure response closely.

AUC = area under curve.

bid dosing, consider increasing the dose or using a tid regimen. Measure blood pressure 2 to 3 hours after dosing for **terazosin** as well. Although **terazosin** usually has once-daily dosing, if the response is diminished, consider bid dosing. When a **diuretic** is added to the treatment regimen of any of these drugs, the dose of the **alpha$_1$-adrenergic antagonist** is reduced for 2 to 3 days and then retitrated to control the blood pressure.

Rational Drug Selection

COST. Prazosin is the least expensive of this drug class. **Terazosin** is the most expensive, and **doxazosin** is in the middle for cost. **Doxazosin** is less likely than the other two drugs to produce postural hypotension and fluid retention, however, and may be used as monotherapy. The overall cost of the treatment regimen for this drug is reduced because an additional drug is unnecessary.

CONVENIENT DOSING. Both **doxazosin** and **terazosin** offer once-daily dosing (Table 12–9). **Prazosin** requires bid or tid dosing. **Doxazosin** is scored to allow the tablet to be broken in half so that dosages can be easily increased without a change in tablet size.

TACHYPHYLAXIS. Although all drugs in this class may exhibit tachyphylaxis to their antihypertensive effects, **prazosin** is especially noted for this problem and frequently requires increased dosages over time.

INDICATIONS. Doxazosin, prazosin, and terazosin are all approved to treat hypertension. Treatment of BPH symptoms is approved FDA only for **doxazosin, tamsulosin,** and **terazosin,** although dosage data for this indication are published for **prazosin.**

Monitoring

Clinical monitoring of symptoms according to guidelines for hypertension (see Chapter 38) and for BPH is the main monitoring parameter. Fluid retention is monitored by weekly weighing and patient education about signs and symptoms of fluid overload to report (e.g., pe-

Table 12–8. Dosage Schedule: Selected Alpha$_1$-Adrenergic Antagonists

Drug	Indication	Initial Dose	Maintenance Dose
Doxazosin	Hypertension	1 mg qd at bedtime	2–16 mg qd. Depending upon standing blood pressure (BP), increase dose in 2-mg increments until target BP is achieved. Doses >4 mg increase risk of postural hypotension.
	BPH	1 mg qd at bedtime	1–8 mg qd. Depending on the urodynamics and BPH symptomatology, the dose is increased to 2 mg and then to 4 mg and 8 mg/d. The recommended maximum dose is 8 mg. The titration interval is 1–2 wk.
Prazosin	Hypertension	Adults: 1–2 mg bid or tid; take first dose at bedtime	Adults: 6–15 mg/d in 2–3 divided doses. Depending upon standing BP, increase dose in 1-mg increments, with the larger dose being given at bedtime until target BP is achieved. Doses >20 mg/d usually do not increase efficacy. Children: 0.5–7 mg tid.
	BPH	Children: 0.5 mg tid 1 mg bid	1–5 mg bid. Depending on urodynamics and BPH symptomatology, increase dose in 1-mg increments. Maximum dose is 7 mg.
Tamsulosin	BPH	0.4 mg qd following a meal	May be increased after 2–4 wk to 0.8 mg qd.
Terazosin	Hypertension	1 mg qd at bedtime	1–5 mg qd. Depending upon standing BP, increase dose in 1-mg increments until target BP is achieved. Doses above 20 mg/d do not increase efficacy.
	BPH	1 mg qd at bedtime	Increased in a stepwise fashion to 2, 5, then 10 mg. Doses of 10 mg are usually required for clinical effect. Dose may be 10–20 mg qd. Four to 6 wk are required to assess for beneficial response, so this is the interval for dosage adjustment.

Table 12–9. Available Dosage Forms of Selected Alpha$_1$-Adrenergic Antagonists

Drug	Dosage Form	Package
Doxazosin (Cardura)	Tablets: 1 mg, 2 mg, 4 mg, 8 mg	In bottles of 100 scored tablets
Prazosin (Minipress)	Generic capsules: 1 mg, 2 mg, 5 mg	In bottles of 30, 60, 90, 100, 120, 250, 500, 1000 capsules
	Minipress capsules: 1 mg, 2 mg, 5 mg	In bottles of 250, 1000 capsules
Tamsulosin (Flomax)	Capsules: 0.4 mg	In bottles of 100, 1000 capsules
Terazosin (Hytrin)	Capsules: 1 mg, 2 mg, 5 mg, 10 mg	In bottles of 100 capsules

ripheral edema, weight gain of more than 1 kg in a 24-hour period). Reduced white blood cell (WBC) counts of 1 to 2.4 percent have been noted, although no patients became symptomatic with these lower counts. A baseline WBC is drawn prior to initiation of therapy and as part of regular physical examinations. This class of drugs is heavily metabolized by the liver, so baseline liver function tests are also recommended.

Cancer of the prostate gland and BPH often coexist and have the same symptoms. Patients who are to begin on **alpha₁-adrenergic antagonist** therapy for BPH should first have digital rectal examinations and prostate-specific antigen (PSA) levels drawn to rule out prostate cancer. Research has indicated that **doxazosin** and **terazosin** do not affect PSA levels in patients treated for less than 3 years (*Drug Facts and Comparisons,* 1998).

Patient Education

ADMINISTRATION.   The drug should be taken exactly as prescribed, at the same time each day, even if the patient is feeling well. The first dose at initiation of therapy and the first dose each time the dosage is increased should be taken at bedtime to minimize the first-dose effect. Missed doses are taken as soon as they are remembered unless it is almost time for the next dose. Doses are not doubled. All drugs in this class may be taken without regard to food intake.

The **NSAIDs** decrease the antihypertensive effects of most drugs in this class. OTC medications that contain **NSAIDs** should be avoided. Advise the patient to consult the health care provider before taking any OTC drug, especially cough, cold, and allergy remedies.

If the drug is given for BPH, teach the patient the signs and symptoms of BPH to monitor (urinary frequency, a feeling of incomplete bladder emptying, interruption of urinary stream, decreased size and force of stream, terminal urinary dribbling, and straining to start the flow of urine). Improvement in these symptoms may take 4 to 6 weeks.

ADVERSE DRUG REACTIONS.   Hypotensive reactions are the most common. In addition to taking the first dose at bedtime, teach patients to rise slowly from a supine position and to dangle their feet over the side of the bed before arising. Not exercising in hot weather and main-

taining a fluid intake of 2 L per day of noncaffeinated fluids can also decrease these reactions.

Larger volumes of fluid may exacerbate another common adverse reaction: fluid retention. The best assessment of excessive fluid is weight gain. Report gains of more than 2 lb in 1 day or swelling of the ankles to the health care provider.

Nasal congestion may occur. It should not be treated with OTC **antihistamines** or other cold remedies without first consulting with the health care provider. Drowsiness and dry mouth are also common. The patient should avoid activities requiring mental alertness until the patient's individual response to the drug is known. Drowsiness frequently subsides after 7 to 10 days of continuous therapy. Dry mouth can be minimized by good oral hygiene, chewing sugarless gum, or sucking on hard candy.

The leading cause of nonadherence to a treatment regimen with **alpha₁-adrenergic antagonists** is inhibition of ejaculation and impotence. These reactions should be reported to the health care provider, who may choose a different drug to treat the disorder or change the dosage.

LIFESTYLE MANAGEMENT.   If the drug is being given for hypertension, encourage the patient to adhere to additional interventions for reduction of blood pressure, such as weight loss, low-sodium diet, smoking cessation, regular exercise, and stress management. Further discussion of patient education is in Chapter 38.

Beta-Adrenergic Antagonists (Blockers)

Beta-adrenergic antagonists (blockers) are mainstays in the treatment of hypertension and cardiac disorders. They are also useful in a variety of other disorders, including glaucoma, migraine headache prophylaxis, and hyperthyroidism. They act by occupying beta receptor sites and competitively preventing occupancy of these sites by catecholamines and other beta agonists. A major difference among these drugs is their selectivity for beta₁ and beta₂ receptor sites, and this difference has important clinical implications. Another clinically useful difference among these drugs is the presence in some of them of intrinsic sympathomimetic activity (ISA), which provides a partial agonist effect.

Clinical Pearl

Patients may have difficulty understanding how best to determine changes in force of urine stream. Try asking if they have to stand closer to the toilet when voiding.

ON THE HORIZON

Alfuzosin

Alfuzosin, an alpha₁ selective quinazoline derivative, is under investigation for use in the treatment of BPH. It is efficacious in blocking alpha₁ receptors in prostate smooth muscle.

The action of these drugs is through blockade of beta-adrenergic receptors, and they are usually referred to in health care literature as **beta blockers.** Because this term is easily recognized, **beta blockers** is used throughout this text to denote **beta-adrenergic antagonists.**

Pharmacodynamics

Blockade of beta-adrenergic receptors produces clinically significant action on the cardiovascular, renal, and respiratory systems and on the eye. This blockade also results in metabolic and endocrine effects.

Cardiovascular Effects

The heart has mainly beta₁ receptors. Blockade of these receptors acts at the sinoatrial (SA) node to decrease heart rate (negative chronotropism), in the atria and ventricles to decrease contractility (negative inotropism) and conduction velocity (negative dromotropism), and at the atrioventricular (AV) junction to decrease automaticity and propagation velocity. Taken together, these effects decrease the incidence of angina, decrease cardiac rhythm disturbances associated with rapid rhythms, decrease both supine and standing blood pressure, and reduce reflex orthostatic tachycardia. In patients whose severely damaged hearts require sympathetic stimulation for adequate ventricular function, beta blockade may worsen the condition.

In the vascular system, beta blockade opposes beta₂-mediated vasodilation and may initially result in a rise in peripheral vascular resistance, but chronic drug administration leads to a fall in peripheral resistance through a central effect that causes reduced sympathetic outflow to the periphery. These effects are central to the use of these drugs in the treatment of hypertension.

Renal Effects

Blockade of the beta₁ receptors in the juxtaglomerular apparatus of the kidney reduces the release of renin. This effect on the RAA system leads to less angiotensin II–mediated vasoconstriction and aldosterone-mediated volume expansion, resulting in decreases in blood pressure.

Respiratory Effects

Beta₂ receptors are located throughout the body. In the lungs, blockade of these receptors interferes with endogenous adrenergic bronchodilator activity, which results in passive bronchial constriction. This increase in airway resistance is particularly problematic for patients with reactive airway diseases such as asthma.

Ocular Effects

Although beta₂ stimulation results in changes in pupil size and accommodation, **beta blockers** administered topically as ophthalmic solutions have little or no effect on pupillary muscles. The exact mechanism by which these drugs reduce intraocular pressure is not established but is thought to be achieved by reduction in the production of aqueous humor. Some studies have shown a slight increase in outflow facility with **timolol (Timoptic).** Topical use of **beta blockers** is discussed in Chapter 24.

Metabolic and Endocrine Effects

Beta₂ blockade effects on the liver lead to inhibition of lipolysis, resulting in increased triglycerides and cholesterol and decreased high-density lipoproteins. For patients with hyperlipidemia, beta₂ blockade may worsen the condition.

Effects on the liver also lead to inhibition of gluconeogenesis. **Beta blocker** action on the pancreas results in decreased insulin secretion. Taken together, these actions may impair recovery from hypoglycemia in patients with diabetes. **Beta₁ selective drugs** are less likely to cause these problems.

Effects on Other Systems

The effect of beta blockade on other body systems is the source of the adverse drug reactions that may cause nonadherence to the drug regimen. These effects include contraction of the detrusor muscle of the bladder that may result in urinary frequency and vascular effects on the male sex organs that may result in impotence. Increased GI motility may contribute to diarrhea.

Pharmacokinetics

Absorption and Distribution

All **beta blockers** are well absorbed when given orally and are widely distributed in body tissues (Table 12–10). All cross the placenta and enter breast milk. CNS penetration varies, based on lipid solubility, from no penetration for **timolol**, to minimal penetration for **acebutolol** and **atenolol**, moderate penetration for **nadolol**, **pindolol**, and **propranolol**, and more penetration for **metoprolol**.

Metabolism and Excretion

All **beta blockers** undergo hepatic metabolism, but some have significant first-pass effects (**acebutolol, pindolol, propranolol, metoprolol, timolol**). Bioavailability also varies significantly. **Propranolol extended release** has the lowest at 9 to 15 percent. Most have bioavailabilities around 50 percent.

All **beta blockers** have renal excretion, and some are also excreted to some degree in feces and bile (**acebutolol, atenolol, timolol**). Those with an alternate route to renal excretion are more appropriately used for patients with renal impairment.

Pharmacotherapeutics

Precautions and Contraindications

Beta blockers are contraindicated for patients with respiratory conditions that include a bronchospastic component. Although there are **beta$_1$ selective drugs** that have less effect on the beta$_2$ receptors in the lungs, to date no **beta blocker** is sufficiently selective to beta$_1$ to completely reduce the risk of beta$_2$ blockade. Even **beta$_1$ selective drugs** show beta$_2$ effects at higher doses. *Drug Facts and Comparisons* (1998) suggests that low doses of **acebutolol, atenolol,** and **metoprolol** may be cautiously used for patients with bronchospastic disease who do not respond to any other hypertensive treatment.

These drugs are also contraindicated for patients with heart failure and AV block, where their actions to decrease heart rate and myocardial contractility result in increased reduction in cardiac output and worsened failure. Decreased cardiac output and the initial vasoconstrictive action of these drugs may also worsen peripheral vascular diseases.

Older adults often have limited cardiac and renal reserves. **Beta blockers** are used to treat conditions common to older adults, but care must be taken with dosing, and closer monitoring of cardiac and renal status is required.

Table 12–10. Pharmacokinetics: Selected Beta Blockers

Drug	Onset	Peak	Duration	Protein Binding	Bioavail-ability	Half-Life	Elimination
Acebutolol*	60 min	4–6 h	24–30 h	26%	<50%	3–4h; (8–13 h for diacetolol, the active metabolite)	30–40% in urine; 50–60% in feces/bile
Atenolol	60 min	2–4 h	24 h	6–16%	50–60%	6–9 h	50% unchanged in urine; rest in feces
Metoprolol	15 min	90 min	13–19 h	12%	50–77%	3–7 h	<5% unchanged in urine
Nadolol	5d**	3–4 h	17–24 h	30%	30–50%	20–40 h	Unchanged in urine
Pindolol*	7d**	1 h	24 h	40%	100%	3–4 h	60–65% metabolites and 35–40% unchanged drug in urine
Propranolol	30 min	60–90 min	6–12 h	90%	30%	3–5 h	<1% unchanged in urine
Propranolol ER	UK	6 h	24 h	90%	9–18%	8–11 h	<1% unchanged in urine
Timolol	UK	1–3 h	12–24 h	10%	75%	4 h	Metabolites and unchanged drug in urine

*Intrinsic sympathomimetic activity. Pindolol more than acebutolol.
** = onset of cardiovascular effects
UK = unknown

Clinical Pearl

For patients with diabetes who must take a **beta blocker,** the diaphoresis associated with hypoglycemia is not masked by these drugs. Patients should be taught to recognize this indication of possible hypoglycemia and test their blood glucose levels whenever unexplained diaphoresis occurs.

Because of their effects on carbohydrate metabolism and their ability to mask the common symptoms of hypoglycemia, **beta blockers** must be used cautiously for patients with diabetes. If **beta blockers** must be used, beta$_1$ selective drugs are less likely to produce these problematic effects.

Beta blockers may also mask clinical signs of developing or continuing thyrotoxicosis, and abrupt withdrawal may precipitate hyperthyroidism, including thyroid storm. They are used with caution in patients at risk for developing or having hyperthyroidism. In contrast, **propranolol** may be useful in decreasing the symptoms of thyrotoxicosis and has been used for this purpose, although it is not FDA approved.

Beta blockers **are Pregnancy Category C. Embryotoxic effects have been identified in animals. All cross the placenta and can cause fetal or neonatal bradycardia, hypotension, hypoglycemia, or respiratory depression. If these drugs must be used, avoid use during the first trimester, use the lowest dose that produces a therapeutic effect, and discontinue the drug at least 2 to 3 days prior to delivery. Beta$_1$ selective drugs or drugs with ISA appear to be somewhat less problematic in this regard, and *acebutolol* and *pindolol* are listed as Pregnancy Category B. Note, however, that neonates of mothers who received these latter drugs had reduced birth weight and decreased blood pressure and heart rate at birth.**

Propranolol is excreted in breast milk, but with a concentration too low to have any significant effect. **Metoprolol** is excreted in very small quantities. All other **beta blockers** are excreted in larger amounts. Although adverse effects to infants have not been demonstrated, nursing mothers should be given these drugs only when benefits clearly outweigh risks.

Safety and efficacy in children have not been established. **Propranolol** does have a pediatric dose schedule for children with hypertension.

Adverse Drug Reactions

Beta blockade affects target organs and nontarget organs and tissues alike. This wide range of effects results in many adverse reactions for these drugs. The discussion here focuses on the adverse reactions on each organ system.

CARDIOVASCULAR. Bradycardia, CHF with concomitant pulmonary edema, peripheral vasoconstriction, and hypotension are the most common cardiovascular adverse reactions. They have been discussed here in the Precautions and Contraindications section.

CENTRAL NERVOUS SYSTEM AND PSYCHIATRIC. Fatigue, weakness, and dizziness are associated with reduced oxygen transport to the brain secondary to excessive hypotension. Anxiety, depression, drowsiness, insomnia, nightmares, and mental status changes are more common in those drugs that have higher CNS penetration and in older adults. These adverse reactions may disappear when a less lipophilic **beta blocker** is substituted.

ENDOCRINE. Alterations in carbohydrate metabolism resulting in hyperglycemia, hypoglycemia, or unstable diabetes have been discussed in the Precautions and Contraindications section.

GASTROINTESTINAL. Dry mouth is common. It may be reduced by good oral hygiene, chewing sugarless gum, or sucking on hard candy. Changes in GI motility may result in anorexia, nausea, vomiting, flatulence, and constipation or diarrhea.

GENITOURINARY. One of the most likely reasons for nonadherence to a treatment regimen that includes **beta blockers** is the risk for impotence and decreased libido, based on the action of the drugs on the male sexual organs. Effects on the detrusor muscle of the bladder may produce urinary frequency.

RESPIRATORY. Bronchospasm and dyspnea have been discussed in the Precautions and Contraindications section. Nasal stuffiness may also occur.

OTHERS. Less common adverse reactions include muscle and joint pain, pruritic rashes, and facial swelling. These are not directly related to the actions of these drugs.

Drug, Food, and Laboratory Test Interactions

DRUG INTERACTIONS. Many drug interactions occur with **beta blockers,** and before they are prescribed, Table 12–11 should be consulted. Common problems include additive hypotension with other **antihypertensives,** acute ingestion of **alcohol** and **nitrates,** brady-

Table 12–11. Drug Interactions: Selected Beta Blockers

Drug	Interacting Drug	Possible Effect	Implications
All beta blockers	Aluminum salts, barbiturates, calcium salts, cholestyramine, colestipol, NSAIDs, ampicillin, rifampin, salicylates	Decrease the bioavailability and plasma levels of beta-adrenergic antagonists, possibly resulting in decreased pharmacological effect	Avoid concurrent use. Separate administration of cholestyramine or colestipol from administration of beta-adrenergic antagonist by 4 h.
	Calcium channel blockers	Potentiate effects of beta-adrenergic antagonists	Do not administer within 24 h of each other. If must give both, monitor for heart failure and decreased peripheral perfusion.
	Ciprofloxacin and other quinolones, cimetidine	Bioavailability of beta-adrenergic antagonists metabolized by CYP-450 may be increased	Select different antibiotic or different beta-adrenergic antagonist.
	Digoxin	Additive bradycardia	Avoid concurrent administration. If must give both, monitor closely for digitalis toxicity. May need to adjust doses of one or both
	Antihypertensives, alcohol, nitrates	Additive hypotension	Avoid acute ingestion of alcohol. Monitor blood pressure (BP) closely.
	Amphetamines, cocaine, ephedrine, epinephrine, norepinephrine, phenyl-ephrine, pseudoephedrine	Concurrent use may result in unopposed alpha-adrenergic stimulation, resulting in excessive hypertension and bradycardia	Avoid concurrent use. Warn patients because many of these are included in OTC cold remedies.
	Prazosin	Concurrent administration may potentiate postural hypotension	Avoid concurrent administration.
	Sulfonylureas	Hypoglycemic effects of sulfonylureas may be attenuated	Select different hypoglycemic or antihypertensive. If they must be given together, monitor blood glucose closely.
	Clonidine	Life-threatening and fatal increases in BP have resulted after discontinuance of clonidine in patients also receiving beta-adrenergic antagonist or after simultaneous withdrawal	
Metoprolol, propranolol	Ranitidine	May increase bioavailability of metoprolol; other beta-adrenergic antagonists not affected	Select different histamine$_2$ blocker, but avoid cimetidine (see above).
	Hydralazine	Additive pharmacological effect	Avoid concurrent use or closely monitor effects.
	MAOIs	Bradycardia may develop	Avoid concurrent use or use within 14 d of MAOI.
	Propafenone	Plasma levels of metoprolol increased	Avoid concurrent use.
	Benzodiazepines (BDZ)	Effects of BDZ increased by lipophilic beta-adrenergic antagonist	Change to atenolol. It does not interact.
Propranolol only	Haloperidol	Hypotensive episodes	Select different antipsychotic.
	Phenothiazines	Propranolol bioavailability and phenothiazine plasma levels increased, with potential toxicity	Selected different beta-adrenergic antagonist.
	Acetaminophen	Decreased acetaminophen clearance	Avoid concurrent use or reduce dose.
	Warfarin	Increased anticoagulant effect	Select different beta-adrenergic antagonist.

cardia with **digitalis glycosides,** and altered effectiveness of **hypoglycemic drugs.** Concurrent use of several drugs found in OTC cold remedies **(ephedrine, phenylephrine, pseudoephedrine)** may result in unopposed alpha-adrenergic stimulation, causing excessive hypertension and bradycardia. **Metoprolol** and **propranolol** have drug interactions in addition to those found with other **beta blockers.** The drug in this category with the fewest interactions is **atenolol.**

Life-threatening and fatal increases in blood pressure have been observed in patients taking **clonidine** and a **beta blocker** concurrently when the **clonidine** was withdrawn or when both the **clonidine** and the **beta blocker** were withdrawn. It is best to avoid using these drugs together, but if they are both given and withdrawal of one or both becomes necessary, withdraw the **beta blocker** first to avoid unopposed alpha stimulation and significant hypertension.

FOOD INTERACTIONS. Food enhances the bioavailability of **metoprolol** and **propranolol.** This effect is not noted with **nadolol** or **pindolol.**

LABORATORY TEST INTERACTIONS. Beta blockers may cause increased blood urea nitrogen (BUN), serum lipoprotein, potassium, triglyceride, and uric acid levels. They may also increase antinuclear antibody (ANA) titers and blood glucose levels.

Clinical Use and Dosing

Regardless of the indication for which a **beta blocker** is given, there is no simple correlation between dose or plasma level and therapeutic effect. The dose sensitivity range in clinical practice is wide because sympathetic tone varies widely among individuals. Proper dosing requires titration.

ANGINA. Atenolol, metoprolol, nadolol, and **propranolol** are indicated for long-term management of angina. They are used alone or in combination with long-acting nitrates. **Beta blockers** affect the myocardial oxygen supply-demand equation on the demand side. Both **beta$_1$ selective** and **nonselective agents** decrease the force of myocardial contractility, heart rate, and conduction velocity. **Nonselective agents** also decrease systemic vascular resistance and blood pressure, reducing afterload. Because they reduce myocardial oxygen demand, **beta blockers** are the drugs of choice for exertional angina. They are especially useful for patients with exertional angina whose lifestyle involves frequent vigorous activity, for patients with resting tachycardia, and for patients who have concomitant disease that might benefit from beta blockade (e.g., hypertension, post MI, migraine headaches). They do not improve myocardial oxygen demand, and **propranolol** has been reported to increase the risk for coronary artery vasospasm in some

patients. Additional discussion of their use in patients with angina is in Chapter 26.

To reduce the risk for adverse drug reactions, doses are started low and increased slowly, usually at no shorter than weekly intervals, based on resolution of symptoms. **Atenolol** and **nadolol** both require dosage adjustment for renal function impairment because principally the kidney excretes both drugs.

HYPERTENSION. Initial drug therapy for hypertension is with a **diuretic** or a **beta blocker** because they have been shown to reduce morbidity and mortality in numerous randomized controlled trials (RCT) (NHBPEP, 1997). **Beta blockers** are also chosen because of reduced cost. They may be used in combination with other **antihypertensives,** largely to mitigate the adverse effects associated with these drugs. **Atenolol, metoprolol, nadolol,** and **propranolol** are the drugs most commonly chosen. **Pindolol** or **acebutolol** can be used when ISA is a consideration because they have fewer myocardial depressant effects and do not increase cholesterol and triglyceride levels. Consideration of renal function is again important for dosing of some drugs. Additional discussion of the use of **beta blockers** in hypertension management is in Chapter 38.

POSTMYOCARDIAL INFARCTION PROPHYLAXIS. Use of **beta blockers** in post MI prophylaxis has been shown to decrease mortality by 30 to 40 percent. They are most effective for patients who have had severe anterior MIs. The mechanism of action in MI prophylaxis appears to be related to limitation of infarct size, prevention of primary arrhythmic events, protection from subsequent ischemia, and prevention of recurrent coronary occlusion. In comparing benefits versus adverse reaction profiles, the most benefits go to older adults and those with tachycardia. These drugs are less beneficial for young patients and those with small MIs. **Atenolol, metoprolol, propranolol,** and **timolol** have been shown to be effective for this indication.

MIGRAINE HEADACHE PROPHYLAXIS. **Propranolol** in doses of 160 to 200 mg/day has proved effective in reducing the incidence of migraine headache in some patients. The mechanism of action is related to prevention of beta receptor–induced vasodilation and promotion of increased extracellular levels of serotonin. **Timolol** with initial doses of 10 mg bid and maintenance doses of 10 to 30 mg/day has also been effective for this indication. For **propranolol,** if a satisfactory response to the maximum dose is not obtained in 4 to 6 weeks, the drug should be gradually withdrawn because a longer trial is not associated with any better outcome. For **timolol,** the trial should be 6 to 8 weeks. **Atenolol** (50 to 100 mg/day), **metoprolol** (50 to 100 mg/day), and **nadolol** (40 to 80 mg/day) have also been tried. The trial time is similar to that for **propranolol.**

ARRHYTHMIAS. Propranolol, pindolol, and acebutolol have indications for the treatment of supraventricular arrhythmias, suppression of premature ventricular contractions, and tachycardia. These indications are useful mainly for inpatients and are not discussed here.

GLAUCOMA. Topical application of **beta blockers** in the treatment of glaucoma is discussed in Chapter 24.

UNLABELED USES. Unlabeled indications for which some evaluation of effectiveness has been made include:

1. Alcohol withdrawal syndrome: **atenolol** 50 to 100 mg/day.
2. Aggressive behavior: **metoprolol** 200 to 300 mg/day and **propranolol** 80 to 300 mg/day.
3. Antipsychotic drug-induced akathisia: **nadolol** 40 to 80 mg/day, **pindolol** 5 mg/day, **propranolol** 20 to 80 mg/day, and **metoprolol** more than 100 mg/day.
4. Essential tremor: **metoprolol** 50 to 300 mg/day, **nadolol** 120 to 240 mg/day, and **timolol** 10 mg/day.
5. Situational anxiety (stage fright): **propranolol** 40 mg and **nadolol** 20 mg. **Propranolol** 40 to 320 mg/day has been used for acute panic syndromes.
6. Enhanced cognitive performance in older adults: **metoprolol** 50 to 200 mg/day.

WITHDRAWAL OF BETA BLOCKERS. For all **beta blockers,** abrupt withdrawal can be life-threatening. It can result in severe angina, MI, ventricular arrhythmias, and death. To withdraw any of these drugs, taper the dose by one-half every 4 days. Patients at high risk for serious consequences to rapid withdrawal include those with angina, coronary artery disease, and migraines. Low-risk patients include those with hypertension and supraventricular tachycardia.

Rational Drug Selection

BETA SELECTIVITY. In selecting the most appropriate **beta blocker,** first consideration is usually given to beta$_1$ selectivity. **Atenolol, acebutolol,** and **metoprolol** are **beta$_1$ selective drugs. Nadolol, pindolol, propranolol,** and **timolol** are **nonselective drugs.**

The clinical significance of selectivity relates to the relative lack of action of **beta$_1$ selective drugs** on the beta$_2$ receptors. This relative lack of action makes **beta$_1$ selective blockers** more appropriate than **nonselective agents** for patients with chronic obstructive pulmonary diseases, asthma, peripheral vascular diseases such as Raynaud's syndrome, and diabetes mellitus who have clear indications for taking a **beta blocker.** Among the **beta$_1$ selective blockers, atenolol** has greater selectivity than **metoprolol,** which has greater selectivity than **acebutolol.**

PHARMACOKINETICS. The best choice of drug based on pharmacokinetics would be one with a long enough half-life to permit once-daily dosing, consistent bioavailability and limited interpatient variability in dosing, limited CNS penetration to reduce adverse reactions, and an excretion mechanism that does not require dosage adjustments, so that extensive laboratory testing prior to initiation of therapy is not required. No one drug meets all these requirements, but several come close.

Atenolol and **metoprolol** have longer half-lives that permit once-daily dosing regimens, although **metoprolol** frequently has its best effects with bid dosing. All other **beta blockers** have half-lives that require at least bid dosing, with **propranolol** having bid and tid dosing. **Propranolol** is sometimes used to treat anxiety symptoms in depressed patients specifically because it clears the system quickly in cases of overdose.

Atenolol and **nadolol** do not have significant hepatic first-pass effects. **Acebutolol, metoprolol, pindolol, propranolol,** and **timolol** have significant first-pass effects and increased interpatient variability in the amount of drug that enters the patient's bloodstream. They also have short half-lives and require more frequent dosing.

Timolol has the least CNS penetration, but it is a **nonselective agent. Acebutolol** and **atenolol** have minimal CNS penetration. The drug with the most CNS penetration is **metoprolol.**

Beta blockers that are excreted primarily by the kidney have increased half-lives in renal failure. Dosage adjustments are necessary. **Atenolol** and **nadolol** fall into this category (see Table 12–12). Although **acebutolol** is excreted through the GI tract, its active metabolite is excreted through the kidneys, and the daily dose is reduced in renal failure. Poor renal function has only minor effects on **pindolol** clearance, and the half-life of **metoprolol** is essentially unchanged.

COST. Generic **propranolol** is the least expensive of the **beta blockers,** followed by **metoprolol** and then **atenolol.** Other **beta blockers** are significantly more expensive.

With all of these parameters taken together, the most cost-effective and convenient **beta blocker** for angina management, hypertension, and post-MI prophylaxis is **atenolol,** which has once-daily dosing, low CNS penetration, a low adverse reactions profile, and beta$_1$ selectivity (Table 12–13).

CONCURRENT DISEASE STATES. Disease processes that contraindicate use of **beta blockers** or require cautious use have been discussed: diseases with a bronchospastic component, heart failure, AV block, and diabetes mellitus. Because of their initial vasoconstriction, they are also poor choices for patients with peripheral vascular disease and Raynaud's syndrome.

Beta blockers are good choices to treat patients who have more than one of the disease processes for which they are indicated. Hypertensive patients who also have angina or who have had a previous MI, for example, are excellent candidates for **beta blockers. Atenolol, meto-**

Table 12–12. Dosage Schedule: Selected Beta Blockers

Drug	Indication	Initial Dose	Maintenance Dose
Atenolol (Tenormin)	Hypertension	50 mg qd	If target blood pressure (BP) not achieved in 1–2 wk, increase to 100 mg qd. Higher doses not likely to help. Reduce dosage to 50 mg if creatinine clearance (CCr) 15–35 cc/min; 50 mg qod if CCr < 15 cc/min.
	Angina	50 mg qd	If symptoms continue, increase to 100 mg. Some patients may need 200 mg. Reduce dosage to 50 mg if CCr 15–35 cc/min; 50 mg qod if CCr < 15 cc/min.
	MI (prophylaxis)	50 mg qd	50–100 mg qd (see note above re CCr).
Metoprolol (Lopressor)	Hypertension	100 mg/d in single or divided doses (extended-release tablets: 50–100 mg qd)	If target BP not achieved, increase at weekly intervals. Maintenance dose usually 100–450 mg/d. Does better in divided doses (extended release tablets: 100–400 mg qd).
	Angina	100 mg/d in two divided doses (extended-release tablets: 100 mg qd)	If symptoms continue, increase in weekly intervals up to 400 mg/d in two divided doses (extended release: up to 400 mg qd).
	MI (prophylaxis)	100 mg/d in two divided doses	100 mg/d in two divided doses.
Nadolol (Corgard)	Hypertension	40 mg qd	Increase in doses of 40–80 mg/d until target BP achieved. Maintenance dose usually 40–80 mg/d. Max dose 320 mg/d. Increase dosage interval in renal impairment: CCr > 50 = q24h; CCr 31–50 = q24–36h; CCr 10–30 = q24–48h; CCr < 10 = q40–60h.
	Angina	40 mg qd	If symptoms continue, increase in 3–7 d intervals to 80–160 mg/d. Max dose is 240 mg/d. Increase dosage interval in renal impairment. CCr > 50 = q24h; CCr 31–50 = q24–36h; CCr 10–30 = q24–48h; CCr < 10 = q40–60h.
Propranolol (Inderal)	Hypertension	40 mg bid (SR = 80 mg qd)	Usual maintenance dose is 120–240 mg bid or tid (SR = 120–160 mg qd); max dose = 640 mg/d.
	Angina	80–320 mg in 2, 3, or 4 divided dose (SR = 80 mg qd)	If symptoms continue; give 160-mg SR tablet; max dose, 320-mg SR.
	MI (prophylaxis)		180–240 mg/d in 2–3 divided doses.
	Migraine prophylaxis	80 mg/d (SR)	160–240 mg/d in divided doses.
Timolol (Blocadren)	MI (prophylaxis)		10 mg bid.
	Migraine prophylaxis	10 mg bid	Maintenance dose 10–30 mg. May take up to 8 wk of maximum daily dose.

SR = sustained release.

prolol, and **propranolol** are useful for all of these indications.

INDICATIONS. Specific agents have been demonstrated to work with specific disorders. Other drugs in the class may not work as well. For example, drugs with ISA (**acebutolol** and **pindolol**) have not been shown to be effective in post-MI prophylaxis. **Propranolol** is the only one proven useful in managing exertional or other stress-induced angina associated with idiopathic hypertrophic subaortic stenosis. The drug chosen should have research to support its use.

Monitoring

Monitoring parameters for **beta blockers** are essentially those used to monitor the disease process they are being

Table 12–13. Available Dosage Forms: Selected Beta Blockers

Drug	Dosage Form	Package
Acebutolol (Sectral)	Capsules: 200 mg	In bottles of 100 capsules and in Redipak 100s
	Capsules: 400 mg	In bottles of 100 capsules
Atenolol (Tenormin)	Tablets: 25 mg, 50 mg, 100 mg	In bottles of 30, 60, 90, 100, 120, 500, 1000 tablets
Metoprolol (Lopressor)	Tablets: 50 mg, 100 mg	In bottles of 100, 1000 scored tablets
Metoprolol (Toprol-XL)	Tablets, extended release: 50 mg, 100 mg, 200 mg	In bottles of 100 film-coated and scored tablets
Nadolol (Corgard)	Tablets: 20 mg and 160 mg	In bottles of 100 scored tablets
	Tablets: 40 mg, 80 mg, 120 mg	In bottles of 100, 1000 scored tablets
Pindolol (Visken)	Tablets: 5 mg, 10 mg	In bottles of 100, 1000 scored tablets
Propranolol (Inderal)	Tablets: 10 mg, 20 mg, 40 mg, 80 mg	In bottles of 100, 500, 1000 scored tablets
	Tablets: 60 mg, 90 mg	In bottles of 100, 500 scored tablets
Timolol (Blocadren)	Tablets: 5 mg, 10 mg, 20 mg	In bottles of 100 tablets; 10-mg tablets are scored

used to treat (e.g., the number of anginal attacks, the lowering of blood pressure). For the drugs requiring dosage adjustments based on renal function, serum creatinine and/or creatinine clearance testing should be done prior to initiation of therapy. For drugs with significant first-pass effects, it may be appropriate to assess liver function before beginning therapy. Because almost 50 percent of people with diabetes are unaware that they have this condition, and the management of diabetes may be compromised by the addition of a **beta blocker,** a serum glucose level should also be drawn prior to therapy.

Patient Education

ADMINISTRATION. The patient should take the drug exactly as prescribed, at the same time each day, even if feeling well. Do not skip or double doses. If a dose of **atenolol, metoprolol,** or **nadolol** is missed, it should be taken, up to 8 hours before the next dose is due. **Pindolol, propranolol,** and **timolol** should be taken up to 4 hours before the next dose. Abrupt withdrawal may precipitate life-threatening arrhythmias, hypertension, and myocardial ischemia. Be certain there is enough drug on hand to cover weekends or traveling. The patient should wear identification describing the disease process and the medication regimen at all times.

Food may enhance the bioavailability of **propranolol** and **metoprolol.** They should be taken consistently either with food or on an empty stomach. **Propranolol** can be crushed and mixed with food, including oral solutions and semisolids, if it is consistently given with food. Food intake does not affect other **beta blockers.**

Consult with the health care provider before taking any OTC drugs, especially cold remedies, while taking a **beta blocker.** Several drugs common in these preparations have drug interactions that result in hypertension and excessive bradycardia.

If these drugs are being taken for angina, **beta blockers** cannot relieve acute anginal attacks. If acute chest pain occurs, the patient should contact the health care provider immediately or go to the nearest hospital.

ADVERSE REACTIONS. Hypotensive reactions and bradycardia are the most common adverse reactions. Arising slowly from a supine position and dangling the feet over the side of the bed before standing will reduce postural hypotension. No exercise in hot weather and intake of at least 2000 cc of noncaffeinated fluid a day will also reduce these problems. Assessment of blood pressure and pulse is necessary on a biweekly basis for those taking these drugs. Teach the patient home blood pressure and pulse monitoring and advise contacting the health care provider if the pulse is less than 50 bpm or if the blood pressure changes suddenly.

Beta blockers may exacerbate diseases with a bronchospastic component. Teach patients to report wheezing or difficulty in breathing to the health care provider immediately. Dizziness and drowsiness may occur with the drugs. Avoid driving or other activities that require mental alertness until response to the drug is known. Insomnia can be reduced by not taking the last dose of the day late in the evening. Dry mouth responds to good oral hygiene, chewing sugarless gum, or sucking on hard candy.

Depression and confusion have been associated with the **beta blockers** that have significant CNS penetration. The patient should report such problems, and a different **beta blocker** or a different class of drugs may be tried.

For diabetics, these drugs may mask the signs and symptoms of hypoglycemia and impair recovery from a hypoglycemic attack. **Beta$_1$ selective drugs** are less likely to cause this problem. The one indication of hypoglycemia that is not masked is diaphoresis. In the event of unexplained diaphoresis, the patient should check the blood glucose level immediately.

Beta blockers are contraindicated in the first trimester of pregnancy and must be withdrawn before delivery. Women of childbearing age should have this warning discussed with them.

Nonadherence to a treatment regimen with a **beta blocker** is often caused by inhibition of ejaculation and impotence. If these occur, the patient should report them to the health care provider, who may choose a different drug to treat the disorder or change the dosage.

LIFESTYLE MANAGEMENT. If the drug is being given for hypertension, encourage the patient to adhere to additional interventions for reduction of blood pressure, such as weight loss, a low-sodium diet, smoking cessation, regular exercise, and stress management. Further discussion of patient education is in Chapter 38. Further discussion of patient education about angina occurs in Chapter 26.

Combined Alpha- and Beta-Adrenergic Antagonists

Drugs that exhibit blockade at both alpha and beta receptors have most of the same effects and adverse reactions as drugs that block only one type of receptor. Because the alpha blockade predominates, however, they are less likely to produce reflex tachycardia or significant reductions in heart rate or cardiac output. Alpha blockade also balances the tendency of beta blockers to produce vasoconstriction and increase peripheral vascular resistance.

There are two main drugs in this class: **carvedilol** (Coreg) and **labetalol** (Normodyne). Both are used to treat hypertension, and **carvedilol** is also used to reduce progression of CHF. This section focuses on aspects of these drugs that are different from **alpha-adrenergic antagonists** and **beta blockers**. Similar aspects of these drugs to the other two classes are discussed only briefly.

Pharmacodynamics

These two drugs combine selective alpha$_1$-adrenergic blocking with nonselective beta blockade. The alpha and beta blockades decrease blood pressure, with standing blood pressure more affected than supine. Single doses of **labetalol** have no significant effect on sinus rate, intraventricular conduction, or QRS duration. AV conduction time is only modestly prolonged. No significant change in cardiac output occurs, and only small changes in peripheral resistance. In addition, **carvedilol** reduces orthostatic hypotension and exercise-induced reflex tachycardia. In hypertensive patients with normal renal function, it also decreases renal vascular resistance. Neither of these drugs demonstrates an effect on serum lipoproteins.

Pharmacokinetics

Absorption and Distribution

Both drugs are rapidly absorbed (Table 12–14). **Carvedilol** is more protein bound than **labetalol**. Both drugs are widely distributed in body tissues.

Metabolism and Excretion

Both drugs undergo rapid hepatic first-pass metabolism, resulting in bioavailabilities between 25 and 35 percent. **Carvedilol** undergoes more excretion in bile and feces than does **labetalol**.

Pharmacotherapeutics

Precautions and Contraindications

Because they include nonselective beta blockade, **alpha-beta blockers** are contraindicated for patients with respiratory conditions that include a bronchospastic component. They are also contraindicated in overt, New York Heart Association (NYHA) class IV heart failure, greater than first-degree AV block, and severe bradycardia. Unlike **beta blockers**, they can be used for patients with mild heart failure (**labetalol**) or even moderate heart failure (**carvedilol**) and bradycardia in the 50 to 60 bpm range because of their limited effects on heart rate and myocardial contractility.

Cautions related to diabetes and thyroid disease and problems with withdrawal are similar to those of **beta blockers**. Although they produce less vasoconstriction, caution is still required when these drugs are administered to patients with peripheral vascular disease.

Table 12–14. Pharmacokinetics: Combined Alpha-Beta Blockers

Drug	Onset	Peak	Duration	Protein Binding	Bioavailability	Half-Life	Elimination
Carvedilol	1 h	1–2 h	12 h	>98%	25–35%	7–10 h	Primarily in bile and feces; <2% unchanged in urine
Labetalol	20 min	1–4 h	8–12 h	50%	25% (increased by food and in older adults)	3–8 h	In bile and feces; 50–60% as conjugates in urine

Hepatic impairment creates issues for both drugs. Like many **beta blockers,** they are heavily metabolized by the liver, and use in patients with clinically manifested liver disease is not recommended. Hepatic injury has occurred with both drugs, and onset of jaundice or hepatic dysfunction indicated by symptoms or elevations of liver function tests necessitates withdrawal of the drug.

Both drugs are also Pregnancy Category C for the same reasons as beta blockers. Small amounts of labetalol (0.004%) are excreted in breast milk, and the amount of carvedilol excreted in breast milk is unknown. Caution should be exercised in giving these drugs to nursing mothers, with careful consideration of benefits versus risks.

Plasma levels of **carvedilol** average 50 percent higher in older adults than in young adults. Although there was no notable difference in adverse reactions in study subjects, it is advisable to monitor older patients more closely for adverse reactions such as dizziness, which places them at risk for falls.

Adverse Drug Reactions

Adverse drug reactions are essentially the same as those seen with **beta blockers,** with the exception of fewer cardiac-related reactions (e.g., bradycardia, decreased contractility) and less incidence of CNS-related reactions. The risk for orthostatic hypotension is higher than with **beta blockers** related to the alpha$_1$-adrenergic blockade.

Drug, Food, and Laboratory Test Interactions

DRUG INTERACTIONS. Drug interactions are similar to those for **beta blockers,** with a few additions (Table 12–15). As with **beta blockers,** drugs that inhibit the CYP-450 2D6 system increase plasma levels of **alpha-beta blockers.** Increased blood levels of **labetalol** and **carvedilol** increase the risk for adverse reactions.

FOOD INTERACTIONS. When **carvedilol** is taken with food, its rate of absorption is slowed, but the bioavailability is not affected. Taking it with food minimizes the risk for postural hypotension.

LABORATORY TEST INTERACTIONS. The presence of a **labetalol** metabolite in the urine may falsely increase urinary catecholamine levels measured by a nonspecific trihydroxyindole reaction. There have also been reversible increases in serum transaminases (4% of patients) and, rarely, reversible increases in BUN. **Labetalol** has also produced a false-positive test for **amphetamine** in a patient whose urine was screened for the presence of drugs.

Clinical Use and Dosing

HYPERTENSION. Both drugs are used to treat essential hypertension. They are used alone or in combination with other **antihypertensive agents,** especially **thiazide-type diuretics.** Cost considerations remove them from first-line choices. Both drugs are begun at a low dose, and dosage is increased until target blood pressure is achieved (Table 12–16). **Carvedilol** begins at 6.25 mg bid (Table 12–17). Adjustments are made at 7- to 14-day intervals, based on standing systolic blood pressure. **Labetalol** is initiated at 100 mg bid and increased in 100-mg increments every 2 to 3 days until target blood pressure is achieved.

CONGESTIVE HEART FAILURE. **Carvedilol** has an indication for treatment of heart failure in a narrow group of patients: mild to moderate (NYHA class II or III) heart failure of ischemic or cardiomyopathic origin, in conjunction with **digitalis, diuretics,** and **angiotensin-converting enzyme (ACE) inhibitors,** to reduce the progression of disease. Treatment is begun at one-half the hypertension dosage, with increases at 2-week intervals. Maximum dose is based on patient weight.

UNLABELED USES. **Labetalol** has been used to treat the withdrawal hypertension associated with **clonidine** with-

Table 12–15. Drug Interactions: Combined Alpha-Beta Blockers

Drug	Interacting Drug*	Possible Effect	Implications
Carvedilol	Inhibitors of CYP-450 2D6 (e.g., cimetidine, ciprofloxacin and other quinolones, quinidine, fluoxetine, paroxetine, propafenone)	Increased blood level of carvedilol	Avoid concurrent use.
	Rifampin	Plasma concentration of carvedilol reduced by 70%	Avoid concurrent use.
Labetalol	Beta agonists, theophylline	Labetalol can blunt the bronchodilator effect	A greater than normal dose of beta agonist may be required.

*Other drug interactions that are the same as for beta blockers: antihypertensives, alcohol, calcium channel blockers, clonidine, digoxin, MAOIs, nitrates, and sulfonylureas. See Table 12–11.

Table 12–16. Dosage Schedule: Combined Alpha-Beta Blockers

Drug	Indication	Initial Dose	Maintenance Dose
Carvedilol	Hypertension	6.25 mg bid; if dose is tolerated using standing systolic blood pressure (BP) measured 1 h after the dose, maintain this dose for 7–14 d	After initial dose, increase to 12.5 mg bid if needed, based on trough BP using same standing systolic BP. Maintain this dose for 7–14 d before increasing to 25 mg if needed. When increasing dose, give first larger dose at bedtime to avoid orthostatic hypotension. Full antihypertensive effect seen in 7–14 d. Maximum dose is 50 mg.
	CHF	3.125 mg bid for 2 wk	Individualize dose and closely monitor during up-titration. If initial dose is tolerated, increase to 6.25 mg bid. Dose can then be doubled every 2 wk to the highest level tolerated by the patient. Maximum dose is 25 mg bid for <85 kg; 50 mg bid for >85 mg. Transient worsening of CHF may be treated by increasing diuretic or reducing carvedilol dose.
Labetalol	Hypertension	100 mg bid alone or added to a diuretic	If target BP is not achieved in 2–3 d, increase in increments of 100 mg bid every 2–3 d. Maintenance dose is usually 200–400 mg bid. Full antihypertensive effect seen within first 1–3 h of initial dose. Maximum dose 2400 mg/d. Older adults require lower doses.

drawal, using the maintenance dose for treating hypertension. **Carvedilol** appears to be beneficial in treating angina (25 to 50 mg bid) and idiopathic cardiomyopathy (6.25 to 25 mg bid)

WITHDRAWAL OF THE ALPHA-BETA BLOCKERS. As with **beta blockers**, abrupt withdrawal can be life-threatening. Angina has not been observed, but withdrawal can result in MI, ventricular arrhythmias, and death. To withdraw either of these drugs, taper the dose by one-half every 4 days over a period of 1 to 2 weeks. Patients at high risk for serious consequences due to rapid withdrawal include those with angina, coronary artery disease, and migraines. Low-risk patients include those with hypertension but no coronary artery disease.

Rational Drug Selection

Rational drug selection is largely related to cost and indications. See the discussion in the Clinical Use and Dosing section.

RACE AND ETHNICITY. For hypertension, **alpha-beta blockers** are effective in the African-American population when lifestyle modification and diuretics are not sufficient to reach the target blood pressure.

AGE. Because of the risk for orthostatic hypotension, these drugs should be used with caution in older adults.

CONCOMITANT DISEASES. **Carvedilol** may be chosen when the patient has concomitant mild to moderate

Table 12–17. Available Dosage Forms: Combined Alpha-Beta Blockers

Drug	Dosage Form	Package
Carvedilol (Coreg)	Tablets: 3.125 mg, 6.25 mg, 12.5 mg, 25 mg	In bottles of 100 tablets
Labetalol (Normodyne)	Tablets: 100 mg, 200 mg, 300 mg	In bottles of 100, 500 film-coated tablets
Labetalol (Trandate)	Tablets: 100 mg, 200 mg, 300 mg	In bottles of 100, 500 scored film-coated tablets

heart failure. **Labetalol** may be chosen when the patient cannot tolerate changes in heart rate but needs beta blockade (e.g., post-MI prophylaxis).

Monitoring

Liver function tests should be performed before initiating therapy, when adjusting dosage, and at the first indication of liver dysfunction (pruritus, dark urine, persistent anorexia, jaundice, upper-right quadrant tenderness, or unexplained flulike syndrome). If the patient has laboratory evidence of liver injury, stop the drug and do not restart it.

Renal function tests should be performed prior to initiating therapy and at regular intervals for any patients with a concomitant disease process that may impair renal function.

Clinical monitoring of the disease process for which the drug was prescribed is also indicated. Discussion of such monitoring for hypertension is discussed in Chapter 38.

Patient Education

ADMINISTRATION. The patient should take the drug exactly as prescribed, at the same time each day, even if feeling well. Do not skip or double doses. If a dose is missed, for **labetalol,** it should be taken up to 8 hours before the next dose is due. For **carvedilol,** it should be taken up to 4 hours before the next dose. Abrupt withdrawal may precipitate life-threatening arrhythmias, hypertension, and myocardial ischemia. Be certain there is enough drug on hand to cover weekends or traveling. The patient should wear identification describing the disease process and the medication regimen at all times.

Take **carvedilol** with food. This slows absorption and reduces the chance of orthostatic hypotension.

The patient should consult with the health care provider before taking any OTC drugs, especially cold remedies, while taking an **alpha-beta blocker.** Several ingredients common in these preparations cause drug interactions that result in hypertension and excessive bradycardia.

ADVERSE REACTIONS. Hypotensive reactions and bradycardia are the most common adverse reactions. Arising slowly from a supine position and dangling the feet over the side of the bed before standing will reduce postural hypotension. No exercise in hot weather and liquid intake of at least 2000 mL of noncaffeinated fluids a day will also reduce these problems. Assessment of blood pressure and pulse is necessary on a biweekly basis for patients taking these drugs. Teach patients home blood pressure and pulse monitoring, and advise them to contact the health care provider if their pulse is less than 50 bpm or if the blood pressure changes suddenly.

Alpha-beta blockers may exacerbate diseases with a bronchospastic component. Teach patients to report wheezing or difficulty in breathing to the health care provider immediately.

Dizziness and drowsiness may occur with these drugs. Patients should avoid driving or other activities that require mental alertness until their response to the drug is known.

For diabetics, these drugs may mask the signs and symptoms of hypoglycemia and impair recovery from a hypoglycemic attack. **Beta$_1$ selective drugs** are less likely to cause this problem. The one indication of hypoglycemia that is not masked is diaphoresis. In the event of unexplained diaphoresis, patients should check their blood glucose levels immediately.

Because alpha-beta blockers contain beta blockers, they are contraindicated in the first trimester of pregnancy and must be withdrawn before delivery. Women of childbearing age should have this topic discussed with them.

A leading cause of nonadherence to a treatment regimen with an **alpha-beta blocker** is inhibition of ejaculation and impotence. If these occur, report them to the health care provider, who may choose a different drug to treat the disorder or change the dosage.

LIFESTYLE MANAGEMENT. Lifestyle management is the same as for **beta blockers.**

Postganglionic Blockers

Unlike the previous blocking drugs discussed here, **postganglionic blockers** do not involve direct receptor blockade. These drugs act indirectly on adrenergic neurons by inhibiting the release of norepinephrine from synaptic nerve endings. The net result is a reduction in stimulation of adrenergic nerves so that the pharmacological effects are similar to other **adrenergic receptor blockers.** Because they do not cross the blood-brain barrier (with the exception of **reserpine**), they have fewer CNS adverse reactions than some of the **alpha and beta blockers.** For the treatment of hypertension, their adverse reactions profile has resulted in their being supplanted by newer drugs, and they are no longer first-line therapy.

Pharmacodynamics

Postganglionic blockers are transported across the sympathetic nerve membrane by the same mechanism that transports norepinephrine. Once they enter the nerve, they are concentrated in transmitter vesicles, where they replace norepinephrine. Because they replace norepinephrine, they gradually deplete norepinephrine stores in the nerve ending. **Reserpine (Serpalan)** depletes stores in the brain and adrenal medulla. **Guanadrel (Hylorel)** and **guanethidine (Ismelin)** do not cross the blood-brain barrier and so act only on peripheral sympathetic neurons. The result in both cases is suppression of responses mediated by both alpha- and beta-adrenergic receptors without actual blockade of these receptors. Sympathetic blockade results in modest decreases in peripheral resistance and cardiac output so that blood pressure is lowered. These drugs also decrease blood pressure by decreasing the sympathetically induced reflex vasoconstriction that occurs on sitting up, so that venous pooling of blood and postural hypotension are both adverse reactions associated with these drugs.

Pharmacokinetics

Absorption and Distribution

Absorption varies among the drugs in this class (Table 12–18). **Guanadrel** is rapidly and well absorbed after oral administration, with peak plasma concentrations occurring within 1.5 to 2 hours after ingestion. **Guanethidine** is incompletely absorbed, with only 30 to 50 percent absorbed after oral ingestion. **Reserpine** is slowly and incompletely absorbed, with only 40 to 50 percent absorbed following oral ingestion.

Distribution also varies among drugs. **Reserpine** is the most widely distributed; it crosses the blood-brain barrier and the placenta and enters breast milk. **Guanadrel** crosses the placenta but not the blood-brain barrier, and its level of entry into breast milk is unknown. **Guanethidine** crosses the placenta and enters breast milk but does not cross the blood-brain barrier.

Half-lives vary among the drugs, from 12 hours for **guanadrel** to 4 to 8 days for **guanethidine** and 11 days for **reserpine**. These differences significantly affect dosing and residual effects after the drug is withdrawn.

Metabolism and Excretion

No definitive studies of the metabolism of **reserpine** have been made, but it is generally accepted that it is metabolized in the liver. At least 50 percent of the drug is lost in feces as unabsorbed drug, and small amounts are excreted unchanged in urine. **Guanadrel** is also metabolized by the liver, and 50 percent is excreted unchanged in urine. **Guanethidine** is partially metabolized by the liver into three metabolites that are less active than the parent drug. The drug and its metabolites are excreted in urine.

Pharmacotherapeutics

Precautions and Contraindications

Mental depression or a history of mental depression, especially with suicidal tendencies, is a contraindication for **reserpine**. **Reserpine** has been known to cause severe mental depression, and the signs and symptoms of this depression may be masked, making recognition difficult. Drug-induced depression may also persist for several months after the drug is discontinued and be severe enough to precipitate suicide.

Because all three drugs increase GI motility and secretion, they are used with caution for patients with history of peptic ulcer disease and are contraindicated for patients with active ulcerative disease. Renal function impairment also requires cautious use of all three drugs in that decreased blood pressure may further compromise renal function. **Guanadrel** requires dosage adjustments for patients with creatinine clearance below 60 cc/minute.

Both **guanadrel** and **guanethidine** are used cautiously for patients with asthma or other bronchospastic disorders because these disorders may be aggravated by catecholamine depletion and **adrenergic agonists** may interfere with the hypotensive effects of these drugs. They are also used cautiously in the presence of cardiovascular or cerebrovascular insufficiency disorders because they tend to cause fluid retention and bradycardia.

Reserpine and *guanethidine* **are Pregnancy Category C. There are no adequate and well-controlled studies in pregnant women, and these drugs cross the placenta. Because other drugs to treat hypertension are approved for use during pregnancy, these drugs should not be used for that purpose.**

Guanadrel **is listed as Pregnancy Category B, but there are no adequate and well-controlled studies of this drug in pregnant women. It should also not be used to treat pregnant women with hypertension.**

The safety and efficacy of all of these drugs have not been established in children.

Adverse Drug Reactions

Adverse drug reactions for this class of drugs are based on their blockade of normal adrenergic stimulation and

Table 12–18. Pharmacokinetics: Postganglionic Blockers

Drug	Onset	Peak	Duration	Protein Binding	Half-Life	Elimination
Guanadrel	2 h	4–6 h	9–12 h	20%	10 h	50% unchanged in urine
Guanethidine	1–3 wk	1–3 wk	2 wk	Minimal	4–8 d	In urine
Reserpine	1–3 wk	3–6 wk	1–6 wk	96%	11 d	50% in feces as unabsorbed drug; small amount in urine

their hypotensive effects. Adverse effects associated with blockade of adrenergic stimulation affect multiple body systems and include drowsiness, dizziness, fatigue, confusion, headaches, nasal stuffiness, visual disturbances, cough, shortness of breath, dry mouth, urinary frequency, and leg cramps. GI adverse effects are often the most problematic. Diarrhea, the most common, may require management with **antidiarrheal agents** such as **diphenoxylate (Lomotil), loperamide (Imodium),** or an **anticholinergic agent.** Ejaculation disturbances and impotence are common reasons for lack of adherence to the treatment regimen.

Cardiovascular effects associated with hypotension include bradycardia, dizziness, fainting, and fluid retention. Postural hypotension can be severe. Blood pressure may fall so low that perfusion of the heart and brain is compromised. Patients with known regional vascular disease (e.g., cerebral or coronary) are at particular risk for this problem. Factors that promote vasodilation (e.g., **alcohol,** warm environments, and strenuous exercise) increase the risk for postural blood pressure changes. Fluid retention usually requires the addition of a **thiazide diuretic.**

All drugs in this class have CNS depression as an adverse reaction, but **reserpine** is especially noted for this problem. It can produce severe depression with suicidal potential. This adverse reaction is discussed in the Precautions and Contraindications section.

Drug Interactions

Neuronal uptake is necessary for the hypotensive action of these drugs. Drugs that block the catecholamine uptake process or displace amines from the nerve terminals (e.g., cocaine, amphetamine, TCAs, and phenothiazines) block their effects. **CNS depressants** have additive effects with **reserpine.** Many other psychotropic drugs have interactions with all three drugs in this class. **Guanethidine** should be discontinued at least 1 week prior to initiating therapy with minoxidil to prevent the profound postural hypotension that occurs when they are given concurrently. Other interactions are included in Tablet 12–19.

Clinical Use and Dosing

HYPERTENSION. **Guanadrel** is recommended as add-on therapy for patients with hypertension who have not responded adequately to **thiazide diuretics** alone. The dose is individualized but usually started at 10 mg/day, which can be given by breaking a scored 10-mg tablet in half for use as 5 mg bid (Table 12–20). Most patients eventually require 25 to 75 mg/day in two divided doses. For larger doses, tid or qid dosing may be needed to reduce adverse reactions. Renal impairment requires dosage adjustment. Because this drug has a substantial orthostatic effect, mon-

itor both supine and standing blood pressure, especially when the dosage is adjusted.

Guanethidine is recommended for moderate to severe hypertension and for renal hypertension secondary to pyelonephritis or renal artery stenosis. **ACE inhibitors** are contraindicated in the presence of renal artery stenosis, and **guanethidine** offers an alternative for these patients. Dosage begins with 10 mg/day and is increased gradually every 5 to 7 days. Blood pressure readings are taken with the patient supine and after standing for up to 10 minutes. Dosage is increased only if there has been no decrease in standing blood pressure. The usual maintenance dose is 25 to 50 mg daily. It is reduced in the presence of excessive postural hypotension or severe diarrhea. **Thiazide diuretics** enhance the effectiveness of **guanethidine** and reduce the incidence of edema. When they are added to the treatment regimen, reduction in the dose of **guanethidine** is often required. Although safety and efficacy in children have not been established, a dosing regimen for children is published.

Reserpine is used for mild hypertension and as adjunct therapy for more severe forms. For patients not receiving other **antihypertensive drugs,** the initial dose is 0.5 mg daily for 1 to 2 weeks (Table 12–21). The dose is then reduced to a maintenance dose of 0.1 to 0.25 mg/day. Higher doses are associated with serious mental depression.

In all cases, this class of drugs is not first-line management for hypertension. These drugs are used only when other **antihypertensive drugs** do not adequately control blood pressure.

AGITATED PSYCHOTIC STATES. **Reserpine** is the only drug in this class with this indication. The usual initial dose is 0.5 mg/day, but it may range from 0.1 mg to 1 mg, depending upon patient response. Dosage adjustments are based on patient response.

Rational Drug Selection

COST. Of the three drugs, **reserpine** is the least expensive, **guanadrel** is the most expensive, and **guanethidine** is in the middle. The difference in cost between the least and most expensive is extensive.

INDICATIONS. Indications were discussed previously. None of these drugs is a first-line drug for hypertension, although **guanethidine** may be used for patients with renal artery stenosis. Only **reserpine** has an indication for agitated psychotic state.

Monitoring

In addition to clinical monitoring of the indication for which the drug was given, renal function assessment with serum creatinine or creatinine clearance is recommended for all three drugs prior to initiation of therapy.

Table 12–19. Drug Interactions: Postganglionic Blockers

Drug	Interacting Drug	Possible Effect	Implications
Guanadrel, guanethidine, reserpine	Adrenergic agonists	Hypotensive effects of the postganglionic blocker (PGB) may be reversed. The PGB may potentiate the effects of direct-acting adrenergic agonists. The action of indirect-acting adrenergic agonists may be inhibited.	Avoid concurrent use. Select a different antihypertensive.
	TCAs and MAOIs	TCAs may block the norepinephrine-depleting and blood pressure–lowering effects of PGBs. If TCA is discontinued abruptly, enhanced PGB effect, resulting in hypotension, may occur.	Avoid concurrent use. Discontinued MAOIs at least 1 wk prior to starting a PGB.
	NSAIDs	Effectiveness of PGB may be decreased by concurrent use of NSAIDs.	Avoid concurrent use. Select a different antihypertensive.
Guanadrel	Beta blockers	Potentiates effects of guanadrel, resulting in excessive postural hypotension.	Select a different antihypertensive.
	Phenothiazines	Effects of guanadrel reversed.	Select a different antihypertensive.
	Vasodilators	May increase risk for postural hypotension.	Avoid concurrent use.
Guanethidine	Anorexiants, haloperidol, methylphenidate, phenothiazines, thioxanthenes	Hypotensive effects of guanethidine reversed or antagonized.	Avoid concurrent use. Select a different antihypertensive.
	Minoxidil	Profound postural hypotension.	Avoid concurrent use or discontinue guanethidine 1 wk before minoxidil is begun.
Reserpine	Antihypertensives, nitrates, alcohol	Additive hypotensive effects.	Select a different antihypertensive.
	Digoxin, quinidine, procainamide	Increased risk for toxicity and arrhythmias.	Select a different antihypertensive.
	CNS depressants (alcohol, antihistamines, antidepressants, opioids, sedative-hypnotics)	Additive CNS depression.	Select a different antihypertensive.

Patient Education

ADMINISTRATION. The patient should take the drug exactly as prescribed, at the same time each day, even if feeling well. Do not skip or double doses. If a dose of **reserpine** is missed, omit it and return to the regular dosage schedule. If a dose of **guanadrel** or **guanethidine** is missed, the patient should take it as soon as it is remembered but not double doses. If two doses in a row are missed, contact the health care provider so that blood pressure may be checked. These drugs treat hypertension but do not cure it, and they should not be discontinued without health care provider consultation.

All three drugs may be administered with food to decrease GI distress. **Guanethidine** may be crushed and taken with thick liquids or soft foods for patients who have difficulty swallowing.

The patient should consult the health care provider before taking any OTC drugs, especially cold remedies, while taking these drugs. Drug interactions may produce additive CNS depression.

ADVERSE REACTIONS. Postural hypotensive reactions are the most common adverse reactions. Arising slowly from a supine position and dangling the feet over the side of the bed before standing will reduce postural hy-

Table 12–20. Dosage Schedule: Postganglionic Blockers

Drug	Indication	Initial Dose	Maintenance Dose
Guanadrel	Hypertension	5 mg bid (may be given by breaking a scored 10-mg tablet in half)	Increase in increments of 5–10 mg/d at weekly intervals until target blood pressure (BP) is achieved. Maintenance dose 20–75 mg/d in 2, 3, or 4 divided doses.
		Impaired renal function: CCr 30–60 cc/min = 5 mg qd CCr < 30 cc/min = 5 mg q48h	Increase dosage at intervals of > 7 d for moderate renal impairment and > 14 d for severe impairment.
Guanethidine	Hypertension	Adults: 10 mg qd	Increase dose gradually at a minimum of 5- to 7-d intervals. Recommended dosing increments: 10 mg/d, 20 mg/d, 30–37.5 mg/d, 50 mg/d.
		Children: 0.2 mg/kg/d	Increase in increments of 0.2 mg/kg/d at 7 to 10-d intervals until target BP is achieved. Max dose is 3 mg/kg/d.
Reserpine	Hypertension Agitated psychotic states	0.5 mg/d for 1–2 wk 0.5 mg/d (may range from 0.1–1 mg/d)	Reduce dose to 0.1–0.25 mg/d. Dosage adjusted according to patient response.

CCr = creatinine clearance.

potension. No exercise in hot weather and noncaffeinated fluid intake of at least 2000 cc/day will also reduce these problems. Biweekly assessment of blood pressure is necessary for patients taking these drugs. Teach patients home blood pressure monitoring, and advise them to contact the health care provider if their blood pressure changes suddenly.

Dizziness and drowsiness may occur with these drugs. Avoid driving or other activities that require mental alertness until response to the drug is known.

Patients should weigh themselves daily and report weight gain of more than 2 kg in 24 hours or swelling of the feet and ankles to the health care provider. A **diuretic** may need to be added to the treatment regimen.

Dry mouth can be managed by good oral hygiene, frequent mouth rinses, and sugarless gum or candy. Other adverse effects associated with adrenergic blockade should be reported and managed as needed.

For **reserpine**, early indications of depression (e.g., despondency, early morning insomnia, loss of appetite, impotence, or self-deprecation) should be reported immediately. The drug may need to be withdrawn.

LIFESTYLE MANAGEMENT. Lifestyle management includes those instructions associated with management of hypertension, which are discussed in Chapter 38.

Cholinergic Agonists

Cholinergic agonists, also known as **parasympathomimetics** or **muscarinic agonists**, promote or mimic the action of ACh. These effects may be achieved either by direct agonist effect or indirectly by preventing the breakdown of ACh by acetylcholinesterase (AChE). As with **adrenergic agonists**, these drugs are not organ-specific; when one organ is targeted for therapeutic reasons, the drug simultaneously produces effects in other organs. The targeted organ effects become the desired drug action, and the other organ effects become the adverse drug effects.

There are three categories of drugs in this class: **muscarinic agonists, cholinesterase inhibitors**, and **ganglionic stimulants**. Each category is discussed separately. The prototypic drug among **ganglionic stimulants** is **nicotine**, which is the only drug discussed in that category.

Table 12–21. Available Dosage Forms: Postganglionic Blockers

Drug	Dosage Form	Package
Guanadrel (Hylorel)	Tablets: 10 mg, 25 mg	In bottles of 100 scored tablets
Guanethidine (Ismelin)	Tablets: 10 mg, 25 mg	In bottles of 100 scored tablets
Reserpine (Serpalan)	Tablets: 0.1 mg, 0.25 mg	In bottles of 100, 1000, 5000 tablets
Reserpine (Ser-Ap-Es)	Combined with hydralazine 25 mg/ hydrochlorothiazide 15 mg/reserpine 0.1 mg	In bottles of 100, 1000 tablets

Muscarinic Agonists

Pharmacodynamics

Muscarinic receptors are located in the eye, heart, blood vessels, lung, GI tract, urinary bladder, and sweat glands. The results of stimulation of these receptors are depicted in Table 12–1. Their activation by **muscarinic agonists** modifies organ function by release of ACh from PNS nerves: (1) to activate muscarinic receptors on target organs to alter organ function and (2) to activate muscarinic receptors on nerve terminals to inhibit the release of their neurotransmitters.

There are five drugs in this group, each with a different susceptibility to breakdown by cholinesterase and different degrees of action at muscarinic and nicotinic receptors. **ACh (Miochol)** is highly susceptible to cholinesterase and very active at both types of receptors. **Carbachol (Isopto Carbachol)**, **pilocarpine (Isopto Carpine)**, and **bethanechol (Urecholine)** have negligible susceptibility to cholinesterase, and all three act at muscarinic receptors. **Carbachol** also acts at nicotinic receptors. **Methacholine** has little susceptibility to cholinesterase and is very active at muscarinic receptors only.

Muscarinic agonists are used clinically to treat glaucoma and to improve GI and urinary bladder tone. **ACh** lacks selectivity to target tissues and is so rapidly destroyed by cholinesterase that its half-life is too short for most clinical applications. Its use is restricted to dilation of the pupil for ophthalmic surgery. **Methacholine** is used only for diagnosis of bronchial airway hyperactivity by specialists familiar with its use for this purpose. Neither of these drugs is discussed here.

Carbachol and **pilocarpine** are used to treat glaucoma. This use is discussed in Chapter 24. **Pilocarpine** comes in an oral form that can be used to increase salivary gland secretion for the management of xerostomia in patients who have undergone radiation therapy of the neck. This use is too restricted for discussion in this text. The only remaining drug in this category is **bethanechol**, and the remainder of this section discusses that drug.

Pharmacokinetics

Absorption and Distribution

Bethanechol can be given orally or subcutaneously (SC). Effects appear in 30 to 90 minutes after oral administration and 5 to 15 minutes after SC administration. The effects peak in 60 minutes for the oral dose and 15 to 30 minutes for the SC dose. Duration of action is approximately 1 hour for the oral dose and 2 hours for the SC dose. The dose required to produce a therapeutic effect is significantly different by these two routes because **bethanechol** is a quaternary ammonium compound carrying a positive charge, which greatly impedes absorption from the GI tract.

Metabolism and Excretion

This drug is inactivated at neuronal synapses and in plasma by cholinesterase. Small amounts of unchanged drug are sometimes excreted in the urine.

Pharmacotherapeutics

Precautions and Contraindications

Bethanechol is contraindicated in the presence of many diseases. It is contraindicated in peptic ulcer disease because at the usual therapeutic doses it can cause excessive secretion of gastric acid that could intensify gastric erosion and precipitate gastric bleeding and possible perforation. Its ability to increase GI peristalsis also contraindicates its use for patients with intestinal obstruction. Because of its ability to contract the bladder and increase pressure within the urinary tract, it is also contraindicated in the presence of urinary tract obstruction or weakness of the bladder wall. Stimulation of the muscarinic receptors in the lungs may result in bronchoconstriction, and it is contraindicated for patients with latent or active bronchospastic disorders. **Bethanechol** can cause hypotension and bradycardia. It is contraindicated for patients with disease processes that would be worsened by low blood pressure or low cardiac output.

Bethanechol is also contraindicated in patients with hyperthyroidism. When initially given **bethanechol**, patients with hyperthyroidism react similarly to other patients by experiencing hypotension and bradycardia. However, the body reacts to the hypotension with the release of increased amounts of norepinephrine from sympathetic nerves, resulting in increased heart rate. Because the heart tissue of patients with hyperthyroidism is highly sensitive to norepinephrine levels, even small increases in the amount of norepinephrine can produce cardiac arrhythmias.

It is not known whether *bethanechol* can cause fetal harm when given to pregnant women or if it can affect reproductive capacity. It is Pregnancy Category C and should be used only when the benefits clearly outweigh the potential risk to the fetus. Whether *bethanechol* is excreted in breast milk is also unknown.

Adverse Drug Reactions

Adverse reactions are rare following oral administration but more common after SC administration. GI, respiratory, and cardiac reactions were discussed in the Precautions and Contraindications section. Additional GI symptoms include abdominal pain, nausea, belching, and diarrhea. Other adverse reactions include increased tearing and miosis of the pupils and flushing that produces a feeling of warmth and a sensation of heat about the face.

TOXICITY. Muscarinic poisoning can occur from overdosage and from ingestion of certain poisonous mushrooms. Early symptoms of poisoning are abdominal cramps, salivation, flushing, nausea, and vomiting. **Atropine** is the specific antidote. The preferred route of administration is SC to provide a rapid response. The recommended dose for adults is 0.6 mg repeated every 2 hours, based on clinical response. The recommended dose for children under the age of 12 is 0.01 mg/kg repeated every 2 hours, based on clinical response. The maximal single dose in children should not exceed 0.4 mg.

Drug Interactions

Additive drug interactions may occur with **cholinesterase inhibitors.** A critical fall in blood pressure may occur with **ganglionic blockers. Quinidine, procainamide, phenothiazine**, and **TCAs** may antagonize the effects of **bethanechol.** Avoid concurrent administration of these drugs.

Clinical Use and Dosing

Bethanechol acts on the PNS to increase the tone of the detrusor urinae muscle, usually producing a contraction strong enough to initiate micturition and empty the bladder. It also stimulates gastric motility, increases gastric tone, and often restores impaired rhythmic peristalsis.

URINARY RETENTION. **Bethanechol** is used in primary care for neurogenic atony of the urinary bladder with retention. Oral dosing begins at 10 to 50 mg tid or qid. The minimum effective dose is determined by giving 5 to 10 mg initially and repeating the dose every hour until a satisfactory response occurs or 50 mg is reached. SC dosing begins with 2.5 mg. The minimum effective dose is determined by injecting 2.5 mg initially and repeating every 15 to 30 minutes until satisfactory response is obtained or adverse reactions appear, but the maximum number of doses is four. The minimum effective dose is then given tid or qid as needed.

REFLUX ESOPHAGITIS. **Bethanechol** has been used on an investigational basis for the treatment of gastroesophageal reflux. The drug is given orally in a dose of 25 mg qid for adults. In infants and children, the oral dose is 3 mg/m$_2$ tid.

Patient Education

ADMINISTRATION. To avoid nausea and vomiting, the patient should take the drug 1 hour before or 2 hours after a meal. The SC form is intended for subcutaneous use only and should never be given intramuscularly (IM) or IV because the resultant high drug levels can cause severe toxicity, evidenced by bloody diarrhea, bradycardia, profound hypotension, and cardiovascular collapse.

ADVERSE REACTIONS. This drug may cause abdominal discomfort, salivation, sweating, or flushing. Teach the patient to notify the health care provider if these occur. The dose may be reduced or the drug discontinued.

Dizziness or lightheadedness may occur when the patient arises from a lying or sitting position. The probable cause is hypotension. Arising slowly from a supine position and dangling the feet over the side of the bed before standing will reduce postural hypotension. No exercise in hot weather and a daily fluid intake of at least 2000 cc of noncaffeinated liquids will also reduce these problems.

Bethanechol may exacerbate diseases with a bronchospastic component. Teach the patient to report wheezing or breathing difficulties to the health care provider immediately.

Cholinesterase Inhibitors

This class of drugs prevents the degradation of ACh by AChE, thereby enhancing the activity of ACh at cholinergic receptors. These drugs act as indirect cholinergic agonists. These inhibitors can intensify ACh activity at all cholinergic junctions (muscarinic, ganglionic, and nicotinic) and so have a wide range of responses and adverse reactions.

There are two basic categories of **cholinergic inhibitors. Reversible inhibitors** produce effects of moderate duration. They include **ambenonium (Myletase), demecarium (Humorsol), donepezil (Aricept), edrophonium (Tensilon, Enlon, Reversol), neostigmine (Prostigmin), pyridostigmine (Mestinon), physostigmine (Antilirium)**, and **tacrine (Cognex).** Drugs in this group used for clinical diagnosis or for treatment of glaucoma are not discussed in this chapter.

Irreversible inhibitors are highly toxic and, although they can be split from AChE, the split takes place extremely slowly, and effects exist until new cholinesterase can be generated. They contain a phosphate atom and are referred to as organophosphate cholinesterase inhibitors. Because they are highly lipid-soluble, they can be absorbed even through the skin. Because of their systemic toxicity, they have only one clinical indication, as a treatment for glaucoma. The irreversible drugs are not discussed in this chapter.

Pharmacodynamics

The **reversible AChE inhibitors** act as poor substrates for AChE. The process by which AChE breaks down ACh into choline and acetic acid takes place in two steps: (1) binding ACh to the active center of AChE and (2) splitting of the ACh, which regenerates free AChE. This reaction is rapid so that one molecule of AChE can break down a large amount of ACh in a relatively short time. The **reversible AChE inhibitors** follow this same process, except that the process takes place slowly; the drug is bound to the active center of AChE for a relatively long time, preventing the regeneration of free AChE, and preventing AChE from catalyzing the breakdown of more ACh. The slowing down of the inactivation of ACh results in an increased intrasynaptic concentration of ACh and intensified neural transmission at virtually all junctions where ACh is the neurotransmitter. In sufficient doses, **neostigmine** and **pyridostigmine** can produce skeletal muscle stimulation and activation of muscarinic, ganglionic, and nicotinic receptors in the CNS. In therapeutic doses, they usually affect only muscarinic and nicotinic receptors at the myoneural junction without altering CNS function.

Tacrine and **donepezil**, used to treat Alzheimer's disease (AD), are designed to alter CNS function. AD is associated with profound cholinergic depletion. **Tacrine** increases the availability of intrasynaptic ACh in the brain. It is also thought to act as a partial agonist at muscarinic receptors by blocking reuptake of dopamine, serotonin, and norepinephrine. **Donepezil** is structurally dissimilar to other **AChE inhibitors**. With a high degree of selectivity, it reversibly and noncompetitively inhibits AChE in the CNS. It has very limited peripheral activity and a longer duration of inhibitory action than **tacrine**.

Pharmacokinetics

Absorption and Distribution

Each of the **AChE inhibitors** differs in its pharmacokinetics (Table 12–22). **Neostigmine** and **pyridostigmine** carry a positive charge. This charge results in poor absorption from the GI tract, and oral doses must be much greater than SC doses to produce a therapeutic effect. Once absorbed, these drugs distribute to sites of action in the myoneural junction and at peripheral muscarinic receptors, but they do not cross the blood-brain barrier.

Tacrine is rapidly absorbed following oral administration, but absorption is significantly reduced when it is taken with food, and a 30 to 40 percent decrease in bioavailability results. Because it is lipid-soluble, it crosses the blood-brain barrier, and its drug concentration is highest in the brain. Women tend to have concentrations that are 50 percent higher than those of men, even when they take the same dose.

Food has no effect on the absorption of **donepezil**. It is well absorbed following oral administration, with a bioavailability approaching 100 percent. Like **tacrine**, it is concentrated in the CNS, with very little peripheral activity.

Metabolism and Excretion

Neostigmine and **pyridostigmine** are degraded by AChE and metabolized by the liver to inactive products. The inactive products are excreted via the kidney.

Tacrine is extensively metabolized by CYP-450 1A2 isoenzymes in the liver. Terpstra and Terpstra (1998) suggest that the higher concentrations of drug in women may be related to decreased CYP-450 1A2 isoenzyme activity in women. Cigarette smoking also reduces this isoenzyme, and smokers have higher concentrations than nonsmokers. The relatively high first-pass effect in the metabolism of tacrine is dependent upon the dose administered. The CYP-450 1A1 system can be saturated at low doses. A larger fraction of a higher dose will escape elimination than a lower dose. Once in the plasma, elimination is not dose dependent. Although studies in patients with liver disease have not been done, it is rea-

Table 12–22. Pharmacokinetics: Selected Acetylcholinesterase Inhibitors

Drug	Onset	Peak	Duration	Protein Binding	Bioavailability (BA)	Half-Life	Elimination
Donepezil	Within 6 wk*	4 h	24 h	94–96%	100%	60–100 h	57% in urine; 15% in feces
Neostigmine	45–75 min	Unknown	2–4 h	15–25%	1–2%	40–60 min	By enzymatic degradation
Pyridostigmine PO	30–35 min	Unknown	3–6 h	UK	11–17%	3.7 h	By enzymatic degradation
Pyridostigmine SR	30–60 min	Unknown	6–12 h	UK	UK	3.7 h	By enzymatic degradation
Tacrine	Within 6 wk*	1–2 h	4–8 h	55%	17%; food reduces BA by 30–40%	2–4 h	1% as unchanged drug in urine

*Observable reduction in clinical symptoms.
UK = unknown.

sonable to expect that hepatic dysfunction reduces clearance of this drug. Pharmacokinetics are unaffected in older adults and in patients with renal insufficiency.

Donepezil is extensively metabolized by CYP-450 2D6 and 3A4 isoenzyme systems in the liver to two active and two less active metabolites. Approximately 57 percent of it is excreted in the urine and 15 percent in feces. Hepatic impairment has been shown to decrease clearance by 20 percent. Pharmacokinetics are unaffected in older adults and in patients with renal insufficiency.

Pharmacotherapeutics

Precautions and Contraindications

The only absolute contraindications for **neostigmine** and **pyridostigmine** are mechanical intestinal and urinary obstruction. The reasons are the same as those given for **bethanechol.** A relative contraindication is a history of reaction to **bromides.** *Neostigmine and pyridostigmine are Pregnancy Category C because they may cause uterine irritability, and neonates may display muscular weakness. Use these drugs only when clearly needed and the benefits clearly outweigh the risks to the fetus. Neostigmine is ionized at physiological pH and is not expected to be excreted in breast milk. Pyridostigmine is excreted in breast milk and should not be used by breastfeeding women.* Safety and efficacy have not been established for children.

Tacrine has been associated with hepatotoxicity. It is contraindicated for patients who have previously been treated with the drug and developed jaundice, and for patients with abnormal transaminase levels or clinical jaundice with a serum bilirubin above 3 mg/dL. Patients who are unwilling or unable to avoid drinking alcohol should also not have this drug prescribed because concurrent use may have additive toxic effects on the liver.

Cholinergic agonists are thought to have some potential to cause generalized seizures. **Tacrine** is also contraindicated for patients with a history of stroke, subdural hematoma, hydrocephalus, or CNS tumor because they are at increased risk for this adverse reaction.

Unlike **tacrine, donepezil** is not associated with hepatotoxicity. The only contraindication is hypersensitivity to **piperidine derivatives.**

All of these drugs should be used with caution for patients with a history of bronchospastic disorders, peptic ulcer disease, cardiovascular diseases that may worsen in the presence of hypotension or bradycardia, and hyperthyroidism. The reasons are the same as for **muscarinic agonists** and are based on the increased activity of ACh.

Both *tacrine* **and** *donepezil* **are Pregnancy Category C, but there are no well-controlled studies in pregnant women. Because these drugs are used to treat AD, they are unlikely to be used for women of childbearing age who are likely to become pregnant.** It is not known if they are excreted in breast milk, and there are no well-controlled trials to document safety and efficacy in any illness occurring in children.

Adverse Drug Reactions

Each of these drugs differs in adverse reactions. **Neostigmine** and **pyridostigmine** are associated with the adverse reactions common to all **cholinergic agonists.** In addition, muscle weakness, fasciculations, cramps, and spasms have been noted.

TOXICITY. The warning signs of overdose are very similar to common adverse reactions, and there is a narrow margin between the first appearance of adverse reactions and serious toxic effects. Adverse reactions such as excessive GI stimulation, excessive salivation, miosis, and fasciculations of voluntary muscles should be reported to the health care provider immediately, and the drug will be temporarily discontinued. **Atropine** 0.5 to 1 mg IV may be required.

The primary adverse reactions associated with **tacrine** are GI related. Tolerance to these reactions can be improved by taking the drugs with meals, although this practice reduces bioavailability. Other cholinergic-associated adverse reactions are usually dose-dependent and can be treated by temporarily reducing the dose.

HEPATOTOXICITY. **Tacrine** has been associated with hepatotoxicity in patients with a history of liver disease. A significant number of patients, even without such a history, develop elevated serum transaminases (ALT and AST). If the drug is promptly withdrawn, clinical evidence of liver injury is rare. To prevent liver injury in patients on this drug, monitor their liver function frequently. This topic is discussed in the Monitoring section.

Donepezil is well tolerated, with few adverse reactions. The most common are headache and diarrhea. Patients with a history of frequent GI complaints may be prone to recurrence of these problems while taking this drug. As with **tacrine,** cholinergic-associated adverse reactions are usually dose-dependent and can be treated by temporarily reducing the dose.

Drug Interactions

Synergistic effects occur between these drugs and other **cholinergic agonists.** Antagonistic effects occur with **anticholinergic drugs. Neostigmine** and **pyridostigmine** have increased risks for neuromuscular blockade with **aminoglycoside antibiotics** and **succinylcholine.** With the latter drug, respiratory support may be needed. These combinations should be avoided. **Atropine** and **belladonna derivatives** suppress many of the early warning symptoms of overdose and toxicity to **neostigmine** and **pyridostigmine.** Given the narrow margin between therapeutic dose and overdose, this increased risk is unacceptable, and these drugs should also not be given together. **Corticosteroids** and **magnesium** also interact with these drugs. Their interactions are presented in Table 12–23.

Their significant metabolism by the CYP-450 enzyme systems of the liver creates many drug interactions for **donepezil** and **tacrine.** Any drug metabolized by the CYP-450 1A2 isoenzymes has interactions with **tacrine,** and those metabolized by 2D6 and 3A4 have interac-

Table 12–23. Drug Interactions: Selected Acetylcholinesterase Inhibitors

Drug	Interacting Drug	Possible Effect	Implications
Donepezil	Anticholinergics	Donepezil antagonizes activity of anticholinergics.	Avoid concurrent administration.
	Bethanechol, succinylcholine	Synergistic cholinergic activity.	Reduce bethanechol dose if they must be given concurrently.
	NSAIDs	Donepezil increases gastric acid secretion.	Monitor for active or occult bleeding.
	Furosemide, digoxin, warfarin	At concentrations of 0.3–10 mg/cc did not affect binding or these drugs.	
	Ketoconazole, quinidine, other drugs metabolized by CYP-450 2D6 and 3A4 isoenzymes	Potentially inhibit donepezil metabolism.	Inhibit in vitro. No clinical studies to date. Choose alternative "azole" or antiarrhythmic.
Neostigmine, pyridostigmine	Succinylcholine	Increase neuromuscular blocking; prolonged respiratory depression with extended periods of apnea.	Provide respiratory support as needed or avoid concurrent use.
	Aminoglycoside antibiotics	Aminoglycosides have mild but definite nondepolarizing blocking action that may accentuate neuromuscular block.	Choose different antibiotic or monitor closely for increased blockade.
	Local and general anesthetics, antiarrhythmics	Decreased effects of neostigmine.	Increase dose of neostigmine while patient is taking these drugs.
	Atropine, belladonna derivatives	Suppress muscarinic symptoms of excessive GI stimulation, leaving only more serious symptoms of fasciculation and paralysis of voluntary muscles as signs of overdose.	Avoid concurrent use. Margin of safety is already quite narrow, and this makes it narrower.
	Corticosteroids	Decrease anti-AChE effects of neostigmine or pyridostigmine. Anti-AChE effects may increase after stopping steroids.	Avoid concurrent use or provide respiratory support as needed. Monitor respiratory status closely after stopping steroid.
	Magnesium	Has direct depressant effect on skeletal muscle; may antagonize beneficial effects of neostigmine or pyridostigmine.	Avoid concurrent use.
	Methocarbamol	A single case report indicates this drug may impair effect of pyridostigmine.	Only one case report. Monitor for possible effect.
Tacrine	All drugs metabolized by CYP-450 1A2 isoenzymes	May inhibit metabolism of tacrine.	Avoid concurrent use, or monitor effects and adjust doses as needed.
	Anticholinergics	Tacrine interferes with anticholinergic activity.	Monitor for anticholinergic activity if they must be given together. Note: Many drugs have anticholinergic-like effects even if not anticholinergic drugs. These should also be watched.

Continued on next page

Table 12–23. Drug Interactions: Selected Acetylcholinesterase Inhibitors (*continued*)

Drug	Interacting Drug	Possible Effect	Implications
	Cimetidine	Increases the peak plasma level of tacrine by 54% and the AUC by 64%.	Choose different histamine₂ blocker.
	Bethanechol, succinylcholine	Synergistic effects. Can cause bladder outlet obstruction.	Avoid concurrent use.
	Theophylline	Coadministration doubles theophylline elimination half-life and average plasma level.	Monitor plasma theophylline levels and reduce theophylline dose if they must be given together.
	NSAIDs	Increased risk for GI bleed.	Monitor for occult bleeding with serial stool guaiac tests and hemoglobin determinations. May need to take antacids while on tacrine therapy.

AUC = area under curve.

tions with **donepezil.** The number of drugs metabolized by the 1A2 isoenzymes is relatively small, but the number metabolized by 2D6 and 3A4 is large. To date, these drug interactions have largely been in vitro and in theory, but as these two drugs are prescribed for larger numbers of patients, the interactions must be monitored for and are likely to occur. **Donepezil** has the positive lack of interaction with **furosemide, digoxin,** and **warfarin,** drugs often prescribed for older adults who are also likely candidates for **donepezil.**

Clinical Use and Dosing

MYASTHENIA GRAVIS. Neostigmine and **pyridostigmine** are used to treat myasthenia gravis. In this disorder, an autoimmune process occurs in which the patient's immune system produces antibodies directed against nicotinic receptors on skeletal muscle, reducing the number of receptors by 70 to 90 percent. The end result is muscle weakness. **Reversible cholinesterase inhibitors** are the mainstay of treatment, preventing ACh inactivation and intensifying the effects of ACh on motor neurons. These drugs do not cure the disorder, but manage its symptoms, so treatment is lifelong.

Establishing an optimum dose for treatment can be a challenge because these drugs do not produce effects only at selected target organs. A small initial dose is administered, followed by other small doses until an optimal dose is reached. Signs of improvement that indicate optimal dosage include improved ability to swallow and to raise the eyelids.

The initial adult dose of **neostigmine** is usually 15 mg/day, and for children it is 2 mg/kg daily in divided doses given every 3 to 4 hours. The interval between dose increases is highly individualized. The average adult dose is 150 mg/day, but the maximum dose may approach 375 mg/day. Larger portions of the daily dose may be given 30 to 60 minutes prior to activities that produce greater fatigue, such as eating or shopping. For **pyridostigmine,**

the initial adult dose is 60 mg/day, and for children it is 7 mg/kg divided into five or six doses daily. Sustained-release tablets are available that require once- or twice-daily dosing. Regular tablets or syrup may be administered with extended-release tablets for optimum control of symptoms. Both of these drugs can be given parenterally if the patient has difficulty swallowing, but it is important to remember that, because of their first-pass effects, oral doses are 30 to 40 times greater than parenteral doses.

REVERSAL OF NONPOLARIZING NEUROMUSCULAR BLOCKADE. By producing increased ACh at the myoneural junction, **neostigmine** and **pyridostigmine** can reverse the effects of **nondepolarizing blocking agents.** They cannot be used to counter the effects of **succinylcholine** because it is a **depolarizing neuromuscular blocker.** The most common application of this role is immediately postoperative and is determined by the anesthesiologist. Because it would probably not be used in primary care or by a nurse practitioner, this use is not discussed further.

ALZHEIMER'S DISEASE. This disease is associated with a significant deficiency in brain levels of choline acetyltransferase, the enzyme responsible for the synthesis of ACh. In addition, cholinergic neurons in the brain's basal ganglia degenerate, resulting in a loss of cholinergic input to the muscarinic receptors in the frontal and temporal lobes of the cerebral cortex. Enhancing cholinergic activity with drugs is designed to counteract the decreased stimulation of the remaining cholinergic neurons. **Donepezil** and **tacrine** are both used to treat AD by increasing the availability of ACh through preventing its degradation by AChE.

Tacrine is a centrally active, noncompetitive, **reversible AChE inhibitor.** According to Terpstra and Terpstra (1998), approximately 30 to 40 percent of AD patients who were able to complete the drug trials demonstrated modest improvement in cognitive and functional measures. Unfortunately, these improvements were not noted to last longer than 30 weeks, and many patients did not complete the trials because of the adverse reactions associated with this drug. The response was dose-related, and adverse reactions increase as the dose increases.

Dosing usually begins with 10 mg given four times daily between meals. Taking the drug with meals makes it more tolerable, but the bioavailability is decreased by 30 to 40 percent, requiring higher doses for the same effect. Doses are increased at 6-week intervals, based on liver function studies, to a maximum of 160 mg/day. The monitoring requirements are discussed later. An adequate response is defined as the lack of apparent disease progression for 6 months, and it requires at least 8 weeks at doses greater than 120 mg/day. The highest-tolerated dose is the most efficacious.

Donepezil is a **piperidine-based derivative** dissimilar from other **AChE inhibitors** in its pharmacokinetics and tolerability. It is also a centrally active, noncompetitive, **reversible AChE inhibitor,** but its duration of inhibitory action is longer than **tacrine**. This longer duration of action permits once-daily dosing, which is a major advantage for this drug. Another advantage for this drug is its better adverse reactions profile. The most problematic adverse reaction is digestive complaints, and this may require dosage reduction.

Clinical trials showed improvement in cognitive function for as long as 2 years, but after this period there were indications that the drug did not prevent further long-term disease progression. The improvement was dose-related, and adverse reactions also increased with the increased dose.

The recommended starting dose is 5 mg daily at bedtime. Doses are increased at 1-week intervals to a maximum of 10 mg daily. The higher dose should be used if tolerated because it is more efficacious. Unlike **tacrine, donepezil** is not likely to cause hepatotoxicity and does not require assessment of liver function in determining dose increases or frequent monitoring of liver function throughout therapy.

Table 12–24 shows the clinical use and dosing schedules for all four of these drugs. Only uses associated with primary care are presented.

Rational Drug Selection

FORMULATION. For **neostigmine** and **pyridostigmine,** formulation is a consideration (Table 12–25). Difficulty in swallowing is a common problem for patients with myas-

Table 12–24. Dosage Schedule: Acetylcholinesterase Inhibitors

Drug	Indication	Initial Dose	Maintenance Dose
Donepezil	AD	5 mg qd at bedtime for 1 wk.	May increase to 10 mg qd. The higher dose should be used if tolerated, because it is more efficacious.
Neostigmine	Myasthenia gravis	Adults: Oral: 15 mg/d divided and given every 3–4 h. Increase dose in 15 mg increments at daily intervals until optimal response is achieved. SC/IM: 0.5 mg every 2–3 h. Children: Oral: 2 mg/kg/d in 6–8 divided doses. SC/IM: 0.01–0.04 mg/kg every 2–3 h.	Usual dose is 150 mg/d divided and given every 3–4 h. Maximum dose is 375 mg/d. Usually needed short term, and dose is 5 mg every 2–3 h. Same maintenance dose. Usually needed short term. Same dose.
Pyridostigmine	Myasthenia gravis	Adults: Oral: 60 mg/d divided and given every 3–4 h. Increase dose in 60-mg increments at daily intervals until optimal dose is achieved. IM: one-third the oral dose. Children: Oral: 7 mg/kg/d divided into 5–6 doses. IM: 0.05–0.15 mg/kg/dose every 2–3 h.	Usual dose is 600 mg/d divided and given every 3–4 h. Maximum dose is 1500 mg/d. Same maintenance dose. Usually needed short term. Same dose.
Tacrine	AD	10 mg qid between meals for 6 wk; may be given with food, but bioavailability is decreased 30–40%.	If ALT remains unchanged, increase by 40 mg/d every 6 wk up to a maximum of 40 mg qid. Usual maintenance dose is 120 mg/d.

ALT = alanine aminotransferase.

Table 12–25. Available Dosage Forms: Acetylcholinesterase Inhibitors

Drug	Dosage Form	Package
Donepezil (Aricept)	Tablets: 5 mg, 10 mg	In bottles of 30 tablets; unit dose blister packs of 100 tablets
Neostigmine (Prostigmin)	Tablets: 15 mg	In bottles of 100 scored tablets
Pyridostigmine (Mestinon)	Tablets: 60 mg	In bottles of 100, 500 tablets
	SR tablets: 180 mg	In bottles of 100 tablets
	Syrup: 60 mg/5 cc	In 480-cc bottles of raspberry-flavored syrup (5% alcohol, sorbitol)
Tacrine (Cognex)	Tablets: 10 mg, 20 mg, 30 mg, 40 mg	In bottles of 120 tablets; unit dose packs of 100 tablets

thenia gravis. **Pyridostigmine** is available in a syrup form that can be used by many patients with this problem without having to resort to an injectable form. In addition, the syrup can be used for children to administer their small and individualized doses based on body weight.

COST. There is not a significant cost differentiation between **neostigmine** and **pyridostigmine**. The cost differential between **tacrine** and **donepezil** is largely related to the monitoring costs. **Donepezil** does not produce hepatotoxicity and requires only routine monitoring of blood chemistries. **Tacrine,** which does produce hepatotoxicity, requires frequent monitoring of liver function. The monitoring guidelines are presented later. The cost of so many tests for so long is high. According to Terpstra and Terpstra (1998), the cost of **tacrine** therapy "is about $1600 per year for the medication, $360 per year for liver function tests for the first year and $120 per year for hepatic monitoring in each of the following years."

DOSING SCHEDULE. The dosing schedules of **neostigmine** and **pyridostigmine** are similar. Those of **donepezil** and **tacrine** are quite different. **Donepezil** has a once-daily dosing regimen. **Tacrine** requires four daily doses, and they are most effective on an empty stomach, which results in their timing being adjusted for meals. For patients who are older adults and who have a disease process that includes memory problems, or for patients whose caregivers are also older adults, this complex regimen may present adherence problems.

ADVERSE REACTIONS PROFILE. **Neostigmine** and **pyridostigmine** have similar adverse reaction profiles. **Donepezil** has fewer adverse reactions than **tacrine**.

TIME TO RECURRENCE OF DISEASE PROGRESSION. **Tacrine** has been associated with loss of beneficial effects after about 30 weeks. **Donepezil** has shown positive effects for at least 2 years.

Monitoring

Monitoring parameters for **tacrine** are complex and, at a minimum, continue for 9 months. Baseline liver function tests (total bilirubin, aspartate transaminase [AST],

and alanine aminotransferase [ALT]) should be done prior to initiation of therapy. ALT levels, the ones most likely to indicate hepatotoxicity, should be monitored every other week for the first 16 weeks of therapy, then monthly for 2 months, and then every 3 months. If the ALT level remains less than double the upper limit of normal, the dose may be left unchanged or titrated upward as needed. If the ALT level is more than double the upper limit of normal, weekly monitoring of liver function is required. If the ALT level is three to five times the upper limit of normal, weekly monitoring of liver function is required, and the dose must be decreased by 40 mg/day. If the ALT level returns to the normal range with the reduced dose, every other week monitoring of ALT levels is sufficient. Treatment is discontinued if the ALT concentration is more than five times the upper limit of normal.

Donepezil requires routine monitoring of blood chemistries and hematology. **Neostigmine** and **pyridostigmine** do not have monitoring parameters beyond those of the disease process they are used to treat.

Patient Education

ADMINISTRATION. Administration education differs for the two groups of drugs. For all of the drugs, the drug should be taken exactly as prescribed. Doses should not be skipped or doubled up.

For **neostigmine** and **pyridostigmine**, patients may need to set a backup alarm to remind them to take a dose when the doses are every 3 to 4 hours. Taking the dose late may cause myasthenic crisis, and taking it early may result in cholinergic crisis. Because drug therapy is lifelong, it is important to establish a regimen that the patient can follow over time.

For **donepezil**, missed doses should be skipped and the schedule resumed the next day. Patients taking **tacrine** should deal with missed doses by taking them as soon as possible unless it is within 2 hours of the next dose. For both **donepezil** and **tacrine**, increasing the dose may not improve the symptoms but it does increase the risk for adverse reactions. Abruptly discontinuing the drug may cause a decline in cognitive function.

ADVERSE REACTIONS. All of these drugs have in common the adverse reactions associated with an increased amount of ACh: dizziness, miosis, lacrimation, excessive secretions in the respiratory and GI tracts, bronchospasm, bradycardia, abdominal cramps, nausea, vomiting, diarrhea, and excessive salivation. Because they have fewer peripheral effects, **donepezil** and **tacrine** have fewer of the peripheral adverse reactions and more of those associated with the CNS. Patients and their caregivers should observe safety precautions related to the dizziness.

Administration of **neostigmine** or **pyridostigmine** with food or milk helps to minimize adverse GI reactions. Patients with myasthenia gravis often have difficulty with swallowing. Sustained-release tablets must be swallowed whole. Regular tablets may be crushed, and syrup forms of **pyridostigmine** are available to facilitate administration in this situation. The mottled appearance of the sustained-release form of **pyridostigmine** does not affect its potency.

Administration with food may reduce GI complaints for **donepezil** and does not affect its bioavailability. Although **tacrine** can also be administered with food, this decreases its bioavailability by 30 to 40 percent and may necessitate increased dosage. The higher the dosage, the higher the risk for adverse reactions. For patients with difficulty in swallowing, **tacrine** capsules can be dissolved in any aqueous solution. Orange juice masks the bitter taste best.

Tacrine has adverse reactions associated with hepatotoxicity. Patients who experience jaundice, rash, or fever should contact the health care provider immediately. The drug will be discontinued.

LIFESTYLE MANAGEMENT. No specific lifestyle modifications are directly related to these drugs. Patients with myasthenia gravis should at all times wear identification describing the disease and the medication regimen.

Nicotine

The major source of **nicotine** use is tobacco products. Although tobacco contains many hazardous products (carbon monoxide, hydrogen cyanide, ammonia, nitrosamines, and tar), the one of major concern and the one associated with the addictive mechanism of the drug is **nicotine.** The focus of this chapter is **nicotine** as a drug. Chapter 41 discusses smoking cessation.

Pharmacodynamics

The actions of **nicotine** are based on their effects on nicotinic receptors. Inhibition or stimulation of the receptor is dose-dependent. Low doses stimulate receptors, and high doses inhibit them. Ingestion of the **nicotine** found in pesticides results in high doses, and as little as 40 mg can be lethal. Most of the **nicotine** in smoked tobacco products is destroyed by burning or escapes in sidestream smoke so that the dose is relatively low. For cigarette, cigar, and pipe smokers, **nicotine** stimulates nicotinic receptors at several locations. The receptors in the autonomic ganglia and the adrenal medulla receive the greatest stimulation. Those in the carotid body, aortic arch, and CNS are also stimulated, with the CNS effects similar to those of cocaine. At the dose produced by smoking, the receptors at the myoneural junction are not affected.

Cardiovascular Effects

Cardiovascular effects result from stimulation of the sympathetic ganglia and the adrenal medulla, promoting the release of epinephrine and norepinephrine. These catecholamines produce vasoconstriction, accelerated heart rate, and increased force of ventricular contraction. The end result is increased blood pressure and increased cardiac output.

Gastrointestinal Effects

The GI effects result from stimulation of the nicotinic receptors in the parasympathetic ganglia, resulting in in-

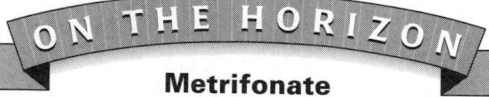

ON THE HORIZON

Metrifonate

FDA approval for **metrifonate,** a third **AChE inhibitor** specifically designed for treatment of AD, was anticipated in 1999. According to Terpstra and Terpstra (1999), it is not metabolized by the CYP-450 enzyme system but is converted nonenzymatically to an active metabolite. Preclinical studies have shown that this enzyme elevates ACh levels by stably binding to the active site of AChE, resulting in inhibition of AChE for long periods of time. The most pronounced effect appears to be in areas of the brain deficient in ACh. Two large double-blind, randomized trials were recently published. Further discussion of this drug is found in the article by Terpstra and Terpstra.

creased secretion of gastric acid and increased tone and motility of the GI smooth muscle. **Nicotine** can also induce vomiting, based on a complex process that involves the receptors in the aortic arch and the CNS. Vomiting often follows tobacco ingestion by infants and children.

Central Nervous System Effects

The effect on the CNS is stimulation, resulting in increased respiratory rate and an arousal pattern on the electroencephalogram. Moderate doses can cause tremors, and high doses can cause convulsions. Psychological effects include increased alertness, facilitation of memory, improved cognitive function, reduced aggression, and suppressed appetite. **Nicotine** also facilitates the release of dopamine at the "pleasure center," producing the same effects as other highly addictive drugs, such as **cocaine, amphetamines,** and **opioids.**

The replacement therapy formulations produce similar but lesser effects because the dose is lower and the pharmacokinetics are different. Depending on the formulation used, the stimulation of the pleasure centers may be significantly different.

Pharmacokinetics

Absorption and Distribution

Three forms of replacement therapy for **nicotine** addiction exist: chewing gum, transdermal patches, and nasal spray (Table 12–26). The **nicotine** in the gum is bound to an exchange resin and released only during chewing. Approximately 68 percent of the **nicotine** in patches is absorbed via the skin. Both of these formulations raise blood levels of **nicotine** slowly, producing less pleasure than cigarettes, but relieving withdrawal symptoms. Each of these systems is labeled by the actual amount of **nicotine** absorbed. Approximately 93 percent of the **nicotine** in the nasal spray is absorbed through the nasal mucosa, and blood levels rise rapidly, much the same as with smoking, producing some subjective pleasure while suppressing withdrawal symptoms.

Nicotine replacement therapy (NRT) by any formulation is widely distributed in the body, crosses the placenta, and enters the breast milk.

Metabolism and Excretion

Nicotine is metabolized mainly by the liver and, to a lesser extent, by the kidney and lung. There is no significant skin metabolism. More than 20 metabolites have been identified, all of which are believed to be less active than the parent compound. The half-life of **nicotine** is 1 to 2 hours, but the half-life of its primary metabolite (cotinine) is 15 to 20 hours, and its concentrations exceed **nicotine** by 10-fold.

Ten to 20 percent of **nicotine** is excreted unchanged in the urine. As high as 30 percent may be excreted with high urine flow rates and urine acidification below pH 5.

Pharmacotherapeutics

Precautions and Contraindications

The effects on the various body systems determine the contraindications. In each case, the decision to use or not

Table 12–26. Pharmacokinetics: Selected Nicotine Replacement Systems

Drug	Onset	Peak	Duration	Protein Binding	Percent Absorbed	Half-Life	Elimination
Nicorette gum	Rapid	15–30 min	Unknown	<5%	Unknown	1–2 h	10% unchanged in urine. Up to 30% with high urine flow rates and pH 5.
Nicoderm patch	Slow	2–4 h	24 h	<5%	68%	1–2 h	10% unchanged in urine. Up to 30% with high urine flow rates and pH 5.
Habitrol patch	Slow	6–12 h	24 h	<5%	68%	1–2 h	10% unchanged in urine. Up to 30% with high urine flow rates and pH 5.
Prostep patch	Slow	9 h	24 h	<5%	68%	1–2 h	10% unchanged in urine. Up to 30% with high urine flow rates and pH 5.
Nicotrol nasal spray	Rapid	4–15 min	Unknown	Unknown	93%	1–2 h	10% unchanged in urine. Up to 30% with high urine flow rates and pH 5.

use **NRT** is based on the likelihood of smoking cessation and its benefits versus the potential adverse effects.

Cardiovascular effects result in contraindicated use of **NRT** for patients with severe cardiovascular disease, life-threatening arrhythmias, severe or worsening angina, or vasospastic diseases and during the immediate post-MI period. **NRT** is used in the presence of hypertension only when the benefits of smoking cessation clearly outweigh the risk for perpetuating the hypertension.

The actions of **nicotine** on the adrenal medulla require cautious use of **NRT** for patients with hyperthyroidism, pheochromocytoma, or type 1 diabetes mellitus. **Nicotine** is extensively metabolized by the liver, and its total clearance is dependent on liver blood flow. **NRT** should be used with caution in the presence of hepatic impairment. Only severe renal impairment is expected to affect the clearance of nicotine or its metabolites. Less severe renal impairment does not preclude the use of **NRT**.

Nicotine delays healing in esophagitis and peptic ulcer disease and should be used for patients with active disease only when the benefits clearly outweigh the risks. Transdermal systems are usually well tolerated by patients with normal skin but may be irritating for patients with some skin disorders.

Administration of *nicotine* during pregnancy can cause fetal harm. It is associated with decreased fetal breathing movements and with decreased placental perfusion, resulting in infants who are small for gestational age. Some forms are Pregnancy Category X (*nicotine polacrilex*), and some are Pregnancy Category D (*transdermal nicotine*). Pregnant women should use them only if the likelihood of smoking cessation justifies the potential risk to the fetus.

Nicotine passes freely into breast milk and has the potential for serious harm to the nursing infant. Replacement therapy should be undertaken only if the likelihood of smoking cessation justifies the potential risk to the nursing infant.

The amount of **nicotine** that can be tolerated by an adult can produce poisoning or be lethal in children. The systems used for replacement therapy are contraindicated for children. Adults using these systems should take every precaution to keep them out of the reach of children.

Adverse Drug Reactions

Adverse reactions are largely based on the actions of **nicotine** on the various body systems. CNS adverse effects include headache, insomnia, and dizziness. Cardiovascular adverse effects include tachycardia and hypertension. GI system effects include abnormal taste, dry mouth, and dyspepsia.

Nicorette gum may produce pharyngitis, belching, increased salivation, hiccoughs, and nausea and vomiting. **Nicotrol** nasal spray may produce nasopharyngeal irritation, rhinitis, sneezing, and watery eyes. Transdermal systems may produce burning, erythema, and pruritus at the patch site. Applying the patch to different sites each day may reduce these symptoms. **Nicotine** kinetics are similar for all sites of application on the upper body and upper outer arm.

Drug Interactions

Smoking cessation, with or without **NRT**, may alter the patient's response to a number of drugs for which smoking is known to increase the metabolism and lower the blood levels. Table 12–27 lists these drugs and the changes in patient response.

Effective absorption of **Nicorette** gum requires slightly alkaline saliva. Coffee, tea, cola, and other drinks and foods may reduce salivary pH. It may be beneficial for patients to not ingest food or drink while or within 15 minutes of using this product.

Clinical Use and Dosing

The only indication for **NRT** is smoking cessation. Choice of route and dose are dependent upon patient wishes, cost, and smoking history (Table 12–28). The Fagerstrom Test for Nicotine Dependence (Andrews, 1998), discussed in Chapter 41, can be used to determine appropriate dose.

Nicorette gum comes in two strengths: 2 mg/piece and 4 mg/piece (Table 12–29). Patients with low to moderate nicotine dependence use the 2 mg/piece strength; patients with high dependence use the 4 mg/piece strength. The average dosage is 9 to 12 pieces of gum/day. The maximum dose is 30 pieces of the 2 mg/piece

Clinical Pearl

Substituting one or more pieces of sugarless gum for pieces of **Nicorette** gum and increasing the number of substitutions may help in reducing the dose during withdrawal.

Table 12–27. Drug Interactions: Nicotine Replacement Therapy
or Smoking Cessation

Interacting Drug	Patient Response with Smoking	Patient Response with Nicotine Replacement Therapy (NRT) or Smoking Cessation	Implications
Acetaminophen, caffeine, imipramine, labetalol, oxazepam, pentazocine, prazosin, propranolol and other beta blockers, theophylline	Increased metabolism and lowered blood levels of these drugs	Reversal of increased metabolism	Dosage reduction at cessation of smoking and onset of NRT may be necessary.
Catecholamines, cortisol	Increased circulating catecholamines and cortisol	Return to normal levels	Dosage of adrenergic agonist and adrenergic antagonists may need to be adjusted.
Furosemide	Reduced diuretic effects and decreased cardiac output	Increased diuretic effects	Dosage reduction may be needed.
Insulin		Increased SC insulin absorption	Monitor blood glucose levels and adjust dosage of insulin.
Propoxyphene	Increased first-pass metabolism	Decreased first-pass metabolism	Dosage adjustments may be needed.

Table 12–28. Dosage Schedule: Nicotine Replacement Therapy

Drug	Dosing	Length of Therapy	Cost
Nicorette gum	9–12 pieces of gum/d. Maximum dose for 2-mg piece is 30/d; for 4-mg piece is 20/d. Low to moderate dependence start with 2 mg; high dependence start with 4 mg.	After 3 mo, withdraw gradually. Use beyond 6 mo not recommended.	2-mg piece: $27.80 for 48 pieces. 4-mg piece: $31.29 for 48 pieces.
Habitrol patch Nicoderm patch	21 mg/d patch for 6 wk; then 14 mg/d patch for 2 wk; then 7 mg/d patch for 2 wk.	8–12 wk.	Habitrol patches: 21 mg/d: $121.75 for 30. 14 mg/d: $115.70 for 30. 7 mg/d: $109.60 for 30. Nicoderm patches: 21 mg/d: $27.80 for 7. 14 mg/d: $27.80 for 7. 7 mg/d: $27.80 for 7.
Nicotrol	15 mg/d patch for 12 wk; then 10 mg/d patch for 2 wk; then 5 mg patch for 2 wk.	14–20 wk.	Each strength costs $25.76 for 7 patches.
Prostep	22 mg/d for 4–8 wk; then 11 mg/d for 2–4 wk.	6–12 wk.	22 mg/d: $34.18 for 7 patches. 11 mg/d: $31.49 for 7 patches.
Nicotrol NS	1 spray each nostril prn. Max doses is 5 doses/h or 40 doses/d.	After 4–6 wk, gradually withdraw.	$36/10 cc.

Table 12–29. Available Dosage Forms: Nicotine Replacement Therapy

Drug	Dosage Form	Package
Nicorette	Gum: 2 mg per square	In packs of 96
Nicorette DS	Gum: 4 mg per square	In packs of 96
Habitrol	Transdermal: 21 mg, 14 mg, 7 mg	In 30 systems per box
Nicoderm	Transdermal: 21 mg, 14 mg, 7 mg	In 14 systems per box
Nicotrol	Transdermal: 15 mg, 10 mg, 5 mg	In 14 systems per box
Prostep	Transdermal: 22 mg, 11 mg	In 7 systems per box
Nicotrol NS	Nasal spray: 10 mg/cc	In 10-cc bottles (100 doses)

strength and 20 pieces of the 4 mg/piece strength. Dosing on a fixed schedule (e.g., one piece every 2 to 3 hours) is more effective than prn dosing. After 3 months, the patient should discontinue **nicotine** use. Withdrawal should be gradual. Gradual reduction is accomplished over 2 to 3 months by decreasing the daily dose by one or more every 4 to 7 days and decreasing the chewing time with each piece from 30 minutes to 10 to 15 minutes every 4 to 7 days. The gum may be discontinued when one or two pieces per day are sufficient to control the craving for **nicotine.** Use of this product beyond 6 months is not recommended.

Patches are applied every morning to clean, dry, hairless skin of the upper body or upper arm and worn for 16 (**Nicotrol**) to 24 (all other patches) hours each day. The site is changed daily and not reused for at least 1 week. Most patients begin with the largest dosage patch and gradually decrease the dose. Patients with cardiovascular disease, those who weigh less than 100 lb, or those who smoke less than one-half pack per day should begin treatment with a smaller patch.

Habitrol and **Nicoderm** patches come in 21 mg/day, 14 mg/day, and 7 mg/day doses. The 21 mg/day patch is worn for 6 weeks, and then the 14 mg/day dose and the 7 mg/day dose are worn for 2 weeks each. The entire course of therapy is 8 to 12 weeks.

Nicotrol patches come in 15 mg/day, 10 mg/day, and 5 mg/day doses. The 15 mg/day patch is worn for 12 weeks, and then the 10 mg/day and 5 mg/day patches are worn for 2 weeks each. The entire course of therapy is 14 to 20 weeks.

Prostep patches come in 22 mg/day and 11 mg/day doses. The 22 mg/day patches are worn for 4 to 8 weeks, and the 11 mg/day patches are then worn for 2 to 4 weeks. The entire course of therapy is 6 to 12 weeks.

Nicotrol NS nasal spray device delivers 0.5 mg of nicotine per activation. Two sprays (one in each nostril) constitute one dose and are equivalent to the nicotine in one cigarette. Initial dosing is 1 to 2 doses per hour but never more than 5 doses per hour or 40 doses per day. After 4 to 6 weeks, the doses are gradually reduced and then stopped completely.

Rational Drug Selection

COST. If cost is calculated on a daily basis, assuming the recommended dose of the patches and the midrange use of the gum, the average daily cost for the gum is about $6.25 per day; for **Habitrol, Nicoderm,** and **Nicotrol** about $4 per day; and for **Prostep** about $4.85 per day. The total cost for the entire course of therapy is higher for **Nicorette** gum at $562 for 3 months of therapy. Among the patches, the daily cost is about the same, but **Nicotrol** has a longer program and **Prostep** a shorter one. Total cost for **Habitrol** and **Nicoderm** is around $278, for **Nicotrol** it is $360, and for **Prostep** it is $200.

CONVENIENCE. The patches are often the preferred method of **NRT** because they provide relatively constant concentrations of serum **nicotine** and they are convenient to use. A new patch is applied on a daily basis. **Nicorette** gum, however, is available OTC and does not require a prescription or the cost of a visit to a health care provider.

SUCCESS RATES. According the Andrews (1998), **nicotine** gum improves smoking cessation rates by 40 to 60 percent at 12 months. Transdermal patches approximately double the 6- to 12-month abstinence rates of a placebo. Lehne (1998) reports "good news, bad news" for abstinence with the nasal spray. Nearly 50 percent of users avoided smoking for 1 year, but many of these people continued to use the spray and were unwilling or unable to give it up.

CONCOMITANT DISEASES. Gum is more likely to produce GI adverse reactions and should be avoided for patients with esophagitis and active peptic ulcer disease. Patches are well tolerated by patients with normal skin but may cause problems for patients with certain skin disorders. Patients who have sinus problems, allergies, or asthma should avoid the sprays.

Monitoring

No specific monitoring is required.

Patient Education

ADMINISTRATION. Nicorette gum is not swallowed. It is chewed for a few seconds until a peppery taste or tingling sensation occurs. It is then "parked" between the cheek and gum until the sensation is almost gone (about 1 minute), and the process of chewing and parking the gum is repeated for approximately 30 minutes. Rapid, vigorous chewing is more likely to result in adverse reactions and is to be avoided. Dosing on a fixed schedule (e.g., one piece every 2 to 3 hours) is more effective than prn dosing. Eating or drinking acidic beverages should be avoided 15 minutes before or during the use of the gum. Gradual reduction of the dose can be accomplished by decreasing the daily dose by one or more every 4 to 7 days, by decreasing chewing time to 15 minutes, or by substituting sugarless gum for one or more of the daily doses.

Transdermal patches (**Habitrol, Nicoderm, Nicotrol, Prostep**) are applied at the same time each day to clean, dry, hairless skin of the upper torso or upper arm. Sites are rotated daily, and the same site should not be used again for at least 1 week. The patch is kept in its sealed pouch until it is applied. It is then pressed firmly in place with the palm for 10 seconds to be sure there is good contact. The patch remains in place while the patient is showering, bathing, or swimming. **Nicotrol** patches remain in place for 16 hours. All others remain in place for 24 hours. Wash hands with plain water after handling the patches because soap increases the absorption of **nicotine.** To prevent children from exposure to the drug in the patch, dispose of patches by folding them in half and wrapping them in aluminum foil.

Nicotrol NS nasal spray is used much like other nasal sprays. Tilt the head back slightly and spray once into each nostril. Do not sniff, swallow, or inhale through the nose as the spray is administered. Replace the child-resistant cap after using and before disposal. Gradual reduction of the dose is accomplished by using one spray at a time, using the spray less frequently, or skipping a dose. A date for stopping the spray should be set.

ADVERSE REACTIONS. The most common adverse reactions vary with the route of administration. For **Nicorette** gum, the most common are increased salivation, sore mouth, and pharyngitis. Substituting sugarless gum for some doses of **Nicorette** not only aids in dosage reduction but also can improve these symptoms. Good oral hygiene and adequate fluid intake are also helpful.

For the transdermal patches, burning, erythema, and itching at the application site may occur. These usually subside within 1 hour. Allergic reactions can occur, including reactions to the adhesive. Teach the patient to report rash or other symptoms of an allergic reaction or failure of these symptoms to resolve. A different brand or a different route of administration may be required.

For the nasal spray, nasopharyngeal irritation, sneezing, rhinitis, and watery eyes may occur. This route should be avoided in patients with sinus problems or asthma.

LIFESTYLE MANAGEMENT. Successful smoking cessation is dependent on more than **NRT.** It often involves counseling and support groups and may involve other drugs such as antidepressants concomitantly. Lifestyle changes associated with addictive substances are never easy. Chapter 41 provides more data on smoking cessation.

Cholinergic Blockers

Cholinergic blockers are also referred to as **parasympatholytics, muscarinic antagonists,** and **anticholinergics.** The term **anticholinergic** can be deceiving because it implies blockade of all cholinergic receptors. In reality, cholinergic blockers produce selective muscarinic blockade against the actions of ACh. Because muscarinic receptors are found in many organs of the body (the eye, heart, blood vessels, lung, GI tract, urinary bladder, and sweat glands), and these drugs cannot be targeted at a single organ, they have many adverse reactions.

There are several subtypes of **cholinergic blockers** based on the organs they are likely to target. **Atropine** is the prototype drug in this class and affects most muscarinic receptors. Its main use orally is as an adjunct to treatment of GI disorders. Other uses are more related to hospital-based care. Its oral use is discussed in this section. **Scopolamine** has actions similar to **atropine** except for increased CNS depression and ability to suppress motion sickness and emesis. It is also covered in this section. The **antispasmodic** group of drugs is indicated for reduction of GI motility and urinary tract smooth muscle spasm. They are covered in this section. **Ipratropium bromide (Atrovent)** is used to treat asthma and other respiratory disease. It is discussed in Chapter 15. **Mydriatic cycloplegics** are used for ophthalmic procedures. This use is covered in the chapter on drugs used to treat eye conditions. Centrally acting **cholinergic blockers** are used to treat Parkinson's disease and to counteract the extrapyramidal adverse reactions associated with some **psychotropic drugs.** They are briefly discussed here, but these uses are covered in Chapter 13.

Pharmacodynamics

Cholinergic blockers competitively block the actions of ACh at muscarinic receptors. They have no direct effect on the receptor. Their actions are based on preventing receptor activation and thereby producing an action that is the opposite of the action associated with stimulation of these receptors. The results of the stimulation of these receptors are depicted in Table 12–1. Blockade produces clinically significant action on the cardiovascular, respiratory, urinary, GI, and central nervous systems, on exocrine glands, and on the eye. Different drugs in the class affect these systems to differing degrees.

Cardiovascular Effects

Because stimulation of muscarinic receptors decreases heart rate, blockade increases heart rate. The effect on contractility and automaticity is minimal.

Respiratory Effects

Blockade of muscarinic receptors in smooth muscle causes relaxation of the bronchial muscle, and blockade in bronchial glands decreases bronchial secretions.

Exocrine Gland Effects

Blockade of other exocrine glands produces decreased secretion from salivary glands, sweat glands, and the acid-secreting cells of the stomach.

Urinary and Gastrointestinal Effects

Blockade of muscarinic receptors in smooth muscle in these systems decreases tone in the urinary bladder and both tone and motility in the GI tract.

Central Nervous System Effects

At therapeutic doses, muscarinic blockade produces mild CNS excitation. At higher doses, it produces hallucinations and delirium. **Scopolamine** is the exception, with its sedating action.

Optic Effects

Blockade of muscarinic receptors on the iris produces mydriasis. Blockade of receptors on the ciliary muscle produces cycloplegia.

The action is also, to some extent, dose-dependent. Some muscarinic receptors can be blocked at relatively low doses, and some require higher doses for blockade to occur. Doses required to block receptors in the stomach and bronchial smooth muscle are higher, for example, than those required to block receptors at other locations. Because treatment with higher doses results in more adverse reactions, and other drugs are more effective, this class of drugs is not used as primary agents to suppress gastric acid secretion or to dilate the bronchi.

Pharmacokinetics

Absorption and Distribution

Cholinergic blockers in the **belladonna alkaloid group** (atropine, scopolamine) are well absorbed from the gut and cross the conjunctival membrane (Table 12–30). When applied in a suitable vehicle, **scopolamine** is absorbed from the skin. In contrast, only about 10 to 30 percent of a dose of the drugs in the **quaternary group** (methantheline [Banthine], propantheline [Probanthine]) is absorbed after oral administration because these drugs have decreased lipid solubility. **Benztropine (Cogentin)**, **oxybutynin (Ditropan)**, and **trihexyphenidyl (Artane)** are all well absorbed following oral administration.

The **belladonna alkaloid group** is widely distributed, with significant levels reaching the CNS within 30 to 60 minutes after administration. The **quaternary group** is widely distributed except to the CNS, where it is poorly taken up. The distribution of **benztropine (Cogentin)**, **oxybutynin (Ditropan)**, and **trihexyphenidyl (Artane)** is not clearly known.

Metabolism and Excretion

Both the **belladonna alkaloids** and the **quaternary groups** are metabolized mostly by the liver and excreted in urine. The metabolism and excretion of the other drugs are not clearly known.

Table 12–30. Pharmacokinetics: Selected Cholinergic Blockers

Drug	Onset	Peak	Duration	Half-Life	Elimination
Atropine PO	30 min	30–60 min	4–6 h	3 h	30–50% unchanged in urine
Benztropine	1–2 h	Several days	24 h	Unknown	Unknown
Dicyclomine	Unknown	Unknown	Unknown	9–10 h	80% in urine; 10% in feces
Propantheline	30–60 min	2–6 h	6 h	3–4 h	Inactivated in upper small intestine
Oxybutynin	30–60 min	3–6 h	6–10 h	Unknown	Unknown
Scopolamine PO	30 min	1 h	4–6 h	8 h	Mostly metabolized by liver
Scopolamine transdermal	4 h	Unknown	72 h	Unknown	Mostly metabolized by liver
Trihexyphenidyl	1 h	2–3 h	6–12 h	5.6–10.2 h	Unknown

Pharmacotherapeutics

Precautions and Contraindications

Absolute contraindications to these drugs are few and based on their effects on various body systems. **Cholinergic blockers** are contraindicated in glaucoma, particularly angle-closure glaucoma, because of their ability to produce mydriasis and cycloplegia, thereby impeding the flow of aqueous humor. Cautious use is necessary in obstructive disorders of the GI and urinary tracts, including bladder outlet obstruction and benign prostatic hypertrophy (BPH), based on the ability of these drugs to decrease tone and motility in these systems. Patients with hypertension and tachycardia or other cardiac arrhythmias require cautious use, based on these drugs' effects on heart rate.

Older adults are particularly susceptible to the CNS effects of **cholinergic blockers,** with an increased risk for cognitive impairment and falls. Other drugs should be chosen when possible, or **cholinergic blockers** should be used with caution.

All drugs in this class except dicyclomine and oxybutynin are Pregnancy Category C. There are no well-controlled studies in pregnant women, and these drugs should be used only when potential benefits clearly outweigh the risk to the fetus. Dicyclomine and oxybutynin are Pregnancy Category B. No risk to the fetus has been shown in animal or human studies.

The **quaternary group** of drugs is not widely distributed in the body and is the least problematic for lactating women. All other **cholinergic blockers** either have wide distribution, including breast milk, or their distribution is not known. They should be avoided in nursing mothers unless clearly needed.

Safety and efficacy of all of these drugs have not been established in children.

Adverse Drug Reactions

Adverse reactions to **cholinergic blockers** are based on their actions on tissues other than the target tissue or organ. The discussion here focuses on the adverse reactions on each organ system.

CARDIOVASCULAR. Cholinergic blockade eliminates the parasympathetic influence on the heart, resulting in tachycardia. This action can be used therapeutically to treat patients with bradycardia below 50 bpm. The **belladonna alkaloids** have the highest incidence of this adverse reaction.

RESPIRATORY. **Cholinergic blockers** are sometimes used to produce relaxation of bronchial smooth muscle for patients with asthma, but their tendency to thicken and dry bronchial secretions can result in ineffective airway clearance and make patients more at risk for respiratory infection.

EXOCRINE GLANDS. Blockade of muscarinic receptors on sweat glands can produce anhidrosis. Because sweating is necessary for cooling the body, patients are at risk for hyperthermia. The effect on salivary glands produces xerostomia (dry mouth). Not only is this irritating but also it can impair swallowing. Oral hygiene, use of sugarless gum, and other methods to reduce this problem should be taught to patients.

GASTROINTESTINAL AND URINARY. Decreased tone and motility in the GI tract can lead to constipation, especially when the secretory function of the intestine is also reduced. Patients are taught to increase their intake of fluids and dietary fiber. Blockade of muscarinic receptors in the urinary tract reduces contractile force and pressure in the urinary bladder and increases tone in the urinary sphincter. These combined effects produce urinary hesitancy and urinary retention and increase the risk for urinary tract infection. Impotence has also been reported.

EYE. Mydriatic and cycloplegic action of **cholinergic blockers** results in increased intraocular pressure, blurred vision, and photophobia.

CENTRAL NERVOUS SYSTEM. Cholinergic blockers that cross the blood-brain barrier produce varied adverse reactions, from mild excitation to dizziness and confusion and, in the case of **scopolamine,** CNS depression. These adverse reactions are more common in older adults.

Drug Interactions

Many drugs that are not **cholinergic blockers** can produce significant muscarinic blockade. These drugs include **antihistamines, disopyramide, quinidine, phenothia-zine antipsychotics,** and **TCAs.** Additive or synergistic antimuscarinic effects occur when these drugs are given with **cholinergic blockers.** Additive CNS depression can occur with **alcohol, antidepressants, opioids,** and **sedative-hypnotics.**

Because **cholinergic blockers** alter transit time through the GI tract, they may alter the absorption of any orally administered drug. For drugs with a narrow therapeutic range or drugs that can reach toxic levels if retained too long in the GI tract, concurrent administration is not recommended. **Antacids** and **adsorbent antidiarrheals** decrease the absorption of **cholinergic blockers.**

Drug interactions specific to each drug are presented in Table 12–31.

Clinical Use and Dosing

PARKINSON'S DISEASE. First-line management of Parkinson's disease is usually accomplished with **dopaminergics** and **dopamine agonists.** Rather than as direct treatment of the disorder, **cholinergic blockers** are useful early in the course of the disease to control tremor by relaxing smooth muscle. They are also useful for middle-aged patients who have tremor but little rigidity or bradykinesia and in controlling salivation and drooling.

Trihexyphenidyl is one **cholinergic blocker** currently used as an adjunct to therapy with **carbidopa/levodopa.** The initial dose is 1 to 2 mg the first day, increased by 2-mg increments at 3- to 5-day intervals until a total of 6 to 10 mg is given daily (Table 12–32). Many patients re-

Table 12–31. Drug Interactions: Selected Cholinergic Blockers

Drug	Interacting Drug	Possible Effect	Implications
Atropine, dicyclomine, propantheline, scopolamine	Other drugs with cholinergic blocking effects: antihistamines, disopyramide, quinidine, phenothiazines, TCAs, MAOIs	Additive cholinergic blocking adverse effects; antipsychotic effects of phenothiazines decreased.	Avoid concurrent use or select drug in each category with the fewest cholinergic blocking properties. Adjust phenothiazine dose.
	Orally administered drugs	Atropine may alter absorption by slowing GI motility.	Separate administration or select drugs that do not have narrow therapeutic ranges for which altered absorption would create a problem.
	Antacids	Decrease the absorption of the cholinergic blocker.	Separate administration. Give cholinergic blocker first and then antacid at least 30 min later.
	Amantadine	Coadministration may result in increased cholinergic blocking adverse effects.	Consider decreasing the dose of the cholinergic blocker.
	Atenolol	Pharmacological effects of atenolol may be increased.	Metoprolol and propranolol not affected. Substitute one of these if possible.
	Oral potassium	May increase GI mucosal lesions.	Take with food and at least 8 oz water.
Benztropine, trihexyphenidyl	Other drugs with cholinergic blocking effects: antihistamines, disopyramide, quinidine, phenothiazines, TCAs	Additive cholinergic blocking adverse effects; antipsychotic effects of phenothiazines decreased.	Additive cholinergic blocking adverse effects. Antipsychotic effects of phenothiazines decreased. Adjust phenothiazine dose.
	Bethanechol	Counteracts the cholinergic effects of bethanechol.	Avoid concurrent use.
	Antacids and antidiarrheals	May decrease absorption.	Separate administration. Give cholinergic blocker first and then antacid or antidiarrheal at least 30 min later.
	Haloperidol	Worsens schizophrenic symptoms, increases risk for tardive dyskinesia, decreases blood levels of haloperidol.	Avoid concurrent use for schizophrenic patients. Increase dose of haloperidol for others.*
	Levodopa	Decreased GI motility, increased deactivation of levodopa, and reduced intestinal absorption.	Effectiveness of levodopa is reduced. May need to alter dose of levodopa if both must be given.
Oxybutynin	CNS depressants: alcohol, antihistamines, antidepressants, opioids, sedative-hypnotics	Additive CNS depression.	Avoid concurrent administration or monitor closely for CNS effects. May need to alter dosage.
	Other drugs with cholinergic blocking effects: antihistamines, disopyramide, quinidine, phenothiazines, TCAs, MAOIs	Additive cholinergic blocking adverse effects; antipsychotic effects of phenothiazines decreased.	Additive cholinergic blocking adverse effects. Antipsychotic effects of phenothiazines decreased. Adjust phenothiazine dose.

Continued on next page

Table 12–31. Drug Interactions: Selected Cholinergic Blockers *(continued)*

Drug	Interacting Drug	Possible Effect	Implications
	Haloperidol	Worsens schizophrenic symptoms, increases risk for tardive dyskinesia, decreases blood levels of haloperidol.	Avoid concurrent use for schizophrenic patients. Increase dose of haloperidol for others.*
	Atenolol	Bioavailability of atenolol increased; increased effects.	Metoprolol and propranolol not affected. Substitute one of these if possible.
	Nitrofurantoin	Increased blood levels and bioavailability of nitrofurantoin.	Choose different antibiotic to treat urinary tract infection if patient already on oxybutynin.
Scopolamine	Alcohol, meperidine	Additive CNS depression.	Unless desired therapeutic effect, may need to alter dose of one or both.

*Administration of these drugs may be a therapeutic choice with phenothiazines to reduce extrapyramidal adverse reactions associated with phenothiazines.

ceive maximum benefits at this dose, but postencephalitic patients often require doses of 12 to 15 mg/day. The drug is best tolerated when the daily dose is divided into three doses and taken at mealtimes. High doses may be divided into four doses and taken at mealtimes and bedtime. Because of the relatively high dosage of sustained-release capsules, they are not used for initial therapy. Once patients have been stabilized on regular formulations, they may be switched to sustained release. Sustained-release capsules are administered in a once-daily dose after breakfast or in bid doses 12 hours apart.

When given concurrently with **levodopa**, the usual dose may need to be reduced. Conversely, **trihexyphenidyl** decreases the total bioavailability of **levodopa**. Careful adjustment of the doses of the two drugs is required, depending upon adverse reactions and degree of symptom control.

Benztropine is also used for this indication. The dose is 1 to 2 mg/day with a range of 0.5 to 6 mg/day. Therapy is initiated with a 0.5- to 1-mg dose and increased in 0.5-mg increments until optimal benefits are achieved. Postencephalitic patients begin with 2 mg/day in one or more doses, which are increased by 0.5 mg/day until optimal benefits are reached.

The long duration of action of this drug makes it especially suitable for a bedtime medication, and some patients experience greatest relief by taking the entire dose at bedtime. Others do better with divided doses, bid to qid. The bedtime dose makes it easier for patients to turn in bed at night and to rise in the morning.

MANAGEMENT OF EXTRAPYRAMIDAL SYMPTOMS (EPS) SECONDARY TO DRUG THERAPY. Cholinergic blockers are the drugs of choice for treating akathisia arising from **antipsychotic drugs**. Both **benztropine** and **trihexyphenidyl** are used for this indication. Size and frequency of dosing are determined empirically.

The initial dose of **trihexyphenidyl** for this indication is 1 mg in a single dose. If symptoms are not controlled within a few hours, the dose is gradually increased until control is achieved. Daily dosages range from 5 to 15 mg, although symptoms have been controlled on as little as 1 mg/day. An elixir form is available for patients who have difficulty with swallowing tablets. Control can be more rapidly achieved by temporarily reducing the dose of the **antipsychotic** drug when **trihexyphenidyl** therapy is initiated and then adjusting both drugs until the desired effects are achieved without EPS reactions.

Benztropine therapy is initiated with 1 to 2 mg daily or bid. Dosage titration is in 0.5-mg increments at 5- or 6-day intervals so that the smallest amount required for symptom relief is used. A dose of 1 to 2 mg bid or tid usually provides symptom relief within 1 to 2 days. The maximum dose is 6 mg/day. Older adults and thin patients often cannot tolerate the higher doses. **Benztropine** also comes in an injectable form that can be used for patients with severe dystonic reactions or for those who cannot swallow a pill. The intramuscular dose is 1 to 2 mg, and relief of symptoms is rapid.

For both of these drugs, after several weeks of therapy, the drug may be withdrawn to see if symptoms return and to determine the need for continued therapy. Some patients' symptoms do not return, and some drug-induced EPS reactions do not respond to these two drugs.

ANTISPASMODIC FOR BLADDER INSTABILITY. **Oxybutynin** exerts direct antispasmodic effects and inhibits the muscarinic action of ACh on smooth muscle. It exhibits only one-fifth the cholinergic blocking activity of **atropine** but has 4 to 10 times the antispasmodic activity.

Table 12–32. Dosage Schedule: Selected Cholinergic Blockers

Drug	Indication	Initial Dose	Maintenance and Maximum Dose
Atropine	Irritable bowel syndrome, peptic ulcer disease	Adults: 400 μg q4–6h. Children: 10 μg/kg q4–6h.	May increase to 600 μg if needed. Not to exceed 400 μg.
Benztropine (Cogentin)	Parkinson's disease	1–2 mg/d. For postencephalitic patients: 2 mg/d.	Increase in increments of 0.5 mg/d gradually at 5- or 6-d intervals until symptom relief. Use smallest dose that achieves effect. Maximum dose is 6 mg/d. Older adults and thin patients may not tolerate higher doses. Giving dose at bedtime is preferred.
	Drug-induced EPS	1–2 mg qd or bid oral or IM.	1–2 mg PO provides relief in 1–2 d and prevents recurrence. If inadequate relief in that time, may increase to 2 mg tid. 1–2 mg IM provides rapid relief. Maximum dose by either route is 6 mg/d.
Dicyclomine	Irritable bowel syndrome	80 mg/d in 4 equally divided doses.	Increase to 160 mg/d in 4 divided doses.
Oxybutynin	Antispasmodic for bladder instability	Adults: 5 mg bid or tid. The XL formulation is given once daily. Children: 5 mg bid.	Adults: 5 mg qid or 10 mg bid of the XL formulation. Children: 5 mg tid.
Propantheline	Peptic ulcer	15 mg 30 min before meals and 30 mg at bedtime.	Same as initial dose.
Scopolamine	Prevention of nausea and vomiting associated with motion sickness	One transdermal disk applied to postauricular skin 4 h before antiemotic effect is desired.	One disk delivers 0.5 mg/d for 3 d. If effect needed for more than 3 d, remove and replace with new disk.
Trihexyphenidyl	Parkinson's disease Drug-induced EPS	1–2 mg/d tablets or elixir. Initial therapy usually not begun with sustained release.	Increase in increments of 2 mg at 3- to 5-d intervals until 6–10 mg/d. Postencephalitic patients may require 12–15 mg/d. All doses tolerated better when given in 3 divided doses with meals. Higher doses given in 4 divided doses with meals and at bedtime. After dosage is stabilized, sustained-release forms may be used. Total daily dose is same as other forms but can be given qd at breakfast or in 2 divided doses 12 h apart.

EPS = extrapyramidal symptoms.

No cholinergic blocking effects occur at the myoneural junction. This combination of effects makes it especially useful to treat bladder spasms. Patients with conditions characterized by involuntary bladder contractions experience increased bladder capacity, diminished frequency of urination, and reduced urgency related to voiding. These effects are strongest for patients with uninhibited neurogenic bladder. It is also extremely effective for patients who experience incontinence. It is well tolerated in long-term administration (more than 2 years). Because it increases blood levels and bioavailability of **nitrofurantoin,** a different **antibiotic** should be chosen to treat any concurrent urinary tract infection that may be associated with urinary retention. Assessment for bladder outlet obstruction should be done prior to prescribing because obstruction contraindicates the use of this drug.

For adults, the initial dose of **oxybutynin** is 5 mg bid or tid of the regular formulation or the syrup and 5 to 10 mg daily for the extended-release (XL) formulation (Table 12–33). Symptom response usually occurs with the first dose but may require up to a week for the full effect. If the desired effects have not occurred in 1 week, the dose is increased. The maximum dose is 20 mg/day. For children, the initial dose is 5 mg bid, with a maximum dose of 15 mg/day. Adverse reactions are more likely with higher doses, and lifestyle modifications should be made concurrently to keep the dose as low as possible. For children and adults who have difficulty in swallowing pills, the drug is available in a syrup form.

PREVENTION OF NAUSEA AND VOMITING ASSOCIATED WITH MOTION SICKNESS. **Scopolamine** in a transdermal form is used for this indication. One disk is applied to the clean, dry postauricular skin at least 4 hours before the antiemetic effect is desired. Over a space of 3 days, 0.5 mg is delivered. If therapy is required for more than 3 days, the original disk is removed and replaced with a new one. Only one disk is worn at a time. After application of the disk, the hands are washed with soap and water to prevent any traces of the drug from coming into direct contact with the eyes.

ADJUNCT THERAPY IN MANAGEMENT OF IRRITABLE BOWEL SYNDROME AND PEPTIC ULCER DISEASE. **Atropine** is used for both indications. **Dicyclomine** is used for the management of irritable bowel syndrome in patients who do not respond to the usual interventions with sedation and diet. **Propantheline** is indicated for its antisecretory activity in the management of peptic ulcer disease.

The initial adult dose of **atropine** for both indications is 400 µg every 4 to 6 hours. Doses may be increased, if necessary, to 600 µg. For children, the dose is 10 µg/kg every 4 to 6 hours. The dose is not to exceed 400 µg. Children are especially sensitive to the adverse reactions associated with **atropine**, and every effort should be made to keep the dose as low as possible. Symptoms of poisoning in infants and children differ from adults'. They include burning sensations in the mouth, difficulty in swallowing, rash, blurred vision, tachycardia, tachypnea, fever up to 109°F, muscle incoordination, and eventually seizure, respiratory paralysis, and death. The antidote for **atropine** poisoning is **physostigmine**.

The only oral dose of **dicyclomine** shown to be effective is 160 mg/day in four equally divided doses. However, because of adverse effects, the initial dose is 80 mg/day in four equally divided doses. The dose is then increased if tolerated. For patients who have difficulty with swallowing, a syrup form is available with the same

Table 12–33. Available Dosage Forms: Selected Cholinergic Blockers

Drug	Dosage Form	Package
Atropine	Tablets: 400 µg	In bottles of 100
	Soluble tablets: 400 µg, 600 µg	In bottles of 100
Benztropine (Cogentin)	Tablets: 0.5 mg, 1 mg, 2 mg	In bottles of 100, 1000, and 100s; Cogentin tablets are scored
	Injection: 1 mg/cc	In 2-cc ampules
Dicyclomine (Anti-spaz, Bentyl, Dibent, Di-Spaz)	Tablets: 10 mg	In bottles of 30, 100, 120, 1000, and 100s
	Tablets: 20 mg	In bottles of 15, 20, 30, 100, 120, 250, 1000, and 100s
	Capsules: 20 mg	In bottles of 100, 1000
	Syrup: 10 mg/5 cc	In 118-cc, 250-cc bottles
	Injection: 10 mg/cc	In 2-cc, 10-cc vials
Oxybutynin (Ditropan, Ditropan XL)	Tablets: 5 mg XL tablets: 5 mg, 10 mg	In bottles of 100, 500, 1000, and 100s
	Syrup: 5 mg/cc	In 473-cc bottles
Propantheline (ProBanthine)	Tablets: 7.5 mg	In bottles of 100 sugar-coated
	Tablets: 15 mg	In bottles of 100, 500, 1000, and 100s
Scopolamine	Transderm-Scop: 1.5-mg disk	In 4-unit blister packs
Trihexyphenidyl (Artane)	Tablets: 2 mg, 5 mg	In bottles of 30, 100, 250, 1000, and 100s; Artane tablets are scored
	Sequels (sustained release): 5 mg	In bottles of 60
	Elixir: 2 mg/5 cc	In 480-cc bottles, lime-mint flavor

dosage range. A formulation for IM administration is also available, but the dose is 80 mg/day in four equally divided doses.

The oral dose of **propantheline** for adults is 15 mg 30 minutes before meals and 30 mg at bedtime. For patients with mild manifestations, older adults, and patients of small stature, the dose is 0.5 mg tid. The safety and efficacy of this drug for treating peptic ulcer in children have not been established. There is a dosage schedule published for antisecretory and antispasmodic use in children, but it is an unlabeled use. The dose for children is 1.5 mg/kg a day in three or four divided doses for antisecretory indications and 2 to 3 mg/kg a day in four to six divided doses given every 4 to 6 hours for antispasmodic indications.

Both **atropine** and **scopolamine** are used as part of preoperative medication to reduce secretions and facilitate induction of anesthesia. **Atropine** is also used in acute care to treat bradyarrhythmias and anticholinesterase poisoning. These indications are not commonly part of primary care and are not discussed here.

Rational Drug Selection

Aside from clinical indications, there are few parameters that assist in deciding which is the best drug to choose. Some are associated with slightly fewer adverse reactions, but all have several reactions that cause patients to not adhere to treatment regimens.

COST. Each indication has a limited number of drugs to choose from, and their costs often do not vary significantly. Generic drugs are, as usual, less expensive than brand names, and oral forms are less expensive than injectables. In the case of **Artane** and **Cogentin**, however, only the brand-name tablets are scored to enable titrating doses more closely. According to the cost index in *Drug Facts and Comparisons* (Cada, 1998), **atropine** tablets produced by Lilly Pharmaceutical are significantly less expensive than other brands. This source also lists **benztropine** as less expensive than **trihexyphenidyl**.

FORMULATION. In addition to these cost data, formulation can be an issue when speed is a major concern (e.g., severe dystonic symptoms in a patient who is taking an **antipsychotic**) or when the patient has difficulty in swallowing for any of a variety of reasons, including the progression of the disease process itself. Several drugs come in injectable or syrup forms.

Monitoring

No specific monitoring parameters are required for **cholinergic blockers** beyond monitoring for adverse reactions and the monitoring parameters that are appropriate for the disease being treated.

Patient Education

ADMINISTRATION. Instruct the patient to take the drugs exactly as prescribed. If a dose is missed, take it as soon as remembered unless it is almost time for the next dose. Do not double doses. **Benztropine** is administered with food or immediately after meals to minimize gastric irritation. The tablet may be crushed and administered with food if the patient has difficulty in swallowing. **Atropine, dicyclomine,** and **propantheline** are administered 30 to 60 minutes before a meal, **oxybutynin** on an empty stomach (may be given with food to minimize GI irritation), and **trihexyphenidyl** is administered after a meal (may be given before a meal for patients with dry mouth or with the meal if GI distress occurs). Extended-release formulations must be swallowed whole and not crushed or chewed. Calibrated measuring instruments such as medicine cups or syringes should be used with liquid formulations to make certain the dose is accurate.

The **scopolamine** disk has specific instructions for its application. The disk is applied to clean, dry skin behind the ear at least 4 hours before the antiemetic effect is desired. It is left in place for up to 3 days. Only one disk at a time is worn. If longer effects are required, the disk is removed and replaced. Hands are washed with soap and water after application to make sure no trace of the drug comes in contact with the eyes. The same procedure is followed when removing the disk.

ADVERSE REACTIONS. Cholinergic blockers have many adverse reactions because their actions are not organ-specific. Cardiovascular reactions include tachycardia. Teach patients to take their own pulses and report heart rates above 100 bpm. Dosage adjustments may be required. This adverse effect is especially problematic for patients who concurrently have coronary artery disease and for older adults.

Cholinergic blockers tend to thicken and dry respiratory secretion. Advise the patient to drink at least 2 quarts of noncaffeinated fluid daily to maintain adequate hydration.

Fluid and fiber intake are also important because these drugs may cause constipation and difficulty in voiding. Dry mouth can be relieved by good oral hygiene, cold drinks, hard candy, or sugarless chewing gum.

The therapeutic goal for many of these drugs is to reduce gastric secretion. Substances that increase gastric acid secretion such as **alcohol**, tobacco, caffeine, and **aspirin** should be avoided.

Activities that require visual acuity, mental alertness, and vigorous activity in warm weather can create problems. **Cholinergic blockers** may result in blurred vision, photophobia, and dizziness, and they reduce the sweating necessary to cool the body during exercise.

LIFESTYLE MANAGEMENT. Several of the disease processes for which these drugs are prescribed require lifestyle modifications. Incontinence can also be treated with a variety of therapies besides drugs. Gallo and colleagues (1997) discuss bladder retraining, Kegel exercises, biofeedback, and other modalities. Carlson (1998) stresses the importance of nonpharmacological therapies in treating irritable bowel syndrome and reports that no study has offered convincing evidence that drug therapy of any kind is consistently effective in treating this disorder.

REFERENCES

Andersen, P., Seljeflot, I., Herzog, A., Arnesen, H., Hyermann, I., & Holme, I. (1998). Effects of doxazosin and atenolol on atherothrombogenic risk profile in hypertensive middle-aged men. *Journal of Cardiovascular Pharmacology, 31*(5), 677–683.

Andrews, J. (1998). Optimizing smoking cessation strategies. *Nurse Practitioner, 23*(8), 47–64.

Barron, H., Viskin, S., Lundstrom, R., et al. (1998). Beta blockers dosages and mortality after myocardial infarction: Data from a large health maintenance organization. *Archives of Internal Medicine, 158,* 449–453.

Cada, D. (Ed.). (1998). *Drug facts and comparisons.* St. Louis: Facts and Comparisons.

Carlson, E. (1998). Irritable bowel syndrome. *Nurse Practitioner, 23*(1), 82–88.

Deglin, J., & Vallerand, A. (1999). *Davis' drug guide for nurses* (6th ed.). Philadelphia: FA Davis.

Frank, T. (1998). Adrenergic inhibitors in the treatment of hypertension. *Clinical Reviews* (Winter), 23–27.

Gallo, M., Fallon, P., & Staskin, D. (1997). Urinary incontinence: Steps to evaluation, diagnosis and treatment. *Nurse Practitioner, 22*(2), 21–43.

Kastsung, B. (1998). *Basic and clinical pharmacology* (7th ed.). Stamford, CT: Appleton & Lange.

Lehne, R. (1998). *Pharmacology for nursing care* (3rd ed.). Philadelphia: Saunders.

Lepor, H., et al. (1996). The efficacy of terazosin, finasteride, or both in benign prostatic hyperplasia. *New England Journal of Medicine, 335,* 533.

Madjlessi-Simon, T., Mary-Krause, M., Fillette, F., Lechat, P., & Jaillon, P. (1996). Persistent transient myocardial ischemia despite beta adrenergic blockade predicts a higher risk of adverse cardiac events in patients with coronary artery disease. *Journal of American College of Cardiology, 27,* 1586–1591.

Messerli, F., Grossman, E., & Goldbourt, U. (1998). Are beta blockers efficacious as first-line therapy for hypertension in the elderly? *Journal of American Medical Association, 279*(23), 1903–1907.

National High Blood Pressure Education Program (1997). *The sixth report of the Joint National Committee on Prevention, Detection, Evaluation, and Treatment of High Blood Pressure* (NIH Publ. No. 98-4080). Rockville, MD: National Institutes of Health, National Heart, Lung, and Blood Institute.

Sadowski, A., & Redeker, N. (1996). The hypertensive elder: A review for the primary care provider. *Nurse Practitioner, 21*(5), 99–112.

Terpstra, T., & Terpstra, T. (1998). Treating Alzheimer's disease with cholinergic drugs: Part 1. *Nurse Practitioner, 23*(11), 90–101.

Terpstra, T., & Terpstra, T. (1999). Treating Alzheimer's disease with cholinergic drugs: Part 2. *Nurse Practitioner, 24*(1), 117–119.

Van Zwieten, P. (1996). From alpha and beta to I1: An overview of sympathetic receptors involved in blood pressure control targets for drug treatment. *Journal of Cardiovascular Pharmacology, 27*(Suppl 3), S5–10.

Vashi, V., et al. (1998). Pharmacokinetic interaction between finasteride and terazosin, but not finasteride and doxazosin. *Journal of Clinical Pharmacology, 38,* 1072–1076.

CHAPTER 13

· · · · · · ·

Drugs Affecting the Central Nervous System

CHAPTER OUTLINE

Alcohol (Ethanol)

*T*raditionally, alcohol abuse and drunkenness were considered to be the result of weak moral character, and alcoholics therefore deserved the painful results of their behavior. In 1987, however, the American Medical Association declared alcoholism to be a disease that has a variety of contributory biopsychosocial factors, prominent among which is heredity.

Although a single gene has not yet been isolated, it is understood that the offspring of one alcoholic parent has approximately a 33 percent chance of developing the disease, and the offspring of two alcoholic parents has a doubled risk. It is also possible to trace the disease through nondrinking parents to alcoholic grandparents.

Pharmacodynamics

The chemical name for **alcohol** is **ethanol**. Although an individual's initial response to **alcohol** may appear to be loss of inhibition, leading to excitation, **ethanol** is a central nervous system (CNS) depressant, and sleep, coma, and death may result from overdose, depending on the amount ingested. Brain cell death occurs in chronic use both because of the poor nutritional status of most alcoholics and as a direct result of the **alcohol.**

Although **ethanol** is a CNS depressant, withdrawal can cause rebound psychomotor irritability, which, in its extreme form, is known as delirium tremens (DTs) and can include both auditory and visual hallucinations. Nausea and vomiting, trembling, sweating, tachycardia, and anxiety are common.

Some researchers think the addictive quality of **ethanol** is due to the interaction of acetaldehyde with neurotransmitters in the brain, resulting in the formation of tetrahydroisoquinolines (TIQs), which are similar to addiction-causing substances in **heroin** and **morphine.**

Tolerance occurs because liver cells that are exposed to steady, long-term, significant **ethanol** intake increase their production of metabolic enzymes, which allows the individual to increase intake. Eventually, however, the damaged liver is unable to function normally, and little **alcohol** is needed to cause intoxication.

Because of hydrogen produced during metabolism of **ethanol,** the body utilizes alcohol for energy, allowing the buildup of fat in the liver, which, in combination with the cirrhotic effects of acetaldehyde, can result in the physical manifestations of end-stage alcoholism, such as jaundice, ascites, and portal hypertension.

Other destructive effects of chronic heavy **alcohol** use are vitamin B deficiency (especially thiamine), peripheral neuropathy, Wernicke-Korsakoff syndrome, gastric and esophageal bleeding and ulcers, cardiac arrhythmias and hypertension, loss of peripheral and night vision, impotence, pancreatitis, and depression.

Pharmacokinetics

Absorption and Distribution

Ethanol is absorbed partially via the stomach lining but primarily in the small intestine. The rate of absorption is dependent on the contents of the stomach and the strength of the **alcohol** ingested, so that an alcoholic drink containing 40 to 50 percent alcohol, such as whiskey, imbibed on an empty stomach, is in the bloodstream within 20 minutes. Beer, containing 4 percent **ethanol,** especially if consumed with or immediately after eating food, is absorbed much more slowly. Following absorption, **ethanol** is distributed initially to areas of the nervous system with the greatest water content, principally the cerebrum and cerebellum. Large people whose body composition contains more water are able to tolerate greater amounts of **alcohol** without intoxication because the **alcohol** is more dilute than in a smaller person. **Ethanol** acts in the spinal cord and vital centers after the cerebrum and cerebellum because those areas contain less water.

Metabolism and Excretion

Ethanol is metabolized in the liver by the action of alcohol dehydrogenase, and its initial by-products are hydrogen and acetaldehyde, which is toxic to the body. The rate of metabolism is constant at 10 mL of **alcohol** every 90 minutes. This means 1 oz, for example, of whiskey, 1 glass of beer, and 3 to 4 oz of wine.

Women become intoxicated more quickly than men because their bodies contain less of the enzyme alcohol dehydrogenase, and they also suffer more rapid damage from chronic, heavy **ethanol** ingestion because of accumulation of acetaldehyde in the liver.

Ethanol is excreted through the kidneys and skin.

Pharmacotherapeutics

Drug Interactions

Because **ethanol** is a CNS depressant, drug interactions of greatest concern are those that lead to an additive depressive effect on respiratory function, the most frequent cause of death in **alcohol** overdose. **Alcohol** use should be absolutely avoided by patients taking **barbiturates, hypnotics, tricyclic antidepressants (TCAs),** and **anticonvulsants.**

Salicylates combined with **ethanol** may cause gastric bleeding; **acetaminophen** and **isoniazid** in combination with **ethanol** may lead to hepatotoxicity.

Table 13–1 presents information on drug interactions.

Table 13–1. Drug Interactions: Alcohol

Drug	Interacting Drug	Possible Effect	Implications
Alcohol	Benzodiazepines, barbiturates, hypnotics, neuroleptics, opiates, muscle relaxants, TCAs, anticonvulsants	Additive CNS, respiratory, and/or cardiac depression, coma, death	Do not use when patient is a known alcoholic. Instruct patient to abstain from alcohol while taking these drugs.
	Salicylates	Gastric bleeding	Use alternative drugs if patient is unable or unwilling to abstain from alcohol use.
	Acetaminophen	Hepatotoxicity	Monitor liver function tests if patient is unwilling to abstain from alcohol use.
	Isoniazid	Hepatotoxicity, hypertensive crisis with tyramine-containing alcoholic beverages	Use alternative drugs if patient is unable or unwilling to abstain from alcohol use.
	Verapamil, histamine₂ (H₂) blockers	Increased alcohol concentration	Warn patient about increased level of intoxication, risk of overdose of alcohol.
	Warfarin	Impaired warfarin metabolism	Monitor bleeding time if patient is unwilling to abstain from alcohol use.
	Metronidazole, cephalosporins	Reaction similar to disulfiram and ethanol	Warn patient to abstain from alcohol use.
	Cocaine	Sudden death	Warn patient of possible risk and refer for treatment.

Monitoring

For the patient using **alcohol**, monitoring is for signs and symptoms of alcoholism, as well as for signs and symptoms of withdrawal in the patient with chronic **alcohol** use.

Common symptoms of acute **alcohol** withdrawal, which can continue for 3 to 5 days following the last intake, include nausea and vomiting, sweating, tremors, tachycardia, irritability, headache, anxiety, insomnia, seizures, confusion, and coma. In addition to supportive measures such as environmental quiet, rest, and adequate fluid intake as tolerated, early treatment may include **anxiolytics** for psychomotor agitation, **neuroleptics** for psychosis, over-the-counter (OTC) **analgesics** for headache, and **diazepam (Valium)** for acute treatment of seizures.

Care must be taken when prescribing **benzodiazepines** because of their potential to replace **alcohol** as the dependent substance. Also of concern is the use of OTC **analgesics**, particularly **acetaminophen** because of its hepatotoxicity and **salicylates** because of the potential for gastric bleeding. Table 13–2 presents the drugs commonly used in the treatment of acute **alcohol** withdrawal.

Long-term measures, as well as directly addressing the issue of chemical dependency, may require vitamin supplementation and mental health evaluation and/or treatment.

Treatment may also include the use of **disulfiram (Antabuse)**. **Disulfiram** interferes with the action of alcohol dehydrogenase, thereby allowing the accumulation of acetaldehyde in the liver. When **ethanol** is ingested orally or absorbed through the skin, even in the extremely small amounts present in some salad dressings and perfumes, the individual experiences an extremely unpleasant reaction of headache, sweating, nausea and vomiting, flushing of the neck and face, dyspnea, and tremors. Death is a potential result if alcoholic beverages are consumed, and it can occur within 15 minutes. Because of these effects, **disulfiram** is used as an **alcohol** deterrent, particularly for those individuals experiencing repeated relapse, and prescribed in the range of 250 to 500 mg daily.

Patient Education

Anyone taking **disulfiram** should be instructed in the avoidance of **ethanol**-containing substances and should not take the initial dose until a minimum of 12 hours has elapsed since the last exposure to such a substance.

Table 13–2. Drugs Commonly Used: Treatment of Acute Alcohol Withdrawal

Drug	Indication	Dose	Notes
Hydroxyzine (Atarax)	Psychomotor agitation, anxiety, nausea, vomiting	50–100 mg PO qid	Adverse effects: dry mouth, urinary retention, blurred vision Onset/duration: 15–30 min/3 h
Lorazepam (Ativan)	Agitation, anxiety, insomnia (short-term use only)	1–2 mg PO q4–6h; max 6 mg/24 h	Adverse effects: sedation
Clorazepate (Tranxene)	Agitation, anxiety, insomnia (short-term use only)	Initial dose 30 mg PO q4–6h, followed by 30–60 qd in divided doses; titrating up to a maximum of 45–90 mg/24 h in divided doses, then titrating down and off by day 5	Adverse effects: may increase CNS depression Onset/peak/duration: 15 min/ 1–2 h/4–6 h
Diazepam (Valium)	Seizures	5–10 mg intravenous (IV) bolus at 5 mg/min; may repeat q 5–10 min; max 30 mg; may repeat in 2–4 h if seizures reappear	Onset/duration: 1–5 min/15 min
Haloperidol (Haldol)	Psychosis	Initial dose 0.5–5 mg bid or tid; increase depending on response to max of 100 mg/24 h	Monitor for extrapyramidal symptoms (EPSs) or neuroleptic malignant syndrome (NMS) Onset/peak/duration: erratic/3–5 h/24 h

Anorexiants

Anorexiants are short-term adjuncts to calorie-limiting, cognitive-behavioral weight loss programs for severely obese individuals. The **anorexiants** commonly in use today are **nonamphetamine** appetite suppressants that are chemically and pharmacologically related to **amphetamines**. Well known among them are **fenfluramine (Pondimin), phentermine (Phentrol, Zantryl, Adipex-P, Ionamin, Obe-Nix 30, Fastin)**, and **dexfenfluramine (Redux)**. Others are **benzphetamine (Didrex), diethylpropion HCl (Tenuate), mazindol (Mazanor, Sanorex)**, and **phendimetrazine tartrate (Bontril, Prelu-2, Rexigen Forte)**.

Pharmacodynamics

These drugs are sympathomimetic amines and are thought to exert their anorexiant action by stimulation of the satiety centers in the hypothalamus and limbic region.

Diethylpropion and **phentermine** act through adrenergic pathways, **mazindol** through both adrenergic and dopaminergic pathways, and **fenfluramine** through serotonergic pathways.

Pharmacokinetics
Absorption and Distribution

After oral administration, **anorexiants** are absorbed in the stomach and small intestine, depending on whether they are the regular or extended-release form. They are lipid-soluble and widely distributed, and they cross the blood-brain barrier. **Diethylpropion** and its metabolites also cross the placental barrier and is **FDA Pregnancy Category C.**

Metabolism and Excretion

Anorexiants are metabolized in the liver and excreted through the kidneys. Duration of action is 4 to 6 hours with the regular form and longer with the extended-release form. Half-lives vary from 8 to 20 hours.

Table 13–3 presents the pharmacokinetics of **anorexiants.**

Pharmacotherapeutics
Precautions and Contraindications

Anorexiants carry a high risk of tolerance and dependence, both physical and psychological, and use in pa-

Table 13–3. Pharmacokinetics: Anorexiants

Drug	Onset	Peak	Duration	Half-Life	Excretion
Fenfluramine	—	Steady state 3–4 d	4–6 h	20 h	Urine
Mazindol	—	—	8–15 h	—	Urine
Phendimetrazine tartrate	—	—	4–6 h	1.9–9.8 h	Urine
Benzphetamine	—	—	4–6 h	—	Urine
Diethylproprion HCl	—	—	4–6 h	—	Urine
Phentermine	—	—	4–6 h	—	Urine

tients with known histories of **alcohol** or drug dependence should be cautious because of the high risk of cross-tolerance. Actively drinking alcoholics taking **anorexiants** have experienced paranoia, psychosis, and depression. Use of **anorexiants** should be limited to a maximum of 6 months and discontinued at any sign of tolerance.

Because these drugs have CNS-stimulant effects, they are contraindicated for individuals taking other **stimulant drugs** and for those whose health history includes cardiac disease, hyperthyroidism, hypertension, and glaucoma. Other contraindications include hypersensitivity to **sympathomimetic amines**, pregnancy, children under age 12, and within 14 days of taking a **monoamine oxidase inhibitor (MAOI)**.

Safety of use in lactating women has not been established.

Adverse Drug Reactions

In 1997, **dexfenfluramine** and **fenfluramine** were removed from the market by the FDA because of potentially fatal cardiac and pulmonary adverse reactions. **Dexfenfluramine, fenfluramine, phentermine,** and the combination **fenfluramine** and **phentermine** (commonly called fen-phen) have been implicated in the development of regurgitant cardiac valve disease and primary pulmonary hypertension.

Seizures have occurred in people with epilepsy who take **diethylpropion.**

Patients taking high doses of **anorexiants** over a long period may experience dizziness, fatigue, and depression if the drug is withdrawn abruptly. Because of its serotonergic effect, patients abruptly withdrawn from **fenfluramine** may have experienced rebound depression.

Patients with diabetes may experience a change in their need for **antihyperglycemics** while taking **mazindol** because of the **anorexiant's** effect of increasing glucose uptake from skeletal muscles.

Other adverse events may include overstimulation and agitation, dry mouth, hypersensitivity, mydriasis, hair loss, dysuria, impotence, bone marrow suppression, and gynecomastia.

Drug Interactions

Anorexiants elevate serotonin levels and should not be prescribed to patients on other serotonergic agents because of the increased risk of serotonin syndrome, the symptoms of which can include hyperthermia, although temperature may be normal; agitation, restlessness, confusion; ataxia, myoclonus, tremor, shivering, rigidity; and hypertension or hypotension, tachycardia, and diaphoresis.

Fenfluramine, because of its CNS-depressant action, could cause sedation when taken with **TCAs** and **furazolidone.**

The actions of **adrenergic blockers, insulin, sulfonylureas,** and **phenothiazines** may be antagonized during concomitant administration of **anorexiants.**

Table 13–4 presents drug interactions.

Clinical Use and Dosing

Anorexiants are indicated for the treatment of morbid exogenous obesity in conjunction with a calorie-restrictive dietary regimen. The course of treatment with **anorexiants** should last no longer than 6 months. An alternative method of treatment is to use the drug for a few weeks followed by no drug for a period, suggested to be half the length of time with the drug, followed by reinstitution of the drug for a few more weeks. Table 13–5 presents the dosage schedule and available dosage forms for **anorexiants.**

Rational Drug Selection

Because of the potential for change of antihyperglycemic demands that occur with **mazindol,** the patient and clinician must be able to closely monitor blood glucose levels during and immediately following treatment with this drug.

Table 13–4. Drug Interactions: Anorexiants

Drug	Interacting Drug	Possible Effect	Implications
All anorexiants	MAOIs	Hypertensive crisis	Do not prescribe during or within 14 d of use of MAOI
	Alcohol	CNS depression	Abstain from alcohol use
	Phenothiazines	Psychosis	Monitor for increased psychotic symptoms
	Insulin, sulfonylureas	Altered requirements	Monitor blood glucose
	Guanethidine	Antagonization of effect	Monitor for increased blood pressure
	Furazolidone	Serotonin syndrome	Monitor for symptoms of syndrome
Fenfluramine	TCAs	CNS depression	Do not use concomitantly
Fenfluramine, phentermine	SSRIs	Serotonin syndrome	Monitor closely during concomitant use of selective serotonin reuptake inhibitor (SSRI) for gastrointestinal (GI) symptoms, elevated temperature and bloodpressure, ataxia, disorientation, dizziness

The patient has a choice between the extended-release form, requiring one daily administration, versus the regular form, which requires administration two to three times daily.

Monitoring

As stated previously, close monitoring for blood glucose levels is required for patients with diabetes who are taking **mazindol.** Patients should be monitored for depression, exacerbation of psychotic symptoms, and tolerance.

Patient Education

Patient education includes telling the patient to abstain from **alcohol** during treatment with **anorexiants;** to monitor for sedation and refrain from hazardous activities if sedation is present; to advise the clinician if psychiatric symptoms such as depression, agitation, or psychosis occur; to increase fluid intake and suck on hard candies if dry mouth occurs; and not to take an **antidepressant** during the course of treatment with **anorexiants.**

Barbiturates

Barbiturates have been used historically as **anxiolytics,** as **sedative-hypnotics,** and for control of seizures. Cur-

rently, because of the problems associated with their use, the indications for short-acting **barbiturates** are limited to preanesthesia sedation, short-term treatment of insomnia, and uncontrollable seizure activity, such as status epilepticus. Long-acting **phenobarbital (Solfoton, Mebaral)** is the drug of choice for some types of epilepsy, the only indication for its long-term use.

Pharmacodynamics

Barbiturates are CNS depressants and can be short- (30 minutes to 4 hours), intermediate- (6 to 8 hours), or long-acting (10 to 12 hours). They produce sedation and sleep by decreasing sensitivity to stimuli in the reticular formation, a primitive area deep in the brainstem through which all the sensorimotor nerve tracts pass.

Pharmacokinetics

Absorption and Distribution

Barbiturates are administered by oral, parenteral, and rectal routes. Their rate of absorption depends on the route of administration, but, generally, salts are absorbed more rapidly than acid forms. They are widely distributed, particularly to brain, kidney, and liver tissue and fluid.

Table 13–5. Dosage Schedule: Anorexiants

Drug	Indications	Dosage	Available Dosage Forms
Benzphetamine (Didrex)	Short-term adjunctive treatment of exogenous obesity	25–50 mg qd; max 150 mg qd	Tablets: 25 mg, 50 mg
Diethylpropion (Tenuate, Tenuate Dospan)	Short-term adjunctive treatment of exogenous obesity	25 mg tid ac* or prn if needed; Sustained release: 75 mg q AM	Tablets: 25 mg Sustained release: 75 mg
Fenfluramine (Pondimin)	Short-term adjunctive treatment of exogenous obesity	20 mg tid ac; may increase at qd intervals by 20 mg to maximum of 120 mg/d Sustained release: 75 mg qd in midmorning	Tablets: 25 mg Sustained release: 75 mg
Mazindol (Mazanor)	Short-term adjunctive treatment of exogenous obesity	1 mg tid 1 h ac or 2 mg qd 1 h before lunch	Tablet: 1 mg, 2 mg
Phendimetrazine tartrate (Bontril PDM, Prelu-2, Rexigen Forte)	Short-term adjunctive treatment of exogenous obesity	35 mg bid or tid 1 h ac Sustained release: 105 mg qd before breakfast	Tablets: 35 mg Capsules: 35 mg Sustained release: 105 mg
Phentermine (Phentrol, Zantryl, Adipex-P, Obe-Nix 30, Ionamin)	Short-term adjunctive treatment of exogenous obesity	8 mg tid, 30 minutes ac or 15–37.5 mg qd before breakfast or 10–14 h before bedtime	Tablets: 8 mg, 30 mg, 37.5 mg Capsules: 15 mg, 18.75 mg, 30 mg, 37.5 mg
Dexfenfluramine (Redux)	Short-term adjunctive treatment of exogenous obesity	15 mg bid with meals	Capsules: 15 mg

*ac = *ante cibum* (before meals).

Metabolism and Excretion

Barbiturates are metabolized by hepatic enzymes and excreted in the urine, although up to 50 percent is eliminated unchanged. **Phenobarbital** actually stimulates the synthesis of hepatic microsomal enzymes, increasing the rate at which the drug is metabolized and thereby increasing tolerance to adverse effects.

These drugs are FDA Pregnancy Category D and should be avoided during pregnancy, although, given no other pharmacological option, careful assessment of the risk-benefit ratio may indicate their use. Infant sedation has occurred when the lactating mother has used *barbiturates.*

Table 13–6 presents the pharmacokinetics of **barbiturates.**

Pharmacotherapeutics

Precautions and Contraindications

Barbiturates combined with **alcohol** have been responsible for many deaths, whether suicide or accident, because of the additive depressive effect each has on the other. Caution should be exercised in prescribing them for patients with a history of depression or suicide attempts. If the clinician has any doubts about the patient's safety and there is no other medication option, no more than a week's worth of the drug should be supplied at a time and for as short a period as possible.

Because of the anxiolytic effect of the short-acting **barbiturates,** known as *downers* on the street, they are drugs of choice for abuse. In addition to the hazard associated with the narrow therapeutic index and the risk from combining them with other CNS depressants, particularly **alcohol,** the short-acting barbiturates **secobarbital (Seconal)** and **pentobarbital (Nembutal)** can cause physiological dependence fairly quickly. Tolerance leads the individual to increase the dose: 1 g can cause toxic adverse effects, and doses of 2 to 10 g can be lethal.

Withdrawal and detoxification are potentially fatal and should be accomplished extremely gradually. Withdrawal symptoms usually begin 8 to 12 hours after the last use and can range from nausea and vomiting, confusion, and tremors to delirium and seizures, with the latter beginning approximately 16 hours after the last use. If untreated, symptoms can last for several days or prove fatal.

Table 13–6. Pharmacokinetics: Barbiturates

Drug	Onset	Peak	Duration	Half-Life	Excretion
Pentobarbital	10–15 min IV immediate	—	3–4 h	15–50 h	Urine, feces
Secobarbital	10–15 min IV immediate	—	3–4 h	15–40 h	Urine, feces
Amobarbital	45–60 min	—	6–8 h	16–40 h	Urine, feces
Aprobarbital	45–60 min	—	6–8 h	14–34 h	Urine, feces
Butabarbital	45–60 min	—	6–8 h	66–140 h	Urine, feces
Phenobarbital	30 min or more IV: less than 5 min	IV: 15 min or more	10–16 h	53–118 h	Urine, feces
Mephobarbital	30 min or more	—	10–16 h	11–67 h	Urine, feces

Barbiturates are not recommended for children younger than 6 years old.

Other contraindications include barbiturate sensitivity, severely impaired liver function, nephritis, impaired pulmonary function with dyspnea or obstruction, and history of dependence on **barbiturates** or **hypnotics.** They should not be administered subcutaneously (SC) or intra-arterially.

Adverse Drug Reactions

Adverse reactions are due to the depressant effects of the drug and can consist of persistent sedation and drowsiness, leading to safety concerns for patients in situations requiring alertness. Although respiratory depression and cardiac depression are dose-related, they are always a concern, especially in combination with other **CNS depressants.**

Other adverse reactions may include agitation, particularly in young children and older adults, confusion, headache, insomnia, ataxia, skin rash, nausea and vomiting, bradycardia, dyspnea, and somnolence.

Rebound status epilepticus may follow abrupt withdrawal of **barbiturates** during daily administration for treatment of seizure disorders.

Drug Interactions

As discussed before, CNS depression may occur with concurrent use of drugs such as **antihistamines, alcohol, benzodiazepines, valproic acid,** and **MAOIs.**

Barbiturates may also decrease the efficacy of **beta blockers, steroids, hormones, doxycycline, theophylline, protease inhibitors,** and **quinidine.**

Table 13–7 presents drug interactions.

Clinical Use and Dosing

Phenobarbitol and **mephobarbital** are effective in the treatment of some types of epilepsy, primarily tonic-clonic, simple partial, and complex partial seizures, because the reduction of response to stimuli raises the threshold of seizure activity.

In addition to epilepsy, other indications for use include preanesthetic sedation and short-term treatment of insomnia. The latter indication, however, is open to controversy because of the risk of dependence and because depression is frequently the etiology of insomnia, raising concerns about suicide.

Other than parenteral administration of **phenobarbital** in medical emergencies such as eclampsia and status epilepticus, **barbiturates** are generally given orally. The short-, intermediate-, and long-acting forms have an onset of action ranging from 10 to 60 minutes, a duration of action from 3 to 16 hours, and half-lives from 24 to 100 hours.

Rational Drug Selection

Although efficacious in the treatment of partial, tonic-clonic, and cortical focal seizures, **phenobarbital** and **mephobarbital** are not considered the first-line treatment of the medical emergencies mentioned previously, which also include seizures associated with meningitis and tetanus. The first choice in such situations is intravenous (IV) **diazepam (Valium).**

Phenobarbital for the treatment of epilepsy is usually prescribed in low doses so that dependence and tolerance are not significant concerns. Adults are treated with 50 to 100 mg two to three times per day, and children are prescribed 3 to 5 mg/kg per day. For uses other than

Table 13–7. Drug Interactions: Barbiturates

Drug	Interacting Drug	Possible Effect	Implications
Barbiturates	Anticoagulants	Induces metabolism of anticoagulants and rebound bleeding when barbiturate stopped	Monitor bleeding times
	Antihistamines, alcohol, benzodiazepines	Increases CNS depression	Avoid concurrent administration
	Neuroleptics	Decreases effect of neuroleptic	Monitor for increase in psychotic symptoms
	Beta blockers, steroids, estrogen, doxycycline, protease inhibitors, valproate, theophylline, griseofulvin, quinidine, phenylbutazone	Induces metabolism and decreases effectiveness of drugs	Monitor blood levels where appropriate and assess effectiveness if concurrent administration unavoidable
	Caffeine	Antagonizes sedation and increases insomnia	Avoid coffee, tea, colas, and chocolate

treatment of tonic-clonic seizures and focal epilepsy, safer drugs are available.

Short-acting **barbiturates** are schedule II controlled drugs and therefore unavailable to nurse practitioners (NPs). **Phenobarbital** is schedule IV and may be included on a state NP Formulary, depending on the individual state's rules and regulations.

Table 13–8 presents the dosage schedule of **barbiturates**.

Monitoring

The difference between therapeutic and toxic plasma levels is not wide, and levels should be monitored frequently. The therapeutic range is 15 to 40 µg/mL.

Patient Education

Patients should be instructed to refrain from **alcohol** while taking **barbiturates** and cautioned about the concomitant use of OTC cold and allergy medications.

Advise patients to exercise caution when they are participating in hazardous activities because of the possibility of sedation.

Table 13–9 presents the available dosage forms of **barbiturates**.

Benzodiazepines

Benzodiazepines have been frequently prescribed to treat anxiety and insomnia. However, because of the increased potential for tolerance and dependence on the newer variations, the CNS depressant–related adverse

effects, and the development of **buspirone**, many clinicians are more cautious in assessing risks versus benefits for their patients than they might have been previously.

Benzodiazepines have also been extensively used for muscle relaxants, preanesthesia sedation, prevention and treatment of panic attacks, acute agitation and dystonia, emergency treatment of uncontrollable seizures, and treatment of restless leg syndrome.

Pharmacodynamics

Benzodiazepines are thought to exert their anxiolytic and sedative effects by increasing the action of gamma-aminobutyric acid (GABA), an inhibitory neurotransmitter, thereby decreasing the effect of neuronal excitation.

Pharmacokinetics

Absorption and Distribution

Benzodiazepines are rapidly and widely distributed following oral administration. **Chlordiazepoxide (Librium)** and **diazepam (Valium)** are slowly and inconsistently absorbed after intramuscular (IM) administration, but **lorazepam (Ativan)** is rapidly absorbed and widely distributed after IM injection.

They are lipid-soluble and highly protein-bound, which means they compete with other protein-bound drugs for receptor sites.

Benzodiazepines are metabolized in the liver and excreted through the urine in inactive conjugate forms.

Table 13–8. Dosage Schedule: Barbiturates

Drug	Indications	Dosage
Amobarbital sodium	Sedation, hypnotic, preanesthetic, acute convulsive episodes	Sedative: 30–50 mg bid to tid Hypnotic: 65–200 mg IM: 65–500 mg IV: do not exceed 50 mg/min Children age 6–12: 65–500 mg Single dose not to exceed 1 g
Aprobarbital	Sedation, hypnotic, preanesthetic, acute convulsive episodes	Sedative: 40 mg tid Insomnia: 40–80 mg hs*; if persists, 80–160 mg hs
Butabarbital sodium	Sedation, hypnotic, preanesthetic, acute convulsive episodes	Sedation: 15–30 mg tid to qid Hypnotic: 50–100 mg hs Preoperative sedation: 50–100 mg 60–90 min before surgery Children: 2–6 mg/kg/d; not to exceed 100 mg
Mephobarbital	Sedation, hypnotic, preanesthetic, acute convulsive episodes, treatment of partial and generalized tonic-clonic and cortical focal seizures	Sedative Adult: 32–100 mg tid–qid; optimal dose is 50 mg Children: 16–32 mg tid–qid Epilepsy Adult: average 400–600 mg daily Children under age 5: 16–32 mg tid–qid Children over age 5: 32–64 mg tid–qid Start low and increase dose gradually over 4–5 d In combination with phenobarbital, use half the average dose of both
Pentobarbital sodium	Sedation, hypnotic, preanesthetic	Adult Sedation: 20 mg tid–qid Hypnotic: 100 mg hs Children Sedation: 2–6 mg/kg/d, not to exceed 100 mg/d Hypnotic: dose based on age and weight Rectal: Adult: 120–200 mg Children: Age 12–14 (80–100 lb): 60 or 120 mg Age 5–12: (40–80 lb): 60 mg Age 1–4 (20–40 lb): 30 or 60 mg Age 2 mo–1 yr (10–20 lb): 30 mg Do not divide suppository IV: Initial dose of 100 mg in adult with proportional decrease of dose for children or debilitated adults. Wait for a full minute to assess effect before adding more. Not to exceed 200–500 mg for healthy adult. IM: Usual adult dose is 150–200 mg Children: 2–6 mg/kg as single injection; not to exceed 100 mg
Phenobarbital	Sedation, hypnotic, preanesthetic, treatment of partial and generalized tonic-clonic and cortical focal seizures, status epilepticus	Epilepsy Adults: 60–100 mg/d Children: 3–6 mg/kg/d Acute convulsions Adults: 200–320 mg IM/IV, repeat q6h prn Children: 4–6 mg/kg/d IM/IV for 7–10 d to blood level of 10–15 μg/mL

Continued on next page

Table 13–8. Dosage Schedule: Barbiturates (*continued*)

Drug	Indications	Dosage
		Sedation Adults: 30–120 mg/d in divided doses; not to exceed 400 mg/24 h Children: 8–32 mg Hypnotic Adult: 100–200 mg Children: dose based on age and weight Preoperative sedation Adults: 100–200 mg IV 60–90 min before surgery Children: 1–3 mg/kg IM or IV Status epilepticus 15–20 mg/kg IV over 10–15 min; may require 15 min or more to achieve peak
Secobarbital sodium	Sedation, hypnotic, preoperative sedation, status epilepticus	Preoperative sedation Adult: 200–300 mg 1–2 h before surgery or 1 mg/kg IM 10–15 min before surgery Children: 2–6 mg/kg not to exceed 100 mg or 4–5 mg/kg IM Hypnotic Adult: 100 mg hs, 100–200 mg IM, or 50–250 mg IV Status epilepticus Children: 15–20 mg/kg IV over 15 min

*hs = *hora somni* (at bedtime).

Table 13–9. Available Dosage Forms: Barbiturates

Drug	Dosage Form	How Supplied
Amobarbital sodium	Powder for injection	In 250 and 500 mg vials
Aprobarbital (Alurate)	Elixir 40 mg/5mL	In pint
Butabarbital sodium	Tablets:15 mg, 30 mg 50 mg, 100 mg Elixir: 30 mg/5mL	In bottles of 100 and 1000 scored tablets In bottles of 100 scored tablets In pint
Mephobarbital (Mebaral)	Tablets: 32 mg, 50 mg,100 mg	In bottles of 250 tablets
Pentobarbital sodium (Nembutal)	Capsules: 50 mg 100 mg Elixir: 20 mg/5mL Suppositories: 30 mg, 60 mg, 120 mg, 200 mg Injection: 50 mg/mL	In bottles of 100 capsules In bottles of 100 and 500 capsules In pints In 12 foil-wrapped In 2-mL Tubex, 2-mL ampules and 20- and 50-mL vials
Phenobarbital	Tablets: 15mg, 30 mg 60 mg, 100 mg 90 mg Elixir: 15 mg/5mL 20 mg/5 mL Injection: 30 mg/mL, 60 mg/mL 65 mg/mL, 130 mg/mL	In bottles of 100, 1000, and 5000 tablets In bottles of 100 and 1000 tablets In bottles of 1000 tablets In 5, 10, and 20 mL; fruit flavored In pint and gallon In 1-mL Tubex In 1-mL vials
Secobarbital (Seconal)	Capsules: 100 mg	In bottles of 100 capsules
Oral combinations (Tuinal)	Capsules: 50 mg amobarital and 50 mg secobarbital 100 mg amobarbital and 100 mg secobarbital	In bottles of 100 capsules In bottles of 100 capsules

Table 13–10. Pharmacokinetics: Benzodiazepines

Drug	Onset	Peak	Duration	Half-Life	Excretion
Alprazolam	Intermediate	1–2 h	Intermediate	6–27 h	Urine
Chlordiazepoxide	Intermediate	0.5–4 h	Long	5–30 h	Urine
Clonazepam	Intermediate	1–2 h	Long	18–50 h	Urine
Clorazepate	Fast	1–2 h	Long	40–50 h	Urine
Diazepam	Very fast	0.5–2 h	Long	20–80 h	Urine
Halazepam	Slow	1–3 h	Intermediate	14 h	Urine
Lorazepam	Intermediate	2–4 h	Intermediate	10–20 h	Urine
Prazepam	Slow	6 h	Long	30–100 h	Urine
Oxazepam	Slow	2–4 h	Intermediate	5–20 h	Urine

Peak effects occur in 0.5 to 4 hours, and half-lives range from 5 to 80 hours.

Table 13–10 presents the pharmacokinetics of **benzodiazepines**.

Pharmacotherapeutics

Precautions and Contraindications

The development of dependence, which can be psychological as well as physical, is of concern. Although dependence is usually related to dose (high) and duration of use (more than a few weeks), it can occur in the absence of these parameters. It is thought that the newer **benzodiazepines, alprazolam (Xanax)** and **lorazepam (Ativan)**, are more likely to cause dependence because of their high potency and rapid, short-term action.

Symptoms of withdrawal, which usually occur 1 to 2 days after the last dose of short-acting **benzodiazepines** and 5 to 10 days after the last dose of the long-acting varieties, resemble withdrawal symptoms of other CNS depressants. Use of the drug should be gradually tapered rather than abruptly discontinued because of the risk of severe withdrawal symptoms.

One strategy for tapering is to decrease the dose by 0.5 mg per week, and then by 0.25 mg per week for the last few weeks. Another is to substitute in an equivalent dose a long-acting **benzodiazepine** such as **clonazepam (Klonopin)** for a short-acting one and then titrate down.

Benzodiazepines are contraindicated in pregnancy and lactation and in the presence of hepatic and renal disease, and they are not recommended for children under age 6. Other contraindications include hypersensitivity to **benzodiazepines** and acute narrow-angle glaucoma.

Geriatric patients should generally be prescribed lower doses because of their decreased rate of metabolism and consequent potential accumulation of the drug.

These drugs are not the treatment of choice for depression or psychosis or in the absence of anxiety signs and symptoms.

Adverse Drug Reactions

Major adverse effects are due to the drugs' action as **CNS depressants.** The same concerns as with other **CNS depressants** apply to their use: excessive sedation, particularly initially, in a situation requiring mental and physical alertness, and the potential for cardiac and respiratory depression, especially in combination with other **CNS depressants.**

Paradoxical anxiety, agitation, and acute rage may result from treatment with **benzodiazepines.**

Clonazepam may increase salivation.

Drug Interactions

Drug interactions of most concern are those involving other **CNS depressants**, such as **barbiturates, alcohol, antihistamines,** and **neuroleptics,** because of their additive CNS-depressant effects. **Benzodiazepines** also increase the blood levels of **TCAs** and **digitalis** preparations.

Table 13–11 presents drug interactions.

Clinical Use and Dosing

Benzodiazepines are indicated for the short-term treatment of anxiety disorders. Unlabeled uses include emergency treatment of status epilepticus, acute alcohol withdrawal syndrome, irritable bowel syndrome, chemotherapy-induced nausea and vomiting, and restless leg syndrome.

Table 13–11. Drug Interactions: Benzodiazepines

Drug	Interacting Drug	Possible Effect	Implications
All benzodiazepines	Digoxin	Increased level of digoxin	Monitor level; take pulse before giving digoxin
	TCAs	Increased plasma level of TCAs	Monitor level of TCA
	Barbiturates, nefazodone, fluoxetine, fluvoxamine, MAOIs, sertraline, alcohol, antihistamines	Increased CNS depression	Avoid concurrent administration
	Clozapine	Increased sedation, salivation, hypotension, delirium, respiratory arrest	Avoid concurrent administration
Alprazolam	Grapefruit juice	Decreased metabolism and increased effect of alprazolam	Use alternative juice
Alprazolam, clonazepam	Carbamazepine	Decreased plasma level of benzodiazepines	Use alternative anticonvulsant
Clonazepam	Lithium	Increased sexual dysfunction	Warn of possible adverse effects
Clonazepam, diazepam, chlordiazepoxide	Phenytoin	Decreased plasma level and toxicity of phenytoin	Use alternative anticonvulsant Monitor phenytoin blood level; may need lower dose
Clonazepam, lorazepam	Valproate	Decreased metabolism and increased effect of benzodiazepines	May require lower dose of benzodiazepine
Diazepam	Phenobarbital	Additive CNS depression; increased metabolism of diazepam	May affect treatment of status epilepticus

Table 13–12 presents the dosage schedule for **benzodiazepines.**

Rational Drug Selection

Diazepam is the treatment of choice for status epilepticus, administered by a parenteral route, preferably IV because of the rapidity of absorption and effect.

In acute alcohol withdrawal, care must be exercised so that cross-tolerance does not develop. Because dependence has occurred after as little as 4 to 6 weeks of use, these drugs should be slowly tapered to avoid withdrawal symptoms.

Monitoring

Increased blood levels of **TCAs** and **digitalis** may occur with concurrent use of **benzodiazepines** and should be monitored.

In long-term use, periodic assessment of liver function and blood counts should be performed.

Patient Education

Advise the patient to avoid **alcohol**. Because drowsiness may be an adverse effect, tell the patient to avoid taking a **benzodiazepine** before or during situations in which mental or physical alertness is required to maintain safety.

Table 13–13 presents the available dosage forms.

Buspirone

Buspirone (BuSpar) is a member of the **azaspirones,** a relatively new group of **anxiolytics** that exert their effects without the CNS depression and sedation of **barbiturates** and **benzodiazepines** but also without the anti-

Table 13–12. Dosage Schedule: Benzodiazepines

Drug	Indications	Dosage
Alprazolam	Anxiety, panic attacks	Anxiety: 0.25–0.5 mg tid; do not exceed 4 mg/d in divided doses Panic attack: 0.5 mg tid; may increase in increments of no more than 1 mg/d every 3–4 d Older or debilitated adult: 0.25 mg bid–tid; decrease by maximum of 0.5 mg every 3 d
Chlordiazepoxide	Anxiety	5–25 mg tid–qid, depending on severity of anxiety Older or debilitated adult: 5 mg bid–qid Children: 5 mg bid–qid; alternatively, 0.5 mg/kg/d every 6–8 h; not recommended in children under age 6
	Acute alcohol withdrawal	50–100 mg PO prn; not to exceed 300 mg/d 50–100 mg IM or IV; may repeat every 2–4 h
Clonazepam	Anxiety, insomnia, restless leg syndrome	Adult: 0.5–10 mg tid, not to exceed 20 mg/d Children under age 10 or 30 kg: 0.01–0.03 mg/kg every 8 h, not to exceed 0.2 mg/kg/d
Clorazepate dipotassium	Anxiety	Adult: 30 mg/d in divided doses Older or debilitated adult: 7.5–15 mg/d Maintenance: 22.5 mg or 11.25 mg as single daily dose
	Acute alcohol withdrawal	Day 1: 30 mg followed by 30–60 mg in divided doses Day 2: 45–90 mg in divided doses Day 3: 22.5–45 mg in divided doses Day 4: 15–30 mg in divided doses Reduce dose gradually to 7.5–15 mg daily and discontinue when condition is stable; maximum dose is 90 mg/d
Diazepam	Anxiety	Adult: 2–10 mg PO bid–qid; 2–10 mg IM or IV, depending on severity of symptoms; may repeat in 3–4 h Older or debilitated adult: 2–2.5 mg PO qd–bid Children: 1–2.5 mg PO tid–qid; no more than 0.25 mg/kg IM or IV over 3 min; may repeat in 15–30 min for severe anxiety; not recommended in children under 6 mo
	Acute alcohol withdrawal	10 mg tid–qid for first 24 h or 10 mg IM/IV initially, then 5–10 mg IM/IV in 3–4 h, depending on severity
	Adjunct for muscle spasms	2–10 mg bid–qid or 5–10 mg IM/IV initially, then 5–10 mg IM/IV in 3–4 h if needed; higher doses may be needed in treating tetanus
	Sedation (preprocedure)	Adults: 2–10 mg PO every 3–4 h as needed; 5–15 mg IM/IV before procedure Children: 0.04–0.2 mg/kg every 2–4 h; not to exceed 0.6 mg in 8-h period
	Adjunct in seizure disorders, status epilepticus	Status epilepticus: IV route if possible; administer slowly Adult: 5–10 mg initially; may repeat every 10–15 min if needed to max of 30 mg; may repeat in 2–4 h if needed Children over age 30 d and under 5 yr: 0.2–0.5 mg every 2–5 min to maximum of 5 mg or 0.2–0.5 mg/kg/dose every 15–30 min for 2 or 3 doses; maximum of 5 mg Newborns: 0.5–1 mg/kg/dose every 15–30 min for 2 or 3 doses
	Tetanus	Infants over age 30 d: 1–2 mg IV or IM slowly; repeat every 3–4 h if needed Children age 5 or older: 5–10 mg every 3–4 h as needed
Halazepam	Anxiety	20–40 mg tid–qid with optimum of 80–160 mg daily Older or debilitated adult: 20 mg qd–bid
Lorazepam	Anxiety	2–6 mg/d in divided doses with largest dose hs Older or debilitated adult: 1–2 mg/d in divided doses

Continued on next page

Table 13–12. Dosage Schedule: Benzodiazepines (*continued*)

Drug	Indications	Dosage
	Insomnia Sedation	2–4 mg hs 0.05 mg/kg IM not to exceed 4 mg; 2 mg or 0.044 mg/kg (0.02 mg/lb) IV Children under age 18: parental route not recommended
Prazepam	Anxiety	30 mg/d in divided doses; range of 20–60 mg or 20 mg hs with range of 20–40 mg Older or debilitated adult: 10–15 mg/d in divided doses
Oxazepam	Anxiety, alcohol withdrawal	10–30 mg tid–qid, depending on severity Older or debilitated adult: 10 mg tid; may cautiously increase to 15 mg tid–qid Children up to age 12: dosage not established Alcoholics with acute anxiety, tremulousness, or acute inebriation: 15–30 mg tid–qid

Table 13–13. Available Dosage Forms: Benzodiazepines

Drug	Dosage Form	How Supplied
Alprazolam	Tablets Oral solution Intensol solution	0.25, 0.5, 1, 2, mg 0.5 mg/5 mL 1 mg/mL concentrated solution to be mixed with liquid or semi-solid food, using only the provided calibrated dropper
Chlordiazepoxide	Tablets Capsules Powder for Injection	10, 25 mg 2, 5, 10 mg 100 mg
Clorazepate	Tablets Capsules	3.75, 7.5, 11.25, 15, 22.5 mg 3.75, 7.5, 15 mg
Clonazepam	Tablets	0.5, 1, 2 mg
Diazepam	Tablets Oral solution Intensol solution Injection	2, 5, 10 mg 5 mg/5 mL 5 mg/mL 5 mg/mL
Halazepam	Tablets	20 mg
Lorazepam	Tablets Intensol solution Injection	0.5, 1, 2, mg 2 mg/mL 2 or 4 mg/mL
Prazepam	Tablets Capsules	5, 10 mg 5, 10, 20 mg
Oxazepam	Tablets Capsules	15 mg 10, 15, 30 mg

convulsant or muscle-relaxant qualities. **Buspirone** has little risk of dependence and few drug interactions, and it is considered relatively safe, even in high doses.

Pharmacodynamics

Although the exact mechanism of action of **buspirone** is not understood, its anxiolytic properties appear to be due to its action on serotonin and dopamine receptor sites. The dopaminergic effect is presynaptic and carries little risk of dystonia or tardive dyskinesia.

Pharmacokinetics

Absorption and Distribution

Buspirone may be taken with food, which may delay absorption but increases bioavailability. It is almost 100 percent absorbed and is 95 percent protein-bound. It is lipid-soluble, therefore having broad distribution in brain and adipose tissue and a longer half-life. The long half-life is also due to the presence of active metabolites.

Metabolism and Excretion

Buspirone is metabolized by oxidation in the liver and is excreted primarily in urine, with approximately one-third excreted in feces. The half-life range is 2 to 11 hours.

Onset, Peak, and Duration

It takes about 1 to 2 weeks for the onset of the effects of **buspirone,** with 3 to 6 weeks for maximum benefit. It peaks in 0.7 to 1.5 hours and has an intermediate duration.

Pharmacotherapeutics

Precautions and Contraindications

Buspirone is contraindicated in patients with hypersensitivity to **buspirone** or in those with severe hepatic or renal disease.

It is considered Pregnancy Category B. The extent of excretion in breast milk is not clear and, because use in children younger than age 18 is not recommended, use during lactation should be avoided.

Although **buspirone** is not commonly thought to be sedating, as with other **anxiolytics**, drowsiness should be assessed prior to use in situations requiring cognitive or motor alertness in order to maintain safety.

Adverse Drug Reactions

Adverse effects are few and usually resolve with continued use. Most common are light-headedness, headache, insomnia, nausea, nervousness, and dry mouth.

Drug Interactions

Interactions between **buspirone** and other **serotonergic drugs** such as **MAOIs** and **selective serotonin reuptake inhibitors (SSRIs)** have the potential to cause serotonin syndrome, with its symptoms of nausea, diarrhea, chills, sweating, elevated temperature and blood pressure, agitation, ataxia, coma, and death.

Another interaction of potential concern is with **neuroleptic drugs** because of the competition with them for metabolism, which could result in higher plasma levels of the neuroleptic.

Clinical Use and Dosing

Used primarily for anxiety, **buspirone's** usual dose is 15 mg per day in two to three doses. The dose may be increased by 5 mg per day at intervals of 3 days. The maximum dose is 60 mg per day. It is available in 5-mg and 10-mg tablets.

Rational Drug Selection

Although **buspirone** can be used as the sole pharmacotherapeutic modality for anxiety, it is frequently used adjunctively with **SSRIs** because of its serotonergic effects, particularly in treatment-resistant depression or when there is a clear anxiety component.

A positive response may begin within 7 to 10 days of starting the drug, but maximum benefits may not become evident for 3 to 6 weeks.

Monitoring

No monitoring other than periodic reassessment of the drug's continued effectiveness is required.

Patient Education

To maintain safety, advise the patient to assess for drowsiness before engaging in situations requiring mental or physical alertness.

Dopaminergics

The **dopaminergics**, also known as **dopamine agonists, amantadine (Symmetrel), bromocriptine (Parlodel), carbidopa-levodopa (Sinemet), selegiline hydrochloride (Eldepryl),** and **pergolide (Permax)** are the pharmacological treatments of choice for Parkinson's disease. **Amantadine** is occasionally used for the parkinsonism-like extrapyramidal symptoms (EPSs) of the **antipsychotic drugs.**

Pharmacodynamics

Dopamine and acetylcholine are the neurotransmitters primarily responsible for balance and coordinated musculoskeletal functioning, and each needs to balance the other for smooth functioning to take place. When dopamine depletion occurs, either idiopathically as in Parkinson's disease or because of inadequate synthesis or impaired storage, transmission, or reuptake, the classic signs of muscular rigidity, tremors, and psychomotor retardation appear. Excessive amounts of dopamine are thought to produce the positive symptoms of schizophrenia, such as hallucinations and delusions.

Amantadine is effective because, in dopamine depletion, it releases from storage the remaining dopamine, whereas the dopamine precursors **levodopa** and **carbidopa-levodopa** increase synthesis. **Bromocriptine** and **pergolide** act as **dopamine agonists** at the postsynaptic receptor sites. The latter four are used in the treatment of true Parkinson's disease.

Pharmacokinetics

Absorption and Distribution

Dopaminergics are administered orally. They are relatively rapidly and completely absorbed.

Table 13–14. Pharmacokinetics: Dopaminergics

Drug	Onset	Peak	Duration	Half-Life	Excretion
Amantadine (Symmetrel)	48 h	4 h	—	18–24 h	Urine
Bromocriptine mesylate (Parlodel)	—	1–3 h	4–8 h	3–8 h	Feces (85–98%) Urine
Carbidopa-levodopa (Sinemet)	—	1–3 h	4–6 h	—	Urine
Selegiline HCl (Eldepryl)	—	0.5–2 h	—	18–20 h	Urine
Pergolide (Permax)	—	—	—	—	Urine

Metabolism and Excretion

Variations occur in metabolism; for example, **bromocriptine** is metabolized in the liver, but **amantadine** is excreted unchanged. **Selegiline** has three active metabolites, including amphetamine and methamphetamine, and deaths have occurred when **selegiline** has been taken concurrently with **meperidine.**

Dopaminergics are excreted through urine and feces. Table 13–14 presents the pharmacokinetics of dopaminergics.

Pharmacotherapeutics

Precautions and Contraindications

Selegiline is contraindicated with concurrent administration of **meperidine** and with hypersensitivity.

Renal impairment should be carefully assessed before using **amantadine** because it is excreted unchanged through the kidneys. **These drugs are Pregnancy Cat-** egories B and C. Their use during lactation and in children has not been evaluated.

Patients with underlying cardiac arrhythmias who have taken **pergolide** have experienced bradycardia and sinus tachycardia.

Adverse Drug Reactions

Adverse effects may include nausea and vomiting, lightheadedness, postural hypotension, abdominal pain, dyspepsia, depression, insomnia, hallucinations, and confusion.

Treatment with the sustained-release form of **levocarbidopa** may cause CNS effects such as dyskinesias.

Drug Interactions

Administration with **MAOIs** may cause hypertensive crisis.

Food with **levodopa** increases the availability and peak plasma level of the drug.

Table 13–15 presents food and drug interactions.

Table 13–15. Food and Drug Interactions: Dopaminergics

Drug	Interacting Drug or Food	Possible Effect	Implications
All	Antihypertensives	Increased antihypertensive effect	Monitor for postural hypotension, blood pressure
	Oral contraceptives	Decreased effectiveness of oral contraceptives	Use backup contraception
	MAOIs, TCAs, opioids	Hypertensive crisis	Avoid concurrent use
Carbidopa-levodopa	Food	Increased plasma level of carbidopa-levodopa with sustained-release form	Avoid taking with food
	Anticholinergics	Increased adrenocorticotropic hormone (ACH) adverse effects and decreased effect of levodopa	Monitor eye pain/vision; effect of dopaminergic
	Haldol, hydantoins	Decreased effect of levodopa	Monitor eye pain/vision; effect of dopaminergic

Clinical Use and Dosing

Table 13–16 presents the indications and dosage schedule of **dopaminergics**.

Rational Drug Selection

Sinemet, a combination of **levodopa** and **carbidopa**, is used in this fashion because **carbidopa** prevents metabolism of **levodopa** and increases its bioavailability. The form is less available and may require higher doses to achieve the desired plasma level.

Other combinations, such as **levodopa** and **amantadine** and **levodopa-carbidopa** with **selegiline**, may provide improved response over a single drug or in cases of deterioration in status.

Monitoring

As indicated previously, renal function must be assessed prior to **amantadine** use, and ongoing evaluation of creatine clearance should be performed when impairment is present.

Patient Education

Advise the patient to exercise care when changing position to prevent postural hypotension and to avoid hazardous activities if dizzy.

Table 13–17 presents the available dosage forms of **dopaminergics**.

Hydantoins

The **hydantoins, phenytoin (Dilantin), mephenytoin (Mesantoin), ethotoin (Peganone)**, and **fosphenytoin (Cerebyx)**, are the first-line treatment of choice for tonic-clonic and partial complex seizures and the least sedating drugs used to treat seizure disorders of any type. Although more than one **hydantoin** is available, **phenytoin** is the most commonly used.

Pharmacodynamics

Hydantoins inhibit and stabilize electrical discharges in the motor cortex of the brain by affecting ion exchanges during depolarization and repolarization They also affect the brain stem's contribution to grand mal seizures and additionally depress cardiac conduction.

Pharmacokinetics

Absorption and Distribution

The usual route of administration is oral. Absorption occurs in the small intestine and is slow, although the rate is dependent upon the form of the drug.

The rate and degree of absorption from IM administration are erratic, generally resulting in lower plasma levels than the oral route. **Hydantoins** are 87 to 93 percent

Table 13–16. Dosage Schedule: Dopaminergics

Drug	Indications	Dosage
Amantadine	Parkinson's disease; drug-induced EPS; parkinsonism syndrome following carbon monoxide poisoning	Adults: 100–200 mg bid; may increase to maximum of 400 mg/d in divided doses after several weeks without response after lower dose In conjunction with levodopa: 100 mg qd–bid
Bromocriptine mesylate	Parkinson's disease	Adult: initial dose 1.25 mg bid with meals; if dosage increase needed after 2 weeks, increase by 2.5 mg/d in divided doses with meals; maintain at lowest dose producing optimal response; usual range 10–40 mg/d
Carbidopa-levodopa	Parkinson's disease; parkinsonism syndrome following carbon monoxide or manganese poisoning	Adult: 1 tab (25 mg carbidopa and 100 mg levodopa) tid or 1 tab (10 mg carbidopa and 100 mg levodopa) tid–qid; may increase by 1 tab qd–qod until maximum of 8 tabs/d. Tablets of various ratios may be used but maintain 70–100 mg carbidopa/d CR form: 1 tab bid with minimum of 6 h between doses; increase as above; do not crush or chew tabs
Pergolide mesylate	Adjunctive treatment of Parkinson's disease with carbidopa-levodopa	Adult: initial dose 0.05 mg/d for 2 d, then increase gradually by 0.1–0.15 mg/d every 3 d over next 12 d; then may increase by 0.25 mg/d every 3 d until optimal response; usually given tid
Selegiline HCl	Adjunctive treatment of Parkinson's disease with carbidopa-levodopa	Adult: 5 mg bid with breakfast and lunch; after 2–3 d, decrease dose of carbidopa-levodopa.

CR = controlled release.

Table 13–17. Available Dosage Forms: Dopaminergics

Drug	Dosage Form	How Supplied
Amantadine	Capsules	100 mg
	Syrup	50 mg/5 mL
Bromocriptine	Tablets	2.5 mg
	Capsules	5 mg
Carbidopa-levodopa	Tablets	10 mg carbidopa/ 100 mg levo- dopa
		25 mg carbidopa/ 100 mg levo- dopa
		25 mg carbidopa/ 250 mg levo- dopa
	Sustained- release tablets	50 mg carbidopa/ 200 mg levo- dopa
		25 mg carbidopa/ 100 mg levo- dopa
Pergolide	Tablets	0.05, 0.25, 1 mg
Selegiline	Tablets	5 mg

protein-bound. The therapeutic plasma level range is 10 to 20 µg/mL and correlates well with treatment effect.

Metabolism and Excretion

Metabolism takes place in the liver; excretion, via the kidneys. Plasma half-lives range from 6 to 24 hours.

Table 13–18 presents the pharmacokinetics of **hydantoins**.

Pharmacotherapeutics

Precautions and Contraindications

Ethotoin is contraindicated in the presence of hepatic or hematologic disorders, and **phenytoin** should be avoided in patients with sinus bradycardia, sinoatrial block, second- and third-degree atrioventricular block, and Stokes-Adams syndrome. **Hydantoins** are contraindicated in hypersensitivity.

Although fetal defects have been associated with use of hydantoins during pregnancy, risk Category D, the majority of fetuses exposed in utero have been born defect-free. Risks to the woman who goes without the drug may outweigh any to the fetus. **Hydantoins** are present in breast milk; their safety during lactation has not been established.

Rebound status epilepticus may result from abrupt discontinuance of these drugs.

Use cautiously in cases of severe myocardial insufficiency and hypotension.

Older adults or those with impaired liver function may manifest signs of toxicity at lower-than-usual doses.

Phenytoin-induced hepatitis is a common hypersensitivity reaction. Other hypersensitive reactions may include fever, rash, arthralgias, and lymphadenopathy and may be mistaken for other medical syndromes. Insulin demands may be altered, and death has resulted from too-rapid IV administration.

Adverse Drug Reactions

Possible adverse effects are multiple and may include CNS effects such as ataxia, nystagmus, dizziness, confusion, drowsiness, and headache; cardiovascular effects such as hypotension and depression; and gastrointestinal (GI) effects such as nausea, vomiting, diarrhea, constipation, and weight gain. Other possible adverse effects include skin rashes, hyperglycemia, tinnitus, gynecomastia, coarsening of facial features and enlargement of the lips, urinary retention, hematopoietic complications, photophobia, and polyarthropathy.

Drug Interactions

Drug interactions consist of those that either increase or decrease the effect of the **hydantoin** and those that decrease the effect of the other drug. Interactions that increase **hydantoin's** effect because of increased metabolism, competition for binding sites, or for unknown reasons occur with **benzodiazepines, cimetidine, disul-**

Table 13–18. Pharmacokinetics: Hydantoins

Drug	Onset	Peak	Duration	Half-Life	Excretion
Ethotoin (Peganone)	—	—	—	3–9 h	Urine
Fosphenytoin (Cerebyx)	—	—	—	—	Urine
Mephenytoin (Mesantoin)	30 min	—	24–48 h	Unknown	Urine
Phenytoin (Dilantin)	slow	4–12 h (extended) 1.5–3 h (rapid)	5 h	22 h	Urine

firam, acute ethanol use, TCAs, salicylates, and valproic acid.

The opposite effect occurs with concurrent administration of barbiturates, chronic ethanol use, rifampin, theophylline, influenza virus vaccine, pyridoxine, and antacids.

Concurrent administration causes the decreased effect of carbamazepine, estrogens, corticosteroids, haloperidol, methadone, levodopa, sulfonylureas, oral contraceptives, and cardiac glycosides.

Table 13–19 presents drug interactions.

Clinical Use and Dosing

Table 13–20 presents the indications and dosage schedules of hydantoins.

Rational Drug Selection

Hydantoins are used for the treatment of grand mal and psychomotor seizures. Mephenytoin use is reserved for refractive tonic-clonic seizures and for the treatment of Jacksonian and focal seizures. Phenytoin has been used instead of magnesium sulfate in severe preeclampsia. Hydantoins are not the first-line treatment of status epilepticus, but IV phenytoin can be used for the control of grand mal types of seizures.

Monitoring

Baseline blood count, urinalysis, and liver function tests should be assessed prior to onset of treatment, with frequent reassessment during the first few months of treatment.

Plasma levels should be monitored, particularly in cases when drugs that increase plasma hydantoin, such as ibuprofen, are also used. Conversely, other drugs negatively affected by concurrent administration with hydantoins may need plasma level monitoring. Phenytoin may alter thyroid hormone demands, which may require monitoring.

Patient Education

Advise the patient not to stop the drug abruptly, to wear a medical identification bracelet, to avoid hazardous situations if drowsiness occurs, and to report adverse effects to the clinician.

Table 13–21 presents the available dosage forms of hydantoins.

Iminostilbenes

Carbamazepine (Tegretol) is an iminostilbene derivative structurally related to TCAs. It is used to treat epilepsy, bipolar affective disorder, aggressive and assaultive behavior, and some neuralgias.

Pharmacodynamics

The method of action of carbamazepine is not fully understood but is thought to exert its effect by inhibiting electroexcitability in the limbic brain. It also has an antidepressant component because of its relationship to the TCAs.

Table 13–19. Drug Interactions: Hydantoins

Drug	Interacting Drug	Possible Effect	Implications
All hydantoins	Allopurinol, cimetidine, diazepam, disulfiram, alcohol (acute intake), phenacemide, succinimides, valproic acid	Increased plasma level of hydantoins	May need to decrease hydantoin dose; monitor plasma level
	Barbiturates, carbamazepine, alcohol (chronic use), theophylline, antacids, calcium	Decreased plasma level of hydantoins	May need to increase hydantoin dose; monitor plasma level
	Corticosteroids, dicumarol, digitoxin, doxycycline, haloperidol, methadone, oral contraceptives, dopamine, furosemide, levodopa	Decreased effect of interacting drug	Monitor plasma levels where possible; monitor signs and symptoms

Table 13–20. Dosage Schedule: Hydantoins

Drug	Indications	Dosage
Ethotoin	Generalized tonic-clonic or psychomotor seizures	Adults: initially 1 g/d or less in 4–6 divided doses, spaced as evenly as possible, taken after food; increase gradually to usual maintenance dose of 2–3 g/d Children: initial maximum dose of 750 mg/d in divided doses as with adult; usual maintenance dose of 500–1000 mg/d
Fosphenytoin	Status epilepticus	IV loading dose: 15–20 mg PE/kg diluted in 5% dextrose or 0.9% saline solution at rate of 100–150 mg PE/min (PE: phenytoin sodium equivalent units) Other measures such as IV diazepam will be needed Nonemergent loading dose and maintenance: loading dose 10–20 mg PE/kg IV or IM; maintenance 4–6 mg PE/kg/d at rate of 150 mg PE/min or less
Mephenytoin	Generalized tonic-clonic or psychomotor seizures; focal seizures refractory to other agents	Adults: initial dose of 50–100 mg/d for first week; increase by 50–100 mg/d at weekly intervals; usual range 400–600 mg/d; maximum of 800 mg/d Children: usual range 100–400 mg/d
Phenytoin	Generalized tonic-clonic, psychomotor, and simple partial seizures; status epilepticus	Adult: initial PO dose 1 g in 3 divided doses, then after 24 h, 300 mg/d in 1 dose (extended release) or tid (rapid acting); IV loading dose of 10–15 mg/kg at rate of 50 mg/min; maintenance dose of 100 mg PO or IV every 6–8 h Children: 4–8 mg/kg/d PO in divided doses; 15–20 mg/kg IV at rate of 50 mg/min

Pharmacokinetics

Absorption and Distribution

Carbamazepine is absorbed through the stomach, the suspension being absorbed more rapidly than the tablet form. The drug is 76 percent bound to plasma protein.

Metabolism and Excretion

Carbamazepine is metabolized in the liver and may induce its own metabolism. Excretion is through urine and feces.

Onset, Peak, and Duration

Peak blood levels occur 1 to 6 hours after administration. Its half-life can be as long as 35 hours with initial dosing but is typically 10 to 20 hours as administration continues. Steady state is attained in 2 to 4 days.

Pharmacotherapeutics

Precautions and Contraindications

Contraindications include hypersensitivity to **carbamazepine** or **TCAs**, history of bone marrow suppression, and concurrent administration with **MAOIs**.

Teratogenic defects have occurred, and *carbamazepine* **is Pregnancy Category C. It is excreted in** human milk but is not contraindicated during lactation.

Safety of use in children under age 6 has not been established.

Use with caution in patients with increased intraocular pressure because of its mild anticholinergic effects. Caution is also indicated in patients with a history of previous adverse hematologic reactions to any drugs and in those with cardiac, renal, or hepatic damage.

Adverse Drug Reactions

Carbamazepine has the potential to cause blood dyscrasias, some potentially lethal. Although a transient decrease of the white cell count can occur and is manageable, **carbamazepine** can depress the bone marrow and lead to leukopenia, thrombocytopenia, agranulocytosis, and aplastic anemia. For that reason, a baseline blood screen that includes a complete blood count (CBC), chemistry, liver function tests, and thyroid-stimulating hormone (TSH) test should be obtained, followed by periodic monitoring. Follow-up studies should be more frequent initially, decreasing to every 3 to 4 months if the results remain normal or the CBC and differential are only minimally lowered.

Other adverse reactions can include hepatic damage and impaired thyroid function. Less serious early adverse events may include drowsiness, dizziness, blurred vision, ataxia, nausea and vomiting, dry mouth, diplopia, and headache.

Table 13–21. Available Dosage Forms: Hydantoins

Drug	Dosage Form	How Supplied
Ethotoin	Tablets	250, 500 mg
Fosphenytoin sodium	Injection	150 mg (100 mg phenytoin) 750 mg (500 mg phenytoin)
Mephenytoin	Tablets	100 mg
Phenytoin sodium Phenytoin	Chewable tablets Injection Oral suspension	50 mg 50 mg/mL 30 mg/5 mL, 125 mg/5 mL
Phenytoin sodium, rapid-acting	Capsules	30, 100 mg
Phenytoin sodium, extended release	Capsules	30, 100 mg
Phenytoin sodium with phenobarbital	Capsules	100 mg/16 mg or 100 mg/32 mg

Drug Interactions

The interactions of most significance are those that increase the plasma level of **carbamazepine** to potentially toxic amounts, such as concurrent administration of **propoxyphene, hydantoins, cimetidine,** some **antibiotics, isoniazid,** and **verapamil.** Interactions that can result in hepatic damage occur with coadministration of some **anesthetics;** interactions that decrease plasma levels of the other drug occur with **beta blockers, succinimides, valproic acid, haloperidol, doxycycline,** and **nondepolarizing muscle relaxants.**

Table 13–22 presents drug interactions.

Clinical Use and Dosing

Table 13–23 presents the indications, dosage schedules, and available dosage forms of **carbamazepine.**

Rational Drug Selection

Carbamazepine is indicated in the treatment of partial complex seizures. For other types of seizures, it should be reserved for refractory seizure activity or for patients experiencing severe adverse effects from other **anticonvulsants.**

The drug is used as a third-line mood stabilizer for bipolar patients who have not responded to **lithium** or **divalproex (Depakote)** and for patients unable to tolerate either of the others.

Although **clonazepam** is the preferred drug, **carbamazepine,** in a dosage range of 100 to 300 mg at bedtime, can be used to treat restless leg syndrome.

Carbamazepine should not be used for pain relief except in the case of trigeminal neuralgia.

Monitoring

As discussed previously, plasma levels should be monitored on a regular basis. The therapeutic range is 4 to 12 μg/mL. Higher levels can lead to toxic symptoms consisting of the initial adverse effects and also possibly hypertension, tachycardia, electrocardiogram (ECG) changes, stupor, agitation, urinary retention, nystagmus, respiratory depression and cyanosis, seizures, and coma.

Children and geriatric patients may develop toxicity at levels below 12.

Patient Education

Patients (or their parents, in the case of children) taking **carbamazepine** should be instructed to report to the clinician any symptoms such as skin lesions, bruising, fever, or sore throat. **Carbamazepine** should then be discontinued and another drug substituted. Also, tell the patient that administration with food may increase absorption, and because **carbamazepine** can be sedating, care should be exercised in situations in which mental and physical alertness is required for safety.

Lithium

Lithium's stabilizing effect on manic individuals was discovered in the mid-1940s, making it the earliest psychotropic drug available for use. It is now considered the mood-stabilizing treatment of choice for classic bipolar affective disorder (BAD) and is used as an adjunct for treatment-resistant unipolar depression.

Table 13–22. Drug Interactions: Carbamazepine

Drug	Interacting Drug	Possible Effect	Implications
Carbamazepine	Anesthetics	Hepatic or renal damage	Ensure anesthetist is aware of carbamazepine use
	Cimetidine, propoxyphene, isoniazid, calcium channel blockers, fluoxetine, valproic acid, erythromycin, paroxetine, fluvoxamine, danazol, grapefruit juice, influenza vaccine, olanzapine, loxapine, ritonavir, nicotinamide	Increased plasma level of carbamazepine	Monitor plasma level
	Hydantoins, barbiturates, primidone, felbamate, rifampin, cisplatin, theophylline	Decreased plasma level of carbamazepine	Monitor level for possible dosage increase; monitor for seizure activity
	MAOIs	Hyperpyretic crisis	Do not give during or within 14 d of MAOI use
	Doxycycline, anticoagulants, warfarin, theophylline, haloperidol, acetaminophen, alprazolam, clozapine, anticonvulsants, clomipramine, phenytoin, primidone	Decreased effect of interacting drug	Monitor plasma levels when able; monitor for signs and symptoms of condition for which interacting drug was prescribed
	Lithium	Increased risk of neurotoxicity	Monitor plasma levels of both drugs; monitor for CNS-related adverse events

Pharmacodynamics

Lithium carbonate (Lithobid, Eskalith) is a naturally occurring substance, similar to sodium in its lack of metabolism, its excretion through the renal system, and its affinity for the same binding sites. Both are widely distributed and interchangeable.

The relationship between sodium, **lithium,** and body fluid is inverse in that when sodium and fluids are depleted, such as can occur during severe vomiting, prolonged heavy sweating, and diuretic use, the level of **lithium** is increased. The opposite also occurs, for example, as a result of water intoxication, which has the effect of decreasing the **lithium** level. Such variations in **lithium's** concentration can also be the product of abrupt dietary changes.

Lithium's mechanism of action is not completely understood but, because of the two substances' ability to substitute for each other, it is possible that **lithium** replaces sodium during depolarization in neuronal pathways, effectively stopping the transmission of electrical impulses.

Pharmacokinetics

Absorption and Distribution

Lithium is absorbed through the GI tract and distributed throughout the body according to water volume.

Metabolism and Excretion

Lithium is not metabolized and is excreted through the kidneys.

Onset, Peak, and Duration

Onset is in 5 to 14 days. Peak plasma levels occur in 1 to 4 hours, and absorption is complete in 8 hours. The half-life is 17 to 36 hours.

Pharmacotherapeutics

Precautions and Contraindications

Because **lithium** is almost completely excreted via the renal system, it is essential that the presence of kidney disease

Table 13–23. Dosage Schedule: Carbamazepine

Drug	Indications	Dosage	Available Dosage Forms
Carbamazepine	Partial complex seizure disorder	Adults and children over age 12: initially 200 mg bid; increase by 200 mg/d at weekly intervals to maximum of 1000 mg/d for children age 12–15; maintenance range: 800–1200 mg/d 3–4 times/d Children under age 12: initially 100 mg bid; increase by 100 mg/d tid–qid at weekly intervals to maximum of 1000 mg/d; may also give at 20–30 mg/kg/d tid–qid; maintenance range 400–800 mg/d	Tablets: 200 mg Chewable tablets: 100 mg Suspension: 100 mg/5 mL
	Trigeminal neuralgia	Adults: 100 mg bid on first day; increase by 200 mg/d at 100 mg every 12 h to maximum of 1200 mg/d; maintenance range 200–1200 mg/d, usually 400–800 mg/d; decrease dosage or discontinue every 3 mo	
	Bipolar disorder, aggressive/assaultive behavior	Same dosage guidelines as above until severe mood swings are stabilized and plasma level is within therapeutic range	

be assessed before a course of treatment is begun. Baseline blood chemistry, including creatinine, blood urea nitrogen (BUN), and TSH levels, should be obtained. In the event of positive findings, a different drug should be used.

Other contraindications are children younger than age 12, pregnancy (Pregnancy Category C) and lactating women, and severe cardiac disease.

Extreme caution should be used when prescribing **lithium** to patients with sodium depletion or to those taking **diuretics.** Hypothyroidism may occur with long-term administration.

Adverse Drug Reactions

Early, transient adverse reactions may occur, including fine tremors of the fingers, nausea, dry mouth, headache, and drowsiness. **Lithium** may be taken with food to minimize GI distress, and the form of the drug may be changed to sustained release to minimize adverse effects associated with dosage peaks.

The index between therapeutic and toxic levels is narrow at the upper end, requiring frequent monitoring initially and in the event of significant changes in fluid balance, as often as daily if necessary. The therapeutic range is 0.5 to 1.5 mEq/L.

Indicators of toxicity, which can also occur at therapeutic levels, are coarse tremors of the hands that impair function, nausea and vomiting, diarrhea, stupor, polydipsia and polyuria, muscle weakness, and ataxia. If the **lithium** level is elevated enough, death can result. Treat-

ment for overdose is supportive, ensuring adequate hydration, but may require dialysis.

Drug Interactions

Drug interactions of particular concern are associated with elevated **lithium** concentration, which increases the potential for toxicity, such as may occur with **SSRIs, nonsteroidal anti-inflammatory drugs (NSAIDs),** and some **antihypertensives** and **anesthetics.**

Decreased **lithium** levels may result with concurrent use of **sodium salts, bulking agents** such as **Metamucil,** and **theophylline.**

Concurrent administration with **anticonvulsants** may cause increased toxicity of both drugs.

Table 13–24 presents drug interactions.

Clinical Use and Dosing

Table 13–25 presents the indications, dosage schedules, and available dosage forms of **lithium.**

Rational Drug Selection

Because of its long half-life, **lithium** takes 10 to14 days to reach maximum efficacy and therefore is not indicated in the treatment of acute mania. Rather, it is indicated for maintenance and prophylaxis when BAD presents with classic symptoms of discrete depressive and manic or hypomanic episodes, followed by return to baseline functioning for the individual.

Table 13–24. Drug Interactions: Lithium

Drug	Interacting Drug	Possible Effect	Implications
Lithium	Angiotensin-converting enzyme (ACE) inhibitors, antibiotics (ampicillin, doxycycline, tetracycline, spectinomycin), antihypertensives, metronidazole, NSAIDs, antimicrobials, diuretics, SSRIs	Increased lithium level	Monitor lithium blood levels and for signs and symptoms of toxicity Avoid NSAIDs
	Caffeine, psyllium, urinary alkalizers, theophylline	Decreased lithium level	Monitor lithium blood level and recurrence of manic signs and symptoms for need to increase dose
	Anticonvulsants, calcium channel blockers, phenothiazines, haloperidol	Increased neurotoxicity	Avoid coadministration
	Benzodiazepines	Sexual dysfunction	Avoid
	SSRIs	Serotonin syndrome	Keep SSRI dose low Monitor for signs and symptoms of serotonin excess

A strategy for responding to acute mania would be to start a patient on **lithium** supplemented initially with a high-potency **neuroleptic** such as **risperidone** and to discontinue the **neuroleptic**, if possible, when the required length of time for **lithium** to become efficacious has elapsed and the mania has abated.

Some clinicians raise the level to 1.2 mEq/L to begin treatment during an acute stage and back down to 0.8 to 0.9 mEq/L for maintenance. As a patient achieves and maintains stability, levels need not be obtained as frequently.

Lithium is also prescribed for patients who have been resistant to adequate trials of the usual **antidepressants**. Adjunctive doses of **lithium** are frequently lower than they would be for BAD, with concomitantly lower risks.

Monitoring

Because signs and symptoms of toxicity may occur even at subtoxic blood levels, patients should always be assessed for tremors, nausea and vomiting, diarrhea, and drowsiness. Lowering the dose will usually be sufficient to resolve the symptoms.

Blood levels should be obtained 14 days after beginning treatment and 14 days after every dosage change. The frequency of routine blood levels after stability is achieved is generally every 3 to 6 months. In the event of patient illness involving severe vomiting, diarrhea, prolonged high fever, or heatstroke, more frequent monitoring is needed.

The procedure for obtaining an accurate **lithium** level

Table 13–25. Dosage Schedule: Lithium

Drug	Indications	Dosage	Available Dosage Forms
Lithium (Lithobid, Eskalith, lithium carbonate, Lithotabs)	Treatment of manic phase of BAD and prevention of manic episodes	Acute mania: 600 mg tid or 900 mg bid extended release Maintenance: 300 mg tid–qid or 450 mg bid extended release	Capsules: 150, 300, 600 mg Tablets: 300 mg Slow-release tablets: 300 mg Controlled-release tablets: 450 mg Syrup: 300 mg/15 mL
	Refractory unipolar depression	300–600 mg qd	

is to have the sample drawn 12 hours after the last dose, usually the bedtime dose, before any morning dose has been taken. The patient need not be fasting, but the timing needs to be accurate within an hour to ensure standardization of interpretation by the clinician.

Routine blood counts with differential and chemistry screens should be obtained yearly.

Patient Education

Patients should be informed of the procedure for obtaining an accurate **lithium** level as just described. Advise the patient to report any illness involving severe vomiting, diarrhea, or prolonged high fever. Also tell patients engaging in activities that produce copious sweating to increase their water intake and maintain an adequate salt intake. The patient's level of drowsiness should be assessed before participation in activities requiring mental or physical alertness in order to maintain safety.

Local Anesthetics

Etidocaine hydrochloride (Duranest), ropivacaine HCl (Naropin), chloroprocaine HCl (Nesacaine), bupivacaine HCl (Sensorcaine), and lidocaine HCl (Xylocaine) are **local anesthetics** similar in their mechanism of action and use. They are discussed here as a group.

Indications for use are **local** or **regional anesthesia** required for surgical or dental procedures, parturition or cesarean section, or peripheral nerve blockage for pain.

Pharmacodynamics

These drugs are primarily **amino amide compounds.** The mechanism of action is the blockade of nerve impulses by inhibition of ion flux across the cell membrane.

Pharmacokinetics

Absorption and Distribution

Local anesthetics are sterile, isotonic solutions that are available with or without **epinephrine.** They are absorbed and distributed to the appropriate neuronal level by venous perfusion.

Metabolism and Excretion

All are metabolized in the liver and excreted via the kidneys.

Onset, Peak, and Duration

Onset of action is rapid, the length of time depending on whether the route of administration is SC, IM, IV, or epidural. Half-lives are from 1.5 to 2 hours.

Pharmacotherapeutics

Precautions and Contraindications

The only absolute contraindication to use is hypersensitivity, but caution should be exercised when **epinephrine** is included in the solution and the patient is currently being treated with a **vasopressor** or when the patient is in shock or heart block.

Pregnancy is a relative contraindication because of the lack of adequate studies demonstrating safety; however, fetal risk versus maternal need must be assessed.

Adverse Drug Reactions

Because of the risk of adverse reactions in the event of incorrect administration technique or of toxicity because of excessively rapid increase or excessive total dose, emergency resuscitative equipment must be immediately available to the patient.

Only technically skilled clinicians should administer **local anesthetics.** Possible skill-related adverse events can include accidental intravascular infusion, fetal intracranial injection during paracervical block, and subarachnoid penetration.

Aspiration without blood or cerebral spinal fluid return must be clearly accomplished before each dose of anesthetic, even through a previously placed catheter. A small test dose of the anesthetic should be injected to assess for hypersensitivity or adverse reaction prior to administration of the full dose.

Symptoms of toxicity include restlessness, anxiety, incoherent speech, light-headedness, perioral numbness or tingling, blurred vision, dizziness, tremors, and drowsiness. Toxicity, if unrecognized or untreated, may progress to respiratory and/or cardiac depression and arrest. Hypotension or hypertension, tachycardia or bradycardia, and hyperthermia are other indicators of trouble requiring immediate intervention, initially by the provision of supplemental oxygen.

Progression of anesthesia is related to the characteristics of the targeted nerve fiber but proceeds in the following direction: pain, temperature, touch, proprioception, and skeletal muscle tone. Adequate time must be allowed to achieve full anesthesia before procedures are begun.

Drug Interactions

The only relevant adverse interaction could be between the **epinephrine** that some **local anesthetics** contain and **vasopressors** because of a possible additive effect.

Clinical Use and Dosing

Table 13–26 presents the indications and dosage of **local anesthetics.**

Table 13–26. Dosage Schedule: Local Anesthetics

Drug	Indications	Dosage
Bupivacine HCl (Sensorcaine)	Peripheral nerve block, local infusion	Local infusion: 0.25% solution to maximum volume and dose Peripheral block: 0.5% solution, 5 mL to maximum volume; 25 mg to maximum dose
Chloroprocaine (Nesacaine)	Peripheral nerve block, digital block, paracervical block	Peripheral block: 2% solution, 2–3 mL; 40–60 mg Digital block: 1% solution, 3–4 mg; 30–40 mg; without epinephrine Paracervical block: 1% solution, 3 mL at each of 4 sites, up to 120 mg
Etidocaine HCl (Duranest)	Peripheral, central, or lumbar nerve block	1% solution, 5–40 mL; total dose 50–400 mg
Lidocaine HCl (Xylocaine)	Percutaneous Infiltration, peripheral, intercostal, paracervical nerve block	Percutaneous block: 0.5–1% solution, 1–60 mL; 5–300 mg Peripheral block: 1.5% solution, 15–20 mg; 225–300 mg Intercostal block: 1% solution; 3 mL, 30 mg Paracervical block: 1% solution; 10 mL, 100 mg each site
Ropivacaine (Naropin)	(same as above)	Major nerve block: 0.5% solution, 35–50 mg; 20–40 mg Field block: 0.5% solution, 1–40 mg; 5–200 mg

Rational Drug Selection

The choice of **anesthetic** depends on the local area to be deadened and its local blood supply. If much bleeding is anticipated, an **anesthetic** with **epinephrine** can be useful to decrease the bleeding by constriction of local vessels.

Monitoring

Monitoring is focused on possible anaphylactic responses such as dyspnea and edema.

Patient Education

Patients should be advised that pain levels may increase as the **anesthesia** wears off. Table 13–27 presents the available dosage forms of local anesthetics.

Monoamine Oxidase Inhibitors

The **MAOIs phenelzine (Nardil), isocarboxazid (Marplan),** and **tranylcypromine (Parnate)** are **antidepressants** infrequently prescribed since the introduction of **SSRIs** because of the **MAOIs'** strong potential for adverse interactions with certain foods and drugs. They are primarily reserved for the treatment of refractory unipolar depression.

Pharmacodynamics

The **MAOIs** exert their effect by inhibition of the hepatic enzymes that metabolize norepinephrine, serotonin, and dopamine, thereby increasing the bioavailability of these neurotransmitters.

Pharmacokinetics

Absorption and Distribution

The **MAOIs** are administered orally and are rapidly and thoroughly absorbed from the GI tract.

Metabolism and Excretion

Metabolism occurs in the liver, and excretion is in the urine.

Onset, Peak, and Duration

Whereas **SSRIs** and **TCAs** have long half-lives, requiring 3 to 4 weeks before full therapeutic benefits are evident, patients taking **MAOIs** may begin to experience relief of their depressive symptoms immediately or within approximately 14 days. Onset is 1 to 2 weeks, the peak for **isocarboxazid** and **tranylcypromine** is 0.7 to 3 hours and 1 to 2 hours for **phenelzine**, and their half-lives are 1 to 3 hours.

Table 13–27. Available Dosage Forms: Local Anesthetics

Drug	Dosage Form	How Supplied
Bupivacaine HCl	Single-dose ampules	5% solution in 5 mL with 1:200,000 epinephrine 0.25%, 0.5%, 0.75% solution in 30 mL without epinephrine 0.5%, 0.75% solution in 30 mL with 1: 200,000 epinephrine
	Multiple-dose vial	0.25%, 0.5% solution in 50 mL with and without 1:200,000 epinephrine
Chloroprocaine	Single-dose ampules	2% solution in 30 mL 3% solution in 20 mL
	Multiple-dose vial	1% solution in 30 mL 2% solution in 30 mL
Etidocaine HCl	Single-dose vials	1% solution in 30 mL without epinephrine 1% solution in 30 mL with 1:200,000 epinephrine 1.5% solution in 20 mL with 1:200,000 epinephrine
Lidocaine HCl	Single- and multiple-dose vials	1% solution in 2, 5, 10, 20, 30, 50 mL without epinephrine, with 1:200,000 and 1:100,000 epinephrine 1.5% solution in 10, 20 mL without epinephrine 1.5% solution in 5, 10, 30 mL with 1:200,000 and 1:100,000 epinephrine 2% solution in 2, 5, 10, 20, 50 mL without epinephrine 2% solution in 10, 20, 50 mL 1:100,000 epinephrine 2% solution in 5, 10, 20 mL with 1:200,000 epinephrine 5% solution in 50 mL with and without 1:200,000 epinephrine
Ropivacaine	Single-dose ampules and multiple-dose vials	7.5, 10 mg in 10 mL 2, 7.5, 10 mg/mL in 20 mL 5, 7.5 mg/mL in 30 mL

Pharmacotherapeutics

Precautions and Contraindications

Contraindications include liver or kidney disease, hypersensitivity, congestive heart failure or arteriosclerotic disease, and age over 60.

These drugs are Pregnancy Category C. They are excreted in breast milk, and safety has not been established. They are not recommended for children.

Postural hypotension and suppression of myocardial pain may occur.

Adverse Drug Reactions

Initial adverse effects may include insomnia, anxiety, and agitation as a result of the delayed metabolism of dopamine, as well as dry mouth, blurred vision, urinary retention, and constipation because of anticholinergic activity.

Drug Interactions

Because **MAOIs** inhibit the metabolism of norepinephrine, hypertensive crisis can occur if they are administered concurrently with other drugs or foods that raise blood pressure, examples of which are **anticholinergics, sympathomimetics, stimulants,** and foods containing tyramine, which is a precursor to dopamine, norepinephrine, and epinephrine. These restrictions apply during use or within 14 days following discontinuance of the **MAOI.**

Symptoms of hypertensive crisis include headache, heart palpitations, stiff or sore neck, chest tightness, tachycardia, sweating, and dilated pupils. The crisis needs to be managed immediately, and the patient should remain standing until it is. Usual treatment is with **phentolamine (Regitine)** 5 mg IV and then 0.25 to 0.5 mg IM every 4 to 6 hours.

The prolonged metabolism of norepinephrine and the pressor effect of other drugs can lead to interactions resulting in hypotension. Heart failure has occurred.

The 14-day restriction discussed previously also applies with the use of **SSRIs.** The increased amount of serotonin available due to inhibition of its metabolism by the **MAOI** leads to a risk of the potentially fatal serotonin syndrome.

As a result of other drug interactions, particularly with **meperidine,** CNS depression can also develop.

Table 13–28 presents drug interactions.

Table 13–28. Drug Interactions: Monoamine Oxidase Inhibitors

Drug	Interacting Drug	Possible Effect	Implications
All MAOIs	Anorexiants, venlafaxine, SSRIs, bupropion, bromocriptine, L-dopa, L-tryptophan, MAO–B inhibitor, sumatriptan	Increased serotonergic Effect, possible serotonin syndrome	Avoid
	CNS depressants, meperidine, antipsychotics	Increased CNS depression	Use cautiously in hazardous situations
	Buspirone, L-dopa, reserpine, stimulants, tetrabenazine, guanethidine, meperidine	Increased blood pressure and possible hypertensive crisis	Monitor blood pressure; avoid if possible
	Antihypertensives, propoxyphene, meperidine, diuretics, nitroglycerin	Hypotension	Monitor blood pressure; avoid concurrent administration if possible
	Insulin, sulfonylureas	Hypoglycemia	Monitor blood glucose and for signs and symptoms of hypoglycemia
	Carbamazepine	Increased carbamazepine level	Monitor level; use alternative anticonvulsant if possible
	TCAs	Seizures and delirium	Avoid

Clinical Use and Dosing

Table 13–29 presents the indications, dosages, and available dosage forms of **MAOIs.**

Rational Drug Selection

Except in treatment-resistant situations in which the patient can be closely monitored or is hospitalized, **MAOIs** are infrequently used.

Monitoring

Periodic liver function tests should be performed and the drug discontinued if any abnormalities are found.

Patient Education

Advise the patient that strict dietary restrictions need to be followed. Foods containing tyramine or vasopressors, including cheese, yogurt, sour cream, meat and meat products, dried fish and herring, alcoholic beverages, fermented vegetables such as sauerkraut, avocados, bananas, raisins, soy sauce, miso soup, bean curd, fava beans, caffeine, chocolate, and ginseng, must be excluded.

Nonphenothiazine Antipsychotics

A number of **nonphenothiazine antipsychotics** have been marketed relatively recently, beginning in 1990.

Table 13–29. Dosage Schedule: Monoamine Oxidase Inhibitors

Drug	Indications	Dosage	Available Dosage Forms
Phenelzine sulfate	Refractory unipolar depression	15 mg tid; may increase to max of 90 mg/d at rapid pace Maintenance: 15 mg/d	Tablets: 15 mg
Tranylcypromine	Refractory unipolar depression	30 mg/d in divided doses; may increase after 2 wk in 10 mg/d increments every 1–3 wk; max 60 mg/d; taper off gradually	Tablets: 10 mg
Isocarboxazid	Refractory unipolar depression	30 mg/d in divided doses Maintenance: 10–20 mg/d	Tablets: 10 mg

These drugs, referred to as *novel, atypical,* or *nonconventional* **neuroleptics,** include **risperidone (Risperdal), olanzapine (Zyprexa), quetiapine (Seroquel),** and **clozapine (Clozaril).**

Pharmacodynamics

Although the mechanism of action for these **antipsychotics** is less well understood than that of the conventional **antipsychotics,** all atypical **antipsychotics** act as postsynaptic dopamine receptor antagonists in the brain. **Clozapine** seems to blockade dopamine at the limbic level rather than in the striatum as the others do, accounting for its relative lack of EPSs. Most of this group also variously affect serotonergic, adrenergic, histaminic, and cholinergic receptors.

Pharmacokinetics

Absorption and Distribution

These drugs are all administered orally and are rapidly and completely absorbed.

Metabolism and Excretion

All are metabolized in the liver and primarily excreted through the renal system.

Onset, Peak, and Duration

Onset is within a few days to a few weeks. These drugs reach their peak activity in approximately 1 to 6 hours and steady state within a few days, and they have half-lives of approximately 9 to 30 hours. **Clozapine** peaks in 2.5 hours and has a half-life of 8 to 12 hours, whereas **olanzapine** peaks in 6 hours and has a half-life of 21 to 54 hours. **Quetiapine** peaks in 1.5 hours and has a half-life of 6 hours; **risperidone** peaks in 1 hour and has a half-life of 3 to 21 hours.

Pharmacotherapeutics

Precautions and Contraindications

Nonphenothiazine antipsychotics **are not recomended in pregnant (Pregnancy Category C) or lactating women or in young children.** Safer medications are available to treat behavior problems in children.

They should be prescribed cautiously, if at all, in the presence of hepatic or renal disease. Analysis of risk versus benefit is particularly indicated in the situation of individuals who have disease but who also have poor quality of life without treatment with a **neuroleptic.** Because of liver function decline, the geriatric population generally requires smaller doses.

An additional contraindication is hypersensitivity.

Adverse Drug Reactions

Because of the risk of potentially fatal agranulocytosis, **clozapine** is reserved for the treatment of severe schizophrenia refractory to complete trials, including full dosing and adequate length of time, of at least two different types of neuroleptics.

Clozapine is available only through a patient management system, such as that offered by the Zenith Goldline **Clozapine** Alert Program, into which a clinician and patient are both registered. A baseline white blood cell (WBC) count with differential is obtained prior to treatment, then monitored weekly or biweekly, depending on the length of time the patient has been taking **clozapine,** before the next week's medication is dispensed by the pharmacy. Monitoring should be continued for 4 weeks after **clozapine** is discontinued. The prescribing clinician and any individuals, including the patient and his or her significant others, must be aware of the possible indications of a falling WBC (fever, lethargy, bruising or other skin lesions, other flulike symptoms). A precipitous onset of agranulocytosis is potentially lethal within 24 to 72 hours and requires immediate attention. Additionally, if a clear response to **clozapine** is not evident within a few months, the medication should be discontinued.

Although risk of developing EPS, tardive dyskinesia (TD), and neuroleptic malignant syndrome (NMS) exist with any **antipsychotic,** it is significantly less with the **nonphenothiazine antipsychotics** than with the first-generation, the **phenothiazine antipsychotics.** There is a significantly reduced risk of EPS, especially with **clozapine.** Dystonias, akathisia, akinesia, dyskinesia, and drug-induced parkinsonism are relatively infrequently seen.

Other potential adverse reactions are sedation, dry mouth, urinary retention, constipation, orthostatic hypotension with concomitant tachycardia, weight gain, and sexual dysfunction.

Drug Interactions

Drug interactions with **atypical antipsychotics** can occur. Notable are those with other drugs that induce hepatic metabolism, such as **carbamazepine,** and with CNS depressants such as **alcohol.**

Smoking increases the rate of metabolism of **antipsychotics,** thereby decreasing their effect.

Combinations of **antipsychotics** may increase the risk of TD, an irreversible event, and NMS.

Table 13–30 presents drug interactions.

Table 13–30. Drug Interactions: Nonphenothiazine Antipsychotics

Drug	Interacting Drug	Possible Effect	Implications
All nonphenothiazine antipsychotics	Antihypertensives CNS depressants	Hypotension Increased CNS depression	Monitor blood pressure Warn patient about drowsiness
Clozapine	Anticholinergics	Increased anticholinergic effect	Increase fluid intake; use hard candies for dry mouth; stool softener if needed; monitor for urinary retention
	Caffeine	Increased effect of clozapine	Monitor CNS depression, WBC
	Lithium	Increased risk of neurotoxicity and agranulocytosis	Monitor lithium level, WBC, and for signs and symptoms of neurotoxicity
Quetiapine	Glucocorticoids	Decreased effect of quetiapine	Avoid concurrent use
Clozapine, quetiapine	Phenytoin	Increased toxicity of phenytoin; decreased antipsychotic effect	Monitor phenytoin blood levels and for increased psychotic symptomatology
	Erythromycin, ketoconazole, itraconazole, fluconazole	Increased effect of antipsychotics	Monitor for increasing CNS depression
Olanzapine, quetiapine	Rifampin, SSRIs	Decreased effect of antipsychotics	Monitor for increased psychotic symptomatology
Olanzapine, quetiapine, risperidone	Carbamazepine	Increased toxicity of carbamazepine	Monitor plasma levels of carbamazepine
	Dopaminergic	Antagonistic to effect of antipsychotics	Do not use if possible; increased dose may be required
Olanzapine, quetiapine, clozapine	Cimetidine	Increased effect of antipsychotics	Monitor for increasing CNS depression

Clinical Use and Dosing

Table 13–31 presents the indications, dosages, and available dosage forms of **nonphenothiazine antipsychotics.**

Rational Drug Selection

Indications for use include schizophrenia, schizoaffective disorder, depression or mania with psychotic features, and severe agitation and delusions due to dementia. It is also used to decrease self-destructive behavior that is nonsuicidal in intent. As with all antipsychotics, positive effects may occur within a few days to a few weeks to a few months.

All **antipsychotics,** whether conventional or novel, with the exception of **clozapine,** are equally effective in the treatment of the positive symptoms of psychosis, that is, hallucinations, delusions, agitation, thought disorganization, and altered perceptions. One distinguishing difference is that the atypical drugs appear to be more ef-

fective in the treatment of negative symptoms: poverty of speech and affect, lack of socialization, and psychomotor retardation.

Changing from one **antipsychotic** to another may be indicated because of the adverse effects or lack of response. Change should be accomplished by slowly titrating off the first medication and onto the second, with a washout period in between if possible. If the presence of acute psychotic symptoms makes a washout period unfeasible, overlap of the medications should be at the lowest doses and for the shortest period of time possible.

Monitoring

No specific blood tests are available to determine the plasma level of these medications. Dosages are adjusted based on subjective information provided by the patient, collateral information sources, and the clinician's objective observations of the patient.

Table 13–31. Dosage Schedule: Nonphenothiazine Antipsychotics

Drug	Indications	Dosage	Available Dosage Forms
Clozapine (Clozaril)	Refractory severe schizophrenia	Initial dose: 25–50 mg/d increasing by 25-mg increments/d until target range of 300–450 mg/d; maximum dose 900 mg/d; can give once daily or in divided doses; do not increase dose until adequate time for response has been provided, usually a few weeks Maintenance: lowest dose possible to resolve psychotic symptoms Discontinuation: taper slowly over 1–2 wk	Tablets: 25, 100 mg
Olanzapine (Zyprexa)	Psychotic disorders, severe agitation	2.5–10 mg daily in single dose; dosage adjustment should occur no less often than once weekly; 5 mg/d in debilitated patients or those with predisposition to hypotension	Tablets: 2.5, 5, 7.5, 10 mg
Risperidone (Risperdal)	Psychotic disorders, severe agitation	Initial dose: 1 mg bid; increase by 1 mg per dose until 3 mg bid is reached; most efficacious in range of 4–6 mg/d; increase in increments of 1 mg/d at no less than weekly intervals; debilitated patients should begin with 0.5 mg bid and the dose increased in 0.5 mg increments	Tablets: 1, 2, 3, 4 mg Solution: 1 mg/1 mL
Quetiapine (Seroquel)	Psychotic disorders, severe agitation	Initial dose: 25–50 mg bid with dosage increases of 25–50 mg bid–tid at intervals of 2 d or more; usual range 300–400 mg/d; do not exceed 800 mg/d	Tablets: 25, 100, 200 mg

Patient Education

Patients taking **clozapine** and their significant others or family members need to be knowledgeable about the possible signs and symptoms of agranulocytosis.

Patients also need to know to avoid hazardous situations if the drugs cause drowsiness.

Advise patients to increase their fluid intake if dry mouth or constipation occurs. Sucking on hard candies may also relieve dry mouth.

Nonopioid Analgesics and Antipyretics

This large group of **analgesics** can be divided according to whether the drug is centrally or peripherally active. Within the first category, the centrally acting, are **methotrimeprazine (Levoprome)** and **tramadol HC1 (Ultram)**. The second, larger group, those that are peripherally acting, contains the **salicylates (aspirin, Arthropan, Doan's, Dolobid)**, **acetaminophen (Tylenol)**, and the NSAIDs (**Motrin, Advil, Nuprin, Orudis, Feldene, Aleve, Naprosyn, Indocin, Clinoril, Tolectin, Meclomen, Ponstel, Lodine, Toradol, Daypro,** Duralt, Ansaid, Nalfon, Relafen, Cataflam, and Voltaren).

Pharmacodynamics

Although **methotrimeprazine** and **tramadol** are not **opioids**, their mechanism of action probably involves opioid receptor sites and is consequently probably similar to that of the **opioids**. Many precautions that apply to the **opioids** also apply to them. The reader is referred to the section on **opioid analgesics** for a review of these precautions.

The exact analgesic mechanism of action of **salicylates, acetaminophen,** and the **NSAIDs** is unclear, but it is thought that the inhibition of prostaglandin synthesis provides relief of pain and swelling. All three types of drugs exert this effect; however, **acetaminophen** is less inhibitory and therefore somewhat less effective in the relief of musculoskeletal pain.

Acetaminophen's antipyretic property is by direct action on the temperature-regulating hypothalamus; the others decrease body temperature by peripheral vasodilation and diffusion of excess heat.

One characteristic unique to the **salicylates** is prolongation of bleeding time because of inhibition of platelet aggregation.

Pharmacokinetics

Absorption and Distribution

Absorption is rapid and complete through the GI tract but less so through rectal suppository.

Methotrimeprazine has a half-life of 15 to 30 hours, tramadol 6 to 7 hours, acetaminophen 1 to 3 hours, salicylates 6 to 12 hours, and NSAIDs similar to the salicylates.

Nonopioid analgesics are relatively rapid acting, with onset of analgesia within 1 hour, peaking in 2 to 3 hours, and lasting 3 to 4 hours. With the exception of methotrimeprazine, all are administered orally or by rectal suppository.

Metabolism and Excretion

Metabolism is by conjugation and excretion through the renal system.

Table 13–32 presents the pharmacokinetics.

Pharmacotherapeutics

Precautions and Contraindications

Contraindications to the use of salicylates include children and adolescents with fever and flulike symptoms because of the risk of Reye's syndrome, as well as sensitivity, hemophilia, and hemorrhagic states. Relative contraindications to all include acute alcoholism and liver and kidney disease.

Individuals with a history of opioid abuse or dependence should use neither methotrimeprazine nor tramadol.

Table 13–32. Pharmacokinetics: Nonopioid Analgesics and Antipyretics

Drug	Onset	Peak	Duration	Half-Life	Excretion
Salicylates (aspirin, salicylic acid)	30–60 min	2–3 h	3–4 h	15–20 min (2–3 h low dose up to 20 h high dose)	Urine
Acetaminophen	30–60 min	0.5–2 h	3–4 h	1–3 h	Urine
Methotrimeprazine	15–30 min	30–90 min IM	4 h	15–30 h	Urine, feces
Tramadol HCl	Within 60 min	2–3 h	3–4 h	6–7 h	Urine
Flurbiprofen	2 d	1–2 h		2–3 h	Urine
Ibuprofen	1–2 h	1–2 h	4–6 h	1.8–2.5 h	Urine
Ketoprofen	—	0.5–2 h	—	2–4 h	Urine
Naproxen	1 h	1–4 h	Up to 7 h	12–15 h	Urine
Etodolac	0.5 h	1–2 h	4–12 h	7.3 h	Urine
Indomethacin	0.5 h	1–2 h 2–4 h SR	4–6 h	4–5 h 4.5–6 h SR	Urine
Ketorolac	10 min IM	0.5–1 h	Up to 6 h IM	2.4–8.6 h	Urine
Nabumetone	—	0.5–1 h	—	22.5–30 h	Urine
Sulindac	—	2–4 h	—	7.8—16.4 h	Urine
Tolmetin	—	0.5–1 h	—	1–1.5 h	Urine
Meclofenamate	—	0.5–1 h	—	2–3.3 h	Urine
Mefenamic acid	—	2–4 h	—	2–4 h	Urine
Piroxicam	1 h	3–5 h	48–72 h	30–86 h	Urine

SR = sustained release.

Acetaminophen can be used safely throughout pregnancy (Pregnancy Category A) and lactation, but *salicylates* (Pregnancy Category D for *aspirin* and C for *salsalate* and *magnesium salicylate*) and *NSAIDs* (Pregnancy Categories B and C) are not recommended. *Acetaminophen* syrups are available for infants and young children, as are suppositories.

Adverse Drug Reactions

Hepatotoxicity may result from exceeding the dosage guidelines of **acetaminophen.**

Both **salicylates** and **NSAIDs** prolong bleeding time, which may cause more extensive bruising than usual.

Some **NSAIDs** can prolong pregnancy if taken before the onset of labor.

Increasing age appears to increase the risk of adverse reactions to **NSAIDs.**

Salicylates and **NSAIDs** can lead to GI distress and bleeding, particularly when combined with alcohol or with long-term use.

Drug Interactions

Many drugs, such as **anticoagulants, angiotensin-converting enzyme (ACE) inhibitors, beta blockers,** and **hydantoins,** may have decreased effects when used concurrently with **NSAIDs.** The combination of **lithium** and **NSAIDs** increases the risk of **lithium** toxicity. **Cimetidine** and **probenecid** may decrease the effectiveness of the **NSAID** they are combined with. **Carbamazepine, barbiturates, hydantoins, alcohol,** and **isoniazid** may decrease the effects of **acetaminophen.**

Corticosteroids, urinary alkalizers, antacids, and **ascorbic acid** may inhibit **salicylate** action, and **salicylates** may have the same effect on **heparin, nitroglycerine, sulfonylureas, exogenous insulin,** and **valproic acid.**

Table 13–33 presents drug interactions.

Clinical Use and Dosing

Table 13–34 presents the indications and dosage schedules for **nonopioid analgesics** and **antipyretics.**

Rational Drug Selection

Methotrimeprazine and **tramadol** are indicated for the relief of moderate to severe pain, with the use of the former limited to IM injections in nonambulatory patients. **Acetaminophen, salicylates,** and **NSAIDs** are used for

Table 13–33. Drug Interactions: Nonopioid Analgesics and Antipyretics

Drug	Interacting Drug	Possible Effect	Implications
Acetaminophen	Barbiturates, carbamazepine, hydantoins, isoniazid, rifampin, sulfinpyrazone, alcohol, charcoal	Decreased effect of acetaminophen	May need higher dose; monitor for hepatotoxicity
Salicylates	Charcoal, ammonium chloride, ascorbic acid, antacids, urinary alkalinizers, carbonyl anhydrase inhibitors, corticosteroids, nizatidine	Decreased effect of salicylates	May need higher dose; monitor for salicylism
	ACE inhibitors, anticoagulants, beta blockers, loop diuretics, methotrexate, nitroglycerin, NSAIDS, probenecid, sulfinpyrazone, saronolactone, sulfonylureas, exogenous insulin, valproic acid	Decreased effect of interacting drug	Dosage adjustment may be required
NSAIDs	Anticoagulants, ACE inhibitors, beta blockers, digoxin, hydantoins, loop diuretics, penicillamine, sympathomimetics, thiazide diuretics, methotrexate, cyclosporine	Decreased effect of interacting drug	Dosage adjustment and plasma level monitoring may be required
	Cimetidine, salicylates, probenecid, dimethyl sulfoxide (DMSO)	Decreased effect of NSAID	May need higher dose
	Lithium	Increased lithium toxicity	Avoid
Methotrimeprazine, tramadol	CNS depressants	Increased CNS-depressant effect	Avoid concurrent administration

Table 13–34. Dosage Schedule: Nonopioid Analgesics and Antipyretics

Drug	Indications	Dosage
Acetaminophen (Tylenol, Feverall, Liquiprin, Acephen, Neopap, Dapa)	Mild to moderate pain, especially useful if NSAIDs or salicylates cannot be used; fever during illness such as flu in children and adolescents	Adults: PO: 325–650 mg to maximum of 4 g/d Suppository: 650 mg every 3–4 h to maximum of 6 g/d Children: PO: 10 mg/kg 4–5 times/d to maximum of 5 times/d Suppository: Age 3–11 mo: 80 mg every 6 h Age 1–3 yr: 80 mg every 4 h Age 3–6 yr: 120–125 mg every 4–6 h to maximum of 720 mg/24 h Age 6–12 years: 325 mg every 4–6 h to maximum of 2.6 g/24 h
Acetylsalicylic acid (aspirin, buffered aspirin)	Mild to moderate pain; fever; arthritis; MI prophylaxis; TIA in men	Adults and children >14 yr: 325–650 mg every 3–4 h Extra strength: 500 mg every 3 h or 600 mg every 6 h TIA: 300–1300 mg/d in divided doses MI prophylaxis: 300–325 mg/d Children <14: 10–15 mg/kg every 4 h to maximum of 60–80 mg/kg/d
Choline salicylate (Arthropan)	Arthritis	Adults and children >12: 870 mg every 3–4 h to maximum of 6 times/d
Indomethacin (Indocin)	Mild to moderate pain; fever	Adults: 25–50 mg bid–tid to maximum of 200 mg/d; SR: 75 mg once daily
Sulindac (Clinoril)	Mild to moderate pain; fever	Adults: 150–200 mg bid
Tolmetin sodium (Tolectin)	Mild to moderate pain; fever	Adults: 400 mg tid to maximum of 1800 mg/d Children >2: 15–30 mg/kg in 3–4 doses to maximum of 30 mg/kg/d
Meclofenamate sodium (Meclomen)	Mild to moderate pain; fever	Adults: 50–100 mg every 4–6 h to maximum of 400 mg/d
Mefenamic acid (Ponstel)	Mild to moderate pain; fever	Adults: 250–500 mg every 6 h to maximum of 1 wk in duration of use
Etodolac (Lodine)	Mild to moderate pain; fever	Adults: 600–1200 mg/d in divided doses to maximum of 1200 mg/d Weight 60 kg or less: maximum of 20 mg/kg
Ketorolac (Toradol)	Mild to moderate pain; fever; intended for pain management up to 5 d following IV use of ketorolac only	Adults <65: 30 mg IM every 6 h or 1-only 60 mg injection; PO 20 mg initially, followed by 10 mg every 4–6 h to maximum of 40 mg/24 h Adults >65: half above dose
Magnesium salicylate (Doan's)	Mild to moderate pain; fever; arthritis	Adults: 650 mg 4 h or 1090 mg tid to maximum of 4.8 g/d in divided doses
Diflunisal (Dolobid)	Mild to moderate pain; fever; arthritis	Adults: 1 g initially, followed by 500 mg every 8–12 h to maximum of 1.5 g/d
Ibuprofen (Motrin, Advil, Nuprin)	Mild to moderate pain; fever; arthritis	Adults: 200–400 mg every 4–6 h to maximum of 3.2 g/d Children age 6 mo to 12 yr: 5–10 mg/kg every 4–6 h to maximum of 40 mg/kg/d; take with milk or meals to avoid GI distress

SR = sustained release.

Continued on next page

Table 13–34. Dosage Schedule: Nonopioid Analgesics and Antipyretics (*continued*)

Drug	Indications	Dosage
Ketoprofen (Orudis)	Mild to moderate pain; fever; arthritis	Adults: 12.5–50 mg every 6–8 h to maximum of 300 mg/d Take with milk or meals
Piroxicam (Feldene)	Mild to moderate pain; fever; arthritis	Adults: 20 mg/d in single dose
Naproxen (Aleve, Naprosyn)	Mild to moderate pain; fever; arthritis	Adults and children >12: 500 mg initially, followed by 250 mg every 6–8 h to maximum of 1.375 g/d Controlled release: 1000 mg once/d
Oxaprozin (Daypro)	Mild to moderate pain; fever; arthritis	Adults: 1200 mg once daily; maximum 1800 m/d
Bromfenac sodium (Duract)	Mild to moderate pain; fever; arthritis	Adults: 25–50 mg every 6–8 h to maximum of 150 m/d
Flurbiprofen (Ansaid)	Mild to moderate pain; fever; arthritis	Adults: 200–300 mg/d in divided doses; maximum of 100 mg/single dose and 300 mg/d
Fenoprofen (Nalfon)	Mild to moderate pain; fever; arthritis	Adults: 200–600 mg tid–qid; take with food
Nabumetone (Relafen)	Mild to moderate pain; fever; arthritis	Adults: 1000 mg/d as single dose to maximum of 2000 mg/d
Diclofenac (Cataflam, Voltaren)	Mild to moderate pain; fever; arthritis	Adults: 50 mg tid to maximum of 225 mg/d
Methotrimeprazine (Levoprome)	Moderate to severe pain in nonambulatory patients; obstetric analgesia; pre-operative sedation	Adults: analgesia: 10–20 mg IM every 4–6 h Older and debilitated adults: initial dose of 5–10 mg Obstetric: 15–20 mg Preanesthesia: 2–20 mg 45 min-3 h before surgery; usual dose 10 mg Postoperative analgesia: 2.5–7.5 mg every 4–6 h Give deep IM; never IV or SC
Tramadol HCl (Ultram)	Moderate to moderately severe pain	Adults: 50–100 mg every 4–6 h to maximum of 400 mg/d

the relief of mild to moderate pain and the treatment of fever.

Because of their inhibition of platelet clumping, **salicylates** are also used to prevent transient ischemic attacks (TIAs) and/or stroke in at-risk males and to prevent recurrent myocardial infarction (MI) and angina in both genders. **Salicylates** have not been demonstrated to be effective in the prevention of cerebral ischemia in women.

Monitoring

Liver function tests and bleeding times may need to be performed, depending on the individual situation.

Patient Education

Advise the patient not to combine these medications with others in the same category or with the heavy use of alcohol and to contact the clinician if excessive bruising or nosebleeds occur.

Table 13–35 presents the available dosage forms.

Opioid Analgesics and Their Antagonists

With the exception of **codeine** products such as **Tylenol #3,** most of this group of drugs are **schedule II narcotics** and therefore unavailable for prescriptive purposes to NPs. They are nevertheless all discussed in this section.

Codeine is currently the only **opioid analgesic** available in NP formularies. The other **opioid analgesics** are **hydromorphone (Dilaudid), meperidine (Demerol), methadone (Dolophine), morphine sulfate, opium (paregoric, opium tincture), oxycodone (Roxicodone,**

Table 13–35. Available Dosage Forms: Nonopioid Analgesics and Antipyretics

Drug	Dosage Form	How Supplied
Acetaminophen	Tablets	160, 325, 500, 650 mg
	Chewable tablets	80 mg
	Capsules	80, 160, 500 mg
	Caplets	160 mg
	Sustained-release caplets	650 mg
	Liquid	160 mg/5 mL, 500 mg/15 mL
	Elixir	80, 120, 130, 160, 325 mg/5 mL
	Solution	100 mg/mL, 120 mg/2.5 mL
	Suspension	80 mg/10.8 mL, 160 mg/5 mL
	Suppository	80, 120, 125, 300, 325, 650 mg
Acetylsalicylic acid	Tablets	325, 500 mg
	Enteric-coated tablets	81, 165, 325, 500, 625, 975 mg
	Sustained-release tablets	650, 800 mg
	Chewable tablets	81 mg
	Buffered tablets	325, 500 mg
	Suppository	120, 200, 300, 600 mg
	Gum	227.5 mg
Choline salicylate	Liquid	870 mg/5 mL
Indomethacin	Capsules	25, 50 mg
	Sustained-released capsules	75 mg
	Suspension	25 mg/5 mL
	Suppository	125 mg
Sulindac	Tablets	150, 200 mg
Tolmetin sodium	Tablets	200, 600 mg
	Capsules	400 mg
Meclofenamate sodium	Capsules	50, 100 mg
Mefenamic acid	Capsules	250 mg
Etodolac	Tablets	400 mg
	Capsules	200, 300 mg
Ketorolac	Tablets	10 mg
	Injection	15, 30 mg/mL
Magnesium salicylate	Tablets	325, 467, 500, 545, 580, 600 mg
Diflunisal	Tablets	250, 500 mg
Ibuprofen	Tablets	100, 200, 30, 400, 600, 800 mg
	Chewable tablets	50, 100 mg
	Suspension	100 mg/5 mL
	Oral drops	40 mg/mL
Ketoprofen	Tablets	12.5 mg
	Capsules	25, 50, 75 mg
	Sustained-released capsules	100, 150, 200 mg
Piroxicam	Capsules	10, 20 mg
Naproxen	Tablets	200, 250, 375, 500 mg
	Sustained-released tablets	375, 500 mg
	Suspension	125 mg/5 mL

Continued on next page

Table 13–35. Available Dosage Forms: Nonopioid Analgesics and Antipyretics (*continued*)

Drug	Dosage Form	How Supplied
Oxaprozin	Tablets	600 mg
Bromfenac sodium	Capsules	25 mg
Flurbiprofen	Tablets	50, 100 mg
Fenoprofen	Tablets Capsules	600 mg 200, 300 mg
Nabumetone	Tablets	500, 750 mg
Diclofenac	Tablets Sustained-release enteric-coated tablets	50, 100 mg 25, 50, 75 mg
Methotrimeprazine HCl	Injection	20 mg/mL
Tramadol HCl	Tablets	50 mg

OxyContin, Roxicodone Intensol), oxymorphone HCl (Numorphan), propoxyphene HCl (Darvon, Dolene), propoxyphene napsylate (Darvon-N), fentanyl (Sublimaze, Duragesic), levorphanol tartrate (Levo-Dromoran), sufentanil citrate (Sufenta), dezocine (Dalgan), pentazocine (Talwin), butorphanol tartrate (Stadol), nalbuphine HCl (Nubain), and buprenorphine HCl (Buprenex).

Fentanyl HCl (Alfenta) and fentanyl transmucosal system (Fentanyl Oralet) are used in hospital settings for anesthetic induction or maintenance only, and levomethadyl acetate HCl (Orlaam) is used only in the management of opiate dependence.

Pharmacodynamics

Narcotic analgesics are active at various opioid receptor sites and act as agonists, partial agonists, or mixed agonist-antagonists. Their action provides analgesia and causes euphoria, hypotension, and respiratory depression. Some are natural opium alkaloids, some synthetic, and some a combination of the two. Mixed agonist-antagonists can cause withdrawal symptoms when given to narcotic-dependent individuals because of their preference at specific opioid receptor sites.

Although not entirely understood, narcotic antagonists block or reverse opioids by competing at their receptor sites and reverse respiratory depression, hypotension, and sedation. Indications for use are accidental narcotic overdose and prolonged surgical use of narcotics.

Pharmacokinetics

Absorption and Distribution

Opioid analgesics are administered orally or parenterally, and their rate of absorption depends on the route used.

Onset of action is rapid and varies from 2 or 3 minutes up to 60 minutes, depending on whether the route of administration is IV, SC, IM, or oral. Half-life is generally up to 6 hours, although levorphanol's is 12 to 16 hours and methadone's is 15 to 30 hours. Meperidine has an active metabolite, normeperidine, whose half-life is 15 to 30 hours.

Nalmefene HCl (Revex), naloxone HCl (Narcan), and naltrexone HCl (ReVia) are indicated for acute crises and are given parenterally. Their onset of action is within 2 to 15 minutes, with duration of action 1 to 4 hours. Because their half-lives can be shorter than the narcotic they are reversing, patients must be closely monitored for symptoms of a recurrence of depression.

Metabolism and Excretion

Opioid analgesics and antagonists are metabolized in the liver and excreted in urine.

Table 13–36 presents the pharmacokinetics.

Pharmacotherapeutics

Precautions and Contraindications

Because of the respiratory depressant effect of these drugs, compromised pulmonary function is a contraindication. Cautious use is indicated in the case of head injury, increased intracranial pressure, and acute abdominal conditions because of the drugs' capacity to mask symptoms and to increase cerebrospinal fluid pressure.

Safety of use in pregnant and nursing women is not established, and they are classified in Pregnancy Category C. Infants born to addicted mothers suffer sedation, respiratory depression, and withdrawal.

Oxycodone, propoxyphene, methadone, oxymor-

Table 13–36. Pharmacokinetics: Opioid Analgesics and Antagonists

Drug	Onset	Peak	Duration	Half-Life	Excretion
Alfentanil	Immediate	—	—	1–2 h	Urine
Codeine	10–30 min	0.5–1 h	4–6 h	3 h	Urine
Fentanyl IM transdermal	7–15 min 6 h	20–30 min 12–24 h	1–2 h 72 h	1.5–6 h	Urine
Hydromorphone	15–30 min	0.5–1 h	4–5 h	2–3 h	Urine
Levorphanol	30–90 min	0.5–1 h	6–8 h	1–16 h	Urine
Meperidine	10–45 min	0.5–1 h	2–4 h	3–4 h	Urine
Methadone	30–60 min	0.5–1 h	4–6 h	15–30 h	Urine
Morphine	15–60 min	0.5–1 h	3–7 h	1.5–2 h	Urine
Oxycodone	15–30 min	1 h	4–6 h	—	Urine
Oxymorphone	5–10 min	0.5–1 h	3–6 h	—	Urine
Propoxyphene	30–60 min	2–2.5 h	4–6 h	6–12 h	Urine
Sufentanil	1.3–3 min	—	—	2.5 h	Urine
Nalmefene	5–15 min	1.5–2.3 h	—	1–10.8 h	Urine
Naloxone	2 min	—	1–4 h	30–81 min	Urine
Naltrexone	Rapid	Within 1 h	—	4–13 h	Urine
Buprenorphine	15 min	60 min	6 h	2.2–3.5 h	Urine
Butorphanol	<10 min	30–60 min	3–4 h	2.5–4 h	Urine
Dezocine	<15–30 min	30–150 min	2–4 h	2–4 h	Urine
Nalbuphine	15–30 min	30–60 min	3–6 h	5 h	Urine
Pentazocine	15–30 min	15–60 min	3 h	2.2–3.5 h	Urine

phone, and **hydromorphone** should not be used in children.

Narcotic analgesics carry the risk of physical tolerance and dependence, as well as having street value, so that the prescribing clinician needs to obtain a clear history and knowledge of current substance use, because of both cross-tolerance and the possibility of additive CNS depression. Some have been implicated in suicide or accidental death, particularly in combination with **alcohol.** Additionally, as indicated previously, **mixed agonist-antagonists** should not be prescribed for narcotic-addicted individuals because of the risk of physical withdrawal. Patients wishing treatment of narcotic addiction with **methadone** should be referred to an appropriate treatment facility.

Naltrexone is particularly hepatotoxic and can be injurious to the liver when used in high doses. Individuals with impaired liver function should be assessed carefully for signs of further damage.

Careful titration of antagonists' dose is required because the blockade of opioids by antagonistic action means the individual may experience withdrawal symptoms, called *acute abstinence syndrome,* at about the time the next **narcotic** dose is due. Achieving a balance between reversing depression and preventing acute withdrawal is delicate and necessitates careful titration in small increments. This situation applies equally to the drug-affected neonate.

In addition to these concerns, attention is also needed in postoperative situations in which the antagonist's action may leave the patient in acute, severe pain.

Adverse Drug Reactions

Common adverse reactions can include sedation, nausea, vomiting, dizziness, euphoria, lethargy, uncoordinated movements, agitation, depression of cough reflex, and paresthesias.

Adverse reactions to antagonists may include nausea and vomiting, tachycardia, hypertension, fever, and dizziness.

Drug Interactions

Some interacting drugs, such as **alcohol, hypnotics, barbiturates,** and **antipsychotics,** can create additive CNS-depressant effects. Others, such **as cimetidine, hydantoins, nicotine,** and **droperidol,** can interfere with narcotic effects. Other drug interactions, for example with **carbamazepine, warfarin,** and **MAOIs,** may decrease the effect of the interacting drug.

Table 13–37 presents drug interactions.

Clinical Use and Dosing

Table 13–38 presents the indications and dosage schedules of **opioid analgesics** and **antagonists.**

Rational Drug Selection

Indications for the use of **opioid analgesics** are the control of pain, primarily acute as in the case of postoperative and obstetric pain; however, **fentanyl** is available in a transdermal patch for the treatment of severe chronic pain requiring a narcotic. Another indication is preoperative sedation for the facilitation of anesthesia.

Monitoring

No specific monitoring is required other than that already discussed.

Patient Education

Patients should be warned about the potential for physical dependence and, while using the amount necessary to adequately provide the desired effect, should be encouraged, when possible, to switch to an analgesic that does not cause dependence.

Opioid analgesics may cause drowsiness and, for safety reasons, should not be used when mental or physical alertness is required.

Table 13–39 presents available dosage forms.

Phenothiazines

Phenothiazines were the first class of **psychotropic medications,** beginning with **chlorpromazine (Thorazine),** that were found to be effective in the treatment of the positive symptoms (hallucinations and delusions) of schizophrenia. They have been widely used since 1954, but, since the advent of newer nonconventional **antipsychotics** such as **risperidone** and **olanzapine,** which are discussed in a different section of this chapter, they are now being prescribed less frequently because of their risk of serious adverse effects.

The **phenothiazine group,** in addition to **chlorpromazine,** includes **promazine (Sparine), thioridazine (Mellaril), fluphenazine (Prolixin), perphenazine (Trilafon), prochlorperazine (Compazine), promethazine (Phenergan),** and **trifluoperazine (Stelazine).** Although not chemically members of this group, **haloperidol (Haldol)** and **thiothixene (Navane)** are considered conventional **antipsychotics** and are included in this discussion.

Pharmacodynamics

The positive symptoms of schizophrenia include hallucinations, delusional thinking, and agitation, which are thought to be the result of an imbalance in the ratio of dopamine and acetylcholine in nerve terminals. Excessive amounts of dopamine lead to these symptoms, and inadequate levels lead to parkinsonism. **Phenothiazines** attempt to correct this imbalance by decreasing the amount of available dopamine.

Less clear is the etiology of negative symptoms of schizophrenia (lack of affect, interpersonal relationships,

Table 13–37. Drug Interactions: Opioid Analgesics and Antagonists

Drug	Interacting Drug	Possible Effect	Implications
Opioids	CNS depressants, alcohol, hypnotics, barbiturates, benzodiazepines, antipsychotics	Additive CNS depression	
	Cimetidine, hydantoins, rifampin, droperidol, charcoal, nicotine	Decreased effect of opioid	Increased doses of opioid may be required
	Carbamazepine, warfarin, MAOIs, furazolidone, nitrous oxide	Decreased effect of interacting drug	Monitor blood levels when possible
Nalmefene	Flumazenil	Seizures	Use with caution
Naltrexone	Thioridazine	Decreased effect of thioridazine	Higher dose may be required

Table 13–38. Dosage Schedule: Opioid Analgesics and Antagonists

Drug	Indications	Dosage
Alfentanil HCl (Alfenta)	Anesthetic adjunct only	—
Codeine	Mild to moderate pain; coughing	Adult: PO, IM, IV, SC: 15–60 mg every 4 h to maximum of 360 mg/24 h; usual dose is 30 mg Children >1 yr: PO, IM, SC: 0.5 mg/kg every 4–6 h
Fentanyl (Sublimaze, Duragesic, Oralet)	Anesthesia; postoperative analgesia; management of chronic pain	Adults: Postoperative analgesia: 0.05–0.1 mg IM every 1–2 h Transdermal: 25, 50, 75, 100, 125, 150, 175, 200, 225, 250, 275, and 300 µg/h system; change once every 72 h Titrate dose upward first time only in 3 d, thereafter at 6-d intervals
Hydromorphone HCl (Dilaudid, HydroStat IR)	Moderate to severe pain	Adults: PO: 2–4 mg every 4–6 h Parenteral: 1–4 mg every 4–6 h; slow IV over 1–5 min Rectal: 3 mg every 6–8 h
Levorphanol tartrate (Levo-Dromoran)	Management of opioid dependence	Adults: PO, SC: 2–3 mg
Meperidine (Demerol)	Moderate to severe pain; preoperative sedation	Adults: PO, IM, SC: 50–150 mg every 3–4 h Children: PO, IM, SC: 1–1.8 mg/kg (0.5–0.8 mg/lb) every 3–4 h
Methadone (Dolophine)	Severe pain; management of opioid dependence	Adults: PO, IM, SC: 2.5–10 mg every 3–4 h; oral dose is half of parenteral
Morphine sulfate (Astramorph PF, Duramorph, Infumorph, MSIR, MS Contin, Oramorph SR, Roxanol, OMS concentrate, MS/L, RMS)	Moderate to severe acute and chronic pain; pre-anesthetic sedation	Adults: PO: 10–30 mg every 4 h Controlled release: 30 mg every 8 h; do not crush or chew SC/IM: 5–20 mg/70 kg every 4 h IV: 2.5–15 mg/70 kg in 4–5 mL water for injection over 4–5 min Continuous IV pump infusion: 0.1–1 mg/mL in 5% dextrose Rectal: 10–20 mg every 4 h Children: SC, IM: 0.1–0.2 mg/kg to maximum of 15 mg every 4 h
Oxycodone (Roxicodone, OxyContin)	Moderate to moderately severe pain	Adults: 5 mg or 5 mL every 6 h
Oxymorphone (Numorphan)	Moderate to severe pain; preanesthetic sedation; relief of anxiety/dyspnea in pulmonary edema and left ventricular failure	Adults: SC, IM: 1–1.5 mg every 4–6 h IV: 0.5 mg Rectal: 5 mg every 4–6 h
Propoxyphene HCl (Darvon)	Mild to moderate pain	Adults: 65 mg every 4 h to maximum of 390 mg/d
Propoxyphene napsylate (Darvon-N)	Mild to moderate pain	Adults: 100 mg every 4 h to maximum of 600 mg/d
Buprenorphine (Buprenex)	Moderate to severe pain	Adults and children >13: IM, IV: 0.3 mg every 6 h; may repeat once 30–60 min later if needed; compatible with most IV solutions

Continued on next page

Table 13–38. Dosage Schedule: Opioid Analgesics and Antagonists (*continued*)

Drug	Indications	Dosage
Butorphanol tartrate (Stadol)	Pain; preanesthesia sedation	Adults: IM: 1–4 mg every 3–4 h to nonambulatory patients IV: 0.5–2 mg every 3–4 h Nasal: 1 mg = 1 spray in each nostril; may repeat if needed in 60–90 min; may repeat 2 dose sequences in 3–4 h
Dezocine (Dalgan)	Pain management	Adults: IM: 5–20 mg every 3–6 h; usual dose 10 mg IV: 2.5–10 mg every 2–4 h; usual dose 5 mg
Nalbuphine (Nubain)	Moderate to severe pain; preoperative sedation	Adults: SC, IM, IV: 10 mg/70 kg every 3–6 h to maximum of 20 mg/dose or 160 mg/24 h
Pentazocine (Talwin, Talwin NX)	Moderate to severe pain; preoperative sedation	Adults: PO: 50–100 mg every 3–4 h to maximum of 600 mg/24 h; initial dose 50 mg IM, SC, IV: 30 mg every 3–4 h to maximum of 360 mg/24 h
Pentazocine combinations	Mild to moderate pain	Adults: 12.5 mg with 325 ASA (Talwin compound caplets): 2 tabs tid–qid 25 mg with acetaminophen 650 mg (Talacen caplets): 1 tab every 4 h to maximum of 6 tabs/24 h
Nalmefene (Revex)	Reversal of opioid effects	Opioid-dependent patients: Initial challenge dose of 0.1 mg/70 kg. If no signs or symptoms of withdrawal within 2 min, use following guidelines: Non-opioid-dependent patients: Initial dose of 0.25 μg/kg followed by 0.25 μg/kg doses at 2–5 min intervals until degree of opioid reversal is attained Give IV; if no IV access is available, give 1 mg SC or IM as single dose
Naloxone (Narcan)	Reversal of opioid depression	Adults: IV, IM, SC For overdose: 0.4–2 mg IV; may repeat at 2- to 3-min intervals Postoperative: 0.1–0.2 mg IV at 2- to 3-min intervals; may repeat in 1- to 2-h intervals if needed Children: For overdose: 0.01 mg/kg IV; may follow with 0.1 mg if needed; if no IV access, give IM or SC in divided doses Postoperative: initial dose of 0.005–0.01 mg IV repeated at 2- to 3-min increments if needed
Naltrexone (ReVia)	Blocks effects of opioids; treatment of alcohol dependence	Alcoholism: 100 mg PO once daily Opioid dependence: do not give until patient has been abstinent for 10 d, then give challenge dose of 25 mg once; if no withdrawal signs and symptoms occur, continue with maintenance dose; if signs and symptoms occur, repeat challenge in 24 h Maintenance: 50 mg every 24 h; dosing may be flexible (e.g., 100 mg on Mon and Wed; 150 mg on Fri)

Table 13–39. Available Dosage Forms: Opioid Analgesics and Antagonists

Drug	Dosage Form	How Supplied
Codeine	Tablets Injection	15, 30, 60 mg 30, 60 mg
Fentanyl	Injection Transdermal patch	0.05 mg/mL 25, 50, 75, 100 µg/h
Hydromorphone HCl	Tablets Injection Suppository Oral liquid	1, 2, 3, 4, 8 mg 1, 2, 3, 4, 10 mg/mL 3 mg 5 mg/mL
Levorphanol tartrate	Tablets Injection	2 mg 2 mg/mL
Meperidine	Tablets Injection Syrup	50, 100 mg 10, 50, 100 mg/mL; 25, 50, 75 mg/dose for injection 50 mg/5 mL
Methadone	Tablets Injection Dispersible tablets Solution Concentrate	5, 10 mg 10 mg/mL 40 mg 5, 10 mg/5 mL, 10 mg/10 mL 10 mg/mL
Morphine sulfate	Tablets Controlled-release tablets Soluble tablets Injection Solution Suppository	15, 30 mg 15, 30, 60, 100, 200 mg 10, 15, 30 mg 0.5, 1, 2, 3, 4, 5, 8, 10, 15, 25, 50 mg/mL 10, 20, 100 mg/5 mL; 10 mg/2.5 mL,; 20 mg/mL 5, 10, 20, 30 mg
Oxycodone	Tablets Controlled-release tablets Solution Concentrate	5 mg 10, 20, 40 mg 5 mg/5 mL 20 mg/mL
Oxymorphone	Injection Suppository	1, 1.5 mg/mL 5 mg
Propoxyphene HCl	Capsules	32, 65 mg
Propoxyphene napsylate	Tablets	100 mg
Buprenorphine	Injection	0.324 mg/mL
Butorphanol tartrate	Injection Nasal spray	1, 2 mg/mL 10 mg/mL
Dezocine	Injection	5, 10, 15 mg/mL
Nalbuphine	Injection	10, 20 mg/mL
Pentazocine	Tablets Injection	50 mg; 50 mg with 0.5 mg naloxone 10, 20 mg/mL
Pentazocine combinations	Tablets	12.5 mg with 325 mg ASA, 25 mg with 650 mg acetaminophen
Nalmefene	Injection	1 mg/mL
Naloxone HCl	Injection	0.4, 1 mg/mL; 0.02 mg/mL neonatal
Naltrexone HCl	Tablets	50 mg

motivation), and treatment with antipsychotics is frequently less successful than it is of positive symptoms.

Pharmacokinetics

Absorption and Distribution

Phenothiazines are usually administered orally, although parenteral versions of **haloperidol** and **fluphenazine** are available. The drugs are absorbed rapidly and distributed widely to adipose tissue. Peak action of oral **phenothiazines** is within 1 hour; IM injections begin action within 10 or 15 minutes.

Metabolism and Excretion

Phenothiazines are metabolized in the liver and excreted in the urine. Their half-life is 10 to 30 hours. Because of their lipid solubility, several weeks may be required before their benefits become evident.

Table 13–40 presents the pharmacokinetics.

Pharmacotherapeutics

Precautions and Contraindications

Treatment of psychotic symptoms is an attempt to correct the chemical imbalance between dopamine and acetylcholine by decreasing the effect of dopamine without causing parkinsonism. Also, because there is an inverse relationship between dopamine and acetylcholine, attempts to correct the imbalance by decreasing dopamine also run the risk of increasing acetylcholine action and producing an additional, different set of adverse effects.

Phenothiazines are grouped according to whether they are high- or low-potency compared with the standard dose of 100 mg of **chlorpromazine**. High-potency drugs like **haloperidol** and **fluphenazine** carry an increased risk of causing parkinsonism-like and various movement-related EPS, whereas low-potency drugs carry less risk of EPS but more risk of anticholinergic adverse reactions. Treatment of psychosis with **phenothiazines, haloperidol,** and **thiothixene,** therefore, involves an attempt to reduce or eliminate the psychotic symptoms while balancing the various possible adverse reactions.

Adverse Drug Reactions

Safety of *phenothiazine* use during pregnancy and lactation has not been established; therefore, they should be avoided if possible. They are classified under Pregnancy Category C.

The only absolute contraindication is hypersensitivity.

Anticholinergic effects include dry mouth, blurred vision, sedation, urinary retention, constipation, tachycardia, orthostatic hypotension, and weight gain. EPSs are more serious and can include dystonias, dyskinesias, akathisia, akinesia, drug-induced parkinsonism, TD, and NMS.

As indicated in the earlier discussion of **dopaminergics,** NMS, although rare, is a potentially life-threatening event that requires an immediate response. The hall-

Table 13–40. Pharmacokinetics: Phenothiazines

Drug	Onset	Peak	Duration	Half-Life	Excretion
Chlorpromazine HCl	Erratic	2–4 h	Up to 6 mo	10–30 h	Urine
Fluphenazine decanoate	1 h; 1–3 d	2–4 h; 2–3 d	6–8 h; up to 4 wk	6.8–14.3 d	Urine
Perphenazine	Erratic	2–4 h	6 h	12–24 h	Urine
Promazine HCl	—	2–4 h	4–6 h	—	Urine
Trifluoperazine	Erratic	2–4 h	4–6 h	13 h	Urine and feces equally
Thioridazine HCl	Erratic	2–4 h	4–6 h	24–36 h	Urine
Thiothixene	Slow	2–8 h	Up to 12 h	34 h	Urine
Loxapine	20–30 min	2–4 h	12 h	5–19 h	Urine
Pimozide	—	6–8 h	—	55 h	Urine
Haloperidol decanoate	Erratic	3–5 h; 4–11 d	Up to 3 wk	12–36 h; 3 wk	Urine, bile
Molindone HCl	Erratic	1.5 h	24–36 h	10–20 h	Urine and feces equally

mark of NMS is hyperthermia, the sequelae of which represent the threat to life. All patients on **antipsychotics** should be monitored for significant temperature increases and routinely assessed for early signs of parkinsonism: body and facial rigidity, stiff movements, and tremor.

TD is an irreversible adverse effect frequently associated with young men and with women over age 70 who are taking high-potency antipsychotics. The abnormal movements indicative of TD are involuntary and are primarily confined to the face and hands. They consist of movements like repeated tongue rolling, pill-rolling movements of the hands, and thrusting, ticklike movements of the face. They are not present during sleep.

Motor function of individuals taking **antipsychotics** should be routinely assessed with the use of the Abnormal Involuntary Movement Scale (AIMS), which rates various movements such as joint rigidity and balance on a numerical scale, thereby enabling the clinician, over time, to detect changes that represent early EPSs. Table 13–41 presents an AIMS checklist the NP may use to evaluate patients.

Drug Interactions

Drug interactions are many and varied, the most serious effect of which is CNS depression. Use of **phenothiazines** in combination with **CNS depressants** should be avoided.

Other interactions involve a decreased effect of the **antipsychotic** or the interacting drug. **Lithium** in combination with a **phenothiazine** increases the risk of neurotoxicity and EPSs.

Table 13–42 presents drug interactions.

Clinical Use and Dosing

Table 13–43 presents the indications and dosage schedules of phenothiazines.

Rational Drug Selection

Usually EPSs can be decreased or eliminated by the addition of drugs such as **benztropine (Cogentin), diphenhydramine (Benadryl), trihexyphenidyl (Artane), atenolol (Tenormin),** or **amantadine (Symmetrel)**. A decrease in the dose or a change to a different type of **antipsychotic** may also counter these effects. Anticholinergic effects can be addressed by nonpharmacological measures such as increased fluid intake and dietary bulk.

The depot form is used if compliance is an issue, whether the patient is an inpatient or an outpatient. It is usually administered every 2 to 4 weeks. IM injections of **prochlorperazine** and **promethazine** are commonly used in inpatient settings, particularly surgical, to provide relief from nausea and vomiting; IM **chlorpromazine** is frequently used when rapid sedation is required.

Monitoring

Plasma levels of hydantoins, lithium, and blood glucose of diabetic patients on **hyperglycemic agents** should be monitored at regular intervals.

Patient Education

Anticipate the need for refills so that required appointments can be arranged before the patient runs out of medications.

Advise patients to tell their clinician of any signs or symptoms indicative of EPS, TD, or NMS.

Table 13–41. Abnormal Involuntary Movement Scale (AIMS) Checklist

Instructions: Rate on a scale from 1 to 5, with 1 being none and 5 being severe. Rate at each appointment initially, then decrease frequency unless patient is a male under age 25 or a female over age 70.

Abnormal Involuntary Movement	Scale	Notes
Holding arms outstretched to sides		
Arms outstretched to front with hands flat and parallel		
Walking in a straight line		
Fluidity of shoulder and elbow joints		
Touching each finger with thumb of both hands		
Sticking tongue out straight		
Rolling head laterally, front and back		

Table 13–42. Drug Interactions: Phenothiazines

Drug	Interacting Drug	Possible Effect	Implications
All phenothiazines	Alcohol, antihistamines, barbiturates, hypnotics, narcotics, benzodiazepines	CNS depression	Avoid; monitor for adverse reactions
	Lithium	Increased risk of neuro-toxicity and EPS	Monitor lithium levels and signs and symptoms of toxicity
	Lithium, antacids, cimetidine	Decreased antipsychotic effect	May require increased antipsychotic dose
	Anticholinergics	Increased anticholinergic effect; increased risk of hyperthermia	Monitor temperature
	Beta blockers	Increased effect of both drugs	Monitor for adverse reactions
	Dopaminergics	Antagonize antipsychotic effect	Avoid concurrent use
	Hypoglycemics	Decreased diabetic control	Monitor blood glucose closely
	Phenytoin	Increased toxicity of phenytoin	Monitor blood level of phenytoin; lower dose of antipsychotic may be needed
	Trazodone	Increased hypotension	Monitor postural hypotension; warn patient to change position slowly
	Diazoxide	Hyperglycemia	Monitor blood glucose
	TCAs	Increased sedation, risk of seizures, anti-cholinergic effect, serum levels of TCA, risk of arrhythmias	Use SSRI

The patient and family members should be informed of any signs or symptoms of decreased effectiveness of the **antipsychotic** and should be helped to understand the chronicity of the patient's disorder, if applicable.

Table 13–44 presents available dosage forms.

Selective Serotonin Reuptake Inhibitors

The following discussion of **SSRIs**, which include **flu-oxetine (Prozac)**, **sertraline (Zoloft)**, **paroxetine (Paxil)**, and **fluvoxamine (Luvox)**, also covers **bupro-pion (Wellbutrin)**, **venlafaxine (Effexor)**, **nefazodone (Serzone)**, **trazodone (Desyrel)**, **citalopram (Celexa)**, and **mirtazapine (Remeron)**. Even though the latter five are not strictly in the **SSRI** category, all these **anti-depressants** are relatively recently available pharmaco-

logical agents and appear to be outstripping the demand for the older **TCAs** by both patients and clinicians.

Pharmacodynamics

These drugs all affect neurotransmitters in the synaptic cleft by preventing presynaptic transmitter reuptake, by blockade of postsynaptive receptors, or both.

Pharmacokinetics

Absorption and Distribution

All are given orally and are thoroughly absorbed. Peak plasma levels vary, ranging from 1 to 8 hours, and have a positive correlation with duration of half-life.

Table 13–43. Dosage Schedule: Phenothiazines

Drug	Indications	Dosage
Chlorpromazine HCL (Thorazine)	Psychosis; acute severe agitation	Adults: PO: 25 mg tid to maximum of 40 mg/d IM: 25 mg initially; may repeat with 25–50 mg in 1 h; maximum 400 mg IM every 4–6 h; substitute with oral as soon as possible; give concentrate with 60 mL or more of diluent Children: PO: 0.5 mg/kg every 4–6 h as needed Rectal: 1 mg/kg every 6–8 h as needed IM: 0.5 mg/kg every 6–8 h as needed
Fluphenazine (Prolixin)	Psychosis; acute severe agitation	Adults: PO: 0.5–10 mg/d in divided doses at 6- to 8-h intervals IM: 5 mg every 6 h to maximum of 30 mg/d Older adults: PO 1–2.5 mg/d; IM one-third to one-half oral dose starting with 1.25 mg Decanoate: 12.5–25 mg deep IM every 1–3 wk
Perphenazine (Trilafon)	Psychosis; acute severe agitation	Adults: 8–16 mg 2–4 times daily to maximum of 64 mg/d Older adults: one-third to one-half adult dose Children >12: lowest adult dose possible
Promazine (Sparine)	Psychosis; acute severe agitation	Adults: 10–200 mg every 4–6 h; maximum dose of 1000 mg/d IM: 50–150 mg; may repeat up to 300 mg total Children >12: 10–5 mg every 4–6 h
Trifluoperazine (Stelazine)	Psychosis; acute severe agitation	Adults: 15–20 mg/d in divided doses to maximum of 40 mg/d IM: 1–2 mg every 4–6 h as needed Older adults: low end of adult dose Children >6 yr: 1 mg 1–2 times daily; adjust according to weight
Thioridazine (Mellaril)	Psychosis; acute severe agitation	Adults: 50–100 mg tid to maximum of 800 mg/d Children >2 yr: 0.5 to maximum of 3 mg/kg/d
Thiothixene (Navane)	Psychosis; acute severe agitation	Adults: 6–60 mg/d in divided doses; maximum 60 mg/d IM: 16–20 mg 2–4 times/d to maximum of 30 mg/d
Loxapine (Loxitane)	Psychosis; acute severe agitation	Adults and children >15: 10 mg bid initially; may increase rapidly to maintenance of 20–60 mg/d IM: 12.5–50 mg every 4–6 h until desired response; then start oral
Pimozide (Orap)	Psychosis; acute severe agitation	Adults and children over age 12: 30 mg/d in divided doses; range 20–60 mg/d Older adults: 10–15 mg/d in divided doses or single hs dose
Haloperidol (Haldol)	Psychosis; acute severe agitation	Adults: 0.5–5 mg 2–3 times daily to maximum of 100 mg/d IM: 2–5 mg; may repeat after 60 min; substitute with oral as soon as feasible. First oral dose should be administered 12–24 h following last IM dose Decanoate: deep IM every 4 wk; initial dose 10–15 times oral dose; not to exceed 100 mg Older adults: lower doses and slower titration Children: 0.05–15 mg/kg/d; may give in divided doses
Molindone HCl (Moban)	Psychosis; acute severe agitation	Adults and children over age 12: 50–75 mg/d to maximum of 225 mg/d Maintenance of nonsevere case: 5–15 mg 3–4 times daily

Table 13–44. Available Dosage Forms: Phenothiazines

Drug	Dosage Form	How Supplied
Chlorpromazine	Tablets	10, 15, 25, 50, 100, 150, 200 mg
	Concentrate	30, 100 mg/mL
Fluphenazine	Tablets	1, 2.5, 5, 10 mg
	Elixir	2.5 mg/5 mL
	Concentrate	5 mg/mL
	Injection	2.5 mg/mL
	Decanoate/ethanoate (SC)	25 mg/mL
Perphenazine	Tablets	2, 4, 8, 16 mg
	Concentrate	16 mg/5 mL
	Injection	5 mg/mL
Promazine HCl	Tablets	25, 50, 100 mg
	Injection	25, 50 mg/mL
Trifluoperazine	Tablets	1, 2, 5, 10 mg
	Concentrate	10 mg/mL
	Injection	2 mg/mL
Thioridazine	Tablets	10, 15, 25, 50, 100, 150, 200 mg
	Suspension	25, 100 mg/5 mL
	Concentrate	30, 100 mg/mL
Thiothixene	Capsules	1, 2, 5, 10, 20 mg
	Concentrate	5 mg/mL
	Injection	2 mg/mL
Loxapine succinate/HCl	Capsules	5, 10, 25, 50 mg
	Concentrate	25 mg/mL
	Injection	50 mg/mL
Pimozide	Tablets	2 mg
Haloperidol	Tablets	0.5, 1, 2, 5, 10, 20 mg
	Concentrate	2 mg/mL
	Decanoate	5, 50, 100 mg/mL
Molindone HCl	Tablets	5, 10, 25, 50, 100 mg
	Concentrate	20 mg/mL

Metabolism and Excretion

They are metabolized in the liver and excreted primarily through the urinary tract.

Table 13–45 presents the pharmacokinetics.

Pharmacotherapeutics

Precautions and Contraindications

Contraindications to use are limited to hypersensitivity to any of the drugs and concurrent or within 14 days of the administration of an **MAOI.** The latter restriction is due to the high risk of hypertensive crisis.

Because **bupropion** lowers the seizure threshold, it carries an additional contraindication for individuals with seizure disorder, a history of it, or factors predisposing to a seizure disorder, such as head trauma, tumor, bulimia, or concurrent use of another drug that lowers the seizure threshold.

The risk of seizure with **bupropion** is dose-related as well; therefore, maximums exist beyond which the risk significantly increases: a maximum of 150 mg per dose and 450 mg total dose per day. With adequate knowledge of medical history and careful dose titration, the risk of seizure is minimal.

Adverse Drug Reactions

Adverse reactions to this group of drugs depend on which receptors are affected but are usually relatively minor and transient. They can include nausea and vomiting,

Table 13–45. Pharmacokinetics: Selective Serotonin Reuptake Inhibitors (SSRIs)

Drug	Time to Reach Steady State	Peak	Duration	Half-Life	Excretion
Desaryl	3–7 d	1–2 h	Long-acting	4–9 h	Urine, feces
Fluoxetine HCl	2–4 wk	6–8 h	Long-acting	2–9 d	Urine
Fluvoxamine maleate	7 d	3–8 h	Long-acting	16 h	Urine
Nefazodone HCl	4–5 d	1 h	Long-acting	2–4 h	Urine, feces
Mirtazapine	5 d	12 h	Long-acting	61 h	Urine, feces
Bupropion HCl	1.5–5 d	2 h	Long-acting	8–24 h	Urine
Paroxetine HCl	10–14 d	5.2 h	Long-acting	10–24 h	Urine
Sertraline HCl	7 d	4.5–8 h	Long-acting	1–4 h	Urine
Venlafaxine	3–4 d	1–3 h	Long-acting	5–11 h	Urine
Citalopram	7 d	4 h	Long-acting	35 h	Urine

diarrhea, headache, light-headedness, sedation, weight gain or loss, and exacerbation of anxiety and agitation.

Although rare, priapism is possible for men taking **trazodone,** and they should be cautioned to discontinue the medication and seek medical attention should this occur.

Another adverse event of note is that patients with bipolar disorder being treated with an **antidepressant** in the absence of a mood stabilizer face an increased risk of precipitation of mania or hypomania or of a rapid cycling of their illness. The risk is particularly present with **fluoxetine** and **bupropion** because these drugs tend to be more activating than other **antidepressants.**

A third significant concern is serotonin syndrome, which occurs in the presence of excessive serotonergic activity. Therefore, maximum recommended doses must be adhered to, combinations of **serotonergic agents** with other **serotonergic agents** must be avoided, and adequate time for titration when changing from one **serotonergic antidepressant** to another must be provided. A safe rule of thumb when making such a change is to allow five half-lives per dose decrease, so that titrating off a 20-mg dose of **fluoxetine** would need 5 days at 10 mg before starting another serotonergic antidepressant. Symptoms of serotonin syndrome are nausea, diarrhea, chills, sweating, hyperthermia, hypertension, myoclonic jerking, tremor, agitation, ataxia, disorientation, confusion, and delirium. It can progress to coma and death.

Although safety of use during pregnancy has not been established, *sertraline* **in particular has been used without adverse consequences. Risk versus benefit needs to be carefully considered, as it does also during lactation. Caution is recommended.** *Fluvoxamine* **is Pregnancy Category C, and the others are Category B.**

Children generally require smaller doses than do adults, although some of these agents are not recommended for use with children. Elderly patients generally are prescribed the same doses as younger patients.

Drug Interactions

Significant drug interactions may occur. As discussed previously, serotonin syndrome may result from the interaction between an **SSRI** and any other **serotonergic drug,** such as **anorexiants** and **tryptophan.**

Another interaction of concern is between **SSRIs** and **TCAs** because the result is an increase in the plasma level of the **TCA,** which increases the risk of cardiac conduction complications.

Table 13–46 presents drug interactions.

Clinical Use and Dosing

Table 13–47 presents the indications, dosage schedules, and available dosage forms of **SSRIs,** as well as the neurotransmitters affected.

Rational Drug Selection

The **SSRIs,** with the exception of **fluvoxamine,** are indicated for the treatment of depressive, anxiety, and panic disorders; obsessive-compulsive disorder (OCD); and bulimia. **Fluvoxamine** is FDA-approved only for the treatment of OCD, although it is likely to be as effective as the others for the listed disorders.

Unlabeled uses include the treatment of anorexia, attention deficit–hyperactivity disorder (ADHD), the de-

Table 13–46. Drug Interactions: Selective Serotonin Reuptake Inhibitors (SSRIs)

Drug	Interacting Drug	Possible Effect	Implications
All (SSRIs)	Anorexiants, ergotamine, tryptophan	Serotonin syndrome	Avoid, or use with caution
	MAOIs	Hypertensive crisis	Contraindicated
	Valproate Carbamazepine	Increased level of anti-convulsant	Monitor plasma levels
	TCAs	Increased level of TCA, increased risk of cardio-toxicity	Monitor blood levels of TCA; use with caution
	Benzodiazepines	Increased plasma level of benzodiazepines with sedation and psychomotor/cognitive impairment	Avoid long-term use of benzodiazepines
	Beta blockers	Bradycardia, syncope	Warn patient
	Insulin	Increased insulin sensitivity	Monitor blood glucose
	Neuroleptics	Increased plasma level of neuroleptic	Monitor for adverse reactions
	Zolpidem	Hallucinations and delirium	Avoid

pressive phase of bipolar disorder, chronic headaches and other types of chronic pain, post-traumatic stress disorder (PTSD), impulse control disorders, trichotillomania, and premenstrual syndrome.

The others are labeled only for the treatment of depression, although **bupropion,** because of its blockade of dopamine receptors, seems to have some efficacy in the treatment of ADHD.

Titration is an issue because too-rapid dosage reduction or abrupt cessation of a serotonergic agent can result in withdrawal symptoms consisting of dizziness, lethargy or agitation, nausea, "electric shocklike" sensations, headache, fever, sweating, insomnia, and incoordination of movement.

Patients newly starting on the **antidepressants** need to be advised that it may take 3 to 4 weeks before they experience relief of their symptoms. During that lag time, depressed patients with suicidal ideation need to be closely monitored because of the increased risk related to psychomotor activation without remission of depression.

If used for the treatment of anxiety, doses may need to be higher than they are for the treatment of depression.

Because of their activating characteristics, with the exceptions of **trazodone** and **fluvoxamine,** these drugs are generally taken in the morning or early afternoon to prevent sleep disruption.

Monitoring

No specific monitoring is required.

Patient Education

Advise the patient that these drugs may take as long as 3 to 4 weeks until their benefits become evident and that the initial adverse reactions, commonly including nausea, intermittent light-headedness, sedation, akathisia, and sleep disruption, should be minor and transient. Also, tell the patient to assess the level of sedation the drug can initially cause before engaging in hazardous activities.

Stimulants

The prototype stimulant drug is **amphetamine,** which has a long history since it was first developed more than 100 years ago. It has been used to treat depression, obesity, narcolepsy, and respiratory depression and as an energizer during World War II. At present, **amphetamines** possess notoriety as street drugs of abuse.

Two types of **amphetamines, dextroamphetamine (Dexedrine)** and **methamphetamine (Desoxyn),** are oc-

Table 13–47. Dosage Schedule: Selective Serotonin Reuptake Inhibitors (SSRIs)

Drug	Indications	Neurotransmitters Affected	Dosage	Available Dosage Forms
Fluoxetine (Prozac)	Depression, OCD, bulimia	Primary: serotonin Secondary: norepinephrine	Adolescents and adults: 20–80 mg/d; may increase slowly at 5-d intervals after 3- to 4-wk trial at lower dose; OCD may require a higher dose Older adults: half dose	Capsules: 10, 20 mg Liquid: 20 mg/5 mL
Sertraline (Zoloft)	Depression, OCD	Primary: serotonin Secondary: norepinephrine	Adolescents and adults: 50–200 mg/d; increase at weekly intervals Children and older adults: half dose	Tablets: 50, 100 mg
Paroxetine (Paxil)	Depression, OCD, panic disorder, social phobia	Primary: serotonin Secondary: norepinephrine	Adolescents and adults: 20–60 mg/d; panic disorder and OCD may require higher doses; taper off slowly Children and older adults: half dose	Tablets: 10, 20, 30, 40 mg
Fluvoxamine (Luvox)	Depression, OCD	Primary: serotonin Secondary: norepinephrine	Adults: 50–300 mg/d; dose >100 mg should be divided; increase in 50-mg increments every 4–7 d Older adults: half dose	Tablets: 50, 100 mg
Trazodone (Desryl)	Depression	Primary: serotonin Secondary: adrenergic	Adults: 50–400 mg/d; increase in 50-mg increments every 3–4 d; take with food	Tablets: 50, 100, 150, 300 mg
Venlafaxine (Effexor)	Depression	Primary: serotonin Secondary: norepinephrine	Adults: 75–225 mg/d in divided doses. When discontinuing, taper off over a 2-wk period; increase in 75-mg increments at 4-d intervals; take with food	Tablets: 25, 37.5, 50, 75, 100 mg
Nefazodone (Serzone)	Depression	Primary: serotonin Secondary: adrenergic	Adults: 200–600 mg/d in 2 divided doses; increase in 100-to 200-mg/d increments at weekly intervals	Tablets: 100, 150, 200, 250 mg
Bupropion (Wellbutrin)	Depression, ADHD (adolescent, adult; unlabeled use)	Dopamine	Adolescents and adults: 75–450 mg/d; give 2–3 times/d with 6-h intervals in between; no single dose to exceed 150 mg; increase at 3- to 4-d intervals	Tablets: 75, 100 mg Sustained-release tablets: 75, 100 mg
Mirtazapine (Remeron)	Depression	Primary: histaminic Secondary: serotonin	Adults: 15–30 mg/d, preferably at bedtime	Tablets: 15, 30 mg
Citalopram (Celexa)	Depression	Primary: serotonin Secondary: norepinephrine and dopamine.	Adults: 20 mg qd; may increase in 20-mg increments at weekly intervals; maximum 60 mg/d Older adults: 20 mg/d	Tablets: 20, 40 mg

casionally still used for the treatment of childhood ADHD, narcolepsy, and extreme obesity, but **methylphenidate (Ritalin)** and **magnesium pemoline (Cylert)** have become more widely used for these disorders.

Other **stimulants**, such as **caffeine** and **phenylpropanolamine** found in OTC cold medicines, are primarily significant because of the additive **stimulant** effect they have in combination with other **stimulants**.

Pharmacodynamics

The **CNS stimulants** are sympathomimetic amines that act as dopamine agonists and indirectly release and prevent the reuptake of dopamine, serotonin, and norepinephrine in the presynaptic nerve ending. This action stimulates the cerebral cortex, brain stem, and the reticular activating system and appears to stimulate the reward center in the brain, which accounts for the drugs' considerable abuse potential.

Pharmacokinetics

Absorption and Distribution

Taken orally, the drugs are quickly and thoroughly absorbed, with a rapid onset of action. Peak plasma levels occur in less than 1 to 4 hours. Their half-lives are from 1 to 12 hours.

Metabolism and Excretion

These **stimulants** are metabolized in the liver and excreted in the urine. Urine acidity influences the rate of excretion of amphetamine in that increased alkalinity increases its half-life, a fact that can be important in drug overdose.

Table 13–48 presents pharmacokinetics.

Pharmacotherapeutics

Precautions and Contraindications

Contraindications to use include arteriosclerotic and symptomatic heart disease, hypertension, hyperthyroidism, hypersensitivity to **sympathomimetic amines**, glaucoma, agitation, history of drug abuse, and during or within 14 days of the use of an **MAOI**.

Stimulants are contraindicated for pregnant (Pregnancy Category C) and lactating women.

Stimulants may cause insomnia and should therefore be taken no closer than 6 hours before bedtime.

Adverse Drug Reactions

Positive effects of the drugs include alertness, increased concentration, improved physical performance, increased purposeful motor activity, improved mood, and anorexia. Undesirable effects would be the extremes of these effects, including insomnia, undesired weight loss and growth retardation in children, tachycardia, palpitations, restlessness, irritability, euphoria, headache, tremor, increased libido with impaired ability, hypertension, and arrhythmias. Some individuals may experience a paradoxical drowsiness.

Drug Interactions

Various undesirable drug interactions may occur, perhaps the most significant being the interaction between **MAOIs** and **stimulants** because of the risk of hypertensive crisis. Others include decreased or increased effects of both the stimulant and the interacting drug.

Table 13–49 presents drug interactions.

Clinical Use and Dosing

Table 13–50 presents the indications, dosage schedules, and available dosage forms of **stimulants**.

Rational Drug Selection

With the exception of **pemoline, stimulants** are DEA schedule II and cannot be prescribed by NPs. To prevent anorexia and growth retardation in children, the drug should be given with or after meals. Additionally, some children may exhibit symptoms of their ADHD as the drug begins to wear off and may do better on the sustained-release form of **methylphenidate**.

As indicated previously, **CNS stimulants** are indicated for the treatment of childhood ADHD, narcolepsy, and ex-

Table 13–48. Pharmacokinetics: Stimulants

Drug	Onset	Peak	Duration	Half-Life	Excretion
Dextroamphetamine	30 min	1–3 h	4–20 h	10–30 h	Urine
Methamphetamine HCl	30 min	1–3 h	3–6 h	4–5 h	Urine
Methylphenidate HCl	30–60 min	1.9–4.7 h	4–6 h	1–3 h	Urine
Magnesium pemoline	—	2–4 h	8 h	12 h	Urine

Table 13–49. Drug Interactions: Stimulants

Drug	Interacting Drug	Possible Effect	Implications
All stimulants	MAOIs	Increased risk of hypertensive crisis and stroke	Avoid
	CNS depressants, alkalinizing agents	Decreased effect of stimulant	Dosage may need adjustment
	Antidepressants	Increased effect of antidepressant, especially with TCAs; increased risk of cardiotoxicity in children	Avoid use of TCAs
	Guanethidine	Increased hypotensive effect	Warn patient about dizziness and syncope
	Hypoglycemic agents	Increased glucose lability and decreased control	Monitor blood glucose
	Acidifying agents	Decreased effect of stimulant	Dosage adjustment may be required
	Phenytoin	Increased plasma level of phenytoin	Monitor plasma level

ogenous obesity refractive to other forms of treatment. The use of **stimulants** in the treatment of adolescent and residual adult ADHD is a matter of some controversy, given the street value of these drugs, the increasing use of drugs of abuse, and their association with violent behavior. Because **pemoline** seems to stimulate the reward center less forcefully than the other two and has a delayed onset of action, it is less useful as a drug of abuse, but it is also probably less effective therapeutically.

Monitoring

No specific monitoring is required, other than that the amount of drug used is consistent with the amounts prescribed and dispensed.

Patient Education

Parents need to be aware that these drugs have street value and should be safely stored in the home.

Succinimides

The **succinimides ethosuximide (Zarontin)**, **methsuximide (Celontin)**, and **phensuximide (Milontin)** are the third major type of **anticonvulsants** and the treatment of choice for childhood absence seizure disorder.

Pharmacodynamics

Ethosuximide, methsuximide, and phensuximide exert their anticonvulsant effect by suppression of the motor cortex and by inhibition of stimuli.

Pharmacokinetics

Absorption and Distribution

Succinimides are administered orally and are thoroughly absorbed from the GI tract.

Metabolism and Excretion

Succinimides are metabolized in the liver and excreted through the urinary tract, although a small amount of **phensuximide** is also excreted in bile.

Onset, Peak, and Duration

There is a wide difference in their half-lives, ranging from 60 hours in adults and 30 hours in children for **ethosuximide**, 2.6 to 4 hours for **methsuximide**, and 4 hours for **phensuximide**. Peak plasma levels are achieved in 1 to 4 hours for **methsuximide** and **phensuximide** and in 3 to 7 hours for **ethosuximide**. **Methsuximide** has an onset of action of 15 to 30 minutes and a duration of 3 to 4 hours.

Pharmacotherapeutics

Precautions and Contraindications

Anticonvulsants in general are associated with fetal defects, but the *succinimides*, with careful monitoring of plasma levels, appear to be safe for use during pregnancy and are Pregnancy Category C. They are contraindicated, as are other *anticonvulsants*, during lactation.

Although uncommon, **succinimides** have caused

Table 13–50. Table 13–50: Dosage Schedule: Stimulants

Drug	Indications	Dosage	Available Dosage Forms
Dextroamphetamine (Dexedrine)	ADHD, narcolepsy, exogenous obesity	Adult: 10 mg daily; may increase by 10-mg increments every week to maximum of 30 mg/d; give individual doses at 4- to 6-h intervals Children age 3–5: 2.5 mg/d; increase by 2.5 mg daily at weekly intervals to range of 0.1–0.5 mg/kg/d; give in morning Children >5: 5 mg 1–2 times/d; may increase in 5-mg increments weekly to maximum of 40 mg/d; usual range 0.1–0.5 mg/kg/d	Tablets: 5, 10 mg Sustained-release capsules: 5, 10, 15 mg
Methamphetamine HCl (Desoxyn); salt mixtures with amphetamine (Adderall)	ADHD, narcolepsy, exogenous obesity	Adults and children >12: 5 mg 1–2 times/d; may increase at 5-mg increments weekly to maximum of 25 mg/d; may be twice-daily dosing or SR once daily; SR dose is 10–15 mg in morning	Tablets: 5 mg Sustained-release tablets: 20 mg
Methylphenidate HCl (Ritalin)	ADHD, narcolepsy,	Adults: 20–30 mg/d in 2–3 divided doses; maximum 60 mg/d Children >6: 5 mg bid with increase of 5-mg increments at weekly intervals; maximum 60 mg/d. Stop drug if no improvement in 4 wk All ages: SR tabs taken in morning may be supplemented with afternoon regular tablets if needed; if insomnia is present, give regular tab no later than 6 PM	Tablets: 5, 10, 20 mg Sustained-release tablets: 20 mg
Magnesium pemoline (Cylert)	ADHD	Adults and children >6: 37.5 mg in morning; may increase by 18.75-mg increments at weekly intervals to maximum of 112.5 mg/d	Tablets: 18.75, 37.5, 75 mg Chewable tablets: 37.5 mg

SR = sustained release.

blood dyscrasias, and their use should be preceded by a CBC with differential, repeated at frequent intervals initially and less often as the patient continues on the medication without adverse effects. Liver function tests should also be obtained prior to instituting treatment.

Adverse Drug Reactions

The most common adverse reactions are GI distress, which can be relieved by administering the medication with food or milk, and CNS depression, consisting of sedation, ataxia, and lethargy. Symptoms of toxicity are a worsening of these adverse reactions.

Drug Interactions

Significant drug interactions are limited to those that increase CNS depression, such as **alcohol** and other **CNS depressants.** The result is additive CNS depression, and the patient should be warned.

Succinimides may be given concurrently with other **anticonvulsants** but may antagonize the other and contribute to tonic-myoclonic breakthrough seizures, therefore indicating the need for a higher dose of the other **anticonvulsant.**

When given with **TCAs,** an antagonistic effect to **succinimides** occurs that may lower the patient's seizure threshold; therefore, avoid concurrent use.

With **estrogen,** the **succinimides** may decrease the

effect of **oral contraceptives**; therefore, warn the patient to use a backup birth control method.

Clinical Use and Dosing

Table 13–51 presents the indications, dosage schedules, and available dosage forms of **succinimides.**

Rational Drug Selection

Succinimides are the treatment of choice for childhood absence seizure disorders and have no other clinical use. Although absence seizures are usually outgrown by adulthood, **valproic acid** becomes the primary treatment, should they persist.

Phensuximide is somewhat less effective in controlling seizure activity than either **ethosuximide** or **methsuximide,** and more genitourinary adverse effects have been reported than with the others. **Methsuximide** is equally effective as **ethosuximide** but is slightly more toxic.

Monitoring

Plasma levels should be monitored. The normal range is 40 to 100 µg/mL.

Patient Education

Advise the patient to avoid **alcohol** and, if sedation occurs, to avoid hazardous activities.

Tricyclic Antidepressants

The development of **TCAs** grew out of work with **phenothiazines,** to which they are structurally related. Prior to their availability in the 1960s, depression had been treated with **stimulants** and **tranquilizers,** both of which had some utility but left the basic mood disorder essentially unchanged. They were not overshadowed until the late 1980s, when the new **SSRIs** began to be widely marketed.

Although now less frequently used than in the past, **amitriptyline (Elavil), nortriptyline (Pamelor, Aventyl), imipramine (Tofranil), doxepin (Sinequan), trimipramine maleate (Surmontil), amoxapine (Asendin), desipramine (Norpramin, Pertofrane), protriptyline HCl (Vivactil),** and **clomipramine (Anafranil)** still have their individual usefulness.

Pharmacodynamics

The **TCAs** act on the neurotransmitters serotonin and norepinephrine by inhibiting their reuptake at the presynaptic neuron. **Amoxapine,** as an active metabolite of the **antipsychotic loxapine,** also has a similar interaction with postsynaptic dopamine.

Pharmacokinetics

Absorption and Distribution

All are administered orally, thoroughly absorbed, and lipophilic. Steady state is achieved in approximately 5 days, but there is a lag time of 2 to 4 weeks before remission of depressive symptoms becomes evident. Half-life ranges from 8 to 90 hours but averages 24 to 36 hours.

Metabolism and Excretion

The **TCAs** are metabolized in the liver and excreted in urine.

Table 13–52 presents the pharmacokinetics.

Table 13–51. Dosage Schedule: Succinimides

Drug	Indications	Dosage	Available Dosage Forms
Ethosuximide (Zarontin)	Absence seizures (petit mal)	Adults and children >6: 500 mg daily or 250 mg bid; may increase by 250 mg every 4–7 d to maximum of 1.5 g/d Children <6: 250 mg daily or 125 mg bid; optimal dose 20 mg/kg/d; maximum dose 1.5 g/d	Capsules: 250 mg Syrup: 250 mg/5 mL
Methsuximide (Celontin)	Absence seizures (petit mal); second choice	Adults and children: initially 300 mg/d; may increase by 300-mg/d increments at weekly intervals to maximum of 1.2 g/d in divided doses	Capsules: 150, 300 mg
Phensuximide (Milontin)	Absence seizures refractory to other drugs	Adults and children: 500–1000 mg 2–3 times daily	Capsules: 500 mg

Table 13–52. Pharmacokinetics: Tricyclic Antidepressants

Drug	Onset	Peak	Duration	Half-Life	Excretion
Amitriptyline HCl	45 min	2–12 h	—	31–46 h	Urine, feces
Amoxapine	—	2–4 h	—	8 h	Urine
Clomipramine	—	2–4 h	—	19–37 h	Urine
Desipramine HCl	—	2–4 h	—	12–24 h	Urine
Doxepin HCl	—	2–4 h	—	8–24 h	Urine
Imipramine HCl	—	2–4 h	—	11–25 h	Urine, feces
Nortriptyline HCl	—	2–4 h	—	18–44 h	Urine
Protriptyline HCl	15–30 min	24–30 h	4–6 h	67–89 h	Urine
Trimipramine maleate	—	—	—	7–30 h	Urine

Pharmacotherapeutics

Precautions and Contraindications

Contraindications include cardiovascular disorders, glaucoma, prostatic hypertrophy, concomitant use of **MAOIs,** and hypersensitivity.

Safety of use in pregnancy is unclear. *TCAs are Pregnancy Category C and are excreted in low doses in breast milk.*

Although rare, TD and NMS have been reported, with the highest risk correlated with the use of **amoxapine.**

The **TCAs** should be titrated gradually in either direction. Nausea, headache, vertigo, malaise, and nightmares have been noted following abrupt discontinuance of the drug or after large dose decreases.

The most significant risks related to **TCA** use are cardiac conduction disorder and, in individuals with a prior history of seizure disorder, seizures. At highest risk of the former are children and the elderly; therefore, baseline ECG and periodic monitoring should be performed.

Another significant concern with **TCAs** is that the index between therapeutic and toxic levels is narrow, which may be crucial when treating a depressed person with suicidal ideation who becomes energized before the affective component of the illness begins to remit. Such patients should be closely monitored and may need to be dispensed only a small amount of the tablets at a time until the suicidal ideation resolves.

Adverse Drug Reactions

Anticholinergic adverse effects are common and can include dry mouth, constipation, urinary hesitancy or retention, blurred vision, sedation, orthostatic hypotension, weight gain, nausea and vomiting, gynecomastia, and changes in libido. Patients newly prescribed a **TCA** should be cautioned about safety in situations in which mental alertness is required until the full effect of the drug has been determined.

Drug Interactions

The most significant drug interactions are those that increase the plasma level of the **TCA** and thereby increase the risk of cardiotoxicity, such as can occur with the concurrent use of **SSRIs, cannabis,** and **sympathomimetics.**

Hyperpyrexia can occur with **MAOIs** and **TCAs.**

Table 13–53 presents drug interactions.

Clinical Use and Dosing

Table 13–54 presents the indications, dosage schedules, and available dosage forms of **TCAs.**

Rational Drug Selection

Indications for the use of **TCAs** are depression, anxiety with sleep disturbance, enuresis in children age 6 or older, OCD (**clomipramine** only), chronic pain, panic disorder, and eating disorders. The latter three are unlabeled uses.

Unlike **SSRIs,** which are generally more activating, **TCAs** are sedating and are therefore usually taken at bedtime.

Monitoring

Plasma levels and ECG should be routinely assessed.

Table 13–53. Drug Interactions: Tricyclic Antidepressants

Drug	Interacting Drug	Possible Effect	Implications
All TCAs	SSRIs, anorexiants, cimetidine, oral contraceptives, charcoal, calcium channel blockers, protease inhibitors, propoxyphene, methylphenidate	Increased plasma level of TCA and increased risk of cardiotoxicity	Use with caution; monitor plasma levels of TCA
	Narcotics, barbiturates, antihistamines, alcohol, benzodiazepines, antipsychotics	Increased CNS depression; increased TCA plasma level; increased risk of cardiotoxicity	Use with caution; monitor plasma level of TCA
	Anticholinergics	Increased anticholinergic adverse reactions	Avoid concurrent use if possible
	Dicumarol	Increased prothrombin time	Monitor
	Carbamazepine, phenytoin	Increased plasma level of anticonvulsant	Monitor blood levels of anticonvulsants
	MAOIs	Hyperpyretic crisis	Avoid concurrent use
	Clonidine, guanethidine	Antihypertensive effect antagonized by TCA	Monitor blood pressure
	Levodopa	Hypertension, dyskinesia	Use different type of antidepressant
	Tamoxifen, nicotine, rifampin	Decreased TCA effect	May require higher dose
	Sympathomimetics	Hypertension, risk of arrhythmias	Avoid if possible
	Cannabis	Increased risk of cardiotoxicity; tachycardia, light-headedness, confusion, mood lability, delirium	Avoid

Patient Education

Advise the patient to avoid engaging in hazardous activities if drowsy or sedated. If the patient develops dry mouth, advise an increase in fluid intake and sucking hard candies. If constipation develops, advise an increase in fluid intake and a bulking agent or stool softener.

Valproates

Valproic acid (Depakene) and its derivatives **divalproex sodium** and **sodium valproate (Depakote)** are another major group of **anticonvulsants**. They are also frequently used agents in the treatment of bipolar disorder.

Pharmacodynamics

Although the mechanism of action of the **valproates** are not completely understood, they are thought to prevent seizure activity and mania by an increase in the inhibitory action of gamma-aminobutyric acid (GABA).

Pharmacokinetics

Absorption and Distribution

Valproates are administered orally, are rapidly and thoroughly absorbed, and are highly protein-bound.

Metabolism and Excretion

Valproates are metabolized in the liver and excreted via the kidneys.

Onset, Peak, and Duration

Peak plasma levels generally occur within 1 to 4 hours, although when administered via syrup, the drug peaks

Table 13–54. Dosage Schedule: Tricyclic Antidepressants

Drug	Indications	Dosage	Available Dosage Forms
Amitriptyline (Elavil)	Depression	Adult: 75 mg/d in divided doses to maximum of 150 mg/d; may give entire dose at bedtime; hospitalized patients may require 200–300 mg/d. Adolescents and older adults: 40–100 mg/d in divided doses or at bedtime; maximum 100 mg/d.	Tablets: 10, 25, 50, 75, 100, 150 mg
Amoxapine (Asendin)	Depression	Adults and children >16: 50 mg bid–tid, gradually increasing to 200–300 mg/d/ if needed; maximum 400 mg/d. If total dose equals 300 mg or more, give in divided doses. Older adults: 25 mg bid–tid; may gradually increase to maximum of 300 mg/d.	Tablets: 25, 50, 100, 150 mg
Clomipramine	OCD	Adults: 25 mg/d initially, increase over 2 wk to maximum or 250 mg/d. Give with food to minimize GI distress. May divide dose initially, give at hs for maintenance. Children and adolescents: 25 mg/d intially; may gradually increase over 2 wk to maximum of 3 mg/kg/d or 100 mg, whichever is smaller, or for adolescents, to maximum of 3 mg/kg/d or 200 mg, whichever is smaller.	Capsules: 25, 50, 75 mg
Desipramine HCI (Norpramin, Pertofrane)	Depression	Adults: 100–200 mg/d in single or divided dose; maximum 300 mg/d. Adolescents and older adults: 25–100 mg/d; maximum 150 mg/d.	Tablets: 10, 25, 50, 75, 100, 150 mg Capsules: 25, 50 mg
Doxepin HCI (Sinequan)	Depression, especially helpful with sleep disruption	Adults: 75–150 mg/d, preferablly at hs; maximum 300 mg/d. Dilute concentrate with 120 mL of milk, water, or juice.	Capsules: 10, 25, 50, 100, 150 mg Concentrate: 10 mg/mL
Imipramine HCI (Tofranil)	Depression, enuresis in children >6 yr	Adults: 50–150 mg/d at hs; maximum 200 mg/d. Hospitalized patients may require 250–300 mg/d. Adolescents and older adults: 30–40 mg/d to maximum of 100 mg/d. Children: 1.5 mg/kg/d tid to maximum of 5 mg/kg/d. Increase by increments of 1–1.5 mg/kg/d at 3- to 5-d intervals.	Tablets: 10, 25, 50 mg Capsules: 75 100, 125, 150 mg
Nortriptyline HCI (Pamelor, Aventyl)	Depression	Adults: 25 mg tid–qid to maximum of 100 mg/d. Adolescents and older adults: 30–50 mg/d in divided doses.	Capsules: 10, 25, 50, 75 mg Solution: 10 mg/5 mL
Protriptyline HCI (Vivactil)	Depression	Adults: 100–200 mg/d in single or divided dose; maximum 60 mg/d. Make increase in AM. Adolescents and older adults: 25–100 mg/d; maximum 150 mg/d.	Tablets: 5, 10 mg
Trimipramine maleate (Surmontil)	Depression	Adults: 75–150 mg/d in divided doses; maximum 200 mg/d. Hospitalized patients may require 250–300 mg/d. Adolescents and older adults: 50–100 mg/d.	Capsules: 25, 50, 100 mg

more rapidly. Conversely, the enteric-coated version delays absorption and peaking. Their half-lives are in the range of 5 to 20 hours.

Pharmacotherapeutics

Precautions and Contraindications

Contraindications include hypersensitivity and hepatic disease.

Use of these drugs during pregnancy is associated with the development of spina bifida. They are Pregnancy Category D. Their use should be restricted to cases in which the woman's life would be endangered without them, and they should be used with caution during lactation.

The plasma level range is 50 to 100 µg/mL. Levels above 100 are thought to be toxic, although symptoms of toxicity can occur at blood levels within the normal range, and patients have been maintained on levels above 100 without apparent toxicity. Symptoms of toxicity include dizziness, hypotension, tachycardia or bradycardia, drowsiness, visual hallucinations, and respiratory depression. Coma and death may result.

Although relatively uncommon, **valproic acid** may impair platelet aggregation so that bleeding time may be prolonged, and it may suppress bone marrow production. For this reason, a CBC with differential should precede use and be repeated with regularity initially and less frequently as the patient continues to take the medication without adverse event.

Rare cases of hepatotoxicity and liver failure have occurred, primarily in children younger than age 2 who have been on combination therapy. Consequently, patients in this population need to be closely monitored and treated with **valproic acid** or its derivatives as single agents only. Liver function tests should be performed prior to use in any age category and repeated at appropriate intervals.

Patients with diabetes taking **valproic acid** may show falsely positive ketone urine tests because the drug is partially excreted in the urine as a ketone metabolite. Any patient may have initially elevated liver enzymes, but this is usually transitory.

Adverse Drug Reactions

Valproic acid is well tolerated, and most adverse effects, such as GI distress and CNS depression, are mild and transient. Safety in situations requiring mental alertness are of concern initially, and the patient should be instructed to avoid potentially dangerous situations until the effect of the drug can be assessed.

Table 13–55. Drug Interactions: Valproates

Drug	Interacting Drug	Possible Effect	Implications
Valproic acid and derivatives	CNS depressants	Increased sedation and disorientation	Warn patient about safety issues; avoid if possible
	Anticoagulants	Increased bleeding time	Monitor bleeding time
	Anticonvulsants	May increase or decrease plasma level of other anticonvulsant	Monitor plasma levels
	TCAs	Increased blood level of TCA and increased risk of cardiotoxicity	Monitor blood level of TCA
	Antibiotics	Increased valproate level	Monitor blood level of valproate; decreased dosage may be required
	Lithium	Increased tremors	Decrease lithium dose
	Neuroleptic	Increased risk of neurotoxicity, sedation, EPS	Monitor for signs and symptoms of toxicity
	Antiviral	Decreased valproate level	Monitor plasma level of valproate
	Cimetidine, salicylates	Increased plasma level and half-life of valproate	Monitor plasma level of valproate

Table 13–56. Dosage Schedule: Valproates

Drug	Indications	Dosage	Available Dosage Forms
Valproic acid (Depakote, Depakene, Depacon)	Complex partial, simple (petit mal), absence seizure epilepsy; mania; migraine headache	Adult: 750 mg daily in divided doses; may increase rapidly to control acute mania to maximum of 60 mg/kg/d For migraine headache: 250 mg bid Children and older adults: reduce dose Sprinkle capsule should not be chewed and not stored for future use once opened; take with food to prevent GI distress For acute mania: 60-mg IV infusion (20 mg/min or less) at same frequency as oral dose	Depakene: 250 mg capsule; 250 mg/5 mL syrup Depakote: 125, 250, 500 mg delayed-release tablets; 125-mg sprinkle capsule Depacon: 5-mg injection

Drug Interactions

Many common drug interactions have to do with competition with protein-binding sites. **Valproates** in combination with other **CNS depressants** can lead to an additive depressant effect. Bleeding time can be increased in combination with **anticoagulants**. Combinations of **TCAs** and **valproates** can lead to increased risk of cardiotoxicity.

Table 13–55 presents drug interactions.

Clinical Use and Dosing

Table 13–56 presents indications, dosage schedules, and available dosage forms of **valproates.**

Rational Drug Selection

Valproic acid is indicated for the treatment of simple and partial complex absence seizures, either singly or adjunctively. It is being increasingly used for tonic-clonic, myoclonic, and generalized seizures and in the treatment of migraine headache.

Valproic acid's psychiatric indications include the treatment of bipolar disorder, particularly the rapid-cycling or mixed types, both for acute mania and prophylaxis.

Other uses include treatment of mood instability, such as that which occurs with borderline personality disorder or PTSD; anger and aggression; and adjunctively in the treatment of resistant unipolar depression.

The usual adult dose is 750 to 3000 mg a day, taken once, most commonly at bedtime, or in divided doses.

Monitoring

Plasma levels should be assessed to help guide dosage adjustments. CBCs and chemistries should be obtained prior to the onset of treatment and then at regular intervals.

Patient Education

Patients should be advised to avoid hazardous activities until their level of sedation is determined. Also, advise patients not to abruptly discontinue the drug.

REFERENCES

American Psychiatric Association. (1998). *Practice guideline for the treatment of patients with panic disorder.* Washington, DC: Author.

Arvanitis, L. A., & Miller, B. G. (1997). Multiple fixed doses of "seroquel" (quetiapine) in patients with acute exacerbation of schizophrenia: A comparison with halperidol and placebo. *Biological Psychiatry, 42,* 233–246.

Bezchlibnyk-Butler, K., & Jeffries, J. (Eds.). (1998). *Clinical handbook of psychotropic drugs* (8th ed.). Toronto: Hogrefe & Huber.

Boyer, W. (1995). Serotonin uptake inhibitors are superior to imipramine and alprazolam in alleviating panic attacks: A meta-analysis. *International Clinical Psychopharmacology, 10,* 45–49.

Brown, C. S., Markowitz, J. S., Moore, T. R., & Parker, N. G. (1999). Atypical antipsychotics: Adverse effects, drug interactions, and cost. *Annals of Pharmacotherapy, 33,* 210–217.

Conley, R. (1997). New pharmacologic treatments. *Journal of the California Alliance for the Mentally Ill, 8,* 1315.

Davidson, J. (1998). *Social anxiety disorder.* Philadelphia: Current Medicine.

Drug facts and comparisons (3rd ed.). (1999). St. Louis: Wolters Kluwer.

Julian, R. (1998). *A primer of drug action: A concise, nontechnical guide to the actions, uses, and side effects of psychoactive drugs* (8th ed.). New York: W. H. Freeman.

Julian, R. (1998). *Attention deficit disorder in adults.* Symposium at the meeting of the Eugene Area Psychiatric Mental Health Nurse Practitioners, Eugene, OR.

Kane, J. (1997). The new antipsychotics. *Journal of Practical Psychiatry and Behavioral Health,* 343–354.

Keltner, N. L. (1997a). Catastrophic consequences secondary to psychotropic drugs, part 1. *Journal of Psychosocial Nursing, 35,* 41–45.

Keltner, N. L. (1997b). Catastrophic consequences secondary to psychotropic drugs, part 2. *Journal of Psychosocial Nursing, 35,* 48–50.

Mavissakalian, M. R., & Prien, R. F. (Eds.). (1995). *Long-term treatments of anxiety disorders.* Washington, DC: American Psychiatric Press.

McIvor, R. J., & Turner, S. W. (1995). Drug treatment in posttraumatic stress disorder. *British Journal of Hospital Medicine, 53,* 501–506.

Nunes, E. V., et al. (1995). Treating anxiety in patients with alcoholism. *Journal of Clinical Psychiatry, 56,* 3–9.

Oregon Health Resources Commission. (1998a). *Technical assessment and recommended clinical guidelines for anti-psychotic drugs.* Salem: Oregon Health Resources Commission.

Oregon Health Resources Commission. (1998b). *Technical assessment and recommended clinical guidelines for anti-depressant drugs in the treatment of depression.* Salem: Oregon Health Resources Commission.

Preskorn, S. (1997). Clinically relevant pharmacology of selective serotonin reuptake inhibitors: An overview with emphasis on pharmacokinetics and effects on oxidative drug metabolism. *Clinical Pharmacokinetics, 32*(Suppl 1), 1–21.

Ravizza, L., et al. (1995). Predictors of drug treatment response in obsessive-compulsive disorder. *Journal of Clinical Psychiatiatry, 56,* 368–373.

Sack, D. (1997). Is this the dawning of real hope? *Journal of the California Alliance for the Mentally Ill, 8,* 1617.

Schatzberg, A., & Nemeroff, C. (Eds.). (1995). *The American Psychiatric Press textbook of psychopharmacology.* Washington, DC: American Psychiatric Press.

Schweizer, E. Generalized anxiety disorder: Longitudinal course and pharmacologic treatment. *Psychiatric Clinics of North America, 18,* 843–857.

Zajecka, J. M., & Ross, J. S. (1995). Management of comorbid anxiety and depression. *Journal of Clinical Psychiatry, 56,* 10–13.

CHAPTER 14

· · · · · · ·

Drugs Affecting the Cardiovascular and Renal Systems

CHAPTER OUTLINE

Angiotensin-Converting Enzyme Inhibitors and Angiotensin II Receptor Antagonists

Angiotensin-converting enzyme inhibitors (ACEIs) and **angiotensin II receptor antagonists (ATRAs)** lower blood pressure (BP) by their action on the renin-angiotensin-aldosterone system. Approximately 20 percent of patients who have essential hypertension (HTN) have abnormally high renin levels and respond well to drugs that lower plasma renin activity. Their mild and usually transient adverse effects and their ease of dosing make them popular drugs in treating a disorder in which the adverse effects of the drugs are often more noticeable to the patient than the symptoms of HTN. The complexity of their mechanism of action results in their having roles in the treatment of congestive heart failure (CHF) and diabetic nephropathy as well. **ATRAs** probably have similar roles in the treatment of CHF and diabetic nephropathy prevention, but to date there have been no large trials and **ATRAs** are not yet approved for these latter roles. There has been one trial with an **ATRA** in the treatment of CHF in older adults (Pitt et al., 1997).

Pharmacodynamics

As shown in Figure 14–1, inhibition of ACE activity results in decreased vasopressor activity, decreased sodium and water retention, and increased vasodilation. Taken together, the result is decreased intravascular volume and peripheral vascular resistance (PVR), which lead to decreased blood pressure. **ATRAs** do not affect

ACE activity but rather act by blocking the angiotensin AT_1 receptor. **ATRAs** have similar action to **ACEIs** on vasoconstriction and aldosterone secretion but no activity related to bradykinin. **ACEIs** and **ATRAs** do not affect cardiac output and so do not produce reflex tachycardia. Their role in the treatment of heart failure is related to their ability to reduce both preload (through the reduction in sodium and water retention) and afterload (through reduction in PVR). PVR is also decreased through reduction in angiotensin's effect on norepinephrine release. New evidence suggests that a parallel system for angiotensin generation exists in several other tissues, including the heart, and this system may contribute to the trophic changes associated with cardiac hypertrophy. **ACEIs** may prevent this hypertrophy. **ACEIs** are the only drug class that has all these functions and are one of only two groups of drugs that have been demonstrated to decrease mortality from CHF by 25 to 31 percent (CONSENSUS, 1987; DHHS, 1994; Pfeffer, 1995; SOLVD, 1991; SOLVD, 1992). **ATRAs** have not yet been approved to treat heart failure, but many clinicians are using them.

The effectiveness of **ACEIs** in preventing diabetic nephropathy probably results from decreased glomerular efferent arteriolar resistance and a reduction in intraglomerular capillary pressure, which causes improved renal hemodynamics, diminished proteinuria, retarded glomerular hypertrophy, and a slower rate of decline in glomerular filtration rate (GFR). These drugs do not affect glucose metabolism or raise serum lipid levels, but they do improve insulin sensitivity; all of these are important issues in type 2 diabetes mellitus. **ATRAs** have not yet been subjected to sufficient research for approval in preventing diabetic nephropathy.

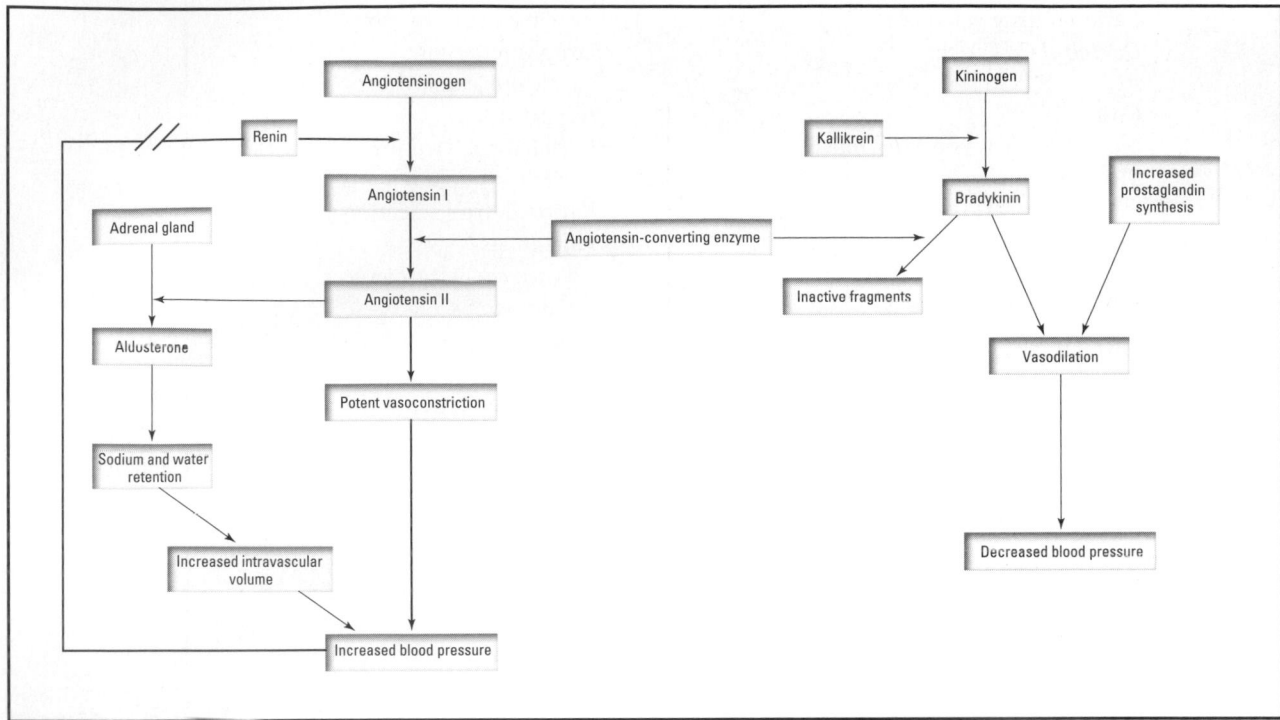

Figure 14–1. Renin-angiotensin-aldosterone system. Renin acts on angiotensinogen to create the inactive decapeptide angiotensin I. Angiotensin I is then converted, primarily in the lung, to angiotensin II, a potent vaso-constrictor, through the activity of angiotensin-converting enzyme (ACE). Angiotensin II stimulates aldosterone secretion, causing retention of sodium and water and loss of potassium by the kidney. ACE is also involved in the inactivation of bradykinin, a vasodilator. Together, these systems help to control blood pressure.

Pharmacokinetics

Absorption and Distribution

The **ACEIs** and **ATRAs** are well absorbed orally, with some variation in bioavailability based on the presence of food in the gut (Table 14–1). **Captopril (Capoten)**, the prototype drug for the **ACEI** class, is rapidly absorbed, with a bioavailability of about 70 percent when taken on an empty stomach. Bioavailability is decreased to 30 to 40 percent if taken with food. **Losartan (Cozaar)**, the prototype drug for the **ATRA** class, undergoes extensive first-pass metabolism, resulting in 33 percent bioavailability. It may be taken without regard to food.

Distribution is to most body tissues except the central nervous system (CNS). **ACEIs** and **ATRAs** cross the placenta and are found in breast milk.

Metabolism and Excretion

Except for **captopril** and **lisinopril (Zestril, Prinivil)**, all **ACEIs** are prodrugs converted to active metabolites by hydrolysis, primarily in the liver. **Losartan** has both an active drug and an active metabolite (5-carboxylic acid) hydrolyzed by the liver. **Captopril** is metabolized by the liver to inactive compounds. The kidney is the primary organ of excretion for all **ACEIs** and **ATRAs** ex-

cept **fosinopril (Monopril)** and **moexipril (Univasc)**, and impaired renal function can significantly prolong their half-lives. **Losartan** and its active metabolite are excreted mainly by the kidney, but some biliary elimination also occurs. **Captopril**, with a half-life of less than 2 hours, is the only short-acting **ACEI**. It requires bid or tid administration, with steady state achieved in 2 to 3 days. All other members of the class have 11- to 12-hour half-lives and require more time to achieve steady state. **Losartan** has a 2-hour half-life, and its active metabolite has a 6- to 9-hour half-life. Dosing may be daily or in two divided doses. Steady state is achieved in 3 to 6 weeks.

Pharmacotherapeutics

Precautions and Contraindications

Only three absolute contraindications to use of **ACEIs** exist: bilateral renal artery stenosis, angioedema, and pregnancy. In bilateral renal artery stenosis, increased vascular pressure and vasoconstriction appear to be required to sufficiently overcome the stenotic blood flow to perfuse the kidney. The vasodilating effect of an **ACEI** or an **ATRA** prevents the kidney from maintaining its perfusion, and ischemic renal failure may develop. Angioedema occurs in approximately 0.2 percent of patients taking

Table 14–1. Pharmacokinetics: Angiotensin-Converting Enzyme Inhibitors and Angiotensin II Receptor Antagonists

Drug	Onset (h)	Peak (h)	Duration (h)	Protein Binding	Bioavail- ability	Effect of Food on Absorption	Active Metabolite	Half-Life	Elimination
Angiotensin-Converting Enzyme Inhibitors									
Benazepril	1	2–4	24	95%	37%	None	Benazeprilat	NRF: 10–11 h IRF: prolonged	Total: nd Unchanged: trace
Captopril	0.25	0.5–1.5	6–12	25–30%	75%	Reduced	—	NRF: <2 h IRF: 3.5–32 h	Total: >95% 40–50% in urine
Enalapril	1	4–6	24	50–60%	60%	None	Enalaprilat	NRF: 1.3 h IRF: nd	Total: 94% in urine and feces Unchanged: 54% in urine
Fosinopril	1	2–6	24	95%	100%	None	Fosinoprilat	NRF: 12 h IRF: prolonged	Total: 50% in urine, 50% in feces Unchanged: negligible
Lisinopril	1	6	24	none	25%	None	—	NRF: 12 h IRF: prolonged	Total: nd Unchanged: 100% in urine
Moexipril	1	3–6	24	50%	15%	Reduced	Moexiprilat	NRF: 2–9 h IRF: prolonged	Total: 13% in urine, 53% in feces Unchanged: 1% in urine, 1% in feces
Quinapril	1	2–4	24	97%	60%	Reduced	Quinaprilat	NRF: 2 h IRF: prolonged	Total: 60% in urine, 37% in feces Unchanged: trace
Ramipril	1–2	4–6.5	24	73%	50–60%	Reduced	Ramiprilat	NRF: 13–17 h IRF: prolonged	Total: 60% in urine, 40% in feces Unchanged: <2%
Angiotensin II Receptor Antagonists									
Candesartan	UK	3–4	UK	79%	15%	None	Inactive metabolite	9 h	33% in urine, 66% in feces
Losartan	Varies	1 h parent, 6 h metabolite	24	98%	33%	Decreases by 10%	5-Carboxylic acid (EXP-3174)	Drug: 2 h; metabolite 6–9 h	4–6% of drug and metabolite unchanged in urine, 60% in feces
Irbesartan	UK	1–3	UK	90%	60–80%	None	Inactive metabolite	11–15 h	20% in urine, 80% in feces
Valsartan	Varies	2–4	UK	95%	25%	Decreases by 40–50%	Metabolite significantly less potent	6 h	13% in urine, 83% in feces

NRF = normal renal function; IRF = impaired renal function; nd = no data; UK = unknown.

ACEIs and can be life-threatening. The physiological reason for this adverse response appears to be related to an increase in bradykinin level associated with inhibition of ACE. It usually occurs with the first dose or within the first month of therapy and is more common in the longer-acting agents. Because this is a class phenomenon, the **ACEI** must be discontinued, and no other drug in this class may be used. **ATRAs** do not affect the bradykinin system and should not cause this adverse response. Angioedema is a very serious adverse response, so administration of an **ATRA** in a patient who exhibited angioedema with an **ACEI** is still a questionable clinical practice.

The **ACEIs** and **ATRAs** should be used cautiously with patients who have impaired renal function, and dosage adjustment may be required. Hypovolemic or hyponatremic states also require cautious use. Adequate hydration is required to maintain an appropriate GFR and must be adequate before starting these drugs to prevent renal dysfunction. Inadequate hydration can also produce hypovolemia based on the vasodilating effects of **ACEIs** and **ATRAs**. Hyperkalemia contraindicates use because reduced aldosterone secretion may worsen this electrolyte imbalance. Hyperkalemia risk increases for patients with CHF because of the reduced blood flow to the kidneys. They should have their serum potassium level checked prior to initiating therapy and within 1 week to note trends. Although these drugs are used with caution in hepatic impairment, it is not an absolute contraindication to their use.

During the SAVE trial (Pfeffer et al., 1992) using **captopril**, mortality was increased in the immediate postmyocardial infarction period. An interval of 3 to 5 days after myocardial infarction (MI) is recommended before **ACEIs** are begun.

Because ACEIs and ATRAs can cause fetal and neonatal morbidity and mortality, they are Pregnancy Category C in the first trimester of pregnancy and Pregnancy Category D in the second and third trimesters and during lactation.

Adverse Drug Reactions

Adverse reactions for both **ACEIs** and **ATRAs** are usually transient, mild, and more common in longer-acting agents. Most common are those associated with hypotension (dizziness, headache, fatigue, orthostatic hypotension). Tachyphylaxis frequently occurs with continued therapy. Also common and often cited as the reason for discontinuance of **ACEIs** is a dry, hacking cough that usually occurs in the first week of therapy. This is a class phenomenon for **ACEIs,** but changing to a different **ACEI** has been associated with less or no cough in some patients. Because the action of bradykinin may be responsible for the adverse reactions of cough and angioedema, **ATRAs** do not produce these effects (Pylypchuk, 1998). Changing to an **ATRA** provides benefits similar to those

of the **ACEI** with less likelihood of cough. Less common adverse reactions with **ACEIs** include a rash that is most common with **captopril** and not a class phenomenon, neutropenia that increases with high doses, renal impairment, and concomitant collagen diseases.

Drug Interactions

Additive hypotensive effects occur with **diuretics,** and this drug interaction is sometimes used clinically. Additive hypotension may also occur with other **antihypertensives, nitrates, phenothiazines,** and acute **alcohol** ingestion. Because of the interference with aldosterone secretion, the concurrent use of **potassium supplements, potassium-sparing diuretics,** or **cyclosporine** may result in hyperkalemia. The antihypertensive response is reduced by nonsteroidal anti-inflammatory drugs **(NSAIDs)** because of their effect on prostaglandins. Cytochrome P-450 (CYP) 2C9 and 3A4 isoenzymes are involved in the metabolism of **losartan.** Drugs that inhibit this system (e.g., **cimetidine**) may cause increased levels of free drug. Other specific drug interactions and the appropriate actions to prevent them are given in Table 14–2.

Clinical Use and Dosing

HYPERTENSION. **ACEIs** and **ATRAs** are the drugs of choice for patients who are young and white and for diabetic patients, for whom they are most effective and have the lowest incidence of adverse reactions. They are generally not effective for black patients. No specific difference related to gender has been shown (National High Blood Pressure Education Program, 1997). Doses for HTN vary with each drug, but adverse reactions increase with higher doses. The first dose may cause a steep drop in BP, especially for patients taking **diuretics. Diuretics** should be stopped for 2 to 3 days to allow rehydration before starting an **ACEI. ACEIs** and **ATRAs** increase in effectiveness when given with a **diuretic,** and **diuretics** may be reintroduced if needed after the **ACEI** or **ATRA** dose has been stabilized. Because reduced aldosterone secretion may result in potassium retention, **thiazide diuretics** make an excellent combination on account of their tendency to foster potassium loss. The best approach is to start low and go slow. Begin with the lowest dose recommended for the **ACEI** or **ATRA** and increase the dose at 1- or 2-week intervals until BP is controlled. For further information, see Chapter 38 on drugs used to treat HTN.

HYPERTENSIVE PROTEINURIC DIABETES. To prevent diabetic nephropathy or slow its progression, **ACEIs** should be used to treat the HTN. Dosages usually used for HTN are appropriate here.

POSTMYOCARDIAL INFARCTION. **ACEIs** should be started early after MI in stable, high-risk patients (ante-

Table 14–2. Drug Interactions: Angiotensin-Coverting Enzyme Inhibitors and Angiotensin II Receptor Antagonists

Drug	Interacting Drug	Possible Effect	Implications
All ACEIs	Diuretics	Hypotension and renal dysfunction	Discontinue 2–3 d before initiating therapy with ACEI or initiate with low dose. Ensure adequate hydration prior to first dose and warn about potential for dizziness.
	Antihypertensives, nitrates, alcohol, phenothiazines	Hypotension	Warn patient. Avoid concurrent use if possible. Avoid or reduce alcohol use.
	Potassium supplements, potassium-sparing diuretics	Hyperkalemia	Avoid concurrent use. Teach patient that salt substitutes often are high in potassium. Read label and check with provider before using.
	NSAIDs	Blunted antihypertensive effects	Avoid concurrent use or monitor for need to increase ACEI dose. Teach patient not to take over-the-counter drugs (OTCs) without informing provider.
	Antacids	Decreased absorption of ACEI; increased risk for digitalis or lithium toxicity	Avoid use or separate doses by at least 1 h.
	Allopurinol	Increased risk of hypersensitivity reactions	Avoid concurrent use.
	Capsaicin	Increased incidence of cough	
Captopril	Probenecid	Decreased elimination and increased levels of captopril	Avoid concurrent use.
Enalapril	Rifampin	Decreased effectiveness of enalapril	Monitor for need to increase dose of enalapril or select a different ACEI.
All ATRAs	Cimetidine	Increased effects of ATRA	Select different histamine$_2$ blocking agent.
	Phenobarbital	May decrease effects of ATRA	If use is necessary, monitor for need to change ATRA dose.
	Diuretics, especially thiazide diuretics	Hypotension	Same as for ACEIs.

rior MI, previous MI, Killip class II). They should be continued indefinitely for all patients with left ventricular dysfunction (ejection fractions less than 40%) or symptoms of heart failure and used as needed to manage BP or symptoms in all other patients (SOLVD, 1991). Dosages usual for treating HTN are used unless heart failure is present (Table 14–3).

CONGESTIVE HEART FAILURE. For symptomatic heart failure, the dose is about half that used for HTN. Start low and go slow also applies here. A common problem is the parameters given for systolic blood pressure (SBP) in patients with CHF. In patients with CHF and low ejection fractions (less than 40%), the vasodilating effect of **ACEIs** provides adequate perfusion even with SBP below 90 mm Hg. For patients who cannot tolerate an **ACEI, hydralazine,** in combination with a **long-acting nitrate,** has been shown to be equally effective in reducing morbidity and mortality from CHF.

Asymptomatic patients who have moderately or severely reduced left ventricular ejection fractions (less than 35%) should be treated with an **ACEI** to reduce

Table 14–3. Dosage Schedule: Selected Angiotensin-Converting Enzyme Inhibitors and Angiotensin II Receptor Antagonists

Drug	Starting Dose	Maintenance Dose	Maximum Dose
Angiotensin-Converting Enzyme Inhibitors			
Benazepril	CHF:* HTN: 10 mg qd	CHF:* HTN; 20–40 mg qd	80 mg/d
Captopril	CHF: 6.25–12.5 mg tid HTN: 25 mg bid or tid	CHF: 25–50 mg tid HTN: 50–100 mg tid	450 mg/d
Enalapril	CHF: 2.5 mg bid HTN: 5 mg qd	CHF: 5–10 mg qd HTN: 20 mg qd	40 mg/d
Lisinopril	CHF: 2.5–5 mg qd HTN: 10 mg qd	CHF: 10 mg qd HTN: 20 mg qd	80 mg/d
Angiotensin II Receptor Antagonists			
Candesartan	16 mg qd	8–32 mg qd or bid in divided doses	32 mg/d
Irbesartan	150 mg qd	150–300 mg qd	300 mg/d
Losartan	25–50 mg qd	25–100 mg qd or bid in divided doses	100 mg/d
Valsartan	80 mg qd	80–160 mg qd or bid in divided doses	320 mg/d

*Not yet approved by FDA for treatment of CHF.
CHF = congestive heart failure; HTN = hypertension.

their chance of developing heart failure. The overall recommendation is that **ACEIs** should be prescribed for all patients with left ventricular systolic dysfunction unless specific contraindications exist (DHHS, 1994).

Rational Drug Selection

SHORT-ACTING VERSUS LONG-ACTING. Adverse reactions such as angioedema and renal dysfunction usually occur within the first few doses. Instituting therapy with **captopril,** a short-acting form, enables rapid onset of action, assessment of patient tolerance, and the ability to clear the drug quickly should an adverse reaction occur. **Captopril** requires frequent dosing, and adherence is less likely with this treatment regimen in the long term. Other **ACEIs** have the advantage of once-daily dosing, and as soon as patient tolerance is determined, patients should be converted to these other agents to improve adherence. **ATRAs** also allow once-daily dosing.

COST. ACEIs and ATRAs are expensive. **Captopril** has recently become generic, which has significantly reduced its cost. **Benazepril (Lotensin)** is the next least expensive to date. Initiate therapy with **captopril** for the reasons given previously, and then change to the least expensive long-acting form or to an **ATRA.** Despite the lack of a formal indication for **benazepril** in CHF, many clinicians use it at one-half the HTN dose because of the cost variable.

DIFFICULTY IN SWALLOWING. For patients who have difficulty in swallowing, **ramipril (Altace)** may be a good choice. The capsules may be opened and sprinkled on applesauce, added to apple juice, or dissolved in 4 oz water with no change in the effectiveness of the drug. **Captopril** may be crushed but may have a sulfurous odor and requires bid or tid dosing.

Monitoring

Baseline BP and pulse reading should be taken before initiating therapy, within 1 hour of first dose (when a

Clinical Pearl

Many **ACEIs** have the same cost for different strengths. It is possible to prescribe a high strength of the drug and have the patient halve it to achieve the desired dose, resulting in considerable cost savings.

Clinical Pearl

If you hear an abdominal bruit in a patient known to have vascular disease, give **captopril,** a short-acting **ACEI,** and measure serum creatinine prior to the dose and within 1 or 2 days after the dose. A rapid rise in the creatinine level suggests renal artery stenosis. A slower rise probably indicates a problem with poor hydration that can be corrected by rehydrating the patient and discontinuing or lowering the dose of any **diuretics** the patient is taking.

steep drop in BP may occur), and with each change in dosage. Weight and other indicators of fluid status should also be monitored. See Chapter 38 for further BP monitoring guidelines.

During administration of **ACEIs** and **ATRAs,** monitoring renal function is important. Serum creatinine levels should be drawn before beginning therapy, after the first week of therapy, monthly during the first 3 months, and when increasing the dose. The **ACEI** dose should be reduced if serum creatinine is more than 2.5 mg/dL (National High Blood Pressure Education Program, 1997).

For patients with renal impairment or receiving more **captopril** than 150 mg/day, assess urine protein prior to initiation, every 2 to 4 weeks for the first 3 months of therapy, and regularly thereafter for up to 1 year. Increased proteinuria suggests reevaluation of **ACEI** therapy. For patients on **losartan,** no change in dosage is required based on renal impairment. Initial doses of 25 mg/day of **losartan** are required for patients with impaired hepatic function. Liver function studies should be performed prior to initiating therapy. The dose may be increased as tolerated. According to drug company literature, no patient has had to discontinue the drug because of increased liver function test values.

For **ACEIs,** the white blood cell (WBC) count with differential should be monitored prior to initiation of therapy, monthly for the first 3 to 6 months, and periodically for up to 1 year for patients at risk for neutropenia (renal impairment, collagen vascular disease, high doses). Therapy should be discontinued if the neutrophil count is less than 1000/mm^3.

Patient Education

Patient education focuses on administration of the drug, adverse reactions to expect and appropriate responses to each, and concomitant lifestyle management (Table 14–4).

ADMINISTRATION. The drug should be taken exactly as prescribed, at the same time each day, even if the patient is feeling well. Missed doses should be taken as soon as remembered unless it is almost the time for the next dose. Doses should not be doubled. The **ACEIs** vary on whether food alters absorption (see Table 14–1). **ATRAs** may be administered without regard to food intake.

Drug interactions occur with some over-the-counter (OTC) and prescription drugs. The patient should consult the health care provider before taking any OTC drugs, especially cold remedies. Because they affect prostaglandins, **NSAIDs** may counteract the effects of **ACEIs.** Salt substitutes often contain potassium and should be avoided unless approved by the health care provider.

ADVERSE REACTIONS. Hypotensive reactions are the most common. Changing position slowly, not exercising in hot weather, and keeping fluid intake at more than 2 L/day (noncaffeinated) will decrease these reactions. There is no effective treatment to date for the cough. Changing to another **ACEI** or to an **ATRA** may help. For the few patients who experience impairment in taste, this generally resolves in 8 to 12 weeks, even with continued therapy. Rash is rare and mostly occurs with **captopril.** It should be reported, and a different **ACEI** may be prescribed.

Clinical Pearl

Patients should be monitored for indications of angioedema. Suspect angioedema in any patient who calls the next morning after taking the first dose and complains of voice changes or swollen tongue. Stop the drug immediately. The symptoms recede as the drug is eliminated. Protection of the airway is rarely needed, but careful assessment of airway status is required.

Table 14–4. Available Dosage Forms: Selected Angiotensin-Converting Enzyme Inhibitors and Angiotensin II Receptor Antagonists

Drug	Dosage Form (tablet/capsule)	Other Forms
Angiotensin-Converting Enzyme Inhibitors		
Benazepril (Lotensin)	5 mg, 10 mg, 20 mg, 40 mg	In combination with amlodipine (Lotrel)
Captopril (Capoten)	12.5 mg, 25 mg, 50 mg, 100 mg	In combination with HCTZ (Capozide)
Enalapril (Vasotec)	2.5 mg, 5 mg, 10 mg, 20 mg	In combination with HCTZ (Vaseretic) In combination with felodipine ER (Lexxel)
Fosinopril (Monopril)	10 mg, 20 mg	
Lisinopril (Zestril)	2.5 mg, 5 mg, 10 mg, 20 mg, 40 mg	In combination with HCTZ (Zestoretic)
Moexipril (Univasc)	7.5 mg, 15 mg	
Quinapril (Accupril)	5 mg, 10 mg, 20 mg, 40 mg	
Ramipril (Altace)	1.25 mg, 2.5 mg, 5 mg, 10 mg	
Angiotensin II Receptor Antagonists		
Candesartan (Atacand)	4 mg, 8 mg, 16 mg, 32 mg	
Irbesartan (Avapro)	75 mg, 150 mg, 300 mg	
Losartan (Cozaar)	25 mg, 50 mg	In combination with HCTZ (Hyzaar)
Valsartan (Diovan)	80 mg, 160 mg	

HCTZ = hydrochlorothiazide.

Serious adverse reactions include angioedema and renal failure. If flushing or pallor of the face; hoarseness; swelling of the face, eyes, lips, or tongue; or difficulty in swallowing or breathing occurs, the patient should discontinue the drug and notify the health care provider immediately. Swelling of the feet and ankles and decreased urine output should also be reported.

The *ACEIs* are contraindicated in pregnancy. In women of childbearing age, this topic should be discussed and effective contraception instituted prior to prescription.

LIFESTYLE MANAGEMENT.   A cardiac-healthy lifestyle includes weight loss, aerobic exercise, tobacco avoidance, decreased dietary saturated fats, and moderation in **alcohol** and dietary sodium. Stress management is also important.

Calcium Channel Blockers

Calcium is a vital component in the excitation-contraction process in muscles, in electrical excitation, and in facilitating myocardial relaxation. Calcium enters cells via three types of voltage-dependent calcium channels (L-type, N-type, and T-type). The L-type, or long-lasting, channels are predominant in cardiac and smooth muscle and the ones blocked by most **calcium channel blockers**

(CCBs). One **T-type channel blocker, mibefradil (Posicor)**, originally approved for clinical use has been withdrawn. **CCBs** have multiple indications, including angina, HTN, and selected tachyarrhythmias. Unlabeled indications include migraine headache prophylaxis, Raynaud's syndrome, cardiomyopathy, and esophageal spasm. Laboratory evidence indicates that **CCBs** may interfere with platelet aggregation and reduce the development of atherosclerotic lesions; however, clinical studies have not yet firmly established roles in blood clotting and atherosclerosis in humans.

Pharmacodynamics

As shown in Figure 14–2, contraction of smooth muscles is triggered by an influx of calcium through transmembrane calcium channels. **CCBs** directly block the influx of calcium at the onset of the cycle, like the sodium channel blockade in local anesthetics. The drugs act from the inner side of the membrane and bind to channels in depolarized membranes, converting the mode of operation of the channel from frequent openings to rare openings. The result is a marked decrease in transmembrane calcium content and prolonged vascular smooth muscle relaxation.

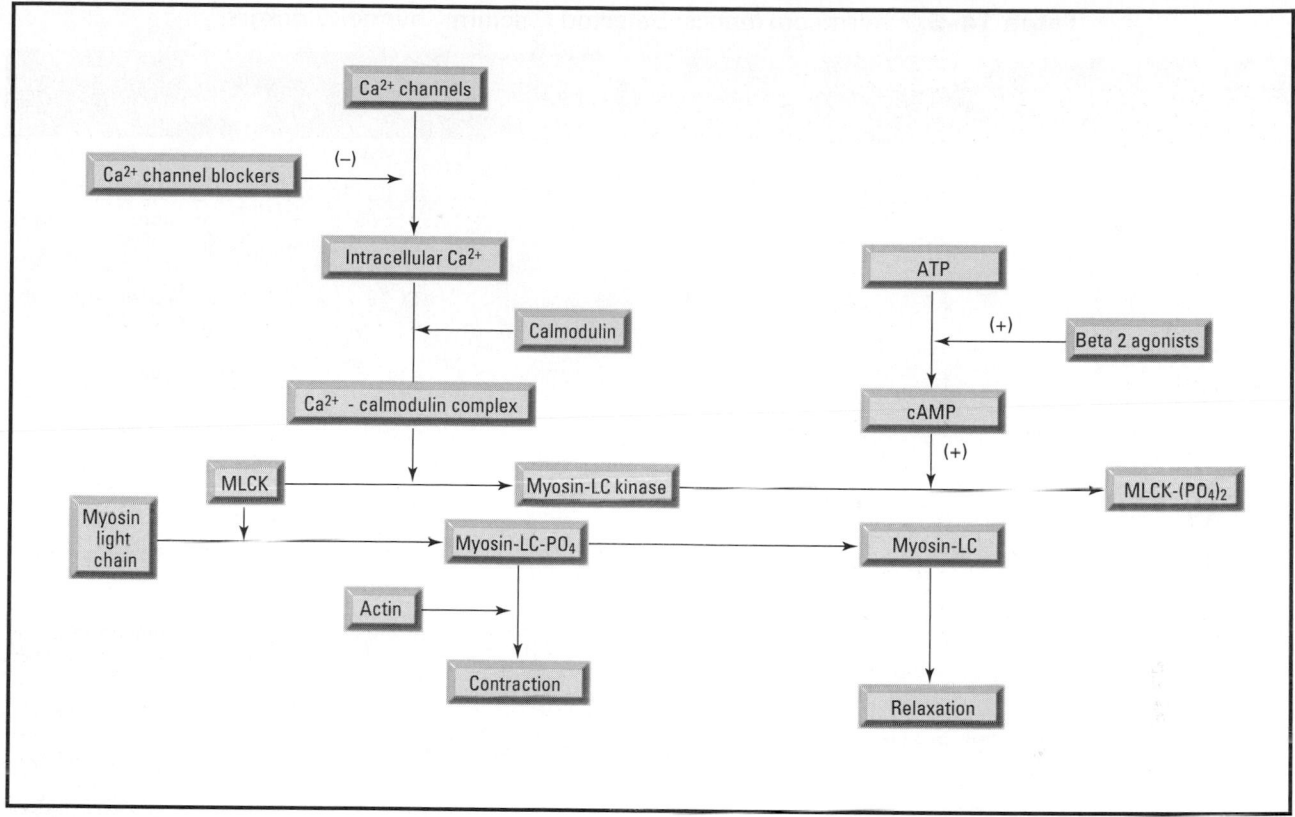

Figure 14–2. Control of smooth muscle contraction. Contraction is triggered by influx of calcium (Ca) through transmembrane calcium channels. The calcium combines with calmodulin to form a complex that converts the enzyme myosin light-chain kinase (MLCK) to its active form. The latter phosphorylates the myosin light chains, initiating the interaction of myosin with actin that produces contraction. Relaxation begins with the re-absorption of calcium, removing it from interaction with the myosin system. Substances that increase cyclic adenosine monophosphate (cAMP), including beta agonists, may cause relaxation in smooth muscle by accelerating the inactivation of MLCK.

The blocking action of **CCBs** occurs via three different receptors: diphenylalkylamine-based and benzothiazepine-based (both type 1 receptors) and dihydropyridine-based (type 2 receptors). The physiological response in the calcium channel is different for these two receptor types, and these differences are important in the clinical choice of **CCB**. All **CCBs** relax arterial smooth muscle but have little effect on venous beds. This results in significant reduction in afterload but limited effect on cardiac preload. In cardiac muscle, reduction in contractility (negative inotropism) and decreases in sinoatrial (SA) and atrioventricular (AV) nodal conduction velocity also occur. Although this is true of all classes of **CCBs**, the greater degree of vasodilation seen in the **dihydropyridines** causes sufficient reflex increase in sympathetic tone to overcome the negative inotropic effects. The effect of a **CCB** on nodal conduction depends on whether it delays slow calcium channel recovery. **Nifedipine (Adalat, Procardia)** and the other **dihydropyridines** do not affect the rate of recovery of these channels. At doses used clinically, they do not affect conduction through the AV node. In contrast, **verapamil (Calan, Isoptin)** not only affects openings of calcium channels but also decreases the rate of recovery, resulting in depression of the SA node firing rate and slowing of AV nodal conduction. This is the basis of its use in treating supraventricular tachycardias. **Verapamil** also has a direct negative inotropic effect.

Pharmacokinetics

Absorption and Distribution

All **CCBs** are well absorbed orally, but there is variance in bioavailability among them (Table 14–5). **Verapamil** and **diltiazem (Cardizem)**, prototype **type 1 CCBs**, are rapidly absorbed but rapidly metabolized to yield bioavailabilities of 20 to 35 percent and 40 to 65 percent, respectively. The **dihydropyridines (type 2 CCBs)** are absorbed at varying rates, and their bioavailabilities vary from 65 to 90 percent for **amlodipine (Norvasc)** to 15 to 20 percent for **felodipine (Plendil)**. The presence of food in the gut does not affect bioavailability in any of these drugs. **Nifedipine** may also be administered sublingually, with slightly more rapid onset of action but with less bioavailability than when bitten and swallowed. **Nifedipine, verapamil,** and **diltiazem** are avail-

Table 14–5. Pharmacokinetics: Selected Calcium Channel Blockers

Drug	Onset	Peak (h)	Duration (h)	Protein Binding	Oral Bioavailability	Half-life (h)	Elimination
CCB: dihydropyridines							
Amlodipine	1 h	6–12	24+	>93%	65–90%	30–50 (56 in hepatic impairment)	10% drug and 60% metabolite in urine
Felodipine	1 h	2.5–5	24	>99%	15–20%	11–16	<0.5% unchanged in urine
Isradipine	<2 h	1.5	12	95%	15–24%	8	Unknown
Nicardipine PO	20 min	1–2	8	95%	35%	2–4	<1% unchanged in urine
Nicardipine SR	2–4 h		12–24				
Nifedipine PO	20 min	0.5–1	6–8	90%	45–70%	2–5	1–2% unchanged in urine
Nifedipine XL	20 min	6–8	24	92–98%	86%	2–5	1–2% unchanged in urine
Nifedipine bite or SL	5–15 min	0.5					
CCB: type 1							
Diltiazem PO	30 min	2–3	6–8	70–80%	40–65%	3–6	2–4% unchanged in urine
Diltiazem SR/CD	30–60 min	6–11	24	70–80%	67%	5–7	2–4% unchanged in urine
Verapamil PO	30 min	0.5–1	3–7	90%	20–35%	4.5–12	3–4% unchanged in urine
Verapamil SR	1–2 h	5–7	24	88–92%		4–12	3–4% unchanged in urine

able in very rapid acting intravenous (IV) forms. This latter form is not used in primary care.

Distribution is to most body tissues, with only **nimodipine (Nimotop)** crossing the blood-brain barrier. All cross the placenta. **Verapamil, diltiazem,** and **nicardipine (Cardene)** are excreted extensively in breast milk. **Nifedipine** is excreted at less than 5 percent in breast milk, making it the drug of choice during lactation.

Metabolism and Excretion

All **CCBs** are extensively metabolized by the liver. **Diltiazem** and its metabolites are eliminated in feces. **Verapamil** is eliminated in both urine and feces. The **dihydropyridines** are eliminated in urine. Dosage reduction based on renal impairment is recommended only for **nicardipine.**

Most **CCBs** have short-acting forms with half-lives between 2 and 8 hours and sustained-release forms with half-lives of 12 to 24 hours. **Amlodipine** is the exception,

with a half-life of 30 to 50 hours. Reduced adverse reactions are seen with the use of sustained-release forms.

Pharmacotherapeutics

Precautions and Contraindications

Verapamil has the strongest negative inotropic effect and should be avoided in CHF, where this effect can worsen the disorder. It also has the strongest effect on nodal conduction and can significantly worsen bradycardia. **Diltiazem** also affects nodal conduction and can worsen or cause bradycardia, although less than verapamil. None of the **CCBs** are drugs of choice immediately after MI, but **diltiazem** has shown some benefit in reducing mortality in non-Q-wave MI for a selected group of patients whose ejection fractions are above 40 percent. For those with ejection fractions below 40 percent and for all other patients early after MI, **type 1 CCBs** are

Clinical Pearl

....

Amlodipine can also be crushed and put down a nasogastric (NG) tube, which is not possible with sustained-release preparations. This provides the clinical advantage of acting as if **amlodipine** were sustained release with less venous pooling, less reflex tachycardia, and once-daily dosing.

....

contraindicated because of their negative inotropic and bradycardic effects. Patients with ventricular dysfunction, SA or AV nodal conduction disturbances, and SBPs below 90 mm Hg should not be treated with **type 1 CCBs** because of the high risk for induction of heart failure and significant hypotension. The **dihydropyridines** are less dependent on the heart for their effects, but they are still not the drugs of choice after MI. **Dihydropyridines** should also be avoided for patients with significant peripheral edema. Their strong peripheral vasodilating effects result in peripheral pooling of blood and may lead to reflex tachycardia. They are also contraindicated in unstable angina because of their potential to cause tachycardia. Short-acting forms more commonly cause these problems, and the short-acting form of **nifedipine** resulted in increased morbidity and mortality when used to treat patients post-MI and with CHF. If it is necessary to give a **dihydropyridine** to a patient who has peripheral edema or a tachyrhythm disturbance, the sustained-release forms are preferred. All **CCBs** should be used cautiously in severe hepatic impairment, with dosage reduction recommended for most agents.

All **CCBs** relax smooth muscle contractions of the esophagus and are sometimes used to treat esophageal spasm. This relaxation makes gastroesophageal reflux disease (GERD) worse, and **CCBs** should be avoided for patients with this disorder.

Based on teratogenic and embryotoxic effects demonstrated in small animals, *CCBs* **are Pregnancy Category C. They should be used only when benefits clearly outweigh risks. Crawford (1995) suggests that** *verapamil* **may be used in pregnant patients who develop atrial fibrillation with rapid ventricular response. Although data on the use of** *verapamil* **in pregnancy are** **limited, he states that no reported adverse fetal effects have been reported with this short-term use.**

Adverse Drug Reactions

The more common adverse reactions of **CCBs** are extensions of their actions. Reduction in BP secondary to vasodilation may result in dizziness, headache, hypotension, and syncope. These reactions occur less often in long-acting formulations. Decreased myocardial contractility may lead to heart failure with congestion, shortness of breath, cough, and palpitations. Gastrointestinal (GI) symptoms are especially disturbing to patients and include dry mouth, nausea, vomiting, and constipation.

Although not common, sexual dysfunction and gynecomastia may occur. Hyperglycemia is also uncommon but may affect the choice of the drug in patients with diabetes. Other common adverse reactions, such as peripheral edema, dysrhythmias, and heart failure, are discussed in the precautions section.

The highest rate of adverse reactions is found in the short-acting **dihydropyridines** (17%), especially **nifedipine,** and the lowest rate in **amlodipine** (less than 1%). All adverse drug reactions for **CCBs** are less common with sustained-release forms because the amount of drug in the system at any given time is more stable.

Drug Interactions

Additive hypotensive effects are major concerns with all **CCBs** given concurrently with other **antihypertensives, nitrates, quinidine,** or **alcohol.** Antihypertensive effects may be decreased with concurrent use of **NSAIDs. Verapamil, diltiazem,** and some **dihydropyridines** have an additive bradycardic effect with **beta-adrenergic block-**

Clinical Pearl

....

Constipation is especially common with **verapamil,** with almost 100% of patients experiencing significant constipation. Patients taking this drug should be encouraged to increase the fiber in their diet and may need to have a stool softener ordered.

....

ers (BBs) or digoxin. Serum **digoxin** levels may be increased with risk of toxicity when it is concurrently used with **verapamil, diltiazem,** or **nifedipine. Verapamil** may decrease the effectiveness of **rifampin,** and the effectiveness of **verapamil** may be decreased by concurrent administration of vitamin D and calcium. **Verapamil** may also alter serum lithium levels. CYP 3A4 isoenzymes are involved in the metabolism of **diltiazem, felodipine, nifedipine,** and **verapamil.** Drugs that inhibit this system, including grapefruit juice, may increase free drug levels. Specific drug interactions and appropriate actions to prevent them are found in Table 14–6.

Clinical Use and Dosing

CHRONIC STABLE ANGINA. Both type 1 and type 2 CCBs are effective in the treatment of stable and exertional angina (Table 14–7). They act on both sides of the supply-demand equation: peripheral vasodilation and negative inotropism reduce oxygen demand; dilation of coronary arteries increases oxygen supply.

Among the **dihydropyridines, nifedipine, nicardipine,** and **amlodipine** are drugs of choice. The long-acting form of **nifedipine (Procardia XL)** is the most often prescribed. Combining this drug with **propranolol (Inderal),** a **BB,** has proved more effective than either agent given alone, possibly because the **BB** suppresses the reflex tachycardia that may occur with type 2 **CCBs.**

Nicardipine is structurally similar to **nifedipine** but less likely to cause hypotension and left ventricular dysfunction. It is useful for patients with angina who also have mild heart failure or borderline HTN. **Amlodipine** is well tolerated, with less venous pooling and minimal

Table 14–6. Drug Interactions: Selected Calcium Channel Blockers

Drug	Interacting Drug	Possible Effect	Implications
All CCBs	Fentanyl, nitrates, anti-hypertensives, acute alcohol ingestion, quinidine	Additive hypotension	Monitor for orthostatic changes. Warn patient. Reduce or avoid alcohol use.
	NSAIDs	Decreased antihypertensive effects	Warn patient. Avoid concurrent use or monitor therapeutic response and adjust CCB dose.
Verapamil, diltiazem, nifedipine	Digoxin	Increased serum digoxin levels	Monitor for digoxin toxicity. Teach signs and symptoms to report to provider.
	CYP-450 3A4 inhibitors (including grapefruit juice)	Decreased hepatic clearance of CCB with increased risk of toxicity to CCB	Monitor for orthostatic changes, rate and rhythm changes.
	Calcium salts, vitamin D	Reduced response to CCB	Avoid concurrent use. If use is necessary, monitor therapeutic response and adjust CCB dose.
	Cyclosporine, prazosin, quinidine, theophylline, carbamazepine	Decreased metabolism of these drugs and increased toxicity risk	Monitor therapeutic levels and signs and symptoms of toxicity.
Verapamil, diltiazem, felodipine, isradipine, nicardipine, nifedipine, nimodipine	Beta-adrenergic blockers, digoxin, disopyramide, phenytoin	Myocardial depression, bradycardia, conduction defects, CHF	Do not administer within 24 h of each other. If you must give both, monitor for heart failure and decreased peripheral perfusion.
Diltiazem	Phenobarbital, phenytoin	Increased metabolism and decreased effect of diltiazem	Avoid concurrent use. Select different anticonvulsant.
	Cyclosporine	Enhanced action of cyclosporine	Monitor renal function with blood urea nitrogen (BUN) and creatinine levels. Monitor cyclosporine levels.
Verapamil	Rifampin	Decreased effect of rifampin	Avoid concurrent use. Select different CCB if rifampin is needed to treat tuberculosis.
	Lithium	Altered serum lithium levels with increased toxicity risk	Avoid concurrent use. Select different CCB.

Table 14–7. Dosage Schedule: Selected Calcium Channel Blockers

Drug	Starting Dose	Maintenance Dose	Maximum Dose
Amlodipine	5 mg qd	5–10 mg qd	10 mg qd
Diltiazem PO	30 mg q6–8h	30–90 mg q6–8h	240 mg/d
Diltiazem CD	120 mg qd	120–180 mg qd	300 mg/d
Diltiazem SR	60 mg q12h	60–120 mg q12h	240 mg/d
Felodipine	2.5 mg qd	2.5–5 mg qd	20 mg/d
Isradipine	2.5 mg q12h	2.5–5 mg q12h	20 mg/d
Nicardipine PO	60 mg tid	60 mg tid	120 mg/d
Nicardipine SR	60 mg q12h	60 mg q12h	120 mg/d
Nifedipine (Adalat CC)	30 mg	30–60 mg qd	90 mg/d
Nifedipine (Procardia XL)	30 mg	30–60 mg qd	120 mg/d
Verapamil PO	80 mg tid	80–160 mg tid	480 mg/d
Verapamil SR	120 mg qd or q12h	120–240 mg qd or q12h	480 mg/d

reflex tachycardia, and is safe to use for patients with significant ventricular dysfunction. In addition, its long half-life means it acts like a sustained-release form. Although sustained-release forms of the other drugs cannot be crushed, **amlodipine** can be crushed so that patients who have difficulty in swallowing or who have nasogastric (NG) tubes can use this drug and still benefit from the reduced adverse effects associated with sustained release. The dose is 5 mg initially, with a maximum dose of 10 mg. Doses higher than 10 mg have not demonstrated any increase in benefit. **Amlodipine** has been used in combination with several **BBs** to produce improved response. The long acting form of each of these drugs offers once-daily dosing, which improves adherence.

Diltiazem, also effective in angina therapy, is less likely to cause hypotension and other adverse responses associated with peripheral vasodilation (reflex tachycardia) than **nifedipine,** and it has less negative inotropic activity than **verapamil.** The reduction in average daily heart rate associated with this drug improves coronary artery filling time and myocardial oxygen supply. Of the type 1 drugs, it is most often chosen because of its low adverse drug response profile. **Diltiazem** is a good choice for patients who need to reduce their heart rate. **Verapamil** is more often prescribed for treatment of arrhythmias because it has the most potent negative inotropic effect and significantly slows AV nodal conduc-

tion. It is not used for patients with compromised left ventricular function, bradycardia, or AV block. **Verapamil** might be chosen for patients with supraventricular tachycardia who also have angina.

VASOSPASTIC (VARIANT, PRINZMETAL'S) ANGINA. CCBs that produce more coronary artery vasodilation and reduce vasospasm are the drugs of choice. **Diltiazem, long-acting nifedipine,** and **amlodipine** are the most commonly used.

UNSTABLE ANGINA. Medical therapy for unstable angina involves **nitrates, BBs,** and **heparin,** which are effective in controlling pain, and **aspirin,** which reduces mortality. When vasospasm is a component of this angina, **CCBs** may offer an additional treatment. There is insufficient evidence at this time, however, to indicate whether this addition decreases mortality. When a **CCB** is chosen, **verapamil** is the drug of choice. **Type 2 CCBs** are contraindicated because they tend to increase heart rate and have less vasospastic protection. Because **verapamil** is often given in combination with other drugs that lower BP, hypotension is a serious potential adverse response.

HYPERTENSION. Initial drug therapy for HTN is monotherapy. Because **diuretics** and **BBs** have been shown to reduce cardiovascular morbidity and mortality in controlled trials, these two classes of drugs are preferred as initial therapy. (National High Blood Pressure Education

Clinical Pearl

The delivery system for **nifedipine (Procardia XL)** is excreted in the feces as a whole orange capsule. This does not mean that the liquid drug inside the capsule was not absorbed. To avoid alarm, the patient should be warned about this.

Program, 1997). **CCBs** are equally effective in reducing BP, but there is insufficient research to date to demonstrate their efficacy in reducing morbidity and mortality, and they should be reserved for special indications or used when **diuretics** and **BBs** have proved ineffective. Special indications include black patients, who, as a group, are more responsive to diuretics and **CCBs** than they are to **BBs** or **ACEIs**. **CCBs** would also be appropriate for patients with certain concomitant pathologies such as asthma, in which **BBs** are contraindicated.

When a **CCB** is chosen, **amlodipine** is especially good for patients with left ventricular dysfunction and CHF. **Long-acting nifedipine, diltiazem,** or **verapamil** may be used for patients with coronary artery disease (CAD). **Long-acting nifedipine** is a good choice as well for patients who also have peripheral vascular disease because of its peripheral vasodilating effect.

For all **CCBs,** older adults usually require a starting dose about half the usual dose, and increases in dosage should be gradual to reduce adverse drug responses. (See Chapter 38 for further discussion.)

SUPRAVENTRICULAR TACHYCARDIA AND ATRIAL FIBRILLA-TION. Type 1 **CCBs** are useful in treating selected supraventricular tachycardias because they slow AV nodal conduction. **Verapamil** (80 to 120 mg orally) can be used to terminate the rhythm. Conversion usually occurs in about 1 hour. **Diltiazem** (40 to 80 mg orally) can also be tried. Prophylaxis with **verapamil** (240 to 480 mg/day) is effective for patients with paroxysmal supraventricular tachycardia (PSVT). It is important to be certain that the rhythm is not ventricular; **verapamil** may worsen ventricular rhythm disturbances because of its negative inotropic effects. **Verapamil** is also used as an alternative to **digoxin** to slow a rapid ventricular response in the treatment of atrial fibrillation through its direct effect on the AV node, prolonging its refractory period and conduction time. Doses are similar to those used for PSVT. If it must be used concurrently with **digoxin,** the **digoxin** level must be evaluated frequently because **verapamil** slows the clearance of **digoxin** and may increase the risk of toxicity.

MIGRAINE HEADACHE PROPHYLAXIS. Migraine prophylaxis is an unlabeled indication for **CCBs.** Of patients with frequent migraines for whom **CCBs** are prescribed, 30 percent report a 30 percent reduction in migraines. The **CCB** used most often is **verapamil** (240 to 480 mg/day). To facilitate adherence, it is best to use the sustained-release form to permit once-daily dosing. The trial to determine effectiveness should last at least 3 months. Failure to give an adequate dose or an adequate trial time is a common reason for failure of migraine prophylaxis.

RAYNAUD'S SYNDROME. This is also an unlabeled indication. **Type 2 CCBs** are the **CCB** choice for this disorder because of their peripheral vasodilating effects and some platelet inhibition. The drug most studied and the first choice is **long-acting nifedipine.** The initial dose is 10 mg orally given in the office to assess the effect on BP. If the patient does not experience a drop in SBP more than 20 mm Hg below baseline or a drop below 90 mm Hg, then 10 mg orally tid is prescribed. The dose may be increased by 10 mg/day every 3 to 4 days to a maximum of 30 mg tid to achieve the desired effect. Monitoring every 2 to 4 months is necessary because the initial response may be transient. If **nifedipine** does not work, **diltiazem** may be tried, beginning at 30 mg qid and increasing every 3 to 4 days until a maximum of 120 mg qid is reached. **Felodipine** and **isradipine (DynaCirc)** are also powerful **vasodilators** and may be tried. Research is absent on their use. Raynaud symptoms are often present only during cold exposure. Drugs may be stopped during the summer months.

ESOPHAGEAL SPASM. Although this is an unlabeled indication, **CCBs** may offer transient improvement for patients with mild spasm. **Short-acting nifedipine** (10 to 30 mg qid) or **diltiazem** (90 mg qid) have been used. Because these drugs make GERD worse, this disorder must be ruled out before a **CCB** is prescribed.

Because these drugs are Pregnancy Category C, female patients capable of childbearing should be made aware of the risks of these drugs, and contraception should be instituted before *CCBs* are prescribed.

Rational Drug Selection

SHORT-ACTING VERSUS LONG-ACTING. Short-acting forms of **CCBs** have been associated with more adverse drug reactions. In several trials, the short-acting form of **nifedipine** was associated with increased mortality at higher doses in post-MI patients. All **type 2 CCBs** cause vasodilation that results in reflex tachycardia and peripheral pooling of blood. These actions are greatly reduced in the long-acting forms. To reduce adverse drug reactions and improve adherence, long-acting forms should be used.

COST. **CCBs** are expensive. **Verapamil** is the least expensive, but its adverse reaction profile includes significant constipation in almost 100 percent of patients. Although this reaction can be mitigated by the concurrent prescription of a stool softener, the cost advantage is lost by the additional cost of the stool softener. The sustained-release form of **diltiazem** is the most expensive **CCB** and must be given bid. The remaining drugs fall between these two. Cost may be a factor in choosing to use a **CCB,** but it is not a major factor in choosing among them.

DIFFICULTY IN SWALLOWING OR NG TUBE PLACEMENT. Only **amlodipine** can be crushed and mixed with food for patients who have difficulty swallowing; it can also be put down an NG tube.

Monitoring

Liver function should be evaluated prior to initiating therapy. Dosage reductions for most **CCBs** are recommended with severe hepatic impairment because of the extensive metabolism of these drugs by the liver.

Patient Education

ADMINISTRATION. The drug should be taken exactly as prescribed, at the same time each day, even if the patient is feeling well. Sustained-release drugs taken once daily are best taken in the morning for therapeutic effect. Missed doses should be taken as soon as remembered unless it is almost the time for the next dose. Doses should not be doubled. Sudden withdrawal may precipitate myocardial ischemia so withdrawal is gradual. **CCBs** cannot relieve acute anginal attacks. If acute chest pain occurs, the health care provider should be contacted immediately or the patient should go to the nearest hospital. For patients taking **isradipine** or **nifedipine**, anginal attacks sometimes occur 30 minutes after administration because of reflex tachycardia. This is usually temporary and not necessarily an indication for stopping the drug, but this symptom should be reported to the health care provider.

Several of the **CCBs** come in more than one form, from short-acting drugs requiring multiple doses daily to long-acting drugs with once-daily dosing (Table 14–8). The patient has to read the label carefully and follow the appropriate dosing schedule. This is especially important if a different form or a different **CCB** is prescribed.

The **CCBs** may be taken without regard to food intake with the exception of **diltiazem**, which is best absorbed if taken before meals.

Drug interactions occur with some OTC and prescription drugs and with **alcohol.** The patient should consult the health care provider before taking any OTC drugs, especially cold remedies.

ADVERSE REACTIONS. Hypotensive reactions are the most common. Changing position slowly, not exercising in hot weather, and keeping intake of noncaffeinated fluids above 2 L/day will decrease these reactions. Bradycardia is also possible, especially for patients on **type 2 CCBs.** Patients should learn how to monitor their own pulse rate and contact the health care provider if the rate is less than 50 beats per minute (bpm) or has irregular beats. Heart failure may also develop. Report dyspnea, pronounced dizziness, or nausea. **Type 1 CCBs** more commonly exhibit peripheral edema. Report swelling of hands and feet or ankles and decreased urine output.

Constipation is especially a problem for **verapamil** but may occur with other **CCBs.** The patient should increase dietary fiber and report this adverse response to the health care provider. Stool softeners may be prescribed prophylactically with **verapamil** and for treatment with other **CCBs.**

Wearing protective clothing and using sunscreen will prevent photosensitivity reactions.

LIFESTYLE MANAGEMENT. See ACEIs.

Cardiac Glycosides

Cardiac glycosides (CG) are among the oldest known drugs. They have been medically recognized in the treatment of heart failure since 1785. Although there are three main glycosides available, **digoxin** is by far the most commonly prescribed because of its convenient

Table 14–8. Available Dosage Forms: Selected Calcium Channel Blockers

Drugs	Dosage Form (tablet/capsule)	Other Forms
Amlodipine (Norvasc)	2.5 mg, 5 mg, 10 mg	In combination with benazepril (Lotrel)
Diltiazem (Cardizem)	30 mg, 60 mg, 90 mg, 120 mg SR: 60 mg, 90 mg, 120 mg CD: 120 mg, 180 mg, 240 mg, 300 mg XR: 180 mg, 240 mg	
Felodipine (Plendil)	ER: 5 mg, 10 mg	In combination with enalapril (Lexxel)
Isradipine (DynaCirc)	2.5 mg, 5 mg	
Nicardipine (Cardene)	20 mg, 30 mg SR: 30 mg, 45 mg, 60 mg	
Nifedipine (Adalat, Procardia)	CC: 30 mg, 60 mg, 90 mg XL: 30 mg, 60 mg, 90 mg	
Verapamil (Calan, Isoptin)	40 mg, 80 mg, 120 mg SR: 120 mg, 180 mg, 240 mg	

pharmacokinetics, the alternative routes of administration, and the techniques for monitoring its serum level. This section focuses on **digoxin** and its use in treating supraventricular tachycardias and heart failure.

Pharmacodynamics

Mechanical Effects on Heart Muscle

All **CGs** are strong and highly selective inhibitors of the sodium-potassium-adenosine triphosphatase (ATPase) system: the "sodium pump." The preferential binding of **CGs** to ATPase occurs following phosphorylation of the alpha subunit of the enzyme. Extracellular potassium promotes dephosphorylation of the enzyme and decreases the affinity of the enzyme for the **CG**. This may explain why increased extracellular potassium reverses some of the toxic effects of these drugs.

The sodium pump is the major determinant of the concentration of sodium in the cell. As shown in Figure 14–3, inhibition of this pump results in sodium and calcium buildup inside the cell. The combination of the changes in sodium and calcium results in increased velocity of the shortening of cardiac muscle, with a shift upward and to the left in the ventricular function curve. This causes an increase in stroke work for a given filling volume or pressure (positive inotropism).

Electrical Effects on Heart Muscle

A mixture of direct and autonomic actions produce the electrical effects (negative chronotropism) seen with **CGs.** At therapeutic levels, **CGs** decrease automaticity and conduction velocity through the AV node via central vagal stimulation and facilitation of muscarinic transmission at the cardiac muscle cell. Because cholinergic innervation is more prevalent in the atria, these actions affect atrial and AV nodal function more than Purkinje or ventricular function.

Other Effects

Several studies suggest that these drugs may also decrease plasma renin activity, reduce plasma norepineph-

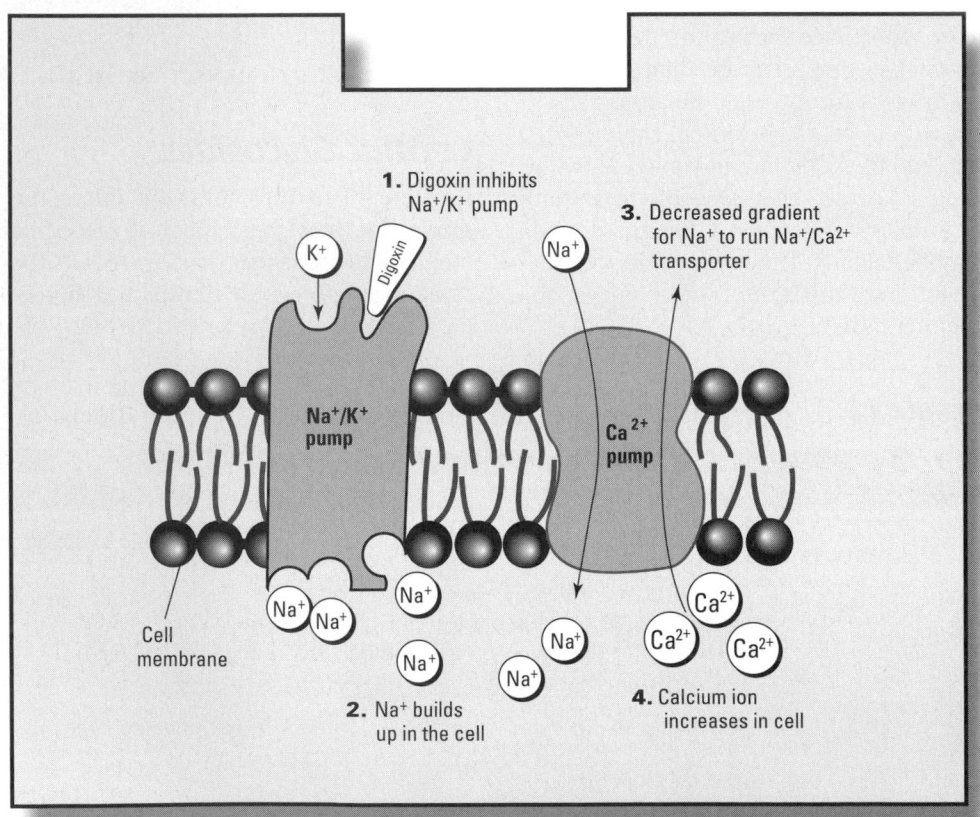

Figure 14–3. Effects of digoxin on the sodium-potassium pump. The sodium pump is the major determinant of the concentration of sodium in the cell. Inhibition of this pump results in sodium buildup inside the cell. The resultant decrease in sodium gradient reduces the sodium-calcium transport mechanism and calcium ions also increase inside the cell. The influx of sodium through voltage-gated channels is a major determinant in cardiac action potentials. This influx is reduced when the sodium gradient is decreased. Ultimately, contraction of cardiac muscle results from the interaction of calcium with the actin-myosin system. Reduced extracellular calcium levels decrease this contraction.

rine levels, and restore baroreceptor sensitivity, all of which are factors in heart failure pathology. **CGs** affect all smooth excitable tissues, including smooth muscle and the CNS. These actions on other tissues explain many of their adverse responses.

Pharmacokinetics

Absorption and Distribution

Digoxin is well absorbed orally (Table 14–9). Approximately 10 percent of individuals, however, have intestinal bacteria that inactivate **digoxin** in the gut, greatly reducing bioavailability and requiring higher-than-average doses to produce a therapeutic response. Treatment of these individuals with antibiotics can cause a sudden increase in bioavailability that results in toxicity. Product formulation may also be a factor in bioavailability. Generic tablet preparations have a bioavailability of 70 to 80 percent; the bioavailability is 90 to 100 percent for **digoxin** elixir and encapsulated gel. The narrow safety margin between therapeutic effect, loss of effect, and toxicity means that even small variations in bioavailability can have serious consequences. It is best to prescribe by brand.

Once absorbed, **CGs** are widely distributed to tissues, including the CNS. **Digoxin's** volume of distribution is large (4 to 7 L/kg) and dependent on plasma protein-binding capacity. Its highest tissue concentration (10 to 50 times that in plasma) is found in heart, kidney, and liver. The principal tissue reservoir is skeletal muscle, so dosing is based on lean muscle mass. Neonates and infants tolerate and seem to require higher doses to achieve a therapeutic effect than older children and adults.

Digoxin crosses the placenta, and drug levels in maternal and umbilical vein blood are similar.

Metabolism and Excretion

Digoxin is not extensively metabolized and is excreted largely unchanged by the kidneys. Its half-life is 36 to 48 hours with normal or near-normal renal function. In the absence of oral or IV loading doses, steady state is achieved in about four half-lives or 1 week. Its clearance rate is proportional to the GFR and is similar for neonates, infants, children, and adults. For patients with elevated serum creatinine levels, drug clearance closely parallels creatinine clearance. Improvement in cardiac output and renal blood flow through therapy with a variety of agents may increase renal **digoxin** clearance and require dosage adjustments. Several drugs (most notably **quinidine, amiodarone, verapamil,** and **diltiazem**) reduce clearance and can double the serum concentration, resulting in toxicity unless the dose of **digoxin** is reduced.

Pharmacotherapeutics

Precautions and Contraindications

CGs are contraindicated in AV blocks and uncontrolled ventricular arrhythmias because their action on the AV node may worsen the arrhythmia. Patients with idiopathic hypertrophic subaortic stenosis (IHSS) may develop worsening outflow tract obstruction with **CG** use because of the action of **CGs** on myocardial contractility. Their use in cor pulmonale is questionable. Although they may be beneficial for some patients, toxicity risk increases in the presence of hypoxia.

Because **digoxin** is excreted essentially unchanged by the kidneys, renal impairment suggests cautious use and close monitoring. Hypothyroidism and chronic renal failure decrease **digoxin's** volume of distribution, necessitating a decrease in both loading and maintenance doses. **Digitoxin** is metabolized in the liver and excreted via bile into the gut and may be a good choice for pa-

Table 14–9. Pharmacokinetics: Cardiac Glycosides

Drug	Onset	Peak	Duration	Protein Binding	Oral Bioavail-ability	Half-Life	Time to Steady State	Volume of Distribution	Elimination
Digoxin PO	1–2 h	6–8 h	2–4 d	20–40%	50–75%	NRF: 36–48 h IRF: prolonged	1 wk or 4 doses	6.3 L/kg	Unchanged by kidney
Digoxin IM	30 min	4–6 h	2–4 d	20–40%	50–75%	NRF: 36–48 h IRF: prolonged	1 wk or 4 doses	6.3 L/kg	Unchanged by kidney
Digitoxin	30 min–2 h	4–12 h	2–3 wk	>90%	>90%	NRF: 4–6 d IRF: not prolonged		0.6 L/kg	Metabolized by liver; excreted into gut via bile

NRF = normal renal function; IRF = impaired renal function.

tients with renal impairment. **Digoxin** may be used safely in renal impairment as long as renal function and necessary dosage adjustments are made.

CGs are used cautiously for patients with electrolyte abnormalities because the concentrations of potassium, calcium, and magnesium in the extracellular compartment affect sensitivity to **CGs** and may result in **digitalis** toxicity. **Digoxin** may exacerbate atrial fibrillation due to Wolff-Parkinson-White syndrome by facilitating conduction through the bypass tract and shortening its refractory period. It should not be used to treat this disorder.

Older adults are particularly at risk for toxic effects because of altered renal clearance; they require slower digitalization and careful monitoring.

Because 20 to 30 percent of **digoxin** is bound to plasma proteins, diseases that lower serum albumin may require alterations in loading doses.

Digoxin **is a Pregnancy Category C drug. Although safety has not been formally established,** *digoxin* **has been used safely in pregnancy for many years without adverse effects to the fetus. Blood levels should be monitored carefully during this time to avoid toxicity.**

Adverse Drug Reactions

The GI tract is the most common site of adverse drug reactions, including anorexia, nausea, vomiting, and diarrhea. These result from CNS actions, including chemoreceptor trigger zone stimulation. Other CNS-based adverse responses include fatigue, disorientation, depression, and hallucinations, especially in older adults, and visual disturbances, including yellow vision and green halos around lights. The visual disturbances are considered classic signs of toxicity but actually occur rarely. Atrial arrhythmias and atrial tachycardia with AV block are the most common signs of toxicity in children. Cardiac adverse reactions are extensions of the therapeutic action of these drugs (bradycardia, junctional and AV block arrhythmias, premature ventricular contractions (PVCs), and bigeminy). Gynecomastia is a rare adverse reaction reported in some men.

TOXICITY. Toxicity is commonly caused by excessive administration of a **CG**, by too much diuresis resulting in hypokalemia, by concurrent development of renal insufficiency, or by administration of drugs that interfere with excretion of **digoxin** (see Drug Interactions). It is especially common in older adults. Each of these common etiologies and the patient's calcium and magnesium levels should be considered in the differential diagnosis.

Diagnosis of toxicity is based on both clinical and laboratory data. Serum levels alone are insufficient to diagnose toxicity because there is considerable overlap in serum concentrations between those with and without evidence of toxicity (see Monitoring for times to draw serum levels). **Toxicity commonly occurs with serum levels above 2 ng/mL.** Recognition of **CG** toxicity is an important differential diagnosis of arrhythmias and neurological and GI symptoms for patients taking **CGs**. The more common arrhythmias were listed previously.

Treatment of toxicity depends on the problem. AV junctional and first-degree block rhythms, ventricular ectopic beats, or an excessively slow ventricular response to atrial fibrillation often requires **CG** dosage adjustment and careful monitoring. Potassium administration should be considered to reduce automaticity, even when serum potassium is in the normal range, unless a high-grade AV block is also present. **Lidocaine** has minimal effects on the AV node and may be used to treat ventricular ectopic beats that threaten hemodynamics. Bradycardia and second- or third-degree AV block usually respond to **atropine.** When toxicity is severe or life-threatening, the antidote for **CG** toxicity is antidigoxin immunotherapy, **digoxin immune fab (Digibind).** Patients who require this medication are hospitalized so that cardiopulmonary resuscitation equipment and medications are available when it is administered.

Any patient who becomes toxic to a **CG** should have the indications for that drug carefully reviewed. In some cases, it is possible to stop the drug altogether. Several studies, however, have shown negative consequences for withdrawal of **digoxin** (Packer et al., 1993; Uretsky et al., 1993), so the decision should be carefully made.

Drug Interactions

Any drug that may cause hypokalemia, hypercalcemia, or hypomagnesemia increases the risk of toxicity. Several **antiarrhythmic drugs (quinidine, amiodarone,**

Clinical Pearl

A full neutralizing dose of **Digibind** is relatively expensive ($2000 to $3000). This cost should be considered in deciding to treat patients with suspected or non-life-threatening toxicity. It should also be remembered that **Digibind** has a half-life of 2 to 6 hours, and during that time the rhythm disturbance for which the **CG** was given may recur and cannot be treated with a **CG**.

verapamil, **diltiazem**, and **propafenone**) increase serum **CG** levels and toxicity risk. Drugs that can have an adverse response of bradycardia can exhibit additive bradycardia when given with **CGs**. This is especially a concern with **BBs**. **Antacids** and **kaolin-pectin** interfere with absorption.

INTERACTIONS WITH POTASSIUM, CALCIUM, AND MAGNESIUM. **Potassium** and **CGs** interact by inhibiting each other's binding to sodium-potassium-ATPase. Hyperkalemia reduces the enzyme-inhibiting actions of **CGs**, and hypokalemia facilitates these actions. Hyperkalemia, however, inhibits the abnormal cardiac automaticity seen in excessive doses of **CGs** so that moderately increased extracellular potassium reduces toxic effects of **CGs**. **Calcium** facilitates the toxic actions of **CGs** by overloading the intracellular calcium stores. Hypercalcemia increases the risk of **CG**-induced arrhythmias. **Magnesium** has the opposite effects to **calcium**. Hypomagnesemia is a risk factor for arrhythmias. Specific drug interactions and the appropriate actions to prevent them are given in Table 14–10.

Clinical Use and Dosing

ATRIAL FIBRILLATION, PAROXYSMAL SUPRAVENTRICULAR TACHYCARDIA. Treatment is aimed at slowing the

Table 14–10. Drug Interactions: Cardiac Glycosides

Drug	Interacting Drug	Possible Effect	Implications
CGs	Phenobarbital, phenytoin, rifampin	Decreases the effect of digitoxin	Increase dose of digitoxin or change to digoxin.
	Thiazide and loop diuretics, mezlocillin, piperacillin, ticarcillin, amphotericin B, glucocorticoids	May cause hypokalemia and increase risk of CG toxicity	Monitor serum potassium levels, and teach patient signs and symptoms of hypokalemia to monitor for and report. Administer potassium supplement prn and encourage diet high in potassium. Where possible, choose alternative drug, especially antibiotic.
	Calcium preparations	Facilitates toxicity by accelerating overloading of intracellular calcium stores	Monitor for indications of toxicity. Avoid concurrent administration. Separate administration of CG and milk intake by at least 30 min.
	Quinidine, cyclosporine, amiodarone, verapamil, diltiazem, propafenone, diflunisal	Increases serum levels of CG and risk of toxicity	Avoid concurrent use or monitor serum levels 5–7 d after adding one of these drugs. Consider reducing CG dose by half if patient has signs of toxicity or a high normal CG level at initiation of interacting drug.
	Spironolactone	Increases digoxin half-life	Reduce dose of digoxin or increase dosing interval.
	Beta-adrenergic blockers, quinidine, disopyramide	Additive bradycardia	Avoid concurrent use or teach patient to monitor pulse rate and report pulse <60 bpm. Monitor electrocardiogram (ECG) regularly.
	Antacids, colestipol, kaolin-pectin, cholestyramine	Decreases absorption of CG if given concurrently	Separate administration by at least 1 h and give CG first.
	Thyroid hormones	May decrease therapeutic effects and cause arrhythmias	Monitor for effectiveness. Monitor ECG at regular intervals.

rate and converting to sinus rhythm if possible. Asymptomatic or mildly symptomatic patients with a rapid ventricular response should be treated with a **CG,** with a goal of a resting ventricular rate between 70 and 80 bpm (Table 14–11). **Digoxin** is preferred because it slows AV nodal conduction, resulting in a slower ventricular rate. It does not convert to sinus rhythm directly. Slowing heart rate yields greater diastolic filling time, permitting improved myocardial oxygenation. Cardiac muscle with an improved supply-demand ratio may return to sinus rhythm. **Digoxin** is less effective at slowing heart rate when vagal tone is low and adrenergic stimulation is high, such as during exercise, and in maintaining sinus rhythm or reducing the incidence of PSVT. Additional **antiarrhythmic drugs** may need to be added for these purposes.

For asymptomatic and mildly symptomatic patients, a loading dose is rarely required. Treatment is started with a maintenance dose if the ventricular response is less than 120 bpm. For young patients and those with normal renal function, the maintenance dose is 0.25 mg to 0.5 mg daily. For older adults and those with renal impairment, the maintenance dose is 0.125 mg daily.

If the ventricular rate is between 120 and 150 and still well tolerated, outpatient digitalization with a loading dose is reasonable. The dose is 10 to 15 µg/kg in divided doses over 24 hours. The usual pattern is 0.25 mg orally q6h for four doses. If creatinine clearance is less than 20 mL/min, give one-half the loading dose and start with 0.125 mg daily for maintenance. Patients who are not hemodynamically stable require rapid digitalization in a hospital.

Drug levels may be drawn at steady state (5 to 7 days), but the best indication of appropriate dosing is an acceptable heart rate. An adequately digitalized patient has a serum level of 1.5 to 2 ng/dL when atrial fibrillation is being treated.

HEART FAILURE. Although no longer the first-line drug for treatment of heart failure, **digoxin** is still central to treatment for patients with severe systolic dysfunction (ejection fractions less than 40 percent and with an audible S3 heart sound). In fact, the presence of S3 is a potent predictor of response to **CG** therapy. **Digoxin** is also beneficial in heart failure resulting from uncontrolled HTN or severe aortic stenosis, although BP reduction and valve surgery are the mainstays of therapy in these disorders. **CGs** are less beneficial with ejection fractions of more than 40 percent or in heart failure secondary to hypertrophic cardiomyopathies. They have no benefit in heart failure due to recurrent transient ischemia. The primary mechanism of action in heart failure is through its positive inotropic action, increasing ejection fraction at a given preload and afterload.

Patients who are hemodynamically stable are treated with an initial dose of 0.125 mg, increasing to 0.25 mg. The DHHS (1994) guidelines suggest, however, that patients with mild-to-moderate heart failure often become asymptomatic on optimal doses of **ACEIs** and **diuretics** and usually do not require **digoxin.** For less stable patients, the treatment regimen includes a loading dose similar to that used to treat atrial fibrillation of 120 to 150 bpm and a maintenance dose of 0.25 to 0.5 mg/day. **Diuretics** are the first drugs in treating patients with heart failure to reduce extracellular fluid (ECF) volume and thereby afterload. **Vasodilators** may be added to reduce preload and afterload. **ACEIs** are the drugs of choice for vasodilation because of their proven beneficial

Table 14–11. Dosage Schedule: Digoxin

Drug	Clinical Use	Patient Status	Loading Dose	Maintenance Dose
Digoxin	Atrial fibrillation with ventricular response <120 bpm or stable CHF	Young adult or normal renal function	None.	0.25–0.5 mg/d for atrial fibrillation; 0.25 mg/d for CHF
		Older adult or impaired renal function	None.	0.125 mg/d
	Atrial fibrillation with ventricular response 120–150 bpm or less stable CHF	Young adult or normal renal function	1–1.5 mg/d in four divided doses 6 h apart.	0.25–0.5 mg/d for atrial fibrillation; 0.25 mg/d for CHF
		Older adult or impaired renal function	If creatinine clearance <20 cc/min, give half the loading dose in four divided doses 6 h apart.	0.125 mg/d

Therapeutic serum level of digoxin: atrial fibrillation, 1.5–2 ng/cc; CHF, 0.8–1.2 ng/cc.

Clinical Pearl

··

1. **CGs** should not be used unless there is clear evidence of severe chronic systolic dysfunction or atrial fibrillation. In older adults, ankle edema is more often due to venous insufficiency than to heart failure. Even if it is related to heart failure, it is more often caused by diastolic dysfunction and better treated with **diuretics** or **ACEIs.**
2. **Digoxin** should not be discontinued unless a reversible cause of the heart failure has been completely corrected or there was no basis for the drug in the first place. Patients who respond appropriately to **digoxin** therapy have a chronic problem and need the drug chronically.
3. ST-T wave changes on the ECG do not correlate directly with serum drug levels and should not be used as an indication of toxicity. Serum drug levels are needed.

··

effects on mortality risk and functional status. **Digoxin** is usually added to this treatment regimen for those patients with severe heart failure whose symptoms persist despite optimal doses of **ACEIs** and **diuretics** (DHHS, 1994). See Chapter 34 for further discussion.

Therapeutic levels usually occur in 5 to 7 days. An adequately digitalized patient has a serum level of 0.8 to 1.2 ng/mL, lower than that needed to treat atrial fibrillation.

Rational Drug Selection

FORMULATION. **Digoxin** is well absorbed orally with a bioavailability of 70 to 80 percent. **Digoxin** elixir in capsules and encapsulated gel (**Lanoxicaps**) have 90 to 100 percent bioavailability and may be useful when careful titration of the dose is important.

BRAND. The best choice of CG is the purified glycoside, **digoxin**. It is well absorbed, can be used parenterally if needed, and has an intermediate duration of action, with a half-life of 36 to 48 hours. Even in the presence of renal failure, it can be used if the dose is adjusted.

COST. **Digoxin** is available in a generic form that reduces the cost.

Monitoring

Routine monitoring of **digoxin** levels is generally overdone. Monitoring should occur in addition to clinical judgment, rather than as a substitute for it. In general, testing should be done when:

1. The patient is taking other drugs that may alter the pharmacokinetics of **digoxin** (see Drug Interactions).
2. Steady state has been achieved (4 to 5 half-lives or 1 to 2 weeks after starting dose).
3. Toxicity is suspected.

4. Confirmation of adequacy of maintenance dose is needed in situations of poor therapeutic response.
5. A reference point is needed in adjusting a dose.
6. Patient adherence to the treatment regimen is questioned.
7. The patient has unstable renal function.

To avoid sampling during the distribution phase of the drug response curve, levels should be drawn at least 6 hours after the last dose. Therapeutic levels vary, based on the reason for treatment, but generally range from 0.8 to 2 ng/mL.

Because of their critical role in sensitivity to toxicity, serum electrolytes (potassium, calcium, magnesium) should be monitored on a regular basis, especially for patients who are taking concurrent **diuretics.** Renal function status is also critical to dosing of **CGs**; therefore, serum creatinine levels should be evaluated periodically and prior to any dosage change.

Patient Education

ADMINISTRATION. The patient should take the drug exactly as prescribed, at the same time each day. The long half-life means that taking it at different times each day would be permissible, but the narrow therapeutic range means that missing a dose or doubling a dose could result in toxicity. Taking the drug at the same time each day lessens the likelihood of nonadherence to the appropriate regimen. When the drug is prescribed on an eccentric schedule (e.g., 0.25 mg MWF and 0.125 mg TTSS), taking at the same time each day reduces the complexity of the schedule. Placing the appropriate dose in a pill container with compartments for each day of the week also reduces the chance of nonadherence. If one dose is missed but remembered within 12 hours, it should be taken. If two doses are missed, the health care provider should be contacted for instructions. The drug should not be stopped or the dosage altered without first contacting the health care provider.

Although the presence of food in the gut does not alter absorption of **CGs,** the ingestion of a high-fiber meal may decrease absorption. Tablets can be crushed and administered with food for patients who have difficulty swallowing. Patients should eat a diet high in potassium (bananas, orange juice, tomato juice, spinach, melons, dates, raisins, soybeans, prunes, potatoes, and molasses), unless also taking a **potassium-sparing diuretic** or an **ACEI,** and eat moderate amounts of calcium (800 to 1000 mg/day).

Do not alternate between dosage forms (Table 14–12). Each form has a different bioavailability, and changing forms may result in toxicity. For the same reason, the patient should check with the pharmacist during each drug refill to make certain the drug comes from the same manufacturer.

Store the drug in its original, tightly covered, light-resistant container. The patient who uses a pillbox for weekly dosing should not mix the **digoxin** with other drugs in the same compartment. Drugs often look alike and can be mistaken for one another.

CGs interact with many prescription and OTC drugs. Patients should avoid concurrent use of other drugs without first consulting the health care provider and not take **antacids** or **antidiarrheal drugs** within 1 hour of taking the **CG.** Milk may have the same effect on absorption, and doses should also be separated by 1 hour.

ADVERSE REACTIONS. Patients should learn to take their own pulse and then contact the health care provider before taking the drug if the pulse rate is less than 60 or more than 100 bpm. Signs and symptoms of toxicity include nausea, vomiting, diarrhea, confusion, depression, irregular pulse, yellow vision, and green halos around lights. Pulse changes and these symptoms should be reported to the health care provider immediately. Some patients can tolerate heart rates as low as 50 bpm without other symptoms and can be taught mainly to report symptoms of toxicity or worsening heart failure. Signs and symptoms of worsening heart failure include persistent cough; shortness of breath; weight gain of more than 2 lb in 1 day or 5 lb in 1 week; swelling of ankles, legs, or hands; and sensation of fullness in the abdomen. Follow-up appointments are also critical to evaluate the effectiveness of these drugs and to monitor for toxicity.

LIFESTYLE MANAGEMENT. Cardiac-healthy lifestyle is discussed under **ACEIs.** Patients should carry identification or wear a medical information bracelet or necklace that describes the disease process and drug regimen at all times.

Antiarrhythmics

Cardiac rhythm disturbances range from benign and asymptomatic to malignant and life-threatening. For some arrhythmias, definitive drug therapy has research support; for many arrhythmias, there is no demonstrated correlation between a particular rhythm disturbance and a particular class of **antiarrhythmic** drug. Selection of a specific drug is often arbitrary and largely based on adverse responses, interactions with other drugs being taken, and concurrent clinical problems. Unfortunately, **antiarrhythmic drugs** can paradoxically cause lethal arrhythmias in some patients. Choosing not to treat may be a better choice, especially in asymptomatic or minimally symptomatic patients. Debate continues about the relative merits of invasive versus noninvasive testing to assist in the selection of a specific **antiarrhythmic.** Given these variables, it is probably best to refer to a cardiologist any patients with rhythm disturbances for which there is no clearly demonstrated appropriate drug choice. When the drug is chosen by the specialist, management in the primary care setting requires understanding both the beneficial effects and adverse effects of these drugs, the monitoring required, and appropriate patient education. The six classes of **antiarrhythmics** are discussed here with that management approach in mind. To be practical in a primary care setting, the drug must be available in oral form and have an effective half-life of at least 6 hours. Drugs that do not meet these criteria are not discussed.

Pharmacodynamics

Arrhythmias are caused either by abnormal pacemaker activity or by abnormal impulse conduction. The goal of therapy with an **antiarrhythmic** is to reduce ectopic pacemaker activity or alter abnormal conduction. The major mechanisms by which **antiarrhythmics** act to do this are: (1) sodium channel blockade, (2) blockade of sympathetic nervous system (SNS) effects on the heart, (3) prolongation of the effective refractory period, and

Table 14–12. Available Dosage Forms: Oral Cardiac Glycosides

Drug	Dosage Form	Other Forms
Digitoxin (Crystodigin)	Tablet: 50 μg, 100 μg, 150 μg, 200 μg	
Digoxin (Lanoxin)	Tablet: 0.125 mg, 0.25 mg, 0.5 mg Capsule: 0.05 mg, 0.1 mg, 0.2 mg Elixir: 0.05 mg/mL	

(4) blockade of the calcium channel. Different classes of **antiarrhythmics** act in one or more of these ways, and drugs in one class may have significant actions associated with a different class. Placement in a given class is based on predominant action.

All pacemakers in the heart, normal and ectopic, depend on appropriate phase 4 diastolic depolarization. Increasing the phase 4 slope may result in accelerated pacemaker discharge. Figure 14–4 depicts the cardiac action potential with slope phases. Potential causes of this increased slope include hypokalemia, beta-adrenergic stimulation, fiber stretch, acidosis, and partial depolarization by currents of injury. Blockade of sodium channels (**class I antiarrhythmics**) or calcium channels (**class IV antiar-**

rhythmics) reduces the permeability ratio of these ions to potassium permeability, making the threshold more negative and reducing the phase 4 slope. **BBs (class II antiarrhythmics)** indirectly reduce the slope by blocking the chronotropic action of norepinephrine. Hyperkalemia stabilizes the membrane potential and also reduces the rate of pacemaker firing. Vagal discharge also reduces phase 4 slope and makes the potential more negative (cardiac glycoside activity).

Disturbances in impulse conduction are either (1) simple blocks related to severely depressed conduction that may sometimes be relieved by the parasympathetic action of atropine or (2) reentry conduction, in which one impulse reenters and excites areas of the heart more

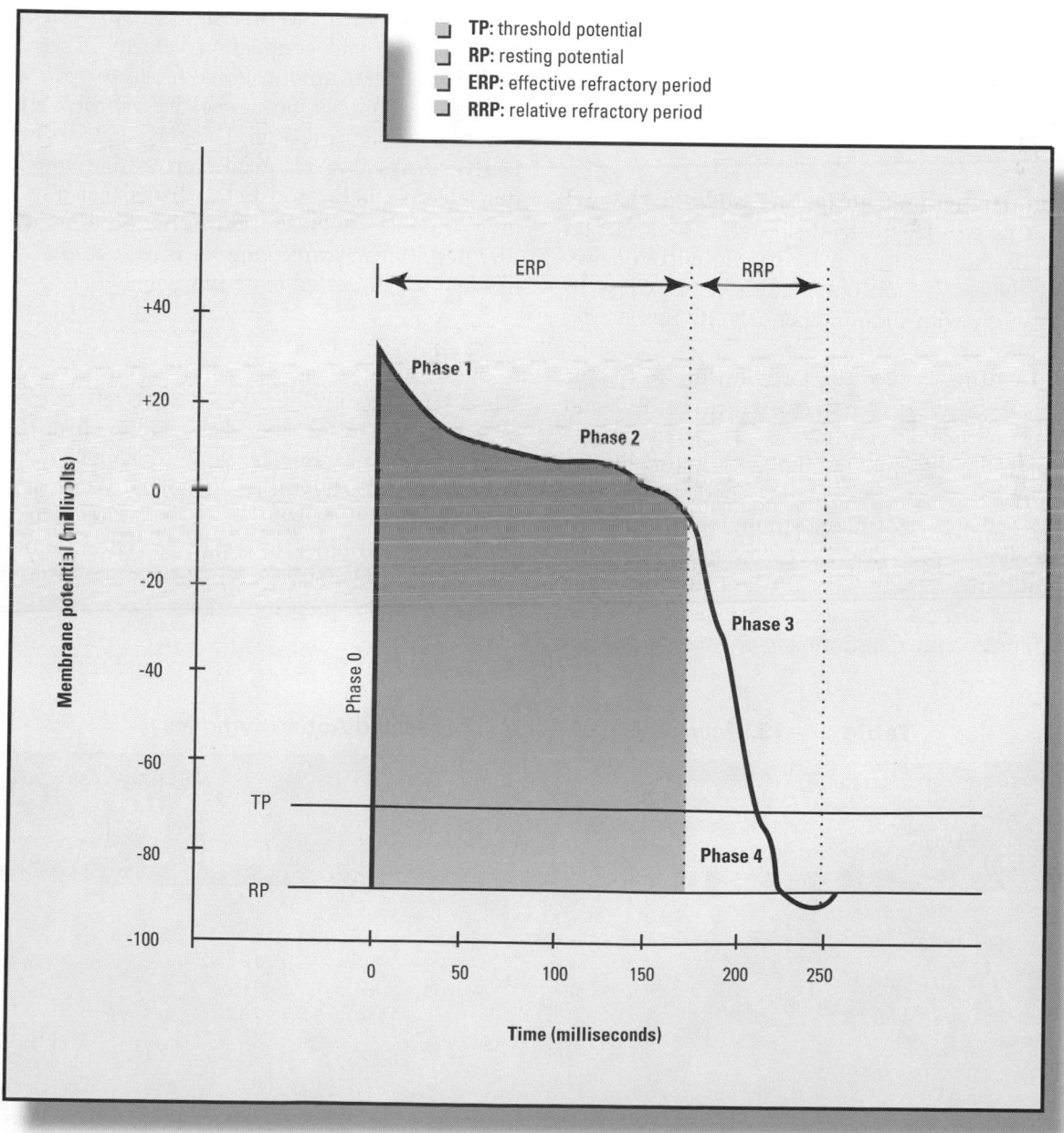

Figure 14–4. Cardiac action potential: ventricles.

than once. Reentry requires (1) an obstacle to normal conduction, (2) unidirectional block in the circuit, and (3) conduction time around the circuit timed so that the impulse does not enter refractory tissue (Table 14–13). Too slow an impulse results in bidirectional block or the impulse collides with the next normal impulse; too fast results in bidirectional conduction or the impulse reaches tissue that is still refractory. Slowing conduction by depressing the sodium current (**class I**) or calcium current (**class IV**) abolishes reentry arrhythmias. Lengthening or shortening the refractory period also makes reentry less likely. Converting unidirectional block to bidirectional block (**class III**) also decreases reentry.

Effective **antiarrhythmics** act more on cardiac tissue being abnormally stimulated than on normal cardiac tissue. These drugs decrease the automaticity of ectopic pacemakers more than the SA node, and they reduce conduction or increase the refractory period more in depolarized tissue than in normally polarized tissue.

Class I

Class I antiarrhythmic drugs are sodium channel blockers. Class IA lengthens the duration of the action potential, **IB** shortens it, and **IC** has no effect or may minimally increase action potential duration. **Class IB** interacts rapidly with sodium channels, **IC** acts slowly, and **IA** is intermediate.

Class IA drugs reduce the rate of firing of ectopic foci, increase the effective refractory period (ERP), and reduce the speed of conduction. They also block parasympathetic nervous discharge, resulting in increased conduction rate at the AV node. This anticholinergic activity can produce serious increases in ventricular rate in the presence of rapid atrial activity, such as that found in atrial fibrillation. **Class IB** drugs block both activated and inactivated sodium channels. The effect is extremely limited in normally polarized tissue but

highly effective in depolarized and injured tissue. They do not affect the automaticity of the SA node or conductivity through the AV node. Their shortening effect on the ERP eliminates unidirectional block and may trigger reentry arrhythmias. **Class IC** drugs primarily block the sodium fast channel during phase 0 of the action potential. Because of their propensity for severe exacerbation of arrhythmias, even in normal doses with post-MI patients (Echt et al., 1991), they are reserved for patients with severe ventricular tachycardias for whom other drugs have not worked.

Class II

Class II drugs (beta blockers) reduce adrenergic activity in the heart. Blockade by these drugs increases threshold potential and prolongs ERP, thereby decreasing heart rate and conduction velocity. These effects probably convert unidirectional block to bidirectional. They also exert a significant negative inotropic effect, reducing force of contraction. This class includes **beta$_1$ selective drugs** that act mainly on cardiac muscle and **nonselective beta$_1$ and beta$_2$ drugs** that also act on lung, arteriole, pancreatic, kidney, adipose, and liver tissues, resulting in a wide range of adverse responses. Beta blockers are discussed more thoroughly in Chapter 12.

Class III

Class III drugs prolong the effective refractory period by some mechanism other than sodium channel blockade, often by blocking potassium channels, which results in a decreased rate of automaticity of ventricular ectopic beats. They may also convert unidirectional block to bidirectional block in reentry arrhythmias but have little effect on depolarization. Most of the drugs in this class also have significant actions associated with other classes.

Table 14–13. Mechanism of Action of Selected Antiarrhythmics

Drug	Effect on Sinoatrial Rate	Effect on Atrioventricular Node Refractory Period	Effect on PR Interval	Effect on QRS Duration	Effect on QT Interval	Sinoatrial Node Automaticity
Amiodarone	–	+	+	+	+ +	–
Disopyramide	± (2)	± (2)	± (2)	+	+ +	±
Flecainide	0	0	+	+ +	0	–
Mexiletine	0 (1)	±	0	0	0	–
Procainamide	±	± (2)	± (2)	+	+	±
Propafenone	0	+	+	+	0	0
Quinidine	± (2)	± (2)	± (2)	+	+	±
Sotalol	– –	+ +	+ +	0	+ +	–
Tocainide	0 (1)	–	0	0	0	0/–

– = suppresses or slows; + = stimulates or increases speed or duration; **(1)** = may suppress diseased sinus nodes;
(2) = anticholinergic effect and direct depressant action.

Class IV

CCBs constitute **class IV.** They were discussed in more detail earlier in this chapter, including their role in arrhythmia management.

Pharmacokinetics

Absorption and Distribution

All classes of **antiarrhythmics** are well absorbed orally, with sustained-release forms and **amiodarone (Cordarone)** having slower absorption times (Table 14–14). Bioavailabilities vary greatly depending upon protein binding, with **propafenone (Rhythmol)** having the lowest at 3 percent bioavailability with 97 percent protein binding and **sotalol (Betapace)** having the highest (90%) with no protein binding. The presence of food in the gut does not affect bioavailability except for **sotalol;** food may reduce its absorption by as much as 20 percent.

Distribution is to most body tissues. **Amiodarone** exhibits high levels of drug in fat, muscle, lung, and spleen tissues. Cardiac tissue concentration is about 30 times higher than plasma concentration. **Amiodarone** and **quinidine** easily cross the placenta. **Disopyramide (Norpace), quinidine,** and **sotalol** are all found in breast milk, and **mexiletine (Mexitil)** is found in breast milk in concentrations similar to those found in plasma. **Tocainide (Tonocard)** is the only one that crosses the blood-brain barrier. **Disopyramide** has an unusual protein-binding curve, with binding sites becoming saturated at increasing dosages leading to a nonlinear rise in free drug and misleading measurements of plasma concentration.

Metabolism and Excretion

All **antiarrhythmics** are metabolized by the liver. Half-lives of these drugs vary from 3 to 4 hours for **procainamide** to 13 or more days for **amiodarone.** As the only **short-acting antiarrhythmic, procainamide** requires frequent dosing administration, with steady state achieved in 2 to 3 days. Other **antiarrhythmics** have longer half-lives and require more time to achieve steady state. Hepatic impairment increases half-life in those drugs eliminated totally or partially in feces. Renal impairment significantly increases half-life in those drugs eliminated all or largely in the urine. Reduced dosages of **procainamide** and **quinidine** are required for patients with CHF or renal impairment that decreases volumes of distribution of these drugs. **Tocainide** dosages should be reduced in renal impairment for similar reasons. Approximately 10 percent of patients are slow metabolizers of **propafenone,** resulting in an increase in half-life from 7 hours to 10 to 32 hours. Because this drug has been associated with proarrhythmia and increased mortality post-MI, the trend is away from its use.

Pharmacotherapeutics

Precautions and Contraindications

Because their mechanisms of action differ, the various classes also have different precautions and contraindications.

CLASS IA. Antimuscarinic actions in the heart common to this class inhibit vagal effects and may lead to increased sinus rate and AV conduction. Use cautiously for patients with cardiac problems, for whom increased heart rate might worsen the condition.

CLASS IB. Use cautiously for patients with heart failure related to the potential for hypotension secondary to decreased myocardial contractility. This occurs mainly with large doses and in fewer than 10 percent of patients. The major extracardiac adverse effects of these drugs are neurological and occur most frequently in older adults, so patients with neurological conditions and older adults should be carefully monitored for these adverse responses.

CLASS IC. No muscarinic effects are present with this class, but severe exacerbations of arrhythmia have occurred in patients with preexisting ventricular tachyarrhythmias and previous MI, even with normal doses of the drugs. These drugs should be reserved for patients unresponsive to less toxic drugs, especially if these patients have CHF, sinus nodal dysfunction, or heart block.

CLASS II. **Beta blockers** are generally contraindicated for patients with bronchospastic disorders such as asthma. They are used with caution for patients with diabetes because they decrease insulin secretion and may mask many of the signs of hypoglycemia. Because of their peripheral vasoconstrictive effects, they are a poor choice for patients with peripheral vascular disease and Raynaud's syndrome.

Clinical Pearl

For patients with diabetes who must take a **beta blocker,** the diaphoresis associated with hypoglycemia is not masked by these drugs, and diabetics should be taught to recognize this indication of hypoglycemia.

Table 14–14. Pharmacokinetics: Selected Antiarrhythmics

Drug	Onset	Peak	Duration	Bioavail-ability	Protein Binding	Half-Life	Active Metabolite	Elimination
Amiodarone	1–3 wk	UK	wk–mo	35–65%	95%	26–107 d	Yes (DEA)	99% in bile
Disopyramide PO	0.5–3.5 h	2.5 h	1.5–8.5 h	50%	35–95%	4–10 h; increased in hepatic, renal impairment	No	10% unchanged in feces, 50% unchanged in urine
Disopyramide CR	0.5–3.5 h	4.9 h	12 h	50%	35–95%	4–10 h; increased in hepatic, renal impairment	No	10% unchanged in feces, 50% unchanged in urine
Flecainide	Days	d–wk	12 h	>80%	40%	20 h	No	30% unchanged in urine
Mexiletine	0.5–2 h	2–3 h	8–12 h	>80%	60–75%	12 h	No	10% unchanged in urine
Procainamide PO	0.5 h	1–1.5 h	3–4 h	75%	15–20%	3–4 h; increased in renal impairment	Yes (NAPA)	40–70% unchanged in urine
Procainamide SR	0.5 h	1–1.5 h	6 h	75%	15–20%	3–4 h; increased in renal impairment	Yes (NAPA)	40–70% unchanged in urine
Propafenone	UK	4–5 d	UK	3–11%	97%	7 h (90% of patients); 10–32 h in slow metabolizers (10%)	Yes	<1% excreted unchanged
Quinidine PO (sulfate)	0.5 h	1–1.5 h	6–8 h		80%	6–8 h; increased in CHF and severe liver impairment	Yes	20% unchanged in urine; urinary excretion enhanced in acid urine
Quinidine PO (sulfate-ER)	0.5 h	4 h	8–12 h		80%	6–8 h; increased in CHF and severe liver impairment	Yes	20% unchanged in urine; urinary excretion enhanced in acid urine
Quinidine PO (gluconate)	0.5 h	3–5 h	6–8 h		80%	6–8 h; increased in CHF and severe liver impairment	Yes	20% unchanged in urine; urinary excretion enhanced in acid urine
Sotalol	Hours	2–3 d	UK	90%	Not bound	7–12 h	No	90% unchanged in urine
Tocainide	0.5–1 h	0.5–2 h	8–12 h		10%	12 h	No	30–50% unchanged in urine

Class II (beta blockers) are covered in Chapter 12; class IV (CCBs) were covered earlier in this chapter.
UK = unknown; CHF = congestive heart failure.

Abrupt withdrawal of **beta blockers** may result in rebound beta stimulation resulting in tachycardia; therefore, they should be tapered by half every 4 hours. Patients at high risk for serious exacerbation of their disease related to abrupt withdrawal include those with angina, CAD with ventricular arrhythmias, and migraines. Hypertensive patients are at lower risk. **Beta blockers** are discussed in more detail in Chapter 12.

CLASS III. **Sotalol** is the major **class III** drug used in primary care. It is a **nonselective beta blocker** that also prolongs action potential. Its precautions are similar to **class II**. **Amiodarone**, also a **class III** drug, has significant properties of several other classes as well. The muscarinic effects associated with sodium-channel blockade suggest cautious use for patients with SA or AV nodal dysfunction, bradycardia, or CHF. **Amiodarone** inhibits the enzyme that converts T_4 to T_3, and iodine is a major component of this drug; therefore, about 5 percent of patients with underlying predisposition to thyroid disease may develop thyrotoxicosis or hypothyroidism. If this drug must be used to treat the rhythm disturbance, careful monitoring and treatment of the thyroid disorder must be undertaken. Potentially fatal pulmonary fibrosis occurs in 5 to 15 percent of patients, and use for patients with pulmonary disease is questioned. At-risk patients should have thyroid and pulmonary function studies done before **amiodarone** therapy is initiated.

CLASS IV. **CCBs** have been discussed earlier in this chapter. All *antiarrhythmics* are **Pregnancy Category C** except *amiodarone*, which is Pregnancy Category D.

Adverse Drug Reactions

The more common adverse reactions of **antiarrhythmics** are extensions of their actions. Reduction in BP may result in dizziness, hypotension, fatigue, and syncope. Decreased myocardial contractility may result in CHF. Each class has the potential to produce rhythm disturbances, often exaggerations of or the reverse of the one being treated. **Class IC** drugs are especially proarrhythmic. GI symptoms, which are especially disturbing to patients, include nausea, vomiting, diarrhea, and constipation. GI symptoms are especially prevalent in **class IA** drugs, occurring in 33 to 50 percent of patients. Although not common, sexual dysfunction and urinary retention may occur in **classes I** and **III**. The **atropine**-like activity of **disopyramide** (urinary retention, dry mouth, and constipation) may require discontinuance of the drug. Adverse neurological reactions of **antiarrhythmics** include tremor, blurred vision, and nervousness. **Amiodarone** has several adverse drug effects not common to other **antiarrhythmics**, including extrapyramidal syndrome (EPS) effects, hepatitis, epididymitis, corneal and skin deposits, peripheral neuropathy, and photosensitivity. These effects increase with cumulative doses and limit its utility for long-term therapy. Adverse effects associated with beta blockade in **class II** drugs and **sotalol** are discussed in Chapter 12. Those relevant to **CCBs** have been discussed earlier in this chapter.

Drug Interactions

Cross-class and intraclass increases in cardiac effects are common between **antiarrhythmics**, increasing serum levels and toxicity risks. Several drugs increase or decrease the metabolism of **antiarrhythmics: cimetidine (Tagamet), phenobarbital, rifampin (Rifadin),** and **phenytoin (Dilantin),** which also has **class IB** antiarrhythmic activity, resulting in alterations in effectiveness and toxicity risk. The anticoagulation effects of **warfarin (Coumadin)** are increased by many **antiarrhythmics**, particularly **amiodarone**. Additive anticholinergic effects occur as an interaction between several **antiarrhythmics** and other drugs that have anticholinergic properties. The metabolism and excretions of several **class I** drugs are significantly affected by urine pH, resulting in altered serum levels and toxicity risk. The CYP-450 3A4 system is involved in the metabolism of **quinidine.** Drugs that inhibit this system, including grapefruit juice, may increase free drug levels. CYP-450 2D6 is involved in **flecainide (Tambocor)** and **propafenone** metabolism. Drugs that inhibit this system may similarly increase free drug levels. Selected **antiarrhythmics** may potentiate the hypotensive effects of **antihypertensives, nitrates,** and **alcohol. Beta blockers** may alter the effectiveness of **insulin** and oral **hypoglycemics.** Specific drug interactions and the appropriate actions to prevent them are given in Table 14–15.

Clinical Use and Dosing

ATRIAL ARRHYTHMIAS (ATRIAL FIBRILLATION/FLUTTER, AV NODAL REENTRANT TACHYCARDIA, WOLFF-PARKINSON-WHITE [WPW] TACHYCARDIAS). All antiarrhythmics have some use in these disorders. **Class IA drugs (quinidine, procainamide)** are especially useful. **Quinidine** has a short-acting form that is given every 4 to 6 hours, a long-acting form for every 8-hour administration, and **Quinidex Extentabs,** which can be given bid (Table 14–16). It has been combined with **mexiletine** to enhance effectiveness and reduce adverse effects. **Procainamide's** half-life is only 3 to 4 hours, requiring frequent dosing. If around-the-clock antiarrhythmic activity is required, a sustained-release preparation must usually be given every 6 hours. Less frequent dosing is sometimes possible in renal disease, where excretion is slowed. **Amiodarone** is very effective against supraventricular arrhythmias, especially in children, in whom it appears to be quite safe. The wide range of adverse reactions seen in adults and its many drug interactions make it a second-

Table 14–15. Drug and Food Interactions: Selected Antiarrhythmics

Drug	Interacting Drug/Food	Possible Effect	Implications
Amiodarone*,†	Digoxin	Increases blood levels and toxicity risk	Decrease dose of digoxin by 50%. Monitor for toxicity.
	Class I antiarrhythmics	Increases blood levels and toxicity risk	Decreases of these drugs by 30–50%.
	Phenytoin	Increases blood levels of phenytoin; may decrease amiodarone blood levels	Avoid concurrent use. If they must be given together, monitor serum levels of both drugs.
	BBs, CCBs	Increases risk for bradyrhythms, sinus arrest, and AV block	Monitor for dizziness and orthostatic and mental status change. Safety issues.
	Cholestyramine	May decrease amiodarone blood levels	Separate doses by 1 h and give amiodarone first.
	Antihypertensives	May produce profound hypotension	Monitor BP. Safety issues.
Disopyramide*,†,‡	Phenytoin, phenobarbital	Decreases blood levels and effectiveness	Monitor pulse, ECG for effectiveness.
	Other antiarrhythmics	Additive cardiac toxic effects (prolonged conduction, decreased cardiac output)	Avoid using disopyramide for 48 h before or 24 h after verapamil.
	Drugs with anticholinergic properties	Additive anticholinergic effects	Monitor for dry mouth, wheezing, urinary retention, orthostatic hypotension.
Flecainide†	CCBs, Disopyramide, BBs, verapamil	Increases arrhythmia risk Additive myocardial depression	Combination should be avoided or given cautiously.
	Amiodarone	Doubles serum flecainide levels	Decrease flecainide dose by 50%.
	Digoxin	Increases serum digoxin levels by small amount	Monitor serum digoxin level and indications of toxicity.
	Alkalinizing agents, foods that increase urine pH to >7§, strict vegetarian diet	Promotes reabsorption, increases blood levels, increases toxicity risk	Monitor serum levels.
	Acidifying agents, foods that decrease urine pH to <5§, acidic juices	Increases renal elimination, decreases effectiveness	Monitor serum levels and clinical indicators of effectiveness.
Mexiletine	Opioid analgesics, atropine, antacids	Slows absorption of mexiletine	Separate adminstration of antacids by at least 1 h.
	Metoclopramide	Speeds absorption	
	Phenytoin, phenobarbital, cigarette smoking	Increases metabolism and decreases effectiveness of mexiletine	Avoid concurrent use.
	Alkalinizing and acidifying agents§	Same as with flecainide	Same as with flecainide.
Procainamide†	Other antiarrhythmics	Additive effect (see amiodarone)	
	Antihypertensives, nitrates	Potentiates hypotensive effects	Monitor BP. Safety issues.
	Drugs with anticholinergic properties¶	Additive anticholinergic effects	Monitor for dry mouth, wheezing, urinary retention, orthostatic hypotension.
	Ranitidine, quinidine, trimethoprim	Increases serum levels and effects of procainamide	Monitor for procainamide toxicity (tachycardia, confusion, drowsiness, nausea, and vomiting).

Continued on next page

Table 14–15. Drug and Food Interactions: Selected Antiarrhythmics *(continued)*

Drug	Interacting Drug/Food	Possible Effect	Implications
Propafenone*,‡	Digoxin	Increases digoxin levels by 35–85%	Dosage reduction required.
	Metoprolol, propranolol	Increases serum levels and effects of these drugs	Dosage reduction may be required.
	Quinidine	Inhibits propafenone metabolism	Avoid concurrent use.
Quinidine*,†,‡	Digoxin	Increases serum levels and toxicity risk	Dosage reduction recommended.
	Amiodarone	See amiodarone	See amiodarone.
	Phenytoin, phenobarbital	Increases metabolism and decreases effectiveness of quinidine	Monitor therapeutic effects.
	Verapamil	Decreases metabolism and increases serum levels of quinidine	Monitor for toxicity.
	Antihypertensives, nitrates, alcohol	Additive hypotension	
	Procainamide, propafenone, tricyclic antidepressants (TCAs)	Increases serum levels and risk for toxicity for each of these drugs	
	Drugs with anticholinergic properties¶	Additive anticholinergic effects	Monitor for dry mouth, wheezing, urinary retention, orthostatic hypotension
	Alkalinizing and acidifying foods and drugs§	See flecainide	
Sotalol	General anesthetics, IV phenytoin, CCBs	Additive myocardial depression	
	Digoxin	Additive bradycardia	
	Antihypertensives, nitrates, alcohol	Additive hypotension	
	Amphetamines, ephedrine, epinephrine, norepinephrine, phenylephrine, pseudoephedrine	Unopposed alpha-adrenergic stimulation, leading to excessive HTN and bradycardia	Avoid concurrent use. Teach patient not to use OTCs without contacting health care provider.
	Amiodarone, disopyramide, procainamide, quinidine	Increases proarrhythmia risk	Avoid concurrent use.
	Clonidine	Potentiates rebound HTN when clonidine discontinued	Use caution and monitor BP closely when discontinuing clonidine.
	Insulin, oral hypoglycemics	May alter effectivenss of diabetic drugs	Dosage adjustment of diabetic drugs may be required.
	Monoamine oxidase inhibitors (MAOIs)	May result in increased HTN	Use cautiously within 14 d of MAOI.
Tocainide†,‡	Other antiarrhythmics	Additive cardiac effects	Avoid concurrent use.
	Beta-adrenergic blockers	Concurrent use may precipitate CHF	

*Interacts with warfarin to increase anticoagulation. Monitor prothrombin time. Dosage of warfarin may need to be decreased. For amiodarone, the decrease may be 33–50%.
†Interacts with cimetidine to increase serum levels of the antiarrhythmic. Choose different histamine$_2$ blocker. Monitor for toxicity if cimetidine must be used.
‡Interacts with rifampin to decrease serum levels and effectiveness of antiarrhythmic. If they must be used together, monitor for decreased therapeutic effect of antiarrhythmic, and adjust dosage as needed.
§Foods that alkalinize urine: all fruits except cranberries, prunes, plums; all vegetables; milk. Foods that acidify urine: cheeses, cranberries, eggs, fish, grains, meats, plums, poultry, prunes.
¶Drugs with anticholinergic properties: antihistamines, atropine, benztropine, haloperidol, phenothiazines, TCAs, trihexyphenidyl.

Table 14–16. Dosage Schedule: Selected Antiarrhythmics

Drug	Clinical Use	Starting Dose	Maintenance Dose	Maximum Dose (Adjusted Dose)	Plasma Concentration
Amiodarone	Ventricular arrhythmias (unlabeled use in PSVT, atrial fibrillation)	400–600 mg tid for 1–2 wk	400–600 mg/d 200 mg/d for PSVT, atrial fibrillation	1000 mg	1–2 μg/cc
Atenolol	Prevent primary arrhythmic event post-MI Insufficient control of atrial fibrillation with digoxin	100 mg qd or 50 mg bid 25–50 mg/d added to digoxin dose	100 mg qd or 50 mg bid for at least 9 d post-MI 100 mg/d; 50 mg/d if severe renal impairment		
Disopyramide	Ventricular arrhythmia (unlabeled use in PSVT)	150 mg q8h *Children:* mg/kg/d in 4 divided doses at q6h intervals: <1 yr = 10–30 1–4 = 10–20 4–12 = 10–15 12–18 = 6–15 *Adults* <50 kg 400 mg/d *Adults* >50 kg 400–800 mg/d in divided doses q6h for standard tablets; q12h for controlled release		For creatinine clearance <40 cc/min, dosage in adults is 100 mg q8h; further reductions as clearance decreases	2–4 μg/cc
Flecainide†	Sustained ventricular tachycardia, PSVT	100 mg q12 h for ventricular tachycardia; 50 mg q12h for PSVT	100–150 mg q12h for ventricular tachycardia; 50–100 q12h for PSVT	Ventricular tachycardia: 400 mg/d; PSVT: 300 mg/d; adjust doses by 50-mg increments; mininum 4 d between adjustments	
Mexiletine	Ventricular arrhythmias	200 mg q8h (if rapid control of arrhythmia is essential, load with 400 mg)	200–300 mg q8h	1200 mg/d; adjust doses by 50–100-mg increments; minimum 2–3 d between adjustments	0.5–2 μg/cc
Procainamide	Ventricular arrhythmias	750 mg q6h *Children:* 15–50 mg/kg/d in divided doses *Young adults:* 50 mg/kg/d in divided doses (q3–4h for tablets; q6h or q8h for sustained release); reduce dose if age >50 or		4 g/d	3–10 μg/cc (risk of cardiac and GI toxicity increases if >8 μg/cc)

Continued on next page

Table 14–16. Dosage Schedule: Selected Antiarrhythmics *(continued)*

Drug	Clinical Use	Starting Dose	Maintenance Dose	Maximum Dose (Adjusted Dose)	Plasma Concentration
		with renal or hepatic impairment			
Propafenone[†]	Ventricular arrhythmias (unlabeled use in PSVT associated with WPW)	150 mg q8h	225–300 mg q8h	900 mg; increases doses at minimum of 3-d intervals	0.2–1.5 µg/cc (nonlinear change in plasma level related to dose increase)
Propranolol	PSVT; atrial fibrillation; tachycardias associated with digitalis toxicity, excessive catecholamines, thyroid dysfunction	10–30 mg tid–qid given ac and hs; for atrial fibrillation uncontrolled by digoxin, add 40–80 mg of propranolol to digoxin dose		240 mg/d	
Quinidine	Premature atrial contraction, PSVT, atrial fibrillation, atrial flutter, atrioventricular nodal reentry; WPW, VC; ventricular tachycardia not associated with complete heart block	Single-dose 200-mg tablet to assess for idiosyncratic reaction	200–300 mg tid or qid for tablets; 300–600 mg q8h for sustained release*		2–6 µg/cc
Sotalol	Ventricular arrhythmias	80 mg bid	240–320 mg/d in 2 divided doses; long half-life makes more than bid dosing unnecessary	640 mg, adjust doses at minimum 2 d interval	
Tocainide	Ventricular arrhythmias	400 mg q8h	1200–1800 mg/d in 3 divided doses	<1200 mg/d in renal and hepatic impairment	4–10 µg/cc

*Because the rate of absorption from various sustained-release formulations may be markedly different, they are not interchangeable.
†Because of proarrhythmic effects, use with lesser arrhythmias is not recommended.
PSVT = paroxysmal supraventricular tachycardia; MI = myocardial infarction; WPW = Wolff-Parkinson-White syndrome.

line drug choice. Reentrant supraventricular tachycardia is the major indication for **verapamil (Calan, Isoptin)**, and it is the preferred drug. It can also be used to decrease the rate in atrial fibrillation/flutter with rapid ventricular response. The long-acting form has the advantage of once-daily administration. The high risk for clot formation associated with atrial fibrillation requires concurrent anticoagulation therapy with either **aspirin** or **warfarin**, depending on the risk profile of the patient.

VENTRICULAR ARRHYTHMIAS (VENTRICULAR ECTOPIC BEATS, VENTRICULAR TACHYCARDIA, VENTRICULAR FIB-RILLATION). Simple ventricular rhythm disturbances such as occasional premature ventricular contractions (PVCs) are rarely treated in primary care. Complex ventricular irritability demonstrated with ventricular rhythm disturbances is associated with increased risk for MI and sudden death. Despite this fact, only symptomatic patients with underlying heart disease, malignant forms of arrhythmia such as recurrent ventricular tachycardia, and poor left ventricular (LV) function seem to benefit from prophylactic **antiarrhythmic** therapy. Controlled trials of **antiarrhythmic** therapy in minimally symptomatic post-MI patients with reduced ejection fractions actually showed increased rates of arrhythmia-associated death in those treated (Echt et al., 1991). **Class IA** agents have moderate efficacy in treating ventricular arrhythmias and are the most commonly prescribed. **Quinidine** remains the first-line drug. The **gluconate** form has a lower adverse effect profile. The bioavailability varies among preparations, making dosage adjustment important if changing forms. **Disopyramide** has a pronounced negative inotropic effect, which limits its usefulness. **Procainamide** requires q6h to q8h dosing, even in its sustained-release form. **Class IB** drugs are fairly weak **antiarrhythmics** for these problems and are either second-line drugs or used with **class IA** drugs. Their relatively long half-lives allow bid or tid dosing. They are well tolerated in heart failure, having little negative inotropic effect, with **mexiletine** more negatively inotropic than **tocainide**. **Class IC** drugs are moderately effective but are reserved for very refractory cases because of their proarrhythmic qualities. **Class II** drugs are useful in exercise-induced ventricular tachycardia but should be monitored with serial exercise testing to check efficacy. They are safe and especially useful in arrhythmias caused by ischemic heart disease because they are among the few drugs proven to reduce CAD mortality. Selection for $beta_1$ receptors reduces many of their adverse reactions. **Atenolol (Tenormin)**, has strong $beta_1$ selectivity, resulting in a low adverse effect profile, and is used for post-MI arrhythmia prophylaxis. **Propranolol (Inderal)**, a **nonselective beta blocker**, is used with several arrhythmias. **Class III** drugs are the best choice for monomorphic ventricular tachycardia.

A common noncardiac cause of tachyarrhythmias is hyperthyroidism. **Propranolol**, a **class II drug**, slows the heart rate by its beta-blocking action, and has the added effect of preventing peripheral conversion of T_4 to T_3, thereby reducing the serum levels of the more active form of thyroid hormone.

Rational Drug Selection

RISK VERSUS BENEFIT.   The choice of **antiarrhythmic** drugs is usually based not only on benefit (correction or prevention of the rhythm) but also on risks (adverse effects and toxicity). Benefits may be assessed and drugs chosen by electrophysiological studies. When no agent meets electrophysiological study criteria for choice, empiric **amiodarone** may be prescribed because of its effects in all classes and because it has been shown to reduce mortality in cardiac arrest survivors from 50 to 20 percent at 2 years post cardiac arrest. The more potentially lethal the arrhythmia, the more acceptable the risks. In terms of prevention, only **beta blockers** have been definitively shown by research to reduce mortality in relatively asymptomatic patients. Risks related to adverse reactions are present in all **antiarrhythmics** and increase with higher doses and longer times of administration.

CONCURRENT DISEASES.   The presence of diseases in other organ systems may dictate the choice of drug, based on the effects of the **antiarrhythmic** on that system (bronchospasm in asthma, urinary retention in benign prostatic hyperplasia).

COST.   All **antiarrhythmics** are expensive. Those requiring frequent monitoring by diagnostic tests need to have the cost of this monitoring factored into their cost. For example, **amiodarone** may require every 3 to 6 months chest x-rays, pulmonary function tests, and ophthalmic examinations, as well as TSH and free T_4 levels, dependent upon the signs and symptoms found in the patient. This significantly raises the cost of this drug. Generic **procainamide** requires q6h to q8h dosing. Cost is increased significantly when generic is switched to the sustained-release form.

DECISION STEPS.   Because the margin between therapeutic efficacy and toxicity is narrow, and the knowledge needed to prescribe these drugs is extensive, it is best to refer patients to a cardiologist for initiation of therapy. Phone consultation may also be required during therapy unless the provider has extensive experience with **antiarrhythmic** therapy. When this is not possible, Katsung (1998) recommends several important steps in deciding on therapy:

1. Any factor that might be precipitating the arrhythmia should be determined and eliminated. Especially relevant are adverse drug reactions, underlying disease states such as thyroid disorders, and potassium levels.
2. A firm arrhythmia diagnosis should be established. Use of inappropriate drugs because of a misdiagnosis of the arrhythmia can be catastrophic in some cases.
3. Establish a reliable baseline on which to judge the efficacy of any subsequent **antiarrhythmic** therapy. Methods include ambulatory monitoring, electrophysiological studies, and treadmill exercises.
4. The mere identification of an arrhythmia does not necessarily require its treatment. An excellent justification for conservative treatment was provided by the CAST trials (Echt et al., 1991).

Monitoring

LABORATORY DATA.   Potassium concentration in the extracellular space is the major determinant of resting membrane potential and membrane stability. **Potassium levels should always be checked and kept more than 4 mEq/L for patients with rhythm disturbances.** Renal and hepatic functions (blood urea nitrogen [BUN], creatinine, transaminases) should be watched because they are the principal routes of excretion for **antiarrhythmic drugs.** Intervals for these tests depend on drug class. **Antiarrhythmics** tend to have narrow therapeutic ranges and are often given to patients who are taking other drugs with which they may interact, increasing the risk of toxicity or lack of efficacy. Serum drug levels should be monitored at regular intervals after steady state is achieved. Timing of the blood draw is critical. The sample is usually drawn 4 to 6 hours after the last oral dose so that a peak serum level is not mistaken for a steady-state level. Anticoagulation studies (PT, INR, aPTT) are discussed in Chapter 16. Laboratory studies related to the underlying disease that may be causing the arrhythmia are not discussed here.

ECG. Monitoring 12-lead electrocardiograms (ECGs) for indications of efficacy and toxicity is essential, especially concerning drugs for which ECG changes are the primary indicators of such problems. The frequency of monitoring depends on the stability of the patient's drug regimen and the presence of symptoms.

OTHER STUDIES. Electrophysiological studies, echo-cardiography, and exercise stress testing are best done in consultation with a cardiologist. Monitoring for **beta blockers** is discussed in Chapter 12 and for **CCBs** earlier in this chapter. Monitoring parameters are further delineated in Table 14–17.

Table 14–17. Monitoring Parameters for Selected Antiarrhythmics

Drug	Parameters	Timing	Comments
Amiodarone	Chest x-ray, pulmonary function studies	Every 3–6 mo	High risk for pulmonary fibrosis. Risk of sudden cardiac death may outweigh risk associated with pulmonary dysfunction. Every effort should be made to rule out other treatable cause of pulmonary problem. Some providers schedule tests based on symptoms after 1 y without problems.
	Thyroid-stimulating hormone (TSH), Free T_4	Every 6 mo	Monitor closely for other indications of thyroid dysfunction as well.
	Ophthalmic exam (slit lamp and fundoscopy)	Every 6 mo	Although rare, visual impairment may progress to permanent blindness. Any symptoms of impairment should result in prompt ophthalmic exam. Corneal microdeposits are reversible with reduction in dose and no reason to stop treatment.
Flecainide*	ECG		Watch for sinus node problems and AV block.
	Liver function studies		Highly metabolized in liver. Liver disease may significantly increase free drug level.
	Serum drug levels		Keep trough <1 μg/cc
Mexiletine*	Liver function studies		Aspartate aminotransferase (AST) elevations >3 times upper limit of normal (ULN) have been observed. Assess for other treatable causes such as CHF or acute MI before stopping drug.
Procainamide†	Complete blood count (CBC)		At initiation of therapy to assess for blood dyscrasias.
	Antinuclear antibody (ANA) titer		At initiation of therapy and at any indication of lupuslike syndrome.
Propafenone	Liver function studies		Highly metabolized by liver. Liver disease may increase bioavailability to 70%.
Quinidine†	CBC, renal and liver function studies		Discontinue drug if blood dyscrasias or hepatic or renal dysfunction occurs.
Sotalol	Fasting blood glucose		May affect insulin secretion and glucose metabolism. May mask indications of hypoglycemia in patients with diabetes.

All require monitoring of potassium level and 12-lead ECG. Most require serum drug levels. Monitoring of renal function is prudent in all.
†ECG changes are the primary indicators of toxicity in these drugs. QRS >25% above normal or prolonged QT intervals suggest reduction in dose by as much as 50%.
*Changes in urine pH can alter drug excretion. Monitor urinalysis on annual visits.

Patient Education

Cardiac rhythm disturbances tend to engender fear. A thin line exists between providing, on the one hand, enough information to have the patient appreciate the seriousness of the disorder (or the lack of seriousness in benign forms of arrhythmia) and therefore adhere to the treatment regimen and, on the other hand, so much information that fear or denial takes over and adherence suffers. Most patients and their families appreciate an honest discussion of the disorder and its treatment, accompanied by assurance of effective treatment for most forms of arrhythmia. Most **antiarrhythmics** have annoying adverse reactions, and patients are more likely to tolerate them when the importance of the drug is explained.

ADMINISTRATION. The patient should take the drug exactly as prescribed. For doses taken more than once daily, evenly space the doses. Abrupt withdrawal of these drugs may result in life-threatening arrhythmias, HTN, or myocardial ischemia. The patient should keep enough medication on hand for weekends, holidays, and vacations. For **amiodarone,** if a dose is missed at its usual time, it should not be taken at all that day, simply the next day's dose. Its very long half-life maintains a stable dose. For **disopyramide, mexiletine, procainamide sustained-release, propafenone,** and **tocainide,** a dose that is missed should be taken as soon as it is remembered unless the next dose is due in 4 hours or less. For **flecainide,** the missed dose should be taken unless the next dose is due in 6 hours, and for **sotalol,** 8 hours. For **quinidine** and standard formulations of **procainamide,** the separation is 2 hours.

Several drugs come in more than one formulation, from standard to sustained release (Table 14–18). The patient should read the label carefully and follow the appropriate dosing schedule, especially if the drug is changed to a different form or a different drug. For sustained-release formulations, the tablets should not be crushed or chewed but must be swallowed whole. Patients who have difficulty in swallowing should be placed on standard formulations that can be crushed.

Food intake is a concern with some of the **antiarrhythmics. Sotalol** absorption is significantly decreased when it is taken with food. It should always be taken on an empty stomach. **Mexiletine, tocainide,** and **quinidine,** however, have uncomfortable GI adverse effects unless they are taken with food. Foods that alter urine pH affect the excretion of **flecainide, mexiletine,** and **quinidine** and should be avoided or taken in consistent amounts. (See Table 14–15 for a list of such foods.)

Drug interactions are frequent with both prescription and OTC drugs. The patient should consult the health care provider before taking any other drugs, including OTC cold remedies.

ADVERSE REACTIONS. Dizziness is the most common adverse response. Changing position slowly, especially when arising from a lying position, decreases this reaction. Caution should be taken in driving or other activities that require alertness until the patient's response is known. Monitoring of pulse rate and rhythm and BP provides early indications of efficacy and toxicity. Patients should learn to take their own pulse and BP and check them whenever symptoms occur. Hypotension and slow, rapid, or irregular heart rates should be reported promptly. Bone marrow is affected in many classes. Pa-

Table 14–18. Available Dosage Forms: Selected Antiarrhythmics

Drug	Dosage Form (tablets and capsules)
Amiodarone (Cordarone)	200 mg
Disopyramide (Norpace)	100 mg, 150 mg Extended release: 100 mg, 150 mg
Flecainide (Tambocor)	50 mg, 100 mg, 150 mg
Mexiletine (Mexitil)	150 mg, 200 mg, 250 mg
Procainamide (Pronestyl) Procainamide (Procan SR)	250 mg, 375 mg, 500 mg Sustained release: 250 mg, 500 mg, 750 mg, 1000 mg
Propafenone (Rythmol)	150 mg, 250 mg
Quinidine sulfate (Quinidex) Quinidine gluconate (Quinalan)	200 mg, 300 mg Extended release: 300 mg Sustained release: 324 mg
Sotalol (Betapace)	80 mg, 160 mg, 240 mg
Tocainide (Tonocard)	400 mg, 600 mg

tients should report fever, chills, sore throat, or unusual bruising to health care provider. Photosensitivity may occur through window glass, thin clothing, and sunscreens for patients who are taking **amiodarone, disopyramide, or quinidine.** Protective clothing and sunblock are recommended during and for 4 months following therapy. Some find wearing dark glasses helpful. With **amiodarone,** a bluish discoloration of the skin in areas exposed to sunlight may occur. It is usually reversible and fades over several months. This drug is also associated with epididymitis. Patients should report pain or swelling in the scrotum. **Procainamide** occasionally is associated with a lupuslike syndrome. Joint swelling and rashes should be reported. Frequent mouth washes, good oral hygiene, sugarless gum, or hard candy may relieve the dry mouth commonly found with **disopyramide.** The patient should notify the health care provider if dry mouth, constipation, difficulty in urinating, or blurred vision persists with this drug. Tremors are an early indication of excessive doses of **mexiletine** and **tocainide** and should be reported promptly.

For all of these drugs, the importance of keeping follow-up appointments to monitor efficacy and adverse reactions cannot be overstated. Failure to discover problems early can result in permanent adverse changes for some drugs, and life-threatening events as well.

Because these drugs are Pregnancy Category C or D, female patients capable of childbearing should be made aware of the risks of these drugs, and contraception should be instituted before prescribing them.

LIFESTYLE MANAGEMENT. Lifestyle management is similar to that discussed for **ACEIs.** The patient should always wear a medical identification bracelet or necklace that states the name of the drug and the disorder for which it is being taken. Patient education related to **beta blockers** is discussed in Chapter 12.

Nitrates

Nitrates were first introduced for the treatment of angina in the nineteenth century. Their ability to affect both oxygen supply and demand and their effectiveness in rapid relief of acute angina have made them central to the treatment of this disorder.

Pharmacodynamics

Nitroglycerin (NTG) and its analogues act largely by providing more nitric oxide (NO) to vascular endothelium and arterial smooth muscle, resulting in vasodilation (Fig. 14–5). All parts of the vascular system, from larger arteries to large veins, relax in response to nitrates. Dilation of venous capacitance vessels results in venous pooling in the periphery and decreased venous return to the heart, which leads to decreased preload. Arterial dilation, which occurs more commonly with higher doses, decreases systemic arterial pressure, resulting in decreased afterload. Together, these effects decrease myocardial oxygen demand.

Nitrates also increase myocardial oxygen supply by increasing the transmyocardial gradient, causing increased blood flow to the myocardium. Their coronary artery vasodilating effect—originally thought to be their primary role in improving myocardial oxygen demand—is now thought to play a limited role because of atherosclerotic changes in the coronary arteries. They have little effect on angina associated with atherosclerotic CAD.

Indirect actions include reflex responses of baroreceptors and hormonal mechanisms to decreased arterial pressure. The primary mechanism is sympathetic discharge, resulting in tachycardia and increased myocardial contractility. Another action of clinical significance

ON THE HORIZON

Class III drugs are **potassium channel blockers,** but they also have effects found in other classes. **Amiodarone, quinidine,** and **sotalol** all have potassium channel-blocking properties in addition to their effects on sodium channels or beta receptors. "Pure" **potassium channel-blocking drugs** are currently entering clinical trials. Potassium channel blockade would result in increased action potential duration, increased refractoriness, and reduced automaticity. They should be effective in treating reentry problems, in inhibiting ventricular fibrillation that is due to myocardial ischemia, and in improving contractility. An investigational D-isomer of the **class III drug sotalol** has no beta-blocking properties and thus no adverse reactions associated with beta blockade. It retains its effect on repolarization and would increase the instances where it could be used.

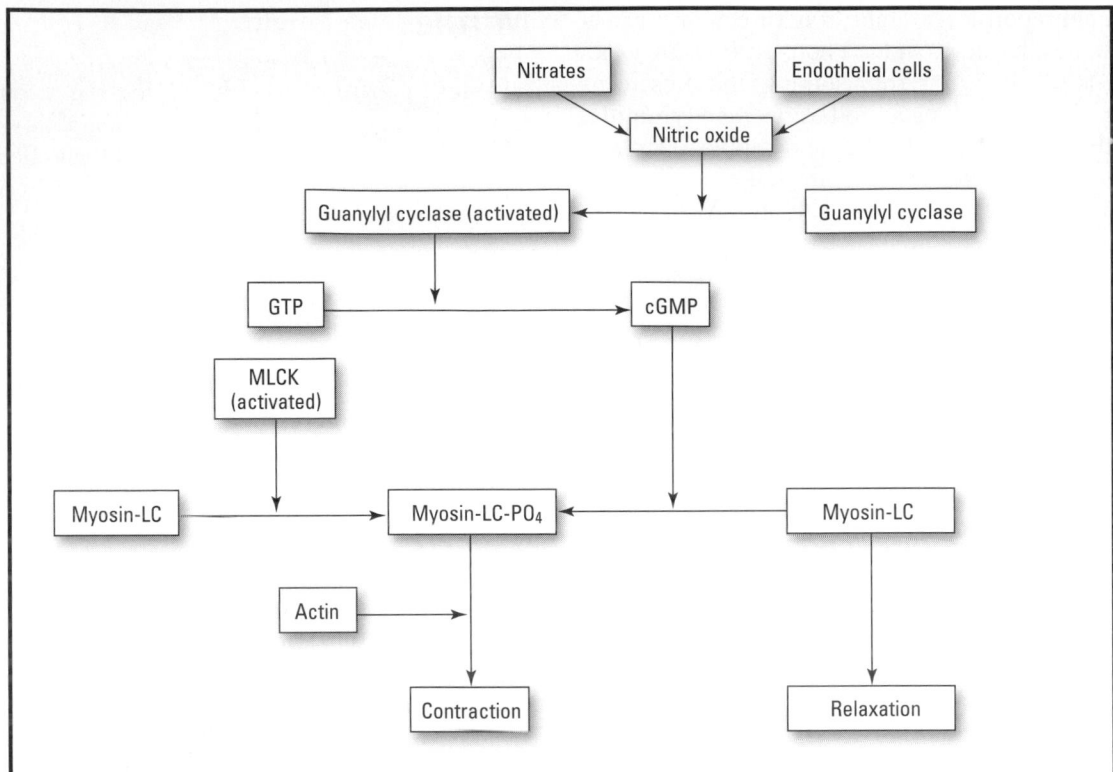

Figure 14–5. Action of substances that increase nitric oxide concentration in smooth muscle cells. Nitrates, nitrites, and other substances that increase nitric oxide concentration in smooth muscle cells potentiate the activation of guanylyl cyclase. Activated guanylyl cyclase then facilitates the production of cGMP. Through a series of not clearly known intermediate steps, the cGMP facilitates the dephosphorylation of the myosin light chain, resulting in muscle relaxation.

is on platelet aggregation. NO released from **NTG** increases cyclic guanosine monophosphate (cGMP), resulting in decreased platelet aggregation. This action is believed to play a role in reduction of infarct size and mortality post-MI for patients given IV **NTG** and may also exist for other forms of **NTG.**

Relaxation of smooth muscle of the bronchi, GI tract, and genitourinary tract also occurs but so briefly that this action is not considered clinically significant.

Pharmacokinetics

Absorption and Distribution

Nitrates are well absorbed by oral, buccal, sublingual, and transdermal routes (Table 14–19). Sublingual absorption is dependent on salivary secretion. Dry mouth (including drug-induced) decreases absorption. **Amyl nitrite** is available in an inhaled form, providing for very rapid absorption.

Metabolism and Excretion

Oral nitrates have a significant hepatic first-pass effect. Hepatic organic nitrate reductase removes nitrate groups from the parent molecule, yielding less potent vasodilators than the parent drug and resulting in low bioavailability for most products. **Oral nitrates** must be given in sufficiently high doses to sustain blood levels despite the first-pass effect. **NTG** has a short half-life (1–4 minutes), but the two major metabolites (1,2 and 1,3 dinitrates) have longer half-lives and appear in substantial concentrations, making them responsible for some of the pharmacological activity. The dinitrates are further metabolized to mononitrates. **Isosorbide dinitrate** is metabolized to active metabolites that accumulate more than the parent drug with long-term therapy. Because **isosorbide mononitrate** is the major active metabolite of **isosorbide dinitrate** and most of the clinical activity is attributed to this metabolite, it is now available as a single-entity product with a bioavailability of nearly 100 percent.

The sublingual route avoids this hepatic first-pass effect and is preferred for achieving a rapid blood level. The inhalation route has the same advantages. The buccal and transdermal routes also avoid the first-pass problems but have slower onsets of action. Total duration of effect by these routes is brief. When longer duration of action is needed, oral preparations are given.

Metabolism of **nitrates** leads to glucuronide derivatives and carbon dioxide excreted by the kidneys and the lungs.

Table 14–19. Pharmacokinetics: Selected Nitrates

Drug	Onset	Peak	Duration	Metabolite	Half-Life	Excretion
Amyl nitrate inhalant	0.5 min		3–5 min	None	UK	⅓ in urine
Isosorbide dinitrate, sublingual	2–5 min	6 min	1–3 h	Isosorbide mononitrate	Drug: 45 min Metabolite: 2–5 h	In urine
Isosorbide dinitrate, oral	20–40 min	6 min	4–6 h	Isosorbide mononitrate	Drug: 45 min Metabolite: 2–5 h	In urine
Isosorbide dinitrate, oral (SR)	up to 4 h	6 min	6–8 h	Isosorbide mononitrate	Drug: 45 min Metabolite: 2–5 h	In urine
Isosorbide mononitrate, oral	30–60 min	UK	7 h	Metabolized to glycerol and CO_2	UK	In urine and lung
Isosorbide mononitrate, oral (SR)	Slow	3–4 h	>12 h	Metabolized to glycerol and CO_2	UK	In urine and lung
NTG, sublingual	1–3 min	4 min	30–60 min	1,2 dinitroglycerol and 1,3 dinitroglycerol	Drug: 1–3 min Metabolites: approx. 40 min	In urine
NTG, translingual spray	2 min	4 min	30–69 min	1,2 dinitroglycerol and 1,3 dinitroglycerol	Drug: 1–3 min Metabolites: approx. 40 min	In urine
NTG buccal tablet	1–2 min	4 min	3–5 h	1,2 dinitroglycerol and 1,3 dinitroglycerol	Drug: 1–3 min Metabolites: approx. 40 min	In urine
NTG oral (SR)	20–45 min	4 min	3–8 h	1,2 dinitroglycerol and 1,3 dinitroglycerol	Drug: 1–3 min Metabolites: approx. 40 min	In urine
NTG topical ointment*	30–60 min	4 min	2–12 h	1,2 dinitroglycerol and 1,3 dinitroglycerol	Drug: 1–3 min Metabolites: approx. 40 min	In urine
NTG transdermal patch	30–60 min	4 min	Up to 24 h	1,2 dinitroglycerol and 1,3 dinitroglycerol	Drug: 1–3 min Metabolites: approx. 40 min	In urine

*Used almost exclusively in the hospital.
All have approximately 60% protein binding.
Half-life of NTG is 1–4 min; others have longer half-lives, with SR preparations up to 12 h.
UK = unknown.

Pharmacotherapeutics

Precautions and Contraindications

Precautions and contraindications are largely related to the actions of these drugs. Vasodilation can result in increased intracranial pressure, so **nitrates** are contraindicated in head trauma or cerebral hemorrhage. Vasodilation can also result in postural hypotension. Patients with volume depletion and anemia should avoid using **nitrates**. *Drug Facts and Comparisons* (1998) states that closed-angle glaucoma is also a contraindication because intraocular pressure (IOP) may be increased. Katsung (1998) states that this is no longer the case, and **nitrates** can be safely used in the presence of increased IOP. Some individuals have hypersensitivity or idiosyncratic responses to **nitrates** and must avoid them. For the transdermal patches, allergy to adhesive may limit their use.

Because the activity of these drugs may compromise maternal-to-fetal circulation, they are Pregnancy Category C. Amyl nitrite is Pregnancy Category X because it markedly reduces system BP and blood flow

on the maternal side of the placenta. Safety and efficacy in children have not been established.

Adverse Drug Reactions

The major adverse reactions are direct extensions of therapeutic vasodilation: orthostatic hypotension with potential for syncope, tachycardia, and throbbing headache. Hypotension may result in decreased diastolic filling pressure, and the tachycardia may result in decreased diastolic filling time, leading to myocardial ischemia, arrhythmias, and rebound HTN. Headache may be severe and persists in up to 50 percent of patients. For patients with severe, persistent headache, it may be necessary to use a different drug group to treat the disease process.

Less common adverse reactions include nausea, vomiting, incontinence of urine and feces, dysuria, impotence, and urinary frequency. Rash and cutaneous vasodilation with flushing may occur with transdermal applications and can be reduced by rotating the site of application.

TOLERANCE. With continuous exposure, smooth muscle develops clinically significant tolerance (tachyphylaxis). In well-controlled clinical trials, **nitrates** were no more effective than placebo after 18 to 24 hours of continuous therapy, particularly for long-acting/sustained-release preparations. The mechanisms by which this occurs are not fully understood. One mechanism proposed is that, over time, decreased substrate (sulfhydryl) results in decreased cGMP, leading to decreased vasodilation. Orally bioavailable compounds containing sulfhydryl groups, such as N-acetylcysteine, may diminish tolerance to the hemodynamic effects of **nitrates** in heart failure (Mehra et al., 1994), but additional research is needed for validation. Attempts to overcome **nitrate** tolerance by increasing dosage, even to doses far in excess of those commonly used, have failed. Only after **nitrates** have been absent from the body for 10 to 12 hours does their effectiveness return. See Clinical Use and Dosing for recommendations to overcome this problem.

Drug Interactions

Additive hypotension is possible with other drug classes that have actions or adverse effects of hypotension: **antihypertensives, beta blockers, CCBs, haloperidol (Haldol),** or **phenothiazines.** Drugs with anticholinergic effects may decrease absorption of sublingual or buccal NTG. **Aspirin** increases **nitrate** serum concentrations and may potentiate their action. **Nitrates** may decrease the pharmacological effects of **heparin.** Specific drug interactions and the appropriate actions to prevent them are given in Table 14–20.

Clinical Use and Dosing

ANGINA. **Nitrates** are the cornerstones of therapy for angina, and for many patients with stable, predictable angina, they are sufficient for control of symptoms. Dosage depends on formulation, with sublingual doses used to treat acute attacks and long-acting forms used for prevention (Table 14–21). Dosing for **sublingual NTG,** a short-acting form, is 0.4 to 0.6 mg every 5 minutes for up to 3 doses. If the angina is not relieved by the second dose, the recommendation is to take the third dose, call 911, and go to the hospital. Dosing for **isosorbide dinitrate,** a long-acting form, is 10 to 40 mg orally bid or tid; the sustained-release form is 40 to 80 mg qd. **Isosorbide mononitrate** dosing is 20 mg bid. For both long-acting forms, twice-daily dosing on an eccentric schedule, with doses separated by 7 hours, is preferred to reduce problems with tolerance. For variant (Prinzmetal's) angina, in which the mechanism may be largely related to vasospasm, long-acting **nitrates** are occasionally sufficient to control symptoms, although **CCBs** are often added to the treatment regimen. Dosing is similar. For unstable angina, the prophylactic value of long-acting nitrates is uncertain, but they may play a role, depending on the underlying pathology. In exertional angina, short-acting forms taken within 5 or 10 minutes of exercise may prevent the anginal episode. Dosing is usually 0.4 mg sublingually.

Table 14–20. Drug Interactions: Nitrates

Drug	Interacting Drug	Possible Effect	Implications
Isosorbide dinitrate, isosorbide mononitrate	Antihypertensives, alcohol, BBs, phenothiazines	Additive hypotension	Monitor BP closely. Teach home BP monitoring.
NTG	Antihypertensives, alcohol, BBs, CCBs, haloperidol, phenothiazines	Additive hypotension	Monitor BP closely. Teach home BP monitoring.
	Agents with anticholinergic properties	May decrease absorption of SL and buccal formulations	Use other formulation if possible.

Table 14–21. Dosage Schedule: Selected Nitrates

Drug	Clinical Use	Starting Dose	Maintenance Dose	Maximum Dose
Isosorbide dinitrate SL, chewable	Treatment of angina	2.5–5 mg SL; 5 mg chewable	Titrate upward until angina relieved or adverse reactions limit.	—
Isosorbide dinitrate, oral	Treatment and prevention of angina; not for acute attack	5–20 mg q6h	10–40 mg bid (eccentric schedule: 8 A.M. and 2 P.M.)	—
Isosorbide dinitrate, oral SR	Same as oral	40 mg bid (eccentric schedule)	40–80 mg bid (eccentric schedule) or qd	—
Isosorbide mononitrate, oral	Treatment and prevention of angina; not for acute attack	5–10 mg bid (eccentric schedule)	20 mg bid (eccentric schedule)	—
Isosorbide mono-nitrate, oral SR	Same as oral	30–60 mg qd	120 mg qd after several days on initial dose	240 mg/d
NTG SL	Prophylaxis	5–10 min prior to activities that might precipitate attack	—	3 tablets in 15 min
	Treatment of acute anginal attacks	0.4–0.6 mg tablet under tongue q 5 min times 3		3 tablets in 15 min
NTG, translingual spray	Prophylaxis	5–10 min prior to activities that might precipitate attack. Do not inhale spray.	—	3 metered sprays in 15 min
	Treatment of acute anginal attacks	1–2 metered sprays onto or under tongue		3 metered sprays in 15 min
NTG, oral SR	"Possibly effective" for prophylaxis or treatment of angina	2.5–2.6 mg tid or qid	Increase by 2.5/2.6 mg increments over a period of days or weeks until adverse reactions limit	2.6 mg qid
NTG, transdermal patch	Prevention of angina	0.2–0.4 mg/h on 12–14 h; off 10–12 h	0.4–0.8 mg/h on 12–14 h; off 10–12 h	—

HEART FAILURE. Their role in reducing ventricular filling pressure and pulmonary and system vascular resistance give **nitrates** a place in the treatment of CHF. **Isosorbide dinitrate** administered chronically has been shown to be effective in improving exercise capacity and in reducing symptoms. Its limited effect of systemic vascular resistance and the problem of tolerance mean that it is rarely single-drug therapy. Combining this drug with **hydralazine** has produced a more sustained improvement than either drug alone. Tolerance limits long-term effectiveness and develops more easily with sustained-release forms. The dosing regimen that produces the most sustained hemodynamic effects and minimizes the development of tolerance appears to be 40 mg q8h. Patients with advanced right-sided heart failure with resultant portal hypertension may have variable ab-

sorption of **oral nitrates.** The sublingual form is recommended for these patients.

INITIATION OF THERAPY. Start low and go slow is appropriate here. If the initial dose is too high, severe vascular headaches and the possibility of orthostatic hypotension may cause patients to stop taking the drug. Beginning low and advancing slowly over a period of 1 to 2 weeks usually results in the desired effects without the headaches.

Dosage increases should be made against the following parameters:

1. Reduced angina or lack of angina with usual activity.
2. Heart rate at rest increases by no more than 15 bpm.

Clinical Pearl

Patients with migraine headaches are especially at risk for **nitrate** headaches. Start them first on a **beta blocker** for migraine prophylaxis, and then add the **nitrate** to prevent the problem.

3. BP does not fall to the point of causing orthostatic hypotension.

Headache or its absence is not a reliable variable by which to judge therapy because tachyphylaxis for this adverse effect is common in a few weeks to 1 month.

PREVENTION OF TOLERANCE.   To prevent or reduce the development of tolerance, a **nitrate**-free interval of 10 to 12 hours/day is required. Sustained-release preparations are more likely to lead to tolerance and should be avoided unless used qd. Short-acting products with bid/tid dosing are less likely to lead to tolerance. For bid dosing, use an eccentric dosing schedule separated by 7 hours (e.g., 7 A.M., 2 P.M.). Patients whose anginal symptoms occur at night may do best with a daytime **nitrate**-free interval, and the reverse holds for those whose symptoms occur during the daytime. If around-the-clock coverage is necessary for anginal symptoms, coverage with a **beta blocker** or **CCB** during the nitrate-free interval may be needed.

Rational Drug Selection

FORMULATION AND COST.   **Sublingual NTG** has rapid action, long-established efficacy, easy use, and low cost. A disadvantage is its short duration of action. It is also volatile and must be kept in a tightly capped, amber container and stored in a cool place. Once a bottle is opened, it is generally effective for only about 6 months. Onset and duration of action of a single metered dose of **translingual spray** is about the same as **sublingual NTG.** Each canister contains 200 doses and retains efficacy for up to 3 years. Some skill is required to use it. Cost per dose is substantially higher than for the sublingual form, but the prolonged shelf life helps reduce total cost. It is a good alternative for patients who wear dentures or have dry mucosa. **Oral NTG** has questionable efficacy and is available only in sustained release, a form associated with increased incidence of tolerance. **Transdermal** delivery systems offer easy use and release **NTG** at a constant rate to maintain steady-state plasma levels. They are also inexpensive, with cost at approximately $1/day. Tolerance is an issue unless a **nitrate**-free interval is provided, and bioavailability varies significantly from patient to patient. Physical exercise and ambient temperatures may increase absorption.

Among the **oral nitrates, isosorbide dinitrate** provides sustained **nitrate** activity and better anginal prophylaxis. Single doses significantly improve hemodynamic parameters and exercise tolerance for up to 4 hours. Its action is not as rapid as **sublingual NTG** but does occur in 15 to 30 minutes, which is appropriate for prevention. Eccentric scheduling appears to balance the need for angina coverage and the avoidance of tolerance. In generic form, its cost is very low. **Chewable** and **sublingual** forms provide more rapid onset of action, but the duration of action falls to about 2 hours. Because there appears to be no clear benefit over **sublingual NTG**, the higher cost of these latter two forms does not seem to justify their use. **Isosorbide dinitrate** is also available in a sustained-release form that requires only bid or qd dosing, but it has highly variable intestinal absorption, and the risk of **nitrate** tolerance is higher unless it is used once daily.

Isosorbide mononitrate offers 100 percent bioavailability and the convenience of once-daily dosing but otherwise appears to have no significant clinical advantage over **isosorbide dinitrate. Nitrate** tolerance occurs less often for the regular formulation. The sustained-release form has the same problems with tolerance as other sustained-release formulations. Cost is significantly higher (approximately 10 times).

Monitoring

No specific monitoring parameters exist for **nitrates.**

Patient Education

ADMINISTRATION.   Take the drug exactly as prescribed. For oral doses taken more than once daily, a **nitrate**-free interval of 10 to 12 hours is necessary to prevent nitrate intolerance. For bid dosing, an eccentric dosing schedule separated by 7 hours (e.g., 7 A.M., 2 P.M.) is best. If anginal symptoms occur at night, it may be best to have a daytime **nitrate**-free interval, with the reverse for symptoms occurring during the daytime. If round-the-clock coverage is necessary for anginal symptoms, coverage with a **beta blocker** or **CCB** during the **nitrate**-free interval may be needed.

Several drugs come in more than one formulation, from standard to sustained release (Table 14–22). The patient should read the label carefully and follow the appro-

Table 14–22. Available Dosage Forms: Nitrates

Drug	Dosage Form
Isosorbide dinitrate, SL	Tablets: 2.5 mg, 5 mg, 10 mg
Isosorbide dinitrate, chewable	Tablets: 5 mg, 10 mg
Isosorbide dinitrate, oral	Tablets: 2.5 mg, 5 mg, 10 mg, 20 mg, 30 mg, 40 mg
Isosorbide dinitrate, oral SR	Tablets: 40 mg
Isosorbide mononitrate, oral	Tablets: 10 mg, 20 mg
Isosorbide mononitrate, oral SR	Tablets: 60 mg
NTG, SL	Tablets: 0.15 mg, 0.3 mg, 0.4 mg, 0.6 mg
NTG, buccal SR	Tablets: 1 mg, 2 mg, 3 mg
NTG, translingual	0.4 mg per spray
NTG, oral SR	Tablets: 2.5 mg, 6.5 mg, 9 mg
NTG, transdermal	0.1 mg, 0.2 mg, 0.3 mg, 0.4 mg, 0.6 mg in boxes of 30, 33, or 100 patches

priate dosing schedule. This is especially important if the drug is changed to a different form or a different drug. For sustained-release formulations, the tablets should not be crushed or chewed but must be swallowed whole. **Sublingual NTG** tablets may lose potency when stored. Store in tightly closed, amber glass containers. Tablets lose potency when exposed to air, heat, or moisture or when mixed with other tablets. Do not open the bottle frequently or keep bottles of tablets next to the body (e.g., in a shirt pocket) or in an automobile glove compartment. A burning sensation under the tongue is not a reliable method of testing potency. Adhere to the expiration date on the bottle, usually 6 months, and write on the bottle the date the bottle was first opened. If ordered for treatment of acute anginal attacks, **sublingual NTG** is the drug of choice. At the first sign of an attack, the patient should sit down and place one sublingual tablet under the tongue and allow it to dissolve. It should not be swallowed. If the pain is not relieved, repeat every 5 minutes for up to three doses. If the angina is not relieved by the second dose, the patient should take the third dose, call 911, and go directly to the hospital. Dry mouth may reduce the effectiveness of **sublingual NTG.** Dry mouth problems should be discussed with the health care provider. Sublingual spray may be used in the same manner as the tablet. Lift the tongue and spray the dose under the tongue. Transdermal patches also required a **nitrate**-free interval of 10 to 12 hours. Follow the same instructions as for oral tablets related to this interval. The site of application should be changed each time, with the best sites the anterior chest and the upper arms in areas not covered with hair. Remove the clear plastic cover over the medication side of the patch before applying. Apply firm pressure over the patch to ensure contact with the skin. Physical exercise and ambient temperatures may increase absorption by this route, resulting in more adverse effects.

For all forms, do not double doses and do not discontinue abruptly, which may result in rebound angina. Avoid concurrent use of alcohol with these drugs. Because some OTC drugs interact with **nitrates** or contain alcohol, do not take any new OTC drugs, including cold remedies, without first discussing this with the health care provider.

ADVERSE REACTIONS. The major adverse reactions are throbbing headaches, rapid heart rates, and decreased BP when arising from a sitting or lying position, with the potential for fainting. Headache may be severe; although it should decrease with continued therapy, it persists in up to 50 percent of patients. It is less likely with lower doses and slow increases in doses. It is best treated with **acetaminophen (Tylenol).** Report headaches to the health care provider, who may alter the dose or change the drug. Rapid heart rates should also be reported right away. They may worsen the condition for which the **nitrate** is prescribed. Making position changes slowly minimizes the BP changes. When arising from lying down, the patient should sit on the edge of the bed for a few minutes before standing to allow the body to adjust to the different position.

The rashes, skin irritation, and flushing/blushing of the skin that may occur with transdermal patches can be reduced by rotating the site of application.

Incontinence of urine and bowel movements, pain on urination, frequent urination, and impotence are rare adverse responses. They should be reported so that a potential cause other than the **nitrate** can be ruled out or alterations in the drug regimen can be undertaken.

Because these drugs are Pregnancy Category C, female patients capable of childbearing should be made aware of the risks of these drugs, and contraception should be instituted before they are prescribed. *Amyl nitrite* **is Pregnancy Category X and should not be prescribed in these circumstances.**

LIFESTYLE MANAGEMENT. See ACEIs.

Peripheral Vasodilators

Peripheral vasodilators are used to treat HTN and peripheral vascular disease (PVD), although significant clinical improvement of PVD rarely occurs with these drugs alone. **Peripheral alpha₁ antagonists** and **central alpha₂ agonists** can be used for these purposes. They are discussed in Chapter 12. The focus of the discussion here is on two drugs, **hydralazine (Apresoline)** and **minoxidil (Loniten)**, and their use in treating HTN.

Pharmacodynamics

Peripheral vasodilators useful in the treatment of HTN act by direct relaxation and dilation of arteriolar smooth muscle, thereby decreasing PVR. They do not dilate the capacitance vessels (epicardial coronary arteries) and do not relax venous smooth muscle.

Pharmacokinetics

Absorption and Distribution

Hydralazine is well absorbed orally. Taking it with food increases absorption. It is widely distributed and crosses the placenta but enters breast milk in minimal amounts. It is compatible with breastfeeding according to the American Academy of Pediatrics. **Minoxidil** is also well absorbed orally and widely distributed. It enters breast milk in larger amounts and should not be used while breastfeeding (Table 14–23).

Metabolism and Excretion

With **hydralazine**, bioavailability is low and variable among patients, based on their genetics. Rapid acetylators have greater hepatic first-pass metabolism, lower bioavailability, and less antihypertensive benefit than do slow acetylators. Although hydralazine's half-life is short, vascular effects persist longer than blood concentrations would suggest, based on the avid binding of this drug to vascular tissue. **Minoxidil** is not protein bound and has a higher bioavailability. Its half-life is also short, but it also has a longer antihypertensive effect because of the persistence of its active metabolite, minoxidil sulfate.

Pharmacotherapeutics

Precautions and Contraindications

Use cautiously in patients with cardiovascular disease. Myocardial ischemia may result from the increased oxy-

gen demand associated with SNS stimulation. Because these drugs do not dilate the epicardial coronary arteries, the peripheral arterial vasodilation may "steal" blood flow from any ischemic region of the heart. If used alone, sodium and water retention may precipitate high-output CHF. Both problems are more likely to occur in older adults.

Cautious use is also recommended for patients with pulmonary HTN related to the potential for severe hypotension.

Both drugs are Pregnancy Category C and should be used only when benefits clearly outweigh risks.

Adverse Drug Reactions

Decreased peripheral resistance triggers compensatory responses in the SNS and in the renin-angiotensin-aldosterone system. These reflexes prevent the orthostatic hypotension and sexual dysfunction caused by many other **antihypertensives**, but they precipitate added tachycardia, increased cardiac contractility and output, sodium and water retention, headache, and tachyphylaxis to the antihypertensive effects. **Hydralazine** sometimes induces a lupuslike syndrome. It appears to be dose-related in that it occurs almost exclusively with doses above 50 mg/day. The incidence is highest in white women. A positive antinuclear antibody (ANA) test is found in these patients, but no renal impairment is seen. Discontinuing the drug reverses the syndrome, but the ANA does not return to normal until 6 to 8 months after the drug is stopped. **Minoxidil** has been associated with elongation, thickening, and enhanced pigmentation of fine body hair. This effect has resulted in an unlabeled use in treating male pattern baldness.

Drug Interactions

Additive effects may occur with other **antihypertensives**. **NSAIDs** may decrease their antihypertensive effects. Interactions with **beta blockers** and **loop diuretics** are positive in that they prevent the adverse effects common to these drugs. Specific drug interactions and the appropriate actions to prevent them are given in Table 14–24.

Clinical Use and Dosing

HYPERTENSION. The usual oral dose of **hydralazine** is 25 to 100 mg bid, which provides smooth control of BP

Table 14–23. Pharmacokinetics: Selected Peripheral Vasodilators

Drug	Onset	Peak	Duration	Protein Binding	Bioavailability	Half-Life	Elimination
Hydralazine PO	45 min	1–2 h	6–12 h	87%	30–50%	3–7 h	12–14% in urine
Minoxidil	30 min	2–3 h	24+ h	None	UK	4.2 h	20% in urine

UK = unknown.

Table 14–24. Drug Interactions: Peripheral Vasodilators

Drug	Interacting Drug	Possible Effect	Implications
Hydralazine	Antihypertensives, alcohol, nitrates*	Additive hypotension	Avoid concurrent use or monitor BP closely.
	MAOIs	Severe hypotension	Avoid concurrent use.
	NSAIDs	Reduced antihypertensive effects	Choose different analgesic or anti-inflammatory.
	BBs	Increased blood levels of hydralazine	Used concurrently to treat adverse reactions. May require reduction of hydralazine dose.
Minoxidil	Antihypertensives, alcohol, nitrates, guanethidine	Additive hypotension	Avoid concurrent use or monitor BP closely.
	NSAIDs	Reduced antihypertensive effects	Choose different analgesic or anti-inflammatory.

*Hydralazine may be prescribed with isosorbide dinitrate to treat CHF.

regardless of acetylator type (Table 14–25). The maximum dose recommended is 200 mg/day to minimize the risk of the lupuslike syndrome. **Minoxidil** is usually started at 5 mg daily and increased at 3-day intervals to 10 mg/day, then 20 mg/day, and then 40 mg/day, each in two divided doses. Effective control of BP may occur at any of these doses.

The SNS stimulation and sodium and water retention problems associated with both of these drugs require the concurrent administration of a **beta blocker** and a **loop diuretic. BBs** prevent the tachycardia, increased cardiac output, and increased renin release; **diuretics** prevent the salt and water retention caused by decreased renal sodium excretion.

HEART FAILURE. **Hydralazine** with concurrent administration of **isosorbide dinitrate** has been used to treat CHF. This combination and **ACEIs** are the only classes of drugs that have been demonstrated to reduce mortality in CHF. The dosage is up to 800 mg tid to reduce afterload. This is not a long-term management solution.

Rational Drug Selection

These drugs are third-line therapy for moderate to severe HTN. **Minoxidil** should be used only in severe renal failure or when no other **antihypertensive** has been effective.

Monitoring

There are no specific monitoring requirements for these drugs beyond those used for patients with HTN. HTN is discussed in Chapter 38.

Patient Education

ADMINISTRATION. Patients should take the drug exactly as prescribed at the same time each day, even if they are feeling well. A missed dose should be taken as soon as it is remembered; doses should not be doubled. If more than two doses in a row are missed, the patient should consult the health care provider. These drugs control but do not cure HTN. The patient should not

Table 14–25. Dosage Schedule and Available Dosage Forms: Peripheral Vasodilators

Drug	Starting Dose	Maintenance Dose	Maximum Dose	Available Dosage Form
Hydralazine (Apresoline)	10 mg qid. After 2 to 4 d, may increase to 25 mg qid for the rest of the first week, then increase to 50 mg qid.	25–100 mg qid. Once maintenance dose is achieved, may go to bid dosing.	400 mg/d. To minimize risk of lupus-like syndrome, keep maximum dose <200 mg/d.	Tablets: 10 mg, 25 mg, 50 mg, 100 mg
Minoxidil (Loniten)	5 mg/d increased at 3-d intervals to 10 mg/d, then 20 mg/d, then 40 mg/d; each in 2 divided doses.	5–40 mg/d in 2 divided doses.	100 mg/d.	Tablets: 2.5 mg, 10 mg

stop or alter the dose without first contacting the health care provider.

Hydralazine should be taken with meals to enhance absorption. **Minoxidil** may be taken without regard to meals or food.

Drug interactions occur with **NSAIDs** and some OTC drugs, especially cough, cold, and allergy remedies. The patient should not take any other drugs without first consulting the health care provider.

ADVERSE REACTIONS. Hypotensive reactions are the most common. Changing position slowly and avoiding exercise in hot weather can decrease these reactions. The patient should learn home BP and pulse monitoring and report decreases in BP by more than 20 mm Hg or increases in pulse of more than 20 bpm above baseline. Dyspnea, pronounced dizziness, or nausea should be reported. Because fluid retention may occur, patients should weigh themselves daily and report weight gain of more than 5 lb in 1 week or more than 1 lb in 1 day, as well as swelling of hands, feet, or ankles or decreased urine output.

Because these drugs are Pregnancy Category C, female patients capable of childbearing should be made aware of the risks of these drugs, and contraception should be instituted before they are prescribed.

LIFESTYLE MANAGEMENT. Adherence with other interventions for HTN, such as weight reduction, low-sodium diet, smoking cessation, moderation of alcohol intake, regular exercise, and stress management, is as important as the drugs.

Antilipidemics

Elevated lipoproteins, especially low-density lipoproteins (LDLs), have been associated with serious and potentially lethal cardiovascular disorders associated with atherosclerosis. High-density lipoproteins (HDLs), by contrast, exert antiatherogenic effects. Lowering LDL levels and raising HDL levels through diet, exercise, and drugs have been shown to decrease the progression of atherosclerosis. Atherosclerosis, with its resultant CAD, is the leading cause of death for both men and women. In the Framingham study, a 10 percent decrease in cholesterol level was associated with a 2 percent decrease in the incidence of CAD morbidity and mortality. Drugs that affect lipid levels differentially affect LDL, HDL, and triglyceride levels. Their clinical application is based on how they affect each of these.

This section focuses on the drugs used to lower plasma lipoprotein levels. The pathophysiology of atherosclerosis, the relationship of hyperlipidemia to atherosclerosis development, and the management of hyperlipidemia based on the National Cholesterol Education Program guidelines are discussed in Chapter 37.

Pharmacodynamics

There are four general classes of **lipid-lowering drugs: niacin, fibric acid derivatives, bile acid–binding resins,** and **competitive inhibitors of HMG-CoA reductase** (Fig. 14–6). Each is discussed separately.

Niacin decreases very low density lopoprotein (VLDL) and LDL levels. The primary mechanism of action is probably inhibition of VLDL secretion, which, in turn, decreases production of LDL levels by 10 to 15 percent. Clearance of VLDL via the lipoprotein lipase pathway also results in lowering of triglyceride levels by 20 to 80 percent. HDL catabolism is concurrently decreased, resulting in elevations of HDL levels by 20 to 30 mg/dL. The drug has no effect on bile acid production. Reduction in circulating fibrinogen levels and increases in tissue plasminogen levels also decrease the risk for thrombogenesis.

Fibric acid derivatives (gemfibrozil [Lopid]) increase lipolysis of triglycerides via lipoprotein lipase, resulting in a decrease of 50 percent or more in triglyceride levels. A decrease in VLDL is also related to decreased secretion by the liver. Only modest reductions in LDL levels (15 to 20%) occur in most patients. Patients with combined hyperlipidemia may actually increase their LDL levels. HDL levels increase by 15 to 25 percent as a direct consequence of decreasing triglycerides.

Bile acid–binding resins (colestipol [Colestid] and **cholestyramine [Questran])** exchange chloride ions for negatively charged bile acids, promoting a 10-fold increase in bile acid excretion. The increased clearance results in enhanced conversion of cholesterol to bile acids by the liver. Increased uptake of LDL from plasma results from up-regulation of high-affinity LDL receptors on cell membranes, especially in the liver. The net result is decreased LDL levels by 10 to 35 percent. HDL levels increase about 5 percent. Triglycerides may also rise initially, but they return to baseline within a few weeks.

Reductase inhibitors (atorvastatin [Lipitor], fluvastatin [Lescol], lovastatin [Mevacor], pravastatin [Pravachol], and **simvastatin [Zocor]** block synthesis of cholesterol in the liver by competitively inhibiting HMG-CoA reductase activity. They induce an increase in high-affinity LDL receptors, resulting in an increased catabolism of LDL and an increase in the liver's extraction of LDL precursors. The net result is decreased LDL levels by 25 to 45 percent. Modest decreases in triglycerides of 10 to 30 percent and increases in HDL of 8 to 10 percent also occur.

Pharmacokinetics

Absorption and Distribution

Absorption and distribution vary greatly among antilipidemics (Table 14–26). **Atorvastatin, niacin, fluvastatin, gemfibrozil,** and **simvastatin** are all well ab-

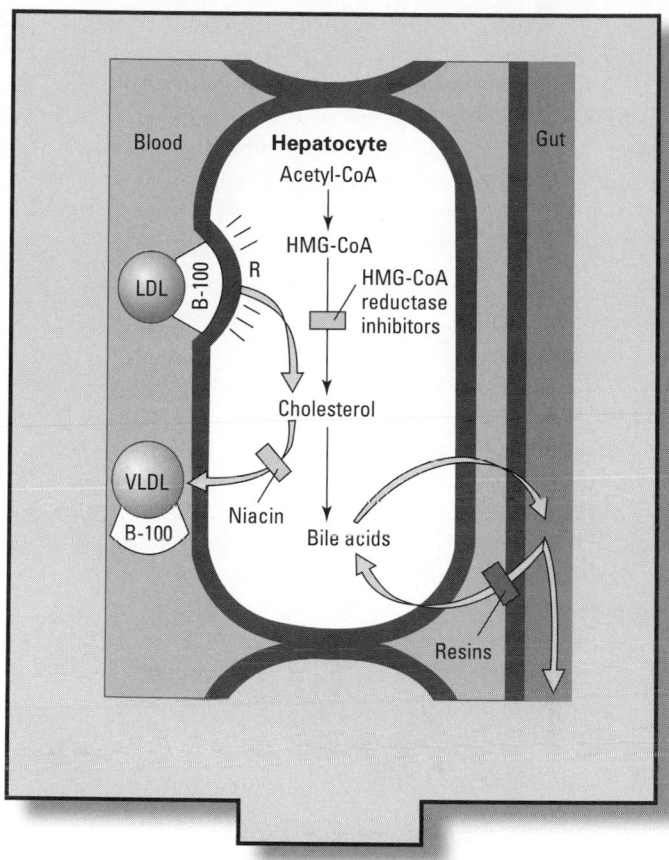

Figure 14–6. Sites of action of antihyperlipidemics.

Table 14–26. Pharmacokinetics: Selected Antilipidemics

Drug	Onset	Peak	Duration	Protein Binding	Bioavailability	Half-Life	Elimination
Atorvastatin	Rapid	1–2 h	20–30 h	>98%	12%	14 h	<2% in urine
Cholestyramine	24–48 h	1–3 wk	2–4 wk	NA	0%	UK	Insoluble complex in feces
Colestipol	24–48 h	1 mo	1 mo	NA	0%	UK	Insoluble complex in feces
Fluvastatin	1–2 wk*	4–6 wk*	Unknown	>98%	<24%	<1 h	5% in urine, 90% in feces
Gemfibrozil	2–5 d*	4 wk*	Months	95%	UK	1.5 h	70% in urine, 6% in feces
Lovastatin	2 wk*	4–6 wk	6 wk	>95%	35%	3–4 h	10% in urine, 83% in feces
Niacin		45 min	Unknown	UK	UK	45 min	88% unchanged in urine
Pravastatin	1–2 wk*	4–6 wk*	Unknown	50%	17%	1.8 h	20% in urine, 70% in feces
Simvastatin	1–2 wk*	4–6 wk*	Unknown	95%	<5%	3 h	13% in urine, 60% in feces

*Effect on plasma lipids.
NA = not applicable; UK = unknown.

sorbed. **Lovastatin** and **pravastatin** are poorly absorbed. With the exception of **atorvastatin**, food decreases the rate of absorption of the reductase inhibitors. Food intake does not affect absorption of the other antilipidemics. Most are widely distributed and enter breast milk in variable amounts. **Cholestyramine** and **colestipol** are not absorbed at all and have no distribution. Their action is entirely related to binding bile acids in the gut.

Metabolism and Excretion

Niacin and **gemfibrozil** have some metabolism by the liver but are excreted mostly unchanged in the urine. These drugs are affected by impaired renal function. The reductase inhibitors are extensively metabolized by the liver, often employing CYP-450 2C6 and 3A4 enzyme systems, and usually on first pass. This explains their universally low bioavailabilities, from less than 5 percent for **simvastatin** to 35 percent for **lovastatin**. Because reductase inhibitors are largely excreted in bile and feces, with only small amounts excreted unchanged in the urine, plasma levels are not significantly affected by renal function but may increase markedly with hepatic failure and chronic alcoholic cirrhosis.

Plasma half-lives are generally short (45 minutes to 3 hours), with the exception of **atorvastatin**, whose half-life is 14 hours.

Pharmacotherapeutics

Precautions and Contraindications

Active liver disease is a contraindication for all **antilipidemics** except the **bile acid–binding resins**. Marked persistent increases in serum transaminases and drug-induced hepatitis have occurred with **reductase inhibitors,** and they should be used with caution in any patient who consumes substantial quantities of **alcohol** or who has a history of liver disease. Cautious use of the **bile acid–binding resins** is suggested for patients with a history of constipation, and phenylketonuria (PKU) is a contraindication for **cholestyramine.** Severe renal impairment warrants cautious use of those drugs excreted largely unchanged in the urine (**niacin, gemfibrozil**). Some **niacin** products contain tartrazine (FDC yellow dye #5) and should be avoided for patients with an **aspirin** allergy. Because of its tendency to GI irritation, **niacin** should also be used cautiously for patients with a history of peptic ulcer disease.

Niacin and *gemfibrozil* are Pregnancy Category C. Risks and benefits should be weighed. All the *reductase inhibitors* are Pregnancy Category X and should not be given to women who have the potential to become pregnant. No Pregnancy Category has been assigned to the *bile acid–binding resins.* All *antilipi-*

demics should be avoided during breastfeeding. With the exception of **niacin**, the safety of **antilipidemics** has not been established for children under age 18 years. Use of **reductase inhibitors** in children is restricted to those with heterozygous or homozygous familial hypercholesterolemias with some residual receptor activity.

Adverse Drug Reactions

Cutaneous flushing, especially of the face and upper body, has been associated with **niacin.** Gradually increasing initial low doses helps to reduce this adverse reaction. **Niaspan,** an extended-release form of **niacin,** can be administered at bedtime, with the smaller amount of cutaneous flushing occurring while the patient is sleeping to make the drug more easily tolerated. **Gemfibrozil** has a few GI symptoms, including dyspepsia, abdominal pain, and diarrhea. The **bile acid–binding resins'** major problems are GI effects, including constipation that may be severe and result in impaction. Other GI symptoms include flatulence, nausea, vomiting, and abdominal pain. Headache is also common. A fairly rare symptom is a burnt odor to the urine.

The **reductase inhibitors** all have headache as a common adverse reaction. **Atorvastatin** and **simvastatin** have the lowest adverse reaction profiles, with myalgia for the former and abdominal pain for the latter as the only adverse reactions besides headaches. **Fluvastatin, lovastatin,** and **pravastatin** all have GI-associated adverse reactions (dyspepsia, abdominal pain, flatulence, constipation, or diarrhea). Generally, these reactions are mild and transient.

Rhabdomyolysis with renal dysfunction secondary to myoglobinuria has occurred with some **reductase inhibitors.** Although it occurs in only 0.1–0.5 percent of patients, when it does occur, it is serious. Myopathy should be considered in any patient with diffuse myalgias, muscle tenderness and weakness, and elevations in creatine kinase (CK) values more than 10 times the upper limit of normal. Consider temporarily withholding or discontinuing drug therapy in patients with a risk factor predisposing them to the development of renal failure secondary to rhabdomyolysis, including hypotension; major surgery or trauma; severe metabolic, endocrine, or electrolyte disorder; or uncontrolled seizures.

Drug Interactions

All **antilipidemics** except **niacin** affect **warfarin** activity: **bile acid–binding resins** decrease its effect, and the other classes increase its effect. **Gemfibrozil** has interactions with several other **antilipidemics**. All **reductase inhibitors**—atorvastatin most of all—increase **digoxin** levels. Systemic **imidazole** and **triazole** therapies increase **reductase inhibitor** levels by 20-fold. **Propra-**

nolol decreases the antilipidemic activity of **reductase inhibitors**. **Niacin, erythromycin,** and **cyclosporine** all increase the risk of rhabdomyolysis when given with **reductase inhibitors.** Taking **lovastatin** with food enhances its blood levels. Specific drug interactions and the appropriate actions to prevent them are given in Table 14–27.

Clinical Use and Dosing

INCREASED LDL. Niacin, bile acid–binding resins, and **reductase inhibitors** all reduce LDL. **Niacin** is an effective and inexpensive first-line drug. A B-complex vitamin, it is available OTC. It has been shown to reduce all-cause mortality for patients with CAD. Because of its many adverse reactions, it is most frequently given as adjunctive therapy with a **bile acid–binding resin** or a **reductase inhibitor** for patients with heterozygous familial hypercholesterolemia. Most patients require 2 to 6.5 g/day of **niacin** for this disease process. For other types of hypercholesterolemia, a dose of 1.5 to 3.5 g/day is usually enough. The daily dose should be divided and given with meals, starting at 100 mg bid or tid and gradually increasing at 5- to 7-day intervals (Table 14–28).

Reductase inhibitors are first-line drugs in monotherapy and in combinations. Because of the diurnal pattern on cholesterol synthesis, **reductase inhibitors** are given in the evening in a single daily dose. **Atorvastatin** is the most potent and has the best adverse reaction profile. The usual dose is 10 mg initially increased at 2- to 4-week intervals up to 80 mg. **Simvastatin** also has an excellent adverse reaction profile and is twice as potent on a weight basis as **lovastatin** and **pravastatin**. The initial dose is 5 to 10 mg, with a maximum of 40 mg. **Lovastatin** has a midrange adverse reactions profile. Because it must be taken with food, it is given with the evening meal. Initial dose is 10 to 20 mg, with dosage increases at 6- to 8-week intervals to a maximum dose of 80 mg. **Pravastatin** is similar in potency and adverse effects profile to **lovastatin**. The initial dose is 10 to 20 mg, with a maximum of 40 mg. **Fluvastatin** is about one-half as potent as **lovastatin** and has a midrange adverse reactions profile. The initial dose is 20 mg, with a maximum dose of 40 mg. Splitting the 40-mg dose into bid doses slightly improves the LDL-lowering ability (Table 14–29).

Bile acid–binding resins have been first-line therapy for years, with a proven safety record. They are best for patients with a low CAD risk profile but who are unable to reduce their LDL by diet alone. Their biggest drawback is their GI adverse effect profile. **Cholestyramine** and **colestipol** come in powdered form. The initial dose is 1 tsp mixed with juice in a slurry. They are never swallowed in dry form. The dose is taken one-half hour before, during, or one-half hour after a meal for several days. Doses are increased gradually, based largely on GI adverse reactions. A common dose is 2 to 3 tsp at breakfast and supper.

ELEVATED VLDL AND ELEVATED TRIGLYCERIDES. **Gemfibrozil** is the most potent **triglyceride-lowering agent** because of its effect on VLDL, and it is generally used only for this purpose. The initial dose is 600 mg/day, increased gradually to 1200 mg/day, taken bid 30 minutes before the morning and evening meals. Data from the Helsinki Heart Study resulted in the recommendation that this drug not be used for patients with combined hyperlipidemia who have CAD symptoms. In severe mixed lipidemia, **niacin**, plus a **bile acid–binding resin** or a **reductase inhibitor**, often produces marked reduction in triglyceride levels. To prevent pancreatitis for patients with marked hypertriglyceridemia, **niacin** in large doses may be used for patients who do not respond to **gemfibrozil**.

DECREASED HDL. **Niacin** is clearly the most effective agent in increasing levels of HDL. **Gemfibrozil** is the next best at increasing HDL, followed by the **reductase inhibitors**. Although they are now recognized as a risk factor in heart disease, HDL levels are not usually treated alone. This factor is a bonus effect when choosing a drug to treat elevated LDL or VLDL levels.

Rational Drug Selection

In addition to the nature of the lipoprotein abnormality and the mechanism of action and adverse reaction profile of the drug, as discussed previously, factors taken into account in selecting the appropriate drug or drug combination include degree of CAD risk, age of the patient, and cost.

DEGREE OF CAD RISK. For all risk groups, dietary reduction in saturated fat and cholesterol is first-line therapy. When drug therapy is a necessary adjunct, the following pattern is helpful.

For high-risk CAD patients as defined by the National Cholesterol Education Program, **niacin** and **reductase inhibitors** are the most cost-effective and should be tried first. If patient response is inadequate after 4 months, switch to a different drug or try a combination of drugs. Combinations of **reductase inhibitors** with **niacin** have shown promise for the highest-risk patients who fail to respond to either of the two first-line drugs classes alone. The combination of a **reductase inhibitor** with **gemfibrozil** is to be avoided because of the risk for rhabdomyolysis. Patients whose response is still inadequate should be referred to a lipid disorder specialist. **Estrogen replacement therapy** should be considered for postmenopausal women with elevated cholesterol because estrogens lower LDL and raise HDL levels. Evidence suggests reduction of CAD risk with estrogen.

For moderate-risk CAD patients, drug therapy is generally not needed if dietary modifications are followed. For isolated low-HDL patients, aerobic exercise, smok-

Table 14–27. Drug Interactions: Selected Antilipidemics

Drug	Interacting Drug	Possible Effect	Implications
All reductase inhibitors	Digoxin	Slight elevation in digoxin levels. Concurrent administration with atorvastatin may increase steady-state levels by 20%.	If unable to choose alternative drug, monitor for digoxin toxicity. Avoid concurrent use of atorvastatin.
	Warfarin	Increased anticoagulant effect.	Monitor PT/INR closely.
	Itraconazole and other azole antifungals	Coadministration increases reductase inhibitor levels 20-fold.	Temporarily interrupt reductase inhibitor if systemic azole antifungals needed.
	Propranolol	Decreases antilipidemic activity.	Choose alternative beta blocker.
Atorvastatin	Maalox TC	Coadministration decreases atorvastatin level by 35%; LDL reduction is not altered.	Separate doses by at least 1 h.
	Norethindrone, ethinyl estradiol	Increases contraceptive levels by 30% and 20%, respectively.	Choose alternative contraceptive or antilipidemic.
	Colestipol	Coadministration decreases atorvastatin levels by 25%; LDL reduction > than either alone.	May be therapeutic choice.
	Erythromycin	Atorvastatin levels increased by 40%; increased myopathy risk.	Choose alternative antibiotic.
	Cyclosporine, gemfibrozil, niacin	Increased myopathy and rhabdomyolysis risk.	Avoid concurrent use.
Cholestyramine	Mycophenolate	Decreases area under curve (AUC) by 40%.	Monitor for indications of rejection.
	Piroxicam	Elimination enhanced.	Choose alternative NSAID.
	Thyroid hormones	Possible loss of efficacy with potential hypothyroidism.	Chose alternative antilipidemic.
	Vitamins A, D, E, K, and folic acid	May interfere with vitamin absorption, with resultant bleeding tendencies.	With long-term therapy, vitamins A and D may be given in water-miscible form; vitamin K can be supplemented parenterally or orally.
	Warfarin	Decreased anticoagulant effect.	Choose alternative antilipidemic, or monitor PT/INR more closely.
Fluvastatin	Alcohol	Daily intake of 20 g more than 2 h after evening meal or within 1 h of fluvastatin dose increases AUC by 30%.	Avoid daily alcohol intake.
	Niacin, propranolol, digoxin	Decreases fluvastatin bioavailability.	Avoid concurrent administration.
	Rifampin	May cause decrease in fluvastatin AUC and plasma clearance.	Choose alternative antilipidemic.
Gemfibrozil	Warfarin	Enhances anticoagulant effect.	Choose alternative antilipidemic or monitor PT/INR closely.
	Colestipol	Bioavaiability of gemfibrozil reduced.	Avoid concurrent use.
	Lovastatin	Severe myopathy or rhabdomyolysis.	Avoid concurrent use.
	Pravastatin	Urinary excretion and protein binding reduced.	Avoid concurrent use.
Lovastatin	Isradipine	Increased lovastatin clearance with reduced effect.	Choose alternative CCB
	Food	Taking on empty stomach decreases absorption by 30%.	Take consistently with food.
Pravastatin	Cholestyramine, colestipol	Decreases pravastatin levels by 40–50%.	Take pravastatin 1 h before or 4 h after bile acid–binding resins.
	Cyclosporine	Coadministration increases pravastatin level 7-fold.	Separate doses as above.

Table 14–28. Dosage Schedule: Selected Antilipidemics

Drug	Clinical Use	Starting Dose	Maintenance Dose	Maximum Dose
Atorvastatin	Increased LDL	10 mg qd in evening dose	5–40 mg qd; increased at 2- to 4-wk intervals	80 mg/d
Cholestyramine, colestipol	Increased LDL	1 tsp (5 g) mixed in juice as slurry; taken 30 min before, during, or 30 min after breakfast and dinner	2–3 tsp (10–15 mg), increased based on GI symptoms	24 g/d
Fluvastatin	Increased LDL	20 mg qd in evening dose	40 mg qd or 20 mg bid	40 mg/d
Gemfibrozil	Increased VLDL and triglycerides	600 mg bid 30 min before breakfast and dinner	600–1200 mg bid	1200 mg bid
Lovastatin	Increased LDL	10–20 mg qd in evening dose	10–40 mg qd; increased at 4- to 8-wk intervals	80 mg/d
Niacin	Increased LDL	100 mg bid–tid with meals	2–6.5 g/d for familial hyperlipidemia, 1.5–3.5 g/d for other types of hyperlipidemia; increase doses at 5–7-day intervals	8 g/d
Niaspan	Increased LDL	375 mg qd at bedtime for 7 d	Increase at 7-d intervals to 500 mg, then 750 mg, based on tolerance	1000 mg/d
Pravastatin	Increased LDL	10–20 mg qd in evening dose	20 mg qd	40 mg/d
Simvastatin	Increased LDL	5–10 mg qd in evening dose	20 mg qd; increase at 4-wk intervals	40 mg/d

Table 14–29. Available Dosage Forms: Antilipidemics

Drug	Dosage Form
Atorvastatin (Lipitor)	Tablets: 10 mg, 20 mg, 40 mg
Cholestyramine (Questran)	Powder: 5-g packets or bulk container with 5-g scoop; 9-g packet or bulk container with 9-g scoop
Colestipol (Colestid)	Granules: 5-g packet or bulk container with 5-g scoop Flavored granules: 7.5-g packets or bulk container with 7.5-g scoop Tablets: 1 g
Fluvastatin (Lescol)	Tablets: 20 mg, 40 mg
Gemfibrozil (Lopid)	Tablets: 600 mg
Lovastatin (Mevacor)	Tablets: 10 mg, 20 mg, 40 mg
Niacin	Tablets: 25 mg, 50 mg, 100 mg, 125 mg, 250 mg, 400 mg, 500 mg Extended-release tablets: 125 mg, 250 mg, 400 mg, 500 mg, 750 mg, 1000 mg Extended-release capsules: 125 mg, 250 mg, 300 mg, 400 mg, 500 mg Elixir: 50 mg/5 cc in pints and gallons
Niacin (Niaspan)	Tablets: 500 mg, 750 mg, 1000 mg Tablets: 21-d starter pack: 375 mg (7 d), 500 mg (7 d), 750 mg (7 d)
Pravastatin (Pravachol)	Tablets: 10 mg, 20 mg, 40 mg
Simvastatin (Zocor)	Tablets: 5 mg, 10 mg, 20 mg, 40 mg

ing cessation, and weight loss if they are obese are added to the dietary therapy. There is to date no evidence that drug treatment to increase HDL levels reduces CAD risk.

Elevated triglycerides are not an independent risk factor for CAD, and no consensus exists about treating these elevations. **Gemfibrozil** is the drug of choice when treatment is chosen. It is also the drug of choice for patients with very high triglyceride levels (more than 800 mg/dL) who are at risk for pancreatitis because of this high level.

AGE. The prevalence of hypercholesterolemia and CAD risk is greatest among people older than age 65 years. Because dietary therapy alone often fails to achieve the LDL goal in older adults, drug therapy is used as an adjunct. **Reductase inhibitors** are the first-line choice. These drugs are well tolerated in the older adult, with minor diarrhea and occasional sleep disturbances the most common problems. Because these drugs may cause an elevation in liver enzymes, it is important to monitor liver function tests in older patients. **Niacin** is effective, but it is not as well tolerated because its adverse reactions profile is more common in the older adult. It may also trigger hypotension and arrhythmias. Multiple daily dosing is required, which may increase the complexity of a drug regimen often already complex. **Niaspan** taken once daily at bedtime may address these problems. **Bile acid–binding resins** are safe for older adults, but their GI problems, especially the risk of constipation and impaction, and their effect on the absorption of many of the drugs older adults are often also taking make them less desirable than **reductase inhibitors.**

COST. Although it is usually not the first factor considered in choosing therapy, cost can be a factor, especially for older patients on fixed incomes. **Niacin** is clearly the least expensive of the **antilipidemics**, with other drugs costing 4 to 14 times as much. The major disadvantage to this drug is its adverse reactions profile, but this can be greatly reduced by starting with 100 mg tid, taking it with meals, administering 325 mg of **aspirin** 30 minutes before taking the drug to decrease its flushing effects, and gradually increasing the dose. **Niaspan** is more expensive than the generic **niacin.** The next least expensive is **gemfibrozil,** but it has limited uses. **Reductase inhibitors** are relatively expensive, but from least expensive to most expensive at this time they are **pravastatin, simvastatin, lovastatin, fluvastatin,** and **atorvastatin. Bile acid–binding resins** are the most expensive. The most common adverse reactions are constipation and bloating, and these can be partially resolved by increasing dietary fiber.

MONOTHERAPY VERSUS MULTIPLE DRUGS. According to Katsung (1998), combined drug therapy is useful when VLDL levels are significantly increased during treatment with a **bile acid–binding resin**, LDL and VLDL levels are both elevated initially, LDL or VLDL levels are not nor-

malized with a single agent, or elevated levels of the lipoprotein Lp(a) coexist with other hyperlipidemias.

Specific cholesterol, LDL, and HDL guidelines and treatment protocols are further discussed in Chapter 37.

Monitoring

Measurement of the LDL cholesterol level is the top priority, although a lipid profile is usually done because it provides more data and is not more expensive. Lipid levels should be measured beginning about 4 to 6 weeks after initiation of therapy and then every 3 to 4 months until control is established. After that, every 6 to 12 months is usually enough.

Monitoring protocols for specific drugs in addition to the standard lipid levels are as follows. For **niacin,** liver function studies (LFTs), uric acid levels, and blood glucose levels are done initially at 4- to 6-week intervals until a stable dose is determined and then at 3- to 4-month intervals. For **reductase inhibitors,** LFTs are done prior to initiating therapy, every 4 to 6 weeks during the first 3 months of therapy, every 6 to 12 weeks for the rest of the first year, and then every 6 months. If aspartate aminotransferase (AST) or alanine aminotransferase (ALT) levels increase to three times normal, reduce the dose or discontinue therapy. CK levels are monitored if muscle tenderness is exhibited. For **gemfibrozil,** LFTs should be assessed prior to initiating therapy and with the same protocol as **reductase inhibitors.**

Patient Education

The importance of patient education in the treatment of hyperlipidemia cannot be overemphasized because, in addition to appropriate drug therapy, lifestyle management is the key to success.

ADMINISTRATION. The patient should take the drug exactly as prescribed and not skip doses or double up on missed doses. **Bile acid–binding resins** are taken before meals mixed and vigorously shaken with 4 to 6 oz water, milk, fruit juice, or other noncarbonated beverage. Rinsing the glass with a small amount of additional liquid ensures that all the dose was taken. For patients who require thick liquids, these drugs can also be mixed with cereals or pulpy fruits such as applesauce. The powder cannot be taken dry. If other drugs are to be taken, administer them 1 hour before or 4 hours after the **bile acid–binding resin. Reductase inhibitors** are best taken in the evening because of their action on cholesterol synthesis. **Lovastatin** is the only **reductase inhibitor** that should be taken with food to improve its absorption; it is best taken with the evening meal. **Atorvastatin** can be taken at any time of the day and without regard to food.

ADVERSE REACTIONS. Cutaneous flushing, especially of the face and upper body, has been associated with **niacin.**

Aspirin 325 mg taken 30 minutes prior to the dose can reduce or eliminate this response; hot fluids taken near the time of the dose make the flushing worse. Taking **niacin** with meals reduces the incidence of adverse reactions. A high-fiber diet or **psyllium** supplement just before a meal usually ameliorates the flatulence, constipation, or abdominal pain associated with **bile acid–binding resins.** Natural laxatives such as prunes or stool softeners can also be helpful. For these drugs and for **gemfibrozil,** the health care provider should be notified of persistent constipation or flatulence. For all **reductase inhibitors,** muscle tenderness or pain may indicate a serious problem that may require discontinuance of the drug. It should be reported immediately to the health care provider. **Fluvastatin, lovastatin,** and **pravastatin** all have GI-associated adverse reactions (dyspepsia, abdominal pain, flatulence, constipation, or diarrhea) and headache. Generally, these effects are mild and transient.

For all of these drugs, the importance of keeping follow-up appointments to monitor efficacy and adverse reactions cannot be overstated. Failure to discover problems early can result in increased risk for CAD and, for some drugs, life-threatening events.

Because the *reductase inhibitors* are Pregnancy Category D or X, female patients capable of childbearing should not take these drugs, and contraception should be instituted before prescribing them. The health care provider should be notified if pregnancy is planned or suspected.

LIFESTYLE MANAGEMENT. For a cardiac-healthy lifestyle, it is important to stress the need for dietary restriction in fat, cholesterol, carbohydrates, and **alcohol**; regular aerobic exercise; and smoking cessation. Medication helps to control hyperlipidemia, but it does not cure it.

Diuretics

Diuretics are first-line therapy in the treatment of CHF and HTN through their reduction in extracellular fluid (ECF) volume. Of the several classes of diuretics, the ones most commonly used in primary care are the **distal tubular (thiazides** and **aldosterone antagonists)** and **loop diuretics.** These drugs are the focus of this discussion.

Pharmacodynamics

Disease processes that increase renal sodium and water retention result in increased ECF volume. This increased volume increases capillary hydrostatic pressure. Taken together, the result is increased afterload, which leads to heart failure. Increased ECF volume also contributes to HTN. **Diuretics** act to reduce this volume in different

ways (Fig. 14–7). The **loop diuretics** inhibit sodium reabsorption in the ascending loop of Henle. These drugs are short acting and cause a large natriuresis. The **thiazide-type diuretics** act on the distal renal tubule to inhibit sodium reabsorption. Their effect is generally longer lasting, and they cause less brisk diuresis. Both of these classes also result in increased potassium excretion. The **potassium-sparing diuretics** include **aldosterone antagonists** and agents that inhibit excretion of potassium distally. These agents are weak **diuretics,** often used in combination with **thiazides** to reduce potassium loss.

Initially, **diuretics** promote natriuresis, decrease plasma volume, and reduce cardiac output. With time, these effects return to baseline, but total peripheral resistance remains decreased. The mechanism behind this additional long-term effect of **diuretics** is not clearly known but may be related to the amount of sodium in the vessel walls themselves. Theoretically, sodium in vessel walls contributes to the ability of the vessels to constrict, and loss of sodium from the vessel walls may contribute to vasodilation, leading to decreased PVR. Decreased PVR reduces afterload to improve cardiac functioning and reduce BP.

Diuretics may also be used as adjunct therapy for disease processes in which the treatment itself may contribute to fluid retention—for example, use of **CCBs** and some **antiarrhythmics.**

Pharmacokinetics

Absorption and Distribution

Absorption and distribution vary among the **diuretics** (Table 14–30). **Thiazide** and **loop diuretics** are all well absorbed orally. Among the **potassium-sparing diuretics, spironolactone (Aldactone)** is well absorbed, **amiloride (Midamor)** is poorly absorbed, and **triamterene (Dyrenium)** has an absorption somewhere between the other two. Food enhances the absorption of **metolazone (Zaroxolyn).** All are widely distributed, cross the placenta, and enter breast milk. The **thiazides** enter intracellular spaces as well, which may explain their preferential use in refractory edema.

Metabolism and Excretion

The liver is the primary site of metabolism for all **diuretics. Furosemide (Lasix)** has nonhepatic and hepatic metabolism. All **diuretics** are excreted mostly unchanged in the urine. **Metolazone, bumetanide (Bumex),** and **spironolactone** have some excretion in feces and bile. Plasma half-lives vary from 30 to 60 minutes for **furosemide** to 24 hours for the active metabolite of **spironolactone.** Impaired renal or hepatic function increases the half-life of **furosemide.**

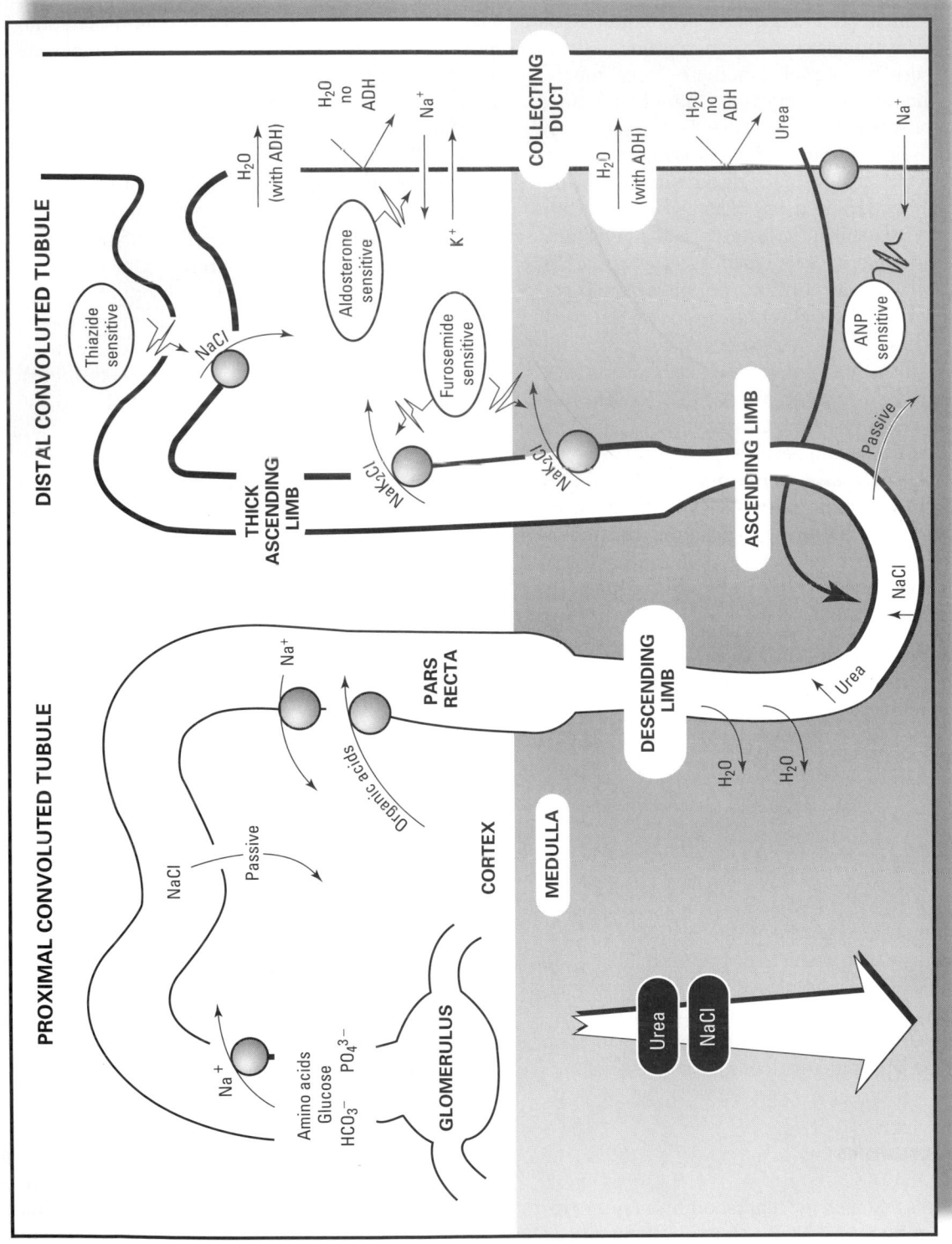

Figure 14-7. Sites of action of diuretics.

Table 14–30. Pharmacokinetics: Selected Diuretics

Drug	Onset (h)	Peak (h)	Duration (h)	Protein Binding	Bioavail-ability	Half-Life (h)	Elimination
Thiazide and Related Diuretics							
Hydrochlorothiazide	2	4–6	6–12	20–80%	65–75%	5.6–14.8	Unchanged in urine
Indapamide	1–2	2	up to 36	71–79%	93%	14	7% unchanged in urine
Metolazone	1	2	12–24	<20%	65%	No data	6–15% in feces, partially excreted unchanged in urine
Loop Diuretics							
Bumetanide	0.5–1	1–2	4–6	94–96%	72–96%	1–1.5	50% in urine, 20% in feces
Furosemide	1	1–2	6–8	91–97%	60–64%	0.5–1 (increased in renal and hepatic impairment and in neonates)	Unchanged in urine
Torsemide	1	1–2	6–8	>90%	80%	3.5	20% in urine
Potassium-Sparing Diuretics							
Amiloride	2	6–10	24	23%	15–25%	6–9	50% in urine
Spironolactone	24–48	48–72	48–72	>98%	>90%	13–24	In urine and bile
Triamterene	2–4	6–8	12–16	50–67%	30–70%	3	21% in urine

Pharmacotherapeutics

Precautions and Contradictions

All **diuretics** affect electrolytes. They should be carefully selected and used cautiously for patients with preexisting electrolyte abnormalities. **Potassium-sparing diuretics** have an absolute contraindication for patients with impaired renal function because of their tendency to produce hyperkalemia. Creatinine clearances less than 25 to 30 cc/minute suggest careful monitoring of electrolytes and cautious use with all **diuretic** classes except **loop diuretics.** Hepatic dysfunction suggests cautious use with all **diuretics,** especially those with some excretion in feces or bile.

For patients with a history of gout or renal calculi, cautious use of **thiazide** and **loop diuretics** and **spironolactone** is suggested because of the potential for hyperuricemia. **Diuretics** should be used cautiously for patients with diabetes, who may require alterations in their hypoglycemic regimen related to glucose intolerance.

Older adults are at increased risk for hypotension with these drugs and require careful BP monitoring and patient teaching about mobility. *Diuretics decrease plasma volume and may decrease placental perfusion. Thiazide and loop diuretics* are Pregnancy Category C and should be used only when benefits clearly outweigh risks. Jaundice and thrombocytopenia may be seen in neonates. *Spironolactone* is Pregnancy Category B, making it the best choice for pregnant women when a diuretic must be used. Safety has been established in children only for **furosemide, hydrochlorothiazide,** and **spironolactone.**

Adverse Drug Reactions

Electrolyte imbalances are common in all **diuretic** classes. **Thiazide** and **loop diuretics** cause hypokalemia and may cause hypercalcemia, hyponatremia, and hypomagnesemia. When it occurs, the hypomagnesemia must be corrected first to permit successful treatment of the hypokalemia. The average potassium loss is 0.6 mEq/L and is dose-related. Increased sodium intake exacerbates the potassium loss. Metabolic alkalosis may be associated with the hypokalemia. **Potassium-sparing diuretics** cause hyperkalemia.

Hyperuricemia may occur with all **diuretics**; **thiazide** and **loop diuretics** and **spironolactone** are the most likely to cause it, and **indapamide (Lozol)** is the least likely. The hyperuricemia itself is usually not treated unless gout or renal calculi develop.

Glucose intolerance is a problem with all diuretic groups; **thiazide** and **loop diuretics** cause the most difficulty, and **metolazone** and **indapamide** have the least effect. This intolerance is directly linked to the serum potassium level, and correcting hypokalemia often relieves the problem.

Hypotension secondary to fluid volume deficits can also occur with all **diuretics**. Starting with a low dose and increasing the dose gradually can reduce this problem.

Hyperlipidemia with increases in cholesterol, LDL, and triglycerides has been seen with **thiazide diuretics**. The elevations are transient and tend to return to baseline in about 6 months.

Gynecomastia occurs in 50 percent of patients receiving **spironolactone**, and impotence occurs in a smaller number. These can be distressing to men. **Loop diuretics** have a small risk for hearing loss and tinnitus.

Drug Interactions

All **diuretics** have potential additive hypotensive effects with other drugs that lower BP. Synergistic hypokalemia is probable between **thiazide** and **loop diuretics**, and additive hypokalemia may occur between these classes and **mezlocillin, piperacillin, ticarcillin, amphotericin B,** and **glucocorticoids.** Hypokalemia may increase the risk of **digitalis** toxicity. Concurrent administration of **potassium-sparing diuretics** and **ACEIs** may lead to significant hyperkalemia. **Potassium** preparations, including nonsodium salt substitutes, may also result in significant hyperkalemia.

Thiazide and **loop diuretics** decrease the renal excretion of **lithium** and may induce lithium toxicity. These two classes may decrease the action of **sulfonylureas** and **insulin. Thiazide diuretics** and **spironolactone** diminish the anticoagulant effects of **warfarin,** whereas **loop diuretics** enhance its anticoagulant effects. Additive ototoxicity occurs between **loop diuretics** and **aminoglycosides** and **cisplatin. NSAIDs** and **salicylates** may decrease the diuretic effectiveness of all classes.

Specific drug interactions and the appropriate actions to prevent them are given in Table 14–31.

Clinical Use and Dosing

Regardless of the clincal use, start with the lowest effective dose, increase the dose gradually to reduce the likelihood of adverse reactions, consider reducing doses where appropriate, and consider **potassium** supplementation or combination with a **potassium-sparing diuretic** when laboratory studies indicate it is appropriate.

HYPERTENSION. Initial drug therapy for HTN is monotherapy. Because **diuretics** have been shown to reduce cardiovascular morbidity and mortality and because of their low cost, they are preferred as initial therapy, especially for sodium-sensitive patients such as blacks, older adults, the obese, and those with renal insufficiency. Patients with diabetes are also sodium sensitive, but **ACEIs** are preferred as initial therapy because of their ability to prevent diabetic nephropathy. **Thiazide diuretics** are generally not the first drugs of choice for patients with hyperlipidemia because of their potential for worsening the hyperlipidemia; however, lipid disorders do not contraindicate the use of **thiazide diuretics.**

All classes of **diuretics** have been used to treat HTN. The most effective class is the **thiazides. Loop diuretics** may be used but are not as effective for this indication. The dose-response curve of diuretics is fairly flat. Increasing the dose produces more adverse reactions with little change in therapeutic benefit. Dosage should be increased no sooner than 4 weeks, which is the length of time usually required to achieve optimal therapeutic effect. When a **thiazide diuretic** is added to an existing **antihypertensive** regimen, reduce the dosage of the other **antihypertensives** to prevent excessive hypotension and orthostasis.

EDEMA ASSOCIATED WITH CHF, HEPATIC CIRRHOSIS, AND RENAL DISEASE. The most effective class for this indication is the **loop diuretics.** They are effective in moderate to severe disease and can be used when creatinine clearance is less than 25 cc/minute. **Indapamide** is also indicated for edema associated with CHF and is effective with these low creatinine clearance levels. **Thiazide diuretics** may be used to treat the edema associated with mild CHF, corticosteroid and estrogen therapy, premenstrual syndrome, and limited renal dysfunction. They are not useful if the creatinine clearance is less than 25 cc/minute. Among the **thiazides, hydrochlorothiazide** is the first choice for this indication. Intermittent dosing may be advantageous and reduce the incidence of adverse reactions. With premenstrual syndrome, the drug should be taken 3 to 5 days before menstruation and discontinued when menstruation begins. Frequent dosage adjustments may be necessary in edematous patients.

Dosages for both indications for each drug are indicated in Table 14–32.

Rational Drug Selection

INDICATIONS. When HTN or symptoms of CHF are mild, diuretic therapy can be initiated with **hydrochlorothiazide** 50 mg. For patients with renal impairment, the addition of **metolazone** 2.5 to 5 mg is helpful. When these conditions are moderate to severe, **furosemide** 20 to 40 mg is necessary. **Potassium-sparing diuretics** are relatively weak agents and are used mainly in conjunction

Table 14–31. Drug Interactions: Selected Diuretics

Drug	Interacting Drug	Possible Effect	Implications
Thiazide diuretics	Allopurinol	Concurrent use may increase incidence of hypersensitivity reactions.	Avoid concurrent use.
	Anticholinergics	Increased diuretic absorption.	Monitor diuretic effect.
	Anticoagulants	Diminished anticoagulant effect.	Monitor PT/INR. Adjust anticoagulant dose prn.
	Antigout agents	Diuretic may increase uric acid levels.	Choose different diuretic or adjust antigout agent dose.
	Antineoplastics	Diuretic may prolong antineoplastic-induced leukopenia.	Monitor WBC. Choose alternative diuretic.
	Bile acid–binding resins	Resins bind thiazides and reduce absorption by up to 85%.	Give thiazide 2 h before or 4 h after bile acid–binding resin.
	Calcium salts	Hypercalcemia may be worsened.	Avoid concurrent use.
	Diazoxide	Hyperglycemia, often with symptoms of frank diabetes.	Choose alternative antihypertensive.
	Digitalis glycosides	Digitalis toxicity and toxicity-induced arrhythmias.	Monitor potassium level and administer supplement as needed.
	Lithium	Decreased renal excretion of lithium, resulting in toxicity.	Monitor lithium level closely, or choose alternative diuretic.
	Loop diuretics	Synergistic diuresis and hypokalemic effects.	Reduce doses of both or one of these unless planned for therapeutic reasons. Monitor electrolytes closely.
	NSAIDs	Some may reduce diuretic effect; concurrent administration of indomethacin has been associated with renal failure.	Monitor diuresis. Avoid concurrent administration of indomethacin.
	Sulfonylureas, insulin	Diuretics induce hyperglycemia and may decrease hypoglycemic effects.	Monitor serum glucose. Adjust dose of hypoglycemic.
	Vitamin D	Biologic actions of vitamin D enhanced, resulting in hypercalcemia.	Monitor serum calcium levels.
Loop diuretics	Aminoglycosides, cisplatin	Increased risk for ototoxicity.	Avoid concurrent use. If you must use aminoglycoside, use different diuretic during time it is administered.
	Anticoagulants	Enhanced anticoagulant activity.	Monitor PT/INR. Adjust dose prn.
	Digitalis glycosides	Digitalis toxicity and toxicity-induced arrhythmias.	Monitor potassium levels and administer potassium supplement prn.
	Hydantoins	Reduces diuretic effect of furosemide.	Monitor diuretic effect and adjust dose prn.
	Lithium	Decreased renal excretion of lithium, resulting in toxicity.	Monitor lithium levels closely or choose different diuretic.
	NSAIDs, salicylates	Reduces effects of diuretic.	Monitor diuretic effect and adjust dose.
	Sulfonylureas	Diuretic-induced hyperglycemia may reduce hypoglycemic effect.	Monitor serum glucose and adjust dose of sulfonylurea, or choose different diuretic.
	Theophylline	Actions of theophylline may be enhanced or inhibited.	Monitor theophylline levels closely, or choose different bronchodilator.
Potassium-sparing diuretics	ACE inhibitors, potassium preparations	Concurrent use may result in hyperkalemia.	Avoid concurrent use. Choose different diuretic.
	Anticoagulants	Decreased anticoagulant effects.	Monitor PT/INR and adjust dose prn.
	Cimetidine	May increase bioavailability and decrease renal clearance of triamterene only.	Choose alternative histamine$_2$ blocker.
	Digitalis glycosides	Interaction complex and difficult to product risk of toxicity.	Monitor digitalis level closely or avoid concurrent use.
	NSAIDs, salicylates	Decreased diuretic effect; interaction with indomethacin has resulted in renal failure.	Monitor diuretic effect. Avoid concurrent use with indomethacin.

Table 14–32. Dosage Schedule: Selected Diuretics

Drug	Clinical Use	Starting Dose	Maintenance Dose	Maximum Dose
Amiloride	Adjunctive therapy for edema of CHF	5 mg qd	10 mg qd or 5 mg bid.	20 mg/d
Bumetanide	Edema of CHF, hepatic cirrhosis, renal disease; useful as alternate for furosemide allergy	0.5 mg qd	2 mg/d; intermittent dosing every other day or 3–4 d with 1–2 d between is safest and most effective.	10 mg/d
Furosemide	Refractory edema of CHF, hepatic cirrhosis, renal disease	20–80 mg qd or bid	Titrate in increments of 20–40 mg q6–8h until desired diuresis; give bid 8 A.M. and 2 P.M.	600 mg/d; for CHF with chronic renal failure, doses of 2–2.5 g/d have been used
	HTN	40 mg bid	Titrate up or down to control HTN.	
	Infants and children	2 mg/kg/d	Titrate in increments of 1 mg/kg q6–8h until desired diuresis.	6 mg/kg/d
Hydrochlorothiazide	HTN	12.5 mg/d	25–50 mg qd or in 2 divided doses.	50 mg/d
	Edema	25–200 mg/d	25–100 mg/d.	200 mg/d
	Infants <6 mo	3.3 mg/kg/d	3.3 mg/kg/d.	
	Infants 6 mo–2 y	12.5 mg/kg/d	Up to 37.5 mg/d.	
	Children 2–12 y	37.5 mg/d	Up to 100 mg/d; all infant and children doses given in 2 divided doses and based on body weight.	Rarely need more than 50 mg/d
Indapamide	HTN	1.25 mg qd	2.5–5 mg qd; increase at 4-wk intervals if needed to control HTN.	5 mg/d
	Edema of CHF	2.5 mg qd	If response not adequate in 1 wk, increase to 5 mg qd.	5 mg/d
Metolazone (Zaroxolyn only)	Adjunct therapy for HTN	2.5 mg qd	5 mg qd.	20 mg qd
	Renal disease, CHF	5 mg qd	10 mg qd.	20 mg qd
Spironolactone	HTN	50 mg qd	50–100 mg qd or in 2 divided doses.	100 mg/d
	Edema of CHF, hepatic cirrhosis, nephrotic syndrome	25–100 mg qd	25–200 mg/d in divided doses; if inadequate diuresis after 5 d, add different diuretic or change diuretics.	>100 mg/d; increased adverse reactions without improved therapy possible
	Children: edema	3.3 mg/kg/d in single or divided doses	3.3 mg/kg/d.	
	Children: HTN	1 mg/kg qd	1–2 mg/kg bid.	
Torsemide	Edema of CHF	10 mg qd	10–20 mg qd.	20 mg qd
	Edema of cirrhosis	5–10 mg qd	10–20 mg qd.	20 mg qd
	Renal failure (if refractory to or requires large doses of furosemide)	20 mg qd	Titrate upward, doubling doses until desired diuresis.	200 mg/d
Triamterene	Edema of CHF, hepatic cirrhosis, steroid use	50 mg qd	50–100 mg bid.	300 mg/d

CHF = congestive heart failure; HTN = hypertension.

with **thiazide** or **loop diuretics** to prevent hypokalemia (Table 14–33).

CONCURRENT DISEASE PROCESSES. Increasing glucose levels can be a problem for patients with diabetes, and hyperuricemia can be a problem for patients with gout. In the order of most likely to have these adverse effects to least likely, the drugs are **thiazides, loops, potassium-sparing, metolazone,** and **indapamide.** Drug choices for patients with diabetes or gout are in the reverse order of this list. Hypokalemia can be a significant problem for patients with cardiac disorders. Drugs likely to have this adverse reaction are the **loop** and **thiazide diuretics.** These drugs are still often chosen for their effects on the edema associated with CHF. Careful monitoring of potassium levels must accompany their use with these patients. Hyperkalemia can be lethal for patients with renal failure and problematic for those with reduced renal function. **Potassium-sparing diuretics** are contraindicated in the former and rarely chosen in the latter. Both **potassium-sparing diuretics** and **thiazides** should be avoided for patients with creatinine clearance less than 25 to 30 cc/minute. **Loop diuretics, metolazone,** and **indapamide** are safe alternatives for these patients. Hyperlipidemia is usually a transient phenomenon, and there is no consensus on the restriction of a drug class because of it. **Indapamide** effectively controls mild to moderate HTN, with no adverse reaction of lipids and minimal impact on potassium, glucose, and uric acid. It appears to address most concerns.

COMBINATIONS. **Metolazone** by itself is not a strong diuretic, but as an adjunct to **loop diuretics,** its synergistic effect frequently overcomes refractory cases or enables dosage reduction of the **loop diuretic,** resulting in fewer adverse reactions. Combining a **potassium-wasting diuretic** with a **potassium-sparing diuretic** can prevent hypokalemia. Some drugs come in this combination (**triamterene and hydrochlorothiazide [Maxzide], spironolactone and hydrochlorothiazide [Aldactazide],** making it possible to take only one tablet.

COST. **Torsemide** is two to four times more potent than **furosemide** yet is in the same class. When a patient is refractory to **furosemide** or requires a very large dose, changing to **torsemide** may not only improve the outcome but also reduce the cost and make the treatment regimen less complex with increased likelihood of adherence. Comparison of monthly cost for the average dosing of one of these diuretics, from most expensive to least expensive, is **indapamide** (with a wholesale cost to the pharmacy of approximately $25 in 1998 terms), **amiloride, torsemide, metolazone, Aldactazide, Maxzide, Aldactone, triamterene, bumetanide, Lasix, Esidrix, spironolactone generic, spironolactone-hydrochlorothiazide generic, furosemide generic,** to **hydrochlorothiazide generic** (with a wholesale cost of approximately $1.04 in 1998

Table 14–33. Available Dosage Forms: Selected Diuretics

Drug	Dosage Form	In Combination with
Amiloride (Midamor)	Tablets: 5 mg	Hydrochlorothiazide 50 mg (Moduretic)
Bumetanide (Bumex)	Tablets: 0.5 mg, 1 mg, 2 mg	
Furosemide (Lasix)	Tablets: 20 mg, 40 mg, 80 mg Oral solutions: 8 mg/cc, 10 mg/cc	

Hydrochlorothiazide (Esidrix, E-zide, HCTZ, Hydrochlor, Hydro-D, HydroDIURIL)	Tablets: 25 mg, 50 mg, 100 mg
	Oral solutions: 10 mg/cc, 100 mg/cc
		Spironolactone (Aldactazide)
		Triamterene
		   (Dyazide, Maxzide)
		Hydralazine (Apresazide)
		Reserpine
		   (Hydropres, Hydro-Serp,
		   Hydroserpine)
		Captopril (Capozide)
		Metoprolol (Lopressor)
		Benazepril (Lotensin HCT)

Indapamide (Lozol)	Tablets: 1.25 mg, 2.5 mg	
Metolazone (Zaroxolyn)	Tablets: 2.5 mg, 5 mg, 10 mg	
Spironolactone (Aldactone)	Tablets: 25 mg, 50 mg, 100 mg	Hydrochlorothiazide (Aldactazide)
Triamterene (Dyrenium)	Capsules: 50 mg, 100 mg	Hydrochlorothiazide (Dyazide, Maxzide)
Torsemide (Demadex)	Tablets: 5 mg, 10 mg, 20 mg, 100 mg	

terms).The generic form of each of these drugs is less expensive than the brand name, and the value of generic diuretics is quite clear!

Monitoring

In addition to monitoring the clinical indicators (BP, heart rate, edema, weight gain, dyspnea, cough, urine output), it is also critical to monitor renal function, glucose level, and electrolytes. Prior to initiating therapy, BUN, creatinine, electrolytes (sodium, potassium, calcium, and magnesium), uric acid, and glucose levels should be drawn. The patient should return to the clinic 1 week after initial prescription for a follow-up visit to check the clinical indicators and their electrolytes. Potassium levels of 3.5 to 4 mEq/L are usually not an indication for supplementation in a noncardiac patient. Patients with cardiac disorders should have their potassium levels maintained at 4 to 4.5 mEq/L. Spacing of monitoring after the first visit depends on lability of symptoms and dosage adjustments. Specific indicators to monitor depend on the common adverse effects of the specific drug(s) being used. This topic is discussed further in Chapters 34 and 38.

Patient Education

ADMINISTRATION. Patients should take the drug exactly as prescribed, even if they are feeling well, and not skip or double doses. For drugs given twice daily, the morning dose should be taken at breakfast and the evening dose no later in the day than 4 P.M. These drugs increase urine output, and taking the drug later may make the patient get up at night to urinate. Some of these drugs come alone or in combination. Check with the pharmacist with each refill to make certain the drug is the correct form.

ADVERSE REACTIONS. Hypotensive reactions are the most common. Changing position slowly, not using **alcohol**, not standing for long periods, and avoiding exercise in hot weather can decrease these reactions. These drugs are used to reduce fluid volume in the body. Weighing daily helps to monitor that fluid. The patient should notify the health care provider if weight loss of more than 1 lb per day or 5 lb per week, excessive thirst, dry skin or mucous membranes, dizziness, muscle pain, weakness or cramps, nausea, vomiting, increased heart rate, or diarrhea occurs. These may indicate an abnormal potassium level.

Potassium-wasting diuretics may cause potassium loss from the body. The health care provider monitors this loss with laboratory work. If instructed by the health care provider, a diet high in potassium may be needed. Foods high in potassium include bananas, dates, figs, fish, citrus juices, melons, molasses, baked potatoes, prunes, soybeans, and tomatoes. If an **oral potassium** supplement is prescribed, powders or liquids can be diluted in at least 4 oz fruit juice to improve the taste. Tablets taken with meals reduce GI irritation.

Potassium-sparing diuretics cause the body to hold potassium. The health care provider monitors this gain with laboratory work. Patients should not take **potassium** supplements or use salt substitutes that have **potassium** in them.

Occasionally, these drugs cause GI upset that may be reduced by taking them with meals. Use of a sunscreen prevents photosensitivity reactions, although these are rare.

Changes in blood sugar and other body chemicals may occur. Follow-up appointments that allow the health care provider to assess levels of these chemicals and progression of the disease process are important.

LIFESTYLE MANAGEMENT. If these drugs are taken for HTN, it is important to continue with the other therapies for HTN, including weight loss, restricted sodium intake, stress reduction, regular aerobic exercise, not using tobacco products, and moderation in **alcohol** intake. These drugs help to control HTN but do not cure it. Patients should not use OTC preparations without first checking with the health care provider. They may interact with these drugs or make the disease process worse.

REFERENCES

Barker, L., Burton, J., & Zieve, P. (1995). *Principles of ambulatory medicine* (4th ed). Baltimore: Williams & Wilkins.

Beta Blocker Heart Attack Trial Research Group. (1982). A randomized trial of propranolol in patients with acute myocardial infarction. *Journal of the American Medical Association, 247,* 1707.

Blacher, J., Raison, J., Amah, G., Schiemann, A., Stimple, M., & Safar, M. (1998). Increased arterial distensibility in postmenopausal hypertensive women with and without hormone replacement therapy after acute administration of the ACE inhibitor moexipril. *Cardiovascular Drugs and Therapy, 12,* 409–414.

Cohn, J., Johnson, G., Ziesche, S., Cobb, F., Francis, G., Tristani, F., Smith, R., Dunkman, B., Loeb, H., Wong, M., Bhat, G., Goldman, S., Fletcher, R., Doherty, J., Hughes, C., Carson, P., Contron, G., Shabetai, R., & Haakenson, C. (1991). A comparison of enalapril with hydralazine-isosorbide dinitrate in the treatment of chronic congestive heart failure. *New England Journal of Medicine, 325,* 300–310.

CONSENSUS Trial Study Group. (1987). Effect of enalapril on mortality in severe congestive heart failure. *New England Journal of Medicine, 316,* 1429–1435.

Crawford, M. (1995). *Current diagnosis and treatment in cardiology* (1st ed.) Norwalk, CT: Appleton & Lange.

Deglin, J., & Vallerand, A. (1998). *Davis's drug guide for nurses* (6th ed.). Philadelphia: F. A. Davis.

Digitalis Investigation Group. (1997). The effect of digoxin on mortality and morbidity in patients with heart failure. *New England Journal of Medicine, 336*(8), 525–533.

Echt, D., Liebsen, P., Mitchell, B., et al. (1991). Mortality and morbidity in patients receiving encainide, flecainide, or placebo: The Cardiac Arrhythmia Suppression Trial. *New England Journal of Medicine, 324,* 781.

Esmail, Z., & Loewen, P. (1998). Losartan as an alternative to ACE inhibitors in patients with renal dysfunction. *Annals of Pharmacotherapy, 32*(10) 1096–1098.

Fish, A. (1994). Angiotensin converting enzyme inhibitors: Inhibition of growth, a novel mechanism of action. *Journal of Cardiovascular Nursing, 8*(4), 57–71.

Gottlieb, S., Dickstein, K., Fleck, E., Kostis, J., Levinee, T., LeJemtel, T., & DeKock, M. (1993). Hemodynamic and neurohormonal effects of the angiotensin II receptor antagonist losartan in patients with congestive heart failure. *Circulation, 88,* 1602–1609.

Hardman, J., Limbird, L., Molinoff, P., & Ruddon, R. (1996). *Goodman and Gilman's: The pharmacological basis of therapeutics* (9th ed.). New York: McGraw-Hill.

Kastrup, E. (Founding Ed.) (1998). *Drug facts and comparisons.* St. Louis: Facts and Comparisons.

Katsung, B. (1998). *Basic and clinical pharmacology* (7th ed.). Stamford,CT: Appleton & Lange.

Levine, A., Muller, C., & Levine, T. (1998). Effects of high-dose lisinopril-isosorbide dinitrate on severe mitral regurgitation and heart failure remodeling. *American Journal of Cardiology, 82*(6), 1299–1301.

Mancia, G., & van Zwieten, P. (1996). How safe are calcium channel antagonists in hypertension and coronary heart disease? *Journal of Hypertension, 14*(1), 13–17.

Mehra, A., Shotan, A., Ostrzega, E., Hsueh, W., Vasquez-Johnson, J., & Elkayam, U. (1994). Potentiation of isosorbide dinitrate effects with N-acetylcysteine in patients with chronic heart failure. *Circulation, 89,* 2595–2600.

National High Blood Pressure Education Program. (1997). *The sixth report of the joint national committee on detection, evaluation, and treatment of high blood pressure* (NIH Publ. No. 98–4080). Rockville, MD:National Institutes of Health, National Heart, Lung, and Blood Institute.

Packer, M., Gheorghiade, M., Young, J., Constantini, P., Adams, K., Cody, R., Smith, L., Van Voorhees, L., Gourley, L., & Joily, M. (1993). Withdrawal of digoxin from patient with chronic heart failure treated with angiotensin-converting enzyme inhibitors. RADIANCE Study. *New England Journal of Medicine, 329,* 1–7.

Pfeffer, M. A., et al., on behalf of the SAVE Investigators. (1992). Effect of captopril on mortality and morbidity in patients with left ventricular dysfunction after myocardial infarction. *New England Journal of Medicine, 327,* 669–677.

Pfeffer, M. A. (1995). ACE inhibition in acute myocardial infarction. *New England Journal of Medicine, 332*(2), 118–170.

Pitt, B., Segal, R., Martinez, F., Meurers, G., Cowley, A., et al. (1997). Randomized trials of losartan versus captopril in patients over 65 with heart failure (Evaluation of Losartan in the Elderly Study, ELITE). *Lancet, 349,* 747–752.

Pylypchuk, G. (1998). ACE inhibitor–versus angiotensin II blocker–induced cough and angioedema. *Annuals of Pharmacotherapy, 32*(10), 1060–1066.

Ross, S., Lev-Ran, A., & Hwang, D. (1995). Effects of enalapril and nitrendipine on the extraction of epidermal growth factor and albumin in hypertensive NIDDM patients. *Diabetes Care, 18*(5), 690–693.

Sadowski, A., & Redeker, N. (1996). The hypertensive elder: A review for the primary care provider. *Nurse Practitioner, 21*(5), 99–112.

Salerno, A., & Zugibe Jr., F. (1994). Calcium channel antagonists: What do the second-generation agents have to offer? *Postgraduate Medicine, 95*(1), 181–188, 190, 201–202.

Simmons, M. (1994). Myocardial infarction: ACE inhibitors for all? forever? *Lancet, 344*(8918), 279–281.

Simon, T., Gelarden, R., Freitag, S., Kassler-Taub, K., & Davies, R. (1998). Safety of irbesartan in the treatment of mild to moderate systemic hypertension. *American Journal of Cardiology, 82*(2), 179–182.

Smith, S., Blair, S., Criqui, M., Fletcher, G., Fuster, V., Gersh, B., Gotto, A., Gould, L., Greenland, P., Grundy, S., Hill, M., Hlatky, M., Houston-Miller, N., Krauss, R., LaRosa, J., Ockene, I., Oparil, S., Pearson, T., Rapaport, E., & Starke, R. (1995). Preventing heart attack and death in patients with coronary disease. *Circulation, 92,* 2–4.

SOLVD Investigators. (1991). Effect of enalapril on survival of patients with reduced left ventricular ejection fraction and congestive heart failure. *New England Journal of Medicine, 325,* 293.

SOLVD Investigators. (1992). Effect of enalapril on mortality and development of heart failure in asymptomatic patients with reduced left ventricular ejection fractions. *New England Journal of Medicine, 327,* 685.

U.S. Department of Health and Human Services. (1994). *Heart failure: Management of patients with left-ventricular systolic dysfunction* (AHCPR Publ. No. 94–0613). Rockville, MD: Author.

Uretsky, B., Young, J., Shahidi, F., Yellen, L., Harrision, M., & Joily, M. (1993). Randomized study assessing the effect of digoxin withdrawal in patients with mild to moderate chronic congestive heart failure: Results of the PROVED trial. *Journal of the American College of Cardiology, 22,* 955–962.

Velussi, M., Brocco, E., Frigato, F., Muollo, B., Maioli, M., Carraro, A., Tonolo, G., Fresu, P., Cernigoi, A., Fioretto, P., & Nosadini, R. (1996). Effects of cilazapril and amlodipine on kidney function in hypertensive NIDDM patients. *Diabetes, 45*(2), 216–222.

Viscoli, C., Horwitz, R., & Singer, B. (1993). Beta-blockers after myocardial infarction. Influence of first-year clinical course on long-term effectiveness. *Annuals of Internal Medicine, 118,* 99.

CHAPTER 15

· · · · · · ·

Drugs Affecting the Respiratory System

CHAPTER OUTLINE

Numerous medications are available to treat disorders of the respiratory system. **Bronchodilators** act on the bronchial smooth muscle to reverse bronchospasm. **Leukotriene receptor agents** are relatively new medications that act to decrease the inflammation in the lungs of patients with asthma. **Antihistamines, decongestants, expectorants,** and **antitussives** are over-the-counter (OTC) medications included in this chapter. **Inhaled anti-inflammatory medications** used for asthma and **intranasal steroids** used for the treatment of seasonal or perennial rhinitis are discussed. Prescribing recommendations for the multiple medications used in the treatment of asthma or chronic obstructive pulmonary disease (COPD) are provided in Chapter 28. Intravenous forms of respiratory medications, which are rarely used in primary care, are not discussed here.

Bronchodilators

Beta$_2$ Receptor Agonists

Beta$_2$ receptor agonist bronchodilator agents are widely used in caring for all ages of patients to treat reversible bronchoconstriction caused by asthma or reactive airway disease (RAD). A variety of **beta-agonist bronchodilators** are available, and the medications come in a variety of forms and delivery systems. **Albuterol (Ventolin, Proventil)** is the most commonly prescribed drug in this class. Other **sympathomimetic bronchodilator medications** used in primary care are **metaproterenol (Alupent), terbutaline (Brethine, Brethaire), bitolterol (Tornalate), pirbuterol (Maxair),** and **salmeterol (Serevent).**

Pharmacodynamics

Bronchodilators act on the smooth muscle of the bronchial tree to reverse bronchospasm, thereby decreasing airway resistance and residual volume and increasing vital capacity and airflow. **Beta agonists** stimulate beta$_2$ adrenergic receptors in the lung to increase production of cyclic adenosine monophosphate (cAMP) by activation of adenyl cyclase, the enzyme that catalyzes the conversion of adenosine triphosphate (ATP) to cAMP. Increased cAMP concentrations relax bronchial smooth muscle and inhibit release of mediators of immediate hypersensitivity from cells, especially from the mast cells.

The perfect **bronchodilator** would work only on the beta$_2$ receptors in the lungs and have no other actions or systemic effects. Unfortunately, all of the currently available preparations have some effects on other body systems, such as the cardiovascular system, skeletal muscles, and central nervous system (CNS).

Albuterol is a **selective beta$_2$ agonist** with some minor beta$_1$ activity. It can increase heart rate by directly stimulating beta$_2$ receptors in the heart and by stimulating beta$_2$ receptors in vascular smooth muscle. The effect on cardiac beta$_2$ receptors is of consequence only at high serum levels of **albuterol** because it has a low affinity for these receptors and there are fewer beta$_2$ receptors in the heart than beta$_1$ receptors. Stimulation of the beta$_2$ receptors in the vascular smooth muscle leads to vasodilation, a decrease in diastolic blood pressure, and therefore a reflex increase in heart rate. **Albuterol** causes beta$_2$ receptor stimulation of skeletal muscle that leads to tremors. **Albuterol** has fewer cardiac and CNS effects than some of the other beta agonists and therefore is often the drug of choice for first-line therapy. **Pirbuterol** is a **selective beta$_2$ agonist** that is structurally identical to **albuterol**, except for the substitution of a pyridine ring for the benzene ring in their chemical makeup.

Terbutaline has a pharmacodynamic profile similar to **albuterol**, in that it is a **selective beta$_2$ agonist** with minor beta$_1$ activity. **Terbutaline** is also noted to inhibit uterine contractions via its beta receptor–mediated action on uterine smooth muscle. **Metaproterenol** is also a **selective beta$_2$ agonist** with some beta$_1$ activity, although it is less selective than **albuterol** or **terbutaline**. **Bitolterol** is hydrolyzed by the esterases in the lung to colterol, or terbutylnorepinephrine, which is a **selective beta$_2$ agonist**.

Salmeterol is unique in that it is a long-acting **inhaled bronchodilator** with a 12-hour half-life. **Salmeterol** is more selective for beta$_2$ receptors than **albuterol** and has minor beta$_1$ activity. **Salmeterol** exerts long-lasting bronchoprotection effects against allergen-, exercise-, histamine-, and methacholine-caused bronchospasm.

Pharmacokinetics

ABSORPTION AND DISTRIBUTION. **Albuterol** most commonly is inhaled and gradually absorbed from the bronchi. The overall systemic concentration remains low following recommended doses. The low systemic concentration is due to the need to use only 5 percent of the dose required orally to achieve the desired effects. Oral forms of **albuterol** are well absorbed from the gastrointestinal (GI) tract, rapidly enter the bloodstream, and are widely distributed in the body fluids and tissues. Extended-release oral **albuterol** is formulated to be absorbed from the stomach more slowly. Breast milk excretion is not known.

Pirbuterol is minimally absorbed from the respiratory tract, with amounts below the limits of serum assay detected after administration via inhalation. Its distribution is unknown.

Terbutaline is available in inhaled, oral, and subcutaneous (SC) forms. The inhaled form of **terbutaline** is minimally absorbed from the respiratory tract. Approximately 33 to 50 percent of the oral form is absorbed from the GI tract and is widely distributed. If administered SC, **terbutaline** is almost completely absorbed and is widely distributed. It crosses the placenta and is excreted in breast milk.

Metaproterenol may be administered via the inhaled route or orally. Approximately 3 percent of the inhaled **metaproterenol** dose is absorbed intact through the lungs. Oral dosing results in approximately 10 percent of the dose being absorbed intact. Distribution of **metaproterenol** is unknown.

Bitolterol absorption is too low to be measured by serum assay; distribution is unknown.

Salmeterol administered via inhaler is absorbed via the lungs in small amounts; undetectable amounts are found in the serum with recommended doses. With chronic administration, **salmeterol** is detected in the serum at very low levels. **Salmeterol** is excreted in breast milk in small amounts, approximately equal to plasma levels.

METABOLISM AND EXCRETION. Most of the common **bronchodilators** are metabolized in the liver and excreted primarily in the urine.

Albuterol is metabolized into albuterol 4′-O-sulfate, which has little or no beta-adrenergic stimulating effect and no beta-adrenergic blocking effect. Approximately 72 percent of inhaled **albuterol** is excreted in the urine within 24 hours of inhalation, 28 percent of this as unchanged drug and 44 percent as the metabolite. Another 10 percent of the inhaled **albuterol** is excreted in the feces. Oral administration of **albuterol** results in 65 to 90 percent of the dose being excreted in the urine over 3 days, the majority in the first 24 hours. About 4 percent of the oral **albuterol** dose is excreted in feces.

Pirbuterol is not metabolized extensively, with 51 percent of the dose excreted in the urine as **pirbuterol** plus its sulfate conjugate. **Terbutaline** is partially metabolized in the liver, primarily to inactive sulfate conjugate, and is excreted in the urine. **Metaproterenol** is metabolized by the liver into its sulfate conjugate and excreted in the urine. **Bitolterol** is a prodrug that is hydrolyzed by esterases in tissue and blood to the active moiety colterol. Within 24 hours, 83 percent of the dose is excreted in the urine. After 72 hours, 85.6 percent of the dose has been excreted in the urine and 8 percent in the feces, as conjugated colterol.

Salmeterol xinafoate, as ionic salt, dissociates so that the **salmeterol** and 1-hydroxy-2-naphthoic acid (xi-nafoate) are metabolized and excreted independently. **Salmeterol** base is extensively metabolized by hydroxylation in the liver. Urinary elimination accounts for 25 percent of the drug, and 60 percent is eliminated in the feces over a period of 7 days. The **xinafoate** moiety has no apparent pharmacological activity, is extensively protein-bound, and has a long elimination half-life of 11 days.

Table 15–1 shows the pharmacokinetic properties of selected **bronchodilators**.

Table 15–1. Pharmacokinetics: Selected Bronchodilators

Drug	Onset	Peak	Duration	Half-Life	Metabolism	Elimination
Beta₂ Agonists						
Albuterol				2.7–5 h	Hepatic	Renal 90%; fecal 10%
Inhalation	5–15 min	0.5–2 h	2–6 h			
Oral short-acting	15–30 min	2–3 h	4–6 h			
Oral extended-release			8–12 h			
Bitolterol				Unknown	Hydrolyzed by esterases in tissues and blood to colterol	Renal
Inhalation	3–4 min	0.5–1 h	5–8 h			
Metaproterenol				Unknown	Hepatic	Renal
Inhalation	1 min	1 h	1–2.5 h			
Nebulization	5–30 min	1 h	4 h			
Oral	15–30 min	1 h	4 h			
Pirbuterol				Unknown	—	Renal
Inhalation	5 min	0.5–1 h	5 h			
Salmeterol	14 min	3–4 h	12 h	Unknown	Hydroxylization	Feces
Inhalation						
Terbutaline				Unknown	Liver (partial)	Renal; small amount in bile, feces
Inhalation	5–30 min	—	3–6 h			
Oral	30 min	—	4–8 h			
Anticholinergic						
Ipratropium				2 h	Ester hydrolysis	Renal
Inhalation	15–30 min	1–2 h	4–5 h			
Xanthine Derivatives						
Theophylline				Children <6 mo: >24 h; >6 mo: 1.1–3.7 h Adult non-smokers: 8.7–2.2 h; adult smokers: 4–5 h; adults with COPD, congestive heart failure (CHF), cor pulmonale, or liver disease may exceed 24 h	Liver	Renal
Immediate-release	—	2 h				
Extended-release		4–7 h	—			
Liquid		1 h				

Pharmacotherapeutics

PRECAUTIONS AND CONTRAINDICATIONS. There are relatively few contraindications to the use of **sympathomimetic bronchodilators.** Cardiac arrhythmias associated with tachycardia, tachycardia or heart block caused by digitalis intoxication, angina, narrow-angle glaucoma, organic brain damage (**epinephrine** only), and shock during general anesthesia with halogenated agents are all contraindications to **beta₂ agonists.** Because of these drugs' effects on the cardiovascular system, patients with hypertension, ischemic heart disease, coronary insufficiency, congestive heart failure, and a history of stroke and/or cardiac arrhythmias should be monitored closely for adverse effects during administration of any of the sympathomimetic bronchodilators. For patients with diabetes mellitus, there is a potential drug-induced hyperglycemia that may result in loss of diabetic control when using any of the **beta₂ agonists**, and their **insulin** dosage may need to be increased. For patients with hyperthyroidism, adverse reactions are more likely to occur with the use of **bronchodilators.** Patients taking **digoxin** require close monitoring when **albuterol** is started because **albuterol** increases the volume of distribution of **digoxin** and can cause up to a 30 percent decrease in blood digoxin levels. Patients with diagnosed or suspected pheochromocytoma should avoid the **beta-adrenergic antagonists** because severe hypertension may occur.

Lower doses of **bronchodilators** may be necessary in older adults because of increased sympathomimetic sensitivity.

Terbutaline **is Pregnancy Category B; the rest of the** *beta-agonist bronchodilators* **are Pregnancy Category C.** No reports linking the use of *albuterol* with human congenital anomalies have been published. *Terbutaline* **is used during pregnancy to prevent contractions related to preterm labor (not an FDA-approved use), and therefore oral forms of the** *beta agonists* **should be used selectively in patients in labor.** Inhaled **forms of the** *beta agonists* **are less likely to affect uterine contractions** (Katstrup, 1999).

Small amounts of **terbutaline** and **salmeterol** can be measured in breast milk. The other **inhaled beta-agonist bronchodilators** cannot be measured in breast milk, probably on account of the low amount of drug that is used and absorbed. The use of **inhaled bronchodilators** during lactation is most likely safe, with careful monitoring of the infant.

Albuterol is used extensively in infants and children with minimal adverse effects. **Metaproterenol** may also be used in young children, although **albuterol** is generally the first-choice medication. The safety of **pirbuterol, bitolterol, terbutaline,** and **salmeterol** for use in children age 12 and under has not been established.

ADVERSE DRUG REACTIONS. Adverse reactions to the **beta-agonist bronchodilators** are usually transient. It is usually not necessary to discontinue the medication, but a temporary reduction in the dose may alleviate some of the side effects. Slowly increase the dose after the reaction to the optimal dosing has subsided.

Supraventricular and ventricular ectopic beats have occurred with **beta-agonist** inhalation, but the incidence is low (**bitolterol** 0.5%, **terbutaline** about 4%, **pirbuterol** less than 1%). Tachycardia and palpitations are reported in 14 percent of patients who use these **sympathomimetic bronchodilators.**

The **beta-agonist bronchodilators** exhibit some CNS excitation effects, with tremors, dizziness, shakiness, nervousness, and restlessness reported in some patients. Headaches may occur with **bronchodilator** use in 2 to 28 percent of patients. Insomnia is rare, reported in 1 to 3 percent of patients.

DRUG INTERACTIONS. Because of the cardiovascular effects of the **bronchodilators,** careful monitoring for drug interactions is necessary. If any of the **beta agonists** are prescribed with **digitalis glycosides,** caution and careful monitoring of the patient's electrocardiogram (ECG) is necessary because there is an increased risk of cardiac arrhythmia.

Beta agonists used with **beta-adrenergic blocking agents** (including ophthalmic preparations) may result in mutual inhibition of therapeutic effects. **Tricyclic antidepressants** and **monoamine oxidase inhibitors (MAOIs)** used with **albuterol, metaproterenol,** or **terbutaline** may potentiate the effects of the **bronchodilator** on the vascular system. Table 15–2 shows drug interaction information.

CLINICAL USE AND DOSING

Bronchospasm. The **bronchodilators** are used primarily in the treatment of bronchospasm associated with asthma, bronchitis (acute or chronic), and COPD.

The dose of **albuterol metered-dose inhaler (MDI)** in adults and children over age 4 is 2 puffs every 4 to 6 hours. The dose of **albuterol (Ventolin, Proventil)** delivered via nebulizer for adults and children over age 12 is 2.5 mg (0.5 mL) in 2 mL normal saline; for younger children up to 15 kg, the dose is 0.1 to 0.15 mg/kg per dose. For children over 15 kg, the dose is the same as for adults, 2.5 mg/dose. Inhaled forms of **albuterol** may be repeated once after 5 to 10 minutes, up to two times (three doses total) during exacerbations. The oral **albuterol** dose in adults is 2 to 4 mg three or four times a day, up to a maximum of 32 mg/day. Children age 6 to 12 are prescribed 2 mg **albuterol** three or four times a day. Children under age 6 are usually prescribed **albuterol** syrup, dosed at 0.1 mg/kg three times a day. **Albuterol** also comes in an inhalation capsule (**Ventolin Rotacaps**) for use in a **Rotahaler** inhalation device. The dose of **albuterol** inhalation capsule for patients age 4 and older is one 200-µg capsule delivered via the **Rotahaler** every 4 to 6 hours.

Table 15–2. Drug Interactions: Selected Bronchodilators

Drug	Interacting Drug	Possible Effect	Implications
Beta₂ Agonists			
Albuterol	Digoxin	Digoxin serum levels may be decreased	Decreased dose of albuterol may be needed
	Other sympathomimetics	Additive effects	Serious adverse cardiac effects; do not use concurrently
	MAOIs	Potentiates albuterol	Severe hypertension, headache, hyperpyrexia, and possible hypertensive crisis; do not use concurrently
	Tricyclic antidepressants	Potentiates the pressor response of sympatho-mimetics	Arrhythmias if used concurrently
	Beta blockers (including ophthalmic agents)	Mutual inhibition of thera-peutic effects	Should not be used together
	Cocaine	Increased CNS stimulation	Observe patients for cardiac and CNS effects
	Thyroid hormones	Cardiac effects of both drugs enhanced	Increased risk of coronary insufficiency from combined use of these drugs; avoid this combination in patients with preexisting cardiac disease
	Ritodrine	Increased CNS stimulation	Avoid concurrent use
Bitolterol	Other sympathomimetics	Additive effects	Serious adverse cardiac effects; avoid concurrent use of sympathomimetics
	MAOIs	Potentiates bitolterol	Severe hypertension, head-ache, hyperpyrexia, and possible hypertensive crisis; do not use together
	Tricyclic antidepressants	Potentiates the pressor response of sympatho-mimetics	May cause arrhythmias; do not use together
	Beta blockers (including ophthalmic agents)	Mutual inhibition of thera-peutic effects	Should not be used together
Metaproterenol	Other sympathomimetics	Additive effects	Serious adverse cardiac effects; avoid concurrent use
	MAOIs	Potentiates metaproterenol	Severe hypertension, head-ache, hyperpyrexia, and possible hypertensive crisis; do not use together
	Tricyclic antidepressants	Potentiates the pressor response of sympatho-mimetics	May cause arrhythmias; do not use together
	Beta blockers (including ophthalmic agents)	Mutual inhibition of thera-peutic effects	Should not be used together
	Inhalation anesthetics	Sensitizes the myocardium to the effects of meta-proterenol	May cause arrhythmias; use with caution and, if possible, avoid concurrent use
	Theophylline or caffeine	Additive toxic effects	CNS stimulation or toxicity a concern; use with caution and close monitoring

Continued on next page

Table 15–2. Drug Interactions: Selected Bronchodilators (*continued*)

Drug	Interacting Drug	Possible Effect	Implications
	Thyroid hormones	Cardiac effects of both drugs enhanced	Increased risk of coronary insufficiency from the combined use of these drugs; use with caution in patients with preexisting cardiac disease
Pirbuterol	Other beta agonists	Additive effects	Increased adverse effects; avoid concurrent use
	MAOIs, tricyclic anti-depressants	Potentiates pirbuterol	Severe hypertension, head-ache, hyperpyrexia, and possible hypertensive crisis; do not use within 14 d of each other
Salmeterol	Beta blockers (including ophthalmic agents)	Mutal inhibition	Avoid concurrent use
	MAOIs, tricyclic anti-depressants	Potentiates vascular effects of salmeterol	Severe hypertension, head-ache, hyperpyrexia, and possible hypertensive crisis; do not use concurrently
Terbutaline	Halogenated anesthetics	Sensitizes the myocardium to the effects of terbutaline	Ventricular arrhythmias; do not use concurrently
	MAOIs, tricyclic antide-pressants, maprotiline	Potentiates vascular effects of terbutaline	Severe hypertension, head-ache, hyperpyrexia, and possible hypertensive crisis; do not use concurrently Decreased antihypertensive effect; should not be used together
	Beta blockers and other antihypertensive agents	Mutual inhibition	Do not use together
	Cocaine	Increased CNS and cardiac stimulation	Observe patients for arrhythmias
	Cardiac glycosides, levodopa	Increased potential for cardiac arrhythmias	Dosage of cardiac glycoside or levodopa should be decreased and the patient closely monitored
Anticholinergics Ipratropium	Cromolyn inhalation solution	Forms a precipitate when mixed together	Do not mix
Xanthine Derivatives Theophylline	Allopurinol, beta blockers, calcium channel blockers, cimetidine, oral contraceptives, corticosteroids, disul-firam, ephedrine, influenza virus vaccine, interferon, macrolides, mexiletine, quinolones, thiabendazole, thyroid hormones, carbamaze-pine, isoniazid, loop diuretics, fluvoxamine, ticlopidine, propafenone, zileuton	Increased serum theophylline levels if taken concurrently	Lower doses of theophylline may be necessary; monitor theophylline level closely when starting, stopping, or changing the dose of these medications; doses of theo-phylline may need to be temporarily decreased after administration of influenza vaccine

Continued on next page

Table 15–2. Drug Interactions: Selected Bronchodilators (*continued*)

Drug	Interacting Drug	Possible Effect	Implications
	Aminoglutethimide, barbiturates, charcoal, hydantoins, ketoconazole, rifampin, smoking (cigarettes, marijuana), sulfinpyrazone, beta agonists, thioamines, carbamazepine, isoniazid, loop diuretics, lansoprazole, primidone, ritonavir	Decreased serum theophylline levels if taken concurrently	Increased doses of theophylline may be necessary; monitor theophylline level closely when starting, stopping, or changing the dose of these medications; theophylline toxicity may occur if these medications are stopped suddenly
	Inhalation anesthetics	Increased risk of cardiac arrhythmias	Avoid or use with caution
	Sympathomimetics	May cause excessive stimulation, nervousness, irritability, and insomnia	Avoid concurrent use or use with caution
	Lithium	Theophylline may increase renal clearance of lithium	Monitor lithium clinical effectiveness if theophylline is prescribed
	Zafirlukast	May increase theophylline levels if added to an existing theophylline regimen	Monitor theophylline levels closely after adding zafirlukast to the treatment regimen

Metaproterenol (Alupent) comes in MDI, inhalation solution, and syrup forms. The dose of **metaproterenol MDI** in adults and children over age 12 is 2 to 3 inhalations every 3 to 4 hours, not to exceed 12 inhalations per day. The dose of **metaproterenol** delivered via nebulizer in adults and children age 12 years and older is 0.1 to 0.2 mL of 5 percent solution diluted in 2.5 mL normal saline up to every 4 hours. **Metaproterenol** is also available in a hand bulb nebulizer, and the dose for adults and children age 12 years and older is 5 to 15 (usually 10) inhalations every 4 hours, or three to four times a day for chronic use. **Metaproterenol MDI** and nebulizer solution are not recommended for children under age 12; oral syrup is the suggested therapy in this age group. **Metaproterenol** syrup dose in children over age 9 or who weigh more than 60 lb is 20 mg (10 mL) three or four times a day. For children age 6 to 9 who weigh less than 60 lb, the dose of **metaproterenol** syrup is 10 mg (5 mL) three or four times a day. The dose of **metaproterenol** in children younger than 6 is 1.3 to 2.6 mg/kg per day in doses divided to take three or four times a day.

Terbutaline is available in MDI (**Brethaire**), oral tablets (**Brethine**), or parenteral form for SC injection. The dose of **terbutaline MDI** in adults and children age 12 and older is 2 puffs every 4 to 6 hours. The dose of oral **terbutaline** for bronchospasm in adults and children age 15 or older is 5 mg three times a day, with a maximum of 15 mg in 24 hours. For children age 12 to 15, the dose of **terbutaline** is 2.5 mg three times a day, with a maximum dose of 7.5 mg in 24 hours. The dose of parenteral **terbutaline** (**Brethine Injection**) in adults

is 0.5 mg SC in the lateral deltoid. The dose may be repeated in 15 to 30 minutes. The maximum dose is 0.5 mg in 4 hours. **Terbutaline** is not recommended for children under age 12.

Pirbuterol is available only in MDI form (**Maxair Autohaler**). The dose of **pirbuterol** in adults and children over age 12 is 1 to 2 inhalations every 4 to 6 hours for a maximum of 12 inhalations in 24 hours.

Bitolterol (Tornalate) is available in MDI form. The adult dose to treat acute bronchospasm is 2 puffs, 1 to 3 minutes apart, followed by a third puff if needed. For prevention of bronchospasm, the adult dose is 2 puffs every 8 hours. **Bitolterol** is not recommended for use in children younger than 12.

Salmeterol (Serevent) is a long-acting **bronchodilator** available in MDI form. The dose for adults and children age 12 and older to control asthma and to prevent bronchospasm is 2 puffs twice a day. **Salmeterol** is not to be used for short-term bronchospasm relief. Patients need to have a short-acting **bronchodilator** also prescribed for them to use for short-term relief, and they need to be educated not to use **salmeterol** for acute exacerbations.

Exercise-induced bronchospasm. **Bronchodilators** used just before exercise can prevent exercise-induced bronchospasm. The two medications recommended by the Expert Panel II Report: Guidelines for the Diagnosis and Management of Asthma (National Asthma Education and Prevention Program, 1997) are inhaled **albuterol** or other short-acting **beta$_2$ agonist** and **salmeterol.** The dose of **albuterol** MDI to prevent exercise-induced bronchospasm is 2 puffs 5 minutes prior to exercise. **Albuterol** used this way should prevent exercise-induced bronchospasm for 2 to 3 hours. The dose of **salmeterol** is 2 puffs 30 to 60 minutes prior to exercise. **Salmeterol** should prevent exercise-induced bronchospasm for 10 to 12 hours. If patients are already taking **salmeterol** twice daily for asthma control, they should not use another dose before exercise, and another medication such as a short-acting bronchodilator or **cromolyn** should be used.

Table 15–3 presents the dosage recommendations.

RATIONAL DRUG SELECTION.   *The Expert Panel II Report* does not differentiate or recommend a specific short-acting **beta$_2$ agonist** for use in asthma. Therefore, the practitioner who is prescribing for adults may choose any of the short-acting **bronchodilators.** Choosing an appropriate **bronchodilator** is a matter of the age of the patient and the cost.

Patient age. The only short-acting **bronchodilators** that can be prescribed for children under age 12 are **albuterol** and **metaproterenol.** **Albuterol** is by far the more often used medication in clinical practice and is safe to use even in infants.

Cost. Of the short-acting **bronchodilators, albuterol** is the least expensive, especially if a generic formula is prescribed. There are no generic formulations of most of the other **beta-agonist bronchodilators.**

MONITORING.   There is no specific monitoring required for **bronchodilators.** As a part of overall asthma management, pulmonary function and response to **bronchodilators** should be monitored with a peak flowmeter. If a patient is on **digitalis,** an ECG should be done prior to starting a **beta agonist** and routinely during therapy to detect cardiac arrhythmias that may occur.

PATIENT EDUCATION

Administration. The **bronchodilator** should be used as prescribed. Overuse of **bronchodilators** will lead to increased adverse effects, and using the **bronchodilator** less than prescribed may lead to increased bronchospasm and decreased pulmonary function.

The administration of **bronchodilators** via MDI can be difficult for most adults and all children. Learning to coordinate the release of the medication from the inhaler with a deep breath is difficult. Written and pictorial instructions are available with the inhaler, but the provider must not assume that the patient understands the proper method of administering inhaled medications. Use verbal instructions as well as actual demonstration with a placebo inhaler to reinforce the written instructions. These instructions and demonstrations should be repeated at follow-up visits.

To properly use an inhaler, the patient should first exhale and then tilt the head slightly back and place the inhaler mouthpiece either about 2 inches from the open mouth or between open lips. While inhaling, the patient should press down on the canister, breathe in slowly and deeply, and hold his or her breath for 10 seconds (count of 10) or as long as comfortable. If 2 puffs are prescribed, then the patient should wait at least 1 full minute between inhalations.

To assist with the delivery of inhaled medications, a spacer can be prescribed. The **Aerochamber** is a tube-like device that has pictures drawn on the outside to remind the patient of the proper technique for using the inhaler. For younger children and adults, the **InspirEase** spacer gives a visual cue of the spacer bag deflating to help in taking a deep-enough breath. Both of these devices emit a whistling sound if the patient is taking too rapid a breath, giving a cue to breathe slowly.

The use of a nebulizer should be demonstrated to the patient either in the clinic or by the home health agency that is providing the device. Specific instructions vary slightly with the manufacturer. The key points that should be covered with nebulizer use are accurate measurement of the medication (if using nebulizer solution) and appropriate cleaning of the equipment.

The use of **Ventolin Rotocaps** via the **Rotahaler** has to be demonstrated to the patient to ensure proper use.

Clinical Pearl

ADMINISTERING MEDICATIONS VIA A NEBULIZER TO INFANTS AND TODDLERS

Administering a medication via nebulizer to an infant or toddler is, at times, a challenge.

One trick is to "blow" the nebulized medication into the patient's face near the nose and mouth. This is achieved by occluding the mouthpiece end of the unit and aiming the "tail" end toward the patient's nose and mouth. This is especially effective if the child is sleeping and needs the medication.

Another suggestion to parents of young children is to either read a book to the child during the treatment or play an appropriate short video to make the time pass more quickly.

Table 15–3. Dosage Schedule: Selected Bronchodilators

Drug	Indication	Dose	Comments
Beta₂ Agonists			
Albuterol	Bronchospasm associated with asthma or COPD	*Inhaled:* 2 puffs q4–6h *Nebulizer* (run over 10–15 min) Adults: dilute 0.5 mL of 0.5% solution in 3 mL normal saline OR give 1 unit dose Children: 0.01–0.03 mL/kg of 0.5% solution diluted in 2 mL normal saline *Oral* Adults: 2–4 mg tid or qid up to a max of 32 mg/day Children 6–12 y old: 2 mg tid or qid Children <age 6 y: 0. 1 mg/kg divided tid	May repeat dose in 5–10 min during exacerbations; check proper inhaler technique with every clinic visit
	Exercise-induced asthma	*Inhaled:* 2 puffs 5 min prior to exercise	
Bitolterol	Acute bronchospasm	*Inhaled* Adults and children >12: 2 puffs 1–3 min apart, followed by a third puff if needed	Not recommended for children under age 12
	Bronchospasm prevention	*Inhaled:* 2 puffs every 8 h	
Metaproterenol	Bronchospasm associated with asthma or COPD	*Inhaler* Adults and children >12: 2–3 inhalations every 3–4 h; do not exceed 12 inhalations/d *Nebulizer* Adults and children >12: 0.1–0.2 mL of 5% solution diluted in 2.5 mL normal saline up to every 4 h *Hand bulb nebulizer* Adults and children >12: 5–15 (usually 10) inhalations every 4 h or 3–4 times/d (chronic use) *Syrup* Children >9 or who weigh >60 lb: 20 mg (10 mL) tid or qid Children age 6–9 who weigh <60 lb: 10 mg (5 mL) tid or qid Children <6: 1.3–2.6 mg/kg/d in doses divided tid or qid	Metaproterenol MDI or nebulizer solutions are not recommended in children <12; oral syrup is the suggested therapy in this age group

Continued on next page

Table 15–3. Dosage Schedule: Selected Bronchodilators (*continued*)

Drug	Indication	Dose	Comments
Pirbuterol	Bronchospasm associated with asthma	*Inhaled* Adults and children >12: 1–2 puffs every 4–6 h; maximum 12 puffs/d	Not recommended for children <12
Salmeterol	Long-acting bronchodilator for preventing broncho-spasm	*Inhaled* Adults and children >12: 2 puffs bid	Not to be used for short-term relief or acute exacerbations; patients need to have a short-acting bronchodilator also prescribed for them. If using salmeterol for asthma control, patients should not use another dose for exercise-induced asthma; a short-acting bronchodilator or cromolyn should be used
	Exercise-induced asthma	*Inhaled* 2 puffs 30–60 min before exercise	
Terbutaline	Bronchospasm associated with asthma or COPD	*Inhaled* 2 puffs every 4–6 h; do not repeat more often than every 4–6 h *Oral* Adults and children >15: 5 mg tid; max 15 mg/24 h Children 12–15: 2.5 mg tid; max 7.5 mg/24 h *Parenteral* Adults: 0.5 mg SC in the lateral deltoid; may repeat in 15–30 min; maximum dose is 0.5 mg in 4 h	Not recommended in children <12 Terbutaline is used to control premature contractions in pregnant women, so use with care in the patient in the third trimester nearing EDC, because it may affect labor
Anticholinergics Ipratropium	Bronchospasm associated with asthma or COPD	*Inhaler* Adults and children >12: 2 puffs qid; maximum 12 puffs/24 h *Nebulizer* 1 unit dose (500 μg)	Contraindicated in patients with soybean or peanut allergy. Ipratropium can be mixed with albuterol 0.5% solution for nebulizer use if used within 1 h
Combination Medications Albuterol/ipratropium (Combivent)	Bronchospasm associated with COPD, not controlled with one bronchodilator alone	*Inhaled* Adults: 2 puffs qid	Primarily used for COPD patients; simplifies medica-tion regimen by combining two commonly prescribed medications; not recom-mended for children

Continued on next page

Table 15–3. Dosage Schedule: Selected Bronchodilators (*continued*)

Drug	Indication	Dose	Comments
Xanthine Derivatives Theophylline	Bronchospasm associated with asthma, COPD, and bronchitis	The dose for asthma and COPD is variable with the patient's weight and serum theophylline levels *Adults* (>16): Initially: 6 mg/kg/24 h or 400 mg/24 h tid or qid; the dose is increased every 3 d in 25% increments until desired serum theophylline levels are achieved (ideally between 10 and 20 μg/mL); max dose: 13 mg/kg/d *Children* Initially: 16 mg/kg/24 h; max 400 mg/d; dosage may be increased by 25% every 3 d to a maximum based on age (age 1–9, max 24 mg/kg/d; age 9–12, max 20 mg/kg/d; age 12–16, max daily dose is 18 mg/kg Monitoring for serum theophylline levels is the same in children as for adults, with a steady-state theophylline level of 5–15 μg/mL the goal	Dosing adjustments are made based on the serum theophylline level: if the level is 5–10 μg/mL, the dose is increased by 25% every 3 d until desired serum concentrations of theophylline are reached; if the serum concentration is between 10 and 15 μg/mL, maintain dosage if tolerated and recheck at 6– to 12–mo intervals; if level is 15–19.9 μg/mL, consider decreasing dose by 10% to provide a greater margin of safety; if the level is 20–25 μg/mL, then decrease dose by 10% and recheck level in 3 d; if serum level is 25–30 μg/mL, then decrease subsequent doses by 25%, and redraw level in 3 d; if theophylline level is >30 μg/mL, then skip next 2 doses, decrease dose by 50%, and recheck in 3 d

Adverse reactions. The patient should be instructed not to exceed the recommended dosage of the medication because excessive use may lead to increased adverse effects. Overuse of the **beta$_2$ agonist bronchodilators** can lead to seizures, hypokalemia, anginal pain, and hypertension. Patients should understand that they may have some stimulant-like effects (e.g., increased heart rate, tremors) when they initially begin the medication, but these effects should lessen if they use it correctly. Some patients may get a headache with the use of **bronchodilators.** Patients who experience GI upset when taking oral medications should take the medications with food. The patient should inform the provider if palpitations, tachycardia, chest pain, muscle tremors, dizziness, headache, or flushing occurs.

Lifestyle management. Lifestyle management issues related to the disease process being treated should be discussed. They often include the following:

1. The patient needs to self-monitor respiratory status with a peak flowmeter to determine the effectiveness of the prescribed medication.
2. The patient should avoid or quit smoking.
3. The patient should avoid environmental triggers for asthma at home, work, and school.

Table 15–4 presents the available dosage forms of selected **bronchodilators.**

Xanthine Derivatives

Methylxanthines have declined in importance in the treatment of asthma, but there are still patients who may benefit from the use of **theophylline.** The other **methylxanthines** that have been used in the past include **caffeine** and **theobromine. Theophylline** and **caffeine** are closely related chemically in that **theophylline** is 1,3-dimethyl-

Table 15–4. Available Dosage Forms: Selected Bronchodilators

Drug	Dosage Form	How Supplied
	BETA₂ AGONISTS	
Albuterol Ventolin	Metered-dose inhaler: 90 μg/puff Syrup: 2 mg/5 mL Tablets: 2 mg, 4 mg Solution for nebulizer: 0.5% (5 mg/mL) Solution for nebulizer: 0.083% in unit-dose vial Rotacaps: 200 μg	17 g (about 200 inhalations) 480 mL 100, 500 20 mL with dropper 3-mL unit dose 24, 96
Proventil	Metered-dose inhaler: 90 μg/puff Tablets: 2 mg, 4 mg Extended-release tabs: 4 mg Syrup: 2 mg/5 mL Solution for nebulizer: 0.5% (5 mg/mL) Solution for nebulizer: 0.083% in unit-dose vial	17 g (about 200 inhalations) 100, 500 100 480 mL 20 mL with dropper 3-mL unit dose
Generic	Tablets: 2 mg, 4 mg Syrup: 2 mg/5 mL Solution for nebulizer: 0.5% (5 mg/mL)	100, 500 480 mL 20 mL with dropper
Bitolterol Tornalate	Metered-dose inhaler: 0.37 mg/puff	15 mL (about 300 inhalations)
Metaproterenol Alupent	Tablets: 10 mg, 20 mg Syrup: 10 mg/5 mL Metered-dose inhaler: 0.65 mg/puff Solution for inhalation: 0.4%, 0.6% Solution for inhalation: 5%	100, 1000 480 mL 5-mL, 10-mL inhaler 2.5 mL 10-mL, 30-mL vials with dropper
Metaprel	Tablets: 10 mg, 20 mg Syrup: 10 mg/5 mL Metered-dose inhaler: 0.65 mg/puff Solution for inhalation: 5%	100 480 mL 10-mL inhaler 10 mL with dropper
Generic	Tablets: 10 mg, 20 mg Syrup: 10 mg/5 mL Solution for inhalation: 0.4%, 0.6% Solution for inhalation: 5%	100, 1000 480 mL 2.5 mL 0.3-mL, 30-mL vials with dropper
Pirbuterol Maxair inhaler	Inhaler: 0.2 mg/puff	25.6 g MDI (about 300 inhalations)
Salmeterol Inhaler Serevent	Inhaler: 25 μg/puff	6.5-g MDI (60 inhalations), 13-g MDI (120 inhalations)
Terbutaline Brethaire	Inhaler: 0.2 mg/puff	10.5-g MDI (about 300 inhalations)
Brethine	Tablets: 2.5 mg, 5 mg Parenteral: 1 mg/mL	100, 1000 2-mL ampule
Bricanyl	Tablets: 2.5 mg, 5 mg Parenteral: 1 mg/mL	100, 1000 2-mL ampule

Continued on next page

Table 15–4. Available Dosage Forms: Selected Bronchodilators (*continued*)

Drug	Dosage Form	How Supplied
ANTICHOLINERGICS		
Ipatropium Atrovent	Inhaler: 18 μg/puff Solution for nebulizer: 500 μg per unit-dose vial	14-g MDI (200 inhalations) 25 unit-dose vials (2.5 mL each) per foil pouch
COMBINATION MEDICATIONS		
Albuterol-ipratropium Combivent	Inhaler: ipratropium 18 μg/puff combined with albuterol 90 μg/puff	14.7-g MDI (200 inhalations)
XANTHINE DERIVATIVES		
Theophylline (immediate release) Slo-Phyllin	Tablets: 100 mg, 200 mg Syrup: 80 mg/5 mL	100 (dye-free) Pint
Theolair	Tablets: 125 mg, 250 mg Solution: 80 mg/15 mL	100 15 mL, 18.75 mL, 30 mL, 500 ml
Generic	Tablets: 100 mg, 200 mg, 300 mg Elixir: 80 mg/15 mL	100, 500, 1000 15 mL, 30 mL, pint, gallon
Theophylline (timed release) Slo-bid Gyrocaps	Timed-release capsules (8–12 h): 50 mg, 75 mg, 100 mg, 125 mg, 200 mg, 300 mg	100, 1000
Slo-Phyllin	Timed-release capsules (8–12 h): 60 mg, 125 mg, 250 mg	100, 1000
Theo-24	Timed-release capsules (24 h): 100 mg, 200 mg, 300 mg	100, 500
Theobid Jr Duracaps	Timed-release capsules (12 h): 130 mg	60
Theo-Dur Sprinkles	Timed-release capsules (12 h): 50 mg, 75 mg, 125 mg, 200 mg	100
Theo-Dur	Timed-release tablets (8–24 h): 100 mg, 200 mg, 300 mg, 400 mg	100, 500, 1000, 5000
Uni-Dur	Timed-release scored tablets (24 h): 400 mg, 600 mg	100
Uniphyl	Timed-release tablets (24 h): 400 mg, 600 mg	100, 500

xanthine and **caffeine** is 1,3,7-triethylxanthine, and they share many of the same effects on the body. Because of the vast consumption of **caffeine** by patients throughout the world in tea, coffee, and cola beverages and because many OTC preparations for analgesia contain **caffeine, caffeine** pharmacodynamics are discussed briefly here.

Pharmacodynamics

Theophylline and the other **methylxanthines** work directly by an unknown mechanism believed to be mediated by selective inhibition of specific phosphodiesterases (PDEs). This, in turn, produces an increase in cAMP, which then leads to bronchial smooth muscle and pulmonary vessel relaxation.

Theophylline and **caffeine** have an impact on most of the major body systems. They both are powerful CNS stimulants, often causing insomnia and excitability. Although both drugs have cardiovascular effects, **theophylline** has a greater effect on the cardiovascular system. **Theophylline** directly stimulates the myocardium and increases myocardial contractility and heart rate. By relaxing vascular smooth muscle, theophylline dilates the coronary, pulmonary, and systemic blood vessels. Both **theophylline** and **caffeine** increase gastric acid secretion and may produce nausea and vomiting, although this reaction is probably due to CNS effects. Both **methylxanthines** stimulate skeletal muscle, causing tremors. **Theophylline** acts directly on the renal tubules to cause increased sodium and chloride excretion. By increasing renal blood flow (from increased heart rate) and the glomerular filtration rate, **theophylline** and **caffeine** also cause diuresis. Often these effects occur even when **theophylline** is within the therapeutic range.

Pharmacokinetics

ABSORPTION AND DISTRIBUTION. **Methylxanthines**, such as **theophylline**, are most commonly used in an oral form that is rapidly and completely absorbed from the GI tract. Delayed-release and extended-release tablets are also available, and their rate of absorption varies among the various formulations. The absorption of slow-release forms of **theophylline** can be significantly altered by gastric pH and food ingestion; therefore, patient education regarding timing these medications is important to the success of the medication. **Theophylline** distributes rapidly in nonadipose tissue and body water, including breast milk and cerebral spinal fluid. **Theophylline** crosses the placenta. The volume of distribution (VD) for **theophylline** averages 0.45 L per kg of body weight (L/kg) and ranges from 0.3 to 0.7 L/kg from infants to adults. The volume of distribution may be altered in premature neonates, elderly patients, adults with cirrhosis, pregnant women during the third trimester, and critically ill patients, probably because of altered protein binding. Serum **theophylline** levels should be monitored closely in these patients. **Theophylline** distributes readily into breast milk with a milk:plasma ratio of 0.7.

METABOLISM AND EXCRETION. **Theophylline** is metabolized primarily in the liver, with very little or no first-pass effect. Metabolism is believed to occur over multiple parallel pathways, mediated by cytochrome P-450 isoenzyme. Medications that induce cytochrome P-450 can significantly increase clearance of **theophylline**. In neonates, several of these pathways are undeveloped but mature slowly over the first year of life. **Caffeine** is a minor active metabolite of **theophylline** in older children

and adults. In premature neonates and children younger than 6 months, **caffeine** has a long half-life because of their immature livers, which results in significant accumulation. As the liver matures, the half-life of **caffeine** shortens and therefore does not accumulate in older children and adults. Table 15–1 outlines the half-life of **theophylline** in various ages of patients with a variety of diseases. Patients with congestive heart failure, cor pulmonale, pulmonary edema, and prolonged fever can have decreased metabolism of **theophylline** and therefore need to be closely monitored. Smoking and high-protein diets can increase the **theophylline** excretion rate, and high-carbohydrate diets can decrease it.

Pharmacotherapeutics

PRECAUTIONS AND CONTRAINDICATIONS. The only true contraindications to **theophylline** are hypersensitivity to any **xanthine**, peptic ulcer disease, and underlying seizure disorder.

Because of its effects on the cardiovascular system, patients with hypertension, ischemic heart disease, coronary insufficiency, congestive heart failure, or a history of stroke and cardiac arrhythmias should be monitored closely for adverse effects while taking **theophylline**.

Excessive doses may lead to toxicity. Incidence of toxicity increases when serum **theophylline** levels are above 20 µg/mL. Toxicity is found if serum **theophylline** levels reach 25 µg/mL in 75 percent of patients. Toxicity should not occur at recommended dosages but may occur if **theophylline** clearance is decreased (hepatic impairment, chronic lung disease, cardiac failure, patients older than age 55, and infants under age 1 year).

Theophylline clearance may be decreased in older patients (over age 55).

Theophylline **is Pregnancy Category C. There are no published reports linking** *theophylline* **with congenital defects.** *Theophylline* **crosses the placenta, and newborn infants may have therapeutic serum levels if maternal serum** *theophylline* **levels are in the high-normal range. Transient tachycardia, irritability, and vomiting can be found in newborns of women consuming** *theophylline.*

With close monitoring, **theophylline** may be used in children. Infants younger than 1 year old have decreased **theophylline** clearance and should have close monitoring of serum **theophylline** levels. **Theophylline** is used to treat apnea in preterm infants, with a therapeutic serum **theophylline** range of 5 to 10 µg/mL. If levels are kept in this range, the neonate should not have signs of toxicity.

ADVERSE DRUG REACTIONS. Adverse drug reactions are uncommon with serum **theophylline** levels below 20 µg/mL, although some patients may show toxic effects between 15 and 20 µg/mL, especially during initiation of therapy. The CNS adverse effects that may be seen include irritability, restlessness, seizures, and insomnia. Gastroesophageal reflux may occur. The cardiovascular adverse effects that may occur include palpitations, tachycardia, hypotension, and life-threatening arrhythmias. Other adverse effects include rash, diuresis, and tachypnea.

At serum **theophylline** levels above 20 µg/mL, patients may experience nausea, vomiting, diarrhea, headache, insomnia, and irritability. At levels above 35 µg/mL the patient may have hyperglycemia, hypotension, cardiac arrhythmias, tachycardia, seizures, brain damage, and death.

DRUG AND FOOD INTERACTIONS. Many medications act to either increase or decrease **theophylline** clearance; these medications are shown in Table 15–2. Of significance is smoking tobacco, which increases **theophylline** clearance. **Theophylline** levels should be monitored closely if the patient begins or quits smoking while on **theophylline**. **Nicotine** replacement products (gum or patch) also affect **theophylline** clearance. Normalization of **theophylline** clearance may not return to normal for 3 months to 2 years after smoking cessation.

The sedative effects of **benzodiazepines** may be antagonized by **theophylline**. Concurrent use of **theophylline** with **beta$_2$ agonist bronchodilators** may result in additive toxicity. **Lithium** levels may be reduced by **theophylline**. The concurrent use of **tetracyclines** with **theophylline** may lead to an increased incidence of **theophylline** adverse reactions. See Table 15–2 for other drugs that affect **theophylline levels** or interact with **theophylline**.

Theophylline elimination may be influenced by the patient's diet. A diet that is low in carbohydrates and high in protein increases the elimination (shortens the half-life) of **theophylline**. A diet that is high in carbohydrates and low in protein decreases the elimination (lengthens the half-life) of **theophylline**. A diet that contains a lot of charcoal-broiled foods accelerates the hepatic metabolism of **theophylline** because of a high polycyclic hydrocarbon content.

CLINICAL USE AND DOSING

Asthma and chronic obstructive pulmonary disease. The National Heart, Lung, and Blood Institute (NHLBI) *Expert Panel Report II* (1997), which gives guidelines for the management of asthma, recommends reserving **theophylline** for long-term control of asthma and for prevention of symptoms, especially nocturnal symptoms. These guidelines recommend that long-acting inhaled or oral **beta$_2$ agonists** be tried before **theophylline** on account of toxicity issues with **theophylline**.

The dose of **theophylline** for asthma and COPD varies with the patient's weight and serum **theophylline** levels. The adult patient (older than age 16) is started on a dose of 6 mg/kg per 24 hours or 400 mg/24 hours,

whichever is less, divided at 6- to 8-hour intervals. The dose is increased every 3 days in 25 percent increments until the desired serum **theophylline** levels are achieved (ideally between 10 and 20 µg/mL). The maximum dose for patients over age 16 is 13 mg/kg per day. Dosing adjustments are made based on the serum **theophylline** level. If the level is 5 to 10 µg/mL, the dose of **theophylline** is increased by 25 percent every 3 days until desired serum concentrations of **theophylline** are reached. If the serum concentration is between 10 and 15 µg/mL, maintain dosage if tolerated and recheck at 6- to 12-month intervals. If the serum **theophylline** level is 15 to 19.9 µg/mL, consider decreasing the dose by 10 percent to provide a greater margin of safety. If the serum **theophylline** level is 20 to 25 µg/mL, then decrease the dose by 10 percent and recheck the level in 3 days. If the serum level is 25 to 30 µg/mL, skip the next dose and decrease subsequent doses by 25 percent; redraw **theophylline** level in 3 days. If the **theophylline** level is above 30 µg/mL, then skip the next two doses and decrease the dose by 50 percent; recheck in 3 days. If the patient has a serum **theophylline** level above 20 µg/mL, consultation with a physician is indicated to determine if hospitalization for **theophylline** toxicity is warranted, based on clinical status.

The Expert Panel Report II guidelines for the management of asthma in children indicate considering **theophylline** as therapy in moderate persistent asthma, after medium-dose inhaled **steroids** and a combination of medium-dose inhaled **steroids** and **nedocromil** have been tried. These guidelines state that **theophylline** should be prescribed as an adjunct to medium-dose inhaled **steroids** (NAEPP, 1997). The initial dose of **theophylline** in children is 16 mg/kg per 24 hours up to a maximum of 400 mg per day. The dosage may be increased by 25 percent every 3 days to a maximum that is based on age. For children age 1 to 9 years, the maximum is 24 mg/kg per day; for 9 to 12 years, the maximum dose is 20 mg/kg per day; for 12- to 16-year-old patients, the maximum daily dose is 18 mg/kg. If the patient is over age 16, then the dosing is the same as for adults, maximum 13 mg/kg per day. Monitoring for serum **theophylline** levels is the same in children as for adults, with a steady-state **theophylline** level of 5 to 15 µg/mL the goal.

RATIONAL DRUG SELECTION. Because **theophylline** is the only **xanthine derivative** that is commonly used, the selection process basically involves choosing between the different forms of **theophylline** that are available on the basis of the cost and convenience of each of them. There are immediate-release, timed-release, and liquid formulas. Capsules that can be opened and sprinkled on soft foods are convenient for some patients.

Immediate release. When therapy is initiated, the daily dose may be changing frequently based on serum **theophylline** levels, and immediate-release tablets or capsules should be prescribed. The variety of dosage tablets available (100 mg, 125 mg, 200 mg, 250 mg, 300 mg) makes titrating the dose easier if incremental increases or decreases are required. Immediate-release **theophylline** requires dosing every 6 to 8 hours. Children usually require every-6-hour dosing, and adults usually require every-8-hour dosing, although this timing may vary by individual. The cost of immediate-release **theophylline** is slightly higher than most of the timed-release formulas because more doses are taken and therefore more tablets need to be dispensed in a month. Many patients are stabilized to a set dose per 24 hours and then switched to a timed-release formula.

Timed release. The variety of available timed-release **theophylline** products are described in Table 15–4. The formulas range from 8- to 24-hour release. It is recommended that patients be stabilized on immediate-release formulas to determine the total 24-hour dose that is required and then switched to a timed-release formula of choice. With some timed-release **theophylline** formulas offering once-daily dosing, there is a definite improvement in convenience with the timed-release products. One caution for the patient is that the dose must be taken at the same time every day to have steady serum **theophylline** levels.

Liquid. The liquid forms of **theophylline** may be used for children or patients who have difficulty in swallowing pills or capsules. The liquid is available in two strengths, 80 mg/15 mL and 150 mg/15 mL.

Sprinkles. **Theophylline** timed-release sprinkles (**Theo-Dur Sprinkle**) are another convenient way to dose **theophylline.** The capsules may be swallowed whole or opened and the contents sprinkled on soft food such as applesauce or pudding. They are available in a range of strengths, 50 mg, 75 mg, 125 mg, and 200 mg. The dose is administered every 12 hours.

MONITORING. The patient who is taking **theophylline** needs to be monitored closely for signs of toxicity. When therapy is initiated, **theophylline** levels should be drawn frequently as the dosage is titrated. If the patient is demonstrating any signs of toxicity, a serum **theophylline** level should be drawn. Once the patient is stabilized and has a steady **theophylline** level, then monitoring should be done every 6 to 12 months. More frequent levels may need to be done if a new medication is added to the patient's regimen (see Table 15–2) or if the patient has a change in overall health that may affect the ability to metabolize or excrete **theophylline. Theophylline** levels need to be timed to measure peak levels of the drug. A serum **theophylline** level should be drawn 1 to 2 hours after immediate-release formulas and 5 to 9 hours after the morning dose of sustained-release formulas. The patient should have a **theophylline** level drawn when changing brands of **theophylline** because there is some variance in the medications between brands.

PATIENT EDUCATION

Administration. The patient should be instructed to take the medication exactly as prescribed. Missed doses or irregular timing of doses can cause wide variations in the serum **theophylline** level, resulting in either subtherapeutic or toxic levels. The patient may take the medication either with or without food, but consistency is important because food can alter the absorption of the medication. The patient should not chew or crush enteric-coated, sustained-release tablets or capsules.

Adverse reactions. Toxicity should be discussed with any patient who is taking **theophylline.** Patients who are having signs of toxicity may mistakenly think they have a viral illness. Instead, patients with any unusual symptoms should contact their provider. The symptoms to report include nausea, vomiting, insomnia, jitteriness, headache, rash, severe GI pain, restlessness, convulsions, or irregular heartbeat.

The patient should avoid large amounts of **caffeine**-containing beverages, which can increase the adverse effects of **theophylline.** Explain that **theophylline** elimination may be influenced by the patient's diet. A diet that is low in carbohydrates and high in protein increases the elimination of **theophylline,** a diet that is high in carbohydrates and low in protein decreases the elimination of **theophylline,** and a diet that contains a lot of charcoal-broiled foods accelerates the hepatic metabolism of **theophylline.** Any drastic changes in patients' diets should be discussed with the provider, and a plan for monitoring developed.

The impact on serum **theophylline** levels that different drugs may have should be discussed with the patient. Any change in the patient's overall medication regimen should warrant a status review and possibly serum **theophylline** levels. The impact of smoking on **theophylline** levels should be discussed and patients advised to notify their provider if they start or stop smoking.

Lifestyle management. Lifestyle management issues related to the disease process should be discussed. They often include the following:

1. The patient needs to self-monitor respiratory status with a peak flowmeter to determine the effectiveness of the medication prescribed.
2. The patient should avoid or quit smoking.
3. The patient should avoid environmental triggers for asthma at home, work, and school.

Anticholinergics

Inhaled anticholinergics are used primarily to treat COPD. **Ipratropium bromide** is a quaternary amine anticholinergic that is structurally similar to **atropine. Ipratropium bromide** is the primary **inhaled anti-**

cholinergic that is used in primary care. It is available as a single medication (**Atrovent**) or combined with **albuterol** (**Combivent**).

Pharmacodynamics

When inhaled, **ipratropium's** actions are confined to the mouth and airways. It acts to block the muscarinic cholinergic receptors by antagonizing the action of acetylcholine. Blocking the cholinergic receptors decreases the formation of cyclic guanosine monophosphate (cGMP), which leads to decreased contractility of the smooth muscle of the lungs, probably because of the actions of cGMP on intracellular calcium. The amount of bronchodilation caused by **ipratropium** inhalation is thought to reflect the level of parasympathetic tone.

Pharmacokinetics

ABSORPTION AND DISTRIBUTION. **Ipratropium**, when inhaled, is poorly absorbed from both the lung and the GI tract. Only 1 to 2 percent of a dose is systemically absorbed. **Ipratropium** penetrates the CNS poorly. It is unknown whether **ipratropium** crosses the placenta. **Ipratropium** is excreted into breast milk in minimal amounts.

METABOLISM AND EXCRETION. Most of the dose (90%) of **ipratropium** is swallowed and excreted in the feces unchanged. The portion of the dose that is absorbed is partially metabolized by ester hydrolysis to inactive metabolites. Approximately 50 percent of the absorbed drug is excreted unchanged in the urine.

Pharmacotherapeutics

PRECAUTIONS AND CONTRAINDICATIONS. **Ipratropium** is contraindicated for patients with soy lecithin hypersensitivity. It is also contraindicated for patients with sensitivities to related foods and legumes, such as peanut oil, soybeans, and peanuts. **Ipratropium** is also contraindicated for patients with hypersensitivity to **atropine** or **atropine derivatives** and for those with **bromide** sensitivity.

Ipratropium should not be used for the treatment of acute bronchospasm.

Ipratropium, even though poorly absorbed systemically, should be avoided for patients with urinary retention, bladder neck obstruction, or prostatic hypertrophy, because of its anticholinergic effects. **Ipratropium** may increase intraocular pressure in patients with closed-angle glaucoma.

Ipratropium bromide **is Pregnancy Category B. Its safety in pregnancy has had limited study; therefore, it should be used in pregnancy only if clearly indicated.** **Ipratropium** is excreted in breast milk in minimal amounts. **Atropine**, a chemically related drug, is considered safe during lactation. Because such small amounts of drug reach the breast milk, **ipratropium** is probably safe for use if needed during breastfeeding.

The safety and effectiveness of **ipratropium** have not been established in children under age 12. Providers may use **ipratropium** in younger children as an adjunct to **beta-agonist** therapy in acute exacerbations of asthma and for acute therapy in bronchiolitis.

ADVERSE DRUG REACTIONS. The most common adverse drug reaction reported with **ipratropium** is cough. Also reported are the related symptoms of hoarseness, throat irritation, and dysgeusia. Nausea, vomiting, and dyspepsia are thought to be related to the local anticholinergic effects that **ipratropium** has on the GI system. Xerostomia (dry mouth) is reported in 2 percent of patients.

Other anticholinergic effects that are reported (in less than 2% of patients) include urinary retention, dizziness, drowsiness, and constipation. Prostate disorders may also be noted (less than 2% reported).

If **ipratropium** is accidentally sprayed in the eyes, the patient may experience temporary eye irritation, pain, mydriasis, blurred vision, cycloplegia (paralysis of the ciliary muscle), irritant conjunctivitis, and visual disturbances.

Rare allergic and anaphylactoid reactions may occur. Reactions include urticaria, maculopapular rash, bronchospasm, pruritus, laryngospasm, oropharyngeal edema, and angioedema of the tongue, lips, and face. The patient's history usually includes sensitivity to other drugs and foods. Allergy to soybeans, legumes, or soy lecithin appears to be correlated with hypersensitivity to **ipratropium bromide.**

DRUG INTERACTIONS. **Ipratropium** is minimally absorbed into the systemic circulation after inhalation, and therefore there are no major drug interactions.

Patients who are concurrently using **cromolyn sodium** and **ipratropium bromide** via nebulizer should be cautioned not to mix the two, because a precipitate will form.

CLINICAL USE AND DOSAGE

Chronic Obstructive Pulmonary Disease. The dose of **ipratropium** from an MDI is 18 μg per spray. The dose of **ipratropium** for adults with COPD is 2 inhalations (36 μg) four times a day, for a total of 8 puffs per day. If needed, the patient may take up to 12 puffs per day (maximum of 216 μg/24 hours.) If using a nebulizer, the dose of **ipratropium** is one unit-dose vial (500 μg) three to four times a day via nebulizer, with doses 6 to 8 hours apart. **Ipratropium** may be mixed with **albuterol** if used within 1 hour.

The **ipratropium-albuterol** combination (**Combivent**) is indicated for second-line use for patients with COPD. It should be prescribed for patients already on a bronchodilator who continue to have bronchospasm that may benefit from a second bronchodilator. Each inhalation of **Combivent** administers 103 μg of **albuterol sulfate** and 18 μg of **ipratropium bromide.** The dose of

Combivent is 2 inhalations four times a day. The patient may take additional inhalations but must not exceed 12 inhalations per 24 hours.

Asthma. The adult dose of **ipratropium** for asthma is 2 inhalations (36 µg) four times a day. It should not be used for exercise-induced asthma. For children age 3 to 14, the dose is 1 or 2 inhalations three to four times a day. The dose of **ipratropium** solution is one unit dose (500 µg) administered via a nebulizer three to four times a day. **Ipratropium** may be mixed with **albuterol** if the combination is used within 1 hour.

RATIONAL DRUG SELECTION. **Ipratropium** is a first-line choice in the treatment of COPD and a second-line bronchodilator in the treatment of asthma. For the practitioner considering prescribing both **ipratropium** and **albuterol,** an appropriate choice would be the combination product **Combivent.**

Cost. The cost of a month's supply of **Atrovent** MDI is $30 to $40. There is no generic **ipratropium** MDI available. The cost of **Atrovent** inhalation solution is $9 to $10 per day, and generic **ipratropium** inhalation solution is $7 to $8 per day. The cost of the combination product **Combivent** is $30 to $40 per month, a significant cost savings over prescribing the two products individually.

MONITORING. There is no specific laboratory monitoring necessary with the use of **ipratropium,** other than monitoring the disease process.

PATIENT EDUCATION

Administration. **Ipratropium** should be used as prescribed. Overuse of **bronchodilators** leads to increased adverse effects, and using the **bronchodilator** less than prescribed may lead to increased bronchospasm and decreased pulmonary function.

The administration of medication via an MDI can be difficult for most adults and all children. Learning to coordinate the release of the medication from the inhaler with a deep breath is difficult. Written and pictorial instructions are available with the inhaler, but the provider must not assume that the patient understands the proper method of administering inhaled medications. Use verbal instructions as well as actual demonstration with a placebo inhaler to reinforce the written instructions.

These instructions and demonstrations should be repeated at follow-up visits.

To properly use an inhaler, the patient should first exhale and then tilt the head slightly back and place the inhaler mouthpiece either about 2 inches from the open mouth or between open lips. While inhaling, the patient should press down on the canister, breathe in slowly and deeply, and hold his or her breath for 10 seconds (count of 10) or as long as comfortable. If 2 puffs are prescribed, then the patient should wait at least 1 full minute between inhalations. If the patient is prescribed other inhalers, advise the patient to use the **ipratropium** first and wait 5 minutes before using the other inhalers as directed.

To assist with the delivery of inhaled medications, a spacer can be prescribed. The **Aerochamber** is a tubelike device that has pictures drawn on the outside to remind the patient of the proper technique to use in administering the inhaler. For younger children and adults, the **InspirEase** spacer gives a visual cue of the spacer bag deflating to help in taking a deep-enough breath. If the patient is taking too rapid a breath, both of these devices emit a whistling sound as a cue to breathe slowly.

Administration of **ipratropium** via nebulizer is per the manufacturer's directions. One unit dose of **ipratropium** is administered every 6 to 8 hours. **Albuterol** can be added to the **ipratropium** if the mixture is used within 1 hour. **Cromolyn** will precipitate if added to **ipratropium** solution, and the patient should be advised of this if both medications are prescribed. The nebulizer medication cup should be rinsed well between drugs if these two medications are to be used concurrently via nebulizer.

Regardless of administration method, patients should rinse their mouths with water after inhaling **ipratropium** to minimize dry mouth.

To prime the MDI, patients using **Combivent** are recommended to "test-spray" the oral inhalation aerosol three times into the air before using the first time. The patient should also prime the MDI in this manner if the medication has not been used in more than 24 hours.

Adverse reactions. The patient should be advised that a cough may develop and that less common complaints of throat irritation, hoarseness, or dry mouth may occur. Using a spacer device and rinsing the mouth with water

Clinical Pearl

SPACERS

Spacer devices usually require a prescription to be dispensed. The provider can often get samples of different spacers from the manufacturers.

after administration will decrease the incidence of these adverse effects.

Patients should be aware of the cross-sensitivity between **ipratropium** and soybean or other legume allergies.

Other adverse effects occur less often, but patients should be aware of the possible adverse effects and be instructed to notify their provider if they begin to have adverse effects from the **ipratropium**.

Lifestyle management. Lifestyle management issues related to the disease process should be discussed. They often include the following:

1. Patients need to self-monitor their respiratory status with a peak flowmeter to determine the effectiveness of the medication prescribed.
2. The patient should avoid or quit smoking.
3. The patient should avoid environmental triggers for asthma at home, work, and school.
4. Patients with COPD should avoid unnecessary exposure to viral respiratory infections.

Leukotriene Modifiers

Leukotriene-receptor agonists and **leukotriene-receptor inhibitors** are two relatively new classes of asthma medications. They were developed with the theory that cysteinyl leukotrienes play a significant role in the chronic inflammation associated with asthma. Leukotrienes are substances that induce numerous effects that contribute to the inflammatory process, including smooth-muscle contractility; neutrophil aggregation, degranulation, and chemotaxis; vascular permeability; and on lymphocytes. There is currently one **leukotriene receptor antagonist** available for use in asthma, **zafirlukast (Accolate)**. **Zileuton (Zyflo)** and **montelukast (Singulair)** are the **leukotriene-receptor inhibitors** currently available. There are at least nine different **leukotriene-receptor antagonists** that have been developed and are currently being evaluated for human use.

Pharmacodynamics

LEUKOTRIENE-RECEPTOR AGONISTS. **Zafirlukast** is a synthetic, selective, and competitive **leukotriene-receptor agonist** (LTRA) of leukotriene D4 and E4 (LTD4 and LTE4). These leukotrienes have been identified as components of slow-reacting substance of anaphylaxis. There is evidence that the cysteinyl leukotrienes contribute to the pathophysiology of asthma, including airway edema, smooth-muscle constriction, and cellular changes associated with the inflammatory process. In vitro studies demonstrated that **zafirlukast** antagonized the contractile activity of three leukotrienes (LTC4, LTD4, and LTE4) in the conducting airway smooth muscle.

LEUKOTRIENE-RECEPTOR INHIBITORS. **Montelukast** is a **selective leukotriene-receptor antagonist** that inhibits the cysteinyl leukotriene (CysLT1) receptor. It binds with high affinity and selectivity to the CysLT receptor. **Montelukast** inhibits the actions of LTD4 at the CysLT1 receptor. Cysteinyl leukotrienes and leukotriene receptor occupation have been correlated with the pathophysiology of asthma.

Zileuton is a specific inhibitor of 5-lipozygenase, which inhibits leukotriene (LTB1, LTC1, LTD1, and LTE1) formation. **Zileuton** inhibits leukotriene-dependent smooth-muscle contractions by blocking cysteinyl leukotriene production. By inhibiting leukotriene production, **zileuton** decreases the effects of leukotrienes in the respiratory tract, which are inflammation, edema, mucus secretion, and bronchoconstriction.

Pharmacokinetics

ABSORPTION AND DISTRIBUTION. **Zafirlukast** is rapidly absorbed from the GI tract following oral administration. Peak plasma concentrations are reached in 3 hours. The bioavailability of zafirlukast may be decreased when taken with food, and it should be taken on an empty stomach. **Zafirlukast** is greater than 99 percent protein-bound, primarily to albumin. **Zafirlukast** is excreted in breast milk in measurable amounts (50 ng/mL) compared with 255 ng/mL in plasma, when administered in healthy women in 40-mg/day dosages.

Zileuton is rapidly absorbed from the GI tract following oral administration. Peak plasma concentrations are reached 1.7 hours after dosing. Although the ingestion of food with **zileuton** results in an increase in mean peak level (27% increase), food does not cause significant changes in the extent of absorption or in time-to-peak plasma concentration. Therefore, the manufacturer states that **zileuton** may be taken with food. **Zileuton** is 93 percent protein-bound. There are no studies regarding **zileuton** in human breast milk, but both **zileuton** and its metabolites are excreted in rat milk.

Montelukast is rapidly absorbed following oral administration, with peak plasma concentration achieved in 3 to 4 hours for the film-coated tablet and in 2 to 2.5 hours after administration of the chewable tablet. **Montelukast** is more than 99 percent protein-bound. There is minimal distribution across the blood-brain barrier in rats; no human studies are available. **Montelukast** crosses the placenta in rats and is excreted in rat milk; there are no human studies available.

METABOLISM AND EXCRETION. **Zafirlukast** is extensively metabolized. In vitro studies using human liver microsomes showed that the hydroxylated metabolites of **zafirlukast** are formed through the cytochrome P-450 2C9 (CYP 2C9) enzyme pathway. Additional studies using human liver microsomes show that **zafirlukast** inhibits cytochrome P-450 CYP 3A4 and CYP 2C9 isoenzymes at concentrations close to the clinically achieved plasma concentrations. The metabolites of **zafirlukast** found in plasma are at least 90 times less potent **LTD4 receptor antagonists** than **zafirlukast**. Following oral administration of **zafirlukast**, urinary excretion accounts for approximately 10 percent of the dose, and the remainder is excreted in the feces. Unmetabolized **zafirlukast** is not found in the urine.

Zileuton is also extensively metabolized by the liver. Liver microsome studies have shown that **zileuton** and its N-dehydroxylated metabolite can be oxidatively metabolized by the cytochrome P-450 isoenzymes CYP IA2, CYP 2C9, and CYP 3A4. The urinary excretion of the inactive N-dehydroxylated metabolite and unchanged **zileuton** each accounted for less than 0.5 percent of the doses.

Montelukast is extensively metabolized by the liver, with no detectable amounts of metabolites found in the plasma. Cytochrome P-450 3A4 and 2C9 are the liver enzymes involved with the metabolism of **montelukast**. **Montelukast** and its metabolites are excreted almost exclusively via the bile, with less than 0.2 percent excreted in the urine.

Table 15–5 presents the pharmacokinetics.

Pharmacotherapeutics

PRECAUTIONS AND CONTRAINDICATIONS. The only true contraindication to the **leukotriene modifiers zafirlukast** and **montelukast** is hypersensitivity to any of the components of the medication. **Zileuton** is contraindicated if the patient has active liver disease (transaminase level more than three times the upper limit of normal). The leukotriene modifiers are not to be used for primary treatment of an acute asthma attack.

Zafirlukast should be used with caution in patients with hepatic dysfunction because it is extensively metabolized by the liver. If a patient has alcoholic cirrhosis, the clearance of **zafirlukast** is reduced about 50 to 60 percent. **Zileuton** may alter liver function, and therefore the patient should have normal liver function studies prior to initiating therapy. **Zileuton** should be used with caution in the patient who consumes large amounts of alcohol or who has a past history of liver disease. There

is no need to adjust the dose of **montelukast** in the patient with mild to moderate hepatic insufficiency because the elimination is only slightly prolonged.

Leukotriene modifiers should not be abruptly substituted for inhaled or oral **steroids**. Caution is advised as systemic **corticosteroids** are reduced. There have been reports that the reduction of oral **steroid** dose in some patients on **zafirlukast** has been followed by eosinophilia, vasculitic rash, worsening pulmonary symptoms, cardiac complications, and/or neuropathy sometimes presenting as Churg-Strauss syndrome, a systemic eosinophilic rash.

Zafirlukast **and** *montelukast* **are Pregnancy Category B, but there are no studies in pregnant women; therefore, use only if clearly needed.** *Zileuton* **is Pregnancy Category C.**

The safety of **zafirlukast** and **zileuton** for use in children younger than age 12 is unknown, and they are not recommended for use in children. **Montelukast** may be prescribed for children as young as 6; safety in younger children is not known.

Caution should be used in prescribing any of the leukotriene modifiers to lactating women because the effects on infants are unknown.

ADVERSE REACTIONS. The most common adverse reaction reported with **zafirlukast** use is headache. GI upset, myalgias, and fever are reported in a small percentage of patients. There is a reported increase in respiratory infections in patients older than age 55 who are taking **zafirlukast**. The respiratory infections were usually mild to moderate and associated with coadministration of **inhaled corticosteroids**.

In 12 percent of study patients taking **zileuton**, alanine aminotransferase (ALT) elevation occurred, with women older than age 65 appearing to be at risk for ALT elevations. Sixty-one percent of the liver enzyme elevation occurred within the first 2 months of treatment.

The reported adverse reactions of those taking **montelukast** are similar to placebo.

DRUG INTERACTIONS. **Zafirlukast** should be used with caution with any drug that is metabolized by cytochrome P-450 2C9 and 3A4 isoenzymes. Coadministration of **aspirin** with **zafirlukast** results in about a 45 percent increase in plasma **zafirlukast** level. **Erythromycin** coad-

Table 15–5. Pharmacokinetics: Leukotriene Modifiers

Drug	Onset	Peak	Duration	Protein Binding	Bioavail-ability	Half-Life	Metabolism	Elimination
Montelukast	—	3–4 h	—	>99%	64%	2.7–5.5 h	Extensive hepatic	Bile
Zafirlukast	3–14 d	2–4 h	—	>99%	Unknown	About 10 h	Extensive hepatic	Feces: 90% Urine: 10%
Zileuton	—	1.7 h	—	93%	Unknown	1–2.3 h	Hepatic	Urine: 87–95%

ministered with **zafirlukast** results in a 40 percent decrease in plasma **zafirlukast** level. Concurrent **terfenadine** use leads to decreased plasma **zafirlukast** levels, and **theophylline** use has a similar profile. When **warfarin** is prescribed to the patient taking **zafirlukast**, there is a clinically significant increase in prothrombin time (PT).

Zileuton potentiates **theophylline**, with a 33 percent decrease in **theophylline** dose recommended when these drugs are used concurrently. **Zileuton** potentiates **warfarin, propranolol,** and possibly other **beta blockers.** Monitor coadministration of any drug that is metabolized by isoenzyme CYP-3A4.

Monitor closely the patient who is taking drugs that are metabolized by cytochrome P-450 (**phenobarbital, rifampin**) concurrently with **montelukast.**

Table 15–6 presents drug interactions.

CLINICAL USE AND DOSING. **Zafirlukast** and **zileuton** are indicated in the treatment of asthma in adults and children age 12 or older. **Montelukast** is indicated for use in the treatment of asthma for patients age 6 or older.

The dose for **zafirlukast** is 20 mg twice daily in adults and children age 12 or older. Because food reduces bioavailability of **zafirlukast**, it must be taken on an empty stomach.

The dosage for **zileuton** is one 600-mg tablet four times daily, for a total daily dose of 2400 mg. **Zileuton** may be taken with food, so an easy dosing schedule is to take **zileuton** with meals and at bedtime.

The adult dosage (patients age 15 or older) of **mon-**

Table 15–6. Drug Interactions: Leukotrine Modifiers

Drug	Interacting Drug	Possible Effect	Implications
Montelukast	Phenobarbital	Decreases area under curve (AUC) of dose by about 40%	Monitor patient closely
	Rifampin	Decreased metabolism of montelukast	Monitor
Zafirlukast	Aspirin	Increased plasma levels of zafirlukast	Monitor
	Erythromycin	Decreased plasma levels of zafirlukast	Use together with caution
	Theophylline	Decreased plasma levels of zafirlukast	Use cautiously
	Warfarin	Increased PT	Closely monitor PT
	Drugs metabolized by CYP 2C9: amitriptyline, diclofenac, ibuprofen, imipramine, phenytoin, tolbutamide	Possible interactions	Until more data known, zafirlukast should be used cautiously in patients stabilized on these medications
	Drugs metabolized by CYP 3A4: alprazolam, astemizole, carbamazepine, cisapride, some corticosteroids, cyclosporine, diazepam, calcium channel blockers (felodipine, isradipine, nicardipine, nifedipine, nimodipine), diltiazem, erythromycin, lidocaine, lovastatin, midazolam, quinidine, simvastatin, triazolam, verapamil	Possible interactions	Until more data known, zafirlukast should be used cautiously in patients stabilized on these medications
Zileuton	Propranolol	Doubles propranolol serum concentrations, AUC, and half-life	Increased beta-blocker activity, bradycardia
	Theophylline	Doubles serum theophylline levels, prolongs theophylline clearance and half-life	Reduce theophylline dosage by 30–50%; monitor closely
	Warfarin	Decreased warfarin clearance, leading to increased prothrombin time (PT)	Monitor PT closely

telukast is 10 mg once a day in the evening. The dose of **montelukast** in children age 6 to 14 is 5 mg once a day in the evening. **Montelukast** may be taken without regard to meals.

Table 15–7 shows the dosage schedule.

RATIONAL DRUG SELECTION. Drug selection is based on the age of the patient and convenience in dosing. Children age 6 to 12 may be prescribed only **montelukast**. **Montelukast** offers once-a-day dosing without regard to meals, which may make it more convenient than the other two **leukotriene modifiers.**

MONITORING. Monitoring of improving or worsening asthmatic symptoms, bronchodilator use, and pulmonary function are necessary to determine the efficacy of the **leukotriene modifiers.**

Because of the effects of **zileuton** on the liver in some patients, liver enzymes must be drawn initially and monitored carefully to track elevated hepatic transaminases. Serum ALT must be drawn before treatment and once a month for the first 3 months of treatment with **zileuton.** Liver function should be monitored every 2 or 3 months for the remainder of the first year and periodically thereafter. If symptoms of liver dysfunction (right upper quadrant pain, nausea, fatigue, lethargy, pruritus, jaundice, or "flulike" symptoms) or elevated liver transaminase occurs, discontinue the medication and monitor liver function until it is back to normal.

PATIENT EDUCATION. Patient education focuses on proper dosing of the medication, adverse reactions, and the general asthma management plan. The incorporation of the **leukotriene** medications into the asthma treatment plan is covered in Chapter 28.

Administration. The patient must take the medication as prescribed, even if symptom-free. These medications are not for acute episodes of asthma. Patients must continue to use the bronchodilator inhaler for acute episodes of bronchospasm. They are not to decrease or discontinue

any of their other asthma medications unless instructed to do so by their health care provider.

Zafirlukast must be taken on an empty stomach, whereas **zileuton** may be taken with food. **Montelukast** may be taken without regard to meals.

Pregnant or nursing women should not take these medications.

Adverse reactions. **Zileuton** can affect liver function. Patients should be aware of the importance of liver function monitoring while on **zileuton** and know the signs of liver dysfunction to report to their health care provider. If patients exhibit right upper quadrant pain, nausea, fatigue, lethargy, pruritus, jaundice, or "flulike" symptoms, they are to notify their health care provider immediately.

Patients should be aware of significant drug interactions with **leukotriene modifiers** because of the way they are metabolized by the liver. Patients should be advised to discuss with their health care provider any new medications that are prescribed or discontinued.

Lifestyle management. Lifestyle management issues related to the disease process should be discussed. They often include the following:

1. The patient needs to self-monitor respiratory status with a peak flowmeter to determine the effectiveness of the medication prescribed.
2. The patient should avoid or quit smoking.
3. The patient should avoid environmental triggers for asthma at home, work, and school.

Table 15–8 presents the available dosage forms.

Respiratory Inhalants

Corticosteroids

The Expert Panel Report II states that **corticosteroids** are the "most potent and effective **anti-inflammatory** med-

Table 15–7. Dosage Schedule: Leukotriene Modifiers

Drug	Indication	Dose	Comments
Montelukast	Prophylaxis and chronic treatment of asthma	Adults: 10 mg once daily in P.M. Children age 6–4: 5 mg once daily in P.M.	Not recommended for children <6
Zileuton	Prophylaxis and chronic treatment of asthma	Adults: 600 mg qid	Not recommended for children <12. Evaluate liver function prior to initiating therapy and routinely during therapy; contraindicated in acute liver disease
Zafirlukast	Prophylaxis and chronic treatment of asthma	Adults: 20 mg bid	Not recommended for children <12; must be taken on an empty stomach

Table 15–8. Available Dosage Forms: Leukotriene Modifiers

Drug	Dosage Form	How Supplied
Montelukast (Singulair)	Tablets: 10 mg Chewable tablets: 5 mg	30, 90, 100
Zafirlukast (Accolate)	Tablets: 20 mg	60, 100
Zileuton (Zyflo)	Tablets: 600 mg	120

ication currently available" (NAEPP, 1997). Their anti-inflammatory effects lead to improvement in the severity of asthma symptoms, increased peak flow readings, and decreased airway hyperresponsiveness. In general, **inhaled steroids** are safe and well tolerated at recommended dosages and can be used by both children and adults. **Corticosteroids** are also used intranasally for the treatment of allergic rhinitis.

The commonly prescribed **inhaled corticosteroids** for asthma are **beclomethasone dipropionate** (Beclovent, Vanceril), **triamcinolone acetonide** (Azmacort), **budesonide** (Pulmicort Turbohaler), **flunisolide** (AeroBid), and **fluticasone** (Flovent). There are significant differences between the different formulations in the amount of **steroid** delivered per inhalation, and they are not interchangeable without adjusting the inhalations per day.

The **corticosteroids** that are available for intranasal use are **beclomethasone** (Beconase, Vancenase), **triamcinolone** (Nasacort), **budesonide** (Rhinocort), **flunisolide** (Nasalide, Nasarel), and **fluticasone** (Flonase).

Pharmacodynamics

In the treatment of asthma and allergic rhinitis, the primary actions of orally **inhaled corticosteroids** are anti-inflammatory. The **inhaled adrenocorticosteroids** inhibit the IgE and mast cell–mediated migration of inflammatory cells into the bronchial tissue (late-phase allergic reaction). The exact mechanism of action by which the **inhaled corticosteroids** inhibit bronchoconstrictor mechanisms and produce smooth-muscle relaxation is not known. The exact mechanism of action of **corticosteroids** on the nasal mucosa is unknown. **Intranasal corticosteroids** applied topically to the nasal tissues exert local anti-inflammatory effects without any systemic glucocorticoid effects.

Pharmacokinetics

ABSORPTION AND DISTRIBUTION. Absorption of **inhaled corticosteroids** occurs from the lungs and from the GI tract. Approximately 10 to 30 percent of the dose from an MDI is delivered to the lungs. If a spacer device is not used, approximately 80 percent of the dose from an MDI is swallowed, with the oral bioavailability differing from drug to drug.

Beclomethasone is rapidly absorbed from the nasal and pulmonary tissues and GI tract. Upon inhalation, 10 to 25 percent of the drug is deposited in the tissues of the mouth, trachea, and lungs, where it is completely absorbed. The remainder of the dose is swallowed. The oral bioavailability of inhaled **beclomethasone** is 20 percent. **Beclomethasone** is highly protein-bound. **Beclomethasone** and its metabolites do not appear to distribute into the tissues, but **beclomethasone** does cross the placenta. With systemic administration, **steroids** are excreted in breast milk; it is not known whether inhaled **beclomethasone** is found in breast milk.

Triamcinolone (Azmacort) MDI is packaged with a built-in spacer to enhance the delivery of the medication to the lungs. **Triamcinolone** (Nasacort) for intranasal use is delivered via intranasal metered-dose pump. **Triamcinolone** is rapidly and completely absorbed from lung tissues and nasal mucosa. It is distributed throughout the hilar areas of the lungs. The oral bioavailability of the swallowed portion of the dose is 10.6 percent. **Triamcinolone** is weakly protein-bound and crosses the placenta. It is not known whether inhaled **triamcinolone** is excreted in breast milk.

Approximately 20 percent of the inhaled dose of **budesonide** reaches the systemic circulation. Once absorbed from the nasal tissues or lungs, the distribution of **budesonide** is extensive. **Budesonide** is 88 percent protein-bound. It is not known if **budesonide** is excreted in breast milk, but it passes through the placenta.

Flunisolide is rapidly absorbed from the bronchial tree, with 10 to 20 percent of the inhaled dose distributing into the lungs. Fifty percent of an intranasal dose of **flunisolide** is absorbed into the systemic circulation. The oral bioavailability of the dose is 20 to 40 percent. **Flunisolide** crosses the placental barrier. Breast milk excretion is unknown.

Fluticasone is primarily absorbed in the lung, resulting in systemic bioavailability of 30 percent of the dose. Intranasal **fluticasone** has a systemic bioavailability of less than 2 percent. It is highly lipid-soluble and is rapidly distributed into the tissues. **Fluticasone** is 91 percent protein-bound. **Fluticasone** crosses the placenta. Breast milk excretion is unknown.

METABOLISM AND EXCRETION. All of the **inhaled corticosteroids** have some portion of the dose that is swallowed. After GI absorption, they all undergo high first-pass liver metabolism.

In the lung, **beclomethasone** is rapidly metabolized to beclomethasone 17-monopropionate, and more slowly to free **beclomethasone**. Metabolites of **beclomethasone** are excreted mainly in the feces, with a small portion excreted in the urine.

Triamcinolone is metabolized into three less active ingredients, 6β-hydroxytriamcinolone acetonide, 21-carboxytriamcinolone, and 21-carboxy-6β-hydroxytriamcinolone acetonide. All of the metabolites of **triamcinolone** are eliminated in the feces.

Budesonide undergoes extensive first-pass metabolism into two main metabolites, 16-alpha-hydroxyprednisolone (24%) and 6-beta-hydroxybudesonide (5%). The metabolites are excreted in the urine (66%) and the feces.

The part of the **flunisolide** dose that is swallowed is absorbed and metabolized by the liver into several metabolites. One of the metabolites has minor glucocorticoid activity. The drug is further metabolized into inactive metabolites. Excretion of inhaled **flunisolide** is not described, but oral doses are excreted equally in the feces and the urine.

Fluticasone is metabolized in the liver primarily by cytochrome P-450 3A4. The only detectable metabolite is a 1-beta-carboxylic acid derivative. Excretion is primarily in the feces, with less then 5 percent excreted in the urine.

Pharmacokinetics are presented in Table 15–9.

Pharmacotherapeutics

PRECAUTIONS AND CONTRAINDICATIONS. All of the inhaled corticosteroid preparations are contraindicated in acute status asthmaticus or when intensive, acute therapy is warranted. They should not be used for relief of acute bronchospasm.

Care should be used when substituting any of the **inhaled corticosteroids** for **oral corticosteroid** therapy. There have been deaths due to adrenal insufficiency in asthmatic patients who were switched from **oral** to **inhaled corticosteroids.**

The risk for hypothalamic-pituitary-adrenal (HPA) suppression is low with **inhaled corticosteroids,** but the risk increases when **inhaled corticosteroids** are administered while the patient is taking **oral steroids.**

Inhaled corticosteroids should be avoided in patients with Cushing's syndrome. They should be used with caution in patients with ocular herpes simplex infections, tuberculosis, oral or nasal surgery or trauma, healing nasal septal ulcers, and untreated respiratory infection (viral, fungal, or bacterial).

All of the inhaled corticosteroids are Pregnancy Category C. There have not been any well-controlled studies of the effects of *inhaled corticosteroids* **during pregnancy.**

The use of high-dose **inhaled steroids** in children may inhibit growth. The safety of **beclomethasone** in children under age 6 has not been determined; doses higher than 400 μg/day warrant close monitoring of growth. **Triamcinolone** inhalant therapy should not be prescribed to children under age 6, because the safety and efficacy have not been established. Dosages of 256 μg/day of **budesonide** have caused a decrease in the rate of lower leg

Table 15–9. Pharmacokinetics: Respiratory Inhalants

Drug	Onset	Peak	Protein Binding	Bioavailability	Half-Life	Metabolism	Elimination
Corticosteroids							
Beclomethasone	Few days to 3 wk	—	—	<5%	15 h	Hepatic	Feces
Budesonide	—	—	88%	10%	2 h	Hepatic	Renal
Flunisolide	Few days to 4 wk	10–30 min	—	20%	1.8–2 h	Hepatic	Renal, feces
Fluticasone	—	—	91%	30%	—	Hepatic	Feces
Triamcinolone	—	—	Weak	10%	0.5–1 h	Hepatic	Feces
Inhaled Antihistamine							
Azelastine	—	2–3 h	88%	40%	22 h	Hepatic	Feces
Anti-inflammatory Agents							
Cromolyn sodium	—	—	—	<1%	—	Not metabolized	Bile, renal
Nedocromil	—	20 min	—	6–9%	1.5–2.3 h	Not metabolized	Renal: 64% Feces: 36%

growth; monitor growth carefully if prescribing. **Budesonide** safety has not been determined for children under age 6. Inhibition of growth has been noted in children on high-dose inhaled **fluticasone**. **Fluticasone** should not be prescribed to children under age 4. The safety of inhaled **flunisolide** in children under age 6 has not been established.

ADVERSE REACTIONS. All of the **inhaled corticosteroids** have associated xerostomia, hoarseness (5 to 50% of patients), tongue and mouth irritation, flushing, and dysgeusia (altered taste sensation). Rash and urticaria have been reported with the use of **flunisolide, beclomethasone,** and **fluticasone.** Dysmenorrhea has been reported in 1 to 3 percent of patients using inhaled **fluticasone.**

Local immunosuppression can lead to oral candidiasis with any of the **inhaled corticosteroids.** Cataracts can be induced with **corticosteroid** use, even with **inhaled corticosteroids.** Bronchospasm may occur with any of the **inhaled corticosteroids.**

With high-dose **inhaled corticosteroid** use, HPA suppression is theoretically possible. Concurrent use of **systemic corticosteroids** with **inhaled corticosteroids** increases the likelihood of HPA suppression, compared with the use of either one alone.

Pulmonary infiltrates with eosinophilia may occur with inhaled **flunisolide,** usually when **inhalation corticosteroid** therapy replaces **systemic corticosteroid** therapy. The cause is unknown.

Intranasal corticosteroid use may cause nasal irritation, itching, sneezing, and nasal dryness. The patient may experience bloody nasal mucus or epistaxis.

DRUG INTERACTIONS. There are no known drug interactions with inhaled **triamcinolone, flunisolide,** or **beclomethasone.**

Ketoconazole increases plasma concentration of **fluticasone** and **budesonide** when coadministered. The interaction is due to inhibition of cytochrome P-450 3A4 (CYP 3A4) isoenzyme, the enzyme that metabolizes **fluticasone** and **budesonide.** There are no other known drug interactions, but close monitoring for **corticosteroid**-related side effects is advisable if coadministered with other drugs that are known to inhibit CYP 3A4. Those drugs include **anastrozole (Arimidex)** in high doses, **delavirdine (Rescriptor), erythromycin, fluconazole (Diflucan), fluoxetine (Prozac), itraconazole (Sporanox), mibefradil (Posicor), nefazodone (Serzone), nelfinavir (Viracept), ritonavir (Norvir),** and **zileuton (Zyflo.)**

Drug interactions are presented in Table 15–10.

CLINICAL USE AND DOSING

Asthma. The **inhaled corticosteroids** are one of the long-term control medications used to manage the inflammatory process associated with asthma. Dosages for the **inhaled corticosteroids** vary with the specific product and the delivery method. The patient is started on **inhaled corticosteroids** according to the expert panel guidelines for the management of asthma (NAEPP, 1997). An adult (or child over age 5) with mild persistent asthma is started on a low dose of **inhaled corticosteroids** or **cromolyn** or **nedocromil** (discussed later in this chapter). If the patient has moderate persistent asthma, then the patient is prescribed daily **inhaled corticosteroids** at a medium dose. Severe persistent asthma requires daily high-dose **inhaled corticosteroids.** See Table 15–11 for dosing **inhaled corticosteroids** for adults and children over age 5. Chapter 28 should be referred to for comprehensive asthma management.

Children under age 5 with persistent asthma require daily **anti-inflammatory** therapy. Young children with mild persistent asthma are usually started on a trial of **cromolyn** or **nedocromil,** before **inhaled corticosteroids.** If needed, low-dose **inhaled corticosteroids** are started, using a spacer or, for infants, a holding chamber with a mask. If the child has moderate persistent asthma, medium-dose **inhaled corticosteroids** are begun. High-dose **inhaled steroids** are prescribed for severe persistent asthma. The provider should be familiar with the differences in dosing young children and adults.

Allergic rhinitis. Allergic rhinitis results when allergens come in contact with the nasal mucosa, causing a hypersensitivity reaction. **Nasal corticosteroids** are used to manage the inflammatory response associated with seasonal or perennial allergies. **Intranasal corticosteroids** may be used once or twice a day, depending on the drug chosen. Once clinical improvement occurs, usually in 3 to 7 days, the dose can be decreased. See Table 15–11 for dosing information.

RATIONAL DRUG SELECTION. The expert panel report (NAEPP, 1997) does not recommend one **inhaled corticosteroid** over another; therefore, the choice is mostly based on ease of dosing and the adverse drug interactions and indications previously addressed. There are no generic equivalent formulas of any of the **inhaled corticosteroids** available at this time; the costs are within a fairly close range and therefore not a major factor.

Dosing. If a patient requires a high dose of **inhaled steroid,** the **beclomethasone** 42 μg/puff dose would be more than 20 puffs per day, whereas the dose of **budesonide** would be 8 or more puffs per day. High-dose **triamcinolone** would also be 20 puffs per day. **Fluticasone** and **flunisolide** have the highest steroid anti-inflammatory effect per puff, which makes dosing high-dose **inhaled steroids** more convenient (see Table 15–11 for dosing). If the patient requires a low dose or if trying to wean the dose, **beclomethasone** or **triamcinolone** would be the first choice.

MONITORING. The patient who is using **inhaled corticosteroids** needs to be monitored for adverse effects of

Table 15–10. Drug Interactions: Respiratory Inhalants

Drug	Interacting Drug	Possible Effect	Implications
Corticosteroids Beclomethasone	None known	—	—
Budesonide	Ketoconazole*	Increased budesonide concentrations and suppression of plasma cortisol levels	Observe the patient for increased corticosteroid-related side effects
Flunisolide	None known	—	—
Fluticasone	Ketoconazole*	Increased fluticasone concentrations and suppression of plasma cortisol levels	Observe the patient for increased corticosteroid-related side effects
Triamcinolone	None known	—	—
Inhaled Antihistamines Azelastine	Cimetidine	The mean maximum concentration (Cmax) and area under the curve (AUC) of azelastine is increased when co-administered with cimetidine	Monitor closely if coadministering
	Ethanol or other CNS depressants	Reduced mental alertness and impairment of CNS performance may occur	Use concurrently with caution
Anti-inflammatory Agents Cromolyn	None known	—	—
Nedocromil	None known	—	—

*There are no other known drug interactions, but close monitoring is advisable if coadministered with other drugs that are known to inhibit CYP 3A4. Those drugs include anastrozole in high doses, delavirdine, erythromycin, fluconazole, fluoxetine, itraconazole, mibefradil, nefazodone, nelfinavir, ritonavir, and zileuton.

the medication, effectiveness of the medication, and the asthma disease process. If high-dose **inhaled corticosteroids** are used for a long time, blood glucose and potassium should be monitored.

PATIENT EDUCATION

Administration. Patients who are concurrently using an **inhaled bronchodilator** should administer the **bronchodilator** first and wait several minutes before using the **inhaled corticosteroid.** This procedure enhances the absorption of the **steroid** in the bronchial tree and decreases the adverse effects of the inhaled fluorocarbon propellants in the two aerosols.

The administration of **inhaled corticosteroids** via an MDI can be difficult for most adults and all children. Learning to coordinate the release of the medication from the inhaler with a deep breath is difficult. Written and pictorial instructions are available with the inhaler, but the provider must not assume that the patient understands the proper method of administering inhaled medications. Use verbal instructions as well as actual demonstration with a placebo inhaler to reinforce the written instructions. These instructions and demonstrations should be repeated at follow-up visits.

To properly use an inhaler, the patient should first exhale and then tilt the head slightly back and place the inhaler mouthpiece either about 2 inches from the open mouth or between open lips. While inhaling, the patient should press down on the canister, breathe in slowly and deeply, and hold her or his breath for 10 seconds (count of 10) or as long as comfortable. If multiple puffs are prescribed, then the patient should wait at least 1 full minute between inhalations.

To assist with the delivery of inhaled medications, spacers can be prescribed. The **Aerochamber** is a tube-like device that has pictures drawn on the outside to remind the patient of the proper techniques. For younger children and adults, the **InspirEase** spacer gives a visual cue of the spacer bag deflating to help in taking a deep-enough breath. Both of these devices cue the patient to breathe slowly by emitting a whistling sound if the patient is taking too rapid a breath.

Table 15–11. Dosage Schedule: Respiratory Inhalants

Drug	Indication	Dose	Comments
Corticosteroids			
Beclomethasone	Asthma	*Adults and children >5:* Low dose: 168–504 µg daily in divided doses either bid, tid, or qid (4–12 puffs of 42 µg) Medium dose: 504–840 µg daily in divided doses (12–20 puffs of 42 µg) High dose: >840 µg daily in divided doses (>20 puffs of 42 µg) *Children <5:* Low dose: 84–336 µg daily in divided doses (2–8 puffs of 42 µg) Medium dose: 336–672 µg daily in divided doses (8–16 puffs/d of 42 µg) High dose: >672 µg daily in divided doses (>16 puffs per day of 42 µg)	Patients should rinse their mouths with water after use; if needed, use inhaled bronchodilator first
	Allergic rhinitis	*Adults and children >6:* 42 µg/spray aqueous nasal spray: 1–2 sprays each nostril bid 42 µg/spray nasal inhaler: 1 spray each nostril 2–4 times/d 84 µg/spray aqueous nasal spray: 1–2 sprays each nostril once a day	Not recommended for use in children <age 6
Budesonide	Asthma	*Adults:* Low dose: 200–400 µg daily (1–2 inhalations daily) Medium dose: 400–600 µg daily (2–3 inhalations daily) High dose: >600 µg daily (>3 inhalations daily) *Children >6:* Low dose: 200 µg daily (1 inhalation daily) Medium dose: 200–400 µg daily (2–3 inhalations daily) High dose: >400 µg/d (>2 inhalations daily)	Rinse mouth after use Has rapid onset for an inhaled steroid Improvement can occur within 24 h of beginning treatment, although maximum benefit may not be achieved for 1–2 wk Not recommended for children <age 6
	Allergic rhinitis	*Adults and children >6:* Initially 2 sprays in each nostril bid or 4 sprays once daily in the A.M. (max 4 sprays/nostril/d)	Blow nose prior to using For perennial rhinitis, gradually reduce over 2–4 wk to lowest effective dose
Flunisolide	Asthma	*Adults:* Low dose: 500–1000 µg daily (2–4 puffs daily divided in bid dose) Medium dose: 1000–2000 µg daily (4–8 puffs divided bid) High dose: >2000 µg daily (>8 puffs divided bid)	Rinse mouth after use If needed, use inhaled bronchodilator first Safety in children <6 has not been established

Continued on next page

Table 15–11. Dosage Schedule: Respiratory Inhalants (*continued*)

Drug	Indication	Dose	Comments
	Allergic rhinitis	*Children >6:* Low dose: 500–750 µg (2–3 puffs daily) Medium dose: 1000–1250 µg daily (4–5 puffs daily divided bid) High dose: >1250 µg daily (>5 puffs divided bid) *Adults:* Initially 2 sprays each nostril bid, maximum 8 sprays each nostril per day *Children 6–14:* Initially 1 spray each nostril tid or 2 sprays each nostril bid; maximum 4 sprays/nostril/d	Blow nose prior to using Safety in children <6 has not been established
Fluticasone	Asthma	*Adults and children >11:* Low dose: 88–264 µg daily (2–6 puffs of 44 µg/puff divided bid) Medium dose: 264–660 µg daily (2–6 puffs of 110 µg/puff daily divided bid) High dose: >660 µg (>6 puffs 110 µg/puff or >3 puffs 220 µg/puff) *Children 4–11:* Low dose: 88–176 µg daily (2–4 puffs of 44 µg/puff divided bid) Medium dose: 176–440 µg daily (2–4 puffs 110 µg/puff divided bid) High dose: >440 µg (>4 puffs 110 µg/puff or >2 puffs 220 µg/puff)	Safety in children under age 4 has not been established
	Allergic rhinitis	*Adults and children >11:* Initially 2 sprays each nostril once a day or 1 spray in each nostril bid; for maintenance, reduce dose to 1 spray each nostril daily *Children 4–11:* Initially 1 spray in each nostril once daily; may increase to 2 sprays in each nostril once daily if needed; for maintenance: 1 spray in each nostril once daily	Safety in children <4 has not been established
Triamcinolone	Asthma	*Adults and children >12:* Low dose: 400–1000 µg daily divided in bid, tid, or qid doses (4–10 puffs) Medium dose: 1000–2000 µg daily in divided doses (10–20 puffs) High dose: >200 µg daily in divided doses (>20 puffs)	Rinse mouth after use Safety in children under age 6 has not been established

Continued on next page

Table 15–11. Dosage Schedule: Respiratory Inhalants (*continued*)

Drug	Indication	Dose	Comments
	Allergic rhinitis	*Children 6–12:* Low dose: 400–800 μg per day in divided doses (4–8 puffs daily) Medium dose: 800–1200 μg daily in divided doses (8–12) High dose: >1200 μg daily in divided doses (>12 puffs) *Adults and children >12:* 2 sprays in each nostril once daily; may increase if needed to a maximum of 8 sprays/d; reduce dose as condition improves *Children 6–12:* 2 sprays each nostril once daily; may reduce as condition improves	Safety in children <6 has not been established
Inhaled Antihistamine Azelastine	Allergic rhinitis	*Adults and children >12:* 2 sprays (137 μg/spray) per nostril bid	Safety in children has not been established The unit must be primed before using for the first time by pumping the activator 4 times, until a fine mist occurs
Anti-inflammatory Agents Cromolyn sodium	Asthma	*Inhaled* *Adults and children >5:* 4 puffs qid initially; wean down to 2 puffs bid to tid; may use 2 puffs prior to exercise or allergen exposure *Nebulizer* *Adults and children >2:* 1 unit dose qid, weaning down to bid	Cromolyn must be used continuously 3–4 wk before maximum effect is achieved Cromolyn is very safe to use in children, with fewer side effects than inhaled steroids
	Allergic rhinitis	*Adults and children >6:* 1 spray in each nostril 3–4 times a day; may increase dosage to 6/d if needed	Begin therapy 1 wk before known exposure; for allergic rhinitis, 2–4 wk of therapy may be needed to produce relief; blow nose prior to administering
Nedocromil	Asthma	*Inhaled* *Adults and children >6:* 2 puffs qid *Nebulizer* *Adults and children >2:* 1 ampule via nebulizer qid	Once control is established, the dose can be reduced to 3 times a day; after several weeks the dose can be further decreased to bid

Patients should rinse their mouths with water after each use to help reduce dry mouth, hoarseness, and candidiasis infection.

The patient should clear the nasal passages of mucus prior to using **intranasal corticosteroids.** If the nasal passages are swollen and blocked, the patient should administer a **topical decongestant** prior to using **intranasal corticosteroids.** The medication is sprayed into the nasal passages. The patient does not need to inhale the medication. The patient should understand that the effects are not immediate and that clinical improvement may take 3 to 7 days. Rinsing the mouth with water after use will reduce the rare chance of candidiasis infection associated with **intranasal corticosteroid** use.

Inhaled steroids are not to be used as abortive asthma medications; they are for preventive therapy only. The provider should have patients bring in all their inhalers and review which are to be used for abortive therapy (**beta-agonists**) and which are for preventive therapy. The patient should be advised to continue to use the **inhaled corticosteroid** even when not having asthma symptoms.

Adverse reactions. The patient should be advised to notify the provider if sore mouth or throat occurs. Oral *Candida* infections are possible, and the patient should get prompt treatment. The patient should be aware of the possibility of dysphonia developing. Rinsing the mouth with water and using a spacer device will decrease its incidence.

Other adverse effects occur less often, but the patient should be aware of them and be instructed to notify the provider if adverse effects begin to develop from the inhaled medication.

Relatively few medications interact with the **inhaled corticosteroids. Ketoconazole** should be avoided for patients who are prescribed **fluticasone** and **budesonide**. Patients should be instructed to notify all providers that they are on **inhaled corticosteroids** to avoid possible interactions.

Lifestyle management. Lifestyle management issues related to the disease process should be discussed. They often include the following:

1. Patients need to self-monitor their respiratory status with a peak flowmeter to determine the effectiveness of the medication prescribed.
2. The patient should avoid or quit smoking.
3. The patient should avoid environmental triggers for asthma at home, work, and school.

Available dosage forms are presented in Table 15–12.

Inhaled Anti-inflammatory Agents

Cromolyn sodium and **nedocromil** are synthetic compounds that inhibit antigen-induced bronchospasm. **Cromolyn** was originally produced to be used as a **bronchodilator** but was found to have no **bronchodilator** activity. Nevertheless, **cromolyn** inhibits antigen-induced bronchospasm, blocks the release of histamine, and is a **mast cell stabilizer. Nedocromil** is similar to **cromolyn** in many ways, but there are distinct differences, which are discussed in this section.

Cromolyn is used in the treatment of asthma (**Intal**) and allergic rhinitis (**Nasalcrom**). **Nedocromil** (**Tilade**) is approved for use in patients with asthma who are not controlled with **beta-agonists** alone.

Pharmacodynamics

Cromolyn and **nedocromil** both act to inhibit mast cell degranulation, which prevents the release of histamine and slow-reacting substance of anaphylaxis (SRS-A).

Neither drug prevents the binding of IgE to the mast cell or the binding of antigen to IgE. **Cromolyn** and **nedocromil** also prevent the release of leukotrienes, which induce numerous effects that contribute to the inflammatory process in the lungs. **Nedocromil** also inhibits and prevents the release of platelet activating factor (PAF). With continued use, **cromolyn** and **nedocromil** reduce bronchi hyperreactivity to stimuli such as cold air, allergens, and environmental irritants.

Neither drug has bronchodilator, antihistamine, or vasoconstrictor activity, and at therapeutic doses they have no systemic activity.

Pharmacokinetics

ABSORPTION AND DISTRIBUTION. Inhaled **cromolyn** is poorly absorbed systemically, with only 8 percent of the dose absorbed. Approximately 5 to 10 percent of the inhaled dose reaches the lungs, with the amount affected by the degree of bronchoconstriction present. Intranasal **cromolyn** is minimally absorbed. Distribution of the absorbed amount of the drug is unknown. Minimal amounts of **cromolyn** cross the placenta and distribute into breast milk.

Inhaled **nedocromil** is slowly absorbed from the lungs, with 6 to 9 percent of the dose having systemic bioavailability. Absorption of **nedocromil** is affected by exercise and decreased forced expiratory volume (FEV) measurements. Distribution is unknown. **Nedocromil** is thought to cross the placenta. It is unknown whether **nedocromil** is excreted in breast milk.

METABOLISM AND EXCRETION. The portion of the dose of **cromolyn** that is absorbed from the lung is rapidly excreted unchanged in the urine and bile. The remaining portion of the dose is exhaled or swallowed and excreted unchanged in the feces. **Nedocromil** is not metabolized and is excreted unchanged in the urine (64%) and feces (36%).

Pharmacotherapeutics

PRECAUTIONS AND CONTRAINDICATIONS. Neither **cromolyn** nor **nedocromil** is a **bronchodilator**, and they are contraindicated in the treatment of acute bronchospasm or status asthmaticus.

Hypersensitivity to **cromolyn** or **nedocromil** is a contraindication to their use.

Both *cromolyn* and *nedocromil* are Pregnancy Category B. These drugs should be used with caution in the lactating mother because their safety has not been established.

Cromolyn is safe for use in children as young as 2 years old (nebulizer solution). Safety and efficacy of **nedocromil** in children under age 12 have not been established.

Table 15–12. Available Dosage Forms: Respiratory Inhalants

Drug	Dosage Form	How Supplied
CORTICOSTEROIDS		
Beclomethasone		
Beclovent	Inhaler: 42 μg/puff	6.7-g (80 inh), 16–8 g (200 inh) canisters
Vanceril	Inhaler: 42 μg/puff	16–8 g (200 inh) canisters
Vanceril Double Strength	Inhaler: 84 μg/puff	12.2-g canisters (120 inh)
Beconase	Nasal inhaler: 42 μg/spray	16.8-g (200 inh) canisters
Beconase AQ	Aqueous nasal inhaler: 42 μg/spray	25-g canister (200 sprays)
Vancenase Pockethaler	Nasal inhaler: 42 μg/spray	7-g (200 sprays) Pockethaler
Vancenase AQ Double Strength	Aqueous nasal inhaler: 84 μg/spray	19-g canister (120 sprays)
Budesonide		
Pulmicort Turbuhaler	Turbuhaler: 200 μg/dose	200-dose Turbuhaler
Rhinocort	Nasal spray: 32 μg/spray	7-g (200 sprays)
Flunisolide		
Aerobid	Inhaler: 250 μg/puff	7-g canister (100 inh)
Nasalide	Nasal solution: 25 μg/spray	25-mL metered pump (200 sprays)
Nasarel	Aqueous nasal spray: 25 μg/spray	25-mL metered pump (200 sprays)
Fluticasone		
Flovent	Inhaler: 44 μg/puff, 110 μg/puff, 220 μg/puff	44 μg/puff in 7.9-(60 inh) and 13-g (120 inh) canisters; 110 μg/puff in 13-g (120 inh) canister; 220 μg/puff in 13-g (120 inh) canister
Flonase	Aqueous nasal spray: 50 μg/spray	16 g (200 inh) canisters
Triamcinolone		
Azmacort	Inhaler: 100 μg/puff	20-g (240 inh) canisters
Nasacort AQ	Aqueous nasal spray: 55 μg/spray	10-g (100 sprays) canisters
INHALED ANTIHISTAMINE		
Azelastine		
Astelin	Aqueous nasal spray: 137 μg/spray	2 × 17-mL bottles (100 sprays/bottle)
ANTI-INFLAMMATORY AGENTS		
Cromolyn Sodium		
Intal	Inhaler: 800 μg/puff Solution for nebulizer: 20 mg/2-mL ampules	8.1-g (112 inh) canister 2-mL ampules (60, 120)
Nasalcrom	Nasal solution: 5.2 mg/spray	13-mL (100 sprays) and 26-mL (200 sprays) metered pump
Nedocromil		
Tilade	Inhaler: 1.75 mg per puff Solution for nebulizer: 11 mg/2.2-mL ampule	16.2-g (104 inh) canister 2-mL ampules (60, 120)

ADVERSE REACTIONS.   **Cromolyn** is generally well tolerated. Inhaled **cromolyn** may cause bronchospasm, which can be avoided by preadministering a **beta-agonist bronchodilator**. Throat irritation and cough are also reported. Intranasal **cromolyn** may produce nasal irritation and cause sneezing.

Nedocromil is well tolerated, with an unpleasant taste the most common (12.6%) reported adverse effect. Altered taste sensation (dysgeusia) has also been reported. Other reported adverse reactions are cough (7%), headache (6%), sore throat (5.7%), rhinitis (4.6%), and nausea (4%).

DRUG INTERACTIONS.   There are no clinically significant drug interactions with either **cromolyn** or **nedocromil**. **Cromolyn** solution for nebulizer use will form a precipitate if mixed with **ipratropium** solution.

CLINICAL USE AND DOSING

Asthma. **Cromolyn** is considered a long-term control drug for the treatment of moderate asthma. It is available in inhaled form, nebulizer solution, and dry powder in a capsule for inhalation with a **Spinhaler** device. The dosage of **cromolyn** MDI for adults and for children older than 5 is 2 sprays (800 μg/spray) inhaled four times a day at regular intervals. The dosage of oral inhalation capsules in adults and children older than 5 is 1 capsule (20 mg) delivered via the **Spinhaler** device four times a day. The dose of nebulizer solution of **cromolyn** is 1 ampule (20 mg) four times a day at regular intervals. The dose of **cromolyn** may be decreased after the patient is stabilized (usually after 4 weeks) to two or three doses a day. If used concurrently with **bronchodilators**, the **bronchodilator** should be administered first. **Cromolyn** may be mixed with **albuterol** in a nebulizer cup to simplify dosing. The patient should understand that the effectiveness of **cromolyn** depends on its regular use.

The dose of **nedocromil** MDI in adults and children age 12 or older is 2 inhalations four times a day at regular intervals. After good control is achieved, which usually takes several weeks, the patient's dose may be weaned to three times a day. After several weeks of good control, the patient may be further weaned to twice-a-day dosing, which is the minimal effective dose. Patients should understand that effective treatment depends on continued use, even if they are having no asthma symptoms.

Bronchospasm prophylaxis. **Cromolyn** is indicated for patients with exercise-induced bronchospasm or individuals who have bronchospasm with known precipitating factors (e.g., pet exposure). The dose of **cromolyn** MDI for adults and children age 5 or older is 2 inhalations 10 to 15 minutes before exercise. If exercise is prolonged, the dose may be repeated. The dose of **cromolyn** inhalation capsules in adults and children age 5 or older is 1 capsule (20 mg) administered via a **Spinhaler** device not more than 1 hour before exercise. Nebulizer dosing

in adults and children age 2 or older is 1 ampule administered via nebulized solution not more than 1 hour prior to exercise. For maximum effectiveness, the time between the use of inhaled **cromolyn sodium** and exercise should be as brief as possible.

Allergic rhinitis. The dosage of **cromolyn sodium** nasal inhalation spray in adults and children age 6 and older is 1 spray in each nostril three to four times a day. The dose may be increased to six times a day if needed. The dose is administered while the patient is inhaling, and the nostrils should first be cleared of mucus. Two to four weeks of therapy may be needed to produce relief from perennial rhinitis.

Concurrent use of corticosteroids. If the patient is using corticosteroids chronically for asthma control, the dosage should remain the same after the introduction of **cromolyn** or **nedocromil** into the treatment regimen. If the patient improves, then the corticosteroid can be weaned slowly. Even if the patient cannot be completely weaned off the corticosteroids, the dose of steroid can often be decreased to avoid some of the effects of chronic steroid use.

RATIONAL DRUG SELECTION.   The decision of which inhaled anti-inflammatory to use is often based on cost and on patient variables such as age or ease of dosing.

Patient variables. **Cromolyn** has dosage forms available for use in children as young as 2 years, whereas **nedocromil** is approved only for patients age 12 and older.

Administration. **Cromolyn** comes in multiple formulations that allow the provider to match the patient's age and lifestyle with an administration form. **Nedocromil** is available only in MDI form.

Cost. The cost of **cromolyn** MDI ($30 to $40 each) is lower than **nedocromil** MDI ($50 to $60 each). The cost of **cromolyn** inhalation capsules is $200 per month if administered four times a day.

MONITORING.   No specific monitoring is required other than monitoring associated with the disease process.

PATIENT EDUCATION

Administration. The administration of **inhaled anti-inflammatory** agents requires the patient to use the medication as prescribed. Neither **cromolyn** nor **nedocromil** is effective if not used at regular intervals. Clarification regarding the use of **inhaled bronchodilators** that can be used as needed and the **inhaled anti-inflammatory** agents will enable the patient to use the medication appropriately, as will a written plan.

The administration of **cromolyn** or **nedocromil** via an MDI can be difficult for adults and children alike. Learning to coordinate the release of the medication from the inhaler with a deep breath is difficult. Written and pictorial instructions are available with the inhaler, but the provider must not assume that the patient understands the proper method of administering inhaled medications. Use verbal instructions as well as actual demonstration with a placebo inhaler to reinforce the written instructions. These instructions and demonstrations should be repeated at follow-up visits. Do not assume that the patient who already is using another medication via MDI is using it correctly. These teaching steps should be used whenever a new medication is introduced.

To properly use an inhaler, the patient should first exhale, then tilt the head slightly back, and place the inhaler mouthpiece either about 2 inches from the open mouth or between open lips. While inhaling, the patient should press down on the canister, breathe in slowly and deeply, and hold her or his breath for 10 seconds (count of 10) or as long as comfortable. If 2 puffs are prescribed, then the patient should wait at least 1 full minute between inhalations.

To assist with the delivery of inhaled medications, a spacer can be prescribed. The **Aerochamber** is a tubelike device that has pictures drawn on the outside to remind the patient of the proper technique to use in administering the inhaler. For younger children and adults, the InspirEase spacer gives a visual cue of the spacer bag deflating to help them take a deep enough breath. If the patient takes a rapid breath, both devices emit a whistling sound to cue the patient to breathe slowly.

The use of **cromolyn** via nebulizer must be demonstrated to the patient in the clinic or by the home health agency that is providing the nebulizer. Because the vials are premeasured, there is no concern about dosing error.

The use of the oral inhalation capsule of **cromolyn** ought to be demonstrated in the clinic to ensure accurate use.

Adverse reactions. At therapeutic dosages, minimal adverse reactions are reported. The patient should be instructed not to exceed the recommended dosage of the medication.

Lifestyle management. Lifestyle management issues related to the disease process being treated should be discussed. They often include the following:

1. The patient needs to self-monitor respiratory status with a peak flowmeter to determine the effectiveness of the medication prescribed.
2. The patient should avoid or quit smoking.
3. The patient should avoid environmental triggers for the asthma at home, work, and school.

Inhaled Antihistamines

Newer inhaled medications are the **inhaled antihistamines**. Azelastine (Astelin NS) is the only **intranasal H_1 blocker** currently available in the United States. **Azelastine** is used for the treatment of seasonal allergic rhinitis.

Pharmacodynamics

Azelastine is an H_1 agonist and a potent inhibitor of histamine release from the mast cell. **Azelastine** and its metabolite desmethylazelastine inhibit the effects of histamine by competing with histamine for H_1 binding sites. **Azelastine** may also interfere with histamine- and leukotriene-induced bronchospasm.

Pharmacokinetics

ABSORPTION AND DISTRIBUTION. **Azelastine**, administered intranasally, has a systemic oral bioavailability of 40 percent. Protein binding of **azelastine** is 88 percent and, for the active metabolite desmethylazelastine, is 97 percent. Peak serum concentrations are reached in 2 to 3 hours. Exact absorption information is not known. Distribution is unknown, but because somnolence is a reported adverse effect, **azelastine** is assumed to enter the CNS. It is not known whether **azelastine** crosses the placenta or is distributed in breast milk.

METABOLISM AND EXCRETION. **Azelastine** is metabolized into the principal active metabolite, desmethylazelastine. Following intranasal dosing of **azelastine** to steady state, plasma concentration of desmethylazelastine is 20 to 30 percent of **azelastine**. Excretion of **azelastine** and desmethylazelastine is via the feces.

Clinical Pearl

STRATEGIES FOR CROMOLYN NEBULIZER TREATMENTS

Appropriate use of **cromolyn sodium** requires qid dosing, which can add up to 2 hours a day of treatments to administer via nebulizer. Strategies should be discussed as to what parents can do to entertain their child during the treatment. Adults and older children can read or watch a TV program or video. Younger children need more creative solutions to enable them to sit still for treatments. One solution is to administer one or two doses per day while the child is sleeping by "blowing" the medication into the mouth and nose.

Pharmacotherapeutics

PRECAUTIONS AND CONTRAINDICATIONS. Some patients using intranasal **azelastine** may experience somnolence and should be cautioned not to drive or operate heavy equipment while using it.

It is unknown whether **azelastine** is excreted in breast milk. Use during lactation with caution. Because seasonal allergic rhinitis is not generally a life-threatening disease, the benefits do not outweigh the unknown risks to the infant.

Azelastine **is Pregnancy Category C. It should be used in pregnancy only if the potential benefits outweigh the risks to the fetus. There are no adequate studies in pregnant women. In animals receiving more than 240 times the normal dose, external and skeletal abnormalities have been noted.**

Safety in children under age 12 has not been established.

ADVERSE REACTIONS. The most commonly reported adverse reaction to **azelastine** is bitter taste (19%). Other reported adverse reactions are somnolence (11%), headache, weight gain (2%), and myalgia (1.5%). Local effects such as nasal irritation, epistaxis, sneezing, and rhinitis are also reported.

DRUG INTERACTIONS. There is an additive impairment of CNS function when **azelastine** is used with **ethanol** or other **CNS depressants.** When **azelastine** is coadministered orally with **cimetidine,** the area under the curve (AUC) and maximum concentration (Cmax) are increased by 65 percent. Data regarding interactions with intranasal **azelastine** and **cimetidine** are not available. **Azelastine** should be used cautiously with other **antihistamines.**

CLINICAL USE AND DOSING

Allergic rhinitis. **Azelastine** is approved for use in seasonal allergic rhinitis. It is used to treat the specific symptoms of rhinorrhea, sneezing, and nasal pruritus. The dose for adults and children older than age 12 is 2 sprays (137 µg/spray) per nostril twice a day.

RATIONAL DRUG SELECTION

Oral versus intranasal antihistamine. The provider may choose to use **intranasal azelastine** rather than a **systemic antihistamine** because of decreased adverse effects or fewer drug interactions noted with the intranasal product.

Cost. The cost of **azelastine** is approximately $40 to $50 for a 2-month supply. This is more expensive than the **first-generation antihistamines** but less expensive than most of the **second-generation antihistamines.**

Patient variables. **Azelastine** should not be prescribed to children under age 12 and should be used with caution in pregnant and lactating patients.

MONITORING. There is no specific monitoring required with the use of **azelastine.**

PATIENT EDUCATION

Administration. The patient should be instructed to prime the medication unit before use by pumping the activator four times, or until a fine mist appears. The patient should keep the sprayer pointed away from the face, other people, and pets when priming the medication. The patient should wipe the tip of the sprayer with a clean tissue after using and replace the cap between uses. To prevent the spread of infection, the sprayer should be used by only one person.

Adverse reactions. The patient should be instructed about the most common adverse reactions. Caution regarding driving or operating heavy equipment while using **azelastine** should be stressed. The bitter taste that some patients experience may be decreased by drinking water or another fluid after administration. The patient should report any unusual adverse reactions to the provider.

The patient should be cautioned not to drink **alcohol** or take any other **CNS depressants** while using intranasal **azelastine.** The patient may not be aware that an intranasal medication can have an interaction with an orally administered medication, and therefore the provider must give careful instructions before prescribing **azelastine.**

Oxygen

Oxygen is a basic element essential for human life, with oxygen deprivation leading to rapid death. Therapy with **oxygen** is necessary for life in several diseases that interfere with normal oxygenation of blood and tissues. **Oxygen** as a therapeutic gas is delivered from steel containers and is 99 percent pure.

Oxygen is prescribed to treat hypoxia, or tissue deprivation of oxygen. Hypoxia can be caused by an inadequate supply of oxygen to the lungs, which can be due to poor ventilation or inadequate partial pressure of inspired oxygen. Inadequate pulmonary function can lead to hypoxia, as in a mismatch between ventilation and perfusion. Tissue hypoxia may occur with inadequate delivery of oxygen to the tissues, such as occurs in low cardiac output. Tissue hypoxia may also occur if the oxygen concentration of the blood is low, as occurs in anemia.

The effects of hypoxia can be observed in all major organ systems. The respiratory system increases the ventilatory rate and depth as a result of stimulation of carotid and aortic chemoreceptors. The heart increases cardiac output by increasing the heart rate. With severe hypoxia, bradycardia develops and ultimately leads to circulatory failure. The CNS is the most sensitive to hypoxia, with initial impaired judgment and psychomotor ability, leading to confusion, restlessness, and ultimately stupor, coma, and death.

Pharmacokinetics

The oxygen content of inhaled air is normally 20.9%, equivalent to a partial pressure of 159 mm Hg. As oxygen is inhaled, it enters the pulmonary airways and travels to the distal airways and alveoli. In the distal airways, the partial pressure of oxygen (PO_2) is decreased by dilution with carbon dioxide and water vapor and by uptake into the blood. The diffusion of oxygen into the pulmonary capillary blood is driven by the gradient between the PO_2 in mixed venous blood and that in the alveolar gas. The pressure gradient increases when 100% **oxygen** is administered, causing increased oxygen diffusion into the pulmonary capillary blood. **Oxygen** is delivered via the circulation to the tissue capillary beds, where oxygen is diffused by its higher partial pressure out of the blood and into the cells.

Oxygen in the blood is carried by the hemoglobin, with a small amount in physical solution in the plasma. The amount of oxygen carried by the hemoglobin depends on the partial pressure of carbon dioxide ($PaCO_2$) and is usually illustrated with the oxyhemoglobin dissociation curve.

PRECAUTIONS AND CONTRAINDICATIONS. The only contraindication to **oxygen** use is concurrent smoking while the **oxygen** is running. **Oxygen** is a flammable gas that will ignite if a flame is too near. This has implications for chronic smokers, who should turn off their **oxygen** to smoke.

Oxygen should be prescribed to patients with chronic carbon dioxide retention with extreme caution and close monitoring. Because hypoxemia may the primary stimulus for respiration in these patients, the lowest possible concentration of **oxygen** to avoid serious tissue hypoxia should be used. In patients with hypercapnia, the sudden increases in $PaCO_2$ produced by **oxygen** may result in cessation of respiration.

ADVERSE DRUG REACTIONS

Dry nasal passages. The most common adverse drug reaction reported in patients who are administered **oxygen** is dry nasal passages from the flow of gas through the nasal cannula. This can be prevented by administering humidified **oxygen** by mask or by keeping the flow rate low (less than 5 to 6 L/minute).

Toxicity. **Oxygen** toxicity occurs when inspired concentrations of **oxygen** exceed those of air for prolonged periods of time. Cell membrane and death are thought to be caused by increased production of reactive species such as superoxide anion, singlet oxygen, hydroxyl radical, and hydrogen peroxide. Some tissues, including the respiratory tract, the CNS, and the retina, are more sensitive to high **oxygen** concentration.

In the respiratory tract, inhalation of 100% **oxygen** for 6 to 8 hours can lead to decreased movement of tracheal mucus. In as little as 12 hours of 100% **oxygen**, the patient may experience tracheobronchial irritation and complain of chest tightness. After 17 hours, there is increased alveolar permeability and inflammation. Overall pulmonary function decreases after 18 to 24 hours of continuous 100% **oxygen**. After 24 hours of 100% **oxygen**, the patient usually has symptoms of nausea, vomiting, and anorexia. The patient may survive 1 week on toxic levels of **oxygen**. Death occurs from pulmonary edema.

Oxygen toxicity of the CNS does not occur until the partial pressure of inspired **oxygen** is greater than 2 atmospheres, which usually occurs in a hyperbaric chamber.

The retina of a premature neonate can be damaged by exposure to high levels of **oxygen** for prolonged periods. The development of retrolental fibroplasia is thought to be related to high levels of PaO_2 administered to the neonate. Adults rarely have **oxygen**-induced retinopathy, even with hyperbaric levels.

DRUG INTERACTIONS. There are no drug interactions with **oxygen**.

CLINICAL USE AND DOSING. **Oxygen** is administered to treat hypoxia as determined by pulse oximetry or arterial or mixed venous blood gases. Hypoxia is usually a symptom or manifestation of an underlying disease and therefore **oxygen** therapy is not curative, but it does provide symptomatic and temporary improvement in the patient's status. The underlying cause of hypoxia needs to be treated.

Correction of hypoxia. To correct hypoxia, **oxygen** is administered to the patient via a variety of **oxygen** delivery systems. The provider chooses a delivery system based on the fraction or percent of **oxygen** (FIO_2) that is desired for treatment. The goal of treatment is to maintain **oxygen** saturation above 90%.

A nasal cannula (NC) will deliver an FIO_2 of 0.24 to 0.35 if the flow of **oxygen** is at 5 to 6 L/minute. Higher flow rates via NC dry out the nasal mucosa and will not achieve higher FIO_2 because the **oxygen** is mixed with ambient air. Humidified **oxygen** can be delivered to decrease nasal passage dryness. The percentage of **oxygen** that can be delivered via NC is 22 to 44%.

Masks cover the mouth and nose and allow for a higher concentration of **oxygen** to be delivered. **Oxygen** delivery via mask requires a flow rate above 5 L/minute to avoid accumulation of exhaled air in the mask. A flow rate of 8 to 10 L/minute is recommended. A simple face mask, which allows room air to dilute the **oxygen**, delivers 40 to 60% **oxygen** to the patient. A face mask with an oxygen reservoir provides a constant flow of **oxygen** at above 60% concentration. If the flow rate of **oxygen** is 6 L/minute, then the **oxygen** concentration is 60%. The **oxygen** concentration increases by 10% for every liter per minute increase in flow. When 10 L/minute of **oxygen is** delivered via a mask with an oxygen reservoir, the percentage of **oxygen** delivered reaches 100%. A Venturi mask allows for controlled percentages of **oxygen** to be delivered to patients. The mask can be adjusted to deliver 24%, 28%, 35%, and 40%. This type of mask is used on patients with chronic hypercapnia (e.g., COPD patients) to tightly control the amount of **oxygen** delivered and avoid respiratory depression associated with high oxygen concentrations in these patients.

Oxygen may also be delivered by hood or tent to provide a known concentration to the patient, with little cooperation required from the patient. Flow rates must be high enough to prevent accumulation of carbon dioxide.

MONITORING.   Monitoring the patient on **oxygen** is necessary to treat hypoxia and to avoid toxicity. The most accurate yet invasive method to monitor blood oxygenation is by arterial or mixed venous blood gas sampling. This procedure can be painful for the patient and requires rapid transport of the specimen to the laboratory. Blood gases have the advantage of providing additional information, besides oxygenation, regarding the patient's status that may assist in the treatment of the underlying cause of hypoxemia. Pulse oximetry is a noninvasive method of monitoring the patient receiving **oxygen** therapy. It measures the difference in absorption of light by oxyhemoglobin and deoxyhemoglobin in an accessible location, such as the finger, toe (in children), or ear. Pulse oximetry measures the hemoglobin saturation and not PO_2.

The need for continuing **oxygen** therapy should be monitored by drawing arterial blood gases after 1, 3, and 6 months of therapy.

PATIENT EDUCATION

Administration. The patient who is receiving home **oxygen** therapy requires knowledge of the appropriate use of **oxygen**, as well as education about safe administration.

The patient should use the **oxygen** as prescribed by the provider. Increasing or decreasing the flow rate of **oxygen** may have adverse effects. Using **oxygen** for fewer hours than prescribed will increase hypoxia and will have detrimental effects.

The patient should understand that **oxygen** is a flammable gas that should be kept away from open flame. Patients who smoke should be cautioned not to smoke while their **oxygen** is running.

Adverse reactions. There are minimal adverse reactions with the use of **oxygen.** The patient should be advised of the potential of developing dry nasal passages. Increasing hydration and increasing the humidity of the home will help somewhat.

Oxygen toxicity should be discussed and the patient advised to use the **oxygen** only as directed. Patients who

begin to exhibit symptoms that may be related to toxicity should contact their health care provider.

Lifestyle management. Lifestyle management issues related to the disease process being treated should be discussed. They often include the following:

1. The patient should avoid or quit smoking.
2. COPD patients should avoid unnecessary exposure to viral respiratory infections.
3. Patients with COPD or other chronic respiratory diseases should avoid high altitudes.
4. Before traveling by air, the patient should contact the provider to formulate a plan of care.

Antihistamines

Antihistamines are used in primary care to treat a variety of allergic conditions. This chapter addresses the **antihistamines** used to treat allergic symptoms specific to the respiratory tract. **Antihistamines** are also called **H_1 receptor antagonists,** which describes the action the medication has at the cellular level. This text uses **antihistamine,** the more commonly used name in clinical practice.

The first **antihistamines** became available in the 1940s, with the still widely used **diphenhydramine** first available in the 1950s. They are referred to as the **first-generation antihistamines.** The 1980s brought a new generation of **nonsedating antihistamines** that provided relief to allergy sufferers without causing the drowsiness of the earlier medications. They are referred to as **second-generation antihistamines.** New **antihistamines** that are longer-acting and have better adverse-effect profiles continue to be developed.

Pharmacodynamics

Antihistamines are **H_1 receptor antagonists** that reduce or prevent most of the physiological effects of histamine at the H_1 receptor site. **Antihistamines** compete with histamine for H_1 receptor sites on the effector cells. They do not prevent histamine release or bind with histamine that has already been released. They prevent, but do not reverse, responses mediated by histamine. The effects of **antihistamines** include inhibition of respiratory, vascular, and GI smooth-muscle constriction by antagonism of the constrictor action on smooth muscle. **Antihistamines** strongly block the action of histamine that results in increased capillary permeability and formation of edema and wheal. They also decrease the flare and itch responses of histamine on peripheral nerve endings. Histamine-activated exocrine secretions (salivary, lacrimal) are decreased with the use of systemic **antihistamines. Antihistamines** with strong anticholinergic (atropine-like) properties may have an increased drying effect by decreasing secretions from cholinergically innervated glands.

The **first-generation antihistamines** competitively antagonize the effects of histamine at the peripheral H_1 receptor sites in the GI tract, uterus, large blood vessels, and bronchial muscle. **First-generation antihistamines** bind nonselectively to the central H_1 receptors and can cause both CNS stimulation and depression. CNS depression is found even with therapeutic doses of the **first-generation antihistamines.** Some of the **first-generation antihistamines** are more likely to depress the CNS than others, and patients vary in their sensitivity to the different preparations. Commonly prescribed **first-generation antihistamines** include the **ethanolamine** drugs **diphenhydramine (Benadryl)** and **clemastine (Tavist)**, the alkylamines **brompheniramine (Dimetane)** and **chlorpheniramine (Chlor-Trimeton)**, the **piperazine hydroxyzine (Atarax, Vistaril)**, and the **piperidine cyproheptadine (Periactin).**

Second-generation antihistamines are selective for peripheral H_1 receptors and therefore as a group are less sedating. They do not cross the blood-brain barrier in appreciable amounts; consequently, very little of the **second-generation antihistamines** gets into the brain. Their effects on performance and on objective measures of sedation vary little from placebo. **Second-generation antihistamines** that are commonly prescribed include the **piperazine** drug **cetirizine (Zyrtec)** and the **piperidines astemizole (Hismanal), fexofenadine (Allegra)**, and **loratadine (Claritin).**

Antihistamines have other pharmacodynamic properties related to their central action rather than their histamine receptor blockade action. Several **first-generation antihistamines** have significant antiemetic and antinausea properties due to strong anticholinergic properties caused by the **antihistamine's** binding to the muscarinic receptors. **Diphenhydramine** can be used to reverse the extrapyramidal adverse effects caused by **phenothiazines.** Probably because of their anticholinergic actions, some of the **antihistamines (diphenhydramine)** have effects on Parkinson's symptoms and may be effective in the early stages of treatment.

Pharmacokinetics

ABSORPTION AND DISTRIBUTION. The **first-generation antihistamines** are stable lipid-soluble amines that are well absorbed from the GI tract. **Diphenhydramine** is widely distributed throughout the body tissues and fluids, including the CNS. It crosses the placenta and is found in breast milk. The distribution of **clemastine** is not known, but the drug does cross the placenta and is distributed in breast milk. **Chlorpheniramine** is approximately 72 percent protein-bound and is widely distributed in body tissue and fluids. **Chlorpheniramine** crosses the placenta and is found in breast milk. Distribution of **hydroxyzine** has not been fully described, and it is not known whether it crosses the placenta or is dis-

tributed in breast milk. The distribution of **cyproheptadine, dimenhydrinate**, and **brompheniramine** is unknown.

The **second-generation antihistamines** are rapidly absorbed from the GI tract, although concurrent food ingestion can decrease or delay absorption. Administration of **astemizole** with food decreases its absorption by 60 percent. **Fexofenadine** is rapidly absorbed, and absorption is not affected by food intake. Administration of **loratadine** with food decreases absorption up to 40 percent for the syrup or tablet and 48 percent for the rapid-disintegrating tablet. **Astemizole** is highly protein-bound and is widely distributed, except in the CNS. **Astemizole** does not cross the blood-brain barrier, but it may cross the placenta and is found in breast milk. Absorption of **cetirizine** is slightly reduced by food intake. **Cetirizine** is widely distributed, except in the CNS, where concentrations are less than 10 percent of the peak serum concentration. It is unknown whether **cetirizine** crosses the placenta, but it has been measured in breast milk. **Fexofenadine** distribution is unknown. **Loratadine** is 97 percent protein-bound and is excreted in breast milk. It is not known if **loratadine** crosses the placenta.

METABOLISM AND EXCRETION. The **first-generation antihistamines** are metabolized primarily in the liver. **Diphenhydramine** is metabolized in the liver, with the unchanged portion of the dose and metabolites excreted in the urine in 24 to 48 hours. **Clemastine** is extensively metabolized by an unknown mechanism. **Clemastine** and its metabolites are excreted primarily in the urine. Metabolism of **chlorpheniramine** is extensive, occurring first in the gastric mucosa and then on the first pass through the liver. Metabolites of **chlorpheniramine** are excreted in the urine, with the excretion rate dependent on the pH of the urine and urinary flow. **Cyproheptadine** is metabolized in the liver into several conjugated metabolites, with excretion in the urine and feces. **Hydroxyzine** is completely metabolized by the liver. Metabolism and excretion of **brompheniramine** and **dimenhydrinate** are unknown.

Most of the **second-generation antihistamines** are metabolized by the liver to active metabolites by the hepatic microsomal P-450 system. Consequently, metabolism of these drugs can be affected by competition for the P-450 enzymes by other drugs. **Astemizole** is eliminated in the feces primarily, with some minimal urinary excretion. **Cetirizine** is minimally metabolized by the P-450 enzymes and is primarily excreted unchanged in the urine. Approximately 5 percent of the dose of **fexofenadine** is metabolized, with 80 percent excreted in the feces and 11 percent excreted in the urine. **Loratadine** has a high first-pass effect and is metabolized in the liver to the active metabolite, descarboethoxyloratadine. Patients with chronic liver disease have higher peak plasma concentrations (double the normal levels) of **loratadine** than healthy patients. Elimination of **loratadine** is through the urine and feces.

Food interactions are possible if patients are taking **astemizole**. Grapefruit juice has components that inhibit the activity of cytochrome P-450 enzymes in cells lining the intestine walls. Inhibition of the CYP-450 enzymes causes increased plasma **astemizole** concentrations, leading to cardiac toxicity.

See Table 15–13 for the pharmacokinetics.

Pharmacotherapeutics

PRECAUTIONS AND CONTRAINDICATIONS

First-generation antihistamines. Although **first-generation antihistamines** are available without prescription and all **antihistamines** are widely prescribed, the provider must be aware of the precautions and absolute contraindications to the **antihistamines**.

The **first-generation antihistamines** are generally safe and effective. **Antihistamines** are contraindicated in patients with the following: narrow-angle glaucoma, lower respiratory tract symptoms (thickens secretions and impairs expectoration), stenosing peptic ulcer, symptomatic prostatic hypertrophy, bladder neck obstruction, pyloroduodenal obstruction, and **MAOI** use.

There are few but significant precautions to the **first-generation antihistamines**. Because of the anticholinergic effects, caution is required for patients with a predisposition to urinary retention, history of bronchial asthma, increased intraocular pressure, hyperthyroidism, cardiovascular disease, or hypertension. **Antihistamines** cause varying degrees of sedation and drowsiness and reduce mental alertness; therefore, patients should not drive or perform other tasks requiring mental alertness while taking **the first-generation antihistamines**. Chil-

Table 15–13. Pharmacokinetics: Selected Antihistamines

Drug	Onset	Peak	Duration	Protein Binding	Half-Life	Metabolism	Elimination
First-Generation Antihistamines							
Brompheniramine	15–30 min	2–5 h	4–6 h	—	25 h	Hepatic	Renal
Clemastine	15–30 min	2–5 h	10–12 h (up to 24 h)	—	—	Probably hepatic	Renal
Chlorpheniramine	30–60 min	2–6 h	4–8 h	72%	Adults: 20–24 h Children: 10–13 h	Gastric mucosa and hepatic	Renal
Cyproheptadine	—	6–9 h	8 h	—	1–4 h	Hepatic	Primary renal; some in feces
Diphenhydramine	15–30 min	2–4 h	4–6 h	98–99%	1–4 h	Hepatic	Renal
Hydroxyzine	15–60 min	—	4–6 h	—	3–20 h	Hepatic	Renal
Second-Generation Antihistamines							
Astemizole	2–3 d	1–4 h; peak 9–12 d	—	97%	20 h (distribution); 168–264 h (elimination)	Hepatic CYP 3A4	Primarily fecal
Cetirizine	Rapid	1 h	—	93%	8.3 h	Minimal 60% excreted unchanged	Renal, feces (10%)
Fexofenadine	1 hr	2.6 h	12 h	60–70%	14.4 h	95% excreted unchanged	Fecal (80%), renal (11%)
Loratadine	1–3 h	8–12 h	>24 h	97%	8.4 h	Hepatic CYP 3A4 and 2D6	Fecal, renal

dren should be supervised when they are taking these medications and performing potentially unsafe activities such as swimming or bicycling.

The first-generation antihistamines *chlorphenira-mine, brompheniramine, diphenhydramine, clemastine,* **and** *cyproheptadine* **are Pregnancy Category B.** *Hydrox-yzine* **is the only first-generation antihistamine classi-fied as Pregnancy Category C.**

First-generation antihistamines are contraindicated in newborns and premature infants, who may have se-vere reactions (convulsions.) Breastfeeding is also a con-traindication for the use of **first-generation antihista-mines** because all of the medications are excreted in breast milk.

Caution should be exercised with the use of **first-generation antihistamines** in young children because a paradoxical CNS stimulation can occur. Do not exceed recommended dosages for each age group of children.

Second-generation antihistamines. The **second-genera-tion antihistamines** have only a few contraindications. The use of **astemizole** is contraindicated in patients with significant hepatic dysfunction and concomitant **eryth-romycin, clarithromycin, troleandomycin, quinine, ketoconazole,** or **itraconazole** therapy. Cases of *torsade de pointes* have been reported following **astemizole** use. Prolonged QT interval is a potential adverse effect of **astemizole,** which is contraindicated in patients with prolonged QT syndrome, hypokalemia, or hypomagne-semia (including patients on diuretics with a potential for causing these electrolyte imbalances). **Astemizole** is also contraindicated in patients on **HIV protease in-hibitors, serotonin reuptake inhibitors, cisapride, sparfloxacin, zileuton,** and **mibefradil. Terfenadine** (**Seldane**) has been removed from the market because of these potentially life-threatening drug interactions.

The **second-generation antihistamines** are generally not recommended during pregnancy, especially during the third trimester, because of a seizure risk to the fetus. **Loratadine and cetirizine are classified Pregnancy Category B. The other second-generation antihista-mines, astemizole and fexofenadine, are Pregnancy Category C, and their use should be avoided.**

Astemizole and **fexofenadine** are not recommended for children under age 12. **Loratadine** may be pre-scribed to children as young as age 6. **Cetirizine** syrup is approved for children as young as age 2.

ADVERSE DRUG REACTIONS. As described previously, the major adverse reaction to **first-generation antihista-mines** is sedation, which can interfere with a patient's ability to function at work or school. Other central adverse effects include dizziness, tinnitus, lassitude, disturbed co-ordination, fatigue, headache, irritability, nervousness, blurred vision, diplopia, and tremors. The next most com-mon adverse effects are GI and include increased or de-creased appetite, nausea, epigastric distress, vomiting,

constipation, and diarrhea. Dry mouth, urinary retention, and dysuria are also adverse effects reported in patients taking **first-generation antihistamines.** The concurrent ingestion of **alcohol** or other **CNS depressants** produces an additive effect that further impairs function.

The **second-generation antihistamines** have few cen-tral adverse effects. The major improvement in the **second-generation antihistamines** is that the incidence of drowsiness is greatly reduced. They are well tolerated by the GI system and have a minimal incidence of dry mouth (5 percent or less). Overall, when patients have adverse re-actions to the **first-generation antihistamines,** a change to a **second-generation drug** often alleviates the problem.

DRUG INTERACTIONS. The **first-generation antihista-mines** should be used with caution concurrently with any medication that has CNS-depressant effects. All of the **first-generation antihistamines** exhibit additive CNS sedation effects if coadministered with **ethanol, anxiolytics, sedatives, hypnotics,** and **barbiturates.** The anticholinergic effects of **antihistamines** may be en-hanced if coadministered with **tricyclic antidepres-sants** and **phenothiazines.** It is recommended that H_1 **agonists** not be used within 2 weeks of **MAOIs** because of increased anticholinergic effects. **Cyproheptadine** may reverse the antidepressant effects of **selective sero-tonin reuptake inhibitors (SSRIs).** Two **antihista-mines** should not be prescribed at the same time to avoid additive anticholinergic and sedative effects.

The **second-generation antihistamines,** although not sedating when used singly, may have additive CNS sedation effects if used with other **CNS depressants (barbiturates, anxiolytics, sedatives, hypnotics, etha-nol,** and **benzodiazepines).** Concurrent use with another H_1 **blocker** may cause sedation. There is a sus-pected interaction between **astemizole** and **fluvoxam-ine (Luvox),** and they should be coadministered with caution and close monitoring.

Astemizole and **loratadine** are extensively metabo-lized by the cytochrome P-450 enzymes, and coadminis-tration of other medications that are also metabolized by these enzymes should be avoided. **Astemizole** and the following drugs are metabolized by cytochrome P-450 3A4: macrolide antibiotics (**clarithromycin, erythromy-cin,** and **troleandomycin**), **mibefradil (Posicor),** qui-nine, protease inhibitors (**indinavir, nelfinavir,** and **ri-tonavir**), SSRIs, some **antifungal agents (ketoconazole, itraconazole),** and **zileuton (Zyflo.)** **Loratadine** is me-tabolized by the cytochrome P-450 3A4 isoenzyme, as are **erythromycin, cimetidine,** and **ketoconazole.**

Table 15–14 presents drug interactions.

CLINICAL USE AND DOSING

Respiratory allergies. Most of the **antihistamines** are ef-fective in the treatment of seasonal allergic rhinitis and conjunctivitis. **Antihistamines** effectively treat the sneezing, rhinorrhea, watery eyes, and itching of eyes, nose, and throat associated with seasonal allergies or hay fever. The treatment decision is often made according to the adverse-effect profile and cost. Although the **first-generation drugs diphenhydramine, chlorpheniramine, brompheniramine,** and **clemastine** are effective, inexpensive, and available without prescription, their adverse effect of drowsiness often prevents pa-

tients from being able to continue their daily activities. The usual adult dose of **diphenhydramine** for respiratory allergies is 25 to 50 mg every 4 to 6 hours. The adult dose of **chlorpheniramine is** 4 mg every 4 to 6 hours or 8 to 12 mg of the extended-release form. **Brompheniramine** is dosed at 4 mg every 4 to 6 hours in adults with respiratory allergies. Pediatric doses for these medications are given in Table 15–15.

Table 15–14. Drug Interactions: Selected Antihistamines

Drug	Interacting Drug	Possible Effect	Implications
First-Generation Antihistamines Brompheniramine	MAOIs	MAOIs can prolong and intensify the effects of antihistamines	Avoid concurrent use
	Ethanol and other CNS depressants	Additive CNS depression	Use with caution
Clemastine	MAOIs	Additive anticholinergic effects	Concurrent use contraindicated
	Antimuscarinics: Tricyclic antidepressants, phenothiazines, ethanolamine-derivative H₁ blockers (clemastine, carbinoxamine, promethazine, trimeprazine) clozapine, cyclobenzaprine, disopyramide	Additive anticholinergic effects	Avoid concurrent use
	CNS depressants: Ethanol, antipsychotics, sedatives, hypnotics, opiate agonists, barbiturates	Enhanced CNS-depressant effect	Avoid concurrent use
Chlorpheniramine	MAOIs	Additive anticholinergic effects	Avoid concurrent use
	Antimuscarinics: Tricyclic antidepressants, phenothiazines, benztropine	Enhanced anticholinergic effects of chlorpheniramine	Chlorpheniramine has moderate anticholinergic effects and is preferable to other H₁ blockers when an H₁ blocker must be used
	CNS depressants	Enhanced CNS-depressant effect	Avoid concurrent use
Cyproheptadine	*Antimuscarinics:* Tricyclic antidepressants, phenothiazines, ethanolamine-derivative H₁ blockers (clemastine, diphenhydramine), benztropine	Increased anticholinergic effects of cyproheptadine	Avoid concurrent use
	CNS depressants: Barbiturates, ethanol, benzodiazepines, tricyclic antidepressants, opiate agonists	Enhanced CNS-depressant effect	Avoid concurrent use
	SSRIs	Reversal of antidepressant effects of SSRIs	Use cyproheptadine only if needed

Continued on next page

Table 15–14. Drug Interactions: Selected Antihistamines (*continued*)

Drug	Interacting Drug	Possible Effect	Implications
Diphenhydramine	MAOIs	Additive anticholinergic effects	Do not use within 2 wk of each other
	Antimuscarinics: Tricyclic antidepressants, phenothiazines, ethanolamine-derivative H₁ blockers (clemastine, carbinoxamine, promethazine, trimeprazine) clozapine, cyclobenzaprine, disopyramide	Additive anticholinergic effects	Avoid or use with caution; monitor closely if coadministration is necessary
	CNS depressants: Ethanol, antipsychotics, sedatives, hypnotics, opiate agonists, barbiturates	Enhanced CNS-depressant effect	Avoid concurrent use
Hydroxyzine	MAOIs	May prolong and intensify the anticholinergic effects of antihistamines	Concurrent use contraindicated; avoid use within 2 wk of each other
	Antimuscarinics: Tricyclic antidepressants, phenothiazines, ethanolamine-derivative H₁ blockers (clemastine, carbinoxamine, promethazine, trimeprazine) atropine, benztropine	Additive anticholinergic effects	Avoid concurrent use
	CNS depressants: Ethanol, antipsychotics, sedatives, hypnotics, opiate agonists, barbiturates	Additive CNS-depressant effects	Avoid concurrent use
Second-Generation Antihistamines Astemizole	*Drugs metabolized by CYP-450 3A4:* Macrolide antibiotics (clarithromycin, erythromycin, azithromycin, troleandomycin), azole antifungals (ketoconazole, itraconazole, fluconazole, miconazole), zileuton, protease inhibitors (indinavir, nelfinavir, ritonavir, saquinavir), SSRIs (fluoxetine, fluvoxamine, nefazodone, paroxetine, sertraline)	Increased plasma levels of astemizole may cause serious cardiac toxicity	Do not coadminister

Continued on next page

Table 15–14. Drug Interactions: Selected Antihistamines (*continued*)

Drug	Interacting Drug	Possible Effect	Implications
Cetirizine	*CNS depressants:* Barbiturates, ethanol, benzodiazepines, tricyclic antidepressants, opiate agonists	Additive CNS-depressant effects and drowsiness	Use with caution
Loratadine	Macrolide antibiotics (clarithromycin, erythromycin, troleandomycin)	Interferes with the metabolism of loratadine, resulting in increased serum concentrations of loratadine	Does not cause cardiac toxicity, but coadminister with caution
	CNS depressants: Barbiturates, ethanol, benzodiazepines, tricyclic antidepressants, opiate agonists	Additive CNS-depressant effects and drowsiness	Avoid or minimize concurrent use

If a patient cannot tolerate the **first-generation antihistamines,** a **second-generation** medication can be prescribed to treat respiratory allergies. The dose of **astemizole** in adults and children over age 12 is 10 mg once a day. The dose of **cetirizine** that should be prescribed for adults and children over 12 is 5 to 10 mg/day given once a day. In children age 6 to 11, the dose of **cetirizine** is 5 to 10 mg once daily. For **cetirizine** syrup prescribed to children age 2 to 5, the dose is 2.5 mg (½ tsp) once daily. The dose of **cetirizine** may be increased to 5 mg/day, delivered as 5 mg once daily or 2.5 mg twice a day. The dose of **fexofenadine** in healthy adults and children age 12 or older is 60 mg twice a day. If a patient has renal impairment (creatinine clearance [CCr] less than 80 mL/minute), the dose of **fexofenadine** is 60 mg once daily. The dose of **loratadine** in healthy adults and children over age 6 is 10 mg once a day. If an adult has renal or liver disease, the dose of **loratatine** is 10 mg every other day.

Hypersensitivity reactions. The **first-generation antihistamine diphenhydramine** is usually the drug of choice for patients with acute hypersensitivity reactions. It is available in oral tablet, capsule, and liquid forms without prescription and in parenteral form for acute intramuscular (IM) or intravenous (IV) use. The adult oral dose of **diphenhydramine** is 25 to 50 mg every 4 to 6 hours for hypersensitivity reactions. In children over 10 kg with hypersensitivity reactions, the dose of **diphenhydramine** is 12.5 to 25 mg every 4 hours. Children age 2 to 6 are prescribed **diphenhydramine** syrup, at a dose of 6.25 mg every 4 hours. In an acute hypersensitivity reaction, IM administration of **diphenhydramine** may be necessary. The adult dose of **diphenhydramine** is 10 to 50 mg deep IM or IV, with a maximum of 400 mg per day. In children, the dose is 1.25 mg/kg per dose given deep IM every 4 hours, with a maximum daily **diphenhydramine** dose of 300 mg. **Cyproheptadine** is also indicated for use in hypersensitivity reactions. The adult dose of **cyproheptadine** is 4 mg three times a day. No second-generation antihistamines are indicated for use in hypersensitivity reactions.

Urticaria and angioedema. In urticaria, histamine is the primary mediator, and therefore the **antihistamines** are the drugs of choice and quite effective. **Clemastine,** a very effective treatment for urticaria, is available in both tablet and liquid form for use with children (older than age 6) and adults. **Hydroxyzine** is effective in the management of pruritus due to allergic conditions such as chronic urticaria and in histamine-mediated pruritus. It is also available in tablet and liquid form. **Hydroxyzine** may be used safely in children younger than age 6 and therefore may be a better choice than **clemastine** in younger children with urticaria. **Astemizole, cetirizine,** and **loratadine** may be prescribed for urticaria. See Table 15–15 for dosing information.

Nighttime sleep aid. **Diphenhydramine** is available without prescription as a sleep aid and is a safe treatment for occasional insomnia. The recommended dose for adults is 50 mg at bedtime. Table 15–15 presents dosing information.

RATIONAL DRUG SELECTION

First- versus second-generation antihistamines. Although many of the **first-generation antihistamines** are readily available without prescription, the common adverse effect

Table 15–15. Dosage Schedule: Selected Antihistamines

Drug	Indication	Dose	Comments
First-Generation Antihistamines Brompheniramine	Allergic and vasomotor rhinitis, pruritus, conjunctivitis	*Adults:* 4 mg PO q4–6h *or* 8–12 mg of sustained-release form 2 to 3 times/d Maximum dose: 12 mg/24 h *Children 6–12 years:* 2 mg q4–6h; maximum 12 mg/24 h *Children <6:* 0.125 mg/kg/d in divided doses every 6–8 h	May be administered with or without food
Clemastine	Allergic rhinitis	*Adults and children >12:* 1 mg bid *Children 6–12:* 0.5 mg bid	May be administered without regard to meals
	Pruritus, mild urticaria, angioedema	*Adults and children >12:* 2 mg bid *Children 6–12:* 1 mg bid	May be administered without regard to meals
Chlorpheniramine	Allergic rhinitis, conjunctivitis, pruritus, urticaria	*Adults and children >12:* 4 mg every 4–6 h; maximum 24 mg/d *Children 6–12:* 2 mg every 4–6 h; maximum 12 mg/d *Children 2–5:* 1 mg every 4–6 h; maximum 4 mg/d *Extended-release form: Adults and children >12:* 8–12 mg bid or tid; maximum 24 mg/d *Children 6–12:* 8 mg once daily; maximum 12 mg/d *Children 2–5:* use other forms	Administer with food or milk to minimize gastric irritation
Cyproheptadine	Allergic rhinitis, conjunctivitis, pruritus, urticaria	*Adults and children >14:* 4 mg q8–12h; usual range 12–16 mg/d; maximum dose 0.5 mg/kg/d *Children 7–14:* 4 mg q8–12h; maximum 16 mg/d *Children 2–6:* 2 mg q8–12h; maximum 12 mg/d	Administered without regard to meals
Diphenhydramine	Upper respiratory allergies	*Adults and children >12:* 25–50 mg every 4–6 h; maximum 300 mg/d *Children 6–12:* 12.5–25 mg q4–6h; max 150 mg/24 h *Children 2–6:* 6.25 mg; max 37.5 mg/24 h	May cause drowsiness; may cause excitability in young children
Hydroxyzine	Allergic and vasomotor rhinitis, pruritus	*Adults:* 25 mg 3–4 times/d *Children >6:* 12.5–25 mg 3–4 times/d; max 50–100 mg/24 h *Children <6:* 12.5 mg 3–4 times/d; max 50 mg/24 h *or* 1–2 mg/kg/d in divided doses	May cause drowsiness
	Nausea/vomiting	*Adults:* 25–100 mg 3–4 times/d *Children 6–12:* 12.5–25 mg every 6 h *or* 1–2 mg/kg/d in divided doses	May cause drowsiness

Continued on next page

Table 15–15. Dosage Schedule: Selected Antihistamines (*continued*)

Drug	Indication	Dose	Comments
	Insomnia	*Children <6:* 12.5 mg every 6 h *or* 1–2 mg/kg/d in divided doses *Adults:* 50–100 mg PO 30–60 min before bedtime	May cause drowsiness
Second-Generation Antihistamines Astemizole	Allergic rhinitis, pruritus, urticaria	*Adults and children >12:* 10 mg once daily	Take on empty stomach; astemizole should not be used prn for the immediate relief of symptoms; do not exceed daily recommended dosage
Cetirizine	Seasonal or perennial rhinitis, chronic urticaria, pruritus	*Adults and children >12:* 5–10 mg once daily *Children >6–11:* 5–10 mg once a day *Children 2–5:* 2.5 mg initially; can increase dose to 5 mg/d (either as one 5-mg dose or 2.5 mg q12h)	May be administered without regard to food, but food may delay absorption by up to 1 h; patients with renal impairment (CCr <31 mL/min) decrease dose to 5 mg once daily
Fexofenadine	Allergic rhinitis	*Adults and children >12:* 60 mg PO bid	Dose without regard to meals; not recommended in children <12; patients with renal impairment (CCr <80 mL/min) reduce starting dose to 60 mg once daily
Loratadine	Allergic rhinitis, chronic urticaria	*Adults and children >6:* 10 mg once daily	Dose without regard to meals; patients with renal impairment (CCr <30 mL/min) reduce starting dosage to 10 mg every other day

of sedation prevents their use during the day by patients who need to be alert for work or school. The **second-generation antihistamines** are well tolerated and do not impair daytime functioning. They are also longer acting, allowing for convenient once- or twice-a-day dosing.

Cost. The **second-generation antihistamines** are much more expensive than the **first-generation antihistamines.** Another factor found with managed care is that some insurance companies will not pay for the cost of the more expensive **second-generation antihistamines.** For the patient, the higher cost is offset by the ability to perform daily functions more easily when taking the **second-generation** medications.

MONITORING. No specific laboratory monitoring is necessary with **antihistamines.**

PATIENT EDUCATION. Patient education focuses on proper use of the medication, adverse reactions, and safety precautions while using the medications.

Administration. Patients should be instructed regarding the proper dosing of the drug. Especially if patients are switching from a shorter-acting **first-generation** to a longer-acting **second-generation antihistamine,** they need to be aware of the dosing schedule. Doses should not be doubled or increased unless prescribed by the health care provider. The long-acting **second-generation antihistamines** should not be taken closer together than prescribed, so missed doses need to be held until the time of the next dose (every 12 or 24 hours).

Some **antihistamines** cause GI upset and need to be taken with food. **Astemizole** and **loratadine** should be taken on an empty stomach because absorption may be decreased by as much as 60 percent.

Patients should be instructed not to crush or chew sustained-release tablets.

Adverse reactions. Some **antihistamines (first-generation)** may cause drowsiness, and patients should observe caution while driving or performing other tasks requiring alertness. Patients should avoid **alcohol** and other **CNS depressants** while taking **antihistamines**. Patients should be instructed to report excessive drowsiness to their health care provider to determine whether another medication would provide therapeutic effects without sedation.

Patients taking **astemizole** or **loratadine** should be aware of the serious interaction between the **antihistamines** and **macrolide antibiotics** and **oral azol antifungals.** Written instructions regarding the specific medications to avoid are the most effective and safest method of ensuring that patients do not accidentally get placed on any new medication that would cause a serious adverse reaction. The additive CNS depression that occurs with the **antihistamine** and other **CNS depressants** (e.g., alcohol) should be addressed and the patient cautioned regarding driving or operating heavy machinery.

Lifestyle management. Lifestyle management related to the disease process needs to be discussed with the patient. Points to discuss often include avoidance of known allergens and using environmental methods to control dust mites and other common allergens.

Available dosage forms are presented in Table 15–16.

Decongestants

Decongestants are widely used for congestion associated with the common cold and allergic rhinitis. Many preparations are available without a prescription, and they are available in many formulations. They come in liquid, tablet, capsule, nasal spray, or drops, providing a variety of methods of administration. Although patients may self-treat with decongestants and the health care provider may rarely prescribe them, they are included here for the provider to learn about the proper dosing and potential adverse effects or drug interactions that may occur with these medications.

Pharmacodynamics

The **decongestants** are **alpha-adrenergic receptor agonists (sympathomimetic)** that produce vasoconstriction by stimulating alpha receptors within the mucosa of the respiratory tract, which temporarily reduces the swelling associated with inflammation of the mucous membranes. These sympathomimetic amines act on the alpha receptors of the vascular smooth muscle, causing vasoconstriction, pressor effects, and nasal decongestion. Other alpha effects include constriction of the GI and urinary sphincters, mydriasis, and decreased pancreatic beta cell secretion. **Pseudoephedrine (Sudafed)**, the most commonly used **systemic decongestant,** is noted to have mild CNS-stimulant effects, especially in patients sensitive to sympathomimetic drugs. **Phenylpropanolamine** is often combined with an **antihistamine (Dimetapp)** in OTC cold medications.

Other effects of the **systemic decongestants** are increased heart rate, force of contraction, and cardiac output (**phenylpropanolamine** more than **pseudoephedrine**). These effects are usually mild in healthy patients, and at appropriate dosages decongestion occurs without dramatic blood pressure changes. **Phenylpropanolamine (Dexatrim)** has mild appetite suppression properties and is marketed as a nonprescription diet aid.

Topical decongestants are sympathomimetic amines that cause intense vasoconstriction when applied directly to swollen mucous membranes of the nasal passage. This shrinks the swollen membranes, causing almost immediate relief from nasal congestion. There are minimal systemic effects from topical use of **nasal decongestants.**

Pharmacokinetics

ABSORPTION AND DISTRIBUTION. The **oral decongestants** are well absorbed from the GI tract and widely distributed. **Pseudoephedrine** is widely distributed and presumed to cross the blood-brain barrier and placenta. Small amounts of **pseudoephedrine** are excreted in breast milk. **Phenylpropanolamine** is rapidly absorbed after oral administration and is widely distributed into the extracellular spaces. **Phenylpropanolamine** is about 20 percent protein-bound. Whether **phenylpropanolamine** crosses the placenta is not known, but it is assumed that it is distributed in breast milk.

Absorption and distribution of the **topical decongestants** have not been described.

METABOLISM AND EXCRETION. **Pseudoephedrine** is partially metabolized in the liver into norpseudoephedrine, an active metabolite. **Pseudoephedrine** and its metabolite are excreted in the urine, with 50 to 75 percent of the dose excreted as unchanged drug. Excretion of **pseudoephedrine** is highly dependent on the pH of the urine. If the urine is acidic (pH near 5), the rate of urinary excretion is increased. If the urine is alkaline (pH of 8), the rate of excretion is slowed, as some of the drug is reabsorbed into the renal tubule.

Phenylpropanolamine is minimally metabolized in the liver to an active metabolite. Approximately 90 percent of the dose of **phenylpropanolamine** is excreted unchanged in the urine. If the urine is acidic (pH of 5 or less), renal excretion of the drug is increased. Alkalinization of the urine decreases renal excretion of **phenylpropanolamine.**

Metabolism and excretion of the **topical decongestants** are not available.

Table 15–17 presents the pharmacokinetics.

Pharmacotherapeutics

PRECAUTIONS AND CONTRAINDICATIONS. There are only a few absolute contraindications to taking **decon-**

Table 15–16. Available Dosage Forms: Selected Antihistamines

Drug	Dosage Form	How Supplied
FIRST-GENERATION ANTIHISTAMINES		
Brompheniramine Dimetapp Allergy	Capsules: 4 mg Scored tablets: 4 mg	24 24
Clemastine Tavist-1	Scored tablets: 1.34 mg (1 mg clemastine)	8, 16
Tavist	Scored tablets: 2.68 mg (2 mg clemastine)	100
Tavist Syrup	Syrup: 0.67 mg (0.5 mg clemastine)/5 mL	4-oz bottles (5.5% alcohol)
Generic	Tablet: 1.34 mg (1 mg clemastine), 2.68 mg (2 mg clemastine)	100
Chlorpheniramine Chlor-Trimeton Allergy 4 hour	Tablets: 4 mg	24, 100
Chlor-Trimeton Allergy 8 hour	Sustained-release tablets: 8 mg	15, 100
Chlor-Trimeton Allergy 12 hour	Sustained-release tablets: 12 mg	10, 24, 100
Chlor-Trimeton Syrup	Syrup: 2 mg/5 mL	4-oz bottles
Chlo-Amine	Chewable tablets: 2 mg	96
Generic	Tablets: 4 mg Syrup: 2 mg/5 mL	100, 1000 4-oz bottles
Cyproheptadine Periactin	Tablets: 4 mg	100
Periactin Syrup	Syrup: 2 mg/5 mL	Pints (5% alcohol)
Generic	Tablets: 4 mg Syrup: 2 mg/5 mL	100, 250. 500, 1000 Pints, gallons
Diphenhydramine Benadryl Allergy	Capsules: 25 mg Tablets: 25 mg	24, 48, 100, 1000 24, 48
Benadryl Dye-Free Allergy Softgels	Capsules: 25 mg	24
Benadryl Allergy Liquid	Liquid: 12.5 mg/5 mL	4-oz , 8-oz bottles (no alcohol)
Benadryl Dye-Free Allergy Liquid	Liquid: 6.25 mg/5 mL	4-oz bottles (no alcohol)
Benadryl Allergy Chewables	Chewable tablets: 12.5 mg	24
Generic	Capsules: 25 mg, 50 mg Tablets: 25 mg Syrup: 12.5 mg/5 mL Liquid: 6.25 mg/5 mL	30, 100, 1000 24, 100 4 oz (5% alcohol) 4 oz, 8 oz (0.5% alcohol)

Continued on next page

Table 15–16. Available Dosage Forms: Selected Antihistamines *(continued)*

Drug	Dosage Form	How Supplied
Hydroxyzine Atarax	Tablets: 10 mg, 25 mg, 50 mg, 100 mg Syrup: 10 mg/5 mL	100, 500 Pints (0.5% alcohol)
Vistaril	Capsules: 25 mg, 50 mg, 100 mg Suspension: 25 mg/5 mL	100, 500 4 oz, pint bottles (no alcohol)
Generic	Tablets: 10 mg, 25 mg, 50 mg Capsules: 25 mg, 50 mg, 100 mg Syrup: 10 mg/5 mL	100, 250, 500, 1000 100, 250, 500, 1000 5-mL unit dose, 12.5 mL, 25 mL, pint
SECOND-GENERATION ANTIHISTAMINES		
Astemizole Hismanal	Scored tablet: 10 mg	30, 100
Cetirizine Zyrtec	Tablets: 5 mg, 10 mg Syrup: 1 mg/mL	100 4 oz and pints (no alcohol)
Fexofenadine Allegra	Capsules: 60 mg	60, 100, 1000
Loratadine Claritin	Tablets: 10 mg Syrup: 1 mg/mL Rapidly disintegrating tablets: 10 mg (Claritin Redi-tabs)	14, 30, 100, 500 Pints 30

Table 15–17. Pharmacokinetics: Selected Decongestants

Drug	Onset	Peak	Duration	Protein Binding	Half-Life	Metabolism	Elimination
Systemic Phenylpropanolamine	30 min	1.5 h 3.5 h (extended release)	3 h 12–16 h (extended release)	20%	3–4 h	Minimally metabolized in liver	90% unchanged in urine; excretion decreased by alkalinization of urine
Pseudoephedrine	30 min	—	4–8 h 12 h (extended release)	—	9–16 h	Hepatic	Renal 55–75% as unchanged drug; excretion affected by urine pH
Topical Phenylephrine	—	—	0.5–4 h	—	—	Hepatic, intestinal	Unknown
Oxymetazoline	—	—	—	—	—	—	—
Tetrahydrozoline			3 h	—	—	—	—

gestants. The **oral decongestants** are absolutely contraindicated for patients on concurrent **MAOI** therapy. Concurrent use of these medications may result in severe headache, hypertension and hyperpyrexia, and possibly hypertensive crisis. **Oral decongestants** are also contraindicated for patients with severe hypertension or coronary artery disease. **Phenylpropanolamine** (sustained-release formula) is contraindicated in nursing mothers. In children younger than 12, sustained-release **phenylpropanolamine** and **pseudoephedrine**, as well as **naphazoline (Privine),** are not to be used. **Topical imidazolines (oxymetazoline)** are to be used with caution in children. **Topical naphazoline** is contraindicated for patients with glaucoma.

ADVERSE DRUG REACTIONS.   Adverse effects are minimal at recommended doses, unless a patient is sensitive to **sympathomimetics.** CNS effects may include anxiety, tenseness, restlessness, headache, light-headedness, dizziness, drowsiness, tremor, insomnia, hallucinations, psychological disturbances, CNS depression, and weakness. Of these CNS effects, the most common adverse effects are restlessness and tremors. Cardiovascular adverse effects include transient hypertension, arrhythmia, and cardiovascular collapse, with hypotension, palpitations, tachycardia, and bradycardia. These adverse reactions are rare at recommended doses in healthy individuals. Other adverse effects are nausea, vomiting, pallor, and, rarely, shortness of breath or respiratory difficulty (at higher doses).

Topical decongestants have adverse reactions related to the intense vasoconstrictor effect of the nasal spray or sensitivity to additives such as **sulfites.** Transient stinging is the most common adverse effect reported with **topical decongestants.** Burning, sneezing, dryness, and local irritation are all reported with topical drugs. The most significant adverse reaction with **topical decongestants** is rebound congestion (rhinitis medicamentosa) with prolonged or chronic use. This does not occur with short-term (3 to 5 days) use.

DRUG INTERACTIONS.   The **MAOIs** and **beta-adrenergic blockers** increase the effects of sympathomimetics; therefore, patients taking these medications should avoid **decongestants.** Sympathomimetics may reduce the antihypertensive effects of **methyldopa, guanethidine, mecamylamine, reserpine,** and *Veratrum* **alkaloids.** See Table 15–18 for further drug interactions.

CLINICAL USE AND DOSING

Nasal congestion. **Oral decongestants** are used for the temporary relief of nasal congestion due to the common cold, sinus infection, and allergic rhinitis. They may be used to promote nasal or sinus drainage and are also indicated in the relief of eustachian tube congestion. The adult dose of **pseudoephedrine** for nasal congestion is 60 mg every 4 to 6 hours. In children age 6 to 12, the dose is 30 mg every 4 to 6 hours, and in children age 2 to 6, the dose of **pseudoephedrine** is 15 mg every 4 to 6 hours. In younger children, the dose of **pseudoephedrine** is 4 mg/kg per day divided in four-times-a-day doses. The adult dose of **phenylpropanolamine** for nasal congestion is 20 to 25 mg every 4 hours. Children age 6 to 12 should be prescribed 10 to 12.5 mg every 4 hours, and children age 2 to 6 years, 6.25 mg every 4 hours. Complete dosing of the different forms of the **oral decongestants** is found in Table 15–19.

Topical decongestants are indicated in the symptomatic relief of nasal congestion due to the common cold, sinus infection, and allergic rhinitis. As previously mentioned, **topical decongestants** are only for short-term (three to five days) use because of the rebound congestion of long-term use. **Nasal decongestants** may also relieve ear block and pressure pain in air travel, especially if a patient is suffering from a common cold or sinus infection. The adult dose of **oxymetazoline** topical nasal spray is 1 or 2 drops or sprays of 0.05% solution in each nostril twice a day or up to every 6 hours if needed. Children age 2 to 5 should use 2 to 3 drops of the 0.025% solution in each nostril. The use of 0.05% **oxymetazoline** should be avoided in children. The dose of topical **phenylephrine** nasal solution in adults is 1 to 2 sprays or drops of 0.25% or 0.5% solution every 4 hours as needed for congestion. Adults with severe congestion can use **phenylephrine** 1% solution. Children age 6 to 12 should use 0.25% solution, 2 sprays in each nostril every 4 hours. If the child is between age 6 months and 6 years, the 0.125% solution should be prescribed. The dose of **phenylephrine** in young children and infants is 1 to 2 drops or sprays every 4 hours. Use **topical nasal decongestants** sparingly in young children.

Table 15–19 presents dosing information.

RATIONAL DRUG SELECTION

Topical versus systemic. **Topical decongestants** are effective and have few adverse effects. Many health care providers recommend them for short-term use for the common cold and sinusitis. A concern is the significant rebound congestion that occurs if the **topical decongestants** are used long term. It can occur in as little as a week of constant use. Therefore, **topical decongestants** for allergic rhinitis, while safe, must be accompanied with strict patient education to prevent rebound congestion. In patients who are sensitive to the drying effects of the **topical decongestants,** the oral form may be better tolerated. The reverse is also true; in patients sensitive to **sympathomimetics,** the **topical decongestants** are usually tolerated.

Short- versus long-acting. There are short- and long-acting forms of both **oral** and **topical decongestants.** In general, the short-acting forms are better tolerated and have fewer adverse effects. The longer-acting forms are useful

Table 15–18. Drug Interactions: Selected Decongestants

Drug	Interacting Drug	Possible Effect	Implications
Systemic Phenylpropanolamine	Indomethacin	Concurrent administration may lead to increased blood pressure (BP)	Use concurrently with caution
	Caffeine	May cause increased serum caffeine levels, leading to toxic effects	Caution patient to minimize caffeine intake while using
	Bromocriptine	Possible exacerbation of bromocriptine side effects and hypertension	Avoid concurrent use
	Caffeine, cocaine, and other sympathomimetic drugs	Additive sympathomimetic activity	Use concurrently with caution
	MAOIs, furazolidone, procarbazine	Concurrent use can prolong and intensify the cardiac stimulation and vasopressor effects, may lead to severe cardiovascular and cerebrovascular response	Avoid use within 14 d of each other
	Ergot alkaloids	Peripheral vasoconstriction, additive vasoconstriction	Avoid concurrent use
	Methyldopa, reserpine	Decreased antihypertensive effects	Monitor BP closely if using concurrently
	Thyroid hormones	Increased effects of both agents on the cardiovascular system	Use concurrently with caution
	Halogenated anesthetics	Cardiac arrhythmias	Use together with caution
Pseudoephedrine	Caffeine, cocaine, and other sympathomimetic drugs	Additive sympathomimetic activity	Use concurrently with caution
	MAOIs, furazolidone, procarbazine	Concurrent use can prolong and intensify the cardiac stimulation and vasopressor effects, may lead to severe cardiovascular and cerebrovascular response	Avoid use within 14 d of each other
	Ergot alkaloids	Peripheral vasoconstriction, additive vasoconstriction	Avoid concurrent use
	Methyldopa, reserpine	Decreased antihypertensive effects	Monitor BP closely if using concurrently
	Thyroid hormones	Increased effects of both agents on the cardiovascular system	Use concurrently with caution
	Urinary alkalinizers: Sodium bicarbonate, sodium citrate, potassium citrate, sodium lactate, sodium acetate	Increased alkalinization of the urine leads to tubular reabsorption of pseudoephedrine	Observe for increased adverse effects; use together with caution
Topical Phenylephrine	MAOIs, tricyclic antidepressants	Hypertensive crisis	Do not use within 14 d of each other
	Beta blockers	May increase vasopressor effects of sympathomimetics	Monitor closely for adverse reaction

Continued on next page

Table 15–18. Drug Interactions: Selected Decongestants (*continued*)

Drug	Interacting Drug	Possible Effect	Implications
Oxymetazoline	MAOIs, tricyclic anti-depressants	Hypertensive crisis	Do not use within 14 d of each other
	Beta blockers	May increase vasopressor effects of sympatho-mimetics	Monitor closely for adverse reaction
Tetrahydrozoline	None reported	—	—
Xylometazoline	None reported	—	—

for patients who require all-day or all-night relief, if they can tolerate them.

Cost. Cost is usually not a major factor in prescribing **decongestants,** which are available OTC, and generic forms of all the medications are available.

MONITORING. There is no specific monitoring required with the **decongestants.**

PATIENT EDUCATION

Administration. The first concern the health care provider should address is self-prescribing and dosing of the nonprescription **decongestants.** Whether a drug interaction is a concern or a patient may be taking an inappropriate dose, it is important for the health care provider to be aware that the patient may be taking a **decongestant.** A thorough history should include any self-prescribed medications and the amount and timing of these medications. Patient teaching should include proper dosing, especially in pediatric patients. Patients with cardiovascular disease, hyperthyroidism, diabetes mellitus, or prostatic hypertrophy should use these products sparingly and only upon the advice of their health care provider.

When **topical decongestants** are recommended, it is imperative that the patient be warned about rebound congestion and cautioned to use the medication for only 3 to 5 days or, for chronic allergic rhinitis use, only 2 of every 7 days.

Parents should be cautioned not to use adult-formula nasal sprays in children. There are children's strength **oxymetazoline** (0.025%) and **phenylephrine HCl** (0.125%) available for children.

Adverse reactions. Patients should notify their health care provider if insomnia, dizziness, weakness, tremor, or irregular heart beat occurs with **topical decongestants.** Patients should be cautioned not to exceed the recommended dosage because higher doses cause nervousness, dizziness, or sleeplessness.

Table 15–20 presents available dosage forms.

Cough Preparations

Antitussives

Antitussives are widely used by patients to self-treat coughs. It is essential for the health care provider to educate the patient on the useful physiological mechanism a cough provides by clearing the airway of secretions and foreign material. Therefore, a cough should not be suppressed if it is protecting the airway. There are times when an **antitussive** is necessary to provide rest or sleep. The cough reflex is complicated, involving both the central and peripheral nervous systems, as well as the smooth muscle of the bronchial tree. The drugs that can affect this complex mechanism are diverse, ranging from **bronchodilators** to drugs that act centrally or peripherally to suppress cough. This section discusses the nonprescription **antitussives dextromethorphan** and **benzonatate. Codeine,** which is also used as an **antitussive,** is covered in the CNS chapter with the other **opioids.** Dosing of **codeine** for **antitussive** use is included here.

Pharmacodynamics

Cough results when sensory stimuli or irritation in the bronchial tree stimulates cough receptors, probably located in the bronchial smooth muscle. A message is sent via the afferent nervous system to the cough centers in the medulla. **Antitussives** work either centrally or peripherally to affect the cough. The exact mechanism of action of antitussives is poorly understood. **Dextromethorphan,** the D isomer of the **codeine** analogue levorphanol, acts centrally in the cough center in the medulla to elevate the threshold for coughing. **Codeine** works as an **antitussive** through direct action on receptors in the cough center of the medulla, at lower doses than is required for analgesia. **Benzonatate (Tessalon)** is related to **tetracaine** and is thought to anesthetize the stretch receptors in the respiratory passages, thereby decreasing their activity and calming the cough peripherally at its source.

Table 15–19. Dosage Schedule: Selected Decongestants

Drug	Indication	Dose	Comments
Systemic Phenylpropanolamine	Nasal congestion	*Adults:* 20–25 mg every 4 h; max 150 mg/d *Children 6–12:* 10–12.5 mg every 4 h; max 75 mg/d *Children 2–6:* 6.25 mg every 4 h; max 37.5 mg/d	*Extended-release formula:* *Adults:* 75 mg every 12 h *Children:* not recommended
Pseudoephedrine	Nasal congestion	*Adults and children >12:* 60 mg every 4–6 h (20 mL of 15 mg/5 mL liquid); max 240 mg/day *Children 6–12:* 30 mg every 4–6 h (10 mL of 15 mg/5 mL liquid); max 120 mg/d *Children 2–6:* 15 mg every 4–6 h (5 mL of 15 mg/5 mL liquid); max 60 mg/d *Children <2:* 1 mg/kg/dose every 4–6 h; max 4 doses *or* 6–11 lb: 0.4 mL (1/2 dropperful) of drops 12–17 lb: 0.8 mL (1 dropperful) of drops 18–23 lb: 1.2 mL (1.5 dropperful) of drops 24–35 lb: 1.6 mL (2 dropperfuls) of drops	*Extended-release (12-h formula):* *Adults and children >12:* 120 mg every 12 h; max 240 mg/d *Children <12:* not recommended *Extended release (24-h formula):* *Adults and children >12:* 1 tablet; max 240 mg/d *Children <12:* not recommended
Topical Phenylephrine	Nasal congestion and eustachian tube congestion	*Adults and children >12:* 1–2 sprays of 0.25% or 0.5% solution in each nostril every 4 h prn congestion; 1% solution can be used in adults with severe congestion *Children 6–12:* 1–2 sprays of 0.25% solution in each nostril every 4 h prn congestion *Children 2–6:* 2 drops or sprays of 0.125% or 0.16% solution to each nostril every 4 h as needed *Children 6 mo–2 yr:* 1–2 drops of 0.16% solution in each nostril every 3–4 h prn	Advise patients to use nasal decongestant spray for a maximum of 2–3 d in a row to avoid rebound congestion
Oxymetazoline	Nasal congestion	*Adults and children >6:* use 1–2 drops or sprays of 0.05% solution in each nostril bid *Children 2–5:* 1–2 drops of 0.025% solution in each nostril bid; do not use 0.05% solution in young children *Children <2:* not recommended	Advise patients to use nasal decongestant spray for a maximum of 2–3 d in a row to avoid rebound congestion
Tetrahydrozoline	Nasal congestion	*Adults and children >6:* 2–4 drops or 3–4 sprays of 0.1% solution in each nostril every 3–4 prn *Children <6:* 2–3 drops of 0.05% solution in each nostril every 3–4 hours prn	

Table 15–20. Available Dosage Forms: Selected Decongestants

Drug	Dosage Form	How Supplied
SYSTEMIC		
Phenylpropanolamine Entex (Rx)	Tablet: phenylephrine 5 mg, phenylpropan- olamine 45 mg, guaifenesin 200 mg	100, 500
Entex LA (Rx)	Sustained-release tablets: phenylpropanola- mine 75 mg, guaifenesin 400 mg	100
Entex Liquid (Rx)	Liquid: phenylephrine 5 mg, phenylpropanol- amine 20 mg, guaifenesin 100 mg/5 mL	Pints (contains alcohol)
Dimetapp (OTC)	Tablets and capsules: phenylpropanolamine 25 mg, brompheniramine 4 mg	12, 24
Dimetapp Elixir (OTC)	Elixir: phenylpropanolamine 12.5 mg, brompheniramine 2 mg	4 oz, 8 oz, 12 oz
Dimetapp Cold & Allergy Quick Dissolve Tabs (OTC)	Quick-dissolve tablets: phenylpropanolamine 6.25 mg, brompheniramine 1 mg	10
Dimetapp Extentabs (OTC)	Extended-release tablets: phenylpropanola- mine 75 mg, brompheniramine 12 mg	12, 24, 48, 100, 500
Pseudoephedrine Sulfate Afrin	Extended-release tablets: 120 mg (60 mg immediate release/60 mg extended release)	100
Drixoral Non-Drowsy Formula	Extended-release tablets: 120 mg (60 mg immediate release/60 mg extended release)	20
Pseudoephedrine HCl Sudafed	Tablets: 30 mg, 60 mg Extended release: 120 mg Liquid: 30 mg/5 mL	24, 48, 100, 1000 10, 20 4 oz
Pediacare	Drops: 7.5 mg/0.8 mL	15 mL w/dropper
Generic	Tablets: 30 mg, 60 mg Liquid: 30 mg/5 mL	24, 100, 1000 120 mL, 240 mL, pint, gallon
TOPICAL		
Phenylephrine Neo-Synephrine	Solution: 0.125%, 0.25%, 0.5%, 1%	30 mL, drops or spray bottle
Generic	Solution: 0.125%, 0.25%, 0.5%, 1%	30 mL, drops or spray bottle
Oxymetazoline Afrin Children's Nose Drops	Solution: 0.025%	20-mL bottle with dropper
Afrin	Solution: 0.05%	15-mL spray bottle and 20-mL drops
4-Way Long Lasting Nasal	Solution: 0.05%	15-mL spray bottle
Dristan Long Lasting	Solution: 0.05%	15mL, 30-mL spray bottle
Neo-Synephrine 12 Hour	Solution: 0.05%	15-mL spray bottle
Generic	Solution: 0.05%	15-mL, 30-mL spray bottle

Continued on next page

Table 15–20. Available Dosage Forms: Selected Decongestants *(continued)*

Drug	Dosage Form	How Supplied
Tetrahydrozoline Tyzine	Solution: 0.1%	15-mL spray, 30-mL drops
Tyzine Pediatric Drops	Solution: 0.05%	15-mL drops

Pharmacokinetics

ABSORPTION AND DISTRIBUTION. Dextromethorphan, codeine, and benzonatate are absorbed well from the GI tract. The distribution of dextromethorphan and benzonatate is unknown. Codeine is 7 percent protein-bound and widely distributed, including in the CNS. Codeine freely crosses the placenta and is distributed into breast milk.

METABOLISM AND EXCRETION. Dextromethorphan is extensively metabolized by the liver and excreted in the urine, mostly as metabolites. Codeine is metabolized in the liver by glucuronidation into morphine and norcodeine. The metabolism of codeine into morphine is mediated by cytochrome P-450 2D6. Codeine is eliminated in the urine as unchanged drug, norcodeine, and free and conjugated morphine. The metabolism and excretion of benzonatate is unknown. See Table 15–21 for the pharmacokinetics.

Pharmacotherapeutics

PRECAUTIONS AND CONTRAINDICATIONS. Antitussives are not to be used for persistent or chronic cough caused by smoking, asthma, or emphysema. In asthma, antitussives may impair expectoration and thus cause increased airway resistance. Expectorants must not be used by patients with excessive respiratory secretions for the same reason. Patients must be cautioned not to self-medicate their cough for long periods (more than 7 days) without seeking the care of their health care provider. If high fever or rash accompanies a cough, patients must be seen by their health care provider.

Benzonatate is contraindicated for patients allergic to tetracaine, procaine, or related compounds.

Dextromethorphan, codeine, and benzonatate can cause drowsiness, dizziness, nausea, and GI upset. In addition, patients taking benzonatate may experience headache, constipation, pruritus, skin eruptions, a sensation of burning eyes, a vague "chilly" sensation, chest numbness, and hypersensitivity.

Patients with hepatic function impairment should be monitored if dextromethorphan is prescribed because metabolism of the drug may be impaired. The metabolism of codeine can be affected by deficiency of cytochrome P-450D or by medications that may inhibit CYP 2D6.

Codeine may cause dependence and should be used with caution in a patient with a history of substance abuse. Although dextromethorphan is not addictive, there have been reports of abuse of dextromethorphan-containing products, especially among teenagers.

Codeine causes decreased gastric motility and therefore should be used cautiously by patients with GI obstruction, ileus, or preexisting constipation. Patients with acute ulcerative colitis may be more sensitive to the constipating effects of codeine.

Dextromethorphan and *codeine* are Pregnancy Category C, but no teratogenic effects have been demonstrated. *Codeine* should be used with caution near term in pregnancy. *Benzonatate* is Pregnancy Category C and is to be given to pregnant women only if

Table 15–21. Pharmacokinetics: Selected Cough Preparations

Drug	Onset	Peak	Duration	Protein Binding	Half-Life	Metabolism	Elimination
Antitussives Dextromethorphan	15–30 min	—	5–6 h	—	11 h	Extensive hepatic	Renal
Codeine (used as an antitussive)	30–60 min	1–2 h	4–6 h	7%	3–4 h	Primarily hepatic (CYP 2D6)	Renal
Benzonatate	15–20 min	—	3–8 h	—	—	—	—
Expectorants Guaifenesin	Rapid	—	—	—	1 h	—	Renal

clearly needed. There are better-studied choices for antitussives in pregnancy, such as *dextromethorphan* or short-term *codeine*.

DRUG INTERACTIONS. Use of **antitussives** with any **CNS depressant** may cause increased CNS depression. Concurrent use of **dextromethorphan** and **MAOIs** is contraindicated.

Codeine should be used with caution concurrently with medications that are metabolized by CYP 2D6 isoenzymes. **Quinidine** has been shown to interfere with the metabolism of **codeine**. Other medications that inhibit CYP 2D6 are **amiodarone (Cordarone), tricyclic antidepressants, metoclopramide (Reglan), SSRIs, cimetidine (Tagamet), thioridazine (Mellaril), propafenone (Rythmol), mibefradil (Posicor),** and **haloperidol (Haldol).**

Drugs interactions are shown in Table 15–22.

CLINICAL USE AND DOSING

Cough. **Dextromethorphan, codeine,** and **benzonatate** are used to control nonproductive cough. **Antitussives** should be used only for the nonproductive, irritant-like cough, after other pathology has been ruled out, specifically asthma or pneumonia. **Antitussives** are not to be used for asthmatic cough or for coughs accompanied by excessive respiratory secretions.

Dextromethorphan is available in many forms and either singly or in combination with **expectorants**. As it is available without prescription, it is widely used by patients to self-medicate their cough, not always appropriately. The adult dose of **dextromethorphan** is 10 to 30 mg every 4 to 8 hours. Children age 6 to 12 are given a dose of 5 to 10 mg every 4 hours or 15 mg every 6 to 8 hours. The dose of **dextromethorphan** in children age 2 to 6 is 2.5 mg to 7.5 mg every 4 to 8 hours.

Benzonatate is available only by prescription and is effective in controlling dry, irritant-like coughs. The dose for adults and children age 10 and older is 100 mg three times a day.

Codeine, a schedule II medication, may be administered alone or in combination with another agent such as **guaifenesin** for cough suppression. The adult dose of **codeine** for cough suppression is 10 to 20 mg every 4 to 6 hours, with the maximum daily dose not exceeding 120 mg. Children older than age 1 year may be prescribed codeine for a nonproductive cough. The dosage is 1 to 1.5 mg/kg per day in divided doses every 4 hours. An alternative dosing schedule is to prescribe 2.5 to 5 mg every 4 hours to children age 2 to 5. Children age 6 to 12 can be prescribed 5 to 10 mg every 4 to 6 hours (maximum 60 mg per day).

Table 15–23 presents dosing information.

RATIONAL DRUG SELECTION. Patients may self-medicate their cough with a nonprescription form of **dex-**

Table 15–22. Drug Interactions: Selected Cough Preparations

Drug	Interacting Drug	Possible Effect	Implications
Antitussives			
Dextromethorphan	MAOIs	Dextromethorphan can block neuronal uptake of serotonin and can increase concentrations of serotonin if combined with MAOIs; hypertensive or hyperpyretic crisis is possible	Use concurrently with caution, if at all; avoid use within 14 d
	SSRIs	SSRIs interfere with dextromethorphan metabolism, leading to toxicity	Use lower doses of dextromethorphan
	CNS depressants	Additive CNS depression	Use with caution
	Amiodarone, quinidine	These drugs inhibit CYP 2D6; dextromethorphan toxicity may occur	Monitor for toxicity if prescribed concurrently
Codeine (used as an antitussive)	CNS depressants, alcohol	Additive CNS depression	Use cautiously and reduce dose to avoid additive effects
	Antihypertensive agents	Antagonizes antihypertensives	Monitor patients closely
	Antidiarrheals	Can lead to severe constipation	Use with caution; monitor the patient
Benzonatate	None known	—	—
Expectorants			
Guaifenesin	None known	—	—

Table 15–23. Dosage Schedule: Selected Cough Preparations

Drug	Indication	Dose	Comments
Antitussives Dextromethorphan	Cough	*Adults and children >12:* 10–30 mg every 4 h or 30 mg every 6–8 h	Do not exceed 120 mg in 24 h
		Children 6–12: 5–10 mg every 4 h or 15 mg every 6–8 h	Do not exceed 60 mg in 24 h
		Children 2–6: 2.5–5 mg every 4 h or 7.5 mg every 6–8 h	Do not exceed 30 mg in 24 h
Codeine (used as an antitussive)	Cough	*Adults:* 10–20 mg every 4 h	Do not exceed 120 mg in 24 h
		Children 6–12: 5–10 mg every 4 h	Do not exceed 60 mg in 24 h
		Children 2–6: 2.5–5 mg every 4 h	Do not exceed 30 mg in 24 h
Benzonatate	Cough	*Adults and children >age 10:* 100 mg tid, up to 600 mg per day	
Expectorants Guaifenesin	Cough	*Adults and children >12:* 200–400 mg every 4 h	Maximum 2.4 gm/24 h
		Children 6–11: 100–200 mg every 4 h	Maximum 1.2 gm/24 h
		Children 2–5: 50–100 mg every 4 h	
		Children <2: 12 mg/kg/d in 6 divided doses	Maximum 600 mg/24 h

tromethorphan, and the health care provider has little to do with the choice of the medication. (Advertising has the largest impact.) The health care provider becomes involved when the patient asks which is the recommended formula or if nonprescription products are not effective.

Cost. Although nonprescription **dextromethorphan** is less expensive than **benzonatate** or **codeine**-containing preparations, patients with good prescriptive coverage may actually pay less out of pocket for the prescription product. Cost must therefore be evaluated on an individual basis.

Effectiveness. Patients might feel that a prescription medication is more effective than nonprescription, but **dextromethorphan** has been found to be as effective as **codeine** in the treatment of cough.

MONITORING. There is no specific monitoring required when prescribing **antitussive** medications.

PATIENT EDUCATION. Patient education centers on proper administration, adverse reactions, and drug interactions with the **antitussive** agents.

Administration. Patients should be aware of the proper dosing of **antitussive** medication. When they are self-medicating, they often are not following the recommended dosing schedule. The health care provider needs to determine if the patient is taking the proper amount, measured with a calibrated measuring spoon (not a silverware tablespoon), and spacing the dosage appropriately. The medications may be taken without regard to food but may be better tolerated if taken with food or milk.

Adverse reactions. CNS depression is the major concern. Some of the **antitussives** are in alcohol-containing syrup form, and others may cause sedation. Driving or operating hazardous machinery should be undertaken with caution, and not at all if the patient is sensitive to the sedating effects of the **antitussives.** Patients should also be aware that long-term (more than 7 days) cough or cough accompanied by fever should be seen by their health care provider.

Patients concurrently taking **MAOIs** should not take **antitussives. Antitussives** should be taken with caution if the patient is concurrently taking any other CNS-sedating medications.

Lifestyle management. The patient with a cough should be encouraged to increase fluid intake to improve the viscosity of the respiratory secretions. The patient should refrain from smoking and, if possible, stop smoking. Avoidance of respiratory irritants and people with respiratory infections will decrease the incidence of cough.

Table 15–24 presents available dosage forms.

Expectorants

Guaifenesin is the only **expectorant** ingredient listed by the FDA panel as having scientific evidence of safety and efficacy. **Guaifenesin** is indicated as an **expectorant** in the symptomatic treatment of cough due to the common cold and mild upper respiratory infections.

Pharmacodynamics

Guaifenesin's main mechanism of action is to increase the output of the respiratory tract by decreasing adhesiveness and surface tension. The increased flow of the

Table 15–24. Available Dosage Forms: Selected Cough Preparations

Drug	Dosage Form	How Supplied
ANTITUSSIVES		
Dextromethorphan Scot-Tussen DM Cough Chasers	Lozenges: 2.5 mg	20
Hold DM	Lozenges: 5 mg	10
Robitussin Cough Calmers	Lozenges: 5 mg	10
Supress	Lozenges: 7.5 mg	1000
Robitussin Pediatric	Liquid: 7.5 mg/5 mL	120 mL, 240 mL
Vicks Formula 44	Liquid: 15 mg/5 mL	120 mL, 240 mL (contains 10% alcohol)
Vicks Formula 44 Pediatric	Liquid: 15 mg/15 mL (1 mg/mL)	120 mL (no alcohol)
Delsym	Sustained-action liquid: 30 mg/5 mL	89 mL
Codeine sulfate (used as an antitussive)	Tablets: 15 mg, 30 mg, 60 mg	100
Benzonatate	Capsules: 100 mg	100, 1000
EXPECTORANTS		
Guaifenesin Robitussin	Syrup: 100 mg/5 mL	30 mL, 60 mL, 120 mL, 240 mL, pint, gallon (contains 3.5% alcohol)
Generic	Syrup: 100 mg/5 mL	120 mL, 240 mL, pint, gallon

thinned secretions promotes ciliary action and facilitates the removal of respiratory mucus. This changes a dry, nonproductive cough into a more productive cough.

Pharmacokinetics

ABSORPTION AND DISTRIBUTION. Guaifenesin is rapidly absorbed from the GI tract after oral administration. Distribution is unknown. It is not known whether **guaifenesin** crosses the placenta or is distributed in breast milk.

METABOLISM AND EXCRETION. The exact mechanism of metabolism of **guaifenesin** is unknown. Its major metabolite, beta (2-methoxyphenoxy) lactic acid is excreted in the urine.

Pharmacotherapeutics

PRECAUTIONS AND CONTRAINDICATIONS. Guaifenesin is not to be used for persistent cough, such as that found with smoking, asthma, or emphysema. Cough related to heart failure or **angiotensin-converting enzyme (ACE)** **inhibitor** therapy should not be treated with **guaifenesin.** Cough accompanied by high fever or lasting longer than 7 days should be evaluated by a health care provider.

Guaifenesin is Pregnancy Category C. There have been no problems documented in breastfeeding women taking this medication. Use in children over 2 years old is considered safe.

ADVERSE DRUG EFFECTS. GI upset, nausea, and vomiting are the most commonly reported adverse effects of **guaifenesin.** Drowsiness, diarrhea, dizziness, rash, and headache have also been reported. **Guaifenesin** is contraindicated only if the patient is hypersensitive to **guaifenesin.**

DRUG INTERACTIONS. There are no drug interactions of significance with **guaifenesin;** however, **guaifenesin** may cause false readings in certain laboratory determinations of 5-hydroxyindoleacetic acid (5-HIAA) and vanillylmandelic acid (VMA).

CLINICAL USE AND DOSING

Dry, nonproductive cough. **Guaifenesin** is indicated in the symptomatic relief of dry, nonproductive cough, with mucus in the respiratory tract. The dose of **guaifenesin** for adults and children over age 12 is 200 to 400 mg every 4 hours. The **guaifenesin** dose in children age 6 to 11 is 100 to 200 mg every 4 hours. Children age 2 to 5 should be dosed with 50 to 100 mg of **guaifenesin** every 4 hours. For younger children, the dose is 12 mg/kg per day in 6 divided doses.

MONITORING. There is no specific laboratory monitoring required with the use of **guaifenesin.**

PATIENT EDUCATION. The patient should be aware of the proper dose of **guaifenesin.** The patient should be using a calibrated medication spoon and taking the appropriate dose per age.

Guaifenesin is an OTC product, and patients may self-medicate, often without proper understanding of the medication. The provider may assist the patient in making the proper choice of cough medication by explaining the difference between the OTC products **guaifenesin** and **dextromethorphan.** An explanation of the many combination products that are available and some guidance about appropriate use will assist the patient in making an informed choice.

REFERENCES

American Medical Association. (1997). *Managing asthma today (1 & 2): Integrating new concepts.* Chicago: AMA.

Autio, L., & Rosenow, D. (1999). Effectively managing asthma in young and middle adulthood. *Nurse Practitioner, 24*(1), 100–111.

Colice, G. L. (1996). Nebulized bronchodilators for outpatient management of stable chronic obstructive pulmonary disease. *American Journal of Medicine, 100*(Suppl 1A), 1A-11S–1A-15S.

Cummins, R. O. (1997). *Advanced cardiac life support.* Dallas: American Heart Association.

Drazen, J. M., Israel, E., Boushey, H. A., Chinchilli, V. M., Fahy, J. V., Fish, J. E., Lazarus, S. C., Lemanske, R. F., Martin, R. J., Peters, S. P., Sorkness, C., & Szefler, S. J. (1996). Comparison of regularly scheduled with as-needed use of albuterol in mild asthma. *New England Journal of Medicine, 335*(12), 841–847.

Drombrowski, M., Thom, E., & McNellis, D. (1999). Maternal-fetal medicine units (MFNIU) studies of inhaled corticosteroids during pregnancy. *Journal of Allergy and Clinical Immunology, 103*(2), S356–S359.

Georgitis, J.W. (1999). The 1997 asthma management guidelines and therapeutic issues relating to the treatment of asthma. *Chest, 115*(1), 210–217.

Kastrup, E. (Founding Ed.). (1999). *Drug facts and comparisons.* St. Louis: Facts and Comparisons.

Katzung, B. (1998). *Basic and clinical pharmacology* (7th ed.). Stamford, CT: Appleton & Lange.

Ladebauche, P. (1997). Managing asthma: A growth and developmental approach. *Pediatric Nursing, 23*(1), 37–44.

Lieu, T. A., Quesenberry, C. P., Capra, A. M., Sorel, M. E., Martin, K. E., & Mendoza, G. R. (1997). Outpatient management practices associated with reduced risk of pediatric asthma hospitalization and emergency department visits. *Pediatrics, 100*(3).

Luskin, A. T. (1999). An overview of the recommendation of the working group on asthma and pregnancy. *Journal of Allergy and Clinical Immunology, 103*(2), S350–S353.

Matthay, R. A., & Arroliga, A. C. (1996). Chronic airway diseases. In J. C. Bennett & F. Plum (Eds.), *Cecil textbook of medicine* (20th ed., pp. 381–390). Philadelphia: WB Saunders.

National Asthma Education and Prevention Program. (1997). *The Expert Panel Report II: Guidelines for the diagnosis and management of asthma* (NIH pub. 97-405 1). Bethesda, MD: National Heart, Lung, and Blood Institute, National Institutes of Health.

National Heart, Lung, and Blood Institute. (1995). *Global strategy for asthma management and prevention NHLBI/WHO report* (NIH pub. 95-3659). Bethesda, MD: National Institutes of Health.

Simmons, M. S., Nides, M. A., Rand, C. S., Wise, R. A., & Tashkin, D. P. (1996). Trends in compliance with bronchodilator inhaler use between follow-up visits in a clinical trial. *Chest, 109*(4), 963–968.

Tashkin, D. P., Bleecker, E., Braun, S., Campbell, S., DeGraff, A. C., Hudgel, D. W., Boyars, M. C., & Sahn, S. (1996). Results of a multicenter study of nebulized inhalant bronchodilator solutions. *American Journal of Medicine, 100*(Suppl 1A), 1A-62S–1A-68S.

VanAndel, A. E., Reisner, C., Menjoge, S. S., & Witek, T. J. (1999). Analysis of inhaled corticosteroid and oral theophylline use among patients with stable COPD from 1987 to 1995. *Chest, 115*(3), 703–707.

Wendel, P. J., Ramin, S. M., Barnett-Hamm, C., Rowe, T. F., & Cunningham, F. G. (1996). Asthma treatment in pregnancy: A randomized controlled study. *American Journal of Obstetrics and Gynecology, 175*(1), 150–154

CHAPTER 16

·······

Drugs Affecting the Hematopoietic System

CHAPTER OUTLINE

Anticoagulants and Antiplatelets

O f the approximately 300,000 patients annually who have a thromboembolus, more than 50,000 die (Goroll, May, & Mulley, 1995). The morbidity and mortality associated with these emboli could be significantly reduced by timely use of **anticoagulation** therapy. **Oral anticoagulation therapy** has been used in primary care for almost 50 years, and the number of indications for its use has steadily increased. The introduction of low molecular weight **heparin** with less bleeding risk has allowed the outpatient use of **injectable anticoagulation therapy** as well. With more selective and reliable laboratory tests to monitor blood levels, the management of **anticoagulation therapy** has become a major tool in the prevention of thrombus formation in primary care.

Pharmacodynamics

Although the exact details of the clotting mechanism are not fully understood, it is generally accepted that clotting occurs when several circulating proteins interact in a cascading series of limited proteolytic actions (Fig. 16–1). At each step, a precursor protein is converted to an active protease that activates the next clotting factor, and finally a solid clot is formed. The components involved at each stage are a protease from the preceding stage, a precursor protein, a protein activator, calcium, and an organizing surface provided by platelets. Fibrinogen is the substrate for the enzyme thrombin (factor IIa). This protease is formed by activation of its precursor protein, prothrombin. Prothrombin is bound by calcium to a platelet surface, where activated factor X (Xa), in the presence of factor V (Va), converts it to circulating thrombin. Thrombin then converts fibrinogen to fibrin to form the clot. **Oral anticoagulants** such as **warfarin**

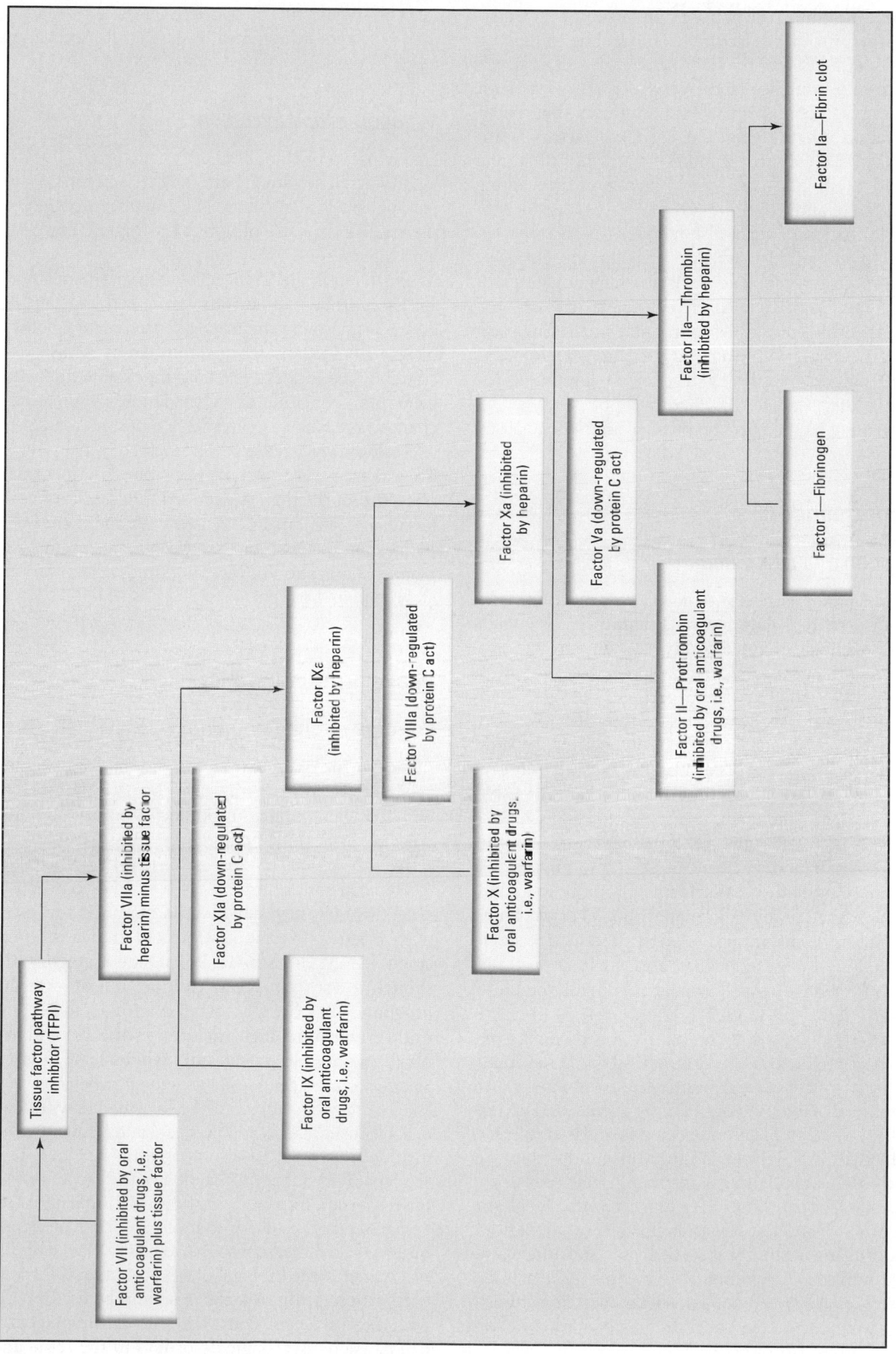

Figure 16–1. The clotting cascade.

(**Coumadin**) inhibit the hepatic synthesis of several clotting factors, including factor X. The decline in clotting factors is a function of the half-life of each factor, which varies from 5 hours for factor VII to 72 hours for factor II. Plasma also contains protease inhibitors that inactivate coagulation proteins. One of these factors is antithrombin III. **Heparin** inhibits the activity of several activated clotting factors through its role in accelerating the activity of antithrombin III.

The formation of a clot also requires that platelets aggregate to form the organizing base for the clot. The prostaglandin thromboxane A_2 is an arachidonate product that causes platelets to change shape, release their granules, and aggregate. **Aspirin** antagonizes this pathway and interferes with platelet aggregation. **Ticlopidine (Ticlid)** reduces platelet aggregation by inhibiting the adenosine diphosphate (ADP) pathway of platelets. Unlike **aspirin**, it has no effect on prostaglandin metabolism.

Pharmacokinetics

Absorption and Distribution

Heparin, including the low molecular weight drugs **ardeparin (Normiflo)**, **dalteparin (Fragmin)**, and **enoxaparin (Lovenox)**, is not absorbed in the gastrointestinal (GI) tract and must be given intravenously (IV) or subcutaneously (SC). The IV route is used in acute care. SC injection of **heparin** results in considerable individual variation in bioavailability. Low molecular weight heparins have less variation, but bioavailability between drugs is not consistent, and these drugs are not interchangeable. Once absorbed, all **heparins** are distributed in plasma and extensively protein-bound (Table 16–1).

The **coumarin derivative** most commonly used is **warfarin (Coumadin)**. **Warfarin** is rapidly and completely absorbed orally. Although serum levels are found in 1 to 2 hours, the anticoagulation effect is dependent on depletion of clotting factors, and the full effect does not occur for 3 to 4 days. **Warfarin** is highly bound to plasma protein.

Aspirin is rapidly and completely absorbed after oral administration. Bioavailability is dependent on the dosage form, the presence of food, gastric emptying time, gastric pH, presence of antacids or buffering agents, and particle size. Bioavailability of enteric-coated forms is erratic. It is partially hydrolyzed during absorption and distributed to all body tissues and fluids, including fetal tissues and breast milk. Protein binding is highest with low plasma concentrations and lower with high concentrations.

Ticlopidine is rapidly absorbed after oral administration. Administration after meals increases the area under the curve (AUC) by 20 percent. Because of its nonlinear pharmacokinetics, clearance decreases markedly with repeated administration. In older adults, half-lives of

12.6 hours after the first dose increased to 4 to 5 days with repeated dosing. Steady-state levels occur in about 14 to 21 days.

Metabolism and Excretion

Heparins are metabolized by the liver and the reticuloendothelial system. There may be a secondary site of metabolism in the kidney. Clearance is nonlinear, and the half-life may be prolonged at higher doses and in liver disease.

Warfarin is metabolized by hepatic microsomal enzymes cyproheptadine (CYP) 1A2 and 2C9 and is excreted primarily in the urine as inactive metabolites.

Aspirin is extensively metabolized by the liver and excreted by the kidney. The amount excreted depends on urine pH. As pH increases, the amount excreted as unchanged drug increases from 2 or 3 percent to 80 percent.

Ticlopidine is extensively metabolized by the liver. Trace amounts of intact drug are found in the urine, and one-third of the dose is excreted in feces and bile as intact drug. Clearance decreases with age. Renal impairment alters plasma levels but does not seem to affect platelet aggregation or bleeding times, except in moderately impaired patients.

Pharmacotherapeutics

Precautions and Contraindications

All **anticoagulants** are contraindicated for patients who are hypersensitive to the drug or actively bleeding or who have hemophilia, thrombocytopenia, severe hypertension, intracranial hemorrhage, infective endocarditis, active tuberculosis, or ulcerative lesions of the GI tract.

Heparins are contraindicated in advanced hepatic or renal disease. They may be used in patients who are actively bleeding to treat disseminated intravascular coagulation (DIC). **Heparin is Pregnancy Category C. Although it does not cross the placenta, its use during pregnancy has been associated with 13 to 22 percent unfavorable outcomes, including stillbirth and prematurity. It should be used only when clearly indicated.** Safety has not been established in newborns. Hyperkalemia may develop, and use for patients with diabetes or renal insufficiency requires care and frequent monitoring of activated partial thromboplastin time (aPTT).

Hepatic dysfunction potentiates the response to **warfarin** through impaired synthesis of coagulation factors. Hypermetabolic states produced by fever or hyperthyroidism also increase responsiveness to **warfarin**, probably by increasing the catabolism of vitamin K–dependent coagulation factors. **Warfarin** should be used cautiously with these patients. **Warfarin crosses the placenta and can cause hemorrhagic disorders in the fetus and se-**

Table 16–1. Pharmacokinetics: Selected Anticoagulants and Antiplatelets

Drug	Onset	Peak	Duration	Protein Binding	Bioavail-ability	Half-Life	Elimination
Anticoagulants							
Ardeparin	—	2.1–3.3 h	—	—	76–108%	Not known	In urine
Dalteparin	—	4 h	up to 24 h	—	81–93%	3–5 h (increased in renal insufficiency)	In urine
Enoxaparin	—	3–5 h	12 h	—	92%	4.5 h	In urine
Heparin (SC only)	20–60 min	2–4 h	8–12 h	Extensive	—	1–3 h (nonlinear and dose dependent; 30 min for doses of 25 μg/kg vs. 150 min for doses of 400 μg/kg); half-life shorter for patients with deep vein thrombosis (DVT) than those with pulmonary embolism; half-life may be prolonged in liver disease	50% unchanged in urine; some urine degradation products have anticoagulant activity; also eliminated by reticuloendothelial system (lymph nodes and spleen)
Warfarin	—	3–5 d	2–5 d	97–99%	—	1–2.5 d	In urine as inactive metabolites
Antiplatelets							
Aspirin	5–30 min	1–3 h	3–6 h	Concentration-dependent low doses: (100 μg/mL) = 90% high doses: (400 μg/mL) = 76%	—	15–20 min	Renal excretion depends on urine pH; as pH increases from 5 to 8, renal clearance increases from 2–3% to more than 80%
Ticlopidine	2 h	8–11 d	2 wk	98%	—	12.6 h for single dose; 4–5 days with repeated dosing	60% in urine, 23% in feces; clearance decreases with age

rious birth defects. It is Pregnancy Category X and should not be administered during pregnancy.

Hypersensitivity to **aspirin** and cross-sensitivity with **nonsteroidal anti-inflammatory drugs (NSAIDs)** may occur, contraindicating the drug. **Aspirin** hypersensitivity is more prevalent in patients with asthma, nasal polyps, or chronic urticaria. Reye's syndrome has been associated with its use in children and teenagers who have influenza or chickenpox. Reversible hepatotoxicity has occurred. Use **aspirin** cautiously in patients who have liver damage, preexisting hypoprothrombinemia, or vitamin K deficiency.

Because patients with severe hepatic disease may have bleeding disorders, **ticlopidine** is not recommended for

these patients. **Ticlopidine is Pregnancy Category B. Despite the lack of evidence of teratogenic potential with this drug, it should be used in pregnancy only when clearly indicated.** Safety and efficacy in children under age 18 have not been established. Clearance increases with age, and older adults' increased sensitivity to this drug requires close monitoring for adverse effects.

Adverse Drug Reactions

All **anticoagulants** can cause excessive bleeding. Several studies have shown that the incidence of bleeding severe enough to require hospitalization or transfusion is less than 5 percent. Risk of this complication is higher early in the initiation of therapy, with wide fluctuations in aPTT or international normalized ratio (INR) and in older adults, especially women above age 60. Patients with laboratory studies within the therapeutic range who exhibit this adverse reaction should be evaluated for underlying pathological processes that may be the source of the bleed before implication of the **anticoagulant.**

Heparins can also cause thrombocytopenia and anemia. The incidence of thrombocytopenia is up to 30 percent and is more likely with bovine than porcine **heparin.** Early thrombocytopenia occurs 2 to 3 days after initiating therapy, and a delayed form occurs 7 to 12 days after initiation. If the platelet count falls below 100,000/mm^3, the **heparin** should be discontinued. **The antidote for enoxaparin overdose is protamine sulfate 1 mg for each mg of enoxaparin; for dalteparin, it is 1 mg for each 100 anti-Xa international unit (IU) of dalteparin.** Both are given by slow IV injection. Because of **heparin's** short half-life, **heparin** overdose is usually treated by withdrawal of the drug. If treatment is required, **protamine sulfate** is also the antidote for **heparin** overdose.

Toxicity and overdose of **warfarin** are usually treated by withholding one or more doses. If it must be treated, **vitamin K 1 to 10 mg is the antidote for warfarin overdose with minor bleeding; 5 to 50 mg may be used for frank bleeding.**

Hemorrhagic skin necrosis in women and cyanotic toes in men have been observed in patients with therapeutic levels of **anticoagulants.** The mechanism appears to be related to a transient inhibition in proteins S and C in patients who are congenitally absent in these clotting factors.

Although rare, allergic reactions do occur with **warfarin.** They are characterized by symmetrical maculopapular erythematous lesions. Some are isolated and some confluent. They tend to occur on the face, neck, and torso. Because of the length of time to therapeutic dose for **warfarin,** the drug reaction does not occur until the patient has been on the drug for 8 to 10 days.

Aspirin can produce gastric erosions that increase the risk of serious upper GI bleeding. This adverse effect is more likely when it is used in combination with other **anticoagulants** such as **warfarin.** Salicylism (tinnitus) associated with the use of **aspirin** occurs at serum levels above 200 µg/mL. In addition to tinnitus, indications of **aspirin** toxicity are headache, hyperventilation, agitation, mental confusion, lethargy, diarrhea, and sweating. Severe toxic effects may occur at levels above 400 µg/mL that occur with high doses. Such high doses are not used for antiplatelet therapy, so the management of severe toxicity is discussed in Chapter 23, which covers the use of **aspirin** for anti-inflammatory therapy.

Reversible neutropenia has occurred 3 weeks to 3 months after the initiation of therapy with **ticlopidine.** Severe neutropenia (less than 450 neutrophils/mm^3) or thrombocytopenia (less than 80,000 plt/mm^3) is an indication to discontinue the drug.

Drug Interactions

Cephalosporins and **penicillins** given parenterally have both been associated with coagulopathies, increasing the risk of bleeding when given with **heparin.** Although not reported for these drugs when they are given orally, there may be an increased risk. Second- and third-generation **cephalosporins** and high doses of **penicillins,** regardless of route of administration, have also been associated with an increased bleeding risk with **warfarin** because they inhibit the cyclic interconversion of vitamin K.

Drugs that affect platelet functioning or cause hypoprothrombinemia, including **aspirin, NSAIDs, dipyridamole, quinidine,** and **valproic acid,** increase the risk of bleeding when used with any **anticoagulant.**

Wells, Holbrook, and Crowther (1994) did a critical analysis of articles reporting a possible interaction between foods or drugs and **warfarin.** They searched the entire MEDLINE and TOXLINE databases and reviewed 751 citations. Of the 81 different foods and drugs appraised, only 39 were judged to have a highly probable interaction: 17 potentiating a **warfarin** effect, 10 inhibiting it, and 12 producing no effect. Drugs potentiating and inhibiting **warfarin** are shown in Table 16–2. Drugs producing no effect were **antacids, atenolol, bumetanide, enoxacin, famotidine, fluoxetine, ketorolac, metoprolol, naproxen, nizatidine, psyllium,** and **ranitidine.** Other drugs have been reported to have interactions, but convincing evidence of a causal association was lacking. Although it may be prudent to carefully monitor patients on these other drugs, these data, reported at the fourth Consensus Conference on Antithrombotic Therapy, should be kept in mind.

Clinical Pearl

To maintain anticoagulation in patients with allergic reactions to **warfarin, enoxaparin** can be given SC long term. The usual dose is 1 mg/kg.

Table 16–2. Drug Interactions: Selected Anticoagulants and Antiplatelets

Drug	Interacting Drug	Possible Effect	Implications
Anticoagulants Ardeparin Dalteparin Enoxaparin	Platelet inhibitors: aspirin, salicylates, NSAIDs, dipyridamole sulfinpyrazone, ticlopidine	Increased risk of bleeding.	Avoid concurrent use.
Heparin	Cephalosporins and penicillins	Altered platelet aggregation and other coagulopathies with increased risk of bleeding.	Mainly related to parenteral administration of these drugs; close monitoring required regardless of route of administration if used concurrently.
	Nitroglycerin	Effect of heparin may be decreased.	Reports are conflicting; monitor drug effects closely.
	Platelet inhibitors: aspirin, salicylates, NSAIDs, dipyridamole, hydroxychloroquine, phenylbutazone, ticlopidine	Increased risk of bleeding.	Avoid concurrent use.
	Digitalis, tetracycline, nicotine, antihistamines	May partially counteract anticoagulant action.	Avoid concurrent use.
Warfarin	Alcohol (if concomitant liver disease), amiodarone, anabolic steroids, cimetidine, clofibrate, cotrimoxazole, erythromycin, fluconazole, isoniazid, metronidazole, omeprazole, phenylbutazone, piroxicam, propafenone, propranolol, sulfinpyrazone	Evidence indicates it is highly probable that these drugs potentiate action with increased risk of bleeding (Wells, Holbrook, & Crowther, 1994).	Avoid concurrent use; if necessary, dosage adjustment of warfarin may be required.
	Acetaminophen, chloral hydrate, ciprofloxacin, propoxyphene, disulfiram, itraconazole, quinidine, phenytoin, tamoxifen, tetracycline, flu vaccine	Evidence indicates these drugs probably potentiate action with increased risk of bleeding (Wells, Holbrook, & Crowther, 1994).	Avoid concurrent use.
	Aspirin	Increases risk of bleeding with higher doses; even low doses of aspirin (100 mg/d) have been associated with increased risk of minor bleeding in one major study.	Avoid concurrent use.
	Oral contraceptives	May decrease the anticoagulant effect.	Use other birth control method.
	Loop diuretics	May increase anticoagulant effect and increase risk of bleeding.	Choose alternative diuretic.
	Barbiturates, carbamazepine, chlordiazepoxide, cholestyramine, dicloxacillin, griseofulvin, nafcillin, rifampin, foods high in vitamin K,* large amounts of avocado	Inhibits anticoagulant action (Wells, Holbrook, & Crowther, 1994).	Avoid concurrent use of drugs. Maintain stable intake of foods high in vitamin K so that diet is balanced.

*Foods high in vitamin K: asparagus, beans, broccoli, brussels sprouts, cabbage, cauliflower, cheese, collards, fish, milk, mustard greens, pork, rice, spinach, turnips, yogurt.

Clinical Use and Dosing

PREVENTION AND TREATMENT OF VENOUS THROMBOSIS, SYSTEMIC THROMBOSIS, AND PULMONARY EMBOLISM; PREVENTION OF EMBOLIC STROKE IN ATRIAL FIBRILLATION OR TISSUE HEART VALVES. **Warfarin** is the drug of choice for this indication. Patients with acute pulmonary emboli, deep vein thrombosis, or acute systemic embolization are admitted to the hospital for **heparin** therapy and then placed on **oral anticoagulation.** All other patients can be safely started on **warfarin** as outpatients. Therapy is initiated with 5 mg daily unless the patient weighs less than 110 pounds, is over age 75, or is at increased risk of bleeding. Patients with these weight, age, and risk parameters are started on 2.5 mg daily. Steady state is achieved in 5 to 7 days, at which time dosage adjustments are made, based on INR laboratory results. The goal of therapy is an INR of 2 to 3. Therapy is continued indefinitely for patients with valvular disease, atrial fibrillation, systemic thrombosis, or artificial heart valves. In deep vein thrombosis and pulmonary embolism, therapy is usually continued for 3 to 6 months. Patients with atrial fibrillation who are successfully treated with elective cardioversion remain on **warfarin** for 2 to 4 weeks, and therapy is then discontinued if they remain in sinus rhythm.

The American College of Chest Physicians' most recent recommendations on the prevention of venous thrombosis include consideration of the use of low molecular weight **heparin** for many high-risk groups (Clagget, Anderson, & Heit, 1995). These recommendations are given in Table 16–3.

RECURRENT SYSTEMIC EMBOLISM OR MECHANICAL HEART VALVES. **Warfarin** is the drug of choice. Therapy is initiated and maintained the same as for prevention of venous thrombosis, except that the goal of therapy is an INR of 3 to 4.5. Some authors recommend an INR of 2.5 to 3.5 for mechanical valves and report a significant reduction in bleeding risk, with little if any reduction in therapeutic value (Katsung, 1998). Therapy is continued indefinitely for mechanical heart valves. For systemic embolization that recurs after 6 months of therapy, therapy is usually continued for an additional 12 months.

PREVENTION OF MYOCARDIAL INFARCTION AND STROKE. **Aspirin** (300 to 325 mg daily) has been demonstrated to significantly decrease the risk for myocardial infarction (MI) and embolic stroke. For patients with sensitive GI tracts, enteric-coated tablets often are used, although their bioavailability is somewhat erratic. Doses of 81 to 100 mg also reduce GI problems, but these low doses require a single daily dose of 300 to 325 mg twice monthly (first and fifteenth day of the month). **Ticlopidine** (250 mg bid) taken with food is also acceptable for this indication. Long-term therapy with **ticlopidine** has yet to be evaluated. Given the significantly increased half-life that occurs with long-term dosing, it is reserved for patients with aspirin intolerance or hypersensitivity.

PREVENTION OF POSTOPERATIVE DEEP VEIN THROMBOSIS OR THROMBOEMBOLISM. Low molecular weight **heparins** have been approved for limited applications in prevention of deep vein thrombosis after hip, knee, and abdominal surgeries. They are used for 14 days or less and are prescribed by the surgeon. SC **heparin** may be used for a similar application in a variety of surgeries and for patients with long-term reduced mobility. The primary care provider is likely to deal with the low molecular weight **heparin** drugs mainly on a short-term basis. Management of patients in extended care facilities may include the use of both low molecular weight and regular **heparin** on a longer basis.

TREATMENT OF PATIENTS ON LONG-TERM WARFARIN THERAPY WHO REQUIRE SURGERY. Two different approaches can be taken in maintaining adequate anticoagulation to prevent thrombotic or embolic events while not increasing the risk of bleeding during a surgical procedure. The first is to stop **warfarin** 4 to 5 days prior to surgery and replace it with high-dose **heparin** therapy (17,500 units [U] every 12 hours) adjusted to maintain the aPTT in the midtherapeutic range. In the hospital, the patient can then be placed on IV **heparin** that can be discontinued 3 hours before surgery, or the SC route can be continued and stopped 12 hours before surgery. The second approach is to continue the **warfarin** but keep the INR around 1.5 during the surgical procedure. This level has been shown to be safe in selected surgeries. In each case, **warfarin** therapy is restarted postoperatively. For patients undergoing dental procedures, tranexamic acid mouthwash can be used without interrupting anticoagulant therapy. It is also recommended that **ticlopidine** and **aspirin** be discontinued 10 to 14 days before surgery. Increased blood loss has occurred with patients on these drugs at the time of surgery.

Rational Drug Selection

COST. Although SC administration of an **anticoagulant** (**heparin**) is usually a short-term measure, cost is still a significant factor. The difference in cost between **heparin** and the newer low molecular weight **heparins** (**ardeparin, dalteparin, enoxaparin**) is significant, with the newer drugs being much more expensive. Of these drugs, **enoxaparin** is the least expensive and has been used longer term in some situations. When the cost of laboratory monitoring is factored into the equation, the difference in cost between the low molecular weight **heparins** and regular **heparin** is less dramatic. All injectable forms are more expensive than oral forms because of the need for equipment to deliver them. Of all the drugs used to prevent clotting, **aspirin** is by far the cheapest.

ROUTE OF ADMINISTRATION. Oral anticoagulation is preferred because it does not require specialized equipment or skills to administer, and it is less expensive. For

Table 16–3. Dosage Schedule: Selected Anticoagulants and Antiplatelets

Drug	Indication	Initial Dose	Maintenance Dose
Ardeparin	Prevention of deep vein thrombosis (DVT) after knee surgery	50 anti-Xa U/kg	50 anti-Xa U/kg qd for <14 days after knee surgery
	High-risk surgical patients (age >40; previous DVT; immobility; cancer; major surgery; obesity; congestive heart failure (CHF); MI; stroke; pelvic, hip, and leg fractures; high-dose estrogen)*	50 anti-Xa U/kg	50 anti-Xa U/kg qd
Aspirin	MI and stroke prevention	300–325 mg qd	300–325 mg qd
Dalteparin	Prevention of DVT after abdominal surgery	2500 IU qd	2500 IU qd for 5–10 d after surgery
	High-risk surgical patients (same as ardeparin)*	2500 IU qd	2500 IU qd for 5–10 d after surgery
Enoxaparin	Prevention of DVT after hip, knee, or abdominal surgery	30 mg bid for hip or knee surgery; 40 mg bid for abdominal surgery	30–40 mg bid for <14 days for hip or knee surgery; 7–10 days for abdominal surgery
	Systemic anticoagulation	1 mg/kg bid	1 mg/kg bid
	Recurrent systemic embolism prevention	40 mg qd	40 mg qd
	High-risk surgical patients (same as ardeparin)*	40 mg bid	30–40 mg bid for 7–10 d
Heparin	Preventive of postoperative thromboembolism	5000 IU 2 h preop	5000 U q8–12h for 7 d after surgery
Ticlopidine	Preventive of stroke in patients intolerant of aspirin	250 mg bid with food	250 mg bid with food
Warfarin	Prevention and treatment of venous thrombosis, systemic embolism, and pulmonary embolism; prevention of embolic stroke in atrial fibrillation	5 mg qd; for patients <110 lb, >age 75, or at increased risk of bleeding: 2.5 mg qd	Measure INR at 5–7 d and adjust to INR of 2–3
	Recurrent systemic embolism and mechanical heart valves		Measure INR at 5–7 d and adjust to INR of 3–4.5
	Total hip replacement or hip fracture surgery*	5 mg qd For patients <110 lb, > age 75, or at increased risk of bleeding: 2.5 mg qd	Measure INR at 5–7 d and adjust to INR of 2–3

*Recommendation of American College of Chest Physicians. They also state that low molecular weight heparin may be used for hip fracture surgery, ischemic stroke with paralysis of lower extremities, and medical patients with clinical risk factors. Specific doses are not given for these indications, but fixed dose bid started postoperatively is recommended for surgical patients.

patients who cannot swallow or for other reasons cannot take an **oral anticoagulant,** SC injections of **heparin** in either standard or low molecular weight formulation can be used. Patients or their family members must be taught correct techniques for administration (Table 16–4).

BRAND. Anticoagulant effects may vary slightly by brand. Because even small variances can cause significant differences in anticoagulation, brands should not be interchanged. **Warfarin** comes in a variety of tablet strengths, making it possible to be exact in dosing, and it is the preferred **oral anticoagulant.** These tablets are color-coded by dose, which also makes it easier to be certain the patient

takes the correct dose, especially if the dose is prescribed over the telephone.

Monitoring

Monitoring for dosage adjustments of **warfarin** is by INR blood tests. Daily INRs are done initially to guard against excessive anticoagulation in unusually sensitive patients and are continued until the therapeutic range is achieved and maintained for at least 2 consecutive days. The testing interval is then lengthened to two or three times weekly for 1 or 2 weeks, then less often, depending on

Table 16–4. Available Dosage Forms: Anticoagulants and Antiplatelets

Drug	Dosage Form (Tablet/Capsule)	Other Forms
Ardeparin (Normiflo)	—	In 0.5 cc in 10-syringe pack with 25 g $\times$ $\frac{5}{8}$-in 5,000 anti-Xa units 10,000 anti-Xa units
Aspirin	81-mg chewable (orange flavor) 165-mg enteric-coated 325-mg tablets Also in film coated and caplets	—
Dalteparin (Fragmin)	—	In 10-syringe pack: 16 mg/ 0.2 cc 32 mg/0.2 cc
Enoxaparin (Lovenox)	—	In 10-syringe pack with 27 g $\times$ $\frac{1}{2}$-in needles: 30 mg/0.3 cc 40 mg/0.4 cc
Heparin sodium	—	In multiple-dose vials: 1000 U/cc (1-, 10-, 30-cc vials) 2000 U/cc (5-, 10-cc vials) 2500 U/cc (5-, 10-cc vials) 5000 U/cc (1-, 10-cc vials) 10,000 U/cc (0.5-, 1-, 4-, 5-, 10-cc vials) 20,000 U/cc (1-, 2-, 4-cc vials) 40,000 U/cc (1-, 2-, 5-cc vials)
Ticlopidine (Ticlid)	250-mg tablets (In 30 and 100 tablets/bottle)	—
Warfarin (Coumadin)	Scored tablets: 1-mg pink 2-mg lavender 2.5-mg green 3-mg tan 4-mg blue 5-mg peach 6-mg teal 7.5-mg yellow 10-mg white (In 100 and 1000 tablets/bottle)	—

the stability of the INR results. If the INR results remain stable, testing is reduced to as seldom as every 6 weeks. Drawing the blood in the morning with the patient taking the drug in the evening provides more stable results and allows rapid dosage changes if necessary.

Protocols for dosage adjustments vary, but to maximize safety and avoid wide swings in anticoagulation, 10 percent changes in weekly doses are best unless the INR is widely out of range. If the INR is too low, the total weekly dose is adjusted upward by 10 percent and the INR is rechecked in 2 weeks. If the INR is too high, the daily dose is held for 1 day and then the weekly dose is adjusted downward by 10 percent and the INR is rechecked in 2 weeks. If the INR is above therapeutic range but less than 6, the patient is not bleeding, and rapid reversal is not indicated for surgical intervention, then two or more doses

can be omitted and daily INRs are drawn. **Warfarin** is then resumed at a lower dose when the INR is within therapeutic range. If the INR is greater than 6 but less than 10 and the patient is not bleeding, or when rapid reversal is indicated, **vitamin K** (1 to 2 mg) can be given SC. After **vitamin K,** the INR usually returns to a 2 to 3 range within 24 hours. INR results above 10 or serious bleeding suggests referral. If the INR has frequent variability, external reasons such as dietary changes, undisclosed drug use, poor adherence, and intermittent **alcohol** consumption are evaluated, and the INR is drawn daily or weekly until a stable INR is reached. Once a stable dose is reached, monitoring may be done every 3 months.

Monitoring for dosage adjustment of **heparin** is by aPTT blood tests. The goal of therapy is 1.5 to 2.5 times the control. Platelet counts and hematocrit are done every 2 or 3 days initially. Thrombocytopenia tends to occur about the fourth day and resolves despite continued **heparin** therapy. Thrombocytopenia severe enough to require discontinuing therapy may occur about the eighth day of therapy. After this time, periodic testing of platelet and hematocrit levels and testing for occult blood in the stool are done during the course of **heparin** therapy regardless of the route of administration. Low doses of SC **heparin** (5000 U bid) do not require monitoring because this regimen does not prolong the aPTT. For the low molecular weight **heparins**, the same periodic monitoring of platelet and hematocrit levels is required, but the likelihood of thrombocytopenia is much less. No monitoring of aPTT is required.

The dose of **aspirin** for antiplatelet therapy is low to moderate. The serum salicylate level is approximately 100 µg/mL. At low doses, no specific monitoring is required, although **aspirin** will prolong bleeding time.

Severe neutropenia and thrombocytopenia have occurred with the administration of **ticlopidine.** The onset of these problems occurred 3 weeks to 3 months after the start of therapy, with no documented cases beyond that time. It is essential that complete blood counts (CBCs) and white blood cell (WBC) differential counts be performed every 2 weeks, starting from the second week to the end of the third month of therapy. More frequent monitoring is necessary for patients whose absolute neutrophil counts consistently decline or are 30 percent lower than baseline counts. After the first 3 months of therapy, CBCs are needed only for patients with signs or symptoms suggesting an infection.

Patient Education: Anticoagulants

ADMINISTRATION. **Anticoagulants** should be taken exactly as prescribed, at the same time each day, even if the patient is feeling well. Missed doses should be taken as soon as remembered the same day. Doses should not be doubled. The health care provider should be informed of missed doses at the time of checkup or laboratory tests. Doses are highly individualized and are determined by the results of laboratory tests (INR for **oral anticoagulants** and aPTT, platelet counts, and hematocrit for **heparin**). Patients should not change the dose unless directed to do so by the health care provider and should have the laboratory tests drawn each time they are ordered.

Difference in anticoagulation effect can occur between brands. The drug is prescribed by brand name and should be consistently filled that way. **Warfarin** tablets are color-coded by dose, and patients should learn the color code for the brand used. For the **heparins,** which are injectable, the patient or a family member must be taught correct SC injection technique.

Oral anticoagulants may be taken without regard to timing of food intake. The type of food, however, is important. Ingestion of large quantities of foods high in vitamin K may antagonize the anticoagulant effect. This does not mean that these foods must be avoided entirely. They are part of a well-balanced diet. They should be eaten in consistent amounts so that anticoagulation levels can be maintained at a consistent level.

Drug interactions may also occur with some over-the-counter (OTC) drugs, particularly **aspirin, NSAIDs,** and cold remedies that contain these products, and with alcohol. Many drugs are also prepared in an alcohol base. Some multivitamins contain vitamin K and should not be taken. The patient should consult with the primary care provider before taking any OTC medications or new prescription medications.

ADVERSE REACTIONS. Unusual bleeding is the most common adverse effect for all **anticoagulants.** To prevent bleeding, the patient should use a soft toothbrush, avoid flossing, shave with an electric razor, and, if cut, apply pressure for 5 to 10 minutes. If the bleeding does not stop, the patient should continue the pressure and contact the health care provider. Whenever possible, intramuscular (IM) injections should be avoided. If they must be given, apply pressure to the injection site for 2 to 5 minutes to prevent bleeding or hematoma formation. Applying ice to the site of an SC injection for about 30 seconds prior to injecting the **heparin** reduces the chances of bleeding and hematoma formation. The following should be reported to the health care provider:

1. Any bleeding that does not stop within 5 minutes
2. Nosebleeds and bleeding gums
3. Red or pink tinged urine
4. Faintness or weakness
5. Headaches
6. Stomach pains
7. Skin rash or unusual bruising
8. Red, black, or tarry stools or diarrhea

Dermal necrosis occurs in a small percentage of patients. Necrotic skin lesions in women and cyanotic toes in men should be reported.

Warfarin is contraindicated in pregnancy. Women who are capable of becoming pregnant should have this topic discussed with them, and contraception should be instituted before prescribing this drug.

To reduce the risk of adverse reactions, the patient should wear an identification bracelet that states the anticoagulant being taken. Inform all health care providers about the anticoagulation therapy so that new prescriptions and any treatments can take it into account. The patient should consult the health care provider before undergoing dental work or elective surgery.

Patient Education: Antiplatelets

ADMINISTRATION. Daily dosing is the usual way **aspirin** is taken for antiplatelet effects. Taking it with a full glass of water reduces the risk of lodging the drug in the esophagus. Because **aspirin** may cause GI upset, it should be taken with food or after meals. Enteric-coated forms are available but have slightly less reliable amounts of drug reaching the bloodstream. Enteric-coated tablets may not be crushed or chewed. For patients with difficulty in swallowing, liquid forms are available. **Aspirin** that has a strong vinegarlike odor should not be used.

Ticlopidine may also cause GI upset and ought to be taken with a full glass of water and with food or after meals.

ADVERSE REACTIONS. Toxicity to **aspirin** may occur even with small doses in some patients, who should immediately report to the health care provider ringing in the ears (tinnitus), unusual headache, hyperventilation, agitation, mental confusion, lethargy, diarrhea, or sweating.

For **ticlopidine,** a decrease in the number of WBCs can occur, especially during the first 3 months of therapy. A severe decrease can increase risk for infection. It is critical that the patient obtain the scheduled blood tests to detect this problem. Report to the health care provider any indications of infection such as fever, chills, or sore throat. **Ticlopidine** can also affect liver function. Promptly report severe or persistent diarrhea, skin rashes, yellow skin or sclerae, dark urine, or light-colored stools.

For both drugs, unusual bleeding is the most common adverse effect. To prevent bleeding, the patient should use a soft toothbrush, avoid flossing, shave with an electric razor, and, if cut, apply pressure for 5 to 10 minutes.

Hematopoietic Growth Factors

Hematopoietic growth factors are glycoprotein hormones that regulate the proliferation and differentiation of hematopoietic progenitor cells in the bone marrow. Produced by recombinant DNA technology, these factors include **erythropoietin, granulocyte colony-stimulating factor (G-CSF),** and **granulocyte-macrophage colony-stimulating factor (GM-CSF).** Anemias due to deficiency in erythropoietin, such as those found in patients with end-stage renal disease or AIDS or patients undergoing chemotherapy, are among the most refractory to treatment. The introduction of these **growth factors** has made effective treatment possible. Their use is also being investigated for anemic patients with normal erythropoietin levels who wish to donate their own blood before surgery for autologous transfusions.

Pharmacodynamics

Stem cells in the hematopoietic bone marrow respond to various colony-stimulating factors and erythropoietin to produce mature erythrocytes and WBCs. Erythrocyte differentiation proceeds from erythroblasts through normoblasts to reticulocytes and finally to mature erythrocytes, based on stimulation from erythropoietin, with additional support from GM-CSF and interleukin-3 (IL-3). Granulocytes (neutrophils, eosinophils, and basophils/mast cells) are fully matured in the bone marrow by stimulation from G-CSF, GM-CSF, and IL-3. The agranulocytes (monocytes and lymphocytes) are produced by the stimulation from GM-CSF, IL-3, and macrophage colony-stimulating factor (M-CSF) and are released into the bloodstream before they mature. Monocytes become mature macrophages within 1 or 2 days, and lymphocytes travel to the lymphoid tissues, where they are stimulated to differentiate into T cells or B cells. The development of these blood cells is shown in Figure 16–2.

Endogenous erythropoietin is produced by the normal kidney in response to tissue hypoxia. In anemia, more erythropoietin is produced, signaling the bone marrow to produce more erythrocytes. Unless there is iron deficiency, a primary bone marrow disorder, or bone marrow suppression from drugs and chronic disease, this stimulation of erythrocyte production corrects the anemia. In addition to iron, erythropoiesis is dependent on sufficient amounts of vitamin B_{12} and folic acid. In end-stage renal disease, the kidney is unable to produce the erythropoietin necessary for the stimulation of erythrocyte growth. **Epoetin alfa (Epogen, Procrit)** has the same biologic effects as erythropoietin.

Endogenous colony-stimulating factors respond to decreased leukocyte counts or the presence of infection to signal the production of leukocytes. G-CSF is lineage-specific, supporting the proliferation and differentiation of neutrophils. GM-CSF is multipotential, stimulating proliferation and differentiation of early and late granulocyte progenitor cells, as well as erythroid and megakaryocyte progenitors. **Filgrastim (Neupogen)** has the same biologic effects as G-CSF. **Sargramostim (Leukine)** has the same biologic effect as GM-CSF.

Pharmacokinetics

Absorption and Distribution

All **hematopoietic growth factors** are well absorbed following SC injection. Their distribution is similar to their endogenous equivalents (Table 16–5).

Metabolism and Excretion

Epoetin alfa is eliminated by first-order kinetics with a circulating half-life of 4 to 13 hours in patients with chronic renal failure. There is no apparent difference in half-life for patients on or not on dialysis. The half-life is

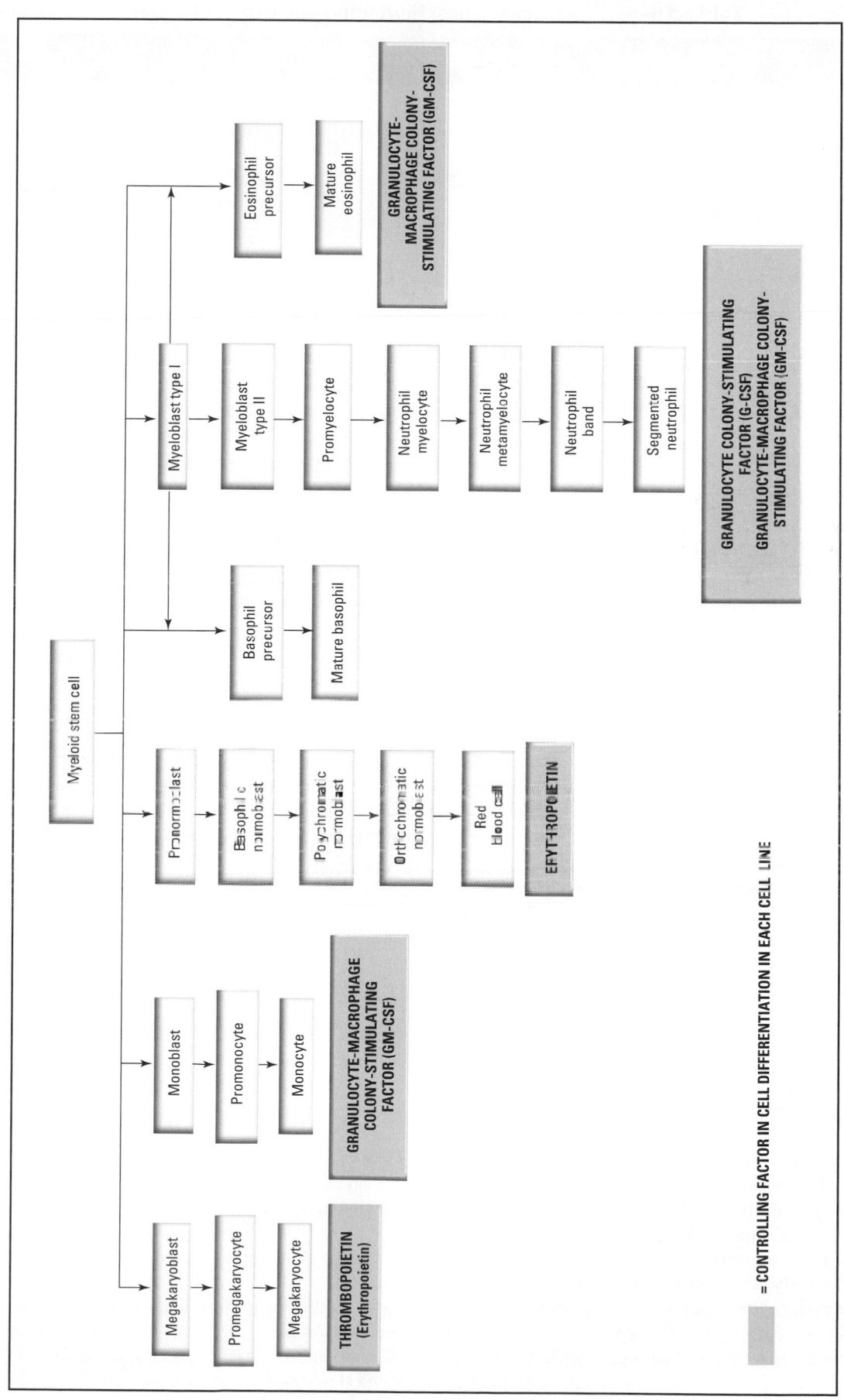

Figure 16-2. Development of blood cells.

Table 16–5. Pharmacokinetics: Hematopoietic Growth Factors

Drug	Onset	Peak	Duration	Half-Life
Epoetin alfa	10 days*	5–24 h	>24 h	4–13 h in chronic renal failure (about 20% shorter in healthy patients)
Filgrastim	—	2–8 h	—	3.5 h
Sargramostim	—	3 h	12 h	1.6–2.6 h

*Increase in reticulocytes.

about 20 percent shorter in healthy patients. **Filgrastim** is also eliminated by first-order kinetics, with an elimination half-life of 3.5 hours in healthy patients and those with cancer. **Sargramostim** has a half-life after SC injection of 2.6 hours.

Pharmacotherapeutics

Precautions and Contraindications

The only contraindication for **epoetin alfa** is uncontrolled hypertension; increases in erythrocyte production may also be accompanied by increases in extracellular fluid (ECF) volume, which can increase blood pressure. Up to 80 percent of patients with chronic renal failure (CRF) have hypertension, which should be controlled before a patient starts **epoetin alfa** therapy and carefully monitored during such therapy. During early phases of therapy, when the hematocrit is increasing, about 25 percent of patients with CRF require initiation of or increases in antihypertensive therapy. Hypertension has been observed rarely in patients with cancer or HIV who are being treated with this drug.

Epoetin alfa is Pregnancy Category C. Adverse effects have occurred in rats, and there are no adequate and well-controlled studies in pregnant women. Use only if the potential benefit clearly outweighs the risk to the fetus. Contraception may be appropriate prior to initiating therapy. Some women's menses have resumed after therapy with this drug. It is not known whether this drug is excreted in breast milk. Caution is advised in prescribing to lactating women. Safety and efficacy have not been established in children.

The only contraindication for **filgrastim** is hypersensitivity to *Escherichia coli*–derived proteins because this drug is derived from DNA manipulation of *E. coli*. *Filgrastim* is Pregnancy Category C. There are no adequate and well-controlled studies in pregnant women. Use only if the potential benefit clearly outweighs the risk to the fetus. Contraception may be appropriate prior to initiating therapy. It is not known whether this drug is excreted in breast milk. Caution is advised in prescribing to lactating women. Serious long-term risks associated with daily **filgrastim** have not been identified in children age 4 months to 17 years with severe chronic neutropenia. The safety and efficacy in neonates and patients with autoimmune neutropenia have not been established.

Contraindications to **sargramostim** include excessive leukemic myeloid blasts in the bone marrow and known hypersensitivity to the product or to yeast-derived products. Occasional transient supraventricular arrhythmias have occurred, especially with patients who have a history of cardiac arrhythmias. Use with caution for patients with such a history. Sequestration of granulocytes in the pulmonary circulation with occasional dyspnea has occurred, especially in patients with preexisting lung diseases. Administer with caution to patients with hypoxia. Fluid retention has occurred in a few patients. Use with caution for patients with preexisting fluid retention, pulmonary infiltrates, or congestive heart failure.

Sargramostim is Pregnancy Category C. There are no adequate and well-controlled studies in pregnant women. Use only if the potential benefit clearly outweighs the risk to the fetus. Contraception may be appropriate prior to initiating therapy. It is not known whether this drug is excreted in breast milk. Caution is advised in prescribing to lactating women. Safety and efficacy in children have not been established.

Adverse Drug Reactions

Seizures have been observed in some patients being treated with **epoetin alfa** (2.5% of patients undergoing dialysis during the first 90 days of therapy). The relationship with seizure is uncertain, and the risk appears to lessen when the rate of increase in hematocrit is slower.

Skin rashes and urticaria are rare, mild, and transient. There is no evidence of antibody formation to **epoetin alfa.**

The major adverse reaction is hypertension. The risk is higher in patients with CRF, and the reaction is discussed in the Precautions and Contraindications section. There have been rare reports of serious or unusual thromboembolic events. A causal relationship has not been established.

Allergic-type reactions have developed with **filgrastim** on initial and subsequent treatment in fewer than 1 in 4000 patients. Skin, respiratory, and cardiovascular systems common to most hypersensitivity reactions are typical. Administration of **antihistamines, steroids, bronchodilators,** or **epinephrine** resulted in resolution. Symptoms recurred in more than 50 percent of the patients who were rechallenged with this drug.

Adverse reactions to **sargramostim** include headache and transient pruritic rashes. Hypersensitivity reactions are rare. Cardiovascular, respiratory, and fluid retention problems are discussed in the Precautions and Contraindications section.

All of the **hematopoietic growth factors** can produce bone pain from the stimulation of the bone marrow. This may require analgesia.

Drug Interactions

Drug interactions for all the **hematopoietic growth factors** are minimal (Table 16–6). Only those drugs such as **lithium** that may potentiate myeloproliferative effects require avoidance of concurrent use or cautious use.

Clinical Use and Dosing

ANEMIA ASSOCIATED WITH CHRONIC RENAL FAILURE. **Epoetin alfa** is the drug of choice to elevate and maintain erythrocyte levels and decrease the need for transfusions. Patients both on dialysis and not on dialysis benefit equally. It is not intended for immediate correction of severe anemia because it takes 10 days to see increases in reticulocyte counts. The starting dose is 50 to 100 U/kg given SC three times weekly. Maintenance doses are based on individual responses, and adjustments are based on hematocrit levels. Table 16–7 shows guidelines for dosage adjustments. Dosage adjustments are not to be made more than once monthly, based on the time it takes for erythroid progenitors to mature and red blood cell (RBC) survival time.

ANEMIA RELATED TO ZIDOVUDINE THERAPY IN PATIENTS WITH HIV INFECTION. **Epoetin alfa** is the drug of choice to elevate and maintain erythrocyte levels and decrease the need for transfusions when the endogenous erythropoietin level is 500 mU/cc or less and the dose of zidovudine is 4200 mg/week or less. The initial dose is 100 U/kg SC three times weekly for 8 weeks. Maintenance doses are based on individual responses, and adjustments are based on hematocrit levels. Table 16–7 shows the general guidelines for dosage adjustments. Dosage adjustments are timed as noted previously.

ANEMIA IN PATIENTS WITH CANCER ON CHEMOTHERAPY. **Epoetin alfa** is the drug of choice to elevate and maintain erythrocyte levels and decrease the need for transfusions. The initial dose is 150 U/kg given SC three times weekly. Patients with lower baseline serum **erythropoietin** levels tend to respond more vigorously to this drug. Treatment is not recommended for patients with serum **erythropoietin** levels below 200 mU/cc. Dosage adjustments are made after 8 weeks of therapy. Table 16–7 shows the general guidelines for dosage adjustments. Dosage adjustments are timed as noted previously.

REDUCTION IN NEED FOR ALLOGENEIC BLOOD TRANSFUSIONS IN SURGERY PATIENTS WITH HEMOGLOBIN LEVELS BETWEEN 10 AND 13. Anemic patients scheduled to undergo elective, noncardiac, nonvascular surgery, with anticipated significant blood loss, benefit from **epoetin alfa** therapy to reduce the need for allogeneic blood transfusions. The recommended dose is 300 U/kg a day SC for 10 days prior to surgery, on the day of surgery, and for 4 days after surgery. An alternative dosing schedule is 600 U/kg once weekly at 21, 14, and 7 days before surgery, plus a fourth dose on the day of surgery. All patients on these regimens must receive adequate **iron** supplementation, beginning no later than the start of the epoetin therapy and continuing throughout the therapy.

DECREASE THE INCIDENCE OF INFECTION IN PATIENTS ON MYELOSUPPRESSIVE THERAPY. Both **filgrastim** and

Table 16–6. Drug Interactions: Hematopoietic Growth Factors

Drug	Interacting Drug	Possible Effect	Implications
Epoetin alfa	Heparin	May increase requirement for heparin anticoagulation during dialysis	Monitor aPTT carefully in dialysis patients.
Filgrastim	Lithium	May potentiate the release of neutrophils	Drug interaction not fully studied; no recommendations at this time.
	Antineoplastic agents	Simultaneous use may have adverse effect on rapidly proliferating neutrophils	Avoid use 24 h before or 24 h after chemotherapy.
Sargramostim	Lithium	May potentiate myeloproliferative effects of sargramostim	Avoid concurrent use or use cautiously.

Table 16–7. Dosage Schedule: Hematopoietic Growth Factors

Drug	Indication	Initial Dose	Maintenance Dose
Epoetin alfa	Anemia in chronic renal failure	50–100 U/kg 3 times weekly	Individualized; reduced dose when hematocrit (Hct) approaches 36% or increases >4 points in any 2-wk period. Increase dose if Hct does not increase by 5–6 points after 8 wk of therapy and remains below target range of 30–36%.
	Zidovudine-treated HIV-infected patients	100 U/kg 3 times weekly for 8 wk	Individualized; when the desired response is attained, titrate to maintain it. If response is too low, increase by 50–100 U/kg three times weekly. Evaluate response every 4–8 wk and adjust by 50–100 U/kg increments. If response is too low at 300 U/kg, response is unlikely. If Hct exceeds 40%, stop dose until Hct is 36%, then resume treatment with a dose reduced by 25%.
	Cancer patients on chemotherapy	150 U/kg 3 times weekly	If response is too low after 8 wk, increase dose up to 300 U/kg three times weekly; higher doses are not likely to produce a response. If Hct exceeds 40%, or increases >4% in any 2-wk period, stop dose until Hct is 36%, then resume treatment with a dose reduced by 25%.
	Presurgery	300 U/kg/d *or*	Given 10 d prior to surgery, day of surgery, and for 4 d after surgery.
		600 U/kg once weekly	Given 21, 14, and 7 d prior to surgery and then day of surgery.
Filgrastim	Myelosuppressive chemotherapy	5 μg/kg/d no earlier than 24 h after or 24 h before next dose of chemotherapy	Dose given daily for up to 2 wk. Discontinue therapy if ANC>10,000 mm^3 after expected nadir of chemotherapy.
	Severe chronic neutropenia: Congenital	6 μg/kg twice daily	Individualized; reduce dose if ANC persistently >10,000 mm^3.
	Cyclic/idiopathic	5 μg/kg daily	

sargramostim have been used for this indication. It is an unlabeled use in the latter. The recommended starting dose for **filgrastim** is 5 μg/kg a day given as a single dose SC. Dosage adjustments are based on CBC and platelet data and are done in increments of 5 μg/kg per day, according to the duration and severity of the absolute neutrophil count (ANC) nadir. It is given daily for up to 2 weeks until the ANC has reached 10,000 mm^3. Clinical trials have shown effective doses to be 4 to 8 μg/kg a day. Because it is an unlabeled use, the dosing schedule for **sargramostim** is not specified in the literature. Because of the specialty use of this drug and the need for IV administration, it is not discussed here.

SEVERE CHRONIC NEUTROPENIA. Severe chronic neutropenia (SCN) can be congenital, cyclic, or idiopathic. Chronic administration of **filgrastim** reduces the incidence and duration of sequelae of neutropenia, such as fever, infection, and oropharyngeal ulcers. The initial dose for congenital SCN is 6 μg/kg twice daily SC. For cyclic or idiopathic SCN, the initial dose is 5 μg/kg every day. Dosage adjustments are based on the patient's clinical course and ANC.

Other indications for the use of these drugs, including bone marrow transplant, are beyond the scope of this book.

Rational Drug Selection

This choice of drug is based on its indication because each drug has very specific uses.

Monitoring

Monitoring parameters are different for each drug and are discussed specific to that drug.

EPOETIN ALFA. Patients with CRF not on dialysis require monitoring of blood pressure and hematocrit no less frequently than patients maintained on dialysis. Hematocrit is monitored twice weekly until it is stabilized in the target zone and the maintenance dose has been established and then for at least 2 to 6 weeks after each dosage adjustment. Maintenance monitoring is individualized, based on patient stability. In some patients, increases in blood urea nitrogen (BUN), creatinine, uric acid, phosphorus, and potassium have been noted. These values are routinely monitored in patients with CRF and require no additional monitoring.

Patients on **zidovudine** therapy for HIV infection require monitoring of hematocrit weekly until it is stabilized. Periodic monitoring thereafter is based on the progression of the disease.

During therapy with **epoetin alfa,** absolute and functional iron deficiency may develop. Functional iron deficiency is presumed to be based on inability to mobilize iron stores rapidly enough to support increased erythropoiesis. Transferrin saturation should be at least 20 percent, and ferritin should be at least 100 ng/cc. Prior to initiating therapy and at regular intervals during therapy, determine transferrin and ferritin levels. Virtually all patients at some point require supplemental **iron.**

Delayed or diminished responses suggest referral to a hematologist. *Drug Facts and Comparisons* (Kastrup, 1998) lists possible common etiologies for patients who fail to respond or to maintain a response to doses within the recommended range:

1. Functional iron deficiency
2. Underlying infectious, inflammatory, or malignant disease
3. Occult blood loss
4. Underlying hematologic diseases, such as thalassemia, refractory anemia, or myelodysplastic disorder
5. Vitamin B_{12} or folic acid deficiency
6. Hemolysis
7. Aluminum intoxication

FILGRASTIM. For patients on myelosuppressive chemotherapy, CBCs and platelet counts are done prior to initiating therapy and twice weekly during therapy. Following therapy, the same indicators are monitored around the time of the nadir of the chemotherapy. **Filgrastim** therapy may be terminated when the ANC is 10,000 mm^3 or greater. For patients with SCN, CBCs with differential, platelet counts, and evaluation of bone marrow morphology and karyotype are done prior to initiating therapy. During the initial 4 weeks of therapy and for 2 weeks after any dosage adjustment, CBCs with differential and platelet counts are done. Once the patient is stable, monthly CBCs with differential and platelet counts are sufficient.

Patient Education

ADMINISTRATION. If the patient can safely and effectively self-administer these drugs, instruction is provided in correct SC injection technique and proper dosage (Table 16–8). Self-administration is common in patients with CRF. Detailed instructions on dilution and storage stability are included in the package insert.

ADVERSE DRUG REACTIONS. Hypertension and allergic reactions are the two most common adverse reactions. Self-monitoring of blood pressure and signs and symptoms of an allergic reaction are taught.

Iron Preparations

Iron is an essential mineral in the production of hemoglobin, myoglobin, and a number of enzymes. Iron-deficiency anemia results in problems with oxygen transport that affect the energy metabolism of every cell in the body. Iron-deficiency anemia is commonly seen in infants, particularly premature infants; in children during rapid growth periods; and in pregnant and lactating women. It may also occur after gastrectomy and with

Table 16–8. Available Dosage Forms: Hematopoietic Growth Factors

Drug	Dosage Form	Other Forms
Epoetin alfa (Epogen, Procrit)	Subcutaneous: (in 1-cc single-dose vials) 2000 U/cc 3000 U/cc 4000 U/cc 10,000 U/cc 20,000 U/cc	—
Filgrastim (Neupogen)	Subcutaneous: (in 1- and 1.6-cc single-dose vials; preservative-free) 300 µg/cc	—

malabsorption disorders, particularly those of the small bowel. The most common cause in adults is blood loss. Menstruation may cause the loss of more than 30 mg of iron with each period. Occult blood loss may occur from GI bleeding and from cancer. Prevention and treatment of this form of anemia are accomplished by administration of supplemental iron.

Pharmacodynamics

Approximately 67 percent of total body iron is bound to heme in red blood cells and muscle cells, and approximately 30 percent is stored bound to ferritin or hemosiderin mononuclear phagocytes and hepatic parenchymal cells. The remaining 3 percent is lost daily in urine, sweat, bile, and epithelial cells shed from the GI tract. Iron not lost is continuously recycled, as shown in Figure 16–3. Recycling is made possible by transferrin.

As iron deficiency develops, storage **iron** decreases and then disappears, followed by decreased serum ferritin and then serum iron. Finally iron-binding capacity increases, resulting in a decrease in transferrin saturation. At this point, anemia develops. Administration of **iron** reverses the process so that eventually not only is serum iron improved but also iron storage is replenished. Management of anemia is discussed in Chapter 25.

Pharmacokinetics

Absorption and Distribution

Only about 10 percent of the average daily dietary intake of **iron** is absorbed (1 to 2 mg/day) in patients with adequate iron stores. Absorption is enhanced in the presence of depleted iron stores and when erythropoiesis is increased. Iron is primarily absorbed in the duodenum and upper jejunum by an active transport mechanism.

The ferrous form is absorbed three times more readily than the ferric form. The common ferrous forms (sulfate, gluconate, and fumarate) are absorbed almost on a milligram-for-milligram basis but differ in the amount of elemental iron each contains.

Factors that significantly affect absorption include sustained-release forms, dose, and the presence of food. Sustained-release or enteric-coated forms have less available **iron** because they transport the **iron** beyond the duodenum before it is released. As dose increases, the amount of **iron** absorbed increases, but the percentage of **iron** absorbed decreases. Food can decrease the absorption of **iron** by 40 to 66 percent, but gastric intolerance often requires administration with food. Concurrent administration of **vitamin C** may enhance absorption, but the literature is still controversial. Eggs and milk inhibit **iron** absorption.

Iron is transported via blood bound to transferrin. The transferrin-ferric iron complex is delivered to maturing erythroid cells, where transferrin receptors pick up and internalize the iron and release it within the cell.

Metabolism, Storage, and Excretion

Iron is stored as either ferritin or hemosiderin. Ferritin is more readily available and is water soluble. Hemosiderin is a particulate substance containing aggregates of ferric core crystals. Both are stored in macrophages in the liver, spleen, and bone marrow. Because the ferritin present in plasma is in equilibrium with stored ferritin, the plasma ferritin level can be used to estimate total-body iron stores.

There is no mechanism for excretion of iron. Iron is lost mainly through shedding of the GI mucosal cells, with small losses in urine, sweat, and bile. These losses total no more than 1 mg of iron per day. Because the body has no mechanism for excretion of iron, iron balance is achieved largely through control of the amount of **iron** absorbed in the gut.

ON THE HORIZON

Interleukin-3, Stem Cell Factor, and Monocyte-Macrophage Colony-Stimulating Factor

IL-3, stem cell factor, and **monocyte-macrophage colony-stimulating factor** are currently in clinical trials. **IL-3** would provide broad-based therapy because it is involved in the generation and stimulation of all progenitor cells. **Stem cell factor** would provide therapy at an even earlier stage in blood cell development. **Monocyte-macrophage colony-stimulating factor** would provide a targeted approach to patients who do not require such a broad stimulation of blood cell growth.

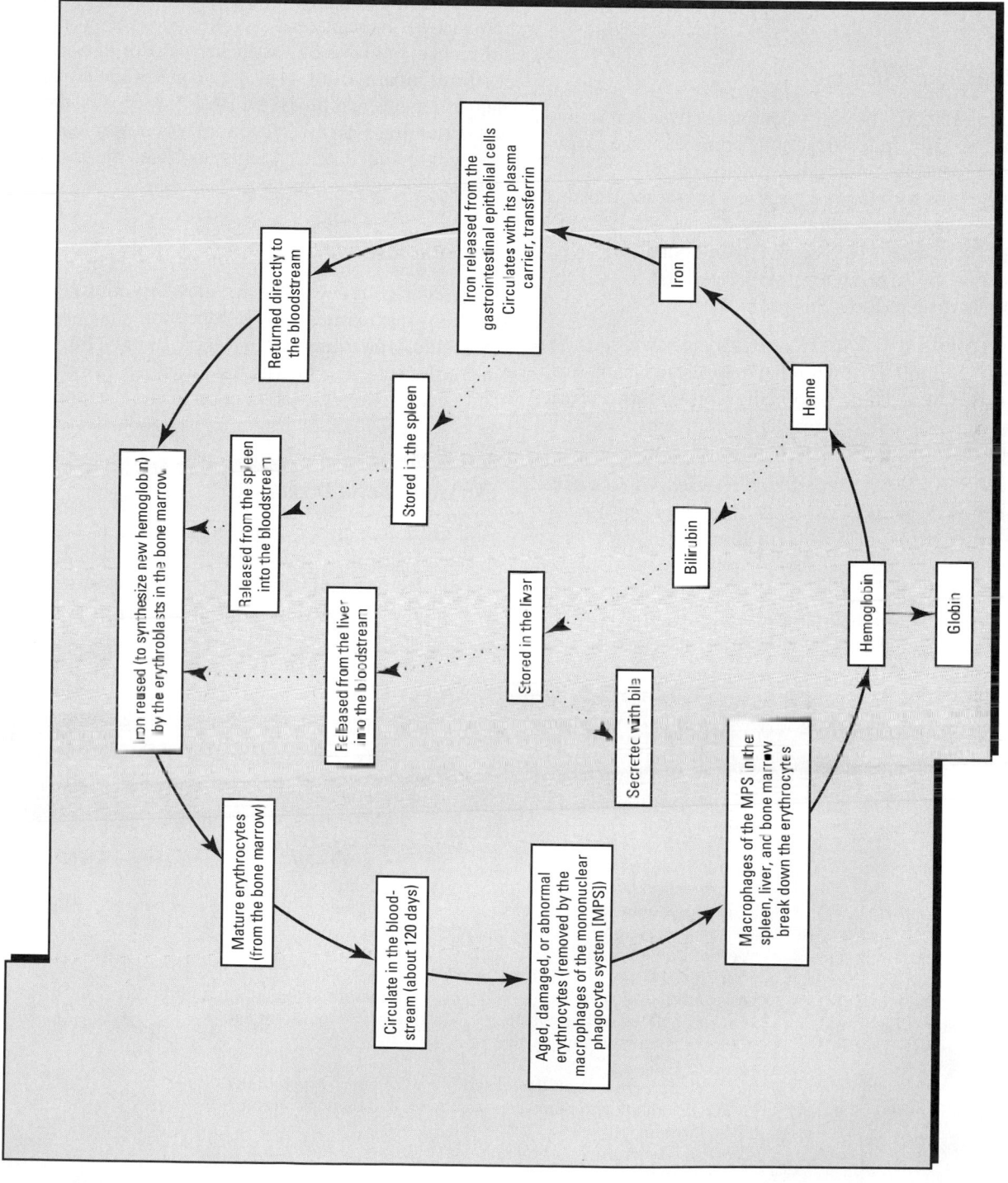

Figure 16–3. The iron cycle.

Pharmacotherapeutics

Precautions and Contraindications

The only contraindications to the use of **iron** are hemochromatosis and hemolytic anemia. Tartrazine and sulfite are found in some **iron** formulations. Patients sensitive to them should not take these formulations.

Adverse Drug Reactions

GI symptoms are the most common adverse reactions and are usually mild. Irritation, anorexia, nausea and vomiting, constipation, or diarrhea may occur. Administering the **iron** with food reduces most of these problems. Stools may appear darker in color, which can present a problem in assessing GI bleeding. **Iron**-containing preparations may cause temporary staining of the teeth. Dilution of the drug reduces this problem.

ACUTE TOXICITY. Acute iron toxicity is seen almost exclusively in children who have ingested many iron tablets. As few as 10 tablets of common oral **iron** preparations can be lethal in young children. Symptoms occur in four stages:

1. Within 1 to 6 hours, lethargy, nausea, vomiting, abdominal pain, tarry stools, weak and rapid pulse, hypotension, acidosis, and coma occur.
2. If not immediately fatal, symptoms may subside for about 24 hours.
3. Symptoms return in 12 to 48 hours and may also include diffuse vascular congestion, pulmonary edema, shock, acidosis, convulsions, anuria, hyperthermia, and death.
4. If the patient survives, in 2 to 6 weeks, pyloric stenosis, hepatic cirrhosis, and central nervous system (CNS) damage may be seen.

Treatment involves maintaining airway, respiration, and circulation. If the patient is a candidate for emesis, **syrup of ipecac,** followed by gastric lavage with 1 to 5 percent **sodium bicarbonate,** is used to convert the ferrous sulfate to ferrous carbonate, which is poorly absorbed and less irritating. Systemic chelation with **deferoxamine** IM is recommended for patients with serum **iron** levels above 300 mg/dL.

Drug Interactions

Drug interactions involve chelation (**levodopa, penicillamine, quinolones**) or competition for absorption (**antacids, cimetidine, methyldopa, tetracyclines**). Food interactions occur with vitamin C (enhances absorption) and calcium (decreases absorption unless calcium carbonate is used). Drug interactions are shown in Table 16–9.

Clinical Use and Dosing

Oral **iron** therapy is used to prevent and treat iron-deficiency anemia. Because they are more efficiently absorbed, **ferrous salts** should be used. Sustained-release and enteric forms should not be used because **iron** is best

Table 16–9. Drug Interactions: Iron

Drug	Interacting Drug	Possible Effect	Implications
Iron	Antacids	Absorption reduced.	Separate administration by at least 2 h.
	Ascorbic acid	Absorption enhanced.	Increase may not be significant; must be given concurrently.
	Calcium	Coadministration decreases absorption of both; calcium carbonate does not decrease iron absorption.	Separate administration by at least 2 h or use calcium carbonate for calcium supplementation and take between meals.
	Chloramphenicol	Serum iron levels may be increased.	—
	Cimetidine	Absorption reduced.	Separate administration by at least 2 h.
	Levodopa	Forms chelates with iron salts, decreasing levodopa levels by up to 90%.	Avoid concurrent use.
	Methyldopa	Methyldopa absorption decreased.	Avoid concurrent use.
	Penicillamine	Marked reduction in penicillamine absorption.	Avoid concurrent use.
	Quinolones	Decreased absorption of quinolones by up to 90%.	Choose different antibiotic.
	Tetracyclines	Coadministration decreases absorption and serum levels of both by up to 90%.	Separate administration by at least 2 h.
	Vitamin C	Absorption enhanced.	May not be significant and requires concurrent administration.

absorbed in the duodenum and jejunum. Different **ferrous salts** provide different amounts of elemental **iron**. In an iron-deficient patient, about 50 to 100 mg of **iron** can be incorporated into hemoglobin daily. About 25 percent of ferrous salt given orally can be absorbed. Given these two facts, Katsung (1998) recommends giving 200 to 400 mg of elemental **iron** daily to correct iron deficiency rapidly. If the patient cannot tolerate this large a dose, lower doses may be given, but resolving the deficiency takes longer. Richer (1997) recommends 150 to 250 mg of elemental **iron** daily. This slightly lower dose has fewer adverse drug effects. The daily dose is divided and given three or four times each day. Table 16–10 shows the dosing schedules for children and adults. Treatment continues for 3 to 6 months to correct the anemia and replenish iron stores.

Rational Drug Selection

COST. *Drug Facts and Comparisons* (Kastrup, 1998) includes a cost index (CI) based on cost per 180 mg of iron. The most expensive **ferrous sulfate** was **Fer-In-Sol**, a liquid form used mostly for infants and small children (CI = 88). Other liquid formulations were also expensive, but the least expensive was **ferrous sulfate elixir** (CI = 7–21, depending on brand). **Ferrous sulfate** tablets varied from **Mol-Iron** (CI = 12) to generic forms (CI = 2.4). The most expensive **ferrous gluconate** was **Fergon** elixir (CI = 34), and the least expensive was generic (CI = 4.6). **Simron** was listed with a CI of 292. **Ferrous fumarate** varied from a suspension (**Feostat**, CI = 50) to tablets (**Femiron**, CI = 24 to generic, CI = 1). Generic **ferrous salts** are clearly less expensive, even though all of these compounds are OTC medications.

FORMULATION. **Ferrous salts** come in tablets, capsules, suspensions, drops, and chewable formulations (Table 16–11). Unless a patient's age or disease process makes swallowing difficult or impossible, the tablets are the cheapest, and they are easily digested and absorbed.

Table 16–10. Dosage Schedule: Iron

Drug	Indication	Initial Dose	Maintenance Dose
Iron	Replacement in iron-deficiency anemia	Adults: Ferrous sulfate 300–325 mg (60–65 mg of elemental iron) daily Ferrous gluconate 300–325 mg (34–38 mg of elemental iron) daily Ferrous fumarate 200 mg (66 mg of elemental iron) daily Ferrous fumarate 325 mg (106 mg elemental iron) daily *Note:* These low doses reduce CI intolerance. Maintenance doses are started initially for severe anemia.	Adults: Ferrous sulfate 300–325 mg (60–65 mg of elemental iron) tid–qid Ferrous gluconate 300–325 mg (34–38 mg of elemental iron) qid Ferrous fumarate 200 mg (66 mg of elemental iron) tid–qid Ferrous fumarate 325 mg (106 mg elemental iron) bid–tid *Note:* Goal is 150–250 mg of elemental iron/d. Children: *2–12 y:* goal is 3 mg/kg/d of elemental iron in 3–4 divided doses. *6 mo–2 y:* goal is up to 6 mg/kg/d of elemental iron in 3–4 divided doses. *Infants:* 10–25 mg of elemental iron daily in 3–4 divided doses. 30 mg elemental iron daily (not taken with meals) during last two trimesters Ferrous sulfate 300–325 mg once daily
	Iron supplement in pregnancy and lactation	—	Adults: Ferrous sulfate 300–325 mg (60–65 mg of elemental iron) tid–qid Ferrous gluconate 300–325 mg (34–38 mg of elemental iron) qid Ferrous fumarate 200 mg (66 mg of elemental iron) tid–qid Ferrous fumarate 325 mg (106 mg elemental iron) bid–tid *Note:* Goal is 150–250 mg of elemental iron/d.

Table 16–11. Available Dosage Form: Iron

Drug	Dosage Form	Other Forms
Ferrous Fumarate (33% Elemental Iron)		
Femiron	Tablets: 63 mg (20 mg iron)	—
Feostat	Tablets: 100 mg (33 mg iron)	Suspension: 100 mg/5 cc (33 mg iron/5 cc) Drops: 45 mg/0.6 cc (15 mg iron/0.6 cc)
Fumerin	Tablets: 195 mg (64 mg iron)	—
Fumasorb	Tablets: 200 mg (66 mg iron)	—
Generic	Tablets: 325 mg (106 mg iron)	—
Hemocyte	Tablets: 324 mg (106 mg iron)	—
Ircon	Tablets: 200 mg (66 mg iron)	—
Nephro-Fer	Tablets: 350 mg (1120 mg iron)	—
Ferrous Gluconate (11.6% Elemental Iron)		
Fergon	Tablets: 320 mg (37 mg iron)	Elixir: 300 mg/5 cc (34 mg iron/5 cc)
Generic	Tablets: 300 mg (34 mg iron) Tablets: 325 mg (38 mg iron)	—
Simron	Capsules: 86 mg (10 mg iron)	—
Ferrous Sulfate (20% Elemental Iron)		
Feosol		Elixir: 220 mg/5 cc (44 mg iron/5 cc)
Feratab	Tablets: 300 mg (60 mg iron)	—
Fer-In-Sol		Syrup: 90 mg/5 cc (18 mg iron/5 cc) Drops: 75 mg/0.6 cc (15 mg/0.6 cc)
Fer-Iron		125 mg/1 cc (25 mg iron/cc)
Generic	Tablets: 324 mg (65 mg iron) Capsules: 250 mg (50 mg iron)	Elixir: 220 mg/5 cc (44 mg iron/5 cc) 75 mg/0.6 cc (15 mg iron/0.6 cc)
Mol-Iron	Tablets: 195 mg (39 mg iron)	—

Monitoring

The reticulocyte count is measured 7 to 10 days after initiation of therapy because it is the first measurable response to **iron** therapy. A significant rise should be noted toward the normal 0.5 to 1.5 percent of the body's RBCs. Hemoglobin levels drawn at 2 weeks from initiation of therapy should indicate a rise in hemoglobin concentration of 0.1 to 0.2 g/100 cc per day of therapy. Normal hemoglobin levels of 14 to 18 g/dL in men and 12 to 16 g/dL in women should be reached in 1 to 3 months. Monitoring of RBC and hemoglobin levels thereafter is based on individual patient risk, response, and symptoms.

Patient Education

PREVENTION. Prevention of iron deficiency is the most important issue. The average American diet contains about 12 mg of iron daily. Twenty percent of this is absorbed in markedly deficient patients, but only 10 percent is absorbed in normal patients. This means that 0.6 to 1.2 mg of elemental iron is taken up under normal circumstances. This is an adequate requirement for men and postmenopausal women; however, menstruating women need 1.5 mg/day, and pregnant and lactating women need 2.5 mg/day. Eating iron-rich foods can prevent the need for **iron** supplements, especially in adults. Red meat is the best source of iron, but fish and iron-enriched breads and cereals are also good sources. The iron in eggs and green vegetables is not absorbed because it is bound to phosphates and phytates in these foods. Nutrition should be discussed, including iron-rich foods that are reasonable in cost. Most people who eat a balanced diet do not need **iron** supplements. Pregnant women, infants, and children during rapid growth periods may need **iron** supplementation.

ADMINISTRATION. Patients should take **iron** as directed. If a dose is missed, they should take it as soon as it is remembered within 12 hours but not double doses. **Iron** should be taken on an empty stomach. If GI upset occurs, **iron** can be taken with food, but the amount absorbed is less. Taking it with vitamin C or citrus juice may enhance absorption. Patients should avoid taking **iron** at the same time as **antacids, tetracycline,** or **quinolones,** which decrease absorption, and drink liquid **iron** preparations in water or citrus juice or through a straw to prevent discoloration of teeth. Do not use sustained-release preparations.

ADVERSE RESPONSES. Constipation is the most common problem. Increase fluids and fiber in the diet, especially iron-rich cereals. Stools may turn dark green or black. This color change is harmless.

Acute **iron** toxicity/poisoning can occur with an overdose. This is especially a problem with children, in whom as few as 10 of the commonly available **iron** tablets can be fatal. Keep **iron** preparations in childproof containers and in a locked medicine cabinet. Do not refer to vitamins or drugs as candy. Contact the local Poison Control Center immediately if overdose is suspected. Keep **syrup of ipecac** available, with enough for at least one dose for each child in the household.

Folic Acid

Folic acid deficiency is most often related to inadequate dietary intake of green vegetables or excessive boiling of these vegetables in cooking. Other sources of folic acid deficiency include impaired absorption because of ileal disease or **phenytoin** use; increased demand during pregnancy, hyperthyroidism, hemolytic anemia, or malignancy; and impaired utilization for patients taking **methotrexate, triamterene,** and **trimethoprim.**

Pharmacodynamics

Exogenous folate is required for nucleoprotein synthesis and maintenance of normal erythropoiesis. Folic acid stimulates the production of erythrocytes, WBCs, and platelets. Folic acid undergoes a series of oxidative-reductive changes that result in the formation of tetrahydrofolic acid, a cofactor in transformation reactions in the biosynthesis of purines and thymidylates. Impaired thymidylate synthesis is thought to be the mechanism behind neural tube defects in the offspring of pregnant women with folic acid deficiency. Within 3 months of inadequate intake of folates, megaloblastic changes and anemia can develop. Supplemental folic acid is useful in preventing **folic acid** deficiency in high-risk patients with high folate requirements and in alcoholics and patients with liver disease, who may have deficient storage of folate.

Pharmacokinetics

Absorption and Distribution

Only about 50 to 200 μg of folate is absorbed from the daily intake of 500 to 700 μg in the average diet. Pregnant women may absorb as much as 300 to 400 μg of folate daily. Oral **folic acid** supplements are well absorbed from the proximal jejunum, and intramuscular or subcutaneous administration also results in excellent absorption.

Metabolism, Storage, and Excretion

Folic acid is converted by the liver to its active metabolite (dihydrofolate reductase). Approximately 5 to 20 mg of folate is stored in the liver and other tissue extensively bound to plasma proteins. Folates are excreted in the urine and stool and destroyed by catabolism so that serum levels fall within days when intake is inadequate.

Pharmacotherapeutics

Precautions and Contraindications

The only contraindication is administration when **vitamin B$_{12}$** is deficient. **Folic acid** in doses greater than 0.1 mg/day may mask the indications of pernicious anemia in that the hematologic symptoms are gone, but the neurological symptoms continue to progress. Except in pregnancy and lactation, daily doses of **folic acid** should not exceed 0.4 mg/day until pernicious anemia has been ruled out.

Folic acid is Pregnancy Category A. Pregnant women are more prone to develop folic acid deficiencies, and their diet should be supplemented. The recommended dietary allowance (RDA) for *folate* during pregnancy is 0.4 mg/day.

Adverse Drug Reactions

Rare transient rashes are the only adverse drug reaction.

Drug Interactions

Sulfonamides, methotrexate, and **triamterene** interfere with the activity of folate reductase and prevent the activation of **folic acid** (Table 16–12). Absorption is decreased if it is given concurrently with **sulfasalazine**. **Folic acid** requirements are increased in the presence of **estrogens, phenytoin,** and **glucocorticoids**.

Clinical Use and Dosing

TREATMENT OF MEGALOBLASTIC ANEMIA DUE TO FOLIC ACID DEFICIENCY. After pernicious anemia has been ruled out, the initial dose is up to 1 mg/day in adults and children. When clinical symptoms have subsided and the laboratory studies have normalized, maintenance doses range from 0.1 mg/day for infants to 0.8 mg/day for pregnant and lactating patients. Table 16–13 shows these dosages by age group.

PREVENTION OF FOLIC ACID DEFICIENCY IN ALCOHOLICS AND PATIENTS WITH LIVER DISEASE. Maintenance doses of **folic acid** may be sufficient to prevent folic acid deficiency in these patients if the upper limit for each age is used.

PREVENTION OF FOLIC ACID DEFICIENCY IN PREGNANCY. Doses of 0.4 mg prior to conception and throughout pregnancy have been associated with risk reductions of up to 50 percent for neural tube defects in the offspring. The U.S. Public Health Service recommends that all women of childbearing age who are capable of becoming pregnant consume 0.4 mg of **folic acid** daily. Because there are risks with higher doses that B_{12} deficiency may be overlooked, total folate intake should not exceed 1 mg/day.

DURING LACTATION TO MEET INFANT REQUIREMENTS. During lactation, **folic acid** requirements are markedly increased. Mothers who are breast-feeding and have folic acid deficiency require doses of 0.8 mg/day to prevent folic acid deficiency in their infants.

Rational Drug Selection

Folic acid is available OTC at less cost than in prescription form (Table 16–14).

Monitoring

The only specific monitoring parameters are those associated with managing the anemia that is being treated.

Patient Education

Although folic acid is part of a normal diet, supplemental **folic acid** should be taken only after consultation with a health care provider. In particular, pregnant women and those who may become pregnant should discuss the need for **folic acid** with their provider. Foods high in folate include green vegetables (especially asparagus, lettuce, spinach, and broccoli), liver, yeast, and mushrooms, which should be included in a balanced diet.

Vitamin B₁₂

Vitamin B_{12} deficiency can be caused by poor intake, impaired absorption, increased demand, or faulty utilization. Poor intake is rare, except in strict vegetarians who do not eat eggs or use dairy products. Impaired absorp-

Table 16–12. Drug Interactions: Folic Acid

Drug	Interacting Drug	Possible Effect	Implications
Folic acid	Aminosalicylic acid	Decreased serum folate levels.	Avoid concurrent use.
	Oral contraceptives	May impair folate metabolism and produce folate depletion, but the effect is mild and not likely to cause anemia.	Monitor for clinical indications of anemia.
	Sulfonamides	Prevent the activation of folic acid by causing a dihydrofolate reductase deficiency.	Avoid concurrent use.
	Methotrexate Triamterene Sulfasalazine	Signs of folate deficiency have been reported.	Monitor for indications of anemia.
	Hydantoins	An increase in seizure activity and a decrease in serum concentrations of the hydantoin to subtherapeutic levels. Phenytoin may cause a decrease in serum folate levels, but clinically important anemia occurs in <1% of patients on long-term therapy.	If folic acid is administered, a higher dose of phenytoin may be needed.

Table 16–13. Dosage Schedule: Folic Acid

Drug	Indication	Initial Dose	Maintenance Dose
Folic acid	Treatment of megaloblastic anemia	Up to 1 mg/d until laboratory studies are normal	Infants: 0.1 mg/d Children <4 y: 0.3 mg/d Adults and children >4 y: 0.4 mg/d Pregnant and lactating women, patients who are alcoholic, and patients with liver disease: 0.8 mg/d
	Prevention of folic acid deficiency		Infants: 0.1 mg/d Children <4 y: 0.3 mg/d Adults and children >4 y: 0.4 mg/d Pregnant and lactating women, patients who are alcoholic, and patients with liver disease: 0.4 mg/d

tion is most often related to the lack of intrinsic factor found in pernicious anemia. Absorption can also be impaired by diseases of the ileum, by bacterial overgrowth from stasis such as occurs with severe constipation, and by altered digestive enzymes associated with gastrectomy. Faulty utilization is associated with rare genetic defects.

Pharmacodynamics

Vitamin B_{12} is critical to two essential enzyme systems. In one system, it is the cofactor in metabolism of methylmalonyl-CoA. When this metabolism does not take place, methylmalonyl-CoA accumulates, and abnormal fatty acids are synthesized. It is believed that these abnormal fatty acids in cell membranes of the CNS are responsible for the neurological manifestations of vitamin B_{12} deficiency. The other system involves folate metabolism. In the presence of vitamin B_{12} deficiency, the final steps in folate metabolism cannot occur, which explains why the megaloblastic anemia found in **vitamin B_{12}** deficiency can be partially corrected by **folic acid** administration. Management of anemia is discussed in Chapter 25.

Pharmacokinetics

Absorption and Distribution

Approximately 1 to 5 μg of the daily dietary intake of 5 to 30 μg is absorbed. In the stomach and duodenum, **vitamin B_{12}** complexes with intrinsic factor secreted by the parietal cells of the gastric mucosa. This complex is then separated in the terminal ileum in the presence of calcium and absorbed by a highly specific receptor-mediated transport system. Patients with intrinsic factor deficits require parenteral administration of B_{12} to bypass this absorption problem. **Vitamin B_{12}** is well absorbed following IM and SC injection. Plasma level peaks within 1 hour after injection.

Once absorbed, **vitamin B_{12}** is distributed throughout the body, bound to a plasma protein, transcobalamin II.

Metabolism, Storage, and Excretion

Excess **vitamin B_{12}** is stored mainly in the liver and released when needed to carry out normal cellular functions. Because the normal daily requirement of vitamin B_{12} is only about 2 μg, it would take approximately 5 years for all the stored **vitamin B_{12}** to be exhausted and megaloblastic anemia to develop if **vitamin B_{12}** absorption stopped. After injection, **vitamin B_{12}** is stored in the liver for approximately 400 days.

Within 48 hours after injection, 50 to 98 percent of the dose appears in the urine. The major portion is excreted within the first 8 hours.

Pharmacotherapeutics

Precautions and Contraindications

The only contraindications to injectable **vitamin B_{12}** are hypersensitivity to **cobalt**, B_{12}, or any component of

Table 16–14. Available Dosage Forms: Folic Acid

Drug	Dosage Form	Other Forms
Folic acid (OTC)	Tablets: 0.4 mg, 0.8 mg	
Folic acid (prescription)	Tablets: 1 mg	Multidose vial for injection (Folvite); 5 mg/cc

these and the presence of Leber's disease, a hereditary optic nerve atrophy. Severe and swift optic nerve atrophy occurs in patients with this disease who are treated with **cyanocobalamin.**

Pulmonary edema, peripheral vascular thrombosis, and congestive heart failure may occur early in treatment with **vitamin B_{12}.** Cautious use and careful monitoring are suggested. Blunted or impeded therapeutic response may occur in the presence of uremia, folic acid deficiency, concurrent infection, or iron deficiency.

Vitamin B_{12} (parenteral) is Pregnancy Category C. Adequate and well-controlled studies have not been done with pregnant women.

Adverse Drug Reactions

Hypokalemia and sudden death have occurred in severe megaloblastic anemia treated intensely. Serum potassium levels should be carefully monitored, and supplementation provided as needed.

Anaphylactic shock and death have occurred after parenteral administration. An interdermal test dose is given to patients sensitive to the **cobalamins.**

Transient diarrhea, urticaria, and pruritus may occur but are not common. Pain is common at the injection site.

Drug Interactions

There are few drug interactions with injectable **vitamin B_{12}.** Several drugs, **extended-release potassium,** and excessive intake of **alcohol** or **vitamin C** may decrease absorption of oral **vitamin B_{12}.** Table 16–15 shows these drug interactions.

Clinical Use and Dosing

PREVENTION OF VITAMIN B_{12} DEFICIENCY IN OTHERWISE HEALTHY PERSONS. Vitamin B_{12} is an essential vitamin,

and needs increase during pregnancy. The National Academy of Sciences recommends oral doses of 2.2 µg/day during pregnancy. Vitamin B_{12} is excreted in breast milk in concentrations that approximate the mother's **vitamin B_{12}** blood level. The Food and Nutrition Board of the National Academy of Sciences—National Research Council recommends 2.6 µg/day during lactation, 0.3 to 0.5 µg/day for infants under age 1 year, and 0.7 to 1.4 µg/day for children age 1 to 10 years (Table 16–16).

PERNICIOUS ANEMIA. Parenteral therapy is required for life for patients with pernicious anemia. Initial dosing is 100 µg daily for 6 or 7 days by IM or deep SC injection. The hematologic response to injected B_{12} is usually rapid. Reticulocytosis begins on the second or third day and is usually maximal by the fifth to tenth day. If there is clinical improvement and an appropriate reticulocyte response has occurred after 7 days of therapy, the same dose (100 µg) is given on alternate days for an additional 7 days. Then the dose is given every 3 or 4 days for another 2 to 3 weeks. By this time, the hematologic values should be normal. Follow this initial regimen with 100 µg monthly for the life of the patient. If neurological symptoms are present, a twice-monthly dose is recommended for 6 months prior to beginning the monthly dose.

PATIENTS WHO DO NOT HAVE PERNICIOUS ANEMIA BUT WHO DO HAVE VITAMIN B_{12} DEFICIENCY. In seriously ill patients, both **vitamin B_{12}** and **folic acid** may need to be administered. Dosages for children vary, based on the presence of hematologic versus neurological signs. Oral doses up to 1000 µg have been used; however, oral therapy is not usually recommended for deficiency states.

UNNECESSARY VITAMIN B_{12} THERAPY. Some well-meaning health care providers have given **parenteral vitamin B_{12}** to patients with fatigue or other vague symptoms. Sometimes these patients report feeling better, in all probability related to a placebo effect. There is no in-

Table 16–15. Drug Interactions: Vitamin B_{12}

Drug	Interacting Drug	Possible Effect	Implications
Vitamin B_{12}	Aminosalicylic acid	Reduced biologic and therapeutic action of B_{12}. Abnormal Schilling test and symptoms of B_{12} deficiency.	Avoid concomitant administration.
	Chloramphenicaol	Hematologic effects of B_{12} may be decreased in patients with pernicious anemia.	Choose a different antimicrobial.
	Colchicine	May cause malabsorption of B_{12} (oral).	If unable to avoid concomitant use, administer B_{12} parenterally.
	Aminoglycosides Extended-release potassium supplements Cimetidine Excessive intake of alcohol or vitamin C		

Table 16–16. Dosage Schedule: Vitamin B$_{12}$

Drug	Indication	Initial Dose	Maintenance Dose
Vitamin B$_{12}$	Pernicious anemia	100 µg/d for 6–7 d IM or deep SC	If clinical improvement and reticulocyte response, give 100 µg on alternate days for 7 doses, then every 3–4 d for 2–3 wk. Then give 100 µg monthly for life of patient. If neurological symptoms are present, a twice-monthly dose is recommended for 6 mo prior to beginning the monthly dose.
	Vitamin B$_{12}$ deficiency without pernicious anemia	Cyanocobalamin: *Parenteral* Adults: 30 µg/d for 5–10 d Children: For hematologic signs: 10–50 µg/d for 5–10 d For neurological signs: 100 µg/d for 10–15 d *Oral** Up to 1000 µg/d	*Parenteral* Adults: 100–200 µg monthly Children: For hematologic signs: 100–250 µg/d every 2–4 wk For neurological signs: 100 µg once or twice weekly for several months, then taper to 250–1000 µg monthly by 1 y *Oral** Maximum that can be absorbed in a single dose is 5 µg. Percent absorbed decreases with increased dose.
		Hydroxocobalamin: Adults: 30 µg/d for 5–10 d Children: 100 µg doses to equal 1–5 mg over 2 wk	Adults: 100–200 µg/mo. Children: 30–50 µg every 4 wk.

*Oral therapy is usually not recommended to treat deficiency. Oral therapy is used mainly for prevention of deficiency.

dication that **vitamin B$_{12}$** is useful for patients who do not have a deficiency state. Although there is little risk in giving this drug, the better approach is to determine the underlying problem that is causing the patient's symptoms, such as depression, anxiety, or the presence of an inflammatory disease or other disorder that may inhibit erythropoiesis.

Rational Drug Selection

Of the two main parenteral forms of **vitamin B$_{12}$**, **cyanocobalamin (Crystamine, Cyanoject, Cyomin)** is less protein-bound and has a shorter duration of action than **hydroxocobalamin (Hydrobexan, Hydro Cobex, Hydro-Crysti-12)** (Table 16–17). The latter form may mean less frequent injections, but antibody reactions are more common with this form. Either one works as well.

Monitoring

During treatment for severe megaloblastic anemia, monitor serum potassium levels closely for the first 48 hours, and replace potassium if needed. Reticulocyte counts, hematocrit, iron, folic acid, and vitamin B$_{12}$ serum levels are obtained prior to treatment, between the fifth and seventh day of therapy, and then frequently until the hematocrit is normal. If folate levels are also low, **folic**

acid may need to be administered. Monitoring for folic acid is discussed in the section on that drug. Relapse of symptoms is not uncommon in the presence of continuing therapy. Hematologic evaluations should continue at regular intervals throughout the patient's lifetime based on the individual response to therapy.

Patient Education

ADMINISTRATION. Oral administration of **vitamin B$_{12}$** is useful only for nutritional deficiencies. It should be taken with meals to increase absorption. It may be taken with fruit juices, but ascorbic acid alters the stability of the drug. There is no evidence that expensive vitamin preparations are any more efficacious than less costly ones. Vitamins are not a substitute for a well-balanced diet.

Monthly parenteral administration is necessary for the rest of the patient's life to treat pernicious anemia. Failure to do so leads to the return of the anemia and the development of incapacitating and irreversible damage to the nerves of the spinal cord. IM injections should be given in large muscles such as the buttock or thigh, and SC injection should be given deeply in these same areas.

ADVERSE DRUG REACTIONS. Diarrhea, itching, and urticaria may sometimes occur but are usually temporary. Hypokalemia has occurred early in the treatment of se-

Table 16–17. Available Dosage Forms: Vitamin B$_{12}$

Drug	Dosage Form	Other Forms
Cyanocobalamin/vitamin B$_{12}$	Tablets: 500 mg, 1000 mg	Multidose vials (30 cc): 100 μg/cc injection; multidose vials (10 cc, 30 cc): 1000/μg/cc injection
Crystamine		Multidose vials (10 cc, 30 cc): 1000 μg/cc injection
Cristi-1000		Multidose vials (10 cc): 1000 μg/cc injection
Cyanoject		Multidose vials (10 cc, 30 cc): 1000 μg/cc injection
Cyomin		Multidose vials (30 cc): 1000 μg/cc injection
Rubesol-1000		Multidose vials (10 cc, 30 cc): 1000 μg/cc injection
Hydroxocobalamin/vitamin B$_{12}$ Hydrobexan Hydro Cobex, Hydro-Cristi-12, LA-12		All injection forms; multidose vials (30 cc): 1000 μg/cc injection

vere anemia. The health care provider should monitor for this problem. A diet high in potassium may be helpful. Although rare, cardiac and pulmonary symptoms have occurred. The patient should report shortness of breath, swelling in the lower legs or ankles, and pain or redness in the calves.

REFERENCES

Ament, P., & Bertolino, J. (1994). Enoxaparin in the prevention of deep venous thrombosis. *American Family Physician, 50*(8), 1763–1768.

Clagget, G., Anderson, F., & Heit, J. (1995). Prevention of venous thromboembolism. *Chest, 108*(4), 312S–334S.

Deglin, J., & Vallerand, A. (1998). *Davis's drug guide for nurses* (6th ed.). Philadelphia: F. A. Davis.

Goroll, A., May, L., & Mulley, A. (1995). *Primary care medicine* (3rd ed.). Philadelphia: Lippincott.

Kastrup, E. (Founding Ed.). (1998). *Drug facts and comparisons.* St. Louis: Facts and Comparisons.

Katzung, B. (1998). *Basic and clinical pharmacology* (7th ed.). Stamford, CT: Appleton & Lange.

Koopman, M., & Buller, H. (1998). Low-molecular weight heparins in the treatment of venous thromboembolism. *Annals of Internal Medicine, 128*(12), 1037–1038.

Levine, M., Gent, M., Hirsh, J., et al. (1996). A comparison of low-molecular weight heparin administered primarily at home with unfractionated heparin administered in the hospital for proximal deep-vein thrombosis. *New England Journal of Medicine, 334*(11), 677–681.

Planes, A., Vochelle, N., Darmon, J., et al. (1996). Risk of deep-venous thrombosis after hospital discharge in patients having undergone total hip replacement: Double-blind randomised comparison of enoxaparin versus placebo. *Lancet, 348,* 224–228.

Richer, S. (1997). A practical guide for differentiating between iron deficiency anemia and anemia of chronic disease in children and adults. *Nurse Practitioner, 22*(4), 82–98.

Selig, P. (1996). Pearls for practice: Management of anticoagulation therapy with the international normalized ratio. *Nurse Practitioner, 8*(2), 77–80.

Wells, P., Holbrook, A., & Crowther, N. (1994) The interaction of warfarin with drugs and food: A critical review of the literature. *Annals of Internal Medicine, 121,* 676–683.

Zamorski, M. (1998). Warfarin and aspirin for prevention of IHD. *Journal of Family Practice, 46*(5), 358–359.

CHAPTER 17

· · · · · · ·

Drugs Affecting the Immune System

CHAPTER OUTLINE

Plague Vaccine
  Pharmacodynamics
  Pharmacokinetics
  Pharmacotherapeutics
  Precautions and contraindications
  Adverse drug reactions
  Drug interactions
  Clinical use and dosing
  Patient education
Rabies Vaccine
  Pharmacodynamics
  Pharmacokinetics
  Pharmacotherapeutics
  Precautions and contraindications
  Adverse drug reactions
  Drug interactions
  Clinical use and dosing
  Patient education

IMMUNE GLOBULIN SERUMS
Pharmacodynamics
Pharmacokinetics
Pharmacotherapeutics
  Precautions and contraindications
  Adverse drug reactions
  Drug interactions
  Clinical use and dosing

Monitoring
Patient education

DIAGNOSTIC BIOLOGICALS
Tuberculin Purified Protein Derivative
  Pharmacodynamics
  Pharmacokinetics
  Pharmacotherapeutics
  Precautions and contraindications
  Adverse drug reactions
  Drug interactions
  Clinical use and dosing
  Monitoring
  Patient education

IMMUNOMODULATORS
Pharmacodynamics
Pharmacokinetics
  Absorption and distribution
  Metabolism and excretion
Pharmacotherapeutics
  Precautions and contraindications
  Adverse drug reactions
  Drug interactions
  Clinical use and dosing
  Monitoring
  Patient education

Primary care providers prescribe immunizations frequently, with pediatric providers prescribing many vaccines daily. Although vaccination is typically associated with children, the U.S. Public Health Service identified an adult immunization rate of at least 60 percent as one of the target goals for Healthy People 2000. In the United States, 45,000 people die each year from influenza, pneumococcal, and hepatitis B disease, all preventable by vaccination (Satcher, 1999).

The immunization schedules may change, but the underlying premise of preventing the spread of infectious disease through mass immunization of susceptible populations does not change. This chapter discusses immunizations, **immune globulin serums**, and the diagnostic drugs used in primary care, such as **purified protein derivative (PPD)** for tuberculosis (TB) screening. The **immunomodulators cyclosporine** and **azathioprine** are addressed. The use of **interferon** is not discussed here because it is usually prescribed by specialty care providers.

Immunizations

Vaccination is the single best technique for preventing infectious disease. **Vaccines** exist for many diseases that affect adults and children. This section of the chapter discusses active immunization with either attenuated or inactivated infective agents, the recommended schedule of immunizations for adults and children, and the true precautions and contraindications to immunization. Issues surrounding immunization such as barriers to immunization are discussed, as well as immunization of special populations and travel immunizations.

Vaccines are divided into two different types: those that are made from attenuated ("modified-live") or inactivated ("killed") infective agents. **Attenuated vaccines** include **measles, mumps, and rubella (MMR); oral polio (OPV); varicella virus vaccines; yellow fever (YF-Vax); and BCG.** Inactivated vaccines include **diphtheria, tetanus, and pertussis (DTP, DTaP, DT, Td), Haemophilus influenzae type b (Hib), hepatitis A and B, influenza (Fluzone),** and **inactivated polio vaccine (IPV). Cholera, Japanese encephalitis virus,** and **plague vaccine** are other **inactivated vaccines. Typhoid vaccine** is available in an inactivated form and an oral live attenuated form. The pharmacodynamics of each **vaccine** is discussed according to its category.

Attenuated Vaccines

Measles, Mumps, and Rubella Vaccine

Pharmacodynamics

Immunization with **measles, mumps,** and **rubella (MMR)** or **measles vaccine** alone stimulates the immune system to produce disease-specific antibodies by inducing a subclinical infection with attenuated virus particles. This subclinical infection is not contagious. The **vaccine**-induced antibodies are capable of virus neutralization by complement activation, induction of cell-mediated immunity, and opsonization. The available **single-agent** and other **combination vaccines** include **measles virus vaccine (Attenuvax), mumps virus vaccine live (Mumpsvax), rubella (Meruvax II), rubella and mumps (Biavax II)**, and **measles and rubella virus vaccine live (M-R-Vax II)**.

Pharmacokinetics

The **MMR vaccine** is administered subcutaneoulsy (SC). Following SC injection, antibodies are detectable in 2 weeks (rubella may take 2 to 6 weeks) in 95 percent of patients vaccinated, and immunity occurs in about 10 days. Immunity persists for 15 years or more, with permanent immunity developing in most patients. More than 99 percent of people who receive two doses of **MMR** separated by at least 1 month develop evidence of immunity to measles, which is why the current recommendation is for 2 doses. Immunity to mumps persists for at least 20 years.

Pharmacotherapeutics

PRECAUTIONS AND CONTRAINDICATIONS. **MMR** contains live, attenuated virus, and virus has been detected for 1 to 4 weeks after vaccination in the pharynx or nose of most patients who receive the **vaccine**; however, this does not appear to cause virus transmission.

According to the Centers for Disease Control and Prevention (CDC), there are relatively few true contraindications to administering **MMR vaccine.** They include previous anaphylactic reaction to the **MMR vaccine** or any component of the **vaccine**, including **neomycin** (topically or systemically administered) or gelatin. A history of contact dermatitis to **neomycin** is not a contraindication to **MMR.** Anaphylactic reaction or hypersensitivity to eggs is no longer a contraindication to **MMR.**

Immunosuppression can potentiate virus production, and therefore **MMR** vaccination is not recommended for immunocompromised patients. In patients with HIV infection, **MMR vaccine** can be administered if the patient is asymptomatic or without evidence of severe immunosuppression. **MMR** should not be given to patients who are severely immunocompromised because of cancer, leukemia, or lymphoma or who are on immunosuppressive drug therapy, including high-dose **steroids** or radiation therapy. **MMR** may be given to close contacts of immunosuppressed patients, including health care workers.

MMR vaccination is generally deferred if a patient has a moderate or severe febrile illness and is given when the patient recovers from the acute phase of the illness. Mi-

nor illnesses, with or without fever (diarrhea, upper respiratory infection, or otitis media), are not contraindications to **MMR** vaccination, and vaccination should not be postponed.

Patients who receive blood products or **immune globulin (IG)** should wait 5 to 6 months before administration of **MMR.**

MMR vaccine **should not be given to pregnant women or women who may become pregnant within 3 months after administration. There is a theoretical possibility of congenital rubella syndrome in the infant if the mother is given** *rubella vaccine* **when pregnant. Women should be asked if they are pregnant before administration of** *MMR* **and advised to avoid pregnancy for 3 months after administration of the vaccine. Pregnancy in the mother of a patient receiving** *MMR* **is not a contraindication.**

MMR may be administered to breastfeeding women.

The **MMR vaccine** may be safely administered to children of all ages, although it may not be immunogenic in infants under age 12 months. If **MMR** or monovalent **measles vaccine** is administered to a child under age 12 months, then the child should be revaccinated with **MMR** at 12 to 15 months of age and receive a third dose of **MMR** at age 4 to 6 years.

ADVERSE DRUG REACTIONS. Approximately 5 to 15 percent of children develop a fever of at least 103°F after vaccination with **MMR.** The fever usually occurs 7 to 12 days after **MMR** vaccination. The fever usually lasts 1 to 2 days, and the patient is otherwise asymptomatic. **MMR** may cause a transient maculopapular rash 7 to 10 days after vaccination in 5 percent of patients.

Thrombocytopenia is a rare adverse reaction that may occur within 2 months of administration of **MMR vaccine.** The incidence of thrombocytopenia is 1 case per 1 million doses upon passive surveillance in the United States and 1 case per 30,000- to 40,000 doses in prospective studies. The clinical course of thrombocytopenia is generally benign and transient.

DRUG INTERACTIONS. **MMR** should not be administered to patients receiving **immunosuppressants,** including **corticosteroids, interferon,** and **antineoplastic drugs,** because there may be insufficient response to immunization. Patients may remain susceptible despite immunization.

The **MMR vaccine** may be inactivated by **IG.** To avoid inactivation of the attenuated virus, administer the **MMR vaccine** at least 14 to 30 days before or 6 to 8 weeks after the **IG.** If **IG** is being given in preparation for international travel, the **MMR vaccine** should be administered at least 2 weeks before **IG.**

MMR is not contraindicated if a **PPD** was done recently. **PPD** should be delayed for 4 to 6 weeks after an **MMR** has been given because it may interfere with the tuberculin skin test.

Administration of the **MMR** and **varicella vaccines** is compatible if done on the same day, with different needles and at separate sites. If the two live **vaccines** are not given at the same time, an interval of 1 month between **MMR** and **varicella vaccine** is indicated.

CLINICAL USE AND DOSING. **MMR** is routinely given SC at 12 to 15 months of age with a repeat dose at age 4 to 6 years. The second dose of **MMR** may be given as soon as 4 weeks after the first dose, which is indicated during an epidemic or before international travel. Those children who have not received their second dose of **MMR** by age 12 should have it at that time. Adults born in 1957 or later who are at least age 18 (including those born outside the United States) should receive at least one dose of **MMR** if there is no serologic proof of immunity or documentation of a dose given on or after the patient's first birthday. Health care workers and other adults in high-risk groups, such as students entering college, military recruits, and international travelers, should receive a total of two doses of **MMR**. Adults born before 1957 are considered immune, but proof of immunity may be desirable for health care workers. See Table 17–1 for further information.

If administering a **single-agent vaccine**, the dosing is as follows: **Measles vaccine** is recommended in times of outbreak if exposure is considered likely. If **measles vaccine** is given before age 12 months, reimmunization with **MMR** is recommended at age 12 to 15 months and again at school entry (age 4 to 6). Mumps vaccination is usually given in the form of **MMR**. If indicated in time of outbreak, the patient may receive one SC dose of **mumps vaccine**. **Rubella virus vaccine** is given as a single SC injection. **Rubella vaccine** is routinely given to nonimmune postpartum women before hospital discharge.

MONITORING. Laboratory monitoring is not necessary after **MMR** administration. Rubella titer may be drawn to determine if a patient is immune.

PATIENT EDUCATION. All patients or the parents or guardians of the patients are required by law to receive Vaccine Information Statements (VISs) that are developed by the CDC. They are available in a variety of languages, and every effort to provide adequate information to the patient or parent before immunization should be made. These statements are available at the CDC Website or at *www.immunize.org* in multiple languages (Table 17–2).

The SC injection of **MMR** may sting the patient. There may be postinjection discomfort.

The VIS states that there is a 5 to 15 percent chance that the patient may experience a fever of up to 103°F approximately 7 to 12 days after administration of **MMR**. The patient may also experience rash, malaise, or sore throat.

Oral Poliovirus Vaccine

Pharmacodynamics

Oral poliovirus vaccine (OPV) stimulates the immune system to produce antipoliovirus antibodies against Sabin poliovirus types 1, 2, and 3. After oral administration, the live, attenuated virus enters the small intestine, where it replicates in the villous epithelial cells. These specialized epithelial cells transport the viral antigens to the B cells and macrophages, which process and produce antipoliovirus antibodies. In 1 to 2 weeks after a dose of **OPV**, antibodies are present. The live, attenuated poliovirus lingers in the gastrointestinal (GI) tract for 4 to 6 weeks, inducing both mucosal and serum antipoliovirus antibodies. The local secretory (intestinal) immune responses to **OPV** are greater than those induced by **inactivated poliovirus (IPV)**. **OPV** induces intestinal immunity against wild strains of poliovirus; **IPV** does not. At least two doses of **OPV** are necessary for intestinal immunity. **OPV** may induce a herd type of immunity because of the spread of attenuated live viruses to susceptible contacts during the viral shedding period of 4 to 6 weeks after dosing. Three doses of **OPV** result in sustained, lifelong immunity.

Pharmacokinetics

After oral administration of **OPV**, antibody stimulation occurs within 7 to 10 days. Poliovirus antibodies have been found in serum, nasal secretions, saliva, duodenal fluids, urine, and feces. Poliovirus antibodies are distributed into breast milk.

Pharmacotherapeutics

PRECAUTIONS AND CONTRAINDICATIONS. An anaphylactic reaction to any previous dose of **OPV** is a contraindication to its use. Patients with **neomycin** or **streptomycin** hypersensitivity also should not receive **OPV** because these agents are contained in **OPV** in small quantities.

OPV should be delayed if a patient has a moderate or severe febrile illness or severe respiratory infection. Administration of **OPV** with current viral GI infection, ongoing diarrhea, or vomiting is contraindicated. Vomiting may prevent the vaccine from reaching the stomach and small intestine. Diarrhea may increase transit time, preventing proper contact of the vaccine viruses with villous intestinal cells, and lead to decreased immune response. **Vaccine** administration should be delayed until the vomiting and diarrhea have been resolved.

There is a risk that immunocompromised individuals may develop poliomyelitis from use of live polio virus, which is in **OPV**. Cancer, leukemia, lymphoma, radiation therapy, and immunodeficiency, including HIV or

Table 17-1. Recommended Childhood Immunization Schedule

Recommended Childhood Immunization Schedule United States, January - December 2000

Vaccines[1] are listed under routinely recommended ages. [Bars] *indicate range of recommended ages for immunization. Any dose not given at the recommended age should be given as a "catch-up" immunization at any subsequent visit when indicated and feasible.* (Ovals) *indicate vaccines to be given if previously recommended doses were missed or given earlier than the recommended minimum age.*

Age ▲ / Vaccine ▼	Birth	1 mo	2 mo	4 mo	6 mo	12 mo	15 mo	18 mo	24 mo	4-6 y	11-12 y	14-16 y
Hepatitis B[2]	Hep B	Hep B	Hep B			Hep B					(Hep B)	
Diphtheria, Tetanus, Pertussis[3]			DTaP	DTaP	DTaP			DTaP[3]		DTaP	Td	
H. influenzae type b[4]			Hib	Hib	Hib	Hib						
Polio[5]			IPV	IPV		IPV[5]				IPV[5]		
Measles, Mumps, Rubella[6]						MMR				MMR[6]	(MMR[6])	
Varicella[7]						Var					(Var[7])	
Hepatitis A[8]									Hep A-in selected areas			

Approved by the Advisory Committee on Immunization Practices (ACIP), the American Academy of Pediatrics (AAP), and the American Academy of Family Physicians (AAFP).

On October 22, 1999, the Advisory Committee on Immunization Practices (ACIP) recommended that Rotashield® (RRV-TV), the only U.S.-licensed rotavirus vaccine, no longer be used in the United States (MMWR, Volume 48, Number 43, Nov. 5, 1999). Parents should be reassured that their children who received rotavirus vaccine before July are not at increased risk for intussusception now

[1]This schedule indicates the recommended ages for routine administration of currently licensed childhood vaccines as of 11/1/99. Additional vaccines may be licensed and recommended during the year. Licensed combination vaccines may be used whenever any components of the combination are indicated and its other components are not contraindicated. Providers should consult the manufacturers' package inserts for detailed recommendations.

[2]**Infants born to HBsAg-negative mothers** should receive the first dose of hepatitis B (Hep B) vaccine by age 2 months. The second dose should be at least 1 month after the first dose. The third dose should be administered at least 4 months after the first dose and at least 2 months after the second dose, but not before 6 months of age for infants.

Infants born to HBsAg-positive mothers should receive hepatitis B vaccine and 0.5 mL hepatitis B immune globulin (HBIG) within 12 hours of birth at separate sites. The second dose is recommended at 1–2 months of age and the third dose at 6 months of age.

Infants born to mothers whose HBsAg status is unknown should receive hepatitis B vaccine within 12 hours of birth. Maternal blood should be drawn at the time of delivery to determine the mother's HBsAg status; if the HBsAg test is positive, the infant should receive HBIG as soon as possible (no later than 1 week of age).

All children and adolescents (through 18 years of age) who have not been immunized against hepatitis B may begin the series during any visit. Special efforts should be made to immunize children who were born in or whose parents were born in areas of the world with moderate or high endemicity of hepatitis B virus infection.

[3]The fourth dose of DTaP (diphtheria and tetanus toxoids and acellular pertussis vaccine) may be administered as early as 12 months of age, provided 6 months have elapsed since the third dose and the child is unlikely to return at age 15–18 months. Td (tetanus and diphtheria toxoids) is recommended at 11–12 years of age if at least 5 years have elapsed since the last dose of DTP, DTaP or DT. Subsequent routine Td boosters are recommended every 10 years.

[4]Three *Haemophilus influenzae* type b (Hib) conjugate vaccines are licensed for infant use. If PRP-OMP (PedvaxHIB® or ComVax® [Merck]) is administered at 2 and 4 months of age, a dose at 6 months is not required. Because clinical studies in infants have demonstrated that using some combination products may induce a lower immune response to the Hib vaccine component, DTaP/Hib combination products should not be used for primary immunization in infants at 2, 4 or 6 months of age, unless FDA-approved for these ages.

[5]To eliminate the risk of vaccine-associated paralytic polio (VAPP), an all-IPV schedule is now recommended for routine childhood polio vaccination in the United States. All children should receive four doses of IPV at 2 months, 4 months, 6–18 months, and 4–6 years. OPV (if available) may be used only for the following special circumstances:
1. Mass vaccination campaigns to control outbreaks of paralytic polio.
2. Unvaccinated children who will be traveling in <4 weeks to areas where polio is endemic or epidemic.
3. Children of parents who do not accept the recommended number of vaccine injections. These children may receive OPV only for the third or fourth dose or both; in this situation, health care providers should administer OPV only after discussing the risk for VAPP with parents or caregivers.
4. During the transition to an all-IPV schedule, recommendations for the use of remaining OPV supplies in physicians' offices and clinics have been issued by the American Academy of Pediatrics (see *Pediatrics*, December 1999).

[6]The second dose of measles, mumps, and rubella (MMR) vaccine is recommended routinely at 4–6 years of age but may be administered during any visit, provided at least 4 weeks have elapsed since receipt of the first dose and that both doses are administered beginning at or after 12 months of age. Those who have not previously received the second dose should complete the schedule by the 11–12-year-old visit.

[7]Varicella (Var) vaccine is recommended at any visit on or after the first birthday for susceptible children, i.e., those who lack a reliable history of chickenpox (as judged by a health care provider) and who have not been immunized. Susceptible persons 13 years of age or older should receive two doses, given at least 4 weeks apart.

[8]Hepatitis A (Hep A) is shaded to indicate its recommended use in selected states and/or regions; consult your local public health authority. (Also see MMWR Oct. 01, 1999/48[RR12]; 1–37).

Table 17–2. Vaccine Information Statements

Vaccine Information Statements (VIS) are available from the Centers for Disease Control and Prevention (CDC) or your local health department for the following vaccines. They have also been translated into the languages listed below. A PDF version of these VISs (English and other languages) can be found at *www.immunize.org*.

Vaccines
Chickenpox
Diphtheria, tetanus, and pertussis
Hib
Hepatitis A
Hepatitis B
Influenza
Lyme disease
Measles, mumps, and rubella
Pneumococcus
Polio
Td

Languages
Arabic
Armenian
Cambodian
Chinese
Croatian
Farsi
French
German
Haitian
Hmong
Japanese
Korean
Portuguese
Romanian
Russian
Samoan
Serbo-Croatian
Somali
Spanish
Tagalog
Vietnamese

AIDS, are contraindications to **OPV** use. Drugs that affect the immune system, including high-dose **steroids**, are also a contraindication to **OPV** use. There is a chance that immunosuppressed individuals may contract OPV-associated poliomyelitis from coming in contact with a patient who is shedding the virus. **IPV** is the drug of choice in immunocompromised patients. **IPV** should also be used if household members are immunocompromised.

Vaccination of pregnant women should be avoided. *OPV* is Pregnancy Category C. If exposure to poliomyelitis is imminent and immediate protection is needed, vaccinate with **OPV** or **IPV** according to the adult dosing schedule.

OPV is safe during breastfeeding and is routinely given during infancy.

ADVERSE DRUG REACTIONS. The administration of **OPV** is associated with a low incidence (1 case per 2.6 million doses) of paralytic poliomyelitis in patients who receive the **vaccine** and in household contacts. **Vaccine**-associated paralytic poliomyelitis (VAPP) is most likely to occur after the first dose of **OPV**. Household contacts are put at risk of developing VAPP because poliovirus is shed in the feces for 6 to 8 weeks after a dose of **OPV**. There is no risk of VAPP with the use of **IPV**, which is why, as of January 2000, **IPV** is the drug of choice for routine childhood immunization against polio.

DRUG INTERACTIONS. **OPV** should not be administered to patients receiving **immunosuppressants**, including **corticosteroids, interferon**, and **antineoplastic** drugs, because there may be insufficient response to immunization. Patients may remain susceptible despite immunization. **IPV** is the recommended drug to use in these patients.

The CDC recommends that administration of live-virus vaccines be separated by intervals of at least 1 month, unless data are available regarding simultaneous vaccination (**MMR, HBV, DTP, DTaP, influenza**, and **Hib** may be given with **OPV**). Concurrent administration of **OPV** and **cholera vaccine, parenteral typhoid vaccine**, or **plague vaccine** should generally be avoided because of increased adverse effects. Concurrent administration of **oral typhoid vaccine live** may result in decreased immune responses to **OPV**. IG may be given with **OPV**.

CLINICAL USE AND DOSING. To eliminate the risk of VAPP, the CDC recommended in January 2000 an all-**IPV** schedule for childhood immunizations. **OPV** may be used only for special circumstances, such as mass vaccination campaigns to control outbreaks of paralytic polio and in unvaccinated children who will be traveling in less than 4 weeks to areas where polio is endemic or epidemic. **OPV** may be used in children who have received at least two doses of **IPV** and whose parents do not accept the recommended number of vaccine injections. VAPP should be discussed with these parents before administering **OPV**. See Tables 17–1 and 17–3 for dosing schedules.

PATIENT EDUCATION. All patients or their parents or guardians are required by law to receive CDC VISs, which are available in a variety of languages. Every effort should be made to provide adequate information to patients and parents before immunization.

If a patient receives **OPV**, the patient and family should be instructed that virus is shed in the stools for 6 to 8 weeks and that good handwashing is crucial to preventing the small chance of contracting VAPP from the infected feces.

As previously mentioned, VAPP should be discussed with the parent or, if applicable, the patient before administering **OPV**.

Table 17-3. Vaccines and Toxoids Recommended for Adults, by Age Group

SUMMARY OF ADOLESCENT / ADULT IMMUNIZATION RECOMMENDATIONS — 5/17/98

AGENT	Tetanus & Diphtheria Toxoids Combined (Td)	Influenza Vaccine	Pneumococcal Polysaccharide Vaccine (PPV)	Measles and Mumps Vaccines**	Rubella Vaccine**	Hepatitis B Vaccine	Poliovirus Vaccine: IPV – Inactivated OPV – Oral (Live)	Varicella Vaccine	Hepatitis A Vaccine
INDICATIONS	All adults. All adolescents should be assessed at 11–12 or 14–16 years of age and immunized if no dose was received during the previous 5 years.	a. Adults 50 years of age and older. b. Residents of nursing homes or other facilities for patients with chronic medical conditions. c. Persons ≥6 mo. of age with chronic cardiovascular or pulmonary disorders, including asthma. d. Persons ≥6 mo. of age with chronic metabolic diseases (including diabetes), renal dysfunction, hemoglobinopathies, immunosuppression or immunodeficiency disorders. e. Women in their second or third trimester of pregnancy during influenza season. f. Persons 6 months–18 years of age receiving long-term aspirin therapy. g. Groups, including household members and caregivers, who can infect high-risk persons.	a. Adults 65 years of age and older. b. Persons ≥2 years with chronic cardiovascular or pulmonary disorders including congestive heart failure, diabetes mellitus, chronic liver disease, alcoholism, chronic CSF leaks, cardiomyopathy, COPD, or emphysema. c. Persons ≥2 years with splenic dysfunction or asplenia, hematologic malignancy, multiple myeloma, renal failure, organ transplantation or immunosuppressive conditions, including HIV infection. d. Alaskan Natives and certain American Indian populations.	a. Adults born after 1956 without written documentation of immunization on or after the first birthday. b. Health care personnel born in 1956 who are at risk of exposure to patients and who should have documentation of two doses of vaccine on or after the first birthday or confirmation of seropositivity. c. HIV-infected persons without severe immunosuppression. d. Persons entering post-secondary educational institutions (e.g., college).	a. Persons (especially women) without written documentation of immunization or of seropositivity. b. Health care personnel who are at risk of exposure to patients with rubella and who may have contact with pregnant patients should have at least one dose.	a. Persons with occupational risk of exposure to blood or blood-contaminated body fluids. b. Clients and staff of institutions for the developmentally disabled. c. Hemodialysis patients. d. Recipients of clotting-factor concentrates. e. Household contacts and sex partners of those chronically infected with HBV. f. Family members of adoptees from countries where HBV infection is endemic, if adoptees are HBsAg+. g. Certain international travelers. h. Injecting drug users: i. Men who have sex with men. j. Heterosexual men and women with multiple sex partners or recent episode of a sexually transmitted disease. k. Inmates of long-term correctional facilities. l. All unvaccinated adolescents.	Routine vaccination of those ≥18 years of age residing in the U.S. is not necessary. Vaccination is recommended for the following high-risk adult: a. Travelers to areas or countries where poliomyelitis is epidemic or endemic. b. Members of communities or specific population groups with disease caused by wild polioviruses. c. Laboratory workers who handle specimens that may contain polioviruses. d. Health care workers who have close contact with patients who may be excreting wild polioviruses. e. Unvaccinated adults whose children will be receiving OPV.	a. Persons of any age without a reliable history of varicella disease or vaccination, or who are seronegative for varicella. b. Susceptible adolescents and adults living in households with children. c. All susceptible health care workers. d. Susceptible family contacts of immunocompromised persons. e. Susceptible persons in the following groups who are at high risk for exposure: – persons who live or work in environments in which transmission of varicella is likely (e.g., teachers of young children, day care employees, residents and staff in institutional settings) or can occur (e.g., college students, inmates and staff of correctional institutions, military personnel) – nonpregnant women of childbearing age – international travelers	a. Persons traveling to or working in countries with high or intermediate endemicity of infection. b. Men who have sex with men. c. Injecting and non-injecting illegal drug users. d. Persons who work with HAV-infected primates or with HAV in a research laboratory setting. e. Persons with chronic liver disease. f. Persons with clotting factor disorders. g. Consider food handlers, where determined to be cost-effective by health authorities or employers.
PRIMARY SCHEDULE	Two doses 4–8 weeks apart, third dose 6–12 months after the second. No need to repeat doses if the schedule is interrupted. **Dose:** 0.5 mL intramuscular (IM). **Booster:** At 10-year intervals throughout life.	**Dose:** 0.5 mL intramuscular (IM). Given annually, each fall.	One dose for most people*. **Dose:** 0.5 mL intramuscular (IM) or subcutaneous (SC). *Persons vaccinated prior to age 65 should be revaccinated at age 65 if 5 or more years have passed since the first dose. For all persons with functional or anatomic asplenia, transplant patients, patients with chronic kidney disease, immunosuppressed or immunodeficient persons, and others at highest risk of fatal infection, a second dose should be given—at least 5 years after first dose.	At least one dose of measles-containing vaccine if in college, in a health care profession or traveling to a foreign country with a second dose at least 1 month after the first. **Dose:** 0.5 mL subcutaneous (SC)	One dose **Dose:** 0.5 mL subcutaneous (SC)	Three doses; second dose 1–2 months after the first, third dose 4–6 months after the first. No need to start series over if schedule interrupted. Can start series with one another. **Dose (Adult):** intramuscular (IM) Recombivax HB®: 10 μg/1.0 mL (green cap) Engerix-B®: 20 μg/1.0mL (orange cap) **Dose (Adolescent):** intramuscular (IM) Recombivax HB®: 5 μg/0.5 mL (yellow cap) Engerix-B®: 10 μg/0.5 mL (light blue cap) **Booster:** None presently recommended.	Unimmunized adolescents/adults. IPV is recommended — two doses at 4–8 week intervals, third dose 6–12 months after second (can be as soon as 2 months). **Dose:** 0.5 mL subcutaneous (SC) or intramuscular (IM). Partially immunized adolescents/adults: Complete primary series with IPV (IPV schedule shown above). OPV is *no longer recommended for use in the United States.*	For persons <13 years of age, one dose. For persons 13 years of age and older, two doses separated by 4–8 weeks. If >8 weeks elapse following the first dose, the second dose can be administered without restarting the schedule. **Dose:** 0.5 mL subcutaneous (SC).	HAVRIX®: Two doses, separated by 6–12 months. Adults (19 years of age and older) – **Dose:** 1.0 mL intramuscular (IM); Persons 2–18 years of age – **Dose:** 0.5 mL (IM). VAQTA®: Adults (18 years of age and older): Two doses, separated by 6 months — **Dose:** 1.0 mL intramuscular (IM); Persons 2–17 years of age: Two doses, separated by 6–18 months — **Dose:** 0.5 mL (IM).
CONTRAINDICATIONS	Neurologic or severe hypersensitivity reaction to prior dose.	Anaphylactic allergy to eggs. Acute febrile illness.	The safety of PPV during the first trimester of pregnancy has not been evaluated. The manufacturer's package insert should be reviewed for additional information.	a. Immunosuppressive therapy or immunodeficiency including HIV-infected persons with severe immunosuppression. b. Anaphylactic allergy to neomycin. c. Pregnancy. d. Immune globulin preparation or blood/blood product received in preceding 3–11 months.	Same as for measles and mumps vaccines.	Anaphylactic allergy to yeast.	IPV: Anaphylactic reaction following previous dose of streptomycin, polymyxin B, or neomycin.	a. Anaphylactic allergy to gelatin or neomycin. b. Untreated, active TB. c. Immunosuppressive therapy or immunodeficiency (including HIV infection). d. Family history of congenital or hereditary immunodeficiency in first-degree relatives, unless the immune competence of the recipient has been clinically substantiated or verified by a laboratory. e. Immune globulin preparation or blood/blood product received in preceding 5 months. f. Pregnancy.	A history of hypersensitivity to alum or the preservative 2-phenoxyethanol
COMMENTS	**WOUND MANAGEMENT:** Patients with three or more previous tetanus toxoid doses: a) give Td for clean, minor wounds only if more than 10 years since last dose; b) for other wounds, give Td if over 5 years since last dose. Patients with less than 3 or unknown number of prior tetanus toxoid doses, give Td for clean, minor wounds and Td and TIG (Tetanus Immune Globulin) for other wounds.	Depending on season and destination, persons traveling to foreign countries should consider vaccination. Any person ≥6 mo. of age who wishes to reduce the likelihood of becoming ill with influenza should be vaccinated.	If elective splenectomy or immunosuppressive therapy is planned, give vaccine 2 weeks ahead, if possible. When indicated, vaccine should be administered to patients with unknown vaccination status. All residents of nursing homes and other long-term care facilities should have their vaccination status assessed and documented.	Women should be asked if they are pregnant before receiving vaccine, and advised to avoid becoming pregnant for 30 days after immunization.	Women should be asked if they are pregnant before receiving vaccine, and advised to avoid pregnancy for 3 months after immunization.	a. Persons with serologic markers of prior or continuing hepatitis B virus infection do not need immunization. b. For hemodialysis patients and other immunocompromised or immunosuppressed patients, vaccine dosage is doubled or special preparation is used. c. Pregnant women should be screened for HBsAg and, if positive, their infants should be given post-exposure prophylaxis beginning at birth. d. Post-exposure prophylaxis: consult ACIP recommendation, or state or local immunization program.	In instances of potential exposure to wild poliovirus, adults who have had a primary series of OPV or IPV may be given 1 more dose of IPV. Although no adverse effects have been documented, vaccination of pregnant women should be avoided. However, if immediate protection is needed, pregnant women may be given IPV, in accordance with the recommended schedule for adults.	Women should be asked if they are pregnant before receiving varicella vaccine, and advised to avoid pregnancy for 1 month following each dose of vaccine.	The safety of hepatitis A vaccine during pregnancy has not been determined, though the theoretical risk to the developing fetus is expected to be low. The risk of vaccination should be weighed against the risk of hepatitis A in women who may be at a high risk of exposure to HAV.

CDC — Centers for Disease Control and Prevention

Adapted from the recommendations of the Advisory Committee on Immunization Practices (ACIP). Foreign travel and less commonly used vaccines such as typhoid, rabies, and meningococcal are not included.
**These vaccines can be given in the combined form measles-mumps-rubella (MMR). Persons already immune to one or more components can still receive MMR.

Varicella Virus Vaccine

Pharmacodynamics

Varicella virus vaccine (Varivax) is a **live vaccine** that produces IgG antibody humoral immune response to varicella zoster virus (VZV). Vaccinated patients also have cell-mediated immune response, with activation of both CD4+ helper T cells and CD8+ T lymphocytes. Vaccination appears to prevent serious disease even in patients who do not seroconvert. Postvaccination cases of varicella are mild.

Pharmacokinetics

A single SC dose of **varicella virus vaccine** given to children age 12 months to 12 years stimulates IgG antibody production and results in seroconversion rates of 97 percent. In those age 13 years and older, seroconversion rates are 78 to 82 percent; a second dose results in 99 percent seroconversion in adolescents and adults. Waning immunity has not been demonstrated, with high antibody levels measured for at least 10 years after vaccination.

Pharmacotherapeutics

PRECAUTIONS AND CONTRAINDICATIONS. Patients with **neomycin** or gelatin hypersensitivity should not receive **varicella vaccine** because there are small quantities in the vaccine.

Varicella vaccine should be delayed if a patient has a moderate or severe illness, with or without fever.

There is a risk that immunocompromised individuals will develop varicella from use of live virus for vaccination. Cancer, leukemia, lymphoma, radiation therapy, and immunodeficiency are contraindications to **varicella vaccine** use. Patients with symptomatic or asymptomatic HIV infection should not receive **varicella vaccine.** Drugs that affect the immune system, including high-dose **steroids**, also contraindicate **varicella vaccine** use.

Varicella vaccine may be given to a patient if there is an immunocompromised person in the household. The patient who develops a rash after vaccination should avoid contact with the immunocompromised person for the duration of the rash.

Vaccination of pregnant women should be avoided. *Varicella vaccine* **is Pregnancy Category C. Pregnancy should be avoided for 1 to 3 months after vaccination.** The manufacturer of **Varivax** has established a pregnancy registry to monitor maternal-fetal outcomes of pregnant women inadvertently administered the **varicella virus vaccine live** 3 months before or during pregnancy. For information about the registry, call 1-800-986-8999. **Varicella vaccine** may be given if there is a pregnant household contact, such as the patient's mother. **Varicella vaccine** may be given to a nurs-

ing mother if the risk of exposure to natural VZV is high. It is not known if it is excreted in breast milk.

ADVERSE DRUG REACTIONS. The reactions reported most frequently in children and adults that can be attributed to **varicella vaccine** include fever, injection site reaction, and a vesicular rash. In healthy children, fever of 102°F or higher is reported in 14.7 percent of vaccine recipients. Pain or discomfort at the injection site is reported in 19.3 percent, with 3.4 percent of patients developing a vesicular rash at the injection site. A generalized vesicular rash developed in 3.8 percent of patients, with the median number of five or fewer lesions in healthy children. The vesicular rash occurs within 26 days of injection with **varicella vaccine.**

Adult and adolescent patients require 2 injections and have similar adverse reactions. Fever in **vaccine** recipients age 12 years and older was defined as a temperature of 100°F or higher. After the first dose of **varicella vaccine,** 10.2 percent reported fever, and 9.5 percent reported fever after the second dose. Localized reaction at the injection site was reported in 3 percent of adolescent and adult patients after the first dose and in 1 percent after the second dose. A generalized vesicular rash was reported by 5.5 percent after the first dose and 0.9 percent after the second dose.

DRUG INTERACTIONS. **Varicella vaccine** should not be administered to patients receiving **immunosuppressants,** including **corticosteroids, interferon,** and **antineoplastic drugs,** because there may be insufficient response to immunization. Patients may remain susceptible despite immunization.

It is not known whether **varicella vaccine** may be inactivated by **IG,** although other **live-virus vaccines** may be inactivated. **Varicella vaccine** should not be given for 5 months after **IG** is administered. The CDC recommends that **IG** preparations should not be administered for 3 weeks after **varicella vaccine** is given; the manufacturer recommends waiting 2 months. If **IG** is given in the interval after vaccination, the recipient should be either revaccinated in 5 months or tested for varicella immunity 6 months later and revaccinated if indicated.

Administration of the **MMR** and **varicella vaccines** is compatible if done on the same day, with different needles and at separate sites. If the two live vaccines are not given at the same time, an interval of 1 month between **MMR** and **varicella vaccine** is indicated. **Varicella vaccine** may be given simultaneously with **DTaP, DT, Td, Hib, IPV, OPV,** or **HBV,** using separate sites of injection.

Although no adverse effects from the use of **salicylates** or **aspirin** have been reported, the manufacturer recommends avoidance of **ASA** for 6 weeks after vaccination. Reye's syndrome, which affects children younger than age 15 exclusively, has been associated with **aspirin** use following active varicella infection. Children who are on therapeutic **ASA** therapy may be vaccinated with the **varicella vaccine,** with close clinical monitoring. According to the CDC, vaccination is thought to present less risk than natural **varicella vaccine** in these children.

CLINICAL USE AND DOSING. The CDC and the American Academy of Pediatrics (AAP) recommend that all healthy children who lack a reliable history of varicella infection be routinely vaccinated at age 12 to 18 months. Administration of one dose of **varicella vaccine** is recommended at any time during childhood, before the 13th birthday if possible, because of the increased severity of natural varicella infection after this age.

Healthy adolescents age 13 years and older, who have no history of varicella infection and who have not previously received **varicella vaccine,** should be administered two doses 4 to 8 weeks apart.

The Advisory Committee on Immunization Practices (ACIP) of the CDC recommends vaccination of susceptible adults. Priority for adult immunization should be given to those at high risk of exposure or transmission of varicella disease. They include adults who live in households with children, live or work in an environment where varicella transmission is likely (teachers, health care workers, day care workers) or could occur (college dorm, correctional institution, military), or have household contact with an immunocompromised person; nonpregnant childbearing women; and international travelers. Performing serologic testing of adults before administering is optional and may be cost effective. The **varicella vaccine** dose for adults is two doses, separated by 4 to 8 weeks.

PATIENT EDUCATION. All patients or their parents or guardians are required by law to receive CDC VISs, which are available in a variety of languages. Every effort should be made to provide adequate information to patients and their parents before immunization.

There may be transient burning or stinging upon administration.

Patients should be informed that there is a small chance that they may develop a fever, reaction at the injection site, or vesicular rash after administration of **varicella vaccine.**

Typhoid

Pharmacodynamics

Typhoid vaccines are used to increase resistance to enteric fever caused by *Salmonella typhi.* **Oral typhoid vaccine (Vivotif Berna)** is a **live attenuated vaccine, Ty21a.** The **oral vaccine** is ingested and works in the small intestine to synthesize a lipopolysaccharide that evokes a protective immune response. It is estimated to be 60 to 70 percent effective in preventing typhoid fever. Efficacy of protective immunity depends on the size of the bacterial inoculum consumed.

Pharmacokinetics

The absorption, distribution, and metabolism of **oral typhoid vaccine** are unknown.

Pharmacotherapeutics

PRECAUTIONS AND CONTRAINDICATIONS. Hypersensitivity to **typhoid vaccine** is a contraindication to its use.

Because **oral typhoid vaccine** is a live attenuated virus, it should not be administered to immunocompromised patients, including those who are HIV infected.

Do not administer it to a patient with acute febrile illness or an acute GI illness (diarrhea).

Oral typhoid vaccine is **Pregnancy Category C. It is not known if the vaccine is harmful to the fetus. If it is necessary to vaccinate a pregnant patient, inactivated vaccine is recommended.**

Oral typhoid vaccine is not recommended for use in children younger than age 6 years. Use **inactivated vaccine** in young children.

Clinical Pearl

....

ADMINISTERING MULTIPLE VACCINES

There are currently six possible injections that a child from age 12 to 18 months should receive. This can be traumatic for patient and parent. Most public health officials recommend giving all the recommended **vaccines** at each visit; therefore, the child who is 15 months old could be getting as many as all six injections in one visit. It is best to spread the administration of the **vaccines** out over two or three visits. If it is necessary to give all the **vaccines** in one visit, as in the case of upcoming international travel or a history of unreliable attendance at well child examinations, two people can administer the **vaccines** simultaneously. Giving the **vaccines** simultaneously makes the process faster and simpler for the patient and the person administering the **vaccine.**

....

ADVERSE DRUG REACTIONS. Adverse effects of **oral typhoid vaccine** are infrequent and transient and resolve with intervention. Abdominal pain, diarrhea, vomiting, fever, headache, and rash have been reported.

DRUG INTERACTIONS. The **antimalarial** drug **mefloquine (Lariam)** can inhibit the growth of the live **Ty21a** strain in vitro. It is recommended that **oral typhoid vaccine** be given either 24 hours before or 24 hours after **mefloquine.**

Immunosuppressants may cause insufficient response to the **vaccine.**

The manufacturer recommends that **oral typhoid vaccine** not be administered to individuals receiving **sulfonamides** and **antibiotics,** which may be active against the **vaccine** strains and prevent a sufficient degree of multiplication to induce a protective immune response.

CLINICAL USE AND DOSING. Oral typhoid vaccine is used for primary immunization against *S. typhi* infection in the following:

1. Travelers to areas where a risk of exposure to *S. typhi* is recognized.
2. People who have household contact with a documented typhoid fever carrier.
3. Laboratory workers who have frequent contact with *S. typhi.*

For primary immunization of patients over age 6 years, the dose is 1 capsule on alternate days (days 1, 3, 5, 7) for a total of 4 doses. The capsule needs to be taken 1 hour before meals with a cold glass of water (not warmer than body temperature). The **vaccine** capsule should be swallowed whole. Ideally, the patient should finish the four doses at least 1 week prior to exposure or travel.

A booster dose of 4 capsules, given every other day, is recommended every 5 years under conditions of repeated exposure.

PATIENT EDUCATION. The medication should be taken exactly as prescribed. It must be taken on an empty stomach with *cold* water. Every-other-day dosing should be explained. The patient must understand that all four doses must be taken, at least 1 week prior to travel, to provide the best protection.

Although the possible adverse effects of the **vaccine** are mild and usually transient, the patient should be informed about them.

The best protection against typhoid fever is food and water precautions to prevent contracting *S. typhi.*

Yellow Fever Vaccine

Pharmacodynamics

Yellow fever is a viral illness spread by some species of mosquitoes in Central and South America and in tropical regions of Africa. **Yellow fever vaccine (YF-Vax)** is a live, attenuated virus that is prepared by culturing the 17D strain virus in a living chick embryo.

Pharmacokinetics

After SC administration of the **vaccine,** active immunity to yellow fever occurs in 7 to 10 days and lasts for 10 years or more.

Pharmacotherapeutics

PRECAUTIONS AND CONTRAINDICATIONS. Yellow fever vaccine should be avoided in any patient with a history of egg hypersensitivity or sensitivity to chicken protein.

Because **yellow fever vaccine** is a live attenuated virus, it should not be administered to immunocompromised patients, including those who are HIV infected.

Defer vaccination with **yellow fever vaccine** for 8 weeks following blood or plasma transfusion.

Yellow fever vaccine **is Pregnancy Category C. It is not known if the vaccine is harmful to the fetus. Vaccinate only those pregnant women who are at high risk of contracting the disease.**

Oral typhoid vaccine is not recommended for use in children younger than age 9 months. Rare cases of encephalitis have occurred in infants of this age who have received **yellow fever vaccine.**

ADVERSE DRUG REACTIONS. Up to 10 percent of patients experience fever or malaise, usually 7 to 14 days after administration of vaccine. Myalgia or headache is reported in 2 to 5 percent of **vaccine** recipients.

DRUG INTERACTIONS. Concurrent vaccination with **yellow fever vaccine** and **cholera vaccine** leads to decreased immune response to each **vaccine.** Separate the two by at least 3 weeks. Concurrent vaccination with **yellow fever vaccine** and **hepatitis B vaccine** reduces the antibody titer expected from the **yellow fever vaccine.**

Immunosuppressants may cause insufficient response to the **yellow fever vaccine.**

Preservatives in diluent may kill the live virus in the **vaccine. Yellow fever vaccine** should be reconstituted with the diluent supplied with the **vaccine.**

CLINICAL USE AND DOSING. Immunization against yellow fever is recommended for all people over age 9 months who are living in or traveling to endemic areas. Vaccination is required by international regulations for travel to certain countries. The dose is a single 0.5-mL dose given SC.

PATIENT EDUCATION. Patients should be educated about the mild transient adverse effects that can occur from **vaccine** administration.

Patients should be instructed regarding protecting themselves against mosquitoes. Insect repellant and proper protective clothing and netting provide the best defense against insect-borne diseases.

Bacillus Calmette-Guérin Vaccine

Pharmacodynamics

Immunization with **bacillus Calmette-Guérin (BCG) vaccine** lowers the risk of serious complications of primary TB in children. **BCG** is an immune stimulant. It is used to stimulate the immune system to produce immunity against TB. Vaccination with **BCG** stimulates natural infection with *Mycobacterium tuberculosis* and results in a cell-mediated immune reaction and immunity against TB. Vaccination with **BCG** causes variable degrees of protection against TB. The protective effect of **BCG** use in children against miliary and meningeal TB is about 80 percent. It is less effective in adults.

Pharmacokinetics

BCG is administered percutaneously. Specific pharmacokinetic information is not available. Duration of protection against TB varies according to the potency of the strain of **BCG** used. TB sensitivity may last up to 10 years.

Pharmacotherapeutics

PRECAUTIONS AND CONTRAINDICATIONS. Patients with active TB should not receive **BCG**. **PPD** skin testing should be performed on all patients over 2 months of age who are receiving **BCG**.

Cancer, leukemia, lymphoma, radiation therapy, and immunodeficiency are contraindications to **BCG** use. Patients with symptomatic or asymptomatic HIV infection should not receive **BCG**. Drugs that affect the immune system, including high-dose **steroids**, are also a contraindication to **BCG** use.

Precautions should be taken to avoid accidental exposure to **BCG** solutions during preparation and administration because these solutions contain live, attenuated *M. tuberculosis*.

BCG **is Pregnancy Category C. The CDC does not recommend the use of *BCG* in pregnant women.**

ADVERSE DRUG REACTIONS. A normal reaction to the **BCG vaccine** is skin lesions that appear within 10 to 14 days after the multiple-puncture disk application of **BCG**. The lesions consist of small red papules at the site of administration. The papules reach maximum diameter (3 mm) after 4 to 6 weeks and then scale away and slowly subside. Six months after vaccination, there is usually no visible sign of vaccination, although faint disk marks may be noted.

Lymphadenopathy may occur in a regional lymph node that resolves spontaneously.

Osteomyelitis is a rare occurrence (1 per 1 million doses). **BCG**-induced osteomyelitis affects the epiphyses of the long bones and can occur from 4 months to 2 years after administration.

Rarely, lupoidlike skin reactions have occurred. It has been recommended that patients who experience lupus-like symptoms after **BCG** administration be treated with **isoniazid (INH)** for 3 months.

Disseminated **BCG** infection and death are very rare (about 1 per 5 million doses) and usually occur in children with impaired immune systems.

DRUG INTERACTIONS. Antituberculosis agents (**rifampin, INH, streptomycin**) and **immunosuppressives** may interfere with the development of an appropriate immune response to **BCG** administration.

BCG administration will cause **PPD** skin tests to give false-positive readings for up to 10 years after administration. After 10 years, a positive **PPD** usually indicates infection with *M. tuberculosis*.

CLINICAL USE AND DOSING. In the United States, **BCG** is administered only in very special circumstances, such as unavoidable risk of exposure to *M. tuberculosis* and failure of other methods of prevention and control of TB. With the reemergence of drug-resistant TB, the use of **BCG** is being reevaluated.

The ACIP has set clear criteria for the use of **BCG** in the United States: "**BCG** vaccination should be considered for infants and children who reside in settings in which the likelihood of *M. tuberculosis* transmission and subsequent infection is high provided no other measures can be implemented (e.g., removing child from the source of infection). In addition **BCG** vaccination may be considered for health-care workers who are employed in settings in which the likelihood of transmission and subsequent infection with *M. tuberculosis* strains resistant to **INH** and **rifampin** is high" (CDC, 1996c).

BCG is given to healthy infants from birth to 2 months without TB skin testing. After that, **BCG** is given only to children with negative Mantoux skin tests.

The administration of **BCG** must be exactly as the manufacturer directs. The **vaccine** is dropped onto clean, dry skin over the deltoid muscle and spread over the area to be punctured, using the edge of the multipuncture disk. The prongs of the disk are coated with the virus by lightly dipping them into the spread **vaccine**. The prongs of the disk are pressed into the skin and held for 5 to 10 seconds. After the disk is removed, the **vaccine** is respread to fill all the puncture areas. Additional **vaccine** may be applied to ensure a "wet" **vaccine** site. The vaccinated area needs to be kept dry for 24 hours. No dressing is required.

The dose for infants 1 month or younger is diluted to 50 percent by adding 2 mL of sterile water to the **vaccine**.

The person administering the **vaccine** should take precautions against coming in contact with the live virus.

PATIENT EDUCATION. The patient or parent should be instructed that the virus contains **live vaccine** and that the site should not be touched. The **vaccine** site should be kept clean until the local reaction has resolved.

Clear instructions regarding the normal skin reaction should be given to the patient or parent prior to administration.

Inactivated Vaccines

Diphtheria, Tetanus, and Pertussis Vaccine

Pharmacodynamics

Various combinations of **diphtheria, tetanus,** and **pertussis vaccines** are available on the market. Regardless of the combination of **vaccines,** the basic pharmacodynamic principles are the same.

Diphtheria toxoid induces the production of antibodies against the exotoxin excreted by *Corynebacterium diphtheriae.* Complete immunization (four doses, then boosters every 10 years) induces specific antibodies and reduces the incidence of diphtheria by more than 95 percent. Immunized persons who develop diphtheria have milder illness. Infection with *C. diphtheriae* does not confer immunity, and previously infected persons should still receive toxoid.

Adsorbed **tetanus toxoid** contains antigens that induce the production of antibodies against the exotoxin excreted by *Clostridium tetani.* The duration of immunity against *C. tetani* is about 10 years. Natural immunity to *C. tetani* does not occur in the United States, and even patients with previous *C. tetani* infection should receive the **tetanus toxoid.**

Pertussis vaccine contains inactivated pertussis antigens. **Acellular pertussis vaccine** contains one or more immunogens derived from *Bordetella pertussis* and, unlike **whole-cell vaccine,** contains little or no endotoxin. Immunization with **pertussis vaccine** produces antibodies against *B. pertussis.* The efficacy of **whole-cell pertussis vaccine** for children exposed to pertussis who received at least three doses of DPT is estimated at 59 to 90 percent. **Acellular pertussis vaccine** has a clinical efficacy of 79 to 93 percent in protecting against clinical pertussis after household exposure. Vaccinated patients who do contract pertussis usually have a milder case. **Pertussis vaccine** is always given in combination with **diphtheria** and **tetanus vaccines** (DTP, DTaP).

Pharmacokinetics

The **DTP** or **DTaP** vaccine is given intramuscularly (IM). Ninety percent of patients who receive three doses develop protective immunity against diphtheria and tetanus. Patients who receive four doses of **DPT** have im-

munity that persists for 10 years or more. In patients who receive four doses of **DPT,** immunity to pertussis begins to wane after 4 to 6 years. Ten years after immunization, fewer than 50 percent of vaccine recipients have protective antibodies against *B. pertussis.*

Pharmacotherapeutics

PRECAUTIONS AND CONTRAINDICATIONS. In the United States, it is currently recommended that **DTaP** be used for primary immunization of infants and children. Therefore, the precautions and contraindications to **DTaP** are discussed here, and **DTP** is not discussed, although the contraindications are the same for each **vaccine.**

The true contraindication to **DTaP** vaccination is a patient who experienced an immediate anaphylactic reaction with a previous dose. Encephalopathy that occurred within 7 days of a previous dose, unexplained by another cause, is a possible contraindication to further **pertussis vaccine** use. In this case, **DT** should be substituted for **DTaP.**

Patients with unstable, progressive neurological problems may have the **vaccine** waived. This is done on an individual basis and determined by the patient's medical condition.

Many **DTaP** products contain **thimerosal;** therefore, if the patient is sensitive, the product label should be checked to determine if **thimerosal** is an ingredient.

Precautions associated with **DTaP** include a previous temperature of 105°F (40.5°C) or higher within 48 hours after a dose, history of continuous crying (more than 3 hours) within 48 hours of a dose, convulsions within 3 days of a previous dose, and collapse or shocklike state (hypotonic-hyporesponsive episode) within 48 hours of a previous dose. Although these precautions were once considered contraindications, they are now considered precautions because they have not been proved to cause permanent sequelae. "The decision to give or withhold immunization should be based on the clinical assessment of the earlier episode, the likelihood of pertussis exposure in the child's community, and the potential benefits and risks of the pertussis vaccine" (Committee on Infectious Diseases, AAP, 1997).

DTaP may be given to immunocompromised patients or patients on **immunosuppressive therapy.** It is possible that the immune response to the **vaccine** may be less than optimal. Patients with HIV infection may be immunized.

Infants born prematurely should begin the **vaccine** series based on their date of birth, with the first vaccine given routinely at age 2 months.

Patients with a minor acute or febrile illness, including otitis media, may be immunized. Immunization should be delayed in cases of moderate or severe illnesses, with or without fever.

The contraindications to **DT** include patients older than age 7 years; give **Td.** The contraindications to **DT** or **Td** include hypersensitivity to any component of the **vac-**

cine and moderate to severe illness, with or without fever. Do not postpone for minor illness, including otitis media.

ADVERSE DRUG REACTIONS. Injection site reactions of mild to moderate pain, erythema, swelling, and induration may last for a few days after injection. Transient low-grade fever, chills, malaise, generalized aches and pains, and headache may occur. Fever is common after **DPT** and less common after **DTaP.** Drowsiness, fretfulness, and GI upset may occur.

Seizures may occur and are more likely in children with a history of seizures. Seizures may be related to fever, and antipyretic prophylaxis is recommended every 4 to 6 hours after administration to decrease the incidence of febrile seizure after vaccination.

DRUG INTERACTIONS. Coadministration of radiation therapy, **antineoplastic agents,** or **immunosuppressives** can decrease the immunologic response to the DtaP vaccine.

Neither **DtaP, DT,** or **Td** should be administered concurrently with **cholera vaccine, typhoid vaccine,** or **plague vaccine;** there may be accentuated adverse effects. **DtaP, DT,** or **Td** may be coadministered with **HBV, Hib, meningococcal,** and **pneumococcal vaccines.**

CLINICAL USE AND DOSING. DtaP is routinely given at age 2 months, 4 months, 6 months, 15 to 18 months, and 4 to 6 years. **DT,** if used, is given on the same schedule.

As a booster, **Td** is recommended at age 11 to 12 years if 5 years have elapsed since the last dose and then every 10 years thereafter. If a patient older than age 7 years has never been immunized, the primary series of **Td** is three doses. The first dose is followed by the second dose 4 weeks later. The third dose is given 6 to 12 months after the second dose. Every adult needs a booster every 10 years after completion of the primary series of three doses.

MONITORING. There is no laboratory monitoring needed with **DtaP, DT,** or **Td vaccine.**

PATIENT EDUCATION. The parent or patient should receive a VIS prior to administration of **vaccine.** Any questions or concerns regarding the **vaccine** should be addressed.

The most common adverse reaction after **DtaP** or **Td** injection is pain and erythema at the injection site. Advise the patient to take **acetaminophen** for discomfort for the first 24 hours after injection.

Postvaccination fever, myalgia, and headache can be treated with **acetaminophen** or **ibuprofen** prophylaxis.

Haemophilus b Conjugate Vaccine (Hib)

Pharmacodynamics

There are four formulations of **Haemophilus b (Hib) conjugate vaccine (Hib)** available. Each **vaccine** con-

sists of the Hib capsular polysaccharide covalently linked to another antigen to increase immunogenicity. **Hib conjugate vaccine** exposure stimulates the immune system to produce Hib capsule-specific antibodies that destroy the capsule. This makes the organism vulnerable to antibody and cell-mediated immunity. **Unconjugated capsule polysaccharide vaccines** cause B-cell stimulation only. By conjugating the capsule polysaccharide, T-cell stimulation occurs as well.

Pharmacokinetics

Hib is administered IM. Antibodies are detected approximately 1 to 2 weeks after administration. The **Hib** is more immunogenic in older children; therefore, only one dose is needed for children receiving their first dose at age 15 months or older.

Ideally, the patient should receive the same **conjugate vaccine** product for all of the primary series of immunizations. However, when different products are given for the series, serum antibodies are similar to those of patients who received all the same formula.

The anticapsular antibodies may cross the placenta and are distributed in breast milk.

Pharmacotherapeutics

PRECAUTIONS AND CONTRAINDICATIONS. Anaphylactic reaction to the **vaccine** or any component (including **thimerosal**) is a contraindication to **Hib.**

Moderate to severe illness, with or without fever, may be a reason to delay **vaccine.** Minor illness, including otitis media, is not a reason to delay administration.

Hib vaccine should be administered only to children under age 6 years.

ADVERSE DRUG REACTIONS. The most common adverse reaction following **Hib** is pain, redness, and swelling at the injection site. These symptoms are mild and usually last less than 24 hours. Systemic reactions are infrequent, and when **Hib** is given with **DtaP,** there is no increased incidence of systemic reaction over **DtaP** given alone.

DRUG INTERACTIONS. There are no known interactions.

CLINICAL USE AND DOSING. Dosing of **Hib** depends on the **vaccine** used. **HibTITER (HbOC)** and **ActHib (PRP-T)** are given at 2 months, 4 months, 6 months, and a booster at 12 to 15 months. **PedvaxHIB (PRP-OMP)** is given at 2 months, 4 months, and a booster at 12 to 15 months. The first dose of **Hib** can be given at age 6 weeks but no earlier. Any **Hib vaccine** can be used for the booster dose at age 12 to 15 months.

If the child is receiving the first dose at age 15 months or older but younger than 5 years, only one dose of **Hib** is needed.

MONITORING. No laboratory monitoring is necessary.

PATIENT EDUCATION. Parents should receive a VIS prior to administration of the **vaccine.** Any questions or concerns regarding the **vaccine** should be addressed.

The most common adverse reaction after **Hib** injection is pain and erythema at the injection site. Advise the parent to give **acetaminophen** for discomfort for the first 24 hours after injection.

Inactivated Poliovirus Vaccine

Pharmacodynamics

IPV vaccine is a parenteral noninfectious suspension of three types of inactivated poliovirus. The **IPV** available in the United States since the late 1980s is of enhanced potency and is highly immunogenic. **IPV** inhibits pharyngeal acquisition of poliovirus and, to a lesser extent, provides gut immunity.

Pharmacokinetics

After IM administration of two doses, approximately 95 percent of patients have antibodies to polio. After three doses, 99 to 100 percent of patients have high antibody titers.

Pharmacotherapeutics

PRECAUTIONS AND CONTRAINDICATIONS. A history of immediate hypersensitivity reaction after receiving **IPV** is a contraindication. Patients with **neomycin, streptomycin** or **polymyxin B** hypersensitivity should not receive the **vaccine** because there are small amounts in the **vaccine.**

IPV is the preferred drug (over **OPV**) in immunosuppressed patients, although a protective immune response cannot be guaranteed. **IPV** can be administered to patients with HIV disease.

If it is needed to protect the patient, *IPV* may be administered during pregnancy. *IPV* is Pregnancy Category C.

IPV can be used in infants as young as 6 weeks of age.

ADVERSE DRUG REACTIONS. Injection site reaction is reported in 13 percent of patients. Systemic reactions are infrequent, and when **IPV** is given with **DtaP** there is no increased incidence of systemic reaction over **DtaP** given alone.

DRUG INTERACTIONS. The immune response to **IPV** may be diminished if the patient is taking immunosuppressant medication. Revaccinate 3 months after discontinuing immunosuppressants.

IPV can be coadministered with all other childhood **vaccines.**

MONITORING. There is no need for laboratory monitoring after administration of **IPV.**

PATIENT EDUCATION. Parents should receive a VIS prior to administration of the **vaccine.** Any questions or concerns regarding the **vaccine** should be addressed.

The most common adverse reaction after **IPV** injection is pain and erythema at the injection site. Advise the parent to give **acetaminophen** for discomfort for the first 24 hours after injection.

Hepatitis B Virus Vaccine

Pharmacodynamics

Hepatitis B virus (HBV) vaccine is produced by recombinant DNA technology from common bakers' yeast that is genetically modified to synthesize HbsAg. Active immunization with **HBV** stimulates the immune system to produce antihepatitis B surface antigen antibodies (anti-HBs).

Pharmacokinetics

Three doses of **HBV** induce protective antibody response in more than 95 percent of infants, children, and adolescents and in more than 90 percent of adults. Anti-HBs appear in the serum 2 weeks after IM administration. The minimum anti-HB titer needed to provide protection against hepatitis B is 10 milli-international units (mIU)/mL.

Clinical Pearl

ADMINISTERING INJECTIONS

A "trick" to help older children, adolescents, or adults who are anxious about receiving injections is to encourage them to take slow, deep breaths. Younger children (5-year-olds) can be told to pretend they are blowing up a balloon. Have the patient inhale and exhale two or three times, and then, on the third or fourth exhalation, administer the injection. It is difficult to exhale and tense the muscles at the same time.

Pharmacotherapeutics

PRECAUTIONS AND CONTRAINDICATIONS. The only true contraindication to **HBV vaccine** is hypersensitivity to yeast or other components of the vaccine.

Moderate or severe illness, with or without fever, is a contraindication to **HBV**.

Patients with renal disease requiring hemodialysis or patients with immunosuppression may require larger doses to achieve adequate serum levels of anti-HBs.

HBV **is Pregnancy Category C. The CDC has stated that** *HBV* **may be given in pregnancy if indicated (1998).**

ADVERSE DRUG REACTIONS. Localized reaction at the injection site is reported by 17 percent of **vaccine** recipients. Approximately 15 percent of patients report systemic complaints, including fatigue, weakness, malaise, fever, headache, nausea or vomiting, diarrhea, and pharyngitis. Serum sickness has occurred days to weeks after administration of **HBV**. A very rare side effect is alopecia (occurs 5 in 1 billion doses).

DRUG INTERACTIONS. Patients who are taking **immunosuppressants** or **antineoplastic agents** may require larger doses or additional doses of **HBV** to achieve adequate anti-HB titers.

CLINICAL USE AND DOSING. Vaccination with **HBV** is recommended for all ages, particularly patients at high risk of contracting hepatitis B. Those at high risk include intravenous (IV) drug users, infants born to mothers who are HbsAg-positive, hemodialysis patients, sexually active people with multiple partners, incarcerated people, international travelers, household contacts of hepatitis B carriers, and sexual contacts of hepatitis B carriers. Patients who are getting tattoos or who share razors, toothbrushes, or body-piercing jewelry are also at risk of contracting hepatitis B. Health care workers, day care staff, and other people who may have exposure to body fluids also have a greater risk of contracting hepatitis B.

The ACIP and the AAP recommend universal vaccination of all infants as a comprehensive strategy to control hepatitis B. The current recommendations for childhood immunizations include administering the three-dose **HBV** series to newborns or at age 11 to 12 years to children not previously vaccinated. The series can be started at any age. Some states are requiring proof of **HBV** series completion for entry to the seventh grade.

Vaccination with **HBV** is recommended for all adults who are at high risk of contracting hepatitis B infection.

The recommended schedule for vaccinating infants is to give the first dose at birth or before age 2 months. The second dose is given at age 1 to 4 months. Dose three is given at age 6 to 18 months. The rules regarding minimum **HBV** dose spacing in older children and adults are that there must be 4 weeks between doses 1 and 2, 2 months between doses 2 and 3, and 4 months between doses 1 and 3, allowing the series to be completed in as little as 4 months. The series is never restarted, no matter how long since the previous dose.

The recommended dosing of **HBV** is provided in Table 17–4.

HBV is generally given IM but may be given SC if IM injections are contraindicated (hemophiliacs). **HBV** should be given IM in the deltoid or anterolateral thigh. The immunogenicity of **HBV** is decreased when given in the buttock. **HBV** should not be given with the same syringe or at the same site as **hepatitis B immune globulin (II-BIG).**

Patients who do not develop a serum anti-HB antibody response (10 mIU/mL or more) after three doses of **HBV** should be revaccinated with one to three doses. If the patient does not respond after three additional doses, they are unlikely to respond to any additional doses.

MONITORING. Susceptibility testing before vaccination is not routinely indicated for children or adolescents. Testing for previous infection may be considered in adults in high-risk groups with high rates of hepatitis B infection, such as users of IV drugs, homosexuals, and household contacts of hepatitis B carriers.

Routine postvaccination testing for anti-HBs is not necessary. Postvaccination testing is advised 1 to 2 months after the third dose of **HBV** for those whose subsequent management is determined by their anti-HB status: (1) those at risk for occupational exposure risk from sharp injuries, (2) those with HIV infection, (3) hemodialysis patients, (4) immunocompromised patients at risk of contracting hepatitis B, (5) regular sexual contact of hepatitis carriers, and (6) infants born to HbsAg-positive mothers.

Clinical Pearl

PATIENTS WITH SHOT PHOBIA

In older children and adults who have a true phobia of injections, use **EMLA cream** to anesthetize the injection area. Have the patient apply the disk or cream 1 hour prior to the scheduled administration time, or the cream can be applied in the clinic and the injection administered after 1 hour.

Table 17–4. Recommended Dosing of Hepatitis B Vaccine

Patient Profile	Recombivax HB Dose in μg (mL)	Engerix-B Dose in μg(mL)
Infants of HbsAg-negative mothers and children <11 y	2.5 (0.5 mL pediatric formulation)	10 (0.5 mL)
Infants of HbsAg-positive mothers*	5 (1.0 mL pediatric formulation)	10 (0.5 mL)
Children and adolescents age 11–19 y	5 (0.5 mL of adult formulation)	10 (0.5 mL)
Adults ≥20 y	10 (1 mL of adult formulation)	20 (1 mL)
Patients undergoing dialysis and other immunosuppressed adults	40 (special formulation for dialysis patients)	40 (2 × 1 mL given at different sites; repeat at 1, 2, and 6 mo after initial dose)

*HBIG is also recommended.

PATIENT EDUCATION. Parents should receive a VIS prior to administration of the **vaccine**. Any questions or concerns regarding the **vaccine** should be addressed.

The most common adverse reaction after **HBV** injection is pain and erythema at the injection site. Advise the parent to give **acetaminophen** for discomfort for the first 24 hours after injection.

Hepatitis A Virus Vaccine

Pharmacodynamics

Hepatitis A virus (HAV) vaccine is used to confer immunity to hepatitis A in people at risk of contracting the disease. With **HAV** administration, stimulation of specific antibodies takes place without producing disease symptoms. Serum antibody titers after **HAV** are lower then those resulting from hepatitis A infection. Serum antibody titer of 20 mIU/mL is considered protective. There are two **HAV** products available. Both provide immunity with a two-dose schedule.

Pharmacokinetics

HAV is administered IM. One dose of **HAV** can induce seroconversion in 88 percent of patients by 15 days and 99 percent of patients by 1 month. This rapid seroconversion from a single dose can provide protection for at least 12 months. Administration of a second dose at 6 to 12 months after the first dose provides 100 percent protection. The duration of the **vaccine** protection has not been determined yet, as long-term efficacy has not been established. The **vaccine** has been studied for 8 years, after which patients still had levels above 20 mIU/mL (CDC, 1999b). Theoretically, antibody levels should last 20 years or more.

Pharmacotherapeutics

PRECAUTIONS AND CONTRAINDICATIONS. **HAV** should not be administered to patients with a previous history of severe reaction to **HAV**.

Moderate or severe illness, with or without fever, is a contraindication to **HAV**.

Patients with immunosuppression may be given **HAV**, but they may have lower antibody titers than immunocompetent people.

HAV is Pregnancy Category C. The CDC has stated *HAV* may be given in pregnancy if indicated and that it poses no risk to the fetus (1999f).

The safety and effectiveness of **HAV** in children under age 2 years have not been established.

ADVERSE DRUG REACTIONS. The most frequently reported adverse reaction to **HAV** is soreness at the injection site (56% in adults and 15% in children). Headache and malaise are other minor adverse reactions that have been reported.

From the time the **vaccine** was first licensed in the United States in 1995 through December 1998, more than 6.5 million doses were given, including more than 2.3 million pediatric doses. During this time, no serious adverse effects could be definitely attributed to **HAV**.

DRUG INTERACTIONS. Patients who are taking **immunosuppressants** or **antineoplastic agents** may have a decreased immunologic response to **HAV**.

CLINICAL USE AND DOSING. **HAV vaccine** provides pre-exposure protection from hepatitis A infection in adults and children. **HAV** is recommended for people who are at increased risk for infection and for any person wishing to obtain immunity.

The children who should be routinely vaccinated or considered for vaccination include those living in areas where rates of **HAV vaccine** are at least twice the national average (10.8 cases/100,000). The CDC recommends vaccination for children living in states where the 1987–1997 annual hepatitis A rate was 20 or more cases per 100,000 population. These states, listed by occurrence rate, are Arizona (48 cases/100,000), Alaska, Oregon, New Mexico, Utah, Washington, Oklahoma, South Dakota, Idaho, Nevada, and California (20 cases/100,000). The CDC also recommends **HAV** vaccination for children living in counties or communities where the average hepatitis A infection rate from 1987 to 1997 was greater than 20 cases/100,000. Children who live in states where the occurrence rate is greater than the national average of 10.8 cases per 100,000, but less than 20 cases per 100,000, should be considered for **HAV**. These states are Missouri, Texas, Colorado, Arkansas, Montana, and Wyoming. The provider who does not know the local occurrence rate can contact the local health department for information.

People at increased risk for hepatitis A infection who should be routinely vaccinated include the following:

1. People over age 2 years who are traveling or working in countries that have high or intermediate endemic infection. All of South America, Africa, Greenland, and Asia have high incidence of hepatitis A infection. Russia and Eastern Europe are areas of intermediate prevalence. IG is recommended for children under age 2 years who are traveling to these areas.
2. Men who have sex with men.
3. Illegal drug users.
4. People who have an occupational risk for infection, including those who work with hepatitis A–infected primates or with hepatitis A in a research laboratory setting.
5. People with clotting factor disorders.
6. People with chronic liver disease.

There are currently two different **HAV** products available, **Havrix** and **VAQTA**. **Havrix** is available in two strengths: 1440 enzyme-linked immunoassay units (EL.U) and 720 EL.U. The adult (age 19 and older) dose is 1440 EL.U administered in a two-dose schedule, 6 to 12 months apart. The pediatric (age 2 to 18 years) dose of **Havrix** is 720 EL.U, administered in a two-dose schedule 6 to 12 months apart. **VAQTA** is available in two strengths: adult, which has 50 antigen U per 1-mL dose, and pediatric-adolescent strength, which has 25 U per 0.5-mL dose. The dose for adults is 50 U administered 6 months apart. The dose for children age 2 to 18 years is 25 U administered 6 to 18 months apart.

HAV is injected IM into the deltoid muscle. Injection in the gluteal region results in suboptimal response. Patients with impaired immune systems may require additional doses to obtain an adequate anti–hepatitis A response.

MONITORING. Preimmunization testing of children for hepatitis A antibodies is generally not recommended.

Pretesting may be cost effective in adults who have a high likelihood of immunity from prior infection, such as those who have lived in areas of high hepatitis incidence, those older than 40, and those with a history of jaundice that potentially may have been hepatitis A infection.

Postimmunization testing is not indicated in immunocompetent persons because of the high seroconversion rates in children and adults who receive **HAV**. Postimmunization testing is warranted in immunocompromised patients who may have suboptimal response to the **vaccine**.

PATIENT EDUCATION. Parents should receive a VIS prior to administration of the **vaccine**. Any questions or concerns regarding the **vaccine** should be addressed.

The most common adverse reaction after **HAV** injection is pain and erythema at the injection site. Advise the patient to take **acetaminophen** for discomfort for the first 24 hours after injection.

Influenza Vaccine

Pharmacodynamics

Influenza vaccine (Fluogen, FluShield, Fluzone) is **multivalent vaccine** that contains three different viral subtypes. Each year, the FDA's Vaccines and Related Biologic Products Advisory Committee recommends what strains will be included in the following year's **vaccine**. Consultation with the World Health Organization (WHO) and data from outbreaks in Asia are used to determine the strains of influenza that are most likely to occur in the United States. Because influenza viruses are constantly changing and immunity wanes over time, annual immunization is required. The previous year's **vaccine** cannot be used for the current year.

Influenza virus vaccine imparts immunity by stimulating production of antibodies that are specific to the disease strain. Patients who receive the **vaccine** are immune only to the strains included in the **vaccine** for that year.

Pharmacokinetics

The **influenza vaccine** is administered IM. The **vaccine** produces protective antibodies within 10 to 14 days. The duration of immunity generally lasts from 6 months to 1 year.

Pharmacotherapeutics

PRECAUTIONS AND CONTRAINDICATIONS. Anaphylactic reaction to the **influenza vaccine**, eggs, or egg products is a contraindication to the use of **influenza vaccine**. If the patient's status is unclear, skin testing for egg allergy can clarify whether the **vaccine** can be given.

Thimerosal is used as a preservative in the **vaccine**; therefore, patients with hypersensitivity to **thimerosal** should not receive the **influenza vaccine.** Some of the **influenza vaccines** contain **sulfites**; care should be taken to check the packaging prior to administering **vaccine** to a patient with **sulfite** hypersensitivity.

Patients with an active neurological disorder should defer the **vaccine** until the condition stabilizes.

Patients with HIV disease may be immunized with **influenza vaccine,** but they may have lower **vaccine**-induced antibody levels.

Patients with an acute febrile illness should defer the **vaccine** until their symptoms subside. *Influenza vaccine is Pregnancy Category C, but according to the CDC Guidelines for Vaccinating Pregnant Women (1998), influenza vaccine may be safely administered to pregnant women in their second or third trimester.* Influenza vaccine may be administered to lactating women with no effect on the infant.

Children under age 13 years should not receive **whole-virus vaccine** because of higher adverse effects. Children age 6 months to 13 years should receive **split-virus vaccine.** The safety of **influenza vaccine** has not been established in children younger than 6 months of age.

ADVERSE DRUG REACTIONS. Adverse reactions to the **influenza vaccine** are usually mild and more common in children than in adults.

Local injection site reaction occurs in about 23 percent of patients.

In addition, 5 to 10 percent of patients experience mild systemic adverse effects, including low-grade fever, malaise, and myalgia.

Rarely, a patient has an immediate hypersensitivity reaction to the **vaccine,** including urticaria, angioedema, bronchospasm, and/or anaphylactic shock. These reactions are most likely the result of hypersensitivity to residual egg protein.

DRUG INTERACTIONS. Patients who are taking **immunosuppressants** or **antineoplastic agents** may have a decreased immunologic response to **influenza vaccine.**

Medications that may have inhibited clearance after administration of **influenza vaccine** include **theophylline, phenytoin,** and **warfarin.** Reports concerning impaired drug clearance are conflicting, and the concurrent administration of **influenza vaccine** to patients taking these medications is not contraindicated.

CLINICAL USE AND DOSING. In the United States, the **influenza vaccine** should be administered annually. The optimal time for organized vaccination programs is October through mid-November.

Influenza vaccine is recommended annually for all adults over age 65 years. It is also recommended for younger patients from age 6 months with chronic medical conditions such as heart or lung disease, diabetes, re-

nal dysfunction, hemoglobinopathies, and immunosuppression and those living in chronic care facilities. All health care providers are recommended for an annual **influenza vaccine. Pregnant women who will be in their second or third trimester of pregnancy or pregnant women with underlying medical conditions should be vaccinated against influenza.**

People who are healthy and who live or work with a person at risk should be vaccinated annually with **influenza vaccine.**

Travelers to areas where influenza is endemic should be vaccinated 2 to 4 weeks prior to travel.

Although the **vaccine** is indicated for patients at increased risk from influenza infection, studies of **vaccine** administration to healthy adults demonstrate cost effectiveness. Therefore, anyone who wishes to reduce the likelihood of contracting influenza should be vaccinated.

The dose of **influenza vaccine** is as follows:

1. Patients age over 12 years may be given whole or split virus, 0.5 mL IM in one dose.
2. Children age 9 to 12 years are given split virus in one 0.5-mL IM dose.
3. Previously vaccinated children age 3 to 8 years are given **split-virus vaccine** in one 0.5-mL dose.
4. Children age 3 to 8 years who have never been vaccinated receive **split-virus vaccine** 0.5 mL, with a repeat dose in 4 weeks.
5. Children age 6 to 35 months who have been previously vaccinated receive 0.25 mL of **split-virus vaccine.**
6. Children age 6 to 35 months who have not been previously vaccinated with **influenza vaccine** receive split virus 0.25 mL, with a second dose in 4 weeks.

PATIENT EDUCATION. Parents should receive a VIS prior to administration of **vaccine.** Any questions or concerns regarding the **vaccine** should be addressed.

The most common adverse reaction after **influenza vaccine** injection is pain and erythema at the injection site. Some patients may also experience low-grade fever and malaise. Advise the patient to take **acetaminophen** for discomfort for the first 24 hours after injection.

Pneumococcal Vaccine

Pharmacodynamics

There are two types of **pneumococcal vaccine (Pneumovax 23, Pnu-Imune 23, Prevnar)** currently available. **Polyvalent pneumococcal vaccine (PPV)** contains 23 highly purified capsular polysaccharides from *Streptococcus pneumoniae.* These are the 23 most prevalent or invasive pneumococcal types, accounting for at least 90 percent of all blood isolates associated with clinical infection.

PPV stimulates the immune system to produce pneumococcus capsule-specific antibodies. These antibodies presumably destroy the capsule, making the pneumococcus vulnerable to antibody and cell-mediated immunity. Clinical trials suggest a protective efficacy of 60 to 90 percent. The **23-valent PPV** has limited immunogenicity in children younger than 2 years. The **23-valent vaccine** was approved by the FDA in 1977.

In February 2000, the FDA approved the first **vaccine** to prevent invasive pneumococcal disease in infants and children, **pneumococcal 7-valent conjugate vaccine (Prevnar)**. The **vaccine** targets the seven most common strains of pneumococcus, which account for 80 percent of invasive disease in infants. The **vaccine** is approved for use in patients up to age 5 years, but it is not meant to replace the **23-valent vaccine**, which is approved for high-risk children over age 2 years.

Pharmacokinetics

PPV is administered either SC or IM. Immunity after SC or IM injection occurs in 2 to 3 weeks. Serotype-specific antibodies decline after 5 to 10 years. Children may decline to prevaccination levels in 3 to 5 years, especially asplenic children and children with sickle cell disease.

Pharmacotherapeutics

PRECAUTIONS AND CONTRAINDICATIONS. Previous anaphylactic reaction to the **vaccine** or any component is a contraindication to its use.

Moderate to severe illness, with or without fever, is a reason to defer the **vaccine** until the patient has improved.

Pneumococcal vaccine should be given at least 10 to 14 days before elective splenectomy, organ transplant, **immunosuppressive therapy,** or chemotherapy. Patients with Hodgkin's disease and immunosuppressed patients have suboptimal antibody response to vaccination.

Use **PPV** cautiously in patients with idiopathic thrombocytopenic purpura (ITP), as **PPV** has been associated with relapse of ITP.

PPV is Pregnancy Category C. Use of the vaccine during the first trimester should be avoided. It is not known if the vaccine is excreted in breast milk.

PPV 23-valent vaccine is not recommended in children under 2 years of age.

Prevnar is not for use in adults.

ADVERSE DRUG REACTIONS. Seventy-two percent of **PPV** recipients report local injection site reactions of erythema, induration, and soreness that last up to 48 hours. Occasionally, low-grade fever and arthralgia have been reported. High fever is rare.

During clinical trials of **Prevnar**, adverse effects were generally mild and included local injection site reaction, irritability, drowsiness, and decreased appetite. Approximately 21 percent of children in the **vaccine** group had a fever of 100.3°F or higher, compared with 14 percent of the control group.

DRUG INTERACTIONS. There are no known drug interactions.

CLINICAL USE AND DOSING. Dosing of **PPV** is based on the age and medical condition of the patient:

1. **PPV** is recommended for all adults age 65 or older. The dose is 0.5 mL IM or SC. Revaccinate (a second dose) if the original vaccination was 5 years or more ago *and* the patient was under age 65 when the dose was given.
2. People age 2 years to 65 years who have chronic illness and who are at increased risk of morbidity or mortality from pneumococcal disease should receive **PPV**. These risk factors include chronic cardiac or pulmonary disease, chronic liver disease or alcoholism, diabetes mellitus, and cerebrospinal fluid leaks. Certain populations are at higher risk (Alaskan Natives and certain American Indian populations). The dose of **PPV** is 0.5 mL given IM or SC once. Revaccination is not recommended in these populations.
3. Immunocompetent patients age 2 to 65 years with functional or anatomic asplenia (including sickle cell anemia) should receive 0.5 mL IM or SC. Revaccination is recommended 5 years or more after the first dose; if the patient is under 10 years old, revaccination should be considered 3 years after the first dose.
4. Immunocompromised patients (including HIV infection); those with chronic renal failure, hematologic malignancy, Hodgkin's disease, lymphoma, or multiple myeloma; patients receiving **immunosuppressive therapy;** and patients who have received an organ or bone marrow transplant should receive a dose of 0.5 mL IM or SC. Revaccination should be considered if the first **vaccine** was 5 years or more ago; in children under age 10 years, revaccination is considered 3 years after the first dose.

The suggested dosing schedule for **Prevnar** is four doses given at 2, 4, 6, and 12 to 15 months of age.

MONITORING. No laboratory monitoring is necessary.

PATIENT EDUCATION. Parents should receive a VIS prior to administration of the **vaccine.** Any questions or concerns regarding the **vaccine** should be addressed.

The most common adverse reaction after **pneumococcal vaccine** injection is pain and erythema at the injection site. Advise the patient to take **acetaminophen** for discomfort for the first 24 hours after injection.

Meningococcal Polysaccharide Vaccine

Pharmacodynamics

Meningococcal polysaccharide vaccine Groups A, C, Y, and W-135 Combined (Menomune-A/C/Y/W-135) is for use against meningococcemia and meningitis caused by some types of *Neisseria meningitidis*. **Menomune** stimulates protection against serogroups A, C, Y, and W-135.

Based on multistate surveillance data from 1989 to 1991, *N. meningitidis* serogroup C accounted for 45 percent of meningococcal disease, serogroup B for 16 percent, and serogroups Y and W-135 for most of the remaining cases. Serogroup A is rare in the United States but the most common cause of epidemics in Africa and Asia.

Meningococcal polysaccharides induce the formation of bactericidal antibodies to meningococcal antigens. Postimmunization seroconversion rates for **Menomune A/C/Y/W-135** reported by the manufacturer in children age 2 to 12 years were group A, 72 percent; group C, 58 percent; group Y, 90 percent; and group W-135, 82 percent. Among 20,000 military recruits under epidemic conditions, the **vaccine** demonstrated 90 percent efficacy against serogroup C.

Pharmacokinetics

Protective antibody levels may be achieved within 7 to 10 days after vaccination. The measurable levels of antibodies to serogroups A and C decrease during the first 3 years following vaccination. This decrease occurs more rapidly in infants and young children than in adults.

Pharmacotherapeutics

PRECAUTIONS AND CONTRAINDICATIONS. Previous anaphylactic reaction to any component of the **vaccine**, including **thimerosal**, is a contraindication to its use.

Moderate to severe illness, with or without fever, is a reason to defer the **vaccine** until the patient has improved.

The expected immune response may not be obtained if the **vaccine** is used in patients on **immunosuppressive therapy**.

Menomune A/C/Y/W-135 should not be given to **pregnant women**. It is not recommended for children under age 2 years.

ADVERSE DRUG REACTIONS. Adverse reactions to the **Menomune vaccine** are mild and consist of pain and tenderness at the injection site for 1 to 2 days.

DRUG INTERACTIONS. There are no known drug interactions to this **vaccine**.

CLINCAL USE AND DOSING. The ACIP recommends that the following high-risk groups receive **Menomune A/C/Y/W-135 vaccine** (1997):

1. Patients with deficiencies in late complement components (C3, C5 to C9).
2. Persons with functional or actual asplenia.
3. Research, industrial, and clinical laboratory personnel who routinely are exposed to *N. meningitidis* in solution that may be aerosolized.
4. Travelers to, and residents of, hyperendemic areas such as sub-Saharan Africa. Epidemics have occurred recently in Saudi Arabia, Kenya, Tanzania, Burundi, and Mongolia.

Military recruits are routinely given **meningococcal vaccine**.

Because recent studies have indicated a slightly higher risk of meningococcal disease among freshman dormitory residents, the ACIP recommends that those who provide care to this group give information to students and their parents about meningococcal disease and the **vaccine** (CDC, 1997a). The American College Health Association is recommending that students consider vaccination against meningococcal disease (American College Health Association, 2000).

The dose of **Menomune A/C/Y/W-135** for all ages is a single SC 0.5-mL dose.

Revaccination may be indicated for persons at high risk for infection (travel to or living in epidemic areas). Children who were vaccinated before they were 4 years old should be considered for revaccination in 2 to 3 years if they remain at high risk. Revaccination of older children and adults may be considered in 3 to 5 years after the first dose.

MONITORING. Laboratory monitoring is not necessary with this **vaccine**.

PATIENT EDUCATION. Parents should receive information regarding the benefits and risks of the **vaccine** prior to administration. Any questions or concerns regarding the **vaccine** should be addressed.

The most common adverse reaction after **Menomune vaccine** injection is pain and erythema at the injection site. Advise the patient to take **acetaminophen** for discomfort for the first 24 hours after injection.

Lyme Disease Vaccine

Pharmacodynamics

Lyme disease is a vector-borne illness caused by ticks infested with *Borrelia burgdorferi*. Recombinant **Lyme disease vaccine (LYMErix, Immulyme)** imparts immunity against *B. burgdorferi* by stimulating production of antibodies to the lipoprotein OspA. OspA is a lipoprotein of the *B. burgdorferi* spirochete. The mechanism by which **Lyme disease vaccine** works is thought to be by antibody killing of the spirochete in the tick. Transmission of the OspA antibody occurs while the tick is feeding on the blood of an immunized host, and the antibodies kill the spirochete even before transmission occurs.

Pharmacokinetics

Lyme disease vaccine is administered in a series of three IM injections. Positive immune response is accomplished in 95 percent of recipients at 1 month after the second dose and 99 percent after the third dose. The long-term rate of protection is unknown.

Pharmacotherapeutics

PRECAUTIONS AND CONTRAINDICATIONS. Previous anaphylactic reaction to any component of the **vaccine** is a contraindication to its use. The packaging of the prefilled syringes of **LYMErix** contains dry, natural rubber; therefore, do not use this **vaccine** in a patient with known latex hypersensitivity.

Moderate to severe illness, with or without fever, is a reason to defer the **vaccine** until the patient has improved.

The expected immune response may not be obtained if the **vaccine** is used in patients on immunosuppressive therapy.

The clinical trials of **Lyme disease vaccine** excluded patients with advanced debilitating disease, joint swelling, rheumatoid arthritis, neurological disease, neuromuscular disease, second- or third-degree AV block, or cardiac disease requiring a pacemaker. Therefore, the efficacy and adverse effects of the **vaccine** in these groups are unknown.

Administration of *Lyme disease vaccine* during pregnancy and lactation is not recommended.

The safety and efficacy of the **vaccine** in children under the age of 15 years have not been established.

ADVERSE DRUG REACTIONS. Adverse reactions to **Lyme disease vaccine** are mild and consist of pain and tenderness at the injection site reported by 24 percent of patients.

DRUG INTERACTIONS. There are no known drug interactions with this **vaccine**. **Lyme disease vaccine** may cause a false-positive enzyme-linked immunosorbent assay (ELISA) for Lyme disease. Do a Western blot test to confirm a positive or equivocal ELISA.

CLINICAL USE AND DOSING. The **vaccine** is recommended for individuals age 15 to 70 years at most risk for contracting Lyme disease, those who live or work in grassy or wooded areas that are infested with *B. burgdorferi*–infested ticks.

Injections of **Lyme disease vaccine (LYMErix)** should be injected deep IM into the deltoid muscle. It is not to be injected into the gluteal muscle. The dose is 0.5 mL of **vaccine** given in a three-dose schedule. The initial dose is followed by a second dose in 1 month and then the third dose in 12 months after the first dose. Time the doses so that the second and third doses are several weeks before the beginning of *Borrelia* tick season.

PATIENT EDUCATION. Parents should receive a VIS prior to administration of the **vaccine**. Any questions or concerns regarding the **vaccine** should be addressed. The VIS for Lyme disease can be found at *www.immunize.org* or through your state health division.

The most common adverse reaction after **Lyme disease vaccine** injection is pain and erythema at the injection site. Advise the patient to take **acetaminophen** for discomfort for the first 24 hours after injection.

Typhoid Vaccine

Pharmacodynamics

Typhoid vaccines (Typhoid Vaccine, Typhim Vi) are used to increase resistance to enteric fever caused by *S. typhi*. The efficacy of protective immunity depends on the size of the bacterial inoculum consumed.

There are two parenteral **typhoid vaccines** available, **a heat- and phenol-inactivated vaccine (Typhoid Vaccine)** and a **purified Vi polysaccharide (Typhim Vi)**. Efficacy of **Typhoid Vaccine** is 71 to 77 percent. The efficacy of **Typhim Vi** is 49 to 87 percent in reducing disease incidence.

Pharmacokinetics

Absorption, distribution, and metabolism of **typhoid vaccine** are unknown.

Pharmacotherapeutics

PRECAUTIONS AND CONTRAINDICATIONS. Hypersensitivity to **typhoid vaccine** is a contraindication to its use.

Do not administer to **a patient with acute febrile illness.**

Typhoid vaccine is Pregnancy Category C. **It is not known if the vaccine is harmful to the fetus. If vaccinating a pregnant patient is necessary, inactivated vaccine is recommended.**

Typhoid Vaccine is not recommended for use in children younger than age 6 months. **Typhim Vi** is not recommended for children under age 2 years.

ADVERSE DRUG REACTIONS. **Vaccine** recipients report local injection site reactions of erythema, induration, and soreness that begin within 24 hours and last 1 to 2 days. Systemic symptoms including low-grade fever, headache, and myalgias have been reported. High fever is rare.

DRUG INTERACTIONS. If possible, **plague vaccine** should not be given at the same time as **typhoid vaccine** to avoid the possibility of accentuated adverse effects.

Immunosuppressants may cause insufficient response to the **vaccine**.

CLINICAL USE AND DOSING. It is for primary immunization against *S. typhi* infection in the following:

1. Travelers to areas where a risk of exposure to *S. typhi* is recognized
2. Persons with household contact with a documented typhoid fever carrier
3. Laboratory workers with frequent contact with *S. typhi*

For primary immunization, the patient should receive two doses of **typhoid** 4 or more weeks apart. The dose in adults and children older than age 10 years is 0.5 mL SC, and in children age 6 months to 10 years the dose is 0.25 mL SC. If administering **Typhim Vi**, the dose for persons 2 years of age or older is one 0.5-mL dose administered IM.

PATIENT EDUCATION. Parents should receive information regarding the benefits and risks of the **vaccine** prior to administration. Any questions or concerns regarding the **vaccine** should be addressed.

The most common adverse reaction after **typhoid vaccination** injection is pain and erythema at the injection site. Advise the patient to take **acetaminophen** for discomfort for the first 24 hours after injection.

The best protection against typhoid fever is food and water precautions to prevent contracting *S. typhi*.

Cholera Vaccine

Pharmacodynamics

Cholera vaccine is a suspension of equal parts inactivated Ogawa and Inuba serotypes of killed *Vibrio cholerae*. **Cholera vaccine** provides active immunity against cholera. The **vaccine** is 50 percent effective in reducing disease in endemic areas.

Pharmacokinetics

Little is known about the pharmacokinetics of **cholera vaccine**. Active immunity lasts for 3 to 6 months after vaccination with two IM or SC doses of **vaccine**.

Pharmacotherapeutics

PRECAUTIONS AND CONTRAINDICATIONS. Hypersensitivity to **cholera vaccine** is a contraindication to its use.

Do not administer to a patient with current or recent febrile illness.

Cholera vaccine is Pregnancy Category C and may be given to children as young as age 6 months.

ADVERSE DRUG REACTIONS. **Vaccine** recipients report local injection site reactions of erythema, induration, and soreness that last a few days. Systemic symptoms, including low-grade fever, headache, and malaise, last for 1 to 2 days after vaccination.

DRUG INTERACTIONS. **Cholera vaccine** and **yellow fever vaccine** should be administered at least 3 weeks apart to provide adequate immune response to both **vaccines**. The **vaccines** can be given simultaneously if necessary.

CLINICAL USE AND DOSING. The World Health Organization (WHO) no longer recommends **cholera vaccine** for travelers to or from cholera-affected areas. It is generally not recommended for international travelers. Cholera generally spreads through uncooked contaminated food and water and generally requires ingestion of a large number of organisms. Disinfection or boiling water prevents transmission, as does thoroughly cooking crabs, oysters, and other shellfish before eating.

If **cholera vaccine** is required for travel to a foreign country (determined by that country's health department or ministry), then the dose is as follows:

1. Adults and children age 10 years and older: 0.5 mL SC or IM, two doses 1 week to 1 month apart. An intradermal dose of 0.2 mL may be substituted. A booster dose of 0.5 mL should be administered every 6 months in areas of high risk.
2. Children age 5 to 10 years: 0.3 mL SC or IM, two doses 1 to 4 weeks apart. The patient may also use an intradermal dose of 0.2 mL. A booster dose of 0.3 mL IM or SC should be administered every 6 months in areas of high risk.
3. Children age 6 months to 4 years: 0.2 mL SC or IM, two doses 1 to 4 weeks apart. Give a booster dose of 0.2 mL IM or SC every 6 months. Do not administer intradermally to this age group.

PATIENT EDUCATION. Parents should receive information regarding the benefits and risks of the **vaccine** prior to administration. Any questions or concerns regarding the vaccine should be addressed.

The most common adverse reactions after **cholera vaccine** injection are pain and erythema at the injection site and low-grade systemic symptoms. Advise the patient to take acetaminophen for discomfort for the first 24 hours after injection.

The best protection against cholera is food and water precautions to prevent contracting *V. cholerae*.

Japanese Encephalitis Virus Vaccine

Pharmacodynamics

Japanese encephalitis (JE) is the most common form of viral encephalitis in Asia and is spread by mosquitoes. JE is usually severe, resulting in death in 25 percent of cases, miscarriage in pregnant women, and serious neurological outcomes in infected patients. **JE virus vaccine (JE-VAX)** is an **inactivated vaccine** derived from infected mouse brain. **JE-VAX** was demonstrated to be 91 percent effective in protecting the recipient against JE in endemic Thailand.

Pharmacokinetics

A three-dose schedule, administered at 0, 7, and 30 days, provides the highest level of immunity against JE. Length of full protection against JE is unknown, although immunity is known to last for 12 months after a three-dose initial series.

Pharmacotherapeutics

PRECAUTIONS AND CONTRAINDICATIONS. Previous anaphylactic reaction to any component of the **vaccine**, including **thimerosal**, is a contraindication to its use.

Pregnancy is a contraindication to JE-VAX use.

ADVERSE DRUG REACTIONS. Overall, 20 percent of recipients experience adverse effects from the **vaccine**. **Vaccine** recipients report local injection site reactions of erythema, induration, and soreness. Systemic symptoms including low-grade fever, headache, rash, chills, dizziness, and malaise. Adverse reactions occur usually within 48 hours but may occur as long as 10 days after vaccination.

Generalized urticaria and angioedema of the face, lips and oropharynx may occur in about 1 to 104 per 10,000 doses. Most patients are successfully treated with **antihistamines** or **corticosteroids**. Patients with a history of allergies are more likely to develop this reaction. Patients should be advised to remain in areas where medical intervention is available for 10 days after administration, as delayed allergic response may occur.

DRUG INTERACTIONS. There are no known drug interactions

CLINICAL USE AND DOSING. JE vaccine is recommended for people who will be residing in areas where JE is endemic or epidemic. The ACIP recommends that **JE-VAX** be administered to those who plan on residing in areas where JE is endemic or epidemic. The probability of JE viral infection and illness increases with the duration of the stay in rural endemic areas. Current information on locations of JE virus transmission can be obtained from the CDC. Detailed recommendations, including country-by-country recommendations, are available from the ACIP and are published in MMWR (CDC, 1993). The full document is available at the CDC Website, *www.cdc.gov/nip/publications/ACIP-list.htm.*

JE-VAX is *not* recommended for all travelers to Asia. The vaccine should be offered to people spending a month or longer in endemic areas during the transmission season, especially if they are traveling to rural areas. It should also be offered to those who will be spending extensive time outdoors during their travel.

The dose of **JE-VAX** for adults and children age 3 years and older is a series of three SC doses of 1 mL each, given on days 0, 7, and 30. An abbreviated dosing schedule may be used if necessary, with dosing at 0, 7, and 14 days (only in special circumstances and not recommended routinely). The dose in children age 1 to 3 years is identical except that the dose is 0.5 mL SC. Safety in infants under age 1 year is not known.

PATIENT EDUCATION. Patients should receive information regarding the benefits and risks of the **vaccine** prior to administration. Any questions or concerns regarding the **vaccine** should be addressed.

The most common adverse reactions after **JE-VAX** injection are pain and erythema at the injection site and low-grade systemic symptoms. Adverse reactions may occur up to 10 days after immunization. Patients are advised not to travel outside the United States for 10 days after administration in case of adverse reaction.

Patients should be advised to protect themselves by wearing long-sleeved shirts and long pants. Use of insect repellant should be encouraged. **Permethrin** should be applied to clothing.

Plague Vaccine

Pharmacodynamics

Plague vaccine is a **whole-cell vaccine** consisting of a suspension of inactivated plague bacilli (*Yersinia pestis*). The **vaccine** promotes the production of plague antibodies to decrease the incidence and severity of infection.

Pharmacokinetics

Within 30 days after administration, antibodies can be measured in 88 percent of patients. Duration of protection is approximately 6 to 12 months.

Pharmacotherapeutics

PRECAUTIONS AND CONTRAINDICATIONS. Previous anaphylactic reaction to any component of the **vaccine**, including beef protein, yeast, agar, soybean, casein, or phenol, is a contraindication to its use.

Do not administer **plague vaccine** to a patient with current febrile illness.

Plague vaccine is Pregnancy Category C. Use during pregnancy is not recommended.

The safety of **plague vaccine** has not been studied in children under age 18 years.

ADVERSE DRUG REACTIONS. **Vaccine** recipients report local injection site reactions of erythema, induration, and soreness. Systemic symptoms, including low-grade fever, headache, and mild lymphadenopathy, have been reported. Symptoms usually resolve in 48 hours.

DRUG INTERACTIONS. There are no significant drug interactions. It is advised that **cholera** and **typhoid vac-**

cines not be given at the same time as **plague vaccine,** if possible.

CLINICAL USE AND DOSING. The ACIP recommends vaccinating people against plague only if they are at high risk of contracting the disease. The recognized high-risk groups include laboratory personnel who routinely perform procedures that involve viable Y. *pestis* and people who have regular contact with wild rodents or their fleas (mammalogists, ecologists, and other field workers). If vaccinees are believed to have been exposed to plague, prophylactic antibiotic use should be considered as a supplement to vaccination. Routine administration of **vaccine** is not necessary for people living in areas where plague is enzootic.

The primary series of **plague vaccine** is three doses. The first dose of 1 mL IM is followed by 0.2 mL IM at 4 weeks, then a third dose of 0.2 mL IM 5 months after the second. A booster dose of 0.2 mL is given at 6-month intervals to people remaining at risk. Booster doses every 1 to 2 years can be considered after three or more booster doses or as determined by passive hemagglutination Y. *pestis* antibody titer of less than 1:128.

PATIENT EDUCATION. Patients should receive information regarding the benefits and risks of the **vaccine** prior to administration. Any questions or concerns regarding the **vaccine** should be addressed. Patients are advised to remain in the clinic for 20 minutes after vaccination to determine if adverse hypersensitivity reaction might occur.

The most common adverse reactions after **plague vaccination** injection are pain and erythema at the injection site and low-grade systemic symptoms. Advise the patient to take **acetaminophen** for discomfort for the first 48 hours after injection.

Rabies Vaccine

Pharmacodynamics

Rabies vaccine (Imovax, RabAvert) is a preparation of inactivated rabies virus, which induces active immunity. The two products available differ only in the cell culture used to develop the **vaccine. Imovax** uses human diploid cell (HDC) culture and **RabAvert** uses purified chick embryo cell culture.

Pharmacokinetics

An antibody response to **rabies vaccine** can be measured in 7 to 10 days after administration. Antibodies persist for 2 years.

Pharmacotherapeutics

PRECAUTIONS AND CONTRAINDICATIONS. Previous anaphylactic reaction to any component of the **vaccine,** including **neomycin,** is a contraindication to its use.

Moderate to severe illness, with or without fever, is a reason to defer the **vaccine** until the patient has improved.

The expected immune response may not be obtained if the **vaccine** is used in patients on immunosuppressive therapy.

Rabies vaccine **is Pregnancy Category C. Pregnancy is not a contraindication to postexposure vaccination of pregnant women.** Safety in children under age 6 years has not been established.

ADVERSE DRUG REACTIONS. Local reactions, including pain, erythema, and swelling of the injection site, have been reported by 30 to 70 percent of **vaccine** recipients. Systemic reactions have been reported by 5 to 40 percent of recipients. Systemic reactions include headache, nausea, abdominal pain, muscle aches, and dizziness. Three cases of a neurological illness resembling Guillain-Barré syndrome have been reported.

A serum sickness–like reaction has been reported among about 6 percent of patients who received booster doses of **Imovax.**

DRUG INTERACTIONS. Long-term therapy with **chloroquine (Aralen)** can interfere with the active antibody response to **rabies vaccine.**

Patients who are taking **immunosuppressants** or **antineoplastic agents** may have a decreased immunologic response to **rabies vaccine.**

Rabies IG (RIG) can partially suppress the antibody response to **rabies vaccine.** Follow the CDC recommendations for simultaneous administration exactly, and give no more than recommended of **RIG.**

CLINICAL USE AND DOSING. **Rabies vaccine** can be given for primary or pre-exposure vaccination or as part of postexposure prophylaxis. Pre-exposure vaccination is recommended to high-risk groups, such as veterinarians, animal handlers, and certain laboratory workers. Postexposure prophylaxis is recommended if the patient has a bite that penetrates the skin from a rabid animal. Postexposure **vaccine** administration should always be accompanied by the use of **RIG.**

Pre-exposure vaccine dosing consists of three 1-mL IM injections of **vaccine** in the deltoid muscle. The doses are given on day 0, day 7, and either day 21 or day 28. A booster dose of 1 mL is given every 2 years to those considered at frequent risk, if their serum antibody titer is less than 1:5. Persons considered at frequent risk include veterinarians, animal control officers, wildlife officers, and staff where rabies is enzootic. In very high-risk patients, those who work in research laboratories or **vaccine** production facilities, a serum rabies antibody test should be done every 6 months and **vaccine** administered if levels are less than 1:5.

Postexposure prophylaxis always includes administration of both passive antibody and **vaccine,** with the exception of those who have previously received complete vaccination (pre-exposure or postexposure). For postexposure vaccination, the ACIP recommends five doses of **rabies vaccine**. The dose is 1 mL given IM on days 0, 3, 7, 14, and 28, with **RIG** given on day 0. For those who have previously been vaccinated, two doses of **rabies vaccine** are given on days 0 and 3, with no **RIG** needed.

PATIENT EDUCATION.   Patients should receive information regarding the benefits and risks of the **vaccine** prior to administration. Any questions or concerns regarding the **vaccine** should be addressed. The need for repeated doses should be discussed.

The most common adverse reactions after **rabies vaccination** injection are pain and erythema at the injection site and systemic symptoms including headache, nausea, abdominal pain, muscle aches, and dizziness. Advise the patient to take **acetaminophen** for discomfort.

Table 17–5 presents issues concerning immunizations.

Table 17–5.   Issues in Immunization

BARRIERS TO IMMUNIZATION

Childhood Immunization

Ideally, immunizations should be given as a part of comprehensive child health care. It is widely recognized that childhood immunizations are the most cost-effective way of preventing infectious diseases in children. Many studies have identified barriers to childhood immunization:

1. Financial, with low socioeconomic status placing a child at risk of underimmunization (CDC, 1998)
2. Family structure issues, such as single or teen parenthood (Bates & Wolinsky, 1998)
3. Perceived attitudes regarding the benefit of immunization
4. Provider policies and practices that lead to missed vaccine opportunities during clinic visits

Standards for pediatric immunization practice from the CDC (1994):

1. Immunization services are readily available.
2. No barriers or unnecessary prerequisites to the receipt of vaccines exist.
3. Immunization services are available free or for a minimal fee.
4. Providers utilize all clinical encounters to screen and, when indicated, immunize children.
5. Providers educate parents and guardians about immunization in general terms.
6. Providers question parents or guardians about contraindications and, before immunizing a child, inform them in specific terms about the risks and benefits of the immunizations their child is to receive.
7. Providers follow only true contraindications.
8. Providers administer simultaneously all vaccine doses for which a child is eligible at the time of each visit.
9. Providers use accurate and complete recording procedures.
10. Providers coschedule immunization appointments in conjunction with appointments for other child health services.
11. Providers report adverse events following immunization promptly, accurately, and completely.
12. Providers operate a tracking system.
13. Providers adhere to appropriate procedures for vaccine management.
14. Providers conduct semiannual audits to assess immunization coverage levels and to review immunization records in the patient populations they serve.
15. Providers maintain up-to-date, easily retrievable medical protocols at all locations where vaccines are administered.
16. Providers operate with patient-oriented and community-based approaches.
17. Properly trained individuals administer vaccines.
18. Providers receive ongoing education and training on current immunization recommendations.

Adolescent Immunization

There are no national data regarding vaccination coverage among adolescents, and adolescents are often overlooked in the discussion of immunizations. Immunizations are routinely given during well child examinations; therefore, adolescents, who have fewer health care visits, often are underimmunized. In 1997, the CDC, the National Coalition for Adult Immunization, and various other groups, including health care professionals who care for adolescents and adolescent advocacy groups, set a goal of 90% vaccination coverage for all recommended adolescent immunizations by 2002.

Interventions that increase adolescent immunization include school vaccination requirements, offering vaccinations in school-based settings, informational mailings to adolescents and their parents, and immunizing adolescents at every clinic visit. Many states have implemented vaccine requirements for entering seventh graders, which should raise the adolescent immunization rate significantly. School-based mass immunization has historically been effective in raising immunization rates, with school-based demonstration projects to vaccinate adolescents against hepatitis B achieving more than 70% vaccination coverage (CDC, 1996a). Some providers mail out an informational letter to all parents of teenagers and/or to the teenagers themselves, recommending an annual routine well-child exam and providing information regarding recommended immunizations. Last, every contact with adolescents in the health care setting should be viewed as an opportunity to immunize them.

Continued on next page

Table 17–5. Issues in Immunization (*continued*)

Vaccine	Indications	Timing of Vaccines	Dosing
Hepatitis B	All adolescents not previously vaccinated for hepatitis B	3 doses; can be started at any age; the #2 dose is given 1 or 2 mo after #1 dose; #3 dose is given 4 to 6 mo after #1	Recombivax 5 µg/ 0.5 mL (yellow cap) Engerix-B 10 µg/ 0.5 mL (light blue cap)
MMR	All adolescents who have not had two doses of MMR A booster dose is recommended at age 11 to 12 y if 5 y have elapsed since last dose	One dose A booster dose is recommended every 10 y	Use Td for patients ≥7 y
Varicella	All adolescents who have no reliable history of disease or vaccination	In patients ≥13 y, two doses are administered 4 to 8 wk apart	
Hepatitis A	Adolescents at risk of contracting hepatitis A, including international travelers, food handlers, injecting illegal drug users, and people residing in high-incidence areas	Havrix is administered in a two-dose schedule 6 to 12 mo apart VAQTA is two doses, administered 6 to 18 mo apart	Havrix pediatric strength (2 to 18 y) is 720 EL.U VAQTA pediatric/adolescent strength has 25 U per 0.5-mL dose
Influenza	All adolescents who are at risk for complications of influenza or who live with a high-risk person	Annually in the fall	
Pneumococcal	Adolescents who are at risk for pneumococcal disease or its complications	One dose (may be repeated in 5 y in high-risk patients)	

Adult Immunization

In a recent letter published in *Needle Tips,* U.S. Surgeon General David Satcher, M.D., stated that "in the United States, 45,000 people die each year from influenza, pneumococcal and hepatitis B disease, all preventable by vaccination" (Satcher, 1999). Pneumococcal disease kills more people in the United States annually (11,000 to 41,000) than any other vaccine-preventable bacterial disease (Oregon Health Division [OHD], CD Summary, 1998).

Health care providers who care for adults need to have an attitude similar to pediatric providers, with a goal of reviewing immunization status at every contact with the health care system. Interventions that increase adult immunization rates include the following:

1. Systemwide immunization standing orders
2. Reminders attached to charts of high-risk patients
3. Previsit screening of charts by clinic staff
4. Review of immunization status by the health care provider during every clinic visit
5. Postcard reminders to high-risk patients, especially those with chronic medical conditions and those over age 65
6. Inclusion of Td, HBV, and pneumococcal vaccine in fall "flu shot" clinics
7. Promotional materials regarding adult immunizations posted prominently in clinic
8. Provide adult patients with a lifetime immunization record for them to carry, documenting their immunization status

IMMUNIZATION IN SPECIAL POPULATIONS

Pregnant Patients

The ACIP has published guidelines for vaccinating pregnant women (CDC, 1998): "The risk from vaccination during pregnancy is largely theoretical. The benefit of vaccination among pregnant women usually outweighs the potential risk for disease when (a) the risk for disease exposure is high, (b) infections would pose a special risk for the mother or fetus, and (c) the vaccine is unlikely to cause harm" (CDC, 1994).

Generally, live-virus vaccines are contraindicated in pregnant women because of the possible risk of transmission to the fetus. If a woman is inadvertently given live-virus vaccine while pregnant, she should be counseled about the potential effects on the fetus. It is not normally an indication to terminate pregnancy.

Recommendations for vaccination during pregnancy include the following:

Continued on next page

Table 17–5. Issues in Immunization (*continued*)

Vaccine	May Be Given If Indicated	Contraindicated during Pregnancy	Comments
Routine			
Hepatitis B	X		
MMR		X	
Td	X		
Varicella		X	
Hepatitis A			The theoretical risk to the fetus is low from the inactivated vaccine.
Influenza	X		
Pneumococcal			The safety of the pneumococcal vaccine in the first trimester of pregnancy has not been determined.
OPV/IPV			Vaccination of pregnant women should be avoided, although no adverse effects have been documented. If immediate protection is required, pregnant women should be given OPV or IPV.
Travel and Others			
BCG		X	
Cholera			No specific information regarding safety in pregnancy is available.
Japanese encephalitis (JE)			The vaccine should not be routinely administered during pregnancy. If a pregnant woman will be moving to an area of high risk of JE, then vaccination should be considered.
Meningococcal	X		
Plague			Pregnant women should be vaccinated only if the potential benefits outweigh the potential risks to the fetus.
Rabies	X		
Typhoid			It is not known if the vaccine is harmful to the fetus. If necessary to vaccinate a pregnant patient, inactivated vaccine is recommended.
Yellow fever			It is not known if the vaccine is harmful to the fetus. Only vaccinate pregnant women who are at high risk of contracting disease.

Immunocompromised Patients
In general, severely immunocompromised persons or people with HIV/AIDS should not receive any live, attenuated virus vaccines (OPV, MMR, BCG, oral typhoid, yellow fever). Severely immunocompromised patients or those with HIV/AIDS may receive inactivated vaccines such as DPT/Td, IPV, Hib, HBV, pneumococcal, and influenza. Patients with asplenia, renal failure, and diabetes may receive DPT/Td, OPV, IPV, MMR, Hib, HBV, pneumococcal, and influenza vaccines (CDC, 1993).

Continued on next page

Table 17–5. Issues in Immunization (*continued*)

TRAVEL IMMUNIZATION

International travel is becoming more common, with jet travel allowing people to travel great distances in a few hours. With international travel comes exposure to infectious diseases not common in the United States. Patients should be advised to begin to prepare for their trip at least 8 wk prior to departure. To determine what vaccines the traveling patient will need, the provider can consult with a local travel clinic or the CDC. The CDC Website has a travel information section, maintained by the National Center for Infectious Disease (*www.cdc.gov/travel/*). The Website allows the provider or patient to inquire into recommendations based on the region the patient will be traveling to. Information on traveling with children, outbreaks, and special needs travelers is also located at this site. The CDC also publishes an annual guide, *Health Information for International Travel*.

In addition to special immunizations required by travel, patients should also have all of the recommended routine immunizations for their age, including influenza vaccine. Patients should have a copy of their current immunizations included with their travel documents.

Immune Globulin Serums

IG serums provide passive immunity to infectious diseases. The choice of **IG** is determined by the types of products available, the type of antibody desired, route of administration, timing, and other considerations. **IG** products that may be used in primary care include **immune globulin IM (IGIM, Gammar)**, **hepatitis B immune globulin (HBIG, BayHep B)**, **tetanus immune globulin (TIG, BayTet)**, **respiratory syncytial virus immune globulin (RSV-IGIV, RespiGam)**, **varicella-zoster immune globulin (VZIG, Iveegam)**, **rabies immune globulin (RIG, BayRab)**, and **$Rh_o(D)$ immune globulin (RhoGAM)**.

Pharmacodynamics

IGs are derived from the pooled plasma of adults, processed by cold ethanol fractionation. It consists primarily of immunoglobulin fraction (95% IgG) and is not known to transmit hepatitis, HIV, or other infectious diseases. The concentrated protein solution contains specific antibodies in proportion to the infectious and immunization experience of the donor population from which the plasma was derived. **IG serums** undergo processing to remove and inactivate viruses, including hepatitis A, B, and C; parvovirus B-19; and HIV. Specific IGs differ from **immune globulin IM (IGIM)**, which is sometimes referred to as **gamma globulin**, in that they have high levels of a specific **IG**.

IGIM is a sterile preparation of concentrated antibodies. **IG** provides protection against hepatitis A and measles through passive transfer of antibody. It may be used for pre-exposure prophylaxis or postexposure prevention in the treatment of hepatitis A; it is used postexposure in measles.

Hepatitis B immune globulin (HBIG) is a sterile solution of **IGs** (10 to 18%) against hepatitis B surface antigens (HbsAg). Anti-HBsAg antibodies are collected from donors with high titers of anti-HBsAg. **HBIG** is used to provide passive immunity to patients following exposure to blood infected with hepatitis B (HBV), sexual and household contacts of HBV-infected people, and infants born to HbsAg-positive mothers.

Tetanus immune globulin (TIG) is prepared from the plasma of adults who are hyperimmunized with tetanus toxoid. **TIG** contains antibodies that neutralize the exotoxin produced by *Clostridium tetani*. The passive immunity bestowed by **TIG** is capable of attenuating or preventing tetanus infection by binding free exotoxin.

Respiratory syncytial virus immune globulin (RSV-IGIV) is a polyclonal human hyperimmune globulin. The product is prepared by extracting IgG antibodies from the plasma of humans who have high titers of antibodies against respiratory syncytial virus (RSV). Resistance to RSV disease is via cellular and humoral immunity. **RSV-IGIV** does not protect the nasal mucosa from RSV and thus does not prevent acquired immunity to RSV.

Varicella-zoster immune globulin (VZIG) is derived from human plasma and consists of IgG, with trace amounts of IgA and IgM. **VZIG** is used primarily for passive immunization of high-risk susceptible patients after exposure to chickenpox or herpes zoster. The administration of **VZIG** has shown to significantly reduce the mortality in untreated patients.

Rabies immune globulin (RIG) is primarily **gamma globulin**. **RIG** is used to provide passive immunity to rabies in patients exposed to the virus. Rabies antibodies neutralize the rabies virus to retard its spread and to inhibit its effectiveness.

$Rh_o(D)$ immune globulin (RhoGAM) is used to prevent isoimmunization in $Rh_o(D)$-negative women exposed to $Rh_o(D)$-positive blood. **RhoGAM** is a solution containing IgG antibodies against erythrocyte antigen $Rh_o(D)$, collected from the plasma of human donors. It is believed that the anti-$Rh_o(D)$-antibodies in **RhoGAM** interact directly with the Rh_o(D)-antigens, preventing interaction between the antigens and the maternal immune system. **RhoGAM** prevents the development of erythroblastosis fetalis in current or subsequent pregnancies.

Pharmacokinetics

IGIM, when used for pre-exposure prophylaxis for hepatitis A, confers protection for less than 3 months. It is greater than 85 percent effective in preventing hepatitis A if given within 2 weeks after exposure. **IGIM** can be given to prevent or modify measles in susceptible persons if used within 6 days of exposure.

HBIG is slowly absorbed, with antibodies appearing in 1 to 6 days and peak levels reached in 3 to 9 days. The antibodies remain in the serum for up to 2 months. **HBIG** probably crosses the placenta and may be distributed in breast milk.

TIG is given IM, with peak levels of IgG noted 2 days after administration. The half-life of IgG in circulation is 3.5 to 4.5 weeks.

RSV-IGIV is administered IV on a monthly basis. The serum half-life of **RSV-IGIV** is 22 to 28 days.

VZIG is administered IM, with peak IgG levels obtained in 2 days after administration. It is the most effective if administered within 4 days of exposure to the varicella zoster virus. Antibody protection lasts 3 weeks.

RIG is administered by infiltrating the wound with half of the dose and giving the other half of the dose IM in a separate limb from the injury.

RhoGAM pharmacokinetics is not well described. Peak antibody levels are reached in 5 to 10 days after IM administration. Anti-Rh_o(D) antibodies are not detectable 6 months after administration of **RhoGAM.**

Pharmacotherapeutics

Precautions and Contraindications

An allergic response to **IGIM** or anti-IGA antibodies is a contraindication to **IG serum** use, as is **thimerosal** allergy.

Patients with IgA deficiency often develop antibodies against IgA and are more likely to have anaphylactic or immune-mediated adverse reaction to pooled **IG** products.

RSV-IGIV is contraindicated in patients with cyanotic congenital heart disease.

Live-virus vaccines should not be administered within 3 months of an **IG serum.**

Pregnancy is not a contraindication to most *IG serums.*

Adverse Drug Reactions

Local reactions include tenderness and pain in the injection site that may last for several hours.

Systemic reactions include urticaria and angioedema. Less frequently reported adverse reactions include emesis, chills, fever, myalgia, lethargy, and nausea.

Drug Interactions

IG serums interfere with the immune response to **live-virus vaccines.**

Clinical Use and Dosing

IG serums are used to prevent disease by either pre-exposure or postexposure administration. The clinical use and dosing of the **IG serums** are detailed in Table 17–6.

Monitoring

Laboratory monitoring is not necessary. The patient's Rh status should be determined prior to administering **RhoGAM.**

Patient Education

Patients should receive information regarding the benefits and risks of the **IG** prior to administration. Any questions or concerns regarding the vaccine should be addressed.

The most common adverse reactions after **IG** administration are pain and erythema at the injection site

Diagnostic Biologicals

Tuberculin Purified Protein Derivative

The diagnostic biologic agent that is commonly used in primary care is **tuberculin PPD. PPD** is used to screen asymptomatic individuals for infection with *M. tuberculosis.*

Pharmacodynamics

PPD is administered intradermally to asymptomatic individuals. Once a person has become sensitized to mycobacterial antigens, a hypersensitivity reaction occurs to the administration of the intradermal **PPD.** In sensitive people, the reaction includes induration and erythema at the site of administration. A positive reaction to **PPD** indicates that the person at some time has had a TB infection. A positive test does not indicate an active infection

Table 17–6. Dosage Schedule: Immunomodulators

Drug	Indication	Dose	Comments
I/gamma globulin	Hepatitis A prophylaxis	Length of stay: <3 mo, give 0.02 mL/kg IM. Prolonged (>3 mo), give 0.06 mL/kg and repeat every 4 to 6 mo.	Effective if given before exposure or within 2 wk of exposure.
	Measles	Give 0.25 mL/kg IM. If child is also immunocompromised, give 0.5 mL/kg IM.	Must be given within 6 d of exposure to measles.
Hepatitis B immune globulin (HBIG)	After exposure to blood infected with hepatitis B (HBV)	Administer 0.06 mL/kg IM within 24 h; repeat in 28 to 30 d.	Give hepatitis B vaccine within 7 d and repeat at 1 and 6 mo.
	Sexual contacts of HBV-infected people	Administer 0.06 mL/kg IM within 14 d of sexual contact.	Give hepatitis B vaccine within 7 d and repeat at 1 and 6 mo.
	Infants born to HbsAg-positive mothers	Administer 0.5 mL IM within 12 h of birth.	Give hepatitis B vaccine within 12 h of birth and repeat at 1 or 2 and at 6 mo.
Tetanus immune globulin (TIG)	Passive immunization against tetanus	Clean minor wounds: No TIG necessary. Give Td/DTaP if indicated. All other wounds (may be contaminated with dirt, feces, soil, saliva, and puncture wounds): Unknown or <3 doses of DTP/Td: Give adults 250 U TIG, children 4 U/kg of TIG, give a booster dose of TD/DTaP. History of >3 doses of tetanus toxoid: No TIG, no Td/DTaP booster.	
Respiratory syncytial virus immune globulin (RSV-IGIV)	RSV prophylaxis in high-risk children	*Children <24 mo with broncho-pulmonary dysplasia or chronic lung disease:* Give 750 mg/kg IV once monthly throughout RSV season. *Infants <6 mo born at 32 wk gestation or earlier or infants <12 mo of age if less than 28 wk gestation:* Give 750 mg/kg IV once monthly throughout RSV season.	Medication should be infused at a rate of 1.5 mL/kg/h for the first 15 min, then increase to 3 mL/kg/h for 15 min, maximum rate of 6 mL/kg/h.
Varicella-zoster immune globulin (VZIG)	Passive immunization for high-risk patients exposed to varicella	Administer VZIG within 96 h of exposure. *Adults and adolescents:* 125 U/10 kg, up to 625 U maximum. *Children and infants:* 125 U/10 kg, rounded to nearest 125 U. >40 kg: 625 U IM 30.1–40 kg: 500 U 20.1–30 kg: 375 U 10.1–20 kg: 250 U ≤10 kg: 125 U	Patients should meet the following CDC criteria for VZIG administration: 1. Not immune to varicella 2. Significant exposure <96 h prior to VZIG administration; significant exposure defined as household contact, playmate contact (>1 h contact), hospital contact (in same room) 3. Age <15 y, or immuno compromised adults and adolescents

Continued on next page

Table 17–6. Dosage Schedule: Immunomodulators *(continued)*

Drug	Indication	Dose	Comments
			4. One of the following: leukemia, lymphoma, bone marrow transplant, congenital or acquired immunodeficiency (including HIV), drug- or radiation-induced immunosuppression, premature infants <28 wk gestation, and infants born to mother who develops varicella within 5 d before or 48 h after delivery
Rabies immune globulin (RIG)	Provides passive immunity to rabies	Previously unvaccinated against rabies: Administer 20 IU/kg up to 7 days after the first dose of rabies vaccine.	Postexposure prophylaxis always includes administration of both passive antibody and vaccine, with the exception of those who have previously received complete vaccination. For postexposure vaccination, the ACIP recommends that 5 doses of rabies vaccine be given, with RIG given at the same time as the first vaccine dose.
Rh$_o$(D) immune globulin (RhoGAM)	Rh isoimmunization prophylaxis	Administer 300 μg IM at 28 wk gestation and/or within 72 h of an Rh-incompatible delivery, miscarriage, abortion, or transfusion accident.	Each vial or syringe (~300 μg) prevents sensitization to a volume of up to 15 mL of Rh-positive red blood cells.

but rather that further testing is indicated. See Chapter 43 for more information regarding TB evaluation.

Pharmacotherapeutics

PRECAUTIONS AND CONTRAINDICATIONS. Do not administer **PPD** to known tuberculin-positive reactors because they may have a severe reaction, including ulceration and necrosis at the site of administration.

SC administration should be avoided, as a general febrile reaction or acute inflammation may occur.

Skin testing of immunodeficient people may not be accurate because skin-test responsiveness may be suppressed.

Skin test responsiveness may be delayed in the older adult patient.

PPD testing is safe in pregnancy, during lactation, and in children of all ages, including infants.

ADVERSE DRUG REACTIONS. In highly sensitive people, vesiculation, ulceration, and necrosis can occur at the administration site. A normal adverse reaction is a minimal amount of bleeding at the administration site.

DRUG INTERACTIONS. Live-virus vaccines (MMR, varicella) can suppress the reaction to **PPD** if given within 4 to 6 weeks prior to the **PPD**. **PPD** can be administered during the same visit as **MMR** and **varicella vaccines.**

Patients who have been vaccinated with **BCG** generally are sensitive to **PPD**.

Immunosuppressant medications can suppress the reaction to **PPD** testing.

CLINICAL USE AND DOSING. The Mantoux **PPD** test containing 5 tuberculin units (TU) is the preferred test because the interpretation of the reaction has been standardized. Previously, multiple puncture tests were used, and there were many problems with the interpretation.

The test consists of injecting 5 TU of **PPD** intradermally. A small white bleb should appear at the injection site if it is done correctly. Reactions are read in 48 to 72 hours after administration. For patients who may be highly sensitized, a test dose of 1 TU is used.

Determining the results of the skin test is based on the likelihood of infection and the risk of active TB if infection has occurred. If the patient is HIV-positive or has fibrotic lesions on chest x-ray, a reaction of 5 mm or more induration is considered positive. A reaction of 10 mm or more induration is considered positive in other at-risk patients, including infants and children. In patients who are not in any high-risk category or high-risk environment, a result of 15 mm or more induration is considered positive.

Patients are considered high risk if they have the following conditions: (1) diabetes mellitus; (2) prolonged therapy with **adrenocorticosteroids**; (3) **immunosuppressive therapy**; (4) hematologic and/or reticuloendothelial diseases, such as leukemia or Hodgkin's disease; (5) injection drug users known to be HIV-seronegative; (6) end-stage renal disease; or (6) any clinical presentation that includes substantial rapid weight loss or chronic malnutrition.

People who are in a high-incidence group with a skin test reaction of 10 mm or more induration are candidates for preventive therapy, even if they do not have any of the risk factors. High-incidence groups include (1) foreign-born persons from high-prevalence countries, (2) medically underserved low-income populations, and (3) residents of facilities for long-term care.

MONITORING. The **PPD** should be read by an experienced health care professional who has been trained in the proper method of interpreting the results.

PATIENT EDUCATION. Patients must have an understanding of the reason for **PPD** testing and why the test must be "read" in 48 to 72 hours.

Adverse reactions are rare in patients who are not already sensitized to TB.

Immunomodulators

Although not generally prescribed by primary care providers, two **immunomodulator medications** commonly prescribed to patients by specialty providers are covered in this chapter. **Cyclosporine (Sandimmune)** is prescribed to organ transplant patients and is used for severe rheumatoid arthritis. **Azathioprine (Imuran)** is also prescribed for transplant patients and severe rheumatoid arthritis.

Pharmacodynamics

Cyclosporine is an oral and parenteral **immunosuppressive agent.** It is believed to act by inhibiting the production or release of various lymphokines. The actions of the T-helper cell, the mediators of cellular immunity and tissue rejection, are impaired. **Cyclosporine** may inhibit T-suppressor cells. **Cyclosporine** also inhibits the synthesis of gamma-interferon. **Cyclosporine** does not cause myelosuppression.

Azathioprine is an oral and parenteral **immunosuppressive** that decreases the metabolism of purines and may inhibit DNA and RNA synthesis. It may interfere with coenzyme functioning, decreasing cellular metabolism. **Azathioprine** has the ability to inhibit the delayed hypersensitivity reaction and cellular cytotoxic activity that occur during renal transplantation.

Pharmacokinetics

Absorption and Distribution

After oral administration, approximately 20 to 50 percent of **cyclosporine** is absorbed. Absorption from the GI tract is highly variable. It is widely distributed throughout the body, crosses the placenta, and is excreted in breast milk.

Azathioprine is well absorbed following oral administration. It is widely distributed and crosses the placenta.

Metabolism and Excretion

Cyclosporine undergoes extensive first-pass metabolism. It is metabolized extensively by the liver cytochrome CYP-450 3A (CYP-450 3A) enzyme system. Elimination of **cyclosporine** and its metabolites is primarily through the bile and feces, with only 6 percent excreted renally.

Azathioprine is metabolized in the liver to its active metabolite, mercaptopurine. The metabolites and some unchanged **azathioprine** are excreted in the urine.

Pharmacotherapeutics

Precautions and Contraindications

Hypersensitivity to the medication or components of the product is a contraindication to its use. Oral **cyclosporine** preparations contain corn, castor oil and/or olive oil, and patients with hypersensitivity to these food products should avoid its use.

Patients with renal dysfunction should be monitored for worsening renal function while taking **cyclosporine.** **Azathioprine** can accumulate in patients with renal impairment, possibly causing toxicity.

Hepatic dysfunction can affect the metabolism of both drugs.

Both *cyclosporine* and *azathioprine* **are contraindicated in pregnancy and breastfeeding.**

Table 17–7. Drug Interactions: Immunomodulators

Drug	Interacting Drug	Possible Effect	Implications
Azathioprine	Live vaccines (MMR, varicella)	Decreased antibody response to vaccine.	Wait 3 mo to 1 y after stopping azathioprine before administering live vaccines.
	Allopurinol	Increased pharmacologic and toxic effects of azathioprine.	Avoid concurrent use, or reduce dose of azathioprine by $1/3$ to $1/2$.
	Angiotensin-converting enzyme (ACE) inhibitors	May induce severe leukopenia or anemia.	
	Methotrexate	May increase plasma levels of azathioprine metabolite 6-MP.	Avoid concurrent use.
	Anticoagulants	Decreased effectiveness of anticoagulants.	Avoid concurrent use.
	Alkylating agents/antineoplastic agents	Prior treatment with alkylating agents puts patient at higher risk of developing neoplasms or infection.	
	Cyclosporine	Cyclosporine plasma levels might be decreased.	
Cyclosporine	*Nephrotoxic drugs:* amphotericin B, acyclovir, aminoglycosides, foscarnet, NSAIDs, vancomycin, ganciclovir	Additive nephrotoxicity.	
	Immunosuppressants	Increased risk of lymphoma and infection.	
	Potassium-sparing diuretics: amiloride, spironolactone, triamterene	Hyperkalemia.	Monitor potassium levels.
	Drugs metabolized by CYP-450 3A isoenzyme inhibitors: calcium channel blockers, androgens, clarithromycin, azole antifungals, methylprednisolone, allopurinol, bromocriptine, danazol, erythromycin, dalfopristin, metoclopramide	Increased cyclosporine levels, leading to cyclosporine toxicity.	Monitor cyclosporine levels.
	Drugs metabolized by CYP-450 3A isoenzyme inducers: nafcillin, modafinil, troglitazone, rifampin, carbamazepine, pentobarbital, phenytoin, octreotide, ticlopidine, primidone	Decreased cyclosporine levels.	Monitor cyclosporine levels if any of these drugs are added or deleted from medication regimen.
	Vaccines	Decreased effectiveness of vaccines.	Wait at least 3 mo after therapy with cyclosporine is completed to administer live vaccines.
	Digoxin	Increased digoxin levels.	Monitor digoxin levels.
	Prednisolone	Increased prednisolone levels.	
	Lovastatin	Increased lovastatin levels.	
	Grapefruit juice	Increased cyclosporine levels.	
	Protease inhibitors	Cyclosporine toxicity.	
	SMX/TMP	Decreased blood levels of cyclosporine.	
	Clonidine	Interferes with clonidine pharmacokinetics.	
	Metoclopramide (oral)	Increases oral bioavailability of cyclosporine by 30%.	Monitor cyclosporine concentrations.
	Colchicine	Nephrotoxicity and azotemia.	Avoid concurrent use.
	Orlistat	Altered bioavailability of cyclosporine.	Monitor if using concurrently.

Adverse Drug Reactions

Nephrotoxicity is the most common adverse effect of **cyclosporine** therapy. **Cyclosporine** may also cause hypertension, headaches, GI upset, hirsutism (50% of patients), gingival hyperplasia (4–16%), hypercholesterolemia, and neurological effects such as seizures, tremor, paresthesias, and mood changes.

Hepatic failure can occur with **azathioprine** use. Nausea and vomiting occurred in 12 percent of patients. Patients taking **azathioprine** should be monitored for bone marrow suppression. Other adverse effects reported are fever, rash, pancreatitis, alopecia, and retinopathy.

Drug Interactions

Cyclosporine interacts with many drugs, especially those metabolized by the hepatic CYP-450 isoenzymes. It also interacts with multiple other drugs, presented in Table 17–7.

Azathioprine suppresses the immune system; therefore, **live or inactivated vaccines** should not be given to patients receiving this drug. **OPV** should not be administered to household contacts of patients taking **azathioprine.** It may take the immune system 3 to 12 months to return to normal after administration of **azathioprine.** Other drug interactions are shown in Table 17–7.

Clinical Use and Dosing

Cyclosporine and **azathioprine** are usually prescribed by specialty providers. If in consultation with a specialist, the primary care provider is prescribing these products for rheumatoid arthritis, the dosing is as follows: **Cyclosporine** is started at 1.25 mg/kg twice daily and may increase by 0.5 to 0.75 mg/kg per day at 8 weeks and at 12 weeks, if indicated. Maximum dose is 4 mg/kg per day. Decrease dose by 25 to 50 percent if adverse effects occur. **Azathioprine** is begun at 1 mg/kg per day in one to two divided doses. The dose can be increased in 6 to 8 weeks, by 0.5 mg/kg per day. The dose can be increased every 4 weeks to a maximum of 2.5 mg/kg per day.

Monitoring

Patients prescribed these medications need monitoring of their blood pressure, renal function, and hepatic function. Patients taking **cyclosporine** also need to have serum **cyclosporine** levels checked periodically. Patients taking **azathioprine** need a CBC and serum amylase drawn periodically.

Patient Education

Patients should be instructed to take the medication exactly as prescribed.

Any symptoms of adverse reactions should be reported to the provider immediately. The patient should be cautioned to report any "flulike" symptoms, which may be a sign of hepatic or renal dysfunction.

REFERENCES

American College Health Association (ACHA). (2000). *Recommendations for institutional prematriculation guidelines.* Baltimore: ACHA. (full document at www.acha.org)

Bates, A. S., & Wolinsky, F. D. (1998). Personal, financial, and structural barriers to immunization in socioeconomically disadvantaged urban children. *Pediatrics, 101*(4), 591–596.

Centers for Disease Control and Prevention (CDC). (1993). Inactivated Japanese encephalitis virus vaccine: Recommendations of the ACIP. *Morbidity and Mortality Weekly Report, 42*(RR-1), 1–22.

CDC. (1993). Recommendations of the Advisory Committee on Immunization Practices (ACIP): Use of vaccines and immune globulins in persons with altered immunocompetence. *Morbidity and Mortality Weekly Report, 42*(RR-4), 1–24.

CDC. (1994). General recommendations on immunization: Recommendations of the ACIP. *Morbidity and Mortality Weekly Report, 43*(RR-1), 1–39.

CDC. (1996a). Immunization of adolescents: Recommendations of the ACIP, the American Academy of Pediatrics, the American Academy of Family Physicians, and the American Medical Association. *Morbidity and Mortality Weekly Report, 45*(RR-13), 1–24.

CDC. (1996b). Prevention of plague: Recommendations of the ACIP. *Morbidity and Mortality Weekly Report 45*(RR-14), 1.

CDC. (1996c). The role of BCG vaccine in the prevention and control of tuberculosis in the United States: A joint statement by the advisory council of the elimination of tuberculosis and the ACIP. *Morbidity and Mortality Weekly Report, 45*(RR-4), 1–18.

CDC. (1997a). Control and prevention of meningococcal disease and control and prevention of serogroup C meningococcal disease: Evaluation and management of suspected outbreaks. Recommendations of the ACIP. *Morbidity and Mortality Weekly Report, 46*(RR-5), 1–21.

CDC. (1997b). Immunization of health-care workers: Recommendations of the ACIP and the Hospital Infection Control Practices Advisory Committee. *Morbidity and Mortality Weekly Report, 46*(RR-18), 1–57

CDC. (1997c). Pertussis vaccination: Use of acellular pertussis vaccines among infants and young children: Recommendations of the ACIP. *Morbidity and Mortality Weekly Report, 46*(RR-7), 1–25.

CDC. (1997d). Pneumococcal and influenza vaccination levels among adults aged greater than or equal to 65 years—United States, 1995. *Morbidity and Mortality Weekly Report, 46*(39), 913–919.

CDC. (1997e). Poliomyelitis prevention in the United States: Introduction of a sequential vaccination schedule of inactivated poliovirus vaccine followed by oral poliovirus vaccine. Recommendations of the ACIP. *Morbidity and Mortality Weekly Report, 46*(RR-3), 1–25.

CDC. (1998a). Vaccination coverage by race/ethnicity and poverty level among children aged 19–35 months—United States, 1997. *Morbidity and Mortality Weekly Report, 47*(44), 956–959.

CDC. (1998b). *Guidelines for vaccinating pregnant women.* (full document at www.immunize.org)

CDC. (1999a). Human rabies prevention—United States, 1999: Recommendations of the ACIP. *Morbidity and Mortality Weekly Report, 48*(RR-1), 1–33.

CDC. (1999b). Prevention of hepatitis A through active or passive immunization: Recommendations of the Advisory Committee on Immunization Practices (ACIP). *Morbidity and Mortality Weekly Report, 48*(RR-12), 1–37.

CDC. (2000). Vaccination coverage among adolescents 1 year before the institution of a seventh grade school entry vaccination requirement: San Diego, California, 1998. *Morbidity and Mortality Weekly Report, 49*(5), 101–102, 111.

CDC Division of Bacterial and Mycotic Diseases. (1999). ACIP modifies recommendations for meningitis vaccination. CDC Website (*www.cdc.gov*) 10/20/99.

Committee on Infectious Diseases, American Academy of Pediatrics. (1997). *Red book 1997: Report of the Committee on Infectious Diseases* (24th ed.). Elk Grove Village, IL: American Academy of Pediatrics.

Freed, G. L., Freeman, V. A., & Mauskopf, A. (1998). Enforcement of age-appropriate immunization laws. *American Journal of Preventive Medicine, 14*(2) 118–121.

Harrison, L. H., Dwyer, D. M., Maples, C. T., & Billman, L. (1999). Risk of meningococcal infection in college students. *Journal of the American Medical Association, 281*(20), 1906–1910.

Immunization Action Coalition. (2000). First pneumococcal vaccine approved for infants and toddlers. *IAC Express 139* (2/19/2000). Found at www.immunize.org.

Kenyon, T. A., Matuck, M. A., & Stroh, G. (1998). Persistent low immunization coverage among inner-city preschool children despite access to free vaccine. *Pediatrics, 101*(4), 612–619.

Minderman, E., Harris, N., & Edwards, K. (1999). Polio vaccines: Time for another change. *Contemporary Pediatrics, 16*(*Suppl*) December, 3–13.

Neiderhauser, V. P. (1999). Varicella: The vaccine and the public health debate. *Nurse Practitioner, 24*(3), 74–92.

O'Donovan, C. (1999). Addressing parent's concerns about injectable polio vaccine. *Contemporary Pediatrics, 16*(*Suppl*) December, 14–16.

Oregon Health Division. (1998). Pneumococcal disease: Common . . . deadly . . . preventable. *CD Summary, 47*(20), 1–2.

Oregon Health Division. (1999). Serological testing for hepatitis B: A short review. *CD Summary, 48*(1), 1–2.

Ott, M. J., & Aruda, M. (1999). Hepatitis B vaccine. *Journal of Pediatric Health Care, 13*(5), 211–216.

Satcher, D. (1999). Letter to Immunization Action Coalition members. *Needle Tips & Hepatitis B Coalition News, 9*(1), 2.

Wadsworth, L. (1999). Polio immunization: Dealing with new recommendation and helping parents understand the changes. *Journal of Pediatric Health Care, (Suppl)13*(6), s21–s30.

CHAPTER 18

....

Drugs Affecting the Gastrointestinal System

CHAPTER OUTLINE

wide variety of drugs are used to treat disorders affecting the gastrointestinal (GI) tract. **Cholinergic drugs** increase gastric acid secretion and increase peristalsis; **anticholinergic drugs** inhibit gastric acid secretion and decrease peristalsis. **Nicotine** increases the risk for ulcer formation through its action on the gastric mucosa. These drugs are discussed in Chapter 12. **Phenothiazines** have antiemetic properties and are **narcotic analgesics;** some of their derivatives are used to treat diarrhea. These drugs are discussed in Chapter 13. Several groups of drugs are used almost exclusively to treat GI disorders, and these drugs are discussed in this chapter. Intravenous forms are not used in primary care and are not discussed.

Antacids

Antacids are weak bases that react with hydrochloric acid (HCl) to form a salt and water. They are used to reduce gastric acidity in the treatment of peptic ulcer disease. Various combinations of metallic cation (aluminum, calcium, magnesium, and sodium) and basic anion (hydroxide, bicarbonate, carbonate, citrate, and trisilicate) can be used. Most **antacids** in current use have as their cation aluminum, calcium, or magnesium, and their anion is usually hydroxide (OH), bicarbonate (HCO_3), or carbonate (CO_3). The buffering capacity of the other two anions is too limited to be clinically effective.

Note: Cisapride (Propulsid) has been taken off the market.

Pharmacodynamics

Antacids neutralize gastric acidity, which causes an increase in the pH of the stomach and duodenal bulb. They also inhibit the proteolytic activity of pepsin and increase lower esophageal sphincter tone. Aluminum-based products inhibit smooth muscle contraction and thus slow gastric emptying. They also bind with phosphate ions in the intestine to form insoluble aluminum-phosphate that is excreted in the feces. This action is used to treat hyperphosphatemia in chronic renal failure. Calcium carbonate also suppresses phosphate concentrations.

Acid-neutralizing capacity (ANC) varies between products and is expressed in milliequivalents (mEq) of HCl required to keep an **antacid** suspension at pH 3.5 for 10 minutes in vitro. **Antacids** must neutralize at least 5 mEq per dose. Those with higher ANC values are more likely to be effective in vivo. **Sodium bicarbonate** and **calcium carbonate** have the highest ANC but are not used for chronic therapy because of their systemic effects. Suspensions have greater ANC than powders or tablets.

Pharmacokinetics

Absorption and Distribution

Aluminum- and **magnesium-based antacids** are not absorbable with routine use. With chronic use, 10 to 30 percent of magnesium and smaller amounts of aluminum may be absorbed. These small amounts that are absorbed are widely distributed, cross the placenta, and appear in breast milk. Aluminum concentrates in the central nervous system. **Calcium-based antacids** require vitamin D for absorption from the GI tract. The small amount that is absorbed enters the extracellular fluid, crosses the placenta, and enters breast milk.

If ingested in a fasting state, **antacids** reduce acidity for approximately 20 to 40 minutes. If taken 1 hour after a meal, acidity is reduced for 2 to 3 hours. A second dose given 3 hours after a meal maintains the reduced acidity for more than 4 hours after the meal.

Metabolism and Excretion

The action of **antacids** occurs locally in the GI tract with minimal absorption, and so there is minimal metabolism. **Aluminum-** and **magnesium-based antacids** are excreted in the urine; **calcium-based antacids** are excreted mainly in feces, with 20 percent eliminated in urine.

Table 18–1 shows the pharmacokinetic properties of selected **antacids**.

Pharmacotherapeutics

Precautions and Contraindications

All **antacids** are contraindicated in the presence of severe abdominal pain of unknown cause, especially if accompanied by fever. **Calcium-based antacids** are contraindicated in the presence of hypercalcemia and renal calculi.

Renal impairment presents several issues for patients who take **antacids**. **Magnesium-based antacids** are contraindicated in patients with renal failure and used with caution for patients with any degree of renal insufficiency because the malfunctioning kidney is unable to excrete magnesium, and hypermagnesemia may result. Prolonged use of **aluminum-based antacids** for patients with renal failure may result in or worsen dialysis osteomalacia. Aluminum is not easily removed by dialysis because it is bound to albumin and transferrin, which do not cross the dialysis membrane. As a result, aluminum is deposited in bone, and osteomalacia occurs. Elevated tissue aluminum levels also contribute to the development of dialysis encephalopathy.

Adverse Drug Reactions

Aluminum- and **calcium-based antacids** cause constipation; **magnesium-based antacids** cause diarrhea. Alkalosis may occur but tends to be a clinically significant problem only for patients with renal impairment.

Drug Interactions

All **antacids** have drug interactions with orally administered weakly acidic and weakly basic drugs, decreasing or increasing their absorption and, therefore, their effects. Enteric coating on drugs is used to protect them from the acid of the stomach, and the coating dissolves in the more basic medium of the duodenum. Concurrent administration of **antacids** with enteric-coated drugs destroys the coating, alters their absorption, and increases the risk for adverse reactions. Some **antacids** adsorb or bind to the surface of other drugs, resulting in decreased bioavailability. **Magnesium hydroxide (Milk of Magnesia, Maalox, Mylanta)** has the greatest ability to adsorb and **calcium carbonate** and **alu-**

Table 18–1. Pharmacokinetics: Selected Antacids

Drug	Onset	Peak	Duration	Acid-Neutralizing Capacity (ANC)	Half-Life	Elimination
Aluminum hydroxide	Slightly delayed	30 min	30 min–1 h on empty stomach; 3 h after meals	3.2 (AlternaGEL) 2.0 (Amphojel)	Unknown	In urine
Magnesium hydroxide	Immediate	30 min	30 min–1 h on empty stomach; 3 h after meals	—	Unknown	In urine
Aluminum hydroxide–magnesium hydroxide combinations	Immediate	30 min	30 min–1 h on empty stomach; 3 h after meals	2.7 (Maalox) 5.7 (Maalox HRF) 5.1 (Mylanta)	Unknown	In urine
Calcium carbonate	Slightly delayed	30 min	30 min–1 h on empty stomach; 3 h after meals	—	Unknown	Mostly in feces; 20% in urine

minum hydroxide (**AlternaGEL, Amphojel**) have intermediate ability to adsorb certain drugs. Increasing urinary pH affects the rate of elimination by inhibiting the excretion of weakly basic drugs and increasing the elimination of weakly acidic ones. Separating the ad-

ministration of the **antacid** and the interacting drug by at least 2 hours and giving the interacting drug first in this sequence often can avoid these problems. Table 18–2 provides specific information on drug interactions with selected **antacids**.

Table 18–2. Drug Interactions: Selected Antacids

Drug	Interacting Drug	Possible Effect	Implications
All antacids	Weakly acidic drugs (e.g., digoxin, phenytoin, chlorpromazine, isoniazid, ketoconazole)	Decreased absorption with possible decreased drug effects	Separate administration by at least 2 h, giving the antacid after the drug.
	Weakly basic drugs (e.g., pseudoephedrine, levodopa)	Increased absorption with possible toxicity or adverse reactions	Separate administration by at least 2 h, giving the antacid after the drug.
	Drugs acidic at the time of excretion (e.g., salicylates)	Enhanced excretion	May be used therapeutically to treat salicylate toxicity. Otherwise, avoid concurrent use or alter dosage of drug.
	Drugs basic at the time of excretion (e.g., quinidine, amphetamines)	Decreased excretion	Avoid concurrent use or alter dosage of drug.
	Drugs with enteric coating	Antacids may destroy the coating, resulting in altered absorption or adverse reactions	Avoid concurrent use or separate administration by at least 2 h, giving the antacid after the drug.
	Buffered aspirin products	Alkalinization of urine accelerates aspirin excretion, and systemic alkalosis and increased sodium load may occur	Caution against use of these antacid-analgesic combinations in chronic pain syndromes. Not an issue if used only intermittently.
Aluminum-based antacids	Allopurinol, chloroquine, corticosteroids, ethambutol, histamine$_2$ blockers, iron salts, phenothiazines, tetracyclines, thyroid hormones, ticlopidine	Decreased pharmacological effect of the drug	Avoid concurrent use or separate administration by at least 2 h, giving the antacid after the drug.
	Benzodiazepines	Increased pharmacological effect of the drug	Avoid concurrent use.
Calcium-based antacids	Fluoroquinolones, hydantoins, iron salts, salicylates, tetracyclines	Decreased pharmacological effect of the drug	Avoid concurrent administration.
	Quinidine	Increased pharmacological effect of the drug	Avoid concurrent administration.

Continued on next page

Table 18–2. Drug Interactions: Selected Antacids (*continued*)

Drug	Interacting Drug	Possible Effect	Implications
Magnesium-based antacids	Benzodiazepines, corticosteroids, histamine$_2$ blockers, hydantoins, iron salts, nitrofurantoin, phenothiazines, tetracyclines, ticlopidine	Decreased pharmacological effect of the drug	Avoid concurrent administration.
	Quinidine, sulfonylureas	Increased pharmacological effect of the drug	Avoid concurrent administration.

Clinical Use and Dosing

HYPERACIDITY. Antacids are used for symptomatic relief of stomach upset associated with the hyperacidity of heartburn, acid indigestion, and "sour stomach." Because they are sold over the counter (OTC), doses vary, as patients choose the amount they think they need to relieve symptoms. Generally, dosing is 1 to 2 tablets or 1 to 2 tablespoons of suspension taken intermittently.

PEPTIC ULCER DISEASE. Although the main factor in most duodenal ulcers and many gastric ulcers is infection with *Helicobacter pylori,* hyperacidity is also a factor in peptic ulcer disease (PUD). Patients with uncomplicated PUD can benefit from 15 to 30 cc of antacid suspension 1 to 3 hours after meals and at bedtime. Additional doses may be used for recurring symptoms. Treatment is continued for 4 to 6 weeks for duodenal ulcers and until healing is complete for gastric ulcers. Because their ANC is higher, combined antacids with both aluminum hydroxide and magnesium hydroxide are best unless the patient also has renal insufficiency or failure. Further discussion of PUD occurs in Chapter 32.

GASTROESOPHAGEAL REFLUX DISEASE. Lifestyle management and drugs to increase lower esophageal sphincter tone are central to the management of gastroesophageal reflux disease (GERD), but there is a role for antacids in mild disease. Suspensions are generally used. For acute management, doses may be given every 30 to 60 minutes until symptoms are relieved; for maintenance, doses are given 1 and 3 hours after meals and at bedtime. Additional doses may be given for recurring symptoms. For infants and children, the dose is 0.5 mL/kg (average 2 to 15 mL per dose) 1 to 2 hours after meals or feedings. For adults, the dose is 5 to 30 cc each dose. Further discussion of GERD occurs in Chapter 32.

HYPERPHOSPHATEMIA. Aluminum carbonate (Basaljel) and aluminum hydroxide have been used, along with a low-phosphate diet, to treat hyperphosphatemia in patients with chronic renal failure. They have also been used to prevent the formation of phosphate urinary stones. The dose is 30 mL of suspension with each meal.

CALCIUM DEFICIENCY. Calcium carbonate (Tums) is routinely used to treat calcium deficiency states associated with chronic renal failure, postmenopause, and osteoporosis. Tablets, often in chewable form, are commonly used. The dose is sufficient to provide 1000 mg/day of calcium for patients with chronic renal failure and 1200 to 1500 mg of calcium per day for postmenopausal women and patients with osteoporosis (Table 18–3).

Rational Drug Selection

In addition to consideration of adverse drug reactions and the indications discussed previously, other major factors used to choose among antacids are ANC, sodium content, and cost.

ACID-NEUTRALIZING CAPACITY. Combination products that contain aluminum hydroxide and magnesium hydroxide have the highest ANC. (See Table 18–1.) When moderate to severe hyperacidity is a factor in the disease process under treatment, these drugs are chosen over other antacids.

SODIUM CONTENT. Sodium content of antacids may be significant. Patients who must restrict sodium intake (e.g., with hypertension, congestive heart failure, or marked renal failure) should use a low-sodium antacid. The sodium content is listed on the product label.

COST. Antacids are sold OTC. In general, they are inexpensive, but the cost of a high-dose regimen varies significantly. Katzung (1998) provides a list of costs based on the *Drug Topics Red Book* for 1996. The least expensive were **Mylanta** and **Gelusil,** combination products with simethicone added, with 1-month treatment costs of $95 and $99, respectively. The next least expensive was **Maalox,** a combination product, at $127 for 1

Table 18–3. Dosage Schedule: Selected Antacids

Drug	Indication	Dosage Schedule
Aluminum hydroxide	Hyperphosphatemia	Tablets or capsules: 500–1500 mg with meals
		Suspension: 30 mL with meals
	Hyperacidity	Tablets or capsules: 500–1500 mg 3–6 times daily between meals and at bedtime
		Suspension: 5–30 mL prn between meals and at bedtime
Calcium carbonate	Calcium deficiency in chronic renal failure	Tablets: 1000 mg/day
	Postmenopause or osteoporosis	Tablets: 1200–1500 mg/day
Magnesium hydroxide	Hyperacidity	*Adults and children >12 y:*
		Tablets: 622–1244 mg up to qid
		Liquid: 5–15 mL up to qid with water
		Liquid concentrate: 2.5–7.5 mL up to qid with water
	Laxative	15–30 mL at bedtime with water
Aluminum hydroxide–magnesium hydroxide combinations	Hyperacidity Peptic ulcer disease	Tablets: 1 or 2 prn
		Suspension: 15–30 mL prn
		Suspension: 15–30 mL 1 h and 3 h after meals and at bedtime
	Gastroesophageal reflux disease	*Adults and children >12 y:*
		Suspension: 5–30 mL every 30–60 min for acute management; 5–30 mL 1 h and 3 h after meals and at bedtime for maintenance
		Infants and children <12 y:
		Suspension: 0.5 mL/kg (average dose 2–15 mL) 1–2 h after meals or feedings

month of treatment. The highest cost was **Amphojel,** an **aluminum hydroxide**–only product, with a 1-month treatment cost of $232.

Monitoring

No specific monitoring is required beyond that related to the disease process for which the patient is being treated. Serum phosphate, potassium, and calcium levels may be monitored periodically during chronic use. These drugs may cause increased serum calcium and decreased serum phosphate.

Patient Education

ADMINISTRATION. Antacids should be taken as prescribed, especially related to mealtimes. For best effects, take 1 to 3 hours after meals and at bedtime. To prevent chewable tablets from entering the small intestine in undissolved form, they must be chewed thoroughly before they are swallowed and followed with half a glass of water. Suspensions should be shaken before administration (Table 18–4).

Antacids have many drug interactions when taken concurrently with other drugs. The dose of **antacid** may need to be separated from the dose of another drug by as much as 2 hours. This is especially a problem for enteric-coated tablets of any drug. Health care providers should instruct the patient in timing the administration of such drugs. Patients should be told not begin taking OTC **antacids** on their own without first consulting their health care provider or the pharmacist to discuss any potential drug interactions.

Calcium-based antacids should not be administered with food containing large amounts of oxalic acid (e.g., spinach, rhubarb) or phytic acid (e.g., bran, cereals). These foods decrease the absorption of calcium. Taking these **antacids** with food that contains phosphorus (milk or other dairy products) may lead to milk-alkali syndrome (nausea, vomiting, confusion, and headache).

ADVERSE REACTIONS. Patients should be told to consult their health care provider before taking **antacids** for more than 2 weeks, if a problem recurs, if relief is not obtained, or if symptoms of GI bleeding (black, tarry stools; coffee-ground emesis) occur.

Aluminum- and **calcium-based antacids** may cause constipation. Methods of preventing constipation such as increased bulk in the diet, greater fluid intake, and more mobility should be recommended. **Magnesium-based antacids** may cause diarrhea. Increased fiber in the diet may help this problem.

Table 18–4. Available Dosage Forms: Selected Antacids

Drug	Dosage Form	How Supplied
Aluminum hydroxide (AlternaGEL)	Liquid: 600 mg/5 mL	In 150-mL and 360-mL bottles
(Amphojel)	Tablets: 300 mg, 600 mg	In bottles of 100 tablets
(Alu-Tab)	Tablets: 500 mg	In bottles of 250 tablets
(Alu-Cap)	Capsules: 400 mg	In bottles of 100 capsules
(Dialume)	Capsules: 500 mg	In bottles of 500 capsules
(Generic)	Suspension: 320 mg/5 mL Concentrated suspension: 450 mg/5 mL Concentrated suspension: 675 mg/5 mL Concentrated liquid: 600 mg/5 mL	In bottles of 360 and 480 mL In bottles of 500 mL (peppermint flavor) In bottles of 180, 500 mL (creamsicle flavor) In bottles of 30, 180, 480 mL
Calcium carbonate (Tums)	Tablets/chewable: 500 mg Extra-strength/chewable: 750 mg Ultra/chewable: 1000 mg	In bottles of 36, 75, 150, 400 tablets In bottles of 24, 48, 96 tablets (assorted flavors) In bottles of 36, 72 tablets (assorted flavors)
(Generic)	Tablets: 500 mg, 600 mg, 650 mg, 1250 mg Suspension: 1250 mg/5 mL	In bottles of varying number 60–1000 In bottles of 500 mL (mint flavor)
Magnesium hydroxide (Phillip's Chewables)	Tablets: 311 mg	In bottles of 100, 200 tablets (mint flavor)
(Phillip's Milk of Magnesia)	Liquid: 400 mg/5 mL Concentrated liquid: 800 mg/5 mL	In bottles of 120, 360, 780 mL In bottles of 240 mL
(Generic)	Liquid: 400 mg/5 mL	In bottles of 360 mL, pint, gallon
Aluminum hydroxide-magnesium hydroxide combinations (Maalox)	Tablets/chewable: 200 mg aluminum, 200 mg magnesium Extra-strength: 350 mg aluminum, 350 mg magnesium Suspension: 200 mg aluminum, 225 mg magnesium/5 mL; and 300 mg aluminum, 600 mg magnesium/5 mL	In bottles of 100 tablets (mint flavor) In bottles of 38, 75 tablets (mint creme flavor) In bottles of 148, 355, and 769 mL (mint creme and cherry creme flavors)
(Mylanta)	Tablets/chewable: 200 mg aluminum, 200 mg magnesium, 20 mg simethicone Double-strength: 400 mg aluminum, 400 mg magnesium Suspension: 200 mg aluminum, 225 mg magnesium/5 mL; and 300 mg aluminum, 600 mg magnesium/5 mL	In bottles of 12, 40, 48, 100, 180 tablets In bottles of 24, 60 tablets (mint and cherry) In bottles of 150, 360, and 720 mL

LIFESTYLE MANAGEMENT. Lifestyle management issues related to the disease process should be discussed. They often include smoking avoidance or cessation, inappropriate body positions while sleeping, foods that irritate the gastric mucosa (e.g., spicy foods) or stimulate acid production (e.g., alcohol), and foods that decrease lower esophageal sphincter tone (e.g., fatty food, chocolate, and caffeine).

Antidiarrheals

Diarrhea is a common reason for self-treatment and for patients to seek treatment from a health care provider. Much of the diarrhea seen in a primary care setting has an infectious etiology, is food- or drug-induced, or is the result of inflammatory bowel disease. Diarrhea that lasts for less than 2 weeks is considered acute; if it lasts more than 2 weeks, it is considered chronic. Most episodes are acute and self-limiting, with few serious consequences. The exception is diarrhea in children, for whom dehydration is a worrisome possibility, even with short-term diarrhea. Chronic diarrhea can result in weight loss, dehydration, perianal skin breakdown, and nutritional deficits.

Diarrhea that is drug-induced may be treated simply by removal of the offending drug. Food-induced diarrhea related to food poisoning and other diarrheas of an infectious etiology require antimicrobial therapy. Drugs used to treat infectious diseases are the subject of Chapter 22. The focus of this chapter is drugs used for symptomatic relief. Some of them are chemically related to opioids. **Opioids** are discussed further in Chapter 13. **Anticholinergic agents** are also sometimes used to treat diarrhea. These drugs are discussed in Chapter 12. This chapter does not discuss the diagnosis of diarrhea.

Pharmacodynamics

Three main classes of drugs are used to treat diarrhea: **absorbent preparations** (kaolin and pectin [Kaopectate] and **bismuth subsalicylate** [Pepto-Bismol]), opiates (**diphenoxylate** with **atropine** [Lomotil] and **loperamide** [Imodium]), and **anticholinergics**. Anticholinergics are useful only for inflammatory bowel disease.

Kaolin and **pectin** decrease stool fluid content by absorbing moisture in the stool. They do not effect total water loss, however. Commonly used to treat simple diarrhea, the combination has no proven benefit but seems to be harmless (Goroll et al., 1995).

Bismuth subsalicylate appears to have antisecretory and antimicrobial effects in vitro and may have some anti-inflammatory effects. The salicylate moiety provides the antisecretory effect, and the bismuth moiety may exert direct antimicrobial effects against bacterial and viral enteropathogens. Because of these effects, it is also used as part of a multidrug regimen for the eradication of *H. pylori*.

Diphenoxylate with **atropine** is a constipating meperidine congener that lacks analgesic activity. High doses (4–60 mg), however, can cause opioid activity, including euphoria, and physical dependence with chronic use. The addition of **atropine** provides anticholinergic effects that decrease secretion in the bowel and slow peristalsis.

Loperamide inhibits peristalsis by a direct effect on the circular and longitudinal muscles of the intestinal wall. It also reduces fecal volume, increases viscosity and bulk, and diminishes the loss of fluid and electrolytes. Although it has opioid-like properties, no opioid-like effects have been observed in humans after more than 2 years of therapeutic doses.

Pharmacokinetics

Absorption and Distribution

Kaolin and **pectin** act locally in the bowel and are not systemically absorbed (Table 18–5). **Bismuth subsalicylate** undergoes chemical dissociation in the GI tract; the salicylate moiety is absorbed, with plasma levels similar to those of **aspirin**. There is only negligible absorption of the bismuth moiety. **Diphenoxylate** with **atropine** is well absorbed from the GI tract. Its distribution is unknown, but it does enter breast milk. Forty percent of **loperamide** is absorbed after oral administration, and it does not cross the blood-brain barrier well, so there are limited central nervous system (CNS) effects.

Metabolism and Excretion

The salicylate portion of **bismuth subsalicylate** is metabolized in the liver and more than 90 percent is excreted in urine. **Diphenoxylate** with **atropine** is rapidly and extensively metabolized to diphenoxylic acid, which is biologically active and its main metabolite. It is excreted in urine and feces. **Loperamide** is partially metabolized by the liver and undergoes enterohepatic recirculation to be

Table 18–5. Pharmacokinetics: Selected Antidiarrheals

Drug	Onset	Peak	Duration	Half-Life	Elimination
Bismuth subsalicylate	—	—	—	2–3 h for low doses; 15–30 h for larger doses	>90% of salicylate in urine
Diphenoxylate with atropine	45–60 m	2 h	3–4 h	2.5 h (12–14 h for the metabolite)	14% of drug and metabolites in urine; 49% in feces
Loperamide	1 h	2.5–5 h	10 h	10.8 h (range 9.1–14.4 h)	25% unchanged in feces; 1.3% in urine as free drug and glucuronic acid conjugate

completely metabolized. Most is eliminated in feces, with a minimal amount excreted in urine.

Pharmacotherapeutics

Precautions and Contraindications

Drugs that reduce intestinal motility or delay intestinal transit time have induced toxic megacolon, especially in patients with inflammatory bowel disease. **Diphenoxylate** with **atropine** and **loperamide** should be used cautiously for these patients and promptly discontinued if abdominal distention occurs. Because of their hepatic metabolism and renal excretion, these two drugs should also be used with extreme caution in patients with advanced hepatorenal disease and in all patients with abnormal liver function studies because hepatic coma may be precipitated.

The **atropine** component of **diphenoxylate** with **atropine** contraindicates its use in narrow-angle glaucoma and requires cautious use in prostatic hyperplasia. Children, especially those with Down syndrome, have increased sensitivity to **atropine**. This drug should be avoided or used with extreme caution in children. It is not recommended for use in children under age 12 years. This drug may prolong or aggravate diarrhea associated with organisms that penetrate the intestinal mucosa, such as *Escherichia coli*, *Salmonella*, and *Shigella* or in pseudomembranous colitis associated with broad-spectrum antimicrobial therapy. It should not be used in these conditions.

The **salicylate** component of **bismuth subsalicylate** contraindicates its use in children or teenagers during or after recovery from chickenpox or flulike illness. It is also contraindicated for patients with **aspirin** hypersensitivity.

All **antidiarrheals** require cautious use in older adults and others in whom impaction is a high risk. Older adults are especially sensitive to **diphenoxylate** with **atropine**.

Pregnancy categories vary among these drugs. All are Pregnancy Category C except *loperamide*, which is Pregnancy Category B. However, there are no adequate and well-controlled studies in pregnant women for any of these drugs, and safety during pregnancy has not been established.

Some of the drugs are excreted in breast milk, and the safety of any of the **antidiarrheals** has not been established in lactating women. They should be avoided or used with extreme caution.

None of the **antidiarrheals** has established safety for children under age 2 years. All have published children's doses. It is important to keep in mind that dehydration may influence younger children's response to these drugs.

Adverse Drug Reactions

The main adverse drug reaction for all **antidiarrheals** is rebound constipation. For **bismuth subsalicylate**, an additional reaction that all patients should be warned about is gray-black stools that are a result of the **bismuth**. Patients should be told to expect this reaction and that it does not indicate GI bleeding.

The adverse reactions associated with the other two drugs are related to their anticholinergic and opioid-like effects. **Diphenoxylate** with **atropine** exhibits anticholinergic adverse reactions such as dry mouth and mucous membranes, flushing, tachycardia, and urinary retention, especially in children. **Loperamide** also exhibits these reactions but to a lesser degree. Both drugs have CNS reactions of dizziness and drowsiness, **loperamide** less so than **diphenoxylate** with **atropine**. Because it crosses the blood-brain barrier better, **diphenoxylate** with **atropine** also exhibits sedation, headache, and, in higher doses or with chronic use, euphoria or depression.

Drug Interactions

Bismuth subsalicylate may potentiate the risk for toxicity if taken with **aspirin** and the risk for hypoglycemia if given in large doses with **insulin** or **oral hypoglycemics**. **Diphenoxylate** with **atropine** and **loperamide** both have additive or potentiating CNS effects with other CNS depressants and additive anticholinergic effects with other drugs that share these effects. There are few other drug interactions (Table 18–6).

Clinical Use and Dosing

SIMPLE, ACUTE DIARRHEA. After the cause of the diarrhea has been determined and, if possible, eliminated, absorbent preparations are commonly used for relief of symptoms. **Kaolin-pectin** or **bismuth subsalicylate** taken after each loose stool may be effective. The majority of acute diarrheal illnesses are self-limiting, and the main concern is to maintain hydration.

Hydration can usually be maintained in adults, even with profuse diarrhea, by the use of oral fluids. Goroll (1995) recommends adding a pinch of table salt and a half-teaspoon of honey to an 8-oz glass of fruit juice as a hydrating solution. Nondiet colas that have been allowed to lose their carbonation may also be used. Alternate these solutions with 8-oz glasses of water to which has been added one-quarter teaspoon of baking soda to replenish the electrolytes commonly lost in acute, infectious diarrhea (sodium, potassium, bicarbonate, and chloride).

Children with severe diarrhea need oral rehydrating solutions (ORS) to prevent dehydration (Schmidt, 1999). Examples include **Infalyte, Kao-Lectrolyte,** or **Pedialyte.** These OTC products are available in pharmacies or supermarkets. If the child does not like the flavor, a bit of Kool-Aid powder may be added. Jell-O, water, or sports drinks should be avoided because they do not contain enough sodium. For infants, a homemade recipe includes one-half cup infant rice cereal mixed with 16 oz of water and one-quarter teaspoon of salt.

Table 18–6. Drug Interactions: Selected Antidiarrheals

Drug	Interacting Drug	Possible Effect	Implications
Bismuth subsalicylate	Aspirin	May potentiate salicylate toxicity	Avoid concurrent use
	Tetracycline	May decrease GI absorption	Separate administration by 2 h
	Thrombolytics, warfarin, heparin	Large doses may increase risk for bleeding	Avoid concurrent use or use small doses; monitor clotting studies closely
	Insulin, oral hypoglycemics	Large doses increase risk of hypoglycemia	Avoid concurrent use or use small doses
Diphenoxylate with atropine	CNS depressants, including alcohol, antihistamines, opioids, sedative hypnotics	Additive/potentiating CNS depression	Monitor patient closely if these drugs must be given concurrently
	Monoamine oxidase inhibitors (MAOIs)	Because chemical structure is similar, concurrent use may precipitate hypertensive crisis	Avoid concurrent use or within 14 d of use of MAOI
	Drugs that have anticholinergic properties	Additive anticholinergic effect	Monitor for toxicity; treat symptoms with good oral hygiene, hard candy, sugarless gum
Kaolin-pectin	Digoxin, chloroquine	Decreases GI absorption	Avoid concurrent use or separate doses by at least 2 h, giving kaolin-pectin last
Loperamide	CNS depressants, including alcohol, antihistamines, opioids, sedative hypnotics	Additive/potentiating CNS depression	Monitor patient closely if these drugs must be given concurrently
	Drugs that have anticholinergic properties	Additive anticholinergic effect	Monitor for toxicity; treat symptoms with good oral hygiene, hard candy, sugarless gum

Children should be given ORS to satisfy their thirst for at least 6 hours and often for 24 hours.

If the **absorbents** do not resolve the diarrhea, **diphenoxylate** with **atropine** or **loperamide** may be added. **Diphenoxylate** with **atropine** is given three to four times daily rather than after each loose stool.

Unlike acute diarrhea, chronic diarrhea requires etiologic diagnosis and specific therapy for that diagnosis. Simply suppressing symptoms is not sufficient.

CHRONIC DIARRHEA ASSOCIATED WITH INFLAMMATORY BOWEL DISEASE. **Steroids** and **sulfasalazine** are needed to control diarrhea in exacerbation of inflammatory bowel disease. **Loperamide** 4 mg initially, followed by doses of 2 to 4 mg qid, may be used as adjunct therapy, and it may lead to substantial clinical improvement, especially if combined with added fiber in the diet and **anticholinergics.** If clinical improvement is not observed with doses of 16 mg/day for at least 10 days, symptoms are unlikely to be controlled by further use of this drug.

Carlson (1998) states that no specific pharmacological treatment has firm research evidence to show that it is effective. Despite the absence of research support, she recommends **loperamide**, as discussed previously, or **diphenoxylate** with **atropine.**

CHRONIC DIARRHEA ASSOCIATED WITH PANCREATIC INSUFFICIENCY. Malabsorption due to pancreatic insufficiency requires use of enzyme supplements. **Antidiarrheal** medications are not generally used for this indication.

TRAVELER'S DIARRHEA. The management of traveler's diarrhea can be divided into prevention and treatment. The most important risk factor for acquiring this disorder is the destination. High-risk areas include Latin America, Africa, certain parts of the Middle East, the Dominican Republic, Haiti, and Asia. Intermittent-risk areas include southern Europe, Israel, South Africa, and a number of the Caribbean islands. "Numerous studies performed around the world have shown that entero-

Clinical Pearl

Evaluation of the effectiveness of oral rehydration is based on at least three wet diapers/24 hours in infants. For children over 1 year of age, avoid all fruit juices and other drinks that contain fructose because they usually make the diarrhea worse. If the infant or child is drinking milk or lactose-based formula, try withholding milk or lactose products. Resolution of the diarrhea strongly suggests lactose intolerance. Lactose intolerance is more commonly found in ethnic people of color.

---

toxigenic *E. coli* (ETEC) is the most common causative organism" (Caeiro & DuPont, 1998). Other organisms have been implicated. Oral **antimicrobials** are used for both prevention and treatment of this disorder. Symptomatic management in adults includes **bismuth subsalicylate** 2 tablets or 30 mL of liquid every 30 minutes for no more than eight doses per day for no longer than 48 hours. **Loperamide** 4 mg initially, followed by 2 mg after each loose stool with no more than 8 mg/day for no longer than 48 hours, may also be used. Doses are smaller for children.

Table 18–7 provides adult and children's doses for all of these indications.

Rational Drug Selection

INDICATION. For acute diarrhea, any of the **antidiarrheals** are appropriate. The more severe the diarrhea, the less likely **absorbent agents** are to help. **Bismuth subsalicylate** and **loperamide** are the only drugs indicated for traveler's diarrhea. **Loperamide** is the only drug with an indication for use with inflammatory bowel disease.

COST. Brand names are more expensive than generic formulations, and there is no significant clinical difference between the two. **Diphenoxylate** with **atropine** and **loperamide** are generally more expensive than the **absorbent agents** but are generally more effective.

Monitoring

There is no specific monitoring beyond that required for the disease process being treated. Patients with chronic diarrhea may benefit from monitoring of hydration status and electrolyte studies.

Patient Education

ADMINISTRATION. Despite the fact that many of these drugs are available OTC, they are not innocuous drugs. Patients need to be informed that they should take the **antidiarrheal** exactly as directed; do not make up missed doses or double doses, and do not exceed the maximum number of doses permitted. The health care provider should be notified if the diarrhea continues beyond 48 hours, or if abdominal pain, fever, or distention occurs.

Tablets may be administered with food if GI irritation occurs (Table 18–8). They may also be crushed and taken with fluid. Chewable tablets may be chewed or allowed to dissolve. Calibrated measuring devices should be used for liquid preparations. Suspensions should be shaken before they are measured and administered.

Drug interactions may occur, especially with **diphenoxylate** with **atropine** and **loperamide**. Patients should be told not to take any OTC **antidiarrheal** if they are taking other drugs, especially **digoxin**, **cephalosporin antimicrobials**, **warfarin** or **heparin**, or **CNS depressants** (including **alcohol**) without first contacting their health care provider.

ADVERSE REACTIONS. All **antidiarrheals** have the potential for rebound constipation. As soon as symptoms of diarrhea are reduced, the dosage of the **antidiarrheal** drug should be reduced; it should be stopped as soon as symptoms resolve.

Bismuth subsalicylate can turn the tongue and stools gray-black. Patients should be told that this reaction can be expected and that it does not indicate GI bleeding. **Diphenoxylate** with **atropine** can cause dry mouth and mucous membranes. These symptoms can be improved by good oral hygiene, sucking hard candy, or chewing sugarless gum. Flushing, tachycardia, and urinary retention may also occur. These symptoms are especially notable in children and in older men. They may necessitate stopping the drug. **Loperamide** also exhibits these reactions but to a lesser degree.

Both of these latter drugs can produce CNS reactions of dizziness and drowsiness, **loperamide** less so than **diphenoxylate** with **atropine**. Driving or other activities requiring mental alertness should be avoided until the patient's response to the drug is known.

LIFESTYLE MANAGEMENT. Adding fiber to the diet and using oral rehydrating solutions were discussed previously. The importance of washing one's hands after each bowel movement should be stressed. Education about maintaining nutritional intake is also important. Sometimes patients think that they can stop their diarrhea by

Table 18–7. Dosage Schedule: Selected Antidiarrheals

Drug	Indication	Initial Dose	Additional Doses
Bismuth subsalicylate*	Acute diarrhea	*Adults:* 524 mg every 30 min or 1048–1200 mg every 60 min as needed	Not to exceed 4.2 g/24 h
		Children 9–12 y: 262–300 mg every 30–60 min as needed	Not to exceed 2.4 g/24 h
		Children 6–9 y: 176 mg every 30–60 min as needed	Not to exceed 1.4 g/24 h
		Children 3–6 y: 88 mg every 30–60 min as needed	Not to exceed 704 mg/24 h
		Children <3 y weighing >13 kg: 88 mg	May repeat q4h; not to exceed 6 doses/24 h
		Children <3 y weighing 6.4–8 kg: 44 mg	May repeat q4h; not to exceed 6 doses/24 h
	Traveler's diarrhea	524 mg (2 tablets or 30 mL of 262 mg/15 mL liquid) every 30 min for up to 8 doses	Not to be used for more than 48 h
Diphenoxylate with atropine	Acute diarrhea	*Adults:* 5 mg tid to qid initially	5 mg qd as needed; not to exceed 20 mg/d
		Children 2–12 y: all doses qid and in liquid form 2 y/11–14 kg: 1.5–3 mL 3 y/12–16 kg: 2–3 mL 4 y/14–20 kg: 2–4 mL 5 y/16–23 kg: 2.5–4.5 mL 6–8 y/17–32 kg: 2.5–5.5 mL 9–12 y/23–55 kg: 3.5–5 mL	Reduce dosage as soon as control of symptoms is achieved; maintenance dosage may be as low as one-fourth of initial daily dose; maximum daily dose 20 mg
Kaolin-pectin	Acute diarrhea	*Adults:* 60–120 mL after each loose stool	—
		Children >12 y: 40–60 mL after each loose stool	
		Children 6–12 y: 30–60 mL after each loose stool	
		Children 3–6 y: 15–30 mL after each loose stool	
Loperamide	Acute diarrhea, traveler's diarrhea	*Adults:* 4 mg initially	2 mg after each loose stool; not to exceed 8 mg/d for OTC use or 16 mg/d for prescription use
		Children 9–11 y or 30–47 kg: 2 mg initially	1 mg after each loose stool; not to exceed 6 mg/24 h; OTC use not to exceed 48 h
		Children 6–8 y or 24–30 kg: 1 mg initially	1 mg after each loose stool; not to exceed 4 mg/24 h; OTC use not to exceed 48 h
	Chronic diarrhea associated with inflammatory bowel disease	*Adults only:* 4 mg initially	2 mg after each loose stool until symptoms resolved; maintenance dose is usually 4–8 mg/d in divided doses; not to exceed 16 mg/d

*The dosage schedule for eradication of *H. pylori* is discussed in Chapter 32.

stopping their food intake. Resting the GI tract briefly (e.g., for 24 hours) may be appropriate, but reducing fluid intake is never appropriate, and food intake should be restarted after the GI rest.

The bananas, rice, applesauce, and toast (BRAT) diet can assist in maintaining nutrition and is also helpful in reducing the diarrhea. Stopping milk or other lactose-based food products for a few days may give an indication whether the diarrhea is associated with lactose intolerance.

Table 18–8. Available Dosage Forms: Selected Antidiarrheals

Drug	Dosage Form	How Supplied
Bismuth subsalicylate (Pepto-Bismol)	Tablets/chewable: 262 mg	In bottles of 30, 42 (cherry flavor); 24, 42 (original flavor); <2 mg sodium
	Liquid: 262 mg/15 mL	In bottles of 120, 240, 360, 480 mL; 5 mg sodium/15 mL
	Liquid: 524 mg/15 mL	In bottles of 120, 240, 360 mL; <5 mg sodium/15 mL
Diphenoxylate with atropine (Lomotil)	Tablets: 2.5 mg diphenoxylate, 0.025 mg atropine sulfate	In bottles of 100, 500, 1000, 2500
	Liquid: 2.5 mg diphenoxylate, 0.025 mg atropine sulfate/5 mL	In bottles of 60 mL (cherry flavor) 15% alcohol; with dropper
(Generic)	Tablets: 2.5 mg diphenoxylate, 0.025 mg atropine sulfate	In bottles of 100, 500, 1000, 2500
	Liquid: 2.5 mg diphenoxylate, 0.025 mg atropine sulfate/5 mL	In bottles of 10, 60 mL
Kaolin-pectin (Kaopectate, Kao-Spen)	Suspension: 5.2 g kaolin plus 260 mg pectin/30 mL; 5.85 mg kaolin plus 130 mg pectin/30 mL Also comes in combinations with paregoric, bismuth, carboxy-methylcellulose, and others	
Loperamide (Imodium A-D)	Tablets: 2 mg Liquid: 1 mg/5 mL	In packets of 6, 12 In bottles of 60, 90, 120 mL (cherry/licorice flavor)
(Imodium)	Capsule: 2 mg	In bottles of 100, 500
(Generic)	Capsule: 2 mg Liquid: 1 mg/5 mL	In bottles of 100, 500, 1000 In bottles of 60, 118 mL

Cytoprotective Agents

Peptic ulceration can be caused by a variety of conditions, some of which are iatrogenic. The administration of **non-steroidal anti-inflammatory drugs (NSAIDs)**, for example, has been associated with gastric mucosal damage and ulcer formation. Ulcer formation and GI bleeding related to **NSAID** use often occur without warning. Patients at high risk are those with previous history of ulcers, also on steroids, on high doses, concurrently taking anticoagulants, or older than age 75. Among the agents used to treat or prevent ulcer formation are two **cytoprotective agents, sucralfate (Carafate)** and **misoprostol (Cytotec)**. These drugs are focus of this section.

Pharmacodynamics

Sucralfate is a basic aluminum salt of a sulfated disaccharide, which is believed to act by polymerization and selective binding to necrotic ulcer tissue, where it covers the ulcer site and acts as a barrier to acid, pepsin,

and bile salts. It has no acid-neutralizing activity, and little is absorbed, although some aluminum salts are released. In controlled trials, the drug was comparable to some **histamine$_2$ blockers** for healing of duodenal ulcers (Goroll, 1995). In addition, the drug may directly absorb bile salts and stimulate endogenous prostaglandin synthesis. Prostaglandins are central to the formation and maintenance of the protective mucosa of the GI tract.

Misoprostol is a methyl analogue of prostaglandin E$_1$. The principal mechanism of action of this drug appears to be inhibition of gastric secretion through inhibition of histamine-stimulated cyclic AMP production. Over a dosage range of 50 to 200 µg, it inhibits basal and nocturnal gastric acid secretion and acid secretion in response to a variety of stimuli, including meals, histamine, and coffee. It has no significant effect on fasting or postprandial gastrin or on intrinsic factor output.

Misoprostol also has mucosal protective qualities. Prostaglandin receptors have a high affinity for **misoprostol** and for its acid metabolite. These receptors facilitate the production of mucus and bicarbonate. They also allow the drug taken with food to be effective topically, despite the lower serum concentration.

Pharmacokinetics

Absorption and Distribution

Sucralfate is minimally absorbed (Table 18–9). Its action is largely topical. **Misoprostol** is rapidly and extensively absorbed after oral administration. Distribution of this drug is unknown.

Metabolism and Excretion

Because it is essentially not absorbed, more than 90 percent of **sucralfate** is excreted in feces. **Misoprostol** is rapidly converted to its free acid, which is responsible for its clinical activity. It does not affect the cytochrome P-450 enzyme systems. The metabolite is excreted in urine.

Pharmacotherapeutics

Precautions and Contraindications

Because its action is topical, there are no specific precautions or contraindications for **sucralfate**. It is **Pregnancy Category B.** Its safety and efficacy have not been established in children.

Misoprostol must be used with caution in renal impairment. Its half-life, maximum concentration, and area under the curve (AUC) double with renal insufficiency. No routine dosage adjustments have been recommended, but dosage may need to be reduced if the usual dose is not tolerated. In older adults (over age 65), the AUC for the acid metabolite of **misoprostol** is increased. The cause may be decreased renal functioning associated with aging, and recommendations are the same as for renal impairment.

Misoprostol is Pregnancy Category X. It has been associated with altered fertility in animal studies and may cause abortion, based on its action on the uterus. In studies of women undergoing elective termination of pregnancy during the first trimester, *misoprostol* caused partial or complete expulsion of the uterine contents in 11 percent and increased uterine bleeding in 46 percent (Kastrup, 1998).

It is unlikely that **misoprostol** is excreted in breast milk because of its rapid metabolism, but it is not known if its active metabolite is excreted in breast milk. As a precaution, it should not be administered to lactating women because it has the potential to cause significant diarrhea in the nursing infant.

Safety and efficacy in children under age 18 have not been established.

Adverse Drug Reactions

Adverse reactions in clinical trials with **sucralfate** were minor and rarely led to discontinuance of the drug. Constipation, the most frequent complaint, occurred in only 2 percent of patients. Other adverse reactions, including dizziness and gastric discomfort, occurred in less than 0.5 percent of patients.

Adverse reactions with **misoprostol** were largely GI or gynecological. Diarrhea is the most common complaint (13 to 40% of patients). Abdominal pain, nausea, and flatulence occur in small numbers of patients and are difficult to separate from the symptoms of the disorder for which the drug was prescribed. Spotting, cramps, and postmenopausal bleeding occur in less than 1 percent of nonpregnant patients. Reactions related to pregnancy were discussed previously.

Drug Interactions

Sucralfate may decrease the absorption of several drugs when given concurrently or prior to their administration (Table 18–10). Separating the administration of the interacting drug by at least 2 hours and giving the interacting drug first can often solve the problem.

The only drug of concern with **misoprostol** is the potential for increased diarrhea risk with **magnesium-based antacids.** Food can decrease maximum plasma concentrations, but this has little clinical significance.

Clinical Use and Dosing

PROPHYLAXIS AND TREATMENT OF DUODENAL ULCERS ASSOCIATED WITH NSAID USE. NSAIDs inhibit prostaglandin synthesis and damage the mucosal lining of the stomach, which may result in ulcer formation. The first choice is to discontinue the **NSAID. Misoprostol** is

Table 18–9. Pharmacokinetics: Cytoprotective Agents

Drug	Onset	Peak	Duration	Protein Binding	Half-Life	Elimination
Misoprostol	Minutes	12–15 min	3–6 h	<90%	20–40 min (doubles in renal impairment)	80% in urine
Sucralfate	30 min	Unknown	5 h	Unknown	6–20 h	90% in feces

Table 18–10. Drug Interactions: Cytoprotective Agents

Drug	Interacting Drug	Possible Effect	Implications
Misoprostol	Magnesium-based antacids	Increased risk for diarrhea	Choose different antacid
	Food	Maximum plasma concentrations of acid metabolite are diminished when taken with food	Little clinical significance, but best taken on empty stomach
Sucralfate	Aluminum-based antacids	Increased constipation risk; increase in total body burden of aluminum	Choose different antacid
	Anticoagulants	Decrease in effect of warfarin	Avoid concurrent use
	Digoxin	Reduced serum levels of digoxin; reduced effects	Avoid concurrent use
	Hydantoins	Absorption may be decreased	Separate administration by 2 h and give hydantoin first
	Ketoconazole, quinolones	Bioavailability decreased	Separate administration by 2 h and give drugs first
	Quinidine	Reduced serum levels of quinidine; reduced effects	Separate administration by 2 h and give quinidine first

approved by the Food and Drug Administration (FDA) for prophylaxis or treatment of duodenal ulcers that are due to use of **NSAIDs** for those patients who must continue **NSAID** use. Dosage is 200 µg qid with food (Table 18–11). The last dose of the day is usually taken at bedtime. If this dose cannot be tolerated, 100 µg can be used. The drug is taken for the duration of **NSAID** therapy.

Because **misoprostol** commonly causes a dose-dependent diarrhea and other GI symptoms, and because its stimulant effect on the uterus contraindicates its use for women with childbearing potential, its use as prophylaxis is reserved for those with high risk for and little tolerance of the GI hazards of **NSAIDs**.

TREATMENT OF DUODENAL ULCERS FROM OTHER CAUSES. **Sucralfate** can be used for short-term (up to 8 weeks) treatment of active duodenal ulcer. Dosage is 1 g qid on an empty stomach, 1 hour before meals and at bedtime. Healing usually occurs within 2 weeks. Maintenance therapy after the ulcer has healed is 1 g bid. **Sucralfate** has unlabeled uses in treating gastric and esophageal ulcers, with the same dosing schedule. It appears to have some advantage over **antacids** and **histamine₂ blockers** in stress ulcer prophylaxis.

Although more effective than placebo, **misoprostol** is less effective than **histamine₂ blockers** for treatment of duodenal ulcers from other causes. In doses greater than 400 µg/day, it has an unlabeled use for treatment of duodenal ulcers not responsive to **histamine₂ blockers**.

Rational Drug Selection

Drug selection is based on indications cited previously (Table 18–12). **Sucralfate** is preferred over **misoprostol** for treatment of active duodenal ulcers not caused by **NSAIDs**. **Sucralfate** is also the drug of choice for women of childbearing age.

Monitoring

No specific monitoring parameters exist for these drugs. Monitoring should relate to the disease process being treated.

Patient Education

ADMINISTRATION. Patients should be taught to take the drug exactly as prescribed. **Sucralfate** is taken on an

Table 18–11. Dosage Schedule: Cytoprotective Agents

Drug	Indication	Dosage Schedule
Misoprostol	Prophylaxis and treatment of duodenal ulcers due to NSAID use	200 µg qid with food. Last dose usually at bedtime. Taken for duration of NSAID therapy. If this dose is not tolerated, 100 µg qid may be used.
Sucralfate	Active duodenal ulcer	1 g qid taken 1 h before meals and at bedtime.
	Maintenance after healing of duodenal ulcer	1 g bid taken on empty stomach.

Table 18–12. Available Dosage Forms: Cytoprotective Agents

Drug	Dosage Form	How Supplied
Misoprostol (Cytotec)	Tablets: 100 μg	In bottles of 60, 100 tablets
	Tablets: 200 μg	In bottles of 60, 100 scored tablets
Sucralfate (Carafate)	Tablets: 1 g	In bottles of 100, 120, 500 tablets
	Suspension: 1 g/10 mL	In bottles of 420 mL

empty stomach, **misoprostol** with food. Advise the patient to continue the therapy even if feeling better. **Sucralfate** is given for 4 to 8 weeks to ensure ulcer healing; **misoprostol** is given for the duration of **NSAID** therapy. Missed doses should be taken as soon as remembered unless it is almost time for the next dose. Doses should not be doubled.

ADVERSE REACTIONS. Increased fluid intake, dietary bulk, and exercise may reduce the incidence of constipation associated with **sucralfate**. Diarrhea may occur with **misoprostol**. If it continues for more than 1 week, the health care provider should be notified. The patient should also report onset of black, tarry stools or severe abdominal pain, which may indicate treatment failure and the onset of GI bleeding.

Women of childbearing age should be informed that **misoprostol** will cause spontaneous abortion. The drug should not be prescribed until contraceptive therapy is established. If pregnancy is suspected, the drug should be immediately stopped and the health care provider notified so that pregnancy testing can be performed.

LIFESTYLE MANAGEMENT. Lifestyle management related to peptic ulcers is discussed in Chapter 32.

Antiemetics

Nausea and vomiting are common complaints in primary care and have a multitude of causes. Treatment is often nonpharmacological, but **antiemetics** may also be used to provide symptom relief and prevent fluid and electrolyte disturbances. This section discusses drugs used for these purposes.

Drug classes with antiemetic properties commonly used include **antihistamines, phenothiazines,** and **sedative hypnotics.** The drugs from these classes most commonly used for these antiemetic properties are **dimenhydrinate (Dramamine), diphenhydramine (Benadryl), hydroxyzine (Vistaril), prochlorperazine**

(Compazine), and **promethazine (Phenergan).** These drugs have other uses in treating disorders of the respiratory and central nervous systems. Their uses for purposes other than to prevent or treat nausea and vomiting are discussed in Chapters 13 and 15. A miscellaneous antiemetic not from the previous classes of drugs is **trimethobenzamide (Tigan).** Each of these drugs is discussed in this section.

Pharmacodynamics

Antihistamines that possess significant antiemetic activity have strong anticholinergic effects as well as histamine$_1$ blocking effects. Blockade of histamine$_1$ receptors results in decreased exocrine gland secretion (e.g., salivary and lacrimal). First-generation **antihistamines** with strong anticholinergic properties bind to central cholinergic receptors and produce antiemetic effects, decreasing nausea and vomiting. They are especially helpful in the nausea associated with motion sickness because of their depression of conduction in the vestibulocerebellar pathway. The **antiemetic drugs** in this class are **dimenhydrinate, diphenhydramine,** and **hydroxyzine.**

Phenothiazines block dopamine receptors in the chemoreceptor trigger zone (CTZ). They also bind to and block cholinergic, alpha$_1$ adrenergic, and histamine$_1$ receptors. Although all **phenothiazines** have these actions to some degree, their use as **antiemetics** is limited by their sedating and extrapyramidal effects. The **antiemetic drugs** in this class are **prochlorperazine** and **promethazine.** They are less sedating and have antiemetic effects at lower doses than some other **phenothiazines. Metoclopramide** also blocks dopamine receptors and has been used as an **antiemetic.** Its main use, however, is as a **prokinetic,** and it is discussed in that section of this chapter.

Trimethobenzamide is a miscellaneous **antiemetic** agent that inhibits emetic stimulation of the CTZ. It is used in children in its suppository form.

Pharmacokinetics

Absorption and Distribution

All of these drugs are well absorbed after oral administration (Table 18–13). Oral liquid formulations provide the most reliable absorption. All of these drugs are also well absorbed after intramuscular (IM) injection. All of these drugs except **diphenhydramine** and **hydroxyzine** have formulations for administration by the rectal route. The IM and rectal routes are commonly used when vomiting is present.

Distribution of **antihistamines** is not clearly known, but **phenothiazines** are widely distributed, cross the

Table 18–13. Pharmacokinetics: Selected Antiemetics

Drug	Onset	Peak	Duration	Protein Binding	Half-Life	Elimination
Dimenhydrinate						In feces via biliary excretion
PO	15–60 min	1–2 h	3–6 h	Unknown	Unknown	
PO ER	Unknown	Unknown	12 h	Unknown	Unknown	
IM	20–30 min	1–2 h	3–6 h	Unknown	Unknown	
PR	30–45 min	Unknown	6–12 h	Unknown	Unknown	
Diphenhydramine						In feces via biliary excretion
PO	15–60 min	1–4 h	4–8 h	98–99%	2.4–7 h	
IM	20–30 min	1–4 h	4–8 h	98–99%	2.4–7 h	
Hydroxyzine						In feces via biliary excretion
PO, IM	15–30 min	2–4 h	4–6 h	Unknown	3 h	
Prochlorperazine						Half in urine; half by enterohepatic circulation
PO	30–40 min	Unknown	10–12 h	>90%	Unknown	
PR	60 min	Unknown	3–4 h	>90%	Unknown	
IM	10–20 min	10–30 min	3–4 h	>90%	Unknown	
Promethazine						Half in urine; half by enterohepatic circulation
PO	10 min	Unknown	4–12 h	65–90%	Unknown	
PR	20 min	Unknown	12 h	65–90%	Unknown	
IM	20 min	Unknown	12 h	65–90%	Unknown	
Trimethobenzamide						In urine
PO	10–40 m	Unknown	3–4 h	Unknown	Unknown	
PR	10–40 m	Unknown	3–4 h	Unknown	Unknown	
IM	15–35 m	Unknown	2–3 h	Unknown	Unknown	

ER = extended release; PR = per rectum.

blood-brain barrier and placenta, and enter breast milk. As a result, they are associated with more adverse reactions.

Metabolism and Excretion

Dimenhydrinate, diphenhydramine, and **hydroxyzine** are extensively metabolized by the liver and eliminated in feces by biliary excretion. **Trimethobenzamide** is also metabolized by the liver but is excreted in urine. The **phenothiazines** are metabolized by the liver into active compounds that persist for prolonged periods. They are eliminated half by the kidney in urine and half through enterohepatic circulation. The fetus, infants, and older adults have diminished capacity to metabolize and excrete **phenothiazines.** Children metabolize them more rapidly than adults.

Pharmacotherapeutics

Precautions and Contraindications

The drug class determines the precautions and contraindications. **Antihistamines** have anticholinergic properties and have precautions and contraindications similar to **anticholinergics.** Cautious use in narrow-angle glaucoma, seizure disorders, pyloric obstruction, hy-

perthyroidism, cardiovascular disease, and prostatic hypertrophy is in order. Because they are metabolized so extensively by the liver, they are contraindicated in severe liver disease. Cautious use is also suggested for older adults, and dosage reductions may be required.

Dimenhydrinate and *diphenhydramine* **are Pregnancy Category B,** and they are safe for use in children. **Hydroxyzine is Pregnancy Category C, but has been used safely during labor.** Safety in lactation and in children has not been established, but it has been used for both, and children's doses are published.

Phenothiazines produce extrapyramidal reactions and are contraindicated in Parkinson's disease. They are also contraindicated in narrow-angle glaucoma, bone marrow depression, and severe cardiovascular or hepatic disease because of their serious adverse reactions. Cautious use is suggested in respiratory impairment caused by acute pulmonary infection or chronic respiratory disorders, such as severe asthma or emphysema. "Silent pneumonia" may develop in these patients when they are treated with **phenothiazines.** Because these drugs suppress the cough reflex, aspiration of vomitus is possible, and they should be used cautiously where aspiration is a risk. Although all of these points are important to consider, they are less likely to be a problem in very short-term use as an **antiemetic.**

The *phenothiazines* are Pregnancy Category C. They have dosing schedules for children.

Adverse Drug Reactions

The most common adverse reactions for **antihistamines** are drowsiness and the common anticholinergic effects of dry mouth, blurred vision, and urinary retention. Paradoxical excitation may occur in children. Pain at the injection site occurs in IM injections.

Phenothiazines produce drowsiness as well, but they also produce serious adverse reactions that sometimes occur even with short-term use and low doses. These reactions include extrapyramidal reactions such as dystonia, akathisia, and tardive dyskinesia. Chapter 13 further discusses these reactions. Other serious concerns are their ability to mask acute symptoms of surgical and neurological conditions and the potential for agranulocytosis 4 to 10 weeks after initiation of therapy.

Other adverse reactions are associated with the anticholinergic effects of these drugs and include dry mouth, dry eyes, blurred vision, constipation, and urinary retention. They also discolor urine pink to reddish brown, and patients should be told that this reaction does not indicate hematuria.

The adverse reactions of all of these drugs, with the exception of drowsiness, are less pronounced when the drug is used for a single dose or for no more than 1 day for the treatment of nausea and vomiting.

Drug Interactions

Antihistamines and **phenothiazines** have additive CNS depression with other drugs that produce CNS depression and additive anticholinergic effects with other drugs that have anticholinergic effects or adverse reactions.

Phenothiazines also have additive hypotensive effects with **antihypertensive agents** or acute ingestion of **alcohol.** Concurrent administration of **lithium** increases the risk for extrapyramidal reactions, and **phenothiazines** may mask the signs of **lithium** toxicity. **Antithyroid** agents increase the risk for agranulocytosis.

These and additional drug interactions are listed in Table 18–14.

Clinical Use and Dosing

The only clinical use presented here is to treat nausea and vomiting. Table 18–15 shows the dosing schedules for each of the drugs for this purpose. Other uses for these drugs are discussed in Chapters 13 and 15.

Rational Drug Selection

SYMPTOMATIC TREATMENT OF NAUSEA AND VOMITING CAUSED BY DRUGS, METABOLIC DISORDERS, AND GAS-
TROENTERITIS. The **phenothiazines** are the best choice for initial and short-term treatment for this indication. **Trimethobenzamide** is also effective. The **antihistamines** can also be used and, because they have less serious adverse reactions, are better for longer-term applications. All are available in a variety of dosage forms so that they need not be taken orally by a patient who is nauseated. All also have dosage schedules for children, but **dimenhydrinate** and **diphenhydramine** are easily taken by children because they come in flavored syrups. They are also the drugs of choice for pregnant women.

MOTION SICKNESS. **Antihistamines** are useful for this indication because they act on the vestibular system and the CTZ to help control the nausea and vomiting associated with vestibular dysfunction. They also provide rapid onset of action and have a prolonged effect. The **phenothiazines** are not effective for motion sickness or vestibular disease because their site of action does not involve the vestibular system.

VOMITING DUE TO GASTROPARESIS. For this indication, **prokinetic drugs** are best. They are discussed later in this chapter.

Monitoring

When these drugs are used for a single dose or very short term, no specific monitoring is required beyond that associated with the disease process and the potential fluid and electrolyte shifts that may result from vomiting. If treatment is needed for longer than a few days, the following monitoring parameters are suggested. **Promethazine** has been associated with bone marrow depression. A complete blood count (CBC) prior to initiation of therapy is appropriate. **Phenothiazines** have also been associated with blood dyscrasias that tend to occur between week 4 and week 10 of therapy. A CBC may be done prior to initiation and after 4 weeks of therapy.

Patient Education

ADMINISTRATION. These drugs should be taken as prescribed (Table 18–16). Each of them has special considerations related to administration, which are presented in Table 18–15. For all of the drugs used to treat motion sickness, take 1 to 2 hours prior to departure, except for extended-release **dimenhydrinate,** which is taken 12 hours before departure. For all liquid formulations, use a calibrated measuring device to attain an accurate dose. For all injections, administer deep into well-developed muscle, and avoid the deltoid and subcutaneous (SC) injections. For **hydroxyzine** also use a Z-track method of injection. All tablets except extended-release ones can be crushed or mixed with food, water, or milk to minimize GI distress and for patients who have difficulty with

Table 18–14. Drug Interactions: Selected Antiemetics

Drug	Interacting Drug	Possible Effect	Implications
Dimenhydrinate, diphenhydramine, hydroxyzine	Alcohol, other antihistamines, opioids, sedative hypnotics, other CNS depressants	Additive CNS depression	Avoid concurrent use or warn patient of drowsiness and its consequences
	Aminoglycosides, ethacrynic acid, other ototoxic drugs	May mask indications of ototoxicity of these drugs	Avoid concurrent use
	Tricyclic antidepressants (TCAs), monoamine oxidase inhibitors, quinidine, and other drugs with anticholinergic properties	Additive anticholinergic effects	Avoid concurrent use or provide patient education about ways to reduce or treat anticholinergic effects
	Azole antifungals	Plasma levels (including metabolites) may be increased	Choose different antiemetic
	Macrolide antibiotics	Plasma levels (including metabolites) may be increased	Choose different antiemetic
	Serotonin reuptake inhibitors	Plasma levels (including metabolites) may be increased	Choose different antiemetic
Prochlorperazine, promethazine	Antihypertensives, nitrates, and acute ingestion of alcohol	Additive hypotensive effects	Avoid concurrent administration or monitor blood pressure closely
	Alcohol, antihistamines, antidepressants, opioids, sedative hypnotics, and other CNS depressants	Additive CNS depression May increase TCA serum levels	Avoid concurrent administration or warn about drowsiness and its risks; select different antiemetic or antidepressant other than TCA
	Antihistamines, antidepressants, atropine, haloperidol, other phenothiazines, and other drugs with anticholinergic properties	Additive anticholinergic effects	Avoid concurrent use or provide patient education about ways to reduce or treat anticholinergic effects
	Lithium	Lithium increases risk of extrapyramidal symptom (EPS) reactions; prochlorperazine may mask indications of lithium toxicity	Avoid concurrent use
	Antithyroid agents	Increased risk for agranulocytosis	Choose different antiemetic
	Antacids	Concurrent administration may decrease absorption	Separate administration or give antiemetic by IM or rectal route
Trimethobenzamide	Alcohol, antihistamines, antidepressants, opioids, sedative hypnotics, and other CNS depressants	Additive CNS depression	Avoid concurrent use or warn patient of drowsiness and its consequences

swallowing. Capsules can be opened and emptied to allow mixing for the same reasons.

ADVERSE REACTIONS. Single-dose or short-term use has relatively few adverse reactions. All are associated with drowsiness, dry mouth, dry eyes, constipation, and urinary retention. **Phenothiazines** turn the urine pink to reddish-brown. Patients need to be told that this effect does not constitute hematuria.

Longer-term administration of **phenothiazines** is not recommended because of potentially serious adverse reactions. Patients should be told the indications of dystonia, akathisia, and tardive dyskinesia and to stop the drug and report these immediately.

LIFESTYLE MANAGEMENT. Nausea and vomiting are often self-limiting disorders. Before drug therapy begins, unless there is clear indication of fluid or elec-

Table 18–15. Dosage Schedule: Selected Antiemetics

Drug	Indications	Dosage Schedule	Notes
Dimenhydrinate	Antiemetic	*Adults and children >12 y:* 50 mg PO/IM or 25 mg ER capsules q4h; not to exceed 400 mg/d PR = 50–100 mg q6–8h *Children 6–12 y:* 25–50 mg (PO/IM) q6–8h; not to exceed 300 mg/d *Children 8–12 y:* PR = 25–50 mg q8–12h *Children 6–8 y:* 12.5–25 PR q8–12h	For motion sickness, give dose 1–2 h prior to departure or ER dose 12 h prior to departure. Use calibrated measuring device when giving liquid doses.
Diphenhydramine	Antiemetic	*Adults:* 25–50 mg q6h PO; 10–50 mg q2–3h IM; not to exceed 400 mg/d *Children:* 1–1.5 mg/kg q4–6h PO; not to exceed 300 mg/d IM – 1.25 mg/kg qid; not to exceed 300 mg/d	For motion sickness, give dose 1–2 h prior to departure or ER dose 12 h prior to departure. Use calibrated measuring device when giving liquid doses. Capsules may be emptied and contents taken with food or water. Give IM into deep, well-developed muscle; avoid SC administration.
Hydroxyzine	Antiemetic	*Adults and children >12 y:* 25–100 mg PO/IM tid or qid *Children 6–12 y:* 12.5–25 mg q6h *Children <6 y:* 12.5 mg q6h (General calculation for children: 0.5 mg/kg q6h)	Tablets may be crushed and capsules opened and administered with food or fluid for patients with difficulty in swallowing. Give IM into deep, well-developed muscle using Z track. Do not use deltoid. Injection is painful. Rotate sites frequently. Avoid SC or IV administration.
Prochlorperazine	Antiemetic	*Adults and children >12 y:* 5–10 mg PO/IM tid or qid; may also give 30 mg once daily or 10 mg bid of ER PR = 25 mg bid; not to exceed 40 mg/d *Children 18–39 kg:* 2.5 mg PO/PR tid or 5 mg bid; not to exceed 15 mg/d *Children 14–17 kg:* 2.5 mg PO/PR bid or tid; not to exceed 10 mg/d *Children 9–13 kg:* 2.5 mg PO/PR qd or bid; not to exceed 7.5 mg/d *Children 2–12 kg:* 132 μg/kg IM in single dose	Do not crush or chew ER capsules. Administer with food or milk or a full glass of water to minimize GI distress. Dilute syrup in citrus or chocolate-flavored drinks. Give IM into deep, well-developed muscle. Keep patient recumbent for at least 30 min following injection to avoid hypotensive effects.
Promethazine	Antiemetic	*Adults:* 25 mg PO/IM/PR q4h *Children >2 y:* 0.25–0.5 mg/kg q4–6h PO/IM/PR	For motion sickness, give dose 1–2 h prior to departure. Administer with food, water, or milk to minimize GI distress. Tablets may be crushed and mixed with food or fluids for patients with difficulty in swallowing. Use calibrated measuring device when giving liquid doses. Give IM into deep, well-developed muscle; SC administration may cause tissue necrosis.

Continued on next page

Table 18–15. Dosage Schedule: Selected Antiemetics *(continued)*

Drug	Indications	Dosage Schedule	Notes
Trimethobenzamide	Antiemetic	*Adults:* 250 mg PO tid/qid; IM/PR = 200 mg tid/qid *Children 15–45 kg:* 100–200 mg PO/PR tid/qid or 15 mg/kg/d in 3–4 divided doses *Children <15 kg:* 100 mg PR tid/qid	Capsules can be opened and contents mixed with food or fluid for patients with difficulty in swallowing. Inject deep into well-developed muscle to minimize tissue irritation.

ER = extended release; PR = per rectum.

trolyte disturbances, nonpharmacological interventions can be tried. Resting the GI tract for a brief time (8 hours) by taking only clear liquids in small amounts is often helpful. Clear liquids are anything you can hold up to light and see through. For infants, ORS (discussed in the section on **antidiarrheals**) such as Pedialyte may be used instead of other clear liquids. Formula and milk should be withheld for these 8 hours. For breast-fed babies, continue breastfeeding, but nurse on only one side at each feeding during the first 8 hours. Older children and adults can take any clear liquid and require ORS only if they appear dehydrated. Remember, this treatment does not mean as much clear liquid as the patient can hold. Start with small amounts and gradually increase the intake.

After 8 hours without vomiting, start with food such as saltine crackers, honey on white bread, bland soup, rice, or mashed potatoes. For babies, start with applesauce, strained bananas, and rice cereal. If the baby takes only formula, give 1 or 2 oz less than usual with each feeding. Breast-fed babies can return to regular breastfeeding after 8 hours without vomiting. Most patients will be back on a regular diet within 24 hours.

Emetics

Poisoning is a serious problem in the United States, despite extensive prevention programs. According to the American Association of Poison Control Centers, nearly 2 million poisoning cases are documented each year, and many more go unreported. Vomiting may be a therapeutic intervention in the case of poisoning, except when the substance is a petroleum distillate or volatile oil. Although many drugs have nausea and vomiting as adverse reactions, the drug most commonly used to produce emesis is **ipecac syrup.** It is the only emetic discussed here, and this section does not include discussion of common substances that result in poisoning or the process of diagnostic reasoning that is central to management of patients who experience poisoning.

Pharmacodynamics

Ipecac syrup produces vomiting by a local irritant effect on GI mucosa and through a central medullary effect, stimulating the CTZ. Emetine and cephaeline, two alkaloids, cause the central effect. An adequate dose causes vomiting within 30 minutes in more than 90 percent of patients.

Pharmacokinetics

Absorption and Distribution

Absorption is minimal. Distribution, if any, is unknown.

Metabolism and Excretion

Excretion of the emetine is very slow and detectable in urine for up to 60 days.

Pharmacotherapeutics

Precautions and Contraindications

Ipecac syrup should not be administered to patients who are semicomatose, inebriated, or unconscious, who have no gag reflex, or who are experiencing seizure activity. It is also contraindicated if the poisoning was with caustic substances, petroleum distillates, or volatile oils. In each of these instances, the risk of aspiration is high.

Safety has not been established in pregnancy or lactation or for children less than 6 months of age.

Adverse Drug Reactions

Adverse reactions are few. The most common are sedation and diarrhea, but the more serious one is cardiotoxicity. **Ipecac syrup** can be cardiotoxic if it is not vomited and is allowed to absorb. Absorption of emetine may occur and cause heart conduction disturbances, atrial fibrillation, and even fatal myocarditis.

Table 18–16. Available Dosage Forms: Selected Antiemetics

Drug	Dosage Form	How Supplied
Dimenhydrinate (Dramamine)	Tablets: 50 mg Chewable tablets: 50 mg Injection: 50 mg/mL Liquid: 12.5 mg/4 mL Liquid: 15.62 mg/5 mL	In bottles of 12, 36, 100 scored tablets In bottles of 8, 24 scored tablets In 1-mL ampules and 5-mL vials In 90 mL (cherry flavor); 5% alcohol In 480 mL
(Generic)	Tablets: 50 mg Injection: 50 mg/mL Liquid: 12.5/4 mL	In bottles of 12, 100, 300, 500, 1000 tablets In 1-mL ampules and 1-, 10-mL vials In pint and gallon
Diphenhydramine (Benadryl)	Soft gels: 25 mg Tablets: 25 mg Chewable tablets: 12.5 mg Liquid: 6.25 mg Injection: 50 mg/mL	In 24 capsules In 24, 100 tablets In 24 tablets (grape-flavored); have phenylalanine In 236 mL (dye-free); 118 mL (cherry flavor) In 1-mL ampules, 10-mL vials, and 1-mL syringe
(Generic)	Soft gels: 25 mg Capsules: 50 mg Syrup: 12.5 mg/5 mL Injection: 50 mg/mL	In 30, 100, 1000 capsules In bottles of 100, 1000 capsules In 118 mL In 1-mL ampules and 10-mL vials
Hydroxyzine (Atarax)	Tablets: 10 mg, 25 mg, 50 mg Tablets: 100 mg Syrup: 10 mg/5 mL	In bottles of 100, 500 tablets In bottles of 100 tablets In pints
(Vistaril)	Capsules: 25 mg, 50 mg, 100 mg Oral suspension: 25 mg/5 mL Injection: 25 mg/mL Injection: 50 mg/mL	In bottles of 100, 500 capsules In 120 mL and 473 mL (lemon-flavored) In 10-mL vials In 1-, 2-, 10-mL vials
(Generic)	Tablets: 10 mg, 25 mg, 50 mg Capsules: 25 mg, 50 mg, 100 mg Syrup: 10 mg/5 mL Injection: 25 mg/mL Injection: 50 mg/mL	In bottles of 100, 250, 500, 1000 tablets In bottles of 100, 500, 1000 capsules In 12.5 mL, 25 mL, and pints In 1 mL and 10 mL vials In 2 mL ampules, 1- and 2-mL syringes, and 1-, 2-, 10-mL vials
Prochlorperazine (Compazine)	Tablets: 5 mg, 10 mg, 25 mg Spansules (SR): 10 mg, 15 mg, 30 mg Syrup: 5 mg/5 mL Injection: 5 mg/mL Suppositories: 2.5 mg, 5 mg, 25 mg	In bottles of 100, 1000 tablets In bottles of 50, 500 SR capsules In 120 mL; fruit flavor In 2-mL ampules, 10-mL vials, and 2-mL syringes In 12s; individually foil wrapped
(Generic)	Tablets: 5 mg, 10 mg, 25 mg Injection: 5 mg/mL	In bottles of 12, 30, 100, 1000 tablets In 2-mL ampules and 2-mL and 10-mL vials
Promethazine (Phenergan)	Tablets: 12.5 mg, 25 mg Tablets: 50 mg Syrup: 6.25 mg/5 mL 25 mg/5 ml Suppositories: 12.5 mg, 25 mg, 50 mg Injection: 25 mg/mL, 50 mg/mL	In bottles of 100 scored tablets In bottles of 100 tablets In 118 and 473 mL In 473 mL In 12s; individually foil wrapped In 1-mL ampules
(Generic)	Tablets: 12.5 mg Tablets: 25 mg, 50 mg Syrup: 6.25 mg/5 mL Suppositories: 50 mg Injection: 25 mg/mL, 50 mg/mL	In bottles of 100 tablets In bottles of 100, 1000 tablets In 118 mL In 12s; individually foil wrapped In 1-mL ampules and 10-mL vials

Continued on next page

Table 18–16. Available Dosage Forms: Selected Antiemetics *(continued)*

Drug	Dosage Form	How Supplied
Trimethobenzamide (Tigan)	Capsules: 100 mg Capsules: 250 mg Pediatric suppositories: 100 mg Suppositories: 200 mg Injection: 100 mg/mL	In bottles of 100 capsules In bottles of 100, 500 capsules In 10 individually foil wrapped In 10, 50 individually foil wrapped In 2-mL ampules, 20-mL vials, and 2-mL syringe
(Generic)	Capsules: 250 mg Pediatric suppositories: 100 mg Suppositories: 200 mg Injection: 100 mg/mL	In bottles of 100, 500 tablets In 10 individually foil wrapped In 10, 50 individually foil wrapped In 2-mL ampules and 20-mL vials

Drug Interactions

Activated charcoal adsorbs **ipecac syrup.** If both are to be used, give the activated charcoal only after the **ipecac syrup** has produced vomiting.

Concurrent administration with milk decreases effectiveness. Concurrent administration with carbonated beverages may produce abdominal distention and increase the risk for aspiration.

Clinical Use and Dosing

POISONING. Ipecac syrup contains 7 percent powdered **ipecac. Do not confuse it with ipecac fluid extract, which is 14 times stronger and has caused some deaths.**

Doses are based on age. For adults, 15 to 30 mL is given initially. If vomiting does not occur within 20 to 30 minutes, a second dose of 15 mL may be given. If vomiting still does not occur, the patient must have gastric lavage done. For children age 1 to 12 years, 15 mL is given initially. If vomiting does not occur with 20 minutes, a second dose may be given. As with adults, failure of the second dose to produce vomiting within 20 more minutes requires gastric lavage. For children less that 1 year of age, 5 to 10 mL may be given in one dose, followed by half a glass of water. No second dose should be given. The child should be taken to an emergency room for gastric lavage.

Ipecac syrup does not work well on an empty stomach. It is most effective when given with water or fruit juice.

Patient Education

ADMINISTRATION. Have the patient sit upright with the head slightly forward to reduce aspiration risk. Administer the drug based on the dosing protocol, and follow immediately with adequate amounts of water or fruit juice. For adults, "adequate" means an 8-oz glass and for children, 4 to 8 oz. Children who are young and frightened may be given water before **ipecac syrup.** Do not administer with milk or carbonated beverages.

Advise patients or their parents that ipecac syrup has a 1-year shelf life and therefore needs to be replaced yearly. Have them check the expiration date when they buy it as well. The suggested amount of drug to keep available in the house is one dose per child over age 1 year. The drug comes in a unit-dose format, which is to be preferred over a large bottle that has to be purchased and discarded each year.

ADVERSE REACTIONS. Inform the patient that **ipecac syrup** must be vomited to prevent cardiac symptoms.

LIFESTYLE MANAGEMENT. Regarding poison prevention, every major city has a poison control center. Patients should be given the phone number, and it should be kept near the telephone at all times. Before initiating therapy with **ipecac syrup,** the poison control center should be called and their advice followed.

Histamine₂ Blockers

Histamine₂ blockers (also known as histamine₂ antagonists) inhibit acid secretion by gastric parietal cells through a reversible blockade of histamine at histamine₂ receptors. They are used to reduce gastric acid in patients who are temporarily not taking anything by mouth and for prophylaxis and management of duodenal and gastric ulcers and GERD. They are also used to treat heartburn, acid indigestion, and "sour stomach."

Pharmacodynamics

Histamine₂ blockers are reversible competitive blockers of histamine at histamine₂ receptors, particularly in the gastric parietal cells. They are highly selective, do not affect histamine₁ receptors, and are not **anticholinergic agents.** They are potent inhibitors of all phases of gastric acid secretion, including that caused by muscarinic agonists and gastrin. Fasting and nocturnal secretions and those stimulated by food, insulin, caffeine, pentagastrin, and betazole are all inhibited.

The volume and hydrogen ion concentration of gastric juice, gastric emptying, and the lower esophageal sphincter pressure are all affected to varying degrees by different drugs in this class. **Cimetidine (Tagamet), ranitidine (Zantac),** and **famotidine (Pepcid)** have no effect on gastric emptying. **Cimetidine** and **famotidine** have no effect on lower esophageal sphincter pressure. **Ranitidine, nizatidine (Axid),** and **famotidine** have little or no effect on fasting or postprandial serum gastrin. **Ranitidine** does not affect pepsin secretion or pentagastrin-stimulated intrinsic factor secretion.

Ranitidine is 5 to 12 times more potent and **famotidine** is 30 to 60 times more potent than **cimetidine** in controlling gastric acid secretion, but there is no clear evidence that greater potency has any clinical advantage. Treatment failures have occurred with each of these drugs, and it is doubtful that treatment failure with one drug in the class can be corrected by changing drugs within the class.

Pharmacokinetics

Absorption and Distribution

All drugs in the class are well absorbed following oral administration (Table 18–17). The absorption of **cimetidine, famotidine,** and **ranitidine** may be decreased by **antacids** but is unaffected by food. The absorption of **nizatidine** is decreased by 10 percent only by **aluminum** and **magnesium hydroxides.** With food, AUC and maximum concentration of **nizatidine** increases by 10 percent. **Cimetidine** and **ranitidine** also have IM routes of absorption. All agents enter breast milk and cerebrospinal fluid.

Metabolism and Excretion

All agents are metabolized to differing degrees by the cytochrome P-450 enzyme system of the liver and excreted in differing percentages as unchanged drug in the urine. **Nizatidine** has at least one metabolite that has histamine-blocking activity. All others are metabolized to inactive compounds.

Pharmacotherapeutics

Precautions and Contraindications

Renal impairment requires cautious use and dosage adjustments. (Dosage adjustments are presented in Table 18–19.) Patients with renal impairment are more subject to the CNS adverse reactions. Older adults may have reduced renal function, and these drugs should be used cautiously with this age group. **Cimetidine** seems to have the most problems with decreased renal clearance, and **ranitidine** the fewest.

Hepatocellular injury may occur with **nizatidine,** as evidenced by elevated liver enzymes (ALT, AST, or alkaline phosphatase). These abnormalities are reversible with discontinuation of the drug. Because of this risk, it should not be used for patients with a history of liver disease.

Occasional reversible hepatitis or hepatocellular disorders have occurred with **ranitidine.** It is contraindicated for patients with a history of liver disease.

Histamine₂ blockers are **Pregnancy Category B;** however, there are no adequate and well-controlled

Table 18–17. Pharmacokinetics: Histamine₂ Blockers

Drug	Onset	Peak	Duration	Protein Binding	Bio-availability	Half-Life	Metabolized	Elimination
Cimetidine	30 min	45–90 min	4–5 h	13–25%	60–70%	2 h	30–40%	48% unchanged in urine
Famotidine	60 min	1–4 h	1–4 h	15–20%	40–45%	2.5–3.5 h	30–35%	25–30% unchanged in urine
Nizatidine	60 min	0.5–3 h	Unknown	35%	>90%	1–2 h	<18%	60% unchanged in urine, <6% in feces
Ranitidine	60 min	1–3 h	1–3 h	15%	50–60%	2–3 h	<10%	30–35% unchanged in urine

studies of these agents in pregnant women. They should be used only when the potential benefits outweigh the potential risks to the fetus.

These drugs vary in their excretion in breast milk. **Cimetidine** is excreted in breast milk in milk:plasma ratios of 5:1 to 12:1. Potential daily dose to the infant is 6 mg. Do not nurse. **Famotidine** is excreted in the breast milk of rats. It is not known whether it is excreted in human breast milk. The decision to discontinue the drug is made based on the need of the mother for the drug. **Nizatidine** is excreted in breast milk in a concentration of 0.1 percent of the oral dose in proportion to plasma concentrations. Once again, the decision to discontinue the drug is made based on the need of the mother for the drug. **Ranitidine** is excreted in breast milk with milk:plasma ratios of 1:1 to 6.7:1. **Exercise caution when giving to nursing mother.**

Safety and efficacy for children has not been established. **Cimetidine** is not recommended for children under age 16 unless benefits clearly outweigh risks. In very limited experience, daily doses of 20 to 40 mg/kg have been used. OTC use is not recommended for any of these drugs for children under age 12.

Adverse Drug Reactions

All of these drugs have similar adverse reaction profiles. **Cimetidine** appears to have the greatest degree of antiandrogenic reactions (e.g., gynecomastia and impotence). Reversible CNS (e.g., mental confusion, agitation, psychosis, depression, and disorientation) adverse reactions have also occurred with this drug.

Hematologic adverse reactions include agranulocytosis, granulocytopenia, thrombocytopenia, and aplastic anemia. These reactions are rare but should be monitored. Other less common adverse drug reactions include drowsiness, dizziness, constipation or diarrhea, and nausea. Adverse drug reactions related to liver function are discussed in the precautions and contraindications section.

Drug Interactions

Many of the drug interactions with this class of drugs are related to their metabolism by the cytochrome P-450 (CYP) enzyme system of the liver. **Cimetidine** is the most problematic because it uses several isoenzymes (CYP 1A2, CYP 2C9, and CYP 2D6). Any drug metabolized extensively by these isoenzymes will have its metabolism inhibited by **cimetidine**, with a risk for increased plasma levels and toxicity for that drug. **Famotidine, nizatidine,** and **ranitidine** have less effect on the CYP system and use a narrower number of isoenzymes in their metabolism. Although they still have drug interactions, they are fewer than with **cimetidine**. Table 18–18 provides a detailed list of drug interactions for the various **histamine₂ blockers.**

Clinical Use and Dosing

GASTROESOPHAGEAL REFLUX DISEASE. GERD in adults is treated with stepped therapy. Step 1 involves lifestyle modifications and **antacids. Histamine₂ blockers** may be added during step 1, or they may be initiated with step 2. Single-agent therapy is the choice for patients with mild grades of endoscopic esophagitis. Grades I and II esophagitis heal in approximately 75 percent to 90 percent of patients on this regimen. Grades III and IV heal in only 40 to 50 percent of patients and usually require the addition of other drugs. Standard dosing is shown in Table 18–19. If no esophageal erosive disease is present, twice-daily dosing is effective. Once-daily dosing is not effective in treating GERD.

Infants and children with GERD have also been successfully treated with **histamine₂ blockers** for several years with good response and few adverse reactions. Infants over age 2 months with mild GI symptoms, who are gaining weight and demonstrating developmentally appropriate behaviors, can be treated empirically with a short trial of **antacids** and **histamine₂ blockers.** Standard dosing may be too low in this age group, and increases up to twice the established dose may be required for optimal acid suppression (Ault & Schmidt, 1998). If the child does not respond to drug therapy or delayed gastric emptying is suspected, a **prokinetic** drug is added. Dosing for infants and children is also shown in Table 18–19. Once again, twice-daily dosing is required.

A more detailed discussion of the management of GERD is found in Chapter 32.

PEPTIC ULCER DISEASE. With the advent of the discovery that the cause of PUD is usually an infection rather than excessive acid due to stress, diet, smoking, alcohol consumption, and **NSAIDs,** the treatment pattern has changed. Currently, there is no single uncontroversial therapy for PUD. Short-term treatment and maintenance therapy for both duodenal and benign gastric ulcers, however, still often include **histamine₂ blockers.** Standard dosing schedules are shown in Table 18–19. Once-daily dosing is appropriate for prophylaxis; twice-daily dosing is required for treatment. No difference in healing rates occurred across drugs after 8 weeks (82 to 95%). The usual length of treatment is at least 6 weeks.

A more detailed discussion of the management of PUD is found in Chapter 32.

HEARTBURN, ACID INDIGESTION, AND "SOUR STOMACH." Relief of symptoms may be provided by OTC use of **histamine₂ blockers.** However, it is important for patients to be informed about the potential for drug interactions.

PROPHYLAXIS AND TREATMENT OF DUODENAL ULCERS ASSOCIATED WITH NSAID USE. **Sucralfate,** previously

Table 18–18. Drug Interactions: Histamine$_2$ Blockers

Drug	Interacting Drug	Possible Effect	Implications
Cimetidine	Benzodiazepines, caffeine, calcium channel blockers, carbamazepine, labetalol, metoprolol, metronidazole, pentoxifylline, propafenone, propranolol, quinidine, quinine, sulfonylureas, tacrine, theophylline, triamterene, tricyclic anti-depressants, valproic acid, warfarin*	Decreased hepatic metabolism of these drugs	Select different histamine$_2$ blocker. Monitor drug levels of those with narrow therapeutic range or potential for cardiac rhythm disturbances.
	Ferrous salts, indomethacin, ketoconazole, tetracyclines	Action of these drugs decreased because of decreased absorption	Avoid concurrent administration; separate doses or select different histamine$_2$ blocker.
	Digoxin	Decreased serum digoxin concentrations during co-administration	Select different histamine$_2$ blocker.
	Flecainide	Increased drug effects of flecainide	Select different histamine$_2$ blocker.
	Narcotic analgesics	Toxic effects (e.g., respiratory depression) may be increased	Select different histamine$_2$ blocker.
	Procainamide	Increased plasma levels of procainamide and its cardio-active metabolite by decreasing renal tubular secretion	Select different histamine$_2$ blocker; ranitidine was shown to have similar action in only one study, so best not to choose that drug.
	Tocainide	Decreased drug effects of tocainide	Select different histamine$_2$ blocker.
	Cigarette smoking	Smoking reverses cimetidine-induced inhibition of nocturnal gastric secretion, hindering ulcer healing	Avoid cigarette smoking.
Famotidine	Ketoconazole	Action of drug decreased by reduced absorption	Separate administration by at least 1 h and give ketoconazole first.
	Food	May increase bioavailability of famotidine	No clinical significance.
Nizatidine	Salicylates	Increased serum salicylate levels when given to patients receiving high doses (3.9 g/d) of salicylate	Monitor salicylate levels or select different histamine$_2$ blocker.
	Food	May increase bioavailability of nizatidine	No clinical significance.
Ranitidine	Diazepam	Decreased drug effects of diazepam due to decreased drug absorption	Separate doses by at least 1 h and give diazepam first.
	Sulfonylureas	Increased hypoglycemic effects of glipizide or glyburide	Dosage adjustments may be needed.
	Warfarin	May interfere with warfarin clearance; data conflicting	Monitor PT/INR more closely; may need dosage adjustment.

Continued on next page

Table 18–18. Drug Interactions: Histamine$_2$ Blockers *(continued)*

Drug	Interacting Drug	Possible Effect	Implications
All histamine$_2$ blockers	Alcohol	May increase blood alcohol levels	Avoid use of alcohol.
	Antacids, anticholinergics, metoclopramide	May decrease absorption of cimetidine, ranitidine; less effect on nizatidine and famotidine	Separate dose by at least 1 h for cimetidine and ranitidine; no special precautions needed for nizatidine and famotidine.

*Although interactions with these drugs are not listed for other histamine$_2$ blockers, some effect is probable, even though it is not to the same extent.

INR = international normalized ratio; PT = prothrombin time.

discussed in the section on cytoprotective agents, is the best choice for this indication, but it is more expensive than **histamine$_2$ blockers** and offers only marginal increases in effectiveness.

ALL USES. Regardless of the reason for which the **histamine$_2$ blocker** is prescribed, consideration of renal function is important in determining dosage. In the presence of renal impairment, dosage intervals need to be increased. For **cimetidine**, the interval is increased if the renal impairment is severe; for **famotidine**, if creatinine clearance (CCr) is less than 10 mL/min; and for **nizatidine** and **ranitidine**, if CCr is less than 50 mL/min.

Rational Drug Selection

No specific **histamine$_2$ blocker** is preferred over another for effectiveness. Choice is based on cost and whether the patient is taking other drugs that might have interactions with the specific **histamine$_2$ blocker**.

COST. Generic formulations are always less expensive than brand names. OTC drugs are usually less expensive than prescriptions, but because their dose is lower, the cost difference is lost in the increased number of pills required.

OTHER DRUGS. **Cimetidine** has the most drug interaction potential. Other **histamine$_2$ blockers** have fewer listed drug interactions.

Monitoring

Because of the potential for hepatocellular damage, patients who require higher doses or more than short-term use of this class of drugs should have laboratory testing of liver function prior to initiation of therapy and at regular intervals throughout therapy.

Renal impairment influences drug dosing for all drugs in this class. Patients who require higher doses or more than short-term therapy or for whom renal impairment is a likely risk (e.g., older adults) should have renal function assessment done prior to initiation of therapy.

Patient Education

ADMINISTRATION. Instruct patients to take the drug as prescribed for the full course of therapy, even if they are feeling better. If a dose is missed, it should be taken as soon as remembered but not if it is almost time for the next dose. Do not double doses.

Histamine$_2$ blockers should be taken with meals or immediately afterward and at bedtime to achieve the best effects. Doses taken once daily are best taken at bedtime (Table 18–20). Oral suspensions are shaken prior to administration, and unused portions are discarded after 30 days. The foil is removed from **ranitidine** effervescent tablets or granules, and they are dissolved in 6 to 8 oz of water before they are taken.

If the patient is also taking **antacids** or other drugs whose interaction with **histamine$_2$ blockers** produces interference with absorption, the drugs' administration should be separated by at least 30 minutes to 1 hour. **Sucralfate** should be taken 2 hours after the **histamine$_2$ blocker.**

Patients taking OTC preparations are not to take the maximum doses continuously for more than 2 weeks without consulting their health care provider. A diagnostic workup is in order under these circumstances.

ADVERSE REACTIONS. **Histamine$_2$ blockers** may cause drowsiness or dizziness. Caution patients to avoid driving or other activities requiring alertness until their response to the drug is known.

For male patients taking **cimetidine**, warn about the potential for gynecomastia and impotence. Because other drugs in the class are less likely to cause these problems, a different drug may be selected.

Advise patients to report the onset of black, tarry stools. They are not adverse reactions to the drug but may indicate GI bleeding. Sore throat, diarrhea, rash, confusion, or hallucinations should also be reported promptly. These adverse reactions may require dosage alteration or discontinuation of the drug. Increasing the fluid and fiber in the diet may minimize constipation.

Table 18–19. Dosage Schedule: Histamine$_2$ Blockers

Drug	Indication	Initial Dose	Maintenance Dose
Cimetidine	Short-term treatment of active duodenal ulcer	*Adults:* 800 mg at bedtime or 300 mg qid with meals and at bedtime or 400 mg bid *Children:* 20–40 mg/kg/d in 4 divided doses	*Adults:* 400 mg at bedtime; dosage not to exceed 2.4 g/d. In severe renal impairment, use 300 mg every 8–12 h. *Children:* 20 mg/kg/d; 10–15 mg/kg/d in renal impairment.
	Duodenal ulcer prophylaxis	*Adults:* 300 mg bid or 400 mg at bedtime	Same.
	Treatment of active benign gastric ulcer	*Adults:* 800 mg at bedtime or 300 mg qid with meals and at bedtime	800 mg at bedtime. In severe renal impairment, use 300 mg every 8–12 h. No information concerning usefulness of treatment periods >8 wk.
	GERD	*Adults:* 800 mg bid in morning and at bedtime or 400 mg qid with meals and at bedtime	*Adults:* Same dose for up to 12 wk. Use >12 wk has not been established. May go as high as 600 mg qid if needed. In severe renal impairment, use 300 mg every 8–12 h.
		Children: 20–40 mg/kg/d in 4 divided doses	*Children:* 20 mg/kg/d; 10–15 mg/kg/d if renal impairment.
	Pathological hypersecretory conditions	*Adults:* 300 mg qid with meals and at bedtime	Individualize dose. Do not exceed 2400 mg/d. Continue as long as clinically indicated.
	Heartburn, indigestion, sour stomach	*Adults:* 200 mg (OTC) with water as symptoms occur	Take up to 400 mg bid. Do not take maximum dose for more than 2 wk without consulting health care provider.
Famotidine	Short-term treatment of active duodenal ulcer	*Adults:* 40 mg/d at bedtime or ≤20 mg bid (in morning and at bedtime)	*Adults:* 20 mg at bedtime for up to 8 wk. Most heal in 4 wk. If CCr <10 mL/min, give 20 mg at bedtime or increase dosing interval to 36–48 h.
		Children: 1–2 mg/kg/d in 1 or 2 divided doses	*Children:* Same dose for up to 8 wk. Most heal in 4 wk.
	Duodenal ulcer prophylaxis	*Adults:* 20 mg at bedtime	Same
	Treatment of benign active gastric ulcer	*Adults:* 40 mg at bedtime	Same dose. If CCr <10 mL/min, give 20 mg at bedtime or increase dosing interval to 36–48 h. No data to support treatment beyond 8 wk.
	GERD	*Adults:* 20 mg bid (in morning and at bedtime)	*Adults:* 20 mg for up to 6 wk. If erosive disease, 20–40 mg bid for up to 12 wk.
		Children: 1–2 mg/kg/d in 1 or 2 divided doses	*Children:* Same dose. Treatment trial for 2–4 wk.
	Heartburn, acid indigestion, and sour stomach	*Adults:* Relief: 10 mg (1 tablet) with water Prophylaxis: 10 mg 1 h prior to meal that is expected to cause symptoms	Can be used up to bid for <2 wk.
Nizatidine	Short-term treatment of active duodenal ulcer	*Adults:* 300 mg at bedtime or 150 mg bid (in morning and at bedtime)	300 mg at bedtime. If CCr 20–50 mL/min, give 150 mg at bedtime. If CCr <20 mL/min, give 150 mg every 2 or 3 d.
	Maintenance of healed duodenal ulcer	*Adults:* 150 mg at bedtime	150 mg at bedtime.
	GERD	*Adults:* 150 mg bid (in morning and at bedtime)	150 mg bid.

Continued on next page

Table 18–19. Dosage Schedule: Histamine$_2$ Blockers *(continued)*

Drug	Indication	Initial Dose	Maintenance Dose
Ranitidine	Short-term treatment of active duodenal ulcer	*Adults:* 100–150 mg bid (in morning and at bedtime) or 300 mg at bedtime	150 mg at bedtime. If CCr <50 mL/min, give 150 mg at bedtime.
	Duodenal ulcer prophylaxis	*Adults:* 150 mg at bedtime	150 mg at bedtime.
	Treatment of benign active gastric ulcer	*Adults:* 150 mg bid (in morning and at bedtime	150 mg at bedtime.
	GERD	*Adults:* 150 mg bid (in morning and at bedtime; if erosive disease, give 150 mg qid	*Adults:* 150 mg bid. If CCr <50 mL/min, give 150 mg at bedtime. If erosive disease, give 150 mg bid.
		Children: 2–4 mg/kg/d in two divided doses	*Children:* 2 mg/kg/d in 2 divided doses.
	Pathological hypersecretory conditions	*Adults:* 150 mg bid (in morning and at bedtime)	Individualize dose; doses up to 6 g/d have been used.
	Heartburn, acid indigestion, and sour stomach	*Adults:* Relief: 75 mg up to bid	Can be used up to bid for <2 wk.

For all children <12 years of age, consultation with pediatric specialist is advised.

Table 18–20. Available Dosage Forms: Histamine$_2$ Blockers

Drug	Dosage Form	How Supplied
Cimetidine (Tagamet)	Tablets: 100 mg	In bottles of 16, 32, 64 tablets
	Tablets: 200 mg, 300 mg	In bottles of 100 tablets
	Tablets: 400 mg	In bottles of 60 tablets
	Tablets: 800 mg	In bottles of 30 tablets
	Liquid: 300 mg/5 mL	In 240 mL (mint-peach flavor)
	Injection: 300 mg/2 mL	In single-dose vials, disposable syringes, and 8-mL multiple-dose vials
(Generic)	Tablets: 200 mg, 300 mg, 400 mg, 800 mg	In bottles of 100, 500, 1000 tablets
	Liquid: 300 mg/5 mL	In 240 mL and 470 mL (mint-peach flavor)
	Injection: 300 mg/2 mL	In 2-mL and 8-mL vials
Famotidine (Pepcid)	Tablets: 10 mg	In packets of 12 tablets
	Tablets: 20 mg, 40 mg	In bottles of 30, 90, 100 tablets
	Powder for oral suspension: 40 mg/5 mL when reconstituted	In bottles of 400 mg (cherry-banana-mint flavor)
	Injection: 10 mg/mL	In 2-mL single-dose and 4-mL multidose vials
Nizatidine (Axid)	Capsule: 150 mg	In bottles of 60 capsules
	Capsule: 300 mg	In bottles of 30 capsules
Ranitidine (Zantac)	Tablets: 150 mg	In bottles of 60, 500 tablets
	Tablets: 300 mg	In bottles of 30, 250 tablets
	Effervescent tablets: 150 mg	In bottles of 30, 60 tablets
	Geldose: capsules: 150 mg	In bottles of 30 capsules
	Syrup: 15 mg/mL	In 480 mL
	Efferdose: granules: 150 mg	In 1.44-g packets
	Injection: 25 mg/mL	In 2-mL, 10-mL, and 40-mL vials and 2-mL syringes
(Generic)	Syrup: 15 mg/mL	In 10 mL

LIFESTYLE MANAGEMENT.   Smoking interferes with the absorption of **histamine₂ blockers** and increases gastric acid secretion. Advise the patient to stop smoking. **Alcohol** and products containing **aspirin** or **NSAIDs** and some foods may also increase gastric acid secretion; they should be avoided. Other lifestyle modifications are discussed in Chapter 32.

Prokinetics

Prokinetic drugs, also known as gastrointestinal stimulants, stimulate the motility of the GI tract without stimulating gastric, biliary, or pancreatic secretions. These drugs are used in the management of a wide range of disorders in which reduced GI motility is a problem, including gastroparesis associated with diabetes mellitus, GERD, and emesis associated with cancer chemotherapy. There are two drugs in this class, **metoclopramide (Reglan)** and **cisapride (Propulsid)**, which are discussed in this section.

Pharmacodynamics

Metoclopramide stimulates motility in the upper GI tract. Its mode of action is unclear but appears to be related to sensitizing tissues to the action of acetylcholine. The action does not depend on an intact vagal innervation system, but **anticholinergic drugs** can reverse the action. This drug increases the tone and amplitude of gastric contractions, relaxes the pyloric sphincter and duodenal bulb, and increases peristalsis of the duodenum and jejunum, resulting in accelerated gastric emptying and increased speed of gastric transit. It has almost no effect on the colon or gallbladder. For patients with GERD secondary to decreased lower esophageal sphincter pressure (LESP), **metoclopramide** produces dose-related increases in LESP. These effects begin at doses as low as 5 mg and continue through 20-mg doses.

This drug also has some actions similar to the **phenothiazines** and **dopamine antagonists** and produces sedation and, rarely, extrapyramidal symptoms (EPS). It also induces release of prolactin and transiently increases circulating aldosterone levels. As mentioned in the antiemetic section, it also has antiemetic properties as a result of its antagonism of central and peripheral dopamine receptors. Dopamine produces vomiting by stimulation of the CTZ, and **metoclopramide** blocks this stimulation.

Cisapride significantly accelerates gastric emptying of both liquids and solids, primarily by the release of acetylcholine at the myenteric plexus. It does not induce muscarinic or nicotinic receptor stimulation, nor does it inhibit acetylcholinesterase activity. It is less potent than **metoclopramide** at dopamine receptor blocking. It does not increase or decrease pentagastrin-induced gastric acid secretion. **Cisapride** also has serotonin (5-HT4) activity that may increase GI motility and heart rate. These effects on the heart have resulted in a warning statement about serious cardiac rhythm disturbances.

For patients with GERD secondary to decreased LESP, **cisapride** produces dose-related increases in LESP. These effects begin at doses as low as 20 mg and continue through doses of 10 mg tid.

Pharmacokinetics

Absorption and Distribution

Both drugs are well absorbed after oral administration (Table 18–21). **Metoclopramide** has an injectable formulation. **Cisapride** has a high degree of protein binding, resulting in 35 to 40 percent bioavailability. The reverse is true of **metoclopramide,** which has low protein binding and high bioavailability.

Both drugs are widely distributed throughout body tissues. **Metoclopramide** crosses the blood-brain barrier and the placenta and enters breast milk in concentra-

Table 18–21. Pharmacokinetics: Prokinetic Agents

Drug	Onset	Peak	Duration	Protein Binding	Bioavailability	Half-Life	Elimination
Cisapride	30–60 m	60–90 m	Unknown	97.5–98%	35–40%	8–10 h	<10% as unchanged drug in urine and feces
Metoclopramide PO IM	30–60 m 10–15 m	1–2 h 1–2 h	1–2 h 1–2 h	30% 30%	65–95% 65–95%	2.5–5 h 2.5–5 h	85% in urine after 72 h (25% as unchanged drug); clearance affected by renal function

tions greater than in plasma. **Cisapride** is not known to cross the blood-brain barrier, but it does cross the placenta and is excreted in breast milk at concentrations approximately one-twentieth those observed in plasma.

Metabolism and Excretion

The liver metabolizes both drugs, but **cisapride** uses the CYP 450 3A4 isoenzyme system with drug interactions based on this site of metabolism. Because **metoclopramide** is excreted in urine, clearance is affected by renal function, and doses are reduced in the presence of renal impairment. **Cisapride** is excreted in urine and feces.

Pharmacotherapeutics

Precautions and Contraindications

Both drugs are contraindicated in the presence of disorders in which stimulation of GI motility might be dangerous (e.g., GI hemorrhage, mechanical obstruction, new surgery on the GI tract, or perforation). The dopamine-associated activity of **metoclopramide** affects the CNS, and the drug is used cautiously with patients who have a history of depression. Depression with symptoms ranging from mild to severe, including suicide ideation, have been reported. Patients who are at risk for EPS also require cautious use of this drug.

Because **metoclopramide** is excreted primarily through the kidney, it should be used with caution for patients with renal impairment. Dosage adjustment may be needed. It undergoes minimal hepatic metabolism and is safe to administer to patients with impaired hepatic function as long as their renal function is normal.

Patients with a history of a variety of cardiac disorders (e.g., baseline prolonged QT interval, *torsades de pointes*, long QT syndrome, sinus node dysfunction, second- or third-degree heart block, ventricular rhythm disturbances, ischemic heart disease, clinically significant bradycardia, or congestive heart failure), uncorrected electrolyte disorders (hypokalemia, hypermagnesemia), or respiratory failure should not use cisapride. There are other specific contraindications in the warning box on the package insert. This warning should be read before this drug is prescribed.

Metoclopramide is Pregnancy Category B; however, there are no adequate and well-controlled studies in pregnant women. Case reports to date have not been associated with fetal harm, but the drug should be prescribed only when the benefits clearly outweigh the risks to the fetus.

Cisapride is Pregnancy Category C. It was embryotoxic and fetotoxic in rats and rabbits at doses 100 times (rats) to 12 times (rabbits) the maximum recommended for humans. Use in pregnancy only when the benefits justify the risk to the fetus.

Metoclopramide is excreted in breast milk and concentrates at about twice the plasma level at 2 hours after taking the dose. However, in a mother taking 30 mg/day, the infant would receive less than 45 mg/day, which is still much less than the recommended maximum dose for infants. Exercise caution when giving to a nursing mother, but recognize that there appears to be little, if any, risk to the infant.

Cisapride is excreted in breast milk at very low concentrations. Although there appears to be no risk to the infant, caution should still be used when prescribing for nursing women.

Infants and children age 21 days to 3.3 years with symptomatic GERD have been treated with **metoclopramide** at a daily dosage of 0.5 mg/kg without difficulty. The safety and efficacy of **cisapride** in children have not been established, and serious adverse events have been reported, including deaths due to cardiovascular events. Other potentially serious adverse effects reported in children include anemia, hemolytic anemia, hypoglycemia with acidosis, unexplained apneic episodes, and confusion. This drug should not be used in children unless there is a clear benefit that outweighs these risks.

Adverse Drug Reactions

Adverse reactions associated with **metoclopramide** include depression (see discussion in precautions and contraindications section), extrapyramidal symptoms, (seen in approximately 0.2 to 1% of patients, and more common in children and older adults), dizziness, diarrhea, and hypoglycemia in patients with diabetes. Less common adverse reactions include galactorrhea, amenorrhea, gynecomastia, and impotence secondary to hyperprolactinemia and fluid retention secondary to transient elevations in aldosterone. Approximately 20 to 30 percent of all patients taking this drug experience some adverse reaction, but it is usually mild, transient, and reversible upon withdrawal of the drug. The incidence correlates with the dose and duration of therapy.

Cisapride has a variety of adverse reactions that including dizziness, headache, pharyngitis, constipation, abdominal pain, and diarrhea. These reactions tend to be mild and transient. They are more common with doses of 20 mg than with 10-mg doses. Although not common, cardiovascular adverse reactions are serious and potentially fatal. Patients with a history of cardiac disease should not use this drug. Taking this drug, for example, is an independent risk factor for the adverse cardiovascular reaction of QT prolongation.

Drug Interactions

Drug interactions with **metoclopramide** are largely related to its cholinergic and dopaminergic activities. Additive CNS depression occurs with other CNS depressants, and increased risk of extrapyramidal effects occurs with other drugs that have the potential for EPS problems. Drugs with anticholinergic effects reverse the action of **metoclopramide,** and the reverse is also true.

Many drug interactions with **cisapride** are related to its metabolism by the CYP-450 3A4 isoenzyme system, which is responsible for the metabolism of a large number of drugs. Some of these interactions may result in serious cardiac arrhythmias. Additive CNS depression and interactions with **anticholinergic drugs** are similar to those of **metoclopramide.**

Table 18–22 provides a more detailed list of these drug interactions.

Clinical Use and Dosing

GASTROESOPHAGEAL REFLUX DISEASE. The principal effect of **metoclopramide** in the management of GERD is on symptoms of postprandial and daytime heartburn. For adults, if symptoms occur throughout the day, 10 mg taken 30 minutes prior to each meal and at bedtime is recommended (Table 18–23). When symptoms are confined to specific situations such as after the evening meal, a single 10- to 20-mg dose 30 minutes prior to that meal or at bedtime is effective in preventing the symptoms. Healing of esophageal ulcers and erosions has been demonstrated by endoscopy to occur by 12 weeks at doses of 15 mg qid.

Occasionally, patients who are more sensitive to the therapeutic dose (e.g., older adults) require only 5 mg per dose. Children require daily doses at 0.4 to 0.8 mg/kg in four divided doses (30 minutes prior to each meal and at bedtime). For patients whose CCr is less than 40 mL/min, initiate therapy at approximately half the recommended dosage.

For adults, **cisapride** 10 mg qid for several days results in a significant increase in LESP and increased esophageal clearance. Maximum effect occurs with 10 mg given at least qid (15 minutes before meals and at bedtime). Intermediate effects occur with a 20-mg single dose in the morning before eating, and the least effect is associated with 10 mg as a single dose in the morning before eating. The minimum effective dose should be used.

Steady-state plasma levels are generally higher in older adults because of moderate prolongation of the drug's half-life. However, therapeutic doses can be similar to those used for younger adults except for the extremely elderly. AUC for patients age 85 (± 6 years) reached 2.7 times the level on the 28th day of therapy versus the first day of therapy in one study (Yamamoto, Takano, Sanaka, Kuyama, Yamanaka, Koike, & Mineshita, 1998). Doses for patients over age 80 should be reduced by half to two-thirds. This reduction is best accomplished by giving the recommended dose for adults but only once or twice daily rather than three to four times daily. Children require doses of 0.15 to 0.3 mg/kg

three to four times daily. Patients with hepatic insufficiency require half the normal daily dose.

DIABETIC GASTROPARESIS. Only **metoclopramide** has an indication for treatment of diabetic gastroparesis. Dosage is 10 mg 30 minutes before meals and at bedtime for 2 to 8 weeks. The route of administration is based on the severity of symptoms. If only the earliest manifestation of gastroparesis is present, oral administration is adequate. If the symptoms are more severe, parenteral therapy with 10 mg intravenously (IV) over 1 to 2 minutes for up to 10 days may be needed before oral therapy can be initiated. Rectal formulations can be made by a pharmacist to avoid the IV route. The suppositories each contain 25 mg of **metoclopramide** in polyethylene glycol. One suppository is administered 30 to 60 minutes before each meal and at bedtime. After symptoms are resolved (no more than 8 weeks of therapy), the drug is stopped and reinstituted at the earliest indications of symptom return.

Diabetics often experience renal impairment. Because **metoclopramide** is excreted principally by the kidney, those patients with CCr below 40 mL/min should have their therapy initiated at approximately half the recommended dosage. Depending on clinical efficacy and safety considerations, the dosage may be increased or decreased as appropriate.

Rational Drug Selection

EFFICACY. Metoclopramide has demonstrated limited symptomatic improvement and endoscopically demonstrated esophageal healing for patients with GERD. Cisapride has demonstrated in randomized trials that its healing potential is equal to that of **histamine₂ blockers.** Given its significantly higher cost, however, it is difficult to justify its use in place of **histamine₂ blockers.** It is effective in combination with a **histamine₂ blocker** in the presence of erosive reflux esophagitis. In addition, because of the risk for serious and sometimes fatal ventricular arrhythmias, **cisapride** should generally be reserved for patients who do not respond adequately to lifestyle modifications and other drugs with less serious adverse reactions.

LENGTH OF THERAPY. Metoclopramide is not used for management of GERD if treatment must be long term. With longer than 8 weeks of therapy, there is a much higher risk for adverse reactions, including EPS. **Cisapride** does not have restrictions on length of therapy.

CONCOMITANT DISEASES. Metoclopramide should be used cautiously for patients with diseases that place them at risk for EPS disorders or for patients taking drugs that place them at risk for these disorders. **Cisapride** has the potential for serious, even lethal, adverse reactions for patients with selected cardiac disorders.

Table 18–22. Drug Interactions: Prokinetic Agents

Drug	Interacting Drug	Possible Effect	Implications
Cisapride	Anticholinergics	Decreased effects of either drug.	Avoid concurrent use.
	Antiarrhythmics classes IA/ III, antidepressants, antipsychotics, azole antifungals, bepridil, clarithromycin, dirithromycin, erythromycin, troleandomycin, protease inhibitors, sparfloxacin, delavirdine	These drugs are known to prolong QT intervals; may decrease metabolism and increase levels of cisapride.	Concomitant use of these drugs is contraindicated.
	Cimetidine, ranitidine	GI absorption of these histamine$_2$ blockers is accelerated; increased peak plasma levels and AUC of cisapride with cimetidine only.	Select different histamine$_2$ blocker or prokinetic.
	Anticoagulants	Increases anticoagulation time.	Check PT/INR within first few days of initiation of cisapride and adjust dose of anticoagulant as needed.
	Digoxin	Alters effects of digoxin.	Monitor serum levels of digoxin more closely.
	Alcohol and other CNS depressants	Additive CNS depression.	Avoid concurrent use or warn of potential CNS depression.
	Grapefruit juice	Coadministration increases bioavailability of cisapride.	Avoid concomitant use.
Metoclopramide	Alcohol, antidepressants, antihistamines, opioids, and sedative hypnotics	Additive CNS depression; increases rate of absorption of alcohol.	Avoid concurrent use or warn of potential CNS depression.
	Haloperidol, phenothiazines, other drugs with EPS effects	Increased risk of extrapyramidal reactions.	Avoid concurrent use; select different prokinetic.
	Anticholinergics and opioids	Effects of metoclopramide on GI motility may antagonize these drugs.	If not used therapeutically, avoid concurrent use.
	Cimetidine	Reduced bioavailability of cimetidine.	Select different histamine$_2$ blocker.
	Digoxin	Decreased absorption, plasma levels, and therapeutic effects.	Capsules, elixir, and tablets with high dissolution rate are least affected; use these formulations if both drugs must be given.
	Levodopa	These drugs have opposite effects on dopamine receptors: bioavailability of levodopa increased; effects of metoclopramide decreased.	Avoid concurrent use; metoclopramide is relatively contraindicated for patients with Parkinson's disease.
	Monoamine oxidase inhibitors (MAOIs)	Metoclopramide releases catecholamines that may produce hypertension in patients taking MAOIs.	Use cautiously concurrently, if at all; monitor blood pressure closely.

INR = international normalized ratio; PT = prothrombin time.

Table 18–23. Dosage Schedule: Prokinetic Agents

Drug	Indication	Dosage Schedule	Notes
Cisapride	GERD	*Adults:* Treatment: 10 mg qid (15 min before meals and at bedtime) Prophylaxis: 10 mg bid (15 min before breakfast and at bedtime) or 20 mg at bedtime *Adults >age 80:* 10 mg qd or bid *Children:* 0.15–0.3 mg/kg tid–qid (15 min before meals and at bedtime)	One-half daily dose for patients with hepatic insufficiency; in some adults, dose may need to be increased to 20 mg qid. Use minimal effective dose.
Metoclopramide	GERD	*Adults:* Treatment: 10–15 mg qid (30 min before meals and at bedtime) Prophylaxis: 20 mg at bedtime	Some patients respond to doses as low as 5 mg. Dose not to exceed 0.5 mg/kg/d. Therapy not to exceed 8 wk. Patients with CCr <40 mL/min, initiate therapy with half the recommended dose.
	Diabetic gastroparesis	*Adults:* 10 mg qid (30 min before meals and at bedtime) *Children:* 0.4–0.8 mg/kg/d in 4 divided doses (30 min before meals and at bedtime)	

Other considerations based on concomitant disorders are discussed in the precautions and contraindications section.

Monitoring

Because of the need to adjust dosage in the presence of renal impairment, renal function should be assessed before therapy with **metoclopramide** is begun. Dosage adjustment is required for patients with hepatic insufficiency who are taking **cisapride.** Liver function should be assessed prior to initiation of therapy with this drug.

No other monitoring is required except that for the disease process being treated. Considering the risk for arrhythmias, an electrocardiogram should be considered before initiation of therapy with **cisapride.**

Patient Education

ADMINISTRATION. Advise the patient to take the drug exactly as prescribed (Table 18–24). **Metoclopramide** is taken 30 minutes before each meal and at bedtime; **cisapride** is taken 15 minutes before each meal and at bedtime. If a dose is missed, it should be taken as soon as the patient remembers unless it is almost time for the next dose. Do not double doses or exceed the recommended dose.

ADVERSE REACTIONS. Both drugs may cause drowsiness. Caution patients to avoid driving or other activities that require alertness until their response to the drug is known. Concurrent use of other **CNS depressants,** including **alcohol,** makes this problem worse and causes additive CNS depression.

Warn patients taking **metoclopramide** to notify their health care provider immediately if involuntary movement of the eyes, face, or limbs occurs, which may be EPS-related.

Warn patients taking **cisapride** to seek medical attention immediately if they faint, experience irregular heartbeats or pulse, or notice any other unusual cardiac symptoms. Serious, even fatal, cardiac rhythm disturbances have been associated with this drug. They are more likely if the patient is also taking a drug metabolized by the CYP-450 3A4 isoenzyme system of the liver or has a cardiac disorder that involves prolonged QT intervals. Some OTC drugs use the CYP-450 3A4 system, including **cimetidine.** Patients should not take any OTC drugs without first consulting their health care provider.

Many prescription drugs also use this system. Patients should notify any health care provider who may prescribe a drug for them that they are taking **cisapride.**

LIFESTYLE MANAGEMENT. Lifestyle modifications are used before any drug in the management of both GERD and diabetic gastroparesis. First, patients should try avoiding **alcohol** and **NSAIDs;** smoking cessation; weight loss; sleeping with the head of the bed elevated; avoiding large meals, fatty foods, chocolate, caffeine, and citrus; and avoiding food or fluid intake within 3 hours of

Table 18–24. Available Dosage Forms: Prokinetic Agents

Drug	Dosage Form	How Supplied
Cisapride (Propulsid)	Tablets: 10 mg Tablets: 20 mg Suspension: 1 mg/mL	In bottles of 100, 500 scored tablets In bottles of 100, 250 tablets In 450 mL (cherry-flavored)
Metoclopramide (Reglan)	Tablets: 5 mg Tablets: 10 mg Syrup: 5 mg/5 mL Injection: 5 mg/mL	In bottles of 100 tablets In bottles of 100 scored tablets In 480 mL and unit dose 10 mL In 2-, 10-mL ampules and 2-, 10-, 30-mL vials
(Generic)	Tablets: 5 mg Tablets: 10 mg Syrup: 5 mg/5 mL Injections: 5 mg/mL	In bottles of 100, 500, 1000 tablets In bottles of 100, 500, 1000, 2500 tablets In 480 mL and unit dose 10 mL In 2-mL ampules and 2-, 10-, 20-, 30-mL vials

going to bed at night. These modifications are discussed in more detail in Chapter 32.

Proton Pump Inhibitors

Proton pump inhibitors are **antisecretory drugs** used to treat gastric conditions characterized by hyperacidity. They are used for erosive gastritis, GERD, and Zollinger-Ellison syndrome and as part of a multidrug regimen for short-term treatment of active PUD, especially duodenal ulcers caused by *H. pylori*. Because these drugs inhibit gastric acid secretion by more than 90 percent and frequently produce achlorhydria, they are reserved for patients who do not respond to less powerful drugs.

Pharmacodynamics

Proton pump inhibitors do not exhibit anticholinergic or histamine$_2$ blockade properties but suppress gastric acid secretion by inhibiting the hydrogen-potassium-ATPase (H^+-K^+-ATPase) system at the secretory surface of the gastric mucosa. They block the final step in gastric acid production. The effect is dose related and inhibits both basal and stimulated acid secretion. The decrease in acid secretion lasts for up to 72 hours after each dose. Gastric acid secretion begins within 3 to 5 days after the drug is discontinued and returns to normal within 1 to 2 weeks with **omeprazole (Prilosec)** and 4 weeks with **lansoprazole (Prevacid).**

Normal physiological effects related to suppression of gastric acid secretion result in decreased blood flow to the antrum, pylorus, and duodenal bulb. Increased serum pepsinogen levels and decreased pepsin activity also occur. As with other drugs that increase gastric pH, related increases in nitrate-reducing bacteria and elevation of nitrate concentration in gastric juice occur in pa-

tients with gastric ulcer. Compensatory increases in serum gastrin levels develop initially, but no further increase occurs with continued treatment, and there are no apparent ill effects from this increase.

Pharmacokinetics

Absorption and Distribution

Both of these drugs are acid-labile and so are formulated as enteric-coated granules (Table 18–25). Absorption is rapid and begins after the granules leave the stomach and reach the less acidic duodenum. Peak plasma concentrations are approximately proportional, but because of a saturable first-pass effect, **omeprazole** has a greater than linear response when given in doses above 40 mg.

Both drugs are distributed to the parietal cells of the stomach. They both cross the placenta. It is not known whether they are excreted in breast milk.

Metabolism and Excretion

The liver extensively metabolizes both drugs, and several metabolites have been identified. These metabolites appear to have little or no antisecretory activity. **Omeprazole** is metabolized by the CYP-450 system and may interact with other drugs also metabolized by this system. **Lansoprazole** is metabolized by the CYP-450 3A4 and 2C19 isoenzyme systems; however, it does not have clinically significant drug interactions related to this metabolic site. The plasma elimination half-life of these drugs does not reflect the duration of suppression of gastric acid secretion, apparently because of prolonged binding to the parietal H^+-K^+-ATPase enzyme.

Little unchanged drug is excreted in the urine, but 33 to 70 percent of metabolites are excreted in the urine.

Table 18–25. Pharmacokinetics: Proton Pump Inhibitors

Drug	Onset	Peak	Duration	Protein Binding	Bioavailability	Half-Life	Elimination
Lansoprazole	1 h	1.7 h	>24 h	97%	>80%	1.5 h; increases to 3.2–7.2 h in hepatic impairment	33% in urine; remainder in feces
Omeprazole	1 h	0.5–3.5 h	>72 h	95%	30–40%; increases to 100% in hepatic impairment	30–60 min; increases to 3 h in hepatic impairment	77% in urine; remainder in feces

The rest is excreted in feces. A significant biliary excretion route is implied, especially for **omeprazole.**

Pharmacotherapeutics

Precautions and Contraindications

Atrophic gastritis has been noted occasionally in patients taking **omeprazole** long term. Because of alterations in the pharmacokinetics of these drugs, they should be used cautiously with older adults and patients with hepatic insufficiency or renal impairment. No dosage adjustments are recommended for any of these patients, however.

Omeprazole is Pregnancy Category C. In animal studies, doses far in excess of those given to humans produced increased fetal lethality. There have been no adequate and well-controlled studies in pregnant women. Use in pregnancy only if the potential benefits outweigh the potential risks to the fetus.

Lansoprazole is Pregnancy Category B, but there have been no adequate and well-controlled studies in pregnant women for this drug, either. Use in pregnancy only if the potential benefits outweigh the potential risks to the fetus.

It is not known if these drugs are excreted in breast milk. The decision to discontinue the drug or discontinue nursing should take into account the importance of the drug to the mother.

The safety and efficacy of these drugs have not been established in children, and no dosage schedules are published for children.

Adverse Drug Reactions

Both of these drugs are generally well tolerated, and the adverse reactions that did occur in more than 1 percent of patients in clinical trials included dizziness, drowsiness, abdominal pain, constipation, diarrhea, and flatulence. It is difficult to determine if the GI-related symptoms were associated with the disease or the drug.

Drug Interactions

Both drugs have few drug interactions. Related to its use of the CYP-450 enzyme system, **omeprazole's** interactions include **benzodiazepines, phenytoin,** and **warfarin.** Both drugs interfere with absorption of drugs given orally that depend on an acidic gastric pH to be effective. These drugs include **ketoconazole, esters of ampicillin, digoxin,** and **iron salts.** These and other interactions are shown in Table 18–26.

Clinical Use and Dosing

DUODENAL AND GASTRIC ULCERS. Both drugs are used for treatment of active duodenal ulcer and active benign gastric ulcer. The once-daily dose is taken before a meal, preferably in the morning (Table 18–27). Treatment is for 4 to 8 weeks, although some patients require an additional 4 weeks for healing.

More than 90 percent of duodenal ulcers and 80 percent of gastric ulcers are thought to be related to infection with *H. pylori*. Eradication of this infection significantly affects healing and recurrence rates. The recurrence rate is 15 percent for patients taking **antimicrobial therapy** versus 60 to 100 percent recurrence for those with conventional **antisecretory therapy.** In light of these findings, the protocols that have been established use a multidrug combination of **antimicrobial** and **antisecretory therapy.** Some of these protocols include a **proton pump inhibitor.** Both **omeprazole** and **lansoprazole** can be used in these protocols. Treatment varies from daily dosing to tid dosing, and the length of therapy is 10 days to 4 weeks, depending on the protocol (Table 18–28). Each dose is taken before a meal.

GASTROESOPHAGEAL REFLUX DISEASE. Patients with GERD who do not respond adequately to lifestyle modification, **antacids,** and **histamine$_2$ blockers** can have their **histamine$_2$ blocker** replaced with a **proton pump inhibitor. Omeprazole** is approved for this indication. The once-daily dosing is taken before breakfast. The

Table 18–26. Drug Interactions: Proton Pump Inhibitors

Drug	Interacting Drug	Possible Effect	Implications
Lansoprazole	Theophylline	10% increase in theophylline clearance	Additional titration of theophylline dosage may be required.
Omeprazole	Clarithromycin	Coadministration may result in increased plasma levels of both drugs	This combination is among the FDA-approved treatment options for *H. pylori* eradication.
	Benzodiazepines, phenytoin, warfarin	103% increase in diazepam half-life; 15% reduced clearance of phenytoin; prolonged elimination of warfarin	Use lansoprazole or select a treatment regimen that does not require a proton pump inhibitor if the interacting drugs must be given.
	Enteric-coated aspirin	Increased rate of absorption of single-unit enteric-coated aspirin; intragastric release of aspirin	Separate doses by at least 1 h.
Both drugs	Sucralfate	Decreased absorption of proton pump inhibitor	Take proton pump inhibitor 30 min prior to sucralfate.
	Ketoconazole, esters of ampicillin, digoxin, iron salts	Proton pump inhibitors decrease absorption of these drugs	Avoid concurrent administration; for digoxin, monitor serum levels closely.

Table 18–27. Dosage Schedule: Proton Pump Inhibitors

Drug	Indication	Initial Dose	Maintenance Dose
Lansoprazole	Duodenal ulcer	15 mg qd for 4 wk *H. pylori:* Triple therapy: Lansoprazole 30 mg bid + amoxicillin 1 g bid + clarithromycin 500 mg tid for 10 d Double therapy: Lansoprazole 30 mg tid + amoxicillin 1 g tid for 14 d	15 mg qd
	Benign gastric ulcer	30 mg qd for <8 wk	
	Erosive esophagitis	30 mg qd for <8 wk	15 mg qd
	Hypersecretory disorders	60 mg qd	Up to 90 mg bid; doses >120 mg/d must be divided
Omeprazole	Duodenal ulcer	20 mg qd for 4–8 wk *H. pylori:* Triple therapy: Omeprazole 20 mg bid + clarithromycin 500 mg bid + amoxicillin 1 g bid for 10 d Double therapy: Omeprazole 40 qd + clarithromycin 500 mg tid for 14 d; then omeprazole 20 mg qd for 14 additional days	
	Benign gastric ulcer	40 mg qd for 4–8 wk	
	Erosive esophagitis	20 mg qd for 4–8 wk	20 mg qd
	GERD	20 mg qd for 4–8 wk	
	Hypersecretory disorders	60 mg qd	Up to 120 mg tid; doses >80 mg/d must be divided

Further discussion of multidrug treatment for *H. pylori* is found in Chapter 32.

Table 18–28. Available Dosage Forms: Proton Pump Inhibitors

Drug	Dosage Form	How Supplied
Lansoprazole (Prevacid)	Capsules, delayed-release: 15 mg, 30 mg	In bottles of 100, 1000 tablets
Omeprazole (Prilosec)	Capsules, delayed-release: 10 mg, 20 mg	In bottles of 100, 1000 tablets

length of therapy is 4 to 8 weeks. In the rare patient whose healing does not occur by then, an additional 4 weeks may be needed. The efficacy of these drugs beyond 8 weeks of therapy has not been established, although some providers do use them for longer periods. In the presence of erosive esophagitis, the dose is higher.

Lansoprazole has no specific indication for GERD, but it does have an indication for erosive esophagitis. The once-daily dosing is taken before breakfast. Treatment is for up to 8 weeks. For patients who do not heal within 8 weeks, an additional 8-week course can be considered.

HYPERSECRETORY CONDITIONS (INCLUDING ZOLLINGER-ELLISON SYNDROME). Both drugs can be used to treat these disorders. Doses are individualized and vary from 60 mg daily to 120 mg tid. Doses above 80 mg must be administered in divided doses. Some patients with Zollinger-Ellison syndrome have been treated continuously for more than 5 years.

Rational Drug Selection

DRUG INTERACTIONS. For patients taking drugs metabolized by the CYP 450 system, **lansoprazole** is a better choice. Although both drugs are metabolized by this system, **lansoprazole** appears to have no clinically significant drug interactions related to this metabolic site.

INDICATION. Only **omeprazole** has a published indication for GERD.

DIFFICULTY IN SWALLOWING. For patients with difficulty in swallowing, **lansoprazole** capsules can be opened and the intact granules sprinkled on 1 tablespoon of applesauce and swallowed immediately. Do not chew or crush the granules. The instructions with **omeprazole** specifically state not to open the capsule.

HELICOBACTER PYLORI TREATMENT. To increase adherence, choose the least complex regimen with the fewest adverse reactions that still has a high eradication rate. Chapter 32 has more discussion of this treatment.

Monitoring

The only monitoring relates to the disease process being treated. However, patients taking **proton pump inhibitors** to treat ulcers may be tested for *H. pylori* infec-

tion by urea breath testing. According to a study published in the *Annals of Internal Medicine* (Laine, Estrada, Trujillo, Knigge, & Fennerty, 1998), patients taking **proton pump inhibitors** should stop therapy for 2 weeks before undergoing urea breath testing to diagnose this infection. **Proton pump inhibitors** alone rarely eradicate *H. pylori* infection, but they can suppress it so that testing during **antisecretory therapy** may lead to false-negative results.

Patient Education

ADMINISTRATION. Patients should take the drug exactly as prescribed, even if they are feeling better. If a dose is missed, it should be taken as soon as the patient remembers it, unless it is almost time for the next dose. Do not double doses.

Both drugs are taken before a meal. Drugs taken once daily are preferably taken in the morning. Both drugs may safely be taken with **antacids**.

For patients with difficulty in swallowing, **lansoprazole** capsules can be opened and the intact granules sprinkled on 1 tablespoon of applesauce and swallowed immediately. Do not chew or crush the granules. Do not chew, crush, or open the **omeprazole** capsule.

ADVERSE REACTIONS. Both drugs may occasionally cause drowsiness or dizziness. Patients should avoid activities that require mental alertness until their response to the drug is known. Advise patients to promptly report to their health care provider the onset of black, tarry stool; diarrhea; abdominal pain; or persistent headache, which may indicate progression of the disease or adverse drug effects.

LIFESTYLE MANAGEMENT. Lifestyle modification is always attempted before drugs are used to treat GERD. They are also often used prior to treatment of the other indications for **proton pump inhibitors**. These modifications are discussed in the **prokinetic** drug section and in more detail in Chapter 32.

Laxatives

Constipation is a common affliction caused by everything from lack of sufficient fluids, fiber, and exercise to serious GI diseases to iatrogenic causes secondary to adverse reactions to drugs. It is among the most frequent reasons for self-medication and is particularly troublesome to older adults.

Treatment often takes the form of **laxative** use. More than $500 million is spent annually in the United States on **laxatives** (Goroll et al., 1995). The pathophysiology of constipation varies with its cause, and the action of the drug chosen to treat the constipation must also vary to match the cause. In light of these differences, six main classes of drugs are used to promote evacuation of the bowel. Each class is discussed in this section. Because each of these drugs has several brand names, only the generic name is used. Brand names are given in Table 18–32, where available dosage forms are presented.

Pharmacodynamics

Stimulants

This class of **laxative** has a direct action on intestinal mucosa by stimulating the myenteric plexus. These drugs facilitate the release of prostaglandins and increase cyclic adenosine monophosphate (cAMP) concentration. This increase in cAMP increases the secretion of electrolytes and stimulates peristalsis. Bile must be present for one of the drugs in this class, **phenolphthalein**, to produce its effects. Other drugs in this class include **cascara, senna, bisacodyl,** and **castor oil.**

This group of drugs is used most often for treatment of constipation associated with reduced mobility, constipating drugs, reduced motility, neurogenic bowel secondary to spinal cord injury, and irritable bowel syndrome. They are also used to prepare the bowel for radiological or surgical procedures.

Osmotics

This class exerts its effects mainly by drawing water into the intestinal lumen to increase intraluminal pressure. These drugs are hypertonic salt-based solutions that cause the diffusion of fluid from the plasma into the intestine to dilute the solution to an isotonic state. The **magnesium salts** also cause an increase in the release of cholecytokinin by the duodenum. **Sulfate salts** are considered the most powerful. Drugs in this class include **magnesium sulfate, magnesium hydroxide, magnesium citrate, sodium phosphate,** and **polystyrene glycol electrolyte solution.**

This group of drugs is used to cleanse the entire GI tract for diagnostic purposes, to flush poisons from the system, and to remove parasites. They are useful for the last purpose because they produce a liquid stool without rupturing the ova of the parasite.

Bulk-Producing

These **laxatives** are the safest and most physiological because their action is similar to that achieved by increasing fiber in the diet. They do not hinder absorption of nutrients and are less likely to be habit-forming. This group of drugs consists of natural and semisynthetic polysaccharides and cellulose. When combined with water in the intestine, they produce mechanical distention resulting in an increase in peristalsis. Drugs in this class include **psyllium, methylcellulose,** and **polycarbophil.**

This group of drugs is used for long-term management of simple, chronic constipation, especially if it is related to low fiber intake in the diet. They are also useful in situations where straining at stool is to be avoided and in the management of chronic, watery diarrhea.

Lubricants

Mineral oil is the only drug in this class. Its action is to retard colonic absorption of fecal water and soften the stool. It does not stimulate peristalsis. It is used to soften stool associated with fecal impaction. A major concern with the use of **mineral oil** is that it may decrease absorption of fat-soluble vitamins.

Surfactants

These drugs are often referred to as "stool softeners" because they facilitate admixture of fat and water into the stool and produce an emollient action that reduces surface tension. Drugs in this class are the **docusate** compounds: **docusate sodium, docusate calcium,** and **docusate potassium.**

They are most beneficial when feces are hard or dry, in anorectal conditions where passage for firm stool is painful, and in situations when straining at stool is to be avoided.

Hyperosmolar

The last class of **laxatives** is often listed as "miscellaneous," but they share a similar mechanism of action. **Glycerin** produces local irritation and, as a hyperosmotic compound, draws water from the extravascular spaces into the lumen of the intestine, resulting in more liquid stool. **Lactulose** is a hyperosmotic disaccharide. In the colon, resident bacteria transform the drug into lactic acid and acetic and formic acids. These acids exert an osmotic effect by drawing water from the extravascular spaces into the intestinal lumen.

Glycerin is used to treat fecal impaction and patients with neurogenic bowel, in which the bowel is filled with feces that cannot be evacuated. **Lactulose** is used to treat chronic constipation in older adults, but it also is the only laxative used to treat hepatic encephalopathy. It lowers the pH of the colon, which in turn inhibits the diffusion of ammonia across colonic membranes.

Pharmacokinetics

Absorption and Distribution

Absorption is highly variable between classes from no absorption for the **bulk-forming laxatives** to 3 percent or less for all other classes except the **magnesium salts**, where up to 30 percent may be absorbed (Table 18–29). **Magnesium salts** are widely distributed, cross the placenta, and enter breast milk. Small amounts of metabolites of **bisacodyl** have been found in breast milk. The remaining drugs in each class have no distribution, with their action local in the intestine.

Metabolism and Excretion

Locally acting drugs have no specific metabolism and are excreted in feces. The liver metabolizes small amounts of **bisacodyl**. **Glycerin** is 80 percent metabolized by the liver and 10 to 20 percent by the kidney. **Magnesium salts** are metabolized by the liver and excreted primarily by the kidney.

Pharmacotherapeutics

Precautions and Contraindications

Precautions and contraindications vary by class of **laxative**, but all share the contraindication of use in the presence of nausea, vomiting, or undiagnosed abdominal pain or if bowel obstruction is suspected or diagnosed. Other precautions and contraindications are specific to a class or a drug.

STIMULANTS. **Bisacodyl** is to be used with caution in the presence of severe cardiovascular disease. **Castor oil** is contraindicated in the presence of fat-soluble worms. The extract of **cascara sagrada** contains **alcohol** and should be avoided by people with **alcohol** intolerance.

Castor oil **is contraindicated in pregnancy because it has been associated with induction of uterine contractions.** *Cascara derivatives* **are Pregnancy Category C.** *Bisacodyl* **is safe to use in pregnancy and is listed as Pregnancy Category B.**

Cascara sagrada is excreted in breast milk and may increase the incidence of diarrhea in the nursing infant.

OSMOTICS. **Magnesium salts** are contraindicated in the presence of any degree of renal insufficiency because the kidney may be unable to excrete excessive magnesium ions. Hypermagnesemia, hypocalcemia, and heart block also contraindicate their use. Because large quantities of **polyethylene glycol** or **electrolyte solution** must be taken, these salts are used cautiously for patients with diminished gag reflex unless it is being administered by nasogastric tube.

Magnesium salts **are Pregnancy Category A.** *Polyethylene glycol* **or** *electrolyte solution* **is Pregnancy Category C.**

BULK-FORMING. These drugs are used with caution for patients with a narrowed esophageal or intestinal lumen. Some dosage forms contain sugar or salt and should be avoided by patients who must restrict these substances.

Bulk-forming agents **are not given a specific preg-**

Table 18–29. Pharmacokinetics: Selected Laxatives

Drug Class	Onset	Peak	Site of Action	Elimination
Stimulants	6–10 h 0.25–1 h bisacodyl PR 2–6 h castor oil	Unknown	Colon Colon Small intestine	Mostly in feces
Osmotics (magnesium salts)	0.5–3 h	Unknown	Small and large intestine	Primarily in urine
Bulk-forming	12–24 h	2–3 d	Small and large intestine	In feces
Lubricants	6–8 h PO 2–15 min PR	Unknown	Colon Colon	In feces
Surfactants	24–48 h PO 2–15 min PR	Unknown	Small and large intestine	Small amount absorbed is eliminated in bile
Hyperosmolar	0.25–0.5 h glycerin 24–48 h lactulose	Unknown Unknown	Colon Colon	Unknown Small amount absorbed is excreted unchanged in urine

PR = per rectum.

nancy category but have been safely used during pregnancy.

LUBRICANTS. Lipid pneumonia has occurred in patients who aspirated **mineral oil.** The very young, older adults, people with dysphagia, and debilitated patients are at highest risk.

Although no specific pregnancy category is listed for *mineral oil,* it should be avoided during pregnancy because chronic use decreases the absorption of fat-soluble vitamins and causes hypoprothrombinemia in the newborn.

SURFACTANTS. **Docusate** compounds have no specific contraindications or precautions. **They have not been given a specific pregnancy category but have been safely used during pregnancy.**

HYPEROSMOLAR. Both **hyperosmolar** agents are used with caution in the presence of volume depletion. Older adults are especially at risk for dehydration. Hyperglycemia has been noted in some patients taking **lactulose,** and it is used with caution in the presence of diabetes mellitus.

Glycerin is Pregnancy Category C; *lactulose* is Pregnancy Category B. It is not known if *lactulose* is excreted in breast milk.

Other general precautions include the following:

1. Abuse and dependency: Chronic use of **laxatives,** particularly **stimulants,** may lead to **laxative** dependency, which in turn may result in fluid and electrolyte imbalances, steatorrhea, osteomalacia, and vitamin and mineral deficiencies. The "laxative abuse syndrome" is most commonly seen in women with depression, personality disorders, or anorexia nervosa. Cathartic colon can also result. The pathology resembles ulcerative colitis.
2. Tartrazine sensitivity: Some of these products contain tartrazine, which may cause allergic types of reactions, including bronchial asthma, in susceptible individuals. Although the incidence of this sensitivity in the general population is low, it is frequently seen in patients who also have **aspirin** sensitivity.

Adverse Drug Reactions

Adverse drug reactions are most commonly extensions of the drug's action and include excessive bowel activity, cramping, flatulence, and bloating. Perianal irritation may also develop.

Allergic reactions such as urticaria, dermatitis, rhinitis, and bronchospasm have occurred when patients accidentally inhaled **bulk-forming laxatives. Phenolphthalein** may cause a skin hypersensitivity characterized by a fixed drug eruption. Discontinue the drug if this occurs.

Drug Interactions

Because most **laxatives** have local activity and limited absorption, few drug interactions occur. Table 18–30 lists those drug interactions.

Clinical Use and Dosing

All **laxatives** are used to treat constipation or to prepare the bowel for a procedure. Specific uses for each class are discussed in the pharmacodynamics section. Table 18–31 lists the dosing schedules for each indication.

Rational Drug Selection

The choice of drug to treat constipation depends on the severity of the constipation, the reason for it, and the speed with which resolution is needed. Drugs are used only after the reason for the constipation has been corrected if possible (e.g., stop or decrease the dose of the drug that induced the constipation). Indications for the use of each class of drug are presented in the pharmacodynamics section.

RAPID RESPONSE AND SHORT TERM. **Stimulants** are the drug of choice when rapid response is needed. All are equally effective. They should be used only for short-term, however. Safer drugs can be used for long-term management when speed is not the main issue. The choice of drug depends largely on cost.

Osmotic and **surfactant laxatives** can also be used in this instance. **Magnesium hydroxide** is generally the preferred **osmotic** because of its milder action. **Docusate sodium** is the preferred **surfactant.**

SLOWER RESPONSE AND LONG TERM. **Bulk-forming laxatives** are the drug of choice when rapid response is not needed and long-term management with the least adverse reactions is desired. They are especially suited to older adults. The choice of product depends upon the patient's acceptance of texture and taste. **Lactulose** can be used if the **bulk-forming laxatives** do not work or are not well tolerated. It works well with older adults.

SPECIAL INDICATIONS. **Polyethylene glycol** or **electrolyte solution** is the best drug for cleansing the bowel in preparation for radiologic or surgical procedures. It is very effective and does not produce electrolyte disturbances.

Lactulose is effective in reducing ammonia levels in the blood and brain with patients who have hepatic encephalopathy. It prevents absorption of ammonia from the intestine and produces diarrhea that flushes the ammonia out. Dietary adjustments to reduce ammonia production are simultaneously implemented.

PREGNANCY. For pregnant women, *bulk-forming laxatives* and *surfactants* are safe and effective for reg-

Table 18–30. Drug Interactions: Selected Laxatives

Drug	Interacting Drug	Possible Effect	Implications
All laxatives	Other orally administered drugs	May decrease absorption of other orally administered drugs because of increased motility and decreased transit time	Separate administration by at least 1 h
Bisacodyl	Antacids, histamine$_2$ blockers, proton pump inhibitors	May remove enteric coating of tablets	Separate administration or select different laxative
Lactulose	Antimicrobials	Concurrent use may decrease effectiveness of lactulose used in hepatic encephalopathy	If concurrent use cannot be avoided, dosage adjustments of lactulose may be required
	Antacids	May decrease the effect of lactulose on colon pH	Separate doses by at least 1 h
Magnesium salts	Fluoroquinolones, nitrofurantoin, tetracycline	May decrease absorption of these drugs	Avoid concurrent administration
Mineral oil	Docusate compounds	Concurrent use may increase mineral oil absorption	Avoid concurrent use
	Foods	May decrease absorption of vitamins A, D, E, K	
Psyllium	Digoxin, salicylates, warfarin	May decrease absorption of these drugs	Separate administration by at least 1 h and give drug before psyllium

ular use throughout pregnancy. *Magnesium salts* are Pregnancy Category A, and can be used intermittently.

The precautions and contraindications section lists the pregnancy categories for other drugs, including those that should not be used during pregnancy.

Monitoring

In general, the monitoring for patients taking **laxatives** for more than 6 months includes laboratory assessment of fluid and electrolyte status, especially potassium. For patients taking **lactulose** for hepatic encephalopathy, the overall management of this disorder requires careful monitoring because it is a serious disease with a high potential for complications. Monitoring includes serum electrolytes (e.g., hypokalemia and hypernatremia). For older adults taking **lactulose** for more than 6 months to manage their constipation, laboratory assessment of potassium, chloride, and carbon dioxide should be done periodically or with any indication of fluid or electrolyte disturbance.

Clinical Pearls

POLYTHYLENE GLYCOL/ELECTROLYTE SOLUTION

The taste is quite salty, and many patients find it difficult to consume the required amount of volume in the required amount of time. Place the container of solution in ice in a basin. Do not pour it over ice, which will melt and increase the volume the patient must consume. Have the patient drink 240 mL of fluid each 10 minutes and give them a Tic-Tac or similar small mint-flavored hard candy to suck on between glasses of the drug. This reduces the salty taste in the mouth and makes the drug more palatable.

Table 18–31. Dosage Schedule: Selected Laxatives

Drug	Indication	Dose	Notes
Bisacodyl	Constipation	*Adults and children >12 y:* Tablets: 10–15 mg once daily PR: 10 mg once daily *Children 2–11 y:* Tablets: 5 mg (0.3 mg/kg) once daily PR: 5 mg once daily *Children <2 y:* PR: 5 mg single dose	Up to 30 mg have been used as preparation for bowel procedure
Cascara sagrada	Constipation	*Adults and children >12 y:* Tablets: 300 mg–1 g once daily Extract tablet: 200–400 mg qd Fluid extract: 0.5–1.5 mL qd Aromatic fluid extract: 2–6 mL qd *Children 2–11 y:* Tablets: 150–500 mg once daily Extract tablet: 100–200 mg once daily Fluid extract: 0.25–0.75 mL once daily Aromatic fluid extract: 1–3 mL once daily *Children <2 y:* Fluid extract: 0.12–0.38 mL once daily Aromatic fluid extract: 0.5–1.5 mL once daily	Tablets and liquids come in combinations with docusate and milk of magnesia
Castor oil	Constipation	*Adults and children >12 y:* 15–60 mL in a single dose *Children 2–11 y:* 5–15 mL in a single dose	
Docusate	Constipation	*Calcium* *Adults:* 240 mg once daily *Children >6 y:* 50–150 mg once daily *Potassium* *Adults:* 100–300 mg once daily *Children >6 y:* 100 mg once daily at bedtime *Sodium* *Adults and children >12 y:* 50–500 mg once daily *Children 6–11 y:* 40–120 mg once daily *Children 3–6 y:* 20–60 mg once daily *Children <3 y:* 10–40 mg Suppository: *Adults:* 50–100 mg or 1 suppository	
Glycerin PR	Constipation	*Adults and children >6 y:* 2–3 g as suppository or 5–15 mg as enema *Children <6 y:* 1–1.7 g as a suppository or 2–5 mL as enema	

Continued on next page

Table 18–31. Dosage Schedule: Selected Laxatives *(continued)*

Drug	Indication	Dose	Notes
Lactulose	Constipation	*Adults:* 15–30 mL once daily *Children:* 7.5 mL once daily	May use up to 60 mg/d; unlabeled use.
	Hepatic encephalopathy	*Adults:* 30–45 mL tid–qid *Children and adolescents:* 40–90 mL daily in divided doses *Infants:* 2.5–10 mL daily in divided doses	May be given q1–2h initially; goal is 2–3 soft stools/d; discontinue if diarrhea develops.
Magnesium salts	Constipation	*Sulfate granules* *Adults and children >12 y:* 10–15 g in glass of water *Children 6–11 y:* 5–10 g in glass of water *Hydroxide (milk of magnesia)* *Adults and children >12 y:* 30–60 mL once daily (in concentrate: 10–20 mL once daily) *Children 6–11 y:* 15–30 mL in single or divided doses *Children 2–5 y:* 5–15 mg in divided doses	
	Bowel prep	*Citrate* *Adults and children >12 y:* 240 mL *Children 6–11 y:* 100 mL	
Phenolphthalein	Constipation	*Adults:* 60–194 mg at bedtime	
Polyethylene glycol/ electrolyte solution	Bowel prep	*Adults:* 240 mL every 10 min (up to 4 L) until fecal discharge is clear with no solid material *Children:* 25–40 mg/kg/h until fecal discharge is clear with no solid material	Tastes salty, making it difficult to take. Ice it. May suck on hard candy or breath mints to make more palatable
Psyllium	Constipation	*Adults:* 1–2 tsp/packet/wafer (3–6 g psyllium) in or with a full glass of liquid bid–tid *Children >6 y:* 1 tsp/packet/wafer (1.5–3 g psyllium) in or with 1/2–1 glass of liquid bid–tid	Up to 30 g daily in divided doses. Up to 15 g daily in divided doses.
Senna	Constipation	*Adults and children >12 y:* 360 mg–2 g at bedtime *Children 6–11 y:* 50% of adult dose *Children 1–5 y:* 33% of adult dose Rectal: *Adults and children >12 y:* 30 mg qd–bid	Fletcher's Castoria lists a children's dose of 10–15 mL (6–15 y) and 5–10 mL (2–5 y)

PR = per rectum.

Table 18–32. Available Dosage Forms: Selected Laxatives

Drug	Dosage Form	How Supplied
Bisacodyl (Dulcagen)	Tablets: 5 mg Suppositories: 10 mg	In bottles of 100 tablets In 12 individually foil wrapped
(Dulcolax)	Tablets: 5 mg Suppositories: 10 mg	In bottles of 10, 25, 50, 100, 1000 tablets In 2, 4, 8, 16 , 50 individually foil wrapped
(Fleet)	Tablets: 5 mg Suppositories: 10 mg	In bottles of 24 tablets In 4 individually foil wrapped
Cascara sagrada	Tablets: 325 mg Aromatic fluid extract	In bottles of 100 tablets In 120 mL and in pints
Docusate calcium (Surfak)	Capsules: 50 mg Capsules: 240 mg	In bottles of 30, 100 capsules In bottles of 7, 30, 100, 500 capsules
Docusate potassium (Diocto-K, Dialose, Kasof)	Capsules: 100 mg Capsules: 240 mg	In bottles of 36, 100 capsules (Dialose), 100 capsules (Diocto-K) In bottles of 30, 60 capsules (Kasof)
Docusate sodium (Colace)	Capsules: 50 mg, 100 mg Syrup: 60 mg/15 mL Liquid: 150 mg/15 mL	In bottles of 30, 60, 250, 1000 tablets In 240 and 480 mL In 30 and 480 mL (with calibrated dropper)
(Generic)	Capsules: 50 mg Capsules: 100 mg and 250 mg Syrup: 50 mg/15 mL Syrup: 60 mg/15 mL	In bottles of 100 capsules In bottles of 100, 1000 capsules In 15 and 30 mL In pints and gallons
Glycerin (Sani-Supp)	Adult suppositories Pediatric suppositories	In 10, 25, 50 individually foil wrapped In 10, 25 individually foil wrapped
(Generic)	Adult suppositories Pediatric suppositories	In 10, 12, 25, 50, 100 individually foil wrapped In 10, 12, 25 individually foil wrapped
Lactulose (Cephulac, Chronulac, Enulose)	Syrup: 10 g lactulose/15 mL	In 480 mL and 1.9 L (Cephulac) In 240 and 960 mL (Chronulac) In pint and 1.89 L (Enulose)
(Generic)	Syrup: 10 g lactulose/15 mL	In 240 and 960 mL
Magnesium sulfate (Epsom salts)	Granules: 40 mEq Mg^{2+} per 5g	In 150- and 240-g packets and 4 lb
Magnesium hydroxide (Milk of Magnesia)	Chewable tablets: 300 mg and 600 mg Liquid: 80 mEq Mg^{2+} per 30 mL Concentrate:	In bottles of 100 and 200 tablets In 180, 360, 480, 960 mL In 100, 400, 480 mL (lemon flavor); 240 mL (strawberry and orange creme flavors)
Magnesium citrate	Liquid: 77 mEq Mg^{2+} per 100 mL	In 240, 296, 300 mL
Phenolphthalein (Ex-Lax)	Tablets: 90 mg Chocolate tablets: 90 mg	In 8, 30, 60 tablets In 6, 18, 48, 72 chewable tablets
(Feen-a-Mint)	Tablets: 97.2 mg Chocolate tablets: 65 mg Gum: 97.2 mg/piece	In 12, 30, 60 regular tablets; 20 chewable tablets In 4, 18, 36 chocolate-mint-flavored chewable tablets In 5, 16, 40 peppermint-flavored pieces of gum

Continued on next page

Table 18–32. Available Dosage Forms: Selected Laxatives *(continued)*

Drug	Dosage Form	How Supplied
Polyethylene glycol/ electrolyte solution (Colyte, GoLYTEly)	In oral solution or powder for oral solution	In gallon containers
Psyllium (Fiberall, Konsyl, Metamucil)	Powder: 3.4 g psyllium/5 mL	In 284 and 426 g (Fiberall) In 210, 420, 630, 960 g and 30, 100 unit-dose packets (Metamucil) In 325, 500 g (Konsyl)
	Powder: 6 g psyllium/5 mL Wafers: 1.7 g psyllium Wafers: 3.4 g psyllium Effervescent powder: 3.4 g/5 mL	In 300, 450 g and 25 unit-dose 6 g packets In 24 wafers (Metamucil) In 14 wafers (Fiberall) In 30, 100 single-dose packets (Metamucil)
Senna (Senokot, Fletcher's Castoria)	Tablets: 187 mg Granules: 326 mg Syrup: 218 mg/5 mL Liquid: 33.3 mg/mL	In 20, 50, 100, 1000 tablets (Senokot) In 60, 170, 340 g (Senokot) In 60, 240 mL (Senokot) In 75, 150 mL

Patient Education

Laxatives should not be taken in the presence of nausea, vomiting, or abdominal pain. These symptoms may indicate serious disorders that may be the cause of the constipation and that require a workup. Patients should not take a **laxative** but instead contact their health care provider.

ADMINISTRATION. Rapid-acting **laxatives** are best taken in the morning; slower-acting ones are best taken at bedtime. Taking a **laxative** on an empty stomach and with a full glass of water will produce more rapid results. Do not crush or chew enteric-coated tablets (Table 18–32). Liquids can be given with fruit juice. For infants, taking liquids with fruit juice or infant formula may mask any unpleasant taste. Suspensions are shaken before taking. Effervescent tablets are dissolved in a full glass of water before taking.

Suppositories are usually given close to the time a bowel movement is desired. Lubricate them with a water-soluble lubricant and insert far enough into the rectum to pass the internal rectal sphincter. Encourage the patient to retain the suppository for 15 to 30 minutes before expelling.

Some liquid **laxatives** have special storage requirements. **Magnesium citrate** is refrigerated to ensure potency and palatability.

ADVERSE REACTIONS. The most common adverse drug reactions are excessive bowel activity, cramping, flatulence, and bloating. Perianal irritation may also occur.

Allergic reactions such as a rash, rhinitis, and bronchospasm have occurred when patients accidentally inhaled **bulk-forming laxatives.** Be careful when pouring the powder to avoid this possibility. **Phenolphthalein** may cause a skin hypersensitivity rash. Advise the patient to notify the health care provider if this occurs. The

drug is discontinued and a different **laxative** chosen if the need for a **laxative** continues.

Teach the patient the indications of a fluid or electrolyte disturbance and have them report these symptoms promptly.

LIFESTYLE MANAGEMENT. Prevention is the key with regard to constipation. Lifestyle management should be a major focus. Stress the need for adequate fluids, fiber, and exercise. **Laxatives** are last-resort and temporary measures. They are not intended for long-term management in most cases.

Misconceptions about bowel function should be corrected. Different people have different bowel patterns, all of which may be normal and not signal pathology. Stressing this point is especially important for older adults, who were often taught in their youth that maintenance of health depended on having one bowel movement every day.

Constipation in children may be a control issue or signal pathology. Discuss this topic with the parents. A trial of a **laxative** concurrently with behavior modification is appropriate, but the child needs to be monitored for the need for referral for a GI workup.

REFERENCES

Ault, D., & Schmidt, D. (1998). Diagnosis and management of gastroesophageal reflux in infants and children. *Nurse Practitioner,* 23(60), 78–100.

Blaser, M. (1999). In the world of black and white, *Helicobacter pylori* is gray. *Annals of Internal Medicine,* 130(8), 695–697.

Caeiro, J., & DuPont, H. (1998). Management of travellers' diarrhea. *Drugs,* 56(1), 73–81.

Carlson, E. (1998). Irritable bowel syndrome. *Nurse Practitioner,* 23(1), 82–91.

Centers for Disease Control and Prevention. (1999). *Helicobacter py-*

lori: Fact sheet for health care providers. *http://www.cdc.gov/nci-dod/dbmd/hpylori.htm*.

Chan, F., Sung, J., Chung, S., To, K., Yung, M., Leung, V., Lee, Y., Chan, C., Li, E., & Woo, J. (1997). Randomized trial of eradication of *Helicobacter pylori* before non-steroidal anti-inflammatory drug therapy to prevent peptic ulcers. *Lancet, 350,* 975–979.

Chiba, N., DeGara, C., Wilkinson, J, & Hunt, R. (1997). Speed of healing and symptoms relief in grade II to IV gastroesophageal reflux disease: A meta-analysis. *Gastroenterology, 112*(6), 1798–1810.

Deglin, J., & Vallerand, A. (1998). *Davis' drug guide for nurses* (6th ed.). Philadelphia: F. A. Davis.

Drewitz, D., Sampliner, R., & Garewal, H. (1997). The incidence of adenocarcinoma in Barrett's esophagus: A prospective study of 170 patients followed 4.8 years. *American Journal of Gastroenterology, 92,* 212–215.

Goroll, A., May, L., & Mulley, A. Jr. (1995). *Primary care medicine* (3rd ed.). Philadelphia: Lippincott.

Kastrup, E. (1998). *Facts and comparisons.* St. Louis: Facts and Comparisons.

Katzung, B. (1998). *Basic and clinical pharmacology* (7th ed.). Stamford, CT: Appleton & Lange.

Khuroo, M., Yattoo, G., Javid, G., Khan, B., Shah, A., Gulzar, G., & Sodi, J. (1997). A comparison of omeprazole and placebo for bleeding peptic ulcer. *New England Journal of Medicine, 336*(15), 1054–1058.

Laine, L., Estrada, R., Trujillo, M., Knigge, K., & Fennerty, M. (1998). Effect of proton-pump inhibitor therapy on diagnostic testing for *Helicobacter pylori. Annals of Internal Medicine, 129*(7), 547–550.

Laine, L., Frantz, J., Baker, A., & Neil, G. (1997). A United States multicenter trial of dual and proton pump inhibitor-based triple therapies for *Helicobacter pylori. Alimentary Pharmacology Therapeutics, 11*(5), 913–917.

Middlemiss, C. (1997). Gastroesophageal reflux disease: A common condition in the elderly. *Nurse Practitioner, 22*(11), 51–59.

Navuluri, R., & Yue, S. (1999). Understanding peptic ulcer disease pharmacotherapeutics. *Nurse Practitioner, 24*(3), 128–132.

Nefesoglu, F., Ayanoglu-Dulger, G., Ulusoy, N., & Imeryuz, N. (1998). Interaction of omeprazole with enteric-coated salicylate tablets. *International Journal of Clinical Pharmacology and Therapeutics, 36*(10), 549–553.

Schmidt, B. (1999). *Instructions for pediatric patients* (2nd ed.). Philadelphia: Saunders.

Tamkin, G. (1998). An approach to diarrhea. *Emergency Medicine, 30*(6), 16–36.

Tucker, K., & Schumann, L. (1999). Gastroesophageal reflux disease. *Clinical Advisor, 2*(4), 52–58.

Van der Hulst, R., Rauws, E., Koycu, B., Keller, J., Bruno, M., Tijssen, J., & Tytgat, G. (1997). Prevention of ulcer recurrence after eradication of *Helicobacter pylori:* A prospective long-term follow-up study. *Gastroenterology, 113*(4), 1082–1086.

Yamamoto, T., Takano, K., Sanaka, M., Kuyama, Y., Yamanaka, M., Koike, Y., & Mineshita, S. (1998). Pharmacokinetic characteristics of cisapride in elderly patients. *International Journal of Clinical Pharmacology and Therapeutics, 36*(8), 432–434.

CHAPTER 19

·······

Drugs Affecting the Endocrine System

Biophosphonates

Bone is dynamic tissue that undergoes a continuous process of resorption and formation (remodeling) throughout life. Under normal physiological states, the two processes are about equal. Skeletal mass is usually maximal at about age 35 and declines in women after age 40 and men after age 50. The rate of decline becomes most rapid in women within 2 years of menopause, with one-third to one-half of all bone that will be lost going during the first 5 years after menopause. As the life expectancy of women reaches the mid-80s, osteoporosis in perimenopausal women takes on epidemic proportions, especially among white women in industrial societies. The femoral neck and lumbar vertebrae lose the most. Cortical (compact) bone, which is 80 percent of the skeleton, is lost less rapidly than cancellous (spongy) bone. It is estimated that 24 million Americans have osteoporosis, of whom 80 percent are women. Chapter 48 discusses this concern as it relates to women's health.

In addition to normal aging, pathophysiological conditions can also alter the balance between resorption and formation. Even a minor imbalance can have devastating effects. For example, if bone resorption exceeds formation by only 2 percent per year, in 20 years 40 percent of skeletal mass will be lost. Malignancy, syndromes of ectopic calcification, and Paget's disease are examples of pathological conditions associated with altered bone remodeling.

Pharmacodynamics

The remodeling cycle is initiated by osteoclastic activity. In response to microfractures and other damage associated with normal wear and tear, osteoclasts are drawn to the damaged area of the trabecula, attach to its surface, and resorb the damaged and surrounding bone, creating a resorption pit (Fig. 19–1). Resorption is accomplished by pseudopodia, which attach tightly to the bone surface and secrete acids and enzymes that dissolve bone. The osteoclasts then leave the area and osteoblasts move in, line up to cover the surface of the pit, and form new bone. **Biophosphonates** adhere tightly to bone and, by inhibiting osteoclastic activity, are potent inhibitors of both normal and abnormal bone resorption. Among this group of drugs, **etidronate (Didronel)** reduces both bone resorption and bone formation because formation is coupled with resorption. **Pamidronate (Aredia)** and **risedronate (Actonel)** inhibit bone resorption without inhibiting bone formation and mineralization. **Alendronate (Fosamax)** is a highly selective inhibitor of bone resorption and is 100 to 500 times more potent than the other drugs. **Tiludronate (Skelid)** inhibits osteoclastic activity through two different mechanisms. It inhibits protein-tyrosine-phosphatase, resulting in detachment of osteoclasts from the bone surface, and it inhibits the osteoclastic proton pump. Because **pamidronate** is available only in parenteral form, it is not discussed here.

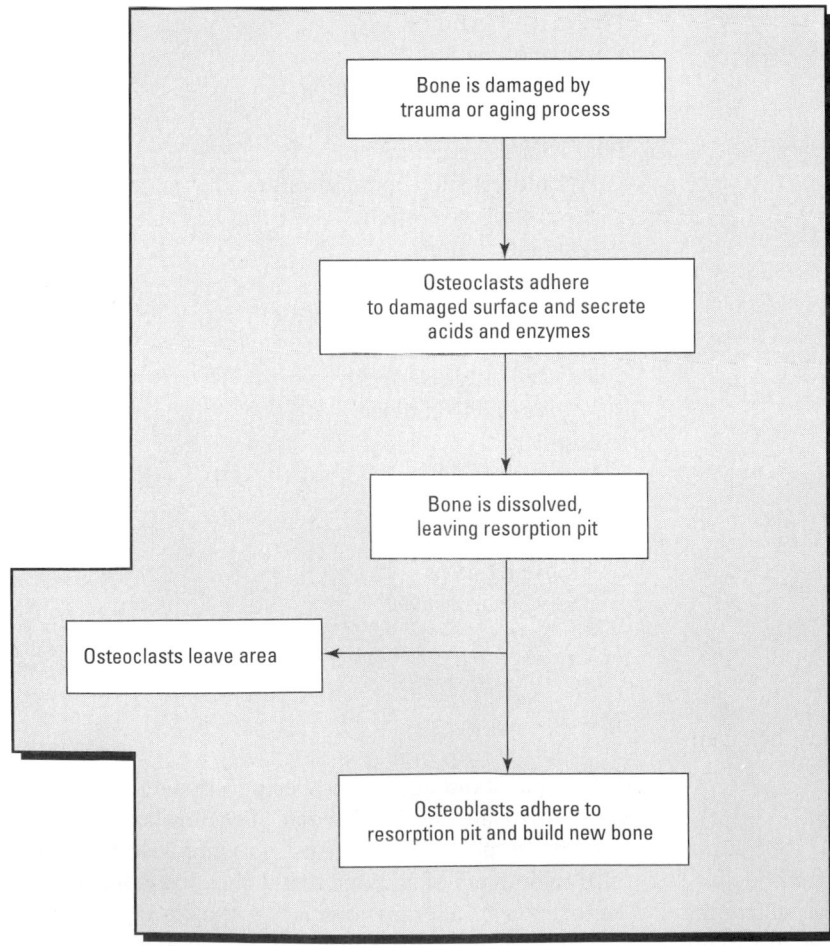

Figure 19–1. Bone remodeling. Damaged bone sections are removed by osteoclasts that use pseudopods to attach to bone surface. Bone is dissolved, leaving a resorption pit. The osteoclasts then leave the site of damage. Osteoblasts enter the resorption pit and build new bone. The process takes 4 to 5 months.

Pharmacokinetics

Absorption and Distribution

Despite the gastric irritation associated with all **biophosphonates,** they must be taken with the patient upright and fasting. Absorption and bioavailability of oral doses are significantly reduced by the presence in the gut of food or other preparations containing divalent cations. To enhance gastric emptying, the patient takes the drug with 8 oz of water. No other food or drink should be ingested, and the patient must remain upright for at least half an hour. Table 19–1 shows the effect of food, coffee, and juice on bioavailability.

These drugs are all mainly distributed to bone. Their terminal half-life in bone is exceedingly long, varying from more than 10 years for **alendronate** to more than 90 days for **etidronate.** The half-life of **risedronate** is much shorter at 220 hours, but this time period is thought to represent the dissociation of this drug from the bone surface, rather than its time within the bone. Their volumes of distribution exclusive of bone vary significantly from 28 L/kg or more for **alendronate** to 1.3 L/kg for **etidronate.**

Etidronate **is listed as Pregnancy Category B; all others are Pregnancy Category C.** *Drug Facts and Comparisons* **(1998) states that there are no adequate and well-controlled studies in pregnant women and recommends use of all** *biophosphonates* **only when they are clearly needed and the benefits to the mother outweigh the potential hazards to the fetus.** It is not known whether these drugs are excreted in breast milk. *Alendronate* is contraindicated in breastfeeding, and the others are to be used with extreme caution.

Safety and efficacy in children have not been established, but children have been treated with **etidronate** at doses recommended for adults to prevent heterotopic ossifications or soft tissue calcifications. The epiphyseal changes that occurred were reversible with discontinuation of the drug.

Metabolism and Excretion

There is no evidence that any of the **biophosphonates** are systemically metabolized. Drug that is not distributed to bone is largely excreted in the urine. Because of the fairly exclusive renal excretion and the high volumes of distribution exclusive of bone, these drugs are not recommended for patients with moderate to severe renal impairment (serum creatinine more than 4.9 and creatinine clearance [CCr] less than 35 cc/min), and dosage adjustments may be necessary if the drug must be given.

Pharmacotherapeutics

Precautions and Contraindications

There are no absolute contraindications. Cautious use is recommended for patients with gastrointestinal (GI) dis-

orders. **Etidronate** has been withheld from patients with enterocolitis because diarrhea has occurred in some patients, particularly at high doses.

Etidronate has also been associated with fractures in patients with Paget's disease when they are given high doses or when therapy lasts longer than 6 months. These patients must be carefully monitored with x-rays and laboratory work to assess for these lesions. **Alendronate** is not recommended for postmenopausal women concurrently on hormone replacement therapy. Because there is a risk for hypocalcemia with all **biophosphonates,** adequate nutrition with special attention to calcium and vitamin D is stressed.

Adverse Drug Reactions

Adverse drug reactions for all **biophosphonates** have been GI, including abdominal pain, nausea, flatulence, constipation/diarrhea, acid regurgitation, and taste perversion. Other GI reactions include esophageal ulcer formation and gastritis. These reactions are seen more often in patients with Paget's disease. Constipation and diarrhea were more common with **risedronate.** Rarely were any of these drugs discontinued because of these adverse reactions.

Another common adverse drug reaction for all biophosphonates is musculoskeletal pain. Once again, it was more common for patients with Paget's disease and more common with **risedronate.** In higher doses, pain incidence also increased to an occurrence of about 20 percent for patients taking **etidronate.** Musculoskeletal pain occurred in about 6 percent of patients taking **alendronate.**

Drug Interactions

Because of these drugs' adverse reactions on the GI tract, drug interactions are most common with other drugs that affect the GI tract. **Ranitidine (Zantac),** for example, doubles **alendronate** bioavailability. It is not known whether other **histamine$_2$ blocking agents** and other **biophosphonates** may have similar interactions. **Calcium supplements** and **antacids** interfere with **biophosphonate** absorption when taken within 1 hour of each other. The risk of GI bleeding is increased when **aspirin** and **nonsteroidal anti-inflammatory drugs (NSAIDs)** are concomitantly taken. Table 19–2 presents these and other drug interactions.

Clinical Use and Dosing

OSTEOPOROSIS. **Alendronate** is the only **biophosphonate** approved for prevention and treatment of osteoporosis is postmenopausal women. Therapy with 10 mg daily can increase bone density by up to 10 percent after 3 years and can decrease vertebral and hip fractures by 50 percent

Table 19-1. Pharmacokinetics: Biophosphonates

Drug	Onset of Effect	Peak	Duration	Bioavailability (with/without Food)	Steady-State V_d Exclusive of Bone	Half-Life ((Normal Renal Function)	Elimination
Alendronate	1 mo	3–6 mo	7 mo (following discontinuation of the drug)	0.7% in females 0.59% in males Reduced by 40% when taken with food; by 60% when taken with coffee or juice	28 L/kg or more	10 y (in bone)	50% in urine
Etidronate	1 mo	Unknown	1 y (following discontinuation of the drug)	1% Reduced when taken with food or juice	1.37 L/kg	More than 90 d (in bone)	Absorbed dose: 50% in urine Unabsorbed dose: in feces
Risedronate	—	—	—	0.63% Reduced by 55% when taken with food or juice	6.3 L/kg	220 h (from bone surface)	50% of absorbed dose in urine; unabsorbed dose in feces
Tiludronate	—	—	—	6% Reduced when taken with food or juice	—	—	—

Table 19–2. Drug and Food Interactions: Biophosphonates

Drug	Interacting Drugs and Food	Possible Effect	Implications
Alendronate	Ranitidine	Bioavailability doubled	Clinical significance unknown
	Aspirin, NSAIDs	Increases risk of GI bleeding with alendronate doses more than 10 mg/d	Avoid concurrent use
	Any food	Bioavailability decreased by 40%	Take 30 min or more before any food intake
	Coffee, orange juice	Bioavailability decreased by 60%	Take 30 min or more before intake
Etidronate	Any food	Bioavailability decreased	Take on an empty stomach 2 h before eating
Risedronate	Any food	Bioavailability decreased	Take 30 min or more before any food intake
Tiludronate	Aspirin	Tiludronate bioavailability decreased when taken 2 h after aspirin	Separate doses by more than 2 h or avoid concurrent use
	Indomethacin	Increases tiludronate bioavailability 2- to 4-fold	Clinical significance unknown
	Any food	Bioavailability decreased by 90%	Take after overnight fast and 4 h before standard breakfast
All biophosphonates	Calcium supplements, antacids	Interferes with biophosphonate absorption. Bioavailability may be decreased by 60% when given within 1 h	Take biophosphonate at least 1 h before

(Table 19–3). Use for this purpose for more than 4 years is currently under study, and no findings have yet been published concerning its efficacy or safety for this length of time. Although its labeled use is treatment of Paget's disease, **etidronate** has been prescribed, as an unlabeled use, to treat postmenopausal osteoporosis and prevent further bone loss in early postmenopausal women. Dosage is 400 mg daily for 14 days, followed by 76 days of elemental **calcium,** 500 mg daily. This drug also has an unlabeled use in the treatment of glucocorticoid-induced bone loss in postmenopausal women. Dosage is 400 mg daily for 1 month and then 400 mg daily for 2 weeks every third month, plus **calcium** and **ergocalciferol. Risedronate** has been used to treat postmenopausal osteoporosis, but it is also an unlabeled use. Dosage is 5 mg daily on a cycle with 2 years on and 1 year off therapy.

PAGET'S DISEASE. All **biophosphonates** are used to treat Paget's disease when the alkaline phosphatase is at least twice the upper limit of normal. It may also be used for those who are asymptomatic or at risk for future complications from their disease. Symptomatic Paget's disease is treated with **etidronate.** Initial dose is 5 to10 mg daily for up to but not exceeding 6 months or 11 to 20 mg/kg daily, not to exceed 3 months. The higher doses are reserved for times when lower doses are ineffective, when there is an overriding need for suppression of in-creased bone turnover, or when prompt reduction of elevated cardiac output is required. Doses greater than 20 mg/kg daily are not recommended. Retreatment for relapse is acceptable only after more than 90 drug-free days and when there is evidence of active disease. Dosage is the same as for initial treatment.

Treatment with **alendronate** uses doses of 40 mg daily for 6 months. Retreatment may be considered after a 6-month post-treatment evaluation period. **Risedronate** treatment is 30 mg daily for 2 months. Retreatment requires a post-treatment evaluation time of 2 months. **Tiludronate** treatment is 400 mg daily for 3 months, with retreatment only after a 3-month post-treatment evaluation. For all of these drugs, indications for retreatment are evidence of active disease or failure to normalize alkaline phosphatase levels.

Patients with Paget's disease benefit from supplemental calcium and vitamin D if their dietary intake is not adequate. Consideration must be given to spacing the administration of the **calcium** supplement and the **biophosphonate** to prevent reduction in bioavailability.

HETEROTOPIC OSSIFICATION. When this is a complication of total hip replacement, **etidronate** may be used at 20 mg/kg daily for 1 month preoperatively and 20 mg/kg daily for 3 months postoperatively. **Etidronate** is also used when this problem occurs secondary to spinal

Table 19–3. Dosage Schedule: Biophosphonates

Drug	Indication	Initial Dose	Maintenance Dose	Renal Use Parameter
Alendronate	Osteoporosis: prevention and treatment in post-menopausal women	10 mg/d	10 mg/d	CCr 35–60: no dosage adjustment CCr 35: use not recommended
	Paget's disease	40 mg/d	40 mg/d for 6 mo; re-treat if needed with same dose only after 6 mo post-treatment evaluation	As above
Etidronate	Paget's disease	5 mg/kg/d	5–10 mg/kg/d not to exceed 6 mo or 11–20* mg/kg/d not to exceed 3 mo; re-treat if needed with same dose only after 3–6 mo post-treatment evaluation	Serum creatinine 2.5–4.9, reduce dose Creatinine more than 5: use not recommended
	Heterotropic ossification: hip replacement	20 mg/kg/d for 1 mo preoperatively	20* mg/kg/d for 3 mo postoperatively	As above
	Spinal cord injury	20 mg/kg/d for 2 wk	10 mg/kg/d for 10 wk	As above
Risedronate	Paget's disease	30 mg/d	30 mg/d for 2 mo; re-treat if needed with same dose only after 2 mo post-treatment evaluation	CCr less than 30: use not recommended
Tiludronate	Paget's disease	400 mg/d	400 mg/d for 3 mo; re-treat if needed with same dose only after 3 mo post-treatment evaluation	CCr less than 30: use not recommended

*Doses in excess of 20 mg/kg/d or for longer than 6 mo have been associated with increased risk for fracture.

cord injury. The dosage then is 20 mg/kg daily for 2 weeks, followed by 10 mg/kg daily for 10 weeks, begun as soon as possible after the injury and prior to evidence of heterotopic ossification.

Other uses of these drugs to treat the hypercalcemia of malignancy are with parenteral dosage forms and are usually reserved for use by specialists. These uses are not discussed here.

Rational Drug Selection

Only one drug (**alendronate**) is approved for prevention and treatment of osteoporosis in postmenopausal women, but some providers have used **etidronate.** There have been no randomized controlled studies comparing these two drugs for this indication, but the same benefit in terms of bone mineral density has not been achieved by cyclic use of **etidronate** as has been achieved by the continuous use of **alendronate.** In addition, studies show a clear fracture-prevention benefit from **alendro-**

nate, and 3- to 4-year studies of **etidronate** are inconclusive with regard to this benefit.

For the treatment of Paget's disease, all **biophosphonates** may be used. **Etidronate** has been used longer for this indication and has midrange adverse drug reactions. Clinical trials reported in *Drug Facts and Comparisons* (1998), however, showed increased efficacy of **alendronate** over **etidronate** in suppression of alkaline phosphatase, with a response rate of 85 percent for **alendronate** as compared with 30 percent for **etidronate** and 0 percent for placebo. In addition, **alendronate** produced mild, transient, and asymptomatic decreases in serum calcium and phosphate as compared with **etidronate.** *Drug Facts and Comparisons* also reported a positive-controlled study conducted in Europe, with treatment groups taking 400 mg/day of **tiludronate** versus 400 mg/day of **etidronate** for 6 months (Table 19–4). **Tiludronate** was more efficacious than **etidronate** in that trial. **Alendronate** and **tiludronate** also have the lowest incidence of musculoskeletal pain. **Risedronate** has the highest ad-

Table 19–4. Available Dosage Forms: Biophosphonates

Drug	Dosage Form
Alendronate (Fosamax)	Tablet: 5 mg, 10 mg, 40 mg (40-mg tablet is triangular)
Etidronate (Didronel)	Tablet: 200 mg, 400 mg (400-mg tablet is scored)
Risedronate (Actonel)	Tablet: 30 mg
Tiludronate (Skelid)	Tablet: 240 mg (equivalent to 200 mg tiludronic acid)

verse drug reaction profile. It is also the newest drug, having been approved in March 1998. Problems can arise with new drugs in phase IV of drug research. With consideration of all these factors, the drugs of choice appear to be **alendronate** and **tiludronate**.

Monitoring

Before beginning treatment, rule out common treatable disorders that can also cause low bone density. These include hyperparathyroidism, vitamin D deficiency, hyperthyroidism, and renal disease. Tests for these disorders are serum calcium and albumin, 25-hydroxy vitamin D, TSH, and serum creatinine levels, respectively. Serum creatinine levels are drawn prior to initiating therapy. Dosage alterations or contraindications to using specific **biophosphonates** occur with serum creatinine levels above 2.5 mg/dL. Because **biophosphonates** inhibit intestinal calcium transport, careful monitoring of serum calcium should be done during therapy. Phosphate, magnesium, and potassium should also be monitored because these electrolytes may be altered by **biophosphonate** administration.

Elevation of alkaline phosphatase is a major indicator of Paget's disease and its reduction is an indicator of the efficacy of treatment. Alkaline phosphatase should be monitored prior to initiating therapy, at the end of each cycle of therapy, and prior to initiating any retreatment.

Measurement of bone mineral density is the most accurate predictor of fracture risk and efficacy of these drugs. Each 10 percent change below peak bone mass is associated with a doubling of the fracture risk for patients with osteoporosis. Dual energy x-ray absorptiometry (DEXA) is the gold standard by which bone mineral density and therapy are monitored, but it is expensive. Initial evaluation with DEXA can also suggest when a disease process other than aging is the probable cause of the bone loss. Once therapy has been established, DEXA is repeated 1 year later to determine progress. Whether to repeat DEXA at later dates is controversial. According to Rosenblatt (1998), DEXA should be used for:

1. Women who are estrogen-deficient, to make decisions about therapy
2. Women who have vertebral abnormalities or osteopenia detected on x-ray, to confirm the diagnosis

3. Patients who are being treated for osteoporosis, to monitor for treatment efficacy
4. Patients receiving long-term **glucocorticoid** therapy, to guide therapy to preserve bone mass
5. Patients with asymptomatic primary hyperthyroidism or other diseases associated with high risk for osteoporosis, to make therapy decisions

Patient Education

ADMINISTRATION. Take the drug first thing in the morning, at least 30 minutes prior to other medications, beverages, or food. Waiting longer than 30 minutes will improve absorption. **Etidronate** and **tiludronate** should be taken 2 hours before any food. **Alendronate, risedronate,** and **tiludronate** should be taken with 8 oz of plain water. Mineral water, coffee, orange juice, and other beverages greatly reduce absorption. If supplemental **calcium** or **antacids** are taken, **biophosphonate** must be administered at least 1 hour before these other drugs. If a dose is missed, skip that dose and resume taking the drug the next morning. Do not double doses or take later in the day. Remaining upright for at least 30 minutes after taking the dose facilitates passage to the stomach and minimizes the risk for esophageal irritation.

ADVERSE REACTIONS. GI distress is the most common adverse reaction. If needed, **aluminum-** or **magnesium-containing antacids** may be taken more than 2 hours after the **biophosphonate**. If diarrhea occurs with **etidronate,** notify the health care provider, who may divide the dose throughout the day to control the diarrhea. Female patients should advise their health care provider if pregnancy is planned or suspected or if they are breastfeeding. The drug may have to be changed or stopped.

LIFESTYLE MANAGEMENT. Eat a balanced diet with adequate amounts of calcium and vitamin D. Consult your health care provider about the need for supplemental **calcium** and **vitamin D.** Participate in regular exercise; it is beneficial for cardiovascular fitness as well as preserving bone mass. Reduce or stop behaviors such as smoking and **alcohol** intake that increase the risk of osteoporosis.

Because relapse is not uncommon, keeping follow-up appointments to monitor progress, even after the drug is discontinued, is important.

Hypothalamic and Pituitary Hormones

A combination of neural and endocrine systems located in the hypothalamus and the pituitary gland mediates control of metabolism, growth, and certain aspects of reproduction. The hormones involved in these hypothalamus-pituitary-hormone axes are adrenocorticotropic hormone, corticotropin-releasing hormone, follicle-stimulating hormone, growth hormone, growth hormone–binding protein, growth hormone–releasing hormone, gonadotropin-releasing hormone, insulin-like growth factor 1, luteinizing hormone, luteinizing hormone–releasing factor, prolactin-releasing factor, prolactin, somatotropin-releasing factor, thyrotropin-releasing hormone, and thyroid-stimulating hormone. The **reproductive hormones** are covered in Chapter 20, the **corticosteroid-related hormones** are covered in Chapter 23, and the **thyroid-related hormones** are discussed later in this chapter. This section discusses the growth hormone axis. Drugs affecting this axis are often prescribed by specialists, and the role of the primary care provider is largely to monitor the drug and its place in the total treatment regimen of the patient.

Pharmacodynamics

The hypothalamus-pituitary–growth hormone axis (Fig. 19–2) begins with growth hormone–releasing hormone (GHRH), which is secreted by the hypothalamus in response to decreased serum glucose levels in the body (hypoglycemia stimulates secretion, and hyperglycemia inhibits it). GHRH then binds to receptors in the anterior pituitary, resulting in the secretion by that gland of growth hormone (GH) (also called somatotropin). GH is a single peptide that attaches to receptors that allow it to pass through the cell membrane. Once inside cells, GH fosters protein synthesis, fat breakdown, and tissue growth. GH also causes hyperglycemia by decreasing glucose utilization by cells and increasing the rate by which glycogen is broken down into glucose. Both **GHRH** and **GH** have now been synthesized by recombinant DNA technology and are available in drug form. They produce the same actions as the natural hormones.

The primary role of **GHRH** at this time is as a diagnostic tool for evaluation of short children with subnormal GH responses to conventional stimuli in order to assess for dysfunction of the hypothalamus or the pituitary. It will not be discussed further.

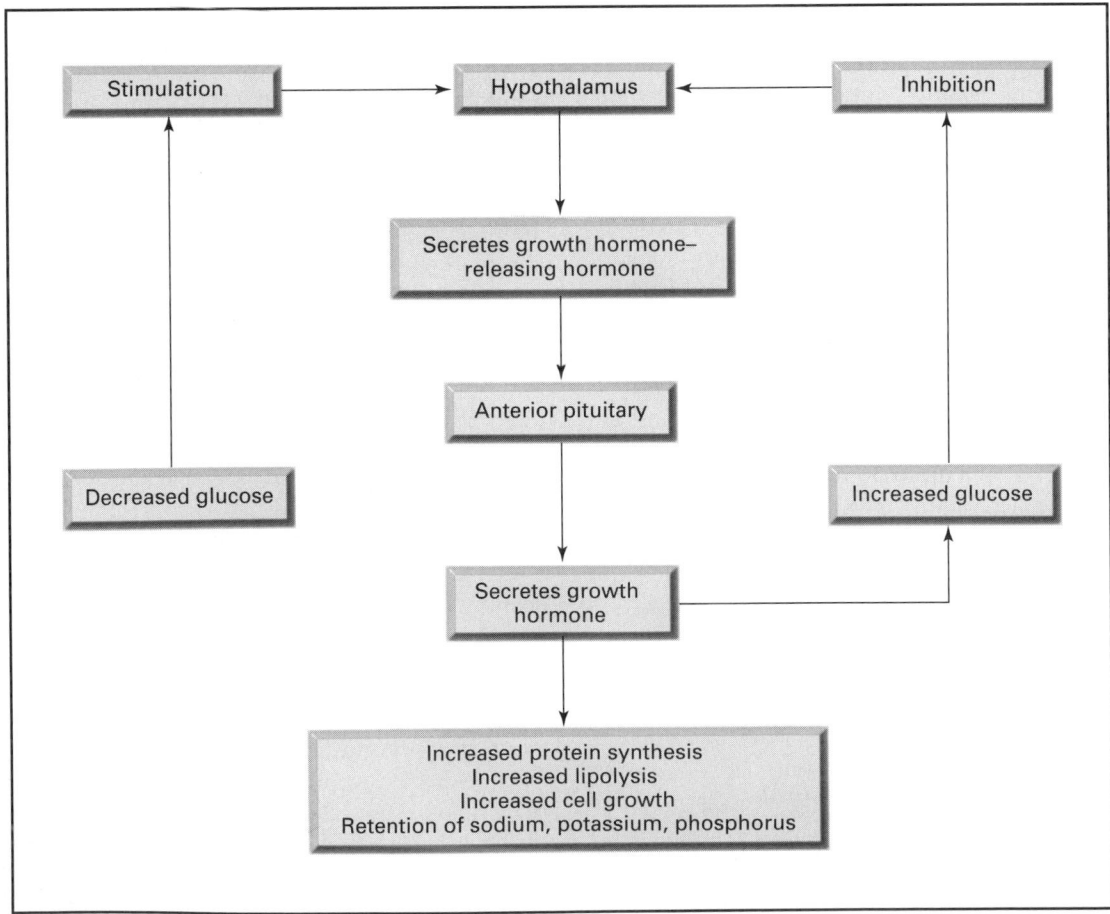

Figure 19–2. Hypothalamus-pituitary–growth hormone axis.

Administration of **somatrem** (Protropin) or **somatropin** (Humatrope, Norditropin, Nutropin), the synthetic **growth hormones**, results in an initial insulin-like effect, with increased tissue uptake of both glucose and amino acids and decreased lipolysis. Within a few hours, there is a peripheral insulin antagonistic effect, with impaired glucose uptake and increased lipolysis. These drugs also stimulate synthesis of somatomedins in the growth plate cartilage and the liver, resulting in increased linear, organ, and skeletal growth and increased cellular protein synthesis. Children with GH deficiency sometimes also experience hypoglycemia that is improved by administration of these drugs. Patients receiving these drugs may also experience reduction in fat stores and decreased mean cholesterol levels, but they are not used specifically for these reasons clinically. The retention of sodium, potassium, and phosphorus that occurs is also not a part of the treatment goal.

Pharmacokinetics

Absorption and Distribution

Somatrem and **somatropin** are both well absorbed after subcutaneous (SC) or intramuscular (IM) administration (Table 19–5). They tend to localize to highly perfused organs, such as the liver and kidney. The area under the curve (AUC) of the two drugs is similar and does not vary based on the injection type or site.

Metabolism and Excretion

Circulating hormone has a half-life of about 20 to 25 minutes and is predominantly cleared by the liver. In the kidney, both drugs are filtered by the glomerulus, reabsorbed in the proximal tubule, and broken down within the renal cells into amino acids that return to the circulation. The total mean half-life of both drugs from administration to elimination is 3.8 to 4.9 hours. Active blood levels persist for up to 36 hours.

Consistent with the role of the liver and the kidney in the elimination of these drugs, there is a reduction in hormone clearance in patients with hepatic or renal dysfunction.

Pharmacotherapeutics

Precautions and Contraindications

Somatrem and **somatropin** are contraindicated in patients with closed epiphyses and those with evidence of active tumor growth. They are used cautiously in growth hormone deficiency due to intracranial tumor because they increase the tumor growth. Patients with coexisting adrenocorticotropic hormone deficiency may experience increased symptoms of this disorder, and **somatrem** or **somatropin** should be used cautiously with these patients.

Serum levels of inorganic phosphorus, alkaline phosphatase, and parathyroid hormone may increase with **somatropin** therapy. Changes in thyroid hormone laboratory measurements have also occurred. This makes management of thyroid disorders more difficult. In addition, untreated hypothyroidism prevents optimal response to **GH** therapy. If **GH** must be used for patients with thyroid dysfunction, frequent monitoring of thyroid function and adequate treatment with **thyroid hormone** is necessary.

Insulin resistance may be induced by **somatrem** or **somatropin** therapy. The drugs are used cautiously with diabetic patients and those with glucose intolerance, and close monitoring of glucose levels is critical.

The safety and efficacy of synthetic *growth hormones* have not been established in pregnancy and lactation. They are Pregnancy Category C and should be used only if clearly needed.

Adverse Drug Reactions

Approximately 30 to 40 percent of patients on **somatrem** and 2 to 4.7 percent of patients on **somatropin** developed persistent antibodies, making them less likely to respond to the drug. Other adverse reactions were rare and included pain at the injection site, hyperglycemia, hypothyroidism, and edema secondary to retained sodium.

Drug Interactions

The only drug interaction was associated with **glucocorticoid therapy**. It may inhibit the growth-promoting effect of the synthetic **growth hormones**.

Table 19–5. Pharmacokinetics: Growth Hormones

Drug	Onset (of Effect)	Peak (Drug in Plasma)	Duration (Drug in Plasma)	Bioavailability	Half-Life (Normal Renal Function)	Elimination
Somatrem, somatropin	Within 3 mo	7.5 h	36 h	75% (SC) 63% (IM)	3.8 h (SC) 4.9 h (IM)	By liver and kidney

Clinical Use and Dosing

GROWTH FAILURE ASSOCIATED WITH CHRONIC RENAL INSUFFICIENCY. Somatropin (Nutropin) is used to treat children with growth failure up to the time of renal transplantation. The weekly dosage is 0.35 mg/kg given SC. No studies have been done to date on its use after transplantation. To optimize therapy for patients receiving hemodialysis, they receive their injections at night, just prior to going to sleep, or at least 3 to 4 hours after dialysis to prevent hematoma formation caused by the heparin. Patients undergoing chronic cycling peritoneal dialysis (CCPD) receive their injections in the morning after they have completed dialysis. Patients undergoing chronic ambulatory peritoneal dialysis (CAPD) receive their injections in the evening at the time of the overnight exchange.

LONG-TERM TREATMENT OF GROWTH FAILURE IN CHILDREN WHO LACK ADEQUATE ENDOGENOUS GH. Somatrem and all forms of somatropin (except Serostim) have been used for this indication. Dosage of somatrem is up to 0.1 mg/kg three times weekly, titrated to individual patient response. Doses in excess of 0.3 mg/kg have resulted in risks of known effects of excess human GH. Dosage of the various forms of somatropin varies by drug, as shown in Table 19–6.

TURNER'S SYNDROME. Nutropin, one brand of somatropin, is the only drug approved for long-term treatment of short stature associated with Turner's syndrome.

The weekly dose is 0.375 mg/kg or less, divided into equal doses three to seven times per week and given SC.

SOMATROPIN DEFICIENCY. Humatrope, one brand of somatropin, is the only drug approved to treat this condition. Patients must meet strict criteria before this drug is prescribed, and tests related to these criteria are usually done by an endocrinologist. For children, the recommended weekly dose is 0.18 mg/kg, divided into equal doses and given either on 3 alternate days or six times per week SC. For adults, the recommended SC dose is started at 0.006 mg/kg given daily and increased to a maximum of 0.0125 mg/kg daily, based on patient response.

Rational Drug Selection

Choice of drug is based on indication and the decision of the endocrinologist.

Monitoring

Prior to initiating and throughout therapy, hepatic and renal function studies are done. Patients with thyroid dysfunction, diabetes mellitus, or glucose intolerance have their disease processes more carefully monitored, as discussed in the section on precautions and contraindications.

Monitoring of bone age by x-ray is done to evaluate growth and to determine epiphyseal closure. The schedule for this assessment is determined by the endocrinologist.

Table 19–6. Dosage Schedule: Growth Hormones

Indication	Drug*	Initial Dose	Maintenance Dose
Growth failure related to chronic renal failure	Nutropin	0.35 mg/kg	0.35 mg/kg/wk (See note in text regarding hemodialysis)
Growth failure due to inadequate endogenous growth hormone	Protropin	0.1 mg/kg	0.1–0.3 mg/kg 3 times/wk; not to exceed 0.3 mg/kg
	Genotropin	0.16 mg/kg	0.16–0.24 mg/kg/wk in equal doses divided into 6–7 injections
	Humatrope	Children: 0.18 mg/kg	0.18–0.3 mg/kg/wk divided into equal doses, given on 3 alternate days or 6 d/wk
		Adults: 0.006 mg/kg	0.006 mg/kg daily
	Norditropin	0.024 mg/kg	0.024–0.034 mg/kg 6–7 times weekly
	Nutropin	0.3 mg/kg	0.3 mg/kg/wk
Turner's syndrome	Nutropin	0.375 mg/kg	0.375 mg/kg/wk divided into equal doses, given 3–7 times/wk
Somatropin deficiency	Humatrope	Children: 0.18 mg/kg	0.18–0.3 mg/kg/wk divided into equal doses, given on 3 alternate days or 6 d/wk
		Adults: 0.006 mg/kg	0.006 mg/kg daily

*Trade names are used because selected brands are the only drugs with FDA approval for a certain use.

Patient Education

These drugs are usually given at home by a family member or self-administered. Education is directed to both the patient and the person who will administer the drug.

ADMINISTRATION. These drugs have specific reconstitution and storage requirements (Table 19–7). Storage for all of them is at temperatures from 2° to 8° Celsius (36° to 46°F). They are not to be frozen. Each brand has a specific reconstitution formula, and the patient or family member should be taught that formula. Reconstituted vials are stable in refrigeration for 14 to 28 days, depending on the brand (except for **Serostim**, which is stable for only 24 hours).

The techniques for SC injection and site selection must be taught. The dosage schedule must be reviewed. **Somatropin** injections should be at least 48 hours apart. Because these drugs are given in weekly schedules, a calendar marked with the days of the week when the drug is to be given may be helpful.

These are injected drugs. Information about proper use and disposal of needles and syringes and cautions against reuse of needles are important.

ADVERSE REACTIONS. Adverse reactions are minimal. Patients and their parents, if appropriate, should be taught to report persistent pain at the injection site and edema. Because of the potential for hyperglycemia, patients should also be taught the signs and symptoms of this disorder and what to do, should it occur.

LIFESTYLE MANAGEMENT. Emphasize the need for regular follow-up visits with the endocrinologist to ensure appropriate growth rate, evaluate laboratory work, and determine bone age by x-ray.

Exocrine Pancreatic Enzymes

The pancreas is both an exocrine gland and an endocrine gland. The exocrine functions of the gland are related to secretion of enzymes into the gut for digestion. Disorders that decrease pancreatic function impair the production and secretion of these enzymes and, therefore, impair digestion. Two major disorders that are characterized by decreased pancreatic functioning are cystic fibrosis and pancreatitis.

Cystic fibrosis affects approximately 30,000 people in the United States. Once a disease of childhood, improved and aggressive management has resulted in a mean survival age of almost 25 years with 25 percent of patients surviving into their 30s and 40s. Initially, this disorder is an obstructive lung disease, but plugging of the pancreatic ducts eventually results in pancreatic insufficiency, with resultant malabsorption of protein, fat, and carbohydrates.

Acute and chronic pancreatitis are characterized by inflammation of the pancreas that results in swelling and obstruction of the pancreatic ducts. This obstruction leads not only to activated enzymes digesting the pancreas itself but also to failure of the enzymes to reach the duodenum and thus the same malabsorption problems.

Treatment for both disorders includes the replacement of pancreatic enzymes in the form of drugs.

Pharmacodynamics

The enzymes secreted by the exocrine pancreas are trypsinogen (protein digestion), chymotrypsin (protein digestion), amylase (carbohydrate digestion), and lipase (fat digestion). These enzymes are secreted into the bowel distal to the stomach because some of them are irreversibly inactivated by pH values of 4 or less. **Pancreatin** (**Donnazyme**) and **pancrelipase** (**Pancrease**) substitute for these enzymes and hydrolyze fats to glycerol and fatty acids, change proteins into proteoses and derived substances, and convert starch into dextrins and sugars.

Pharmacokinetics

Absorption and Distribution

These agents exert most of their effects in the duodenum and upper jejunum. Because they are permanently inactivated by gastric acid and pepsin secretion, problems in delivery by the oral route drugs may occur. Enteric coating may prevent destruction or inactivation by gastric

Table 19–7. Available Dosage Forms: Growth Hormones

Drug	Dosage Form
Somatrem (Protropin)	Powder for injection: 5-mg vial, 10-mg vial
Somatropin (Genotrope)	Powder for injection: 1.5-mg vial
Somatropin (Humatrope)	Powder for injection: 5-mg vial
Somatropin (Norditropin)	Powder for injection: 4-mg vial
Somatropin (Nutropin)	Powder for injection: 5-mg vial

acid but inhibit enzyme delivery to the duodenum. For this reason, it is important to synchronize the delivery of the drug with gastric emptying, and the drug must be taken immediately before or with a meal.

Distribution is local into the GI tract. There is limited if any systemic distribution.

Metabolism and Excretion

Because these drugs are simply enzyme delivery systems and there is limited if any systemic distribution, there is no metabolism or excretion beyond that which would normally occur in the body with the secretion of these enzymes.

Pharmacotherapeutics

Precautions and Contraindications

Pancrelipase is derived from a porcine source. Patients with hypersensitivity to pork proteins should not use this drug. **Pancreatin** is derived from porcine, bovine, or vegetable sources, depending on the brand. Patients with hypersensitivity to hog or beef protein may benefit from the products derived from vegetable sources.

These drugs are contraindicated during acute exacerbations of chronic pancreatitis. During this time, patients receive nothing by mouth to rest the GI tract and have no need for these enzymes. The presence of these enzymes during that time would only exacerbate the pancreatic disorder.

It is not known whether these drugs can cause fetal harm when administered to a pregnant woman. They are Pregnancy Category C and should be given only if the benefit to the mother outweighs any risk to the fetus.

Adverse Drug Reactions

High doses have been associated with GI symptoms such as nausea, cramping, abdominal pain, and diarrhea. Extremely high doses may cause hyperuricosuria and hyperuricemia.

Irritation of the skin and mucous membranes occurs less commonly. Powder spilled on the hands may cause local irritation. The dust of finely powdered concentrates irritates the nasal mucosa and respiratory tract. Inhalation of airborne powder can precipitate an asthma attack.

Drug and Food Interactions

Calcium- and **magnesium-based antacids** may decrease the effectiveness of the enzymes (Table 19–8). The ability of **oral iron** to increase serum iron levels may be reduced by concomitant administration of **pancreatin** or **pancrelipase**. Alkaline foods destroy the coating of enteric-coated products, resulting in destruction of the enzymes by gastric acids.

Clinical Use and Dosing

ENZYME REPLACEMENT IN PATIENTS WITH DEFICIENT EXOCRINE PANCREATIC SECRETIONS, CYSTIC FIBROSIS, CHRONIC PANCREATITIS, PANCREATIC INSUFFICIENCY AND STEATORRHEA OF MALABSORPTION SYNDROMES, AND POSTGASTRECTOMY. The dosing and schedule is the same for each of these conditions. Although each drug is specified in lipase, protease, and amylase units, the drugs are prescribed in units of lipase. Children age 6 months to 1 year initiate therapy with 2000 U of lipase per meal (Table 19–9). Because only two brands of **pancreatin (Entozyme** and **Donnazyme)** tablets are available in doses less than 4000 U and capsules cannot be divided, these two brands or a powdered form of pancrelipase (0.7 g) must be used for this age group. Children age 1 to 6 years initiate therapy with 4000 to 8000 U of lipase. Several brands of both drugs have dosage forms that can deliver this dose. Initial doses for children age 7 to 12 years are 4000 to 12,000 U of lipase. Initial therapy for adults is 4000 U of lipase with each meal or snack. Dosages may be increased as needed, based on patient response.

POSTPANCREATECTOMY AND DUCTAL OBSTRUCTIONS CAUSED BY CANCER OF THE PANCREAS OR COMMON BILE DUCT. The dosing and schedule for these indications is 8000 to 16,000 U of lipase at 2-hour intervals. In severe

Table 19–8. Drug and Food Interactions: Pancreatic Enzymes

Drug	Interacting Drug	Possible Effect	Implications
Pancreatin, pancrelipase	Calcium carbonate, magnesium hydroxide	Decreases effectiveness of pancreatin and pancrelipase	Avoid concurrent administration
	Oral iron	Decreases the serum iron response	Avoid concurrent administration
	Alkaline foods	Destroys coating on enteric-coated products	Give enzymes first and separate administration by at least 1 h

Table 19–9. Dosage Schedule: Pancreatic Enzymes

Drug	Indication	Initial Dose	Maintenance Dose
Pancreatin, pancrelipase	Enzyme replacement in patients with deficient exocrine pancreatic secretions, cystic fibrosis, chronic pancreatitis, pancreatic insufficiency and steatorrhea of malabsorption syndromes, and post-gastrectomy	Children less than age 6 mo: dosage not established Children age 6 mo–1 y: 2000 U of lipase per meal Children age 1–6 y: 4000–8000 U of lipase Children age 7–12 y: 4,000–12,000 U of lipase Adults: 4,000–48,000 U of lipase with each meal or snack	Maintenance dose is within dosage range stated for initial therapy, based on end points of growth curves and minimized symptoms
Pancrelipase powder	Cystic fibrosis	0.7 g with meals	0.7 g with meals
Pancrelipase	Postpancreatectomy and ductal obstructions caused by cancer of the pancreas or common bile duct	8,000–16,000 U of lipase at 2-h intervals	Dose may remain same or be increased to 64,000–88,000 U of lipase with meals, or frequency may be increased to hourly intervals unless nausea, cramps, or diarrhea occurs

deficiencies, the dose may be increased to 64,000 to 88,000 U of lipase with meals, or the frequency of administration may be increased to hourly intervals unless nausea, cramps, or diarrhea occurs.

Rational Drug Selection

COST. There are many available dosages and brands of these drugs (Table 19–10). The least expensive **pancrelipase** is **Viokase** tablets; other brands are anywhere from 2 to 10 times more expensive. Drugs with higher lipase units are more expensive but are about as expensive as it would be to take enough of the lower-dose tablets to gain the higher dose. Given this fact, the dose per unit of lipase is about the same across brands. The least expensive **pancreatin** is over-the-counter (OTC) **Dizyme** tablets, but the cost difference between the least and most expensive is minimal. With this drug, it is actually less expensive to purchase the higher-dosage brands when these doses are required than it is to double or triple the lower-dose brand.

BRAND. It is important to remember that the various brands are not bioequivalent. Each drug varies in the number of units of lipase, protease, and amylase present. Despite cost variables, it is not possible to change brands solely because the dosage has changed. When it is necessary to change brands, the health care provider should monitor the effect of the new drug on end points.

Monitoring

Assessment of the efficacy of **pancreatic enzyme replacement** and the dosage of drug required is accomplished by determining which dose minimizes steatorrhea and maintains good nutritional status. The assessment of the end points in children is aided by charting growth curves. Other data include skinfold thickness, arm muscle circumference, and laboratory values such as albumin, cholesterol, glucose, hemoglobin, hematocrit, transferrin, and electrolytes. Because these drugs may produce elevated uric acid levels, serum and urine are tested for uric acid at regular intervals. Stools are monitored for fat content (steatorrhea), and the patient is told to report foul-smelling and frothy stools.

Patient Education

ADMINISTRATION. All doses are taken immediately before or with meals or snacks. Capsules may be opened and sprinkled on food. Capsules with enteric-coated beads should not be chewed. They may be sprinkled on soft food that is not hot and that can be swallowed without chewing, such as applesauce or gelatin. Swallow immediately because the proteolytic enzymes may irritate the mucosa. Following with a glass of water or juice or eating immediately after taking the drug helps to ensure that the medication is swallowed and does not remain in contact with the mouth and esophagus for long periods.

Table 19–10. Available Dosage Forms: Pancreatic Enzymes

Drug	Lipase (U)	Protease (U)	Amylase (U)	How Supplied
Pancreatin				
Dizyme tablets	6,750	41,250	43,750	Enteric-coated tablets
Entozyme tablets	600	7,500	7,500	Tablets
Donnazyme tablets	1,000	12,500	12,500	Tablets
Pancrezyme 4× tablets	12,000	60,000	60,000	Tablets
4× Pancreatin 600-mg tablets	12,000	60,000	60,000	Tablets
Hi-Vegi-Lip tablets	4,800	60,000	60,000	Tablets
8× Pancreatin 900-mg tablets	22,500	180,000	180,000	Tablets
Creon capsules	8,000	13,000	30,000	Enteric-coated microsphere
Pancrelipase				
Pancrease MT4 capsules	4,000	12,000	12,000	Enteric-coated microtablets
Pancrease capsules	4,000	25,000	20,000	Enteric-coated microsphere
Pancrelipase capsules	4,000	25,000	20,000	Enteric-coated pellets
Protilase capsules	4,000	25,000	20,000	Enteric-coated spheres
Cotazym-S capsules	5,000	20,000	20,000	Enteric-coated spheres
Cotazym capsules	8,000	30,000	30,000	Capsules
Ku-Zyme HP capsules	8,000	30,000	30,000	Capsules
Viokase tablets	8,000	30,000	30,000	Tablets
Pancrease MT 10 capsules	10,000	30,000	30,000	Enteric-coated microtablets
Ilozyme tablets	11,000	30,000	30,000	Tablets
Zymase capsules	12,000	24,000	24,000	Enteric-coated spheres
Ultrase MT 12 capsules	12,000	39,000	39,000	Capsules
Pancrease MT 16 capsules	16,000	48,000	48,000	Enteric-coated microtablets
Viokase powder	16,800	70,000	70,000	Powder
Ultrase MT 20 capsules	20,000	65,000	65,000	Capsules
Ultrase MT 24 capsules	24,000	78,000	78,000	Capsules

Pancrelipase is destroyed by acid. **Sodium bicarbonate** or **aluminum-based antacids** may be used with preparations without enteric coating to neutralize gastric pH. **Calcium-** and **magnesium-based antacids** should not be used for this purpose because they interfere with drug action. Enteric-coated beads are designed to withstand the acid pH of the stomach. Enteric-coated formulations should not be mixed with alkaline food prior to ingestion, or the coating will be destroyed.

The various brands of these drugs are not bioequivalent. Use the same brand consistently unless told to change by the health care provider. This is especially important for OTC brands.

ADVERSE REACTIONS. Adverse reactions are usually GI in nature. Report to the health care provider nausea, stomach cramps, abdominal pain, or diarrhea. Dosages or brands may need to be changed. Irritation of the skin and mucous membranes can also occur. Powder spilled on the hands may cause local irritation. Wash it off immediately. There is no other treatment required. The dust of finely powdered concentrates may irritate the nasal mucosa and respiratory tract. Inhalation of airborne powder can precipitate an asthma attack. If you have asthma or any other chronic lung condition, notify the health care provider.

LIFESTYLE MANAGEMENT. **Pancreatic enzyme replacement** is only part of the treatment regimen. It will not be successful without adherence to the rest of the treatment regimen. Dietary recommendations depend on the reason **enzyme replacement** is needed, but generally the diet is high calorie, high protein, and low fat. For children with cystic fibrosis, the diet is high calorie, high protein, and high fat. The dosage of the **enzyme replacement** is based on fat content of the diet, so the amount of fat in each meal should be fairly consistent. Small, frequent meals are often better tolerated than three large meals, especially when the reason for the **enzyme replacement** is cystic fibrosis or postoperative gastrectomy.

Endocrine Pancreatic Hormones

(Insulins)

Insulin is a small protein molecule secreted by the beta cells of the pancreas. It is essential to the utilization of glucose by all body cells. Disorders of insulin secretion and utilization are found in diabetes mellitus, and the primary use of **insulin** as a drug is treatment of this disorder. Chapter 31 discusses the treatment of both type 1 and type 2 diabetes, including the use of **insulin.** This chapter discusses the drug itself.

Pharmacodynamics

Insulin is normally released from pancreatic beta cells at a constant low basal rate with intermittent bursts in response to a variety of stimuli, including stress, vagal activity, and high blood glucose levels. Figure 19–3 shows one mechanism for the stimulation of insulin release from beta cells. Once the insulin has arrived at an insulin-sensitive cell, it is bound to specialized receptors that are found on the cell membrane.

These receptors foster changes within the cell membrane that result in translocation of certain proteins, such as the glucose transporter from sequestered sites within the cell to the cell surface. Once on the cell surface, the transporter facilitates the intake of glucose by the cell. Several hormonal agents such as **corticosteroids** lower the affinity of the insulin receptor, and others such as GH increase this affinity. Insulin promotes the storage of fat as well as glucose and influences cell growth and metabolic functions in a wide variety of tissues.

Action on Glucose Transporters

The GLUT 1 insulin transporter is found in all tissue, especially in red blood cells and in the brain. It is associated with basal uptake of glucose and transport of glucose across the blood-brain barrier. The GLUT 2 transporter is found in the beta cells of the pancreas and in the liver, kidney, and gut. It regulates insulin release and glucose homeostasis. Defects in this receptor are thought to contribute to the reduced insulin secretion seen in type 2 diabetes. The GLUT 3 transporter is located in the brain, kidney, and placenta and is related to uptake of glucose in neurons and some other tissues. The GLUT 4 transporter is located in muscle and adipose tissue. It is the transporter most associated with lowering blood glucose (BG) levels and is the primary influence in glucose uptake, especially during exercise. It is also the one most associated with insulin resistance in type 2 diabetes. GLUT 5 transporters are found in the gut and the kidney. They are associated with intestinal absorption of fructose.

The total number of insulin receptors can be down-regulated by such factors as obesity and long-standing hyperglycemia. This may explain why weight loss can be a significant factor in diabetes management.

Action on the Liver

Insulin acts on the liver to increase storage of glucose as glycogen and resets the liver after food intake by reversing the amount of catabolic activity. Insulin also decreases urea production, protein catabolism, and cAMP in the liver; promotes triglyceride synthesis; and increases potassium and phosphate uptake by the liver.

Action on Muscle Cells

Insulin promotes protein synthesis by increasing amino acid transport and by stimulating ribosomal activity. It also promotes glycogen synthesis to replace glycogen stores used during muscle activity.

Action on Adipose Tissue

Finally, insulin reduces the circulation of free fatty acids and promotes the storage of triglycerides in adipose tissue. This process is accomplished, in part, by suppression of cAMP production and dephosphorylation of the lipases in fat cells.

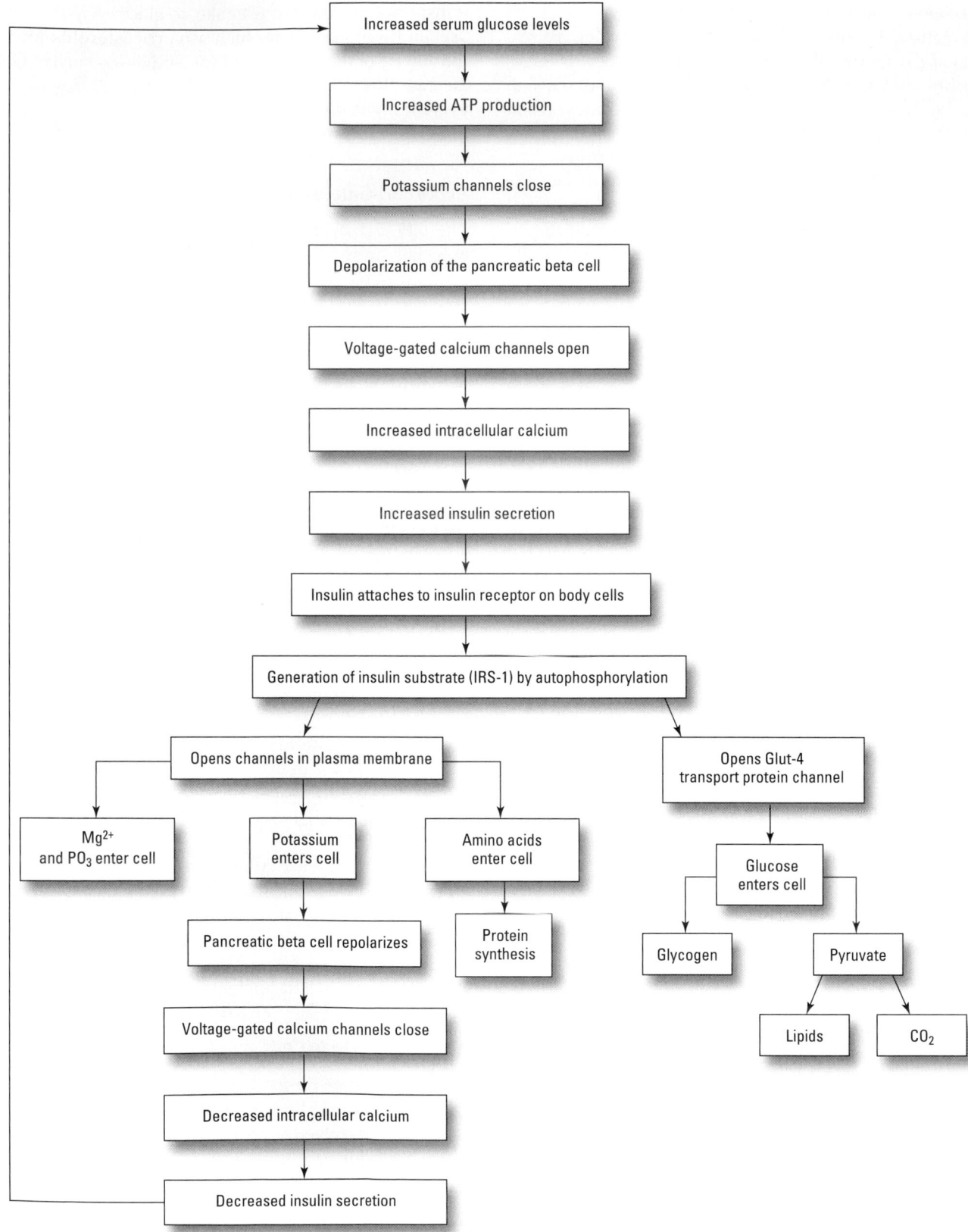

Figure 19–3. Mechanism of insulin release from beta cells.

Administration of **insulin** acts on each of these receptors to produce the same effect as the naturally occurring hormone. Although it is given largely to control BG in patients with diabetes, that is not its only effect on the body.

Pharmacokinetics

Absorption and Distribution

Insulin is absorbed from SC or IM injection sites. Absorption rate is determined by type of **insulin**, injection site, and volume injected. It may also be given intravenously (IV); the drug is placed directly into circulation without the need for absorption. **Insulin** preparations are divided into four types, based on onset, duration, and peak intensity of action. Table 19–11 presents each

of these types. For each, **human insulins** have a more rapid onset of action and shorter duration of activity than **pork insulins**, whereas **beef insulins** have the slowest onset of action and the longest duration of activity (American Diabetes Association, 1998). Injection sites in the abdomen have as much as 50 percent more absorption than the arm, followed by the thighs and buttocks (American Diabetes Association, 1998).

TYPES OF INSULIN. **Lispro** is an **insulin** analogue produced by recombinant DNA technology. This ultra-short-acting **insulin** has the same method of binding to insulin receptors, the same circulating half-life, and the same immunogenicity as **regular insulin**. Its onset of action, however, is much shorter—15 minutes—and it reaches its peak within 1 hour. Clinical trials have demonstrated that optimal time for preprandial injection of this **insulin** is 15 minutes rather than the 30-minute

Table 19–11. Pharmacokinetics: Insulins

Drug	Onset (h)	Peak (h)	Duration (h)*	Metabolism	Excretion
Ultra-short-Acting					
Lispro	0.25	0.5–1.5	6–8	All preparations are metabolized by the liver, the kidney, and muscle tissue	Very little unchanged insulin is excreted in the urine
Short-Acting					
Regular	0.5–1	2–4	8–12	All preparations are metabolized by the liver, the kidney, and muscle tissue	Very little unchanged insulin is excreted in the urine
Semilente	1–1.5	5–10	12–16	All preparations are metabolized by the liver, the kidney, and muscle tissue	Very little unchanged insulin is excreted in the urine
Intermediate-Acting					
NPH	1–1.5	4–8	24	All preparations are metabolized by the liver, the kidney, and muscle tissue	Very little unchanged insulin is excreted in the urine
Lente	1–2.5	7–10	24	All preparations are metabolized by the liver, the kidney, and muscle tissue	Very little unchanged insulin is excreted in the urine
Long-Acting					
PZI	4–8	14–24	36	All preparations are metabolized by the liver, the kidney, and muscle tissue	Very little unchanged insulin is excreted in the urine
Ultralente	4–8	10–30	More than 36	All preparations are metabolized by the liver, the kidney, and muscle tissue	Very little unchanged insulin is excreted in the urine

*Clinically significant duration of action is shorter than the pharmacokinetic duration of action. The clinically significant duration of action for short-acting insulins is approximately 4 h; for intermediate-acting insulins, it is approximately 6–8 h; and for long-acting insulins, it is approximately 12 h.

interval used for **regular insulin.** The duration of action of this **insulin** is not increased with a larger dose.

Regular insulin is a short-acting form whose effect appears within 30 minutes of injection and generally lasts for 8 to 12 hours. The clinically significant duration of action is slightly less, at 4 hours. **Semilente** is also a short-acting form, but its production except for use in the manufactured **Lente insulin** has been discontinued.

Neutral protamine Hagedorn or **isophane** (NPH) is an intermediate-acting **insulin.** The onset of action is delayed by combining the **insulin** with protamine. After SC injection, proteolytic enzymes degrade the protamine in **NPH** to permit absorption of the insulin. Its onset of action is 1 hour, and its duration is 24 hours. **Lente** is also considered an intermediate-acting **insulin,** but it actually is a combination of a short-acting formulation (**Semilente**) and a long-acting formulation (**Ultralente**) to provide a combination of rapid absorption and long duration of action. The clinically significant duration of action for intermediate-acting **insulins** is approximately 6 to 8 hours.

Ultralente is a long-acting **insulin.** The only formulation available is made with **human insulin.** The onset is 4 to 8 hours. The duration of action of the previously available beef and pork formulations was greater than 36 hours. The **human insulin** formulation has a less sustained action than the previous beef and pork forms, with a clinically significant duration of action of about 12 hours.

Insulin is widely distributed to most body tissues.

Metabolism and Excretion

Insulin is metabolized by the liver, the kidney, and muscle cells. Almost all of it is metabolized, and a very small amount is excreted unchanged in the urine.

Pharmacotherapeutics

Precautions and Contraindications

The only contraindications to **insulin** are hypoglycemia and hypersensitivity to any of the ingredients in the product. **Human insulin** derived by recombinant DNA technology from *Escherichia coli* bacteria or yeast rarely poses hypersensitivity problems. Although not so commonly used today, there are **insulin** products derived from porcine or bovine sources. Patients sensitive to pork or beef proteins should not use these **insulins.**

Some studies with **human insulin** have shown increased circulating levels of insulin in patients with renal failure (*Drug Facts and Comparisons,* 1998). Because renal insufficiency and failure are not uncommon complications of diabetes, careful glucose monitoring and dose adjustments are needed for patients with renal dysfunction.

Studies have also shown increased circulating levels of insulin in patients with hepatic function impairment who are taking **human insulin.** Hepatic failure is uncommon in diabetes, but careful glucose monitoring and dose adjustments are needed for these patients as well.

Pregnancy requires careful diabetes management. *Human insulin* **does not cross the placenta and is the drug of choice for pregnant women and those considering pregnancy (American Diabetes Association, 1998).** *Insulin* **is Pregnancy Category B. Because** *insulin* **is given by injection, it is not absorbed intact by the breastfeeding infant. Inadequate or excessive** *insulin* **treatment of mothers with diabetes, however, reduces milk production.** *Insulin* **can be used safely in infants and children.**

Hypothyroidism may delay **insulin** turnover, requiring less **insulin** to treat diabetes. Hyperthyroidism may cause an increase in the renal clearance of **insulin.** Patients with either of these concurrent diseases require more frequent monitoring of glucose levels than other patients with diabetes when **insulin** management is required.

Insulin resistance occurs more commonly in patients with type 2 diabetes, but patients with either type of diabetes who have this problem may require more than 1.5 U of **insulin** per kg of body weight each day in the absence of ketoacidosis or acute infection. Patients who may exhibit this resistance include obese patients; patients with acanthosis nigricans, ketoacidosis, or endocrinopathies; and patients with insulin receptor defects, who may need to have their diabetes managed by an endocrinologist.

Adverse Drug Reactions

Two life-threatening adverse reactions are central to patient management with **insulin:** hypoglycemia and diabetic ketoacidosis. One is associated with too much **insulin** or not enough food and the other with too little **insulin.**

HYPOGLYCEMIA. Hypoglycemia may result from an excessive **insulin** dose, excessive work or exercise without eating, food that is not absorbed in the usual manner because of a postponed or omitted meal, or an illness that results in vomiting or diarrhea. It may also be associated with concurrent administration of another drug that increases the hypoglycemic effects of **insulin. Alcohol** is especially risky in this regard because it not only induces hypoglycemia but also masks the signs and symptoms of the disorder. Table 19–12 shows these drug interactions. Signs and symptoms of hypoglycemia include decreased levels of consciousness, hunger, diaphoresis, weakness, dizziness, and tachycardia. The peak of action for each type of **insulin** is the most likely time for a hypoglycemic reaction. This is especially important when more than one type of **insulin** is being used and the peaks of the different types of **insulin** coincide. Mild episodes of hypoglycemia can be treated with oral glucose. Adjustments in **insulin** dosage, meal patterns, or exercise may be needed.

Table 19–12. Drug Interactions with Insulin

Interacting Drug	Possible Effects	Implications
Acetazolamide, AIDS antivirals, asparaginase, calcitonin, corticosteroids, cyclophosphamide, dextrothyroxine, diazoxide, diltiazem, dobutamide, epinephrine, estrogens, ethacrynic acid, isoniazid, lithium carbonate, morphine sulfate, niacin, phenothiazines, phenytoin, nicotine, thiazide diuretics, thyroid hormones	Decreases hypoglycemic effect of insulin	Close monitoring of blood glucose levels is required if concurrent administration
Alcohol, anabolic steroids, beta-adrenergic blockers*, chloroquine, guanethidine, lithium carbonate, monoamine oxidase inhibitors, mebendazole, octreotide, pentamidine, phenylbutazone, pyridoxine, salicylates, sulfinpyrazone, sulfonamides, tetracyclines	Increases hypoglycemic effect of insulin	Close monitoring of blood glucose levels is required if concurrent administration

*Cardioselective beta-adrenergic blockers (those affecting only or mainly beta₁ receptors) are less likely to affect insulin's hypoglycemic effect and may be acceptable alternatives for patients who must take beta-adrenergic blockers.

More severe episodes, with coma, seizure activity, or neurological impairment, require treatment with IM or SC glucagon or concentrated IV glucose. Additional carbohydrate intake and observation are necessary because hypoglycemia may recur after apparent clinical recovery.

DKA. Diabetic ketoacidosis (DKA) may result from stress, illness, infection, or **insulin** omission. It may also develop slowly after a long period of adequate control of BG. Children with undiagnosed type 1 diabetes may present with DKA at the time of diagnosis. Signs and symptoms of DKA include drowsiness, dim vision, and Kussmaul's respiration. Indications of hyperglycemia that may precede DKA and give warning of its impending occurrence include polyuria, polydipsia, polyphagia, weight loss and fatigue, vomiting, dehydration, ketone odor to the breath, and abdominal pain. Treatment requires hospitalization and is directed at the acid-base and fluid imbalances that result, as well as the elevated BG. IV fluids, correction of the acidosis and hypotension, and low-dose **regular insulin** given SC or by IV infusion are required.

Adverse reactions that are not life-threatening include lipodystrophy, lipohypertrophy, and localized urticaria and itching at the injection sites. These are more common with **pork** and **beef insulin.**

Drug Interactions

Many drugs either decrease or increase the effects of **insulin** because of their effects on BG. Table 19–12 shows these interactions. **Beta-adrenergic blockers** are especially problematic because they can increase insulin resistance, producing hyperglycemia, but can also mask most of the signs and symptoms of hypoglycemia. The one indication of hypoglycemia that **beta-adrenergic blockers** do not mask is diaphoresis, and people with diabetes who must take **beta-adrenergic blockers** for a concurrent disease or condition should be taught to test their blood sugar level whenever they experience diaphoresis.

Clinical Use and Dosing

TYPE 1. Because patients with type 1 diabetes mellitus (formerly called insulin-dependent) do not produce insulin, they must receive **insulin** replacement. A wide variety of regimens are used in this treatment, including **regular insulin** only delivered via insulin pump and mixtures of short-acting and intermediate-acting or short-acting and long-acting **insulins** given in multiple doses from two to four times daily (Table 19–13). Chapter 31 discusses the management of type 1 diabetes mellitus in more detail.

TYPE 2. Patients with type 2 diabetes (formerly called non-insulin-dependent) produce insulin, but they may not produce enough to meet the body's needs. They also have insulin receptor defects, insulin resistance, and altered hepatic glucose metabolism. **Insulin** is prescribed when their disease process cannot be adequately controlled by diet, exercise, weight reduction, and oral agents. Chapter 31 also discusses the pharmacological management of type 2 diabetes mellitus.

Table 19–13. Dosage Schedule: Insulins*

Indication	Drug	Initial Dose	Maintenance Dose
Type 1 diabetes mellitus	Possible combinations: regular, regular and NPH, Lente, lispro, lispro and NPH, mixed insulin, Ultralente, Ultralente and regular,† Velosulin or regular if using pump	Children and adults: 0.5–1 U/kg/d Adolescents during rapid growth: 0.8–1.2 U/kg/d	Based on blood glucose pattern over last 3–7 d. Adjust dose in 2-U increments or maximum of 10% of total daily dose. Adjust one insulin and one administration at a time. Target is fasting blood glucose 80–140 mg/dL.
Type 2 diabetes mellitus not controlled by diet, weight loss, exercise, and sulfonylurea or sulfonylurea and other agent(s) with fasting hyperglycemia	NPH or Lente or mixed insulin All given at bedtime in addition to daytime oral agent	10 U at bedtime	Increase by 2-U increments until fasting blood glucose within target range for patient. Target is fasting blood glucose 80–140 mg/dL.
Type 2 diabetes mellitus not controlled by sulfonylurea or sulfonylurea and other agent(s) with postprandial hyperglycemia	Lispro immediately prior to meals	Based on postprandial BG readings	Individualized
Type 2 diabetes mellitus with poor control even with multiple oral agents	Intensive insulin therapy	Individualized	Individualized
Ketoacidosis	Regular insulin only	Adults: 0.1 U/kg/h as a continuous infusion Children: individualized based on body surface area	Individualized

*Different patterns can be used for individual insulins and combinations. The patterns are shown in Chapter 31. Doses are based on individual fasting blood glucose and glycosylated hemoglobin (HbA$_1$C) levels. Doses in this table are usual total daily doses of insulin of all types.
†Requires two injections because these drugs are incompatible in syringe.

Mixing **insulins** is common practice in diabetic regimens, but not all **insulins** are compatible with each other or make good combinations. The Clinical Practice Recommendations (American Diabetes Association, 1998) state that **regular insulin** and **Ultralente** may be mixed with no blunting of the onset of action of the **regular insulin**. *Drug Facts and Comparisons* (1998) states that **NPH** is preferred to **Lente** as the intermediate-acting formulation in **insulin** mixtures because the excess zinc in **Lente** and **Ultralente** can precipitate some of the soluble **regular insulin** and retard the absorption and biologic effects of the **regular insulin** unless it is injected immediately after mixing. To prevent this problem with **NPH,** all the manufacturers have reduced the protamine content. All premixed formulations of **insulin** (**70/30 Novolin, 70/30 Humulin,** and **50/50 Humulin**) contain **NPH** (percentage is first number) and **regular** (percentage is second number) **insulin.** These premixed **insulins** remain stable at room temperature for 1 month or for 3 months under refrigeration. **NPH** and **regular insulin** mixed in plastic or glass syringes may be stored for 1 week at room temperature and 14 days if refrigerated. All forms of **Lente insulin** may be mixed together. They are chemically identical and differ only in the size and structure of the **insulin** particles.

With the increasing use of **lispro,** an ultra-short-acting **insulin,** there have been attempts made to mix it with a longer-acting **insulin** to provide sustained insulin activity. It can be mixed with **NPH** or **Lente** immediately before injection without affecting its rapid absorption. Premixtures have proved unstable. This is discussed further in the On the Horizon section. Regardless of the **insulin** mixture used, the patient should standardize the interval between mixing the **insulins** and injecting them.

HYPERKALEMIA. IV infusions of glucose and **insulin** produce a shift of potassium into cells and lower serum potassium levels. This treatment is usually reserved for hospitalized patients with very high potassium levels or those at risk for cardiac arrhythmias.

SEVERE KETOACIDOSIS OR DIABETIC COMA. Regular **insulin** given IV is used for rapid effect in severe ketoacidosis or diabetic coma. Because there is a high risk for inducing hyperosmolar coma with this therapy, these patients are also hospitalized.

PREGNANCY. For treatment of gestational diabetes and for management of patients with diabetes who become pregnant, **insulin** is the drug of choice. *Oral hypoglycemic agents* are contraindicated in pregnancy. Any of the insulin treatment regimens used for people with diabetes may be used. Special care must be taken to avoid hypoglycemic episodes.

Rational Drug Selection

BEEF OR PORK VERSUS HUMAN PREPARATIONS. Beef and **pork insulins** have been available commercially for some time. Both are antigenic, beef slightly more so than pork. **Human insulin** is a more recent development, and mass production by recombinant DNA technique has reached the level where **human insulin** production exceeds **beef** and **pork insulin** production in the world. Because of mass production, **human insulin** is now priced lower than either **beef** or **pork insulin.** In addition, **human insulin** is less likely to cause antigenic or lipodystrophic reactions. Given all these parameters, **human insulin** is preferred unless the patient has been taking **beef** or **pork insulin** for some time, is being managed well with them, and does not want to change, or the longer duration of action of **beef** and **pork insulins** is a determining clinical factor.

METHOD OF DELIVERY. Concerning method of delivery, most patients with diabetes inject their **insulin** based on a specific regimen. Any **insulin** shown in Table 19–14 except **velosulin** is appropriate for this use. **Velosulin** is a **human insulin** formulation that contains a phosphate buffer that reduces aggregation of regular **insulin** molecules when used in infusion pumps. It is the only **insulin** currently recommended for pump use. **Lispro** is being tried in some pumps.

RESPONSE TO INTERMEDIATE-ACTING INSULIN. Approximately one-third of patients have either a delayed or early response to intermediate-acting **insulin.** Although these patients may be placed on any **insulin** regimen that includes intermediate-acting **insulin,** in the design of the regimen, this response should be considered.

Half of these patients with altered responses are early responders who experience their peak insulin effect at the early time in the range for that **insulin** (e.g., in 4 hours for **NPH** and 7 hours for **Lente**). They are at high risk to become hypoglycemic, often in the early afternoon after a morning dose. They should have their intermediate-acting **insulin** dose split into two-thirds in the morning and one-third before dinner. The half that are delayed responders experience their peak effect in the late time in the range for that insulin and may experience hypoglycemia in the late evening to early night hours. These patients require a reduction in intermediate-acting **insulin** dose and the addition of a short-acting **insulin** in the morning. These regimens are among those discussed in Chapter 31.

LEVEL OF INTENSITY OF CONTROL. Results of the Diabetes Control and Complications Trial (DCCT, 1993) indicate that tighter controls to lower BG levels significantly reduced the risk of complications associated with diabetes. This trial conclusively demonstrated, in patients with type 1 diabetes, that the risk for development or progression of retinopathy was reduced by 76 percent, for nephropathy by 50 percent, for neuropathy by 60 percent, and for cardiovascular disease by 35 percent. These benefits were observed with an average glycosylated hemoglobin (HbA_1C) of 7.2 percent. The reduction in risk correlated continuously with reduction in HbA_1C. "This relationship implies that complete normalization of glycemic levels may prevent complications" (American Diabetes Association, 1998, p. 23). Although these benefits have not yet been demonstrated for patients with type 2 diabetes, trials to test this benefit are under way. DCCT patients on tight control used combinations of short-acting and intermediate-acting **insulin** given three to four times per day. Those on very tight control used long-acting **insulin** at night with short-acting **insulin** before each meal or more frequently, based on self-monitored glucose measurements. A third group used an insulin pump. Patients who are intelligent, well motivated, and reliable can be taught to regulate their blood sugar with this degree of control. Less capable patients risk hypoglycemic reactions on this regimen and might not be appropriate candidates or may need higher fasting blood sugar targets than the more capable patients. The DCCT trial and management based on it are discussed in detail in Chapter 31.

PRESENCE OF COMPLICATIONS SUCH AS RETINOPATHY AND NEUROPATHY. Patients with complications such as retinopathy and neuropathy may find it difficult to draw up their own **insulin.** Premixed **insulin** may assist with this problem. Choice of **insulin** is based on the commercial availability of premixed **insulin** or those that can be safely stored for some time after mixing.

TYPE 2 DIABETES MELLITUS UNABLE TO CONTROL. Patients with type 2 diabetes who are not controlled on oral agents and have postprandial hyperglycemia can have **lispro** added immediately prior to meals. Patients who

Table 19–14. Available Dosage Forms: Insulin

Drug	Dosage Form
Ultra-short-Acting Insulin	
Lispro/Humalog	100 U/cc in 10-cc vials and 1.5-cc cartridges
Short-Acting Insulin	
Regular/Iletin I (beef and pork)	100 U/cc in 10-cc vials
Regular/Iletin II (pork)	100 U/cc in 10-cc vials
Regular/Purified Pork	100 U/cc in 10-cc vials
Regular/Novolin R (human)	100 U/cc in 10-cc vials
Regular/Novolin R PenFill (human)	100 U/cc in 1.5-cc cartridge (for NovoPen)
Regular/Novolin R PenFill (human)	100 U/cc in 1.5-cc prefilled syringes
Regular/Humulin-R (human)	100 U/cc in 10-cc vials and 1.5-cc cartridges
Regular/Velosulin BR (human)	100 U/cc in 10-cc vials (for pump)
Intermediate-Acting Insulin	
NPH/Iletin I (beef and pork)	100 U/cc in 10-cc vials
NPH-N (pork)	100 U/cc in 10-cc vials
NPH/Iletin II (pork)	100 U/cc in 10-cc vials
NPH/Humulin-N (human)	100 U/cc in 10-cc vials and 1.5-cc cartridges
NPH/Novolin-N (human)	100 U/cc in 10-cc vials
NPH/Novolin PenFill (human)	100 U/cc in 1.5-cc cartridge (for NovoPen)
NPH/Novolin Prefilled (human)	100 U/cc in 1.5-cc prefilled syringes
Lente/Iletin I (beef and pork)	100 U/cc in 10-cc vials
Lente Iletin II (beef)	100 U/cc in 10-cc vials
Lente-L	100 U/cc in 10-cc vials
Lente/Humulin-L	100 U/cc in 10-cc vials
Lente/Novolin-L	100 U/cc in 10-cc vials
Mixed Insulin	
NPH & Regular/Humulin 70/30 (human)	100 U/cc in 10-cc vials and 1.5-cc cartridges
NPH & Regular/Novolin 70/30 (human)	100 U/cc in 10-cc vials
NPH & Regular/Novolin 70/30 PenFill (human)	100 U/cc in 1.5-cc cartridge (for NovoPen)
NPH & Regular/Novolin 70/30 Prefilled (human)	100 U/cc in 1.5-cc prefilled syringes
NPH & Regular/Humulin 50/50 (human)	100 U/cc in 10-cc vials
Ultra-long-Acting Insulin	
Ultralente/Humulin U	100 U/cc in 10-cc vials

have fasting hyperglycemia can have bedtime **NPH** or **Lente** added. If they have overall poor control, intensive **insulin** therapy is used. Although combinations of **insulin** and several different oral agents have been used, the only oral agents that have formal FDA approval for use with insulin are **glimepiride (Amaryl)** and **troglitazone (Rezulin)**. Table 19–13 provides more information on dosing.

Monitoring

Two categories of monitoring are needed for diabetics: (1) control of BG and (2) signs of complications.

CONTROL OF BLOOD GLUCOSE. For patients with type 1 and 2 diabetes, the goals of therapy are prandial BG levels of 80 to 120 mg/dL, bedtime glucose levels of 100 to 140 mg/dL, and HbA$_1$C levels of less than 7 (American Diabetes Association, 1998). Patients with comorbid

diseases, the very young, older adults, and others with unusual conditions or circumstances may warrant different treatment goals. HbA$_1$C levels of 7 correspond roughly to a BG level of 150 mg/dL when it is referenced to a nondiabetic value of 6. HbA$_1$C values can be increased by iron-deficiency anemia, **alcohol** use, and lead toxicity and can be decreased by chronic blood loss, chronic renal failure, and pregnancy when performed by some techniques. These potential confounding variables should be considered in assessing changes in HbA$_1$C levels.

Preprandial BG can be assessed by self-monitoring as often as before every meal and at bedtime. Preprandial BG level assessment should be augmented by monitoring HbA$_1$C because this value reflects the average BG level over a period of 120 days. Assessment intervals by health care providers are based on the degree of control, medication regimen, and other variables, such as financial resources and insurance coverage. For patients with type 1 diabetes, assessment of HbA$_1$C is usually done quarterly. It is done at least every 6 months for patients with type 2 diabetes. Intervals between testing are based on clinical variables, including the long-term degree of glycemic control.

SIGNS OF COMPLICATIONS. The most common complications of diabetes are nephropathy, retinopathy, peripheral and GI neuropathies, hypertension, cardiovascular disease, dyslipidemia, and skin breakdown, especially on the feet. DKA may occur in patients with type 1 diabetes, and hyperosmolar hyperglycemic nonketotic syndrome may occur in patients with type 2 diabetes. All patients with diabetes may experience hypoglycemic episodes. Tight glycemic control with the use of **insulin** is one way to prevent or reduce these complications. All patients with diabetes should be taught how to monitor for and manage these complications. Providers need to be aware of the physical examination and laboratory evaluations that are appropriate to determine the degree of glycemic control and define associated complications and risk factors. Prevention, evaluation, and management of these complications as they relate to pharmacological therapies are discussed in the American Diabetes Association clinical practice recommendations (1998) and in Chapter 31.

Patient Education

ADMINISTRATION. The number, type, and amount of daily **insulin** administrations depends on BG levels, diet, and exercise. The primary care provider must work with the patient to establish the diet-exercise-**insulin** glucose monitoring regimen with active patient participation.

Each type of **insulin** has a specific pattern of onset, peak, and duration. **Lispro** is injected within 15 minutes before a meal. **Regular insulin** is injected 30 to 60 minutes before a meal. For **insulin** suspensions (**NPH, Lente, NPL, Ultralente**), ensure uniform dispersion of **insulin** by rolling the vial gently between the hands until the color is even. Avoid vigorous shaking, which produces air bubbles or foam. **Lispro** and **regular insulins** are clear solutions and do not require dispersion of suspended particles. Do not use them if they are cloudy, discolored, or unusually viscous, which may indicate loss of potency.

Vials of **insulin** not in use should be refrigerated. Extreme temperatures (more than 36°F or less than 2°C) and excessive agitation should be avoided to prevent loss of potency, clumping, frosting, or precipitation. **Insulin** in use may be kept at room temperature.

Maintenance doses of **insulin** are administered SC. The patient must be taught the technique for drawing up the correct dose and for SC injection. Only insulin syringes should be used to draw up **insulin** dosages. Sites should be rotated, but because the abdomen, arm, and leg have different absorption rates, rotation should occur within one general area (e.g., the abdomen). As a general rule, do not administer within 1 inch of the same site for 1 month. **Regular insulin** given IV or IM is reserved for severe DKA and diabetic coma.

Exercise increases the rate of absorption from injection sites (American Diabetes Association, 1998) and increases glucose recycling (Giacca, Groenewoud, Tsui, McClean, & Zinman, 1998), both of which may result in increased risk for hypoglycemia if the dose of **insulin** is unchanged. Exercise should be planned and consistent within a treatment regimen.

When different types of **insulin** are mixed, always draw clear **insulin** into the syringe first. The order of mixing and the procedure used, including the model or brand of syringe and needle, should not be changed from dose to dose. Patients stabilized on a mixture of **insulins** should have a consistent response if the procedure is the same each time. Premixed **insulin** is available commercially and may be used if the type and concentration mix fit the patient.

Most **insulin,** including premixed types, is stable at room temperature for 1 month and for 3 months if refrigerated. Mixtures involving **lispro** that patients mix themselves must be given immediately after they are mixed. Other mixtures (e.g., **regular** and **NPH**) are stable for 7 days at room temperature and 14 days if refrigerated. Patient should be taught storage requirements for their specific **insulin.**

Different brands of **insulin** are not bioequivalent. The patient should not change brands without first consulting the health care provider, who will arrange for close monitoring if the change is appropriate.

ADVERSE REACTIONS. The most common adverse drug reactions are actually an extension of the action of the **insulin.** Hypoglycemia can be life-threatening and has a higher risk of occurrence as the intensity of therapy increases. The patient should be taught the signs and symptoms of hypoglycemia and the appropriate treatment for it, based on whether it is mild, moderate, or severe. Diet and exercise affect **insulin** dosage. Decreased food intake, increased time between the injection of **insulin** (especially short-acting formulations) and food intake, or increased activity may decrease **insulin** requirements and increase the risk for hypoglycemia.

Alcohol intake is especially dangerous for patients with diabetes. The effect of **alcohol** on BG is dependent on the amount ingested and the relationship to food intake. **Alcohol** is not metabolized to glucose and inhibits gluconeogenesis. If it is ingested without food, hypoglycemia can result, even at levels that do not exceed mild intoxication. Not only can it cause hypoglycemia but also it can mask the signs and symptoms of the disorder. For patients using **insulin,** the Clinical Practice Recommendations (American Diabetes Association, 1998) recommend no more than two alcoholic beverages (one alcoholic beverage equals 12 oz beer, 5 oz wine, or 1.5 oz distilled spirits) with and in addition to the regular meal plan. The calories from this **alcohol** must be calculated as part of the total caloric intake and substituted as one alcoholic beverage equals two fat exchanges. Reduction of or abstinence from **alcohol** is preferable.

Hyperglycemia is less immediately life-threatening than hypoglycemia but still an indication of poor control of BG, and it may be life-threatening if it is high enough to produce ketosis. Patients should be taught to recognize early indications of hyperglycemia and the treatment for it.

Accurate monitoring of BG levels is central to managing dosages of **insulin** and to monitoring for adverse drug reactions. The patient should be taught fingerstick BG self-monitoring.

LIFESTYLE MANAGEMENT. Management of type 1 or type 2 diabetes involves diet, exercise, weight control, and self-monitoring of BG, as well as administration of **insulin.** Further patient teaching related to management of diabetes is discussed in Chapter 31.

Oral Diabetic Agents

Ninety-five percent of patients with diabetes mellitus have type 2 diabetes. Type 2 diabetes mellitus has four primary alterations in glucose metabolism: (1) insufficient production of endogenous insulin by the beta cells of the pancreas, (2) tissue insensitivity to insulin, (3) impaired response of the beta cells to BG levels, and (4) excessive production of glucose by the liver. These patients do not have an absence of insulin secretion, although some may eventually develop absence of insulin. They are managed with oral agents that address the alterations in glucose metabolism of type 2 diabetes with the addition of **insulin** during episodes when glycemic control is not possible with oral agents alone.

Sulfonylureas

The first class of oral drugs developed to manage patients with type 2 diabetes mellitus were the **sulfonylureas.** They are true **oral hypoglycemics** and are useful only for patients with some endogenous insulin secretion.

Pharmacodynamics

Sulfonylureas cause an increase in endogenous insulin secretion by the beta cells of the pancreas related to increased cAMP generation. They may improve the binding between insulin and insulin receptors or increase the number of receptors, thereby having a limited ability to improve insulin utilization by the tissues. Hypoglycemic effects appear to be due to increased endogenous insulin production and to improved beta cell sensitivity to BG levels or suppression of glucose release by the liver. **Sulfonylureas** also potentiate the effect of antidiuretic hormone and may produce a mild diuresis. They are useful for patients with type 2 diabetes who are not controlled with lifestyle modifications alone. They are efficacious in about 50 percent of patients with type 2 diabetes for total control of BG and about 30 percent of patients for improved glucose levels without total control, but their use fails to continue to manage BG levels for the long term in about 36 percent of patients.

Pharmacokinetics

Absorption and Distribution

All **sulfonylureas** are well absorbed after oral administration and all except **glipizide (Glucotrol)** can be taken with food (Table 19–15). Absorption of **glipizide** is delayed by the presence of food in the gut and is more effective when taken 30 minutes prior to a meal. **Tolazamide (Tolinase)** is absorbed more slowly than the other **sulfonylureas.**

ON THE HORIZON

Insulin

Premixed preparations of **lispro** and the usual intermediate-acting **insulins** have proved unstable. Trials are under way in Europe for a mixture of **lispro insulin** with **NPL (neutral protamine lispro)** in which **lispro** instead of **regular insulin** is used to make the intermediate-acting insulin. It is being tested in premixed combinations of **NPL** and **lispro** 75:25, 50:50, and 25:75.

Nasal **insulin** delivery systems are also being tested. To date, the mixture of **insulin** and a detergent administered via aerosol has not been proved to provide a reliable and reproducible absorption on the **insulin.** The efficiency of absorption is also low (8% bioavailability), making the delivery system prohibitively expensive.

Table 19–15. Pharmacokinetics: Sulfonylureas

Drug	Onset (h)	Peak (h)	Duration (h)	Half-Life (h)	Metabolism	Elimination
First Generation Acetohexamide	1	Unknown	12–14	6–8	Metabolized in liver to potent active metabolite	Excreted primarily in the urine
Chlorpropamide	1	3–6	25–60	36 (prolonged by renal disease)	80% metabolized in liver; activity unknown	Renal elimination may be increased by increased urine pH
Tolazamide	4–6	1–6	12–24	7	Metabolized in liver to several mildly active metabolites	Excreted primarily in the urine
Tolbutamide	1	4–6	6–12	4.5–6.5	Oxidized in liver to inactive metabolites	Excreted primarily in the urine
Second Generation Glipizide	1–1.5	1–2	10–16	2–4	Metabolized in liver to inactive metabolites	Excreted primarily in urine
Glyburide					Metabolized in liver to weakly active metabolites	Excreted as metabolites in bile and urine, approximately 50% by each route
Nonmicronized	2–4		24	10		
Micronized	1	1.5–3	24	4		
Glimepiride	2	2–3	24	5	Completely metabolized by liver	Excreted 60% in urine and 40% in feces

Although the mechanisms of action are similar for all **sulfonylureas,** the first and second generations differ in absorption. Second-generation compounds are more nonpolar and lipophilic. Therapeutically effective doses and serum concentrations are lower because of their intrinsic potency and ability to cross plasma membranes. All **sulfonylureas** are highly bound to plasma proteins, especially albumin, but the first-generation binding is ionic whereas the second-generation binding is not. Because they have ionic bonds, first-generation drugs are more likely to be displaced from their binding sites by drugs that competitively bind to proteins (e.g., **warfarin, phenylbutazone**). Displacement would result in a greater hypoglycemic effect and may account for the increased risk for hypoglycemia found with first-generation drugs.

Chlorpropamide (Diabinese) and **tolbutamide (Orinase)** enter breast milk. **Glyburide (DiaBeta, Micronase)** reaches high concentrations in bile and crosses the placenta.

Metabolism and Excretion

All **sulfonylureas** are metabolized in the liver to active and inactive metabolites. The hypoglycemic effects of these drugs may be prolonged by severe liver disease because of reduced metabolism. Differences exist among the **sulfonylureas** in the duration of hypoglycemic effects, in part because of their metabolism. **Tolbutamide** is short acting because it is rapidly metabolized to an inactive metabolite by the liver. The active metabolite of **acetohexamide (Dymelor)** is 2.5 times more potent than the parent compound. **Tolazamide** has two active metabolites that are less potent than the parent compound.

All **sulfonylureas** are excreted primarily in the urine. **Glyburide** is excreted as metabolites in bile and urine, approximately 50 percent by each route. The renal elimination of **chlorpropamide** may be sensitive to changes in urine pH, with urinary alkalinization increasing its excretion. The half-life of this drug is prolonged in renal disease.

Pharmacotherapeutics

Precautions and Contraindications

All **sulfonylureas** are contraindicated for patients with hypersensitivity to the drugs or the compounds in which they are mixed. Cross-sensitivity may occur with other **sulfonamides**, including **thiazide diuretics**.

Although the *sulfonylureas* are listed as Pregnancy Category C (*glyburide* is Pregnancy Category B), insulin is the drug of choice for management of diabetes during pregnancy, and *oral hypoglycemic agents should not be used*. All *sulfonylureas* except *glyburide* are teratogenic in animals. There are no adequate studies in pregnant women. Prolonged severe hypoglycemia has occurred in neonates born to mothers on a *sulfonylurea* at the time of delivery. If these drugs must be used during pregnancy, discontinue use 2 to 4 weeks before the expected delivery date. Chlorpropamide and tolbutamide are known to enter breast milk; it is not known if other **sulfonylureas** are also excreted in breast milk. Because of the potential for hypoglycemic reactions in nursing infants, **sulfonylureas** are contraindicated in nursing mothers. Safety and efficacy of these drugs in children have not been established.

Other conditions in which **sulfonylureas** should not be used include type 1 diabetes, DKA or diabetic coma, and uncontrolled infection, burns, or trauma. Patients with adrenal or pituitary insufficiency are especially susceptible to hypoglycemia, and **sulfonylureas** should be used cautiously and patients monitored more frequently if they have these comorbid conditions. Severe hepatic impairment may cause inadequate hepatic release of glucose in response to hypoglycemia. Renal impairment may cause decreased elimination, leading to accumulation of these drugs and resulting in hypoglycemia. All **sulfonylureas** should be used with extreme caution for patients with hepatic or renal impairment, and liver and renal function should be monitored frequently if they must be used.

Older adults and debilitated patients are particularly susceptible to the hypoglycemic action of **sulfonylureas,** and the signs and symptoms of hypoglycemia may be difficult to recognize. Long-acting agents should be avoided, and short-acting ones should be used with caution with these patients.

A bolded warning in all **sulfonylurea** material states that the administration of **oral hypoglycemic drugs** has been reported to be associated with increased cardiovascular mortality as compared to treatment with diet alone or diet plus **insulin**. This warning is based on the study conducted by the University Group Diabetes Program. Patients who were treated for 5 to 8 years with diet plus **tolbutamide** had a rate of cardiovascular mortality approximately 2.5 times that of patients treated with diet alone. A significant increase in total mortality was not observed. Although only one drug in the **sulfonylurea class** was shown to produce this problem, this warning was extended to the entire class because of their close similarities in mode of action and chemical structure. Later studies have not replicated this finding, but the warning has remained.

Adverse Drug Reactions

All **sulfonylureas** may produce severe hypoglycemia. Second-generation drugs are less likely than first-generation drugs to have this adverse reaction. Others at high risk have been discussed in the Precautions and Contraindications section. Hypoglycemia may be difficult to recognize with patients who are concurrently taking **beta-adrenergic blockers** because these drugs mask the signs and symptoms of hypoglycemia, with the exception of diaphoresis. Hypoglycemia is also more likely when caloric intake is reduced, after severe or prolonged exercise, when **alcohol** is consumed, or when more than one glucose-lowering agent is used.

Gastrointestinal disturbances (nausea, epigastric fullness, and heartburn) are the most common adverse reactions. They tend to be dose-related and disappear when the dose is reduced. Diarrhea been associated with **glipizide** use, and taste alteration with **tolbutamide** use. Cholestatic jaundice is rare but requires discontinuation of the drug.

Dermatologic reactions include rashes, pruritus, erythema, and urticaria. These tend to be transient and may disappear despite continued use of the drug. Photosensitivity can also occur, and patients should use sunblock and wear covering clothing when exposed to sunlight.

Syndrome of inappropriate secretion of antidiuretic hormone (SIADH) has occurred after administration of **sulfonylureas**, especially with patients who also have congestive heart failure or hepatic cirrhosis. These drugs stimulate ADH release, augmenting hypothalamic-pituitary release of ADH. The result is excessive water retention and dilutional hyponatremia. **Glipizide, acetohexamide, tolazamide,** and **glyburide** are mildly diuretic.

Hemolytic anemia, agranulocytosis, leukopenia, and thrombocytopenia have occurred but are rare. Patients should have initial and annual complete blood counts done.

The increased insulin secretion generated by **sulfonylureas** has been associated with weight gain and hyperinsulinemia. Combination with **metformin (Glucophage)** reduces these adverse effects.

Drug Interactions

Sulfonylureas interact with a large number of drugs that either increase or decrease their hypoglycemic effect (Table 19–16). **Alcohol** interacts with these drugs to

Table 19–16. Drug Interactions: Sulfonylureas

Drug	Interacting Drug	Possible Effect	Implications
All sulfonylureas	Androgens, anticoagulants,* chloramphenicol, fluconazole, gemfibrozil, histamine₂ blockers, magnesium salts, methyldopa, MAO inhibitors, NSAIDs (except diclofenac), phenyl-butazone, probenecid, salicylates, sulfonamides, tricyclic antidepressants, urinary acidifiers	Enhance the hypoglycemic effect of the sulfonylurea	Avoid concurrent administration or monitor blood glucose levels closely if drug must be given
All sulfonylureas	Beta-adrenergic blockers, cholestyramine, diazoxide, hydantoins, rifampin, thiazide diuretics, urinary alkalinizers	Decrease the hypoglycemic effect of the sulfonylurea	Avoid concurrent administration or monitor blood glucose levels closely
Glimepiride*	In addition to drugs with all sulfonylureas: corticosteroids, phenothiazines, thyroid products, estrogens, oral contraceptives, nicotinic acid, sympathomimetics, and isoniazid	May cause loss of glucose control because these drugs can cause hyper-glycemia	If concurrently administered, monitor closely for loss of glucose control; when they are withdrawn, monitor closely for hypoglycemia

*Concurrent administration of glimepiride and warfarin did not alter the pharmacokinetic properties of warfarin. The changes in prothrombin time/international normalized ratio (PT/INR) were so small that they are unlikely to be clinically significant.

produce a disulfiram-like syndrome, characterized by facial flushing and occasional breathlessness but without the nausea, vomiting, and hypotension seen in a true **alcohol-disulfiram** reaction. This reaction occurs in about 33 percent of patients concurrently ingesting **alcohol** and **chlorpropamide**. It is uncertain whether this reaction occurs with **glyburide** and **glipizide**. No cases have been reported with **glimepiride (Amaryl)**.

Clinical Use and Dosing

TYPE 2 DIABETES MELLITUS. Both first- and second-generation **sulfonylureas** are used to treat type 2 diabetes. They are effective as initial drug therapy, including therapy with patients who have previously used diet, exercise, and weight control alone. Equivalent therapeutic doses vary from 1 mg to 1000 mg, depending on the drug (Table 19–17). Micronized **glyburide** 3-mg tablets provide serum concentrations that are not bioequivalent to those from the conventional formulations. When transferring patients from any **sulfonylurea** to micronized **glyburide**, the dose must be retitrated. Although all the drugs are listed as once-daily doses, many of the drugs work equally well when the daily dose is divided and given bid, especially when higher doses are required. The dose is highly individualized, based on BG readings. Start with the lowest dose and increase every 4 to 7 days, based on glucose control. In general, one-half

the maximum dose is usually the maximally efficient dose for glucose control. If the **blood glucose** level goal is not achieved on one-half the maximum dose, consider adding a drug from a different class.

Maturity onset diabetes of the young (MODY) is a relatively rare subtype of type 2 diabetes, characterized by an early age of onset and autosomal dominant inheritance. Unlike type 2 diabetes, MODY is caused by a primary defect in pancreatic beta cell function, resulting in a decrease in insulin secretion, as well as insulin resistance (Cabanas, 1998). **Sulfonylureas** and **insulin** may be required, depending on the degree of dysfunction of the beta cells.

NEUROGENIC DIABETES INSIPIDUS. For neurogenic diabetes insipidus, **chlorpropamide** in doses of 200 mg to 500 mg has been used. This is an unlabeled use.

Rational Drug Selection

AGE. **Chlorpropamide** and **glyburide** should be avoided in older adults. They are associated with more severe hypoglycemia in this age group. Use a shorter-acting agent such as **glipizide** or **tolazamide**. **Chlorpropamide** should be suitable for a young patient with no renal dysfunction, on no other medication, and not using **alcohol**.

COST. With the most expensive drug, **chlorpropamide**, as a reference of 1, the remaining **sulfonyl-**

Table 19–17. Dosage Schedule: Sulfonylureas

Drug	Initial Dose	Maintenance Dose	Maximum Dose
First Generation Acetohexamide	250 mg	500–1000 mg/d before morning meal 1000–1500 mg/d, divide dose and give bid before morning and evening meals	1500 mg/d
Chlorpropamide	Moderately severe, middle-aged stable adults: 250 mg Older adults: 100–125 mg Severe disease: 250 mg	250 mg/d before morning meal 100–250 mg/d before morning meal 500 mg/d before morning meal	750 mg/d
Tolazamide	100 mg	If fasting blood glucose (FBS) less than 200 mg/dL give 100 mg/d before morning meal If FBS more than 200 mg/dL give 250 mg/d before morning meal If patient malnourished, under-weight, or elderly, give 100 mg/d before morning meal If more than 500 mg/d, divide dose and give bid before morning and evening meal	1000 mg/d
Tolbutamide	1000 mg	500–3000 mg/d, divide dose and give bid before morning and evening meal	2000 mg/d
Second Generation Glipizide Glucotrol	5 mg Older adults, liver disease: 2.5 mg	5–15 mg/d 30 min before morning meal 15–40 mg/d. Doses more than 15 mg/day: divide and give bid before morning and evening meal; adjust doses in 2.5–5 mg increments several days apart	40 mg/d
Glucotrol XL	5 mg	10–20 mg/d 30 min before morning meal; adjust doses in 2.5–5 mg increments several days apart	40 mg/d
Glyburide DiaBeta, Micronase	2.5 mg	1.25–20 mg/d before morning meal. Dose more than 10 mg/d: divide and give bid; adjust dose in increments of 2.5 mg at weekly intervals	20 mg/d
Glynase	1.5 mg	0.75–6 mg/d before morning meal. Dose more than 10 mg/d: divide and give bid before morning and evening meal; adjust dose in increments of 1.5 mg at weekly intervals	12 mg
Glimepiride	1 mg	1–4 mg/d before morning meal. After reaching 2-mg dose, increase in increments of no more than 2 mg at 1–2 wk intervals	8 mg/d

ureas are all less expensive, with generic brands less expensive and brand names more expensive. Among the brand names, **Amaryl (glimepiride)** is the least expensive and compares favorably with generic forms of the other drugs in terms of cost (*Drug Facts and Comparisons,* 1998). Table 19–18 includes available dosage forms with the cost index for each of these drugs.

CONCURRENT DISEASE. In the presence of renal impairment, **glipizide** and **tolbutamide** are reasonable choices because they are oxidized in the liver to inactive metabolites. **Glyburide** is also a reasonable choice because 50 percent of it is excreted in bile, which gives an alternative route for excretion. **Tolazamide** is also safe to use, with creatinine clearance (CCr) less than 30 cc/minute.

Table 19–18. Available Dosage Forms: Sulfonylureas

Drug	Dosage Form	Cost Index*
Acetohexamide (generic)	260 mg in 100-tablet bottles	0.3
	500 mg in 100-tablet bottles	0.5
Dymelor	250 mg (scored) in 200-tablet bottles	0.2
	500 mg (scored) in 50- and 200-tablet bottles	0.5
Chlorpropamide (generic)	100 mg in 100-, 250-, 500-, and 1000-tablet bottles	1
	250 mg in 100-, 500-, and 1000-tablet bottles	2
Diabinese	100 mg (scored) in 100- and 500-tablet bottles	15
	250 mg (scored) in 100-, 250-, and 1000-tablet bottles	17
Glimepiride (Amaryl)	1 mg in 100-tablet bottles	0.2
	2 mg in 100-tablet bottles	0.4
	4 mg in 100-tablet bottles	0.7
Glipizide (generic)	5 mg in 100- and 500-tablet bottles	0.3
	10 mg in 100- and 500-tablet bottles	0.6
Glucotrol	5 mg (scored) in 100- and 500-tablet bottles	0.3
	10 mg (scored) in 100- and 500-tablet bottles	0.8
Glucotrol XL	5 mg in 100- and 500-tablet bottles	0.3
	10 mg in 100- and 500-tablet bottles	0.5
Glyburide (generic)	1.25 mg in 50- and 100-tablet bottles	0.6
	2.5 mg in 100-, 500-, and 1000-tablet bottles	0.3
	5 mg in 100-, 500-, and 1000-tablet bottles	0.4
DiaBeta	1.25 mg (scored) in 50-tablet bottles	0.4
	2.5 mg (scored) in 60-, 100-, and 500-tablet bottles	0.3
	5 mg (scored) in 30-, 60-, 100-, 500-, and 1000-tablet bottles	0.5
Glynase (micronized)	1.5 mg (scored) in 100-tablet bottles	1.5
	3 mg (scored) in 100-, 500-, and 1000-tablet bottles	0.4
	6 mg in 100- and 500-tablet bottles	0.7
Micronase	1.25 mg (scored) in 100-tablet bottles	0.4
	2.5 mg (scored) in 30-, 60-, and 100-tablet bottles	0.3
	5 mg (scored) in 30-, 60-, 90-, 100-, 500-, and 1000-tablet bottles	0.5
Tolazamide (generic)	100 mg in 100- and 250-tablet bottles	0.1
	250 mg in 100-, 200-, 500-, and 1000-tablet bottles	0.2
	500 mg in 100-, 250-, and 500-tablet bottles	0.4
Tolinase	100 mg (scored) in 100-tablet bottles	0.2
	250 mg (scored) in 200- and 1000-tablet bottles	0.5
	500 mg (scored) in 100-unit doses	1
Tolbutamide (generic)	500 mg in 100-, 500-, and 1000-tablet bottles	0.2
Orinase	500 mg (scored) in 200-tablet bottles	0.2

*Cost index based on cost per 100 mg of chlorpropamide.

Clinical Pearl

....

Tolazamide has the added advantage that it may be crushed and put down a nasogastric tube or sprinkled on applesauce or other soft food for patients who have difficulty in swallowing tablets.

....

TAKING MULTIPLE MEDICATIONS. Second-generation **sulfonylureas** are best for patients who are taking multiple medications to minimize potential drug interactions. **Second-generation sulfonylureas** also have the advantage of once-daily administration, thereby reducing the complexity of the drug regimen and improving adherence. Among this group of drugs, **glimepiride** binds to different insulin receptors than other **sulfonylureas** and may be effective when others are not. It is also associated with a lower incidence of hypoglycemic reactions.

CONCURRENT ADMINISTRATION WITH INSULIN. Sulfonylureas have been concurrently administered with **insulin** with some success for patients who are not controlled on diet, exercise, and weight control, plus an oral agent. The drugs most commonly used are **second-generation sulfonylureas.** The only drug that has had the research necessary to obtain formal FDA approval for this indication is **glimepiride.** There is further discussion in the **insulin** section of this chapter and in Chapter 31.

Monitoring

HbA_1C is the preferred tool for monitoring long-term BG control. As discussed in the insulin monitoring section, it provides an indication of the average BG level over the last 120 days. Standards vary from laboratory to laboratory, but in general, each 1 percent change in HbA_1C equals a change in BG of about 30 mg/dL. The goal for patients with type 2 diabetes is the same as the goal for type 1. Glycated albumin (fructosamine) is also sometimes used for monitoring, although it is not recommended as a substitute for HbA_1C except in situations such as hemolytic anemias in which HbA_1C cannot be used (American Diabetes Association, 1998). It indicates the average BG for the past 1 to 3 weeks and is used to assess short-term control. The minimum goal for fructosamine levels is 325 mmol or less, with a goal for intensive therapy of 287 mmol or less. All decreases in these monitoring parameters are beneficial, even if the goal is not met.

The American Diabetes Association (1998) recommends that patients with type 2 diabetes be tested by HbA_1C every 6 months if they are meeting glycemic goals and at least every 3 months if their therapy has changed or they are not meeting glycemic goals. Patients who have gestational diabetes should be encouraged to do self-monitoring of capillary BG. Patients who do not want to do self-monitoring should be monitored with HbA_1C testing, following the same schedule as patients with type 2 diabetes.

The goal for patients with type 2 diabetes in terms of preprandial and fasting blood glucose (FBS) levels is 80 to 120 mg/dL, and bedtime glucose levels should be 100 to 140 mg/dL. Fair control is considered to be 120 to 180 mg/dL, and anything higher is unacceptable control. Self-monitoring of preprandial BG by fingerstick is usually done less often than for patients on **insulin** because the drugs have different pharmacokinetic profiles. Patients are taught to keep a diet, drug, and BG level diary, and these diaries are reviewed at each health care provider visit.

Patient Education

ADMINISTRATION. Patients are taught to take the medication exactly as prescribed, at the same time each day, preferably before or with the morning meal. All **sulfonylureas** except **glipizide** may be taken with food. **Glipizide** must be taken 30 minutes before a meal to prevent a reduction in absorption. If a dose is missed, instruct the patient to take it as soon as remembered unless the timing of the dose will produce a risk for hypoglycemia. Doses should not be taken if the patient is unable to eat.

ADVERSE REACTIONS. The most common adverse reactions are GI. If GI upset is a problem, notify the health care provider. The dose may be divided and given twice daily to reduce this adverse effect. The most serious potential adverse reaction is hypoglycemia. Teach the patient the signs and symptoms of hypoglycemia and how to treat it. The treatment is the same as that discussed in the **insulin** patient teaching section. Caution the patient to avoid concurrent administration of other drugs without first discussing them with the health care provider. Many drugs increase or decrease the effectiveness of **sulfonylureas** and can produce hypoglycemia or hyperglycemia. This is especially a problem with **alcohol** because it both produces hypoglycemia and masks the indications of this adverse reaction. **Alcohol** may also produce a disulfiram-like reaction when combined with some **sulfonylureas.**

Because these drugs may produce alterations in red and white blood cell and platelet formation, patients should notify their health care provider promptly if they experience sore throat, rash, or unusual bruising or bleeding. **Sulfonylureas** may also produce an antidiuretic effect, and patients should promptly report unusual weight gain, swelling of the ankles, drowsiness, or shortness of breath.

LIFESTYLE MANAGEMENT. Management of type 2 diabetes involves diet, exercise, weight control, and self-monitoring of BG, as well as administration of **oral hypoglycemics.** Further patient teaching related to management of diabetes is discussed in Chapter 31.

Biguanides

The **biguanides** are **oral antihyperglycemic drugs** used in the treatment of type 2 diabetes mellitus. Their pharmacology and chemistry are different from the **oral hypoglycemics** so that they form a different class. Monotherapy with **metformin (Glucophage)** has proved effective in patients who have not responded to **sulfonylureas,** who have had only a partial response to **sulfonylureas,** or who have ceased to respond to these drugs. If monotherapy is not effective, they have proved very successful as added therapy for patients who cannot be controlled by lifestyle modifications and **sulfonylureas. Metformin** was first released in the United States in September 1995 and to date is the only drug in this class used clinically. This section discusses that drug.

Pharmacodynamics

Metformin increases peripheral glucose uptake and utilization, improves hepatic response to BG levels so that the liver produces appropriate amounts of glucose, and decreases intestinal absorption of glucose. Taken together, these actions improve glucose tolerance and lower both basal and postprandial plasma glucose levels. Unlike the **sulfonylureas, metformin** does not stimulate insulin release from the pancreatic beta cells and so does not produce hypoglycemia in diabetic or nondiabetic patients except in specific circumstances (see Adverse Effects). **Metformin** also does not cause hyperinsulinemia.

The magnitude of decline in fasting BG concentrations with **metformin** therapy is directly proportional to the level of fasting hyperglycemia. Patients with higher BG levels experience a greater percentage of decrease in BG and HbA$_1$C levels than those with lower BG levels.

Metformin also has a modestly favorable impact on lipids because of its actions in the liver. In clinical studies, **metformin** alone or in combination with a **sulfonylurea** lowered mean fasting serum triglycerides, total cholesterol, and low-density lipids (LDL) and had no adverse effect on high-density lipids (HDL) (Bailey & Turner, 1996).

In contrast to patients taking **sulfonylureas,** patients taking **metformin** do not gain weight. In fact, they often lose weight. Because obesity is a major factor in the pathogenesis of type 2 diabetes, this is an important drug action.

Pharmacokinetics

Absorption and Distribution

Metformin is 50 to 60 percent absorbed after oral administration under fasting conditions (Table 19–19). Food decreases the extent and slightly delays the absorption. Absorption is also not linearly related to dose. The higher the dose, the lower the percentage that is absorbed, so that increased doses do not result in proportionally increased amounts of drug in the body.

Metformin is negligibly bound to plasma proteins. Some studies suggest that red blood cells may be a compartment for distribution. The apparent volume of distribution is very high and averages 654 following single doses of 850 mg.

Metabolism and Excretion

There is no hepatic metabolism for this drug, and it is excreted unchanged in the urine. There is no biliary excretion. Renal clearance is 3.5 times that of CCr, indicating that renal tubular secretion is the major route of elimination.

Pharmacotherapeutics

Precautions and Contraindications

There are two major contraindications to **metformin** use: (1) renal disease or dysfunction and (2) metabolic acidosis. Males with serum creatinine levels 1.5 or higher, females with levels 1.4 or higher, and patients of either gender with abnormal CCr rates should not receive **metformin** because of its heavy dependence on renal function for elimination. Patients with acute or chronic metabolic acidosis and patients at high risk for lactic acidosis because of tissue hypoperfusion or hypoxia (e.g., severe dehydration, heart failure, respiratory failure, and chronic alcoholism with severe liver damage) also should not receive this drug. Lactic acidosis is a rare, but serious complication that can occur with **metformin** because of its accumulation during treatment. When it occurs, it is fatal 50 percent of the time. The risk for lactic acidosis in-

Table 19–19. Pharmacokinetics: Antihyperglycemic Drugs

Drug	Onset*	Peak*	Duration*	Bioavailability	Half-Life	Excretion
Metformin	Days	2–4 wk	Unknown	50–60% if taken fasting; non-linear; reduced by food intake	Adults: 2–3.3 h Older adults: 2.7 h Renal impairment: CCr 61–90: 3.2 h CCr 31–60: 3.75 h CCr 10–30: 4 h	100% excreted unchanged in urine
Acarbose	0.5–1 h	1 h	2–3 h	Less than 2% in plasma	2 h	In feces
Miglitol	0.5–1 h	1 h	2–3 h	100% in extra-cellular fluids at 25 mg; 50–70% at higher doses	Normal renal function: 2 h Renal impairment: CCr < 25: 4 h	In urine
Pioglitazone	UA	2–4 h	UA	99%	3–7 h	15–30% in urine
Repaglinide	0.5 h	1 h	1.4 h	100%	1–1.4 h	90% in feces; 8% in urine
Rosiglitazone	UA	1–3 h	UA	99%	3–4 h	64% in urine; 23% in feces

*Of antihyperglycemic effect.
UA = Data unavailable.

creases in the presence of renal dysfunction, making the interaction of these two contraindications more serious than either one alone.

Although there is no specific contraindication for hepatic dysfunction, it has been associated with some cases of lactic acidosis. **Metformin** should not be used for patients with clinical and laboratory evidence of hepatic disease.

Cautious use is suggested with patients over age 80 because of the probability of decreased renal function. Limited data suggest that total plasma clearance is decreased and half-life is prolonged in healthy older adults as compared with healthy young subjects (*Drug Facts and Comparisons,* 1998). These data suggest that the change in pharmacokinetics is primarily accounted for by change in renal function. For older adults, CCr should be tested before beginning and at least annually during therapy.

Metformin should also be temporarily withheld (48 hours before to 48 hours after the procedure) from patients undergoing radiologic studies that involve an iodine-based contrast medium because such materials may result in altered renal function. It should also be temporarily withheld from patients undergoing surgical procedures in which fluid will be withheld because of the risk for dehydration and hypoperfusion that may result in lactic acidosis. The time frame for withholding the drug is the same.

A decrease in vitamin B_{12} levels to subnormal without clinical manifestations has been observed in about 7 percent of patients receiving **metformin.** This decrease is probably due to interference with vitamin B_{12} absorption from the intrinsic factor–vitamin B_{12} complex. Patients with or at risk for anemia associated with altered vitamin B_{12} utilization should have the disorder treated and under control before beginning **metformin** therapy.

Metformin **is listed as Pregnancy Category B, but it is not recommended for use during pregnancy. The consensus among experts is that** *insulin* **should be used to control BG during pregnancy. Studies in rats indicate that** *metformin* **is excreted in breast milk in levels approximately the same as in the plasma. Similar studies have not been conducted in nursing mothers, but it is prudent to avoid this drug in lactating women.**

The safety and efficacy of **metformin** in children have not been established. Studies in MODY children have not been conducted.

Adverse Drug Reactions

The most common adverse reaction involves GI disturbances (e.g., abdominal bloating, diarrhea, nausea, vomiting, and an unpleasant metallic taste). These adverse reactions are usually transient and resolve in about 2 weeks without a change in dose. They may be reduced by initiating therapy with a low dose and titrating the dose up slowly.

Lactic acidosis is rare and was discussed in Precautions and Contraindications. Hypoglycemia is also rare unless there is a concurrent reduction in caloric intake, an increase in strenuous exercise not compensated for with increased caloric intake, or concurrent use of another **glucose-lowering drug** or **alcohol.** Older adults, debilitated and malnourished patients, and those with adrenal or pituitary insufficiency are also at increased risk for hypoglycemia.

Drug Interactions

Cationic drugs that are eliminated by renal secretion (e.g., **amiloride, digoxin, morphine, procainamide, quinidine, ranitidine, triamterene, trimethoprim,** and **vancomycin**) may compete with **metformin** for its elimination pathway (Table 19–20). Dosage adjustments may be needed in **metformin** or the interacting drugs.

Cimetidine increases the peak **metformin** plasma level by 60 percent, with an increase of 40 percent in its AUC. **Furosemide** increases these levels by 15 percent without any significant change in renal clearance. Both of these drugs may increase the effects of **metformin** because of these alterations. Dosage adjustment for **metformin** may be necessary.

Nifedipine increases absorption and may increase the effects of **metformin.** It concurrently increases the amount excreted in the urine, however, so that the total effect may be small.

Clinical Use and Dosing

TYPE 2 DIABETES MELLITUS. **Metformin** is indicated as monotherapy and as added therapy for patients with type 2 diabetes who cannot achieve adequate BG control on diet, exercise, weight control, and a sulfonylurea alone. It is especially useful for obese patients because it is not associated with weight gain and may produce some weight loss. Its positive effect on lipids creates a clear advantage for patients with hyperlipidemia. The pharmacodynamics of **metformin** are different from those of sulfonylureas so that the two drugs taken together potentiate each other's actions. In clinical trials, both the fasting and the postprandial BG levels of patients decreased by 20 to 30 percent. Because this drop is so dramatic, it is important to monitor BG levels closely when **metformin** is added to the treatment regimen to avoid hypoglycemia.

Metformin is available in 500-mg and 850-mg tablets. Begin therapy with 500 mg bid with the morning and evening meal or 850 mg daily with the morning meal (Table 19–21). The dose is increased in increments of 500 mg at weekly intervals or 850 mg every other week. The most common adverse reactions are GI disturbances. If they occur, the dose should be held at that level and not increased. The symptoms will most likely resolve in about 2 weeks, at which time the dosage can

Table 19–20. Drug Interactions with Metformin

Interacting Drug	Possible Effect	Implications
Alcohol	Potentiates the effect of metformin on lactate metabolism	Warn patients against excessive alcohol intake while taking metformin.
Amiloride, digoxin, morphine, procainamide, quinidine, ranitidine, triamterene, trimethoprim, vancomycin	May compete for elimination pathway	Dosage adjustments may be needed for metformin or interacting drug.
Beta-adrenergic blockers	May mask signs and symptoms of hypoglycemia	Does not affect diaphoresis as indicator of hypoglycemia; teach patient to check blood glucose level if experiencing diaphoresis.
Cimetidine, furosemide	Increases plasma levels of metformin without concurrent increase in renal excretion	Dosage adjustments of metformin may be needed.
Iodine-based contrast media	May affect renal function and increase the risk for lactic acidosis	Withhold metformin for 48 h before and after procedure in which contrast is used.
Nifedipine	Enhances absorption of metformin and may increase effects	Dosage adjustments of metformin may be needed.

Clinical Pearl

When **metformin** is added to a **sulfonylurea** in a diabetic regimen, the increased sensitivity to **insulin** caused by **metformin** results in less need for the insulin secretion generated by the **sulfonylurea**. If the BG level drops too much, the dose of the **sulfonylurea** should be reduced.

be increased again until target BG levels are reached. The maximum dose recommended is 2550 mg/day. The maximum dose should be divided and given tid to reduce GI reactions.

Monitoring

Before initiating therapy and at least annually thereafter, assess renal function. Assessment is by serum creatinine and CCr initially and then by serum creatinine annually. For patients with increased risk for developing altered renal function, the assessment should be more often. Patients who have been previously well controlled on **metformin** who are no longer controlled or who develop illnesses that place them at risk for metabolic acidosis should be assessed for evidence of ketoacidosis or lactic acidosis. Assessment includes serum electrolytes and ketones, BG, and, if indicated, blood pH and lactate levels. Lactic acidosis is characterized by elevated blood lactate levels (more than 5 mmol/L), decreased blood pH, and electrolyte disturbances with an increased anion gap. Because impaired hepatic function may significantly decrease the ability to clear lactate, liver function studies should be done before therapy is initiated.

Response to **metformin** therapy is assessed by daily to weekly monitoring of fasting and postprandial BG and by monitoring HbA$_1$C every 2 to 3 months or monitoring fructosamine every 1 to 2 months. During initial therapy and with each incremental increase, fasting BG is used to evaluate response. After the patient is stabilized on a specific dose, monitoring with fasting BG and HbA$_1$C levels every 3 to 6 months is sufficient.

Some patients with inadequate vitamin B$_{12}$ or calcium intake or absorption may be predisposed to developing subnormal vitamin B$_{12}$ levels. Assessment for this problem is done by red blood cell indices drawn at initiation of therapy and every 2 to 3 years thereafter.

Patient Education

ADMINISTRATION. Patients are taught to take the drug at the same time each day exactly as prescribed. Because the titrating doses will change weekly or every other week, a card or calendar is helpful to remind them of the schedule. If a dose is missed, it is taken as soon as it is remembered unless it is about time for the next dose. Do not double doses. Explain to the patient that **metformin** helps to control hyperglycemia, but it does not cure diabetes. The therapy will be long term.

ADVERSE REACTIONS. The most common adverse reactions are GI disturbances. If they occur, they may be reduced by taking the drug with food rather than before the

Table 19–21. Dosage Schedule: Metformin

Drug	Dosage Schedule	Dosage Form

Metformin (Glucophage) 500-mg tablets	Initial dose: Week 1:500 mg bid
	Continuing dose:
	    Week 2: 1000 mg q AM and 500 mg at evening meal
	    Week 3: 1000 mg q AM and 1000 mg at evening meal
	    Week 4: 1500 mg q AM and 1000 mg at evening meal
		500-mg tablets in 100-tablet bottles

Metformin (Glucophage) 850-mg tablets	Initial dose: Weeks 1 and 2: 850 mg at morning meal
	Continuing dose:
	    Weeks 3 and 4: 850 mg q AM and 850 mg at evening meal
	    Week 5: 850 mg at breakfast, 850 mg at lunch, and 850 mg at evening meal
		850-mg tablets in 100-tablet bottles

meal. The health care provider should be notified of GI disturbances so that the dose may be kept at the current level until they resolve. Even with the same dose, GI disturbances will usually resolve in about 2 weeks. If the GI disturbances include vomiting or diarrhea or the patient develops a fever, the drug is stopped and the health care provider notified. Dehydration may result and presents a risk for developing lactic acidosis and decreased renal function. Patients are taught the signs and symptoms of lactic acidosis (e.g., chills, dizziness, low blood pressure, muscle pain, sleepiness, trouble breathing, slow heart rate, and weakness) and to report them immediately.

Lactic acidosis may also result from any incident that results in hypoperfusion or hypoxia. A patient who is to undergo a procedure with an iodine-based contrast medium or surgery in which fluid will be withheld will be temporarily taken off **metformin;** the health care provider should be notified if one of these procedures is anticipated.

Hypoglycemia is less common than with other **glucose-lowering drugs** but may occur when **metformin** is given with one of these drugs. Patient instruction for hypoglycemia has been discussed in the Insulin and Sulfonylurea sections.

Metformin may cause an unpleasant or metallic taste. This reaction usually resolves spontaneously in a few weeks.

LIFESTYLE MANAGEMENT. Type 2 diabetes is a chronic illness managed with diet, exercise, weight control, and self-monitoring of BG, as well as drug therapy. Further patient teaching related to management of diabetes is discussed in Chapter 31.

Alpha-Glucosidase Inhibitors

The **alpha-glucosidase inhibitors** are **oral antihyperglycemic** drugs used in the treatment of type 2 diabetes mellitus. Their pharmacodynamics are different from those of the **sulfonylureas** and the **biguanides.** The action of this class has proved to reduce blood glucose both as added therapy for patients who cannot achieve control on diet alone and as added therapy for patients whose blood glucose cannot be controlled by lifestyle modifications and other **oral antidiabetic agents. Acarbose (Precose)** was first released in January 1996; **miglitol (Glyset)** was approved in 1998 and released in 1999. Material related to **miglitol** in this section is based on the initial approval as presented in *Drug Facts and Comparisons* (1998).

Pharmacodynamics

Alpha-glucosidase inhibitors do not act directly on any of the defects in metabolism seen in type 2 diabetes mellitus. They competitively inhibit the absorption of complex carbohydrates (CHO) from the small bowel. Their chemical structure is a pseudotetrasaccharide that binds to alpha glucosidase. Because this structure is so similar to the CHO molecule, digestive enzyme activity is partially diverted from CHO digestion while it is trying to digest **acarbose.** This effectively delays the digestion of CHO and permits CHOs that would normally have been digested in the upper small bowel to move further down in the bowel. The lower parts of the bowel have the necessary enzymes to digest this CHO, but, because they are not normally active in this process, enzyme induction is required. The process of induction takes weeks to months, and during this time patients may experience intestinal flatus and abdominal distention. **Alpha-glucosidase inhibitors** have no inhibitory activity against lactase and do not induce lactose intolerance.

Alpha-glucosidase inhibitors lower BG levels after meals. The higher the postprandial BG level, the larger the reduction with this drug. As a consequence of plasma glucose reduction, they also reduce glycosylated hemoglobin levels. The mean reduction in HbA_1C is 0.77 percent, postprandial BG reduction is approximately 50 mg/dL, and fasting BG reduction is 20 mg/dL (*Drug Facts and Comparisons,* 1998).

Unlike the **sulfonylureas,** they do not enhance pancreatic beta cell secretion of insulin and so do not produce hypoglycemia in diabetic or nondiabetic patients, except in special situations. Like **metformin,** they are not associated with weight gain and diminish the weight-increasing effects of **sulfonylureas** when given in combination with them. Their activity is effective on any CHO food intake, including liquid diets taken via nasogastric tube.

Pharmacokinetics

Absorption and Distribution

Less than 2 percent of **acarbose** is systemically absorbed as active drug. The remainder is active in the GI tract with no systemic distribution. **Miglitol** is completely absorbed in the GI tract at 25-mg doses, and 50 to 70 percent is absorbed at higher doses. Its volume of distribution of 0.18 is consistent with distribution primarily into extracellular fluids.

Metabolism and Excretion

Acarbose and **miglitol** are metabolized exclusively by intestinal bacteria and digestive enzymes. The minimal amount of drug absorbed is excreted by the kidney. The plasma elimination half-life of both drugs is about 2 hours, so drug accumulation does not occur with tid dosing. The mean steady-state AUC and maximum concentration of this drug were 1.5 times higher in older adults taking **acarbose,** but this was neither statistically

Clinical Pearl

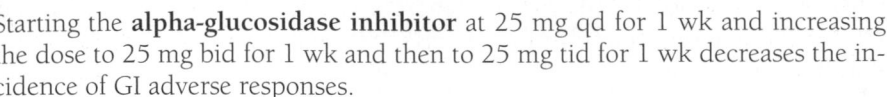
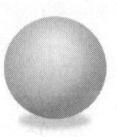

Starting the **alpha-glucosidase inhibitor** at 25 mg qd for 1 wk and increasing the dose to 25 mg bid for 1 wk and then to 25 mg tid for 1 wk decreases the incidence of GI adverse responses.

nor clinically significant. This change was not seen with **miglitol**.

Pharmacotherapeutics

Precautions and Contraindications

Alpha-glucosidase inhibitors should not be used for patients with bowel diseases such as inflammatory bowel disease, bowel obstruction or risk factors for it, chronic intestinal disease associated with marked digestive disorders, or conditions that may deteriorate as a result of increased gas in the intestine.

Plasma concentrations of **alpha-glucosidase inhibitors** were 5 times higher in patients with severe renal impairment (CCr less than 25 cc/min) (*Drug Facts and Comparisons,* 1998). Long-term studies with patients with diabetes have not been conducted. Therefore, treatment with these drugs is not recommended for these patients.

The safety of *alpha-glucosidase inhibitors* in pregnant women has not been established. Although they are listed as Pregnancy Category B, they should not be used in pregnancy unless clearly needed. In a study, a small amount of *acarbose* was excreted in the breast milk of rats. It is not known if it is excreted in human breast milk, and it should not be used in lactating women. *Miglitol* is excreted in human breast milk to a small degree. Total excretion in breast milk accounts for 0.02 percent of a 100-mg maternal dose. Although the levels in breast milk are exceedingly low, it also should not be used for lactating women.

Safety and efficacy in children have not been established for either drug.

Adverse Drug Reactions

GI symptoms are the most common adverse reactions. Approximately 77 percent of patients taking **acarbose** and 41 percent of patients taking **miglitol** experience flatulence, and this is the leading reason for discontinuance of the drug. Approximately 33 percent of patients taking **acarbose** and 29 percent of patients taking **miglitol** experience diarrhea, whereas 21 percent report abdominal pain while taking **acarbose** and 12 percent

while taking **miglitol**. These adverse effects can be reduced by slow titration to maximal dose.

Because of their mechanism of action, **alpha-glucosidase inhibitors** alone do not cause hypoglycemia but may do so in combination with other drugs that lower blood glucose, such as **sulfonylureas**. Treatment of this hypoglycemia cannot be accomplished with the usual ingestion of sucrose (hard candy or soft drinks), fructose, or starches because **alpha-glucosidase inhibitors** delay the absorption of these disaccharides. Because there is no inhibitory activity against lactase or monosaccharides, milk, lactose, and glucose can be used to treat the hypoglycemia.

Reversible increases in serum transaminases (ALT and AST) have occurred with doses greater than 200 mg tid of **acarbose**. Hepatic abnormalities improved or resolved with discontinuance of the drug. This laboratory change has not been reported with **miglitol**.

Drug Interactions

The literature on drug interactions related to **acarbose** is contradictory. The package insert reports no interference with the pharmacokinetics or pharmocodynamics of **digoxin, nifedipine, propranolol,** or **ranitidine.** *Drug Facts and Comparisons* (1998), however, states that **acarbose** interferes with **digoxin** absorption, resulting in decreased serum concentration that may diminish the therapeutic effects of the **digoxin**.

Miglitol has drug interactions with several drugs, including **digoxin, propranolol,** and **ranitidine.** Both **acarbose** and **miglitol** may have their therapeutic effects reduced by concurrent administration with digestive enzymes or intestinal absorbents. Table 19–22 shows drug interactions for these two drugs as reported in *Drug Facts and Comparisons* (1998).

Clinical Use and Dosing

Management of type 2 diabetes mellitus is the only indication for these drugs. They are useful for patients with high postprandial BG levels. The initial dose of both drugs is 25 mg tid taken with the first bite of each meal (Table 19–23). Taking the dose with the first bite is critical; a space between administration of the drug and in-

Clinical Pearl

The delayed absorption of carbohydrates caused by **alpha-glucosidase inhibitors** results in less need for the insulin secretion generated by a **sulfonylurea**. If the BG level drops too much, the dose of the **sulfonylurea** should be reduced.

gestion of food decreases its effect, and no effect occurs if it is taken after a meal. The dose is increased in increments of 25 mg with each meal (75 mg/day) at 4- to 8-week intervals. The maintenance dose is usually 50 mg tid. If no further reduction in postprandial BG is achieved at the higher dose, consider reducing the dose back to 50 mg tid.

Because patients with low body weight are at higher risk for elevations in serum transaminase, the dose should be not be higher than 50 mg tid for patients weighing less than 60 kg, and the 100-mg tid dose should be reserved for patients weighing more than 60 kg. The maximum dose is 100 mg tid.

When given in combination with a **sulfonylurea** or **metformin,** the drop in postprandial BG may be significant. It is important to monitor BG levels closely when **alpha-glucosidase inhibitors** are added to the treatment regimen to avoid hypoglycemia.

Rational Drug Selection

ADVERSE REACTIONS. There have been no reported hepatic adverse reactions and no reported changes in liver function tests with **miglitol** in clinical trials; however, such reactions may be reported later when it is marketed and more patients use it. Patients with mild hepatic impairment might be given **miglitol** with careful monitoring.

The percentage of patients experiencing GI adverse effects in clinical trials is slightly lower with **miglitol.** Patients at risk for this adverse effect might be tried first on **miglitol.**

DRUG INTERACTIONS. **Miglitol** has reported drug interactions with **propranolol** and **ranitidine.** Patients who must take these medications might benefit from choosing **acarbose.**

Monitoring

Before initiating therapy and at least annually thereafter, assess renal function. For patients with increased risk beyond their diabetes for developing altered renal function, the assessment timing should be related to the disease process that produces the added risk. **Alpha-glucosidase inhibitors** are not recommended for patients with renal impairment. Assessment of renal function includes serum electrolytes, blood urea nitrogen (BUN), and serum creatinine. A similar assessment is required related to hepatic function for patients taking **acarbose.** Because **acarbose** has been associated with reversible elevations in serum transaminase, these values should be assessed every 3 months for the first year.

Response to **alpha-glucosidase inhibitor** therapy is assessed by regular monitoring of fasting and postprandial BG. During initial therapy and with each incremental increase, fasting BG is used to evaluate response. After the patient is stabilized on a specific dose, monitoring with fasting BG and HbA$_1$C levels every 3 to 6 months is sufficient.

Patient Education

ADMINISTRATION. Patients are taught to take these drugs with the first bite of each meal. The need for this

Table 19–22. Drug Interactions: Alpha-Glucosidase Inhibitors

Drug	Interacting Drug	Possible Effect	Implications
Acarbose, miglitol	Digoxin	Serum digoxin concentrations may be reduced with reduced therapeutic effect	Choose another antihyperglycemic drug
	Digestive enzymes and intestinal absorbents	Reduced effect of alpha-glucosidase inhibitor	Do not take concomitantly
Miglitol	Propranolol	Reduces bioavailability of propranolol by 40%	Avoid current use
	Ranitidine	Reduces bioavailability of ranitidine by 60%	Avoid current use

Table 19–23. Dosage Schedule: Alpha-Glucosidase Inhibitors

Patient Population	Initial Dose	Incremental Dosage Increases
Weight more than 60 kg (most patients)	25 mg tid with the first bite of each meal for 4 wk	Weeks 5–8: 50 mg tid with first bite of each meal Weeks 9–12: 100 mg tid with first bite of each meal
Weight less than 60 kg	25 mg tid with the first bite of each meal for 4 wk	Weeks 5–8: 50 mg tid with first bite of each meal; then maintain this dose
Patients with poor GI tolerance	25 mg qd with first bite of evening meal for 2 wk	Weeks 3–4: 25 mg bid with first bite of morning and evening meal Weeks 5–12: 25 mg tid with first bite of each meal Week 13: Begin 50 mg tid with first bite of each meal; then maintain this dose

timing of administration must be stressed because taking it too soon reduces its effect and taking it after a meal means no effect. Because the titrating doses may change at 4- to 8-week intervals, a card or calendar is helpful to remind them of the schedule. Explain to the patient that **alpha-glucosidase inhibitors** help to control hyperglycemia, but they do not cure diabetes. The therapy is long term.

ADVERSE REACTIONS. The most common adverse reactions are GI disturbances. If they occur, the health care provider should be notified so that the dose may be adjusted. These effects can be reduced or prevented by slow titration of the dose. Even without changing the dose, GI disturbances usually resolve in about 2 weeks.

Hypoglycemia is less common than with other **glucose-lowering drugs** but may occur when **alpha-glucosidase inhibitors** are given with **insulin, sufonylureas,** or **repaglinide (Prandin).** The usual treatment for hypoglycemia with sucrose, fructose, or starches does not resolve the problem for patients on **alpha-glucosidase inhibitors** because it interferes with the absorption of these carhydrates. An 8-oz glass of milk or lactose tablets can be used to treat the hypoglycemia because **alpha-glucosidase inhibitors** do not affect lactose metabolism. Severe hypoglycemia may need to be treated with intravenous **glucose** or **glucagon.** Patients should wear identification that states they are taking an **alpha-glucosidase inhibitor** and the source of simple carbohydrate that should be used in case of hypoglycemia.

LIFESTYLE MANAGEMENT. Type 2 diabetes is a chronic illness managed with diet, exercise, weight control, and self-monitoring of BG, as well as drug therapy. Further patient teaching related to management of diabetes is discussed in Chapter 31.

Thiazolidinediones

The **thiazolidinediones** are **oral antihyperglycemic** drugs used in the treatment of type 2 diabetes mellitus. Their actions have lowered BG levels as monotherapy for patients who cannot achieve BG control with diet alone, and they have proved very successful as added therapy for patients who cannot be controlled by lifestyle modifications and **sulfonylureas. Troglitazone (Rezulin)** was first released in March 1997. It was removed from the market in 1999 because of the adverse reactions associated with liver damage. **Pioglitazone (Actos)** and **rosiglitazone (Avandia)** are newer drugs in this class. They have been associated with less

Table 19–24. Available Dosage Forms: Alpha-Glucosidase Inhibitors

Drug	Dosage Form
Acarbose (Precose)	50 mg (scored) in 100-tablet bottles 100 mg in 100-tablet bottles
Miglitol (Glyset)	25 mg in 100-tablet bottles 50 mg in 100- and 1000-tablet bottles 100 mg in 100- and 1000-tablet bottles

risk of liver damage. This section discusses these two drugs.

Pharmacodynamics

Thiazolidinediones activate a nuclear receptor that regulates gene transcription, resulting in expression of proteins that improve insulin action in the cell. This action leads to increased utilization of available insulin by the liver and muscle cells and also in adipose tissue. In addition, these drugs reduce hepatic glucose production so that the liver produces appropriate amounts of glucose. Taken together, these actions improve glucose tolerance and lower both basal and postprandial plasma glucose levels. Unlike the **sulfonylureas**, **thiazolidinediones** do not produce hypoglycemia in diabetic or nondiabetic patients, except in special situations, and do not cause hyperinsulinemia because they do not stimulate insulin release from the pancreatic beta cells. Like **metformin**, they have a modest impact on lipids because of their actions in the liver. In clinical studies, these drugs lowered serum triglyceride levels and increased HDL levels. Although total cholesterol and LDL levels increased slightly, the LDL fractions became larger and less dense and so actually reduced coronary heart disease risk. The end result was no change in the serum HDL to total cholesterol ratio, so this risk factor for cardiovascular disease did not improve.

Pharmacokinetics

Absorption and Distribution

Pioglitazone and **rosiglitazone** are rapidly absorbed after oral administration. Food does not alter the extent of absorption. Both drugs are extensively bound to plasma proteins, with a mean volume of distribution ranging from 0.63L/kg for **pioglitazone** to 17.6 L/kg for **rosiglitazone**.

Metabolism and Excretion

Both drugs are highly metabolized by the liver into metabolites. Hepatic function impairment increased C_{max} for both drugs and AUC levels for **rosiglitazone**. The **pioglitazone** site of metabolism in the liver results in inhibition of the CYP-450 3A4 enzyme system. Drugs using this enzyme system are likely to have drug interactions. In vitro drug studies suggest that **rosiglitazone** does not inhibit any of the major CPY-450 enzyme systems. It is predominantly metabolized by CYP-450 2C8 and to a lesser extent 2C9.

Mean plasma elimination half-life ranges from 3 to 7 hours, with 23 percent of **rosiglitazone** and its metabo-

lites recovered in the feces and 64 percent in the urine. **Pioglitazone** is excreted 15 to 30 percent in the urine.

Pharmacotherapeutics

Precautions and Contraindications

The metabolites of these drugs have been found in increased concentrations in patients with chronic liver disease. Although available clinical data to date show no evidence of hepatotoxicity induced by **pioglitazone or rosiglitazone**, it is prudent to remember that these drugs are in the same class as **troglitazone** and may demonstrate similar problems with time. Serum transaminase levels must be checked at the start of therapy and frequently during therapy. Specific monitoring times are discussed in the Monitoring section. These drugs should not be initiated in patients with ALT levels greater than 2.5 times the upper limit of normal. They should be discontinued if the patient develops jaundice or has laboratory measurements suggesting liver injury (e.g., ALT greater than 3 times the upper limit of normal).

An increase in plasma volume with a resultant decrease in hemoglobin of less than or equal to 1 percent with **rosiglitazone** and 2 to 4 percent with **pioglitazone** has been noted in some patients. This may not present a problem for patients with New York Heart Association class I or II heart disease, but these drugs should be used with caution if administered to class III or IV heart disease patients.

In premenopausal anovulatory patients with insulin resistance, **thiazolidinedione** treatment may result in resumption of ovulation. If pregnancy is not desired, a birth control method should be instituted prior to beginning therapy.

There are no adequate and well-controlled studies of the use of *pioglitazone* or *rosiglitazone* in pregnant women. Some animal studies have shown fetal death and growth retardation. Although listed as Pregnancy Category B, *thiazolidinediones* should not be used during pregnancy unless the potential benefit clearly outweighs the risk. *Insulin* is the drug of choice for treatment of diabetes during pregnancy.

It is not known whether these drugs are excreted in breast milk. They are secreted in the milk of lactating rats. Do not administer these drugs to lactating women.

Safety and efficacy in children have not been established.

Adverse Drug Reactions

Thiazolidinediones are generally well tolerated, and all reported adverse reactions (except those associated with hepatic injury discussed in Precautions and Contraindications) have been no more common than those seen with placebo.

Drug Interactions

Administration of **pioglitazone** with an **oral contraceptive** that contains **ethinyl estradiol** and **norethindrone** reduces the plasma concentrations of both components by 30 percent. These changes, added to the resumption of ovulation that occurs in some anovulatory women, could result in loss of contraception. A higher dose of **oral contraceptive** or an alternative birth control method may be needed.

Pioglitazone is metabolized by the CPY-450 3A4 isoenzyme system. Specific formal pharmacokinetic interaction studies have not been conducted with other drugs also metabolized by this system (e.g., **erythromycin, calcium channel blockers, corticosteroids, cyclosporine, HMG-CoA reductase inhibitors**). In vitro, **ketoconazole** appears to significantly inhibit **pioglitazone** metabolism. Until data are available, it is prudent to avoid these drug combinations or to carefully monitor patients concurrently taking **pioglitazone** and any of the drugs also metabolized by the CYP-450 3A4 isoenzyme system.

Table 19–25 presents drug interactions with **thiazolidinediones**.

Clinical Use and Dosing

The only approved indication for these drugs is as therapy for type 2 diabetes mellitus patients not controlled by diet alone or diet and a **sulfonylurea** or **insulin**.

MONOTHERAPY. Clinical trials have been conducted to study the use of both **pioglitazone** and **rosiglitazone** as monotherapy for patients previously treated only with diet. Doses of 15 to 30 mg/day of **pioglitazone** were associated with decreased fasting BG by 39 mg/dL for the 15-mg dose and 58 mg/dL for the 30-mg dose. Glycosylated hemoglobin (HgA$_{1c}$) was reduced by 0.9 percent for the 15-mg dose and 1.3 percent for the 30-mg dose.

The initial dose of **pioglitazone** may be either 15 mg or 30 mg and the dose may be increased in 15-mg increments to a maximum dose of 45 mg/day (Tables 19–26 and 19–27). Because effectiveness of therapy is best evaluated by HgA$_{1c}$ values, it is recommended that the adequate time period for evaluation of drug effectiveness is 3 months unless glycemic control deteriorates.

Rosiglitazone in doses of 8 mg/day reduced fasting BG by 40.8 mg/dL and HgA$_{1c}$ by 0.53 percent. Four-milligram doses reduced fasting BG by 25.4 percent and HgA$_{1c}$ by 0.27 percent. **Rosiglitazone** is usually initiated at 4 mg/day as a single dose. If single-dose therapy is not effective, the dose may be divided into twice-daily dosing or increased incrementally to a maximum dose of 8 mg/day (see Tables 19–26 and 19–27). As with **pioglitazone**, evaluation of adequacy of response requires 12 weeks of therapy.

Thiazolidinediones should not be used as monotherapy for patients previously well controlled on a **sulfonylurea** alone. They should be added to, not substituted for, the **sulfonylurea**.

COMBINATION THERAPY WITH SULFONYLUREAS. When used as added therapy to management with a **sulfonylurea**, initiate **pioglitazone** with either the 15- or 30-mg dose. For **rosiglitazone**, initiate therapy at 4 mg/day in single or divided doses. Continue the current dose of the **sulfonylurea**. If the response in terms of glycemic control is inadequate, increase the dose of the **thiazolidinedione** at 8 to 12 weeks, not to exceed the maximum mg/day (see Table 19–26).

The pharmacodynamics of **thiazolidinediones** are different from **sulfonylureas** so that the two drugs taken together potentiate each other's actions. Both fasting and postprandial BG levels of patients decrease. It is important to monitor BG levels closely when **thiazolidinediones** are added to the treatment regimen to avoid hypoglycemia.

COMBINATION THERAPY WITH INSULIN. As of this printing, approval for the use of **pioglitazone** or **rosiglitazone** in combination with insulin has not been approved. (See Table 19–26 for the clinical use and dosing regimens for **thiazolidinediones**.)

Table 19–25. Drug Interactions with Thiazolidinediones

Drug	Interacting Drug	Possible Outcome	Implications
Pioglitazone	Oral contraceptives	Oral contraceptives with ethinyl estradiol and norethindrone show reduced plasma contraceptive components	May result in loss of contraception; consider higher dose of contraceptive or alternative method
Pioglitazone and rosiglitazone	Bile acid sequestrants	Pharmacological effects of thiazolidinedione may be decreased; bile acid sequestrant reduces absorption	Avoid concurrent use; separate doses by 4 h, giving thiazolidinedione first

Clinical Pearl

When **thiazolidinediones** are added to a **sulfonylurea** in a diabetic regimen, the increased sensitivity to insulin caused by the **thiazolidinedione** results in less need for the insulin secretion generated by the **sulfonylurea**. If the BG level drops too much, the dose of the **sulfonylurea** should be reduced.

Monitoring

Serum transaminase (ALT) levels must be checked at the start of therapy. **Thiazolidinediones** are not started if the pretreatment serum ALT level is more than 2.5 times the upper limit of normal (ULN). Once therapy is started, ALT is checked every 2 months for the first 12 months and periodically thereafter. If the ALT increases to more than 1.5 to 2 times the ULN, liver function tests are done every week until levels return to normal. The drug is discontinued if the ALT level is more than 3 times the ULN. The cost of this amount of monitoring must be considered in the total cost of therapy with these drugs.

If any patient develops symptoms suggesting hepatic dysfunction, the decision whether to continue the therapy with **pioglitazone** or **rosiglitazone** is guided by clinical judgment pending laboratory evaluation. If jaundice is observed, therapy is discontinued.

Response to **thiazolidinedione** therapy is assessed by regular monitoring of fasting BG and HgA$_{1c}$. During initial therapy and with each incremental increase, fasting BG is used to evaluate response. After the patient is stabilized on a specific dose, monitoring with fasting BG and HgA$_{1c}$ levels every 3 to 6 months is sufficient.

Patient Education

ADMINISTRATION. **Pioglitazone** is to be taken once daily in the morning. If it is missed, it can be taken as soon as remembered. If the dose is missed for the entire day, the dose should not be doubled the next day. Explain to the patient that **pioglitazone** helps to control hyperglycemia, but it does not cure diabetes. The therapy is long term.

Rosiglitazone may be taken once daily or twice daily in divided doses. The dosing schedule should not be changed without consultation with the health care

Table 10 26. Dosage Schedule: Thiazolidinediones

Drug	Indication	Initial Dose	Maintenance Dose
Pioglitazone	Monotherapy (see text for more discussion)	15–30 mg qd	May increase in increments up to maximum dose of 45 mg/d.
	Combined with sulfonylurea	15–30 mg qd	Continue current sulfonylurea dose; decrease dose of sulfonylurea if hypoglycemia results. Maximum dose of pioglitazone 45 mg/d.
	Combined with metformin	15–30 mg qd	Continue metformin dose. Maximum dose is 45 mg/d.
Rosiglitazone	Monotherapy	4 mg/d in single dose or in divided doses twice daily	If inadequate response in 12 wk, increase to 8 mg/d in single or divided doses. Maximum dose is 8 mg/d.
	Combined with metformin	4 mg/d in single dose or in divided doses twice daily	May be increased to 8 mg if inadequate control after 12 wk. Maximum dose is 8 mg/d.

Table 19–27. Available Dosage Forms: Thiazolidinediones

Drug	Dosage Form
Pioglitazone (Actos)	15 mg in 30-, 90-, and 500-tablet bottles 30 mg in 30-, 90-, and 500-tablet bottles 45 mg in 30-, 90-, and 500-tablet bottles
Rosiglitazone (Avandia)	2 mg in 30-, 60-, 100-, and 500-tablet bottles 4 mg in 30-, 60-, 100-, and 500-tablet bottles 8 mg in 30-, 60-, 100-, and 500-tablet bottles

provider. If the dose is missed for the entire day, the dose should not be doubled the next day. Explain to the patient that **rosiglitazone** helps to control hyperglycemia, but it does not cure diabetes. The therapy is long term.

ADVERSE REACTIONS. Thiazolidinediones are generally well tolerated and adverse reactions are rare. The one adverse reaction of concern is hepatocellular injury. Advise the patient to report immediately any signs of hepatic dysfunction such as nausea, vomiting, abdominal pain, fatigue, anorexia, jaundice, or dark urine. Explain to the patient that hepatic function must be carefully monitored and that it is essential to keep follow-up appointments for laboratory work.

Hypoglycemia is not a risk with monotherapy, but may occur when thiazolidinediones are given with another **glucose-lowering drug.** The usual treatment for hypoglycemia with sucrose, fructose, or starches will resolve the problem. Mangement of hypoglycemia is discussed in the Patient Education sections of **insulin** and **sulfonylureas.**

Female patients using **oral contraceptives** for birth control and premenopausal anovulatory patients should be informed about the possible need to increase the dose of **oral contraceptive** or choose an alternative birth control method.

LIFESTYLE MANAGEMENT. Type 2 diabetes is a chronic illness managed with diet, exercise, weight control, and self-monitoring of BG, as well as drug therapy. Further patient teaching related to management of diabetes is discussed in Chapter 31.

Meglitinides

The **meglitinides** have a different mechanism of action than any of the other drugs used to treat type 2 diabetes. They are short-acting insulin secretagogues. Their action has proved helpful in lowering BG levels as monotherapy for patients who cannot achieve BG control with diet alone, and they have proved successful in combination with **metformin** for patients who cannot be controlled by

lifestyle modifications or either agent taken alone. **Repaglinide (Prandin)** was first released in April 1998, and to date it is the only drug in this class used clinically. This section discusses that drug.

Pharmacodynamics

Repaglinide closes ATP-dependent potassium channels in the beta cell membrane by binding at specific receptor sites. This potassium channel blockade depolarizes the beta cell and leads to an opening of calcium channels. The resultant influx of calcium increases the secretion of insulin. Because its time in the plasma is less than 2 hours, the effect is very short. The ion channel mechanism is highly tissue-selective, with low affinity for heart and skeletal muscle, which reduces the potential adverse effects of these tissues.

The end result of **repaglinide** stimulation of insulin secretion is lower postprandial BG levels. It does not directly affect fasting BG levels or any of the other defects in metabolism seen in type 2 diabetes mellitus.

Pharmacokinetics

Absorption and Distribution

After oral administration, **repaglinide** is rapidly and completely absorbed from the GI tract. It is highly bound to albumin for distribution, primarily to beta cell membranes. Peak plasma level occurs within 1 hour. The presence of food in the gut decreases absorption. **Repaglinide** is taken before a meal.

Metabolism and Excretion

Repaglinide is completely metabolized by oxidative biotransformation and direct conjugation with glucuronic acid. The CYP-450 enzyme system, particularly 3A4, is involved in metabolism.

This drug is rapidly eliminated from the plasma, with

a half-life of about 1 hour. Within 96 hours after administration, 90 percent of the drug and its metabolites are recovered in the feces and 8 percent in the urine.

Pharmacotherapeutics

Precautions and Contraindications

In clinical trials, patients with moderate to severe hepatic impairment had higher and more prolonged serum concentrations of both total and unbound **repaglinide** than healthy subjects. This drug should be used cautiously with patients who have hepatic impairment, and longer intervals between dosage adjustments should be used.

Repaglinide is Pregnancy Category C. Nonteratogenic skeletal deformities occurred in test animals. Safety in pregnant women has not been established, and *insulin* is the drug of choice for treating diabetes in pregnant women.

Repaglinide was excreted in the breast milk of test animals. It is not known if it is excreted in human breast milk. Because the potential exists for hypoglycemia in nursing infants, it should not be used with lactating women.

No studies have been done to test this drug's safety and efficacy in children.

Adverse Drug Reactions

The risk for hypoglycemia with **repaglinide** is about the same as with **glyburide** and **glipizide**. Patients with hepatic insufficiency, older adults, and debilitated and malnourished patients are at higher risk for hypoglycemia. The frequency of hypoglycemia is also greater for patients who have not been previously treated with **oral hypoglycemic agents** or whose HbA₁C is less than 8 percent. Careful timing of administration with regard to meals lessens the likelihood of this adverse reaction.

Drug Interactions

Because the CYP-450 3A4 enzyme system is involved in metabolism, drugs that induce this enzyme system (e.g., **troglitazone, rifampin, barbiturates, carbamazepine**) may increase **repaglinide** metabolism (Table 19–28). This enzyme system is among the most used widely by drugs for metabolism, and other drug reactions may be found as this drug is used.

Antifungal agents like **ketoconazole** and **miconazole** and **antimicrobial agents** like **erythromycin** inhibit **repaglinide** metabolism and may increase the risk for hypoglycemia by raising blood levels of the drug.

Any drug that alters BG levels has the potential to alter the glycemic control effects of repaglinide. Other **oral hypoglycemics** can potentiate the action of drugs that are highly protein bound by competing for these binding sites (e.g., **NSAIDs, salicylates, sulfonamides, warfarin, beta-adrenergic blockers**, and **monoamine oxidase inhibitors**) This interaction may cross over to **repaglinide**, but to date it is only a potential interaction.

Clinical Use and Dosing

MONOTHERAPY. For monotherapy, if the patient has not previously been treated with oral agents or if the HbA₁C is less than 8 percent, the initial dose is 0.5 mg tid 30 minutes or less before each meal. If the HbA₁C is 8 percent or more or the patient is being switched from another oral agent, the initial dose is 1 to 2 mg tid.

COMBINATION WITH METFORMIN. Initial **repaglinide** dosing in combination with **metformin** is the same as with monotherapy if there is inadequate control with **metformin** and **repaglinide** is being added. **Metformin** can also be added to **repaglinide** therapy if there is inadequate control with **repaglinide** alone. Follow the initial dosing regimen for **metformin**.

Table 19–28. Drug Interactions with Repaglinide

Interacting Drug	Possible Effect	Implications
Drugs that induce CYP-450 3A4	Increases metabolism and may decrease effect of repaglinide	Closely monitor blood glucose levels and patient response
Ketoconazole, miconazole, and potentially other "azoles"	Inhibits repaglinide metabolism and may increase risk for hypoglycemia	Closely monitor blood glucose levels and patient response Choose a different antifungal
Erythromycin and potentially other macrolides	Inhibits repaglinide metabolism and may increase risk for hypoglycemia	Closely monitor blood glucose levels and patient response Choose a different class of antimicrobial
Any drug that increases or decreases BG levels	May alter glycemic effects of repaglinide and increases risk for lack of control or hypoglycemia	Closely monitor blood glucose levels and patient response

FOR BOTH USES. Doses are always administered 0 to 30 minutes prior to each meal (Table 19–29). The patient who does not eat does not use the drug. If extra meals are eaten, extra doses are taken. Dosage changes are based on fasting BG and HbA₁C levels. The preprandial dose should be doubled, up to 4 mg, until satisfactory BG response is achieved. Allow at least 1 week to assess patient response before adjusting a dose. The maximum daily dose is 16 mg. No dosage adjustments are required based on age, race, or gender.

Monitoring

The only monitoring required with this drug is periodic monitoring of fasting BG and HbA₁C. These values should be determined prior to initiation of therapy to determine baseline values and contribute to the decision about initial dose. Thereafter, they are used to monitor patient response.

Patient Education

ADMINISTRATION. Timing of the drug in relation to food is critical. The drug may be taken 30 minutes or less before a meal. If a meal is omitted, the drug should not be taken. If a meal is added to the patient's usual eating pattern, an additional dose of **repaglinide** should be taken. The total daily dose, however, should not exceed 16 mg. The preprandial dose should not be altered without first consulting the health care provider.

ADVERSE REACTIONS. The only adverse effect associated with this drug is hypoglycemia. The risk is about the same as for patients taking **glipizide** or **glyburide.** Patients should be taught how to recognize and manage hypoglycemia, should it occur, as was discussed earlier in the patient teaching sections on **insulin** and **oral hypoglycemics.**

LIFESTYLE MANAGEMENT. Type 2 diabetes is a chronic illness managed with diet, exercise, weight control, and self-monitoring of BG, as well as drug therapy. Further patient teaching related to management of diabetes is discussed in Chapter 31 (Table 19–30).

Glucagon

Glucagon is a hormone secreted by the pancreas. It has several actions, but its primary use clinically is in elevating BG levels for diabetic patients who have hypoglycemia or **insulin** overdose. It is also used to reverse the hypoglycemia induced by **insulin** shock therapy in psychiatric patients.

This drug is administered SC, IM, or IV. Most of the drugs in this book are oral preparations because that is the route most used in primary care. **Glucagon,** however, is used in urgent care and primary care settings in its IM or IV form, so it is included.

Pharmacodynamics

Glucagon is a polypeptide hormone produced by the alpha cells of the pancreas. It accelerates liver glucogenolysis by stimulating cAMP synthesis and increasing phosphorylase kinase activity. This results in increased breakdown of glycogen to glucose and inhibition of glycogen synthesis. The end result is an elevation in BG levels. Glucagon also stimulates hepatic gluconeogenesis by promoting the uptake of amino acids and converting them to glucose precursors. When administered parenterally, **glucagon** also produces relaxation of the smooth muscle of the GI tract, decreases gastric and pancreatic secretions, and increases myocardial contractility. These latter actions are not the primary reason for its clinical use, however.

Table 19–29. Dosage Schedule: Repaglinide

Indication	Initial Dose	Maintenance Dose
Monotherapy for patient not previously managed with oral agent and HbA₁C less than 8%	0.5 mg taken 30 min or less before each meal	Double preprandial dose, up to 4 mg, until blood glucose reaches target level Dose increases at 1-wk intervals Maximum dose 16 mg/d
Monotherapy for patient switching from other oral agent and HbA₁C 8% or more	1–2 mg taken 30 min or less before each meal	Double preprandial dose, up to 4 mg, until blood glucose reaches target level Dose increases at 1-wk intervals Maximum dose 16 mg/d
Combination therapy adding metformin	If HbA₁C less than 8%, dose is 0.5 mg If HbA₁C is 8% or more, dose is 1–2 mg Dose taken 30 min or less before a meal	Double preprandial dose, up to 4 mg, until blood glucose reaches target level Dose increases at 1-wk intervals Maximum dose 16 mg/d

Table 19–30. Available Dosage Forms: Repaglinide

Drug	Dosage Form
Repaglinide (Prandin)	0.5 mg in 100-, 500-, and 1000-tablet bottles 1 mg in 100-, 500-, and 1000-tablet bottles 2 mg in 100-, 500-, and 1000-tablet bottles

Pharmacokinetics

Absorption and Distribution

Glucagon is well absorbed after parenteral administration. Its distribution is unknown.

Metabolism and Excretion

It is extensively metabolized by the liver and kidney and degraded in the plasma. Plasma half-life is about 3 to 6 minutes.

Pharmacotherapeutics

Precautions and Contraindications

The only contraindication to **glucagon** is hypersensitivity to it. It should be given with caution to patients with insulinoma or pheochromocytoma. It may produce an initial increase in BG in these patients, but because of its insulin-releasing effect, it may subsequently cause hypoglycemia. It also stimulates catecholamine release, causing a marked increase in blood pressure in patients with pheochromocytoma.

Glucagon is Pregnancy Category B, but there are no adequate and well-controlled studies in pregnant women. Use in pregnancy should be only if clearly indicated. Because *insulin* is the drug of choice in managing gestational diabetes and other diabetic patients during their pregnancy, the potential for a hypoglycemic reaction exists. The rapid resolution of any moderate to severe hypoglycemia is clearly in the best interests of the fetus and would override any concerns about potential risk from exposure to *glucagon*. It is not known whether this drug is excreted in breast milk. Caution should be used in giving it to a nursing mother.

Adverse Drug Reactions

The most frequent adverse reactions are nausea and vomiting, and these may occur because of the hypoglycemia. Rare allergic reactions resulting in urticaria, respiratory distress, and hypotension have been reported.

Drug Interactions

The anticoagulant effects of **oral anticoagulants** may be increased, with the possibility of bleeding. This interaction may occur after several days of therapy and appears to be dose-related. This interaction is not associated with single-dose therapy to resolve a hypoglycemic reaction.

Clinical Use and Dosing

Reversal of hypoglycemia is the main use for this drug (Table 19–31). **Glucagon** counteracts severe hypoglycemic reactions in diabetic patients and in psychiatric patients recovering from **insulin** shock. BG levels of patients with type 1 diabetes do not respond as well as those of patients with type 2, and patients with type 1 di-

Table 19–31. Dosage Schedule: Glucagon

Indication	Initial Dose	Additional Doses
Hypoglycemia	Children, weight less than 20 kg: 0.5 mg SC, IM, or IV Adult and children, weight more than 20 mg: 1 mg SC, IM, or IV	If response not adequate in 5–15 min, administer 1–2 additional doses; accompany with IV glucose if patient fails to respond
Hypoglycemia in infants	0.3 mg/kg	0.3 mg/kg may be repeated q4h as needed
Insulin shock	After 1 h of coma: inject 0.5–1 mg SC, IM, or IV	If no response in 10–25 min, repeat dose Upon awakening, feed patient orally as soon as possible

abetes often require concurrent administration of carbohydrates. Because all of its actions depend on the presence of glycogen in the liver, **glucagon** is of little or no help in states of starvation, adrenal insufficiency, or chronic hypoglycemia.

An unlabeled use for **glucagon** is in the treatment of **propranolol** overdose and cardiovascular emergencies. Its use in these situations is based on its effects on smooth muscle and myocardial contractility.

Monitoring

Monitoring of BG immediately prior to and after the injection is the only requirement.

Patient Education

Because this drug is administered by the provider when the patient has a decreased level of consciousness, no patient education specific to this drug is required. Patients with diabetes who are at high risk for hypoglycemia may keep this drug on hand to be mixed and injected by a family member. In those circumstances, education of the family member would include recognition of and testing for hypoglycemia and the procedure for mixing and administering **glucagon** parenterally (Table 19–32).

Thyroid Agents

Thyroid hormones include both natural and synthetic compounds. The natural hormones are derived from beef and pork thyroid glands. Because their content and bioavailability are not consistent from dose to dose, they have largely been replaced with the synthetic compounds. This section discusses the **synthetic thyroid hormones.**

Pharmacodynamics

The hypothalamus-pituitary-thyroid hormone axis begins with the secretion of thyrotropin-releasing hormone (TRH) by the hypothalamus in response to cold, stress, and decreased levels of thyroxine (T_4). TRH stimulates the synthesis and release of thyroid-stimulating hormone (TSH) by the anterior pituitary. TSH, in turn, stimulates an adenylyl cyclase mechanism in the thyroid cells to (1) im-

mediately increase the release of stored thyroid hormones, (2) increase iodine uptake and utilization, (3) increase the synthesis of the two thyroid hormones, tri-iodothyronine (T_3) and T_4, and (4) increase the synthesis and secretion of prostaglandins by the thyroid gland. When thyroid hormones are secreted, they create a negative feedback loop, inhibit TRH and TSH secretion, and decrease further thyroid hormone synthesis and secretion. Figure 19–4 depicts the hypothalamus-pituitary-thyroid hormone axis.

As shown in Figure 19–4, thyroid hormones increase all the metabolic processes of the body and are central to the growth and differentiation of body tissues. The mechanism by which thyroid hormones exert their effect is not well understood, but it is believed that most of their effects are exerted through control of DNA transcription and protein synthesis. Administration of **synthetic thyroid hormones—levothyroxine (T_4), liothyronine (T_3), and liotrix (a 4:1 mixture of T_4 and T_3)**—produces the same effects on body tissues as the body's own thyroid hormones and produces the negative feedback loop to reduce further secretion of TSH and thyroid hormones.

Pharmacokinetics

Absorption and Distribution

Levothyroxine (T_4) is variably absorbed, with 48 to 79 percent of the dose absorbed after oral administration (Table 19–33). Fasting increases its absorption, and malabsorption syndromes cause excessive fecal loss of this drug. **Liothyronine (T_3)** is 95 percent absorbed within 4 hours after administration. More than 99 percent of the circulating hormones are bound to serum proteins, including thyroid-binding globulin (TBg), thyroid-binding prealbumin (TBPA), and albumin (TBa). The higher affinity of T_4 for TBg and TBPA as compared with T_3 partially explains the higher serum levels and longer half-life of T_4. T_4 and T_3 exist in the body in equilibrium between bound and free drug, but only the free drug produces the hormone's effects.

Metabolism and Excretion

Thyroid hormones are distributed to most body tissues. They do not readily cross the placenta, and minimal amounts are excreted in breast milk.

Under normal body functioning, the ratio of T_4 to T_3

Table 19–32. Available Dosage Forms: Glucagon

Drug	Dosage Form
Glucagon	1 mg powder for injection in vial with 1 cc of diluent 10 mg powder for injection in vial with 10 cc of diluent (Use immediately after reconstitution; may be kept at 5°C for 48 h)

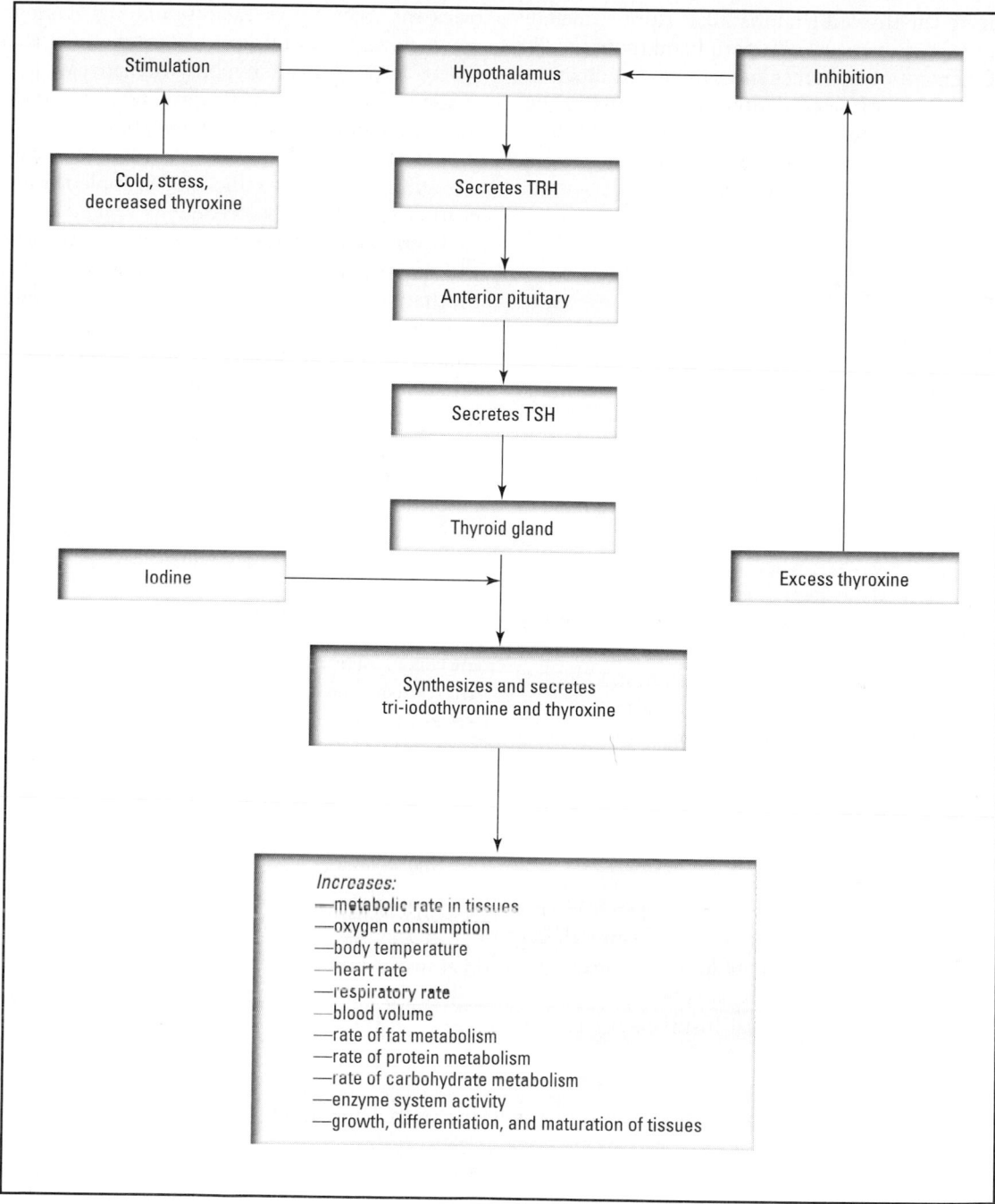

Figure 19–4. Hypothalamus-pituitary-thyroid hormone axis.

Table 19–33. Pharmacokinetics: Oral Thyroid Hormones

Drug	Onset*	Peak*	Duration*	Biologic Potency	Half-Life	Excretion
Levothyroxine (T$_4$)	48 h	1–3 wk	1–3 wk	1	6–7 d†	In feces via bile
Liothyronine (T$_3$)	48 h	24–72 h	72 h	4	1–2 d	In feces via bile

*Effects on thyroid function tests.
†3–4 d in hyperthyroidism; 9–10 d in myxedema.

released from the thyroid gland is 20:1. Approximately 35 percent of T_4 is converted in peripheral tissues to T_3 so that 80 percent of T_3 comes from monodeiodination of T_4. This process of deiodination of T_4 occurs in the liver, kidney, and other body tissues. The conjugated hormones then reenter the hepatic circulation, where they are excreted in the feces via bile.

Pharmacotherapeutics

Precautions and Contraindications

Thyroid hormone replacement is contraindicated after recent myocardial infarction (MI) or in thyrotoxicosis uncomplicated by hypothyroidism. When hypothyroidism is a complicating or causative factor in MI or heart disease, judicious use of small doses of **thyroid hormone** may be called for. Cardiovascular disease, particularly coronary artery disease, may worsen when **thyroid hormones** are given. The increased heart rate associated with **thyroid hormone** administration increases oxygen demand by the heart muscle and decreases oxygen supply by reducing diastolic filling time. If **thyroid hormone** is required for patients who have cardiovascular disease, the lowest dose possible is used and with careful monitoring of signs and symptoms of worsening cardiovascular disease.

Long-term **levothyroxine** therapy has been associated with decreased bone density in the hip and spine in both premenopausal and postmenopausal women. To avoid this problem, the drug should be used only after appropriate clinical evaluation. When the drug is necessary, use only the lowest dose possible to achieve the desired effects, and periodically monitor the patient for osteoporosis.

Thyroid hormone therapy for patients with concomitant diabetes insipidus or adrenal insufficiency exacerbates the intensity of their symptoms. Dosage adjustments downward in **thyroid hormone** may be required. Severe or prolonged hypothyroidism can lead to decreased adrenocortical function. When thyroid replacement therapy is begun, the metabolism increases at a greater rate than adrenocortical activity and can precipitate adrenocortical insufficiency. Supplemental **adrenocorticosteroid** may be needed.

Thyroid hormones **are Pregnancy Category A. Clinical experience does not indicate any adverse effects on the fetus when** *thyroid hormones* **are administered to pregnant women. Do not discontinue ongoing thyroid replacement therapy during pregnancy. Minimal amounts are excreted in breast milk, and it has not been associated with any adverse effects. Caution, however, should be exercised when administering them to nursing mothers.**

Children born with thyroid hormone deficiency may be safely treated with **thyroid hormones.** Failure to do so can have devastating results.

Adverse Drug Reactions

Adverse reactions other than those associated with hyperthyroidism due to overdose are rare. If the patient experiences indications of hyperthyroidism (increased heart rate, cardiac arrhythmias, chest pain, tremors, nervousness, insomnia, irritability, diarrhea, vomiting, weight loss, menstrual irregularities, or heat intolerance), the TSH level should be assessed and appropriate dosage adjustments made.

Drug Interactions

Cholestyramine and **colestipol** decrease the absorption of orally administered **thyroid** preparations because they are **bile acid sequestrants** (Table 19–34). **Estro-**

Table 19–34. Drug Interactions with Thyroid Hormones

Interacting Drug	Possible Effect	Implications
Beta-adrenergic blockers	Actions of beta-adrenergic blocker may be impaired when patient is converted to euthyroid state.	Monitor response to beta-adrenergic blockers; assess for continued need for drug or for dosage adjustment.
Cholestyramine, colestipol	Interferes with thyroid hormone absorption with loss of efficacy.	Administer at least 4 h apart.
Digoxin	Serum levels of digoxin reduced when hypothyroid patient is converted to euthyroid state.	Monitor response to digoxin and serum levels; assess for need for dosage adjustment.
Estrogens	Increases TBg and may decrease response to thyroid hormone.	Monitor therapeutic response.
Warfarin	Increased anticoagulant action.	May need to decrease dose of warfarin; monitor PT/INR carefully.

INR = international normalized ratio; PT = prothrombin time.

Clinical Pearl

Increasing the dose by 25 percent usually results in adequate coverage during pregnancy. Recheck TSH levels in 4 weeks to determine any dosage adjustment.

gens increase TBg and may therefore decrease the response to **thyroid hormones. Thyroid hormones** may decrease the effectiveness of **warfarin, digoxin,** and **beta-adrenergic blockers.**

Many drugs affect thyroid function tests and may interfere with correct assessment of thyroid status. These drugs are discussed in Chapter 39.

Clinical Use and Dosing

HYPOTHYROIDISM. Treatment of hypothyroidism follows the start low and go slow principle to avoid excessive increase in metabolism before the body has a chance to adapt to the increase. For adults, **levothyroxine** is started at 50 µg daily and is increased in increments of 25 µg/day at 2- to 4-week intervals to 100 to150 µg/day. The target dose is based on TSH levels and is usually approximately 1.6 µg/kg. Lower doses and longer intervals for changing doses are required for patients with cardiovascular impairment or long-standing hypothyroidism. In these cases or in severe hypothyroidism, the initial dose is 12.5 to 25 µg/day, increased by 25 µg/day at the 4-week intervals. The target dose is also based on TSH levels. Most patients require no more than 200 µg/day. Failure to respond adequately to doses of 300 µg/day suggests lack of adherence or malabsorption.

Liothyronine is started at 25 µg/day. Dosage is increased by 12.5 to 25 µg/day at 1- to 2-week intervals until a maintenance dose of 25 to 50 µg is reached.

Liotrix is started with 50 µg of **levothyroxine**/12.5 µg of **liothyronine** per day. Doses are increased by 50/12.5 µg at 4-week intervals until a maintenance dose of 50 to 100/12.5 to 25 is reached. For patients with myxedema or hypothyroidism with cardiovascular disease, the doses are reduced.

For all of these drugs, dosages are different for infants, children, and geriatric patients. Table 19–35 presents the dosing schedules for all of these age groups.

HASHIMOTO'S THYROIDITIS. Approximately 70 percent or more of patients with this disorder go on to develop permanent hypothyroidism. If hypothyroidism develops, the treatment regimen is the same as for other causes of hypothyroidism, as discussed previously.

TSH SUPPRESSION IN THYROID CANCER, NODULES, AND EUTHYROID GOITER. The required maintenance dosage for these indications is larger than that for hypothyroidism. The initial dose of **levothyroxine** is 50 to 100 µg/day, and the dose is increased until the TSH level declines to 0.05 to 0.3 mU/L. This therapy is relatively contraindicated in older adults and in patients with cardiovascular disease.

THYROID SUPPRESSION THERAPY. The dose is 2.5 µg/kg daily for 7 to 10 days for this indication. These doses usually yield normal serum T_4 and T_3 levels without a response to TSH.

CONGENITAL HYPOTHYROIDISM. The recommended doses for this indication are based on the infant's weight. Full doses are started immediately upon diagnosis of the condition.

Inappropriate Use of Thyroid Hormones

OBESITY. In euthyroid patients, hormone replacement doses are ineffective for weight reduction. Larger doses may produce serious or even life-threatening toxicity, particularly when given with anorexiants. Use of **thyroid hormones** for this indication is *not* justified.

INFERTILITY. **Thyroid hormone** therapy is *not* justified for the treatment of infertility in male or female patients unless the condition is accompanied by hypothyroidism.

Clinical Pearl

Levothyroxine tablets can be crushed and suspended in a small amount of formula or water for infants who cannot swallow whole tablets. For children who cannot swallow the intact tablet, it may be crushed and sprinkled over a small amount of food such as cooked cereal or applesauce. The suspension cannot be stored for any period of time. The tablet should be crushed, mixed to form a suspension, and given immediately.

Table 19–35. Dosage Schedule: Thyroid Hormones

Drug	Indication	Initial Dose	Maintenance Dose
Levothyroxine	Hypothyroidism and congenital hypothyroidism	Adults: 50 μg qd	Increase dose by 25 μg at 4- to 6-wk intervals to maintenance dose of 100–150 μg qd
		Older adults: 12.5–25 μg qd	Increase dose by 25 μg daily at 6-wk intervals to maintenance dose of 100–150 μg qd
		Children over age 10 y: 2–3 μg/kg qd	Increase in increments of 2 μg/kg/d at 4- to 6-wk intervals to maintenance dose of 150–200 μg qd
		Children 6–10 y: 4–5 μg/kg qd	Increase in increments of 4 μg/kg/d at 4- to 6-wk intervals to maintenance dose of 100–150 μg qd
		Children 1–5 y: 3–5 μg/kg qd	Increase in increments of 3 μg/kg/d at 2- to 4-wk intervals to maintenance dose of 75–100 μg qd
		Children 6–12 mo: 5–6 μg/kg qd	Increase in increments of 5 μg/kg/d at 2- to 4-wk intervals to maintenance dose of 50–75 μg qd
		Infants less than 6 mo: 5–6 μg/kg qd	Increase in increments of 5 μg/kg/d at 4- to 6-wk intervals to maintenance dose of 25–50 μg qd
		Infants less than 2000 g or at risk for cardiac failure: 25 μg qd	Dosage may be increased after 4–6 wk to 50 μg qd
			For infants with congenital hypothyroidism, initiate therapy with full dose as soon as diagnosis is made
Liothyronine	Mild hypothyroidism	Adults: 25 μg qd	Increase in increments of 12.5–25 μg qd at 1- to 2-wk intervals to maintenance dose of 25–75 μg qd
		Older adults or patients with cardiovascular disease: 5 μg qd	Increase in increments of no more than 5 μg qd at 2-wk intervals
	Congenital hypothyroidism	5 μg qd	Increase in increments of 5 μg every 3–4 d until desired response
			Maintenance dose for infants a few months old is 20 μg qd; for children age 1 y, dose is 50 μg qd; above 3 y, use adult dose
	Simple nontoxic goiter	5 μg qd	Increase in increments of 5 μg every 1–2 wk
			When dose of 25 μg qd is reached, increase by 12.5–25 μg qd every 1–2 wk
			Usual maintenance dose is 75 μg qd
	Myxedema	5 μg qd	Increase in increments of 5 μg every 1–2 wk
			When dose of 25 μg qd is reached, increase by 12.5–25 μg qd every 1–2 wk
			Usual maintenance dose is 50–100 μg qd
Liotrix	Hypothyroidism	Adults: 30 mg qd	Increase in increments of 15 mg every 2–3 wk to maintenance dose of 60–120 mg qd
		Children and infants with congenital hypothyroidism	Follow dosage recommendations for levothyroxine (see available dosage forms table for T_4 equivalents for liotrix)

Rational Drug Selection

PHARMACOKINETICS. Levothyroxine (T_4) is the drug of choice for thyroid replacement and suppression therapy because of its longer half-life. This means that it can safely be withheld for up to 2 weeks, if necessary, without altering the patient's thyroid status. Because T_4 is converted to T_3 in the body, use of this drug produces both hormones. Both **levothyroxine** and **liothyronine** (T_3) have content stability, but **liothyronine** is 3 to 4 times more active than **levothyroxine**, and this greater potency increases the risk for cardiotoxicity. **Levothyroxine** should be used with patients who have cardiovascular disease.

COST. Generic forms of all the **thyroid hormones** are less expensive than brand names; however, bioequivalence does not exist between brands and cannot be assumed between generic forms. Cost varies between brands and also between strengths of the same brand. A cost index based on the cost per 600 μg (1 grain) of **thyroid** is included in Table 19–36 on available dosage forms.

MONITORING. **Levothyroxine** is the easiest to monitor via TSH and free T_4 laboratory measurements of thyroid function. The monitoring of therapy with these laboratory tests is more difficult with **liothyronine**. Its best use is for TSH suppression.

Liotrix offers no clear benefit over either of the other drugs on any of these parameters.

Monitoring

Thyroid function is monitored with TSH and free T_4 levels. Because of the negative feedback loop between TSH and **thyroid hormones**, elevations in TSH indicate insufficient **thyroid hormone**, and TSH levels below desired levels indicate excessive **thyroid hormone**. TSH and free T_4 levels are checked initially and at 6 weeks after each dosage adjustment. Recheck them 4 months after achieving target dose, and adjust the dose to keep TSH within normal limits. Once the patient is stable on an appropriate dose, TSH can be checked only annually.

Table 19–36. Available Dosage Forms: Thyroid Hormones

Drug	Dosage Form	Cost Index*
Levothyroxine Generic	100 μg, 150 μg, 200 μg	15, NA, 1
Levo-T	25 μg, 50 μg, 75 μg, 100 μg, 125 μg, 150 μg, 200 μg, 300 μg	NA
Levothroid	25 μg, 50 μg, 75 μg, 88 μg, 100 μg, 112 μg, 125 μg, 137 μg, 150 μg, 175 μg, 200 μg, 300 μg	76, 42, 30, NA, 24, NA, 22, NA, 20, 20, 18, 16
Levoxyl	25 μg, 50 μg, 75 μg, 88 μg, 100 μg, 112 μg, 125 μg, 137 μg, 150 μg, 175 μg, 200 μg, 300 μg	32, 18, 12, 12, 10, 10, 10, NA, 8, 28, 8, 6
Synthroid	25 μg, 50 μg, 75 μg, 88 μg, 100 μg, 112 μg, 125 μg, 150 μg, 175 μg, 200 μg, 300 μg	50, 38, 28, 38, 22, 34, 20, 18, NA, 16, 14
Eltroxin	50 μg, 100 μg, 200 μg, 300 μg	NA
Liothyronine Generic	25 μg	8+
Cytomel	5 μg, 25 μg, 50 μg	96, 24, 18
Liotrix Euthroid (each grain = 60 μg T_4 and 15 μg T_3)	0.5 grain, 1 grain, 2 grains, 3 grains	5, 3, 2, 1.5
Thyrolar (each grain = 50 μg T_4 and 12.5 μg T_3)	0.25 grain, 0.5 grain, 1 grain, 2 grains, 3 grains	15, 8.3, 5.2, 3, 2.5

*Cost index based on cost per 600 μg (1 grain) of thyroid hormone.
NA = not available.

Patient Education

ADMINISTRATION. Thyroid hormones are taken as a single daily dose in the morning before breakfast to prevent insomnia. Taking levothyroxine on an empty stomach enhances absorption. Other types may be taken without regard to food. If a dose is missed, it may be taken that same day as soon as it is remembered. If more than three doses are missed, the health care provider should be informed. Depending on the drug being used, evaluation of thyroid function may be needed. Dosage of the drug is based on laboratory evaluation of thyroid function. The dose should not be altered without first consulting the health care provider.

Caution patients not to change brands of thyroid preparation. They may not be bioequivalent. Although some health food stores may sell dessicated thyroid preparations OTC at a lower cost, these formulations do not have consistent amounts of thyroid hormone in them and should not be substituted for the prescribed drug.

ADVERSE DRUG REACTIONS. Teach the patient how to measure pulse rate. If the pulse rate is greater than 100 beats per minute, the dose should be withheld and the health care provider notified. This may indicate excessive amounts of hormone. Other signs or symptoms that require notification of the health care provider because they may indicate excessive amounts of thyroid hormone (e.g., nervousness, chest pain, weight loss of more than 2 lb in 1 week) should also be taught to the patient.

Some children on thyroid hormone therapy may experience partial hair loss. This is usually temporary, but parents and children should be informed.

LIFESTYLE MANAGEMENT. Thyroid disorders are usually chronic illnesses managed with self-monitoring of symptoms as well as drug therapy. Emphasize the importance of keeping follow-up appointments for evaluation of thyroid function. For children, evaluation of physical and psychomotor growth and development is also central to their management. Explain to the patient that replacement therapy must be taken for life (except in cases of transient hypothyroidism). The drug will treat the disorder but not cure it. Further patient teaching related to management of thyroid disorders is discussed in Chapter 39.

Antithyroid Agents

Antithyroid agents function by either inhibiting the synthesis of thyroid hormones or destroying thyroid gland tissue. Because the drugs used include radioactive iodine 131, issues related to radioactivity will be discussed briefly.

Pharmacodynamics

Propylthiouracil (PTU) and methimazole (Tapazole) inhibit the synthesis of thyroid hormones. They do not inactivate existing thyroxine and tri-iodothyronine that are stored in the thyroid gland or that are circulating in the blood, nor do they interfere with the effectiveness of exogenous thyroid hormones. Propylthiouracil partially inhibits the peripheral conversion of T_4 to T_3. Both drugs are concentrated in the thyroid gland.

Neither of these drugs treats the underlying pathology in hyperthyroidism, and only about 20 percent of patients treated with at least 1 year of therapy go into spontaneous remission.

Radioactive iodine (^{131}I) concentrates in the thyroid gland and is incorporated into storage follicles. There it emits beta rays that result in destruction of the thyroid parenchyma. Approximately 50 percent of patients who receive this therapy become euthyroid, and 50 percent become hypothyroid. This latter group requires thyroid hormone replacement.

Pharmacokinetics

Absorption and Distribution

Propylthiouracil is rapidly absorbed after oral administration, reaching a peak serum level within 1 hour (Table 19–37). This drug is highly protein bound (75 to 80%) and concentrates in the thyroid gland. Concentrations in

Table 19–37. Pharmacokinetics: Antithyroid Drugs

Drug	Onset*	Peak*	Duration*	Bioavail-ability	Protein Binding	Placental Transport and Breast Milk Levels	Half-Life	Excretion
Methimazole	1 wk	4–10 wk	Weeks	80–95%	0%	High	6–13 h	Less than 10% in urine
Propylthiouracil	10–21 d	6–10 wk	Weeks	80–95%	75–80%	Low	1–2 h	35% in urine

*Effect on thyroid function.

breast milk are low, and it crosses the placenta in very low concentrations.

Methimazole is completely absorbed after oral administration but at variable rates. This drug is not protein bound and also concentrates in the thyroid gland. Concentrations in breast milk are high, and it readily crosses the placenta in high concentrations.

Radioactive iodine is readily absorbed after oral administration. Following absorption, it is primarily distributed within the extracellular fluids. It crosses the placenta and enters breast milk. Upon reaching the thyroid, it is rapidly converted to protein-bound iodine. It is not protein bound in the GI tract or salivary glands.

Metabolism and Excretion

Propylthiouracil is completely metabolized by the liver with a significant first-pass effect. **Methimazole** is mostly metabolized by the liver, but some drug (10%) is excreted unchanged in the urine. Both drugs have a short half-life, but this has little influence of the duration of antithyroid action or the dosing intervals because they are concentrated in the thyroid gland.

The nonbound portion of **radioactive iodine** is rapidly excreted in the urine. The protein-bound drug concentrated in the thyroid gland decays by beta and gamma emission with a physical half-life of 8 days. Following oral administration, about 40 percent of the drug has an effective half-life of 0.34 days, and 60 percent has an effective half-life of 7.6 days.

Pharmacotherapeutics

Precautions and Contraindications

Pregnancy creates a serious cautionary condition for the use of *antithyroid drugs*. *Propylthiouracil (PTU)* and *methimazole* are Pregnancy Category D and *radioactive iodine* is Pregnancy Category X. *PTU* and *methimazole* cross the placenta and can induce goiter and even cretinism in the fetus. When it is clinically necessary to administer an *antithyroid drug* to a pregnant woman, *PTU* is the safest of the group because it crosses the placenta in very low concentrations.

Radioactive iodine can cause permanent damage to the fetal thyroid gland. The drug is contraindicated in women who are or may become pregnant. Before initiating therapy with this drug in women with childbearing potential, effective birth control should be instituted. Because *iodine* is excreted in breast milk, it should not be given to nursing mothers.

Patients under age 30 are not usually treated with **radioactive iodine** unless circumstances preclude other therapies or the patient failed to respond adequately on other **antithyroid drugs**.

Iodine allergies are not infrequent. Before administering **radioactive iodine**, assessment of iodine allergy is important.

Adverse Drug Reactions

The potentially most serious adverse reaction to therapy with **propylthiouracil, methimazole,** and **radioactive iodine** is agranulocytosis. This risk is higher for patients who already have decreased bone marrow reserve, for those over age 40, and those receiving more than 40 mg/day. The patient's bone marrow function must be monitored, and the patient taught to report symptoms of this disorder. These drugs must be discontinued, should this adverse reaction occur. It is important to remember that about 10 percent of patients with untreated hyperthyroidism have leukopenia (white blood cell count less than 4000/mm³), often with related granulocytopenia.

Less serious and less frequent adverse reactions to **propylthiouracil** and **metimazole** include drowsiness, headache, paresthesias, vertigo, diarrhea, nausea, arthralgia, and a pruritic skin rash. The nausea and skin rash are more common with **propylthiouracil**. Drug-induced hepatitis and abnormal hair loss may rarely occur with either drug.

Radiation sickness with some degree of nausea and vomiting may occur with the administration of **radioactive iodine**. Tenderness and swelling of the neck, pain on swallowing, sore throat, and cough may occur around the third day after treatment and are usually amenable to analgesics. Temporary thinning of the hair may occur 2 to 3 months after treatment.

Fears of radiation-induced genetic damage, leukemia, and other cancers have been raised. However, after 30 years of clinical experience with **radioactive iodine**, no evidence of long-term negative effects have been found. Patients also express concerns about exposure of family members to radiation. Because such a low dose (4 to 10 microcuries [mCi]) is given for most indications, no radiation safety precautions are required. It is prudent to avoid holding small infants in positions that place them near the patient's neck for the first 1 or 2 days.

Drug Interactions

Any drugs that produce bone marrow depression have an additive effect with **antithyroid drugs** (Table 19–38). Additive antithyroid effects occur with **lithium, potassium iodide,** or **sodium iodide** given with **propylthiouracil**. **Potassium iodide** and **amiodarone** decrease antithyroid effects when given with **methimazole**. The risk of agranulocytosis is increased with concurrent administration of **phenothiazines** with **methimazole** and **propylthiouracil**. The anticoagulant activity of **warfarin** may be potentiated by the anti–vitamin K activity attributed to **propylthiouracil**. Stable **iodine** in any form, **thyroid**

Table 19–38. Drug Interactions with Antithyroid Drugs

Drug	Interacting Drug	Possible Effect	Implications
Methimazole, propylthiouracil, radioactive iodine	Any drug that produces bone marrow depression	Additive bone marrow depression	Monitor white blood cell counts with differential; dosage adjustments or discontinuance of one of the drugs may be needed.
Propylthiouracil	Lithium, potassium iodide, sodium iodide	Additive antithyroid effects	Avoid concurrent administration.
	Warfarin	Anticoagulant effects potentiated	Monitor PT/INR closely.
Methimazole	Potassium iodide, amiodarone	Decreased antithyroid effects	Avoid concurrent administration.
Methimazole, propylthiouracil	Phenothiazines	Increased risk for agranulocytosis	Avoid concurrent administration.
Radioactive iodine	Stable iodine in any form, thyroid drugs, other antithyroid drugs	Affect the uptake of radioactive iodine	Question the patient about recent radiology procedures that have used contrast media and about any other drugs being taken.

INR = international normalized ratio; PT = prothrombin time.

drugs, and other **antithyroid drugs** affect the uptake of **radioactive iodine.**

Clinical Use and Dosing

HYPERTHYROIDISM/GRAVES' DISEASE. Any of the **antithyroid drugs** may be used. **Methimazole** is usually initiated at a dose of 20 to 30 mg/day divided into three equal doses given 8 hours apart. For mild hyperthyroidism, doses of 15 mg/day may be effective. Because of its longer half-life, once-daily dosing may be tried. One small study found either single or divided doses to be equally effective, but further research is needed to make this a recommendation. Maintenance doses are 5 to 15 mg/day. **Propylthiouracil** is initiated with 300 mg/day in three equally divided doses given 8 hours apart. Patients with severe hyperthyroidism may have initial doses of 400 mg/day. Maintenance doses are 100 to 150 mg/day. There are children's doses of both drugs. Treatment is for 6 to 18 months, with most patients being treated for 1 year. Table 19–39 shows the clinical use and dosing for both drugs for adults and children.

The amount of **radioactive iodine** needed to achieve clinical remission without destruction of the entire gland varies widely. The dosage range is 4 to 10 mCi. The dose for total destruction (ablation) of the thyroid gland is 50 mCi, with subsequent doses of 100 to 150 mCi as needed until the gland is completely destroyed.

TOXIC GOITER. Patients with toxic goiter require higher doses of **antithyroid drugs. Methimazole** is initiated at dose of 60 mg/day divided into three equal doses given 8 hours apart. **Propylthiouracil** is initiated with 600 to 900 mg/day in three equally divided doses given 8 hours apart. Maintenance doses are the same as for hypothyroidism.

Some treatment regimens give **methimazole** or **propylthiouracil** for 1 month to "calm" the thyroid and then administer a dose of **radioactive iodine** that is either at the higher end of the dosage range (10 mCi) or that totally destroys the gland (50 mCi). Most patients become euthyroid after the **radioactive iodine.**

Rational Drug Selection

PREGNANCY AND LACTATION. Because the amount of drug that crosses the placenta is low with *propylthiouracil,* the lowest effective dose of this drug is selected if one must be used. In many pregnant women, the thyroid dysfunction diminishes as the pregnancy continues, so that the drug's dose can be reduced. In some cases, the drug can be withdrawn 2 to 3 weeks prior to delivery. Postpartum patients receiving *antithyroid drugs* should not nurse their infants. If it is necessary, however, *propylthiouracil* is the preferred drug.

COST. There is a significant difference in cost between **methimazole** and **propylthiouracil.** Unless the provider is willing to try once-daily dosing and sees this as an advantage, **propylthiouracil** is about 10 percent of the cost of **methimazole.** A cost index is included in Table 19–40 that shows available dosage forms of these two drugs.

Table 19–39. Dosage Schedule: Antithyroid Drugs

Drug	Indication	Initial Dose	Maintenance Dose
Methimazole	Hyperthryoidism	Adults: 15 mg/d for mild; 30 mg/d for moderate; 60 mg/d for severe hyperthyroidism and toxic goiter Children: 0.4 mg/kg/d (alternative dose 0.5–0.7 mg/kg/d or 15–20 mg/m²/d) All doses in 3 equally divided doses given 8 h apart	5–15 mg/d Half the initial dose (alternative dose 1/3–2/3 the initial dose when patient is euthyroid) Maximum dose 30 mg/24 h All doses in 3 equally divided doses given 8 h apart
Propylthiouracil	Hyperthyroidism	Adults: 300 mg/d for mild; 400 mg/d for moderate; 600–900 mg/d for severe hyperthyroidism and toxic goiter Children over age 10 y: 150–300 mg/d Children 6–10 y: 50–150 mg/d (alternative dose is 5–7 mg/kg/d or 150–200 mg/m²/d) All doses in 3 equally divided doses given 8 h apart	100–150 mg/d Maximum dose 1200 mg/24 h Determined by patient response (alternative dose 1/3–2/3 the initial dose when patient is euthyroid) All doses in 3 equally divided doses q8h
Radioactive iodine	Hyperthyroidism Thyroid cancer	4–10 mCi; larger doses for toxic goiter 50 mCi	Subsequent doses of 100–150 mCi

Monitoring

The same thyroid function tests used to evaluate hypothyroidism are used here.

TSH and free T₄ levels are evaluated prior to beginning therapy and whenever symptoms recur, whenever dosages are adjusted and every 2 to 3 months throughout therapy.

To monitor for the risk for agranulocytosis, a complete blood count, including white blood cell count and differential, is done prior to initiating therapy, if symptoms suggestive of this disorder occur, and periodically throughout therapy. This adverse reaction may develop rapidly, usually within the first 2 months of therapy. During that time, both the provider and the patient should be especially vigilant. It is more common in persons over age 40 and those who are receiving more than 40 mg/day. Monitoring may be more frequent for these patients.

Drug-induced hepatitis is not common, but liver function tests should be done prior to therapy and if there is an indication of this disorder.

In addition to laboratory assessment, both the provider and the patient should regularly assess for signs and symptoms of hyperthyroidism (too low a dose) or hypothyroidism (too high a dose)

Patient Education

ADMINISTRATION. The drug should be taken every 8 hours around the clock. It is not necessary to awaken at night to take the drug at exactly 8-hour intervals because the drug is concentrated in thyroid tissue. If a dose is

Table 19–40. Available Dosage Forms: Antithyroid Drugs

Drug	Dosage Form	Cost Index
Methimazole (Tapazole)	5-mg (scored) tablet 10-mg (scored) tablet	25 20
Propylthiouracil (PTU)	50-mg tablet	2.3
Radioactive iodine (Idotope)	8 mCi, 15 mCi, 30 mCi, 50 mCi, 100 mCi	NA
Sodium iodine (¹³¹I)	Range from 0.75 mCi to 100 mCi in capsules Range from 3.5 mCi to 150 mCi in oral solution	NA NA

NA = information not available.

missed, the patient should take it as soon as remembered. If it is almost time for the next dose, the two doses may be taken together. The health care provider should be notified if more than one dose is missed so that an assessment of thyroid function can be done.

Dietary sources of iodine should be discussed and reduced or eliminated. They interfere with the action of the **antithyroid drugs.** Many OTC drugs, especially those used to treat colds, also have **iodine** in them. Teach the patient to read the labels.

ADVERSE REACTIONS. The most serious potential adverse reaction related to **propylthiouracil** and **methimazole** is agranulocytosis. Patients are taught to report sore throat, fever, chills, rash, and unusual bleeding or bruising, as well as the reason for it.

Another potential adverse reaction is drug-induced hepatitis. Patients are also taught to report headache, malaise, weakness, and yellowing of the eye or skin and the reasons for it.

The patient should be told that any abnormal hair loss is probably temporary.

The main concern for patients taking **radioactive iodine** is often fear of radiation damage. It is important to explain that no evidence exists of long-term negative effects and that family members are not being exposed to doses of radiation that require any precautions. At the same time, it must be explained that this exposure is a problem for a fetus, and pregnant women should not receive **radioactive iodine.**

Patients should also be informed about the potential for temporary radiation sickness, with some degree of nausea and vomiting, tenderness and swelling of the neck, pain on swallowing, sore throat, and cough that may occur around the third day after treatment. These problems should be reported, as they can be treated. Temporary thinning of the hair may also occur 2 to 3 months after treatment. Patients should be warned.

LIFESTYLE MANAGEMENT. Hyperthyroidism and goiter are often chronic illnesses managed with self-monitoring of symptoms as well as drug therapy. Emphasize the importance of keeping follow-up appointments for evaluation of thyroid function. For children, evaluation of physical and psychomotor growth and development is also central to their management. Explain to the patient that **antithyroid drug** therapy will be required for 6 to 18 months and perhaps longer, in that recurrence of hyperthyroidism happens in 70 percent of patients. The drug will treat the disorder but may not cure it. Further patient teaching related to management of thyroid disorders is discussed in Chapter 39.

REFERENCES

American Diabetes Association (1998). Clinical practice recommendations. *Diabetes Care, 21*(Supp 1), 1–98.

Bailey, C., & Turner, R. (1996). Drug therapy: Metformin. *New England Journal of Medicine, 334*(9), 574–579.

Bartol, T. (1998, October). Pharmacotherapy for type 2 diabetes: New treatments for an old disease. Presentation at the 21st Annual Education Conference, Oregon Nurses Association–Nurse Practitioners Oregon, Eugene, OR.

Bernstein, G. (1998). The diabetic patient in your practice. *Emergency Medicine, 30*(7), 66–75.

Black, D. (1996) Randomized trial of effect of alendronate on risk of fracture in women with existing vertebral fractures. *Lancet, 348,* 1535–1541.

Blonde, L., Guthrie, R., & Sandberg, M. (1996). Metformin: An effective and safe agent for initial monotherapy in patients with non-insulin-dependent diabetes mellitus. *The Endocrinologist, 6*(6), 431–438.

Burkhardt, K. (1998). When does hypoglycemia develop after sulfonylurea ingestion? *Annals of Emergency Medicine, 31*(6), 771–772.

Cabanas, E. (1998) Maturity-onset diabetes of the young: Recent findings indicate insulin resistance/obesity are not factors. *The Diabetes Educator, 24*(4), 477–480.

Campbell, R.K. (1998). Glimepiride: Role of a new sulfonylurea in the treatment of type 2 diabetes mellitus. *Annals of Pharmacotherapy, 32*(10), 1044–1052.

DeFronzo, R., Goodman, A., & the Multicenter Metformin Study Group. (1995). Efficacy of metformin in patients with non-insulin-dependent diabetes mellitus. *New England Journal of Medicine, 333*(9), 541–549.

Diabetes Control and Complications Trial Research Group. (1993). The effect of intensive treatment of diabetes on the development and progression of long-term complications in insulin-dependent diabetes mellitus. *New England Journal of Medicine, 329,* 997.

Eastman, R., Javitt, J., Herman, W., Dasbach, E., Copley-Merriman, C., & Maier, W. (1997). Model of complications of NIDDM II: Analysis of the health benefits and cost-effectiveness of treating NIDDM with the goal of normoglycemia. *Diabetes Care, 20,* 735–744.

Flick, M., & Schumann, L. (1997). Non-insulin dependent diabetes. *Journal of the American Academy of Nurse Practitioners, 9*(7), 337–343.

Giacca, A., Groenewoud, Y., Tsui, E., McClean, P., & Zinman, B. (1998). Glucose production, utilization and cycling in response to moderate exercise in obese subjects with type 2 diabetes and mild hyperglycemia. *Diabetes, 47*(11), 1763–1770.

Kastrup, E. (Founding Ed.). 1998. *Drug facts and comparisons.* St. Louis: Facts and Comparisons.

Katzung, B. (1998). *Basic and clinical pharmacology* (7th ed). Stamford, CT: Appleton & Lange.

Kummer, S., Boulton, A., Beck-Nielsen, H., Berthezene, F., Muggeo, M., Persson, B., Spinas, G., Donoghue, S., Lettis, S., & Stewart-Long, P., for the Troglitazone Study Group. (1996). Troglitazone, an insulin action enhancer, improves metabolic control in NIDDM patients. *Diabetologia, 39,* 701–709.

Liberman, U., et al. (1995). Effect of oral alendronate on bone mineral density and the incidence of fractures in postmenopausal osteoporosis. *New England Journal of Medicine, 333,* 1437–1443.

Mattock, M., Barnes, D., Viberti, G., Keen, H., Burt, D., Hughes, J., Fitzgerald, A., Sandhu, B., & Jackson, P. (1998). Microalbuminuria and coronary heart disease in NIDDM. *Diabetes, 47*(11), 1786–1789.

Rosenblatt, M. (1998). Osteoporosis: Current status or screening, prevention and therapy. *Primary Care, 10*(3), 53–59.

Schwartz, S., Raskin, P., Fonseca, V., & Graveline, J. (1998). Effect of troglitazone in insulin-treated patients with type II diabetes mellitus. *New England Journal of Medicine, 338*(13), 861–866.

Smits, P., & Thien, T. (1995). Cardiovascular effects of sulphonylurea derivatives: Implications for the treatment of NIDDM. *Diabetologia, 38,* 116–121.

Szlatenyi, S., Capes, K., & Wang, R. (1998). Delayed hypoglycemia in a child after ingestion of a single glipizide tablet. *Annals of Emergency Medicine, 31*(6), 773.

CHAPTER 20

·······

Drugs Affecting the Reproductive System

CHAPTER OUTLINE

OTHER DRUGS AFFECTING THE
REPRODUCTIVE SYSTEM
Drugs Commonly Used in Fertility Clinics
  GnRH
  Follicle-stimulating hormone

Luteinizing hormone and human
  chorionic gonadotropin
Lactation Inhibitors
  Bromocriptine
Drugs Used in Erectile Dysfunction
  Sildenafil citrate

Androgens and Antiandrogens

The androgens (aqueous testosterone [Testandro], testosterone propionate [in oil], testosterone enanthate [in oil, Andro L.A. 200], testosterone cypionate [in oil, Depo-Testosterone], methyltestosterone [Android-10], fluoxymesterone [Halotestin]) have been used to treat both male and female reproductive systems. **Androgens** are used (1) as replacement for deficiency states, (2) as **anabolic therapy** for disorders such as cancer and HIV, and (3) for enhanced athletic performance. The focus of this discussion is the primary care use of these drugs rather than those used by nurse practitioners (NPs) in specialized practices. For information on **antiandrogens,** see Table 20–1.

Pharmacodynamics

Testosterone is by far the most important androgen in humans. A small portion (2%) is found free in plasma and converted to dihydrotestosterone in the skin, prostate, seminal vesicles, and epididymis. Testosterone is produced in the interstitial or Leydig cells, located in the spaces between the seminiferous tubules. The testis, like the ovary, has both reproductive and endocrine functions. Women produce small amounts in the menstruating ovary and the adrenals, and both sexes produce testosterone peripherally from androstenedione, dehydroepiandrosterone (DHEA), and dehydroepiandrosterone sulfate (DHEAS). Research is currently investigating the effects of DHEA and DHEAS on inhibiting atherosclerosis. At puberty, the normal male produces testosterone that causes penile and scrotal growth. The skin changes are pubic, axillary, and beard hair growth. The sebaceous glands make the skin thicker and oilier. Even the vocal cords become thicker, with the resulting lower-pitched voice. More growth occurs in all bones, with epiphyseal closure about age 21. Androgens are crucial for stimulation and maintenance of sexual potency. During adolescence, testosterone increases lean body mass and growth of body hair. Androgen levels remain stable until age 55, when a gradual decline begins. At age 70, a more rapid decline in hormone levels occurs, and men experience decreased muscle mass, strength, and libido. Androgens have metabolic effects in protein metabolism, liver synthesis of clotting factors, and renal production of erythropoietin Androgens affect lipoprotein metabolism, resulting in lower high-density lipoprotein (HDL). For example, men have HDLs of 20 to 40 mg/dL, and women have HDLs in the range of 40 to 60 mg/dL (Katzung, 1998). When men attempt to improve athletic prowess by taking large doses of exogenous testosterone, spermatogenesis is reduced through suppression of follicle-stimulating hormone (FSH).

Pharmacokinetics

Absorption and Distribution

Oral **testosterone** is rapidly metabolized by the gut as methyltestosterone and fluoxymesterone and is converted in its target tissues by the enzyme 5-alpha-reductase. The further conversion of **testosterone** to estradiol by P-450 aromatase occurs in adipose tissue, the liver, and the hypothalamus. Buccal administration lengthens the half-life. Intramuscular (IM) administration (esters) in depot preparations can last 2 to 4 weeks.

Metabolism and Excretion

Degradation of **testosterone** (44%) proceeds in the liver, where it is inactivated to androsterone and etiocholanolone, and then conjugated and excreted in the urine. Six percent is excreted in the feces.

Onset, Peak, and Duration

Oral administration reaches peak levels in 2 hours, buccal in 1 hour, and IM in 8 days to 2 weeks. About 98 percent of circulating testosterone is bound to sex hormone–binding globulin (SHBG). SHBG is increased in plasma by estrogen, thyroid hormone, and cirrhosis of the liver. It is decreased by androgens, growth hormone, and obesity. The final 2 percent remains free to enter the cell (Katzung, 1998). Table 20–2 presents the pharmacokinetics of **androgens** and **antiandrogens.**

Pharmacotherapeutics

Precautions and Contraindications

The areas of clinical usage that are more controversial include stimulating growth in boys with delayed puberty, in aging men to increase strength and muscle mass, and in

Table 20–1. Antiandrogens

The problems of reduced potency in the oral form and the virilizing side effects of androgens led investigators to develop drugs that inhibit synthesis and block sex hormone production receptors. This approach of countering the effects of undesirable androgen excess has enabled therapy at higher dosages. Dihydrotestosterone is the essential androgen in the prostate. The effect of androgens can be reduced by inhibiting 5-alpha-reductase in its target tissues.

Finasteride (Propecia, Proscar)

This steroidlike inhibitor of 5-alpha reductase is orally active and produces a reduction in dihydrotestosterone within 8 hours of administration and lasts for about 24 hours. Forty to 50% is metabolized and excreted through the GI tract. The FDA granted approval for finasteride to treat benign prostatic hypertrophy at 5 mg/day. Finasteride has been used to suppress metastatic prostate cancer. There have also been some successes with this drug in treating hirsute women, although it has not been approved for that use either (Hansen, 1997). In 1998, finasteride became available in a 1-mg dose for male pattern baldness, for men only. Dermatologists are currently prescribing the 1-mg dose for women with alopecia. The main undesirable effects at 1- and 5-mg doses are decreased libido and impotence.

Leuprolide acetate (Lupron)

Leuprolide is a luteinizing hormone–releasing agonist. This drug produces gonadal suppression when blood levels are continuous in the treatment of prostate cancer. It may be given in a dose of 1 mg subcutaneously daily or intramuscularly every 3 months in the depot formulation. Mean plasma levels are achieved in 4 hours and are maintained after an initial drop in concentration. It has even greater suppression when used with flutamide. In pediatric patients, its use is to treat central precocious puberty. In gynecology, its use is in reducing uterine fibroids, endometriosis, and polycystic ovary syndrome. Approximately 90% of women with unstaged endometriosis have relief of pain, and 50% regain fertility with leuprolide. Opposition to medical treatment to restore fertility comes from surgeons, who argue that higher fertility rates can be achieved by laparoscopy with ablation of endometrial implants (Gambone & DeCherney, 1997).

Flutamide (Eulexin, Euflex)

Flutamide behaves like a competitive antagonist at the androgen receptor site, although it is truly a nonsteroidal agent. It has been used with leuprolide for the treatment of stage B2-C prostate cancer, but the most success has been with female androgen excess syndrome. The adverse effects in men are gynecomastia and reversible liver toxicity. Flutamide is rapidly absorbed orally. It is metabolized into six compounds and bound 97% to plasma proteins, reaching a steady state by the fourth dose. Flutamide is excreted in the urine but has not required changes in dose unless renal function is less than 29 mL/min.

Spironolactone (Aldactone)

Another competitive inhibitor of dihydrotestosterone, aldosterone interferes with the androgen receptors in the prostate. It also reduces 17-alpha-hydroxylase activity, lowering plasma levels of testosterone and androstenedione. Refer to Chapter 14 for its uses as a diuretic. Spironolactone is absorbed orally, reaches peak levels in 2 hours, and is metabolized by the liver and excreted through the portal system. Spironolactone has short-term use for primary hyperaldosteronism in patients preoperatively. It is used long-term for those patients who are not good candidates for surgery or those with idiopathic hyperaldosteronism. There are also edematous conditions that require potassium conservation, such as congestive heart failure and cirrhosis of the liver associated with ascites. An unlabeled use is in females with androgen excess for the treatment of hirsutism and acne in dosages of 50 to 200 mg per day. Adverse reactions are usually dose-related and reversible when the drug is discontinued. The commonest adverse reactions are GI upset, drowsiness, gynecomastia, impotence, cutaneous eruptions, and urticaria. Early animal chronic toxicity studies demonstrated tumorigenicity; therefore, use should be balanced against risk. This drug is contraindicated in pregnancy, yet the American Academy of Physicians has stated that it is compatible with breastfeeding. Although this drug is classified as a diuretic, its use in premenstrual syndrome is probably effective because of its antiandrogen effect, even at low doses (25 to 50 mg daily).

athletes to improve competitive performance. In this last area, there has been abuse by coaches and athletes alike. The adverse effects far outweigh the potential benefits.

Because of the abuse potential of **anabolic steroids,** NPs must supply their federal narcotic identification number (DEA number) on all prescriptions written for hormone combinations with **androgens.**

Adverse Drug Reactions

The **androgens** as a class are very potent and can have serious or even fatal reactions if used improperly. Both **testosterone** and **anabolic steroids** have been abused. The use of these drugs by NPs is discouraged because of serious complications. The **anabolic steroids** have a high anabolic, low androgenic ratio of activity. The FDA warns that **androgens** may cause peliosis hepatis. *Peliosis* is the replacement of normal liver tissue with bloody cysts. This vascularity may cause silent fatal abdominal hemorrhage. Liver tumors that are benign and malignant may develop. The lipoprotein changes with these **steroids** may hasten coronary artery disease. Drugs classified as **anabolic steroids** are **oxymetholone, stanozolol, oxandrolone, nandrolone phenpropionate,** and **nandrolone decanoate.**

Less dangerous adverse reactions that occur to females, as well as female fetuses, is clitoral enlargement. This is not reversible when the drug is stopped. Deepening of the voice and male hair patterns may be reversible. Menstrual irregularities may occur through suppression of gonadotropin secretion. Men may develop gynecomastia and reduced sperm levels that threaten fertility. Acne and baldness may occur, even

Table 20–2. Pharmacokinetics: Androgens and Antiandrogens

Drug	Onset	Peak	Duration	Effect of Food on Absorption	Half-Life	Elimination
Androgens Testosterone (short-acting)	NA	1 h	2–3 d	NA	Normal renal function: 10–100 min Impaired renal function: no effect	Total: hepatic metabolism, 90% excretion Unchanged: inactive
Testosterone (long-acting)	NA	2 h	2–4 wk	NA	As above	As above
Testosterone (transdermal)	NA	2–4 h	24 h	None	Normal renal function: 8 d Impaired renal function: no effect	As above
Antiandrogens Finasteride	NA	1–2 h	24 h	None	Normal renal function: 4.8–6 h Impaired renal function: no effect	Total: extensive hepatic Unchanged: NA
Leuprolide	NA	Depot: 4 h	4 wk	NA	NA	NA
Flutamide	NA	2 h	6 h	None	Normal renal function: 8 h Impaired renal function: slightly more than 8 h	Total: mainly in urine Unchanged: 4.2% in feces
Spironolactone (unlabeled use)	24–28 h	48–72 h	48–72 h	Increases absorption	Normal renal function: 20 h Impaired renal function: do not use if blood urea nitrogen (BUN) >30 mg/dL	Total: renal Unchanged: NA

NA = not available.

with short-term therapy. Gastrointestinal (GI) symptoms include nausea and cholestatic jaundice. Suppression of clotting factors, as well as increased red blood cell production, can contribute to hemorrhage and thrombus formation simultaneously. Men can paradoxically have decreased libido, depression, and headache with exogenous administration of **androgens.**

Drug Interactions

The interaction of **anticoagulants** such as **warfarin (Coumadin)** with the 17-alkyl testosterone derivatives has the most significant potential problem. The drugs are the methyl and fluoxy forms used for hypogonadism and male climacteric. The interaction with **tricyclic antide-**

pressants is worrisome enough to switch to a different class of **antidepressants** because four of five patients had paranoid delusions. Although **testosterone** has been used for breast tenderness in the past, its use is discouraged because of lack of proven efficacy and the masculinizing effect on females. Laboratory values of decreasing protein-bound T_4 and increased T_3 uptake need to be mentioned, but because the free T_4 levels are not affected, no deficiency state occurs. Table 20–3 presents drug interactions.

Clinical Use and Dosing

Replacement or augmentation of endogenous androgen for primary hypogonadal males or hypogonadotropic hypogonadism and for male climacteric are the primary

Table 20–3. Drug Interactions: Androgens and Antiandrogens

Drug	Interacting Drug	Possible Effect	Implications
Androgens Testosterone	Anticoagulants	Increased anticoagulant effect	More frequent monitoring of prothrombin time
	Imipramine	Paranoid response	Consider switching to another class of antidepressants
Antiandrogens Finasteride	Theophylline	Not clinically significant; decreases half-life of theophylline by 10%	Check peak flow, consider other drug classes (e.g., albuterol)
Leuprolide	Pituitary, gonadotropic, and gonadal function Lab tests	Misleading results	Consider if lab test reports show unexpected values
Flutamide	None listed	None listed, but flutamide is highly protein-bound	Drug is new enough that there is potential for interactions
Spironolactone	Anticoagulants	Decreased hypothrombinemic effect	Monitor potassium levels in young patients with reduced renal function and in patients over age 65
	Digitalis	May increase or decrease digitalis half-life	As above
	Potassium	Hyperkalemia	As above

clinical uses. **Testosterone enanthate** demonstrated 30 years of clinical use, and the World Health Organization (WHO) selected it as the prototype hormone in its contraceptive efficacy studies (Waites, 1993). In rare situations, **androgens** are used in endometriosis, in refractory anemia, and with **estrogen** for osteoporosis and loss of libido. **Androgens** have anabolic effects with food and exercise for postoperative trauma patients and with some types of metastatic breast cancer. The masculinizing effect on females detracts from wider usage. **Testosterone** is controversial in pediatrics as a height stimulator and in sports as a performance enhancer. NPs in primary care prescribe **androgens** for replacement therapy, and for that reason this discussion is limited. The use of **testosterone** with **estrogen** for osteoporosis and symptomatic treatment of hot flashes and decreased libido can be found in Chapter 36. Table 20–4 presents the dosage schedule for **androgens** and **antiandrogens**.

Rational Drug Selection

SLOW-ACTING VERSUS LONG-ACTING FORM. IM forms have longer half-lives than oral, but less uniform absorption. IM aqueous preparations need to be administered two to three times per week. The patient or a family member can be taught to administer these long-term medications to simplify daily routines. Preparations in oil can be administered at 2- to 4-week intervals. Oral preparations cause less discomfort to administer but may cause gastric irritation.

COST. Oral **testosterone** products are less expensive, in part because equipment and technical skills are not required for administration. Buccal preparations avoid the 44 percent metabolism in the liver, but the tablets are more costly. Transdermal patches are the most recent addition to hormone replacement therapy for men and women, and the convenience is more costly. It seems the best route of administration for children because there are no taste issues or painful injections, and older adults with poor eyesight or swallowing problems would have less difficulty with patch application. Frequently, the patient's third-party payer limits available formulations. Table 20–5 presents the available dosage forms.

Monitoring

Considerable monitoring is necessary when higher doses are administered. In replacement therapy, high dosage would be 400 mg every 2 weeks. In palliation of breast cancer, 100 mg three times per week is a high dosage. Calcium levels in serum and urine may become abnormal in patients with metastatic breast cancer. **Methyltestosterone** and **fluoxymesterone** are apt to cause hepatic toxicity, and liver function tests should be drawn every 6 months. When using **testosterone** in prepubertal males, perform an x-ray every 6 months for bone mat-

Table 20–4. Dosage Schedule: Androgens and Antiandrogens

Drug	Indication	Dose
Androgens Testosterone (short-acting)	Androgen replacement therapy	IM: 25–50 mg 2–3 times wk; generally lower doses for 4–6 mo
	Delayed puberty	Oral: 25–50 mg/d Buccal: 5–10 mg/d
	Growth stimulation in Turner's syndrome	IM: 40–50 mg/m²/dose monthly for 6 mo
Testosterone (long-acting)	Male hypogonadism Males with delayed puberty	IM: 50–400 mg every 2–4 wk IM: 50–200 mg every 2–4 wk
Testosterone (transdermal)	Replacement therapy in males for conditions associated with a deficiency or absence of endogenous testosterone	Topical: use one system nightly, every 24 h
Antiandrogens Finasteride	Benign prostatic hyperplasia Androgenic alopecia	Oral: 5 mg qd, with or without meals Oral: 1 mg qd, with or without meals
Leuprolide	Unlabeled use: treatment for metastatic prostatic carcinoma in combination with flutamide	SC: 1 mg daily
Flutamide	Prostatic carcinoma	Oral: 2 capsules 3 times/d at 8-h intervals for a total daily dosage of 750 mg
Spironolactone (unlabeled use)	Hirsutism	Oral: 50–200 mg/d; 50 mg bid on days 4–21 of the menstrual cycle may help reduce risk of menorrhagia that occurs with higher doses

uration to avoid early closure of epiphyseal centers. Check hemoglobin and hematocrit every 6 months to avoid excessive polycythemia in patients receiving high doses of **androgens.**

Patient Education

ADMINISTRATION. Avoid coadministering with other medications that cause gastric irritation. With buccal forms, food or liquids reduce absorption. Do not swallow buccal tablets; instead, park the tablet between gums and teeth. If the skin is sensitive to the patch adhesive, a small application of aerosolized **cortisone** (e.g., **Asthmacort** or **Nasocort**) to the skin will reduce irritation without loss of efficacy. This topical treatment of the skin can be used for both men and women.

ADVERSE REACTIONS. Caution women to report signs of virilization such as hoarseness, hair thinning, and menstrual disruption. Some adverse effects are reversible if the drug is reduced or temporarily stopped. Keep appointments to monitor serum electrolyte disturbances. An increase in symptoms of angina may be a result of extremely high serum cholesterol. Warn patients to report

any increase in the severity or frequency of chest pain. The **anabolic androgens** may precipitate or worsen glucose intolerance. Monitor blood sugars closely. Older men may develop prostatic hypertrophy with secondary urinary retention while on **androgen** therapy. Ask questions about urine stream and nighttime voiding patterns.

LIFESTYLE MANAGEMENT. Children and young adults with hypogonadism need to treat their chronic problem cautiously because long use of **androgens** can precipitate adverse reactions. If managed early and carefully, males with hypogonadism may be able to raise normal families. Teens requiring therapy need to know that **testosterone** replacement is far different than **anabolic steroid** use by the athlete looking for a competitive edge in an upcoming sports event. Older patients need to reduce sodium in their diets to avoid congestive heart failure while on **androgen** therapy.

Estrogens and Antiestrogens

The **estrogens** include **Premarin, Estrace, Ogen,** and **ethinyl estradiol.** The first **estrogens** prescribed were for replacement therapy. These were conjugated equine

Table 20–5. Available Dosage Forms: Androgens and Antiandrogens

Drug	Dosage Form	How Supplied
Androgens		
Testosterone (short-acting)	Injection	25 mg/mL, 50 mg/mL, 100 mg/mL in 10-mL and 30-mL vials
	Injection (in oil)	100 mg/mL in 10-mL vials
	Tablet	10 mg, 25 mg
	Buccal	10 mg
	Capsule	10 mg
Testosterone (long-acting)	Injection (enanthate in oil)	100 mg/mL, 200 mg/mL in 5-mL and 10-mL vials; 1-mL single-dose syringe
Testosterone (transdermal)	Transdermal	4 mg/24 h; 6 mg/24 h; 2.5 mg/24 h
Antiandrogens		
Finasteride	Oral tablet	1 mg, 5 mg
Leuprolide	Injection	5 mg/mL in 2.8-mL multidose vial
	Lyophilized for injection	7.5 mg, 11.25 mg, 15 mg, 22.5 mg, 30 mg in single-use kit
Flutamide	Capsule	125 mg
	Tablet	250 mg
Spironolactone (unlabeled use)	Tablet	25 mg, 50 mg, 100 mg

estrogens. Later **estrogens** were esterified (80% estrone sulfate and 15% sodium equilin sulfate). **Estradiol** was synthesized into oral and IM preparations, vaginal creams, transdermal patches, and vaginal rings for 3 month administration. Ethinyl forms of **estradiol** became the primary forms for use in oral contraception. **Ethinyl estradiol** is approximately 10 times the potency of **estradiol**. Phytoestrogens and estrogen-like herbal preparations have shown symptomatic improvement with perimenopausal symptoms. Studies are still needed to prove that herbal preparations can be used to prevent such disorders as osteoporosis and cardiac disease.

Information about **antiestrogens** is presented in Table 20–6.

Pharmacodynamics

Estrogens are primarily responsible for the development of the secondary sexual characteristics of the developing female. Estrogens cause proliferation of vaginal and uterine mucosa, increased secretion of the cervix, and glandular development in the breast. Control of estrogen secretion is by the hypothalamus through the pituitary gland. Gonadotropin-releasing hormone (GnRH) from the hypothalamus controls FSH and luteinizing hormone (LH) from the anterior pituitary. FSH and LH stimulate follicular development in the ovary. In the presence of adequate estrogen, LH surge is responsible for ovulation. Primary hormone pathways in the reproductive system are modulated by both negative and positive feedback loops.

The direct effects of estrogen on vasculature promote dilation and inhibit the progression of atherosclerosis. The nonvascular effects of estrogen may offset its beneficial vascular effects. For example, estrogens cause a clotting phenomenon during parturition and in the first 2 to 3 weeks postpartum. Pulmonary embolism and deep vein thrombosis account for the greatest morbidity and mortality associated with pregnancy.

Pharmacokinetics

Absorption and Distribution

Approximately 80 percent of **estradiol** binds strongly to the sex hormone–binding globulin (SHBG) in the target tissues and 18 percent to albumin with less affinity. The 2 percent free fraction is physiologically active. Oral **estrogens** are completely absorbed from the GI tract but rapidly metabolized. Transdermal forms of **estradiol** are only slightly metabolized so that a smaller dose is needed. Vaginal delivery varies in absorption. More hormone is absorbed if the degree of atrophy is great in the surrounding tissues.

Table 20–6. Antiestrogens

Although naturally occurring hormones such as progesterone and testosterone may modify the action of estrogen, the following discussion focuses on the synthetic estrogen antagonists. Drugs in this class may have limited use by most practitioners in primary care. Clomiphene is used for ovulation stimulation by infertility clinics. Danazol is primarily used for endometriosis by gynecologists, and tamoxifen is used for female cancers by oncologists.

Clomiphene (Clomid)

Clomiphene was the first chemical used to initiate ovulation in normogonadotropic, normoprolactinemic, and anovulatory patients. It has also been used as a component in the management of luteal-phase dysfunction, oligo-ovulation, artificial insemination, unexplained infertility, and in vitro fertilization. Although clomiphene has been used for 30 years, it is still a drug that remains in a specialized practice setting. The list of adverse side effects are hot flushes, multiple gestation, visual symptoms, cervical mucus abnormalities, luteal-phase defect, luteinized unruptured follicle syndrome, ovarian cancer, teratogenicity, enlargement of ovarian cysts, and liver disease (Derman & Adashi, 1994).

The agonist-antagonist characteristics of clomiphene depend on the hormone climate. Clomiphene initiates ovulation in the presence of high estrogen levels in anovulatory females. It does this as long as other endogenous mechanisms trigger an LH surge and follicle rupture (Baker & Jaffe, 1995). Clomiphene blocks endogenous estrogen-negative feedback at the level of the hypothalamus. It also elevates estrogen and progesterone levels higher than normal. Its function may even affect the ovary and pituitary glands. Clomiphene also decreases serum insulin-like growth factors and increases SHBG, which assists those infertile women with polycystic ovary (PCO) disease. It has direct antiestrogenic effects on the endometrium and cervical mucus–producing glands. Elevated estrogen levels of women in the reproductive years can override the direct antiestrogen effects on the endometrium and cervical mucus.

This compound is active when taken orally, but little is known about its metabolism. Half of the compound is excreted in the feces within 5 days of administration. The hypothesis is that it is excreted through a slow enterohepatic pathway (Katzung, 1998).

Danazol (Danocrine)

Although the major use of danazol has been to treat endometriosis, it has been employed in severe fibrocystic breast changes, hematologic disorders, and idiopathic thrombocytopenic purpura. Danazol must be used with great caution in hepatic dysfunction. The list of adverse effects is long, which is, in part, why this drug is not indicated for most primary care settings.

Danazol inhibits the midcycle surge of LH and FSH to suppress ovarian function. It has weak progestational and androgenic properties, as does its major metabolite, ethisterone. Danazol binds to androgen, progesterone, and glucocorticoid receptors and translocates the androgen receptor into the nucleus to initiate androgen-specific RNA synthesis. It does not inhibit aromatase, the enzyme required for estrogen synthesis. It also increases the clearance rate of progesterone by competing with the hormone for binding proteins (Katzung, 1998). Danazol is taken orally and is slowly metabolized by the liver and kidneys, being excreted in the feces and urine after a 15-hour half-life.

Tamoxifen (Nolvadex)

The first of possibly many selective estrogen receptor modulator (SERM) drugs to treat conditions that respond to adding or withdrawing estrogens. Used primarily as part of adjuvant therapy for breast cancer in patients with estrogen-receptor (ER)-positive tumors. Recent studies have demonstrated a reduction in breast cancer in those individuals at high risk for developing the disease within 5 years. In the Gail Model, age, family history, medical history of premalignant biopsies, and age at first live birth calculate the patient's absolute risk.

An antiestrogen in mammary tissue, tamoxifen has direct antigrowth activity of its own in the absence of estrogen. The mechanism may be that it blocks estradiol-induced cancer cell growth by altering the local production of growth factors and/or inhibiting the development of the tumor's blood supply (Baker & Jaffe, 1995). Tamoxifen causes hyperplasia in the postmenopausal woman's endometrium and vagina. But in the presence of estrogen, the premenopausal uterus and vagina atrophy. There are currently three large-scale trials under way to evaluate its effectiveness in preventing disease in high-risk women. The results will try to address its potential benefits on bone and lipids while reducing the risk on breast tissue.

This is a nonsteroidal agent that is given orally. Peak plasma levels are reached in a few hours with an initial half-life of 7 to 14 hours. The liver extensively metabolizes tamoxifen, and 65% of the drug is excreted through the gut within 2 weeks.

Raloxifene (Evista)

Raloxifene is the second in a series of SERM drugs. Indications initially were for osteoporosis prevention in women who cannot or will not take hormone replacement therapy. Postmarketing studies have shown a positive lipid effect, which may improve cardiovascular disease risk (Walsh, 1998). Results from the recent MORE randomized trial demonstrated a 76% reduced risk of invasive breast cancer among the women taking raloxifene for osteoporosis. This was attributed to the effect of the drug on ER-positive tumors. (Cummings et al., 1999). This drug can be used only in women past menopause who have never had thromboembolic problems.

Continued on next page

Table 20–6. Antiestrogens *(continued)*

Raloxifene is a selective estrogen receptor modulator similar to tamoxifen with different degrees of estrogen agonist or antagonist activity in different tissues. It is an estrogen agonist on bone and an antagonist on breast and uterus. It appears to be neutral on the vaginal tissues. A comparison of the beneficial effect on bone mineral density is slightly less than that of estrogen. Whether this bone effect will decrease the incidence of fractures has yet to be proved (Raloxifene, 1998).

Raloxifene is taken orally without regard to meals, with a 60% absorption rate. It is highly bound to plasma proteins. The drug is glucuronidated but not further metabolized in the first pass through the liver. It is excreted though the GI tract with a half-life of 27 hours.

Raloxifene is not indicated for pediatric patients or with premenopausal women. Concomitant hormone replacement therapy is not recommended.

Patients who stopped taking raloxifene during the study reported hot flashes that lasted up to 6 months and leg cramps.

Because raloxifene is highly bound (95%) to plasma proteins, close monitoring is recommended when it is used in combination with drugs such as clofibrate, cholestyramine, NSAIDs, diazepam, diazoxide, and warfarin.

One short-term trial indicates that it might be effective for prevention of postmenopausal bone loss without the risk for breast or uterine cancer. It may also have a beneficial effect on lipid metabolism. More studies are indicated to prove that the effect on lipids confers a cardioprotective effect. This drug may be useful for NPs in primary care practices, but at this time the long-term safety effects are not known. It does have some known drug interactions already with cholestyramine and warfarin. Like estrogens, there is some increase in thromboembolic disease, and it is teratogenic for women at risk of pregnancy. Raloxifene cannot be used with any progesterone because progesterone can be converted into estrogen.

If used with anticoagulant therapy, draw prothrombin times frequently early in therapy. Supplemental calcium and vitamin D are necessary if diet does not include 1200 to 1600 mg of calcium and 400 international units of vitamin D.

Raloxifene can be administered orally without regard to food. Patients need to know that hot flashes can sometimes occur at the beginning of therapy, even in postmenopausal women.

If patients have warning prior to necessary surgery, raloxifene needs to be discontinued 72 hours ahead of time. When traveling, patients should get up and move around every hour to avoid long periods of inactivity. The risk of thromboembolic disease (1%) is the same as it is for estrogen users. At this time, studies comparing raloxifene to placebo demonstrate deep vein thrombosis (DVT) and pulmonary embolism (PE) as the most serious of complications.

Metabolism and Excretion

The liver converts **estradiol** into less potent metabolites, estrone and estriol, which are excreted in the bile. A significant portion is reabsorbed in the liver, resulting in undesirable side effects such as increased clotting factors and plasma renin substrate. The water-soluble forms that result from reabsorption are acidic, favoring renal excretion.

Onset, Peak, and Duration

Naturally occurring estradiol levels vary during the menstrual cycle from 50 picograms on day 2 to 350 to 850 picograms on day 14. Patients report symptoms of estrogen deficiency after missing several days of therapy. The literature does not report specific hours of pharmacological effect. Table 20–7 presents the pharmacokinetics of estrogens.

Pharmacotherapeutics

Estrogens have been synthesized for several decades and used in the primary care setting for replacement after oophorectomy and in natural menopause for treatment of hot flashes, vaginal atrophy, and irregular menstrual bleeding. The more potent **estrogen** used for contraception became available in the 1960s. The potency ratio of **replacement estrogens** to **contraception estrogens** is approximately 1:10. Chapter 36 goes into greater detail about **replacement estrogens**, and Chapter 29 deals with its use as a **contraceptive**. Many NPs commonly prescribe the noncontraceptive use of **oral contraceptives** for dysmenorrhea. By contrast, **oral contraceptives** may be more often prescribed to treat amenorrhea and hirsutism associated with polycystic ovary disease in specialty practices.

Precautions and Contraindications

Estrogens have been implicated in the risk of endometrial cancer. The rates have increased dramatically since 1969. At the same time, the survival of endometrial cancers has been higher in **estrogen** users. "Natural" and synthetic **estrogens** have the same risks for users. **Use of *estrogens* during pregnancy is contraindicated because of the high rate of teratogenicity in male and female offspring.** Estrogens were used empirically to treat women who habitually aborted. Most research has proved that there is no benefit in using **estrogens** for preventing miscarriages. The absolute and relative contraindications for **estrogen** use are listed in Chapter 29. These precautions are the same for the **menopausal estrogens, estradiol,** and the more potent hormone **ethinyl estradiol** used for **oral contraceptive.** The exception is that **ethinyl estradiol** is contraindicated in

Table 20–7. Pharmacokinetics: Estrogens and Antiestrogens

Drug	Effect of Food on Absorption	Site of Metabolism	Active Metabolite	Half-Life (Normal Renal Function)	Half-Life (Impaired Renal Function)	Elimination
Estrogens Ethinyl estradiol	None	Liver	Less active estrogenic compounds	NA	No effect	Total: urinary inactive drug Unchanged: NA
Conjugated estrogens	None	Liver		NA		Unchanged: NA
Estradiol transdermal system	None	Skin		NA		Unchanged: NA
Estradiol vaginal ring	None	Vagina		NA		Unchanged: NA
Antiestrogens Clomiphene	None	NA	NA	NA	None (prolonged in renal failure)	Total: feces Unchanged: NA
Danazol	None	NA	NA	NA	NA	NA
Tamoxifen	None	NA	N-desmethyl-tamoxifen	14 d (metabolite)	No effect	Total: <30% feces Unchanged: NA
Toremifene	None	NA	N-demethyl-toremifene	4–6 d	Renal: no effect Hepatic: increased	Total: feces Unchanged: NA
Raloxifene	None	NA	Glucuronide conjugates	27.7–32.5 h	No effect	Total: feces Unchanged: <0.2% in urine

NA = not available.

patients who smoke and are over age 35, but smoking patients may use **postmenopausal hormone replacement therapy (HRT).** The interaction of **estrogens** and smoking showing dose-related morbidity and mortality has been well documented.

Adverse Drug Reactions

Most of the adverse reactions to **estrogens** are dose-related. As a result, the majority of adverse effects are seen in patients on **oral contraceptives.** See Chapter 29 for managing migraine headaches, mood changes, eye discomfort, skin pigmentation, breast changes, weight gain, change in vaginal secretion, and leg discomforts. The adverse reactions more common with **menopausal estrogens** are elevation of systemic blood pressure, gall bladder disease, and irregular bleeding. See Chapter 36 for managing the undesirable adverse effects of **menopausal estrogens.** Women who have estrogen-dependent tumors may have worsening of their cancer while on any form of **estrogen** therapy.

Drug Interactions

Estrogens interfere with laboratory measurements of endocrine and liver function tests and thyroid-binding globulin. In addition, the prothrombin time and factors VII, VIII, IX, and X show increased levels in patients taking **estrogens** at the time of testing. Women may experience impaired glucose tolerance and increased triglycerides when **oral estrogens** are administered. The most common drug interactions are with **anticoagulants, tricyclic anti-**

depressants, barbiturates, antituberculosis drugs, corticosteroids, seizure control medication, and **drugs for spasticity.** Table 20–8 presents drug interactions.

Clinical Use and Dosing

Labeled clinical use ranges from treatment of menopausal deficiency states to palliation of genital cancers in both men and women. The areas of use currently discussed in professional as well as lay journals are osteoporosis, cardiovascular disease, and Alzheimer's disease (both primary and secondary prevention). The unlabeled uses are for postcoital contraception and with Turner's syndrome. See Chapter 29 for the exact dosing of emergency contraception and the choice of products tested for efficacy in this treatment. Table 20–9 presents the dosage schedule of **estrogens.**

Rational Drug Selection

SHORT ACTING VERSUS LONG ACTING. Most women receive oral daily doses of **estrogen.** In this manner, a consistent and expected level is maintained. Some women may have problems remembering or difficulty in swallowing the oral form, and parenteral administration is possible. Giving injections every 3 to 4 weeks is uncomfortable, and the daily levels may vary, depending on the circulation in the muscle into which the dose is injected. If skin sensitivity is not a problem, transdermal preparations may be applied weekly or biweekly to the hip and thigh areas. Vaginal instillation is also possible for patients unable to tolerate oral medications or for severe urethral and urogenital atrophy, as in vulvar dystrophies and dyspareunia.

COST. Oral preparations have been available in the generic form the longest and are the least expensive. Next lowest in price are the vaginal creams. The latest products on the market and also more costly are the transdermal preparations and the vaginal ring. Products that are more convenient are usually more costly, such as prepackaged punch-out cards or dial packs.

ROUTE OF ADMINISTRATION. Oral preparations are easy for most patients and can be taken at mealtime or bedtime. Transdermal patches allow caregivers to assist patients with less dexterity and an inability to swallow. A small percentage of women experience elevated triglycerides with **oral estrogens,** and these patients can avoid the liver metabolism through dermal absorption. Vaginal application reduces liver metabolism but is absorbed less after severe vaginal atrophy is treated. The levels are not as high after the first 6 months of therapy. Some older women lack the finger dexterity to fill an applicator and instill the cream. Cost is definitely an issue with women on Medicare, who often have multiple medications and have to choose which prescriptions they can afford each month. Table 20–10 presents the available dosage forms of **estrogen.**

Monitoring

Oral contraception and **HRT** are chronic medications that are taken for months or years. If the patient has a coexisting medical condition such as one of those listed in Chapter 29, then monitoring of adverse effects is necessary. Schedule 3-month, 6-month, or annual evaluation appointments, depending on the degree of illness or the severity of symptoms. Teaching patients to report potentially worrisome adverse effects is necessary at the institution of therapy. Drawing baseline blood tests such as a lipid panel and ordering mammograms prior to **HRT** are examples of monitoring and screening simultaneously. Patients with diabetes need to perform daily blood sugar measurements. Patients with hypertension need monthly blood pressure readings, and patients with seizures need drug levels measured every 6 months.

Patient Education

ADMINISTRATION. Patients taking **oral contraceptives** need to take them daily at about the same time to avoid breakthrough bleeding. They may experience transient adverse effects such as mild nausea and breast tenderness or midcycle spotting in the first month or two that resolves later. They need to be reassured that this is normal. Sometimes taking the medication at bedtime solves the nausea problem. Some women find it easier to put the birth control packet by the toothbrush to avoid forgetting the medication. Advise the patient that oral tablets may be administered vaginally if the patient is nauseated or vomiting and cannot tolerate the oral route. Also advise the patient that a dry topical spray (e.g., **triamcinolone**) to prepare the skin before applying the transdermal patch eliminates skin sensitivity to the patch adhesive.

ADVERSE REACTIONS. Patients need to know the target organs of **estrogen** therapy. The breasts, uterus, and vagina are more obvious organs dependent on estrogen. Deep blood vessels in the legs, visual disturbances, and severe headache could herald thromboembolic phenomena that could be life-threatening. Patients who smoke and those who are diabetic are at increased risk for this type of complication. Abnormal bleeding patterns or genital pain needs to be reported in all age groups. In younger women who experience irregular bleeding, infection or pregnancy is suspect, but bleeding in a postmenopausal woman may be the first symptom of uterine or ovarian cancer.

LIFESTYLE MANAGEMENT. Patients who smoke have to stop **oral contraceptives** by age 35 because of the inter-

Table 20–8. Drug Interactions: Estrogens and Antiestrogens

Drug	Interacting Drug	Possible Effect	Implications
Estrogens Estrogens	Oral anticoagulants	Estrogens may reduce the hypothrombinemic effect of anticoagulants.	Monitor PT more frequently.
	Antidepressants	Estrogens may alter pharmacological effects of these agents; effects may be dose-dependent; an increased incidence of toxic reactions may also occur.	Monitor cardiac status and blood pressure in patients over age 65.
	Barbiturates, rifampin	Barbiturates, rifampin, and other agents that induce hepatic microsomal enzymes with concomitant estrogens may produce lower estrogen levels than expected.	Use a backup birth control method.
	Corticosteroids	Estrogen coadministration may reduce the clearance and increase the elimination half-life of corticosteroids.	It may be necessary to lower steroid dosage if there is an increase in adverse effects.
	Dantrolene	Definite drug interaction with dantrolene not established; observe caution with concomitant use. Hepatotoxicity occurred more often in women >age 35 receiving dantrolene and estrogen.	Check liver function tests after first 4 wk of therapy in women >age 35.
	Hydantoins	Breakthrough bleeding, spotting, and pregnancy have resulted when these medications were used concurrently. A loss of seizure control has also been suggested and may be due to fluid retention.	Check blood levels of seizure medications after first 2 wk of therapy. Spotting in this patient may indicate less birth control effect. Use a backup birth control method or switch to an IUD.
Antiestrogens Clomiphene	Bromsulphalein (BSP) lab studies	BSP retention of >5% reported in 10–20% of patients; retention is usually minimal but elevated during prolonged clomiphene administration or with apparently unrelated liver disease. In some, preexisting BSP retention decreased even though clomiphene was continued. Other liver function tests usually normal.	Use other liver function tests when patient is taking clomiphene.
Danazol	Insulin	Insulin requirements may increase in patients with diabetes; abnormal glucose tolerance tests may be seen.	More frequent glucose monitoring; repeat glucose tolerance tests when off danazol.
	Warfarin	Prolongation of PT reported with concomitant use.	Measure PT more frequently.

Continued on next page

Table 20–8. Drug Interactions: Estrogens and Antiestrogens *(continued)*

Drug	Interacting Drug	Possible Effect	Implications
Tamoxifen	Anticoagulants	Hypoprothrombinemic effect may be increased by concurrent tamoxifen administration.	Monitor PT more frequently.
	Bromocriptine	Bromocriptine may elevate serum tamoxifen and *N*-desmethyl tamoxifen.	Patient may be toxic; decrease dose if adverse reactions occur.
	Laboratory studies	T_4 elevations occurred in a few postmenopausal patients but not accompanied by clinical hyperthyroidism.	Measure TSH instead of T_4.
Toremifene	Enzyme inducers	Increased toremifene metabolism and lowered serum steady-state concentration.	Make dose adjustments; check drug levels.
	Warfarin	Increased PT.	Measure PT more frequently.
Raloxifene	Ampicillin	Peak raloxifene levels and overall absorption reduced 28% and 14%, respectively, by concurrent ampicillin administration; consistent with decreased enterohepatic cycling associated with antibiotic reduction of enteric bacteria. However, systemic exposure and elimination rate of raloxifene not affected; therefore, raloxifene can be concurrently administered with ampicillin.	Consider prescribing amoxicillin (also has fewer diarrhea adverse effects).
	Cholestyramine	Raloxifene absorption and enterohepatic cycling reduced 60%; avoid coadministration.	Consider statins to decrease cholesterol.
	Warfarin	In single-dose studies, 10% decreases in PT have been observed.	Monitor PT closely.

action effects of smoking and the dosage of the more potent **ethinyl estradiol.** If they can become motivated to quit smoking for at least 1 year, then they can be considered nonsmokers. Ask during each office visit if they would like help in quitting tobacco use.

Progesterones and Progesterone Antagonists

The **progesterones** include Provera, Aygestin, Cyrin, Prometrium, Norplant, depo medroxypro-

---

ON THE HORIZON

Estrogens and Antiestrogens

Several large studies have reported that **estrogen** therapy may delay the onset and progression of Alzheimer's disease.

The question of whether **raloxifene** will act as an **estrogen agonist** or an **estrogen** in the brain is now undergoing clinical trials (Khovidhunkit & Shoback, 1999).

gesterone acetate (DMPA), and **Megace.** Progestin reverses the endometrial tissue buildup that estrogens stimulate. This knowledge has made HRT safer for menopausal patients. Progesterone levels may be lower in perimenopausal women as a result of anovulatory cycles. As a result, "late luteal defect" has been empirically treated with **progesterone.** There are four generations of **synthetic progestins.** Most are used in **oral contraceptives** and for **HRT.** Many formulations of **progesterone** have been developed because many women experience unacceptable mood changes.

Table 20–9. Dosage Schedule: Estrogens and Antiestrogens

Drug	Indication	Dosage
Estrogens		
Ethinyl estradiol	Moderate to severe vasomotor symptoms associated with menopause	0.02–0.05 mg/d
	Female hypogonadism	0.05 mg 1–3 times/d for first 2 wk of theoretical menstrual cycle; follow with progestin during last half of cycle
	Breast cancer (female)	1 mg 3 times/d chronically (palliation)
	Prostate cancer	0.15–2 mg/d chronically (palliation)
Conjugated estrogens	Moderate to severe vasomotor symptoms associated with menopause	1.25 mg/d cyclically
	Atrophic conditions caused by deficient endogenous estrogen production such as atrophic vaginitis and kraurosis vulvae	0.3–1.25 mg or more daily cyclically
	Female hypogonadism	2.5–7.5 mg daily, in divided doses for 20 d, followed by rest period of 10 d
	Female castration; primary ovarian failure	1.25 mg/d
	Osteoporosis	0.625 mg/d cyclically
	Mammary carcinoma (palliation)	10 mg 3 times/d for at least 3 mo
Estradiol transdermal system	Moderate to severe vasomotor symptoms associated with menopause; female hypogonadism; female castration; primary ovarian failure; atrophic conditions caused by deficient endogenous estrogen production such as atrophic vaginitis and kraurosis vulvae; prevention of osteoporosis/loss of bone mass	Menopause: start 0.05 mg applied twice weekly; adjust dose as necessary to control symptoms; attempt to taper or discontinue at 3- to 6-mo intervals; apply on clean, dry area on trunk of body but not breasts
Estradiol vaginal ring	Atrophic vaginitis	Insert ring as deeply as possible in upper third of vaginal vault; remains in place for 3 mo
Estradiol	Moderate to severe vasomotor symptoms associated with menopause; female hypogonadism; female castration; primary ovarian failure; atrophic conditions caused by deficient endogenous estrogen production, such as atrophic vaginitis and kraurosis vulvae; prevention of osteoporosis/loss of bone mass	Menopause symptoms: 1–2 mg/d Osteoporosis prevention: 0.5 mg/d cyclically
	Prostate cancer	1–2 mg 3 times/d
	Breast cancer (inoperable)	10 mg 3 times/d for at least 3 mo
Antiestrogens		
Clomiphene	Treatment of ovulary failure in patients desiring pregnancy whose partners are potent and fertile	First course: 50 mg/d for 5 d Second course: 100 mg/d for 5 d
	Unlabeled uses: Treatment of male infertility; however use is controversial and further study is needed	50–400 mg/d for 2–12 mo

Continued on next page

Table 20–9. Dosage Schedule: Estrogens and Antiestrogens (*continued*)

Drug	Indication	Dosage
Danazol	Endometriosis	800 mg/d in 2 divided doses; consider downward titration
	Fibrotic breast disease	100–400 mg/d in 2 divided doses
	Hereditary angioedema	Starting dose: 200 mg 2–3 times/d; after favorable response, decrease dose by 50% or less at 1- to 3-mo intervals
	Unlabeled uses: precocious puberty, gynecomastia, menorrhagia	None given
Tamoxifen	Breast cancer (adjuvant therapy; advanced disease therapy) Unlabeled use: mastalgia, preventative therapy in high-risk breast cancer	10–20 mg twice daily (A.M. and P.M.) or 20 mg daily; some studies have used dosages of 10 mg 2–3 times/d for 2 y and 10 mg twice daily for 5 y; the reduction in recurrence and mortality was greater in those studies that used the drug for 2 y than in those that used it for <2 y; there was no indication that doses >20 mg/d were more effective; optimal duration of adjuvant therapy unknown
Toremifene	Breast cancer; metastatic in postmenopausal women with estrogen-receptor (ER)-positive or ER-unknown tumors	60 mg once daily; generally continued until disease progression is observed
Raloxifene	Prevention of osteoporosis in postmenopausal women	60 mg daily, which may be administered any time of the day without regard to meals

Table 20–11 presents information on **progesterone antagonists.**

Pharmacodynamics

Progesterone serves as a precursor to estrogens, androgens, and adrenal steroids. It is synthesized in the ovary, testes, and adrenals from circulating cholesterol. The placenta synthesizes and releases large amounts during pregnancy. Progesterone stimulates lipoprotein lipase activity that favors fat deposition. In the liver, progesterone promotes glycogen storage. Its competition with aldosterone in the kidney decreases sodium reabsorption. The respiratory center is also affected, with a resulting increase in respiratory effect to decrease carbon dioxide. Last, progesterone is responsible for secretory changes in the breast and endometrium during pregnancy and menstruation.

Pharmacokinetics

Absorption and Distribution

Oral progestins are rapidly absorbed from the GI tract and quickly undergo hepatic degradation. IM long-acting forms can be maintained for 3 to 6 months. Gel formulation has sustained-release properties, so absorption can be lengthened to 50 hours.

Progesterone is rapidly absorbed following any route of administration.

Metabolism and Excretion

Oral progesterone is rapidly metabolized in the first pass through the liver. In the liver, progesterone is metabolized to pregnanediol and with the glucuronide metabolites conjugated with glucuronic acid. It is excreted in the urine. IM **progesterone** is extensively bound to serum proteins, and its metabolites are excreted 60 percent by the kidney and 10 percent through the bile and feces. The gel formulation is bound primarily to serum albumin and corticosteroid-binding globulin. It is also eliminated through the renal route.

Onset, Peak, and Duration

After oral administration, peak concentrations occur after 1 to 2 hours. Duration of action is 6 to 9 hours. IM preparations reach peak levels by 24 hours and have a half-life of approximately 10 weeks. The liver quickly metabolizes the gel formulation, but the long absorption half-life provides the steady serum concentrations. The absorption half-life of the vaginal gel has been extended to 25 to 50 hours. Table 20–12 presents the pharmacokinetics of **progesterones.**

Table 20–10. Available Dosage Forms: Estrogens and Antiestrogens

Drug	Dosage Form	How Supplied
Estrogens		
Conjugated estrogens	Tablets	0.3 mg, 0.625 mg, 0.9 mg, 1.25 mg, 2.5 mg
	Parenteral (IV/IM)	25 mg in vials with 5 mL sterile diluent
	Vaginal cream	0.625 mg conjugated estrogens in 42.5-g tube with applicator
Estradiol	Tablets	0.5 mg, 1 mg, 2 mg
	Parenteral (IM)	10 mg/mL: 5-mL and 10-mL vials
	(valerate in oil)	20 mg/mL: 5-mL and 10-mL vials and 1-mL unimatic single-dose syringe
		40 mg/mL: 5-mL and 10-mL vials
	Parenteral (IM) (cypionate in oil)	5 mg/mL in 5-mL and 10-mL vials
	Vaginal cream	0.1 mg estradiol/g in 42.5-g tube with applicator
	Vaginal ring	2 mg estradiol in single packs
Ethinyl estradiol	Tablets	0.02 mg, 0.05 mg, 0.5 mg
Estradiol transdermal system	Transdermal system	3.28 mg, 4 mg, 4.33 mg, 6.57 mg, 8 mg, 8.66 mg (calendar packs of 8 and 24 systems)
		3.9 mg, 7.8 mg (packages of 4)
Estropipate	Tablets	0.625 mg, 1.25 mg, 2.5 mg
	Vaginal cream	1.5 mg estropipate/g in 42.5-g tube with applicator
Antiestrogens		
Clomiphene	Tablets	50 mg
Danazol	Capsules	50 mg, 100 mg, 200 mg
Tamoxifen	Tablets (as citrate)	10 mg, 20 mg
Toremifene	Tablets	60 mg
Raloxifene	Tablets	60 mg

Pharmacotherapeutics

Precautions and Contraindications

Progestins have been used empirically to sustain habitual first-trimester abortions, but subsequent studies have shown a fourfold increase in limb defects in babies born to mothers exposed to female hormones. Most first-term abortions are due to a defective ovum. Patients with thromboembolic disease or a history of it should not use **progestins.** Breast cancer may be worsened under hormone influence. Patients with impaired liver function would have trouble metabolizing exogenous hormones. Lactation has been enhanced by **medroxyprogesterone,** although the effects on the infant have not been determined.

Table 20–11. Progesterone Antagonists

Mifepristone (RU 486)
This compound has a long half-life and may prolong the follicular phase of the subsequent cycle. It binds strongly to the progesterone and inhibits the action of progesterone. In 85% of women, it will act as an abortifacient when used in conjunction with misoprostol during the first 7 weeks of pregnancy.

Its initial use would be in a specialty practice and not primary care. Mifepristone's effect in treating endometriosis, Cushing's syndrome, and breast cancer makes it a potentially valuable drug to treat several serious diseases if its controversial introduction into this country can be overcome. This drug is currently in drug studies in Planned Parenthood Clinics across the country, and NPs may be involved with the drug, but only under research protocols.

Table 20–12. Pharmacokinetics: Progesterones and Progesterone-Antagonists

Drug	Peak	Effect of Food on Absorption	Active Metabolite	Half-Life (Normal Renal Function)	Half-Life (Impaired Renal Function)	Elimination
Progesterones						
Progesterone	1–2 h	No effect	5B-pregnan-3A,20A-diol glucoronide	8–9 h	NA	50–60% in urine, 10% in bile and feces; small amount un-changed in bile
Progesterone gel		No effect	5B-pregnan-3A,20A-diol glucoronide	34.8 h	NA	50–60% in urine, 10% in bile and feces; small amount un-changed in bile
Medroxyprogesterone acetate		No effect	5B-pregnan-3A,20A-diol glucoronide	IM: 10 wk	NA	50–60% in urine, 10% in bile and feces; small amount un-changed in bile
Megestrol acetate	2.2 h	No effect	5B-pregnan-3A,20A-diol glucoronide	34.2 h (mean)	NA	50–60% in urine, 10% in bile and feces; small amount un-changed in bile
Progesterone Antagonists						
Mifepristone (RU 486)	1–3 h	No effect	3 active metabolities	20–54 h	NA	NA

NA = not available.

Adverse Drug Reactions

Mental depression has been associated with both short-acting and long-acting **progestins**. Acne and chloasma have occurred with several of the more **androgenic progestin** products. Atypical bleeding patterns have occurred during **progestin** administration. Effects have ranged from spotting to amenorrhea. Patients report increased breast tenderness and galactorrhea.

Drug Interactions

The two drugs known to have specific interactions are **aminoglutethimide** and **rifampin.** The primary result is to decrease effectiveness, and the result can be unplanned pregnancy. In addition to drug-drug interactions, **progesterone** can cause erroneous laboratory results in testing hepatic function, coagulation, thyroid, metyrapone, and other endocrine functions. Table 20–13 presents drug interactions.

Clinical Use and Dosing

The major uses of **progestational hormones** are for perimenopausal and postmenopausal hormonal therapy and as a contraceptive alone and in combination with **estrogen**. The FDA approved the use of **medroxyprogesterone acetate (DMPA)** for contraception in 1993. Its association with reduced bone density after chronic administration is still under study and debate. Other unlabeled uses are in the treatment of dysmenorrhea, endometriosis, hirsutism, and, when **estrogen** is contraindicated, bleeding disorders. **Levonorgestrel** contraceptive implants are a set of six capsules made of Silastic material and filled with 36 mg **levonorgestrel** that are inserted in the medial aspect of the patient's upper arm. The gel form of **progesterone** was released to assist in fertility programs for women with **progesterone** deficits. Refer to Chapter 29 for a more detailed discussion of **progesterone** as contraception and to Chapter 36 for its use in conjunction with **estrogen** for postmenopausal hormone therapy. Table 20–14 presents the dosage schedule of **progesterones** and **progesterone** antagonists.

Rational Drug Selection

SHORT ACTING VERSUS LONG ACTING. Oral products are dosed in a convenient dial pack. These products are short acting, and the patient chooses when to stop and become fertile again. **Progesterone** is available for contraception in two parenteral forms, and both have greater than 99 percent theoretical efficacy. Patient preference is the primary concern. Remembering to take the medication daily is difficult for many women, who frequently choose a long-acting method like **DMPA** or **Norplant**. Some women use **norgesterel** implants because they want to delay fertility longer, and a product such as **Norplant** provides 5 years of contraceptive coverage. Table 20–15 presents the available dosage forms.

Monitoring

Pretreatment physical examinations to assess health and possible contraindications to **progestins** are mandatory. Examination should be age-specific. Patients with seizure disorders need monitoring of their symptoms because increased fluid retention may lower the seizure threshold. Women with migraines are vulnerable to any changes in physiological states, and fluid retention may give them cyclic migraines. Depression should be assessed early in therapy for those women with a history of previous affective disorders. Patients with diabetes may see changes in blood glucose levels, indicating more frequent measurement.

Patient Education

ADMINISTRATION. Most hormone regimens require daily dosing for efficacy, especially for the **progestin**-only oral contraceptive. The most common adverse effect is breakthrough bleeding, especially if doses are missed.

Table 20–13. Drug Interactions: Progesterones and Progesterone Antagonists

Drug	Interacting Drug	Possible Effect	Implications
Progesterones Progesterone	Lab studies	Results of hepatic function, coagulation tests (increase in prothrombin; factors VII, VIII, IX, and X), thyroid, metyrapone test, and endocrine functions may be affected by progestins	Anticipate that laboratory levels of liver function and hormonal assays may not be accurate while the patient is taking these drugs.
Medroxyprogesterone acetate (DMPA)	Aminoglutethimide	Aminoglutethimide may increase the hepatic metabolism of DMPA	Chemotherapy drug used for metastatic cancer. If spotting occurs, give DMPA earlier than 12 wk.
Progesterone Antagonists Mifepristone (RU 486)	No information	No information	No information; currently under study in U.S.

Table 20–14. Dosage Schedule: Progesterones and Progesterone Antagonists

Drug	Indication	Dosage
Progesterones		
Progesterone	Amenorrhea (primary and secondary)	5–10 mg daily for 6–8 consecutive d
	Abnormal uterine bleeding caused by hormonal imbalance in the absence of organic pathology	5–10 mg daily for 6 doses
	Infertility (gel only)	90 mg vaginally once daily (twice daily if complete ovarian failure)
	Unlabeled uses: premature labor, premenstrual syndrome (PMS) (suppositories)	
Medroxyprogesterone acetate	Secondary amenorrhea	5–10 mg daily for 5–10 d
	Abnormal uterine bleeding caused by hormonal imbalance in the absence of organic pathology	5–10 mg daily for 5–10 d, beginning on the 16th or 21st day of menstrual cycle
	Unlabeled use: treatment of menopausal symtoms	10 mg/d
Megestrol acetate	Appetite enhancement in patients with AIDS (suspension only); treatment of anorexia, cachexia, or an unexplained significant weight loss in patients with AIDS; tumors (tablets only); palliative treatment of advanced carcinoma of the breast or endometrium	Initial dose is 800 mg/d (20 mL/d); shake the suspension well before using; in clinical trials evaluating different dose schedules, daily doses of 400 and 800 mg/d were clinically effective
Progesterone Antagonists		
Mifepristone (RU 486)	Abortifacient in early pregnancy (<58 days of amenorrhea)	Dosages from 25 mg twice daily for 4 d to 50 mg 3 times daily for 4 d (success rates of 61–85%); 50–100 mg/d for 7 d (successful in 60–73% of cases); single 600-mg dose (success rate 72–100%); menses typically begins within 5 d of initiation of therapy and continues for 1–2 wk
	Cushing's syndrome	20 mg/kg/d
	Tamoxifen resistant breast cancer with progesterone receptors	200 mg/d

Table 20–15. Available Dosage Forms: Progesterones and Progesterone Antagonists

Drug	Dosage Form	How Supplied
Progesterones		
Progesterone	Tablets	
	Injection (IM)	Powder, micronized in 1, 10, 25, 100, and 1000 g
	Injection (IM) (in oil)	50 mg/mL in 10-mL vials
	Vaginal gel	8% (90 mg) in single-use disposable applicator delivering 1.125 g
Medroxyprogesterone acetate	Tablets	2.5 mg, 5 mg, 10 mg
Megestrol acetate	Injection (IM)	100 mg/mL in 5-mL vials; 400 mg/mL in 2.5- and 10-mL vials and 1-mg Uject
	Tablets	20 mg, 40 mg
	Oral suspension	40 mg/mL (lemon-lime flavor)
Progesterone Antagonists		
Mifepristone (RU 486)	Not available in U.S.	

ADVERSE REACTIONS. **Progestins** should not be used in the first 12 weeks of gestation because of masculinization of the female fetus. Depression and mood swings are common and represent a significant factor in post-menopausal **HRT** cessation. Irregular menstrual patterns and unpredictable spotting contribute to a proportion of women stopping **progestin-only oral contraceptives.** Breast tenderness and galactorrhea are the third most common reason women switch from a **progesterone** contraceptive and another reason that postmenopausal women stop **HRT** altogether.

LIFESTYLE MANAGEMENT. Wearing sunscreen may prevent skin changes such as blotchy pigmentation while using **progestins.** The increase in body weight sometimes seen with **DMPA** use may require some women to increase their frequency or intensity of physical activity. Smoking cessation is encouraged in all patients, but especially in young women using hormonal contraception. The association of both **estrogen** and **progesterone** with morbidity and mortality in patients over age 35 who smoke should be a powerful motivator to quit smoking.

Other Drugs Affecting the Reproductive System

Other drugs affecting the reproductive system include those that are commonly used in fertility clinics (**GnRH, FSH, LH,** and **human chorionic gonadotropin (hCG)**), those used as **lactation inhibitors (bromocriptine),** and those used in erectile dysfunction.

Drugs Commonly Used in Fertility Clinics

GnRH

GnRH is produced in the arcuate nucleus of the hypothalamus and controls the release of FSH and LH for both males and females. See Figure 20–1 for primary and feedback pathways. **GnRH** is used as a stimulant in pulsatile doses if the patient has a functional pituitary gland and an ovary to produce the LH surge initiating ovulation. The pulsate effect is like an artificial hypothalamus (Pearlstein, 1995). **Leuprolide** may be used in pulsate form to stimulate ovulation and continuously to suppress genital cancer. The natural drug **(GnRH)** may be administered intravenously (IV) or subcutaneously (SC), and its analogues may be used SC, IM, or intranasally. The last two routes of administration have 3-hour half-lives. Degradation occurs in the hypothalamus and pituitary.

When used to treat primary hypothalamic amenorrhea, **GnRH** is given 5 µg every 90 minutes (range 1 to 20 µg) via the Lutrepulse pump.

Follicle-Stimulating Hormone

FSH has an analogue, **human menopausal gonadotropin (hMG) (follitropin [Fertinex], menotropins [Pergonal, Humegon]).** It is extracted from the urine of postmenopausal women and standardized as to the FSH and LH content. The drug is used in fertility clinics for both men and women. A hyperstimulation syndrome that can occur with this drug may cause ovarian enlargement, ascites, hydrothorax, hypovolemia, hemoperitoneum, fever, or arterial thromboembolism. It has also been used to test young males for undescended testicle. The testicle will descend temporarily during administration of this drug. The alternative is surgery. When boys have a constitutional delay in puberty, their serum testosterone and estradiol levels will rise under **hCG** stimulation. This drug is produced by the placenta and excreted in urine. It is given IM, peaks in 15 to 27 hours, and has a half-life of 8 hours, compared with 30 minutes for LH. Its site of metabolism is unknown. This drug represents another treatment used in specialty practices.

When used for polycystic ovary syndrome, the dosage is 75 IU per day, given SC, with a dosage adjustment considered after 5 to 7 days.

For follicle stimulation, the dosage is 150 IU per day SC in the early follicular phase. Its use should not exceed 10 days.

ON THE HORIZON

Progesterone

Progesterone alone could have a significant effect on the prevention and management of osteoporosis. Other studies suggest a role for **progesterone** in the management of affective disorders, allergic symptoms, and benign breast disease (Murray, 1998).

Luteinizing Hormone and Human Chorionic Gonadotropin

LH has the analogue **hCG (A.P.L.,** Chorex-5, **Profasi).** Like FSH, LH is produced in the anterior pituitary and used in conjunction with FSH to stimulate ovulation. It also stimulates the corpus luteum to produce progesterone and androgens. No LH preparation is available for use clinically. Instead, a similar preparation, **hCG,** is substituted successfully.

When used to induce ovulation and pregnancy, the dosage of **hCG** is 5,000 to 10,000 USP units 1 day following the last dose of **menotropins.**

For hypogonadotropic hypogonadism in males, the dosage of **hCG** is (1) 500 to 1000 USP units three times weekly for 3 weeks; (2) 1000 to 2000 USP units three times weekly; or (3) 4000 USP units three times weekly for 6 to 9 months, then 2000 USP units three times weekly for an 3 additional months.

For prepubertal cryptorchidism that is not due to anatomic obstruction, the dosage of **hCG** is (1) 4000 USP units three times weekly for 3 weeks, (2) 5000 USP units every second day for 4 injections, (3) 15 injections of 500 to 1000 USP units given over 6 weeks, or (4) 500 USP units three times weekly for 4 to 6 weeks. If this course is not successful, start another course 1 month later, with 1000 USP units per injection.

Lactation Inhibitors

Bromocriptine

Although not a true hormone, **bromocriptine (Parlodel)** has an inhibitory effect on the pituitary gland that produces prolactin. It is widely used for shrinking pituitary prolactin-secreting tumors and reducing the prolactin levels of idiopathic prolactinemia. **Bromocriptine** is an ergot derivative with dopamine agonist properties. Its absorption from the GI tract can be increased by the concomitant use of caffeine. It can be administered by the rectum, by the buccal mucosa, and intranasally. **Bromocriptine** is metabolized in the body through both hydroxylation and demethylation. A small amount of the metabolized drug is excreted in the urine, with most (84%) in the feces. The absorbed drug is excreted via the bile.

When used for hyperprolactinemic indications, the initial dosage is 0.5 to 2.5 mg daily with meals; 2.5 mg may be added as tolerated every 3 to 7 days or until optimal therapeutic response is achieved. Therapeutic dosage is usually 5 to 7.5 mg, with a range of 2.5 to 15 mg per day.

For acromegaly, the initial dose is 1.25 to 2.5 mg for 3 days on retiring. Add an additional 1.25 to 2.5 mg as tolerated every 3 to 7 days. Therapeutic dosage is usually 5 to 7.5 mg, with a range of 20 to 30 mg per day.

Drugs that interact with **bromocriptine** include erythromycin, phenothiazines, sympathomimetics, isometheptene, and phenylpropanolamine.

Drugs Used in Erectile Dysfunction

Sildenafil Citrate

Sildenafil citrate (Viagra) was originally studied as a selective **vasodilator** for use in angina. Although not effective in the coronary arteries, it was effective as a selective inhibitor of cyclic guanosine monophosphate (cGMP), specific phosphodiesterase type 5 (PDE5). This PDE5 has a tenfold selectivity for the enzyme that produces smooth muscle relaxation in the corpus cavernosum of the penis. It has been approved for use in impotence related to erectile dysfunction in men. There is no drug effect without sexual stimulation. It is rapidly absorbed after oral administration and eliminated by hepatic metabolism (mainly cytochrome P-450 3A4). It is converted to an active metabolite that also has a half-life of 4 hours. Ingestion of food reduces its rate of absorption. The peak onset is 30 to 120 minutes, with a duration of 1 to 2 hours. About 80 percent is eliminated in the feces, with most of the remaining eliminated in the urine.

For erectile dysfunction, the dosage is 50 mg (25 to 100 mg, based on effectiveness) taken as needed approximately 1 hour before sexual activity. The maximum recommended frequency is once a day.

The potential drug interactions are many, including **antifungals, macrolide antibiotics** (such as **erythromycin**), **cimetidine, rifampin, nonspecific beta blockers,** and **diuretics.** An absolute contraindication is the use of any form of **nitrates** because of potentiation of a blood pressure–lowering effect, possibly up to 00 mm Hg.

At this point, there are no studies to assess the drug effects on women and libido. Eighty-eight percent of men questioned had improvement in erectile dysfunction. More long-term studies are necessary to demonstrate safety with coadministration of the chronic disease medications. As a result, this drug is not yet recommended for routine use in primary care, but it may be in the near future.

REFERENCES

Baker, V., & Jaffe, R. (1995). Clinical uses of anti-estrogen. *Obstetrical and Gynecological Survey, 51*(1), 45–49.

Cummings, S., Eckert, K., Grady, D., Powles, T., Cauley, L., Norton, L., Nickelsen, N., Bjarnason, N., Morrow, M., Lippman, D., Glusman, J., Costa, A., & Jordan, V. (1999). The effect of raloxifene on risk of breast cancer in postmenopausal women. *Journal of the American Medical Association, 281*(23), 2189–2197.

Derman, S., & Adashi, E. (1994). Adverse effects of fertility drugs. *Drug Safety, 11*(6), 408–421.

Drug Facts and Comparisons (52nd ed.). (1998). Montvale, NJ: Medical Economics.

Gambone, J., & DeCherney, A. (1997). Surgical treatment of minimal endometriosis. *New England Journal of Medicine, 337*(4), 269–270.

Hansen, K. (1997). Hirsutism: Options for treating the whole patient. *Female Patient, 22,* 11–12, 15–17.

Hatcher, R., Stewart, F., Trussell, J., Kowal, D., Guest, F., Stewart, G., & Cates, W. (1998). *Contraceptive technology* (16th ed.). New York: Irvington.

Kastrup, E. (Founding Ed.). (1998). *Drug facts and comparisons.* St. Louis: Facts and Comparisons.

Kastrup, E. (Founding Ed.). (2000). *Drug facts and comparisons.* St. Louis: Facts and Comparisons.

Katzung, B. (1998). Basic and clinical pharmacology (7th ed.). Norwalk, CT: Appleton & Lange.

Kauffman, R., & Bryant, H. (1995). Selective estrogen receptor modulators. *Drug News and Perspectives, 8*(9), 531–539.

Khovidhunkit, W., & Shoback, D. (1999). Clinical effects of raloxifene hydrochloride in women. *Annals of Internal Medicine, 130*(5), 431–439.

Mendelsohn, M., & Karas, R. (1999). The protective effects of estrogen on the cardiovascular system. *New England Journal of Medicine, 340*(23), 1801–1810.

Murray, J. (1998). Natural progesterone: What role in women's health care? *Women's Health in Primary Care,* 1(8), 671–680.

Paganini-Hill, A. (1998). Alzheimer's disease in women: Can estrogen play a preventive role? *The Female Patient,* 23(2), 12–18.

Pearlstein, T. (1995). Hormones and depression: What are the facts about premenstrual syndrome, menopause, and hormone replacement therapy? *American Journal of Obstetrical Gynecology, 173*(2), 646–653.

Raloxifene for postmenopausal osteoporosis. (1998). *Medical Letter, 40*(1002), 29–30.

Shaywitz, S., Shaywitz, B., Pugh, K., Skudlarski, P., Mencl, W., Constable, R., Naftolin, F., Palter, S., Marchione, K., Katz, L., Shankweiler, D., Fletcher, J., Lacadie, C., Keltz, M., & Gore, J. (1999). Effect of estrogen on brain activation patterns in postmenopausal women during working memory tasks. *JAMA, 281*(13), 1197–1202.

Waites, G. (1993). Male fertility regulation: The challenge for the year 2000. *British Medical Bulletin, 49*(1), 210–221.

Walsh, B., Kuller, L., Wild, R., Paul, S., Farmer, M., Lawrence, J., Shah, A., & Anderson, P. (1998). Effects of raloxifene on serum lipids and coagulation factors in healthy postmenopausal women. *JAMA, 279*(18), 1445–1451.

CHAPTER 21

. . . .

Drugs Affecting the Integumentary System

CHAPTER OUTLINE

Monitoring
Patient education
   ADMINISTRATION
   ADVERSE REACTIONS
**MISCELLANEOUS TOPICAL
MEDICATIONS**

Bath dermatologicals
Wet dressings and soaks
Astringents
Sunscreens
Skin protectant

*T*his chapter discusses a wide variety of medications used to treat disorders of the skin or integumentary system, including **topical anti-infective medications** used to treat bacterial, fungal, and viral infections of the skin; **topical corticosteroids** used for a variety of inflammatory diseases; and **topical antipsoriatic** and **acne medications.** Systemic medications used for skin disorders are discussed here only if not covered in another chapter. **Systemic antibiotics** and **antifungal medications** used to treat more serious skin infections, with the exception of **griseofulvin** and **terbinafine**, are discussed in Chapter 22. Systemic medications used for acne are discussed in this chapter, with the exception of systemic antibiotics, which are also covered in Chapter 22.

Anti-infectives

Topical Antibacterials

Bacterial infections of the skin are common with patients of all ages. **Antibacterial medications** commonly used in primary care include topical agents and oral **antibiotics.** The most common pathogens seen in bacterial skin infections are *Staphylococcus aureus* and *Streptococcus pyogenes*. Skin infections with gram-negative bacilli are rare, but they may occur in patients who are immunocompromised or patients with diabetes. These patients usually require intravenous (IV) **antibiotic** therapy for their infections. Impetigo is usually treated topically unless it is a moderate to severe case. Commonly used drugs for impetigo are **mupirocin (Bactroban)** and other topical agents, including **neomycin, bacitracin,** and **polymyxin B.** A combination product that is available over the counter (OTC) combines **neomycin, bacitracin,** and **polymyxin B (Neosporin).** Moderate to severe impetigo, a boil or abscess, perianal streptococcal infections, and cellulitis all require prompt treatment with appropriate **systemic antibiotics.**

Pharmacodynamics

Topical or **systemic antibacterial agents** may be either bacteriostatic or bactericidal. **Mupirocin** is bacteriostatic at low concentrations and bactericidal at high concentrations. **Mupirocin** is structurally unrelated to other **topical antibiotic agents.** It acts by binding to bacterial isoleucyl-tRNA synthetase. It thus inhibits bacterial protein synthesis. **Bacitracin** is bacteriostatic but may also be bactericidal, depending on the antibiotic concentration and the susceptibility of the organism. **Bacitracin** inhibits the cell wall synthesis of the organism. **Erythromycin** binds to the 50 S ribosomal subunit, inhibiting bacterial protein synthesis. It is effective against a wide range of microorganisms. Information regarding the pharmacodynamics of the topical agents **neomycin** and **polymyxin B** is unavailable.

Pharmacokinetics

ABSORPTION AND DISTRIBUTION. The topical agents commonly used to treat bacterial skin infections are minimally absorbed through normal skin. **Mupirocin** has minimal absorption of 0.3% when administered topically. If it is applied to large areas of abraded skin, it may allow for deeper penetration into the epidermal layers. **Mupirocin** may be applied intranasally, and there is no evidence of systemic absorption if used this way. Distribution of **mupirocin** is unknown.

   Bacitracin, when used topically, is minimally absorbed. However, **bacitracin** is readily absorbed through large areas of denuded or burned skin. Topical preparations of **bacitracin** that include **neomycin** and **polymyxin B** are minimally absorbed through normal skin. Distribution of **bacitracin, neomycin,** and **polymyxin B** is unknown. Absorption and distribution of the **oral antibiotics** used to treat skin infections are discussed in Chapter 22.

METABOLISM AND EXCRETION. Metabolism and excretion of the **topical antibacterial agents mupirocin, bacitracin, neomycin,** and **polymyxin B** are unknown. Information regarding the metabolism and excretion of topical **erythromycin** is also unavailable.

Pharmacotherapeutics

PRECAUTIONS AND CONTRAINDICATIONS. True contraindications include hypersensitivity reactions to any components of any of the products. **Mupirocin** should not be used on burns, especially extensive burns, open wounds, or other damaged skin. Increased absorption of polyethylene glycol, the vehicle for **mupirocin** ointment, may occur. Increased absorption of polyethylene glycol should be avoided, especially if there is evidence of moderate to severe renal impairment. **Mupirocin** is not recommended for use over long periods because of possible overgrowth of resistant organisms, including fungi. This overgrowth can lead to superinfection. **Mupirocin** should not be used intranasally in neonates or children younger than 12 years.

Bacitracin should not be used over large areas of the body. **Bacitracin** or **bacitracin** combined with **neomycin** or **polymyxin B** should not be used if there is sensitivity to any of the components. They should not be used for serious burns, deep wounds, or animal bites. **Bacitracin** or the combination product **Neosporin** should not be used for long periods (more than 1 week) because of the possibility of overgrowth of organisms.

ADVERSE DRUG REACTIONS. Adverse drug reactions to **topical antibiotics** are uncommon and generally mild. The most frequently reported adverse reaction to topical **mupirocin** is skin irritation and pruritus. Patients using intranasal **mupirocin** have reported the following: headache (9%), rhinitis (6%), upper respiratory congestion (5%), throat irritation (4%), nasal irritation or stinging (2%), and cough (2%). Adverse reactions to **bacitracin** are rare. Overgrowth of nonsusceptible organisms may occur. Other adverse reactions have not been reported. Adverse reactions to **erythromycin** are also rare, with irritation the most commonly reported reaction. There is a possibility of nephrotoxicity and ototoxicity if **neomycin** is used over large portions of the body (more than 20% of body surface area) or over large burn areas.

DRUG INTERACTIONS. There are no known drug interactions with **mupirocin** (Table 21–1). Intranasal **mupirocin** should not be used concurrently with any other nasal product. Topical **bacitracin, neomycin, polymyxin B, and erythromycin** have no known drug interactions.

CLINICAL USE AND DOSING

Impetigo. Impetigo is a superficial skin infection caused by *S. aureus, S. pyogenes,* or both. Treatment with an **antibiotic** that is effective against both organisms, either topical or oral, ensures successful treatment. Bullous impetigo is usually pure *S. aureus* and should be treated with an **antibiotic** that has good staph coverage.

If only one or two lesions are present, the patient may be treated with topical OTC **antibiotic** ointments such as **bacitracin** or a combination product that combines **bacitracin, polymyxin B,** and **neomycin** (**Polysporin, Neosporin, Triple Antibiotic Ointment**). Either **bacitracin** alone or the **combination antibiotic product** is applied to affected area two to five times per day until the lesions clear. If the patient has up to five singular lesions, topical **mupirocin** ointment may be applied tid until the lesions

are healed (5 to 14 days). **Mupirocin** is considered the most effective **topical antibiotic. Mupirocin** is available only by prescription.

Oral antibiotics are indicated if the patient has more than five lesions or if the lesions continue to worsen after 2 or 3 days of **topical antibiotic** treatment. **Antibiotics** that are effective against *S. aureus* or *S. pyogenes* include **cephalexin (Keflex), amoxicillin/clavulinic acid (Augmentin),** and **dicloxacillin.** A **macrolide antibiotic** such as **erythromycin** or **azithromycin (Zithromax)** can be used if the patient is penicillin-allergic. There is some resistance of *S. aureus* to **erythromycin.** The patient treated with **systemic antibiotics** should be treated for 10 days (5 days with **azithromycin**).

Furuncle. Furuncle, commonly known as a boil or abscess, is usually caused by *S. aureus.* Treatment of a small abscess may include warm packs and **systemic antibiotics** that are effective against *S. aureus.* A larger abscess usually requires incision and drainage, as well as **systemic antibiotics** that provide coverage for *S. aureus.* Gram's stain and culture of the drainage from the abscess can determine if the organism will be sensitive to the **antibiotic** of choice. Prior to Gram's stain results, an appropriate first-line **antibiotic** would be **cephalexin, amoxicillin-clavulinic acid,** or **dicloxacillin.** Length of treatment should be 10 days, unless longer treatment is indicated by clinical progress.

Cellulitis. Cellulitis is a painful bacterial infection involving the soft tissue. The patient may become septic if left untreated. The causative organisms are most commonly *Streptococcus pneumoniae, S. aureus,* or, in children, *Haemophilus influenzae.* Treatment with **systemic antibiotics** that are effective against these organisms is essential. If the clinical picture warrants it, an initial dose of an **intramuscular** (IM)-administered **antibiotic** such as **ceftriaxone** may be given, followed by **oral antibiotic** treatment. **Oral antibiotic** therapy with a broad-spectrum **antibiotic** such as **amoxicillin-clavulanate** or a broad-spectrum **cephalosporin** is indicated. Tissue aspirate cultures can guide the practitioner in determining if the organism is sensitive to the **antibiotic** of choice.

Nasal MRSA Carrier. Eradication of nasal methicillin-resistant *S. aureus* (MRSA) colonization in adult patients and health care workers may be achieved with intranasal **mupirocin.** Intranasal **mupirocin** is supplied in 1-g single-use tubes and should be used twice a day. The patient applies approximately half the ointment from a single-use tube of nasal ointment into one nostril and the other half into the other nostril in the morning and evening for 5 days. Children may require smaller amounts of ointment.

Table 21-1. Drug Interactions: Selected Anti-infectives Used for Skin Disorders

Drug	Interacting Drug	Possible Effect	Implications
Antibacterial Bacitracin	None reported		
Mupirocin	None reported with topical use Other nasal products	Decreased effectiveness of intranasal mupirocin	Avoid use of other nasal products concurrently with intranasal muprirocin.
Neomycin	None reported		
Polymyxin B	None reported		
Antifungal Butenafine	None reported		
Ciclopirox olamine	None reported		
Clotrimazole	Nystatin and amphotericin B	The azole antifungals could interfere with the action of either amphotericin B or nystatin by depleting polyene binding sites; this appears to be the most significant when the azole antifungal is given prior to ampho-tericin B	Do not use concurrently.
	Spermicides (nonoxynol-9 and octoxynol)	Clotrimazole intravaginal preparations should not be administered concur-rently with nonoxynol-9 and octoxynol; clotrima-zole may inactivate the spermicides, leading to contraceptive failure	Do not use concurrently.
Econazole	Topical corticosteroids	Corticosteroids may inhibit the antifungal activity of econazole against *Candida albicans* in a concentration-dependent manner	Avoid the use of topical steroids with econazole. Choose another topical antifungal.
Gentian violet	None reported		
Ketoconazole	None reported		
Miconazole	None reported		
Naftifine	None reported		
Nystatin	Topical clotrimazole (theoreti-cally, all azoles)	Topical azoles compete for binding sites with nystatin	Do not use concurrently.
Oxiconazole	None reported		
Sulconazole	None reported		
Terbinafine	None reported		
Tolnaftate	None reported		
Antivirals Acyclovir	None reported		
Penciclovir	None reported		

RATIONAL DRUG SELECTION

Antibacterial Activity. The choice of a **topical antibiotic** is based on susceptibility. **Mupirocin** is considered a broad-spectrum **topical antibiotic. Bacitracin** and the combination of **bacitracin, neomycin,** and **polymyxin B** are OTC products that combine different antimicrobial spectrums to provide a single broad-spectrum product. **Mupirocin** is considered a broader spectrum **antibiotic** than the **triple-antibiotic** formula. If resistance to the topical product is suspected or if the infection is not responding to **topical antibiotics,** then **systemic antibiotics** are warranted.

Cost. The OTC **topical antibiotic** products are relatively inexpensive. **Bacitracin** is usually sold as a generic product and is quite inexpensive. The combination product of **neomycin, polymyxin B,** and **bacitracin** is available in name brands (**Neosporin, Polysporin**), which are slightly more expensive than the generic product (**triple-antibiotic ointment**). The brand name products are usually less than $10 per 30-g tube, and the generic product approximately $5 for a 30-g tube. **Mupirocin** is somewhat more expensive: A 30-g tube is $20 to $30.

MONITORING. No specific monitoring is required beyond that related to the disease process for which the patient is being treated.

PATIENT EDUCATION

Administration. Patients should be taught how to appropriately apply the **topical antibiotic** ointment. They should be instructed to wash their hands prior to applying the ointment or to use a gloved hand. The **antibiotic** ointment should be applied sparingly only to the affected infection area. Overapplication of the **antibiotic** ointment can increase adverse effects. Patients should not use the **antibiotic** ointment for longer than 1 week unless instructed by their provider. To avoid contamination of the **antibiotic** ointment, care must be taken not to touch the tip of the **antibiotic** ointment container to the infected area or to any other surface.

Adverse Reactions. The patient should be instructed that adverse reactions to **topical antibiotics** are rare but that skin irritation is possible with any topical ointment. Any adverse reactions should be reported to the provider as soon as possible, and the **antibiotic** ointment should then not be used until the patient is instructed otherwise. The patient should not use the **antibiotic** ointment over large surface areas (more than 20% of the body surface) without prior instruction from the provider.

Lifestyle Management. Patients need to be instructed on general infection control measures, especially if the patient has impetigo, a highly contagious disease. Patients should wash their hands after any contact with the infected area. Within the family, the patient infected with impetigo should use care not to share towels or other utensils with other family members to prevent the spread of infection to other family members. The patient should be instructed to wash the impetigo lesions twice a day with antibacterial soap.

Antifungals

Fungal infections of the skin are common in all age groups. Infants and immunocompromised patients may have thrush and *Candida* infections in the diaper area. Tinea corporis, also known as *ringworm,* can be found in patients of all ages. Tinea capitis is most common in children. Tinea pedis, also known as *athlete's foot,* can be found at any age but generally in postpubertal patients. Fungal overgrowth occurs in immunocompromised patients or patients on **antibiotics.**

Antifungal medications are used to treat superficial fungal infections caused by dermatophytic fungi and yeast. The **topical azoles,** which include **clotrimazole (Lotrimin), ketoconazole (Nizoral), miconazole (Monistat), econazole (Spectazole),** and **sulconazole (Exelderm),** are active against common dermatophytes and yeasts. **Ciclopirox olamine (Loprox)** is a broad-spectrum **antifungal. Tolnaftate (Tinactin)** is an OTC product used to treat superficial fungal infections. **Nystatin** is an **antifungal antibiotic** that is both fungistatic and fungicidal and is active against a wide variety of yeasts and yeastlike fungi. **Systemic antifungals** are used to treat tinea capitis and onychomycosis. **Griseofulvin (Grifulvin V, Grisactin)** is the first-line drug choice in the treatment of tinea capitis. Onychomycosis may be treated with systemic **griseofulvin, ketoconazole (Nizoral), itraconazole (Sporanox),** or **terbinafine (Lamisil).** The pharmacological management of systemic fungal infections is discussed in Chapter 30.

Pharmacodynamics

The **topical antifungal medications** can be roughly divided into three major categories and two medications that are not classified. The three major categories are **polyene antibiotic antifungals,** the **topical azoles,** and the **allylamine antifungals. Ciclopirox olamine** and **tolnaftate** do not fit into these categories. **Gentian violet,** an older **antifungal,** is also not classified.

TOPICAL ANTIFUNGALS. **Nystatin** is a **topical antifungal antibiotic** that is nearly identical to **amphotericin B** in structure. **Nystatin** is a **polyene antifungal.** It is effective only against *Candida.* **Nystatin** binds to sterols in the cell membranes of both fungal and human cells. When the **nystatin** binds to the sterols in the cell membrane of the fungus, it causes a change in membrane permeability that allows leakage of intracellular components.

Gentian violet is bactericidal to gram-positive organisms in very high concentration. It inhibits the growth of *Candida* and *Candida albicans.*

The **topical azole antifungals** all act in a similar fashion. They appear to alter the fungal cell membrane by inhibiting ergosterol synthesis through interacting with 14-alpha demethylase, an essential component of the membrane. This causes leakage of cellular contents, such as potassium- and phosphorus-containing compounds. **Clotrimazole** is active against a wide variety of fungi, yeasts, and dermatophytes. Organisms that are susceptible to **clotrimazole** include *Aspergillus fumigatus, C. albicans, Cephalosporium, Malassezia furfur, Trichophyton rubrum,* and some strains of *S. aureus* and *S. pyogenes.* **Miconazole** inhibits the growth of common dermatophytes *T. rubrum, Trichophyton mentagrophytes, C. albicans,* and the active organism in tinea versicolor, *M. furfur.* **Ketoconazole** is a broad-spectrum **antifungal** agent that is active against the dermatophytes *T. rubrum, T. mentagrophytes, Trichophyton tonsurans, Microsporum canis, Epidermophyton floccosum,* and the yeast organisms *C. albicans, Candida tropicalis, Pityrosporum ovale,* and *Pityrosporum orbiculare,* also known as *M. furfur,* the organism responsible for tinea versicolor. **Econazole** and **oxiconazole** have activity similar to **ketoconazole.**

Terbinafine is an **allylamine antifungal** that probably exerts its antifungal effectiveness by inhibiting squalene epoxidase, a key enzyme in sterol biosynthesis in fungi. This results in the accumulation of squalene within the fungal cell and causes fungal cell death. **Terbinafine** has fungicidal activity against dermatophytes. It is less active, however, against *Candida.*

Tolnaftate distorts hyphae and stunts mycelial growth in susceptible fungi.

Butenafine is the first of a new class of **topical antifungal agents,** the **benzylamines. Butenafine** is effective against *C. albicans.* It acts to inhibit fungal ergosterol biosynthesis by interfering with the conversion of squalene into 2,3-oxidosqualene. At higher concentrations, **butenafine** may exert a direct membrane-damaging effect on fungal cell membranes. It is also active against *T. rubrum* and *T. mentagrophytes.*

Ciclopirox olamine is a broad-spectrum **antifungal** agent. It acts on the cell membrane to block transmembrane transport of amino acids into the fungal cell. At higher concentrations, the fungal cell membrane integrity is altered, allowing leakage of intracellular material. It inhibits the growth pathogenic dermatophytes, yeasts, and *M. furfur.*

SYSTEMIC ANTIFUNGALS. The **systemic antifungal agents** used in the treatment of fungal infections of the skin include **griseofulvin,** the **azoles itraconazole** and **fluconazole,** and the **oral allylamine terbinafine.**

Griseofulvin is an **antifungal antibiotic** produced by certain species of *Penicillium.* **Griseofulvin** exerts its fungistatic activity by disrupting the mitotic spindle

structure of the fungal cell. This arrests metaphase cell division. **Griseofulvin** may also produce defective DNA. **Griseofulvin** has an affinity to keratin precursor cells. It is deposited in the keratin precursor cells, which are gradually exfoliated and replaced by uninfected tissue. **Griseofulvin** has a greater affinity for diseased tissue than for healthy tissue. It is tightly bound to the new keratin, which becomes highly resistant to fungal infections.

Fluconazole is a synthetic, broad-spectrum **triazole antifungal** agent of the **imidazole** class. **Fluconazole** has a broader spectrum than the other **imidazole antifungals. Fluconazole** exerts its effect by altering the fungal cell membrane. It is a highly selective inhibitor of fungal cytochrome P-450 and sterol 14-alpha demethylase. This inhibition results in increased cellular permeability, causing leakage of cellular contents.

Itraconazole is a synthetic **triazole antifungal** medication that is closely related to **ketoconazole.** Similar to **ketoconazole,** it exerts its effect by altering the fungal cell membrane. **Itraconazole** inhibits the cytochrome P-450–dependent synthesis of ergosterol, which increases cellular permeability and causes leakage of cellular contents.

Terbinafine is an **allylamine antifungal** that exerts its antifungal effect through interfering with fungal sterol biosynthesis by inhibiting the enzyme squalene monooxygenase. This causes accumulation of squalene, which weakens the cell membrane in sensitive fungi. The accumulation of squalene within the fungal cell causes fungal cell death. **Terbinafine** has fungicidal activity against dermatophytes. It is less active against *Candida.*

Pharmacokinetics

ABSORPTION AND DISTRIBUTION

Topical Antifungals. **Topical antifungals** are poorly absorbed from intact skin. **Nystatin** is not absorbed from intact skin or mucous membranes. Absorption information on **gentian violet** is unavailable. The **topical azoles** have little or no systemic absorption following topical application. When applied topically, **ciclopirox olamine** is minimally absorbed (an average of 1.3%). **Butenafine,** when applied topically, is absorbed through the skin into the systemic circulation in amounts that have not been quantified. Absorption and distribution of **tolnaftate** have not been described. **Terbinafine** may be systemically absorbed when applied topically. Systemic absorption of topically administered **terbinafine** is much lower than that of orally administered **terbinafine.**

Systemic Antifungals. **Griseofulvin** and **terbinafine** are the two **systemic antifungals** discussed in this chapter, as they are primarily used in dermatologic diseases. See Chapter 22 for further information on **systemic antifungal medications.**

Griseofulvin is poorly absorbed, and therefore oral

formulations have been developed in an attempt to increase bioavailability. Microsize **griseofulvin** has a variable and unpredictable oral absorption. Ultramicrosize **griseofulvin** has almost complete absorption. Oral **griseofulvin** is absorbed mainly from the duodenum. Absorption of oral microsize **griseofulvin** may be increased by intake of high-fat food. **Griseofulvin** is widely distributed and concentrates in the skin, hair, nails, fat, and skeletal muscles. **Griseofulvin** does cross the placenta. Distribution in breast milk is unknown but should be assumed because of **griseofulvin's** affinity for fat.

Terbinafine, when administered orally, is well absorbed from the gut. Bioavailability is approximately 40 percent. Administration with food increases the serum area under the curve (AUC) of **terbinafine** by 20 percent. **Terbinafine** is widely distributed, including the central nervous system (CNS), hair, and nailbeds. Following 2 weeks of therapy at recommended doses, **terbinafine** remains in the skin for up to 3 months. The drug may be detected in the nails for up to 90 days following treatment. It is unknown whether **terbinafine** crosses the placenta, but **terbinafine** is excreted in the breast milk of nursing mothers with a milk:plasma ratio of 7:1.

METABOLISM AND EXCRETION

Topical Antifungals.   **Topical antifungals** are either not absorbed or absorbed minimally. Therefore, metabolism information regarding **nystatin, tolnaftate, oxiconazole, sulconazole, butenafine, ciclopirox olamine**, and topical **ketoconazole** is not available. Topically administered **miconazole** is minimally absorbed following application to intact skin, with 1 percent of a dose applied six times daily for 14 days recovered in urine and feces. Metabolism of **oral miconazole** occurs mainly in the liver, and the small amount of topical medication that is absorbed is assumed to be also metabolized in this manner. Topical application of **econazole** results in lower systemic absorption. Less than 1 percent of an applied dose is recovered in urine and feces. Metabolism of **econazole** is unknown. There is little systemic absorption of **clotrimazole** following topical application. The small amounts absorbed are metabolized in the liver and excreted in the bile.

Systemic Antifungals.   **Griseofulvin** is metabolized in the liver, mainly through oxidative demethylation and conjugation with glucuronic acid. The major metabolite is inactive. **Griseofulvin** is excreted through the urine, feces, and perspiration.

Terbinafine is metabolized in the liver through oxidation and hydrolysis to five inactive metabolites. Seventy percent of the oral **terbinafine** dose is excreted in the urine as conjugated and unconjugated metabolites. Clearance of **terbinafine** is decreased by approximately 50 percent in patients with renal impairment or hepatic cirrhosis.

Pharmacotherapeutics

PRECAUTIONS AND CONTRAINDICATIONS

Topical Antifungals.   There are few contraindications to the **topical antifungal medications.** Hypersensitivity to the **antifungal** agent or any of the components of the formulation is a contraindication. Patients with **azole** hypersensitivity are often sensitive to all **azole** derivatives. The **antifungal** agent should be discontinued if sensitization occurs. The use of **antifungals** around the eyes should be avoided. **Gentian violet** is contraindicated in ulcerated areas and in patients with porphyria. **Ketoconazole** cream contains sulfites that may cause allergic types of reactions, including anaphylactic symptoms and life-threatening or less severe asthmatic episodes in susceptible persons.

The *topical antifungals* that are classified **Pregnancy Category B** are *clotrimazole, oxiconazole, ciclopirox olamine, naftifine,* and *butenafine.* The *topical antifungals* classified as **Pregnancy Category C** are *nystatin, ketoconazole, gentian violet, sulconazole, tolnaftate, miconazole,* and *econazole.* Of these, only *ketoconazole* and *econazole* have demonstrated teratogenic effects in animal tests with doses 10 times the maximum recommended human dose. Therefore, *ketoconazole* and *econazole* should be used in pregnant women only when potential benefits to the mother outweigh the potential risk to the fetus. Although systemic absorption following topical application is extremely low, caution is advised in prescribing **econazole** or **ketoconazole** to breastfeeding women. The use of **topical antifungals** on the breast during lactation is not advised. If **antifungal** medication is needed to treat such a topical infection in a lactating woman, application of oral **nystatin** suspension to the affected area on the breast is suggested for safety.

The safety of **topical antifungals** for infants and children varies from product to product. **Nystatin, gentian violet,** and **miconazole** are all safe for use in infants and children. **Econazole** is safe for topical use in children as young as 3 months. **Tolnaftate,** topical **ketoconazole,** and topical **clotrimazole** are contraindicated in children under age 2 years, although topical **clotrimazole** is used for short periods in children under age 2 without adverse effects. The safety of **ciclopirox olamine** for use in children under age 10 has not been established. **Butenafine, oxiconazole,** and **naftifine** have not had safety and effectiveness established for children under age 12.

Systemic Antifungals.   **Griseofulvin** should be used cautiously in patients with hepatic disease. It may be hepatotoxic on rare occasions. Patients with systemic lupus erythematosus (SLE) or lupuslike syndromes should use **griseofulvin** with caution because it has been known to exacerbate lupus. **Griseofulvin** is contraindicated in patients with porphyria or hypersensitivity to **griseofulvin.** There is a possibility of cross-sensitivity to **griseofulvin** in patients with **penicillin** hypersensitivity because **griseo-**

fulvin is produced by a species of *Penicillium*. This cross-sensitivity is theoretical, and patients have been treated with **griseofulvin** without adverse effects.

Griseofulvin **is Pregnancy Category C. Its use should be avoided in pregnant women because some women who received the drug during pregnancy reportedly have had spontaneous abortions or delivered infants with congenital abnormalities.** Griseofulvin may be used safely in children as young as age 2 years.

Terbinafine is contraindicated in patients who have known hypersensitivity to **terbinafine** or any of its components. **Terbinafine** should be used with caution in patients with hepatic disease or renal impairment (creatinine clearance = 50 mL/minute). Dosage adjustment may be needed in these patients. *Terbinafine* **is rated Pregnancy Category B.** *Terbinafine* **should be used in pregnancy only if the potential benefit to the mother outweighs the potential risk to the fetus; treatment of onychomycosis can be postponed until after pregnancy is completed. It is recommended that** *terbinafine* **not be used during pregnancy.** Oral **terbinafine** treatment is not recommended during lactation. After oral administration, **terbinafine** is excreted into the breast milk and can be found in the breast milk in a milk:plasma ratio of 7:1. A decision should be made whether to discontinue breast-feeding or to discontinue **terbinafine**.

ADVERSE DRUG REACTIONS

Topical Antifungals. Adverse reactions are minimal with **topical antifungal medications. Nystatin** may cause mild skin irritation when applied topically to some patients, usually related to the preservative (parabens) in the formulation. The main adverse reaction seen in **gentian violet** is staining of the skin and clothing, which can be significant. It may also cause local burning and skin reactions when used on the oral mucosa or other mucous membranes. The **topical azoles** may all cause itching, stinging, burning, or general skin irritation. Note that cross-sensitization among the **topical azoles** has been reported. Adverse reactions to **topical azoles** occur in approximately 1 to 3 percent of patients treated. The only adverse reaction reported with **tolnaftate** is mild skin irritation. The **allylamine antifungals butenafine** and **naftifine** may cause burning, stinging, dryness, erythema, pruritus, local irritation, and rash. **Ciclopirox olamine** may cause skin irritation, pruritus at the application site, redness, pain, burning, and worsening of clinical symptoms.

Systemic Antifungals. The most common adverse reaction with **griseofulvin** is hypersensitivity, such as skin rashes, urticaria, and rarely angioedema. Less commonly reported adverse reactions are oral thrush, nausea, vomiting, epigastric distress, and diarrhea. Several CNS effects have been reported. Headache occurs frequently in the beginning of therapy but often disappears with con-

tinued therapy. Other CNS adverse effects include fatigue, dizziness, insomnia, confusion, and impaired performance of routine activities. Hepatitis and elevated hepatic enzymes have been reported in a few patients after prolonged use or high doses of **griseofulvin**. A rare adverse effect of granulocytopenia or leukopenia has been reported from prolonged use of high doses of **griseofulvin**. **Griseofulvin** should be discontinued if the patient exhibits these conditions. When rare serious reactions occur with **griseofulvin**, they are usually associated with high doses or long periods of therapy.

Approximately 17 percent of patients taking oral **terbinafine** experience adverse reactions. The most common adverse reactions with oral **terbinafine** are gastrointestingal (GI) symptoms such as diarrhea (5.6%), dyspepsia (4.3%), abdominal pain (2.4%), nausea (2.6%), and flatulence. Two to three percent of patients taking oral **terbinafine** reported headache, dizziness, rash (unspecified), urticaria, and pruritus. Elevated liver enzymes occurred in 2 to 3 percent of patients taking **terbinafine**. Dysgeusia occurs in 2 percent of patients. Rare but serious adverse reactions observed with oral **terbinafine** include serious skin reactions (Stevens Johnson syndrome and toxic epidermal neurolysis). Rare cases of blood dyscrasia have been reported with **terbinafine** use. Severe neutropenia, lymphopenia, thrombocytopenia, and agranulocytosis have all been reported with oral **terbinafine** use. In clinical trials, 1 to 2 percent of patients treated with oral **terbinafine** developed decreased absolute lymphocyte cells (less than 1000/mm^3). These hematologic adverse reactions are reversible with discontinuation of oral **terbinafine**.

DRUG INTERACTIONS

Topical Antifungals. There are few drug interactions found with **topical antifungal medications**. The only significant interactions noted for **topical antifungals** are with **clotrimazole** and **econazole**. **Clotrimazole** and theoretically the other **azole antifungals** inhibit the synthesis of the fungal sterol ergosterol; the **polyene antifungals**, such as **amphotericin B** and **nystatin**, act by binding to ergosterol. Therefore, the **azole antifungals** could interfere with the action of either **amphotericin B** or **nystatin** by depleting polyene-binding sites. This appears to be the most significant when the **azole antifungal** is given prior to **amphotericin B**. **Clotrimazole** intravaginal preparations should not be administered concurrently with **nonoxynol-9** and **octoxynol**. **Clotrimazole** may inactivate the **spermicides**, leading to contraceptive failure. **Corticosteroids** may inhibit the antifungal activity of **econazole** against *C. albicans* in a concentration-dependent manner. When the concentration of **corticosteroid** is equal to the concentration of **econazole**, the antifungal activity of **econazole** is inhibited. When the **corticosteroid** concentration is 10 percent of that of **econazole**, there is no inhibition of antifungal activity.

Systemic Antifungals. **Systemic antifungal medications** have a number of drug interactions. **Griseofulvin** can increase some of the effects of ethanol, causing the patient to experience tachycardia, diaphoresis, and flushing. **Griseofulvin** can accelerate the hepatic metabolism of some medications. **Griseofulvin** may also decrease the hypoprothrombinemic activity of **warfarin,** which decreases its anticoagulant effect. Prothrombin time should be monitored closely if **griseofulvin** is either added or discontinued from **warfarin** therapy. **Estrogens** or **estrogen**-containing **oral contraceptives** can be affected by coadministration of **griseofulvin.** Patients may experience breakthrough bleeding, amenorrhea, or unintended pregnancy. They should use an alternative or second form of contraception while they are taking **griseofulvin** and for 1 month after **griseofulvin** is discontinued. **Griseofulvin** may reduce **cyclosporine** levels, resulting in decreased pharmacological effects. An increase in **cyclosporine** dose may be necessary if **griseofulvin** is added. A second dosage adjustment may be necessary if **griseofulvin** is discontinued. Serum salicylate concentrations may be decreased with **griseofulvin** use. Certain medications, including **barbiturates** and **primidone,** may impair the absorption of **griseofulvin,** resulting in decreased serum concentrations. Food can also affect the absorption of **griseofulvin.** Eating a high-fat meal at the time of dosing may increase microsize **griseofulvin** absorption.

Terbinafine clearance is affected by a number of medications. It is decreased by **cimetidine** and **terfenadine** and increased by **rifampin. Caffeine** clearance is decreased by **terbinafine. Cyclosporine** clearance is increased by **terbinafine. Theophylline** clearance is decreased by **terbinafine.** Patients taking **theophylline, aminophylline,** or **cyclosporine** concurrently with **terbinafine** should be monitored closely for increased or decreased effects of these medications with a narrow therapeutic window. **Terbinafine** may affect the metabolism of **warfarin,** leading to bleeding and coagulopathy.

CLINICAL USE AND DOSING

Candidiasis. There are more than 150 recognized species of *Candida* that can cause a variety of clinical syndromes that are termed *candidiasis* and usually categorized by the site of involvement. The most common sites for mucocutaneous candidiasis are the mouth, where it causes stomatitis or thrush; the esophagus, where it causes esophagitis; and the vagina, where it causes yeast vaginitis. *Candida* can also be invasive or systemic, aspects that are not discussed in this chapter. In most patients, candidiasis is opportunistic disease. *C. albicans* is the most common pathogen in humans; another common pathogen in humans is *C. tropicalis. C. albicans* is part of the normal human flora of the mouth, GI tract, and vagina. It normally lives in balance with other microorganisms within the body. When drugs or conditions, such as broad-spectrum **antibiotics, corticosteroids,** diabetes mellitus, or HIV infection, offset this balance, *C. albicans* may become a pathogen and cause mucocutaneous disease. *Candida* species may be transmitted from person to person, by direct contact either by hands or sexual contact, or during birth from colonized vagina to neonatal oropharynx. Candidiasis has emerged as the most common opportunistic fungal disease.

The first-line treatment for cutaneous *Candida* infections are the OTC **azoles, miconazole** and **clotrimazole,** which are applied twice daily to the affected skin area until clear (Table 21–2). For thrush in patients over age 3 years, a 10-mg **clotrimazole** troche is slowly and completely dissolved in the mouth five times a day for 14 days. Longer therapy may be needed in immunosuppressed patients.

For the patient who does not tolerate the **azole antifungals, nystatin** can be prescribed. **Nystatin** in cream, ointment, or powder formulation can be applied to the affected area two to three times per day until clear (see Table 21–2). Cream is preferred to ointment in intertriginous areas. Treatment should continue for at least 2 weeks. For thrush, the dose in adults and children is 4 to 6 mL of **nystatin** suspension, which is swished around the mouth and swallowed four times per day. The dose in infants is 2 mL, with 1 mL applied on each side of the mouth four times per day. The dose of **nystatin** for neonates is 0.5 mL applied to each side of the mouth four times per day. Adults and older children can use **nystatin** troches, which are slowly dissolved in the mouth. Treatment should continue until symptoms have been resolved for 48 hours.

For refractory oral candidiasis, **gentian violet** may be used. The dose in infants is 3 to 4 drops of a 0.5 percent solution under the tongue or on the inner cheeks after feeding twice per day. In adults and older children, a 1 or 2 percent solution may be applied to the affected area twice daily. The patient is to avoid swallowing the solution. Care should be used when applying **gentian violet,** which will stain any skin or clothing that it touches.

Second-line treatment for cutaneous *Candida* infections includes other prescription **azole antifungal medications. Econazole** is applied to the affected area twice daily for at least 2 weeks. **Oxiconazole** is applied to the affected and immediately surrounding areas once or twice daily until clear. **Sulconazole** may be gently massaged into the affected areas and surrounding skin once daily until clear.

Other **antifungals** effective against *Candida* species include **ciclopirox olamine, naftifine,** and **butenafine. Ciclopirox olamine** is gently massaged into the affected skin and surrounding area twice daily until clinical improvement occurs. **Naftifine** is gently massaged into the affected area once a day for the cream formulation and twice a day for the gel formulation, until clinical clearing is observed. Topical **butenafine** is used in adults and

Table 21–2. Dosage Schedule: Selected Anti-infectives Used to Treat
Skin Disorders

Drug	Indication	Dosage
Antibacterial Bacitracin	Minor cuts, wound, impetigo (1 or 2 lesions only)	Apply a small amount to the affected area once or twice daily; do not use >1 wk
Mupirocin	Impetigo Nasal colonization with MRSA	Apply a small amount to the lesions tid; may cover with gauze Half the ointment from a single-use tube of nasal ointment into one nostril, and the other half into the other nostril bid for 5 d; children may require smaller amounts of ointment
Neomycin	Minor cuts, wounds, impetigo (1 or 2 lesions only)	Apply a small amount to the affected area 1–2 times daily; do not use >1 wk
Polymyxin B	Minor cuts, wounds, impetigo (1 or 2 lesions only)	Apply a small amount to the affected area 1–2 times daily; do not use >1 wk
Triple-antibiotic ointment (polymyxin B, neomycin, bacitracin)	Minor cuts, wounds, impetigo (1 or 2 lesions only)	Apply a small amount to the affected area 1–3 times daily; do not use >1 wk
Antifungals Butenafine	Tinea corporis, tinea cruris	Apply to affected and immediately surrounding area once daily for 2 wk
Ciclopirox olamine	Tinea corporis, tinea cruris	Massage into affected skin bid for at least 2 wk Treat tinea pedis for 4 wk
Clotrimazole	Oral candidiasis Fungal skin infections, including candidiasis Tinea pedis	Adults and children >3 y: 1 troche 5 times daily for 14 consecutive d; dissolve slowly in mouth Children <3 y: Not recommended Apply to affected area bid for 2 wk Treat tinea pedis for 4 wk
Econazole	Tinea corporis, tinea cruris Tinea pedis	Apply to affected area once/d for 2 wk minimum Apply once daily; treat for 4 wk minimum
Gentian violet	Oral candidiasis	All ages: apply with cotton swab to entire inner surface of the mouth 2 times/d until clear
Ketoconazole	Tinea corporis, tinea cruris Tinea pedis	Apply once daily to affected area for 2 wk Apply once daily; treat for 6 wk
Miconazole	Fungal skin infections, including candidiasis Tinea pedis	Apply to affected area 2–3 times/d for 2 wk Treat tinea pedis for 4 wk minimum
Naftifine	Tinea corporis, tinea cruris, tinea pedis	Apply cream once daily until clear, up to 4 wk; gel is applied bid until clear
Nystatin oral suspension	Oral candidiasis	Adults and children: 2–3 mL in each inner cheek (total dose 4–6 mL) qid; have patient hold medication in mouth as long as possible before swallowing; treat for 48 h after clinical cure to prevent relapse

Continued on next page

Table 21–2. Dosage Schedule: Selected Anti-infectives Used to Treat Skin Disorders *(continued)*

Drug	Indication	Dosage
		Infants: 1 mL each cheek qid (2 mL/dose total), until 48 h after clinical cure; may apply medication to inner cheeks and tongue with cotton swab prior to administering the 1-mL dose via dropper
Nystatin cream or ointment	Cutaneous *Candida* infections	All ages: apply to affected areas 2 or 3 times/d until clear
Oxiconazole	Tinea corporis, tinea capitis	Apply to affected area once or twice/d for 2 wk Apply 1 or 2 times daily; treat for 4 wk
Sulconazole	Tinea corporis, tinea cruris Tinea pedis	Massage medication into affected area once or twice a day for 3 wk Apply bid for 4 wk
Terbinafine	Tinea corporis, tinea cruris Tinea pedis	Apply to affected and immediate surrounding areas bid until clinical symptoms are significantly improved, usually 1 wk Apply to affected and immediately surrounding area bid until symptoms are significantly improved, usually 2 wk
Tolnaftate	Tinea pedis	Apply to affected area bid for 2–3 wk; if skin is thickened, treatment may take 4–6 wk; apply sparingly and massage in well; for maintenance or prophylaxis, apply powder once daily
Antivirals Acyclovir	Initial herpes genitalis Mucocutaneous herpes simplex virus (HSV) infections in immunocompromised patients	Apply to lesion every 3 h, 6 times daily for 7 d
Penciclovir	Recurrent herpes labialis (cold sores) on lips and face	Apply q2h while awake for 4 d; begin treatment at earliest sign or symptom

children over age 12, and it is applied to the affected areas once daily until clear. Safety in children under age 12 has not been established.

An optional second-line treatment for oropharyngeal candidiasis (thrush) is systemic **fluconazole.** The dosage in adults is 200 mg orally (PO) on the first day, then 100 mg PO once daily for 14 days. Dosing in children, infants, and neonates older than age 14 days is 6 mg/kg PO on the first day, followed by 3 mg/kg PO once daily for 14 days. Neonates up to age 14 days have the same dose as infants, except it should be given every 72 hours instead of once daily until age 2 weeks. Clinical improvement is rapid with **fluconazole,** with lesions on the inner cheeks often clearing within the first 1 or 2 days of treatment, but treatment should continue for the full 14 days. This point should be stressed to patients.

Tinea Capitis. Tinea capitis is commonly called ringworm of the scalp. The causative organisms are *Microsporum* species and *T. tonsurans. Microsporum* presents usually with broken hairs and a fine gray scale. *Trichophyton* causes "black dot" tinea, which presents with tiny black dots that are the remains of broken hair shafts. Definitive diagnosis is obtained by fungal culture. As fungal cultures may take 2 to 4 weeks for results, treatment is begun while awaiting results.

Treatment of tinea capitis consists of **oral antifungal** therapy with **griseofulvin** and biweekly shampooing with **sporicidal** shampoo. Tinea capitis should always be treated with a **systemic antifungal.** The treatment of choice is **griseofulvin,** with treatment to continue for 6 to 8 weeks or until 2 weeks after potassium hydroxide (KOH) or culture is negative. The dosing for **griseofulvin**

Table 21–3. Available Dosage Forms: Selected Anti-infectives Used to
Treat Skin Infections

Drug	Dosage Form	How Supplied
Antibacterials		
Bacitracin (OTC)		
• Baciguent	500 U/g ointment	In 15- and 30-g tubes
• Generic	500 U/g ointment	In 1-, 15-, and 30-g tubes, 1-lb tub
Mupirocin (Rx)		
Bactroban	2% ointment	In 15- and 30-g tubes
Neomycin (OTC)		
• Myciguent	3.5 mg/g ointment or cream	In 15- and 30-g tubes
• Generic	3.5 mg/g ointment	In 15- and 30-g tubes
Triple-antibiotic ointment (polymyxin B, neomycin, and bacitracin) (OTC)		
• Neosporin Maximum Strength	Polysporin 10,000 U/g, neomycin 3.5 mg/g, bacitracin 400 U/g	In 15-g tubes
• Generic	Polysporin 5,000 U/g, neomycin 3.5 mg/g, bacitracin 400 U/g	In 2.4-, 9.6-, 15-, and 30-g tubes
Antifungals		
Butenafine (Rx)		
Mentax	1% cream	In 15 and 30 g
Ciclopirox olamine (Rx)		
Loprox	1% cream	In 15, 30 and 90 g
	1% lotion	In 30 and 60 mL
Clotrimazole		
• Lotrimin (Rx)	1% cream	In 15, 30 and 90 g
	1% lotion	In 30 mL
	1% solution	In 10 and 30 mL
• Lotrimin AF (OTC)	1% cream	In 12 g
	1% lotion	In 10 mL
• Generic	1% cream	In 30 g
Econazole (Rx)		
Spectazole	1% cream	In 15, 30, and 85 g
Gentian violet (OTC)	1% and 2% solution	In 30 mL
Ketoconazole		
• Nizoral	2% cream	In 15, 30, and 60 g
	2% shampoo	In 4 oz
• Nizoral A-D Shampoo (OTC)	1% shampoo	In 4 and 7 oz
Miconazole		
• Monistat Derm (Rx)	2% cream	In 15, 30, and 90 g
	2% cream	In 15, 30, and 90 g
• Micatin (OTC)	2% powder	In 90 g
	2% spray	In 105 mL
	2% cream	In 30 g
• Generic		
Naftifine (Rx)		
Naftin	1% cream	In 15, 30, and 60 g
	1% gel	In 20, 40, and 60 g

Continued on next page

Table 21–3. Available Dosage Forms: Selected Anti-infectives Used to
Treat Skin Infections *(continued)*

Drug	Dosage Form	How Supplied
Nystatin (Rx)		
• Nilstat	100,000 U/g cream (topical)	In 15 and 30 g
	100,000 U/g ointment (topical)	In 15 and 30 g
• Mycostatin	100,000 U/mL suspension (PO)	In 60 mL with dropper, 16 oz
	Pastilles 200,000 U each (PO)	In 30s
		In 15 g
		In 15 and 30 g
		In 15 and 30 g
• Generic	100,000 U/g powder (topical)	In 15 and 30 g
	100,000 U/g cream (topical)	In 15 and 30 g
	100,000 U/g ointment (topical)	
	100,000 U/g cream (topical)	
	100,000 U/g ointmont (topical)	
Oxiconazole (Rx)		
Oxistat	1% cream	In 15, 30, and 60 g
	1% lotion	In 30 mL
Sulconazole (Rx)		
Exelderm	1% cream	In 15, 30, and 60 g
	1% solution	In 30 mL
Terbinafine		
• Lamisil AT (OTC)	1% cream	In 12 and 24 g
• Lamisil Solution	1% solution	In 30 mL
Tolnaftate (OTC)		
• Tinactin	1% cream	In 15 g
	1% solution	In 10 mL
	1% powder	In 45 g
	1% spray powder	In 100 and 150 g
	1% spray liquid	In 120 mL
• Aftate	1% gel	In 15 g
• Generic	1% cream	In 15 g
	1% solution	In 10 ml
	1% powder	In 45 g
	1% spray powder	In 105 g
Antivirals		
Acyclovir (Rx)		
Zovirax	5% ointment	In 3- and 15-g tubes
Penciclovir (Rx)		
Denavir	1% cream	In 2 g

microsize for adults is 500 mg daily in one or two doses. For children, the dose of **griseofulvin** microsize is 11 mg/kg/day in a single dose. For ultramicrosize **griseofulvin**, the adult dose is 330 to 375 mg/day, and the pediatric dose is 7.3 mg/kg/day in a single dose. **Griseofulvin** is absorbed better with a high-fat meal (whole milk, cheese, or ice cream), and the patient should be instructed about this point when beginning treatment.

The patient should also be treated with a **sporicidal** shampoo such as **selenium sulfide** or **ketoconazole**. The patient should shampoo with either the **selenium** sulfide 2.5 percent shampoo or **ketoconazole** 2 percent shampoo twice weekly until clear. Close contacts should be empirically treated with **sporicidal** shampoo twice per week.

If the patient is not responding to therapy, a culture should be obtained if it has not already been started. Cases resistant to **griseofulvin** may be treated with systemic **terbinafine, fluconazole,** or **itraconazole,** based on the sensitivity of the organism as determined by culture. Resistance to **griseofulvin** is not common, but by culturing the patient at the beginning of therapy, the provider will have sensitivity studies on which to base the treatment decision if there is no response after 4 weeks of treatment. Dosing information regarding systemic **terbinafine, fluconazole,** and **itraconazole** can be found in Chapter 22.

Tinea Corporis.   Tinea corporis is a superficial fungal infection of the skin, also known as *ringworm*. The causative organism is *M. canis, T. tonsurans,* or *E. floccosum*. Tinea corporis presents as an annular lesion with raised borders and a clear center. There may be scaling and usually some erythema. It is spread by direct contact with an infected person or animal. Diagnosis is made by KOH scrapings, Wood's lamp, or fungal culture. Treatment is **topical antifungal** cream, with **miconazole, tolnaftate,** or **clotrimazole** the most common medications used. Other **topical antifungals** may be used, including **terbinafine, sulconazole, ciclopirox olamine, ketoconazole,** and **econazole.**

Tinea Cruris.   Tinea cruris is also known as "jock itch." It is a superficial fungal infection of the groin, upper thighs and intertriginous folds. It is more common in males and rarely occurs before adolescence. The causative fungal organisms are *E. floccosum, T. rubrum,* and *T. mentagrophytes*. *C. albicans* may also be a causative organism. The lesions are scaly with a raised border, erythematous, and slightly brown in color. The treatment for tinea cruris is the same **topical antifungal** medications that are used for tinea corporis, with the same dosing schedule.

Tinea Pedis.   Tinea pedis is a superficial fungal infection of the skin of the feet, commonly called "athlete's foot." It is caused by the dermatophytes *E. floccosum, T. rubrum,* and *T. mentagrophytes*. *C. albicans* may also be a causative organism. Tinea pedis is more common in males and rarely occurs before puberty. Diagnosis is made by the classic clinical presentation of scaling, maceration, fissuring, and inflammation on the feet, especially in the inner digital areas. Treatment for tinea pedis is the same topical agents used for tinea corporis. Length of treatment is extended with tinea pedis, often with 4 weeks of treatment needed.

Tinea Versicolor.   Tinea versicolor is a superficial fungal infection of the skin caused by *P. orbiculare*. Clinically, tinea versicolor appears as multiple scaling, oval maculae that may be hypopigmented or hyperpigmented. The treatment for tinea versicolor consists of topical application of **selenium sulfide** shampoo or a **topical antifungal. Selenium sulfide** shampoo is applied to the tinea versicolor patch and left on for 10 to 15 minutes every day for 1 week. **Selenium sulfide** can be used prophylactically once a month. The **topical azoles miconazole, clotrimazole,** and **econazole** may be used twice a day for 2 to 4 weeks in the treatment of tinea versicolor.

Onychomycosis.   Onychomycosis, also known as Tinea unguium, is a fungal infection of the nail, either fingernail or toenail. Treatment of onychomycosis usually involves months of a **systemic antifungal** medication. Topical treatment is usually not effective. The most commonly prescribed systemic medications for onychomycosis are **griseofulvin, ketoconazole, itraconazole,** and **terbinafine.**

Griseofulvin has been used extensively in the treatment of onychomycosis and has a proven safety profile in adults and children. The medication should be administered for at least 4 months for onychomycosis of the fingernail. Treatment of the toenail should last at least 6 months. Renal, liver, and hematopoietic functions should be measured at least every 8 weeks during therapy. The adult dose of **griseofulvin** microsize for onychomycosis is 750 mg to 1 g/day in divided doses; the dose for ultramicrosize is 660 mg to 750 mg/day. The dose for children is 11 mg/kg/day of microsize **griseofulvin** and 7.3 mg/kg/day of ultramicrosize **griseofulvin.** The medication should be taken with a high-fat meal.

Ketoconazole may be used to treat onychomycosis but is usually not a first-line choice because of the associated possibility of hepatotoxicity. The dose of **ketoconazole** in adults is 200 mg daily for 4 to 6 months. The dose for children is 3.3 to 6.6 mg/kg/day in a single dose. Liver function tests should be done prior to beginning therapy and monthly for the whole course of therapy.

Itraconazole may be used for first-line therapy in adult patients with onychomycosis if a patient cannot tolerate **griseofulvin. Itraconazole** may be dosed in one of two methods, either daily dosing or pulse dosing. The daily dosing regimen for adults with toenail onychomycosis is 200 mg daily for 12 weeks. The pulse regimen for adults with toenail involvement is 400 mg/day for 1 week per month for 3 to 4 consecutive months. If only the fingernail area is involved, the adult dose is 200 mg bid for 7 days, then 3 weeks without treatment, and then 200 mg bid for 1 additional week. Safety in children has not been established, but multiple studies in children over age 3 have reported no serious adverse affects (Suarez & Friedlander, 1998). For onychomycosis, the pediatric pulse dose is 5 mg/kg/day for 1 week per month for 3 to 4 consecutive months. For any patient who takes **itraconazole** for more than 8 consecutive weeks, liver enzymes and electrolytes should be drawn prior to and every 8 weeks during treatment. *Itraconazole* should not be administered to pregnant women or women considering pregnancy.

Systemic **terbinafine** has shown to be useful in the treatment of onychomycosis in both pediatric and adult trials. **Terbinafine** has an extremely long half-life, with persistence due to binding to lipophilic keratinocytes, and it can be found in toenails for 6 months after the start of a 3-month period of therapy. The dose for treating onychomycosis of the fingernail is 250 mg daily for 6 weeks. To treat an infected toenail, the dose is 250 mg daily for

12 weeks. Liver enzymes and complete blood count (CBC) should be monitored every 6 weeks if treatment lasts longer than 6 weeks. Because onychomycosis is not a serious or life-threatening disease, therapy in pregnant women should be deferred until the pregnancy is over.

RATIONAL DRUG SELECTION

Indication. For the treatment of thrush or oral candidiasis, the drug of choice is generally **nystatin,** with its low adverse effect profile and high efficacy. For treating topical dermatophyte infections, generally the OTC **azoles** are the first-line therapy because they are easily available without prescription and low cost. If OTC products are not effective, then a broader spectrum **antifungal** can be prescribed with little difference found in efficacy in treating common organisms that cause tinea infections. If treating tinea capitis or onychomycosis, **griseofulvin** is generally the drug of choice on account of its proven safety profile in both adults and children. If the patient is unable to tolerate **griseofulvin** and a culture-confirmed dermatophyte has been identified, then **itraconazole** and **ketoconazole** are appropriate second-line medications.

Cost. The cost of medication varies greatly among the **antifungals.** Generally, OTC products are less expensive than prescriptions. In the treatment of thrush, **nystatin** is a low-cost, effective therapy for topical fungal infections and is usually covered by insurance plans. When treating cutaneous fungal infections, the OTC products **clotrimazole** and **miconazole** should be the first medications used because of their low cost and their safety profile. If they are ineffective, then a prescription product with a broader spectrum may be used, but it is generally more expensive. In the treatment of tinea pedis, **tolnaftate** is available OTC in a variety of formulations; the generic products are generally the least expensive. **Griseofulvin** is the least expensive **systemic antifungal.**

MONITORING. The patient being treated for oral candidiasis should be monitored for efficacy of treatment, with no laboratory monitoring necessary. The patient being treated for tinea capitis will need monitoring for adverse effects from the **systemic antifungals.** All of the **systemic antifungal agents** can possibly cause some alteration in hepatic function. If the patient is to be on continuous therapy, then baseline and ongoing monitoring of liver function is necessary. If liver enzymes become elevated, the medication should be discontinued. The patient being prescribed **griseofulvin** will require renal, liver, and hematopoietic function measurements every 8 weeks during therapy. Patients receiving **ketoconazole** require liver function tests prior to beginning therapy and monthly for the whole course of their treatment. Patients on **itraconazole** need liver enzyme and electrolyte studies if the medication is prescribed for longer than 8 consecutive weeks. In that case, liver function and electrolytes should be monitored prior to beginning therapy and every

8 weeks during treatment. Liver enzymes and CBC should be monitored every 6 weeks in the patient receiving **terbinafine** who is treated for longer than 6 weeks.

PATIENT EDUCATION

Administration. Instruct patients to take the drug as prescribed for the full course of their treatment, even if they note clinical improvement. In the treatment of oral candidiasis, the patient should be instructed to continue therapy until 2 days after symptoms have disappeared. When treating infants with thrush, all pacifiers and bottle nipples should be washed in warm, soapy water and soaked in hot or boiling water for 20 minutes between each use. This step is important to prevent reinfection of the infant with candidiasis. If treated with **gentian violet,** the patient should be warned that **gentian violet** will stain skin and clothing. If oral candidiasis is treated with **clotrimazole** troche, patients should be instructed to slowly dissolve the troche in their mouth, not chew.

Patients using **topical antifungals** for dermatophyte infections of the skin should be instructed to apply the medication to the infected area and the immediate surrounding area for the full length of treatment. Treatment is often continued beyond the point of clinical clearing to prevent recurrence of the infection. Generally, avoid occlusive dressings, which provide favorable conditions for yeast growth.

The treatment of tinea capitis or onychomycosis involves long-term therapy with **oral antifungal medications.** The patient should be encouraged to continue the medication for the full length of treatment and take the medication as prescribed. **Griseofulvin** must be taken with a high-fat meal to ensure adequate absorption of the medication. **Itraconazole** should be taken with food. **Ketoconazole** and **terbinafine** may both be taken without regard to meals.

In treating topical dermatophyte infections such as tinea corporis or ringworm, family members and pets should be checked for signs of infection and be treated also.

Adverse Reactions. The patient should be given written and oral instructions regarding the adverse drug reactions that may be expected with the medication that is being prescribed. If the patient is prescribed **systemic antifungal** medication, then an explanation of the possible adverse effects and the necessity for laboratory monitoring should be discussed. Patients should be instructed to immediately report to their provider any "flu-like" symptoms, which may be a sign of hepatic toxicity.

Topical Antivirals

Topical antivirals are used to treat herpes simplex virus (HSV) and herpes zoster. The **oral antiviral medications** used to treat these conditions and varicella are discussed in Chapter 22. The two herpes simplex virus infections that are treated with topical medications are HSV-1 and HSV-2, with HSV-1 generally associated with nongenital infection and HSV-2 with genital infection. There are two **topical antiviral medications: acyclovir** (**Zovirax**) and **penciclovir** (**Denavir**).

Pharmacodynamics

Both **acyclovir** and **penciclovir** must be phosphorylated to be active against herpes simplex virus. Intracellularly, both medications are converted to monophosphate forms by viral thymidine kinases, then further converted to diphosphate and finally to triphosphate by various cellular enzymes. **Acyclovir** triphosphate competes with deoxyguanosine triphosphate for a position in the DNA chain of the herpes virus. Once incorporated in the DNA chain, it terminates DNA synthesis. **Penciclovir** triphosphate selectively inhibits viral DNA polymerase by competing with deoxyguanosine triphosphate. This inhibits viral replication. In vitro, **penciclovir** triphosphate is retained inside the HSV-infected cells for 10 to 20 hours, compared with 0.7 to 1 hour for **acyclovir**.

Pharmacokinetics

ABSORPTION AND DISTRIBUTION. After topical application of **acyclovir** or **penciclovir**, there is minimal absorption, and no drug is detected in the blood or urine after application.

Pharmacotherapeutics

PRECAUTIONS AND CONTRAINDICATIONS. The only true contraindication to both **acyclovir** and **penciclovir** is hypersensitivity to the product or any of its components. **Acyclovir** should be used with caution in patients with **ganciclovir** hypersensitivity in that these two drugs have similar chemical structures, and there may be cross-sensitivity.

Acyclovir **is classified as Pregnancy Category C, although no complete or well-controlled pregnancy studies have been performed in humans.** *Penciclovir* **is classified as Pregnancy Category B. No adverse effects on pregnancy outcomes or fetal development are found in animal studies. However, there have been no adequate or well-controlled studies in pregnant women.**

Orally administered **acyclovir** is excreted in breast milk. It is unknown whether topical **acyclovir** is excreted in breast milk. Because topical **acyclovir** cannot be measured in the serum, it is assumed that it is not excreted in breast milk. It is not known if **penciclovir** is excreted in human milk after topical administration. Both medications should be used with caution in a nursing mother until further studies clarify their safety.

Safety and effectiveness in pediatric patients have not been established for either **acyclovir** or **penciclovir**.

ADVERSE DRUG REACTIONS. Although **systemic acyclovir** has extensive adverse reactions, **topical acyclovir** has only transient local adverse reactions. The most common reaction to **topical acyclovir** use is mild pain with transient burning or stinging in 28.3 percent of patients. Pruritus is reported by 4.1 percent of patients, with rash and local edema found in less than 1 percent.

Double-blind, placebo-controlled trials of **penciclovir** cream found no difference in the frequency of adverse events for both treatment groups. When 5 percent **penciclovir** cream (not currently available in the United States) was used, mild erythema was reported in 50 percent of subjects.

DRUG INTERACTIONS. There are no known drug interactions identified with either topical **acyclovir** or topical **penciclovir**.

CLINICAL USE AND DOSING

Herpes Simplex. **Acyclovir** is indicated in the management of initial episodes of herpes genitalis and in limited, non–life-threatening, mucocutaneous HSV infections in immunocompromised patients. There is no clinical evidence for the benefit of using **acyclovir** in the immunocompetent patient, although decreased viral shedding may be noted. Topical **acyclovir** is applied to cover all lesions every 3 hours six times a day for 7 days. The dose size per application should be approximately a ½- to 1-inch ribbon of ointment per 4 square inches of surface area. A glove or finger cot should be used to apply the medication to prevent autoinoculation of other body sites and transmission of infection to other people.

Penciclovir is indicated in the treatment of recurrent herpes labialis (cold sores) on the lips and face. Application to mucous membrane is not recommended. In adults, **penciclovir** 1 percent cream is applied every 2 hours while awake, with treatment started as early as possible (during the prodrome or when lesions appear).

Herpes Zoster. Neither topical **acyclovir** nor topical **penciclovir** is indicated in the treatment of herpes zoster.

Varicella. Although **oral acyclovir** is used in the treatment of varicella, **topical acyclovir** does not have this indication. **Penciclovir** is not used in the treatment of varicella.

RATIONAL DRUG SELECTION

Efficacy. **Penciclovir** is the first **topical antiviral** medication that has been clinically proved to be effective in the treatment of herpes labialis (cold sores). Although **acyclovir** may be used for herpes labialis, it has not been clinically proved to be effective in the treatment of HSV infections in immunocompetent patients. In genital herpes, **acyclovir** is the drug of choice for primary lesions in immunocompromised patients.

Cost. Because topical **acyclovir** and **penciclovir** are both unique **antiviral agents,** their cost is not generally used as part of the decision of whether to use the drug in treatment.

MONITORING. There is no laboratory monitoring necessary for patients treated with topical **acyclovir** or **penciclovir.** Monitoring for the adverse reactions noted previously is the only monitoring needed.

PATIENT EDUCATION

Administration. The patient should be instructed to start therapy with **acyclovir** as early as possible after the onset of the signs and symptoms of HSV infection. When applying **acyclovir,** patients should first wash their hands thoroughly and use a finger cot or rubber glove to apply the ointment to prevent the spread of infection. They should apply enough ointment to thoroughly cover all lesions. Patients should be instructed that **acyclovir** may cause transient burning, stinging, itching, and rash. They should notify their primary care provider if these symptoms become pronounced or persist.

Patients should be instructed to begin therapy with **penciclovir** as soon as symptoms begin, during the prodrome or when lesions appear. They should wash their hands thoroughly after applying **penciclovir** to prevent the spread of infection. Patients should avoid application on or near the eyes or mucous membranes. Although adverse reactions are rare, patients should be instructed to report any skin irritation to their provider.

Agents Used to Treat Acne

Acne is the number one diagnosis seen by dermatologists, accounting for 18 percent of visits (Feldman, Fleischer, & McConnell, 1998). Approximately 85 percent of adolescents have acne to some degree, although acne can also occur in adult patients, accounting for 4.4 percent of visits to internists. Acne is classified as mild, moderate, or severe, and pharmacological intervention is based on the severity of acne.

The medications used in the treatment of acne may be either topical agents or systemic. The topical agents used for acne can be divided into two categories: **retinoids** and **antibiotics.** Oral medications for systemic use are divided into three categories: **oral antibiotics** (discussed in Chapter 22), **hormonal therapy** (discussed in Chapter 30), and **isotretinoin,** an **oral retinoid. Oral antibiotics** are prescribed for moderate to severe acne, and **isotretinoin** is prescribed for severe nodulocystic acne.

The pharmacological management of acne is discussed in Chapter 30.

Pharmacodynamics

TOPICAL RETINOIDS. Tretinoin is a naturally occurring derivative of vitamin A that is structurally related to **isotretinoin.** After topical administration, **tretinoin** appears to prevent horny cell cohesion and to increase epidermal cell turnover. It effects mitotic activity through irritation of the follicular epithelium. This decreases microcomedo formation. The increased turnover of follicular epithelial cells causes extrusion of comedones that have already formed. Formation of new comedones is prevented through sloughing and expulsion of horny cells from the follicle. **Tretinoin** reduces the cell layers of the stratum corneum from 14 to 5 layers. **Tretinoin** does not affect the bacteria found in *Propionibacterium acnes.* Topical **tretinoin** is also used in the treatment of fine wrinkling, mottled hyperpigmentation, roughness, and laxity of the skin associated with sun damage.

Adapalene is a topical retinoid-like drug used for the treatment of mild to moderate acne vulgaris. **Adapalene** binds to specific retinoic acid nuclear receptors but does not bind to the cytosolic receptor protein. Although the exact mode of action of **adapalene** is not known, it is suggested that topical **adapalene** may normalize the differentiation of follicular epithelial cells, resulting in decreased microcomedo formation. It is also a modulator of cellular differentiation, keratinization, and inflammatory processes, all of which represent important features in the pathology of acne vulgaris.

Tazarotene is a **retinoid** prodrug that is converted to its active form, AGN 190299, which is the cognate carboxylic acid of **tazarotene.** The exact mechanism of action of **tazarotene** in the treatment of acne is not well defined, but it is believed that the drug works by normalizing epidermal differentiation and by reducing the influx of inflammatory cells into the skin.

TOPICAL ANTIBIOTICS. Benzoyl peroxide has antibacterial activity against *P. acnes,* the predominant organism in sebaceous follicles and comedones of acne vulgaris. This antibacterial activity is presumably due to the release of active or free-radical oxygen capable of oxidizing bacterial proteins. **Benzoyl peroxide** also has a drying effect, removes excess sebum, causes mild desquamation, and has a sebostatic effect.

Erythromycin is a bacteriostatic **macrolide antibiotic** but may be bactericidal in high concentrations. The mechanism by which topical **erythromycin** acts in reducing inflammatory lesions of acne vulgaris is unknown, but it is presumably due to its antibiotic actions.

Topical **clindamycin** demonstrates in vitro activity against isolates of *P. acnes,* the common bacteria found in acne vulgaris. **Clindamycin** also inhibits lipase-producing organisms, reducing the concentration of free fatty acids in sebum from approximately 14 percent to 2 percent after application. These free fatty acids are possibly a cause of the inflammatory lesions associated with acne.

The mechanism of action by which **tetracycline** improves acne is unknown. **Systemic tetracycline** seems to decrease the amount of free fatty acids present in acne lesions. It appears that **topical tetracycline** has a localized effect in which the medication is delivered to the pilosebaceous apparatus and adjacent tissues. **Tetracycline** is active against *P. acnes,* but there are reports of resistance developing.

Metronidazole is classified as an **antiprotozoal** and **antibacterial** agent. The mechanism by which topical **metronidazole** acts in reducing the inflammatory lesions in acne rosacea is unknown.

The mechanism of action for **azelaic acid** in acne vulgaris is its antimicrobial effect against *P. acnes* and *Staphylococcus epidermidis.* The mechanism of action may be due to inhibition of microbial cellular protein synthesis. **Azelaic acid** decreases the inflammation associated with acne lesions by reducing the concentration of bacteria present in the skin. **Azelaic acid** may also cause normalization of keratinization, leading to an anticomedomal effect. It may also decrease microcomedo formation by reducing the number and size by of keratohyalin granules and the amount and distribution of filaggrin in epidermal layers. **Azelaic acid** does not effect sebum excretion.

SYSTEMIC RETINOIDS. **Isotretinoin** is an isomer of all-*trans* retinoic acid, a metabolite of retinol (vitamin A). Its actions include normalization of the keratinizing process of the follicular epithelium and reduction of sebocyte number with decreased sebum synthesis. Sebum lipid production and composition are altered during **isotretinoin** therapy, with sebum production reversibly reduced to 10 percent of pretreatment levels. **Isotretinoin,** if given in high doses, can reduce the concentration of *P. acnes* bacteria through decreased sebum production.

Pharmacokinetics

ABSORPTION AND DISTRIBUTION

Topical Retinoids. **Tretinoin,** administered topically, is minimally absorbed systemically. Prolonged treatment or administration to large body surface areas can increase systemic absorption. **Adapalene,** when applied topically to the skin, has minimal absorption. Trace amounts of **adapalene** have been found in the plasma of acne patients after chronic topical application. **Tazarotene,** when administered topically to the skin, has minimal systemic absorption because of its rapid metabolism in the skin to the active metabolite. In clinical trials, topical use of **tazarotene** determined that systemic absorption of the total dose was less than 1 percent without occlusion. Even treating psoriasis by applying **tazarotene** to 20 percent of the total body surface area led to systemic absorption of less than 1 percent after 7 days of treatment.

Topical Antibiotics. **Benzoyl peroxide** is absorbed by the skin in unknown amounts. Absorption of topical **erythromycin** is unknown. **Clindamycin,** when applied topically, does exhibit some systemic absorption, depending on the surface area covered. Following multiple topical applications at a concentration equivalent to 10 mg, very low levels of **clindamycin** are present in the serum. Topically applied **tetracycline** does not appear to be absorbed through the skin in sufficient quantities to be detected systemically. **Metronidazole** is absorbed when applied topically but in very small amounts. When 1 mg is applied to the face, the resulting serum concentration is approximately 100 times less than one 250-mg tablet taken orally. Approximately 4 percent of topically applied **azelaic acid** is absorbed systemically.

Systemic Retinoids. The oral bioavailability from oil-filled capsules of **isotretinoin** is approximately 23 to 25 percent. Increased plasma levels may be found if the drug is taken with food. **Isotretinoin** is 99.9 percent plasma protein–bound. Although severe fetal abnormalities have been noted, it is not known whether **isotretinoin** crosses the placenta. Distribution of **isotretinoin** is unknown.

METABOLISM AND EXCRETION

Topical Retinoids. A minimal amount of **tretinoin** is absorbed systemically. This trace amount is metabolized by the cytochrome P-450 hepatic enzyme system. Approximately 1 to 5 percent of a topically applied dose is excreted in the urine within 24 hours. The metabolism of topically applied **adapalene** is unknown. Excretion appears to be primarily by the biliary route. **Tazarotene** is rapidly metabolized in the skin to the active metabolite, tazarotenic acid, which is systemically absorbed and further metabolized by the liver to sulfoxides, sulfones, and other metabolites. Elimination of the metabolites is via fecal and renal pathways.

Topical Antibiotics. **Benzoyl peroxide** metabolism and excretion are unknown. Although topical **erythromycin** absorption is minimal, oral administration demonstrates that **erythromycin** is metabolized in the liver to several inactive metabolites. Excretion of **erythromycin** is mainly via the bile. Topical **clindamycin** is absorbed and metabolized into two active metabolites, clindamycin sulfoxide and N-demethylclindamycin, as well as other inactive metabolites. Following oral dosage, only about 10 percent is excreted in the urine as active drug and metabolites and 3.6 percent in the feces; the remainder is excreted as inactive metabolites. Approximately 80 percent of a dose of **oral metronidazole** is metabolized by side-chain oxidation and glucuronide conjugation into inactive metabolites. The major route of elimination of **metronidazole** and its metabolites is through the urine. Topically applied **azelaic acid** is minimally absorbed and is mainly excreted unchanged in the urine.

Systemic Retinoids. **Isotretinoin** is metabolized in the liver primarily via oxidation. It is unknown whether its metabolite is pharmacologically active. The metabolites are eliminated renally, and unchanged drug and metabolites are excreted in the feces.

Pharmacotherapeutics

PRECAUTIONS AND CONTRAINDICATIONS

Topical Retinoids and Topical Antibiotics. **Topical retinoids** should be avoided in patients with eczema, sunburn, or skin abrasions at the site of application. **Topical retinoids** are contraindicated in lactating women. Safety and efficacy in children below age 12 years have not been established. **All three topical retinoids—***tretinoin, adapalene,* **and** *tazarotene***—are classified as Pregnancy Category C.**

Topical antibiotics used in acne treatment have few true contraindications. **Benzoyl peroxide** may exhibit cross-sensitivity with benzoic acid derivatives. **Erythromycin,** when applied topically, is contraindicated only when the patient is hypersensitive to **erythromycin** or to any component of the preparation. Topical **clindamycin** is contraindicated in any patient who is hypersensitive to **clindamycin** or **lincomycin.** It is also contraindicated in patients with a history of regional enteritis, ulcerative colitis, or antibiotic-associated colitis. Topical **tetracycline** preparations contain sodium sulfites and are contraindicated in patients sensitive to sulfites or **tetracycline. Azelaic acid** has not been well studied in patients with dark skin and should be used cautiously in these patients to avoid hypopigmentation. **Metronidazole** for topical use contains parabens, and therefore any patient who is sensitive to parabens or **metronidazole** should not use it. *Azelaic acid* **is classified as Pregnancy Category B.** Because small amounts of **azelaic acid** are absorbed systemically and may be excreted in breast milk, caution should be exercised in administering it to lactating women. Safety and efficacy of **azelaic acid** in children under age 12 years have not been established.

Systemic Retinoids. **Isotretinoin** should be avoided in patients with **retinoid** hypersensitivity, including vitamin A, **tretinoin,** and **etretinate.** Patients with parabens hypersensitivity should avoid **isotretinoin** because the drug is prepared with parabens, a preservative. *Isotretinoin* **is classified Pregnancy Category X and is** *absolutely contraindicated in pregnancy.* **It may cause severe malformations of the craniofacial, cardiac, thymic, and CNS structures. Many such infants have several malformations. Spontaneous abortions and premature births have also been reported. The drug should not be administered to any woman of childbearing age until after pregnancy has been excluded and appropriate birth control measures are used for at least 1 month. Patients should also avoid pregnancy for at least 1 month after discontinuation of** *isotretinoin.* Breastfeeding is not recommended during **isotretinoin** treatment because of the potential adverse affects to the nursing infant. Caution should be exercised in administering **isotretinoin** to patients with hyperlipidemia; patients may have increased lipids during therapy. **Isotretinoin** should be prescribed cautiously to patients with psychotic disorders; it may cause major depression, psychosis, and, rarely, suicidal ideation.

ADVERSE DRUG REACTIONS

Topical Retinoids. **Topical retinoids** all cause some degree of skin irritation. Burning or pruritus immediately after applying a **topical retinoid** is common. All three **retinoid** products cause erythema, scaling, xerosis, and peeling. These symptoms occur frequently and appear to be necessary for the therapeutic effect. Because photosensitivity may occur with **topical retinoid** use, patients should use sunscreen to prevent severe sunburn. Both **tretinoin** and **tazarotene** may cause skin discoloration, hyperpigmentation, or hypopigmentation, which will resolve after discontinuation of the medication.

Topical Antibiotics. **Topical antibiotics** used in the treatment of acne all cause some dryness, erythema, burning, peeling, and itching. **Benzoyl peroxide** may also cause marked peeling and desquamation, which appears to be a necessary component of the therapeutic effect. **Benzoyl peroxide** may also cause photosensitivity. Allergic contact sensitization may occur with any of the **topical antibiotics** used in the treatment of acne vulgaris. In patients with dark complexions, skin hypopigmentation may occur with the use of topical **azelaic acid.**

Systemic Retinoids. **Isotretinoin** has multiple reported significant adverse reactions. The most commonly reported adverse reactions involve mucocutaneous effects. Cheilitis (inflammation of the lips) occurs in more than 90 percent of patients. Dry skin, pruritus, and skin fragility occur in approximately 80 percent of patients. Conjunctivitis is reported by 40 percent of patients, with facial skin desquamation and drying of mucous membranes reported by approximately 30 percent of patients treated with **isotretinoin.** Patients also report xerosis, xerostomia, and epistaxis. These mucocutaneous drying effects of **isotretinoin** are dose-related and are usually reversible after discontinuation of therapy.

Isotretinoin administration has resulted in alteration of lipid profiles in 25 percent of patients treated, including elevated triglyceride concentrations, a decrease in high-density lipoproteins (HDL) in 15 percent of patients, and hypercholesterolemia in 7 percent of patients. Alcohol consumption may potentiate serum triglyceride elevations. Lipid alterations occur most frequently at dosages greater than 1 mg/kg/day and are reversible upon discontinuation of **isotretinoin.**

Elevation of serum glucose and fasting serum blood glucose has been reported. Exacerbation of diabetes mellitus can occur. Decreases in hemoglobin and hematocrit concentrations have been reported in 10 to 20 percent of patients. Forty percent of patients prescribed **isotretinoin** may have increased sedimentation rates. Patients may also experience anemia and thrombocytopenia.

CNS effects include headache (5%), lethargy, and fatigue. **Isotretinoin** has also been associated with pseudotumor cerebri (benign increased intracranial pressure). Symptoms include headache, visual disturbances, and papilledema. In the postmarketing period, depression has been reported, as have psychosis and, rarely, suicidal indication. If patients report depression, immediate discontinuation of therapy is indicated. Depression appears to subside with discontinuation of therapy and to recur upon reinstitution of therapy.

Adverse GI reactions include anorexia, nausea and vomiting, increased appetite, and thirst. Eighty percent of patients report dry mouth when taking **isotretinoin**. Inflammatory bowel disease, including regional enteritis, may occur.

Musculoskeletal adverse effects such as arthralgia and myalgia are reported in approximately 16 percent of patients taking **isotretinoin**. Skeletal abnormalities have been reported in adults and children receiving excessive doses (greater than 2 mg/kg/day for prolonged periods, 6 months to 2 years). Musculoskeletal symptoms rarely persist after drug discontinuation.

Isotretinoin has been associated with rare cases of hepatitis. Transient increases in alkaline phosphates, lactate dehydrogenase, AST, ALT, GGTP, and LDH have been reported in 10 to 20 percent of patients. If elevated hepatic enzymes persist or if symptoms of hepatitis develop, **isotretinoin** should be discontinued.

Ophthalmic adverse effects including corneal opacification have been reported in patients receiving **isotretinoin** for acne. This ocular effect is reversible with complete resolution or continuing resolution at 6 to 7 weeks following discontinuation of therapy. Of patients taking **isotretinoin**, 25 percent report visual disturbances, including blurred vision, decreased visual acuity, tunnel vision, photophobia, and diplopia.

Isotretinoin may cause transient changes in urinalysis findings, with increased white cells in urine (10 to 20%), proteinuria, microscopic or gross hematuria (less than 10%), and nonspecific urogenital findings in 5 percent of patients. Less than 1 percent of patients have abnormal menses.

DRUG INTERACTIONS

Topical Retinoids and Topical Antibiotics. **Topical retinoids** should not be used concomitantly with other topical medications that have strong drying effects, such as **benzoyl peroxide, salicylic acid,** or **lactic acid** (Table 21–4). Medicated or abrasive soaps or cleaners should also be avoided because they can potentiate the skin irritation caused by **topical retinoids.** Products that contain alcohol, lime, menthol, spices, or perfumes can further dry and irritate the skin and should not be used with **topical retinoids.** Before **topical retinoids** are begun, the effects

of strong topical drying agents need to subside to prevent significant skin irritation. Patients using **tazarotene** should exercise caution with other medications causing photosensitization (**tetracycline**) because severe sunburn may occur. **Topical retinoids** should not be used in the same areas of skin at the same time as **benzoyl peroxide** or **topical antibiotics.** A physical incompatibility between the medications or a change in pH may reduce the efficacy of **topical retinoids** if used simultaneously. When used together for clinical effect, these medications should be used at different times of the day, such as morning and night, to minimize possible skin irritation. **Topical antibiotics** have fewer significant drug interactions than **systemic antibiotics. Benzoyl peroxide** can interact with **topical retinoids,** as noted previously. PABA sunscreens may transiently discolor the skin if used concurrently with **benzoyl peroxide.** All of the **topical antibiotics** may have possible additive irritation when used with other **topical acne agents** (especially abrasives or keratolytics). **Azelaic acid** has no known drug interactions.

Systemic Retinoids. Concomitant use of **isotretinoin** and other sources of vitamin A can potentiate the toxic effects of **isotretinoin. Alcohol** may also potentiate the toxic effects of **isotretinoin. Tetracycline** may increase the incidence of pseudotumor cerebri. Simultaneous use of **isotretinoin** and other drying agents, such as **benzoyl peroxide** or other medicated or abrasive soaps or alcohol-containing products, can potentiate the drying effects of **isotretinoin.** Ethanol can increase the hypertriglyceridemic effects of **isotretinoin.** Lipid determinations should be postponed for at least 36 hours after ethanol consumption.

CLINICAL USE AND DOSING

Acne Vulgaris. **Topical retinoids** are applied to the skin once daily (Table 21–5). A thin film of medication is applied after washing with a gentle cleaner, in the evening before retiring. Care should be taken to avoid the eyes, lips, and mucous membranes. It is recommended that the patients wait 20 to 30 minutes after cleaning before applying **tretinoin.** Patients should wash their hands immediately after applying **topical retinoids.**

Topical antibiotics are applied to affected acne areas twice daily in a thin film. Patients should wash their skin with a gentle cleanser and pat dry before applying. **Benzoyl peroxide** cleanser may be used for cleaning once or twice daily. Patients should wet the skin areas to be treated prior to administration, rinse thoroughly after cleaning, and pat dry. With other dosage forms of **benzoyl peroxide,** patients may gradually increase application to two or three times daily if tolerated. If bothersome or excessive dryness or peeling occurs, patients should reduce the number of applications per day. **Clindamycin** should be applied with a pledget to all of the affected areas twice daily. More than one pledget may be

Table 21–4. Drug Interactions: Selected Acne Medications

Drug	Interacting Drug	Possible Effect	Implications
Topical Acne Medications Retinoids • Adapalene	Benzoyl peroxide Salicylic acid Lactic acid Medicated or abrasive soaps or cleaners Products that contain alcohol, lime, menthol, spices, or perfumes	Increased skin irritation Potentiate the skin irritation caused by topical retinoids Dry and irritate the skin	Avoid concurrent use of topical medications that have strong drying effects, such as benzoyl peroxide, salicylic acid, or lactic acid Concurrent use should be avoided Should not be used with topical retinoids Before beginning adapalene, the effects of strong topical drying agents need to subside to prevent significant skin irritation
Tazarotene	Photosensitizers (tetracycline) Skin irritants (products that contain alcohol, lime, menthol, spices, or perfumes; medicated or abrasive soaps or cleaners)	Increased photosensitivity Potentiate the skin irritation caused by topical retinoids	Avoid concurrent use because severe sunburn may result Concurrent use should also be avoided Before beginning tazarotene, the effects of strong topical drying agents need to subside to prevent significant skin irritation
Tretinoin	Benzoyl peroxide and topical antibiotics Topical sulfur, resorcinol, benzoyl peroxide, or salicylic acid Abrasive soaps and cleansers Products that contain alcohol, lime, menthol, spices, or perfumes	A physical incompatibility between the medications or a change in pH may reduce the efficacy of topical retinoids if used simultaneously Potentiate the skin irritation caused by topical retinoids Increased skin irritation	Tretinoin should not be used in the same areas of skin at the same time as benzoyl peroxide or topical antibiotics; separate use in the same areas by many hours (A.M.-P.M. dosing) Concurrent use should be avoided
Topical antibiotics • Azelaic acid • Benzoyl peroxide	No known interactions Topical retinoids PABA-containing sunscreens Other topical acne agents	A physical incompatibility between the medications or a change in pH may reduce the efficacy of topical retinoids if used simultaneously May transiently discolor skin Additive irritant effects	Avoid use in the same area of skin at the same time Avoid concurrent use If using concurrently, observe for severe skin irritation
• Clindamycin • Erythromycin	Erythromycin Clindamycin Other topical acne agents (especially abrasives and keratolytics)	Antagonize each other Antagonize each other Additive irritant effects	Do not use concurrently Do not use concurrently Avoid concurrent use

Continued on next page

Table 21–4. Drug Interactions: Selected Acne Medications *(continued)*

Drug	Interacting Drug	Possible Effect	Implications
Metronidazole	Oral anticoagulants	May potentiate effects of anticoagulant	Drug interaction less likely with topical metronidazole use but should be kept in mind in concurrent use
Systemic Acne Medication Isotretinoin	Vitamin A	Potentiate the toxic effects of isotretinoin	Do not take concurrently
	Alcohol	Potentiate the toxic effects of isotretinoin	Avoid concurrent use
	Tetracycline	May increase incidents of pseudotumor cerebri	Avoid concurrent use
	Drying agents, such as benzoyl peroxide, or other medicated or abrasive soaps or alcohol-containing products	Can potentiate the drying effects of isotretinoin	Observe for skin irritation if using concurrently
	Ethanol	Can increase the hypertriglyceridemic effects of isotretinoin	Postpone lipid determinations for at least 36 h following ethanol consumption, if patients are taking isotretinoin
	Carbamazepine	Reduced carbamazepine levels with concurrent use	Monitor closely if using concurrently

used. Patients should remove the pledget from the foil just before use and discard after a single use. Patients should be instructed to wash their hands thoroughly after the use of any **topical antibiotic.**

Benzamycin, a product that combines **benzoyl peroxide** and **erythromycin** gel, is a unique product in that the medication is supplied in a package in which the two medications are separate and are mixed immediately prior to dispensing. This combination product forms a gel and should be stirred prior to application. **Benzamycin** should be stored in the refrigerator and expires 3 months after reconstitution. The product should not be allowed to freeze. Patients should apply **Benzamycin** to clean, dry skin twice daily. If irritation occurs, patients may decrease application to once daily. It must be pointed out that **Benzamycin** bleaches fabrics and hair, and care should be taken when handling this product.

Because of the severe adverse effects, **isotretinoin** is usually prescribed only by dermatologists. It must be stressed that, on account of the safety issues, primary care providers usually do not prescribe this medication.

Acne Rosacea.   The topical treatment of rosacea consists of application of topical **metronidazole. Metronidazole** 0.75 percent cream or gel (**MetroGel**) or 1 percent emollient cream (**Noritate**) is applied in a thin film twice a day after washing with a gentle cleanser. There may be some mild skin irritation associated with topical **metronidazole** use. Significant therapeutic results should be noticed within 3 weeks. Clinical studies have demonstrated continuing improvement through 9 weeks of therapy. Patients may use cosmetics after application of topical **metronidazole.** If irritation occurs, patients should reduce frequency, interrupt therapy, or discontinue use. Avoid getting **metronidazole** in the eyes.

RATIONAL DRUG SELECTION

Severity.   The choice of acne medications is generally dependent on the severity of the acne on presentation. Mild acne is generally treated with **benzoyl peroxide,** which is available by prescription and in OTC preparations. **Benzoyl peroxide** alone often treats mild acne. Mild to moderate acne may be treated with the combination of **benzoyl peroxide** and another **topical antibiotic** such as Benzamycin, which contains **benzoyl peroxide** and **erythromycin. Topical retinoids** are used for moderate to severe acne. In the treatment of moderate acne, a combination of **oral antibiotics** and either **topical antibiotics** or **topical retinoids** may be used. Hormonal therapy is indicated in mild to moderate acne (**Ortho-Tri-Cyclen**). **Isotretinoin** is used in the treatment of recalcitrant nodulocystic acne, with its use reserved for the most severe patients.

Table 21–5. Dosage Schedule: Selected Acne Medications

Drug	Indication	Dosage	Notes
Topical Acne Medications Retinoids			
• Adapalene	Acne vulgaris	Apply to affected acne areas once daily at bedtime after washing with gentle cleanser	
• Tazarotene (0.1%)	Mild to moderate facial acne vulgaris	Apply a thin film of tazarotene in the evening, after washing with a gentle cleaner	Avoid eyes, lips, and mucous membranes; patients should wash their hands immediately after applying medication; women of childbearing age should begin the medication during their normal menses
• Tretinoin	Acne vulgaris	Apply sparingly to affected acne areas once daily at bedtime; adjust frequency or strength as tolerated	Wait 20 to 30 min after cleaning with a gentle cleanser before applying tretinoin; patients should wash their hands immediately after applying medication
Topical antibiotics			
• Azelaic acid	Mild to moderate inflammatory acne vulgaris	Massage thin film into affected areas bid	Apply to clean, dry skin; wash hands after application; if persistent irritation occurs, may decrease dose to once daily
• Benzoyl peroxide	Mild to moderate acne vulgaris	Cleansers: wash affected areas once or twice daily Other forms: apply to affected acne areas once daily; may increase to 2–3 times daily if tolerated	Wet areas to be washed with benzoyl peroxide cleanser, cleanse, rinse well, then pat dry If excessive dryness or peeling occurs, patient should reduce the number of applications per day
• Benzoyl peroxide and erythromycin gel (Benzamycin)	Acne vulgaris	Apply to affected acne areas bid	Apply to clean, dry skin; may decrease application to once daily if excessive irritation occurs
• Clindamycin	Acne vulgaris	Apply thin film bid to affected acne areas Pledget: apply to all affected areas bid	Wash hands after applying medication More than one pledget may be used; remove the pledget from the foil just before use and discard after single use
• Erythromycin	Acne vulgaris	Apply a thin layer to affected acne areas bid	Wash hands after applying medication
• Metronidazole	Acne rosacea	Apply to affected areas bid	Wash hands after applying; improvement should be noted in 3 wk

Continued on next page

Table 21–5. Dosage Schedule: Selected Acne Medications *(continued)*

Drug	Indication	Dosage	Notes
Systemic Acne Medication Isotretinoin	Severe, recalcitrant nodulocystic acne, unresponsive to conventional therapy including systemic antibiotics	Initially: 0.5–1 mg/kg/d divided bid; severe acne may require 2 mg/kg/d; treatment continues for 15–20 wk; may discontinue if nodule count decreases by 70% before end of treatment	Isotretinoin is rarely prescribed by primary care providers; its use is usually reserved for specialty dermatology practice because of multiple adverse effects; on account of the extremely high risk of adverse outcomes in the fetus, including deformities and fetal death, written consent should be obtained from the childbearing-age female patient before prescribing isotretinoin; two reliable forms of contraception should be used by childbearing-age patients; monthly pregnancy testing before, during, and 1 mo after therapy is discontinued is required in female patients

Cost. The least expensive topical acne medications are **benzoyl peroxide**, which is available OTC, and topical **erythromycin** and **clindamycin**. Of the **retinoids**, the least expensive is **tretinoin**, at a cost of $10 to $20 for a 15-g tube. **Tazarotene** is quite expensive, with the cost of a 30-g tube ranging from $60 to $70. **Adapalene** costs approximately $20 to $30 for a 15-g tube. The cost of **isotretinoin** ranges from $100 to $500 per month, based on the dose prescribed.

MONITORING. There is no special laboratory monitoring required with the use of **topical antibiotics** or **topical retinoids**. The primary care provider may be involved in the monitoring of the patient who is started on **isotretinoin** by the dermatologist. Monitoring required for this patient includes baseline CBC, both baseline and monthly liver function tests throughout treatment, baseline and monthly pregnancy testing throughout treatment, and serum lipid profile. Serum electrolytes should be drawn as baseline and after 4 to 6 weeks of treatment. An ophthalmologic examination is also required for prescribing **isotretinoin**. If visual difficulties occur, an ophthalmologic examination is required, with a second exam 6 to 7 weeks after discontinuation of the medication.

PATIENT EDUCATION

Administration. When **retinoids** are applied topically, it should be explained that the increased turnover of follicular epithelial cells causes extrusion of comedones, even comedones that may not be seen on the skin surface. Clinically, this causes an initial worsening of acne, as comedones that were previously under the skin are extruded. This "worsening" of acne is not a reason for discontinuation of treatment, and patients should be reassured that the face will clear after approximately 6 to 8 weeks of treatment. The patient should also be instructed to use the medication as prescribed; there is no improved response to **topical retinoids** if they are used more often than recommended, but there is a dramatic increase in skin irritation (Table 21–6).

The manufacturer has developed an extensive patient education curriculum for the prescriber of **isotretinoin** to use with patients. This kit includes written and video information, as well as the consent forms that are required when treating patients with **isotretinoin**. It is recommended that any provider who is prescribing **isotretinoin** use this extensive curriculum prior to and during treatment.

Table 21–6. Available Dosage Forms: Selected Acne Medications

Drug	Dosage Form	How Supplied
TOPICAL ACNE MEDICATIONS		
Retinoids		
Adapalene (Rx)		
Differin	0.1% gel	In 15 and 45 g
	0.1% solution	In 30 mL with applicator
Tazarotene (0.1%) (Rx)		
Tazorac	0.1% aqueous gel	In 30 and 100 g
Tretinoin (Rx)		
• Avita	0.025% cream	In 20 and 45 g
	0.025% gel	In 20 and 45 g
• Retin-A	0.025%, 0.05%, 0.1% cream	In 20 and 40 g
	0.025%, 0.01% gel	In 15 and 45 g
	0.05% liquid	In 28 mL
• Retin-A Micro	0.1% aqueous gel in microspheres	In 20 and 40 g
Topical Antibiotics		
Azelaic acid (Rx)		
Azelex	20% cream	In 30 g
Benzoyl peroxide	2%, 5%, 10% cleansing solution	In 240 mL
• Benzac-AC Wash (Rx)	5%, 10% cleansing solution	In 120 and 240 mL
• Benzac-W Wash (Rx)	2.5% gel	In 60 and 90 g
• Benzac-AC 2½ (Rx)	5% gel	In 60 and 90 g
• Benzac-AC 5 (Rx)	10% gel	In 60 and 90 g
• Benzac-AC 10	2.5%, 5%, 10% aqueous gel	In 1.5 and 3 oz
• Benzac-W (Rx)	5%, 10% gel	In 60 and 90 g
• Benzagel (Rx)		
• Desquam-X 5 Wash (Rx)	5% cleansing solution	In 150 mL
• Desquam-X 10 Wash (Rx)	10% cleansing solution	In 150 mL
• Desquam-E (Rx)	2.5% gel (water based)	In 42.5 g
• Desquam E 5 (Rx)	5% gel (water based)	In 42.5 g
• Desquam-E 10 (Rx)	10% gel (water based)	In 42.5 g
• Desquam-X (Rx)	2.5% gel (water based)	In 42.5 g
• Desquam-X 5 (Rx)	5% gel (water based)	In 42.5 and 85 g
• Desquam-X 10 (Rx)	10% gel (water based)	In 42.5 and 85 g
• Dryox Wash 5 (OTC)	5% cleansing solution	In 240 mL
• Dryox Wash 10 (OTC)	10% cleansing solution	In 240 mL
• Dryox 2.5 (OTC)	2.5% gel	In 30 and 60 g
• Dryox 5 (OTC)	5% gel	In 30 and 60 g
• Dryox 10 (OTC)	10% gel	In 30 and 60 g
• Dryox 20 (OTC)	20% gel	In 30 and 60 g
• Oxy 10 Wash (OTC)	10% cleansing solution	In 120 mL
• Oxy 5 Advanced Formula for Sensitive Skin (OTC)	5% gel	In 30 g
• Oxy 10 Maximum Strength Advanced Formula (OTC)	10% gel	In 30 mg
• Fostex 10% Wash (OTC)	10% cleansing solution	
• Fostex Bar	10% bar	106 g

Continued on next page

Table 21–6. Available Dosage Forms: Selected Acne Medications *(continued)*

Drug	Dosage Form	How Supplied
Benzoyl peroxide Generic (OTC and Rx)	5% mask 10% lotion 5% gel 10% gel	In 30 mL In 30 mL In 45 g In 45 and 90 g
Benzoyl peroxide– erythromycin gel (Benzamycin) (Rx)	Erythromycin 3% and benzoyl peroxide 5% gel	In 23.3 and 46.6 g
Clindamycin (Rx) • Cleocin T	10 mg/mL gel 10 mg/mL lotion 10 mg/mL topical solution 1 mL solution/pad	In 7.5 and 30 g In 60 mL In 30 and 60 mL with applicator In 60s (pledgets)
• C/T/S	10 mg/mL solution	In 30 and 60 mL with applicator
• Generic	10 mg/mL gel 10 mg/mL lotion 10 mg/mL topical solution	In 30 g In 60 mL In 30 and 60 mL
Erythromycin (Rx) • A/T/S	2% solution 2% gel	In 60 mL In 30 g
• Emgel • Erygel • Erycette • T-Stat	2% gel 2% gel 2% saturated swabs 2% saturated swabs 2% solution	In 27 and 50 g In 5, 30, and 60 g 60 swabs 60 swabs In 60 mL, applicator optional
• Akne-Mycin • Generic	2% ointment 2% solution	In 25 g In 60 mL
Metronidazole (Rx) MetroGel	0.75% gel	In 28.4 g
SYSTEMIC ACNE MEDICATIONS		
Isotretinoin (Rx) Accutane	10-, 20-, 40-mg capsules	In 100s

Adverse Reactions. It is important to instruct patients that all **topical antibiotics** used in the treatment of acne may cause skin irritation to some degree. **Benzoyl peroxide** may cause excessive drying, photosensitivity, and allergic contact sensitization. **Tetracycline** may cause discoloration of the skin; patients should inform their provider immediately and discontinue the medication. **Azelaic acid** may cause skin hypopigmentation in patients with dark complexions. Patients should be instructed to notify their provider if this problem develops.

Isotretinoin has many significant adverse reactions, as previously described. Patients should be fully informed about these adverse reactions prior to beginning therapy and should have written information to refer to at home if any adverse effects occur.

Lifestyle Management. The nonpharmacological management of acne includes gentle facial cleansers such as mild soaps or facial washes. Scrubbing, picking, and squeezing of comedones should be avoided. Patients should be advised to use skin products that will not aggravate their acne. That includes oil-based cosmetics, hair spray, mousse, and facial creams and moisturizers. Sunscreens that are oil-free should be used at all times because of the increased photosensitivity due to acne preparations.

Topical Corticosteroids

Topical corticosteroids are adrenocorticosteroid derivatives incorporated into a vehicle suitable for application to the skin. The chemical structure is often modified to make them more lipid-soluble and to increase potency. Structural changes also decrease mineralocorticoids' effects.

Pharmacodynamics

The therapeutic effects of **topical corticosteroids** are due to their nonspecific anti-inflammatory effects. They act against most causes of inflammation, including mechanical, chemical, microbiologic, and immunologic. At the cellular level, they appear to inhibit the formation, release, and activity of endogenous mediators of inflammation, such as prostaglandins, kinins, histamine, liposomal enzymes, and the complement system. When applied to inflamed skin, **steroids** inhibit the migration of macrophages and leukocytes into the area by reversing vascular dilatation and permeability. This results in decreasing edema, erythema, and pruritus by suppressing DNA synthesis. **Corticosteroids** applied topically have an antimitotic effect on epidermal cells. This is its primary action in proliferative disorders such as psoriasis.

At the molecular level, unbound **corticosteroids** readily cross the cell membrane and bind with high affinity to specific cytoplasmic receptors. Inflammation is reduced by diminishing the release of leukocytic acid hydrolyses. **Corticosteroids** also prevent macrophage accumulation at inflamed sites. Interference with leukocyte adhesion to the capillary wall and reduction of capillary membrane permeability and subsequent edema also reduce inflammation.

Pharmacokinetics

ABSORPTION AND DISTRIBUTION. Absorption of **topical corticosteroids** varies, depending on the drug used, the vehicle used, the amount of skin surface area the medication is applied to, and the condition of the skin. Absorption is enhanced by increased skin temperature, hydration, and application to denuded areas, intertriginous areas, or skin surfaces with a thin stratum corneum layer (face or scrotum). Occlusive dressings enhance skin penetration and therefore increase drug absorption. Infants and children have more body surface area to body weight, and therefore proportionally more medication is absorbed into their system.

The penetration of **topical steroid** through the skin varies with the vehicle the medication is in. Ointments are more occlusive and therefore more potent. Creams are less occlusive and usually less potent. Lotions are usually the least potent. Gels, aerosols, lotions, and solutions are useful in hairy areas.

Occlusive dressings such as plastic wrap increase skin penetration approximately tenfold by increasing the moisture content of the stratum corneum. This may be beneficial in resistant cases but may also lead to increased adverse effects because increased absorption of the **corticosteroid** may produce systemic side effects. The relative potency of a product depends on several factors, including the characteristics and concentration of the drug, the vehicle used, and the vasoconstrictor assay. The vasoconstrictor assay is developed by applying an agent to skin under occlusion and assessing the area of skin blanching. Other assays of **steroid** potency involve suppression of erythema and edema following experimentally induced inflammation. **Corticosteroids** distribute into breast milk and cross the placenta.

METABOLISM AND EXCRETION. Following topical administration, **corticosteroids** enter the bloodstream and are metabolized and excreted via the same pathways as systemic steroids. **Corticosteroids** are metabolized in the liver, although some topical preparations are partially metabolized in the skin. Inactive metabolites, as well as a small portion of unchanged drug, are excreted in the urine.

Pharmacotherapeutics

PRECAUTIONS AND CONTRAINDICATIONS. **Corticosteroids** are contraindicated in any patient with a history of hypersensitivity to other **corticosteroids** or any ingredient in the preparation.

Corticosteroids are contraindicated as monotherapy in primary bacterial infections, treatment of rosacea, or acne vulgaris. Use of high-potency or very-high-potency agents on the face, groin, or axilla is contraindicated. Ophthalmic use should be reserved for specialty practice only, because prolonged ocular exposure may cause steroid induced glaucoma and cataracts. When applied to the eyelids or the skin near the eyes, the drug may enter the eyes.

Corticosteroids are Pregnancy Category C. *Corticosteroids* **are teratogenic in animals when administered systemically at relatively low dosages. There are no adequate and well-controlled studies of** *topical steroid* **use in pregnant women. Therefore, use during pregnancy only if the potential benefits outweigh the potential hazards to the fetus. In pregnant patients, do not use extensively.**

Systemic corticosteroids are excreted into breast milk in quantities not likely to have an adverse effect on the infant. Nevertheless, exercise caution when administering **topical steroids** to a nursing mother.

Children may be more susceptible to topical corticosteroids' effects because of their larger body surface area compared to weight. Therefore, in infants and young children, the lowest effective strength of **topical steroid** should be used to prevent systemic corticosteroid effects. Use of high-potency or very-high-potency agents should be avoided. Hypothalamic-pituitary-adrenal (HPA) axis suppression, Cushing's syndrome, and intracranial hypertension have been reported in children receiving **topical corticosteroids**. Chronic **corticosteroid** therapy in children may interfere with growth and development.

The normal inflammatory response to local infections may be masked by **topical corticosteroids.**

ADVERSE DRUG REACTIONS. Topical corticosteroid preparations may all cause localized skin irritation (pruritus, dryness, burning, and dermatitis). Use of **topical corticosteroids** also increases the risk for secondary infection due to immunosuppression. Other localized effects include acneiform rash, allergic contact dermatitis, folliculitis, hypertrichosis, miliaria, and maceration of the skin. Skin atrophy, hypopigmentation, striae, and xerosis may occur. Tolerance may occur with prolonged use of **topical corticosteroids.** Tolerance is reversible and may be prevented by interrupted or cyclic schedules of application for chronic dermatologic conditions.

Systemic absorption may produce reversible HPA axis suppression, Cushing's syndrome, hyperglycemia, and glycosuria. They are more likely to occur with occlusive dressings and with more potent steroid preparations. Patients with liver failure or children may be at higher risk for systemic steroid effects.

Following prolonged application of **topical corticosteroid** around the eyes, cataracts and glaucoma may develop.

Changing to a less potent **topical corticosteroid** preparation may minimize the risk of adverse reactions.

DRUG INTERACTIONS. There are no significant drug interactions noted with **topical corticosteroid** use.

CLINICAL USE AND DOSING

Inflammatory Skin Diseases. **Topical corticosteroids** are used for numerous inflammatory or pruritic dermatoses. Some of the conditions for which **topical corticosteroids** have been proved effective are contact dermatitis, atopic dermatitis, nummular eczema, lichen planus, lichen simplex chronicus, insect bite reactions, discoid lupus erythematosus, and seborrheic dermatitis. Low-dose **topical corticosteroid** may also be used in the treatment of first- and second-degree localized burns and sunburns. The usual dose of a **topical corticosteroid** is to apply it sparingly to affected areas two to four times per day (Table 21–7). **Topical corticosteroids** have a repository effect; with continuous use, one or two applications per day may be as effective as three or more. One dosing schedule that may be used is to apply the medication twice daily until clinical response is achieved, and then only as frequently as needed to control symptoms.

Another dosing schedule that may be used to achieve therapeutic response with fewer adverse effects is short-term or intermittent therapy with high-potency agents for a short period (3 or 4 consecutive days per week or once per week). This may be more effective and cause fewer adverse effects than continuous use of lower potency products.

It must be stressed that **topical corticosteroids** should not be abruptly discontinued. After long-term use or after using a high-potency agent, a rebound effect may occur. To prevent a rebound effect, switch to a less potent agent or alternate **topical corticosteroids** and emollient products.

In children, low-potency agents should be used. Low-potency **topical corticosteroids** should also be used on body sites with a thinner stratum corneum layer (face, scrotum, axilla, and skin folds). If treating large surface areas, a lower-potency agent should be used. Higher-potency agents should be used for areas such as the palms and soles, which are more resistant to treatment. Higher-potency agents are also used for crusting and thickened conditions, which are also more resistant to treatment.

Treatment with very-high-potency **topical corticosteroids** should not exceed 2 consecutive weeks. The total dosage should not exceed 50 g/week because of potential HPA axis suppression.

To increase absorption of **corticosteroids**, occlusive dressings may be used. The technique for properly using occlusive dressings is as follows: First, the area must be soaked in water and gently washed. While the skin is still moist, the medication is gently rubbed into the affected area. The area is then covered with plastic wrap. For hands, a plastic glove may be used; for feet a plastic bag may be used; or a shower cap may be used for the scalp. After the plastic is applied, the edges should be sealed with tape to ensure that the wrap adheres closely to the skin. Do not use for more than 12 hours in a 24-hour period. This technique should not be used with very-high-potency **topical corticosteroids.**

Psoriasis. **Topical corticosteroids** are used to treat psoriasis because of their anti-inflammatory effects on the plaques. Moderate- to high-potency steroids are used because the psoriasis lesions are generally steroid-resistant. Occlusion with plastic may be necessary for best results. The **steroid** cream or ointment is applied two to three times per day. Intermittent or "pulse" therapy minimizes some of the adverse effects and has the best long-term outcome. If using **topical corticosteroids** in the intertriginous areas or on the face, a low-dose medication should be chosen. Regardless of the **topical corticosteroid** preparation, 3 weeks of continuous use is the limit, and patients should be discouraged from using steroids for longer periods. **Topical corticosteroids** should be reserved for psoriasis flare, with other medications used for ongoing therapy.

RATIONAL DRUG SELECTION

Potency. The choice of **steroid** based on potency is determined by the area of skin to be treated, the condition of the area, and the patient's condition. (Table 21–8). In general, low- to mid-potency **topical corticosteroids** are used on children. On the face or other areas with thin skin, low-

Table 21–7. Dosage Schedule: Selected Topical Corticosteroids

Drug	Dosage	Notes
Low Potency		
Hydrocortisone 1% or 2.5%	Apply a thin layer 2–4 times daily	May be used in children
Triamcinolone acetonide 0.025%	Apply a thin layer 3–4 times daily	May be used in children
Intermediate Potency		
Hydrocortisone valerate 0.2%	Apply a thin layer 2–3 times daily	Should be used with caution on face; use lower potency on face
Triamcinolone acetonide 0.1%	Apply a thin layer 3–4 times daily	Should be used with caution on the face; choose lower potency for face
Betamethasone valerate 0.12%	Apply a small amount of foam bid; massage into affected areas until foam disappears	Dispense a small amount of foam onto a clean plate or other cool surface (not on the hand)
Desoximetasone 0.05%	Apply thin film and massage in bid	Not recommended for use in children <10 y
Mometaxone furoate 0.1%	Apply thin film once daily	Do not occlude
High Potency		
Betamethasone dipropionate, augmented 0.05% (cream or lotion)	Apply thin film 1–2 times/d until clear; maximum of 45 g of cream or 50 mL of lotion/wk	Avoid abrupt cessation if used for chronic conditions; not recommended in children
Triamcinolone acetonide 0.5% (Aristocort, Kenalog)	Apply sparingly to affected area 2–3 times daily until clear	Avoid abrupt cessation if used for chronic condition; use with caution and sparingly in children
Halcinonide 0.1%	Apply sparingly 2–3 times/d	Avoid abrupt cessation if used for chronic condition; use with caution and sparingly in children
Super-High Potency		
Betamethasone dipropionate, augmented 0.05% (ointment or gel)	Apply thin film 1–2 times daily	Maximum of 45 g/wk; do not occlude
Clobetasol propionate 0.05%	Apply thin layer and rub in gently bid	Maximum of 50 g/wk and maximum therapy length 2 wk; doses as low as 2 g/d may cause HPA axis suppression
Flurandrenolide 4-μg/cm² tape	Apply tape to clean, dry skin every 12 h	Do not use tape with intertrigo or serum-exuding lesions

potency agents should be used. High-potency agents may be used for brief periods, up to 2 weeks, in areas that are resistant to lower-potency treatment. There are many available **topical steroid** preparations, and it is impossible for any practitioner to be familiar with all of them. It is reasonable for the practitioner to be familiar with one or two agents in each potency category. Each provider needs to be familiar with what medications are allowed from each category in the formulary they are using.

Vehicle. The vehicle used may increase or decrease the potency of the **corticosteroid**. As previously mentioned,

ointments are more occlusive and are effective for dry or scaly lesions. Creams may be used more frequently on oozing lesions on intertriginous areas, where the occlusive effects of ointments may cause increased adverse effects. Gels, aerosols, lotions, and solutions are used on hairy areas. The urea that is added to some products may enhance the penetration of **hydrocortisone** and other **steroids** by hydrating the skin. **Steroid**-impregnated tape (**Cordran**) is useful for occlusive therapy in small areas.

Cost. In general, lower-potency and generic products are less expensive than higher-potency and name-brand prod-

Table 21–8. Available Dosage Forms: Topical Corticosteroids

Drug	Potency	Dosage Form	How Supplied
Alclometasone dipropionate Aclovate	Low	0.05% ointment and cream	In 15, 45, and 60 g
Amcinonide Cyclocort	High	0.1% ointment, cream 0.1% lotion	In 15, 30, and 60 g In 20 and 60 mL
Augmented betamethasone dipropionate	High	0.05% emollient cream 0.05% lotion	In 15 and 45 g In 30 and 60 mL
Diprolene	Super high	0.05% ointment and gel	In 15 and 45 g
Betamethasone dipropionate • Diprosone • Generic	High Intermediate High Intermediate	0.05% cream and ointment 0.05% lotion 0.05% cream and ointment 0.05% lotion	In 15 and 45 g In 20 and 60 mL In 15 and 45 g In 20 and 60 mL
Betamethasone valerate • Luxiq • Valisone • Generic	Intermediate High Intermediate High Intermediate	0.12% foam 0.1% ointment 0.1% cream 0.1% ointment 0.1% cream	In 100 g In 15 and 45 g In 15 and 45 g In 15 and 45 g In 15 and 45 g
Clobetasol propionate Temovate	Super high	0.05% ointment, gel 0.05% scalp application	In 15, 30, and 45 g In 25 and 50 mL
Clocortolone pivalate Cloderm	Intermediate	0.1% cream	In 15 and 45 g
Desonide • DesOwen • Tridesilon	Intermediate Intermediate	0.05% cream, ointment 0.05% lotion 0.05% cream, ointment	In 15 and 60 g In 60 and 120 mL In 15 and 60 g
Desoximetasone • Topicort • Topicort-LP	High Intermediate	0.05% gel 0.25% cream, ointment 0.05% cream	In 15 and 60 g In 15 and 60 g In 15 and 60 g
Dexamethasone Decaspray	Low	0.04% spray	In 25 g
Dexamethasone sodium phosphate Decadron phosphate	Low	0.1% cream	In 15 and 30 g
Diflorasone diacetate Psorcon	High	0.05% emollient cream and ointment 0.05% cream	In 15, 30, and 60 g In 15, 30, and 60 g
Psorcon	Super high	0.05% gel	In 15, 30, and 60 g
Fluocinolone acetonide Synalar	Intermediate	0.025% cream	In 15 and 60 g
Fluocinonide • Lidex • Lidex-E	High High	0.05% cream, ointment, gel 0.05% solution 0.05% emollient cream	In 15, 30, and 60 g In 20 and 60 mL In 15, 30, and 60 g

Continued on next page

Table 21–8. Available Dosage Forms: Topical Corticosteroids *(continued)*

Drug	Potency	Dosage Form	How Supplied
Flurandrenolide Cordran	Super high	4-μg/cm^2 tape	Rolls: 3 in × 24 in, 3 in × 80 in Patch 2 in × 3 in: In 12s
Fluticasone propionate Cutivate	Intermediate	0.05% cream 0.005% ointment	In 15, 30, and 60 g In 15 and 60 g
Halcinonide • Halog-E • Halog	High High	0.1% emollient cream 0.1% cream, ointment 0.1% solution	In 15, 30, and 60 g In 15, 30, and 60 g In 20 and 60 mL
Halobetasol propionate • Ultravate	Super high	0.05% cream, ointment	In 15 and 45 g
Hydrocortisone • Hytone • Cortisone 10 (OTC) • Cortisone 5 (OTC) • Generic	Low Low Low	1% cream, ointment 1% lotion 2.5% cream, ointment 2.5% lotion 1% cream, ointment 0.5% cream 1% cream, ointment 2.5% cream, ointment	In 30 and 120 g In 120 mL In 30 and 60 g In 60 mL In 30 g In 60 g In 20, 30, and 120 g, 1 lb In 20, 30, and 120 g, 1 lb
Hydrocortisone acetate • Maximum Strength Cortaid (OTC)	Low	1% cream, ointment	In 15 and 30 g
Hydrocortisone butyrate • Locoid	Intermediate	0.1% ointment, cream 0.1% solution	In 15 and 45 g In 20 and 60 mL
Hydrocortisone valerate • Westcort	Intermediate	0.2% cream or ointment	In 15, 45, and 60 g
Mometasone furoate • Elocon	Intermediate	0.1% ointment, cream 0.1% lotion	In 15 and 45 g In 27.5 and 55 mL
Triamcinolone acetonide • Aristocort • Kenalog • Generic	Low Intermediate High Low Intermediate High Low Intermediate High	0.025% cream, ointment 0.1% cream, ointment 0.5% cream 0.025% cream, ointment 0.025% lotion 0.1% cream 0.1% lotion 0.2% aerosol 0.5% cream 0.025% cream, ointment 0.1% cream, ointment 0.5% cream	In 15 and 60 g, 1 lb In 15, 60, and 240 g In 15 and 240 g In 15, 80, and 240 g In 60 mL In 15, 60, 80, and 240 g In 60 mL In 23 and 63 g In 20 g In 15, 80, and 454 g In 15 and 80 g, 1 lb In 15 g

ucts, although this difference may be offset by increased efficacy in short-term burst therapy with some dermatoses. Therefore, cost must be evaluated, and the practitioner must determine whether it will be a part of the drug-selection process. Cost must also come into effect when pre-

scribing off-formulary. If possible, prescribe medications that will be covered by the patient's insurance.

MONITORING. Adrenal function should be monitored in children if a high-potency **steroid** or an occlusion is used. Adrenal function should also be assessed in adults who are applying more than 50 g weekly of a high-potency **steroid** preparation. Growth should be monitored in children who are using mid- or high-potency **topical corticosteroids.** The patient should also be monitored for adverse effects, as noted previously. Laboratory studies that should be obtained for patients on high-dose **steroids** are blood glucose and serum potassium levels.

PATIENT EDUCATION

Administration. The patient should be instructed to use the **topical corticosteroid** *exactly* as prescribed. Demonstration of the amount of medication that should be applied will be helpful for most patients. The provider can use a sample-size dose in the area to be treated to show the amount of medication to use. Demonstrate applying a pea-sized amount of **topical corticosteroids** and spreading it thinly over the affected area. The patient should also understand the serious adverse effects that may occur with overuse of **topical corticosteroids.** If mid- or high-potency **topical steroids** are prescribed, the patient must understand that these medications are much stronger than, for example, **hydrocortisone** 1 percent cream, and that these medications therefore have more significant adverse effects associated with them if they are not used appropriately. If occlusion is to be used, clear directions regarding it need to be provided to the patient, preferably in writing.

Adverse Reactions. The patient should have written information regarding the adverse effects that may occur with overuse of **corticosteroids.** Patients should report any adverse effects, including worsening of their condition. When prescribing **topical corticosteroids** to children, the provider must clearly outline the course of treatment for the parent. If mid-potency **steroids** are used in children, the parent should understand the concern about growth in children. Patients should also be instructed not to abruptly discontinue their **topical steroid** medications, which also may cause adverse effects.

Lifestyle Management. Patients who are using **topical corticosteroids** often can benefit from nonpharmacological management. Many conditions require the use of moisturizers or emollients to provide optimal outcome in the disease process. Patients should be encouraged to use these nonpharmacological measures, in addition to the prescribed **topical corticosteroid,** to have the most optimal management of their skin condition. Bathing may improve the outcome with some skin conditions, but this must be individualized based on the patient and the condition.

Topical Antipsoriasis Agents

The management of psoriasis consists of topical medication and phototherapy for mild to moderate psoriasis (less than 20% of the body involved) and for severe psoriasis (more than 20% of the body involved) the addition of systemic medications. Patients with severe disease are usually referred to a dermatologist, and therefore systemic treatment is not covered in this chapter.

Topical therapy for psoriasis consists of **topical steroids, tar** or **keratolytic shampoos** for scalp involvement, and **keratolytic agents** (**anthralin** and **calcipotriene**) for thick plaques, applied topically.

Pharmacodynamics

Calcipotriene, a vitamin D_3 derivative, regulates cell differentiation and proliferation and suppresses lymphocyte activity. In humans, the natural supply of vitamin D depends mainly on exposure to the ultraviolet rays of the sun for conversion of 7-dehydrocholesterol to vitamin D_3 in the skin. After entering the bloodstream, it is metabolized in the liver and kidneys to its active vitamin D form. Vitamin D_3 receptors occur in many parts of the body, including the skin cells known as keratinocytes. **Calcipotriene** has a similar affinity for the vitamin D receptor in the keratinocyte.

Anthralin is an antimitotic agent that is used for chronic psoriasis. It has an antiproliferative effect. The mechanism for the antipsoriasis effect of **anthralin** is unknown, but it inhibits cellular respiration by inactivation of mitochondria.

Coal tar affects psoriasis by enzyme inhibition and antimitotic action. It is manufactured as a by-product of the processing of coke and gas from bituminous coal and is extremely complex, rich in polycyclic hydrocarbons, and variable in composition. Little is known about its mechanism of action. It is used mainly in combination with ultraviolet B (UVB) for this indication.

Tazarotene is a **topical retinoid** prodrug that is used in the treatment of psoriasis. The exact mechanism of action is unclear at this time. Following topical application, **tazarotene** undergoes esterase hydrolysis to the active form, AGN 190299, which is the cognate carboxylic acid of **tazarotene.** It is believed that the drug works by normalizing epidermal differentiation, reducing hyperproliferation, and reducing the influx of inflammatory cells into the skin.

Pharmacokinetics

ABSORPTION AND DISTRIBUTION. Approximately 6 percent of **calcipotriene** is absorbed systemically when it is applied topically to psoriasis plaques. Distribution of **calcipotriene** is unknown. There is evidence that **calcipotriene** does cross the placenta. It is not known whether **calcipotriene** is excreted in breast milk.

Absorption and distribution of **anthralin** are unknown, as is the absorption of coal tar.

Tazarotene, when administered topically to the skin, has minimal systemic absorption because of its rapid metabolism in the skin to the active metabolite, tazarotenic acid, which is systemically absorbed and further metabolized. There is no apparent accumulation of **tazarotene** within body tissues. **Retinoids** may cross the placenta, and therefore it is assumed that **tazarotene** is also harmful to the fetus. It is not known if **tazarotene** is distributed into human breast milk; however, animal studies show that single topical doses of radiolabeled **tazarotene** are detected in maternal milk.

METABOLISM AND EXCRETION.   Approximately 6 percent of a topical dose of **calcipotriene** is systemically absorbed when it is applied to psoriatic skin. Once absorbed, **calcipotriene** is rapidly and extensively metabolized in the liver into inactive metabolites. **Calcipotriene** is excreted in the bile.

Tazarotene is rapidly metabolized in the skin to the active metabolite, tazarotenic acid, which is absorbed and further metabolized. Tazarotenic acid is hydrophilic and quickly metabolized systemically. It is more than 99 percent plasma protein–bound. Metabolism of **tazarotene** to tazarotenic acid occurs via esterase hydrolysis in the skin. After systemic absorption, it is hepatically metabolized to sulfoxides, sulfones, and other metabolites. Elimination is via the fecal and renal routes.

The metabolism and excretion are unknown for **anthralin** and **coal tar**.

Pharmacotherapeutics

PRECAUTIONS AND CONTRAINDICATIONS.   **Calcipotriene** should not be prescribed to any patients with pre-existing hypercalcemia or evidence of vitamin D toxicity. It should also not be used in any patient with hypercalciuria, as this may increase renal calculi formation. **Calcipotriene** should not be applied to the face, as there have been several reports of facial dermatitis following application of this drug to the face. **Calcipotriene** is contraindicated in any patient with known hypersensitivity to any components of the preparation.

The safety and efficacy of **calcipotriene** in children have not been established. Children are at a greater risk of developing systemic adverse effects. **Calcipotriene** should be used cautiously in the elderly because patients over age 65 have significantly more severe skin-related reactions than younger patients treated with topical medication.

Calcipotriene is classified as Pregnancy Category C. **Calcipotriene** should be avoided during breastfeeding because adverse effects on the nursing infant may occur.

Anthralin is contraindicated in any patient with known hypersensitivity to **anthralin** or any component of the product. It should not be used on the face. Use of **anthralin** on acutely or actively inflamed psoriasis eruptions is contraindicated.

Coal tar preparations should not be applied to abraded skin. They should also be avoided on skin that is inflamed, broken, or infected because exacerbation of the condition can occur and systemic absorption of the drug can be increased. Sunlight (UV) exposure should be avoided for at least 24 hours after application of **coal tar** products unless patients are otherwise directed by their care provider. Exposure to sunlight causes a photosensitivity reaction. *Coal tar* **is classified as Pregnancy Category C. It is not known what effects** *coal tar* **may have on the fetus.** Whether **coal tar** is distributed into breast milk is unknown, although it is advised that **coal tar** should be used by lactating women only when clearly needed.

Tazarotene should not be used on eczematous skin because it may cause severe irritation and worsen eczema.

Tazarotene should be used cautiously in patients with known **retinoid** hypersensitivity reactions. Exposure to sunlight should be avoided, as well as UV exposure (including sun lamps). Patients must be warned of their increased photosensitivity and their increased potential for sunburn while using **tazarotene**. *Tazarotene* **is classified as Pregnancy Category X and is contraindicated in women who are pregnant or may be considering pregnancy. Adequate pregnancy prevention is essential when childbearing-age women are prescribed** *tazarotene*. It is not known if **tazarotene** is distributed into human breast milk; however, it should be used cautiously for breastfeeding women. The safety and efficacy of **tazarotene** in children under age 12 have not been established.

ADVERSE DRUG REACTIONS.   The most common reactions reported by patients using topical **calcipotriene** are skin irritation, burning, and pruritus, which affect up to 20 percent of patients during therapy. One to ten percent of patients report erythema, xerosis, and exfoliative dermatitis. There are also rare reports of allergic contact dermatitis. Hypercalcemia and hypercalciuria occur almost exclusively when the recommended dosage of 100 g/week is exceeded. A significant increase in urine calcium is seen when **calcipotriene** is administered at the maximum weekly dose (100 g/week) for 4 weeks.

The most significant adverse reaction noted in the use of **anthralin** is staining and discoloration of the uninvolved skin. Skin irritation is also noted. Permanent staining of clothes and bathroom fixtures may occur.

Coal tar may stain hair or fabrics. Excessive or long-term use may cause folliculitis, sensitization, and photosensitivity.

The most commonly reported adverse reactions from **tazarotene** topical use are burning, stinging, xerosis, and erythema. Worsening of psoriasis may occur. Skin irritation and skin pain may also develop. Reactions reported in fewer than 10 percent of patients include rash, desquamation, irritant contact dermatitis, and skin inflammation. Photosensitivity may occur with **tazarotene**.

DRUG INTERACTIONS.   No drug interactions with **calcipotriene** have been reported (Table 21–9). However, concurrent administration of high-dose **calcipotriene**

Table 21–9. Drug Interactions: Selected Psoriasis Medications

Drug	Interacting Drug	Possible Effect	Implications
Anthralin	Topical corticosteroids	Long-term use of corticosteroids may destabilize psoriasis, and withdrawal may cause rebound phenomenon	A withdrawal period of 1 wk from topical corticosteroid is necessary before beginning therapy with anthralin.
Calcipotriene	Agent that may cause hypercalcemia: vitamin D, vitamin D analogues, calcium supplements	Concurrent administration of *high-dose* calcipotriene may produce hypercalcemia	Avoid using large doses of calcipotriene in patients taking vitamin D analogues or calcium supplements.
Coal tar products	Tetracycline	Increased photosensitivity	Avoid concurrent use.
	Psoralens	Increased photosensitivity, severe sunburn	Avoid concurrent use.
	Topical retinoids	Increased photosensitivity	Avoid concurrent use.
Tazarotene	Photosensitizers (tetracycline)	Increased photosensitivity	Avoid concurrent use; severe sunburn may result.
	Skin irritants (products that contain alcohol, lime, menthol, spices, or perfumes; medicated or abrasive soaps or cleaners)	Potentiates the skin irritation caused by topical retinoids	Concurrent use should also be avoided.

with other agents may produce hypercalcemia. Those agents include vitamin D or vitamin D analogues or **calcium** supplements. Avoid prescribing large doses of **calcipotriene** to patients taking vitamin D analogues or **calcium** supplements.

Anthralin may not be used concurrently with **topical corticosteroid**. A withdrawal period of 1 week from **topical corticosteroid** is necessary before beginning therapy with **anthralin**.

Coal tar preparations may interact with **tetracycline**, psoralens, and **topical retinoids**, and concomitant use should be avoided.

Concomitant use of **tazarotene** and other topical medications that have strong drying effects, such as **benzoyl peroxide, salicylic acid** or sulfur preparations, should be avoided. The manufacturer suggests that a patient's skin "rest" until the effects of such preparations subside before using **tazarotene**.

CLINICAL USE AND DOSING
Psoriasis. **Calcipotriene** is applied in a thin film to the affected psoriasis plaques and rubbed into the skin gently and completely (Table 21–10). In adults, the ointment is applied twice daily in the morning and evening. It is important that the patient does not exceed 100 g/week of **calcipotriene** applied to the skin. Safety and efficacy in children have not been established. For the treatment of mild to moderate scalp psoriasis, the patient applies the topical solution twice daily. Improvement

will be noted as soon as 1 to 2 weeks after treatment has begun. The patient should be reevaluated after 6 to 8 weeks.

When prescribing **anthralin** to a patient who has never used the medication, use a low-concentration product (0.1%). The medication is applied to the psoriatic lesions and rubbed gently until the medication is absorbed. Take care not to get the **anthralin** on the healthy surrounding skin. It is important not to apply excessive medication, which increases the staining of skin and clothes. After the medication is rubbed in, it is left on 10 to 20 minutes, then washed off in the shower. After 1 week, the length of time the medication is in contact with the skin can be increased to 15 to 20 minutes. The strength of **anthralin** can be increased in increments (0.25%, 0.5%, 1%) as tolerated. Some patients require the medication to be applied and left on for 60 minutes to have improvement in their psoriatic lesions. Treatment should be continued until the lesions are completely healed (when nothing is felt with the fingers and the texture of the skin is completely normal).

There are a variety of **tar** preparations, including creams, shampoos, ointments, lotions, gels, and oils. The **tar** preparation is applied to the affected psoriatic lesions once or twice daily. For cream or ointment preparations, the patient should apply enough to cover the affected area and rub in gently. Shampoo should be applied to wet hair, massaged in, and then rinsed. The application is then repeated and left on for 5 minutes.

Table 21–10. Dosage Schedule: Topical Psoriasis Medications

Drug	Dosage	Notes
Anthralin	Begin with 0.1% strength. Apply a small amount to psoriasis lesions and rub in gently, avoiding healthy surrounding skin. Leave on for 10 min and wash off thoroughly. After 1 wk, contact time can be increased to 15–20 min. Increase strength of medication in incremental steps. Scalp cream should be applied to scalp after combing hair to remove scale. Leave on for 10–20 min and rinse well. Begin with 0.25% strength and use daily for at least 1 wk. Increase strength if needed.	Anthralin may stain skin and clothes. May alternate anthralin with other therapies (retinoids, topical steroids, UV light). Discontinue when lesions are healed and skin looks and feels normal.
Calcipotriene	Apply bid to affected area; rub in gently and completely. Treat for 6–8 wk.	Improvement is usually noted after 1 to 2 wk.
Coal tar products	Cream or ointment preparations: Apply enough to cover the affected area and rub in gently, once or twice daily. Shampoo: Apply to wet hair, massage in, and rinse; repeat application and leave on for 5 min. Rinse thoroughly after application. Cleansing bar or gel formulas: Apply to the affected area, rub in gently, leave on for 5 min, and then remove excess. Coal tar solution: May be used full strength or diluted in 3 parts water and applied to a cotton or gauze pad, then massaged gently into the affected area. Baths: The solution may also be used as a bath by adding 4 to 6 tbsp coal tar solution to a tub of lukewarm water. The patient should be immersed into the bath to soak for 10–20 min. Bathing should be performed once daily to once every 3 d; the usual duration of therapy is 30–45 d. The patient must rinse skin thoroughly after a coal tar bath if exposure to UV or sunlight is to follow.	All products are staining.
Tazarotene	The 0.05% or 0.1% gel is applied in a thin film once daily, in the evening, to psoriatic lesions.	Apply to clean, dry skin. No more than 20% of body surface area should be covered.

The shampoo should be rinsed out thoroughly after application. The cleansing bar or gel formulas should be applied to the affected area, rubbed in gently, and left on for 5 minutes; then the excess is removed. **Coal tar** solution may be used full strength or diluted in three parts water, applied to a cotton or gauze pad, and then massaged gently into the affected area. The solution may also be used as a bath by adding 4 to 6 tablespoons of **coal tar** solution to a tub of lukewarm water. The patient should be immersed into the bath to soak for 10 to 20 minutes. Bathing should be performed once daily to once every 3 days; the usual duration of therapy is 30 to 45 days. Patients must rinse their skin thoroughly after a **coal tar** bath if exposure to UV or sunlight is to follow.

Tazarotene should be applied to clean, dry skin. The 0.05 percent or 0.1 percent gel is applied once daily in the evening to psoriatic lesions. The patient should use enough to cover only the lesions with a thin film. No more than 20 percent of body surface area should be covered. Because unaffected skin may be more susceptible to irritation, avoid application of **tazarotene** to these areas. **Tazarotene** was investigated for up to 12 months during clinical trials for psoriasis.

RATIONAL DRUG SELECTION

Potency. With multiple medications available for treatment of psoriasis, the provider must decide which medication provides the most improvement to psoriatic lesions without severe adverse effects (Table 21–11). Response to **antipsoriatic medications** is highly individualized; therefore, different medications may be needed for similar presentation of psoriasis.

Table 21–11. Available Dosage Forms: Selected Psoriasis Medications

Drug	Dosage Form	How Supplied
Anthralin (Rx)		
• Drithrocreme	0.1%, 0.25%, 0.5%, 1% cream	In 50 g
• Drithro-Scalp	0.25%, 0.5% scalp cream	In 50 g
• Lasan	0.4% ointment	In 60 g
	0.1%, 0.2%, 0.4%, 1% cream	In 65 g
Calcipotriene (Rx)		
Dovonex	0.005% ointment, cream	In 30, 60, and 100 g
	0.005% solution	In 50 mL
Coal tar products (OTC)		
• Zetar	30% coal tar emulsion	In 177 mL and 6 oz
	1% shampoo	In 6 oz
• Medotar	1% coal tar ointment	In 480 g
• MG217 Medicated	2% coal tar ointment	In 108 and 480 g
• Fototar	2% cream	In 85 and 480 g
• MG217 Dual Treatment	5% coal tar lotion	In 120 mL
• Tegrin for Psoriasis	5% coal tar lotion	In 177 mL
• Oxipor VHC	48.5% coal tar lotion	In 57 and 118 mL
• Various generic	20% coal tar	In 120 mL, pint, and gal
Tazarotene		
Tazorac	0.05%, 0.1% gel	In 30 and 100 g

Vehicle. The patient's clinical presentation often determines which **antipsoriatic** medication should be first used. Large surface areas may respond to bath emulsions of **coal tar** solutions, where large surface areas can be treated. For scalp psoriasis, **coal tar** shampoo may be used or **anthralin** cream applied to the scalp. **Anthralin** can be irritating to the skin at higher strengths; therefore, lower-strength products should be begun, and the strength increased in increments.

Cost. Of the psoriasis medications, **coal tar** and **topical corticosteroid** are the least expensive. **Anthralin** is quite expensive.

MONITORING. The patient who is being treated for psoriasis should be monitored for the effectiveness of therapy and for adverse effects of the medication. There is no laboratory monitoring required unless treatment levels of **calcipotriene** approach 100 g/week. At that point, serum and urine calcium should be measured to determine the patient's risk for hypercalcemia or hypercalciuria.

PATIENT EDUCATION
Administration. Patients should be instructed to use their psoriasis medications exactly as prescribed. Medications such as **coal tar** or **anthralin** may cause staining or discoloration of the skin, especially if not used correctly. Use of **tazarotene** on healthy skin increases adverse reaction. The patient should be advised to not increase the number of doses per day, which increases adverse effects.

Adverse Reactions. The patient should be instructed that **anthralin** may stain skin, bathroom fixtures, and clothes. Proper application of topical medications will not only optimize treatment but also decrease the adverse effects of the medication. The provider should review the use of medication prior to any change in therapy. Some psoriasis medications cause photosensitivity; therefore, the patient should be instructed to apply sunscreen or avoid sun exposure during therapy.

Topical Antiseborrheic Medications

The mainstay of treatment for seborrheic dermatitis is topical **antiseborrheic** shampoos, with **topical steroid** preparations used for nonhairy areas such as the face. **Selenium sulfide** and **pyrithione zinc** shampoos are commonly used. Tar shampoo is another therapy choice. **Sulfacetamide sodium** is available in lotion form and in combination with other **antiseborrheic** medications, in many formulations.

Pharmacodynamics

Seborrhea is an inflammatory dermatitis that produces erythematous patches and scales. **Selenium sulfide (Selsun)** appears to have a cytostatic effect on the cells of the epidermis and follicular epithelium, leading to reduced corneocyte production. **Pyrithione zinc (Head & Shoulders)** is a cytostatic agent that reduces the cell turnover rate. Its mechanism of action is thought to be a nonspecific toxic effect on the epidermal cells. **Tar derivatives** treat seborrhea by correcting abnormal keratinization and by decreasing epidermal proliferation and dermal infiltration. **Tar derivatives** also decrease pruritus. **Ketoconazole** shampoo (**Nizoral**) may be active against dandruff and seborrheic dermatitis because of reductions of *P. ovale*. **Sulfacetamide sodium (Sebizon)** is an **antibacterial** agent that exerts a bacteriostatic effect against gram-positive and gram-negative microorganisms, which are the common organisms isolated from secondary cutaneous infections.

Pharmacokinetics

ABSORPTION AND DISTRIBUTION. Absorption and distribution of topical **selenium sulfide, pyrithione zinc, ketoconazole,** and **sulfacetamide sodium** are unknown.

METABOLISM AND EXCRETION. Metabolism and excretion of topical **selenium sulfide, pyrithione zinc, ketoconazole,** and **sulfacetamide sodium** are unknown.

Pharmacotherapeutics

PRECAUTIONS AND CONTRAINDICATIONS. **Selenium sulfide** is contraindicated in patients with acute inflammation and exudate, as absorption can be increased. It is also contraindicated in patients who are sensitive to any ingredients. There are no contraindications to the use of **pyrithione zinc. Tar** preparations should not be used on open or infected lesions or on areas of acute inflammation. **Ketoconazole** is contraindicated only for patients who are hypersensitive to any component of the product. It also contains sulfites, and patients who are sensitive to sulfites should be advised not to use **ketoconazole** shampoo. **Sulfacetamide sodium** should not be prescribed if sensitivity to **sulfonamides** is present, because cross-reactions to **topical sulfa** preparations may occur.

Selenium sulfide is Pregnancy Category C, as is *sulfacetamide sodium*. Some *tar* preparations (*Zetar*) are **Pregnancy Category C, and others have no pregnancy warnings listed. Tar** preparations should not be used in children younger than age 2 years. *Ketoconazole* shampoo is Pregnancy Category C.

ADVERSE DRUG REACTIONS. Skin irritation can occur with any of the topical **antiseborrheic** products. They may also cause greater-than-normal hair loss, hair discoloration, and scalp and hair oiliness or dryness. **Ketoconazole** shampoo may interfere with permanent wave solution.

DRUG INTERACTIONS. There are no identified drug interactions with any of the topical **antiseborrheic** products.

CLINICAL USE AND DOSING

Seborrhea and Dandruff. **Selenium sulfide** shampoo is available as an OTC product, which is 1% **selenium sulfide (Selsun Blue, Head & Shoulders Intensive)**, or by prescription, which contains 2.5% **selenium sulfide (Excel, Selsun)**. **Selenium sulfide** shampoo is massaged into wet hair and left on for 2 to 3 minutes before rinsing thoroughly (Table 21–12). It should be applied twice a week until the dandruff is under control, usually within 2 weeks, and then weekly to maintain control. **Tar** shampoos are available OTC and range in strength from 0.5% (**DHS Tar**) to 12% (**Extra Strength Denorex**) coal tar (Table 21–13). The different products vary in their application instructions from daily to weekly, and the patient should be advised to follow the label instructions. **Pyrithione zinc** is the active ingredient in OTC dandruff shampoos such as **Head & Shoulders**. A bar soap containing **pyrithione zinc (ZNP Bar)** is available for use on body areas with seborrheic dermatitis. **Pyrithione zinc** is applied to wet skin or hair, lathered, rinsed, and repeated; the treatment is repeated once or twice weekly to maintain control of dandruff or seborrhea. **Ketoconazole** shampoo is applied to wet hair, lathered, rinsed, and then repeated. It should be used every 3 to 4 days for up to 8 weeks.

Cradle Cap. Cradle cap in infants is treated with low-strength **selenium sulfide** shampoo (1%), which is applied in small amounts to the infant's scalp, massaged in, and rinsed well. The shampoo should not be allowed to get in the infant's eyes, and it should be rinsed out well. Apply twice weekly, with resolution of cradle cap usually occurring after 2 weeks of treatment.

RATIONAL DRUG SELECTION. There is little clinical data to suggest that one **antiseborrheic** product is better than another. **Selenium sulfide** 2.5% shampoo is commonly prescribed or 1% shampoo purchased OTC. **Ketoconazole** shampoo is available OTC (**Nizoral A-D**) and has comparable results to **selenium sulfide** in the treatment of dandruff. Generic **selenium sulfide** is less expensive than **ketoconazole**, but the cost of the brand name (**Excel**) is similar to **ketoconazole**.

MONITORING. There is no laboratory monitoring necessary for any of the topical **antiseborrheic** agents.

PATIENT EDUCATION

Administration. The patient should be instructed to use the medication exactly as directed. Overuse increases adverse effects, without clinical improvement in seborrhea. Seborrheic dermatitis cannot be cured, only controlled; therefore, continued use of the medication will be necessary to maintain control. All of the medications should be rinsed well after use.

Adverse Reactions. Patients should be advised to notify their provider if they have an adverse reaction to the medication prescribed.

Table 21–12. Dosage Schedule: Topical Antiseborrheic Medications

Drug	Indication	Dosage	Notes
Ketoconazole shampoo	Dandruff	Apply to wet hair. Apply and massage into scalp for 1 min, rinse, and repeat, leaving on scalp for 3 min. Use twice weekly for 4–8 wk, with at least 3 d between shampooing.	Ketoconazole shampoo is available in 1% (OTC) or 2% (Rx) formulas. There is no information regarding efficacy of choosing one over the other.
Pyrithione zinc	Dandruff	Shampoo is applied to wet hair, lathered, rinsed, and repeated. Repeat once or twice weekly to maintain control of dandruff.	Keep out of eyes.
	Seborrheic dermatitis	Use pyrithione zinc bar or shampoo. Wet skin, lather, rinse, and repeat. Repeat once or twice weekly to maintain control of seborrhea.	
Selenium sulfide	Dandruff/seborrheic dermatitis	Shampoo is massaged into wet hair, left on for 2–3 min, and rinsed well. Apply twice a week until the dandruff is under control, usually within 2 wk, then once a week to maintain control.	Avoid getting in eyes.
	Cradle cap	Apply shampoo (1%), to the infant's scalp, massage in, and rinse well. Apply twice weekly. Resolution of cradle cap usually occurs after 2 wk of treatment.	The shampoo should not be allowed to get in the infant's eyes, and it should be rinsed out well.
Sulfacetamide sodium	Dandruff/seborrheic dermatitis	Apply lotion to affected areas at bedtime. Apply by parting the hair and squeezing a small amount of medication on the scalp. Once scalp is completely moistened, massage in medication for 2–3 min. Allow medication to remain on overnight, and rinse well or shampoo with a gentle cleanser. Apply medication at bedtime for 8–10 nights. Once seborrhea is under control, lotion can be applied once or twice weekly to maintain control.	If scalp is oily or greasy, shampoo hair before application of sulfacetamide sodium lotion. In severe cases (thick crusts or scaling), twice-daily application may be needed initially.
Tar derivative shampoos	Dandruff, seborrheic dermatitis, cradle cap, and other oily, itchy skin conditions.	Refer to specific product labeling. Apply to wet hair, lather, rinse, and repeat, leaving on for 5 min the second time. Rinse well.	Refer to product label for frequency of use. For severe cases, use daily until control is reached, then once or twice/wk.

Drugs Affecting the Integumentary System ── **605**

Table 21–13. Available Dosage Forms: Antiseborrheic Medications

Drug	Dosage Form	How Supplied
Ketoconazole shampoo		
• Nizoral (Rx)	2% shampoo	In 4 oz
• Nizoral A-D (OTC)	1% shampoo	In 4 and 7 oz
Pyrithione zinc		
• Head & Shoulders	1% shampoo	In 120, 165, 210, 330, and 450 mL
• Zincon	1% shampoo	In 118 and 240 mL
• Danex	1% shampoo	In 120 mL
• DHS Zinc	2% shampoo	In 180 and 360 mL
• Sebulon	2% shampoo	In 120 and 240 mL
• ZNP Bar	2% soap	In 119-g bar
Selenium sulfide shampoo		
• Selsun Blue (OTC)	1% shampoo	In 120, 240, and 330 mL
• Selsun (Rx)	2.5 % shampoo	In 120 mL
• Head & Shoulders Intensive	1% shampoo	In 120, 240, and 330 mL
Treatment (OTC)	2.5 % shampoo	In 120 mL
• Excel (Rx)	1% shampoo (Rx)	In 120 mL
• Generic	2.5 % shampoo (OTC)	In 120 mL
Sulfacetamide sodium		
Sebizon (Rx)	10% lotion	In 85 g
Tar-derivative shampoos (OTC)		
• Zetar	1% coal tar	In 6 oz
• Theraplex T	1% coal tar	In 240 mL
• Ional T Plus	2% coal tar	In 120 and 240 mL
• Neutrogena T/Gel Shampoo	2% coal tar	In 132, 255, and 480 mL
• Neutrogena T/Gel Conditioner		
• Tegrin Medicated Shampoo	5% coal tar	Gel: In 71 g
		Lotion: In 110 and 198 mL
• Tegrin Medicated Extra Conditioning	7% coal tar	In 110 and 198 mL
• Denorex	9% coal tar	In 120, 240, and 360 mL
• Extra Strength Denorex	12.5% coal tar	In 120, 240, and 360 mL

Topical Antihistamines and Antipruritics

The **topical antihistamine** commonly used is **diphenhydramine (Benadryl)**. It may be combined with a variety of other ingredients such as **calamine** and **zinc oxide (Caladryl, Ziradryl)** in OTC products used to treat itching associated with minor skin disorders. **Doxepin (Zonalon)** cream can be used for moderate to severe pruritus associated with atopic dermatitis.

Pharmacodynamics

Topical **diphenhydramine** provides local relief from pruritus and edema because its local effect on the H_1-receptors suppresses the formation of edema, flare, and pruritus. It may also provide local anesthetic activity by decreasing the permeability of the nerve cell membrane to sodium ions, thus blocking the transmission of nerve impulses.

Doxepin's topical mechanism of action is unclear but probably related to its H_1- and H_2-receptor blocking action. **Histamine-blocking drugs** appear to compete at histamine receptor sites and inhibit the activation of histamine receptors.

Pharmacokinetics

ABSORPTION AND DISTRIBUTION. Diphenhydramine is not absorbed in sufficient quantities to produce measurable serum concentrations.

Significant amounts of **doxepin** for topical use can be absorbed systemically if it is used over 10 percent of the body surface area or for long periods. Absorption is increased by occlusion. Serum levels may reach one-third the level of **doxepin** taken orally. It is unknown whether **doxepin** crosses the placenta. **Doxepin** is excreted in breast milk.

METABOLISM AND EXCRETION. Metabolism and excretion of topical **diphenhydramine** are unknown. Negligible amounts are absorbed.

Absorbed **doxepin** is metabolized in the liver, into an active metabolite, *N*-desmethyldoxepin. Parent drug and metabolite are excreted in gastric juice. *N*-desmethyldoxepin is reabsorbed and further metabolized. Primary excretion is renal. **Doxepin** and its metabolites are known to be excreted in breast milk.

Pharmacotherapeutics

PRECAUTIONS AND CONTRAINDICATIONS. Topical **diphenhydramine** is contraindicated if the patient is sensitive to the medication in any form. It is for external use only, and contact with the eyes should be avoided. Prolonged use of topical **diphenhydramine** (more than 7 days) should be avoided.

Drowsiness occurs in more than 20 percent of patients using **doxepin** cream, especially on more than 10 percent of body surface area. Patients with untreated narrow-angle glaucoma and urinary retention should not use doxepin orally or in topical form because of its anticholinergic effect, even in the topical form. *Doxepin* **cream is contraindicated for use in children and is classified Pregnancy Category B. Doxepin** should be used with caution in breastfeeding; one case of apnea and drowsiness has occurred in an infant whose mother was taking oral **doxepin.**

ADVERSE DRUG REACTIONS. Topical **diphenhydramine** may cause skin irritation if used for prolonged periods.

Topical **doxepin** cream may cause excessive drowsiness if used over more than 10 percent of the body surface area. It may also cause dry mouth and lips, thirst, headache, fatigue, or dizziness (occurring in 1 to 10% of patients). Up to 21 percent of patients report burning and stinging upon application of topical **doxepin**, with 25 percent of those patients classifying the burning as "severe." Pruritus, dry skin, and eczema exacerbation are reported in fewer than 10 percent of patients.

DRUG INTERACTIONS. There are no known drug interactions with topical **diphenhydramine** (Table 21–14).

Doxepin cream interacts adversely with alcohol, **cimetidine,** and **monoamine oxidate inhibitors (MAOIs),** and these drugs should be avoided during therapy. **Doxepin** may also interact with any drug that is metabolized by the cytochrome P-450 2D6 enzymes.

CLINICAL USE AND DOSING
Local Reactions to Insect Bites, Stings, and Minor Skin Disorders (Poison Ivy, Sumac, and Oak). Topical **diphenhydramine** is applied to the affected area three to four times a day for up to 7 days (Table 21–15).

Severe Pruritus. **Doxepin** cream is applied in a thin layer four times a day in 3- to 4-hour intervals for up to 8 days of treatment. Treatment for longer than 8 days may result in higher systemic levels of **doxepin.** Other available topical **antipruritics** that are safer to use than **doxepin** are **Aveeno** cream (colloidal oatmeal–based) and **Moisturel** emollient cream or lotion (petrolatum, glycerin-based).

RATIONAL DRUG SELECTION. Selection of a **topical antihistamine** is based on the severity of the pruritus, with **doxepin** reserved for severe cases.

MONITORING. There is no laboratory monitoring necessary with the use of topical **diphenhydramine.**

There is no laboratory monitoring necessary with short-term use of topical **doxepin,** although serum **dox-**

Table 21–14. Drug Interactions: Topical Antihistamine and Antipruritic Medications

Drug	Interacting Drug	Possible Effect	Implications
Diphenhydramine	No known drug interactions		
Doxepin	Alcohol	Increased sedative effects of doxepin.	Use together with caution. Advise patients to limit alcohol use when using topical doxepin.
	Cimetidine	May affect serum doxepin levels.	Avoid concurrent use.
	MAOIs	Serious side effects and death reported with the use of MAOIs and drugs related to doxepin.	Separate use of 2 medications by at least 2 wk.
	Medications metabolized by CP450 2D6 enzymes	Decreased metabolism of doxepin, leading to increased plasma levels.	Monitor closely. May need to adjust dosage of doxepin or other drug. Use together with caution.

Table 21–15. Dosage Schedule: Topical Antihistamine and Antipruritic Medications

Drug	Indication	Dosage	Notes
Diphenhydramine	Local reactions to insect bites, stings, and minor skin disorders (poison ivy, oak, sumac)	Apply to affected area 3 to 4 times/d for up to 7 d.	
Doxepin	Short-term management of moderate to severe pruritus	Apply a thin film qid in at least 3- to 4-h intervals. May use for ≤8 d.	If excessive drowsiness occurs, do one of the following: 1. Decrease body surface area treated 2. Reduce the number of applications per day

epin levels may be necessary for use over prolonged periods.

PATIENT EDUCATION

Administration. The patient should be instructed to use the medication exactly as prescribed (Table 21–16). Overuse or incorrect use may increase the adverse effects of these topical medications.

Adverse Reactions. Patients who are prescribed **doxepin** should be told about the potential for drowsiness and be warned against driving or operating hazardous machinery until they are reasonably certain that **doxepin** does not affect their ability to operate safely.

Lifestyle Management. Patients should be encouraged to use nonpharmacological measures to control their pruritus, including avoidance of sensitizing agents and the use of OTC emollient products such as **Aveeno** to treat their pruritus.

Table 21–16. Available Dosage Forms: Topical Antihistamine and Antipruritic Medications

Drug	Dosage Form	How Supplied
Diphenhydramine (OTC)		
• Benadryl	1% cream	In 15 g
	1% spray	In 60 mL
• Maximum Strength Benadryl 2%	2% cream	In 15 g
	2% spray	In 60 mL
• Generic	1% cream	In 15 and 45 g
Doxepin Zonalon	5% cream	In 30 and 45 g

Moisturizers, Emollients, and Lubricants

Moisturizers, lubricants, and **emollients** help to retain water in the skin. They are composed of petrolatum, lanolin, or other agents such as colloidal oatmeal in an emulsion.

Pharmacodynamics

Emollients, moisturizers, and **lubricants** are applied after the patient bathes. This procedure acts to trap the moisture in the skin. Ointments provide the most occlusive barrier; creams are the next best. Lotions offer the convenience of easy application over large areas of skin but are not as occlusive as ointments and creams.

Pharmacokinetics

Topical **emollients** interact only with the outermost layers of the skin and are not absorbed systemically.

Pharmacotherapeutics

PRECAUTIONS AND CONTRAINDICATIONS. There are no true contraindications to **emollients,** other than to avoid the eyes. Patients who are allergic to wool should avoid **Eucerine** and other lanolin-containing products.

ADVERSE DRUG REACTIONS. There are minimal to no adverse drug reactions reported with the use of **emollients.**

DRUG INTERACTIONS. There are no known drug interactions with emollients.

CLINICAL USE AND DOSING

Dry Skin. To treat dry skin, the **emollient** is applied after patients bathe, one to four times per day. Patients pat their skin dry and then liberally apply the lotion or cream to all affected areas. This procedure acts to trap the moisture in the skin. Ointments provide the most occlusive barrier; creams are the next best. Lotions offer the convenience of easy application over large areas of skin but are not as occlusive as ointments and creams. Before using a lotion, make sure it does not contain alcohol, which is drying and irritating.

There are many **emollient** products available, but many are eliminated by their additives of perfumes or other chemicals, to which many eczema patients are sensitive. Commonly used **emollients** are **Aveeno** cream or lotion, **Eucerine** cream or lotion, **Lubriderm** lotion, and **Moisturel** lotion. White petrolatum (**Vaseline**) or vegetable shortening (Crisco) can be used in severe cases.

RATIONAL DRUG SELECTION

Cost.   Expense can play a role in choosing an **emollient,** as large amounts, over a long period, are needed to be effective. White petrolatum is inexpensive and a good treatment choice for eczema patients who have limited resources. Discussing the cost of **emollients** prior to recommending them to the patient will determine if the provider needs to assist the patient in finding resources to pay for **emollients,** which are usually not covered by health insurance plans. The use of generic equivalents will decrease the cost of **emollients.**

MONITORING.   No laboratory monitoring is necessary with the use of **emollients.** Ongoing monitoring of clinical status is necessary to determine if the **emollient** is effective.

PATIENT EDUCATION

Administration.   The patient should be instructed to apply liberal amounts of the **emollient** to the areas of dry skin. The **emollient** is most effective if applied just after bathing. Daily use offers the best results.

Lifestyle Management.   Nonpharmacological measures used to treat dry skin include hydrating baths and avoidance of offending agents that cause exacerbations. Patients should be told to use rubber or plastic gloves when their hands may be exposed to harsh chemicals or detergents, which may increase dryness. They should avoid wearing irritating fabrics such as wool. Soft cotton clothing allows the skin to breathe.

Baths hydrate the skin. The patient should take a warm—not hot—bath for 20 minutes. The skin is patted dry, and **emollients** are applied immediately to maintain the skin's hydration. The patient should use mild soap to cleanse the groin and axilla and avoid harsh deodorant soaps. After the bath is also a good time to apply **corticosteroid** creams or ointments, if needed.

Agents Used in the Treatment of Burns

In primary care, the most commonly prescribed burn preparation is **silver sulfadiazine (Silvadene).** Other products used to treat second- and third-degree burns include **nitrofurazone (Furacin)** and **mafenide (Sulfamylon),** although they are not commonly used in primary care and are not discussed in depth here.

Pharmacodynamics

Silver sulfadiazine is a **topical anti-infective** active against both bacteria and yeast. It is bactericidal, as it acts on the cell membrane and cell wall to produce a toxic effect on bacteria. It is active against both gram-positive and gram-negative organisms. The organisms that are generally susceptible to **silver sulfadiazine** include *S. aureus, S. epidermidis,* β-hemolytic streptococci, *C. albicans, Klebsiella* species, *Escherichia coli, Enterobacter* species, *Proteus, Pseudomonas, Clostridium perfringens, Morganella morganii, Serratia* species, and *Providencia* species.

Mafenide is bacteriostatic against many gram-positive and gram-negative bacteria, including *Pseudomonas.* It is active in the presence of pus and serum.

Nitrofurazone is a synthetic **nitrofuran,** with a broad spectrum of antibacterial activity, including the following organisms: *S. aureus, Streptococcus* species, *E. coli, C. perfringens,* and *Proteus.*

Reduction of bacterial growth after a deep partial-thickness burn promotes spontaneous healing by preventing conversion of partial-thickness burns to full thickness by sepsis.

Pharmacokinetics

ABSORPTION AND DISTRIBUTION.   Silver sulfadiazine is not absorbed through intact skin. On burns, up to 10 percent of the **sulfadiazine** may be absorbed from **silver sulfadiazine,** with only 1 percent of the silver absorbed. Serum concentrations of 10 to 20 μg/mL of **sulfadiazine** have been reported when large surface areas have been treated. Once absorbed, **sulfadiazine** is distributed into most body tissues. It is not known whether it crosses the placenta or is excreted in breast milk.

METABOLISM AND EXCRETION.   The portion of **sulfadiazine** that is absorbed is metabolized in the liver and excreted renally.

Pharmacotherapeutics

PRECAUTIONS AND CONTRAINDICATIONS.   Silver sulfadiazine is contraindicated in patients sensitive to any of the contents of the preparation, including **sulfa**-sensitive patients.

Silver sulfadiazine **is Pregnancy Category B but is considered Pregnancy Category D in the near-term pregnancy. Pregnant women at or near term should not use** *silver sulfadiazine.* **It is also contraindicated in premature infants and infants age 2 months or younger because the **sulfonamide** displaces bilirubin and causes kernicterus. Use with caution in breastfeeding women.**

Silver sulfadiazine should be used cautiously in patients with G6PD deficiency because **sulfonamides** may cause hemolytic anemia in these patients.

Silver sulfadiazine should be used with caution in patients with hepatic or renal disease, as well as patients with thrombocytopenia, leukopenia, or other hematologic disorders. **Sulfonamides** may worsen these disorders.

Sulfonamides should be used with caution in patients with porphyria, as they may precipitate porphyria.

ADVERSE DRUG REACTIONS. Leukopenia (white blood cell [WBC] count less than 5000) can occur in up to 20 percent of patients, especially if large surface areas are treated. This occurs within 2 to 4 days of beginning therapy and resolves spontaneously upon discontinuation of the medication.

Patients may also experience burning or pruritus at the site of application. Skin discoloration may occur.

Systemic **sulfonamide** reactions have also been reported.

CLINICAL USE AND DOSING. Silver sulfadiazine is applied to burns once or twice daily, in a sterile fashion. It is applied to a thickness of 1/16 inch. The wound should be clean and debrided. **Silver sulfadiazine** should cover the burn at all times; reapply if the medication is removed. Dressings are not necessary but are helpful to prevent the medication from getting on the patient's clothing. **Silver sulfadiazine** should be used until the burn is completely healed.

MONITORING. If the area that the **silver sulfadiazine** is applied to is large or if treatment is prolonged, the patient's CBC, platelet count, liver function, and renal function need to be monitored. The burn should also be monitored for signs of superinfection or delayed separation.

PATIENT EDUCATION
Administration. Patients can treat small partial-thickness burns themselves and apply the **silver sulfadiazine** at home, although the first one or two applications are best done by a trained health care provider to teach the patient the proper technique for applying the medication in a sterile fashion.

Adverse Reactions. Patients should be informed of the possible adverse drug reactions that may occur with the use of **silver sulfadiazine** and report any adverse symptoms to their provider.

Scabicides and Pediculicides

Skin and hair infestation is a frequently seen problem in primary care, with arthropods, scabies, and lice the most common. The pharmacological management of scabies and lice consists of **ectoparasiticides.** The specific medication used varies according to the type of infestation and the age of the patient. There is a choice of OTC products (**permethrin, pyrethrins**) for the treatment of head lice. Prescription-strength **permethrin (Elimite)** and **lindane** are the commonly prescribed **ectoparasiticides.** Crotamiton is another prescription choice for scabies. Nonpharmacological, environmental measures are a key part of the treatment of any infestation, as patients can reinfect themselves or other family members and restart the infestation cycle. **Malathion** is no longer a recommended treatment for infestations, and therefore it is not discussed here.

Pharmacodynamics

Pyrethrins are derived from chrysanthemums and are found in combination with piperonyl butoxide in OTC pediculicide products (**RID, Pronto, A 200**). **Pyrethrins** are 100 percent insecticidal and 70 to 80 percent ovicidal. **Pyrethrins** kill lice in 10.5 to 18.6 minutes. There is no residual activity.

Permethrin is a synthetic compound that is related to **pyrethrins.** It acts on the nerve cell membrane to disrupt the sodium channel current. This disrupts the sodium channel polarization, leading to paralysis. **Permethrin** is 97 percent insecticidal and 70 to 80 percent ovicidal. **Permethrin** cream rinse has residual activity against lice for up to 10 days.

Lindane is absorbed through the exoskeleton of parasites, causing CNS excitation, which leads to convulsions and death. It is 67 percent insecticidal and 45 to 70 percent ovicidal. **Lindane** has no residual activity against head lice.

Crotamiton is **scabicidal** and **antipruritic.** Its mechanism of action is unknown.

Pharmacokinetics

The pharmacokinetics of **pyrethrins** and **crotamiton** is unknown.

Permethrin is absorbed in unknown amounts, although it is thought to be less than 2 percent of the dose. It is then rapidly metabolized by ester hydrolysis into inactive metabolites, which are excreted in the urine. It is unknown whether **permethrin** crosses the placenta or is excreted in breast milk.

Lindane is slowly and incompletely absorbed through intact skin. Absorption is increased though damaged or occluded skin. There are measurable amounts of **lindane** absorbed. Lindane is stored in the body fat. It is metabolized by the liver and excreted in the urine and feces. It is unknown whether **lindane** crosses the placenta. **Lindane** is excreted in breast milk.

Pharmacotherapeutics

PRECAUTIONS AND CONTRAINDICATIONS. Hypersensitivity to any component of the products is a contraindication to their use. Sensitivity to chrysanthemums is a contraindication to the use of **permethrin.**

Although all of the head lice and scabies treatments are relatively safe, they are classified as neurotoxic agents, and they should be used exactly as directed. To limit exposure, the medication should be washed off at a sink, rather than in a shower. Cool or lukewarm water should be used to minimize absorption caused by vasodilatation (Chesney & Burgess, 1998).

Lindane should be avoided in patients with a known seizure disorder.

Permethrin should not be used near the eyes. If it gets in the eyes, they should be flushed with water immediately.

Lindane should not be used on abraded or inflamed skin, which increases the absorption of the medication.

Lindane **is neurotoxic and should not be used in pregnant women more than twice during the pregnancy or in infants younger than 2 years. Permethrin** should not be used on infants younger than 2 months.

There are no contraindications to the use of **crotamiton.**

ADVERSE DRUG REACTIONS. All of the topical **ectoparasiticides** can cause skin irritation, some burning, or pruritus. Contact dermatitis can occur, usually from incorrect use.

CNS toxicity can occur with **lindane**, but this is almost always associated with ingestion or misuse of the product.

CLINICAL USE AND DOSING
Head Lice. Treat only those family members who are actively infested (lice or nits seen on head). Do not treat head lice prophylactically.

Pyrethrin shampoo is applied to *dry* hair and left on for 10 to 20 minutes, with the time varying by brand (Table 21–17). It is important for the product to be applied to dry hair to enable the **pediculicide** to enter the insect's body better. The patient should be re-treated in 1 week, regardless of whether there is evidence of infestation.

Permethrin is a cream rinse that is applied after shampooing (Table 21–18). It is important that the shampoo not have any conditioners in its formula, which makes the **permethrin** less effective. The cream rinse is left in the hair for 10 minutes and then rinsed out. Treatment should be repeated in 1 week, regardless of whether signs of infestation are present.

Lindane is applied to dry hair, working small quantities of water in to create a good lather. The shampoo is left on for 4 minutes. The amount of shampoo prescribed for short hair is 1 oz; for long hair, prescribe 2 oz. The shampoo should be rinsed well.

Nonpharmacological treatments for head lice are an option. With the growing problem of resistance and concern over exposing children to repeated doses of **pediculicides,** there are growing anecdotal reports about the success of various nonmedicated therapies. Popular and safe remedies are mayonnaise (full-fat variety), olive oil, and petroleum jelly. It is thought that they asphyxiate the lice by blocking their breathing apparatus or immobilize them and affect their ability to feed. If the family would like to try these treatments, they should apply a thick layer of the product and cover with a shower cap. The product is left on from 1 hour to overnight, then shampooed out.

Body Lice. Because body lice live on clothing and underwear and come to the skin only to feed, instruct patients to wash all clothing and bedding in hot water to kill lice and nits that are on it, as well as treat their bodies with a pediculicide.

Permethrin 5 percent (**Elimite**) is massaged into skin from head to soles of feet, left on for 8 hours (overnight), and then showered off. Dispense 30 g for an average adult.

Lindane is applied to the total body as a cream or lotion and left on 8 to 12 hours (overnight). The amount needed for an adult is 2 oz.

Pubic Lice. Pubic lice are treated with an application of **lindane** 1 percent cream, lotion, or shampoo. A thin layer of cream or lotion is applied to the hair and skin surrounding the pubic area and left on for 12 hours. If **lindane** shampoo is used, the shampoo is massaged into dry pubic hair and left on for 5 to 10 minutes. If axillary or thigh hair is also infested, then use the cream or lotion. Reapply in 7 days if there is evidence of live lice. Sexual partners should be treated concurrently, and bedding and clothes should also be washed.

Scabies. All family members should receive treatment, even those who are asymptomatic. Family members may be in the incubation period, and so all members of the household need treatment to prevent recurrence.

Permethrin 5 percent cream (**Elimite, Acticin**) is the drug of choice for the treatment of scabies in young children and pregnant women. It is 90 percent effective against the scabies mite and can be used in infants as young as 2 months and in pregnant women. The cream is massaged into the skin from the neck to the soles of feet. It should be left on for 8 to 14 hours and then washed off in the shower. Infants require special application of **permethrin** to the scalp, temple, forehead, hands, and feet. One ounce of **permethrin** per family member is prescribed.

Lindane 1 percent lotion or cream is used for scabies in children over 6 months of age and in nonpregnant adult patients. It is applied in a thin layer from the neck down to the soles of the feet, left on for 8 to 12 hours (overnight), and then washed off thoroughly. If there are crusted lesions present, a tepid bath should be taken prior to application to soften the lesions. Patients should dry the skin thoroughly before applying **lindane.** Two ounces of **lindane** per family member should be prescribed.

Table 21–17. Dosage Schedule: Ectoparasiticides

Drug	Indication	Dosage	Notes
Permethrin	Head lice	Apply permethrin 1% cream rinse after shampooing. Leave in hair for 10 min, then rinse off. Repeat treatment in 1 wk.	It is important that the shampoo formula contain no conditioners, which make the permethrin less effective. Treatment should be repeated in 1 wk, regardless of whether signs of infestation are present.
	Body lice	Permethrin 5% is massaged into skin from head to soles of feet and left on for 8 h (overnight), then showered off.	Dispense 30 g for an average adult. Should not be used in children <2 mo.
	Scabies	Apply 5% cream to entire body and leave on for 8–14 h, then shower off.	All family members must be treated. Dispense 30 g per adult.
Pyrethrins	Head lice	Pyrethrin shampoo is applied to *dry hair* and left on for 10–20 min, with the time varying by brand. Re-treat in 1 wk.	It is important for the product to be applied to dry hair to enable the pediculicide to better enter the insect's body. The patient should be re-treated in 1 wk regardless of whether there is evidence of infestation.
Lindane	Head lice	Lindane is applied to dry hair, working small quantities of water in to create a good lather. Leave shampoo in hair for 4 min.	The amount of shampoo prescribed for short hair is 1 oz; for long hair, prescribe 2 oz. The shampoo should be rinsed well.
	Body lice	Apply cream or lotion to the total body and leave on for 8–12 h (overnight). Shower off.	Dispense 2 oz for an adult.
	Pubic lice	Use lindane cream, lotion, or shampoo. Apply a thin layer of cream or lotion to the hair and skin surrounding the pubic area, and leave on for 12 h. The shampoo is massaged into dry pubic hair and left on for 5–10 min. If axillary or thigh hair is also infested, use cream or lotion. Treat again in 7 d if there is evidence of live lice.	Sexual partners should be treated concurrently. Bedding and clothes should be washed.
	Scabies	Apply cream or lotion from the neck down, and leave on for 8–2 h. Shower off.	All family members should be treated. Dispense 2 oz per adult.

Treat only family members who are actively infested (lice or nits seen on head). Do not treat head lice prophylactically.

Topical corticosteroids are used *after scabies treatment* to treat the pruritus and inflammation associated with the scabies mite. **Hydrocortisone** 1 percent or 2.5 percent or a stronger **corticosteroid**, if indicated, is applied to affected areas twice a day until the lesions are healed.

RATIONAL DRUG SELECTION

Cost. The relative costs of the different **ectoparasiticides** are similar, so cost is not usually a consideration in the treatment.

Adverse Effects. The provider may choose the drug based on the patient's age and the toxicity of the agent. **Lindane should be avoided in pregnant patients, and it is contraindicated in children under age 2 years.**

MONITORING. No specific laboratory monitoring is necessary with the use of **ectoparasiticides.**

PATIENT EDUCATION

Administration. Patients should be instructed to use the prescribed medication exactly as directed. Treatment failure due to incorrect use of the medication is common. Give *written* instructions about how to apply the medication and the length of time that the medication should be left on the skin or hair.

Adverse Reactions. When used as directed, there are minimal adverse effects from the use of **ectoparasiticides.** Skin irritation may occur, but the incidence increases if patients use the medication incorrectly.

Table 21–18. Available Dosage Forms: Ectoparasiticides for the Treatment of Scabies and Lice

Drug	Dosage Form	How Supplied
Permethrin		
• Elimite (Rx)	5% cream	In 60 g
• Nix (OTC)	1% cream rinse	In 60 mL with comb
Pyrethrins (OTC)		
• RID	0.3% shampoo	In 60, 120, and 240 mL
• Pronto	0.33% shampoo	In 60 and 120 mL
• A-200	0.33% shampoo	In 60 and 120 mL
Lindane Generic	1% cream	In 60 g
	1% lotion	In 30 and 60 mL, pint, gal
	1% shampoo	In 30 and 60 mL, pint, gal

Lifestyle Management. Environmental measures should be discussed, and written instructions given to patients or family members to take home to refer to as they delouse the home.

Cauterizing and Destructive Agents

The **cauterizing agents** used in primary care are **silver nitrate** and **chloroacetic acid.** The are three **chloroacetic acid** preparations: **monochloroacetic acid, dichloroacetic acid,** and **trichloroacetic acid. Podophyllum resin (podophyllin)** is used for genital warts.

Pharmacodynamics

Silver nitrate is a strong caustic agent and escharotic. The silver acts as antiseptic, astringent, and germicide. The silver attaches to the protein ion and decreases the protein's solubility. The local effects of silver are self-limiting, and the spread of damage occurs only when the dose of silver overwhelms the capacity of the tissues to fix the ion at the site of application.

Chloroacetic acid rapidly penetrates and cauterizes the skin, keratin, and other tissues. **Monochloroacetic acid** is more deeply destructive than **trichloroacetic acid.**

Podophyllum resin contains podophyllotoxin, which binds to the microtubules in the cell, causing mitotic arrest in metaphase. **Podophyllum** is considered cytotoxic to the wart cells.

Pharmacotherapeutics

PRECAUTIONS AND CONTRAINDICATIONS. Cauterizing agents should be used with great care because they damage any skin they touch.

Silver nitrate used for prolonged periods discolors the skin. It also stains any clothing or linens it contacts.

If wet dressings containing **silver nitrate** are used over large surface areas, electrolyte imbalances may occur, specifically hyponatremia and hypochloremia.

Chloroacetic acids are contraindicated in the treatment of malignant or premalignant lesions.

Only a health care provider should apply **podophyllum resin,** a powerful caustic and severe irritant that must be handled carefully.

Podophyllum resin should not be used in pregnancy because it has lead to birth defects, fetal death, and stillbirth. It is also contraindicated in breast-feeding women.

Podophyllum resin is contraindicated in diabetic patients and other patients with poor circulation. **Podophyllum resin** is also contraindicated in the treatment of malignant or premalignant lesions, bleeding warts, and warts with hair growing from them. The use of **podophyllum** should be avoided if the wart or surrounding tissue is inflamed or irritated.

ADVERSE DRUG REACTIONS. Cauterizing agents are powerful **keratolytics** and **cauterants.** Use with caution to avoid contact with healthy skin. To prevent **chloroacetic acid** from spreading to healthy skin, apply petrolatum around the area to be treated as a barrier to the acid.

Irritation and ulcerative local reactions are the major side effects of **podophyllum. Podophyllum** may cause paresthesias. Serious neuropathy and death have occurred from the use of **podophyllum** in large amounts on multiple lesions.

CLINICAL USE AND DOSING
Umbilical Granuloma. Use a **silver nitrate** stick and touch to granulomatous area. One treatment is usually curative.

Aphthous Ulcer, Vesicular, or Bullous Lesion. Touch lesion with a **silver nitrate** stick. One treatment is usually all that is necessary to provide styptic action.

Poorly Healing Wounds or Ulcers. Apply cotton pad dipped in **silver nitrate** solution to the affected area. A **silver nitrate** stick may also be used.

Verruca (Warts). Remove the callus. Apply a layer of petrolatum to the normal skin around the wart. Apply either **monochloroacetic** or **trichloroacetic acid** to the wart, and cover with a bandage for 5 days. The wart should be removed with the bandage when it is removed.

If using **dichloroacetic acid,** apply it with a pointed wooden applicator or a cotton-tipped applicator. There should never be a large excess drop of acid on the applicator stick. Prevent this by drawing the stick over the lip of the acid container. Touch the applicator stick to the wart. Cauterization progress is determined by a change of the color of the wart to gray-white. Three or four treatments may be necessary for heavy growths.

Podophyllum resin is applied by a health care provider. It is not to be dispensed to the patient. After the area is cleansed, **podophyllum resin** is applied sparingly to the lesion. Avoid contact with healthy skin. The first treatment should be left in place for 30 to 40 minutes and then washed off thoroughly with soap and water. Later treatments may require 1 to 4 hours of contact to produce the desired result. Do not treat numerous lesions or large areas in one treatment, which increases the incidence of neuropathy occurring from **podophyllum** use. Multiple treatments may be necessary.

Keratolytics

Keratolytic agents are used to treat a variety of hyperkeratotic and scaling cutaneous lesions, such as corns, calluses, and warts. **Salicylic acid** is the only OTC product considered safe and effective by the FDA. **Lactic acid** is used to treat xerosis and ichthyosis vulgaris.

Pharmacodynamics

Salicylic acid produces desquamation of the horny layer of the skin without affecting the viable epidermis. It acts by dissolving the intercellular cement substance in the stratum corneum.

Lactic acid is thought to diminish corneocyte cohesion by interfering with the formation of ionic bonds.

Pharmacotherapeutics

PRECAUTIONS AND CONTRAINDICATIONS. **Salicylic acid** products are contraindicated if the patient is sensitive to **salicylic acid.** Prolonged use in infants and patients with decreased renal or hepatic function is contraindicated, as it may lead to salicylism. Topical **salicylic acid** use is contraindicated patients with diabetes or impaired circulation.

Lactic acid should be used carefully on the face or in patients with fair skin, as irritation may occur. Minimize the exposure to UV light or sun when using **lactic acid** topically. *Lac-Hydrin (12% lactic acid)* **is Pregnancy Category C and is not recommended for use in nursing mothers.**

ADVERSE DRUG REACTIONS. Local irritation can occur from **salicylic acid** contact with normal skin surrounding the wart or callus.

Transient stinging or burning has been reported with the use of topical **Lac-Hydrin (12% lactic acid).** Erythema, peeling, dryness, or hyperpigmentation may also occur. **Lac-Hydrin (12% lactic acid)** may cause an eczema flare.

CLINICAL USE AND DOSING
Warts, Corns, and Calluses. There are many **salicylic acid** products available. Products that are 5 to 17 percent in collodion are used for safe, effective removal of common and plantar warts. Transdermal patches are available in 40 percent and 15 percent strengths for use on warts, corns, and calluses. Patients should refer to the individual product's label for instructions for use. To ensure successful treatment, patients should soak the affected area in warm water for at least 5 minutes before applying **salicylic acid.** Loose tissue or dried wart tissue is removed with a washcloth or emery board. In the treatment of warts, improvement should occur in 1 to 2 weeks, with complete resolution taking 4 to 6 weeks.

Xerosis, Dry Skin, and Ichthyosis. **Lac-Hydrin (12% lactic acid)** is applied to the affected area twice a day. The lotion or cream should be rubbed in when applied.

PATIENT EDUCATION
Administration. When instructing patients to use OTC **salicylic acid,** the provider should instruct them to soak the affected area in warm water for at least 5 minutes or to bathe just before applying the medication. This will soften the area and allow better penetration of the medication. Improvement will take at least 1 to 2 weeks, and patients should be advised that total healing may take several weeks.

Topical Anesthetics

This section discusses the use of **EMLA (lidocaine-prilocaine)** for local anesthesia. **EMLA** is unique in that it bridges the gap between **topical** and **infiltration anesthesia.** It is useful in preparing for painful procedures such as bone marrow biopsies, IV starts, and blood draws.

Pharmacodynamics

This product is a unique mixture of **lidocaine** 2.5 percent and **prilocaine** 2.5 percent. The combination has a lower melting point than either agent alone. **EMLA** cream produces anesthesia to a depth of 5 mm. **Local anesthetics** inhibit conduction of nerve impulses from sensory nerves because of an alteration in the cell membrane permeability to ions. When applied to intact skin and covered with an occlusive dressing, local anesthesia is achieved in 1 hour.

Pharmacokinetics

ABSORPTION AND DISTRIBUTION. The **EMLA** cream is absorbed systemically, with greater amounts absorbed based on the amount of medication applied to skin. Absorption is increased across abraded skin or mucous membranes. Once absorbed, **lidocaine** and **prilocaine**

are widely distributed. They most likely cross the placenta and are excreted in breast milk.

METABOLISM AND EXCRETION. The metabolism and excretion of **lidocaine** and **prilocaine** are unknown.

Pharmacotherapeutics

PRECAUTIONS AND CONTRAINDICATIONS. In the patient with methemoglobinemia, **EMLA** is contraindicated. **EMLA** increases the risk of methemoglobinemia if used in patients with G6PD deficiency or in young infants. It is contraindicated in patients with known hypersensitivity to **lidocaine** or other **local anesthetics**.

If instilled into the middle ear, **EMLA** can be ototoxic. Therefore, use in the ear near the tympanic membrane is contraindicated.

In patients with severe hepatic disease, older adults, or debilitated and acutely ill patients, **EMLA** should be used with caution. The minimal effective dose should be used to prevent adverse effects. *EMLA* is Pregnancy Category B. It should be used with caution in nursing mothers.

ADVERSE DRUG REACTIONS. Adverse reactions are generally dose-related and usually result from high plasma levels of anesthetic due to excessive dosage or rapid absorption.

The patient may experience local adverse effects, such as paleness of the area, erythema, and changes in temperature sensation.

DRUG INTERACTIONS. Do not prescribe **EMLA** cream to be used in children younger than 12 months old who are concurrently taking methemoglobinemia-inducing drugs (**acetaminophen, sulfonamides, nitrates, phenytoin, phenobarbital**).

Class I antiarrhythmic agents (**tocainide** and **mexiletine**) may potentiate the toxicity of **EMLA**.

CLINICAL USE AND DOSING
Topical Anesthetic. To provide local anesthesia for minor procedures such as IV cannulation, venipuncture, or circumcision, the dose of **EMLA** varies by the age of the patient. For adults and children over 1 year, an **EMLA** disk can be applied for 1 hour or cream applied and occluded for 1 hour. If the patient is to self-administer the medication before a procedure, for ease of administration **EMLA** disks can be prescribed or a 5-mg tube dispensed and the patient instructed to apply half of the tube to the site or sites. For IV cannulation or venipuncture anesthesia, two sites may be treated. Dosing of cream for younger infants is determined by age, and the provider must refer to the dosing schedule for accurate dosing to prevent adverse effects. Higher dosing is used to harvest skin grafts, which is rarely done in primary care.

MONITORING. The patient being treated with **EMLA** should be monitored for adverse effects, such as methemoglobinemia.

PATIENT EDUCATION
Administration. Patients who are to self-administer **EMLA** should have clear instructions as to the correct use. The patient should clearly understand how to apply the cream and occlude the area with the occlusive dressing. If possible, the first dose can be applied by a health care provider to demonstrate proper use.

Minoxidil

Topical **minoxidil** (**Rogaine**) is the first FDA-approved medication for stimulating hair growth. Alopecia androgenetica, also known as male pattern baldness, affects men and some women. It involves hair loss from the frontal, vertex, and occipital regions of the scalp in men and thinning of the hair in the frontoparietal area or diffuse hair loss in women.

Pharmacodynamics

The exact mechanism of action is unknown, but it does produce growth of epithelial cells near the base of the hair follicle. It may also induce vasodilatation of the scalp blood vessels, which also promotes hair growth. It does not appear to have an antiandrogen effect.

Pharmacokinetics

ABSORPTION AND DISTRIBUTION. Topical **minoxidil** is poorly absorbed (2% of the dose) from an intact scalp. It is widely distributed in body tissues. It is not known whether **minoxidil** crosses the placenta or is distributed in breast milk.

METABOLISM AND EXCRETION. The small portion of topical **minoxidil** that is absorbed is extensively metabolized in the liver. Both the unchanged drug and the metabolites are excreted in the urine.

Pharmacotherapeutics

PRECAUTIONS AND CONTRAINDICATIONS. Minoxidil topical solution used as directed has minimal cardiac effects, but if large amounts are applied, there is a potential for cardiac side effects.

Absorption of **minoxidil** is increased through abraded or irritated skin, leading to a slightly higher risk for cardiac side effects.

Minoxidil should not be used by pregnant patients (Pregnancy Category C) or by children under age 18 years.

ADVERSE DRUG REACTIONS. Minoxidil is generally well tolerated. The topical solution contains alcohol and therefore may be irritating upon application. Patients may be sensitive to **minoxidil** and develop contact dermatitis.

DRUG INTERACTIONS. **Topical steroids, retinoids,** and other drugs that increase blood flow to the area may increase the absorption of **minoxidil,** leading to increased hypotension. Avoid using these topical medications concurrently on the scalp. **Guanethidine** use concurrently with **minoxidil** may cause orthostatic hypotension. There is a possible additive effect if **minoxidil** is used concurrently with **antihypertensives.**

CLINICAL USE AND DOSING

Alopecia Androgenetica. **Minoxidil** is available OTC for the treatment of alopecia androgenetica (male pattern baldness). It is important to note that **minoxidil** does not treat balding of the frontoparietal areas in men, only women. **Minoxidil** is effective in treating balding on the *vertex* of the scalp in men.

Minoxidil 2 percent topical solution is applied to the scalp twice daily for the entire length of treatment. Men may use the 5 percent solution if needed. The patient applies 1 mL directly to the affected area of the scalp (vertex area in men and frontoparietal area in women). The medication should be applied to a dry scalp. Patients should be instructed to wash their hands after using their fingers to rub medication into the scalp. Twice-daily application for at least 4 months may be needed to obtain observable hair growth. If the medication is discontinued, the hair in the treated area will shed in 3 to 4 months.

MONITORING. There is no specific laboratory monitoring needed when topical **minoxidil** is used.

PATIENT EDUCATION. Realistic expectations of therapy should be addressed. **Minoxidil** does not treat patients with predominantly frontal hair loss. It may take 3 to 4 months for the effects of treatment to be noticed. Treatment needs to be continued for there to be a continued effect, and the new hair will shed if the medication is discontinued. Effectiveness is variable among patients. New hair may initially be fine and almost colorless. With continued treatment, the hair should be the same color and thickness as the hair on the rest of the scalp.

Table 21–19. Drug Interactions: Miscellaneous Topical Medications

Drug	Interacting Drug	Possible Effect	Implications
EMLA	Methemoglobinemia-inducing drugs: • Acetaminophen • Sulfonamides • Nitrates • Phenytoin • Phenobarbital	Methemoglobinemia	Methemoglobinemia can occur in very young (<12 mo) or patients with G6PD deficit, so do not use concurrently. Monitor other patients closely if using concurrently.
	Class I antiarrhythmic drugs: • Tocainide • Mexiletine	Additive toxic effects	Use concurrently with caution.
Minoxidil	Topical steroids	Increased absorption of minoxidil	Avoid concurrent use.
	Topical retinoids	Increased absorption of minoxidil	Avoid concurrent use.
	Guanethidine	Increased orthostatic hypertension	Avoid concurrent use.
	Antihypertensives	Possible additive effect	Monitor closely if using concurrently.
Wet dressings and soaks	Collagenase	May be inhibited by aluminum acetate solution	Cleanse site with repeated washing of normal saline before applying the enzyme ointment.
Aluminum chloride (Drysol)	No known drug interactions		
Bentoquatam	No known drug interactions		

Table 21–20. Dosage Schedule: Miscellaneous Topical Medications

Drug	Indication	Dosage	Comments
Lidocaine-prilocaine (EMLA)	Topical anesthesia	*Adults:* Minor dermal procedures: Apply 1 disk or 2.5 g cream in a thick layer with occlusion over 20–25 cm^2 for 1 h. Major dermal procedures: Apply 2 g/10 cm^2 in a thick layer with occlusion for 2 h. For male genital skin as adjunct before local anesthetic infiltration: Apply 1 g in thick layer with occlusion for 15 min. *Children age birth–3 mo (<5 kg):* Maximum of 1 g applied/10 cm^2 for up to 1 h. *Age 3–12 mo (>5 kg):* Maximum of 2 g applied/ 20 cm^2 for up to 4 h. *Age 1–6 y (>10 kg):* Maximum of 10 g applied/ 100 cm^2 for up to 4 h. *Age 7–12 y (>20 kg):* Maximum of 20 g applied/ 200 cm^2 for up to 4 h.	Apply to clean skin. Avoid eyes, mucous membranes, tympanic membrane and application to large areas. Not recommended for children <37 weeks gestation.
Minoxidil	Male pattern baldness	Men: Use minoxidil 5%. Apply 1 mL with dropper or sprayer (6 sprays) bid directly to affected scalp areas.	Do not exceed recommended dose. Continue use or hair loss will begin again.
	Diffuse hair loss or frontoparietal thinning in women	Women: Use minoxidil 2%. Apply 1 mL with dropper bid directly to affected scalp areas.	
Wet dressings and soaks (Burow's Solution, Domeboro)	Relief of inflammatory conditions of the skin (athletes foot, poison ivy, allergy, insect bites)	Burow's Solution: Apply wet dressing of 4 treatments/d, each lasting 30 min. Domeboro: Dissolve 1–2 packets in 16 oz water. Apply wet dressing 4 times/d for 30 min each.	
Aluminum chloride (Drysol)	Hyperhidrosis	Solution is applied once daily to the affected area at bedtime, then washed off in the morning. Excessive sweating may stop after 2 or more treatments.	Once control of hyperhidrosis is achieved, the medication is applied once or twice weekly.
Bentoquatam	Skin protection against rash caused by poison oak, ivy, and sumac	Apply as a wet film to exposed skin at least 15 min prior to possible exposure. Reapply every 4 h to maintain protective barrier. Remove with soap and water.	Must be applied before contact with plant oils. Bentoquatam is not to be used in children under age 6 y.

Table 21–21. Available Dosage Forms: Miscellaneous Topical Medications

Drug	Dosage Form	How Supplied
Lidocaine 2.5%–prilocaine 2.5%	Cream	In 5 g with dressings In 30 g
EMLA	1-g disk	In 2s and 10s
Minoxidil • Rogaine Extra Strength for Men • Rogaine for Women	5% solution 2% solution	In 60 mL In 60 mL
Wet dressings and soaks • Aluminum acetate solution (Burow's Solution) • Aluminum sulfate and calcium acetate (Domeboro)	Solution Powder packets	In 480 mL In 12s and 100s
Aluminum chloride Drysol	20% solution	In 35 mL
Bentoquatam IvyBlock	5% lotion	In 120 mL

Administration. Caution the patient to use the medication exactly as prescribed or, for OTC **minoxidil**, as the instructions indicate.

Adverse Reactions. Adverse effects of the medication should be discussed, and the patient instructed to use the medication exactly as recommended to decrease adverse effects.

Miscellaneous Topical Medications

Bath Dermatologicals

Bath dermatologicals contain colloidal solids and oils that act as **emollients** (Table 12–19). They are used to treat dry skin and the pruritus associated with dry skin and common dermatologic conditions. **Emollient** baths that contain **colloidal oatmeal solids (Aveeno)** or **oils (Alpha Keri Bath Oil, Lubriderm Bath Oil)** can be used to provide relief from pruritus associated with contact dermatitis. These products are available OTC, and the patient should be instructed to use them according to the label instructions. Baths may be used as needed for comfort. Caution the patient to be careful when using bath oils to prevent slipping in the tub.

Wet Dressings and Soaks

Wet dressings or soaks are used to provide comfort from inflammatory conditions of the skin, such as contact dermatitis, insect bites, and athlete's foot. **Burow's** or **Domeboro solution (aluminum acetate solution)** is an astringent wet dressing for relief of the inflammation

associated with contact dermatitis. It can be applied as a wet dressing for 30 minutes four times a day (Table 21–20).

Astringents

Aluminum chloride hexahydrate (Drysol) is an **astringent** used for the management of hyperhidrosis (Table 21–21). The solution is applied once daily to the affected area at bedtime and then washed off in the morning. Excessive sweating may stop after two or more treatments. Once control of hyperhidrosis is achieved, the medication is applied once or twice weekly. **Aluminum chloride hexahydrate** solution should be applied to clean, completely dry skin to prevent irritation. Avoid use on broken, irritated, or recently shaved skin.

Sunscreens

Sunscreens provide either a chemical or physical barrier to sunlight. Chemical **sunscreens** are transparent and absorb portions of ultraviolet light. Some chemical **sunscreens** block UVA (**avobenzone**) and others UVB (**PABA** and others). **Oxybenzone** and **dioxybenzone** block both UVA and UVB light. Multiple-chemical **sunscreens** are usually combined in commercial products to provide broad-spectrum coverage. Physical barrier **sunscreens** contain large particulate ingredients (titanium dioxide, red petrolatum, or zinc oxide) that reflect and scatter UVA, UVB, and visible light.

Efficacy of **sunscreens** is determined by their sunscreen protective factor (SPF). Theoretically, a **sunscreen** with an SPF of 15 should allow the person to remain out in the sun 15 times longer before burning than if the skin is unprotected. SPF is affected by sweating, reflection, and wind. Waterproof formulas maintain sunburn protection for 80 minutes in the water, whereas water-resistant formulas protect for only 40 minutes.

Sunscreens must be applied liberally 30 minutes before sun exposure to allow penetration and binding to skin and must be reapplied after swimming.

Do not use **sunscreens** on children younger than 6 months of age. Do not use **sunscreen** with SPF as low as 2 or 3 on children age 2 years or younger. Sensitivity to **sunscreen** can occur. Contact dermatitis may occur with the use of **PABA** or its esters. **PABA** may permanently stain clothing yellow.

Skin Protectant

Bentoquatam (IvyBlock) is an OTC product that provides a protective barrier against contact dermatitis caused by exposure to poison ivy, oak, or sumac when it is applied before contact. The lotion is applied as a wet film to exposed skin at least 15 minutes prior to possible exposure. Reapply every 4 hours to maintain the protective barrier. Remove with soap and water. **Bentoquatam** is not to be used in children under age 6 years.

REFERENCES

Barber, N. (1996). Dermatological diseases. In C. E. Burns, N. Barber, M. A. Brady, & A. M. Dunn (Eds.), *Pediatric primary care: A handbook for nurse practitioners* (pp. 744–758). Philadelphia: Saunders.

Brady, M. A. (1996). Atopic disorders and rheumatic diseases. In C. E. Burns, N. Barber, M. A. Brady, & A. M. Dunn (Eds.), *Pediatric primary care: A handbook for nurse practitioners* (pp. 491–512). Philadelphia: Saunders.

Chesney, P. J., & Burgess, I. F. (1998). Lice: Resistance and treatment. *Contemporary Pediatrics, 15*(11), 180–190.

Cooper, K. D., Menter, M. A., Ritchlin, C. T., Taylor, J. R., & Zanolli, M. D. (1999). Psoriasis: New clues to causation, new ways to treat. *Patient Care for the Nurse Practitioner, 2*(5), 42–50.

Facts and Comparisons Staff. (1999). *Drug facts and comparisons.* St. Louis: Facts and Comparisons.

Feldman, S. R., Fleischer, A. B., Jr., & McConnell, R. C. (1998). Most common dermatologic problems identified by internists, 1990–1994. *Archives of Internal Medicine, 158*(7), 726–730.

Guzzo, C. A., Lazarus, G. S., & Werth, V. P. (1996). Dermatological pharmacology. In J. G. Hardman & L. E. Limbird, (Eds.), *Goodman & Gilman's the pharmacological basis of therapeutics* (9th ed., pp. 1593–1616). New York: McGraw-Hill.

Hansen, R. C., Krafchik, B. R., Lane, A. T., Odio, M. R., & Schachner, L. A. (1998). Dealing with diaper dermatitis. *Contemporary Pediatrics, 15*(May suppl.), 5–10.

Krinsky, W. L. (1996). Arthropods. In J. C. Bennett & F. Plum, (Eds.), *Cecil textbook of medicine* (20th ed., pp. 1946–1949). Philadelphia: Saunders.

Landow, K. (1997). Dispelling myths about acne. *Postgraduate Medicine, 102*(2),94–99, 103–104, 110–112.

Mallon, E., Newton, J. N., Klassen, A., Stewart-Brown, S. L., Ryan, T. J., & Finlay, A. Y. (1999). The quality of life in acne: A comparison with general medical conditions using generic questionnaires. *British Journal of Dermatology, 140*(4), 672–676.

Murphy, J. L. (Ed.) (1999). *Nurse practitioner prescribing reference.* New York: Prescribing Reference.

Parker, F. (1996). Skin diseases of general importance. In J. C. Bennett & F. Plum, (Eds.), *Cecil textbook of medicine* (20th ed., pp. 2197–2217). Philadelphia: Saunders.

Resnick, S. D. (1998). Principles of topical therapy. *Pediatric Annals, 27*(3), 171–176.

Suarez, S., & Friedlander, S. F. (1998). Antifungal therapy in children: An update. *Pediatric Annals, 27*(3), 177–184.

Whitley, R. J. (1996). In J. C. Bennett & F. Plum, (Eds.), *Cecil textbook of medicine* (20th ed., pp. 1770–1776). Philadelphia: Saunders.

CHAPTER 22

·······

Drugs Used in Treating Infectious Diseases

CHAPTER OUTLINE

Many disease processes once incurable are now treatable with **antibacterial, antifungal,** or **antiviral drugs.** These **anti-infective agents** have made a significant difference in morbidity and mortality throughout the world. In the 1980s, new pathogens began to emerge, and organisms previously susceptible to therapy developed resistance. Factors that contribute to this phenomenon include larger populations of immunocompromised patients, increases in the number and complexity of invasive medical procedures, and increased survival of patients with chronic diseases (Schaad, 1997). Spread of resistant organisms in the community has been associated with daycare for young children, overcrowding, and travel (Helwig, 1997; Roman et al., 1997).

Excessive and inappropriate use of anti-infectious agents is a major factor in drug resistance (Cohen et al., 1997; Schwartz, Mainous, & Marcy, 1998). Lack of knowledge on the part of health care providers and their patients, willingness to prescribe **antibiotics** when pressured by patients, and concerns generated by managed care have all contributed to the vast overuse of **antimicrobial agents** (Bauchner, Pelton, & Klein, 1999; Mangione-Smith, McGlynn, Elliott, Krogstad, & Brook, 1999.) Some experts speculate that we are approaching the end of the **antibiotic** era, when many common organisms will no longer be susceptible to **antibiotics,** multidrug therapy will be required to treat most infections, and patients may die from once curable infections (Levin, Lipsich, & Perrot, 1997). Unless novel drug mechanisms are developed, a prospect many experts find less than likely (Katzung, 1998), providers will be dependent on the current classes of drugs to treat infectious disease. At the same time that **antimicrobial drugs** are becoming less effective for familiar infections, new indications for **antimicrobial drugs** such as peptic ulcer, diabetes, myocardial infarction, and rheumatoid arthritis have been identified or proposed (O'Dell, 1999; Schussheim & Fuster, 1999). Thus, it behooves us to improve our knowledge in this area and to use these drugs wisely.

This chapter focuses on systemic applications of drugs that are active against bacterial, fungal, viral, or parasitic organisms. Topical applications associated with dermatologic conditions are presented in Chapter 21. Although many of these drugs are available in intravenous (IV) formulations, oral (PO) and intramuscular (IM) formulations are more commonly used in primary care and are the focus of this chapter.

Antibiotics: Beta-Lactams

Penicillins

The discovery of **penicillins** initiated the **antibiotic** era. Penicillins are classified as **beta-lactam drugs** because their chemistry includes a unique four-member lactam ring. They share features of chemistry, mechanism of action, and clinical effects with the other **beta-lactam antibiotics: cephalosporins, monobactams, carbapenems,** and **beta-lactamase inhibitors. Cephalosporins** are discussed in the next section, and **beta-lactamase inhibitors** are described with the **penicillins** because they are usually used together in combination products. **Monobactams** and **carbapenems** are used to treat serious infections in the hospital and are not included here.

Penicillins are characterized chemically by the 6-aminopenicillanic acid joined to the beta-lactam ring. Attachment of different substitutes to 6-aminopenicillanic acid in the chemical compound results in different pharmacological and antibacterial characteristics, which are the basis for four **penicillin** subclasses: (1) **penicillinase-sensitive** or **natural penicillins,** (2) **penicillinase-resistant** or **antistaphylococcal penicillins,** (3) **aminopenicillins,** and (4) **antipseudomonal** or **extended-spectrum penicillins.**

Pharmacodynamics

Penicillins hinder bacterial growth by inhibiting the biosynthesis of bacterial cell wall mucopeptide (also called murein or peptidoglycan). This action is dependent on the drug's reaching the penicillin-binding proteins (PBPs), which include transpeptidase, carboxypeptidase, and endopeptidase enzymes involved in the terminal stages of forming the cell wall. When penicillins bind to the PBPs, the wall is weakened, and lysis of the bacterial cell wall occurs. Because human cells lack a cell wall, there is virtually no action against host cells. **Penicillins** are bactericidal against sensitive organisms when adequate concentrations are achieved and are most effective during active cellular multiplication. Less than adequate concentrations may result in only bacteriostatic effects.

Sensitivity

The natural **penicillinase-sensitive group** is active against aerobic, gram-positive organisms, including *Streptococcus* species such as pneumoniae and group A beta-hemolytic (GABHS), some *Enterococcus* strains, and some non-penicillinase-producing *Staphylococcus*. Only about 5 to 15 percent of community-acquired *Staphylococcus aureus* remains susceptible to **natural penicillins,** principally because the majority of strains produce penicillinase. There is growing concern about the increasing resistance of *Streptococcus pneumoniae* to **penicillins.** This organism is the most common bacterial pathogen in upper respiratory infections such as otitis media and sinusitis. **Penicillin**-resistant strains are also commonly resistant to **tetracyclines, macrolides,** and **sulfonamides;** they are commonly called drug-resistant *S. pneumoniae* (DRSP) (Kaplan, 1997; Klein, 1995).

Penicillin G is also active against some gram-negative organisms such as *Neisseria gonorrhoeae* and *Neisseria meningitidis*, although penicillinase-producing strains resistant to **natural penicillin** have become widespread. **Natural penicillins** are highly effective against *Actinomyces israelii, Bacillus anthracis,* oropharyngeal *Bacteroides* species, *Borrelia burgdorferi, Pasteurella multocida, Listeria monocytogenes, Clostridium* species and several other gram-positive anaerobes, and *Treponema pallidum.*

Penicillinase-resistant group, also called **antistaphylococcal penicillins,** has an even narrower spectrum of activity than the **natural penicillins.** They are active against penicillinase-producing *S. aureus* and *Staphylococcus epidermidis* organisms. However, resistance mediated by a mechanism other than penicillinase production is manifested by **methicillin** resistant *S. aureus* (MRSA) and *S. epidermidis* (MRSE). **Methicillin**-resistant strains are resistant to all drugs in the **penicillinase-resistant** group, as well as all **penicillins** and **cephalosporins. Vancomycin,** which is not a **penicillin,** is currently the only single **antibiotic** consistently effective against serious MRSA and MRSE infections, but **vancomycin** resistance has recently been reported (CDC, 1997). **Penicillinase-resistant penicillins** are much less potent against gram-negative bacteria than are **natural penicillins.**

Aminopenicillins are broad-spectrum drugs that are active against many of the same organisms as the **penicillinase-sensitive group,** but they have greater activity against gram-negative bacteria because of their enhanced ability to penetrate the outer membrane of these organisms. They are especially useful for gram-negative urinary and gastrointestinal (GI) pathogens such as *Escherichia coli, Proteus mirabilis, Salmonella,* some *Shigella* species, and *Enterococcus faecalis*. **Aminopenicillins** are also active against the common gram-negative respiratory pathogens *Moraxella catarrhalis* (formerly *Branhamella catarrhalis*) and *Haemophilus influenzae,* type B. Many strains of *H. influenzae,* Enterobacteriaceae, *Salmonella,* and *Shigella* are beta-lactamase producers and therefore resistant to **aminopenicillins,** and resistance due to beta-lactamase production of *E. coli* is increasing.

The **antipseudomonal group** has enhanced activity against gram-negative bacilli, especially *Pseudomonas aeruginosa, Enterobacter, Morganella,* and *Providencia* species, and other gram-negative rods, while retaining activity against the organisms sensitive to the **aminopenicillins,** although they are less active against *Streptococcus* and *Enterococcus*. The **antipseudomonal mezlocillin** has the greatest activity against *Klebsiella* species and *Bacteroides fragilis.*

The combination of **beta-lactamase inhibitors** (e.g., **clavulanate, sulbactam,** and **tazobactam**) with certain **aminopenicillins** and **antipseudomonal penicillins** has broadened their spectrum to include beta-lactamase–producing strains. The oral combination of **amoxicillin** and **clavulanate** is effective against beta-lactamase producing *S. aureus, N. gonorrhoeae, H. influenzae,* and *M. catarrhalis.*

Many texts and references (e.g., Gilbert, Moellering, & Sande, 1999; Kastrup, 1999) have tables that list the organisms generally susceptible to various **penicillins.**

Resistance

Resistance to **penicillins** is due to (1) inactivation by beta-lactamases, (2) alteration in target PBPs on the bacterial cell wall, or (3) a permeability barrier preventing penetration of the antibiotic to the target cell. Beta-lactamase production is the most common mechanism. Beta-lactamases include a large group of enzymes called penicillinases and cephalosporinases. More than 100 different beta-lactamases have been identified, with varying degrees of specificity for various **beta-lactam drugs.** Beta-lactamases produced by *S. aureus, Haemophilus* species, and *E. coli* have narrow specificity for **penicillins;** those produced by *P. aeruginosa* and *Enterobacter* species have broader specificity and will hydrolyze both **penicillins** and **cephalosporins. Beta-lactamase inhibitors (clavulanate, sulbactam,** and **tazobactam)** have weak antibacterial activity but irreversibly inactivate beta-lactamase enzymes produced by bacteria by binding to their active site and protecting the **antibiotic** from inactivation.

Alteration in PBPs is responsible for **methicillin** resistance in staphylococci and **penicillin** resistance in pneumococci. Drug penetration problems are associated with the cellular outer membrane, which is present in gram-negative but not gram-positive organisms. This barrier becomes important only when beta-lactamase is also acting to hydrolyze the **antibiotic** as it slowly enters the membrane.

Pharmacokinetics

Absorption and Distribution

Oral penicillin formulations are generally well absorbed from the GI tract, but several are unstable in acid, resulting in the majority of the dose being destroyed in the stomach. To produce acceptable drug levels, the doses of these acid-labile drugs must be three to four times that of the parenteral formulation and be taken on an empty stomach. Thus, **oral penicillins** are not reliable enough to use for serious systemic infections. **Penicillin V** has less individual variation in absorption than **Penicillin G** and is virtually the only **oral natural penicillin** in use. **Nafcillin's** oral absorption is so poor that the oral route is rarely used, whereas **dicloxacillin** is best absorbed of the **penicillinase-resistant group,** producing blood levels twice that of **oxacillin** or **cloxacillin. Amoxicillin** is more completely absorbed than **ampicillin** and may be given without regard to food. **Carbenicillin,** the only **oral antipseudomonal penicillin,** is not adequately absorbed to attain blood levels effective for systemic infections, so it is indicated only for urinary tract and prostatic infections.

All subclasses of **penicillin** have agents that can be given IM, but different **penicillin salts** have different absorption rates. The IM route is unreliable and erratic, as well as irritating to the tissue, and repeated dosing by this route should be avoided. Because the **penicillin G procaine** and **penicillin G benzathine** formulations are slowly absorbed, they are used as depot agents for IM use only. *IV injection of these depot formulations can be lethal.*

Penicillins are bound to plasma proteins to varying degrees and are well distributed to most tissues and body fluids. Inflammation enhances penetration of the meninges, joints, and eye fluids, which are otherwise poorly penetrated. **Penicillins** cross the placenta and enter breast milk.

Metabolism and Excretion

Excluding **nafcillin** and **oxacillin, penicillins** undergo negligible metabolism and are excreted primarily as unchanged drug in the urine, achieving high concentrations of active drug in the urine. Ninety percent of the renal excretion of **penicillin** is by active tubular secretion, and most other **penicillins** undergo extensive tubular secretion. **Probenecid,** which competes with **penicillins** for the tubular secretion carrier, will prolong the half-life and raise the peak plasma concentration of **penicillins.** Thus, concurrent administration of oral **probenecid** is used to treat some serious infections. Renal insufficiency prolongs the half-life and increases the risk for toxicity of **penicillins.** Table 22–1 shows the pharmacokinetic properties of each of the **penicillin** subclasses.

Pharmacotherapeutics

Precautions and Contraindications

Although fewer than 10 percent of patients taking these drugs have an allergic reaction, **penicillins** are the most likely class of drugs to cause an allergic reaction. History of a serious hypersensitivity reaction (e.g., anaphylaxis, serum sickness, exfoliative dermatitis, hemolysis or other blood dyscrasia) to a **penicillin** contraindicates the use of any **penicillin** on account of the total cross-reactivity

Table 22–1. Pharmacokinetics: Penicillins

Drug	Onset	Peak	Duration	Protein Binding	Bioavail-ability	Half-Life	Penicillinase Resistance	Acid Stability	Elimi-nation
Penicillinase-sensitive									
Penicillin G sodium (IM)	Rapid	0.5–3 h	4–6 h	60%	0	0.7 h	No	NA	Unchanged by kidney
Penicillin G benza-thine (IM)	Delayed	12–24 h	3 wk	UA	0	0.5–1h	No	NA	Unchanged by kidney
Penicillin G procaine (IM)	Delayed	1–4 h	12 h	UA	0	0.5–1 h	No	NA	Unchanged by kidney
Penicillin G potassium (PO)	1 h	1 h	4–6 h	UA	UA	0.5–1 h	No	No	Unchanged by kidney
(IM)	Rapid	15–30 min	4–6 h	UA	0	0.5–1 h	No	NA	Unchanged by kidney
Penicillin V (PO)	Rapid	0.5–1 h	4–6 h	80%	60%	0.5 h	No	No	Unchanged by kidney
Penicillinase-resistant									
Cloxacillin (PO)	30 min	0.5–1.5 h	6 h	93–95%	49%	0.5 h	Yes	Yes	9–22% by liver; 30–45% by kidney
Dicloxacillin (PO)	30 min	1–2 h	6 h	96–98%	UA	0.8 h	Yes	Yes	6–10% by liver; 60% unchanged in urine
Methicillin (IM)	Rapid	0.5–1 h	4–6 h	40%	Minimal	0.4 h	Yes	NA	Unchanged by kidney
Nafcillin (PO)	Rapid	30 min	1–2 h	80–90%	Low	0.5–1.5 h	Yes	Yes	60% by liver; rest un-changed in urine
(IM)	Rapid	30 min	1–2 h	80–90%	0	0.5–1.5 h	Yes	NA	
Oxacillin (PO)	Rapid	0.5–1 h	4–6 h	90–94%	33%	0.5–1 h	Yes	Yes	49% by liver; rest un-changed in urine
(IM)	Rapid	0.5 h	4–6 h	90–94%	0		Yes	NA	
Aminopenicillins									
Amoxicillin (PO)	30 min	1–2 h	8 h	20%	80%	1–1.3 h	No	Yes	30% by liver; 70% un-changed in urine
Ampicillin (PO)	Rapid	1.5–2 h	4–6 h	20%	50%	1–1.5 h	No	Yes	25–60% in urine
(IM)	Rapid	1 h	4–6 h	20%	0	1–1.5 h	No	NA	50–85% in urine
Antipseudomonals									
Carbenicillin (PO)	30 min	0.5–2 h	6 h	50%	UA	0.8–1 h	No	Yes	36% un-changed in urine

Continued on next page

Table 22–1. Pharmacokinetics: Penicillins *(continued)*

Drug	Onset	Peak	Duration	Protein Binding	Bioavail-ability	Half-Life	Penicillinase Resistance	Acid Stability	Elimi-nation
Mezlocillin (IM)	Rapid	1–1.5 h	4–6 h	16–42%	0	0.7–1.3 h	No	NA	55–60% unchanged in urine; 15–30% in bile
Piperacillin (IM)	Rapid	0.5–1 h	4–6 h	16%	0	0.5–1.2 h	No	NA	90% un-changed in urine; 10% in bile
Combinations Amoxicillin/ clavulanate (PO)	30 min	1–2 h	8 h	18–25%	80%	1–1.3 h	Yes	Yes	30% by liver; 70% un-changed in urine
Ampicillin/sulbactam (IM)	Rapid	1 h	6–8 h	20–38%	0	1–1.3 h	Yes	NA	Variable by liver and kidney
Piperacillin/ tazobactam (IM)	Rapid	0.5–1 h	4–6 h	16–30%	0	0.7–1.2 h	Yes	NA	Variable; tazobac-tam 80% by kidney

UA = Information unavailable.
NA = Not applicable

among the **penicillins.** Allergic reactions to **cephalosporins, imipenem,** or **beta-lactamase inhibitors** may contraindicate use of **penicillins.** Cross-sensitivity between these drugs occurs in 5 to 16 percent of patients. Patients with a history of allergy to other substances (e.g., atopic skin conditions) should also use these drugs with caution.

Mezlocillin, carbenicillin (parenteral), and **piperacillin** may induce hemorrhagic manifestations, and they should be used with extreme caution by patients who have anemia, thrombocytopenia, granulocytopenia, or bone marrow depression or who are receiving anticoagulants.

Penicillins are Pregnancy Category B, but there are not adequate and controlled studies in women. They should be used only when clearly indicated.

The safety and efficacy of **carbenicillin** and the **piperacillin-tazobactam** combination have not been established for children under 12 years old. Dosage adjustment of **penicillins** may be required for infants because of their undeveloped renal function. (See the Clinical Use and Dosing section for further discussion.)

Adverse Drug Reactions

Serious and occasionally fatal immediate hypersensitivity reactions (type I hypersensitivity) have occurred, with an incidence of anaphylactic shock of 0.015 to 0.04

percent (Kastrup, 1998). These reactions usually occur within 2 to 30 minutes after administration and are characterized by nausea, vomiting, urticaria, pruritus, tachycardia, severe dyspnea, diaphoresis, stridor, vertigo, and eventually loss of consciousness and circulatory collapse. Treatment is the same as for any anaphylactic reaction. Skin testing may be used to identify those at risk for **penicillin** allergy, but the commercially available skin test antigen (penicilloyl polylysine) does not predict anaphylactic reactions (Gilbert, Moellering, & Sande, 1999). Patients with a known allergy or a positive skin test can be given desensitization therapy. Other hypersensitivity reactions include skin rashes, a serum sickness–like reaction (skin rash, joint pain, fever), exfoliative dermatitis (red, scaly skin), and blood dyscrasias (hemolytic anemia, neutropenia, leukopenia).

A maculopapular rash that does not represent a true allergy occasionally occurs with **ampicillin** (9%) or **amoxicillin.** It is more common with patients who have mononucleosis (43 to 100%), chronic lymphocytic leukemia (90%), or concurrent **allopurinol** therapy (15 to 20%). This measleslike, pruritic, generalized rash typically appears 7 to 10 days after initiation of therapy and remains for a few days after the drug in discontinued. This rash does not contraindicate subsequent use of **aminopenicillins.**

As with many **antibiotics,** common adverse reactions include GI symptoms such as nausea, vomiting, diarrhea, and epigastric distress. **Amoxicillin** produces these symptoms less often than **ampicillin** and can be taken with food, which will further decrease incidence of these adverse effects. Addition of **clavulanate** to form **amoxicillin-clavulanate** doubles the incidence of diarrhea to 10 percent, but new formulations with lower concentrations of **clavulanate** have reduced this uncomfortable side effect. The **penicillinase-resistant penicillins** are the most likely group to cause hepatotoxicity, especially when administered with other hepatotoxic drugs.

Use of broader spectrum **penicillins,** or prolonged or repeat therapy with any broad-spectrum **antibacterial,** may result in bacterial or fungal overgrowth (i.e., super-infection) of nonsusceptible organisms. The patient should be monitored for this possibility and treated with appropriate measures. *Clostridium difficile* colitis is a superinfection that manifests as severe abdominal cramps and pain, watery severe diarrhea that may be bloody, and fever, occurring up to several weeks after discontinuation of the drug. This pseudomembranous colitis or antibiotic-associated colitis is a serious sequela that may abate with supportive therapy and discontinuance of the **antibiotic,** but severe cases require treatment with oral **metronidazole,** oral **vancomycin,** or **cholestyramine.**

Patients who are HIV-positive are more susceptible to hepatotoxicity resulting from **cloxacillin, dicloxacillin,** and **oxacillin** than are HIV-negative patients. Although interstitial nephritis was commonly seen with **methicillin,** which is no longer used, it still occurs occasionally with **oxacillin, nafcillin,** or any other **penicillin.** High doses of **procaine penicillin G** can cause transient mental disturbances, including combativeness, irritability, and hallucinations. Platelet dysfunction is primarily associated with parenteral **carbenicillin, piperacillin,** and **ticarcillin.** Irritability and seizures have occurred with high doses of **penicillin G,** especially in patients with renal insufficiency.

Drug Interactions

The main drug interactions with **penicillins** are shown in Table 22–2. Of interest is the potential for reduced efficacy of **oral contraceptives,** particularly with **aminopenicillins.** It is difficult to tie contraceptive failure to concurrent use of any **antibiotic,** in that no **oral contraceptive** is 100 percent efficacious. There are few case reports of such failures. When the slight risk of pregnancy is unacceptable to the patient, an additional form of contraception should be considered. For drug interactions specific to a particular **penicillin,** selecting a different **penicillin** may be acceptable, but often a different **antibiotic** class that will treat the infection is preferable. Food and acid juices decrease absorption of **penicillin V** and the **penicillinase-resistant group.**

Clinical Use and Dosing

Antibiotics are among the most frequently prescribed drugs in primary care practice, amounting to 12 to 14 percent of all outpatient prescriptions. An **antibiotic** from the **penicillin** family is usually the drug of choice for a susceptible organism because the toxicity of this class is minimal in the nonallergic individual. The most common infections treated with **penicillins** in ambulatory care have been upper respiratory infections (URIs) (pharyngitis, otitis media, sinusitis, bronchitis), pneumonia, sexually transmitted diseases, urinary tract infections, and wound infections. Other important indications for **penicillins** are endocarditis prophylaxis, eradication of *Helicobacter pylori* in gastritis and peptic ulcer disease, and Lyme disease. Serious infections that require hospitalization for monitoring and IV therapy are not included in this discussion, although **penicillins** are an important component of treatment for the 30 to 50 percent of hospitalized patients who receive **antibiotics.**

COLD, ACUTE BRONCHITIS, AND UPPER RESPIRATORY INFECTION. Recently, there has been growing concern that overuse and misuse of **antibiotics** for URIs contribute to **antibiotic** resistance. Gonzales, Steiner, and Sande (1997) found that 51 percent of patients diagnosed as having colds, 52 percent of patients diagnosed as having a URI, and 66 percent of patients diagnosed with acute bronchitis received a prescription for **antibiotics.** Among children, **antibiotics** were prescribed to 44 percent with a common cold, 46 percent with a URI, and 75 percent with acute bronchitis (Nyquist, Gonzales, Steiner, & Sande, 1998). Because the common cold, URI, and acute bronchitis are seasonal, self-limiting illnesses usually caused by viruses, **antibiotics** have no role in management of uncomplicated cases, even though many **antibiotics** are approved for use in bronchitis. Symptomatic treatment, rest, and proper nutrition should be instituted to support the patient while these self-limiting disorders progress through their natural course. Inhaled **albuterol** may improve patient comfort in acute bronchitis (Hueston & Mainous, 1998; Oeffinger, Snell, Foster, Panico, & Archer, 1998). Bronchitis requires **antimicrobial** therapy only if there is prolonged cough with a diagnosed etiology of a specific infection, such as pertussis or *Mycoplasma pneumoniae,* or an underlying pulmonary disease such as cystic fibrosis, bronchopulmonary dysplasia, or severe asthma. **Penicillins** are generally not appropriate for the infecting organisms in these complicated cases of bronchitis. During the common cold, mucopurulent rhinitis (thick, opaque, or discolored nasal discharge) is *not* an indication for **antimicrobials** unless it persists without improvement for more than 10 to 14 days (Dowell, 1998).

CHRONIC BRONCHITIS. It is important to distinguish acute bronchitis from an acute exacerbation of chronic bronchitis. Chronic bronchitis, a condition largely con-

Table 22–2. Drug Interactions: Penicillins

Drug	Interacting Drug	Possible Effect	Implications
Penicillins	Diuretics	Potassium-wasting diuretics may have increased risk for hypokalemia; the reverse is true for potassium-sparing diuretics.	If they must be given together, monitor serum potassium levels and for indications of these electrolyte imbalances.
	Oral contraceptives	Evidence is contradictory. The efficacy of oral contraceptives may be reduced, and increased breakthrough bleeding may occur. Although infrequently reported, contraceptive failure is possible.	It is difficult to tie contraceptive failure directly to penicillin use because no oral contraceptive is 100% efficacious. The use of an additional form of contraception during penicillin therapy should be considered.
	Probenecid	Delays renal elimination and increases blood levels.	Monitor for penicillin toxicity. Rarely used therapeutically anymore.
	Tetracyclines	Bacteriostatic action of tetracyclines may impair bactericidal effects of penicillins.	Avoid coadministration.
Ampicillin	Beta blockers	May reduce bioavailability of atenolol. Beta blockers may potentiate anaphylactic reactions of penicillin.	Select a different penicillin if patient is taking atenolol.
	Allopurinol	Higher incidence of ampicillin-induced rash.	Avoid coadministration.
Mezlocillin, piperacillin	Lithium	May alter excretion of lithium.	Avoid concurrent administration.
Nafcillin	Cyclosporine	Concurrent administration produces subtherapeutic cyclosporine levels.	If they must be used concurrently, monitor cyclosporine levels more closely.
Nafcillin, oxacillin, cloxacillin, dicloxacillin	Food and acidic juices	Decreased absorption of these penicillins.	Avoid concurrent administration.
Penicillin G	Aspirin, phenylbutazone, sulfonamides, thiazide diuretics, indomethacin, furosemide	These drugs compete with penicillin G for renal tubular secretion and thus prolong the serum half-life of penicillin.	Consider altered pharmacokinetics when prescribing or select a different penicillin.
	Colestipol, cholestyramine	May decrease absorption of oral penicillin G.	Separate doses. Give penicillin G 1 h before or 4 h after colestipol or cholestyramine.

fined to smokers, is defined as a recurrent daily cough with sputum production that persists for at least 3 months at a time in at least 2 consecutive years. Patients with underlying chronic bronchitis may periodically become infected with a wide variety of organisms, most commonly viruses, *S. aureus, Haemophilus pneumoniae,* or *M. catarrhalis.* Although some studies show benefit for acute bacterial exacerbations of chronic bronchitis (ABECB), other studies are less supportive, so the management of ABECB is controversial (Gilbert, Moellering, and Sande, 1999; Hueston & Mainous, 1998). Gram's stain and culture are unreliable in patients with ABECB because the respiratory tract is normally colonized below the vocal cords. The decision to use **antimicrobial drugs** may be based on presence of at least two of the three cardinal symptoms: increased sputum volume, increased sputum purulence, and increased dyspnea. The patient reports feeling sicker than usual and may have a fever. A radiograph of the chest may be required to rule out bronchopneumonia. Recovery usually begins 3 to 4 days after **antibiotics** are initiated. Therapy usually continues 5 to 10 days, depending on the drug used (Niederman, Skerett, Yamauchi, & Pinkowish, 1998). If cost is an issue, first-line therapy for ABECB is **doxycycline** or **trimethoprim-sulfamethoxazole.** If cost is not an issue, **amoxicillin-clavulanate** in doses of 875/125 mg twice daily or

500/125 mg three times daily is considered first-line therapy, as are comparably priced third-generation oral **cephalosporins,** newer **macrolides,** and **fluoroquinolones.**

OTITIS MEDIA. Acute otitis media (AOM) is the most common indication for **antibiotic** prescribing in the United States and accounts for nearly half of all pediatric diagnoses and office visits (Carlson & Deay; Kozyrskyj et al., 1998). In assessing middle ear symptoms, it is important to distinguish between AOM and otitis media with effusion (OME). AOM is defined as the presence of fluid in the middle ear in association with signs or symptoms of acute local illness (otalgia, otorrhea, immobile bulging tympanic membrane that may be red) and/or systemic illness (e.g., fever). OME is the presence of fluid in the middle ear in the absence of signs or symptoms of acute illness. OME often follows resolution of AOM and may not abate for several months after the infection.

Antimicrobial drugs are indicated for AOM, although the treatment effect is small, with 80 to 90 percent of untreated cases resolving clinically by 7 to 14 days. Viral etiology is assumed for 35 percent of AOM, and the three most common bacterial etiologies are *S. pneumoniae* (30 to 35%), *H. influenzae* (20 to 25%), and *M. catarrhalis* (10 to 15%). Because culture of AOM requires tympanocentesis, AOM is usually treated empirically. **Amoxicillin** is the first-line drug of choice for AOM in the nonallergic patient in initial doses of 875 mg twice daily or 500 mg three times daily for adults. The pediatric dose is 20 to 50 mg/kg divided into three doses daily. About 90 percent of *M. catarrhalis* strains and 20 to 40 percent of *H. influenzae* strains produce beta-lactamase, and 2 to 33 percent of *S. pneumoniae* are drug resistant (DRSP). However, **amoxicillin** is still highly effective, safe, and inexpensive for AOM, compared with other **antimicrobials.** The traditional course of treatment for AOM is 7 to 10 days, although recent research and guidelines support a 5- to 7-day course for individuals over age 2 without perforation of the tympanic membrane (Kozyrskyj et al., 1998: Pichichero & Cohen, 1997). Perforated tympanic membrane requires at least 10 days of **antimicrobial** treatment (Dowell, 1998). Because of the increased risk of DRSP associated with daycare attendance and recent or recurrent **antibiotic** therapy, patients with these characteristics are appropriately treated for at least 10 days with **amoxicillin** at 80 to 90 mg/kg daily divided into two or three doses (Gooch & Golantly, 2000).

If there is no response after 72 hours of **amoxicillin** alone, it is likely that the causal organism is a beta-lactamase–producing strain of *H. influenzae* or *M. catarrhalis.* If possible, tympanocentesis should be performed for culture and sensitivity. If this is not feasible, empiric treatment with **amoxicillin-clavulanate** in adult doses of 875 mg **amoxicillin** and 125 mg **clavulanate** twice daily is recommended for persistent or recurrent AOM. Children should receive the amount of **amoxicillin-clavulanate** that supplies 80 to 90 mg/kg of **amoxicillin** and 6.4 mg **clavulanate** per day divided into two doses (Tiggs, 2000). The alternative to **amoxicillin-clavulanate** is third-generation **cephalosporins** (Gooch & Golantly, 2000).

Persistent OME after therapy for AOM is expected and does not require treatment. OME should be treated with **antimicrobials** only if bilateral effusions, accompanied by documented hearing loss, persist for 3 or more months, although insertion of tympanostomy tubes is probably more effective therapy. If a child experiences three or more well-documented, distinct occurrences of AOM within 6 months, or four in a year, prophylactic **antimicrobial** therapy for no more than 6 months should be considered. **Sulfonamides** are the preferred drug class for prophylaxis of AOM.

SINUSITIS. Sinus inflammation can be a response to viruses, allergy, pollution, or other irritation. Viral rhinosinusitis is 20 to 200 times more common than bacterial sinusitis, which complicates 5 percent or fewer cases of viral URI. Clinical diagnosis of acute bacterial sinusitis requires prolonged nonspecific upper respiratory signs such as rhinosinusitis and cough without improvement for more than 10 days, or more severe upper respiratory signs and symptoms such as substantial fever, facial swelling, or facial pain. Acute bacterial sinusitis is caused by the same pathogens as otitis media (*S. pneumoniae, H. influenzae, M. catarrhalis*) and often resolves without **antibiotics. Amoxicillin,** in doses listed for otitis media, is often successful for initial treatment. If there is no response in 48 hours, **amoxicillin-clavulanate,** an oral **cephalosporin, clindamycin,** or high-dose **amoxicillin** should be substituted. Treatment should be continued 7 days beyond substantial improvement or resolution of signs and symptoms, usually 10 to 14 days (Dowell, 1998). **Antimicrobial drugs** have little efficacy in treatment of chronic sinusitis.

PHARYNGITIS. The pathogen in pharyngitis is usually a virus, and concurrent rhinorrhea, cough, hoarseness, conjunctivitis, and diarrhea strongly suggest a viral etiology. Most bacterial pharyngitis is self-limiting and will subside without sequelae. The exception is group A beta-hemolytic streptococci (GABHS; *Streptococcus pyogenes*), which is associated with rheumatic fever if not treated. An antigen detection ("rapid strep") test should be used to confirm the diagnosis, with negative results backed up with a throat culture. **Antibiotic** therapy started within 9 days of pharyngitis onset will avoid rheumatic fever. The drug of choice is **penicillin V** in adult doses of 500 mg twice daily or 250 mg four times daily for 10 to 14 days. The dose for children is 25 to 50 mg/kg per day divided into four doses administered every 6 hours for 10 days. Because the taste of the suspension or solution of **penicillin V** may not be acceptable to small children, **amoxicillin** 40 mg/kg per day divided into three doses for 10 days may be used. Because the broader spectrum drug may promote resistance, **penicillin V** is preferred over **amoxicillin.** If nonadherence is anticipated, **penicillin G benzathine** as a single IM dose of 1.2 million U for adults, or a pediatric dose of 25,000 U/kg, may be substituted.

URINARY TRACT INFECTIONS.   *E. coli,* the most common pathogen in community-acquired urinary tract infections (UTIs), has become increasingly resistant to oral **penicillins** because of beta-lactamase production. Consequently, monotherapy with a **penicillin** is no longer first-line treatment for most UTIs in nonpregnant adults. **Amoxicillin-clavulanate** is recommended for empirical treatment of uncomplicated cystitis-urethritis in doses of 500 mg **amoxicillin** and 125 mg **clavulanate** or 875 mg **amoxicillin** and 125 mg **clavulanate** twice daily for 3 days (Orenstein, 1999). For acute uncomplicated pyelonephritis, a 14-day duration of therapy is required. Complicated infections require parenteral therapy. Because of its excellent safety profile, a 3- to 7-day course of **amoxicillin** 250 mg three times daily is still a first-line therapy for treating asymptomatic bacteriuria during pregnancy. **Amoxicillin** is also used to treat UTI during pregnancy in doses of 250 mg every 8 hours for 3 to 7 days (Orenstein, 1999) and for UTI in children (Ogle, 1999).

SEXUALLY TRANSMITTED DISEASES.   Because of beta-lactamase production by many strains of *N. gonorrhoeae,* **penicillins** no longer have a role in treatment of gonococcal infections. However, *T. pallidum* retains susceptibility to **natural penicillins,** so recommended treatment for adults with early primary, secondary, or latent syphilis of less than 1 year's duration is one 2.4-million-U dose of **penicillin G benzathine** IM. For pregnant women, some clinicians administer a second dose 1 week after the first. If latent syphilis is over 1 year's duration or of indeterminate duration, three doses at weekly intervals are required. Because **penicillin G benzathine** does not attain adequate concentrations in the brain, neurosyphilis and congenital syphilis are treated with IV **penicillin G** or IM **penicillin G procaine** (2.4 million U daily for 10 days) plus oral **probenecid** (1 g daily for 10 days). An accepted use of **amoxicillin** is the treatment of chlamydial infections in pregnant women unable to tolerate **erythromycin,** although the mechanism of this cell wall–inhibiting drug for an organism that lacks the cell wall is unexplained (USPDI, 1999).

SKIN AND TISSUE INFECTIONS.   **Amoxicillin-clavulanate** is indicated as first-line therapy for prophylaxis of infection following bites of a variety of mammals, including humans, and for infected postoperative or posttraumatic wounds. Oral **penicillinase-resistant penicillins, oxacillin,** and **dicloxacillin** are indicated for bullous impetigo caused by *S. aureus* and erysipelas of the extremities. **Penicillin V** and **penicillin G benza-**thine are used in the treatment of impetigo caused by group A streptococci. Wounds accompanied by sepsis and severe tissue involvement require hospitalization and intravenous treatment.

BACTERIAL ENDOCARDITIS PROPHYLAXIS.   **Antibiotic** administration has traditionally been recommended for susceptible patients prior to certain oral, GI, and pulmonary invasive procedures when bacteria may be released into the circulation. The American Heart Association recently reevaluated prophylactic **antibiotic** therapy and currently recommends therapy only for those with prosthetic heart valves or previous endocarditis who are undergoing dental extractions or gingival surgery (Gilbert, Moellering, & Sande, 1999). **Penicillins** that are first-line therapy for prophylaxis include **amoxicillin** (adults 2 g and children 50 mg/kg orally 1 hour before procedure) and **ampicillin** (adults 2 g and children 50 mg/kg IM or IV within 30 minutes before procedure). **Penicillin**-allergic patients should use **cephalosporins, clindamycin,** or the newer **macrolides** for prophylaxis.

PNEUMONIA.   Although the pattern of causal organisms in pneumonia varies by age, whether community or hospital acquired, and other risk factors (e.g., smoking, HIV, **alcohol** abuse, IV drug abuse, airway obstruction, use of **corticosteroids**), the most common pathogens in community-acquired pneumonia (CAP) are *S. pneumoniae, M. pneumoniae, Chlamydia pneumoniae, H. influenzae,* and *M. catarrhalis. M. pneumoniae* and *C. pneumoniae* lack a cell wall and are naturally resistant to **penicillins.** Acquired resistance is common in strains of the other organisms that cause pneumonia, so oral or IM **penicillins** have a minimal role in the empiric treatment of pneumonia. **Amoxicillin-clavulanate** in doses of 872/125 mg twice daily is an alternative to **macrolides** and **fluoroquinolones** for CAP, but it is not active against *Mycoplasma, Legionella,* or *Chlamydia* species. The American Thoracic Society recommends **amoxicillin-clavulanate** for CAP patients older than 60 with no comorbidities, because the pneumococcus is the most common pathogen in this group (Gleason, Kapoor, & Stone, 1997). **Natural penicillins** or **aminopenicillins** are appropriate in other populations when culture and sensitivity document susceptible strains of *S. pneumoniae* or other organisms.

***H. PYLORI* ERADICATION.**   Antral gastritis and peptic ulcer of the stomach or duodenum are associated with colonization of *H. pylori.* Eradication of the organism decreases recurrence of ulcer and promotes resolution of gastritis. Although there are myriad treatment regimens for *H. pylori* eradication, twice-daily treatment with **amoxicillin** 1 g, **omeprazole** 20 mg or **lansoprazole** 30 mg, and **clarithromycin** 500 mg for 10 to 14 days is one regimen approved by the Food and Drug

Administration (FDA). Because there is greater than 90 percent eradication with 7-day therapy with this combination, selection pressure for resistance and adverse effects may be reduced by limiting therapy to 1 week. Other **antimicrobials** used in *H. pylori* eradication include **metronidazole, tetracycline,** and **bismuth subsalicylate.** Some experts recommend *H. pylori* eradication prior to initiation of nonsteroidal anti-inflammatory drugs (NSAIDs) to prevent NSAID-induced peptic ulcers, but further research is needed to confirm the efficacy of this prophylaxis.

LYME DISEASE. Lyme disease is caused by *B. burgdorferi* and other *Borrelia* species, transmitted by tick bite. Diagnosis is primarily clinical, although serological testing of positive findings on both the ELISA and Western blot tests provides confirmatory evidence. **Amoxicillin** 500 mg three times daily for 14 to 21 days is used in early stages of the disease, characterized by erythema chronicum migrans, isolated facial nerve paralysis, or arthritis. Alternative treatments for the early stage include **doxycycline, clarithromycin,** or **cefuroxime axetil.**

GROUP B STREPTOCOCCAL DISEASE PREVENTION. Group B streptococci sepsis is among the most important causes of neonatal morbidity and mortality, with a U.S. incidence of approximately 2 cases per 1000 live births (Locksmith, Clark, & Duff, 1999). The Centers for Disease Control and Prevention (CDC) (1996) endorsed one of two strategies for prevention of this infection, although the recommendations are controversial. Use of intrapartum **antibiotics** according to the guidelines has markedly decreased early-onset neonatal infections and death (Schrag et al., 2000). The universal screening strategy includes **antimicrobial** therapy for all women with positive lower genital tract cultures obtained between 35 and 37 weeks of gestation, as well as for women with unknown culture results at the time of labor who have one or more risk factors. About 30 percent of women have positive cultures at 37 weeks. The risk-based strategy does not include routine genital cultures but indicates treatment for any woman in labor with one or more of the risk factors: gestation less than 37 weeks, duration of membrane rupture more than 18 hours, temperature greater than 38°C, or a previous infant with group B streptococcal sepsis. For positive culture or risk factors in the woman with intact membranes, prophylaxis during labor is IV aqueous crystalline **penicillin G** (5-million-U loading dose and 2.5 million U every 4 hours until delivery) or IV **ampicillin** (2-g loading dose and then every 4 hours until delivery). For premature rupture of the membranes, broader spectrum therapy such as **ticarcillin-clavulanate** or IV **ampicillin** plus IV **erythromycin** has been recommended. Following 48 hours of these parenteral drugs, oral **amoxicillin** in doses of 500 mg three times daily, alone or with **erythromycin** 333 mg

base, may be used as maintenance therapy for 5 days or until delivery (Gilbert, Moellering, & Sande, 1999; Locksmith, Clark, & Duff, 1999). Table 22–3 presents the dosage schedule of **penicillins.**

Rational Drug Selection

INDICATION. The first consideration in drug selection is whether **antimicrobial** therapy is indicated. **Antimicrobial** therapy is indicated only when the benefits of therapy (prevention of sequelae or death, more rapid recovery, patient comfort, limitation of transmission) outweigh the costs and risks of the treatment (e.g., antibiotic resistance, allergic response, adverse effects, economic burden). For self-limiting infections, the balance always favors symptomatic and supportive treatment, rather than **antimicrobial** therapy. If the benefit-to-risk balance favors **antimicrobial** therapy, there are two major approaches to drug selection. The definitive or directed method is based on defining tests to identify the organism and drug, and the empiric method is based on previous experience with similar cases. (See Table 22–4.)

Four steps characterize both the empiric and definitive approaches, beginning with making the clinical diagnosis that identifies the infection, such as pharyngitis, urinary cystitis, or cervicitis. Collection of specimens for culture or laboratory test follows the clinical diagnosis. For some infections such as otitis media or pelvic inflammatory disease, specimens are not available without invasive procedures, so they are usually not obtained. Additionally, specimens for culture are not helpful if the site is commonly colonized, such as acute exacerbation of chronic bronchitis. Microbiologic testing is an important tool in the rational prescribing of **antibiotics,** although delay in obtaining results, misinterpretation of colonization as infection, quality control (mislabeling of specimen or using wrong procedure), and cost are disadvantages of routine culture and sensitivity (Kolmos & Little, 1999). Near-patient testing procedures such as the group A streptococci antigen test, urine dipsticks, and microscopy are widely used and have the advantages of moderate cost and immediate results. When the result is negative and immediate, it is much easier for the prescriber to refuse to give in to patients' demands for an **antibiotic.** However, urine dipsticks and microscopy are not considered definitive of the causal organism, and the definitive method is often an unrealized ideal in ambulatory practice. However, even with the empiric method, culture results can confirm the empiric diagnosis or allow appropriate adjustment of therapy.

The final two steps, making the microbial diagnosis and drug selection, differ for definitive and empiric therapy. In definitive therapy, the microbial diagnosis is based on valid and reliable tests such as culture or antigen assays, and drug selection is based on results of sensitivity testing or laboratory tests such as beta-lactamase

Table 22–3. Dosage Schedule: Penicillins

Drug	Indications	Initial Dose	Maximal Dose and Comments
Amoxicillin (Amoxil, Trimox, Polymox, Wymox, generic)	Antibacterial	*Adult* PO: 250–500 mg q8h, 875 mg q12h *Children* PO: <6 kg: 25–50 mg q8h 6–8 kg: 50–100 mg q8h 8–20 kg: 6.7–13.3 mg/kg q8h	Maximal daily dose 4.5 g. Duration of therapy depends on site of infection. Continue treatment 5–14 d, depending on site of infection. Suspensions retain potency after reconstitution for up to 14 d at room temperature or refrigerated, depending on manufacturer.
	Suspected resistant *S. pneumoniae* (DRSP) (off-label)	*Children* PO: 70–90 mg/kg/d divided into 2–3 doses	
	Endocarditis prophylaxis, pre-procedural	*Adult* 3 g 1 h before procedure 1.5 g 6 h after initial dose	
	Chlamydia (in pregnant women; off-label)	500 mg q8h for 7–10 d	
	Gastritis or peptic ulcer due to *H. pylori*	*Adult* PO: For 7–14 d as component of multiantibiotic treatment; 500 mg qid, 750 mg tid, or 1000 mg bid	
	Lyme disease	*Adult:* Duration of therapy 3–4 wk; re-treat if treatment failure PO: 250–500 mg qid *Children:* Duration of therapy 10–30 d, depending on clinical response PO: 6.7–13.3 mg/kg q8h	
	Gonorrhea, endocervical and urethral, uncomplicated	*Prepubertal children* 50 mg/kg plus probenecid 25 mg/kg as single dose (Not for penicillinase-producing strains)	
Amoxicillin and potassium clavulanate (Augmentin)	Antibacterial	*Adults and children >40 kg* PO: 250 mg amoxicillin and 62.5 mg clavulanate q8h for 7–10 d *Children <40 kg* PO: 6.7–13.3 mg/kg amoxicillin and 1.7–3.3 mg/kg clavulanate q8h for 7–10 d	Suspensions maintain potency after reconstitution for 10 d if refrigerated. Pediatric dose equivalent to 20–40 mg/kg amoxicillin divided into 3 doses. Less diarrhea if daily dose in bid therapy because of lower amount of clavulanate.
	Antibacterial, pneumonia, serious or resistant infections	*Adults and children >40 kg* PO: 500 mg amoxicillin and 125 mg clavulanate q8h *or* 875 mg amoxicillin and 125 mg clavulanate q12h *Children <40 kg* PO: 23.3–30 mg/kg amoxicillin and 5.8–7.5 mg/kg clavulanate q8h *or* 35–45 mg/kg amoxicillin and 8.8–11.2 mg/kg clavulanate q12h	Pediatric dose equivalent to 70–90 mg/kg amoxicillin/d in 2–3 divided doses. Using 875 mg amoxicillin and 125 mg clavulanate/5 mL formulation bid decreases clavulanate-related diarrhea.

Continued on next page

Table 22–3. Dosage Schedule: Penicillins *(continued)*

Drug	Indications	Initial Dose	Maximal Dose and Comments
Ampicillin (Polycillin, Principen, Totacillin, generic)	Antibacterial	*Adults and children≥20 kg* PO: 250–500 mg q6h *Children <20 kg* PO: 12.5–25 mg/kg q6h *or* 16.7–33.3 mg/kg q8h	Maximum dose: parenteral 14 g/d; oral 4 g/d. Take on empty stomach. Suspensions retain their potency after reconstitution for 7 d at room temperature or 14 d in refrigerator, depending on manufacturer.
Ampicillin and sulbactam (Unasyn)	Antibacterial	*Adult* IM: 1.5–3 g q6h *Children <12 y* IM: 300–600 mg/kg/d divided into 3–4 doses	After reconstitution, the IM solution loses potency in 1 h. Equivalent to 1–2 g amoxicillin and 0.5–1 g sulbactam. Off-label dosage for children. Equivalent to 200–400 mg/kg/d amoxicillin and 100–200 mg/kg/d sulbactam.
	Gonorrhea	*Adult* IM: 1.5 g (1 g ampicillin and 500 mg sulbactam) as single dose with 1 g probenecid orally	
Carbenicillin indanyl sodium (Geocillin)	UTI and prostatitis	*Adult* PO: 500–1000 mg q6h	Not effective in severe renal impairment (creatine clearance [CCr] <10 mL/min).
Cloxacillin sodium (Cloxapen, generic)	Antibacterial	*Adults and children >20 kg* PO: 250–500 mg (base) q6h *Children <20 kg* PO: 6.25–12.5 mg/kg (base) q6h	Maximum 6 g (base)/d. Suspension stable 14 d in refrigerator. Shake suspension well before measuring. Take on empty stomach, preferably 1 h before meals.
Dicloxacillin sodium (Dynapen, Dycill, Pathocil, generic)	Antibacterial	*Adults and children ≥40 kg* PO: 125–500 mg q6h *Children <40 kg* PO: 3.125–6.25 mg/kg (base) q6h	Maximum adult dose 6 g (base)/d. Shake suspension well before measuring. Take on empty stomach, preferably 1 h before meals.
	Infections in cystic fibrosis patients	*Children <40 kg* PO: 12.5–25 mg/kg (base) q6h	
Mezlocillin (Mezlin)	UTI, uncomplicated	*Adults and children >12 y* IM: 25–31.25 mg/kg q6h *or* 1.5–2 g q6h	Maximum adult dose 24 g/d. Renal impairment (CCr <30 mL/min requires decreased dose. May use sterile water or 1% lidocaine (without epinephrine) as diluent. Retains potency for 24 h at room temperature.
	Other bacterial infection	IM: 33.3–58.3 mg/kg q4h; 50–87 mg/kg q6h; *or* 3–4 g q4–6h *Children >1 mo–12 y* IM: 50 mg/kg q4h	
Oxacillin (Bactocill, Prostaphlin)	Antibacterial	*Adults and children ≥40 kg* PO: 500 mg–1 g (base) q4–6h IM: 250 mg–1 g (base) q4–6h *Children <40 kg* PO: 12.5–25 mg/kg (base) q6h	Maximum adult daily dose 6 g. Take oral forms on empty stomach, preferably 1 h before meals. After reconstitution, IM solution

Continued on next page

Table 22–3. Dosage Schedule: Penicillins *(continued)*

Drug	Indications	Initial Dose	Maximal Dose and Comments
		IM 12.5–25 mg/kg (base) q6h *or* 16.7 mg/kg q4h	retains potency for 4 d at room temperature or 7 d if refrigerated. After reconstitution, oral solution retains potency for 7 d at room temperature or 14 d if refrigerated.
Penicillin G, benzathine (Bicillin L-A)	Prophylaxis for streptococcal infections in patient with rheumatic fever history	*Adult* IM: 1,200,000 U q3–4wk *Children* IM: 1,200,000 U q2–3wk	For deep IM use only into large muscle mass. IV injection causes embolic or toxic reaction. Intra-arterial injection causes necrosis of extremity or organ, especially in children. Maximum daily adult dose 2,400,000 U. Inject at slow, steady rate to avoid blockage of the needle.
	Pharyngitis, group A streptococci	*Adults and adolescents* IM: 1,200,000 U as single dose *Children >27.3 kg* IM: 900,000 U as single dose *Children <27.3 kg* IM: 300,000–600,000 U as single dose	
	Syphilis (primary, secondary, early latent)	*Adults and adolescents* IM: 2,400,000 U as single dose *Children* IM: 50,000 U/kg up to 2,400,000 units as single dose	
	Syphilis (late latent or latent of unknown duration)	*Adults and adolescents* IM: 2,400,000 U weekly for 3 wk *Children* IM: 50,000 U/kg weekly up to 2,400,000 U as single dose for 3 wk	
Penicillin G, procaine	Antibacterial	*Adult* IM: 600,000–1,200,000 U/d	For deep IM use only into large muscle mass. After large doses, some patients may experience a CNS syndrome of transient anxiety, confusion, agitation, combativeness, depression, seizures, hallucinations, expressed fear of impending death.
	Neurosyphilis	*Adult* IM: 2,400,000 U and 500 mg probenecid qid for 10–14 d	
	Congenital syphilis	Children 50,000 U/kg/d for 10–14 d	
	Diphtheria	*Adult* IM: 300,000–600,000 U/d as adjunct to diphtheria antitoxin	
	Rat bite fever	*Adult* IM: 600,000 U every 12 h	

Continued on next page

Table 22–3. Dosage Schedule: Penicillins *(continued)*

Drug	Indications	Initial Dose	Maximal Dose and Comments
Penicillin G benzathine and procaine combined (Bicillin-CR)	Antibacterial	*Adults and children >27 kg* IM: 2,400,000 U as single dose *Children 14–27 kg* IM: 900,000–1,200,000 U as single dose *Children <14 kg* IM: 600,000 U as single dose	See comments for penicillin G benzathine and penicillin G procaine. May be dosed with half of dose on day 1 and half on day 3. For deep IM use only into large muscle mass. Continue until afebrile for 48 h.
	Pneumococcal infections (excluding meningitis)	*Adults* IM: 1,200,000 U every 2–3 d *Children* IM: 600,000 U every 2–3 d	
Penicillin V (Beepen-VK, Betapen-VK, Ledercillin-VK, Pen Vee K, Veetids, V-Cillin K, generic)	Antibacterial	*Adults and children >12 y* 125–500 mg q6–8h *Children <12 y* 2.5–8.3 mg/kg q6h *or* 5–16.7 mg/kg q8h	Maximum adult dose 7.5 g/d. Solution retains potency for 14 d if refrigerated. Shake solution well before measuring.
	Continuous prophylaxis of streptococcal infection in patients with history of rheumatic heart disease	*Adults and children >12 y* 125–250 mg q12h	
	Erysipelas	*Adults and children >12 y* PO: 500 mg q6h *Children <12 y* See antibacterial	
	Gingivitis, acute necrotizing	*Adults* PO: 500 mg q6h	
	Rat bite fever	*Adults and children >12 y* 500 mg q6h for 14 d *Children <12 y* See antibacterial	
	Lyme disease	*Adults and children >12 y* 250–500 mg 3–4 times daily for 3–4 wk *Children <12 y* 5–12.5 mg/kg qid for 3–4 wk	Duration dependent on response. Treatment failures have occurred and retreatment may be necessary.
Piperacillin (Pipracil)	Antibacterial	*Adults and children >12 y* IM: 3–4 g q4–6h	Maximum adult daily dose 24 g. CCr <40 mL/min requires reduced dosage and/or frequency. IM injection should not exceed 2 g per site.
	Urinary tract infection, uncomplicated	*Adults* IM: 1.5–2 g q6h or 3–4 g q12h	

assay. The goal of susceptibility testing is to identify a nontoxic **antimicrobial** drug that will resolve the infection. Although this goal is not always achieved, susceptibility testing can often identify a narrower spectrum or less toxic agent than would be identified by the empiric method of drug selection.

Susceptibility tests measure the concentration of the drug required in vitro to inhibit the growth of the organism (called minimum inhibitory concentration, or MIC) or the concentration required to kill the organism (minimum bactericidal concentration, or MBC). Usually only the MIC is determined, although when bactericidal action is required, such as for immunocompromised patients, endocarditis treatment, and meningitis treatment, the MBC is determined. The MIC or MBC can be correlated with concentrations of the drug attainable by vari-

Table 22–4. Steps in Antimicrobial Drug Selection

Step 1	Make clinical diagnosis
Step 2	Obtain cultures and/or specimens
Step 3	Make microbial diagnosis Results of culture and/or lab test *or* most likely pathogen, references
Step 4	Select drug Results of sensitivity *or* usual susceptibility

ous doses and routes in various compartments of the body where the organism may exist (e.g., middle ear fluid, serum, synovial fluid, cerebrspinal fluid [CSF]). There are two approaches to susceptibility testing: the disk or agar diffusion (Kirby-Bauer) method and the broth dilution method. In the agar diffusion approach, a disk containing a standard amount of the antimicrobial agent is placed on agar lightly seeded with the **antimicrobial** drug. After incubation, susceptibility is determined by the diameter of the visible area of growth inhibition around the disk. The broth dilution method consists of inoculating the organism into a series of liquid media containing increasing concentrations of the **antimicrobial**. The MIC is the lowest concentration that inhibits growth. The broth dilution method is preferred if there is no sharp distinction between sensitivity and resistance on the disk method (Lampris & Maddix, 1998). Sensitivity and resistance represent a continuum rather than a dichotomy. For example, *S. pneumoniae* strains are defined as **penicillin**-susceptible if the MIC is less than 0.1 µg/mL, intermediate if the MIC is 0.1 µg/mL to 1 µg/mL, and resistant if the MIC is greater than 2 µg/mL.

In empiric testing, the microbial diagnosis and drug regimen are determined based on epidemiologic studies. References that compile and update these data annually or biannually include *The Sanford Guide to Antimicrobial Therapy* (Gilbert, Moellering, & Sande, 1999) and the *Handbook of Antimicrobial Therapy* (2000), and periodic updates are given in the biweekly *Medical Letter on Drugs and Therapeutics.* These references identify the drug with the narrowest spectrum that covers the most likely microbiologic pathogens for a specific clinical diagnosis. Clinicians should also consult local sources of information on pathogens and susceptibility, such as the public health department or infectious disease departments of local hospitals. For example, it is useful to know the prevalence of beta-lactamase production by local strains of *H. influenzae.* If rates are high (e.g., above 40%), **amoxicillin** might not be the best choice for initial therapy in otitis media or sinusitis.

ALLERGY HISTORY. Susceptibility, whether empirically or definitively derived, is not the sole determinant of drug selection. Allergy history is important because cross-reactivity to **penicillins** is total; that is, the patient allergic to any **penicillin** will be allergic to all other **penicillins.** In addition, the risk for cross-allergy to related drugs, such as **cephalosporins** and **beta-lactamase inhibitors,** is a consideration. References for empiric therapy provide an alternative nonpenicillin agent whenever the drug of choice is a **penicillin.** For example, **erythromycin** is an alternative to **penicillin V** for treatment of pharyngitis caused by GABHS.

AGE, PREGNANCY, AND GENETIC FACTORS. Age is important in drug selection and dosing, primarily because renal elimination of penicillins changes with age. Neonates and elderly patients often have poor renal function and are more prone to drug toxicity. Highly plasma protein–bound drugs such as **sulfonamides** and the **penicillinase-resistant penicillins** should be avoided in late pregnancy and neonates because these agents may displace bilirubin from plasma proteins of the newborn, causing kernicterus, a central nervous system (CNS) disorder.

Pregnancy contraindicates several classes of *antibiotics* such as *tetracyclines* and *fluoroquinolones,* so *aminopenicillins* may be used for gravid women, even though another agent is the drug of choice in the nonpregnant state.

For some drugs, genetic factors predispose patients to adverse effects.

SITE OF INFECTION. The anatomic site of the infection affects drug selection, as well as dose, route, and duration of therapy. For example, **penicillins** enter CSF poorly, so a CNS infection may require a different agent, higher doses, IV and/or intraventricular administration, or prolonged therapy. When the meninges are inflamed as in meningitis, **penicillin** attains higher concentrations in the CSF. By contrast, **penicillins** enter the urine in high concentrations, permitting single-dose or short-course therapy for susceptible organisms.

IMMUNOCOMPROMISED STATUS. One of the most important factors in drug selection is the immunocompetence of the patient. Patients with immunodeficiency syndromes or neutropenia require bactericidal drugs and extended therapy (Thielman & Neu, 1998).

AFFORDABILITY. Affordability is another consideration in drug selection, although existing data contradict the common assumption that newer, more expensive agents are more effective than established, inexpensive agents (Berman, Byrns, Bondy, Smith, & Lezotte, 1997). One reason **amoxicillin** is the preferred drug of choice for several common URIs is its low cost, combined with its high efficacy and long history of safe use. The highly effective **amoxicillin-clavulanate** is costly and less palatable in suspension, and it causes more adverse effects, particularly diarrhea. As a result, some clinicians and formularies select inexpensive **trimethoprim-sulfamethoxazole** as the preferred agent for treating **amoxicillin** failures in otitis media and sinusitis.

TASTE AND CONVENIENCE. Taste is a significant factor in patient acceptance of a liquid product, affecting adherence to the prescribed regimen (Steele, Thomas, Begue, & Despinasse, 1999). The use of **amoxicillin** suspension rather than **penicillin V** suspension for group A streptococcal infections is an example of drug selection based on taste and convenience. **Amoxicillin** requires two or three doses daily, whereas **penicillin V** requires four doses per day. Frequent dosing decreases compliance and may be particularly problematic when the patient is away from home, such as at work or daycare, especially when the drug requires refrigeration or cannot be taken with food (Pichichero, 1997).

Monitoring

Both microbiologic and clinical responses are used to evaluate the therapeutic outcome of **antimicrobial** therapy. Serial cultures of specimens from infected sites become sterile with successful treatment. Follow-up cultures may detect superinfection or development of resistance. All patients with early or congenital syphilis should have a quantitative VDRL test at 3, 6, 12, and 24 months after therapy.

For most infections treated in outpatient settings, it is sufficient to monitor clinical response alone. Local signs of heat, redness, swelling, tenderness, or discharge usually abate after 48 to 72 hours. Specific indicators of improvement such as the resolution of pulmonary infiltrates and normalization of pulse oximetry in pneumonia are important outcomes to monitor. Systemic signs such as fever, malaise, and leukocytosis also improve. The patient should be advised to call the prescriber if there is not improvement in 48 to 72 hours, when consideration should be given to adjusting the treatment; alternatively, the provider can initiate telephone contact to evaluate progress and improvement. Compliance is monitored throughout the course of therapy, particularly if there is therapeutic failure, as well as after symptoms resolve and the patient is less motivated to complete the therapy.

Signs of allergic reactions may occur from minutes to weeks after the **antimicrobial** drug is initiated, and even after the course of therapy is completed. Although immediate hypersensitivity reactions are more likely to be life-threatening, delayed reactions can also be serious. Superinfection often presents with subtle and nonspecific symptoms such as mouth or throat pain (oral candidiasis) or perineal itching or discharge (vaginal candidiasis), so it is important to attend to these minor complaints. Distinguishing between antibiotic diarrhea and pseudomembranous colitis is at times difficult, but more than four to six watery stools per day or blood in the stool warrants stool cytotoxin assay to detect *C. difficile*.

Other adverse effects are almost exclusively associated with high-dose parenteral therapy, protracted oral therapy, or impaired renal function. During parenteral therapy, periodic urinalysis, blood urea nitrogen (BUN), and creatinine determinations should be performed, especially with agents from the **penicillinase-resistant group** or the **antipseudomonal group.** Monitor serum potassium in patients receiving **mezlocillin, piperacillin, potassium penicillin G,** or other parenteral agents. Patients with low potassium reserves, especially if they are taking cytotoxic drugs or diuretics, can develop hypokalemia. Hyperkalemia has occurred with high doses of **potassium penicillin G** in patients with impaired renal function. The partial thromboplastin time (PTT) and prothrombin time (PT) should be assessed at baseline and during therapy with parenteral **carbenicillin, piperacillin,** or **ticarcillin,** particularly for patients with renal impairment.

Patient Education

ADMINISTRATION. The most critical information to provide to patients who will self-administer **antibiotics** is the importance of completing the full course of therapy. They should understand that failure to complete therapy may result in resistant infections that can be passed on to family and friends or cause the patient to be more seriously ill. Doses of the medication should be spaced as evenly as possible without sleep disruption throughout the 24 hours of a day. Missed doses should be taken as soon as they are remembered, but the dose should not be doubled by taking two doses at the same time.

Oral **penicillins** that should be taken on an empty stomach, 1 hour before a meal or 2 hours after meals, include **ampicillin, carbenicillin,** and the **penicillinase-resistant agents cloxacillin, oxacillin, nafcillin,** and **dicloxacillin. Amoxicillin** may be mixed with milk, fruit juice, water, or ginger ale, but the entire volume should be consumed as soon after mixing as possible. Chewable tablets must be crushed or chewed, or the drug may not absorb adequately. Oral tablets and chewable tablets of **amoxicillin-clavulanate** have different **clavulanate** content and should not be considered interchangeable. The available dosage forms are shown in Table 22–5.

Many **penicillins** are available as solutions or suspensions. Suspensions must be shaken to disperse the particles of drug immediately before measurement. Refrigerated liquid formulations maintain full activity for 14 days after reconstitution, except **amoxicillin-clavulanate** suspension, which lasts for 10 days in the refrigerator. **Amoxicillin** suspension maintains full activity for 14 days whether refrigerated or not, although some manufacturers specify refrigerated storage. Instruct patients not to use **antibiotics** beyond the expiration date. Liquid formulations should always be dispensed with a calibrated measuring device. Because household teaspoons vary from 2 mL to 10 mL in volume, they are unreliable

Table 22–5. Available Dosage Forms: Penicillins

Drug	Dosage Form	How Supplied
Amoxicillin	Tablets (chewable): 125 mg	In bottles of 40, 60, 100, and 500 tablets
	(chewable): 250 mg	In bottles of 30, 40, 60, 100, and 500 tablets
	Capsules: 250 mg	In bottles of 21, 30, 100, 250, 500, and 1000 capsules
	500 mg	In bottles of 21, 30, 50, 100, 250, and 500 capsules
	Powder for oral suspension: 125 mg/5 cc (reconstituted), 250 mg/5 cc (reconstituted)	In 80-, 100-, 150-, and 200-cc bottles
(Amoxil)	Tablets (chewable): 125 mg	In bottles of 60; cherry-banana-peppermint flavor
	(chewable): 250 mg	In bottles of 30 and 100; cherry-banana-peppermint flavor
	Capsules: 250 mg, 500 mg	In bottles of 100 and 500 capsules
	Powder for oral suspension: 50 mg/cc (reconstituted)	In 15- and 30-cc bottles
	125 mg/5 cc (reconstituted), 250 mg/5 cc (reconstituted)	In 80-, 100-, and 150-cc bottles
(Trimox)	Capsules: 250 mg, 500 mg	In bottles of 30, 100, and 500 capsules
	Powder for oral suspension: 50 mg/cc (reconstituted)	In 15-cc bottles
	125 mg/5 cc (reconstituted); 250 mg/5 cc (reconstituted)	In 80-, 100-, and 150-cc bottles
(Wymox)	Capsules: 250 mg	In bottles of 100 and 500 capsules
	500 mg	In bottles of 50 and 500 capsules
	Powder for oral suspension: 125 mg/5 cc (reconstituted), 250 mg/5 cc (reconstituted)	In 100- and 150-cc bottles
Amoxicillin and potassium clavulanate (Augmentin)	Tablets: 250 mg amoxicillin/125 mg clavulanate	In 30 and 100 tablets
	500 mg amoxicillin/125 mg clavulanate	In 20 and 100 tablets
	875 mg amoxicillin/125 mg clavulanate	In 20 and 100 tablets
	Tablets (chewable):125 mg amoxicillin/ 31.25 mg clavulanate	In 30, lemon-lime flavor tablets
	(chewable): 200 mg amoxicillin/28.5 mg clavulanate	In 20, cherry-banana flavor tablets
	(chewable): 250 mg amoxicillin/62.5 mg clavulanate	In 30, lemon-lime flavor tablets
	(chewable): 400 mg amoxicillin/57 mg clavulanate	In 20, cherry-banana flavor tablets
	Powder for oral suspension: 125 mg amoxicillin/31.25 mg clavulanate per 5 cc	In 75-, 100-, and 150-cc bottles banana flavor
	200 mg amoxicillin/28.5 mg clavulanate per 5 cc	In 50-, 75-, and 100-cc bottles orange-raspberry flavor
	250 mg amoxicillin/62.5 mg clavulanate per 5 cc	In 75-, 100-, and 150-cc bottles orange flavor
	400 mg amoxicillin/57 mg clavulanate per 5 cc	In 50-, 75-, and 100-cc bottles orange-raspberry flavor
Ampicillin sodium	Capsules: 250 mg	In bottles of 20, 30, 40, 100, 500, and 1000 capsules
	500 mg	In bottles of 16, 20, 28, 40, 100, 500, and 1000 capsules
	Powder for oral suspension: 125 mg/5 cc (reconstituted), 250 mg/5 cc (reconstituted)	In 80-, 100-, 150-, and 200-cc bottles

Continued on next page

Table 22–5. Available Dosage Forms: Penicillins *(continued)*

Drug	Dosage Form	How Supplied
	Powder for injection: 125 mg, 250 mg, 500 mg, 1 g, 2 g	In multidose vials
(Omnipen)	Capsules: 250 mg 500 mg Powder for oral suspension: 125 mg/5 cc (reconstituted), 250 mg/5 cc (reconstituted) Powder for injection: 125 mg, 250 mg, 500 mg, 1 g, 2 g	In bottles of 500 capsules In bottles of 100 and 500 capsules In 100-, 150-, and 200-cc bottles In multidose vials
(Principen)	Capsules: 250 mg, 500 mg Powder for suspension: 250 mg/5 cc (reconstituted), 250 mg/5 cc (reconstituted)	In bottles of 100 and 500 capsules In 100-, 150-, and 200-cc bottles
Ampicillin sodium and sulbactam sodium (Unasyn)	Powder for injection: 1.5 g (1 g ampicillin/ 0.5 g sulbactam) 3 g (2 g ampicillin/1 g sulbactam)	In multidose vials
Carbenicillin (Geocillin)	Tablets: 382 mg	In bottles of 100 tablets
Cloxacillin sodium	Capsules: 250 mg, 500 mg Powder for oral solution: 125 mg/5 cc	In bottles of 100 capsules In 100- and 200-cc bottles
(Cloxapen)	Capsules: 250 mg 500 mg	In bottles of 100 capsules In bottles of 30 and 100 capsules
Dicloxacillin sodium	Capsules: 250 mg 500 mg	In bottles of 40, 100, and 500 capsules In bottles of 30, 40, 50, 100, and 500 capsules
(Dynapen)	Capsules: 125 mg, 250 mg 500 mg Powder for oral suspension: 62.5 mg/5 cc (reconstituted)	In bottles of 24 and 100 capsules In bottles of 50 capsules In 100- and 200-cc bottles
(Dycil)	Capsules: 250 mg, 500 mg	In bottles of 100 capsules
(Pathocil)	Capsules: 250 mg 500 mg Powder for oral suspension: 62.5 mg/5 cc (reconstituted)	In bottles of 100 capsules In bottles of 50 capsules In 100-cc bottles
Mezlocillin (Mezlin)	Powder for injection: 1 g, 2 g, 3 g, 4 g	In multidose vials
Oxacillin sodium	Capsules: 250 mg, 500 mg Powder for oral solution: 250 mg/5 cc (reconstituted) Powder for injection: 250 mg, 500 mg, 1 g, 2 g, 4 g	In bottles of 100 capsules In 100-cc bottles In multidose vials
(Bactocill)	Powder for injection: 500 mg, 1 g, 2 g, 4 g	In multidose vials
Penicillin G, procaine (Wycillin)	Injection	600,000 U per dose in 1-cc Tubex 1,200,000 U per dose in 2-cc Tubex 2,400,000 U per dose in 4-cc disposable syringe
Penicillin G, benzathine (Bicillin L-A)	Injection	300,000 U per cc in 10-cc vials 600,000 U per dose in 1-cc Tubex 1,200,000 U per dose in 2-cc Tubex 2,400,000 U per dose in 4-cc syringe

Continued on next page

Table 22–5. Available Dosage Forms: Penicillins *(continued)*

Drug	Dosage Form	How Supplied
(Permapen)	Injection:	1,200,000 U per dose in 2-cc Isoject
Penicillin G, benzathine-procaine combined (Bicillin C-R)	Injection	300,000 U (150,000 U of each) per dose in 10-cc vials 600,000 U (300,000 U of each) per dose in 1-cc Tubex 1,200,000 U (600,000 U of each) in 2-cc Tubex 2,400,000 U (1,200,000 U of each) in 4-cc syringe 1,200,000 U (900,000 U of benzathine and 300,000 U of procaine) per dose in 2-cc Tubex
Penicillin V (Penicillin VK)	Tablets: 250 mg 500 mg Powder for oral solution: 125 mg/5 cc (reconstituted) 250 mg/5 cc (reconstituted)	In bottles of 20, 30, 40, 80 100, 500, and 1000 tablets In bottles of 20, 30, 40, 100, 500, and 1000 tablets In 80-, 100-, 150-, and 200-cc bottles
Penicillin V (Pen Vee K)	Tablets: 250 mg, 500 mg Powder for oral solution: 125 mg/5 cc (reconstituted) 250 mg/5 cc (reconstituted)	In bottles of 100-mg and 500-mg scored tablets In 100- and 200-cc bottles In 100-, 150-, and 200-cc bottles
Penicillin V (Veetids)	Tablets: 250 mg, 500 mg Powder for oral solution: 125 mg/5 cc (reconstituted), 250 mg/5 cc (reconstituted)	In bottles of 100 and 1000 tablets In 100- and 200-cc bottles
Piperacillin (Pipracil)	Powder for injection: 2 g, 3 g, 4 g	In multidose vials

for medication measurement. Clinicians should tell the patient whether there will be liquid remaining at the end of the course of therapy and urge disposal of unused medication.

Very concentrated oral forms of **amoxicillin** (50 mg/mL) or **ampicillin** (100 mg/mL) in suspension are called **antibiotic** drops. It is important to explain that the drops are for oral use, describe how to measure and administer the medication appropriate to the patient's developmental and physical capabilities, and specify that an appropriate measuring device be dispensed.

Medications mixed for injection also lose potency with time, although refrigeration after reconstitution will extend the period of full potency. Consult the package insert for proper mixing and storage of reconstituted parenteral **penicillins**. Some of these agents (e.g., **mezlocillin, piperacillin**) can be prepared with **lidocaine** to decrease pain on IM injection. Adhere to the manufacturer's limits on volume of injection at one site. IM injection should be slow and steady, extended over 12 to 15 seconds to minimize pain and avoid blockage of the needle, especially with **procaine** and **benzathine** preparations that are very thick. Because IV extravasation of **nafcillin** causes tissue necro-

sis, IM injection should be avoided, and Z-track injection technique used if this route is unavoidable.

ADVERSE REACTIONS. Patients should be taught to distinguish allergic reactions from other adverse effects, so that they can provide an accurate drug allergy history. Many patients claim **penicillin** allergy because they experienced diarrhea during therapy. Patients with immediate or type I allergies of the anaphylactic type should wear an identification bracelet.

If severe diarrhea occurs, the patient should contact the prescriber before initiating any treatment. For mild diarrhea, they can use adsorbent **antidiarrheal agents** containing attapulgite (e.g., Kaopectate, Donnagel) but should avoid **antiperistaltic agents** that promote the retention of toxins.

Aminopenicillins and **clavulanate** cause false positives on glucose urine testing by the copper sulfate technique (Clinitest). Diabetics on these **penicillins** should use blood glucose monitoring or urine testing based on the glucose enzymatic tests (Clinstix, TesTape).

LIFESTYLE MANAGEMENT. Most infections are self-limiting and resolve with symptomatic treatment, rest, fluids, and nutritious diet. Instead of seeking **antibiotics** for every minor illness, people must learn to trust the natural healing capacity of the human body. Prevention of infection by good handwashing, shunning crowded environments, avoiding cigarette smoke including passive smoke, safe sexual practices, and generally healthy lifestyle will limit the need for **antibiotics**. Other risk-reduction counseling specific to otitis media includes breastfeeding of infants, avoidance of passive smoke, elimination of the pacifier in children over age 1 year, enrollment in daycare with small class size if daycare in unavoidable, and pneumococcal and influenza vaccine (Tiggs, 2000). Because pain has been shown to inhibit the immune system, comfort measures and pain management of patients with infections will promote the antibiotic action.

Cephalosporins

Cephalosporins are **beta-lactam antimicrobial agents,** structurally and chemically related to the **penicillins.** Cefoxitin and cefotetan are actually **cephamycins** and **loracarbef** is a **carbacephem,** but they are usually included with the **cephalosporins** because of their clinical and chemical similarity.

This class of drugs is divided into four generations, based on the order of development and spectrum of antibacterial activity. In general, as the designation increases from first to third generation, there is increased activity against gram-negative organisms and anaerobes, less activity against gram-positive organisms, and increased ability to withstand destruction by beta-lactamases. However, the distinctions among the generations have progressively become blurred as more agents are marketed. Compared to third generation agents, **fourth generation cephalosporins** have increased activity against gram-positive cocci and gram-negative bacilli.

Pharmacodynamics

Cephalosporins inhibit mucopeptide synthesis in the bacterial cell wall, making the bacterium osmotically unstable. As with **penicillins,** this action involves **cephalosporins** binding with PBP involved in the terminal stages of cross-linking peptidoglycans at the cell wall. **Cephalosporins** are usually bactericidal, depending on organism susceptibility, dose, tissue concentration, and the rate of organism multiplication. They are most effective against rapidly growing organisms forming cell walls.

Sensitivity

First-generation cephalosporins are active against gram-positive cocci, including *S. aureus* and *S. epidermidis,* excluding **methicillin**-resistant strains. Agents in this group are also active against group A beta-hemolytic *S. pyogenes* and *S. pneumoniae,* except DRSP. The **first-generation cephalosporins** have limited activity against aerobic gram-negative organisms, such as *E. coli, P. mirabilis,* and *Klebsiella pneumoniae,* and do not enter the CSF.

Second-generation cephalosporins are active against the same organisms as the first generation, with increased activity against *Klebsiella, Proteus,* and *E. coli.* This group is active against beta-lactamase–producing strains of *H. influenzae* and *M. catarrhalis,* as well as intermediate-resistant *S. pneumoniae.* Each of the drugs in this generation has a slightly different spectrum of activity, so susceptibility tests for each must be performed, rather than assuming consistency within the group. This group is not active against *Pseudomonas* and does not reach effective concentrations in the CSF.

Third-generation cephalosporins are active against the same organisms as the first two generations, with added spectrum of activity against gram-negative organisms. They are also active against unusual strains of enteric organisms such as *Morganella, Providencia,* and *Serratia,* with increased activity against *Enterobacter.* Parenteral **cefoperazone, cefotaxime, ceftazidime, ceftizoxime,** and **ceftriaxone** are active against *P. aeruginosa.* Drug resistant strains tend to develop, however, if these drugs are used as monotherapy to treat *Pseudomonas.* Several drugs in this group are active against beta-lactamase–producing strains of *N. gonorrhoeae.* Some agents in this group reach clinically effective concentrations in the CSF.

There is only one fourth-generation cephalosporin **(cefepime)** at this time. This drug has a broader spectrum of activity and is resistant to beta-lactamases that inactivate third generation agents. It is active against both gram-positive and gram-negative organisms and against resistant strains of *Enterobacter* and *Pseudomonas.*

Many texts and references (e.g., Gilbert, Moellering, & Sande, 1999; Kastrup, 1999) have tables that list the organisms generally susceptible to various **cephalosporins** for each of the **cephalosporin** generations.

Resistance

First-generation cephalosporins are generally inactivated by beta-lactamase–producing organisms. **Cefonicid, cefdinir, loracarbef,** and **cefixime** have a high degree of stability to some beta-lactamases. **Cefoxitin, cefuroxime, ceftriaxone, cefotaxime, ceftizoxime, cefmetazole,** and **cefotetan** are highly stable even in the presence of both penicillinases and cephalosporinases produced by both gram-negative and gram-positive organisms. **Cefoperazone, cefpodoxime,** and **ceftazidime** are highly stable in the presence of beta-lactamases produced by gram-negative pathogens. **Cefaclor** is stable in the presence of some beta-lactamases. Changes of PBPs that prevent **cephalosporin** from binding to receptors are accountable for resistance of MRSA, DRSP, *E. faecalis,* and *Enterococcus faecium* to **cephalosporins.**

Pharmacokinetics

Absorption and Distribution

Cephalosporins that have oral formulations are well absorbed from the GI tract. Except for **cefadroxil** and **cefprozil,** absorption is delayed by food, but the amount absorbed is not affected. The absorption of oral ester prodrugs **cefpodoxime proxetil** and **cefuroxime axetil** is increased when given with food. All IM formulations are well absorbed from muscle tissue. Differences in bioavailability exist for the suspension and tablet formulations of both **cefpodoxime proxetil** and **cefixime,** so the formulations should not be substituted.

All **cephalosporins** are widely distributed to most tissues and fluids. Protein binding varies, but **ceftriaxone** is so highly bound to albumin that it should be avoided in neonates at risk for hyperbilirubinemia, especially preterm infants. The penetration of CSF varies by generation. Except for **cefuroxime,** first- and second-generation drugs do not readily enter the CSF, even when the meninges are inflamed. Third-generation drugs and **cefuroxime** readily enter the CSF in the presence of meningeal inflammation. The CSF levels of **cefoperazone,** however, are relatively low. Therapeutic levels are reached in bone at usual doses for most **cephalosporins,** and they are used prophylactically and therapeutically in orthopedic disorders. **Cefazolin** penetrates inflamed bone at higher concentrations than it penetrates normal bone, and it is the drug of choice in preventing and treating bone infection associated with orthopedic surgery.

High concentrations of **ceftriaxone** and **cefoperazone** are found in bile. Bile levels of **cefazolin** can exceed serum levels by up to five times in patients with obstructive biliary disease.

Metabolism and Excretion

Cephapirin is metabolized to less active compounds; however, one of its metabolites contributes to the drug's antibacterial activity. A metabolite of **cefotaxime** increases its spectrum of activity and extends the dosing intervals because of its prolonged metabolic half-life. **Cefuroxime** and **cefpodoxime** are prodrugs metabolized to active metabolites.

Most **cephalosporins** are excreted via the kidney in varying degrees as unchanged drug. Increased cephalosporin plasma concentrations may occur when **probenecid** blocks renal tubular secretion of **cephalosporins.** The combination of oral **probenecid** and

cephalosporins is used in serious infections and single-dose therapy of sexually transmitted diseases. Renal impairment significantly extends the half-life of these drugs. **Cefoperazone** is excreted mainly in bile, and its half-life is unchanged, even in severe renal insufficiency. **Ceftriaxone** also includes an extrarenal route of excretion so that its half-life is affected to a limited degree by severe renal insufficiency. In hepatic dysfunction, the half-life and urinary excretion of both of these drugs are increased. This extra-renal excretion makes these drugs relatively safe in significant renal insufficiency.

Changes Related to Pregnancy and in Children

The pharmacokinetic properties of **cephalosporins** change during pregnancy, tending toward shorter half-lives, lower serum levels, larger volumes of distribution, and increased clearance.

In neonates, accumulation of these drugs due to undeveloped renal function results in prolonged half-lives. In children over 3 months of age, higher doses of **cefoxitin** have been associated with increased incidence of eosinophilia and elevated AST. In children over age 6 months, **ceftizoxime** has been associated with transient elevated levels of AST, ALT, and CPK.

Table 22–6 depicts the pharmacokinetics of selected **cephalosporins.** Half-life alterations associated with end-stage renal disease are included.

Pharmacotherapeutics

Precautions and Contraindications

Like the **penicillins, cephalosporins** may produce hypersensitivity reactions in a small percentage of patients. Cross-sensitivity with **penicillins** increases the risk and occurs in 5 to 16 percent of patients. **Cephalosporins** cannot be assumed to be an absolutely safe alternative to **penicillin** in the **penicillin**-allergic patient and is generally not recommended for those who have had a type I (immediate, anaphylactic) reaction to any penicillin. Skin testing is not helpful for identifying individuals likely to experience anaphylactic reactions to **cephalosporins.**

Cephalosporins and other broad-spectrum **antibiotics** should be prescribed with care for patients with a known history of GI disease, especially colitis, because of the risk for the development of pseudomembranous colitis.

Renal function impairment significantly affects the half-life of most of these drugs, and they may also be nephrotoxic. Use in the presence of markedly impaired renal function (creatine clearance CCr less than 50 mL/minute) is undertaken with extreme caution. Older adults and patients with known or suspected renal impairment are monitored carefully prior to and during therapy. Dosage adjustments are often required based on renal function.

Table 22–6. Pharmacokinetics: Cephalosporins

Drug	Onset	Peak	Duration	Protein Binding	Bioavai-lability	Half-Life NRF/ESRD*	Elimination (% unchanged in urine)
FIRST GENERATION							
Cefadroxil (PO)	Rapid	1.5–2 h	12–24 h	20%	90%	78–96 min/20–25 h	>90%
Cefazolin (IM)	Rapid	1–2 h	6–12 h	80–86%	0	90–120 min/3–7 h	60–80%
Cephalexin (PO)	15–30 min	1 h	6–12 h	10%	UA	50–80 min/19–22 h	>90%
Cephradine (PO) (IM)	Rapid Rapid	1–2 h	6–12 h	8–17%	>90% >90%	48–80 min/8–15 h 48–80 min/8–15 h	>90% >90%
SECOND GENERATION							
Cefaclor (PO)	15 min	0.5–1 h	6–12 h	25%	>90%	35–54 min/2–3 h	60–85%
Cefamandole (IM)	Rapid	0.5–2 h	4–8 h	65–75%	0	30–60 min/2.1 h	UA
Cefonicid (IM)	Rapid	1 h	12–24 h	90%	0	270 min/11 h	99%
Cefotetan (IM)	Rapid	1–3 h	12 h	88–90%	0	180–276 min/13–35 h	51–81%
Cefoxitin (IM)	Rapid	0.5 h	4–8 h	73%	0	40–60 min/20 h	85%
Cefprozil (PO)	UA	1–2 h	12–24 h	36%	95%	78 min/5.2–5.9 h	60%
Cefuroxime (PO) (IM)	UA Rapid	2 h 15–60 min	8–12 h 6–12 h	50% 50%	UA	80 min/16–22 h 80 min/16–22 h	66–100% 66–100%
Loracarbef (PO)	Rapid	0.5–1.2 h	12 h	25%	79%	60 min/32 h	>90%
THIRD GENERATION							
Cefdinir (PO)	Slow	2–4 h	UA	60–70%	20–25%	100 min/18 h	12–18%
Cefixime (PO)	15–30 min	2–6 h	25 h	65%	30–50%	180–240 min/11.5 h	50%
Cefoperazone (IM)	Rapid	1–2 h	12 h	82–93%	0	120 min/1.3–2.9 h	20–30%
Cefotaxime (IM)	Rapid	0.5 h	4–12 h	30–40%	0	60 min/3–11 h	60%
Cefpodoxime (PO)	UA	2–3 h	12 h	21–29%	UA	120–180 min/9.8 h	29–33%
Ceftazidime (IM)	Rapid	1 h	6–12 h	<10%	0	114–120 min/14–30 h	80–90%
Ceftibuten (PO)	Rapid	2–3 h	24 h	65%	UA	144 min/13.4–22.3 h	56%
Ceftizoxime (IM)	Rapid	0.5–1.5 h	6–12 h	30%	0	102 min/25–30 h	80%
Ceftriaxone (IM)	Rapid	1–2 h	12–24 h	85–95%	0	348–522 min/15.7 h	33–67%
FOURTH GENERATION							
Cefepime (IM)	30 min	1–2 h	12 h	20%	0	102–138 min/17–21 h	85%

NRF = normal renal function; ESRD = end-stage renal disease.

Hepatic function impairment is a concern for **cefoperazone** and **ceftriaxone**. If doses above 4 g are used per day, serum concentrations must be monitored.

Cephalosporins are Pregnancy Category B; however, their use during pregnancy should always be based on a risk-benefit determination because relatively few controlled studies exist. All of these drugs cross the placenta with maternal to fetal serum ratios of 0.16 to 1.

The safety and efficacy in children vary by drug. Safety and efficacy have not been established for children under age 1 month for **cefazolin** and **cefaclor**; under age 3 months for **cefuroxime, cephapirin,** and **cefoxitin**; under age 6 months for **cefpodoxime, cefdinir, loracarbef, cefixime, ceftizoxime,** and **cefprozil;** under age 9 months for oral **cephradine;** and under age 1 year for **cefepime** and parenteral **cephradine.**

Adverse Drug Reactions

In addition to type I immediate anaphylactic-type hypersensitivity (see Precautions and Contraindications), serum sickness–like reactions, consisting of erythema multiforme, other skin rashes, arthralgia, and fever, have been reported. This type III delayed reaction usually occurs following a second course of therapy and may be delayed up to 10 or more days after initiation of the drug. Between 0.1 and 1 percent of patients who receive **cefaclor** have this reaction. **Antihistamines** and **corticosteroids** may help to manage symptoms.

Several parenteral **cephalosporins** have been associated with induction of seizure activity, especially in the presence of renal impairment when the dose was not adjusted downward or in intraventicular administration. Discontinuance of the drug resolved the problem in most cases.

Coagulation abnormalities have occurred in conjunction with administration of parenteral **cephalosporins** containing a particular chemical group, **cefamandole, cefmetazole, cefoperazone, cefotetan,** and **moxalactam.** Patients at risk appear to be those with renal impairment, cancer, impaired vitamin K synthesis, malnutrition, or low vitamin K stores. These **cephalosporins** are also associated with the disulfiram-like reaction in patients who consume or, less frequently, inhale **alcohol** (such as aftershave or alcohol swabs).

Immune hemolytic anemia has also been observed with **cephalosporins** in rare instances. Patients who develop anemia within 2 to 3 weeks of the initiation of **cephalosporin** therapy should be evaluated for the role the **cephalosporin** may play in this disorder, and the drug should be stopped until the etiology is determined.

Pseudomembranous colitis is a potentially serious adverse reaction to **cephalosporins** and other broad-spectrum **antibiotics.** Detection and management are described in the discussion of the adverse effects of **penicillins.** Use of **cephalosporins,** especially prolonged or repeat therapy, may result in bacterial or fungal overgrowth of nonsusceptible organisms. The patient should be monitored for this superinfection and treated with appropriate measures.

Incidence of non–*C. difficile* diarrhea is high with some oral **cephalosporins,** including **cefdinir** (16%), **cefixime** (16%), and **cefpodoxime** (7%). There have been reports with **cefpodoxime** of acute liver injury, bloody diarrhea, and pulmonary infiltrates with eosinophilia. **Ceftriaxone** has caused accumulation of biliary sludge or pseudolithiasis, which clears on discontinuation of the drug.

Drug Interactions

Drug interactions vary by drug. Table 22–7 shows specific drugs and their interactions. Drugs that interact with all **cephalosporins** include **probenecid,** which increases plasma levels of cephalosporins, and **loop diuretics,** which increase the risk for nephrotoxicity.

Clinical Use and Dosing

EXACERBATION OF CHRONIC BRONCHITIS. For acute bacterial exacerbations of chronic bronchitis, which are treated empirically, **second-** or **third-generation cephalosporins** cover the most common pathogens (*S. pneumoniae, H. influenzae,* and *M. catarrhalis*). (See discussion of guidelines for initiating treatment in the Clinical Use and Indications section for **penicillins.**) Second-generation agents have greater activity against the pneumococcus. Treatment is continued for 5 to 10 days at dosages shown in Table 22–8.

ACUTE OTITIS MEDIA. Although **amoxicillin** is the recognized first-line drug of choice for otitis media (see the discussion in the Clinical Use and Indications section for **penicillins**), **cephalosporins** play an important role in the management of this common infection. For therapeutic failures of **amoxicillin,** the CDC (Gooch & Golantly, 2000) recommends **amoxicillin-clavulanate, cefuroxime axetil** at 30 mg/kg daily, or **ceftriaxone** 50 mg/kg as a daily IM dose for 1 to 3 days. **Ceftriaxone** is approved as a single injection for first-line therapy, but three daily doses are recommended for children who have recently failed therapy with another **antimicrobial.** A concern about this use of **ceftriaxone** is that there is relatively little clinical experience with this powerful **antibiotic** in treating AOM, and the effect of widespread use on resistance is unpredictable. **Cefuroxime axetil** has diminishing effectiveness against drug-resistant *S. pneumoniae* in the high-intermediate and highly resistant categories, so its long-term effectiveness is also unpredictable. Although other **second-** and **third-generation cephalosporins** may be effective for acute otitis media, compelling research-based evidence is lacking for their effectiveness after **amoxicillin** failure.

SINUSITIS. Second- and **third-generation cephalosporins** with beta-lactamase stability and activity against

Table 22–7. Drug Interactions: Cephalosporins

Drug	Interacting Drug	Possible Effect	Implications
All cephalosporins	Probenecid	Probenecid may increase and prolong cephalosporin plasma levels by competitively inhibiting renal tubular secretion.	Avoid concurrent administration unless planned for therapeutic reasons.
	Loop diuretics	Increased risk of nephrotoxicity.	Use with caution and monitor renal function.
Cefazolin, cefoperazone, cefotetan	Ethanol	Alcoholic beverages consumed concurrently or within 72 hours after these cephalosporins may produce an acute disulfiram-like reaction within 30 min of alcohol ingestion. This reaction may occur ≤3 d after last antibiotic dose.	Warn patients to avoid concurrent ingestion of alcohol.
	Anticoagulants	Hypoprothrombinemic effects of anticoagulants may be increased. Bleeding complications may occur. This interaction is also reported with some other cephalosporins.	Select a different antibiotic class for patients taking anticoagulants. If they must be given together, monitor PT more closely.
Cefaclor, cefdinir, cefpodoxime	Antacids	Extended-release tablets may have reduced plasma concentration when given with antacids.	If both must be given, separate administration by at least 2 h. Cefprozil and ceftibuten do not appear to be affected by antacids and may be substituted if appropriate.
Cefpodoxime, cefuroxime	Histamine$_2$ blockers	Plasma concentrations of the cephalosporin may be reduced by coadministration.	Cefaclor does not appear to be affected and may be substituted if appropriate.
Cefdinir	Iron supplements	Iron supplements and foods fortified with iron reduce absorption of cefdinir by 80% and 30%, respectively.	If iron must be taken, separate administration by 2 h. Iron-fortified infant formula has no effect.

S. pneumoniae are indicated for the treatment of bacterial sinusitis. (See the discussion of guidelines for initiating treatment in the Clinical Use and Indications section for **penicillins**.) **Cefuroxime axetil** 250 mg twice daily for 10 days, **cefprozil** 250 to 500 mg twice daily for 10 days, or **cefpodoxime proxetil** 200 mg twice a day for 10 days is recommended for treatment of sinusitis. Other first-line drugs used in the treatment of sinusitis include **amoxicillin-clavulanate**, **amoxicillin**, and **trimethoprim-sulfamethoxazole**.

PHARYNGITIS. Penicillin V is the drug of choice for treatment of pharyngitis caused by GABHS. (See the discussion of guidelines for initiating treatment in the Clinical Use and Indications section for **penicillins**.) First- and **second-generation cephalosporins** are indicated

as an alternative for this infection as a 10-day course of treatment. A growing number of studies indicate that a 4- to 6-day course of **second-** or **third-generation cephalosporins** will effectively prevent rheumatic heart disease, although the narrower spectrum of second-generation drugs is more appropriate for streptococcal pharyngitis. Recommended pediatric dosages for this indication include **cefuroxime axetil** 20 mg/kg a day divided into two doses for 4 days and **cefprozil** 15 mg/kg a day for 10 days. Adult dosage recommendations include **cefuroxime axetil** 250 mg twice daily for 4 days and **cefprozil** 500 mg daily for 4 to 10 days (Gilbert, Moellering, & Sande, 1999).

URINARY TRACT INFECTION. Oral **cephalosporins** are used as alternatives to first-line empiric therapy in

Table 22–8. Dosage Schedule: Cephalosporins

Drug	Indications	Initial Dose	Maximal Dose and Comments
FIRST GENERATION			
Cefadroxil (Duricef)	Endocarditis prophylaxis	*Adult* PO: 2 g 1 h prior to surgery *Children* PO: 50 mg/kg 1 h prior to surgery	Maximum adult daily dose 4 g. Decrease dose frequency if CCr <50 mL/min.
	Pharyngitis/tonsillitis, impetigo (children)	*Adult* PO: 500 mg q12h *or* 1 g once daily for 10 d *Children* PO: 15 mg/kg q12h *or* 30 mg/kg once/d for 10 d	
	Pneumonia	*Adult* PO: 500 mg–2 g q12h	
	Skin and soft tissue infection	*Adult* PO: 500 mg q12h *or* 1 g once daily *Children* PO: 15 mg/kg q12h	
	Urinary tract infection, uncomplicated	*Adult* PO: 500 mg–1 g q12h *or* 1–2 g once daily *Children* PO: 15 mg/kg q12h	
Cefazolin (Kefzol, Ancef)	Endocarditis prophylaxis	*Adult* IM: 1 g 30 min prior to surgery *Children* IM: 25 mg/kg 30 min prior to surgery	Maximum adult daily dose 6 g, although up to 12 g/d have been used in rare instances. Reconstituted IM solution stable for 24 h at room temperature and 10 d if refrigerated.
	Pneumonia	*Adult* IM: 500 mg q12h *Children* See antibacterial	
	Urinary tract infection, uncomplicated	*Adult* IM: 1 g q12h	
	Antibacterial, mild to moderate infections	*Adult* IM: 250 mg–1 g q6–8h *Children* IM: 6.25–25 mg/kg q6h *or* 8.3–33.3 mg/kg q8h	
Cephalexin (Keftab, Keflex)	Antibacterial, mild to moderate infection	*Adults and children >40 kg* PO: 250 mg q6h *Children ≥1 y* PO: 12.5–25 mg/kg q12h *or* 6.25–12.5 mg/kg q6h *Infants <1 y* PO: 6.25–12.5 mg/kg q6h	Adult maximum daily dose 4 g. If adult dose >4 g/d is needed, substitute parenteral therapy. Shake suspension well before measuring. Potency of suspension maintained after reconstitution for 14 d if refrigerated.
	Antibacterial, severe infection	*Adults and children >40 kg* PO: 1 g q6h *Children ≥1 y* PO: 25–50 mg/kg q12h *or*	

Continued on next page

Table 22–8. Dosage Schedule: Cephalosporins *(continued)*

Drug	Indications	Initial Dose	Maximal Dose and Comments
	Endocarditis prophylaxis (off-label use)	12.5–25 mg/kg q6h *Infants <1 y* See mild to moderate bacterial infections *Adults and children >40 kg* PO: 2 g as single dose 1 h prior to surgery *Children ≥1 y* PO: 50 mg/kg as single dose 1 h prior to surgery	
	Pharyngitis, skin and soft tissue infection, tonsillitis	*Adults and children >40 kg* PO: 500 mg q12h *Children ≥1 y* PO: 12.5–25 mg/kg q12h	
	Cystitis, uncomplicated	*Adults and adolescents >15 y* 50 mg q12h for 7–14 d	
	Otitis media	*Adults and children >40 kg* See mild to moderate bacterial infections *Children ≥1 y* PO: 18.75–25 mg/kg q6h	
Cephradine (Velosef)	Antibacterial, serious or chronic infections	*Adults and children* PO: up to 1 g q6h *Adults* PO: 250–500 mg q6h *or* 500 mg–1 g q12h *Children ≥9 mo* PO: 6.25–12.5 mg/kg q6h or 12.5–25 mg/kg q12h *Infants <9 mo* PO: 6.25–12.5 mg/kg q6h	Maximum adult daily dose 4 g. Adults with impaired renal function (CCr <200 mL/min) require decreased dosage. Shake suspension well before measuring. After reconstitution, retains potency 7 d at room temperature or 14 d if refrigerated.
	Otitis media due to *H. influenzae*	*Children ≥9 mo* PO: 18.75–25 mg/kg q6h or 37.5–50 mg/kg q12h *Infants <9 mo* PO: 18.75–25 mg/kg q6h	
	Urinary tract infection, uncomplicated	*Adults* PO: 500 mg q12h	
	Skin and soft tissue infection and upper respiratory tract infections	*Adults* PO: 250 mg q6h *or* 500 mg q12h *Children* See mild to moderate bacterial infections	
	Pneumonia or prostatitis	*Adults* PO: 500 mg q6h *or* 1 g q12h *Children* See mild to moderate bacterial infections	
SECOND GENERATION			
Cefaclor (Ceclor)	Bacterial infections, pharyngitis, pneumonia, skin infections due to *S. aureus* or *S. pyogenes,* tonsillitis, or urinary tract infection	*Adults* PO: 250–500 mg q8h *or* 375–500 mg extended-release tablet q12h *Infants >1 mo* PO: 6.7–13.4 mg/kg q8h	Adult maximum dose 2 g/d, although 4 g/d have been used in rare cases. Extended-release formulation should be taken with food and not crushed or chewed.

Continued on next page

Table 22-8. Dosage Schedule: Cephalosporins *(continued)*

Drug	Indications	Initial Dose	Maximal Dose and Comments
		or 10–20 mg/kg q12h	Cefaclor extended-release 500 mg bid is equivalent to capsules 250 mg tid, but not to other formulations at doses of 500 mg tid. Shake suspension well before measuring. After reconstitution, the suspension maintains potency for 14 d if refrigerated.
Cefamandole (Mandol)	Pneumonia or skin and soft tissue infections	*Adults* IM: 500 mg q6h	Maximum adult daily dose 12 g. Adults with impaired renal function (CCr <80 mL/min) require decreased dosage and/or frequency of administration. After reconstitution, the solution maintains potency for 24 h at room temperature and 96 h if refrigerated. Carbon dioxide is formed after reconstitution and may cause leakage if syringes are not used immediately.
	Urinary tract infections Severe bacterial infections	IM: 500 mg–1 g q8h *Adults* IM: 1 g q4–6h *Infants and children >1 mo* IM: 25–50 mg/kg q4–8h	
Cefonicid (Monocid)	Urinary tract infections, uncomplicated	*Adults* IM: 500 mg once q24h	Renal impairment (CCr <80 mL/min) requires dosage adjustment. Maximum geriatric dose (>75 y) is 250 mg/d. Stable after reconstitution for 24 h at room temperature and 72 h if refrigerated. Discoloration does not affect potency.
	Antibacterial, mild to moderate infections	IM: 1 g once q24h	
Cefprozil (Cefzil)	Bronchitis, exacerbation	*Adults and children >12 y* PO: 500 mg q12h for 10 d	Patients with impaired renal function (CCr <30 mL/min) require decreased dosage. Maximal pediatric dose 1 g/d. Shake suspension well before measuring. After reconstitution, the suspension maintains potency for 14 d if refrigerated. High ranking for oral solution on palatability. Consider for phenylketonurics that oral solution contains 28 mg phenylalanine/5 mL.
	Pharyngitis, tonsillitis	*Adults and children >12 y* PO: 500 mg q24h for 10 d *Children 2–12 y* PO: 75 mg q12h for 10 d	

Continued on next page

Table 22–8. Dosage Schedule: Cephalosporins *(continued)*

Drug	Indications	Initial Dose	Maximal Dose and Comments
	Sinusitis, acute	*Adults and children >12 y* PO: 250–500 mg q12h for 10 d *Children 6 mo–12 y* PO: 7.5–15 mg/kg q12h for 10 d	
	Skin and soft tissue infection	*Adults and children >12 y* PO: 500 mg q24h for 10 d *Children 2–12 y* PO: 20 mg/kg q24h for 10 d	
	Otitis media	*Children 6 mo–12 y* PO: 15 mg/kg q12h for 10 d	
	Urinary tract infection	*Adults and children >12 y* PO: 500 mg q24h for 10 d	
Cefotetan (Cefotan)	Skin and soft tissue infections, mild to moderate	*Adults* IM: 1–2 g q12h for 5–10 d	Lidocaine (0.5–1%) without epinephrine can be used as diluent for preparing IM injection. Solutions maintain potency 24 h at room temperature, 96 h if refrigerated, and 1 wk if frozen. Dosage should be decreased if CCr <30 mL/min.
	Urinary tract infections	*Adults* IM: 500 mg q12h *or* 1–2 g q12–24h for 5–10 d	
	All other bacterial infections, mild to moderate	*Adults* IM: 1–2 g q12h for 5–10 d	
Cefuroxime axetil (Ceftin)	Pharyngitis, sinusitis, tonsillitis	*Adults and children >12 y* PO: 250 mg bid for 10 d *Children 3 mo–12 y* PO: 10 mg/kg q12h for 10 d	Studies indicate 4- to 6-day treatment effective for group A streptococcal pharyngitis Suspension is not as well absorbed as tablets. Oral forms should be taken with food to increase absorption. Suspension does not require refrigeration and maintains potency for 10 d after reconstitution. Single-dose packets for suspension can be mixed with 10 mL or more cold water; apple, grape, or orange juice; or lemonade. Mix and consume entire volume immediately. Low rating for palatability of suspension.
	Otitis media or impetigo	*Children 3 mo–12 y* PO: 15 mg/kg q12 h up to 1000 mg/d for 10 d	
	Bronchitis, skin and soft tissue infections	*Adults and children >12 y* PO: 250–500 mg bid for 10 d	
	Gonorrhea, uncomplicated	*Adults and children >12 y* PO: 1000 mg as single dose	

Continued on next page

Table 22–8. Dosage Schedule: Cephalosporins *(continued)*

Drug	Indications	Initial Dose	Maximal Dose and Comments
	Lyme disease, early	*Adults and children >12 y* PO: 500 mg bid for 20 d	
	Pneumonia	500 mg bid	
	Urinary tract infection, uncomplicated	125–250 mg for 7–10 d	
Loracarbef (Lorabid)	Bronchitis, exacerbation	*Adults* PO: 200 mg q12h for 7 d	Shake suspension well before measuring. Refrigeration of the suspension is not necessary. Palatability of suspension is rated very high. Dosage reduction required if CCr <50 mL/min.
	Pharyngitis, streptococcal	*Adults* PO: 200–400 mg q12h for 10 d	
	Pneumonia (*S. pneumoniae* or *H. influenzae*)	*Adults* PO: 400 mg q12h for 14 d	
	Sinusitis	*Adults* PO: 400 mg q12h for 10 d	
	Urinary tract infection, uncomplicated cystitis	*Adults* PO: 200 mg q24h for 7 d	
	Uncomplicated pyelonephritis	*Adults* PO: 400 mg q12h for 14 d	
THIRD GENERATION			
Cefdinir (Omnicef)	Bronchitis, exacerbation; sinusitis; otitis media	*Adults* PO: 300 mg q12h *or* 600 mg q24h for 10 d *Children* PO: 7 mg/kg q12h *or* 14 mg/kg q24h for 10 d	
	Community-acquired pneumonia, skin and soft tissue infection	*Adults* PO: 300 mg q12h *or* 600 mg q24h for 10 d *Children* PO: 7 mg/kg q12h for 10 d	
	Pharyngitis, tonsillitis	*Adults* PO: 300 mg q12h for 5–10 d *or* 600 mg q24h for 10 d *Children* PO: 7 mg/kg q12h for 5–10 d *or* 14 mg/kg q24h for 10 d	
Cefixime (Suprax)	Bronchitis, exacerbation; pharyngitis; tonsillitis; or urinary tract infection	*Adults and children >50 kg* PO: 200 mg q12h *or* 400 mg q24h *Children 6 mo–12 y, <50 kg* PO: 4 mg/kg q12h *or* 8 mg/kg q24h	Palatability of suspension rated high. Oral suspension results in higher blood level than tablets, so do not substitute tablets for suspension in otitis media. Shake suspension well before measuring. Refrigeration not required. After reconstitution, it maintains potency for 14 d at room temperature.

Continued on next page

Table 22–8. Dosage Schedule: Cephalosporins *(continued)*

Drug	Indications	Initial Dose	Maximal Dose and Comments
	Gonorrhea, cervical or urethral	*Adults* PO: 400 mg as a single dose	Dosage reduction required if CCr <60 mL/min.
Cefoperazone (Cefobid)	Mild to moderate infection	*Adults* IM: 1–2 g q12h	Adults with impaired liver function should not receive more than 4 g/d. Adults with combined hepatic and renal impairment should receive no more than 1–2 g/d. Lidocaine without epinephrine may be added when preparing injection.
Cefotaxime (Claforan)	Gonorrhea, cervical, urethral, or rectal in females	*Adults and children >50 kg* 500 mg as a single dose	IM doses should not exceed 2 g per site. After preparation, the solution retains potency for 12 h at room temperature and 5 d if refrigerated in syringe and 7 d if refrigerated in original container.
	Gonorrhea, rectal in males Antibacterial, uncomplicated infection	1 g as a single dose *Adults and children >50 kg* IM: 1 g q12h *Children >1 mo <50 kg* IM: 8.3–30 mg/kg q4h *or* 12.5–45 mg/kg q6h	
Cefpodoxime proxetil (Vantin)	Gonorrhea, cervical, urethral, or rectal in females	*Adults* PO: 200 mg as a single dose	Palatability of suspension rated low. Shake suspension well before measuring. Take suspension with food or alone. Tablets should be taken with food. After reconstitution, maintains potency for 14 d if refrigerated.
	Urinary tract infection	*Adults* PO: 100 mg q12h for 7 d	
	Pharyngitis, tonsillitis	*Adults and children >12 y* PO: 100 mg q12h for 5–10 d *Children 5 mo–12 y* PO: 5 mg/kg, up to 400 mg, q12h for 10 d	
	Otitis media	*Children 5 mo–12 y* PO: 10 mg/kg, up to 400 mg, q24h for 10 d *or* 5 mg/kg, up to 200 mg, q12h for 10 d	
	Pneumonia, community acquired Skin and soft tissue infection	*Adults and children >12 y* PO: 200 mg q12h for 14 d PO: 400 mg q12h for 7–14 d	

Continued on next page

Table 22–8. Dosage Schedule: Cephalosporins *(continued)*

Drug	Indications	Initial Dose	Maximal Dose and Comments
Ceftibuten (Cedax)	Bronchitis, exacerbation; otitis media; pharyngitis; tonsillitis	*Adults and children >12 y* PO: 400 mg q24h for 10 d *Children 6 mo–12 y* PO: 9 mg/kg q24h for 10 d	Maximal daily adult dose 400 mg. Renal impairment (CCr <50 mL/min) requires dosage decrease. Shake suspension well before measuring. Maintains potency for up to 14 d if refrigerated.
Ceftizoxime (Cefizox)	Gonorrhea, uncomplicated	*Adults and children >12 y* IM: 1 g as a single dose	After reconstitution, IM solution retains potency at room temperature for 24 h and for 48–96 h if refrigerated. Yellow to amber discoloration does not affect potency. Renal impairment (CCr <80 mL/min) requires dosage decrease.
	Urinary tract infection	*Adults and children >12 y* IM: 500 mg q12h	
	Antibacterial, mild to moderate infection	*Adults and children >12 y* IM: 1 g q8–12h *Children 6 mo–6 y* IM: 50 mg q6–8h	
Ceftriaxone (Rocephin)	Gonorrhea, uncomplicated	*Adults* IM: 250 mg as a single dose	Maximal daily dose is 4 g for adults and 2 g for children (except meningitis is 4 g). Dose should not exceed 2 g/d in patients with both hepatic and renal impairment. After reconstitution, IM solution retains potency for 24 h at room temperature and 48–96 h if refrigerated. Yellow to amber discoloration does not affect potency.
	Otitis media	*Children* IM: 50 mg/kg, up to 1 g, as a single dose	
	Skin and soft tissue infection	*Children* IM: 50–75 mg/kg q24h *or* 25–37.5 mg/kg q12h, up to 2 g/d	
	All other serious infections	*Adults* IM: 1–2 g q24h *or* 500 mg–1 g q12h *Children* IM: 25–37.5 mg/kg q12h up to 2 g/d	

UTI in adults. (See the Clinical Use and Indications section for **fluoroquinolones.**) Duration of therapy for cystitis-urethritis in adults is 3 days; uncomplicated pyelonephritis requires 14 days of treatment. Children require 10 to 14 days of therapy for UTI because it is difficult to distinguish cystitis and pyelonephritis in young children. Oral **cephalosporins** from any generation are effective in the treatment of UTIs in adults and are first-line therapy in children for whom **fluoroquinolones** are not approved. **Cefpodoxime proxetil** is used in adult dosages of 100 mg twice daily for urethritis-cystitis, 200 mg twice daily for pyelonephritis, and pediatric dosages of 10 mg/kg/day divided into two doses. **Cefixime** is used in adult dosages of 400 mg once daily for urethritis-cystitis and pyelonephritis; pediatric dosages are 8 mg/kg/day divided into two doses. Dosage of other agents for adults and children are listed on Table 22–8. UTI is a common cause of unexplained fever in infants and young children 2 months to 2 years of age. In this population, diagnosis requires culture obtained by suprapubic aspiration (Committee on Quality, 1999). The child who is toxic, dehydrated, or unable to retain oral intake should be hospitalized for empiric parenteral therapy with **cephalosporins** or other agents and supportive care until cultures are reported.

SEXUALLY TRANSMITTED DISEASES. Third-generation **cephalosporins** are the first-line treatment for cervicitis, urethritis, pharyngitis, and proctitis due to *N. gonorrhoeae*. Recommended adult dosages as a single dose are **ceftriaxone** 125 mg IM or **cefixime** 400 mg orally. Because *Chlamydia* is commonly associated with genital gonorrhea, **azithromycin** 1 g as a single dose or **doxycycline** 100 mg twice daily for 10 days should be prescribed concurrently (Gilbert, Moellering, & Sande, 1999). **Ceftriaxone** is also used in the treatment of chancroid (250 mg as a single IM dose); early primary, secondary, or latent syphilis (125 mg daily IM for 10 days or 250 mg IM every other day for 5 doses); pelvic inflammatory disease (250 mg IM as a single dose plus **doxycycline** 100 mg daily for 14 days); epididymo-orchiditis (250 mg IM as a single dose plus **doxycycline** 100 mg daily for 10 days); and gonococcal conjunctivitis in the adult (1 g IM as single dose plus saline lavage of eye).

SKIN AND TISSUE INFECTIONS. First-generation **cephalosporins** are first-line agents in the treatment of primary and secondary skin infections, including cellulitis, erysipelas, impetigo, traumatic wound infection, and surgical incision infection. Dosages are listed in Table 22–8. Cat bites, 80 percent of which become infected with *P. multocida* and/or *S. aureus*, can be treated with **amoxicillin-clavulanate** or **cefuroxime axetil** 500 mg twice daily. **Cephalexin** and other **first-generation cephalosporins** should not be used for cat bite infections.

COMMUNITY-ACQUIRED PNEUMONIA. Although many **cephalosporins** are indicated for the treatment of pneumonia, **beta-lactam antibiotics** currently have a declining role in the treatment of CAP. (See the Clinical Use and Indications section for **penicillins**.) Although not active against important pathogens in pneumonia, *Mycoplasma, Legionella,* or *Chlamydia,* **oral second-generation cephalosporins** are an alternative

to **fluoroquinolones** and **macrolides** for empiric treatment of CAP. The American Thoracic Society recommends a **second-generation cephalosporin** for CAP patients older than 60 with no comorbidities because the pneumococcus is the most common pathogen in this group (Gleason, Kapoor, & Stone, 1997). Adult dosages of these agents include **cefuroxime axetil** 250 to 500 mg every 12 hours and **cefprozil** 250 mg every 12 hours, usually for 10 to 14 days; pediatric dosages are listed in Table 22–8.

OTHER USES. Although an off-label use, oral and parenteral **first-generation cephalosporins** are effective in dosages listed on Table 22–8 for endocarditis prophylaxis prior to surgery for patients with a history of rheumatic heart disease. **Cefuroxime axetil** in adult doses of 500 mg twice a day for 21 days is used in early Lyme disease characterized by erythema migrans. **Ceftriaxone** in adult doses of 2 g daily for 14 to 28 days has been used for facial nerve involvement and arthritis of Lyme disease.

Rational Drug Selection

The general principles of rational **antimicrobial** selection, using the definitive and empiric approaches, are presented in the section on **penicillins**. Because there is so much variability within each generation of the **cephalosporins**, sensitivity testing is valuable in drug selection. Selection of **cephalosporins**, like selection of any **antimicrobial**, is based on the organism that is present (in the definitive approach) or most likely present (in the empiric approach), site of infection, resistance patterns, adverse effects, pharmacokinetics, cost, and convenience.

The **oral first-generation cephalosporins** are interchangeable in terms of efficacy and safety, although the wholesale price for **cephradine** is less than for **cephalexin** or **cefadroxil** (Gilbert, Moellering, & Sande, 1999). Parenteral **cefazolin** has good tissue penetration and is the drug of choice for surgical prophylaxis. Oral first-generation agents are good alternatives to **penicillinase-resistant penicillins** in the **penicillin**-allergic patient, unless the allergy is a type I hypersensitivity reaction. An off-label use is endocarditis prophylaxis prior to surgical procedures; **first-generation cephalosporins** have the advantage of a fairly narrow spectrum and may be used by most **penicillin**-allergic individuals.

Second-generation oral cephalosporins are slightly less active against gram-positive cocci than **first-generation oral cephalosporins,** so the latter are the preferred empiric treatment for skin and tissue infections. **Cefaclor** is more susceptible to beta-lactamases than other **oral second-generation cephalosporins. Cefaclor** and **locarabef** have less activity against *H. influenzae* than **amoxicillin** (Tiggs, 2000). **Cefuroxime axetil** has the most consistent activity of the **second-generation**

cephalosporins against **penicillin** intermediate-resistant pneumococci. Consequently, although all **second-generation oral cephalosporins** are approved for URIs, the resistance pattern favors **cefuroxime axetil** for oral therapy for otitis media unresponsive to **amoxicillin,** for sinusitis, and for pneumonia if *S. pneumoniae* is suspected. For other indications including UTIs, all second-generation agents apparently have comparable efficacy. Generic **cefuroxime axetil** is among the less expensive **oral cephalosporins,** but the suspension formulation has been rated one of the least palatable liquid preparations. In one study of **antibiotic** suspensions, **loracarbef** was the least expensive of the **cephalosporins** and had the highest palatability rating of all **antibiotic** suspensions (Steele, Thomas, Begue, & Despinasse, 1999). Although relatively high in cost, **cefprozil** suspension was rated as moderate to high on palatability. With the exception of **cefaclor,** which requires three doses daily, the oral second-generation agents are dosed twice daily. Extended-release **cefaclor** (Ceclor-CD) has the advantages of twice-daily dosing and daily cost comparable to other **second-generation cephalosporins.**

Because of the enhanced beta-lactamase resistance and extended gram-negative spectrum of **third-generation cephalosporins,** agents in this class are indicated for infections where resistance mediated by beta-lactamase is a major consideration, such as gonorrhea infections and resistant otitis media. Although the incidence of GI intolerance would be expected to be lower with the parenteral route of single-dose IM **ceftriaxone,** diarrhea has been observed in up to 25 percent of patients who receive **ceftriaxone** for otitis media. Additionally, IM injections may be poorly accepted by children and their parents, so the convenience and improved compliance expected with **ceftriaxone** may be offset by these liabilities. **Cefdinir** and **cefpodoxime proxetil** are oral agents that share similar antibacterial activity. **Cefixime** and **ceftibuten** are much less active than **cefpodoxime proxetil** against pneumococci, are completely inactive against **penicillin-**resistant pneumococcal strains, and have poor activity against *S. aureus*. **Cefixime** and **cefpodoxime proxetil** are the most active oral agents against *N. gonorrhoeae*. Parenteral **ceftriaxone** and **cefotaxime** are effective against resistant strains of pneumococcus and are used empirically in serious infections presumed to be caused by these strains. Because they cross the blood-brain barrier, **third-generation parenteral cephalosporins** are used to treat meningitis. Unfortunately, this class of drugs is commonly misused for infections that could be treated by a narrower spectrum agent. Because of long half-lives, **ceftriaxone, ceftibuten,** and **cefixime** can be dosed once daily for most infections; **cefpodoxime proxetil** and **cefdinir** require two doses daily. **Third-generation cephalosporins** are expensive relative to other **antimicrobials.** The palatability of **cefixime** suspension was rated moderate to high, whereas **cefpodoxime proxetil** suspension had one of the lowest ratings of all suspensions tested (Steele, Thomas, Begue, & Despinasse, 1999).

Monitoring

Monitoring for therapeutic and adverse responses to **antimicrobials** requires clinical, microbiologic, and laboratory data. (See the section on Monitoring for the **penicillins.**) Because the **cephalosporins** have a broad spectrum, signs and symptoms of pseudomembranous colitis associated with *C. difficile,* as well as other superinfections, should be noted. Diarrhea is common with some **cephalosporins** and must be distinguished from pseudomembranous colitis. Obtain a *C. difficile* cytotoxin assay of the stool if there are more than six watery stools per day or if there is blood in the stool. Although hemolytic anemia is rare with the **cephalosporins,** signs of tiredness or weakness, yellow skin, or yellow eyes require a red blood cell (RBC) count with indices. During prolonged therapy, periodic urinalysis, BUN, and creatinine determinations should be performed to evaluate renal function. If the CCr indicates renal impairment, dosage should be decreased according to the schedule in the package insert or drug reference. The majority of older patients require dosage adjustment because of age-related decrements in renal function. Patients who are receiving protracted courses of **cefamandole, cefmetazole, cefoperazone, cefotetan,** or **moxalactam,** which are parenteral **cephalosporins** that affect clotting, require baseline and periodic assessment of PT. Administer exogenous vitamin K (**phytonadione; AquaMephyton**) 10 mg IM if PT time is prolonged. Patients taking these agents should also be observed for **disulfiram** reaction (abdominal cramping, facial flushing, headache, hypotension, palpitations, shortness of breath, sweating, tachycardia, vomiting) if exposed to **alcohol.**

Patient Education

ADMINISTRATION. Emphasize to the patient or caregiver the importance of completing the entire course of **antibiotic** therapy. Available dosage forms are shown in Table 22–9. IM **cephalosporins** may be irritating and painful. Inject the medication deep into a large muscle mass, and avoid repeated injection by initiating IV access for therapy requiring more than a few injections. Medications mixed for injection will lose potency with time, although refrigeration after reconstitution will usually extend the period of full potency. Consult the package insert for proper mixing and storage of reconstituted parenteral **cephalosporins.** Adhere to the manufacturer's limits on volume of injection at one site. (See also Table 22–8.)

Usually, **oral cephalosporins** should be taken with food or milk if they cause stomach irritation. **Ceftibuten** is the exception because it is poorly absorbed unless

Table 22–9. Available Dosage Forms: Cephalosporins

Drug	Dosage Form	How Supplied
FIRST GENERATION		
Cefadroxil	Capsules: 500 mg Tablets: 1 g	In bottles of 100 capsules In bottles of 24, 50, 100, and 500 tablets
(Duricef)	Capsules: 500 mg Tablets: 1 g Powder for oral suspension: 125 mg/5 cc, 250 mg/5 cc 500 mg/5 cc	In bottles of 20, 50, and 100 capsules In bottles of 50 and 100 tablets In bottles of 50 and 100 cc, orange- pineapple flavored In bottles of 50, 75, and 100 cc, orange- pineapple flavored
Cefazolin	Powder for injection: 250 mg, 500 mg, 1 g, 5 g	In multidose vials
(Ancef, Kefzol)	Powder for injection: 500 mg, 1 g, 5 g	In multidose vials
Cephalexin	Capsules: 250 mg 500 mg Tablets: 250 mg, 500 mg 1 g Powder for oral suspension: 125 mg/5 cc, 250 mg/5 cc	In bottles of 100, 500, and 1000 capsules In bottles of 100, 250, 500, and 1000 capsules In bottles of 20, 100, and 500 tablets In bottles of 24 tablets In 100- and 200-cc bottles
(Keflex)	Capsules: 250 mg 500 mg Powder for oral suspension: 125 mg/5 cc, 250 mg/5 cc	In bottles of 20 and 100 capsules In bottles of 20 capsules In 100- and 200-cc bottles
(Keftab) (monohydrate)	Tablets: 500 mg	In bottles of 100 tablets
Cephradine	Capsules: 250 mg, 500 mg Powder for oral suspension: 125 mg/5 cc, 250 mg/5 cc	In bottles of 24, 40, 100, and 500 capsules In 100- and 200-cc bottles
(Velosef)	Capsules: 250 mg, 500 mg Powder for oral suspension: 125 mg/5 cc, 250 mg/5 cc Powder for injection: 250 mg, 500 mg, 1 g	In bottles of 12 capsules In 100-cc bottles, fruit flavored In multidose vials
SECOND GENERATION		
Cefaclor	Capsules: 250 mg 500 mg Powder for oral suspension: 125 mg/5 cc 187 mg/5 cc 250 mg/5 cc 375 mg/5 cc	In bottles of 30, 100, 500, and 1000 capsules In bottles of 15, 100, and 500 capsules In 75- and 150-cc bottles In 50- and 100-cc bottles In 75- and 150-cc bottles In 50- and 100-cc bottles
(Ceclor)	Pulvules: 250 mg 500 mg CD extended-release: 375 mg, 500 mg Powder for oral suspension: 125 mg/5 cc 250 mg/5 cc	In bottles of 15 and 100 capsules In bottles of 15, 30, and 100 capsules In bottles of 60 tablets In 50- and 100-cc bottles, strawberry flavored In 75- and 150-cc bottles, strawberry flavored

Continued on next page

Table 22–9. Available Dosage Forms: Cephalosporins *(continued)*

Drug	Dosage Form	How Supplied
	375 mg/5 cc	In 50- and 100-cc bottles, strawberry flavored
Cefamandole (Mandol)	Powder for injection: 1 g 2 g	In 10-cc vials In 20-cc vials
Cefonicid (Monocid)	Powder for injection: 1 g	In multidose vial
Cefotetan (Cefotan)	Powder for injection: 1 g, 2 g	In ADD-Vantage vials
Cefprozil (Cefzil)	Tablets: 250 mg 500 mg Powder for oral suspension: 125 mg/5 cc, 250 mg/5 cc	In bottles of 100 film-coated tablets In bottles of 50 and 100 film-coated tablets In 50-, 75-, and 100-cc bottles, bubblegum flavored
Cefuroxime	Powder for injection: 750 mg 1.5 g	In 10-cc multidose vials In 20-cc multidose vials
(Ceftin)	Tablets: 125 mg, 500 mg 250 mg Suspension: 125 mg/5 cc, 250 mg/5 cc	In bottles of 20 and 60 film-coated tablets In bottles of 10, 20, and 60 film-coated tablets In 50- and 100-cc bottles, tutti-frutti flavored
(Kefurox)	Powder for injection: 750 mg 1.5 g	In 10- and 100-cc multidose vials In 20- and 100-cc multidose vials
(Zinacef)	Powder for injection: 750 mg, 1.5 g	In multidose vials
Loracarbef	Pulvules: 200 mg, 400 mg	In bottles of 30 capsules
(Lorabid)	Powder for oral suspension: 100 mg/5 cc, 200 mg/5 cc	In 50-, 75-, and 100-cc bottles, strawberry-bubblegum flavored
THIRD GENERATION		
Cefdinir	Capsules: 300 mg	In bottles of 60 capsules
(Omnicef)	Oral suspension: 125 mg/5 cc	In 60- and 100-cc bottles, strawberry flavored
Cefixime	Tablets: 200 mg	In bottles of 100 scored tablets
(Suprax)	400 mg Powder for oral suspension: 100 g/5 cc	In bottles of 50 and 100 scored tablets In 50-, 75-, and 100-cc bottles, strawberry flavored
Cefoperazone (Cefobid)	Powder for injection: 1 g, 2 g	In multidose vials
Cefotaxime (Claforan)	Powder for injection: 500 mg, 1 g, 2 g	In multidose vials
Cefpodoxime (Vantin)	Tablets: 100 mg, 200 mg Granules for suspension: 50 mg/5 cc, 100 mg/5 cc	In bottles of 20 and 100 tablets In 50-, 75-, and 100-cc bottles, lemon crème flavor

Continued on next page

Table 22–9. Available Dosage Forms: Cephalosporins *(continued)*

Drug	Dosage Form	How Supplied
Ceftazidime	Powder for injection: 500 mg	In multidose vials
(Fortaz)	1 g, 2 g	In multidose and ADD-Vantage vials
(Tazidime)	Powder for injection: 500 mg 1 g 2 g	In 10-cc multidose vials In 20- and 100-cc ADD-Vantage vials In 50- and 100-cc ADD-Vantage vials
(Ceptaz)	Powder for injection: 1 g, 2 g	In multidose vials
(Tazicef)	Powder for injection: 1 g, 2 g	In multidose and ADD-Vantage vials
Ceftibuten	Capsules: 400 mg	In bottles of 20 and 100 capsules
(Cedax)	Powder for oral suspension: 90 mg/5 cc 180 mg/5 cc	In 30-, 60-, 90-, and 120-cc bottles, cherry flavored In 30-, 60-, and 120-cc bottles, cherry flavored
Ceftizoxime	Powder for injection: 500 mg	In 10-cc single-dose fliptop vials
(Cefizox)	1 g, 2 g	In 20-cc single-dose fliptop vials
Ceftriaxone (Rocephin)	Powder for injection: 250 mg, 500 mg, 1 g, 2 g	In multidose vials

taken on an empty stomach; it should be taken 1 hour before or 2 hours after meals. **Cefuroxime axetil,** particularly the suspension formulation, and **cefpodoxime proxetil** should be taken with food to enhance absorption. Tablets and suspension forms of **cefuroxime axetil** and **cefixime** should not be used interchangeably because they have different bioavailability. **Cefuroxime** tablets are more completely absorbed than the suspension; however, the suspension of **cefixime** is better absorbed than the tablets. **Cefdinir** must be taken 2 hours before or 1 hour after **antacids** that contain magnesium or aluminum, which impair its absorption. Patients with phenylketonuria should avoid **cefprozil,** which contains phenylalanine.

Suspensions and **antibiotic** solutions must be shaken to disperse or dissolve particles of drug immediately before measurement. Adhere to the manufacturer's specifications for storage after reconstitution, and advise the patient not to use the drug after the expiration date. Describe to the patient whether there will be liquid remaining at the end of the course of therapy and urge disposal of unused medication. Ask the pharmacist to dispense a measuring device with every liquid preparation.

ADVERSE REACTIONS. If severe diarrhea occurs, the patient should contact the prescriber before initiating any treatment. For mild diarrhea, adsorbent **antidiarrheal agents** containing attapulgite can be used, but **antiperi**staltic agents that would promote the retention of *C. difficile* toxins must be avoided.

Other signs and symptoms of adverse effects that patients should be advised to report include vaginal itching or discharge, sore mouth or throat, white patches on mucous membranes of mouth, easy bruising or bleeding, altered urine output, yellow skin or eyes, or unusual lethargy commencing after the drug is started. Development of skin rash, aching joints, hives, or respiratory problems may signal allergic response and should also be reported. **Cephalosporins** cause false positives on urine testing for glucose when the copper sulfate technique (Clinitest) is used. Diabetics taking **cephalosporins** should use blood glucose monitoring or urine testing based on the glucose enzymatic tests (e.g., Clinstix, TesTape). Anorexia, epigastric pain, nausea, and vomiting in a patient taking a course of **ceftriaxone** may indicate development of biliary sludge or pseudolithiasis, which abates when the drug is discontinued.

LIFESTYLE MANAGEMENT. Practicing infection control and good health hygiene, such as safe sex practices and healthy lifestyle, helps to prevent infections. Supportive nutrition, adequate rest, appropriate fluids, and comfort measures promote recovery from an infection. Maintaining a clean, dry wound site free of excess necrotic tissue and foreign bodies is essential to resolution of a wound infection and wound healing.

Fluoroquinolones

The **fluoroquinolones** are synthetic, broad-spectrum **antibiotics** chemically related to the **quinolone nalidixic acid (NegGram)**, a narrow-spectrum **antibiotic** used to treat UTIs. **Fluoroquinolones** are the newest class of **antibiotics**. Because **trovafloxacin (Trovan)** caused several cases of fulminate liver failure and now has an FDA indication for hospital use only, it is not discussed in this section.

Pharmacodynamics

Fluoroquinolones are bactericidal through interference with enzymes required for the synthesis and repair of bacterial DNA. Addition of two chemical moieties, including a fluorine-containing group and a piperazine group, to the structure of the **quinolone nalidixic acid** resulted in the greatly enhanced antimicrobial efficacy of the **fluoroquinolones**. The fluorine molecule added to create the **fluoroquinolones** provides increased potency against gram-negative organisms and broadens the spectrum to include gram-positive organisms as well. The added piperazine moiety is responsible for the antipseudomonal activity of **fluoroquinolones**. **Levofloxacin**, the pure L-isomer of racemic **ofloxacin**, has a broader gram-positive spectrum than the racemate.

Fluoroquinolones inhibit bacterial topoisomerase II (DNA gyrase) and topoisomerase IV. Inhibition of DNA gyrase prevents the relaxation of positively supercoiled DNA that is required for normal transcription and replication. Inhibition of topoisomerase IV probably interferes with separation of replicated DNA into the daughter cells during replication.

Sensitivity

Fluoroquinolones are notable for their extensive gram-negative activity against *E. coli*, *Klebsiella* species, *Enterobacter*, *Salmonella*, *Shigella*, *Proteus vulgaris*, *Serratia*, *Haemophilus* species, *N. gonorrhoeae*, *N. meningitidis*, *M. catarrhalis*, *Legionella*, and many others. Excepting **trovafloxacin** and **moxifloxacin**, **fluoroquinolones** have little activity against anaerobic organisms but are active against atypical organisms such as *Chlamydia*, *Mycobacterium*, and *Mycoplasma* species. Only **ciprofloxacin** and **levofloxacin** have full activity against *P. aeruginosa*. **Fluoroquinolones** can be divided into two subgroups. **Fluoroquinolones** with limited gram-positive activity (**ciprofloxacin, enoxacin, lomefloxacin,** and **ofloxacin**) have the spectrum previously listed. **Fluoroquinolones** with enhanced gram-positive activity have this spectrum plus considerable activity against *Streptococcus* and *Enterococcus* species, as well as some activity against **methicillin**-resistant *Staphylococcus* species (MRSA and MRSE). **Fluoroquinolones** with enhanced gram-positive activity include **levofloxacin, sparfloxacin,** and two new agents: **moxifloxacin** and **gatifloxacin**. **Grepafloxacin** and **trovafloxacin**, agents recently removed from the market and placed under restricted indications, respectively, were also **fluoroquinolones** with enhanced gram-positive activity. **Trovafloxacin** and **moxifloxacin** have the greatest potency against pneumococci and anaerobes (Andriole, 1999).

Resistance

Resistance is mediated by mutations in the quinolone-binding region of the target enzyme or by a change in the permeability of the organism (Piddock, 1999). Some strains of *P. aeruginosa* developed resistance to **ciprofloxacin** fairly rapidly by expressing genes that promoted efflux of the **fluoroquinolone** from the bacterial cell. **Ofloxacin** treatment of patients with multidrug-resistant pulmonary tuberculosis has resulted in the selection of **quinolone**-resistant mutants in a few patients (Jacobs, 1999). Many scientists and clinicians are concerned that overuse of these agents has already eroded the utility of this new group of drugs. *Staphylococcus*, *Streptococcus*, and *Enterococcus* species once susceptible have now developed increasing resistance. To prevent increased development of resistance to this group of drugs, **fluoroquinolones** should not be used for upper and lower respiratory infections or for skin and soft tissue infections where other inexpensive and safe drugs are still effective. Rather, **fluoroquinolones** should be reserved for uses where the alternative is costlier and more hazardous (Chambers & Jawetz, 1998).

Pharmacokinetics

Absorption and Distribution

All drugs in this class are well absorbed after oral administration. Food only marginally affects absorption of other drugs in this class, but not all agents have been studied for food effects on absorption. Therefore, the manufacturers recommend taking some of these drugs on an empty stomach.

All drugs in this class are widely distributed, with high tissue and urinary levels. For most **fluoroquinolones**, tissue concentrations are usually higher than plasma concentrations. Plasma protein binding is variable. **Fluoroquinolones** are also found in saliva, nasal and bronchial secretions, sputum, bile, lymph, and peritoneal fluid. They cross the blood-brain barrier poorly into uninflamed meninges, but **ciprofloxacin, ofloxacin,** and **trovafloxacin** penetrate to a moderate extent in the presence of inflammation. All appear to cross the placenta. Although **ciprofloxacin, ofloxacin,** and **sparfloxacin** are known to enter breast milk, this property has not been adequately studied for other **fluoroquinolones**.

Metabolism and Excretion

The predominant route of elimination varies widely between **fluoroquinolones**. Ofloxacin, **levofloxacin, lomefloxacin,** and **gatifloxacin** have predominant renal excretion with minimal (less than 10%) metabolism. In contrast, **nalidixic acid, sparfloxacin,** and **moxifloxacin** undergo extensive metabolism (more than 35%). The other drugs undergo modest metabolism but have significant renal excretion as well. A few of them are also excreted in feces. Renal impairment results in increased half-lives of those with substantial excretion of unchanged drug. For patients with CCr 50 cc/minute or less, dosage adjustments may be needed. This is especially of concern with older adults, who are likely to have some degree of reduced renal function (Gatifloxacin and Moxifloxacin, 2000; Turnbridge, 1999).

Table 22–10 depicts the pharmacokinetics of selected oral fluoroquinolones.

Pharmacotherapeutics

Precautions and Contraindications

Preexisting QTc prolongation or concurrent use of other drugs producing this cardiac conduction change produces additive effects with **sparfloxacin** and **moxifloxacin.** This adverse effect resulted in the voluntary withdrawal of **grepafloxacin** from the market in 1999. Although other **fluoroquinolones** produce slight prolongation of the QTc interval, the increase is not considered to be clinically significant.

Cautious use is required for patients with renal impairment. Dosage adjustments of all **fluoroquinolones** except **moxifloxacin** are needed for patients with impaired renal function. (See Table 22–12 later in this section.) **Enoxacin** plasma concentrations are 50 percent higher in older adults than in younger adults, and this difference is related in part to reduced renal function.

Seizures, increased intracranial pressure, and toxic psychoses have occurred with this class. CNS stimulation, including tremors, restlessness, sleeplessness, tiredness, dizziness, lightheadedness, bad dreams, confusion, and hallucinations, may also occur. These symptoms are dose dependent and tend to resolve with continued use. Some studies indicate **fluoroquinolones** inhibit bonding of gamma-aminobutyric acid (GABA) to its receptor, which may be the mechanism of CNS stimulation. Slight decreases in magnesium concentration amplify the effect (Stahlmann & Lode, 1999). Patients with known or suspected CNS disorders and other factors that predispose to

Table 22–10. Pharmacokinetics: Fluoroquinolones

Drug	Onset	Peak	Duration	Protein Binding	Bioavailability	Half-Life*	Elimination
Ciprofloxacin	1 h	1–2 h	12–24 h	20–40%	70%	3–4.8 h	40–50% unchanged in urine; remainder in feces
Enoxacin	Rapid	1–3 h	12 h	40%	90%	3–6 h	>40% unchanged in urine; 20% metabolized by liver
Gatifloxacin	Rapid	1–3 h	24 h	20%	96%	7–8.4 h	70% unchanged in urine
Levofloxacin	Rapid	1–2 h	24 h	24–38%	99%	6–8 h	87% unchanged in urine; eliminated by tubular secretion
Lomefloxacin	Rapid	1.5 h	12–24 h	10%	95–98%	6–8 h	60–80% unchanged in urine; 5% metabolized; 28–30% biliary excretion
Moxifloxacin	Rapid	1–3 h	24 h	30–45%	86%	11–16 h	20% unchanged; 10% metabolized
Norfloxacin	Rapid	2–3 h	12 h	10–15%	30–40%	6.5 h	30% unchanged in urine; 30% in feces; 10% metabolized by liver
Ofloxacin	Rapid	1–2 h	12 h	20–25%	89%	5–7 h	70–80% unchanged in urine
Sparfloxacin	Rapid	3–6 h	24 h	45%	92%	20 h	10% unchanged in urine; partially metabolized by liver

*Half-life is increased in renal impairment, and dosage adjustments may be needed.

seizures should use these agents with caution and careful monitoring.

Older adults and dialysis patients have increased risk of tendon rupture and adverse CNS reactions. Use **fluoroquinolones** cautiously with these populations.

Fluoroquinolones are Pregnancy Category C. Use is not recommended in pregnant women because there are no adequate, well-controlled studies in this population, and teratogenesis has been demonstrated in animals. Use during pregnancy only if there is clear benefit that justifies the risk to the fetus.

Norfloxacin was not detected in breast milk following a 20-mg dose to nursing mothers; however, this dose was low. **Ciprofloxacin** and **sparfloxacin** are excreted in breast milk, but the dose ingested by the infant is small. Concentration of **ofloxacin** in breast milk is similar to maternal plasma, and it is presumed that its L-isomer, **levofloxacin**, also enters breast milk. Other drugs in this class do not have available data. Because **fluoroquinolones** have caused lesions of cartilage of weight-bearing joints in young animals, lactating women should use **fluoroquinolones** only if there is no safer alternative.

The safety and efficacy of this drug class have not been established in children. **Fluoroquinolones** are not recommended for children under the age of 18. Arthropathy and osteochondrosis have been demonstrated in all species of immature animals tested. **Nalidixic acid, norfloxacin,** and **ciprofloxacin** have been used in children without evidence of arthropathy or osteochondrosis, but it should be noted that these three agents have poorer tissue penetration than other **fluoroquinolones.**

Adverse Drug Reactions

Pseudomembranous colitis has been reported with nearly all **antibacterial agents,** including **fluoroquinolones,** and may be mild to life-threatening. It is important to consider this diagnosis in patients who present with diarrhea subsequent to administration of **fluoroquinolones,** especially if this diarrhea contains blood, pus, or mucus. Other common GI adverse reactions include abdominal pain, nausea and, altered taste, which are the most frequent adverse drug reactions.

Serious and occasionally fatal hypersensitivity reactions including Stevens-Johnson syndrome have occurred with **fluoroquinolones.** Some of the reactions occurred following the first dose, presumably due to cross-allergy with other chemicals in the environment. Reactions that were anaphylactic in nature have also occurred.

Use of **fluoroquinolones,** especially in prolonged or repeat therapy, may result in bacterial or fungal overgrowth of nonsusceptible organisms. The patient should be monitored for this superinfection and treated with appropriate measures.

Unique, rare adverse effects have been associated with individual **fluoroquinolones. Ciprofloxacin** has also been associated with acidosis, renal failure, polyuria, urinary retention, and renal calculi. Cardiovascular adverse reactions including angina, atrial flutter, cardiopulmonary arrest, cerebral thrombosis, myocardial infarction, and ventricular ectopy have also been seen. None of these adverse reactions occurs commonly. **Norfloxacin** has rarely been associated with erythema multiforme, hepatitis, pancreatitis, and arthralgia. **Ofloxacin** has been associated with vaginal discharge and genital pruritus. CNS symptoms such as sleep disorders, nervousness, and vertigo have also been seen uncommonly. **Enoxacin** causes more GI distress and dermatologic adverse reactions than other drugs in the class. Crystalluria has been reported with **ciprofloxacin** and other **fluoroquinolones,** especially in patients with alkaline urine (pH above 7.0). **Levofloxacin** and other **fluoroquinolones** have increased or decreased blood sugar in treated diabetics.

Phototoxicity has been observed with all **fluoroquinolones.** Clinical manifestations range from mild erythema to severe bullous eruptions in the sun-exposed areas. **Fluoroquinolones** with high phototoxic potential include **lomefloxacin** and **sparfloxacin.**

Fluoroquinolone tendinitis begins with inflammatory edema that manifests as painful and swollen tendons that are bilateral in 50 percent of cases. Failure to take appropriate measures to rest the tendon can result in rupture. Time from initiation of the drug to onset of tendinitis has varied from 1 to 152 days. Achilles rupture has occurred after drug withdrawal. Most patients who develop tendinitis are elderly (70%), and some (10%) were taking concurrent **corticosteroids,** which also adversely affect tendons (Stahlmann & Lode, 1999).

Ophthalmologic abnormalities, including cataracts and multiple punctate lenticular opacities, have occurred during therapy with some **fluoroquinolones.** A causal relationship has not been clearly established.

Additional adverse reactions are listed in the Precautions and Contraindications section.

Drug Interactions

Drug interactions vary somewhat by drug. Table 22–11 shows the various drug interactions. Several drugs interact with all **fluoroquinolones** to decrease their absorption. **Cimetidine** interferes with the elimination of **fluoroquinolones.** Some **fluoroquinolones** inhibit drug metabolism by CYP-3A4, one of the most important enzymes in hepatic drug metabolism. **Cyclosporine's** nephrotoxic effects are increased by concurrent administration with most **fluoroquinolones,** but especially with **ciprofloxacin** and **norfloxacin. Caffeine** interacts with several drugs in this class and, as with many other drugs that inhibit hepatic enzymes, **warfarin** has increased effects when administered to a patient receiving **fluoroquinolones.**

Food may decrease the absorption of **norfloxacin** and

Table 22–11. Drug Interactions: Fluoroquinolones

Drug	Interacting Drug	Possible Effect	Implications
All fluoroquinolones	Antacids, bismuth subsalicylate, iron salts, sucralfate, zinc salts	Interfere with GI absorption of the fluoroquinolone, resulting in decreased serum levels.	Avoid simultaneous use; administer antacids 2–4 h before or after the fluoroquinolone.
	Anticoagulants	Effects of anticoagulant may be increased.	Monitor PT/INR.
	Antineoplastic agents	Serum levels of fluoroquinolone may be decreased.	Select different antibiotic or monitor serum levels.
	Cimetidine	Cimetidine may interfere with elimination of fluoroquinolones.	Select different histamine$_2$ blocker.
	Cyclosporine	Nephrotoxic effects increased.	Closely monitor renal function.
	Glucocorticoids	Concurrent use may increase risk for tendon rupture.	Select different antibiotic.
	Theophylline	Decreased clearance, increased plasma levels, and toxicity of theophylline have occurred with concurrent use of ciprofloxacin and enoxacin. Data on norfloxacin and ofloxacin contradictory.	Monitor theophylline levels.
Ciprofloxacin	Caffeine	Total body clearance on caffeine reduced, with possible increased pharmacological effects.	Avoid concurrent use.
	Hydantoins	Phenytoin levels may be reduced, producing decreased therapeutic effects.	Avoid concurrent use.
	Probenecid	Renal clearance of ciprofloxacin reduced 50%; serum concentrations increased 50%.	Avoid concurrent use.
Enoxacin	Caffeine	Total body clearance of caffeine reduced. Plasma trough levels of enoxacin 20% higher.	Ofloxacin does not appear to affect caffeine.
	Digoxin	Digoxin serum levels may be increased.	Monitor serum digoxin levels.
Norfloxacin	Caffeine	Total body clearance on caffeine reduced, with possible increased pharmacological effects.	Ofloxacin does not appear to affect caffeine.
	Nitrofurantoin	Antibacterial effect of norfloxacin in urinary tract may be antagonized.	Avoid concurrent use.
Levofloxacin	NSAIDs	Concurrent use increases CNS stimulation and seizures.	Avoid concurrent use.
	Antidiabetic drugs	Increase or decrease blood sugar.	Carefully monitor blood sugar.
Sparfloxacin, moxifloxacin	Amiodarone, disopyramide, quinidine, bepridil, sotalol	Increased risk of serious adverse cardiovascular effects.	Avoid concurrent use.

INR = international normalized ratio; PT = prothrombin time.

enoxacin. Food delays the absorption of **ciprofloxacin,** although total absorption is not changed. Dairy products reduce the absorption of **ciprofloxacin** and should not be used concurrently. **Antacids, bismuth subsalicylate, iron salts, sucralfate,** and **zinc salts** form an insoluble chelate with **fluoroquinolones,** preventing the absorption of the **antimicrobial** drug.

Clinical Use and Dosing

EXACERBATIONS OF CHRONIC BRONCHITIS. In that culture and sensitivity are unreliable because of bronchial colonization in ABECB, empiric therapy is selected to cover the most likely pathogens, which are *S. pneumoniae, H. influenzae,* and *M. catarrhalis.* The treatment of ABECB is described in the Clinical Use and Indications section for **penicillins.** Although considered first-line therapy for ABECB, **fluoroquinolones** are more expensive and have a less favorable safety profile than other agents that cover the likely pathogens, so reserving **fluoroquinolones** for patients who have failed therapy with other agents is prudent. Only **fluoroquinolones** with enhanced activity against *S. pneumoniae,* which include **levofloxacin, sparfloxacin, moxifloxacin,** and **gatifloxacin,** are appropriate for treating ABECB, using dosages summarized in Table 22–12. **Lomefloxacin,** although approved for ABECB, lacks sufficient activity against pneumococci and should not be used in ABECB.

COMMUNITY-ACQUIRED PNEUMONIA. In dosages listed in Table 22–12, **fluoroquinolones** with enhanced gram-positive activity, such as **levofloxacin, sparfloxacin, moxifloxacin,** and **gatifloxacin,** are active against strains of *S. pneumoniae.* In addition, **fluoroquinolones** cover *Legionella,* as well as *M. pneumoniae* and *C. pneumoniae,* which are the most common pathogens in CAP patients without comorbidity. These organisms are resistant to **beta-lactam antibiotics** used for CAP, such as **ampicillin-clavulanate** and second-generation oral **cephalosporins,** but susceptible to **macrolides.** However, **fluoroquinolones** should be reserved for CAP diagnosed by culture and sensitivity, when the patient has failed therapy with **macrolides,** or when there is another reason to believe the organism is resistant to **beta-lactam** and **macrolide antimicrobial drugs.** For older patients or those with underlying disease, **levofloxacin** may be the best choice of the first-line agents. **Fluoroquinolones** are also indicated for CAP following airway obstruction or alcoholic stupor where anaerobic or coliform bacteria are likely pathogens. Usual duration of therapy for CAP is 7 to 14 days. Higher dosages of some **fluoroquinolones** are required for more serious infections.

URINARY TRACT INFECTION. Because of their extensive gram-negative coverage, **fluoroquinolones** are first-line agents in the treatment of infections of the urinary tract and related structures in nonpregnant adults, particularly because resistance to the other first-line therapy, **trimethoprim-sulfamethoxazole,** is increasing. Most UTIs acquired in the community are caused by Enterobacteriaceae, particularly *E. coli,* but *Enterococcus* and *Staphylococcus saprophyticus* are less common causal organisms. **Norfloxacin, nalidixic acid, lomefloxacin,** and **enoxacin** are primarily approved for infections of the urinary tract. **Fluoroquinolones** with enhanced gram-positive activity should be reserved for UTIs requiring the extended spectrum, such as enterococcal and staphylococcal infections diagnosed by culture. **Ciprofloxacin** has the greatest activity against *P. aeruginosa.* Dose and duration of treatment (Table 22–12) depend on the site and severity of the infection and whether it is complicated by obstruction, kidney stones, or other factors. Uncomplicated cystitis and urethritis are treated with **oral fluoroquinolones** for 3 days. Complicated UTI and pyelonephritis require 7 to 14 days of therapy. Dosages of some **fluoroquinolones** for acute cystitis are lower than dosages for more serious urinary tract and kidney infections.

SEXUALLY TRANSMITTED DISEASES AND GENITAL INFECTIONS. **Ofloxacin, norfloxacin, enoxacin, gatifloxacin,** and **ciprofloxacin** are approved for single-dose treatment of uncomplicated gonorrhea manifested as cervicitis, urethritis, pharyngitis, or proctitis. Unfortunately, strains of gonococci resistant to **fluoroquinolones** have been identified worldwide. Because *Chlamydia trachomatis* is associated with genital gonorrhea, **azithromycin** 1 g as a single dose or **doxycycline** 100 mg twice daily for 10 days should be prescribed to follow treatment of genital gonorrhea (Gilbert, Moellering, & Sande, 1999). Although **ofloxacin** is approved for *Chlamydia,* treatment requires 7 days of twice-daily therapy, so the single-dose therapy used for gonorrhea is not sufficient. Syphilis, which may coexist with gonorrhea, is not cured by **fluoroquinolones,** although the symptoms of the disease may be masked. Therefore, it is important to conduct serological tests for syphilis whenever the diagnosis of gonorrhea is made.

On account of good penetration of the prostate, **ofloxacin,** as an initial dose of 400 mg, followed by 300 mg twice daily, is first-line therapy for prostatitis in men less than 35 years old, in whom the most common pathogens are *N. gonorrhoeae* and *C. trachomatis.* Duration of therapy is controversial, but at least 7 days are required. For older men, the most common pathogens for prostatitis are coliforms, and **ofloxacin** is also first-line therapy in doses of 300 mg twice daily for 10 days.

SKIN AND TISSUE INFECTIONS. Although approved for skin and tissue infections, use of **fluoroquinolones** in these infections should be avoided to decrease selection pressure for bacterial resistance. Most skin and tissue infections treated in outpatient settings respond to **beta-**

Table 22–12. Dosage Schedule: Fluoroquinolones

Drug	Indications	Initial Adult Dose	Comments
Ciprofloxacin (Cipro)	Bone and joint infections, mild to moderate	PO: 500 mg q12h for at least 4–6 wk	Maximal adult daily dose 1.5 g. Renal impairment (CCr <50 mL/min) requires dosage reduction. Not recommended for children, but doses of 10–20 mg/kg q12h have been used where no alternative existed. Oral suspension stable for 14 d at room temperature or in refrigerator. Shake well before measuring. Take with full glass of water. Oral and parenteral routes are bioequivalent.
	Bone and joint infections, severe or complicated	PO: 750 mg q12h for at least 4–6 wk	
	Bacterial diarrhea	PO: 500 mg	
	Gonorrhea, cervical and urethral	PO: 250 mg as a single dose	
	Intra-abdominal infections	PO: 500 mg q12h for 7–14 d in combination with oral metronidazole	
	Meningococcal carrier (off-label use)	750 mg as a single dose	
	Prostatitis	500 mg q12h for 28 d	
	Sinusitis	PO: 500 mg q12h 10 d	
	Typhoid fever	PO: 500 mg q12h for 10 d	
	Skin and soft tissue infections, mild to moderate	500 mg q12h for 7–14 d	
	severe or complicated	750 mg q12h for 7–14 d	
	Urinary tract infection, acute, uncomplicated	100 mg q12h for 3 d	
	mild to moderate	250 mg q12h for 7–14 d	
	severe or complicated	500 mg q12h for 7–14 d	
Enoxacin (Penetrex)	Gonorrhea	PO: 400 mg as a single dose	Not for use in children. Avoid caffeine-containing food and beverages. Take 1 h before or 2 h after meals. Renal impairment (CCr < 30 mL/min) requires dosage reduction.
	Urinary tract infection, complicated	PO: 400 mg q12h for 14 d	
	uncomplicated	PO: 200 mg q12h for 7 d	
Gatifloxacin (Tequin)	Acute sinusitis	400 mg daily	Not for use in children. Renal impairment requires dosage reduction.
	Acute exacerbation of chronic bronchitis	400 mg daily	
	Community-acquired pneumonia	400 mg daily	
	Uncomplicated gonorrhea	400 mg as a single dose	
	Uncomplicated skin and soft tissue infection	400 mg daily	
	Uncomplicated urinary tract infection	400 mg daily for 3 d	
	Complicated urinary tract infection	400 mg daily for 7–14 d	

Continued on next page

Table 22–12. Dosage Schedule: Fluoroquinolones *(continued)*

Drug	Indications	Initial Adult Dose	Comments
	Acute pyelonephritis	400 mg daily for 7–14 d	
Levofloxacin (Levaquin)	Bronchitis, acute exacerbation of chronic	500 mg q24h for 7 d	Not recommended for use by children. Renal impairment (CCr <50 mL/min) requires dosage reduction. Take with full glass of water. Oral and parenteral routes are bioequivalent and interchangeable.
	Community-acquired pneumonia	500 mg q24h for 7–14 d	
	Pyelonephritis treatment	250 mg q12h for 10 d	
	Sinusitis	500 mg q24h for 10–14 d	
	Skin and soft tissue infection	500 mg q24h for 7–10 d	
	Urinary tract infection, complicated	250 mg q24h for 10 d	
Lomefloxacin (Maxaquin)	Bronchitis, bacterial exacerbation	400 mg daily for 10 d	Not recommended for use by children. Renal impairment (CCr <40 mL/min) requires dosage reduction. Take with full glass of water with or without food.
	Urinary tract infection, prophylaxis	400 mg as a single dose 1–8 h before surgery	
	Urinary tract infection, complicated	400 mg daily for 14 d	
	uncomplicated due to *E. coli*	400 mg daily for 3 d	
	uncomplicated, due to *P. mirabilis, K. pneumoniae, S. saprophyticus*	400 mg daily for 10 d	
Moxifloxacin (Avelox)	Acute sinusitis	400 mg daily for 10 d	Not for use by children.
	Acute exacerbation of chronic bronchitis	400 mg daily for 5 d	
	Community-acquired pneumonia	400 mg daily for 10 d	
Norfloxacin (Noroxin)	Gonorrhea	800 mg as a single dose	Maximal adult daily dose 800 mg (1.2 g infectious diarrhea). Take on empty stomach with full glass of water (1 h before or 2 h after food or milk). Not recommended for use by children.
	Gastroenteritis (off label)	400 mg q8–12h for 5 d	
	Prostatitis, acute or chronic	400 mg q12h for 28 d	
	Urinary tract infection, uncomplicated, due to *E. coli, K. pneumoniae, P. mirabilis*	400 mg q12h for 3 d	
	uncomplicated, due to other organisms	400 mg q12h for 7–10 d	

Continued on next page

Table 22–12. Dosage Schedule: Fluoroquinolones *(continued)*

Drug	Indications	Initial Adult Dose	Comments
Ofloxacin (Floxin)	Bronchitis, bacterial exacerbations or community-acquired pneumonia	400 mg q12h for 10 d	Maximal adult daily dose 400 mg. Not recommended for use by children. Renal impairment (CCr <50 mL/min) requires dosage reduction. Take with a full glass of water.
	Skin and soft tissue infection	400 mg q12h for 10 d	
	Chlamydia, endocervical or urethral	300 mg q12h for 7 d	
	Gonorrhea, uncomplicated	400 mg as a single dose	
	Pelvic inflammatory disease, acute	400 mg q12h for 10–14 d	
	Prostatitis	300 mg q12h for 6 wk	
	Urinary tract infection, complicated	200 mg q12h for 10 d	
	Cystitis due to *E. coli, K. pneumoniae*	200 mg q12h for 3 d	
	Cystitis due to other organisms	200 mg q12h for 7 d	
Sparfloxacin (Zagam)	Bacterial exacerbation of bronchitis or pneumonia	400 mg on the first day, then 200 mg daily for 10 d	Maximal daily dose for impaired renal function (CCr <50 mL/min) is 400 mg on the first day, followed by 200 mg q48h for a total of 9 d of therapy. Take with a full glass of water. Not recommended for use by children.

lactam antibiotics, except wounds that have been exposed to fresh water, such as ponds, lakes, and swimming pools, that may be infected with *Pseudomonas* and *Aeromonas* species.

INFECTIOUS DIARRHEA. Fluoroquinolones are first-line therapy in treatment of traveler's diarrhea and severe diarrhea not associated with **antibiotic** therapy. Recommended self-treatment for traveler's diarrhea is 3 days of twice-daily therapy with oral **ciprofloxacin** (500 mg), **norfloxacin** (400 mg), or **ofloxacin** (300 mg), combined with **loperamide** 4 mg initially and 2 mg after each stool.

For mild bacterial diarrhea not associated with **antibiotics,** characterized by three or fewer stools per day and minimal associated symptomatology, supportive therapy is usually adequate. For moderate infectious diarrhea, evidenced by four or more stools per day or fewer stools with systemic symptoms, an **antiperistaltic** drug (e.g. **loperamide**) may be added to supportive therapy. Severe infectious diarrhea not associated with **antibiotics** is manifested by six or more unformed stools per day and/or a temperature 101°F or more, tenesmus, blood, or fecal leukocytes. Presence of blood may be indicative of *E. coli* 0157:H7 infection, which has serious sequelae and requires hospitalization. Most common

pathogens in severe infectious diarrhea not associated with **antibiotics** are *Shigella, Salmonella, Campylobacter jejuni,* and *E. coli* (0157:H7 strains). Drugs of choice for severe bacterial diarrhea (not associated with **antibiotics**) are **ciprofloxacin** 500 mg every 12 hours or **norfloxacin** 400 mg every 12 hours. Therapy is continued for 3 to 5 days.

OTHER USES. **Ciprofloxacin** is approved for bone and joint infections, but with the exception of bone infections in cystic fibrosis, many typical pathogens are no longer susceptible to this drug. Use should be reserved for proven susceptibility on culture and sensitivity. Although several **fluoroquinolones** are approved for use in sinusitis, these agents are probably best reserved for other indications because of the nature of this infection. (See Clinical Use and Dosing section for **penicillins.**) **Ciprofloxacin** may be indicated for sinusitis resulting from nasogastric or nasotracheal intubation, where gram-negative bacilli are the likely pathogens. **Levofloxacin, gatifloxacin,** and **moxifloxacin** are indicated for treatment of sinusitis due to highly **penicillin**-resistant pneumococcal infections. Although an off-label use, **ciprofloxacin** as a single 750-mg dose is accepted for eradicating the meningococcal carrier state. **Ciprofloxacin** is also a first-line treatment of typhoid fever in doses of 500 mg twice daily for 10 days. If the patient is in shock or has impaired mental status, mortality will be decreased by initiating **dexamethasone** (3 mg/kg initially, followed by 1 mg/kg every 6 hours for 8 doses) a few minutes prior to **anti-infective** therapy for typhoid.

Rational Drug Selection

Both definitive drug selection and empiric drug selection follow the same principles described in the Rational Drug Selection section for the **penicillins**, regardless of the infection or drug class involved. Specific implications to consider in selecting **fluoroquinolones** are cost, resistance, and adverse effect profile. **Fluoroquinolones** are relatively high-cost agents, with wholesale costs for a course of therapy averaging $70 to $85. Comparable wholesale costs for a typical course of low-cost alternative agents used to treat many of the same infections, such as generic **doxycycline** or **trimethoprim-sulfamethoxazole**, are approximately $2 or $3. The cost of **fluoroquinolones** is comparable to other newer broad-spectrum agents such as **amoxicillin-clavulanate** ($70), **clarithromycin** ($70), and **cefuroxime axetil** ($81 to $149). Another reason to use **fluoroquinolones** judiciously is to prevent resistance. **Ciprofloxacin** is unique as an oral agent effective for *P. aeruginosa*, and the agents with enhanced gram-positive spectrum (**levofloxacin, sparfloxacin, gatifloxacin,** and **moxifloxacin**) have activity against highly **penicillin**-resistant strains of *S. pneumoniae* that are also resistant to **cephalosporins, tetracyclines, macrolides,** and **sulfonamides**. It behooves us to guard these susceptibilities as long as possible by using definitive drug selection based on culture and sensitivity and by selecting agents with the narrowest spectrum. Within the **fluoroquinolones**, agents with an enhanced gram-positive spectrum are the most costly, and agents indicated primarily for genitourinary infections (e.g., **norfloxacin**) are least expensive.

Selection between agents with similar spectrums of bacterial activity may depend on the comparative adverse effects and drug interactions profile. Because **enoxacin** may increase caffeine serum concentrations fivefold, it is seldom selected. **Norfloxacin** has much less effect on caffeine metabolism; **lomefloxacin** and **ofloxacin** appear devoid of effects on caffeine metabolism. Treated diabetics should avoid **fluoroquinolones** if other equally effective **antimicrobial drugs** are available. The patient with prolonged QTc interval or taking drugs that increase the QTc interval should avoid **sparfloxacin** and **moxifloxacin**. Unless there are compelling reasons, **fluoroquinolones** should not be used by children and pregnant women. Renal impairment requires decreased dosage of all agents except **moxifloxacin**. Other **antibacterial drugs** are also preferable for patients with severe cerebral arteriosclerosis or who are otherwise seizure prone (e.g., epilepsy, **alcohol** abuse, **theophylline** or **antipsychotic** drug use).

Monitoring

Monitoring for therapeutic response to **antimicrobial drugs** is described in the Monitoring section for **penicillins**. Patients on prolonged therapy with **fluoroquinolones** should have periodic assessment of organ function, including renal, hepatic, and hematopoietic function. Renal function should be measured or estimated with standard formulas prior to initiation of a **fluoroquinolone**. It is prudent to obtain a baseline electrocardiogram (ECG) prior to prescription of **sparfloxacin** or **moxifloxacin**. The drugs should be withheld and the ECG repeated if syncope occurs, which may indicate development of torsades de pointes, a potentially lethal arrhythmia. Patients taking **theophylline** and **cyclosporine** should have determinations of the plasma concentrations ("blood levels") of these agents, which are metabolized by CYP-3A4, a hepatic drug-metabolizing enzyme inhibited by **fluoroquinolones**. Patients on **warfarin** who are started on **fluoroquinolones** should have their PT monitored closely. When either **ofloxacin** or **enoxacin** is administered for gonorrhea, it may mask, but not cure, coexisting syphilis. Obtain serological testing for syphilis whenever a diagnosis of gonorrhea is made, with repeat testing at 3 months after treatment. Patients with epilepsy, **alcohol** abuse, or concurrent **theophylline** use should be monitored for CNS irritability (agitation, irritability) and seizure activity. Many of the adverse effects have been linked to low serum magnesium, so the patient with, or at risk for, hypomagnesemia should be monitored diligently for adverse effects of **fluoroquinolones** (Stahlmann & Lode, 1999).

Patient Education

ADMINISTRATION. Available dosage forms are shown in Table 22–13. As with all **antimicrobial drugs,** the patient must understand the significance of taking all doses and completing the full course of therapy. **Enoxacin** and **norfloxacin** should be taken on an empty stomach. Although the effect of food on absorption is unknown, the manufacturer suggests that the optimal time for administration of **ciprofloxacin** is 2 hours after meals. All **fluoroquinolones** should be taken with a full glass of water to help avoid dehydration, which can lead to crystalluria. **Fluoroquinolones** should not be taken within 2 to 6 hours of drugs that may chelate them (including **antacids, sucralfate, iron preparations,** and **zinc salts**) and prevent absorption. Dairy products hamper absorption of **norfloxacin**.

ADVERSE REACTIONS. Although **lomefloxacin** and **sparfloxacin** are most likely to cause photosensitivity or phototoxicity, all patients on **fluoroquinolones** should be taught to avoid direct sunlight, sunlamps, and tanning beds from the first dose until several days after therapy is completed. They should withhold the drug and report any

Table 22-13. Available Dosage Forms: Fluoroquinolones

Drug	Dosage Form	How Supplied
Ciprofloxacin (Cipro)	Tablets: 250 mg, 500 mg 750 mg	In bottles of 100 tablets In bottles of 50 tablets
Enoxacin (Penetrex)	Tablets: 200 mg, 400 mg	In bottles of 50 tablets
Gatifloxacin (Tequin)	Tablets: 200 mg, 400 mg	In bottles of 30 and blister packs of 100 In bottles of 50 and blister packs of 100
Levofloxacin (Levaquin)	Tablets: 250 mg, 500 mg	In bottles of 50 and 100 tablets and unit dose
Lomefloxacin (Maxaquin)	Tablets: 400 mg	In bottles of 20 film-coated tablets and unit dose
Moxifloxacin (Avelox)	Tablets: 400 mg	In bottles of: UA
Norfloxacin (Noroxin)	Tablets: 400 mg	In bottles of 100 tablets
Ofloxacin (Floxin)	Tablets: 200 mg, 300 mg, 400 mg	In bottles of 50 tablets
Sparfloxacin (Zagam)	Tablets: 200 mg	In bottles of 55 film-coated tablets

blister, rash, or itching that occurs. With **sparfloxacin** and **lomefloxacin,** severe phototoxic reactions have occurred in spite of sunscreen use and through glass. Recovery was prolonged and the reaction tended to recur if the patient was exposed to sunlight again before recovery. Sunscreens, hats, and long-sleeved clothing should be suggested for even short exposure.

Fluoroquinolones often cause dizziness or lightheadedness, so driving and hazardous activities should be avoided until the individual patient's reaction is known. Adequate fluid intake to maintain urine output of 1500 mL per day will avoid crystalluria. Minimize use of urinary alkalinizers such as citrus drinks and avoid baking soda and **antacids.** If tenderness or inflammation occurs in any tendon, the patient should immediately discontinue the **fluoroquinolone,** notify the prescriber, rest, and refrain from exercise of the affected joint. Diabetics should immediately report any signs or symptoms of hypoglycemia and should perform home blood glucose testing regularly. The drug should be discontinued at any sign of an allergic reaction (hives, itching, yawning, dyspnea) because serious anaphylactic reactions have occurred during first exposure to a **fluoroquinolone.**

LIFESTYLE MANAGEMENT. See the Lifestyle Modification section for the **penicillins.**

Lincosamides

The original drug in this class was **lincomycin.** Although structurally different, it resembled **erythromycin** in activity. Unfortunately, it was too toxic and is no longer in use. **Clindamycin (Cleocin)** is a chlorine-substituted derivative of **lincomycin** and the only remaining drug in the class. Although less toxic, its indications are still limited because of its potential to cause severe **antibiotic-**associated colitis.

Pharmacodynamics

Clindamycin binds to the 50S subunit of the bacterial ribosomes and suppresses protein synthesis. This is the same as the receptor for **macrolides,** so combined use with **erythromycin** and related drugs may decrease the effectiveness of both drugs. The action of **clindamycin** is usually bacteriostatic, but it may produce bactericidal effects if the target tissue is especially sensitive.

Sensitivity

Susceptible organisms are primarily gram-positive, including *S. pneumoniae, S. pyogenes,* and *Streptococcus viridans; S. aureus, S. epidermidis,* and *Staphylococcus albus;* and *Corynebacterium diphtheriae* and *Corynebacterium acnes.* It is also effective against selected anaerobic pathogens: *Bacteroides, Fusobacterium, Actinomyces, Peptococcus, Clostridium perfringens,* and *Clostridium tetani.* A primary indication of **clindamycin** is hospital treatment of serious intra-abdominal infections caused by anaerobic bacteria. In primary care, **clindamycin** is used for infections by gram-positive cocci in **penicillin**-allergic patients and infections by drug-resistant *S. pneumoniae* infections, such as pneumonia, sinusitis, and otitis media.

Resistance

Enterococci and gram-negative aerobic organisms are resistant to **clindamycin.** *C. difficile,* an important cause of **antibiotic**-associated pseudomembranous colitis (AAPMC), is resistant, which explains the prevalence of this disorder as an adverse effect of the drug. Mechanisms of resistance include mutation or modification of the ribosomal receptor site and enzymatic inactivation of **clindamycin**. Resistance to **clindamycin** commonly confers cross-resistance to **macrolides**.

Pharmacokinetics

Absorption and Distribution

Oral administration of **clindamycin** results in complete absorption, and it is not affected by gastric acid. It distributes to pleural and peritoneal fluids, with high concentrations in bile, bone, and urine, but poor penetration of CSF. Plasma protein binding is high. It readily crosses the placenta and is found in breast milk.

Metabolism and Excretion

Clindamycin is metabolized by the liver to active and inactive metabolites. Both the parent drug and its metabolites are excreted in the bile and in urine. Dosage modification is not usually required for renal impairment unless it is very severe, but hepatic impairment may require a decreased dose. Table 22–14 shows the pharmacokinetics of this drug.

Pharmacotherapeutics

Precautions and Contraindications

Use with caution in patients with a history of asthma or significant allergies. Hypersensitivity may occur.

Cautious use is also recommended for the patient with severe renal or hepatic impairment accompanied by severe metabolic aberrations. The routes of excretion include both hepatic and renal.

Clindamycin is Pregnancy Category B. However, it **crosses the placenta in amounts approximating 50 percent of maternal serum levels. It also appears in breast milk. Breastfeeding is probably best discontinued when taking this drug, but the American Academy of Pediatrics considers it to be compatible with breastfeeding.**

Dosages are given for infants and children. It is important to monitor their organ system functions.

Adverse Drug Reactions

The main adverse reactions with this drug are GI, including nausea, vomiting, and a bitter or metallic taste. The most serious is the risk for AAPMC or pseudomembranous colitis. It is important to consider this diagnosis in patients who present with diarrhea subsequent to administration of **clindamycin,** especially if the diarrhea involves six or more stools per day and contains blood, pus, or mucus.

Other adverse effects include dizziness, vertigo, headache, hypotension, and rare cardiac arrhythmias. Jaundice and other indications of hepatic dysfunction and oliguria and other indications of renal dysfunction occasionally occur.

Drug Interactions

There are few drug interactions with **clindamycin.** Table 22–15 lists them.

Clinical Use and Dosing

Because of its anaerobic activity, **clindamycin** is first-line therapy for several serious infections treated parenterally in the hospital. Oral use in primary care settings is restricted to second-line therapy for treatment of infections caused by gram-positive cocci when less toxic agents are contraindicated. Despite the controversy about whether **clindamycin** causes a higher incidence of AAPMC than other **antimicrobials**, research shows that limiting its use decreases prevalence of AAPMC and decreases **clindamycin** resistance (Climo et al., 1998).

INFECTIONS IN PENICILLIN-ALLERGIC PATIENTS. **Clindamycin** is used for bacterial endocarditis prophylaxis as an alternative to **penicillins** in individuals allergic to **penicillin**. It also could be substituted for **penicillin** in treatment of pneumococcal pneumonia and skin and tissue infections, although there are other effective agents that patients with **penicillin** allergies can use.

DRUG-RESISTANT PNEUMOCOCCAL INFECTIONS. Although many strains of *S. pneumoniae* are resistant (DRSP) to **penicillins, cephalosporins, macrolides, tetracyclines**, and **sulfonamides, clindamycin** retains good activity against resistant strains of this organism. **Clindamycin** is recommended for second-line therapy for upper and lower respiratory infections (pneumonia, si-

Table 22–14. Pharmacokinetics: Lincosamides

Drug	Onset	Peak	Duration	Protein Binding	Bioavailability	Half-Life	Elimination
Clindamycin	Rapid	45 min	6–8 h	93%	>90%	2–3 h	>90% hepatic; 10% unchanged in urine; 3.6% in feces

Table 22–15. Drug Interactions: Lincosamides

Drug	Interacting Drug	Possible Effect	Implications
Clindamycin	Erythromycin	Antagonistic effects have occurred for both oral and topical formulations.	Avoid concurrent use.
	Kaolin-pectin	GI absorption is delayed when coadministered.	Give 2 h before or 3–4 h after clindamycin, or avoid concurrent use.
	Neuromuscular blockers	Enhanced neuromuscular blockade that may cause severe respiratory depression.	Avoid concurrent use.

nusitis, otitis media) due to DRSP. Because it does not cover other common pathogens (*H. influenzae* and *M. catarrhalis*), **clindamycin** should be reserved for definitive therapy for DRSP or used in otitis media for nonresponse after at least 72 hours of therapy with a drug that covers *H. influenzae*.

INFECTIONS IN SPECIAL POPULATIONS. **Clindamycin** is indicated for pregnant women and children to treat infections when the first-line agent may be harmful or is not tolerated. For example, **clindamycin** has been used for bacterial vaginosis in pregnancy in doses of 300 mg twice daily for 7 days. Because the first-line agent **metronidazole** is now recognized as safe for use in pregnancy, use of **clindamycin** will probably decline. **Clindamycin** is also used in treatment of malaria and other protozoal infections in pregnant women, children, and those unable to tolerate first-line therapy.

Table 22–16 presents the dosage schedules of **lincosamides**.

Rational Drug Selection

Both definitive drug selection and empiric drug selection follow the same principles described in the Rational Drug Selection section for the **penicillins**, regardless of the infection or drug class involved. Specific implications for selection of **clindamycin** are spectrum of activity and adverse effects. Because **clindamycin** has a narrow spectrum of aerobic activity and lacks activity against *H. influenzae,* it cannot be substituted for other agents typically used to treat URIs, but must used when there is reasonable certainty that the organisms are susceptible to **clindamycin**. On account of the high incidence of pseudomembranous colitis associated with **clindamycin,** patients with a history of colitis and older patients who tolerate colitis poorly should probably not receive this agent. Severe hepatic impairment requires careful monitoring of drug response.

Monitoring

Monitoring for therapeutic response to **antimicrobial drugs** is described in the Monitoring section for **penicillins**. If significant diarrhea occurs (six or more stools daily and/or blood, mucus, or watery diarrhea), the drug should be discontinued. Cytotoxin assay may be used to detect the presence of *C. difficile* and its toxin. If the original infection for which **clindamycin** was prescribed is severe, therapy can continue with observation in the hospital and proctosigmoidoscopy. Mild colitis usually responds to stopping the drug, although fluid, electrolyte, and protein supplements may be required. Systemic **corticosteroids** or **corticosteroid** enemas have sped resolution of mild colitis. Severe AAPMC requires treatment with **metronidazole** or oral **vancomycin,** possibly combined with **cholestyramine** to adsorb the toxins.

Prolonged therapy with **clindamycin** requires assessment of liver function, renal function, and blood counts. Because **clindamycin** contains tartrazine, patients with asthma or **aspirin** allergy are at risk to develop an allergic response and should be assessed for allergic reaction.

Patient Education

ADMINISTRATION. Available dosage forms are given in Table 22–17. The patient should be advised of the necessity of completing the full course of therapy. Because **clindamycin** requires multiple daily doses, the patient should be guided in planning mnemonic strategies to promote adherence. The drug can be taken without regard to meals, but taking the drug with food and a full glass of water will avoid esophageal irritation. Sitting or standing for a full 30 minutes after the dose will also decrease risk of esophageal irritation.

ADVERSE REACTIONS. If severe diarrhea develops, the patient should check with the prescriber before initiating any **antidiarrheal** treatment. **Antiperistaltic agents,** which may worsen the symptoms, should not be used. For mild diarrhea, the patient may use an attapulgite-containing **antidiarrheal** (e.g., **Kaopectate, Donnagel**) at least 2 hours before or 3 to 4 hours after the **clindamycin.** If surgery or general anesthesia is planned during or within a day or so after therapy, the anesthetist or anesthesiologist must be advised, in that **clindamycin** can intensify neuromuscular blockade.

LIFESTYLE MANAGEMENT. See the Lifestyle Management section for the **penicillins**.

Table 22–16. Dosage Schedule: Lincosamides

Drug	Indication	Initial Dose	Comments
Clindamycin (Cleocin)	Serious bacterial infections	*Adults* PO: 150–300 mg q6h *Children* PO: 8–16 mg/kg/d in 3–4 equal doses	Maximal daily adult dose is 2.7 g. Take with food and a full glass of water to decrease esophageal irritation. Sit or stand for 30 min after dose. Dosing for clindamycin palmitate HCl (Cleocin Pediatric) oral solution varies slightly from tablets for children: *Severe infection:* 8–12 mg/kg/d in 3–4 equal doses. *Serious infection:* 13–25 mg/kg/d in 3–4 equal doses. Shake solution well before measuring. Dispense with calibrated measuring device. Do not refrigerate solution because it will become thick and hard to pour.
	Severe bacterial infection	*Adults* PO: 300–450 mg q6h *Children* PO: 16–20 mg/kg/d in 3–4 equal doses	
	Endocarditis prophylaxis (off label)	*Adults* PO: 2 g 1 h before procedure *Children* PO: 20 mg/kg 1 h before procedure	
	Malaria treatment	*Adults* PO: 900 mg tid for 3 d *Children* PO: 6.7–7.3 mg/kg tid for 3 d	
	Bacterial vaginosis in pregnancy (off label)	*Adults* PO: 300 mg bid for 7 d	
	Pneumocystis carinii pneumonia (off label)	*Adults* PO: 1200–1800 mg/d in divided doses with 15–30 mg primaquine daily	
	Toxoplasmosis of CNS treatment (off label)	*Adults* PO: 1200–2400 mg/d in divided doses with 50–100 mg pyrimethamine daily	
	Otitis media	*Children* PO: 20–30 mg/kg/d divided into 4 equal doses	

Macrolides and Azalides

The **macrolides** are another early **antibiotic** group. The prototype drug in this group, **erythromycin**, was discovered in 1952. The drugs in the class (**erythromycin, clarithromycin [Biaxin], dirithromycin [Dynabac],** and **troleandomycin [Tao]**) are compounds characterized by a macrocyclic lactone ring with deoxy sugars attached. A closely related drug, **azithromycin (Zithromax)**, is chemically an **azalide** derived from **erythromycin** by the addition of a methylated nitrogen to the lactone ring. It is generally included with the **macrolide group** and is discussed in the same section here. **Troleandomycin** has little antibacterial activity and is not considered in this chapter.

Pharmacodynamics

This group of drugs reversibly binds to the P site of the 50S ribosome subunit of susceptible organisms and may inhibit RNA-dependent protein synthesis by stimulating the dissociation of peptidyl t-RNA from ribosomes. These drugs may be bacteriostatic or bactericidal, depending on drug concentration.

Macrolides are weak bases, and their activity increases in alkaline media.

Erythromycin is inactivated by acid, and **erythromycin** base is marketed in acid-resistant enteric-coated form to retard gastric inactivation. **Erythromycin** is also formulated as acid-stable salts and esters to improve

Table 22–17. Available Dosage Forms: Lincosamides

Drug	Dosage Form	How Supplied
Clindamycin	Capsules: 75 mg, 150 mg	In bottles of 100 capsules
Cleocin	Capsules: 75 mg, 150 mg, 300 mg Granules for oral suspension: 75 mg/5 cc	In bottles of 16 and 100 capsules In 100-cc bottles
Clinda-Derm	Topical Vaginal	1% lotion, gel solution, and suspension 2% cream

bioavailability. These salts include **erythromycin ethylsuccinate, erythromycin estolate,** and **erythromycin stearate. Dirithromycin** is a prodrug that is converted nonenzymatically during intestinal absorption into a form of **erythromycin. Azithromycin** and **clarithromycin** are semisynthetic derivatives of **erythromycin.**

Sensitivity

Macrolides are active against gram-positive organisms such as pneumococci and other *Streptococcus* species, **methacillin**-sensitive staphylococci, and *Corynebacterium.* Atypical and intracellular organisms commonly resistant to **beta-lactam antibiotics** are also susceptible, such as *Mycoplasma, Legionella, Chlamydia, Helicobacter, Listeria,* and certain strains of *Mycobacterium.* The gram-negative spectrum of the oral **macrolides** includes *Neisseria* species, *Bordetella pertussis, Bartonella quintana,* some *Rickettsia* species, *T. pallidum,* and *Campylobacter* species. *H. influenzae* is somewhat less susceptible.

Among the **macrolides,** there is some variability of spectrum. **Azithromycin** has the greatest activity of the **macrolides** against gram-negative organisms such as *H. influenzae, M. catarrhalis,* and *N. gonorrhoeae.* It is more active than **erythromycin** against anaerobes and has activity similar to **erythromycin** against gram-positive organisms. **Clarithromycin** has broad anaerobic activity and greater activity than **erythromycin** or **azithromycin** against gram-positive organisms such as *Streptococcus* species and **methicillin**-sensitive *Staphylococcus.* Its activity against *H. influenzae* is greater than that of **erythromycin** but less than that of **azithromycin. Dirithromycin** has the narrowest spectrum of the **macrolides.**

Resistance

Resistance to **erythromycin** is usually plasmid-encoded by (1) reduced permeability of the cell membrane or active efflux, (2) production of esterase by Enterobacteriaceae that hydrolyze **macrolides,** or (3) modification of the ribosomal binding site by chromosomal mutation or by a **macrolide**-inducible methylase. Cross-resistance is

nearly complete between **erythromycin** and the other **macrolides.** Cross-resistance may also develop with other **antibiotics** that share the same ribosomal binding site, such as **clindamycin.**

Pharmacokinetics

Absorption and Distribution

All of the **macrolides** are well absorbed from the duodenum following oral administration. Food decreases the amount of absorption of **azithromycin** tablets by 23 percent and the rate of suspension absorption by 56 percent, so these formulations should be taken on an empty stomach. Absorption of enteric-coated products of **erythromycin** is delayed by food. Food also delays the absorption of **clarithromycin,** although bioavailability is not affected, so this drug may be taken without regard to meals. **Dirithromycin** is best absorbed when taken with food or within an hour of having eaten. **Erythromycin base** or **stearate** must be taken on an empty stomach, but the absorption of the **estolate** and **ethylsuccinate** forms are not affected by food intake. Minimal absorption occurs after topical or ophthalmic use.

Macrolides distribute readily to body tissues and enter pleural fluid, ascitic fluid, middle-ear exudates, and sputum. When meninges are inflamed, **macrolides** enter the CSF. Because of high intracellular concentrations, particularly in phagocytic cells, tissue levels are higher than serum levels.

Metabolism and Excretion

Macrolides are partially metabolized by the liver, and **clarithromycin** and **dirithromycin** are converted to active metabolites. This class of drugs is excreted mainly unchanged in bile, with little excreted unchanged drug in urine. **Clarithromycin** and its active metabolite are substantially eliminated by the kidneys, so reduced dosages are required in renal impairment.

Table 22–18 presents the pharmacokinetics.

Table 22–18. Pharmacokinetics: Macrolides and Azalides

Drug	Onset	Peak	Duration	Protein Binding	Bioavailability	Half-Life	Elimination
Azithromycin	Rapid	2.5–3.2 h	24 h	7–50%	40%	11–14 h after single dose; 68 h after multiple doses	6% unchanged in urine; remainder unchanged in bile
Clarithromycin	UA	2 h	12 h	40–70%	55%	3–4 h for 250-mg dose; 5–7 h for 500-mg dose	20–30% unchanged in urine
Dirithromycin	UA	2–4 h	6–8 h	15–30%	10%	2–36 h	81–97% fecal/hepatic
Erythromycin	1 h	1–4 h	UA	7–90%	35–60%	1.4–2 h	5% unchanged in urine; remainder largely in bile

Pharmacotherapeutics

Precautions and Contraindications

Hypersensitivity to any of the **macrolides** and patients' use of **pimozide** contraindicate use of **macrolides**. The removal of **terfenadine** and **cisapride** from the market was related to serious dysrhythmic reactions that frequently were triggered by inhibition of cytochrome P-450 3A4 drug metabolism by **erythromycin** and other drugs.

Known, suspected, or potential bacteremia contraindicates use of **dirithromycin** because serum levels are inadequate to provide antibacterial coverage of the plasma.

RENAL AND HEPATIC IMPAIRMENT. **Azithromycin** is principally excreted via the liver. Patients with impaired hepatic function require cautious use of this drug. There are no data about use with renal impairment, so cautious use is also recommended in decreased renal function.

Clarithromycin is excreted via the liver and the kidney. Dosage adjustments are not required for hepatic impairment in the presence of normal renal function. Renal impairment with CCr less than 30 cc/minute with or without hepatic impairment requires dosages be halved or the dosing interval doubled.

Erythromycin is contraindicated for patients with preexisting liver disease. **Erythromycin estolate** has been associated with the infrequent (one case per 1000 patients) occurrence of cholestatis hepatitis. This has also occurred with other **erythromycin** salts but is rarer in children. Laboratory findings include abnormal liver function tests, peripheral eosinophilia, and leukocytosis. Symptoms include malaise, nausea, vomiting, abdominal cramps and fever. Jaundice may or may not be present. These symptoms tend to occur after 1 to 2 weeks of continuous therapy, disappear if the drug is discontinued, and reappear within 48 hours if the drug is readministered.

Erythromycin may aggravate the weakness of patients with myasthenia gravis. This drug should be avoided in these patients.

OLDER ADULTS. Although maximum plasma concentrations and area under the curve (AUC) of **clarithromycin** and **dirithromycin** increase in older adults, no specific dosage adjustments or precautions are recommended for older adults with normal renal and hepatic function. Younger and older adults appear to have the same pharmacokinetics for **azithromycin**.

Azithromycin and *erythromycin* are Pregnancy Category B and safe to use during pregnancy. *Clarithromycin* and *dirithromycin* are Pregnancy Category C. Animal studies with *clarithromycin* have shown adverse effects on pregnancy outcome and on fetal development. Animal studies with *dirithromycin* have shown significantly decreased fetal weight and incomplete ossification of fetal bone. These latter two drugs should not be used during pregnancy except in clinical circumstances where no alternative therapy is appropriate.

The American Academy of Pediatrics considers **erythromycin** compatible with breastfeeding. Data are not available for the other drugs in this class, and they should be used with extreme caution in nursing mothers.

Safety and efficacy of **azithromycin** by the oral route have been established for children as young as age 6 months for otitis media and CAP. It has been established for children over age 2 years for pharyngitis-tonsillitis. **Clarithromycin** also has established safety and efficacy for children over age 6 months. The safety and efficacy of **dirithromycin** have not been established for children under age 12 years.

Adverse Drug Reactions

The most common adverse reactions to **macrolides** are dose-related GI symptoms, including nausea, vomiting, abdominal pain, cramping, and diarrhea, as well as headache. In general, these reactions are transient, mild to moderate in nature, and reversible when the drug is discontinued. **Erythromycin** is most likely to produce them, whether given orally or parenterally, because it stimulates the motilin receptor in the GI tract. In fact, an off-label use of **erythromycin** for the treatment of gastroparesis derives from this receptor activity. Diarrhea may also be secondary to pseudomembranous colitis, a serious superinfection that requires discontinuation of the drug that has been described for **penicillins**, **cephalosporins**, and **lincosamides**.

Hyperkinesia, dizziness, and agitation have occurred in fewer than 1 percent of children taking **azithromycin**. Stomatitis, dry mouth, and dysphagia have occurred in a small number of adults for all **macrolides**.

Erythromycin has been associated with urticaria, bullous eruptions, eczema, and Stevens-Johnson syndrome. Isolated cases of reversible hearing loss have also been reported with this drug, particularly with parenteral administration.

Laboratory abnormalities include elevated liver function studies (**azithromycin**), increased platelet counts (**dirithromycin** and **erythromycin**) and elevated potassium levels (**dirithromycin**). In each case, fewer than 6 percent of patients were affected.

Drug Interactions

Clarithromycin and **erythromycin** have more drug interactions than the other two drugs in this class because they are strong inhibitors of the cytochrome P-450 enzymes, particularly CYP 3A4. Object drugs in these interactions include such common drugs as **warfarin**, **theophylline**, **carbamazepine**, selected **benzodiazepines**, and **digoxin**. Combination of either of these **macrolides** with **pimozide** can result in serious dysrhythmia; the inhibited metabolism causes prolonged QTc interval of the cardiac cycle, predisposing to potentially fatal cardiac dysrhythmias. Similar interactions occurred with **cisapride (Propulsid)**, **terfenadine (Seldane)**, and **astemizole (Hismanal)**, which were withdrawn from the market on account of these interactions. Table 22–19 lists the various drug interactions by specific drug. Although **azithromycin** has fewer drug interactions than other **macrolides**, confirmed interactions with drugs with narrow therapeutic margins include **digoxin, cyclosporine,** and **pimozide,** which have enhanced effects when given concurrently. In addition, **antacids** containing aluminum or magnesium slow absorption of **macrolides** and **azalides,** so they should be taken 1 hour before or 2 hours after the **antimicrobial** drug, particularly with **azithromycin**.

Clinical Use and Dosing

Macrolides are drugs of choice only for primarily empiric treatment of CAP and chlamydial infections. They are first- or second-line agents for numerous infections. Relative safety in children and convenient dosing schedules have made the newer **macrolides, azithromycin** and **clarithromycin,** popular in primary care practice. In particular, **azithromycin** has a 5-day dosing schedule, with a loading dose on the first day and single daily doses for the subsequent 4 days. **Clarithromycin** usually requires twice-daily dosing but is now available in a delayed-release formulation that can be administered once daily. Although bioavailability varies by **erythromycin** salt, the dosage of base, stearate, and estolate salts are the same for an indication. The dosage of **erythromycin ethylsuccinate** is higher because of the mass of the ethylsuccinate component. The equivalent of 250 mg base is 400 mg ethylsuccinate. Specific dosages are included in the tables.

COMMUNITY-ACQUIRED PNEUMONIA. Pathogens in CAP that are naturally resistant to **beta-lactam antibiotics** are the atypical organisms *C. pneumoniae, M. pneumoniae,* and *Legionella pneumophila.* Other common pathogens in CAP are *S. pneumoniae, H. influenzae,* and *M. catarrhalis. S. aureus* is occasionally the pathogen in postbronchitic pneumonia. Because they have activity against all these organisms, the newer **macrolides** are drugs of choice for empiric treatment of CAP in adults and children over 5 years old. Usual dosages are **azithromycin** 500 mg once on day 1, followed by 250 mg daily on days 2 to 5, or **clarithromycin** 500 mg twice daily for 7 to 14 days. Outpatient treatment of infants and children for CAP is **erythromycin** 10 mg/kg orally four times daily or **clarithromycin** 7.5 mg/kg twice daily. It is desirable to obtain sputum for culture and Gram's stain so that the treatment may be more directed, but it is impossible to identify a pathogen in up to 50 percent of patients with CAP. Consequently, treatment often proceeds empirically. **Macrolides** have high cross-resistance (60%) for highly **penicillin**-resistant *S. pneumoniae* strains. If the patient's condition deteriorates or is not improving by 48 to 72 hours, a switch to a **fluoroquinolone** with extended gram-positive spectrum (e.g., **levofloxacin**) is indicated. The American Thoracic Society recommends **amoxicillin-clavulanate** or a **second-generation cephalosporin** for CAP patients older than 60 with no comorbidities, in that the pneumococcus is the most common pathogen in this population (Gleason, Kapoor, & Stone, 1997).

SEXUALLY TRANSMITTED DISEASES. Nongonococcal and postgonococcal urethritis or cervicitis is most commonly caused by *C. trachomatis* (50%) or *Mycoplasma hominis.* Other etiologies such as *Ureaplasma, Trichomonas, Mycoplasma genitalium,* and viruses account for 10 to 15 percent of cases. **Azithromycin** 1 g as a single oral dose is a

Table 22–19. Drug Interactions: Macrolides and Azalides

Drug	Interacting Drug	Possible Effect	Implications
All macrolides	Pimozide	Two sudden deaths occurred when clarithromycin was added to ongoing pimozide therapy.	Coadministration is contraindicated.
Azithromycin, dirithromycin, erythromycin	Antacids	Aluminum- and magnesium-based antacids reduce peak serum levels but not extent of absorption of azithromycin; when given immediately following antacids, dirithromycin absorption is slightly enhanced; when given immediately prior to antacids, elimination rate of erythromycin may be slightly decreased.	Consider outcomes in patient education.
Azithromycin, clarithromycin, erythromycin	HMG-CoA reductase inhibitors	Increased risk of severe myopathy or rhabdomyolysis.	Avoid concurrent use.
	Cyclosporine	Elevated cyclosporine concentration with increased risk for toxicity.	Dirithromycin is not expected to react.
	Digoxin	Digoxin levels may be elevated based on effect of macrolide on gut flora that metabolizes digoxin in 10% of patients.	Carefully monitor digoxin levels in any patient taking a macrolide.
Clarithromycin, erythromycin	Rifabutin, rifampin	Antibiotic effects of macrolide reduced; adverse GI effects increased.	Select different macrolide.
	Alprazolam, diazepam, midazolam, triazolam	Plasma levels of benzodiazepine elevated, increasing and prolonging CNS depression effects	Azithromycin and dirithromycin not expected to react
	Buspirone	Plasma levels of buspirone elevated, increasing pharmacological and adverse effects.	Azithromycin and dirithromycin not expected to react.
	Carbamazepine	Increased concentration of carbamazepine.	Azithromycin and dirithromycin not expected to react.
	Cisapride	Serious cardiac arrhythmias, including ventricular tachycardia, ventricular fibrillation, torsades de pointes, and QT interval prolongation.	Coadministration contraindicated. Azithromycin and dirithromycin not expected to react.
	Disopyramide	Plasma levels of disopyramide increased. Arrhythmias and prolonged QTc have occurred.	Avoid concurrent administration.
	Ergot alkaloids	Acute ergot toxicity, characterized by severe peripheral vasospasm and dysesthesia, has occurred.	Carefully monitor any patient receiving both drugs.
	Oral anticoagulants	Potentiates anticoagulant effects.	Carefully monitor anticoagulant effects for patients receiving any macrolide.

Continued on next page

Table 22–19. Drug Interactions: Macrolides and Azalides (*continued*)

Drug	Interacting Drug	Possible Effect	Implications
	Theophylline	Concurrent use associated with increased serum theophylline levels.	Avoid concurrent use. Azithromycin and dirithromycin not expected to interact.
Clarithromycin	Fluconazole	Increased mean steady-state trough levels (33%) and AUC (18%) of clarithromycin.	Avoid concurrent use.
	Omeprazole	Increased plasma levels of both drugs and 14-OH clarithromycin.	Select different drug combination.
Dirithromycin	Histamine$_2$ blockers	Dirithromycin absorption slightly enhanced when given immediately after H$_2$ blocker.	Separate doses by at least 1 h or select different macrolide.
Erythromycin	Alfentanil	Alfentanil clearance decreased and elimination half-life increased.	Select different macrolide.
	Bromocriptine	Bromocriptine levels increased; increased pharmacological and adverse effects.	Select different macrolide.
	Felodipine	Felodipine levels increased; increased pharmacological and adverse effects.	Select different macrolide.
	Grepafloxacin, sparfloxacin	Risk for life-threatening cardiac arrhythmias, including torsades de pointes.	Absolute contraindication for sparfloxacin; relative contraindications for grepafloxacin (requires cardiac monitoring and hospitalization).
	Clindamycin, penicillins	Antagonistic effects. Synergism also reported for penicillins.	Select different macrolide.
	Methylprednisolone	Clearance of methylprednisolone greatly reduced.	May be used therapeutically to reduce methylprednisolone dose.

drug of choice for nongonococcal urethritis and cervicitis. If the condition is recurrent or persistent, therapy includes **metronidazole** 2 g as a single oral dose to cover *Trichomonas*, plus either **erythromycin base** 500 mg four times daily for 7 days or **erythromycin ethylsuccinate** 800 mg four times daily for 7 days. **Azithromycin** is also first-line treatment of chancroid as a single oral dose of 1 g. An alternative is **erythromycin base** 500 mg orally four times daily for 7 days. **Azithromycin** is commonly prescribed as part of the treatment of gonococcal urethritis and cervicitis as a 1-g oral dose to cover the chlamydial infections that often coexist with gonorrhea. Although **azithromycin** is active against *N. gonorrhoeae,* 2 g is required to eradicate gonococcal urethritis or cervicitis. This higher dose is more expensive than other treatments and causes a high incidence of GI adverse effects.

Azithromycin is indicated in the treatment of pelvic inflammatory disease due to *C. trachomatis, M. hominis,* or *N. gonorrhoeae.* **Erythromycin** is approved for syphilis caused by *T. pallidum* in **penicillin**-allergic patients but is less effective than other recommended therapies. **Erythromycin** in pregnancy failed to prevent congenital syphilis.

MYCOBACTERIUM AVIUM COMPLEX. Infections with the nontuberculous mycobacterial organism *Mycobacterium avium* complex (MAC) occur in up to 40 percent of patients with AIDS. Advanced immunosuppression is the major risk factor for MAC. Patients with AIDS are thought to acquire this organism usually resident in water and soil by respiratory or GI routes. The syndrome presents with high fever, diarrhea, night sweats, weight loss, anemia, and neutropenia. Diagnosis is usually based on blood culture, although it is sometimes identified on biopsy of the liver, bone marrow, or lymph nodes. MAC prophylaxis is now strongly recommended for HIV-infected adults with a mean CD4 lymphocyte count of fewer than 50 cells/µL. The first-line drugs are either **azithromycin** or **clarithromycin** at dosages listed in Table 22–20. Before prophylaxis is initiated, patients should be evaluated to assure they do not have active MAC or *Mycobacterium tuberculosis*. National guidelines indicated that treatment of MAC should include at least two **antimicrobials**, one of which should be either **clarithromycin** or **azithromycin** (Fletcher, Kakuda, & Collier, 1999). Of these, **clarithromycin**, 500 mg twice daily, has the greatest evidence for efficacy. **Ethambutol** is commonly the second drug, and many expert clinicians add **rifabutin** as a third agent.

PEPTIC ULCER DISEASE. Most patients with peptic ulcer who are not taking NSAIDs, as well as many who are taking NSAIDs, have evidence of *H. pylori*. Although 15 percent of people with *H. pylori* actually develop clinical manifestations of peptic ulcer disease, eradication of *H. pylori* in the individual with peptic ulcer disease markedly decreases ulcer recurrence. Eradication is recommended for all peptic ulcer disease patients with an active ulcer, a history of ulcer complications, or a need for maintenance therapy (Berardi, 1999). **Clarithromycin** is included in many of the multiantimicrobial regimens proven effective for *H. pylori* eradication. Approved combinations include:

1. Twice-daily therapy with **omeprazole** 20 mg, **amoxicillin** 1 g, and **clarithromycin** 500 mg for 14 days
2. **Clarithromycin** 500 mg three times daily with **omeprazole** 40 mg daily for 14 days, followed by **omeprazole** 20 mg daily for 14 days
3. **Clarithromycin** 500 mg three times daily with **ranitidine bismuth citrate (Tritec)** 400 mg twice daily for 14 days, followed by **ranitidine bismuth citrate** 400 mg twice daily for 14 more days

Other combinations with shorter durations (7 to 10 days) have also proved effective. Results of studies on *H. pylori* eradication for patients with dyspepsia or prior to initiating NSAID therapy have been conflicting (Hawkey, Tlassay, & Szczepanski, 1998; Talley, Vakil, Ballard & Fennerty, 1999), so most experts do not recommend *H. pylori* eradication for these indications.

ENDOCARDITIS PROPHYLAXIS. Although the effectiveness of endocarditis prophylaxis has not been established in controlled trials, **antimicrobial** prophylaxis prior to invasive procedures that may cause transient bacteremia allegedly prevents endocarditis in patients with acquired valvular heart disease (such as rheumatic heart disease), previous endocarditis, bioprosthetic and homograft prosthetic heart valves, and complex cyanotic congenital heart anomalies. Recent studies indicate that some cardiac conditions and procedures previously treated derive no benefit from endocarditis prophylaxis, so it is anticipated that the American Heart Association will narrow indications for prophylaxis for dental, respiratory, and genitourinary procedures over the next few years (Gilbert, Moellering, & Sande, 1999). For patients who can take oral medications but are allergic to **penicillins,** a single dose of 500 mg of **azithromycin** or **clarithromycin** for adults or 15 mg/kg for children is indicated for endocarditis prophylaxis 1 hour before the procedure (Prevention of Bacterial Endocarditis, 1997). Although **erythromycin** is approved for endocarditis prophylaxis, the broader spectrum and lower rate of gastrointestinal adverse effects of the newer **macrolides** make them the preferred agents.

EXACERBATIONS OF CHRONIC BRONCHITIS. Although **antibiotic** treatment of ABECB is controversial, the newer **macrolides, azithromycin** and **clarithromycin,** are active against the most common pathogens, *S. pneumoniae, H. influenzae,* and *M. catarrhalis,* and are used empirically to treat this condition. Although **erythromycin** is approved for treatment of ABECB, its narrower spectrum of activity, especially against *H. influenzae,* makes it less desirable, in spite of lower cost.

UPPER RESPIRATORY INFECTIONS. Controlled trials have not demonstrated consistent benefit of **macrolides** or other **antimicrobial drugs** in acute bronchitis (Hueston & Mainous, 1998). However, bronchitis due to *B. pertussis* responds to **erythromycin. Macrolides** are active against *S. pneumoniae, H. influenzae,* and *M. catarrhalis,* the most common bacterial pathogens in AOM and acute sinusitis. However, **erythromycin** is not currently recommended as monotherapy for AOM and acute sinusitis, on account of inadequate coverage of *H. influenzae.* The combination of **erythromycin** and **sulfisoxazole (Pediazole)** is effective for most common URIs. Although both **clarithromycin** and **azithromycin** have adequate coverage for *H. influenzae,* **azithromycin** is the most active. An increasing resistance of *S. pneumoniae* to both of these popular agents has been noted (Bishai & Chaisson, 1999). Recent studies show bacteriologic failure rates in otitis media above 50 percent for **azithromycin** and above 40 percent for **clarithromycin,** compared with 18 to 25 percent for **amoxicillin** (Dagan et al., 2000). **Azithromycin** and **clarithromycin** are no longer considered first-line agents for AOM (Tiggs, 2000). The **macrolides** are also used for treatment of GABHS pharyngitis in **penicillin**-allergic patients. Dosages for URIs are shown in Table 22–20.

Table 22–20. Dosage Schedule: Macrolides and Azalides

Drug	Indication	Dose	Comments
Azithromycin (Zithromax)	Community-acquired pneumonia, otitis media, uncomplicated skin and soft tissue infection, acute bacterial exacerbation of chronic bronchitis	*Adult* 500 mg as single dose on day 1, followed by 250 mg daily on days 2–5 *Child* 10 mg/kg as a single dose on day 1 (not to exceed 500 mg/d), followed by 5 mg/kg as a single dose on days 2–5	Take capsules and pediatric suspension on empty stomach. Tablets and adult single-dose packets may be taken without regard to meals. Store pediatric oral suspension at room temperature after reconstitution. Stable for 10 d. Discard excess after dosing is complete. Shake suspension before measurement, using calibrated dosing device. Pediatric dosing limits: 500 mg daily for pharyngitis, tonsillitis, and first day of dosing for otitis media and pneumonia; 250 mg daily for days 2–5 for otitis media and pneumonia. Do not use adult single-dose packet formulation for doses >1000 mg.
	Pharyngitis/tonsillitis	*Adult* Same as community-acquired pneumonia *Child* 12 mg/kg daily for 5 d (not to exceed 500 mg daily)	As above.
	Chancroid, genital ulcer disease, nongonococcal urethritis caused by *Chlamydia trachomatis*	*Adult* Single 1-g dose	As above.
	Gonococcal urethritis or cervicitis	*Adult* Single 2-g dose	As above.
	Mycobacterium avium complex (MAC)	*Adult* 1.2 g/wk	As above.
Clarithromycin (Biaxin)	Pharyngitis, tonsillitis, otitis media, or skin and soft tissue infection	*Adult* 250 mg bid for 10 d *Child* 15 mg/kg/d divided into 2 doses administered q12h for 10 d	May be given without regard to food. If CCr <30 mL/min, dose should be halved or dosing interval doubled. Store suspension at room temperature after reconstitution. Stable for 14 d. Do not refrigerate. Shake suspension well before measurement with calibrated measuring device.
	Acute maxillary sinusitis	*Adult* 500 mg bid for 14 d *Child* Same as above for 10–14 d	As above.
	Acute exacerbation of chronic bronchitis caused by *S. pneumoniae* or *M. catarrhalis*	*Adult* 250 mg bid for 7–14 d	As above.
	Acute exacerbation of chronic bronchitis caused by *H. influenzae*	*Adult* 500 mg bid for 7–14 d	As above.

Continued on next page

Table 22–20. Dosage Schedule: Macrolides and Azalides *(continued)*

Drug	Indication	Dose	Comments
	M. avium complex (MAC) treatment	*Adult* 500 mg twice daily *Child* 7.5 mg/kg up to 500 mg bid; give in conjunction with other antimycobacterial drugs	As above.
	MAC prophylaxis	*Adult* 500 mg bid	As above.
	Community-acquired pneumonia	*Adult* 250 mg q12h for 7–14 d	As above.
	Active duodenal ulcer associated with *H. pylori* infection in combination with bismuth citrate	*Adult* 500 mg tid with ranitidine bismuth citrate 400 mg bid for days 1–14; followed by bismuth citrate 400 mg/d days 15–28	As above.
	Active duodenal ulcer associated with *H. pylori* infection in combination with omeprazole	*Adult* 500 mg tid with omeprazole 40 mg bid for 14 d; followed by omeprazole alone 20 mg/d for 14 d	As above.
	Active duodenal ulcer associated with *H. pylori* infection, in combination with amoxicillin and lansoprazole	*Adult* 500 mg clarithromycin, 1000 mg amoxicillin, and 30 mg lansoprazole q12h for 14 d	As above.
Erythromycin dose in mg erythromycin base Estolate (Ilosone) Ethylsuccinate (EryPed, E.E.S.) Base (E-Mycin, E-Base, Ery-Tab, Eryc) Stearate (Eramycin)	Antibacterial, mild infection, usual dose	*Adult* 250 mg base (400 mg ethylsuccinate) q6h; *or* 500 mg (800 mg ethylsuccinate) q12h; or 333 mg q8h *Child* 30–50 mg/kg/d of base in divided doses (or 50–80 mg/kg/d ethylsuccinate)	Maximum adult daily dose is 4 g. Take with 180–240 mL of water. Taking with food may decrease effectiveness of erythromycin stearate and certain formulations of erythromycin base. Check package insert for erythromycin base. Take erythromycin stearate and most erythromycin base at least 2 h before or after a meal. Erythromycin estolate, erythromycin ethylsuccinate, and some enteric-coated formulations of base can be taken without regard to meals. Should be taken with meals if GI upset occurs. Do not chew or crush erythromycin base. Suspensions should be shaken before measurement, using a calibrated dispensing spoon.
	Erysipelas or nonbullous impetigo due to *S. pyogenes*	*Adult* 250–500 mg qid for 10 d *Child* 20–50 mg/kg/d in divided doses for 10 d	As above.
	Bullous impetigo or cellulitis due to *S. aureus*	*Adult* 250 mg q6h or 500 mg q12h to maximum of 4 g/d	As above.

Continued on next page

Table 22–20. Dosage Schedule: Macrolides and Azalides *(continued)*

Drug	Indication	Dose	Comments
	Community-acquired pneumonia, mild to moderate	*Child* 20–50 mg/kg/d in divided doses *Adult* 250–500 mg q6h for 10–14 d; treat severe mycoplasma pneumonia with higher dose up to 21 d	As above.
	Upper respiratory tract infection, mild to moderate due to *S. pyogenes* or *S. pneumoniae*	*Child* 20–50 mg/kg/d in divided doses for 10–14 d *Adult* 250–500 mg qid for 10 d *Child* 20–50 mg/kg/d in divided doses for 10 d	As above.
	Pertussis (whooping cough) due to *B. pertussis*	*Adult* 500 mg qid for 10 d *Child* 40–50 mg/kg/d in divided doses for 10 d	As above.
	Newborn conjunctivitis, pneumonia of infancy due to *C. trachomatis*	*Child* 50 mg/kg/d in 4 divided doses for 14 d (conjunctivitis) or 21 d (pneumonia)	As above.
	Urethral, endocervical, or rectal infections due to *C. trachomatis*	*Adult* 500 mg qid for 7 d or 250 mg qid for 14 d (in pregnancy)	As above.
	Nongonococcal urethritis; urethral, endocervical, or rectal infections due to *N. gonorrhoeae*	*Adult* 500 mg qid for at least 7 d	As above.
	Primary syphilis	*Adult* 20 g in divided doses over 10 d or 500 mg qid for 14 d	As above.
	Endocarditis prophylaxis	*Adult* 1 g 2 h before procedure, 500 mg 6 h after procedure *Child* 20 mg/kg 2 h before procedure, 10 mg/kg 6 h after procedure	As above.
Dirithromycin (Dynabac)	Acute bacterial exacerbations of chronic bronchitis; uncomplicated skin and soft tissue infection due to methicillin-sensitive *S. aureus*	*Adult* 500 mg/d for 7 d	Take with food or within 1 h of eating. Do not crush or chew tablets.
	Community-acquired pneumonia caused by *M. catarrhalis* or *S. pneumoniae* (not for empiric therapy)	*Adult* 500 mg/d for 14 d	As above.
	Pharyngitis/tonsillitis caused by *S. pyogenes*	*Adult* 500 mg/d for 10 d	
Erythromycin ethylsuccinate and sulfisoxazole (Pediazole, Eryzole)	Acute otitis media	*Child* 50 mg/kg/d erythromycin and 150 mg/kg/d (to a maximum of 6 g/d) sulfisoxazole in 4 evenly divided doses for 10 d	May be taken without regard to meals. Not for use in infants under age 2 mo.

SKIN OR SOFT TISSUE INFECTIONS. **Macrolides** are indicated for minor infections of skin and soft tissues caused by *S. aureus* or *Streptococcus* species, including impetigo, erysipelas, cellulitis, and wounds of the extremities. Oral and topical **erythromycin** has been used in the treatment of acne. **Macrolides** are primarily indicated for skin and soft tissue infections in **penicillin**-allergic patients, using dosages listed in Table 22–20.

OTHER USES. An accepted off-label use for **erythromycin** is Lyme disease in individuals who are allergic to **penicillin** and in children under 9 years old. However, **erythromycin** may be less effective than **amoxicillin** or **doxycycline**, possibly because of erratic absorption. Other accepted off-label uses for **erythromycin** include treatment of actinomycoses, anthrax, lymphogranuloma venereum, and relapsing fever caused by *Borrelia* species. **Erythromycin** and **azithromycin** are considered drugs of first choice for *C. jejuni*. **Erythromycin** is indicated in the treatment of listeriosis caused by *L. monocytogenes* and in diphtheria prophylaxis and treatment. It has been used in conjunction with oral-local **neomycin** for preoperative preparation of the bowel. **Erythromycin** is indicated in chlamydial conjunctivitis in newborns and chlamydial pneumonia in infants caused by *C. trachomatis*. This agent is also approved for treatment of erythrasma caused by *Corynebacterium minutissimum*. **Erythromycin** is an agonist at the motilin receptor and has been effective in the treatment of gastroparesis.

Rational Drug Selection

Both definitive drug selection and empiric drug selection follow the same principles described in the Rational Drug Selection section for the **penicillins**, regardless of the infection or drug class involved. **Macrolides** are often selected for susceptible organisms as alternatives in **penicillin**-allergic patients. **Azithromycin** and **clarithromycin** have a slightly broader spectrum than **erythromycin** and additional indications, such as MAC. Because of its long history, **erythromycin** has accumulated indications for which the newer agents have not been tested. Increasing resistance of *H. influenzae, Staphylococcus,* and *S. pneumoniae* may increasingly limit the utility of **macrolides** for common bacterial infections. In addition to spectrum of action, the indications for selection of a specific **macrolide** are cost, convenience, and adverse effect profile. **Erythromycin** salts are substantially less expensive than **azithromycin** and **clarithromycin** but have more GI adverse effects. The good bioavailability and milder GI effects of the **erythromycin estolate** salt is offset by the risk of cholestatic jaundice in adults. This agent should not be prescribed for individuals with liver impairment. Patients with history of cardiac arrhythmia or QT prolongation should avoid **erythromycin** or be carefully monitored. **Azithromycin** may be selected over **erythromycin** or **clarithromycin** if the patient is taking interacting drugs whose hepatic metabolism is subject to inhibition. **Erythromycin** is generally preferred over the newer agents during pregnancy and for very young infants because of greater accumulated clinical experience. A major reason for selection of **azithromycin** over other **macrolides** is the enhanced compliance caused by its convenient dosing schedule. However, with its once per day dosing and short duration of 5 days, a single missed dose could jeopardize the successful outcome. There are no indications for **dirithromycin** or **troleandomycin** over other **macrolides**.

Monitoring

Monitoring for therapeutic response to **antimicrobial drugs** is described in the Monitoring section for **penicillins**. Because **erythromycin** and **clarithromycin** inhibit the metabolism of many drugs, observation for altered response to concurrent medications metabolized by cytochrome P-450 3A4 is essential, beginning with the first dose and continuing for several half-lives of the **macrolide** after it is discontinued. Patients taking drugs with narrow therapeutic margins require extra scrutiny if they are taking any **macrolides**, including **azithromycin**. Individuals with a history of hearing loss may be at increased risk for further hearing loss, especially if they have hepatic or renal impairment and are taking high doses (more than 4 g/d) of **erythromycin**. These risk factors may indicate audiometric testing at baseline and whenever there is clinical evidence of hearing loss (e.g., dizziness, fullness in the ears). The hearing loss is usually reversible; it occurs from 36 hours to 8 days after treatment is initiated and begins to recover 1 to 14 days after the drug is discontinued. ECG monitoring of QT interval is particularly recommended for high-dose parenteral therapy. If the patient develops malaise, nausea, vomiting, skin rash, abdominal pain, or jaundice within 1 to 2 weeks after therapy is initiated, the drug should be discontinued and liver function tests initiated to assess for cholestatic jaundice.

Patient Education

ADMINISTRATION. Doses of **macrolides** should be evenly spaced for the best effect. The available dosage forms are shown in Table 22–21. Suspensions must be shaken thoroughly before administration, and excess medication should be discarded after the prescribed therapy is administered and never used by another individual or by the same patient for a different episode. Because it is irritating to the GI mucosa, **erythromycin** should be taken with a full 8-oz glass of water by adults and with at least 4 to 6 oz by children. Food interactions are complex for the

macrolides. **Azithromycin** tablets, the adult single-dose **azithromycin** packet, **clarithromycin**, and **erythromycin estolate** can be taken without regard to meals. **Erythromycin stearate**, most brands of **erythromycin base**, **erythromycin ethylsuccinate**, **azithromycin** capsules, and **azithromycin** suspension must be taken on an empty stomach, 1 hour before or 2 hours after eating. **Dirithromycin** should be taken with food or within an hour of a meal. **Erythromycin ethylsuccinate** has improved bioavailability if taken with food. Because the requirements for administration with respect to food may vary by brand, the package insert is the best guide for **erythromycin base**. Tablets of **erythromycin base**, **erythromycin stearate**, and **dirithromycin** should not be chewed or crushed. If chewable tablets of **erythromycin ethylsuccinate** are prescribed, the necessity for chewing the dosage form should be stressed. If pediatric drops of **erythromycin estolate** (100 mg/mL) or **erythromycin ethylsuccinate** are prescribed, the prescription should specify dispensing a calibrated dropper, and the parent should be instructed on proper measurement and oral administration technique; parents have occasionally assumed drops were meant to be administered in the ear. The adult single-dose **azithromycin** packet should be thoroughly mixed with 2 oz (60 mL) of water and consumed immediately. An additional 2 oz of water should be added to the container, mixed, and ingested to ensure consumption of the entire dose. This form should not be used for doses greater than 1000 mg.

ADVERSE REACTIONS. Taking **erythromycin** with a full glass of water decreases the GI symptoms that are the most common adverse effects. Because patients often discontinue the medication if adverse effects are intolerable, they should be urged to call the prescriber if GI distress becomes severe so that an alternative drug can be prescribed. Patients who experience signs of liver impairment (malaise, nausea, vomiting, abdominal cramps, skin rash, fever, with or without jaundice) should discontinue the **macrolide** and call the prescriber immediately. Syncope may indicate torsades de pointes related to cardiac QT interval prolongation and should also be reported. Other patient education includes information about symptoms of superinfection that is part of the education for all **antibacterial drugs**.

LIFESTYLE MANAGEMENT. See the Lifestyle Management section for the **penicillins**.

Sulfonamides, Trimethoprim, and Nitrofurantoin

The **sulfonamides** were once major **antibacterials**, but the development of resistant strains of bacteria and the incidence of allergic reactions to sulfa drugs resulted in their largely being relegated to treatment of UTIs, otitis media, and some sexually transmitted diseases. **Sulfasalazine (Azulfidine)** is used in the treatment of ulcerative colitis and rheumatoid arthritis for its anti-inflammatory properties rather than for treatment of infection. **Mafenide (Sulfamylon)** and **silver sulfadiazine (Silvadene)** are used to prevent infection in patients with burns. Topical applications such as those for burns are not discussed in this chapter. Included in this section are drugs commonly used in combination with **sulfonamides**, such as **trimethoprim (Proloprim, Trimpex)**, and agents used to treat UTIs, such as **nitrofurantoin (Furadantin, Macrodantin)**. The combination formulation **trimethoprim-sulfamethoxazole (Bactrim, Septra, TMP-SMZ)** is also considered in this section.

Pharmacodynamics

Sulfonamides

Sulfonamides exert their bacteriostatic action by competitive antagonism of para-aminobenzoic acid (PABA), required by susceptible organisms for an essential step in the production of purines and the synthesis of nucleic acids, thereby blocking folic acid synthesis. Microorganisms that use exogenous folic acid and do not synthesize folic acid are not susceptible to **sulfonamides.**

SENSITIVITY. **Sulfonamides** inhibit both gram-positive and gram-negative bacteria. Susceptible organisms include *E. coli, S. pyogenes, S. pneumoniae, H. influenzae, Actinomyces, Nocardia, C. trachomatis, N. gonorrhoeae,* and some protozoa (*Pneumocystis carinii* and toxoplasmosis).

RESISTANCE. The increasing frequency of resistant organisms limits the use of these drugs in chronic and recurrent UTI. Mutations that result in excessive production of PABA cause organisms to develop resistance. Dihydropteroate synthetase with a low **sulfonamide** affinity may be encoded on a plasmid that is transmissible and can be disseminated rapidly and widely. Cross-resistance between **sulfonamides** is common. Initiating therapy promptly with adequate doses for sufficient time can minimize resistance.

Trimethoprim

Trimethoprim inhibits bacterial dihydrofolic acid reductase. Dihydrofolic acid reductases convert dihydrofolic acid to tetrahydrofolic acid, a stage leading to the synthesis of purine and ultimately to DNA. Given with **sulfonamide**, it produces a sequential blocking in this metabolic sequence, resulting in synergistic activity of both drugs. This combination is often bactericidal. The widely used

Table 22–21. Available Dosage Forms: Macrolides and Azalides

Drug	Dosage Form	How Supplied
Azithromycin (Zithromax)	Tablets: 250 mg 600 mg Powder for oral suspension: 100 mg/5 cc 200 mg/5 cc	In bottles of 30 tablets and Z-pak with 6 tablets In bottles of 30 tablets In 300-mg bottles, cherry, crème de vanilla, and banana flavors In 600-, 900-, and 1200-mg bottles, same flavors
Clarithromycin (Biaxin)	Tablets: 250 mg, 500 mg Granules for oral suspension: reconstituted 125 mg/5 cc, 250 mg/ 5 cc	In bottles of 60 film-coated tablets In 50- and 100-cc bottles, fruit punch flavor
Dirithromycin (Dynabac)	Tablets: 250 mg	In bottles of 60 enteric-coated tablets
Erythromycin base	Tablets: 250 mg 500 mg Capsules: 250 mg	In bottles of 100 and 500 film-coated tablets In bottles of 100 film-coated tablets In bottles of 60, 100, and 500 delayed-release capsules
(E-Base)	Tablets: 333 mg 500 mg	In bottles of 100, 500, and 1000 delayed-release, enteric-coated tablets In bottles of 100 and 500 enteric-coated tablets
(Eryc)	Capsules: 250 mg	In bottles of 100 delayed-release capsules
(E-Mycin)	Tablets: 250 mg 333 mg	In bottles of 40, 100, and 500 enteric-coated tablets In bottles of 100 and 500 enteric-coated tablets
(Ery-Tab)	Tablets: 250 mg, 333 mg	In bottles of 100 and 500 delayed-release, enteric-coated tablets
(PCE Dispertab)	Tablets: 333 mg 500 mg	In bottles of 60 tablets with polymer-coated particles In bottles of 100 tablets with polymer-coated particles
Erythromycin estolate	Capsules: 250 mg Suspension: 125 mg/5 cc, 250 mg/5 cc	In bottles of 100 capsules In 480-cc bottles
(Ilosone)	Tablets: 500 mg Capsules: 250 mg Suspension: 125 mg/5 cc 250 mg/5 cc	In bottles of 50 tablets In bottles of 100 capsules In 480-cc bottles, orange flavor In 100- and 480-cc bottles, cherry flavor
Erythromycin stearate	Tablets: 250 mg 500 mg	In bottles of 100, 500, and 1000 film-coated tablets In bottles of 100 and 500 film-coated tablets
(Erythrocin stearate)	Tablets: 250 mg, 500 mg	In bottles of 100, 500, and 1000 film-coated tablets
Erythromycin ethylsuccinate	Tablets: 400 mg Suspension: 200 mg/5 cc, 400 mg/5 cc	In bottles of 100 and 500 tablets In 480-cc bottles
(EryPed)	Tablets: 200 mg Suspension: 200 mg 400 mg Drops/suspension: 100 mg/2.5 cc	In bottles of 40 chewable tablets, fruit flavor In 100- and 200-cc bottles, fruit flavor In 60-, 100-, and 200-cc bottles, banana flavor In 50-cc bottle, fruit flavor
(E.E.S.)	Tablets: 400 mg Suspension: 200 mg/5 cc, 400 mg/5 cc	In 100, 500, and 1000 film-coated tablets In 100- and 480-cc bottles, orange flavor

Continued on next page

Table 22–21. Available Dosage Forms: Macrolides and Azalides *(continued)*

Drug	Dosage Form	How Supplied
	Granules/powder for oral suspension: 200 mg/5 cc (reconstituted)	In 100- and 200-cc bottles, cherry flavor
Erythromycin ethylsuccinate and sulfisoxazole	Granules for oral suspension 200 mg erythromycin base activity and 600 mg sulfisoxazole/5 mL	In 100, 150, and 200 mL
(Eryzole)	Granules for oral suspension 200 mg erythromycin base activity and 600 mg sulfisoxazole/5 mL	In 100, 150, and 200 mL, strawberry flavor
(Pediazole)	Granules for oral suspension 200 mg erythromycin base activity and 600 mg sulfisoxazole/5 mL	In 100, 150, and 200 mL, strawberry-banana flavor

formulation **trimethoprim-sulfamethoxazole** (TMP-SMZ) illustrates the synergy of the combination.

SENSITIVITY. **Trimethoprim** is active against both gram-positive and gram-negative organisms. Gram-positive organisms include *S. pneumoniae,* some staphylococci, and *Enterococcus.* Its spectrum of gram-negative organisms includes *Acinetobacter, Citrobacter, Enterobacter, E. coli, K. pneumoniae, P. mirabilis, Salmonella,* and *Shigella.* Some *Serratia* and the protozoon *P. carinii* are also susceptible.

RESISTANCE. Resistance results from reduced cell permeability, overproduction of dihydrofolate reductase, or production of an altered reductase with less drug-binding ability. Mutation is possible, but the most common cause is plasmid-encoded resistant reductases. As with the **sulfonamides,** dissemination of resistance is rapid and widespread.

Nitrofurantoin

Nitrofurantoin is a synthetic **nitrofuran** that is bacteriostatic in low concentrations and bactericidal in high concentrations. The mechanism of action for this drug is not clearly known, but it may inhibit acetyl coenzyme A, interfering with bacterial carbohydrate metabolism. It may also disrupt bacterial cell wall formation.

SENSITIVITY. **Nitrofurantoin** is active against most gram-positive cocci and gram-negative bacilli that cause UTIs. These include *E. coli, Klebsiella* and *Enterobacter* species, *E. faecalis,* and *S. aureus.* Some strains of *Enterobacter* and *Klebsiella* are resistant. It has no activity against *Pseudomonas* species or *S. saprophyticus.*

Although in vitro susceptibility of *Salmonella, Shigella, Neisseria, S. pneumoniae,* and many anaerobes has been

demonstrated, **nitrofurantoin** does not appear to have clinically significant activity against these organisms.

RESISTANCE. Among susceptible organisms, resistant mutants are rare. Some plasmid-mediated resistance transferable to susceptible organisms has been demonstrated. There is no cross-resistance between this drug and other **antibacterial agents.**

Pharmacokinetics

Absorption and Distribution

Oral **sulfonamides** are absorbed readily from the GI tract. They are distributed widely throughout the body and found in all body tissues, and they readily enter the CSF, pleura, synovial fluids, and the eye. They cross the placenta and enter breast milk. They are bound to plasma proteins in varying degrees. "Free" serum levels of 5 to 15 mg/dL are therapeutically effective for most infections.

Trimethoprim is also well absorbed following oral administration. It is widely distributed in body tissues and crosses the placenta. Distribution into breast milk occurs with high concentrations.

Nitrofurantoin is readily absorbed via oral administration. The macrocrystalline form is absorbed more slowly because of slower dissolution and causes less GI distress, and the monohydrate crystals are so slowly absorbed that twice-daily dosing is effective. Bioavailability is enhanced by taking **nitrofurantoin** with food. Because it undergoes rapid tubular secretion, therapeutic serum and tissue concentrations are achieved only in the urinary tract at usual oral doses. It is not effective in patients with severe renal impairment.

Metabolism and Excretion

Metabolism of **sulfonamides** occurs in the liver by conjugation and acetylation to inactive metabolites. Patients who are slow acetylators have increased risk for toxicity. Renal excretion is mainly by glomerulofiltration, with some acetylated metabolites being less soluble. Acetylated metabolites may produce crystalluria unless the urine is sufficiently alkaline and adequate fluid intake (more than 2500 cc/day) is maintained. **Sulfadiazine** is especially prone to this problem. Small amounts are excreted in feces, bile, breast milk, and other secretions.

Liver metabolism of **trimethoprim** is less than 20 percent. Eighty percent of this drug is excreted unchanged in the urine. Because it is so dependent on the kidney for excretion, elimination is delayed and its half-life is increased in patients with renal impairment.

Approximately 50 to 70 percent of **nitrofurantoin** is rapidly metabolized by body tissues. Distribution is to most body tissues, and it crosses the placenta and enters breast milk. Renal excretion is via glomerulofiltration and tubular secretion. Acid urine enhances antibacterial activity in urine and enhances tubular reabsorption, which increases its activity in renal tissues. Serum half-life is increased in patients with severe renal impairment. Usual doses produce therapeutic urinary levels in patients with normal renal function. If CCr is less than 40 cc/minute, urinary concentrations are not therapeutic, and the increased serum levels may produce toxicity.

Table 22–22 presents the pharmacokinetics of **sulfonamides, trimethoprim,** and **nitrofurantoin.**

Pharmacotherapeutics

Precautions and Contraindications

BLOOD DYSCRASIAS AND GLUCOSE-6-PHOSPHATE DEHYDROGENASE DEFICIENCY. **Sulfonamides** are contraindicated for patients who have blood dyscrasias and G6PD deficiency. Serious adverse reactions secondary to direct toxic effects on the bone marrow have sometimes resulted in death. They include agranulocytosis, aplastic anemia, and other blood dyscrasias. Acute hemolytic anemia resulting in increased destruction of RBCs has resulted in patients whose RBCs have been sensitized because of G6PD deficiency. Sore throat, fever, pallor, purpura, or jaundice may be early indications of these serious blood disorders. These problems occur only rarely with **trimethoprim** and with **nitrofurantoin** only in conjunction with G6PD deficiency.

RENAL IMPAIRMENT. **Sulfonamides** are used cautiously for patients with mild renal impairment and are contraindicated if CCr is less than 50 cc/minute. The more soluble drugs in this class (**sulfisoxazole** and **sulfamethoxazole**) are less likely to result in renal complications. Adequate hydration (more than 2500 cc/day) helps to prevent crystalluria and stone formation. Cautious use of **trimethoprim** is recommended for patients with renal impairment. Renal impairment increases the risk of toxicity of **nitrofurantoin,** which is not effective in severe renal impairment.

FOLATE DEFICIENCY. Because of its effect on folic acid synthesis, **trimethoprim** should be used with caution for patients with folate deficiency. Folate supplementa-

Table 22–22. Pharmacokinetics: Sulfonamides, Trimethoprim, and Nitrofurantoin

Drug	Onset	Peak	Duration	Protein Binding	Bioavailability	Half-Life	Elimination
Nitrofurantoin	UA	0.5 h	6–12 h	60%	UA	20 min*	30–50% unchanged in urine
Sulfadiazine	Varies	3–6 h	6–12 h	32–56%	70–100%	13 h	Mainly in urine; small amount in feces
Sulfamethoxazole	1 h	2–4 h	12 h	65%	70–100%	7–12 h	Mostly by liver; 20% unchanged in urine
Sulfamethoxazole/ trimethoprim	Rapid	2–4 h	6–12 h	65/50%	UA	8–13 h	20% by liver; remainder unchanged in urine
Sulfisoxazole	1 h	2–4 h	4–6 h	90%	70–100%	5–8 h	Mostly by liver
Trimethoprim	Rapid	1–4 h	12–24 h	50%	UA	8–11 h	80% unchanged in urine; 20% by liver

*Increased in renal impairment.

tion may be administered concomitantly without interfering with antibacterial action.

Sulfonamides are Pregnancy Category C. These drugs cross the placenta, and fetal levels average 70 to 90 percent of maternal serum levels. Significant levels may persist if they are given near term. *Sulfonamides* are highly bound to plasma albumin and compete for binding sites with bilirubin, resulting in increased free bilirubin concentrations. In utero, the fetus clears free bilirubin through the placental circulation. After birth, this route is no longer available, and unbound bilirubin may cross the blood-brain barrier. Do not use near term. Jaundice, hemolytic anemia, and kernicterus have occurred. Teratogenicity has occurred in animal studies.

Trimethoprim is also Pregnancy Category C. It crosses the placenta, producing similar levels in fetal and maternal plasma. Teratogenicity has occurred in animal studies. Because it may interfere with folic acid metabolism, it should be used only when its benefits clearly outweigh fetal risks.

Nitrofurantoin is Pregnancy Category B. Use for women of childbearing potential only when it is clearly needed. The incidence of fetal changes in animal studies was low and the alterations minor. It should not be given, however, to pregnant patients with G6PD deficiency because of the risk of hemolysis for both mother and fetus. Do not use at term on account of the possibility of inducing hemolytic anemia in the newborn because of immature enzyme systems. For this reason, *nitrofurantoin* is contraindicated in infants less than 1 month old.

Because they are excreted in breast milk in low concentrations and milk:plasma ratios are as low as 0.5 to 0.6, the American Academy of Pediatrics considers breastfeeding safe during administration of **sulfonamides**. However, premature infants or those with hyperbilirubinemia or G6PD deficiency should not be breast-fed while these drugs are being taken. **Trimethoprim** milk:plasma ratios are 1.25, indicating the drug concentrates in breast milk. Because it may interfere with folic acid metabolism, it should be used cautiously for nursing women. **Nitrofurantoin** is excreted in breast milk in very low concentrations. Infants with G6PD deficiency, however, should not nurse while the mother is receiving this drug.

Sulfonamides are contraindicated in infants under 2 months of age (except as adjunctive therapy with **pyrimethamine** for congenital toxoplasmosis). Insufficient clinical data are available on prolonged or recurrent therapy with **sulfamethoxazole** in children under 6 years with chronic renal disease. It is best to avoid its use in these patients.

Safety for use in infants under 2 months old has not been established for **trimethoprim**, and efficacy has not been established for children under age 12 years. **Nitrofurantoin** is contraindicated in infants under 1 month of age.

Adverse Drug Reactions

As with most **antibiotics**, the most common adverse reactions for all these drugs are in the GI tract. Anorexia, nausea, vomiting, diarrhea, stomatitis, and abdominal pain are the main adverse reactions.

Rashes and generalized skin eruptions are also common adverse reactions for **sulfonamides** and **trimethoprim**. The incidence is dose-related and may include exfoliative dermatitis and Stevens-Johnson syndrome.

Hypersensitivity reactions may occur with **sulfonamides**. Cholestatic jaundice is the indication of the adverse reaction. For the **sulfonamides**, cross-hypersensitivity may occur with chemically related drugs such as **sulfonylureas, thiazide** and **loop diuretics, carbonic anhydrase inhibitors,** and sunscreens with PABA.

Photosensitivity reactions can occur with **sulfonamides**. Measures such as sunscreens and protective clothing may reduce these problems.

Peripheral neuropathy may develop and become severe and irreversible with **nitrofurantoin**. Predisposing conditions include renal impairment, anemia, diabetes, electrolyte imbalances, vitamin B deficiency, and debilitating disease. Less severe peripheral neuropathy has also occurred with **sulfonamides**. CNS adverse effects including headache, dizziness, and drowsiness have occurred with both of these drug classes.

Other serious adverse reactions are discussed in the Precautions and Contraindications section.

Drug Interactions

Trimethoprim and **nitrofurantoin** have very few drug interactions. **Sulfonamides** interact with several commonly used drugs, including **salicylates, warfarin,** and **hydantoins.** Specific drug interactions are listed in Tablet 22–23.

Clinical Use and Dosing

URINARY TRACT INFECTIONS. The most common pathogens in UTIs, including cystitis and pyelonephritis, are *E. coli* and other Enterobacteriaceae, *S. saprophyticus,* and *Enterococcus.*

TMP-SMZ is active against these pathogens and has long been considered the drug of first choice for UTI. Three days of oral **antimicrobial** therapy is recommended for uncomplicated cystitis. If 3-day empiric therapy fails, urine should be sent for culture and subsequent therapy continued for 14 days. Seven-day therapy is recommended for cystitis during pregnancy. Pyelonephritis requires longer therapy than cystitis, usually 7 days with **fluoroquinolones** and 14 days with other agents. In 1996, 18 percent of *E. coli* were resistant to **TMP-SMZ,** so many experts now consider **fluoroquinolones** the primary regimen for UTIs (Gilbert,

Table 22–23. Drug Interactions: Sulfonamides, Trimethoprim, and Nitrofurantoin

Drug	Interacting Drug	Possible Effects	Implications
Nitrofurantoin	Anticholinergics	Increase nitrofurantoin bioavailability by delaying gastric emptying and increasing absorption.	Monitor for adverse reactions and toxicity.
	Magnesium salts	May delay or decrease nitrofurantoin absorption.	Avoid concurrent administration.
	Probenecid	High doses decrease renal clearance and increase serum levels of nitrofurantoin.	Monitor for increased risk for toxicity.
All sulfonamides	Oral anticoagulants	Enhance action of warfarin. Hemorrhage could occur.	Monitor PT/INR closely.
	Cyclosporine	Increased cyclosporine concentration and risk of nephrotoxicity.	Select different antibacterial.
	Hydantoins	Increased serum hydantoin levels.	Monitor serum levels closely.
	Sulfonylureas	Increased sulfonylureas half-life and risk of hypoglycemia.	Avoid concurrent use or monitor blood glucose closely.
	Probenecid and other uricosurics, salicylates, indomethacin	Sulfonamides may be displaced from plasma albumin resting in increased free drug. Sulfonamides may potentiate action of uricosurics.	Unless planned for therapeutic reasons, avoid concurrent administration.
	Thiazide diuretics	May cause increased incidence of thrombocytopenia with purpura.	Avoid coadministration.
Trimethoprim	Phenytoin	Inhibition of hepatic metabolism may result in increased effects of phenytoin.	Avoid concurrent administration or monitor phenytoin levels closely.

INR = international normalized ratio; PT = prothrombin time.

Moellering, & Sande, 1999). However, **fluoroquinolones** are contraindicated in children and pregnancy. **Trimethoprim (Trimpex), TMP-SMZ, nitrofurantoin macrocrystals (Macrodantin)**, and **nitrofurantoin mono-hydrate (Macrobid)** are first-line agents in uncomplicated cystitis and can be used in all but the last few weeks of pregnancy. Of these, only **TMP-SMZ** is effective for pyelonephritis. Twice-daily doses of one double-strength **TMP-SMZ**, containing 160 mg **trimethoprim** and 800 mg **sulfamethoxazole**, is used for both cystitis and pyelonephritis. Dosages of the other agents for cystitis are shown in Table 22–24. Low-dose **nitrofurantoin** at bedtime (50 to 100 mg) is used for chronic suppression of UTI. **TMP-SMZ** (40 mg **TMP** and 200 mg **SMZ** or one-half a single-strength tablet) has also been used at bedtime a minimum of three times weekly and postcoitally to prevent recurrent UTIs in women. Pregnant women with asymptomatic bacteriuria detected during routine screening during the first pregnancy can be treated with **TMP-SMZ, nitrofurantoin,** or **trimethoprim,** as well as **amoxicillin** or oral **cephalosporins.** Other genitourinary indications for **TMP-SMZ** are treatment of acute prostatitis in men over age 35 years, chronic prostatitis, recurrent UTI (more than three in a year), and prophylaxis before and after invasive urologic procedures. Although infrequently used, the **sulfonamides sulfadiazine, sulfamethizole,** **sulfamethoxazole,** and **sulfisoxazole** are approved for treatment of cystitis and uncomplicated pyelonephritis.

OTITIS MEDIA. Because of decreased activity against *S. pneumoniae,* **TMP-SMZ** is no longer considered first-line therapy for AOM (Tiggs, 2000). Because of the low cost of **TMP/SMZ**, it is still used by some in doses of 8 mg/kg a day (based on the **TMP** component) in divided doses every 12 hours for children who fail therapy with **amoxicillin.** The fixed-dose combination of **erythromycin ethylsuccinate** and **sulfisoxazole (Pediazole, Eryzole)** is used as an alternate agent in treatment of AOM, particularly for those allergic to **amoxicillin.** **Sulfisoxazole (Gantrisin)** in doses of 50 to 75 mg/kg a day divided into two doses can be used for suppressive therapy in children with a history of three AOM episodes in 6 months or four episodes in 12 months. Because of increasing resistance, prophylactic **antibiotics** should be used judiciously. See the section on otitis media under **penicillins** for management of otitis media with effusion.

UPPER RESPIRATORY INFECTION. Although many experts fear failure of **TMP-SMZ** in the treatment of sinusitis because of the increasing resistance of *H. influenzae, M. catarrhalis,* and drug-resistant *S. pneumoniae,* which are the major pathogens, it is considered a primary agent for sinusitis. In addition, treatment of acute sinusitis is contro-

Table 22–24. Dosage Schedule: Sulfonamides, Trimethoprim, and Nitrofurantoin

Drug	Indication	Dose	Comments
Nitrofurantoin (Furadantin) Nitrofurantoin macrocrystals (Macrodantin)	Urinary tract infection	*Adult* 50–100 mg qid with meals and at bedtime for 3–7 d or more *Child* 5–7 mg/kg/d in 4 divided doses for at least 7 d	Maximum daily dose 600 mg for adult or 10 mg/kg for children. Take all nitrofurantoins with food or milk to decrease GI distress. All nitrofurantoins are contraindicated in infants under age 1 mo. Suspension should be shaken well before measurement, using a calibrated measuring device. Store at room temperature. The oral suspension can be mixed with water, milk, fruit juice, or infant formula, although it may discolor.
	Long-term suppression of urinary tract infection	*Adult* 50–100 mg at bedtime *Child* 1 mg/kg/24 h in 1 or 2 divided doses	As above.
Monohydrate macrocrystals (Macrobid)	Urinary tract infections	*Adult* 100 mg q12h for 3–7 d	As above.
Sulfadiazine	Antibacterial or antiprotozoal	*Adult* 2–4 g as initial dose, then 1 g q4–6h *Child* 75 mg/kg as initial dose, then 37.5 mg/kg q6h or 25 mg/kg q4h	Take with a full glass of water.
Sulfamethoxazole (Gantanol)	Antibacterial or antiprotozoal, mild to moderate infections	*Adult* Initial dose of 2 g, followed by 1 g q8–10h *Child age >2 mo* 50–60 mg/kg to maximum of 2 g initially, followed by 25–30 mg/kg q12h	Maximum dose for children is 75 mg/kg. Fluid intake should be sufficient to maintain urine output of at least 1200 mL/d. Most crystalluria prone sulfonamide. Take with full glass of water.
Sulfisoxazole (Gantrisin)	Recurrent acute otitis media	*Child* 50 mg/kg at bedtime	Maximum adult daily dose 8 g; maximum daily pediatric dose 6 g. Take with full glass of water. Fluid intake should be sufficient to maintain urine output of at least 1200 mL/d. Shake suspension well before measurement, using calibrated dosing device. Store at room temperature.
	Rheumatic fever prophylaxis (secondary)	*Adult* With carditis, 1 g/d for 10 y or until age 25 Without carditis, 1 g/d for 5 y or until age 18	As above.
	Antibacterial or antiprotozoal	*Adult* 2–4 g initially, then 750 mg-1.5 g q4h; 1–2 g q6h *Child age >2 mo* 75 mg/kg or 2 g/m² initially, followed by 25 mg/kg q4h or 37.5 mg/kg q6h	As above.

Continued on next page

Table 22-24. Dosage Schedule: Sulfonamides, Trimethoprim, and Nitrofurantoin *(continued)*

Drug	Indication	Dose	Comments
Trimethoprim (Polytrim, Trimpex)	Urinary tract infection, treatment	*Adult* 100 mg q12h for 10 d or 200 mg daily *Child age >2 mo* 3 mg/kg bid	May be taken on an empty stomach or with food to decrease GI distress. Doses >600 mg daily have been used to treat *P. carinii*.
	Urinary tract infection, prophylaxis	*Adult* 100 mg/d	As above.
Trimethoprim (TMP)-Sulfamethoxazole (SMZ) (Bactrim, Septra)	Urinary tract infection, shigellosis, acute otitis media	*Adult* 160 mg TMP and 800 mg SMZ q12h for 10–14 d (5 d for shigellosis) *Child age >2 mo* 8 mg/kg/d TMP and 40 mg/kg/d SMZ q12h for 10–14 d (5 d for shigellosis)	Shake suspensions well before measurement, using calibrated measuring device. May be stored at room temperature. Take with full glass of water and ensure adequate fluid intake to maintain urine output of at least 1200 mL daily. If CCr is between 15 and 30 mL/min, dose should be halved; avoid TMP-SMZ if CCr <15 mL/min. Total daily dose in children should not exceed 320 mg TMP and 1600 mg SMZ.
	Traveler's diarrhea	*Adult* 160 mg TMP/800 mg SMZ q12h for 5 d	As above.
	Acute exacerbation of chronic bronchitis	*Adult* 160 mg TMP and 800 mg SMZ q12h for 14 d	As above.
	P. carinii pneumonia prophylaxis	*Adult* 160 TMP and 800 SMZ orally q24h *Child* 150 mg/m² TMP and 750 mg/m² SMZ/d in 2 divided doses on 3 consecutive d	As above.

versial (see Sinusitis in **penicillin** section). Although **TMP-SMZ** is effective in vitro against group A beta-hemolytic *S. pyogenes*, it does not eradicate the organism or protect against rheumatic fever. Thus, it should not be used to treat streptococcal pharyngitis.

EXACERBATIONS OF CHRONIC BRONCHITIS. Although treatment of ABECB is controversial, **TMP-SMZ** may be a good choice for patients who have not taken **antibiotics** recently and therefore are less likely to be infected with a resistant strain (Niederman et al., 1998). Another advantage of this formulation is low cost. However, with repeated use of **TMP-SMZ**, resistant organisms are likely to prevail.

TRAVELER'S DIARRHEA. TMP-SMZ, one double-strength tablet every 12 hours for adults (or 8 mg/kg/day based on the **TMP** component in two divided doses) for 3 days is a first-line alternative to **fluoroquinolones** for treatment of traveler's diarrhea. Routine prophylaxis of traveler's diarrhea is no longer recommended.

OTHER. TMP-SMZ is approved for treatment of shigellosis enteritis in adults and children. It also is used for the prevention and treatment of pneumonia caused by the protozoon *P. carinii* in immunocompromised patients. Malaria is another protozoal infection that **sulfonamides** are used to treat as part of multidrug therapy. **Sulfonamides** are inexpensive agents used primarily outside North America to treat trachoma, inclusion conjunctivitis, toxoplasmosis, chancroid, and meningitis.

Rational Drug Selection

Both definitive drug selection and empiric drug selection follow the same principles described in the Rational

Drug Selection section for the **penicillins**, regardless of the infection or drug class involved. Although no longer primary agents for any infectious disease, the **sulfonamides, trimethoprim**, and **nitrofurantoin** are useful, low-cost alternatives for pregnancy, children, and individuals with **penicillin** allergy. Because **trimethoprim** and **nitrofurantoin** are indicated as monotherapy only for UTI, use of these agents does not contribute as much to selection pressure that promotes resistance to drugs used for other infections. **Sulfonamides** are the most allergenic drug groups and should be avoided in those with hypersensitivity to other **sulfonamides** (e.g., **loop diuretics, thiazide diuretics, sulfonylurea antidiabetic drugs**) and used with caution in patients with severe allergy or bronchial asthma. Both **nitrofurantoin** and **sulfonamides** should be avoided in individuals with a personal or familial history of G6PD deficiency. **Trimethoprim** and **sulfonamides** can worsen folic acid deficiency and should be used cautiously in the presence of megaloblastic anemia; folates can be administered concurrently without interfering with the antibacterial action. **Nitrofurantoin** is available as microcrystals, macrocrystals, and monohydrate macrocrystals. Microcrystals (**Furadantin**) cause excessive GI irritation and should not be used. Monohydrate macrocrystals (**Macrobid**) form a gel that gradually releases the drug, requiring only twice-daily dosing, whereas macrocrystals (**Macrodantin**) require administration every 6 hours. **Nitrofurantoin** should be used with caution in those predisposed to its adverse effects: older patients and those with anemia, renal impairment, electrolyte imbalance, diabetes, vitamin B deficiency, and debilitating diseases.

Monitoring

Monitoring for therapeutic response to **antimicrobial drugs** is described in the Monitoring section for **penicillins**. Culture of the urine to follow up a UTI will verify eradication of the infection. If a patient is on long-term therapy of **nitrofurantoin, trimethoprim**, or a **sulfonamide**, periodic assessment of the complete blood cell (CBC) count, hepatic function, and renal function should be conducted. For **nitrofurantoin**, there should also be periodic evaluation of pulmonary function for signs of fibrosis, physical examination for indications of peripheral neuropathy, and urine culture; superinfections with *Pseudomonas* or *Candida* sometimes occur with chronic therapy. Elderly patients on **nitrofurantoin** should be monitored closely because serious adverse effects like acute pneumonitis and peripheral neuropathy occur more commonly in this population. Any patient on **nitrofurantoin** who develops cough, dyspnea, chest pain, or fever should receive a chest x-ray, sedimentation rate, and CBC to detect the signs of hypersensitivity and pulmonary fibrosis. Patients on long-term **sulfonamide** therapy should also have periodic urinalysis to check for crystalluria or urinary calculi formation. Patients with AIDS are prone to adverse effects of **sulfonamides**.

Patient Education

ADMINISTRATION. Patient counseling for all **antimicrobials** includes advice to complete the entire course of therapy, take the medications as prescribed on a regular schedule, and abstain from sharing medications with others. Available dosage forms are shown in Table 22–25. **Sulfonamides** and solid or liquid forms of **trimethoprim-sulfamethoxazole** should be taken with a full glass of water and sufficient daily fluid intake to maintain 1200 mL urine output in the adult. **Nitrofurantoin** causes less GI distress and is better absorbed if taken with food or milk. Suspensions should be shaken before measurement and taken with a specially marked measuring spoon or comparable device.

ADVERSE REACTIONS. Patients taking **sulfonamides** and **trimethoprim** or combinations containing these agents should be counseled to avoid photosensitivity or photoallergy by wearing protective clothing and sunscreens. They should not expose their skin to ultraviolet light from sun or tanning lamps more than a few minutes until tolerance is determined. The patient who develops a rash while taking these agents should discontinue the drug and contact the health care provider; rash may develop into Stevens-Johnson syndrome. Patients on **sulfonamides** should also report signs of crystalluria (blood in urine) and blood dyscrasias (sore throat, fever, chills, pale skin, unusual bleeding or bruising). **Sulfonamides** may cause dizziness that can make operation of machinery and automobiles dangerous.

Counseling for patients on **nitrofurantoin** includes similar cautions for signs of blood dyscrasias (sore throat, fever, chills, pale skin, unusual bleeding or bruising). Patients should know that the drug may cause brownish discoloration of the urine and elicit a false positive on copper sulfate urine tests for glucose. Patients should call the health care provider if there are signs of acute pulmonary fibrosis (sudden onset of chest pain, dyspnea, cough, fever) or subacute pulmonary fibrosis (dyspnea, nonproductive cough, malaise after 1 to 6 months of therapy). Because rechallenge with **nitrofurantoin** could cause rapid return of the pulmonary condition, the patient should be provided with written information to warn future health care providers of the reaction. Other symptoms to report are signs of peripheral neuropathy (numbness, tingling, pain in extremities) and intolerable GI upset.

LIFESTYLE MANAGEMENT. See the Lifestyle Management section for the **penicillins**.

Table 22–25. Available Dosage Forms: Sulfonamides, Trimethoprim, and Nitrofurantoin

Drug	Dosage Form	How Supplied
Nitrofurantoin (Furadantin)	Oral suspension: 25 mg/5 cc	In 60- and 470-cc bottles
Nitrofurantoin macrocrystals	Capsules: 50 mg, 100 mg	In bottles of 100, 500, and 1000 capsules
(Macrodantin)	Capsules: 25 mg 50 mg, 100 mg	In bottles of 100 capsules In bottles of 100, 500, and 1000 capsules
(Macrobid)	Capsules: 100 mg	In bottles of 100 capsules
Sulfadiazine	Tablets: 500 mg	In bottles of 100 and 1000 tablets
Sulfamethoxazole (Gantanol)	Tablets: 500 mg	In bottles of 100 tablets
Trimethoprim and sulfamethoxazole	Tablets: 400 mg/80 mg 800 mg/160 mg Oral suspension: 200 mg/40 mg/5 cc	In bottles of 100 and 500 tablets In bottles of 100 and 500 double-strength tablets In 150-, 240-, and 480-cc bottles
(Bactrim)	Tablets: 400 mg/80 mg 800 mg/160 mg Oral suspension: 200 mg/40 mg/5 cc	In bottles of 100 tablets In bottles of 150, 250, and 500 tablets In 480-cc bottles, cherry flavor
(Cotrim)	Tablets: 400 mg/80 mg 800 mg/160 mg Oral suspension: 200 mg/40 mg/5 cc	In bottles of 100 and 500 tablets In bottles of 100 and 500 double-strength tablets In 473-cc bottles
(Septra)	Tablets: 400 mg/80 mg 800 mg/160 mg Oral suspension: 200 mg/40 mg/5 cc	In bottles of 100 tablets In bottles of 100 and 250 double-strength tablets In 20-, 100-, 150-, 200-, and 473-cc bottles, cherry flavor; in 473-cc bottles, grape flavor
(Sulfatrim)	Oral suspension: 200 mg/40 mg/5 cc	In 473-cc bottles
Sulfisoxazole (Gantrisin)	Tablets 500 mg	In bottles of 100 and 500 tablets
Trimethoprim	Tablets: 100 mg 200 mg	In bottles of 14, 30, and 100 tablets In bottles of 100 tablets
(Proloprim)	Tablets: 100 mg, 200 mg	In bottles of 100 tablets
(Trimpex)	Tablets: 100 mg	In bottles of 100 tablets

Tetracyclines

Tetracyclines are broad-spectrum **antibiotics** that are used extensively throughout the world. Originally introduced in 1948, they are used in the United States mainly for uncommon infections because newer **antibiotics** can treat common susceptible infections with fewer adverse reactions and drug-drug and drug-food interactions. The second-generation drug **doxycycline (Doxy, Doxychel, Vibramycin)** has fewer problems with drug-food interactions and is frequently used to treat sexually transmitted diseases and as one of four drugs in the treatment of *H. pylori* infection. **Tetracycline (Sumycin)** is used both topically and orally to treat acne. Topical application is discussed in Chapters 21 and 30.

Pharmacodynamics

Tetracyclines include a group of drugs with a common basic structure and activity. Hydrochloride forms of these drugs are more soluble, and **doxycycline** and **minocycline (Dynacin, Minocin)** are highly lipid soluble. The hydrochloride forms are acidic and fairly stable. **Tetracyclines** chelate divalent and trivalent ions, which can interfere with their absorption and activity.

These drugs enter microorganisms by passive diffusion and energy-dependent active transport. Susceptible cells concentrate the drug intracellularly. Once inside the cell, they bind reversibly to the 30S subunit of the bacterial ribosome, eventually preventing the addition of amino acids to growing peptides. They are bacteriostatic for many gram-positive and gram-negative organisms, including anaerobes, rickettsiae, chlamydiae, mycoplasmas, and some protozoa, including amebae.

Sensitivity

Tetracyclines are active against rickettsiae (Rocky Mountain spotted fever, typhus, Q fever, rickettsial pox and tick fever), *M. pneumoniae, Borrelia recurrentis* (relapsing fever), and the agents responsible for psittacosis, lymphogranuloma venereum, and granuloma inguinale.

Gram-negative organisms that **tetracyclines** are effective against include *Haemophilus ducreyi* (chancroid), *Yersinia pestis, Francisella tularensis, Bartonella bacilliformis, Bacteroides* species, *Acinetobacter, Vibrio cholerae,* and *Brucella.* Although not first-line therapy, they also are active against *E. coli, Shigella, H. influenzae,* and *Klebsiella* respiratory and urinary infection.

When **penicillin** is contraindicated, **tetracycline** may be used as an alternative for treatment of infections due to *N. gonorrhoeae, T. pallidum, Treponema pertenue* (yaws), *Clostridium,* and *B. anthracis.*

Because extensive use of **tetracyclines** in the past has resulted in bacterial resistance that may be as high as 74 percent in some organisms, these drugs should not used for common infections unless the organism has been shown by culture and sensitivity testing to be sensitive.

Doxycycline is considered first-line therapy for *N. gonorrhea, C. trachomatis,* and *Ureaplasma urealyticum.* **Minocycline** is used for treatment of asymptomatic nasopharyngeal carriers of *N. meningitidis.* **Tetracycline** appears to inhibit the growth of *Propionibacterium acnes* on the skin surface and reduce the concentration of free fatty acids in sebum.

Resistance

The mechanisms of resistance to **tetracyclines** are (1) decreased intracellular accumulation due to impaired influx or increased efflux of an active transport protein pump, (2) ribosome protection by proteins that interfere with drug binding, and (3) enzymatic inactivation (Katzung, 1998). The most important is the pump activity. The pump protein is encoded on a plasmid and may be transmitted to other organisms. Cross-resistance may occur with **aminoglycosides, sulfonamides,** and **chloramphenicol.**

Pharmacokinetics

Absorption and Distribution

Tetracyclines are adequately but incompletely absorbed in the fasting state. The percentage of oral dose absorbed is highest for **doxycycline** and **minocycline**

(95 to 100%) and intermediate for **oxytetracycline** (Terramycin) and **tetracycline** (60 to 70%). Achlorhydria has no effect on absorption of **tetracyclines.** Food and polyvalent cations (Ca^{2+}, Mg^{2+}, Fe^{2+}, and Al^{3+}) decrease absorption of **tetracycline** but have little effect on **doxycycline** or **minocycline.**

Doxycycline and **minocycline** are highly lipid soluble, readily penetrate the CSF, brain, eye, and prostate, and cross placental membranes. Fetal plasma concentrations reach 60 percent of maternal serum levels. **Minocycline** displays good penetration of saliva. **Tetracycline** has intermediate lipid solubility, and **oxytetracycline** has the least. **Oxytetracycline** readily diffuses across the placenta into fetal circulation and into pleural fluid.

Metabolism and Excretion

This class of drugs undergoes enterohepatic recirculation, is concentrated by the liver in the bile, and is excreted in both urine and feces, largely unchanged. Dosage adjustments of **tetracycline** and **oxytetracycline** are required for renal impairment. **Doxycycline** is secreted in an inactive form into the intestinal lumen and eliminated in feces. Its half-life does not significantly increase in renal impairment, so no dosage adjustments are required. **Minocycline** is metabolized and its half-life is prolonged in oliguria. Because it also uses nonrenal routes of excretion, however, dosage adjustments are not required in renal impairment.

Table 22–26 depicts the pharmacokinetics of selected tetracyclines.

Pharmacotherapeutics

Precautions and Contraindications

RENAL IMPAIRMENT. Extreme caution should be used in the presence of renal impairment. Even usual doses of **tetracyclines** (except **doxycycline** and **minocycline**) may lead to excessive accumulation of the drugs and possible hepatotoxicity, so lower than normal doses are required in renal impairment. If therapy is prolonged, assay of drug serum concentration may be advisable. The antianabolic actions of **tetracyclines** (except **doxycycline**) may cause an increase in BUN and lead to azotemia, hyperphosphatemia, and acidosis in the presence of severe renal impairment.

HEPATIC IMPAIRMENT. There are serious concerns related to hepatotoxicity for intravenous forms of **tetracycline.** This is not a major concern with oral administration, but liver function studies are advisable during long-term management with **doxycycline** or **minocycline.**

Doxycycline is Pregnancy Category D. Others are Pregnancy Category X and should not be used during

Table 22–26. Pharmacokinetics: Tetracyclines

Drug	Onset	Peak	Duration	Protein Binding	Bioavailability	Half-Life	Elimination
Doxycycline	1–2 h	1.5–4 h	12 h	80–95%	93%	15–25 h	30–42% unchanged in urine; some inactivation in intestine; remainder excreted in bile and feces.
Minocycline	Rapid	2–3 h	6–12 h	70–80%	90%	11–18 h	12–16% unchanged in urine; some metabolism by liver; remainder excreted in bile and feces.
Oxytetracycline	1–2 h	2–4 h	6–12 h	20–40%	UA	12–16 h	70% unchanged in urine.
Tetracycline	1–2 h	2–4 h	6–12 h	65%	60–80%	12–16 h	60% unchanged in urine.

pregnancy. **They readily cross the placenta in concentrations up to 60 percent of maternal plasma. *Tetracyclines* are found in fetal tissue and can produce retardation of skeletal development in the fetus and staining of deciduous teeth.**

Tetracyclines are excreted in breast milk. A dosage of 2 g a day for 3 days has achieved a milk:plasma ratio of 0.6 to 0.8. Because of the potential for serious adverse reactions, these drugs are not recommended during lactation.

Children under 8 years of age generally should not use any **tetracycline.** These drugs form a stable calcium complex in any bone-forming tissue, decreasing bone growth. They also may cause permanent yellow-gray-brown discoloration of deciduous and permanent teeth. Enamel hypoplasia has also been reported. **Doxycycline** is less likely to produce these problems, but the risk outweighs any potential benefit for most indications.

Adverse Drug Reactions

As with other **antibiotics,** the most common adverse reactions are associated with the GI tract. Anorexia, nausea, vomiting, and diarrhea are caused by direct irritation of the intestinal mucosa. Taking the drug with food, reducing the dose, or discontinuing the drug usually controls them. Esophageal ulcers have occasionally occurred but can be avoided by taking the drug with a full glass of water and remaining upright for at least 1 to 2 minutes after taking the drug. As broad-spectrum **antibiotics, tetracyclines** can cause AAPMC, previously discussed in the sections on **penicillins, cephalosporins,** and **clindamycin.**

Lightheadedness, dizziness, and vertigo have been reported in 35 to 70 percent of patients taking **minocycline** and in some patients taking **doxycycline.** Pseudotremor cerebri (benign intracranial hypertension) has also been associated with **tetracycline** use. Symptoms are headache and blurred vision and bulging fontanels in infants. Dis-

continuing the drug usually resolves these problems, but the possibility for permanent sequelae exists.

Dermatologic adverse reactions include photosensitivity manifested by an exaggerated sunburn reaction, as well as maculopapular and erythematous rashes. Blue-gray pigmentation of skin and mucosa has been reported with **minocycline.**

Under no circumstances should outdated tetracyclines be administered. The degradation products of these drugs are highly nephrotoxic, and reversible nephrotoxicity including a Fanconi-like syndrome has been reported.

Drug Interactions

The main drug-drug and drug-food interactions associated with **tetracyclines** are with **antacids, iron salts,** and dairy products, based on the formation of poorly soluble chelated compounds. The result is a decrease in **antibiotic** activity. Separation of these products from the administration of **tetracyclines** by at least 2 hours, taking the **tetracycline** first, is recommended. **Doxycycline** and **minocycline** have less affinity for these products and are not significantly affected. Whether **tetracyclines** cause a decrease in efficacy of **oral contraceptives** is controversial, but the alleged mechanism is related to the enterohepatic recirculation of **tetracycline** and **oral contraceptives.** It does seem prudent to suggest the use of a barrier contraceptive method while the patient is taking the **tetracycline** and until the next menses. These and other interactions of the **tetracyclines** are presented in Table 22–27.

Clinical Use and Dosing

GENITOURINARY INFECTIONS. One of the most important indications for **doxycycline** is treatment of genital *C. trachomatis* infections and nongonococcal urethritis

Table 22–27. Drug Interactions: Tetracyclines

Drug	Interacting Drug	Possible Effects	Implications
Tetracyclines	Antacids, dairy foods, iron salts, and sodium bicarbonate	Impair absorption because of formation of a poorly soluble chelate.	Take on empty stomach or separate doses by 2 h and take tetracycline first. Doxycycline and minocycline have low affinity for these and are not significantly affected by food or dairy products.
	Oral anticoagulants	Tetracyclines may increase hypoprothrombinemic effects.	Avoid concurrent administration or monitor PT/INR closely.
	Barbiturates, carbamazepine, hydantoins	Increase metabolism and decrease half-life and serum levels of doxycycline.	Antibacterial activity decreased. Avoid concurrent administration.
	Cimetidine	Decreased GI absorption of tetracyclines because of pH-dependent inhibition of dissolution.	Antibacterial activity decreased. May be true for other histamine$_2$ blockers. Avoid concurrent administration.
	Digoxin	Serum levels of digoxin increased in 10% of patients with risk for toxicity.	Effects last for months after tetracycline discontinued. Select different antibiotic class.
	Insulin	May reduce insulin requirements.	Further study needed. Monitor blood glucose closely.
	Lithium	May increase or decrease lithium levels.	Monitor serum levels closely.
	Oral contraceptives	May decrease effectiveness; breakthrough bleeding may occur.	Controversial. Suggest barrier method for women taking tetracyclines.
	Penicillin	May interfere with bactericidal action of penicillins.	Avoid concomitant administration.

INR = international normalized ratio; PT – prothrombin time.

and cervicitis. **Doxycycline** in doses of 100 mg twice daily for 7 days is a primary first-line agent because of its low cost, but it may have lower compliance than the more expensive **azithromycin**, which requires a single dose in these infections. Sexual partners should be evaluated and treated. In pregnancy, the drug of choice for these conditions is **amoxicillin** or **erythromycin**; **doxycycline** is contraindicated. **Doxycycline** (100 mg twice daily for 14 days) or **tetracycline** (500 mg four times daily for 14 days) is an alternative to **penicillin** for treatment of early primary, secondary, or latent syphilis of less than 1 year's duration. For latent syphilis of more than 1 year's duration without neurosyphilis, a longer course of treatment (28 days) is required. **Doxycycline** (100 mg twice daily for 10 days) is also indicated empirically for epididymo-orchiditis in heterosexual men less than 35 years of age where the likely pathogens are *C. trachomatis* or *N. gonorrhoeae*. Chronic prostatitis, the most common form of prostatitis, is a chronic pain syndrome of unknown etiology. Studies suggest it may have a microbial etiology, and **doxycycline** (100 mg twice daily for 14 days) is used empirically for treatment.

ACNE. Although not indicated for comedonal and mild inflammatory acne vulgaris, which are the less severe stages, **doxycycline** (100 mg twice daily), **minocycline** (50 mg twice a day), or **tetracycline** is adjunct to topical therapy in severe inflammatory acne vulgaris, manifested by comedones, papules, pustules, and possibly deep cysts. Studies have found higher prevalence of resistant organisms in households of teenagers using **oral antibiotics** for acne, so experts have recommended restriction of **oral antibiotics** in acne vulgaris to the most severe cases unresponsive to topical therapy. **Doxycycline** is an oral alternative to topical **metronidazole** in the treatment of acne rosacea.

RESPIRATORY INFECTIONS. Although treatment of ABECB is controversial, **antibiotic** treatment is recommended if the patient has two of the three cardinal symptoms: increased sputum volume, increased sputum purulence, and increased dyspnea (Niederman et al., 1998). **Doxycycline** 100 mg twice daily for 5 to 10 days may be a cost-effective treatment choice for patients who have not had recent **antibiotic** therapy and are therefore less likely to be infected with resistant organisms. In younger healthy outpatients, CAP is likely to be caused by *S. pneumoniae, M. pneumoniae, C. pneumoniae,* or *H. influenzae.* Although the pneumococcus is showing increased resistance, **tetracyclines** have activity against most likely pathogens, and **doxycycline** may be considered an alternative to **fluoroquinolones** or **macrolides** in CAP.

PEPTIC ULCER DISEASE. **Tetracycline** is a component of the first successful **multiantibiotic** regimen used for the eradication of *H. pylori* associated with peptic ulcer disease. The regimen involved 14 days of therapy with **bismuth subsalicylate** (525 mg four times daily), **metronidazole** (250 mg four times daily), and **tetracycline** (500 mg four times daily), accompanied by an H$_2$-receptor blocker for 28 days. Other **antibiotic** combinations including **tetracycline** (see Table 22–27) have also been effective in eradicating *H. pylori*. Eradication *of H. pylori* has been found to decrease the recurrence of peptic ulcer.

LYME DISEASE. **Doxycycline**, 100 mg twice daily, is a primary drug of choice for early treatment of Lyme disease, a tickborne infection caused by *B. burgdorferi*. Duration of oral treatment varies by the presenting signs: early erythema migrans (14 to 21 days), mild cardiac involvement (21 days), arthritis (28 days), and isolated facial paralysis (21 to 28 days). **Amoxicillin** is the alternative for pregnant women and children less than 8 years old, for whom **doxycycline** is contraindicated.

OTHER. **Doxycycline** is an alternative for **penicillin**-allergic patients for prophylaxis of rat, bat, raccoon, and skunk bites (Gilbert, Moellering, & Sande, 1999). The primary drug of choice for ehrlichiosis and rickettsial infections (e.g., Rocky Mountain spotted fever, typhus, Q fever, trench fever caused by *B. quintana*) is **doxycycline**. **Minocycline**, 100 mg twice daily for 6 to 8 weeks, is the drug of first choice for infections by *Mycobacterium marinum*, an infection associated with contamination by water from aquariums. **Minocycline** is also recommended for treating the meningitis carrier state, as an alternative to **sulfonamides** in nocardiosis, and in the treatment of rheumatoid arthritis (100 mg twice daily). **Tetracyclines** are first-line therapy for a number of diseases rarely seen in North America, including trachoma, cholera, and granuloma inguinale. **Doxycycline** is indicated for specific therapy when *B. anthracis* has been identified by culture and for postexposure prophylaxis to anthrax, particularly in **penicillin**-allergic patients. **Doxycycline** is also used in prophylaxis and treatment of falciparum malaria and as an adjunct in treatment of intestinal amebiasis.

Table 22–28 presents the dosage schedule of **tetracyclines.**

Rational Drug Selection

Both definitive drug selection and empiric drug selection follow the same principles described in the Rational Drug Selection section for the **penicillins**, regardless of the infection or drug class involved. When a patient with renal impairment requires a **tetracycline, doxycycline**

is preferred; it does not require dosage adjustment and lacks the antianabolic effects that increase azotemia when other **tetracyclines** are used. Another advantage of **doxycycline** and **minocycline** is decreased chelation with polyvalent cations, which allows them to be taken with meals if necessary. Additionally, these two agents also require fewer daily doses than other **tetracyclines.** Unfortunately, **tetracyclines** are contraindicated in children younger than 8 years old and during pregnancy because of bone and teeth abnormalities in the fetus and young child, as well as increased risk of hepatotoxicity during pregnancy. Besides age and pregnancy, reasons to choose alternative agents over **tetracyclines** are concurrent administration of other hepatotoxic drugs and risk of noncompliance with the complex scheduling required to avoid drug-food interactions.

Monitoring

Monitoring for therapeutic response to **antimicrobial** drugs is described in the Monitoring section for **penicillins.** All patients treated for early syphilis should have quantitative VDRL at 3, 6, 12, and 24 months after therapy, with retreatment if clinical signs recur, a fourfold increase in VDRL is sustained, or an initially high titer fails to decrease to less than 1:8 at 12 months. Long-term therapy with **tetracyclines** exceeding several weeks requires periodic hematopoietic, hepatic, and renal function tests. Because **doxycycline** is metabolized by cytochrome P-450–dependent enzymes, other drugs can induce or inhibit its metabolism. Patients should be assessed for potential interactions of other drugs with **doxycycline**, particularly inducers such as **rifampin, phenytoin, carbamazepine,** and **barbiturates** that accelerate **doxycycline** metabolism and may result in therapeutic failure. Additionally, **digoxin** assays should be obtained when a patient takes broad-spectrum **antibiotics** concurrent with **digoxin.**

Patient Education

ADMINISTRATION. Available dosage forms are given in Table 22–29. Oral solid dosing forms of **tetracyclines** should be stored in a tightly closed container in a dry environment to avoid accelerated decomposition that might result in toxic constituents. The patient should note the expiration date and dispose of outdated **tetracycline** that can cause serious toxicity. The entire prescription should be taken, with doses evenly spaced. Suspension products should be shaken before measurement of the dose with a calibrated dosing device. Although some **tetracyclines** come in liquid formulations for use by adult patients who cannot swallow solids, it should not be assumed they are indicated for children less than 8 years old. **Tetracyclines** can be particularly dangerous during pregnancy. Administer **tetracyclines** 1 hour before or 2 hours after

Table 22–28. Dosage Schedule: Tetracyclines

Drug	Indication	Dose	Comments
Doxycycline (Vibramycin)	Antibacterial	*Adult* 50–100 mg q12h *Child age >8 y* 2.2–4.4 mg/kg/d divided into 2 doses q12h	Maximal daily adult dose 500 mg for 5 d for acute gonococcal infection; 300 mg for all other infections. Shake suspension well before measurement with calibrated device. Store at room temperature for up to 14 d. Do not take this drug within 1 h of other medicines; separation of 3 h preferable. May be administered without regard to meals.
	Endocervical, rectal, or urethral infection caused by *C. trachomatis*	*Adult* 100 mg q12h for 7 d	As above.
	Epididymo-orchitis caused by *C. trachomatis* or *N. gonorrhoeae;* nongonococcal urethritis	*Adult* 100 mg q12h for 10 d	As above.
	Gonococcal infections, uncomplicated (exluding anorectal infections in men)	*Adult* 100 mg q12h for 7 d *or* 300 mg initially, then 300 mg 1 h later	As above.
	Lyme disease	*Adult* 100 mg q12h *Child age >8 y* 1–2 mg/kg q12h	As above.
	Malaria prophylaxis	*Adult* 100 mg daily beginning 1–2 wk before travel, continued through visit and for 4 wk after traveler leaves the malarious area *Child age >8 y* 2 mg/kg daily, up to 100 mg daily on same schedule as adult	As above.
	Early syphilis in penicillin-allergic patient	*Adult* 100 mg q12h for 14 d (extend to 4 wk if >1 y duration)	As above.
	Acne vulgaris	*Adults and adolescents* 100 mg bid for inflammatory form	As above.
	Acne rosacea	*Adult* 100 mg q12h	As above.
	Acute exacerbation of chronic bronchitis	*Adult* 100 mg q12h for 5–10 d	As above.
	Bite of rat, bat, raccoon (prophylaxis)	*Adults and adolescents* 100 mg q12h	As above.
Minocycline (Dynacin, Minocin)	Uncomplicated gonococcal infection	*Adult* 100 mg bid for 5 d for urethral infections in men; for other infections, 200 mg q12h for at least 4 d	Adult maximum daily dose 350 mg on day 1; then 200 mg/d. Shake oral suspension well before measuring, using calibrated device. Keep container tightly closed at room temperature.

Continued on next page

Table 22–28. Dosage Schedule: Tetracyclines *(continued)*

Drug	Indication	Dose	Comments
			Not for children <8 y. Do not take within 1–3 h of other medicines. May be taken with food if GI effects are bothersome.
	Nongonococcal urethritis caused by *C. trachomatis* or *U. urealyticum*	*Adult* 100 mg q12h for at least 7 d	As above.
	Meningococcal carrier	*Adult* 100 mg q12h for 5 d	As above.
	M. marinum	*Adult* 100 mg q12h for 6–8 wk	As above.
	Rheumatoid arthritis (off label)	*Adult* 100 mg bid	As above.
	Syphilis	*Adult* 200 mg base initially, then 100 mg q12h for 10–15 d; *or* 100–200 mg initially, then 50 mg q6h for 10–15 d	As above.
	Antibacterial, other infections	*Adult* 200 mg base initially, then 100 mg q12h; *or* 100–200 mg initially, then 50 mg q6h *Child >8 y* 4 mg base/kg initially, then 2 mg/kg q12h	As above.
Oxytetracycline (Terramycin)	Brucellosis	*Adult* 500 mg q6h for 6 wk, given concurrently with 1 g streptomycin IM q12h the first wk and once/d the second wk	Maximum daily adult dose 4 g; maximum daily pediatric dose 250 mg. Take with full glass of water. Keep container tightly closed in a dry place. Store at room temperature. Parenteral dose must be given by deep IM injection; do not administer IV. Change to oral form as soon as possible.
	Gonorrhea, uncomplicated	*Adult* 1.5 g initially, then 500 mg q6h for total of 9 g	As above.
	Syphilis	*Adult* 500 mg–1 g q6h for 10–15 d for total of 30–40 g	As above.
	Other bacterial infections	*Adult* 250–500 mg q6h *Child >8 y* 6.25–12.5 mg/kg q6h	As above.
Tetracycline (Achromycin V)	Acne	*Adult* 500 mg–2 g/d in divided doses for severe cases; gradually reduce to maintenance dose of 125 mg–1 g/d in divided doses. Alternate-day dosing or intermittent	Shake suspension well before measurement with calibrated device. Not for children <8 y. Keep container tightly closed in a dry place. Store at room temperature. Heed expiration date.

Continued on next page

Table 22–28. Dosage Schedule: Tetracyclines *(continued)*

Drug	Indication	Dose	Comments
		therapy possible if in remission.	Dispose of excess or leftover drug. Do not take within 1–3 h of other drugs. Take with full 8-oz glass of water, and stand for at least 90 s after swallowing. Take drug at least 1 h before bedtime.
	Brucellosis	*Adult* 500 mg qid for 3 wk in combination with streptomycin 1 g bid for the first wk and 1 g/d for second wk	As above.
	Gonorrhea	*Adult* 1.5 g initially, then 500 mg q6h for 4 d for total dose of 9 g	As above.
	Lyme disease (off-label use)	*Adult* 250–500 mg qid *Child >8 y* 6.25–12.5 mg/kg qid	As above.
	Syphilis	*Adult* 30–40 g over 10–15 d	As above.
	Uncomplicated rectal, urethral, or endocervical infections by *C. trachomatis*	*Adult* 500 mg qid for at least 7 d	As above.
	Other bacterial infections	*Adult* 250–500 q6h *or* 500 mg–1 g q12h *Child >8 y* 6.25–12.5 mg/kg q6h *or* 12.5–25 mg q12h	As above.
	Eradication of *H. pylori* in peptic ulcer disease	*Adult* 500 mg qid with (1) bismuth subsalicylate 525 mg qid, metronidazole 250 mg qid for 14 d, plus H$_2$ blocker for 28 d, *or* (2) metronidazole 500 mg qid for 14 d and sucralfate for 14–28 d, *or* (3) bismuth subsalicylate 525 mg qid, metronidazole 250 mg qid, and omeprazole 20 mg/d for 7–10 d	As above.

meals and give **tetracyclines** 2 hours before **antacids.** However, **doxycycline** and **minocycline** can be taken with meals if they cause GI upset when taken on an empty stomach. To avoid esophageal irritation, take **tetracyclines** at least 1 hour before meals with a full 240-mL glass of water and remain standing for at least 90 seconds after swallowing the drug.

ADVERSE REACTIONS. **Tetracyclines** can cause phototoxicity, so sunlight and tanning lights should be avoided. Wear sunscreen, hats, and protective clothing if it is necessary to be in the sun for more than a few minutes. Avoid hazardous activities and driving if dizziness, lightheadedness, or unsteadiness develops, which is most common with **minocycline.** Contact the prescriber if these symptoms interfere with activities of daily living. The patient should stop taking the **tetracycline** and contact a health care provider if headache and blurred vision develop; these are the symptoms of pseudotumor cerebri. Signs of superinfection that should be reported to the

Table 22–29. Available Dosage Forms: Tetracyclines

Drug	Dosage Form	How Supplied
Doxycycline	Capsules: 50 mg 100 mg Tablets: 100 mg	In bottles of 50, 60, 100, and 500 capsules In bottles of 10, 11, 14, 20, 50, 100, 200, and 500 capsules In bottles of 20, 28, 30, 32, 50, 200, and 500 tablets
(Doxy Caps)	Capsules: 100 mg	In bottles of 50 capsules
(Doxychel Hyclate)	Capsules: 50 mg, 100 mg Tablets: 50 mg, 100 mg	In bottles of 50 and 500 capsules In bottles of 50 and 500 tablets
(Vibramycin)	Capsules: 50 mg 100 mg Tablets: 100 mg Powder for oral suspension: 25 mg/5 cc (reconstituted) Syrup: 50 mg/5 cc	In bottles of 50 capsules In bottles of 50 and 500 capsules In bottles of 50 and 500 film-coated tablets In 60-cc bottles, raspberry flavored In 60-cc bottles
Minocycline	Capsules: 50 mg 100 mg	In bottles of 100 capsules In bottles of 50 capsules
(Dynacin)	Capsules: 50 mg 100 mg	In bottles of 100 capsules In bottles of 50 capsules
(Minocin)	Capsules: 50 mg 100 mg Oral suspension: 50 mg/5 cc	In bottles of 100 pellet-filled capsules In bottles of 50 pellet-filled capsules In 60-cc bottles, custard flavor
Oxytetracycline	Capsules: 250 mg	In bottles of 100 and 1000 capsules
(Terramycin)	Capsules: 250 mg	In bottles of 100 and 500 capsules
Tetracycline	Oral suspension: 125 mg/5 cc Capsules: 100 mg 250 mg 500 mg Tablets: 250 mg, 500 mg	In 60- and 480-cc bottles In bottles of 1000 capsules In bottles of 20, 28, 30, 40, 60, 100, 500, and 1000 capsules In bottles of 20, 28, 40, 50, 100, 500, and 1000 capsules In bottles of 30 and 60 tablets
(Sumycin)	Oral suspension: 125 mg/5 cc Capsules: 250 mg 500 mg Tablets: 250 mg 500 mg	In 473-cc bottles, fruit flavor In bottles of 100 and 1000 capsules In bottles of 100 and 500 capsules In bottles of 100 and 1000 tablets In bottles of 100 and 500 tablets

prescriber include pruritus ani, hoarseness, glossitis, sore throat, dysphagia, or vaginal itching and discharge. The patient should also report symptoms of hepatotoxicity that include upper abdominal pain, nausea, vomiting, dark urine, clay-colored stools, or yellowing of skin or eyes. Diarrhea involving six or more stools per day and blood or mucus in the stool could indicate AAPMC and require discontinuation of the **tetracycline** and consultation with the prescriber. Women of childbearing age would be prudent to use a backup barrier method of contraception during **tetracycline** therapy and until the next menses. Women on **hormone replacement** should know that broad-spectrum **antibiotics** can cause exacerbation of hot flashes and menopausal symptoms during

therapy. **Tetracyclines** can cause reversible pigmentation of skin and mucous membranes, which is more common with **minocycline.**

LIFESTYLE MANAGEMENT. See the Lifestyle Management section for the **penicillins.**

Vancomycin

Vancomycin is a narrow-spectrum **antibiotic** that forms its own class. Use of this drug has increased because of the development of organisms resistant to other drugs. Unfortunately, its widespread use led to the development of strains of **vancomycin**-resistant *Enterococcus*

(VRE) and **vancomycin**-intermediate *Staphylococcus aureus* (VISA), greatly reducing treatment options for some infections, especially nosocomial infections in hospitals. These resistant strains are being managed with combinations of **antibiotics** and recently marketed novel agents **linezolid (Zyvox)** and the streptogramin combination **quinupristin-dalfopristin (Synercid)**. Only the oral use of **vancomycin** is discussed here, although it is often used IV in hospitals.

Pharmacodynamics

Vancomycin is a tricyclic glycopeptide **antibiotic** that inhibits cell wall synthesis by binding firmly to the D-Ala-D-Ala terminus of nascent peptidoglycan pentapeptide. The end result is a weakened cell wall susceptible to lysis. The cell membrane is also damaged, contributing to the antibacterial effects.

Sensitivity

Vancomycin is active only against gram-positive bacteria, especially staphylococci. It is bactericidal for gram-positive organisms (streptococci, pneumococci, *Corynebacterium, Listeria, Lactobacilli, Actinomyces,* and *Clostridium*) and most pathogenic staphylococci, including those producing beta-lactamase, and those resistant to **nafcillin** and **methicillin** are killed by a concentration of 4 µg/mL or less. It kills staphylococci relatively slowly and only if cells are actively dividing.

Resistance

Resistance is due to a modification of the binding site of the peptidoglycan building block. This results in loss of a critical hydrogen bond that facilitates high-affinity binding of **vancomycin** to the target organism. To reduce the development of resistant strains, the CDC has recommended limiting this drug to the following uses only:

1. Avoid or minimize use in the empiric treatment of febrile patients with neutropenia unless the prevalence of MRSA or MRSE is high.
2. **Metronidazole** is the preferred initial treatment for *C. difficile* colitis.
3. Avoid or minimize use of **vancomycin** as surgical prophylaxis and for low-birth-weight infants, intravascular catheter colonization or infection, and peritoneal dialysis.

Although most of these recommendations are related to hospitalized patients, primary care providers should also limit the use of this drug.

Pharmacokinetics

Absorption and Distribution

Absorption from the GI tract is poor, although clinically significant serum concentrations have occurred. Onset of action is rapid, with peak concentrations in 1 hour and a duration of 12 hours. It is 52 to 56 percent protein bound and has less than 1 percent bioavailability by the oral route. Its half-life is 4 to 6 hours. Distribution is wide, with 20 to 30 percent penetration of the CSF. The drug crosses the placenta.

Metabolism and Excretion

Oral doses are excreted primarily in feces. IV forms are eliminated more than 90 percent by glomerulofiltration.

Pharmacotherapeutics

Precautions and Contraindications

Because of poor absorption, oral forms are unlikely to cause systemic adverse effects. However, clinically significant serum concentration may occur in some patients who have inflammatory conditions of the intestinal mucosa. Extreme care should be taken if this drug must be administered to these patients. **Vancomycin** is ototoxic, with increased risk for these problems in older adults, who may have an underlying hearing loss. It should be used with extreme caution in this population.

Oral *vancomycin* is listed as Pregnancy Category B; however, the only studies done were with IV *vancomycin*, and they did not show fetal harm. Given the lack of studies with the oral form, *vancomycin* should be given only when clearly needed.

Vancomycin is excreted in breast milk, although concentrations in breast milk during oral administration are low. Exercise caution when giving to a nursing mother. Its safety and efficacy in children have not been established.

Adverse Drug Reactions

Vancomycin therapy can lead to serious ototoxicity that may be transient or permanent. It has occurred most often in patients with IV high doses, who have underlying hearing loss, or who are receiving concomitant therapy with another ototoxic drug. Serial test of auditory function may be helpful to minimize this adverse reaction. Reversible neutropenia has occurred. Skin rash is the most common adverse effect with oral therapy.

Drug Interactions

The only significant interaction between oral **vancomycin** and drugs used in primary care occur with drugs that also have ototoxic or neurotoxic effects. The concomitant administration increases the risk and is to be avoided.

Clinical Use and Dosing

Vancomycin (Vancocin) is used to treat **antibiotic-associated diarrhea or AAPMC** caused by *C. difficile*. It is also used to treat staphylococcal enterocolitis. It is not effective in any other intestinal infections or in systemic infections. Adult dosages are 125 to 500 mg every 6 hours for 7 to 10 days. The maximum daily adult dosage is 2 g. Studies have indicated that the higher dosages result in fecal concentrations far in excess of the MIC and that the 125-mg dose is as effective as higher doses. Dosage for children is 10 mg/kg, up to 125 mg, every 6 hours. Recurrences, which develop in approximately 25 percent of treated patients, may be treated with a second course of oral **vancomycin**, oral **metronidazole**, or oral **bacitracin**.

Because of the cost and potential for resistance with **vancomycin**, the CDC recommends **metronidazole** as the first choice for treating AAPMC. **Cholestyramine** resin has been shown to bind *C. difficile* toxins in vitro and may be used as monotherapy or in conjunction with **antibiotics**.

Vancomycin is available for oral administration in pulvules at 125-mg and 250-mg formulations. It is also available as a powder for reconstitution as a solution of 250 mg/5 mL or 500 mg/6 mL. The more concentrated solution contains ethanol. The solution must be refrigerated after reconstitution and will maintain potency for 14 days. It should be dispensed with a calibrated measuring device.

Monitoring

Positive response to therapy will be manifested in cessation of diarrhea and associated symptoms. Proctosigmoidoscopy and/or colonoscopy may be useful to document the presence of pseudomembranous colitis or relapse in patients with persistent symptoms. Enzyme immunoassay of stool samples for the presence of *C. difficile* toxins may remain positive after treatment, so follow-up cultures and toxin assays are not recommended if clinical improvement is complete. Renal function determinations may be warranted periodically during therapy in patients with renal function impairment or inflammatory disorders of the intestinal mucosa. In these patients, a white blood cell (WBC) count or audiometry may also be monitored during extended or repeat therapy to detect neutropenia.

Patient Education

ADMINISTRATION. If **cholestyramine** is used in conjunction with **vancomycin**, the medications should be administered several hours apart because **cholestyramine** also binds oral **vancomycin** and prevents its effectiveness. The oral solution can cause a bitter or unpleasant taste and mouth irritation and should be followed by a full glass of water. Oral **vancomycin** can be taken without regard to meals. If the patient is too ill for oral therapy, **vancomycin** solution may be administered by enema, long intestinal tube, or directly into a colonoscopy or ileostomy. **Vancomycin** can also be administered IV for colitis because 6 to 15 percent of parenteral **vancomycin** is excreted in the feces. However, IV **vancomycin** is considerably more dangerous than oral-local use.

ADVERSE REACTIONS. Skin rashes may occur and, if serious, should be reported to the health care provider. Patients with renal impairment or inflammatory colitis should report evidence of ototoxicity (loss of hearing; ringing, buzzing or fullness in ears; dizziness), neutropenia (chills, coughing, difficult breathing, sore throat, fever), or nephrotoxicity (altered frequency or amount of urine, nausea or vomiting, increased thirst, difficult breathing, weakness).

LIFESTYLE MANAGEMENT. Mild cases of *C. difficile* colitis may respond to discontinuation of medication alone. Moderate to severe cases require fluid, electrolyte, and protein replacement. If diarrhea is present, administration of an **antiperistaltic antidiarrheal** (e.g., **atropine** and **diphenoxylate, loperamide, opioids**) is contraindicated because it may delay the elimination of toxins from the colon, thereby prolonging or worsening the condition. Good perianal hygiene will improve patient comfort during this illness.

Antimycobacterials

Mycobacterial infections are among the most difficult to cure because mycobacteria (1) grow slowly and are relatively resistant to drugs that are largely dependent on how rapidly cells are dividing, (2) have a lipid-rich cell wall relatively impermeable to many drugs, (3) are usually intracellular and inaccessible to drugs that do not have good intracellular penetration, (4) have the ability to go into a dormant state, and (5) easily develop resistance to any single drug. Tuberculosis, an example of mycobacterial infection, is a worldwide public health issue. In addition to drug-organism issues, adherence is often poor to treatment regimens that include multiple drugs and last for months.

Despite these problems, drug combinations have proved effective in the treatment of mycobacterial disease. Drugs used to treat tuberculosis include first-line drugs (**isoniazid [INH], rifampin [RIF, Rifadin, Ri-**

mactane], ethambutol [EMB, Myambutol], pyrazinamide [PZA], and **streptomycin**) and second-line drugs used for retreatment or recurrent disease (**para-aminosalicylic acid [PASA], ethionamide [Trecator-SC], and capreomycin [Capastat]**). Rifabutin (Mycobutin) is used mainly to treat or prevent MAC. Each of these drugs is discussed in this section. Management of tuberculosis is further discussed in Chapter 43, and HIV infection is discussed in Chapter 35.

Pharmacodynamics

Sensitivity

Isoniazid is the most active drug for the treatment of tuberculosis. It interferes with lipid and nucleic acid biosynthesis in growing organisms. It is also thought that **isoniazid** and **ethambutol** inhibit synthesis of mycolic acids. These acids are important constituents for mycobacteria cell walls but are not found in mammalian cells, which explains this high selectivity. This drug is bactericidal against susceptible mycobacteria.

Rifampin binds to the beta subunit of mycobacteria DNA-dependent RNA polymerase and inhibits RNA synthesis. Antimycobacterial action results in destruction of both multiplying and inactive bacilli. It readily penetrates most tissues and can kill bacteria that are poorly accessible to many other drugs. This drug is bactericidal against susceptible mycobacteria. Rifampin also has activity against *N. gonorrhoeae, Staphylococcus, Mycobacterium leprae* (the cause of leprosy), MAC, and *H. influenzae* type b.

Ethambutol inhibits synthesis of arabinogalactan, an essential component of mycobacteria cell walls. It also arrests cell multiplication, causing cell death. **Ethambutol** enhances the activity of lipophilic drugs such as **rifampin** and **ofloxacin** that cross the mycobacteria cell wall primarily in lipid portions of this wall. It is bacteriostatic against susceptible mycobacteria.

Pyrazinamide, an analogue of **nicotinamide**, is among the least expensive of the drugs in this class. The mechanism of action is unknown, but, although inactive in a neutral pH, at a pH of 5.5 it is bactericidal against tubercle bacilli and some other mycobacteria at concentrations of approximately 20 µg/cc.

Streptomycin is an **aminoglycoside** used now almost exclusively to treat *M. tuberculosis* infections. It is added as a fourth drug to the treatment regimen because up to 80 percent of patients treated with this drug harbor resistant bacilli after 4 months of treatment. Other mycobacteria except MAC and *Mycobacterium kansasii* are resistant to **streptomycin.** This drug is an irreversible inhibitor of protein synthesis. It penetrates cells poorly but is bactericidal in an alkaline extracellular environment.

Para-aminosalicylic acid, structurally similar to para-aminobenzoic acid (PABA) and the **sulfonamides,** is a folate synthesis antagonist that is active almost exclusively against *M. tuberculosis*. It is bacteriostatic. It is not used frequently because primary resistance is common and newer drugs are better tolerated. It will not be discussed further.

Ethionamide is chemically related to **isoniazid** and also blocks the synthesis of mycolic acids. It is bacteriostatic against *M. tuberculosis,* and this drug also inhibits some other *Mycobacterium* species.

Capreomycin, a peptide **antibiotic,** inhibits RNA synthesis, thereby decreasing the replication of tubercle bacilli. Because resistance easily develops when it is given alone, it is given as part of a multidrug regimen. It is bactericidal to susceptible mycobacteria.

Rifabutin is a semisynthetic **ansamycin antibiotic** derived from **rifamycin.** It inhibits DNA-dependent RNA polymerase in susceptible mycobacteria and some other organisms. Prevention of disseminated MAC in HIV-infected patients is its main use. Up to 25 percent of **rifampin** resistant strains of *M. tuberculosis* will be susceptible to **rifabutin,** and it may also be used in this instance.

Resistance

Resistance to **isoniazid** has been associated with excessive production of the product of the *inhA* gene and with mutation or deletion of *katG*, which encodes mycobacterium catalase. *InhA* mutants have low-level resistance and cross-resistance to **ethionamide.** The *katG* mutants have high-level resistance but no cross-resistance. Resistant mutants occur with a frequency of about 1 per 10^6 bacilli. Resistant mutants are selected out if this drug is given alone. Single-drug therapy with **isoniazid** has resulted in 10 to 20 percent prevalence of resistant strains in clinical isolates from the Caribbean and Southeast Asia. Only about 8 to 10 percent of organisms in the United States are resistant to this drug.

Resistance to **rifampin** and **rifabutin** results from point mutations that prevent binding of the drug to RNA polymerase. Cross-resistance often exists between these **rifamycins.**

The mechanism of resistance is unknown for **ethambutol,** but it develops rapidly when used as monotherapy. Resistance to **ethionamide** also develops rapidly when it is used as monotherapy.

Resistance also develops rapidly to **pyrazinamide,** but there is no cross-resistance to other **antimycobacterial drugs** so that it can be given to patients exposed to a case of multidrug-resistant tuberculosis. **Capreomycin** is also useful for treatment of drug-resistant tuberculosis because of its lack of cross-resistance to first-line drugs.

Point mutation that alters the ribosomal binding site is the mechanism of resistance for **streptomycin.**

Pharmacokinetics

Absorption and Distribution

All oral **antimycobacterials** are rapidly and well absorbed in the GI tract after oral administration. **Rifampin** and **rifabutin** need to be taken on an empty stomach. High-fat meals slow the rate of absorption but not the extent. The injectable drugs are rapidly absorbed in muscle tissue but not from the GI tract.

Isoniazid readily diffuses into all body fluid including CSF (90% of serum levels), pleural, and ascitic; tissues; organs; and saliva, sputum, and feces. It also crosses the placenta and enters breast milk.

Rifampin and **ethambutol** also penetrate and concentrate in most body fluids. Adequate penetration of CSF occurs only in the presence of inflamed meninges. They both cross the placenta and enter breast milk.

Pyrazinamide is widely distributed in body tissues and fluids including the liver and lung, and it reaches high concentrations in CSF. It enters breast milk.

Streptomycin and **capreomycin** are widely distributed through extracellular fluid, cross the placenta, and enter breast milk in small amounts. They have poor CSF penetration except in the presence of inflamed meninges.

Ethionamide is widely distributed to body tissues and fluids. CSF concentrations are equal to those in the serum.

Rifabutin is highly lipophilic and distributes in most body fluids and intracellular tissues.

Metabolism and Excretion

The metabolism of **isoniazid** is highly variable and dependent on acetylator status. The liver, in a process that is genetically controlled, primarily acetylates it. Fast acetylators metabolize this drug five to six times faster than slow acetylators do. Approximately 50 percent of blacks and whites are slow acetylators, and the rest are rapid acetylators. The majority of Alaskan natives and Asians are rapid acetylators. The rate of acetylation does not alter effectiveness but may increase the risk for toxic reactions in slow acetylators. Rapid clearance is of no consequence when the drug is given daily but may result in subtherapeutic doses when given once weekly. **Isoniazid** metabolites and unchanged drug are excreted in the urine. Elimination is largely independent of renal function.

Rifampin is also metabolized in the liver by deacetylation, and the metabolite is also active against *M. tuberculosis.* With repeated administration, the half-life decreases. It is excreted mainly through the liver into bile; then, through enterohepatic recirculation, the remainder is excreted in feces, with a small amount excreted in urine.

About 20 percent of **ethambutol** is metabolized by the liver, and it is mainly excreted as unchanged drug in the urine. Marked accumulation may occur in renal failure.

Pyrazinamide is hydrolyzed by the liver to a metabolite that also has antimycobacterial activity. Its half-life may be significantly prolonged in the presence of impaired renal or hepatic function. Approximately 70 percent of the oral dose is excreted in urine by glomerular filtration. **Streptomycin** and **capreomycin** are excreted almost exclusively by the kidney.

Approximately 35 percent of **ethionamide** is metabolized by the liver, and the majority of the drug is excreted in urine as inactive metabolites. Less than 1 percent is excreted as unchanged drug.

Hepatic insufficiency or the age of the patient alters the pharmacokinetics of **rifabutin** only slightly. Somewhat reduced drug distribution and faster drug elimination are seen in renal insufficiency and may result in decreased drug concentrations.

Table 22–30 presents the pharmacokinetics of selected **antimycobacterials.**

Pharmacotherapeutics

Precautions and Contraindications

Cautious use in renal impairment is recommended for **isoniazid, ethambutol, streptomycin,** and **capreomycin.** Dosage adjustments may be required and are discussed in the Clinical Use and Dosing section. Special monitoring is also discussed in that section.

Cautious use in the presence of hepatic impairment is recommended for **isoniazid, rifampin** (hepatotoxic), **pyrazinamide,** and **ethionamide** (hepatotoxic). Black and Hispanic women, women postpartum, and patients older than 50 are at special risk for the development of hepatitis while taking **isoniazid.**

Ethionamide should be given cautiously to patients with diabetes mellitus. Management may be more difficult and hepatitis is more likely in these patients. Hematologic alterations including various anemias and thrombocytopenia have been seen with the use of **isoniazid** and **rifampin.** These drugs should be used cautiously in patients prone to these problems for other reasons. **Ethambutol** and **pyrazinamide** each may precipitate gouty arthritis attacks and should be used cautiously in the presence of this disorder.

Pregnancy categories vary by drug. *Ethambutol* **is Pregnancy Category B and has been used in pregnant women without adverse effects on the fetus. The others are Pregnancy Category C. Often the effect of the drug on the fetus is unknown, or the problem has occurred in animal studies. Using any of the Pregnancy Category C drugs requires consideration of the benefit to the woman patient versus the potential risk to the fetus.** *Streptomycin* **may cause congenital deaf-**

Table 22–30. Pharmacokinetics: Selected Antimycobacterials

Drug	Onset	Peak	Duration	Protein Binding	Bioavailability	Half-Life	Elimination
Capreomycin (IM)	Rapid	1–2 h	UA	UA	UA	4–6 h	52% unchanged in urine within 12 h
Ethambutol	Rapid	2–4 h	24 h	UA	69–85%	3–4 h*	50% metabolized by liver; 50% unchanged in urine
Ethionamide	Rapid	3 h	UA	10%	100%	2–3 h	Metabolized by liver; <1% unchanged in urine
Isoniazid (PO/IM)	Rapid	1–2 h	24 h	80%	UA	1–4 h	50% metabolized by liver; 50% unchanged in urine
Pyrazinamide	Rapid	2 h	UA	UA	UA	9–10 h*	70% metabolites in urine within 24 h
Rifampin	Rapid	2–4 h	24 h	88–90%	90–95%	1–5 h†	40–60% in bile and by enterohepatic circulation
Rifabutin	Rapid	2–4 h	24 h	85%	20%	45 h	30% in feces; 53% as metabolites in urine
Streptomycin (IM)	Rapid	0.5–1.5 h	UA	34–62%	UA	2–3 h*	>90% in urine

*Increased in renal or hepatic impairment.
†Varies by dose and averages 2–3 h after repeated doses.

ness if given to pregnant women and is Pregnancy Category D.

For the drugs that appear in breast milk, the infant should be observed for any evidence of adverse effects. Discontinuing the drug must take into account the importance of the drug for the mother. The drugs that enter breast milk in smaller amounts include **rifampin** and **pyrazinamide**. **Capreomycin** is excreted in such small amounts as to be undetectable in some women.

Use in children varies by drug. Pediatric doses are listed for all of these drugs, but the age under which they should not be used varies. No age restrictions are provided for **isoniazid, rifampin,** and **pyrazinamide. Ethambutol** is not recommended for use by children under age 13 years. Safety and optimal dosage have not been determined for children for **ethionamide** and **capreomycin.** Ototoxicity risk precludes use of **streptomycin** in neonates and in older adults or patients with diminished hearing.

Adverse Drug Reactions

All of the **antimycobacterial drugs** have risks for hypersensitivity reactions, some of which may be severe. The usual management associated with these reactions applies here as well.

Peripheral neuropathy is the most common adverse reaction with **isoniazid.** It occurs in about 2 percent of patients taking 5 mg/kg a day. Prevalence is higher for patients taking higher doses, up to about 44 percent for patients taking 24 mg/kg a day. The symptoms include symmetrical numbness and tingling in the extremities. Patients predisposed to this adverse reaction include the malnourished, slow acetylators, pregnant women, older adults, diabetics, and patients with chronic liver disease, including alcoholics. **Pyridoxine (B_6)** prevents the development of peripheral neuropathy and is recommended at minimum for patients in these at-risk categories. Some providers use **pyridoxine** for all patients on **isoniazid.** Recommended prophylactic doses range from 6 to 50 mg daily, with the lower doses of 6 to 25 mg more common. Treatment of established neuropathy requires 50 to 200 mg daily.

Hepatotoxicity occurs in 10 to 20 percent of patients taking **isoniazid.** Patients at risk were discussed previously. The symptoms are those usually associated with the development of hepatitis, including abnormal liver function studies, jaundice, and fatigue. The frequency of progressive liver damage increases with age. Concurrent **alcohol** use increases the risk. When **rifampin** is given concurrently, the risk is increased fourfold.

Other adverse reactions associated with **isoniazid** include blood dyscrasias, metabolic acidosis, gynecomastia, and hypocalcemia related to altered vitamin D metabolism.

The most common adverse reactions associated with **rifampin** are GI in nature: anorexia, nausea, vomiting, diarrhea, flatulence, and abdominal pain. Although less common than with **isoniazid,** hepatotoxicity leading to hepatitis also occurs with the use of **rifampin.** A harmless orange-red discoloration of body fluids including tears, saliva, urine, sweat, CSF, and feces also occurs. Hematuria should not be confused with this discoloration because it may be an indication of a hypersensitivity reaction.

Other adverse reactions associated with **rifampin** include blood dyscrasias, headache, drowsiness and inability to concentrate, a pruritic rash (1 to 5% of patients), visual disturbances, and exudative conjunctivitis.

Ethambutol also has the usual GI disturbances, but the most serious adverse reaction is optic neuritis, which appears to be dose-related. Signs and symptoms include decreased visual acuity, red-green color blindness, diminished visual fields, and sometimes loss of vision. These adverse reactions are generally reversible when the drug is discontinued promptly. In rare cases, recovery may take up to 1 year. Vision testing should be done before and throughout therapy.

Other adverse reactions include precipitation of gouty arthritis related to elevated uric acid levels, transient impairment of liver function, and infrequent peripheral neuropathy.

The principal adverse reaction with **pyrazinamide** is dose-related hepatotoxicity that may appear anytime during therapy. Patients at risk for this adverse reaction are the same ones mentioned in the Precautions and Contraindications section. Discontinuing the drug may be required. Because this drug inhibits the renal excretion of urates, hyperuricemia also often occurs. It is often asymptomatic but may precipitate acute gouty arthritis. Baseline serum uric acid levels should be drawn.

The most serious adverse effect associated with **streptomycin** and **capreomycin** is ototoxicity. Damage to the eighth cranial nerve results in vertigo, nausea, vomiting, and hearing loss. The risk is increased with higher doses and longer duration of therapy. Nephrotoxicity is also a serious risk for patients on any **aminoglycoside.** Risk for this adverse reaction increases for patients with renal insufficiency and for older adults with age-related decreased renal function. Dosage adjustments are made based on renal function studies to reduce the risk for this adverse reaction. Doses taken two or three times weekly rather than daily doses also reduce the risk for toxicity.

Ethionamide has few adverse reactions, but it is often poorly tolerated because of its most common adverse reaction, GI distress. Some patients develop a metallic taste in their mouths. Other common adverse reactions include hepatitis (rare), optic neuritis, and peripheral neuritis (common). Neurological symptoms can be alleviated by **pyridoxine.**

Rifabutin has been associated with neutropenia and thrombocytopenia. Other adverse reactions include rash (4%) and GI intolerance (3%).

Drug Interactions

Drug interactions and drug-food interactions vary by drug. Many are associated with increasing the common adverse reactions for the particular **antimycobacterial.** Some are associated with reduced effectiveness of the interacting drug. **Rifampin** is an inducer of cytochrome P-450–dependent enzymes and speeds the metabolism of many drugs, resulting in therapeutic failure. Table 22–31 provides a list of the drug interactions.

Clinical Use and Dosing

Resistance to **antimycobacterial drugs** has a frequency of about 1 bacillus in 10^6. However, with 10^8 bacilli lesions in an infected person, resistant mutants are selected out when only one drug is given. For this reason, multiple drugs with independent actions are given so that prevalence of resistance is low with drug combinations. Drug selection and dosing for mycobacterial disease is discussed in Chapters 35 and 43.

Table 22–32 presents the dosage schedule for selected **antimycobacterials.**

Rational Drug Selection

Rifampin is used to treat several nonmycobacterial infections. It is used as prophylaxis for close contacts of people with meningococcal infections caused by *N. meningitidis,* including household members, children and personnel in nurseries and daycare centers, and closed populations such as college dormitories and military recruits. Health care personnel with intimate exposure to index cases (such as mouth-to-mouth resuscitation) should receive prophylactic therapy. Prophylaxis for adults is oral **rifampin** 600 mg every 12 hours for four doses. The dose for children is 10 mg/kg every 12 hours for four doses. **Rifampin** is also indicated for prophylaxis for close contacts of people with actual or suspected infections with *H. influenzae* type b. If one of the contacts in a household is an unvaccinated child age 4 years or younger, it is recommended that all contacts in the household except pregnant women receive prophylaxis. In daycare attended by unvaccinated children younger than age 2 years, prophylaxis with **rifampin** 20 mg/kg up to 600 mg for four doses for all contacts and vaccination of all unvaccinated children should be considered. If all contacts are older than 2 years, prophylaxis is not indicated. If there have been two or more cases in the center within 60 days and unvaccinated children at-

Table 22–31. Drug Interactions: Selected Antimycobacterials

Drug	Interacting Drug	Possible Effect	Implications
Capreomycin	Aminoglycosides and other ototoxic and nephrotoxic drugs	Additive ototoxicity and nephrotoxicity.	Avoid concurrent use.
	Isoniazid, ethionamide	Additive CNS effects; increased risk for peripheral neuropathy.	If symptoms occur, discontinue one of the drugs.
	Phenytoin	Inhibition of phenytoin metabolism; increased toxicity risk.	Monitor serum levels of phenytoin.
Ethambutol	Other neurotoxic drugs	Additive neurotoxicity.	Avoid concurrent use.
	Aluminum salts	Reduced absorption of ethambutol.	Administer ethambutol 1–2 h before aluminum salt.
Isoniazid	Alcohol	Daily ingestion increases risk for hepatitis.	Avoid concurrent use.
	Aluminum salts	Reduced oral absorption of isoniazid.	Administer isoniazid 1–2 h before aluminum salts.
	Oral anticoagulants	Enhanced anticoagulant activity.	Avoid concurrent use or monitor PT/INR.
	Benzodiazepines (BDZs)	Isoniazid may inhibit metabolic clearance of BDZs that undergo oxidative metabolism (e.g., diazepam, triazolam).	Avoid concurrent use.
	Carbamazepine	Toxicity or hepatotoxicity may occur.	Monitor carbamazepine drug levels and liver function.
	Disulfiram	Acute behavioral and coordination changes.	Avoid coadministration.
	Hydantoins	Increased serum hydantoin levels because of inhibition of CYP-450 enzymes. Most significant in slow acetylators.	Monitor hydantoin levels and adjust doses as needed.
	Ketoconazole	Decreased serum ketoconazole levels; decreased antifungal activity.	Select different antifungal.
	Meperidine	Hypotension or CNS depression.	Select different pain management.
	Rifampin	Increased risk for hepatotoxicity.	If alterations in liver function tests, discontinue one of these drugs.
	Tyramine-containing foods	Isoniazid has slight monoamine oxidase inhibition activity.	Teach patient foods to avoid.
	Histamine-containing foods	Diamine oxidase may be inhibited.	Teach patient foods to avoid (e.g., tuna, sauerkraut, yeast extract).
Pyrazinamide	Laboratory interactions	Has been reported to interfere with Acetest and Ketostix urine tests to produce a pink-brown color.	Select different method of determining ketoacidosis.
Rifampin, rifabutin	Acetaminophen, oral anticoagulants, barbiturates, BDZs beta blockers, chloramphenicol, clofibrate, oral contraceptives, corticosteroids, cyclosporine, digitoxin, disopyramide, estrogens, hydantoins, methadone, mexiletine, quinidine, sulfonylureas, theophylline, tocainide, verapamil	Rifampin induces CYP-450 enzyme systems that metabolize these drugs. Therapeutic effects of these drugs decreased.	If patient must take one of the interacting drugs, select different antimycobacterial.

Continued on next page

Table 22–31. Drug Interactions: Selected Antimycobacterials *(continued)*

Drug	Interacting Drug	Possible Effect	Implications
	Digoxin	Decreased serum levels of digoxin.	Monitor serum levels or select different antimycobacterial.
	Enalapril	Significant increase in blood pressure.	Occurred in 1 patient. Monitor.
	Isoniazid	Increased risk for hepatotoxicity.	See isoniazid above.
	Ketoconazole	Decreased ketoconazole levels; decreased antifungal activity.	Select different antifungal.
	Laboratory interactions	Therapeutic levels of rifampin interfere with standard assays of serum folate and B_{12}.	Consider alternative methods for determining concentrations.
Streptomycin	Cephalosporins, vancomycin	Increased risk of nephrotoxicity.	Monitor renal function.
	Loop diuretics	Increased risk for ototoxicity. Hearing loss may be irreversible.	Avoid concurrent use.
	Polypeptide antibiotics	Increased risk of respiratory paralysis and renal dysfunction.	Avoid concurrent use. Select different antimycobacterial.

INR = international normalized ratio; PT = prothrombin time.

tend, prophylaxis is recommended for children and personnel. **Rifampin** is also used off label in the treatment of leprosy and concurrently with other antistaphylococcal agents in the treatment of serious infections in hospitalized patients caused by *Staphylococcus,* including **methicillin**-resistant and multidrug-resistant strains.

Patient Education

Use of **rifampin** and other **antimycobacterial agents** in mycobacterial infections is described in Chapters 35 and 43. Because of the long duration of therapy in tuberculosis infections, instruction and support are essential. Multidrug therapy, essential to prevent development of resistance, presents serious challenges for adherence. Directly observed therapy (DOT), in which each dose is observed by a health care provider or other designated person, has proved very effective in promoting compliance and improving response to therapy. Lifestyle implications of tuberculosis include general health promotion strategies such as good nutrition, rest, and appropriate exercise. Dosages, monitoring, and patient education are summarized in Table 22–32; available dosage forms are given in Table 22–33.

Antivirals

Viral infections range from the annoying but short-lived and self-limiting "common cold" to the progressive and, to date, incurable HIV. Discussion in this section focuses on **nucleoside analogues** used to treat herpesvirus infections and agents used to prevent and treat influenza. Chapter 35 discusses drugs to treat HIV.

Viruses are obligate intracellular parasites that depend on use of the host cell's genetic material for replication. As a result, **antiviral drugs** must either block entry into the cells or be active inside host cells to be effective. The activity of these drugs is usually nonselective to viral components, and so damage to host cells as well as virus results. To further complicate treatment, replication of the virus peaks at or before clinical symptoms appear in many viral infections, so that optimal clinical efficacy depends on early recognition and treatment or prevention. Finally, many viruses depend on enzymes to reproduce and can quickly mutate in the presence of drug therapy.

Viral replication consists of several steps: (1) adsorption to and penetration into susceptible cells, (2) uncoating of viral nucleic acid, (3) synthesis of early, regulatory proteins, (4) synthesis of RNA or DNA, (5) synthesis of late, structural proteins, (6) assembly of viral particles, and (7) release from the cell. **Antiviral drugs** are targeted at these steps. Many of the currently available **antiviral agents** act on synthesis of purine and pyrimidine (step 4).

Nucleoside Analogues

Pharmacodynamics

The **nucleoside analogues** are used mainly to treat herpes infections. **Acyclovir (Zovirax)** is an acyclic guanosine derivative that requires three phosphorylation steps for activation. It is first converted to the monophosphate derivative by the *virus-specific* thymidine kinase and then to the

Table 22–32. Dosage Schedule: Selected Antimycobacterials

Drug	Indication	Initial Dose	Comments
Capreomycin (Capastat)	Tuberculosis, as part of combined drug therapy	1 g IM daily for 60–120 d, then 1 g 2–3 times/wk	Maximum adult daily dose 20 mg/kg. Monitor renal function tests, audiograms, vestibular function, and sites of injection at baseline and at least weekly. Serum potassium should be measured at baseline and monthly during daily therapy. Administer deep IM into large muscle mass because superficial injections associated with pain and sterile abscess. Administer within 24 h of reconstitution. Store in refrigerator after reconstitution. Darkening of reconstituted drug from initial nearly colorless or straw color does not affect potency. Renal impairment requires decreased dose (see package insert). Educate patients to report altered hearing, dizziness, imbalance; altered urination, nausea, vomiting, or thirst. Patients should advise prescribers they are taking capreomycin because of its potential for drug interactions.
Ethambutol (Myambutol)	Tuberculosis, as part of combined drug therapy	*Adult* Orally 15–25 mg/kg/d; *or* 50 mg/kg up to 2.5 g twice/wk; *or* 25–30 mg/kg 3 times/wk *Child* <13 y No dosage established, but should be considered for children with organisms resistant to other drugs and susceptible to ethambutol; not recommended for children <6 y in whom visual acuity cannot be monitored	Maximum adult daily dose 2.5 g. Impairment of renal function may require a decreased dosage. Monitor visual fields and red-green discrimination prior to and monthly during treatment, especially for prolonged therapy or >15 mg/kg daily. Periodic uric acid and renal function tests. Educate about importance of vision monitoring. Blurred vision, eye pain, vision loss, or problems with red-green discrimination should be reported. Other reportable symptoms include evidence of peripheral neuropathy (numbness, tingling, burning pain, weakness in hands or feet), gout (chills, pain and swelling of joints, hot skin over affected joints), and hypersensitivity (rash, fever, joint aches). Take drug with food if GI irritation occurs.

Continued on next page

Table 22–32. Dosage Schedule: Selected Antimycobacterials *(continued)*

Drug	Indication	Initial Dose	Comments
	Atypical mycobacterial infections (off label)	Orally 15–25 mg/kg/d	As above.
Ethionamide (Trecator-SC)	Tuberculosis, as part of combined drug therapy	*Adult* 250 mg q8–12h for 1–2 y or more *Child* 4–5 mg/kg q8h	Maximal daily adult dose 1 g. Children have required 20 mg/kg/d, but maximal daily dose for children is 750 mg. For the approximately 30% of patients unable to tolerate therapeutic dose, dosage is reduced by 2 to 1. Monitor liver function tests periodically. Ophthalmic examinations if symptoms of visual impairment. Orthostatic blood pressure checks. Thyroid function tests if signs of hypothyroidism; serum glucose if signs of hypoglycemia. Neurological exam for peripheral neuritis. Pyridoxine decreases risk of peripheral neuropathy. Report signs of hepatitis (yellow eyes or skin, upper abdominal pain, malaise), peripheral neuritis (numbness, tingling, burning pain, weakness in hands or feet), optic neuritis (blurred vision, eye pain), hypoglycemia (poor concentration, tachycardia, hunger, shakiness), or hypothyroidism (weight gain; dry, puffy skin; coldness; irregular menses). Administer with or after meals if GI irritation occurs. Usually administered after evening meal or at bedtime as a single dose. Serum concentrations may be higher with divided doses, but GI irritation may worsen. Rectal suppositories cause fewer adverse effects, but may cause local irritation.
	Atypical mycobacterial infections (off label) or leprosy (off label)	*Adult* 250 mg q8–12h	As above.
Isoniazid (Laniazid)	Tuberculosis prophylaxis	*Adults* PO or IM 300 mg/d *Child* 10 mg/kg, up to 300 mg, once daily	Maximal adult daily dose 300 mg. Renal impairment does not usually require dosage adjustment if serum creatinine is <6 mg/dL and patient is fast acetylator. For slow acetylators, adjust dose to maintain plasma concentration <1 μg/mL at 24 h after last dose. Monitor liver function tests

Continued on next page

Table 22–32. Dosage Schedule: Selected Antimycobacterials *(continued)*

Drug	Indication	Initial Dose	Comments
			monthly, or more often if liver impairment or clinical signs of hepatitis or prodromal symptoms. CBC and platelet count periodically or at signs of blood dyscrasia (fever, sore throat, bleeding or bruising, tiredness). Ophthalmic exam if signs of optic neuritis. Educate to report signs of clinical hepatitis (dark urine, yellow eyes or skin), hepatitis prodromal symptoms (anorexia, nausea and vomiting, unusual tiredness), optic neuritis (blurred vision or loss of vision, with or without eye pain), or peripheral neuropathy (numbness, clumsiness, burning pain of hands or feet). High risk for peripheral neuropathy (pregnant, high alcohol use, taking anticonvulsants, poor diet, malnourished, history of neuritis, chronic renal failure, diabetes, and over 65) indicates 25 mg pyridoxine/d. May be taken with meals or antacids if GI irritation occurs, but do not take within 1 h of aluminum-containing antacid. Measure syrup with calibrated measuring device. Crystals may form at low temperatures, but they redissolve upon warming to room temperature.
	Tuberculosis, as part of combined drug therapy	*Adults* PO or IM 300 mg once daily *or* 15 mg/kg, up to 900 mg, given 2–3 times/wk *Child* 10 mg/kg, up to 300 mg, once daily, *or* 20–40 mg/kg, up to 900 mg, given 2–3 times/wk	As above.
Pyrazinamide	Tuberculosis, as part of combined drug therapy	*Adults and children* 15–30 mg/kg once daily *or* 50–70 mg/kg 2–3 times/wk; patients with HIV take 20–30 mg/kg/d for first 2 mo	Maximal adult and pediatric daily dosage is 2 g when taken daily, 3 g when taken 3 times/wk, 4 g when taken twice/wk. Monitor liver function tests prior to and every 2–4 wk during treatment. Uric acid determinations may be needed. Educate that arthralgia is usually mild and self-limiting and to report signs of hepatotoxicity (dark urine, anorexia, nausea, vomiting, yellow skin or eyes) and gout (pain, swelling, heat over joints). May be taken without regard to meals.

Continued on next page

Table 22–32. Dosage Schedule: Selected Antimycobacterials *(continued)*

Drug	Indication	Initial Dose	Comments
Rifampin	Tuberculosis, as part of combined drug therapy	*Adult* 600 mg PO once daily *or* 10 mg/kg up to 600 mg 2–3 times/wk *Infants <1 mo* 10–20 mg/kg PO once daily *or* 10–20 mg/kg 2–3 times/wk	Maximum adult or pediatric daily oral dose should not exceed 600 mg. Severe hepatic impairment requires 50% reduction in dosages. Monitor hepatic function prior to and at least monthly during treatment; CBC if signs of blood dyscrasia (sore throat, bleeding, bruising). Advise patients to report signs of hepatotoxicity (dark urine, anorexia, nausea, vomiting, yellow skin or eyes), flulike syndrome, or blood dyscrasias. Reddish-orange or reddish-brown discoloration may stain clothes or soft contact lenses but is otherwise harmless. Avoid alcohol, which can increase hepatotoxicity. Advise health care providers of rifampin use because of high risk of drug interactions. May be taken without regard to meals. Shake suspension before measurement, using calibrated dosing device. Store suspension at controlled room temperature and discard remaining liquid 30 d after reconstitution.
	Meningococcal meningitis prophylaxis	*Adult* 600 mg PO once/d for 4 d *Child* 5 mg/kg q12h for 2 d	As above.
	H. influenzae meningitis prophylaxis (off label)	*Adult* 600 mg PO once/d for 4 d *Child* 20 mg/kg once daily for 4 d (10 mg/kg if <1 mo old)	As above.
Rifabutin (Mycobutin)	MAC disease prophylaxis	*Adult* 300 mg once daily	May need to monitor platelet count and WBC. Before rifabutin increases rate of metabolism of many drugs, including anti-HIV agents, monitor drug response and/or blood levels, if available. Also, dose of rifabutin may need to be adjusted up or down because of drug interactions. Counsel patient to report allergic reaction, GI intolerance, or asthenia. May turn secretions reddish brown that can stain clothing and soft contact lenses. May be administered without

Continued on next page

Table 22–32. Dosage Schedule: Selected Antimycobacterials *(continued)*

Drug	Indication	Initial Dose	Comments
			regard to food. If unable to tolerate single dose, split into 2 equal doses with food. May need to adjust dose up or down for patient taking antiretrovirals.
Streptomycin	Tuberculosis, as part of combined drug therapy	*Adult* 1 g once daily IM. Reduce to 1 g 2–3 times/wk as soon as clinically feasible. *Child* 20 mg/kg once daily IM, not to exceed 1 g/d *Elderly* 500–750 mg once daily IM Duration of therapy may be 1–2 y	Maximum adult daily dose 4 g daily. Maximum pediatric daily dose 1 g. Renal impairment requires reduced dosage. Monitor serum concentrations: peak concentrations >50 µg/mL are associated with nephrotoxicity and should not be >20–25 µg/mL in patients with preexisting renal damage. Caloric stimulation tests may be required before, during, and after prolonged therapy to detect vestibular toxicity. Do audiograms and renal function tests periodically and frequent urinalysis to detect albumin, casts, cells, and decreased specific gravity. Educate patient to report signs of hypersensitivity (skin itching, rash, swelling), vestibular ototoxicity (clumsiness, dizziness, nausea, vomiting), auditory ototoxicity (hearing loss: fullness, ringing, buzzing in ears), peripheral neuritis (burning of face or mouth, numbness, tingling), and nephrotoxicity (altered frequency or amount of urination, thirst, anorexia, nausea and vomiting) Administer deep IM, alternating injection sites. Concentration of solution should not exceed 500 mg/mL. After reconstitution, solution retains potency for 2–28 days at room temperature and 14 days in refriger-ator, depending on manufacturer. See package insert. Darkening of solution does not affect potency.

d- and triphosphate compounds by the *host's* cellular enzymes. Because it requires the viral kinase for the first step, it is selectively activated only in infected cells. The final step, **acyclovir** triphosphate, inhibits viral DNA synthesis. **Valacyclovir (Valtrex)** is the L-valyl ester of **acyclovir**. It is rapidly converted after oral administration to **acyclovir**. Its mechanism of action is then that of **acyclovir**. Serum levels, however, are three to five times higher than those achieved with **acyclovir** and approximate those achieved by IV administration of **acyclovir**.

Famciclovir (Famvir) is the diacetyl ester prodrug of 6-deoxy **penciclovir**, an acyclic guanosine analogue. It is rapidly converted to **penciclovir** by first-pass metabolism. **Penciclovir** has similar pharmacodynamics to **acy-**

Table 22–33. Available Dosage Forms: Selected Antimycobacterials

Drug	Dosage Form	How Supplied
Capreomycin (Capstat)	Powder for injection: 1 g	In 10-cc multidose vials
Ethambutol (Myambutol)	Tablets: 100 mg 400 mg	In bottles of 100 coated tablets In bottles of 1000 scored, film-coated tablets
Ethionamide (Trecator-SC)	Tablets: 250 mg	In bottles of 100 sugar-coated tablets
Isoniazid	Tablets: 50 mg 100 mg 300 mg Syrup: 50 mg/5 cc Injection: 100 mg/cc	In bottles of 100, 500, and 1000 tablets In bottles of 100 and 1000 tablets In bottles of 30, 100, and 1000 tablets In pint, orange flavor In 10-cc multidose vials
(Laniazid)	Tablets: 50 mg Syrup: 50 mg/5 cc	In bottles of 100 and 500 scored tablets In 480-cc, raspberry flavor
(Nydrazid)	Injection: 100 mg/cc	In 10-cc multidose vials
Isoniazid combinations (Rifater)	Tablets: 120 mg rifampin, 50 mg isoniazid, 300 mg pyrazinamide	In bottles of 60 tablets
(Rifamate)	Capsules: 150 mg isoniazid, 300 mg rifampin	In bottles of 60 tablets
Rifabutin (Mycobutin)	Capsules: 150 mg	In bottles of 100 capsules
Rifampin (Rifadin)	Capsules: 150 mg 300 mg	In bottles of 30 capsules In bottles of 30, 60, and 100 capsules
(Rimactane)	Capsules: 300 mg	In bottles of 30, 60, and 100 capsules
Pyrazinamide	Tablets: 500 mg	In bottles of 100 and 500 scored tablets
Streptomycin sulfate	Injection: 400 mg/cc	In 2.5-cc ampules

clovir. Activation is catalyzed by *virus-specified* thymidine kinase in infected cells, resulting in competitive inhibition of the viral DNA polymerase and inhibition of DNA synthesis. It has lower affinity for the viral DNA polymerase than **acyclovir**, but it achieves higher intracellular concentrations and has a more prolonged intracellular effect.

Two other **nucleoside analogues** are **ganciclovir (Cytovene)**, which is used to treat serious cytomegalovirus (CMV) ocular infections, and **ribavirin (Virazole)**, which is active against a wide-range of DNA and RNA viruses, including influenza A and B, parainfluenza, respiratory syncytial virus (RSV), paramyxoviruses, herpes C virus (HCV), and HIV-1. Oral doses of **ribavirin**, however, have not proved to be beneficial for RSV, HCV, or HIV-1 infections. Neither of these agents is considered further in this chapter.

Sensitivity

Acyclovir is active against herpes simplex virus (HSV) 1 and 2, varicella-zoster virus (VZV), and, to a lesser extent, Epstein-Barr virus (EBV), CMV, and herpesvirus 6.

Famciclovir is active against HSV-1 and HSV-2, VZV, EBV, and hepatitis B virus. **Valacyclovir** is converted to **acyclovir** after oral administration and is active against the same viruses.

Resistance

Resistance to **acyclovir** can develop in herpes simplex virus and varicella-zoster virus through alteration is either the viral thymidine kinase or viral DNA polymerase. Because most resistance is based on deficient thymidine kinase activity, cross-resistance occurs with **valacyclovir** and **famciclovir**.

Pharmacokinetics

Absorption and Distribution

Absorption following oral administration varies by drug. **Acyclovir** is poorly absorbed orally (15 to 20%), although therapeutic levels are achieved. Topical formulations produce local concentrations that may exceed 10 µg/kg in herpetic lesions, but systemic concentrations are undetectable. **Famciclovir** is absorbed in the intestine for conversion to its active form, **penciclovir**. **Penciclovir** is marketed as a topical preparation only. **Valacyclovir** is a prodrug converted to **acyclovir** and is 54 percent bioavailable as **acyclovir** after oral administration.

Acyclovir, **famciclovir**, and **valacyclovir** are widely distributed. CSF concentrations are 50 percent of plasma for **acyclovir** and **valacyclovir**. All cross the placenta and are known to enter breast milk.

Metabolism and Excretion

Acyclovir is 90 percent eliminated in the urine as unchanged drug, primarily by glomerular filtration and tubular secretion. The liver metabolizes the rest. The kidneys also excrete the active metabolite of **famciclovir** (**penciclovir**). **Valacyclovir** is rapidly converted to **acyclovir** and has the same excretion pattern. Dosage adjustments are required for each of these drugs in the presence of renal impairment because of prolonged half-lives.

Table 22–34 presents the pharmacokinetics of **nucleoside analogues** for herpesvirus infections.

Pharmacotherapeutics

Precautions and Contraindications

For all drugs in this group, cautious use for patients with renal impairment is recommended, with dosage adjustments based on CCr. This caution is also important in older adults, who commonly have diminished renal function. They should also be used with caution by patients with serious hepatic or electrolyte abnormalities. Although dosage adjustments are not required, alterations in pharmacokinetics have been observed in the presence of hepatic impairment.

Acyclovir is listed as Pregnancy Category C; however, there are no adequate well-controlled studies in pregnant women. *Famciclovir* and *valacyclovir* are listed as Pregnancy Category B; however, *valacyclovir*

converts to *acyclovir* and should be used with the same precautions as *acyclovir*. To monitor maternal-fetal outcomes of pregnant women exposed to *valacyclovir*, Glaxo Wellcome maintains a pregnancy registry. Providers can register their patients by calling (800) 722-9292, extension 58465.

Acyclovir (from the parent drug and from the metabolite of **valacyclovir**) concentrations in breast milk following oral administration have varied from 0.6 to 4.1 times maternal plasma levels. These concentrations could potentially expose the infant to doses of up to 0.3 mg/kg a day. It is appropriate to exercise caution in prescribing these drugs to nursing mothers. **Famciclovir** has been associated with tumorigenicity. The decision to discontinue nursing or avoid the drug is based on the importance of the drug to the mother

Among these drugs, **acyclovir** is the safest for children and can be used in children over 2 years of age. **Famciclovir** does not have established safety and efficacy for children under age 18 years. The safety and efficacy of **valacyclovir** have not been established for children.

Adverse Drug Reactions

Adverse drug reactions vary by drug. **Acyclovir** has few reactions when given orally. Those associated with short-term administration include headache (0.6%), skin rash (0.3%), nausea and vomiting (2.7%), and diarrhea (0.3%). The prevalence of each of these reactions increases with long term use. The most frequent adverse reactions associated with **famciclovir** are headache (9%), dizziness (1%), somnolence, and paresthesias (both 1%). Because it is converted to **acyclovir**, the adverse reactions for **valacyclovir** are the same as for **acyclovir**. Valacyclovir does have a higher incidence of adverse reaction, including serious ones (thrombocytopenia purpura, hemolytic uremic syndrome) in immunocompromised patients.

Drug Interactions

Drug interactions are minimal for **acyclovir**, **famciclovir**, and **valacyclovir**. Table 22–35 presents the few drug interactions that exist for **nucleoside analogues**.

Table 22–34. Pharmacokinetics: Nucleoside Analogues for Herpesvirus Infections

Drug	Onset	Peak	Duration	Protein Binding	Bioavailability	Half-Life	Elimination
Acyclovir	UA	1.5–2.5h	4 h	9–33%	15–20%	3–4 h; 20 h in anuria	>90% in urine; rest metabolized by liver
Famciclovir	Rapid	1 h	8–12 h	20%	77%	2–3 h; prolonged in renal impairment	Mostly in urine
Valacyclovir	UA	1.5–2.5 h	8–24 h	13–18%	54%	2.5–3h; 14 h in anuria	>90% in urine; rest metabolized by liver

Table 22–35. Drug Interactions: Nucleoside Analogues

Drug	Interacting Drug	Possible Effect	Implications
Acyclovir, famciclovir	Probenecid	Increased bioavailability and terminal half-life of acyclovir; decreased renal clearance.	Avoid concurrent use.
	Nephrotoxic drugs	Increased risk for renal toxicity.	Avoid concurrent use or monitor renal function closely.
Famciclovir	Cimetidine	Penciclovir AUC and urinary recovery increased 18% and 12%, respectively.	No clinical significance.
	Theophylline	Penciclovir AUC increased 22%. Renal clearance decreased 12%.	No clinical significance.
	Digoxin	C_{max} of digoxin increased 19% in healthy male volunteers.	Probably of no clinical significance, but to be prudent, monitor digoxin levels closely.

Clinical Use and Dosing

The most important variable in selecting the dosage of **nucleoside analogues** is renal function. The dosing interval, dosage, or both are adjusted for patients with impaired renal function, depending on the dosage and degree of impairment. For example, the usual dose of **valacyclovir** for herpes zoster treatment in a patient with CCr greater than 50 mL/minute is 1 g every 8 hours, whereas the dosage for a CCr less than 10 mL/minute is 500 mg every 24 hours. The prescriber should consult the package insert or a comprehensive reference for specific dosing guidelines.

The **nucleoside analogues** are recommended for the treatment of infections by the herpes simplex virus commonly seen in primary care, specifically genital herpes, herpes zoster (shingles), and varicella (chickenpox). The **nucleoside analogues** do not cure herpes infections but may shorten duration, decrease severity, and reduce the incidence of sequelae of the infection. Oral forms of **acyclovir, valacyclovir,** and **famciclovir** are all indicated for primary genital herpes; they increase the rate of healing but do not prevent recurrences. Although topical **acyclovir** is also approved for treatment of initial herpes genitalis infections, it is less effective than the oral **nucleoside analogues** and is not recommended. The oral **nucleoside analogues** should be initiated as soon as possible after the onset of a recurrent episode. Patients are usually provided with a prescription that can be filled at the first sign of recurrence. Topical **acyclovir** has no benefit in recurrent disease in immunocompetent patients, although it has some value in suppression of mucocutaneous herpes in immunocompromised individuals. Patients with frequent recurrences can be placed on suppression therapy, which decreases subclinical shedding between active episodes and the number of symptomatic recurrences. The definition of frequent recurrence is

somewhat arbitrary, varying from 6 to 10 recurrences per year, depending on the author. However, development of drug resistance is likely to accelerate with increasing chronic use, and suppressive therapy is costly, averaging between $1000 and $2500 annually. In untreated patients, the number of recurrences tends to decrease over time during the first 5 years of the disease. By 3 to 5 years after the initial episode, the number of recurrences may have declined to the point that episodic treatment of recurrences may be preferable. Therefore, the need for suppressive therapy should be reconsidered annually.

Oral **acyclovir** is indicated for the treatment of varicella in immunocompetent patients when started within 24 hours of the chickenpox rash. For immunocompromised patients, parenteral **acyclovir** should be used. The American Academy of Pediatrics does not recommend **acyclovir** for the treatment of uncomplicated chickenpox in healthy children. **Acyclovir** is recommended for healthy, nonpregnant patients age 13 or older, children older than 12 months with a chronic cutaneous or pulmonary disorder, and children receiving short, intermittent, or aerosolized courses of **corticosteroids.** If possible, the **steroids** should be discontinued after known exposure to varicella. The CDC recommends aggressive treatment of varicella in adults 20 years of age and older, in that the majority of deaths from chickenpox occur in this age group. **Varicella-zoster immune globulin** should be given within 96 hours of known exposure of a susceptible adult. If prophylaxis fails, early initiation of **acyclovir** within 24 hours of onset of varicella rash is urged. Susceptible adults at high risk (e.g., immunosuppressed, HIV, **corticosteroid** users) should be vaccinated. Varicella is the leading cause of vaccine-preventable deaths in the United States, so vaccination of children is recommended before the age of 12 to 18 months.

Therapy with **nucleoside analogues** should be initiated within 3 days of the outbreak of the rash in herpes zoster. Therapy is most effective if initiated within 48 hours of the outbreak of the rash. Drug therapy speeds healing and reduces the duration of postherpetic neuralgia.

Other recommended uses of oral **acyclovir** include prophylaxis of herpes simplex and herpes zoster in immunocompromised patients, Bell's palsy, and primary gingivostomatitis in children. Parenteral **acyclovir** is used to treat herpes encephalitis, perinatal herpes simplex of mother and neonate, herpes pneumonia, and Herpes simiae from a monkey bite.

Table 22–36 presents the dosage schedule for **nucleoside analogues** for herpesvirus infections.

Rational Drug Selection

All three of the **nucleoside analogues** used to treat herpes simplex infections have shown equal efficacy in the treatment of genital herpes. Hence, the selection of the specific agent is based on cost and convenience. **Acyclovir** is available as a generic preparation and is generally less expensive than the other **nucleoside analogues.** However, it must be dosed three to five times daily, which may be disruptive and promote noncompliance. **Famciclovir** is dosed two to four times daily, and **valacyclovir** requires one to two doses daily, depending on the indication.

Because of long experience and more extensive research, only **acyclovir** is approved for some indications, such as use by children, varicella treatment, and prevention of oral labial mucocutaneous lesions in immunocompromised patients. Many experts consider **valacyclovir** to be the drug of choice for treatment of herpes zoster because clinical trials have indicated that it decreased the duration of postherpetic neuralgia in patients over 50 years of age more than **acyclovir** did.

Monitoring

The characteristic herpetic lesions of genital herpes, herpes zoster, and chickenpox should be evaluated for resolution or signs of secondary bacterial infection. Temperature and general condition also reflect resolution. BUN and serum creatinine may be assessed prior to therapy in those with risk factors for renal impairment and periodically during prolonged therapy to detect changes in renal function.

Patient Education

ADMINISTRATION. The **nucleoside analogues** can all be taken without regard to meals, in that food does not alter absorption. The available dosage forms are shown in Table 22–37. All forms should be taken with a full glass of water. It is important that the drug be initiated at the earliest sign of recurrence of genital herpes simplex, so the patient must be taught the symptoms of recurrence and how to self-initiate the medication. Early initiation of drug therapy also increases its efficacy for treatment of varicella and herpes zoster, so public education needs to emphasize the treatability of these infections. It is particularly important for adolescents or adults with chickenpox to seek treatment at the first sign of rash or in the prodromal period if they know they are susceptible and have been exposed.

ADVERSE REACTIONS. Although acute renal failure from precipitation of **acyclovir** in the tubules is most common with parenteral **acyclovir**, patients on oral agents have developed acute renal failure and should drink sufficient fluids to remain well hydrated during therapy. Signs of declining renal function that should be reported include abdominal pain, decreased frequency or amount of urination, thirst, anorexia, and nausea or vomiting. Other reportable signs and symptoms include encephalopathic changes (coma, confusion, hallucinations, seizures, tremor), blood dyscrasias (unusual tiredness, chills, fever, sore throat, black stools, unusual bleeding, pinpoint red spots on skin, bruising), and skin reactions like Stevens-Johnson syndrome (peeling, blistering, or loosening of skin; muscle cramps, pain, or weakness; red eyes; rash, itching, or hives).

LIFESTYLE MANAGEMENT. Keeping herpetic lesions clean and dry promotes healing. Wearing loose clothing that does not rub on the lesions decreases pain and enhances healing. Herpes genitalis may be sexually transmitted even if the partner is asymptomatic. Sexual activity should be avoided whenever either partner has symptoms of herpes genitalis. Oral or topical drug therapy does not prevent transmission of the virus. A male or female condom may decrease the risk of transmission, but spermicides and diaphragms have no effect on transmission. Women with a history of genital herpes are more likely to develop cervical cancer; annual or more frequent Pap tests are required. Those who develop postherpetic neuralgia following herpes zoster should be provided with appropriate pain management for this neuropathic pain syndrome.

Other Antivirals for Influenza

Amantadine (Symadine, Symmetrel) and **rimantadine (Flumadine)** are used for prevention and treatment of respiratory infections due to influenza A virus. **Zanamivir (Relenza)** and **oseltamivir phosphate (Tamiflu)** are approved for treatment of acute illness in adults and adolescents over 12 years old who have been symptomatic less than 48 hours, but they also have been used off label in the prevention of influenza. Each of these drugs is reserved for patients at high risk for complications from influenza infections, when vaccination is contraindicated, or to protect the patient until active immunity can develop following vaccination. These drugs should not be considered a substitute for vaccination.

Table 22–36. Dosage Schedule: Nucleoside Analogues for Herpesvirus Infections

Drug	Indication	Initial Dose	Comments
Acyclovir (Zovirax)	Genital herpes, initial episode (mild to moderate)	*Adult* 200 mg q4h while awake, 5 times/d for 10 d; accepted off-label dose: 400 mg PO 3 times/d for 10 d	Severe cases and infections in immunocompromised patients require hospitalization and IV therapy. Acute or chronic renal impairment may require dosage adjustment, depending on CCr and dose. Suspension should be well shaken before measurement, using a calibrated device. Take with water. Suspension retains its potency for 24 mo from date of manufacture. Does not require reconstitution or refrigeration. May be taken without regard to meals. Cross-allergy to valacyclovir.
	Genital herpes, intermittent therapy for recurrent infections (<6 episodes/y)	*Adult* 200 mg q4h while awake, 5 times/d for 5 d; accepted off-label dose: 400 mg PO 3 times daily for 5 d	As above.
	Genital herpes, chronic suppressive therapy (≥6–10 episodes/y)	*Adult* 400 mg PO twice/d or 200 mg 3–5 times/d for up to 12 mo	As above.
	Herpes zoster (shingles)	*Adult* 800 mg PO q4h while awake, 5 times/d, for 7–10 d	As above.
	Varicella (chickenpox) Initiate at earliest sign of the infection (treatment of chickenpox in children 2–12 y not recommended by American Academy of Pediatrics)	*Adults and adolescents* 800 mg PO q4h for 5 d *Child <2 y* Safety and efficacy have not been established, but doses of 3000 mg/m² or 80 mg/kg PO in divided doses have been used *Child 2–12 y and <40 kg* 20 mg/kg up to 800 mg/dose, 4 times/d for 5 d *Child 2–12 y and >40 kg* Same as adult dose	As above.
	Herpes simplex, mucocutaneous prophylaxis (off label)	*Adult* 400 mg PO q12h	As above.
	Bell's palsy due to herpes simplex virus 1 or 2	*Adult* 400 mg PO 5 times/d for 10 d	As above.
Famciclovir (Famvir)	Genital herpes, initial episode (mild to moderate)	*Adult* (off label) 250 mg PO 3 times/d for 5–10 d	Renal impairment may require decreased dosage. May be taken without regard to meals. Initiate as soon as possible after onset of signs or symptoms.
	Genital herpes, intermittent therapy for recurrent infections (<6 episodes/y)	*Adult* 125 mg twice/d for 3–5 d	
	Genital herpes, chronic suppressive therapy (≥6–10 episodes/y)	*Adult* 250 mg PO twice/d or 500 mg once/d for up to 1 y	

Continued on next page

Table 22–36. Dosage Schedule: Nucleoside Analogues for Herpesvirus Infections (*continued*)

Drug	Indication	Initial Dose	Comments
	Herpes zoster (shingles)	500 mg q8h for 7 d	
Valacyclovir (Valtrex)	Genital herpes, initial episode (mild to moderate)	*Adult* 1 g PO twice/d for 10 d	Renal impairment may require dosage adjustment. Hepatic impairment may slow rate, but not extent, of conversion to acyclovir, but dosage adjustment is not required for hepatic impairment. Not indicated for immunocompromised patients (bone marrow transplant, human immunodeficiency syndrome, renal transplantation) because of risk of thrombotic thrombocytopenic purpura/hemolytic uremic syndrome. May be taken without regard to meals. Cross-allergy to acyclovir.
	Genital herpes, intermittent therapy for recurrent infections (<6–10 episodes/y)	*Adult* 500 mg PO twice/d for 5 d	
	Genital herpes, chronic suppressive therapy (≥6 episodes/y)	*Adult* 1 g PO once/d for up to 1 y	
	Herpes zoster (shingles)	1 g PO 3 times/d for 7 d	

Pharmacodynamics

Sensitivity

The exact mechanism of antiviral action by **amantadine** and **rimantadine** is not fully understood. It appears to be the prevention of uncoating and release of infectious viral nucleic acid into the host cells. The reaction is virus-specific to influenza A. It does not appear to interfere with the immunogenicity of inactivated influenza A **vaccine**.

The proposed mechanism of action for **zanamivir** is selective inhibition of influenza A and B virus neuraminidase. This enzyme is essential for viral replication, allows viral release from infected cells, prevents viral aggregation, and possibly decreases the ability of the respiratory mucus to inactivate the influenza virus. Vacci-

Table 22–37. Available Dosage Forms: Nucleoside Analogues for Herpesvirus Infections

Drug	Dosage Form	How Supplied
Acyclovir	Tablets: 400 mg 800 mg Capsules: 200 mg	In bottles of 100, 500, and 1000 tablets In bottles 100 and 500 tablets In bottles of 100 capsules
(Zovirax)	Tablets: 400 mg 800 mg Capsules: 200 mg Suspension: 200 mg/5 cc	In bottles of 100 tablets In bottles of 100 tablets and in Shingles Relief Pak of 35 tablets In bottles of 100 capsules In 473-cc bottles, banana flavor
Famciclovir (Famvir)	Tablets: 125 mg, 250 mg, 500 mg	In bottles of 30 tablets
Valacyclovir (Valtrex)	Tablets: 500 mg	In bottles of 42 film-coated caplets

nation does not appear to alter the activity of **zanamivir** or **oseltamivir** (Two Neuraminidase Inhibitors, 1999).

Resistance

Emergence of resistance to **amantadine** and **rimantadine** is common in treated patients, with a prevalence of 50 percent within 4 to 6 days. The mechanism of resistance appears to be mutations in the RNA sequence coding for the structural M2 protein. Transmission of resistance to household contacts has been demonstrated.

Resistance to **zanamivir** and **oseltamivir** is associated with mutations that result in amino acid changes in the viral neuraminidase or viral hemagglutinin or both. This mutation reduced the neuraminidase response to **zanamivir** by 1000-fold. This drug has not been available for a sufficient length of time to determine its prevalence of resistance or its transmission to household contacts.

Pharmacokinetics

Absorption and Distribution

Amantadine, rimantadine, and **oseltamivir** are well absorbed after oral administration. **Oseltamivir** is a prodrug of the active compound GS4071. Approximately 4 to 17 percent of the inhaled dose of **zanamivir** is systemically absorbed. **Amantadine** is widely distributed to various body tissues including saliva and nasal secretions, and it concentrates in lung tissue. CSF concentrations are half of those in the serum. It crosses the placenta and enters breast milk. Distribution of the other drugs is not known. Protein binding is highest for **amantadine** (67%), midrange for **rimantadine** (40%), and low for **zanamivir** (10%).

Metabolism and Excretion

Amantadine, oseltamivir, and GS4071, the active form of **oseltamivir,** are renally excreted as unchanged drug, and no metabolites have been detected. **Rimantadine** is metabolized by the liver, and less than 25 percent is excreted as unchanged drug in the urine.

Table 22–38 presents the pharmacokinetics of **antivirals** for influenza.

Pharmacotherapeutics

Precautions and Contraindications

Most of the adverse reactions to **amantadine** and **rimantadine** are CNS or psychic disturbances. This drug should be used cautiously for patients with seizure disorders or psychoses. Congestive heart failure (CHF) and peripheral edema have developed in patients taking **amantadine.** Careful observation and dosage titration are required for patients with cardiac disease. Because **acyclovir** is extensively excreted by the kidney, renal impairment can result in significant accumulations in plasma and body tissues. Dosage adjustments are required based on CCr, and it should be used with caution by patients with renal dysfunction. These cautions are especially true for *older adults*, who may have age-related diminished renal function.

The liver metabolizes **rimantadine,** and apparent clearance of the drug in patients with severe liver dysfunction was 50 percent lower than that reported for healthy subjects. Because of the potential for accumulation of this drug and its metabolites, it should be used cautiously in the presence of severe hepatic impairment. Although it is less dependent on renal excretion, dosage adjustments are still required and cautious use is recommended for patients with renal impairment, including *older adults.*

Amantadine and *rimantadine* are Pregnancy Category C. Embryotoxicity and teratogenesis have been observed in animal studies, and there are no adequate well-controlled studies in pregnant women. Use only when clearly needed and when the potential benefits outweigh the fetal risks. *Zanamivir* is listed as Pregnancy Category B. Although it crosses the placenta, fetal blood concentrations in animal studies were significantly lower than maternal plasma. *Oseltamivir* is Pregnancy Category C. With no adequate well-controlled studies in pregnant women, cautious use of both agents is recommended.

Amantadine is excreted in breast milk. Use caution when administering to a nursing mother. It is not known whether **zanamivir** or **oseltamivir** is excreted in human milk. Caution is also recommended with these agents. **Rimantadine** has been associated with adverse effects in the offspring of animals treated with this drug during the nursing period. The drug concentrates in breast milk at approximately twice the levels in maternal serum. It should not be given to nursing mothers.

The safety and efficacy of **amantadine** and **rimantadine** for children under 1 year of age have not been established. For **zanamivir** and **oseltamivir,** safety and efficacy have not been established for children under 12 years of age.

Adverse Drug Reactions

The most frequent adverse reactions for all of these drugs are GI (nausea, vomiting, constipation) and CNS-related (dizziness, depression, insomnia). **Amantadine** has a higher incidence than the others. **Amantadine** is also approved for treatment of Parkinson's disease because it increases the availability of dopamine in certain areas of the brain. This is thought to be the mechanism for the

Table 22–38. Pharmacokinetics: Antivirals for Influenza

Drug	Onset	Peak	Duration	Protein Binding	Bioavailability	Half-Life	Elimination
Amantadine	48 h	1–4 h	UA	67%*	67%	9–37 h	Excreted unchanged in urine
Oseltamivir	Rapid	2.5–6 h	UA	UA	80%	6–10 h	Prodrug; active metabolite GS4071 excreted unchanged in urine
Rimantadine	Rapid	6–7 h	UA	40%	UA	20–65 h	<25% unchanged in urine
Zanamivir	Rapid	1–2 h	UA	<10%	UA	2.5–5.1 h	Excreted unchanged in urine

*In hemodialysis patients, 59%.

high incidence of CNS symptoms and nausea with **amantadine.**

Amantadine is also associated with a less frequent (1 to 5%) incidence of an unusual skin disorder (livedo reticularis) in which there is a semipermanent bluish mottled appearance of the skin of the legs and hands that may result from abnormal capillary permeability associated with vasoconstriction. Occasionally, orthostatic hypotension, peripheral edema, and leukopenia have been reported.

Bronchitis, cough, and shortness of breath are associated with **rimantadine** and **zanamivir.** For **zanamivir**, these problems are related to irritation from inhalation of the drug. **Zanamivir** also is associated with ear, nose, and throat infections.

For all of these drugs, adverse reactions are most common and more severe in older adults.

Drug Interactions

Drug interactions are minimal. **Zanamivir** is not a substrate, nor does it affect any of the CYP-450 isoenzyme systems. No drug interactions are reported for **oseltamivir** and **zanamivir.** Table 22–39 lists the few existing drug interactions.

Clinical Use and Dosing

Rimantadine and **amantadine** are approved for the prophylaxis and treatment of influenza type A, whereas **zanamivir** and **oseltamivir** are approved for only the treatment of both influenza types A and B. Indications for prophylactic therapy include short-term prophylaxis in institutions such as nursing homes, as an adjunct to immunization after the influenza season has commenced, as a supplement to vaccination for those with impaired immunity, to reduce the spread of influenza by unvaccinated health care workers, the prevention of disease in workers in critical service positions such as firefighters and police,

and chemoprophylaxis in those who cannot take the **vaccine** because of allergy to one of the **vaccine** constituents.

Some clinicians prefer the **neuraminidase inhibitors** for prophylaxis, particularly when an unvaccinated high-risk patient is exposed to type B or an unknown type of influenza. The individual is vaccinated immediately and started on **neuraminidase inhibitors** for 4 weeks to allow the antibody response to the **vaccine** to achieve protective concentrations.

Indications for treatment include unvaccinated individuals who contract influenza. However, vaccinated individuals can also get influenza and should be offered treatment, particularly if they are at high risk for pneumonia and other sequelae of influenza.

Lower dosages of **amantadine** and **rimantadine** are required for patients with renal impairment and for older patients who are likely to have an age-related decrement in renal function, such as those who reside in nursing homes. The recommended dosage for those over age 65 is half the dosage for younger adults. The active components of both **zanamivir** and **oseltamivir** are excreted primarily unchanged in the urine. Recommendations for dosage reduction in renal impairment are not available for either agent. However, because **zanamivir** is an inhaled drug that is only 20 percent absorbed systemically, the risk of accumulation is slight. The active metabolite of **oseltamivir** is excreted in the urine, so renal impairment will impede its excretion and predispose a patient to toxicity. However, this drug is new, and the clinical significance of accumulation in older and debilitated patients is not known.

Table 22–40 presents the dosage schedule for **antivirals** used for influenza.

Rational Drug Selection

The benefit of influenza drugs is tempered by the need to initiate treatment within 48 hours of the onset of the illness. Although the presence of fever, cough, myalgia, and

Table 22–39. Drug Interactions: Antivirals for Influenza

Drug	Interacting Drug	Possible Effect	Implications
Amantadine	Anticholinergic drugs (antihistamines, phenothiazines, quinidine, disopyramide, and tricyclic antidepressants)	Increased anticholinergic effects (dry mouth, blurred vision, constipation)	Reduce dose of amantadine or the interacting drug.
	Hydrochlorothiazide with triamterene	Decreased urinary excretion of amantadine with increased plasma concentrations	Avoid concurrent use.
Rimantadine	Acetaminophen, aspirin, cimetidine	Peak concentrations and AUC of rimantidine decreased by 10% to 16%	Probably not clinically significant.

known influenza activity in the community provide the basis for clinical diagnosis, these symptoms are not definitive, and the lack of timely laboratory testing causes both patient and prescriber to hesitate to initiate therapy. However, three new rapid diagnostic office tests that detect influenza and influenza B were recently approved (Rapid Diagnostic Tests, 1999). These include **Flu OIA, Quickvue Influenza Test,** and **Zstatflu.** Another office diagnostic test for influenza A only, **Directigen Flu A,** has been on the market for several years. These tests take no more than 20 minutes, cost between $15 and $20, and have acceptable sensitivity and specificity. However, the tests do not distinguish between influenza A and influenza B.

The selection of an **anti-influenza agent** depends on the spectrum, adverse effect profile, cost, and convenience. The cost of **rimantadine** and **amantadine** is considerably lower than the cost of the **neuraminidase inhibitors,** but they cover only influenza A. Another problem with these agents has been the rapid emergence of resistance. Although **rimantadine** has considerably fewer central nervous system effects than **amantadine,** both appear to have more adverse drug reactions that the **neuraminidase inhibitors.** Because **zanamivir** and **oseltamivir** are both new drugs, the full extent of adverse effects and drug interactions may be unknown. The inhaled route of administration of **zanamavir** has the advantage of decreased systemic effects compared with **oseltamivir,** but the inhalation procedure may contribute to noncompliance.

Monitoring

Baseline evaluation of renal function should be considered for older and debilitated patients who are taking **anti-influenza prophylactic** therapy, which averages several weeks rather than the 5 to 7 days required for treatment. All patients taking **amantadine** or **rimantadine** should be assessed for irritability and seizure activity, and older patients should also be evaluated for confusion, hallucinations, and cognitive impairment. For older and debilitated patients, monitoring should include breath sounds (for evidence of heart failure or development of pneumonia), heart sounds, and weight. Vital signs will also evidence resolution of the influenza and development of adverse effects or sequelae.

Patient Education

ADMINISTRATION. As with all **antimicrobials,** the importance of taking the full course of therapy and following the labeled direction should be stressed. The available dosage forms are shown in Table 22–41. Patients on **zanamivir** require instruction on the proper use of the diskhaler. The oral **anti-influenza drugs** can be taken without regard to meals, although taking the medication with food may decrease GI adverse effects.

ADVERSE REACTIONS. If asthmatics on **zanamavir** experience severe bronchospasm after using the diskhaler, an alternative treatment may be needed. Because the **neuraminidase inhibitors** represent a new drug group, patients should be encouraged to report their experiences with these agents. As with all drugs, serious occurrences should be reported to MedWatch (800-FDA-0178), the Food and Drug Administration's voluntary reporting system for adverse events and product problems.

Amantadine and, to a lesser extent, **rimantadine** have potentially serious adverse effects. Patients should be advised that the drugs can cause dizziness and blurred vision and that patients should defer hazardous activities until they know how they react to the medication. **Alcohol** should be avoided during therapy, as it would compound hypotension and dizziness. Patients and family members should be advised to report signs of CHF (swelling of feet or legs, shortness of breath), neurological and mental status changes (depression, suicidal ideation, hallucinations, confusion, seizures, clumsiness), and anticholinergic effects (dry mouth, blurred vision, constipation, difficult urination). Dry mouth can be relieved by sucking on ice or

Table 22–40. Dosage Schedule: Antivirals for Influenza

Drug	Indications	Initial Dose	Comments
Amantadine (Symmetrel)	Influenza A prophylaxis or treatment	*Young adults and children >12 y* 100–200 mg PO once daily *or* 100 mg PO q12h *Older adults* 100 mg PO once daily *Neonates and infants* Safety and efficacy not established *Children 1–9 y* 1.5–3 mg/kg PO q8h *or* 2.2–4.4 mg/kg PO q12h *Children 9–12 y* 100 mg PO q12h; for child <45 kg dosage of 2.2 mg/kg q12h may be advisable	Maximum daily dose for child 1–9 y, 150 mg; for child 9–12 y, 100 mg; for adults >65 y, daily doses >100 mg should be used with caution, and reduced further if there is renal impairment, seizure disorder, altered mental/behavioral function. Renal impairment at any age may require dosage reduction. Syrup should be stored at room temperature and dispensed with a calibrated liquid measuring device. May be taken without regard to meals.
Oseltamivir (Tamiflu)	Influenza A and B treatment	*Adult* 75 mg PO twice daily for 5 d; start within 48 h of onset of symptoms	Not FDA-approved for influenza prophylaxis, although studies have indicated efficacy. For prophylaxis after exposure, immunize with flu vaccine and administer 75 mg PO once daily for 4 wk. Less nausea if taken with food.
Rimantadine (Flumadine)	Influenza A prophylaxis	*Adults and children >10 y* 100 mg PO twice daily *or* 200 mg PO once daily *Children <10 y* 5 mg/kg PO once daily, not to exceed 150 mg per dose	In adults with impaired renal function (CCr ≤10 mL/min), severe hepatic dysfunction, or elderly nursing home patients, a dose of 100 mg once daily is recommended. After exposure, give flu vaccine followed by 4 wk at prophylactic doses. Although the manufacturer recommends twice-daily dosing, the half-life is sufficiently long that once-daily dosing has proved effective. May be taken without regard to meals. The syrup should be measured with a calibrated liquid dosing device.
	Influenza A treatment	*Adults* 100 mg PO twice/d *or* 200 mg PO once/d for 5–7 d after initial onset of symptoms	
Zanamivir (Relenza)	Influenza A or B treatment	*Adults* 2 (5-mg) inhalations twice daily for 5 d; take 2 doses on day 1 if at least 2 h apart, and start within 48 h of initial onset of symptoms	Not FDA-approved for influenza prophylaxis, although studies have indicated efficacy. For prophylaxis after exposure, immunize with flu vaccine and administer 2 inhalations once/d for 4 wk.

Table 22–41. Available Dosage Forms: Antivirals for Influenza

Drug	Dosage Form	How Supplied
Amantadine	Capsules: 100 mg	In bottles of 100, 250, and 500 capsules
(Symmetrel)	Capsules: 100 mg Syrup: 50 mg/5 cc	In bottles of 100, 250, and 500 capsules In 480-cc bottles, raspberry flavor
Rimantadine (Flumadine)	Tablets: 100 mg Syrup: 50 mg/5 cc	In bottles of 20, 100, 500, and 1000 film-coated tablets In 60-, 240-, and 480-cc bottles, raspberry flavor
Oseltamivir (Tamiflu)	Tablets: 75 mg	UΛ
Zanamivir (Relenza)	Blisters of powder for inhalation: 5 mg	In 4s with 5 Rotadisks and 1 diskhaler

sugarless candy, good oral hygiene, and use of an over-the-counter saliva substitute.

By the time a patient gets influenza, it is too late to educate him or her about the importance of taking the medication within the first 36 hours after onset of symptoms. Therefore, this has to be part of the anticipatory guidance given at the time of the annual influenza shot. Duration of influenza therapy is 5 days for the **neuraminidase inhibitors** and about 5 to 8 days for **amantadine** and **rimantadine**.

LIFESTYLE MANAGEMENT. The single most important factor in influenza prevention is the annual vaccination of individuals at risk and those in service positions. Public health officials are increasingly promoting influenza **vaccine** for broader segments of the population. Most candidates for prophylactic therapy should probably have received vaccination. The wholesale cost of a course of therapy with a **neuraminidase inhibitor** is approximately $45 to $55, exclusive of diagnostic testing, whereas the cost of annual vaccination is $7. Other components of prevention include good handwashing, disposing of contaminated tissues properly, and encouraging infected individuals to convalesce at home rather than in crowded schools and workplaces.

Systemic Azoles and Other Antifungals

Fungi are free-living, highly organized cells with a nucleus bound by a nuclear membrane and a rigid cell wall. Their life cycle includes a dormant spore stage. They occur naturally in soil, water, and air and on plants. Few of them are capable of causing disease in humans, but the incidence of human fungal infections has increased dramatically in recent years, largely because of increased use of **immunosuppressive drugs** and **antibiotics**. *Candida albicans*, a member of the yeast family of fungi, is now the fourth most common organism found in blood cultures in the United States.

Most fungi are completely resistant to conventional **antibiotics**, and new classes of drugs have been created to treat them. There are four main classes of **antifungal drugs**. **Polyene macrolides** include **amphotericin B** and **nystatin (Micostatin, Nilstat)**. The azole group includes two subgroups. The **imidazoles** include **butoconazole (Femstat)**, **clotrimazole (Gyne-Lotrimin, Lotrimin, Mycelex)**, **econazole (Spectazole)**, **ketoconazole (Nizoral)**, **miconazole (Micatin, Monistat)**, **terconazole (Terazol)**, and **tioconazole (Vagistat)**. The **triazoles** include **fluconazole (Diflucan)**, and **itraconazole (Sporanox)**. **Allylamines**, the third main class, include **naftifine (Naftin)** and **terbinafine (Lamisil)**. The last main class, **nuclear acid synthesis inhibitors**, consists of only one drug, **flucytosine (Ancobon)**. **Griseofulvin** is a miscellaneous **antifungal**. Other **antifungals** used topically include **ciclopirox (Loprox)**, **haloprogin (Halotex)**, **oxiconazole (Oxistat)**, and **tolnaftate (Tinactin, Absorbine, Aftate)**.

The topical use of **antifungals** to treat dermatologic infections is discussed in Chapters 21 and 30, and their use in treating vaginal infections is discussed in Chapter 42. This section discusses the systemic use of **antifungals** and the oral route of administration. The classes used orally in primary care by this route are three **azoles** and **terbinafine**, the oral **allylamine**.

Pharmacodynamics

Both subgroups of **azoles (imidazoles** and **triazoles)** reduce fungal ergosterol synthesis in cell membranes by inhibition of fungal CYP-450 enzymes. The specificity of these drugs results from greater affinity for fungal CYP-450 rather than human CYP-450. **Imidazoles** are less specific than **triazoles**, resulting in a higher incidence of drug interactions and adverse reactions.

Among the **imidazoles, ketoconazole** is the least specific to fungal CYP-450, resulting in more drug interactions and adverse reactions than the other **azoles**, and **fluconazole** is the most specific. In general, the **azoles** are fungistatic in low to moderate doses and fungicidal in higher doses.

Human cells and fungal cells share many anatomic and functional characteristics, so it is difficult to identify drugs that will harm the fungal pathogen without harming the human host. However, because fungi contain ergosterol as the essential lipid in the cell membrane and because in human cells this vital function is fulfilled by cholesterol, many antifungal agents are directed at ergosterol. The **allylamines**, represented by **terbinafine** as an agent in the class with an oral formulation, interfere with the synthesis of ergosterol in the cell membranes of fungi at an earlier step than the **azoles** do, by inhibiting the enzyme squalene epoxide. This results in an intracellular accumulation of squalene, disruption of cell membrane function and cell wall synthesis, and fungal cell death.

Sensitivity

The **azoles** have a broad spectrum of activity that includes *Candida* species, *Cryptococcus neoformans,* the endemic mycoses (blastomycosis, coccidioidomycosis, histoplasmosis), and the dermatophytes. **Itraconazole** is also active against *Aspergillus.*

Terbinafine (Lamisil) has in vitro activity against yeasts and a wide range of dermatophyte, filamentous, and dimorphic fungi. It is fungicidal against dermatophytes, such as *Trichophyton* species, *Microsporum* species, and *Epidermophyton floccosum.* It is fungistatic only against *C. albicans,* although it is 65 percent effective in mycologic cure of skin infections by this organism. **Terbinafine** is approved only for treatment of onychomycosis (fungal infection of the nails) but is used off label for tinea capitis (ringworm of the scalp), tinea corporis (ringworm of the body), tinea pedis (ringworm of the feet; athlete's foot), and tinea cruris (ringworm of the groin; jock itch). **Terbinafine** is not effective in the treatment of pityriasis versicolor; the concentrations attained by oral **terbinafine** in the stratum corneum are not adequate to treat this infection.

Resistance

Resistance to **azoles** occurs through a variety of mechanisms. Although still rare, the incidence of resistance is increasing as these drugs are used for prophylaxis as well as therapy. Resistant strains of *C. albicans* have been recovered from patients with AIDS. There is no evidence of resistance to **terbinafine.**

Pharmacokinetics

The pharmacokinetics of the different **azoles** and of **terbinafine** vary significantly. Table 22–42 depicts these pharmacokinetic differences.

Absorption and Distribution

Fluconazole is well absorbed after oral administration, with excellent bioavailability (more than 90%). It is widely distributed with good penetration into CSF, the eye, and the peritoneum.

The absorption of **itraconazole** is enhanced when it is taken with food, resulting in a bioavailability of 55 percent. The absorption of the oral solution is not affected by food, and it is given without regard to food. The bioavailability of the oral solution is different from that of the capsule, and they should not be used interchangeably. Tissue concentrations are higher than plasma concentrations. **Itraconazole** does not enter the CSF but does enter breast milk.

Absorption of **ketoconazole** from the GI tract is pH dependent, with increasing pH resulting in decreasing absorption. Administration with food may decrease absorption. It is widely distributed, but CSF penetration is unpredictable and minimal. Detectable concentrations are found in urine, saliva, sebum, and cerumen. **Ketoconazole** crosses the placenta and enters breast milk.

Terbinafine is well absorbed after oral administration, with bioavailability of 70 to 85 percent, and is not affected by the presence of food. It is lipophilic and extensively distributed. It concentrates in the stratum corneum, attaining concentrations 25 times that in plasma. It is also distributed via the sebum to hair follicles, skin, and nails. It is not known whether **terbinafine** crosses the placenta, but it does enter breast milk.

Metabolism and Excretion

Fluconazole is cleared primarily by renal excretion, with 80 percent appearing as unchanged drug in the urine and 11 percent as metabolites. Half-life is markedly affected by renal impairment, with an inverse relationship between the elimination half-life and CCr. Dosage adjustments are required for patients with impaired renal function.

Itraconazole is extensively metabolized by the liver into several active metabolites, and fecal excretion varies from 3 to 18 percent of the dose. About 40 percent of the dose is excreted in urine as metabolites.

Ketoconazole is also extensively metabolized by the liver, but to inactive metabolites. Excretion is mainly in feces via bile. Renal failure does not alter dosing requirements.

Terbinafine undergoes extensive first-pass metabolism. Metabolism involves only a small fraction (less than 5%) of the hepatic cytochrome P-450 capacity, so the drug interactions that are common with the **azoles** do not affect **terbinafine.** Fifteen metabolites have been identified, but none is active. About 80 percent of a dose is excreted in the urine as metabolites, and 20 percent is

Table 22–42. Pharmacokinetics: Systemic Antifungal Agents

Drug	Onset	Peak	Duration	Protein Binding	Bioavailability	Half-Life	Elimination
Fluconazole	Slow	1–2 h	24 h	11–12%	>90%	30 h*	>80% unchanged in urine; 11% as metabolites in urine
Itraconazole†	Rapid	1.5–5 h	12–24 h	99%	55%	21 h–64 h	40% in urine as inactive metabolites; 3–18% in feces
Ketoconazole	Rapid	1–4 h	24 h	99%	75%	8 h	85–90% in bile and feces; 10–15% in urine
Terbinafine	Slow	2 h	UA	>99%	70–80%	11–17 h	80% in urine as metabolites; 20% in feces

*Increased in renal impairment.
†First number represents capsule, and second number represents oral solution.

eliminated in the feces. Both liver impairment and renal impairment require dosage reduction.

Pharmacotherapeutics

Precautions and Contraindications

All of the **azoles** and **terbinafine** have been associated with hepatotoxicity and with rare cases of hepatitis that are usually reversible with discontinuance of the drug. The **azoles** and **terbinafine** are used cautiously for patients with hepatic impairment. For the ones excreted primarily by the kidney, cautious use is required for patients with renal impairment. With both hepatic and renal impairment, dosage adjustments may be required. Because of the burden on the liver, **terbinafine** should be used with caution by patients with alcoholism, either active or in remission.

Ketoconazole should not be given to patients with prostatic cancer. High doses of **ketoconazole** are known to suppress adrenal cortical function, and patients with prostatic cancer have died when given this drug. This drug is used with caution for patients with a history of achlorhydria or hypochlorhydria because of the effect of pH on its absorption.

All of the *azoles* are Pregnancy Category C. Both *ketoconazole* and *itraconazole* have teratogenic effects in animals. There are no adequate well-controlled studies in pregnant women. These drugs should be used during pregnancy only when the potential benefits to the mother clearly outweigh the risks to the fetus. *Terbinafine* is Pregnancy Category B; animal studies show no effects on fertility or fetal toxicity, but adequate studies in humans have not been conducted.

All of the **azoles** and **terbinafine** are excreted in breast milk. After a single 500-mg dose of **terbinafine**, 0.2 to 0.7 mg of **terbinafine** were detected in breast milk. In spite of these low concentrations, it is prudent to avoid administration of **antifungal drugs** to nursing mothers.

The safety and efficacy of these drugs in children vary. **Ketoconazole** is contraindicated for children under 2 years old and not recommended as first choice among **azoles** for any pediatric patient. The safety and efficacy of **itraconazole** have not been established for children. Children 3 to 16 years of age, however, have been treated with 100 mg/d for systemic fungal infections without report of serious adverse reactions. One study with the oral solution was conducted on 26 pediatric patients receiving doses of 5 mg/kg a day for 2 weeks. No serious adverse reactions were reported (Drug Facts and Comparisons, 1999). **Fluconazole** has safe and effective doses for infants and children. Experience with neonates is limited, but there is a dosage schedule. Although the safety and efficacy of **terbinafine** have not been established in children, it has been used in a small number of children 3 to 16 years of age and was well tolerated.

Adverse Drug Reactions

Azoles are relatively nontoxic, and the most common adverse reactions are relatively minor GI symptoms. Patients taking **fluconazole** and **itraconazole** have rarely developed exfoliative skin disorders. Patients who develop rashes should be carefully monitored, and the drug discontinued if the lesion progresses. The inhibition of human CYP-450 enzymes by **ketoconazole** interferes with the biosynthesis of **adrenal** and **gonadal steroid hormones**, producing gynecomastia, infertility, and menstrual irregularities (Groll, Piscitelli, & Walsh, 1998).

The most common adverse reactions with **terbinafine** are also GI and include nausea, vomiting, and diarrhea. Reversible loss or change of taste has occurred after 5 to 8 weeks of therapy, requiring 2 to 6 months to recover after the drug was discontinued. Other adverse effects reported include hypersensitivity, hepatitis, blood dyscrasias, and Stevens-Johnson syndrome (Amichai & Grunwald, 1998).

Drug Interactions

Drug interactions are more common for the drugs with greater human CYP-450 activity. **Ketoconazole** interacts with drugs that increase gastric pH to produce decreased absorption of **ketoconazole**. Additive hepatotoxicity is also possible with other hepatotoxic drugs. Serious arrhythmias have occurred with concurrent use of **cisapride**.

Itraconazole has many drug interactions. Concurrent use of **cisapride** also increases the risk for ventricular arrhythmias and torsades de pointes. Both of these drugs interact with **rifampin, histamine₂ blockers,** and **warfarin. Fluconazole** has slightly fewer drug interactions but also interacts with **rifampin** and **warfarin.**

Additive hepatotoxicity may occur with concurrent administration of **terbinafine, alcohol,** or other hepatotoxins. Because **terbinafine** is hepatically metabolized by cytochrome P-450, drugs that induce or inhibit these enzymes may alter the clearance of **terbinafine.** Those interactions that have been documented for the **azoles** and **terbinafine** are listed in Table 22–43.

Clinical Use and Dosing

Because of its long half-life, **fluconazole** does not achieve steady state for 5 to 10 days with the usual oral doses, but steady state can be achieved in 2 days with a loading dose of twice the usual dose on the first day. Hence, most dosage regimens for **fluconazole** include a loading dose. Because it may undergo saturation metabolism at higher plasma concentrations, the initial dose of **itraconazole** is often doubled, resulting in a threefold increase in the plasma concentration. However, patients with hepatic or renal insufficiency may need reduced maintenance doses of **fluconazole** and **terbinafine.**

Oral **antifungal drugs** are used to treat superficial infections by yeasts (*Candida,* pityriasis versicolor) and dermatophytes (tinea infections) and to treat invasive systemic mycoses (e.g., paracoccidioidomycosis, blastomycosis, histoplasmosis, aspergillosis, candidiasis). Indications and dosages of the oral **antifungal drugs** are summarized in Table 22–44.

Rational Drug Selection

Antifungal drug selection is based on susceptibility, pharmacokinetics, and adverse effects. The spectrum of **terbinafine** includes dermatophytes, and it is recommended for treatment of onychomycosis and tinea infections. The spectrum of the **azoles** includes dermatophytic and superficial fungi, as well as invasive systemic fungi. **Fluconazole** has more reliable bioavailability than the other **azoles** and is generally recommended for the treatment of mild to moderate systemic fungal infections. **Fluconazole** also has fewer drug interactions than other **azoles** and is preferred by many clinicians for this reason.

Monitoring

Prompt recognition of liver injury is essential with oral **antifungal drugs,** particularly **ketoconazole.** AST, ALT, alkaline phosphatase, and bilirubin should be monitored prior to initiation of therapy, monthly for 3 to 4 months, and frequently thereafter during treatment. Even modest elevations in liver enzymes require discontinuation of **ketoconazole.** Because of the numerous drug interactions with **azoles,** it is important to monitor the drug response of concurrent medications. Therapeutic response should be evaluated at 6 to 8 weeks after initiation of drug therapy for tinea infections, 4 to 6 months for fingernail onychomycosis, and 8 to 9 months for toenail mycoses.

Patient Education

ADMINISTRATION. The available dosage forms are shown in Table 22–45. **Itraconazole** capsules and **ketoconazole** should be taken with food to alleviate GI symptoms and promote absorption. **Antacids** should not be used in conjunction with these agents. **Itraconazole** solution should be taken on an empty stomach; **fluconazole** and **terbinafine** can be taken without regard to meals.

ADVERSE REACTIONS. Ketoconazole can cause drowsiness, so patients should not perform hazardous tasks until their response to the medication is established. Because hepatotoxicity is common to all the oral **antifungals,** concurrent use of **alcohol** is discouraged. **Ketoconazole** may cause phototoxicity, so sunscreen and protective clothing are advisable outdoors. Patients should report signs of liver toxicity (unusual tiredness, anorexia, nausea and vomiting, jaundice, pale stools, dark urine), Stevens-Johnson syndrome (rash, blisters, loosening of skin, red joints), and leukopenia (sore throat or fever). Patients on **terbinafine** should know that loss of taste is a reversible adverse effect.

LIFESTYLE MANAGEMENT. Factors that have contributed to the rise of fungal infections are overuse of **antibiotics,** increased numbers of immunocompromised patients, and increased environmental exposure. Patients and providers should work together to limit **antibiotic** use, which will decrease the emergence of bacterial resistance, as well as fungal superinfection.

Anthelminthics

Infestation with parasitic worms is a major health problem throughout the world. In the United States, approximately 60 million people are estimated to harbor a helminthic parasite (VandeWaa, Henderson, White, & Nowatzke, 1998). The worms are divided into four groups: intestinal nematodes (roundworms), tissue nematodes (roundworms), cestodes (flatworms and tape-

Table 22–43. Drug Interactions: Selected Antifungal Agents

Drug	Interacting Drug	Possible Effect	Implications
Fluconazole	Cimetidine	Reduced fluconazole AUC.	Separate doses.
	Hydrochlorothiazide	Significant increase in fluconazole AUC, possibly because of reduced renal clearance.	Avoid concurrent use.
	Phenytoin	Increased phenytoin AUC.	Monitor serum phenytoin levels.
	Rifampin	A single dose of fluconazole after chronic rifampin resulted in a decrease in AUC and a shorter half-life for fluconazole.	If both must be taken, monitor effectiveness of fluconazole and adjust dose if needed.
	Sulfonylureas	Significant increase in AUC of tolbutamide, glyburide, and glipizide. Several patients experienced hypoglycemic episodes, some requiring oral glucose treatment.	If both must be used, monitor blood glucose levels closely while azole is taken.
	Theophylline	Theophylline AUC and half-life increased and clearance decreased. Increased toxicity risk.	Monitor serum theophylline levels. Dosage adjustment may be needed.
	Warfarin	A single warfarin dose after 14 d of fluconazole resulted in an increase in PT/INR.	Monitor PT/INR closely while taking azole.
Itraconazole	Benzodiazepines	Elevated plasma concentrations of oral midazolam and triazolam. Prolonged sedative-hypnotic effects.	Select different benzodiazepine.
	Buspirone	May elevate buspirone levels, increasing the pharmacological and adverse effects.	Closely monitor clinical response to buspirone. Prudent to start with conservative dose and adjust dose of buspirone as needed.
	Calcium channel blockers	Edema with concurrent use of dihydropyridines.	Monitor cardiac status.
	Phenytoin, phenobarbital, isoniazid, carbamazepine	Increased metabolism of itraconazole. Decreased metabolism of phenytoin.	Increased dosage of azole may be needed. Monitor phenytoin levels; dosage adjustments may be needed.
	Cyclosporine, tacrolimus, oral hypoglycemic agents, and warfarin	Itraconazole decreases metabolism of these drugs. Increased risk for toxicity, hypoglycemia, and anticoagulant effect.	Monitor cyclosporine levels. Monitor for indications of hypoglycemia. Monitor PT/INR.
	Digoxin	Increased digoxin levels.	Monitor digoxin levels closely.
	Antacids, histamine₂ blockers, and other drugs that increase gastric pH	Reduced plasma itraconazole levels.	Much less of a problem with oral solution than with capsules.
	Cisapride	Itraconazole inhibits metabolism of cisapride. Possible ventricular arrhythmias.	Concomitant administration contraindicated.
Ketoconazole	Cisapride	Ketoconazole inhibits metabolism of cisapride. Possible prolonged QT interval.	Concomitant administration contraindicated.
	Antacids, histamine₂ blockers, proton-pump inhibitors, and other drugs that increase gastric pH	Inhibit ketoconazole absorption.	Avoid concurrent use. Fluconazole absorption is not affected.

Continued on next page

Table 22–43. Drug Interactions: Selected Antifungal Agents *(continued)*

Drug	Interacting Drug	Possible Effect	Implications
	Rifampin, isoniazid	Bioavailability and serum levels of either drug may be affected.	Avoid concurrent use.
	Hepatotoxic drug	Additive hepatotoxicity.	Avoid concurrent use.
	Cyclosporine, corticosteroids, warfarin	Ketoconazole decreases metabolism of these drugs. Increased risk for toxicity, anticoagulant effect.	Monitor serum levels. Monitor PT/INR more closely. Because the effect on cyclosporine levels is consistent and predictable, this combination has been used therapeutically to reduce cyclosporine dosage.
	Theophylline	Decreased serum theophylline levels.	Monitor theophylline levels. Dosage adjustment may be needed.
Terbinafine	Alcohol, hepatotoxins	Additive liver damage.	Avoid concurrent use or monitor hepatic function closely.
	Cimetidine	Decreased metabolism of terbinafine.	Avoid concurrent use.
	Phenytoin, rifampin	Increased metabolism of terbinafine.	Avoid concurrent use or monitor response to terbinafine.
	Caffeine	Decreased metabolism of caffeine.	Prudent use of caffeinated beverages.
	Cyclosporine	Increased clearance of cyclosporine, possibly leading to organ rejection.	Avoid concurrent use or monitor cyclosporine levels.

INR = international normalized ratio; PT = prothrombin time.

worms), and trematodes (flukes). The only common helminthic infections in the United States are intestinal nematodes: *Enterobius vermicularis* (pinworm), *Trichuris trichiura* (whipworm), *Ascaris lumbricoides* (roundworm), *Strongyloides stercoralis* (threadworm), and the hookworms *Ancylostoma duodenale* and *Necator americanus*. Only those drugs used to treat these infections are discussed in this chapter.

Pharmacodynamics

The **benzimadoles (mebendazole [Vermox], thiabendazole [Mintezol], albendazole [Albenza])** act in different ways directly on the parasite. **Mebendazole** inhibits the formation of the worm's microtubules and irreversibly blocks glucose uptake, depleting endogenous glycogen storage. The worm "starves to death." **Thiabendazole** suppresses production of eggs or larvae and their subsequent development. **Albendazole** inhibits tubulin polymerization, resulting in loss of cytoplasmic microtubules.

Pyrantel (Pin-Rid, Reese's Pinworm, Antiminth) is a depolarizing **neuromuscular blocking agent** that creates spastic paralysis in the worm. It also inhibits cholinesterases. **Ivermectin (Stromectol)** increases the permeability of the cell membrane, resulting in loss of extracellular calcium and increase in intracellular calcium and also producing massive contractions and paralysis of the worm's neuromusculature.

Drugs of choice for treating intestinal nematodes include **mebendazole, pyrantel,** and **thiabendazole.** Tissue nematodes are best treated with **mebendazole, thiabendazole, albendazole,** or **ivermectin.**

Pharmacokinetics

Absorption and Distribution

Thiabendazole is well absorbed from the GI tract after oral administration. The other drugs are poorly absorbed following oral administration. The oral bioavailability of **albendazole** and **mebendazole** appears to be enhanced (up to fivefold) when taken with a fatty meal.

Albendazole is widely distributed and has been detected in urine, bile, liver, cyst wall, cyst fluid, and CSF. **Ivermectin** has a wide tissue distribution. It apparently enters the eye slowly and to a limited extent. The distribution of **mebendazole, pyrantel,** and **thiabendazole** is not known.

Metabolism and Excretion

Albendazole is rapidly converted by the liver to the primary metabolite, albendazole sulfoxide, which is further converted to other metabolites. These metabolites are excreted primarily in the urine.

Ivermectin is metabolized by the liver. The parent

Table 22–44. Dosage Schedule: Selected Antifungal Agents

Drug	Indication	Initial Dose	Comments
Fluconazole (Diflucan)	Vaginal candidiasis	*Adult* 150 mg as single PO dose	Maximal daily pediatric dose 600 mg. Shake suspension well before measurement, using calibrated liquid dosing device. Store suspension in refrigerator or at room temperature. Dispose of unused suspension 2 wk after reconstitution. May be taken without regard to meals.
	Oropharyngeal candidiasis	*Adult* 200 mg PO on first day, followed by 100 mg once daily for 2 wk *Child* 6 mg/kg PO on first day, followed by 3 mg/kg once daily for at least 2 wk	
	Esophageal candidiasis	*Adult* 200 mg PO on first day, followed by 100 mg once daily for 2 wk *Child* 6 mg/kg PO on first day, followed by 3 mg/kg once daily for at least 3 wk and 2 wk beyond resolution of symptoms; doses up to 12 mg/kg/d have been used	
	Other candidal infections	*Adult* 50–400 mg/d PO *Child* 6–12 mg/kg/d PO have been used	
Ketoconazole (Nizoral)	Candidiasis, vulvovaginal	*Adult* 200–400 mg PO once daily for 5 d *Child >2 y* 5–10 mg/kg PO once daily for 5 d *Child <2 y* Dosage not established	Maximal adult daily dosage is 1 g. Therapy should be continued 1–2 wk in candidiasis (3–5 d in vaginal candidiasis); for 1–8 wk in dermatophytic infections and mycoses of hair and scalp; for 3 mo–1 y for paracoccidioidomycosis; and for 6 mo in other systemic mycoses. Chronic mucocutaneous candidiasis following a remission usually requires indefinite maintenance treatment to prevent relapse. Take with food to promote absorption and decrease GI irritation. In patients with hypochlorhydria or achlorhydria take with acid drink. May be dissolved in cola or seltzer water or taken with these fluids.

Continued on next page

Table 22–44. Dosage Schedule: Selected Antifungal Agents *(continued)*

Drug	Indication	Initial Dose	Comments
			Shake suspension well before measurement using a calibrated liquid measuring device. Store at room temperature.
	Paronychia	*Adult* 400 mg PO once daily *Child >2 y* 5–10 mg/kg PO once daily *Child <2 y* Dosage not established	
	Pityriasis versicolor	*Adult* 200 mg PO once daily for 5–10 d	
	Fungal pneumonia or septicemia	*Adult* 400 mg–1 g PO once daily *Child >2 y* 5–10 mg/kg PO once daily *Child <2 y* Dosage not established	
	All other antifungal indications	*Adult* 200–400 mg PO once daily *Child >2 y* 3.3–6.6 mg/kg PO once daily *Child <2 y* Dosage not established	
Itraconazole (Sporanox)	Onychomycosis	*Adult* 200 mg PO once daily with meal for 12 consecutive wk	Safety and efficacy not established for children. A small number of children age 3–16 y with systemic infections have taken itraconazole capsules, 100 mg daily, without serious adverse effects. In life-threatening conditions a loading dose of 200 mg 3 times/d (600 mg/d) is given for first 3 d. Continue treatment for minimum of 3 mo until clinical parameters indicate fungal infection has subsided. Take capsules with food or cola beverage for better absorption. Oral solution should be vigorously swished in mouth, 10 mL at a time, for several seconds and swallowed. Solution should be taken on an empty stomach. Dispense solution with calibrated liquid measuring device.
	Aspergillosis	*Adult* 200–400 mg PO once daily with meal	
	Blastomycosis or histoplasmosis	*Adult* 200 mg PO once daily with meal; if no improvement or progression, increase in 100-mg increments to 400-mg maximum daily dose. Give doses >200 mg daily in 2 divided doses.	

Continued on next page

Table 22–44. Dosage Schedule: Selected Antifungal Agents *(continued)*

Drug	Indication	Initial Dose	Comments
	Candidiasis, esophageal	*Adult* For solution: 100 mg PO (swish and swallow) once daily for minimum of 3 wk (2 wk after resolution of symptoms); off label: 100–200 mg capsules PO once daily after a meal for 14 d; dose for AIDS and neutropenic patients is 200 mg for 4 wk	
	Candidiasis, oropharyngeal	*Adult* For solution 200 mg PO (swish and swallow) once daily for 7–14 d; if refractory to fluconazole, use 100 mg twice/d for 2–4 wk; off label: 100–200 mg capsules PO once daily after a meal for 14 d; dose for AIDS and neutropenic patients is 200 mg for 4 wk	
	Candidiasis, vulvovaginal (off label)	*Adult* 200 mg PO once daily with meal for 3 d	
	Coccidioidomycosis (off label)	*Adult* 200 mg PO twice daily with meals for 6 wk	
	Histoplasmosis suppression (off label)	*Adult* 200 mg PO twice daily with meals	
	Paracoccidioidomycosis (off label)	*Adult* 100 mg PO once daily with meal for 6 wk	
	Tinea corporis or cruris (off label)	*Adult* 100 mg PO once daily with meal for 15 d	
	Tinea manus or pedis (off label)	*Adult* 100 mg PO once daily with meal for 30 d	
Terbinafine (Lamisil)	Onychomycosis, fingernail	*Adult* 250 mg PO once daily for 6 wk	May be taken without regard to meals. Patients with preexisting stable liver disease, impaired renal function (CCr <50 mL/min), or serum creatinine <3.4 mg/dL should receive 50% reduction in dosage. Safety and efficacy for children and children's dosage not established. Following dosages have been use in treatment of children age 3–16 y: Children 12.5–18.5 kg: oral 62.5 mg once daily Children 18.5–25 kg: 125 mg once daily Children >25 kg: 250 mg once daily

Continued on next page

Table 22–44. Dosage Schedule: Selected Antifungal Agents *(continued)*

Drug	Indication	Initial Dose	Comments
	Onychomycosis, toenail	*Adult* 250 mg PO once daily for 12 wk; extensive toenail infections may take longer	
	Tinea capitis (off label)	*Adult* 250 mg PO once daily for 4–6 wk	
	Tinea corporis or cruris (off label)	*Adult* 250 mg PO once daily for 2–4 wk	
	Tinea pedis (plantar or interdigital) (off label)	*Adult* 250 mg PO once daily for 2–6 wk	

drug and its metabolites are excreted almost exclusively in feces over an estimated 12 days.

Absorbed **mebendazole** is mostly metabolized by the liver. More than 95 percent is excreted in feces, and the remainder by the kidney. **Thiabendazole** is also extensively metabolized by the liver, and the inactive metabolites are excreted in the urine.

Pyrantel pamoate undergoes limited metabolism, and more than 50 percent is excreted as unchanged drug in the feces. Less than 7 percent is found in urine as parent drug and metabolites.

Table 22–46 presents the pharmacokinetics of selected **anthelminthics**.

Pharmacotherapeutics

Precautions and Contraindications

Because the activity of these drugs is specific to the parasites, precautions and contraindications are minimal. Drugs extensively metabolized by the liver require cautious administration to patients with hepatic impairment. Drugs excreted extensively by the kidney may require careful monitoring of renal function.

Pregnancy Category C is given to all of these. There are no adequate well-controlled studies in pregnant women, however, for any of these drugs. *Albendazole* **and** *ivermectin* **have demonstrated teratogenic and embryotoxic effects in some animal studies and should not be given to pregnant women.**

It is not known whether **albendazole, mebendazole, pyrantel pamoate,** or **thiabendazole** is excreted in breast milk. Caution should be exercised when giving them to a nursing mother. Deciding to discontinue the drug or the nursing should take into account the importance of the drug to the mother. **Ivermectin** is known to be excreted in breast milk. Nursing can begin 1 week after the last dose of **ivermectin.**

The safety and efficacy of these drugs in children vary by drug. **Mebendazole** and **pyrantel pamoate** are not recommended for children under 2 years old, and **albendazole** is not recommended for children under 6 years old (although no adverse reactions have been found in studies of children as young as 1 year old). Weight is the determination for some drugs, with **thi-**

Table 22–45. Available Dosage Forms: Selected Oral Systemic Antifungal Agents

Drug	Dosage Form	How Supplied
Fluconazole (Diflucan)	Tablets: 50 mg, 100 mg 150 mg 200 mg Powder for oral suspension: 10 mg/cc 40 mg/cc	In bottles of 30 tablets In single units In bottles of 30 tablets In 35-cc bottles when reconstituted In 35-cc bottles when reconstituted
Itraconazole (Sporanox)	Capsules: 100 mg Oral solution: 10 mg/cc	In bottles of 30 capsules In 150-cc bottles
Ketoconazole (Nizoral)	Tablets: 200 mg	In bottles of 100 tablets
Terbinafine (Lamisil)	Tablets: 250 mg	In bottles of 30 or 100 tablets

Table 22–46. Pharmacokinetics: Selected Anthelminthics

Drug	Onset	Peak	Protein Binding	Bioavailability	Half-Life	Elimination
Albendazole	UA	2–5 h	70%	UA	8–12 h	Mainly in urine; small amount in feces
Ivermectin	UA	4 h	UA	UA	16 h	Fecal elimination; <1% in urine
Mebendazole	UA	2–4 h	95%	2–3%	2.5–5.5 h	>90% fecal elimination; 2% in urine
Pyrantel pamoate	UA	1–3 h	UA	UA	UA	50% unchanged drug in feces; <7% in urine
Thiabendazole	Rapid	1–2 h	UA	UA	1.2 h	5% in feces; 90% in urine

Duration of action of all of these drugs is unknown.

abendazole not recommended for children under 13.5 kg and **ivermectin** contraindicated for children under 15 kg.

Adverse Drug Reactions

Adverse reactions vary by drug, with the most common being nausea, vomiting, diarrhea, transient abdominal pain, fever, pruritus, and skin rash. Reversible neutropenia has occurred with **mebendazole,** and CNS symptoms with **thiabendazole.**

Some patients taking **ivermectin** experience the Mazzotti reaction (fever, headache, dizziness, somnolence, weakness, rash, pruritus, diarrhea, joint pain and muscle spasms, hypotension, tachycardia, lymphadenitis, and peripheral edema), which starts the first day and peaks the second day of therapy. It is due to the killing of the microfilariae and not to toxicity. This reaction diminishes with repeated dosing. **Corticosteroids** may be needed for several days to suppress the inflammatory response.

Drug Interactions

There are few drug-drug interactions with any of these drugs. Table 22–47 lists these interactions.

Clinical Use and Dosing

The five common intestinal helminthic infections in the United States are described here, with indication of the usual **antimicrobial agents.** Dosages of the **anthelminthic drugs** are summarized in Table 22–48.

***ENTEROBIUS VERMICULARIS* (PINWORM).** The pinworm is named for the morphology of the posterior of the female. As many as 50 million people in the United States, primarily children, are infected with pinworm. The primary symptoms of pinworm, perianal itching

and sleep disruption, are related to the fact that the female lays eggs nocturnally in the perianal area. Drugs used to treat pinworms include **pyrantel pamoate, albendazole,** and **mebendazole.**

***TRICHURIS TRICHIURA* (WHIPWORM).** Some 80 million people worldwide and 2.2 million in the United States are infected with whipworm. People acquire whipworm by ingesting uncooked vegetables from soil contaminated by human feces. The infection is usually asymptomatic, although heavy infestations may produce anemia, bloody diarrhea, and growth retardation. Drugs used for whipworm infections include **pyrantel pamoate, albendazole,** and **mebendazole.**

***ASCARIS LUMBRICOIDES* (ROUNDWORM).** The roundworm is the most common helminthic parasite worldwide and affects 4 million people in the United States, primarily in the Southeast. Infection generally is derived from eating feces-contaminated raw vegetables. The parasite has a larval stage that migrates through the lungs, causing seasonal pneumonitis, but GI symptoms are more common. Massive infections can cause intestinal obstruction.

***ANCYLOSTOMA DUODENALE* OR *NECATOR AMERICANUS* (HOOKWORM).** Hookworms comprise pathogens from two genera, *A. duodenale* and *N. americanus.* The larvae live in the soil and must penetrate the skin to enter the circulation, where they are carried to the lungs. Here they penetrate the alveoli, crawl up the pharynx, and are swallowed. They attach to the intestinal wall and can cause anemia. Drugs used for hookworm infections include **pyrantel pamoate, albendazole,** and **mebendazole.**

***STRONGYLOIDES STERCORALIS* (THREADWORM).** The larvae of the threadworm are found in warm, moist soil in the tropics and the southern United States. The larvae may penetrate the skin or be ingested. Pulmonary and GI symptoms are common. The drugs used for threadworm

Table 22–47. Drug Interactions: Selected Anthelminthics

Drug	Interacting Drug	Possible Effect	Implications
Albendazole	Dexamethasone	Steady-state trough of main metabolite 50% higher	Avoid coadministration.
	Cimetidine	Metabolite concentrations in bile and cystic fluid higher	May be used therapeutically.
Mebendazole	Carbamazepine, phenytoin	May reduce plasma levels of mebendazole; possible decrease in therapeutic effects	Avoid concomitant use.
	Cimetidine	Increased plasma concentrations of mebendazole	May be used therapeutically.
Pyrantel pamoate	Theophylline	May increase serum levels of theophylline	Further study needed. Only one case noted.
Thiabendazole	Xanthines	Thiabendazole may compete with these drugs for metabolism sites; may elevate serum levels of xanthine with increased toxicity risk	Monitor serum levels of xanthine closely.

infections are **ivermectin** and **thiabendazole**. **Ivermectin** is the drug of choice because it has fewer adverse effects, but **thiabendazole** has the added benefit of promoting immune function in patients with AIDS.

Rational Drug Selection

Drugs are selected for helminthic infections based on research and previous clinical experience, published by the CDC. Drug selection is modified by specific patient characteristics. For example, **albendazole** is contraindicated in pregnancy. Because it is available as a liquid formulation, **pyrantel pamoate** may be preferred for children when the organism is susceptible. It is also available over the counter, which may reduce inconvenience and promote compliance.

Monitoring

Evaluation of the efficacy of the **anthelminthic drugs** includes assessing the eradication of the helminth. For *E. vermicularis*, cellophane tape swabs of the perianal area should be obtained before starting and 1 week after drug therapy, especially in patients with persistent symptoms. The swab should be obtained every morning prior to defecation and bathing for at least 3 days to determine proof of cure.

For roundworms, hookworms, ascariasis, trichuriasis, and whipworms, stool samples are obtained before and 1 to 3 weeks following treatment to determine proof of cure. For strongyloidiasis, routine stool examinations and special examinations such as the Baermann tech-

nique may be required prior to treatment and repeated at intervals of 3 months, beginning at 6 weeks after treatment, to establish proof of cure.

Patients taking prolonged therapy with these agents should have periodic evaluation of hepatic function and CBCs. These tests should also be repeated whenever there is clinical evidence of hepatotoxicity or blood dyscrasias.

Patient Education

ADMINISTRATION. The available dosage forms are shown in Table 22–49. **Albendazole** should be swallowed whole with a small amount of water and a high-fat meal to decrease GI effects and increase absorption. **Mebendazole** is also taken with a high-fat meal, but it can be chewed or crushed before it is swallowed. **Ivermectin** must be taken with a full glass of water on an empty stomach 1 hour before breakfast. **Pyrantel pamoate** can be taken without regard to meals, at any time of the day. **Thiabendazole** must be chewed or crushed before swallowing and taken after a meal.

ADVERSE REACTIONS. Women of childbearing capacity should take **albendazole** after a negative pregnancy test in the first 7 days following the onset of menses and should use a backup barrier method of contraception for 1 month after completing the therapy. **Albendazole** should not be used in conjunction with over-the-counter or prescription **cimetidine**, which decreases clearance of **albendazole**. Patients who have recently taken **albendazole** should also report signs of neutrope-

Table 22–48. Dosage Schedule: Selected Anthelminthics

Drug	Indication	Initial Dose	Comments
Albendazole (Albenza)	Ascariasis Enterobiasis Hookworm infections Trichuriasis	*Adults and children >2 y* 400 mg PO once daily for 3 d; may repeat in 3 wk *Children <2 y* 200 mg PO as single dose; may repeat in 3 wk	Maximal daily dose for adults and adolescents <60 kg is 800 mg. Take with food containing fat. Swallow tablets whole with small amount of liquid. Shake suspension well before measurement with calibrated liquid measuring device. Store at room temperature.
	Strongyloidiasis	*Adults and children >2 y* 400 mg PO once daily for 3 d; may repeat in 3 wk *Children <2 y* 200 mg PO once daily for 3 d; may repeat in 3 wk	
	Giardiasis	*Adults* 400 mg PO daily for 5 d	
Ivermectin (Stromectol)	Strongyloidiasis	*Adults and children >15 kg* 200 µg/kg as single dose	Take with full glass of water 1 hr before breakfast
Mebendazole (Vermox)	Ascariasis Trichuriasis Hookworm Roundworms Enterobiasis	*Adults and children >2 y* 100 mg PO twice daily, morning and evening, for 3 d; may repeat in 2–3 wk if required *Adults* 100 mg PO as single dose; may repeat in 2–3 wk if required	Take with high-fat meals. Tablets may be chewed, crushed, or swallowed whole.
Pyrantel pamoate (Pin-Rid)	Enterobiasis Ascariasis Trichuriasis Hookworm	*Adults and children* 11 mg/kg as single dose	Maximum daily dose 1 g. May be taken with milk, food, or juice at any time of day. Shake suspension well, and measure with calibrated liquid measuring device. Store at room temperature.
Thiabendazole (Mintezol)	Strongyloidiasis, uncomplicated	*Adults and children >13.6 kg* 25 mg/kg twice daily for 2 d	Maximum adult daily dose 3 g. Chew or crush tablets before swallowing. Take after meals. Shake suspension well before measurement with calibrated liquid dosing device. Take after meals.
	Strongyloidiasis, hyperinfection	*Adults and children >13.6 kg* 25 mg/kg twice daily for 5–7 d; may be repeated if required	

nia (sore throat, fever, unusual tiredness). **Mebendazole** should also be avoided during pregnancy.

Ivermectin and **thiabendazole** can cause lightheadedness, so hazardous activities should be avoided during therapy. Patients should be warned of the asparagus-like odor of urine during **thiabendazole** therapy, which may be unpleasant but is harmless. Both of these agents may be associated with a skin rash or itching during treatment of strongyloidiasis because of the death of microfilariae in the skin. If serious, this syndrome may require short-term therapy with **corticosteroids** to suppress the inflammatory response. Patients on **thiabendazole** should report any evidence of neurotoxicity (numbness or tingling of the hands, delirium, disorientation, hallucinations), crys-

Table 22–49. Available Dosage Forms: Selected Anthelminthics

Drugs	Dosage Form	How Supplied
Albendazole (Albenza)	Tablets: 200 mg	In bottles of 112 tablets
Ivermectin (Stromectol)	Tablets: 6 mg	In 10-unit doses
Mebendazole (Vermox)	Tablets: 100 mg	In 12 tablets
Pyrantel pamoate (Pin-Rid)	Capsules: 180 mg (62.5 mg of pyrantel base) Liquid: 50 mg/cc	In bottles of 24 soft-gel capsules In 60-cc bottles, cherry flavor
(Pin-X)	Liquid: 50 mg/cc	In 30-cc bottles, caramel flavor
(Reese's Pinworm)	Capsules: 180 mg (62.5 mg of pyrantel base) Liquid: 50 mg/cc	In bottles of 24 soft-gel capsules In 30-cc bottles
(Antiminth)	Oral suspension: 50 mg/cc	In 30-cc bottles
Thiabendazole (Mintezol)	Tablets: 500 mg Oral suspension: 50 mg/cc	In bottles of 36 scored, chewable tablets, orange flavor In 120-cc bottles

talluria (back pain, burning on urination), or Stevens-Johnson syndrome (rash, blistering, loose skin, peeling, aching joints and muscles, chills, and fever).

LIFESTYLE MANAGEMENT.   Patients with hookworm and whipworm infections may require **iron** replacement therapy. Eradication of pinworm infections usually requires simultaneous treatment of all household contacts; a vigorous hygiene program of cleaning bedlinens, nightwear, and underwear; and good handwashing habits. Contrary to popular belief, treatment of helminthic infections does not require special diets or purging with laxatives before or after the **antimicrobial** drug.

Metronidazole

Metronidazole (**Flagyl, Metric 21, Protostat**) is a drug that crosses classes—that is, it is effective in parasitical and bacterial infections—so its systemic use is discussed in this separate section. Topical applications are discussed in Chapter 21 and 30 for skin conditions and in Chapter 42 for vaginal disorders.

Pharmacodynamics

Metronidazole is a **nitroimidazole** that disrupts DNA and protein synthesis of susceptible organisms. With anaerobic bacteria and sensitive protozoal cells, the nitro group of this drug is chemically reduced to ferredoxin, which is bactericidal by reacting with intracellular macromolecules.

Metronidazole possesses direct trichomonicidal and amebicidal activity against *Trichomonas vaginalis and Entamoeba histolytica.* It is also active against *H. pylori* and against anaerobic bacteria including *Bacteroides* and *Clostridium.* Although an unlabeled use, it is active against *Giardia lamblia, and Gardnerella vaginalis.* It is now the recommended drug for treatment of pseudomembranous colitis associated with *C. difficile* overgrowth secondary to use of **antibiotics.**

Pharmacokinetics

Absorption and Distribution

Oral **metronidazole** is readily absorbed and widely distributed into most tissue and fluids, including CSF, breast milk, alveolar bone, liver abscesses, vaginal secretions, and seminal fluid. It also crosses the placenta. Intracellular concentrations approach extracellular levels. Onset of action is rapid after oral administration, with peak plasma levels obtained in 1 to 3 hours. Duration of activity is 8 hours. Protein binding is low (less than 20%). The half-life of the unchanged drug is 7.5 hours.

Metabolism and Excretion

Partially metabolized by the liver (30 to 60%), the drug and its metabolites are excreted in feces (6 to 15%), with the rest excreted in urine.

Pharmacotherapeutics

Precautions and Contraindications

Cautious use is recommended for patients with a history of blood dyscrasias. Seizures have occurred as an adverse reaction, and patients with a history of seizure disorder or neurological problems should use this drug with caution. Severe hepatic dysfunction may decrease plasma clearance, and **metronidazole** should be used cautiously with these patients.

Metronidazole **is listed as Pregnancy Category B, but many experts believe it should not be used in the first trimester of pregnancy. It has been used to treat trichomoniasis in the second and third trimester of pregnancy, but not as a single-dose regimen. Although this drug has been used for more than 20 years with no increase in congenital abnormalities, stillbirths, or low birth weight reported, as with any drug given during pregnancy, prudence suggests that it be used only when clearly indicated.**

A nursing mother who needs **metronidazole** should interrupt nursing for 24 hours and use a single-dose regimen. Its safety and efficacy in young children have not been established.

Adverse Drug Reactions

Anorexia, nausea, abdominal pain, dizziness, and headache commonly occur with this drug. Dry mouth and a metallic taste may also develop. Although irritating, these adverse reactions are mild and transient. Infrequent adverse reactions include diarrhea, glossitis, rashes, leukopenia, and peripheral neuropathy. Taking the drug with meals lessens the GI irritation. One rare but serious adverse reaction is seizures.

Drug Interactions

Drug interactions are few. **Cimetidine** may decrease the plasma clearance of **metronidazole,** increasing serum levels; **phenobarbital** and **phenytoin** may accelerate excretion, decreasing serum levels. **Metronidazole** potentiates the anticoagulant effects of **warfarin** so that close monitoring of prothrombin time/international normalized ratio (PT/INR) is required. A disulfiram-like reaction may occur with **alcohol** ingestion, and patients are warned not to consume **alcohol** while taking this drug and for 48 hours after completing it. Leukopenia risk is increased if it is given concurrently with **fluorouracil** or **azathioprine.** Concurrent use should be avoided.

Clinical Use and Dosing

Metronidazole has antiparasitic and antibacterial properties. It is used against the common protozoal infections by *T. vaginalis, G. lamblia,* and *E. histolytica.* **Metronidazole** is also used to treat less common parasites, such as the protozoon *Balantidium coli* (with an oral dose of 750 mg three times daily for 5 days), as an alternative to **tetracycline,** and to treat the helminth *Dracunculus medinensis* or

guinea worm (with an oral dose of 250 mg three times daily for 10 days). **Antibacterial** uses of **metronidazole** include treatment of anaerobic bacterial infections, bacterial vaginosis, AAPMC, and eradication of *H. pylori* in gastritis and peptic ulcer disease. Most of the anaerobic bacterial infections treated with **metronidazole** are serious, even life-threatening, and are treated in the hospital. Dosages of **metronidazole** for these diverse conditions are summarized in Table 22–50. In severe hepatic disease, the dosage of **metronidazole** may need to be decreased; increased dosages might be required for successful therapy of patients taking inducers of hepatic cytochrome P-450, such as **phenobarbital** and **phenytoin.**

TRICHOMONAL VAGINITIS. Trichomonal vaginal infection often occurs during or shortly after menses and is characterized by copious foamy discharge with a pH greater than 5.0, positive "whiff test," punctate hemorrhages of vaginal mucosa, and vaginal irritation. Although it is generally sexually transmitted, the organism can live for weeks on wet towels and toilet seats, so fomite transfer is theoretically possible. In the male, the infection may cause urethral discharge, but it is usually mild, if present at all. Both partners should be treated and a condom used during intercourse for a week to prevent reinfection. Short treatment requires 2 g as a single dose; long treatment is 500 mg three times daily for 7 days. If the infection occurs in the first trimester of pregnancy, deferral of treatment is recommended. Experts disagree over whether the long or short treatment is preferable during pregnant and nonpregnant states. Single-dose therapy promotes compliance, especially if administered under supervision. However, the 7-day therapy may be more effective and may minimize reinfection of the woman long enough to treat sexual contacts.

GIARDIASIS. The life cycle of the protozoon *G. lamblia* involves two stages: a cyst and a trophozoite. The cyst form can live in cold water for months and is ingested by the human hosts. It can also be transmitted during sexual activity. The trophozoite, or actively metabolizing, motile form, lives in the upper two-thirds of the small intestine, and they can be so numerous that they mechanically interfere with digestion. *Giardia* infections may be asymptomatic or cause disease ranging from self-limiting diarrhea to a severe chronic syndrome with malnutrition. In the United States, **metronidazole,** 250 mg three times daily for 5 to 7 days, is the drug of choice for treating giardiasis, although it is not approved for this indication. Asymptomatic cyst passers should also be treated.

AMEBIASIS. Several species of *Entamoeba* infect humans, but *E. histolytica* is the only species known to cause disease. Like many protozoa, *Entamoeba* has two life stages: the cyst and the trophozoite. Infection of the human usually involves ingestion of cysts from fecally

Table 22–50. Dosage Schedule: Metronidazole

Drug	Indication	Initial Dose	Comments
Metronidazole (Flagyl, Metric 21, Protostat)	Anaerobic bacterial infection	*Adults* 7.5 mg/kg PO q6h for 7 d or longer *Child* 7.5 mg/kg PO q6h *or* 10 mg/kg q8h	Maximum adult daily dosage is 4 g. Reduction in dosage may be required for patients with severe hepatic impairment. May be taken with meals or a snack to decrease GI irritation. Avoid alcoholic beverages during therapy and for 48 h after completing it. Sexual partners of patients with *T. vaginalis* should be treated even if asymptomatic. Abstain from sexual contact or use condom for 7 d after therapy begins. Antimicrobial drugs used with metronidazole to eradicate *H.pylori* include bismuth subsalicylate, amoxicillin, tetracycline, plus acid-reducing drug if disease is active. Oral forms: Generic: 250 mg in bottles of 100, 250, 500, and 1000 tablets; 500 mg in bottles of 100, 200, 250, and 500 tablets. Flagyl: 250 mg in bottles of 50, 100, 250, 1000, and 2500 tablets; 500 mg in bottles of 50, 100, and 500 tablets; 375 mg in bottles of 50 and 100 capsules. Metric 21: 250 mg in bottles of 100 tablets. Protostat: 250 mg in bottles of 100 scored tablets; 500 mg in bottles of 50 scored tablets.
	Antibiotic-associated pseudomembranous colitis (*C. difficile*) (off label)	*Adult* 500 mg PO 3 times daily *or* 250 mg PO 4 times daily for 10–14 d	
	Bacterial vaginosis associated with *G. vaginalis* (off label)	*Adult* 500 mg PO twice daily for 7 d	
	Giardiasis (*G. lamblia*) (off label)	*Adult* 250 mg PO 3 times daily for 5–7 d *Child* 5 mg/kg/dose PO 3 times daily for 5–7 d	
	Amebiasis (*E. histolytica*) dysentery	*Adult* 750 mg PO 3 times daily for 5–10 d *Child* 35–50 mg/kg/24 h PO in 3 divided doses for 10 d *or* 11.6–16.7 mg/kg/dose PO 3 times daily for 10 d	

Continued on next page

Table 22–50. Dosage Schedule: Metronidazole *(continued)*

Drug	Indication	Initial Dose	Comments
	Amebiasis *(E. histolytica)* liver abscess	*Adult* 500–750 mg PO 3 times daily for 5–10 d *Child* 35–50 mg/kg/24 h PO in 3 divided doses for 10 d *or* 11.6–16.7 mg/kg/dose PO 3 times daily for 10 d	
	Balantidiasis (off label) *(B. coli)*	*Adult* 500–750 mg PO 3 times/d for 5–10 d *Child* 11.6–16.7 mg/kg/dose 3 times daily for 10 d	
	Gastritis or peptic ulcer, *H. pylori*–associated	*Adult* In combination with antibiotic therapy (see comments): 500 mg PO 3 times daily for 7–14 d	
	Trichomoniasis *(T. vaginalis)*	*Adult* 2 g PO as a single dose *or* 2 divided doses in 1 d; alternative: 250 mg PO 3 times/d for 7 d *Child* 5 mg/kg/dose PO 3 times daily for 7 d	
	Anthelminthic	*Adult* 250 mg PO 3 times daily for 10 d *Child* 8.3 mg/kg/dose PO, up to a maximum of 250 mg, 3 times/d for 10 d	

contaminated food, water, or hands. Transmission of cysts and trophozoites can also occur with fecal exposure during sexual contact. In the intestine, cysts undergo excystation into the trophozoite form and multiply. In many cases, the cysts remain in the intestinal lumen (noninvasive infection), resulting in asymptomatic carriers and cyst passers. In some patients, the cysts invade the intestinal lumen (invasive intestinal disease), resulting in diarrhea or dysentery. Trophozoites also can travel through the bloodstream to form abscesses in the liver, brain, or lung (extraintestinal disease) that are manifested by local signs such as hepatomegaly or cholestasis. Drugs administered for presumptive treatment (broad-spectrum **antibiotics, kaolin, bismuth,** soapsuds enema, **barium**) can suppress shedding of amebae into the stool and delay diagnosis. For invasive intestinal amebiasis, **metronidazole,** 750 mg orally three times daily for 5 to 10 days, is the drug of choice. **Metronidazole** can be used to treat the extraintestinal form of the disease IV or orally. **Metronidazole** is so well absorbed that it is not effective against the noninvasive infection, and it may be necessary to add a luminal agent like **paromomycin** (Hu-

matin), 500 mg PO three times daily for 7 days. **Paromomycin** is an unabsorbable **aminoglycoside** similar to **neomycin.** If the intestinal mucosa is not intact, as in concomitant inflammatory bowel disease, **paromomycin** can be absorbed and cause ototoxicity and nephrotoxicity.

BACTERIAL VAGINOSIS. Bacterial vaginosis develops when the bacterial flora are altered, with loss of the normally predominant lactobacilli and overgrowth of strict and facultative aerobic species such as *Bacteroides, Peptococcus, Mobiluncus, Gardnerella, Streptococcus,* and *Mycoplasma.* The infection manifests with foul-odored, clear, copious vaginal discharge with a pH greater than 4.5, positive "whiff test," and few WBCs. Untreated bacterial vaginosis has been associated with pelvic inflammatory disease, cervicitis, abnormal PAP smear cytology, preterm labor, and low birth weight. During pregnancy, symptomatic women are screened and treated if they are at high risk for preterm delivery. Treatment of low-risk and symptomatic women during pregnancy is controversial. **Metronidazole,** 500 mg orally twice daily for 7 days, or **metronidazole intravaginal gel,** 1 full applicator twice daily for 5 days, is the drug of first choice for bacterial vaginosis. The 2-g single dose is not as effective for bacterial vaginosis as these two regimens. **Metronidazole** is avoided in the first trimester of pregnancy, although the alternative for bacterial vaginosis, **clindamycin,** has not been shown to prevent preterm birth and is no longer recommended by the CDC. It is not necessary to treat sexual partners of women with bacterial vaginosis unless balanitis is present.

Rational Drug Selection

For most of the infections for which **metronidazole** is used, it is the drug of choice because it is clearly more efficacious than the alternatives. Issues in drug selection for these conditions are the lack of effective alternatives for use in the first trimester of pregnancy, comparative efficacy of the long- and short-term oral dosing regimen, and the choice between topical and oral forms for vaginal infections. These issues have been covered in previous sections.

Monitoring

For most of the conditions treated with **metronidazole,** resolution of symptoms indicates effective treatment, and further evaluation is not required. For giardiasis, symptoms may persist for weeks or months after the organism is eradicated because of the lactose intolerance brought on by the infection. If symptoms persist, three stool samples should be collected several days apart about 3 to 4 weeks after completion of treatment. If signs of leukopenia develop (sore throat and fever), a white blood cell count should be collected.

Patient Education

ADMINISTRATION. Although oral **metronidazole** can be taken without regard to meals, it should be taken with food or snacks to decrease GI irritation. If vaginal or topical preparations are used, the patient should be provided with instruction and the opportunity to manipulate a model applicator in the office. Use of the extended-release form of **metronidazole** that can be administered once daily should be considered if nonadherence is an issue, although the vaginal gel and delayed-release oral form are considerably more expensive than other oral forms.

ADVERSE REACTIONS. Chewing sugarless gum or sucking on ice or candy can help to overcome the dry mouth and metallic taste that **metronidazole** can cause. Alcoholic beverages should be avoided during therapy and for 48 hours after the last dose because of the disulfiram-like reaction that about 40 percent of patients on the drug experience if exposed to **alcohol.** Because the drug can cause dizziness or lightheadedness, hazardous activities should be avoided until the patient's response to the medication is established. Headache is a common adverse effect that can be treated with **acetaminophen** or a **NSAID. Metronidazole** causes a harmless darkening of urine. Female patients should be counseled about the symptoms of vaginal candidiasis superinfection, which can complicate therapy and could be mistaken for recurrence of the original infection. The patient and family members should know to report CNS symptoms (ataxia, mood and mental changes, clumsiness, ataxia, seizures), peripheral neuropathy (numbness, tingling, pain, or weakness in hands or feet), and leukopenia (sore throat or fever).

LIFESTYLE MANAGEMENT. Many of the infections treated with **metronidazole** are sexually transmitted. Male or female condom usage may decrease transmittal of some, but not all, infections. For amebiasis and giardiasis, which are not usually considered sexually transmitted, identification of a sexual mode of transmission is helpful in preventing recurrent infections caused by the "ping-pong" of the infection between partners. Patients should be advised of the route of transmission and practices that promote transmittal of the infection. Concurrent treatment and refraining from sexual activity until the treatment is complete may be necessary to resolve the infections. Foreign travel and wilderness travel are other sources of exposure to *Giardia* and amebae that should be considered in the history for diagnosing these conditions.

REFERENCES

Amichai, B., & Grunwald, M. H. (1998). Adverse drug reactions and the new oral antifungal agents: Terbinafine, fluconazole, and itraconazole. *International Journal of Dermatology, 37,* 410–415.

Andriole, V. T. (1999). The future of quinolones. *Drugs,* (Suppl 2)58, 1–5.

Bauchner, H., Pelton, S. I., & Klein, J. O. (1999). Parents, physicians, and antibiotic use. *Pediatrics, 103,* 395–401.

Berardi, R. R. (1999). Peptic ulcer disease. In J. T. DiPiro, R. L. Talbert, G. C. Yee, G. R. Matzke, B. G. Wells, & L. M. Posey (Eds.), *Pharmacotherapy: A pathophysiologic approach* (4th ed., pp. 548–570). Stamford, CT: Appleton & Lange.

Berman, S., Byrns, P. J., Bondy, J., Smith, P. J., & Lezotte, D. (1997). Otitis media-related antibiotic prescribing patterns, outcomes, and expenditures in a pediatric Medicaid population. *Pediatrics, 100,* 585–592.

Bishai, W. R., & Chaisson, R. E. (1999). Drug resistance and the treatment of upper respiratory infections. *American Journal of Managed Care, 5*(15), S943–S962.

Carlson, W., & Deay, R. Acute otitis media program focuses on antibiotic usage. *Drug Benefit Trends, 11*(5), 40–42, 45–47.

Centers for Disease Control and Prevention. (1996). Prevention of perinatal group B streptococcal disease: A public health perspective. *MMWR: Morbidity and Mortality Weekly Report, 45*(SS6), 25–32.

Centers for Disease Control and Prevention. (1997). *Staphylococcus aureus* with reduced susceptibility to vancomycin—United States, 1997. *MMWR: Morbidity and Mortality Weekly Report, 46,* 765–766.

Chambers, J. F., & Jawetz, E. (1998). Sulfonamides, trimethoprim, and quinolones. In B. G. Katzung (Ed.), *Basic and clinical pharmacology* (7th ed., pp. 761–769). Stamford, CT: Appleton & Lange.

Climo, M. W., Israel, D. S., Wong, E. S., Williams, D., Coudron, P., & Markowitz, S. M. (1998). Hospital-wide restriction of clindamycin: effect on incidence of *Clostridium difficile*–associated diarrhea and cost. *Annals of Internal Medicine, 128,* 989–995.

Cohen, R., Bingen, E., Varon, E., de la Roque, F., Brahimi, N., Levy, C., Boucherat, M., Langue, J., & Geslin, P. (1997). Change in nasopharyngeal carriage of *Streptococcus pneumoniae* resulting from antibiotic therapy for acute otitis media in children. *Pediatric Infectious Disease Journal, 16,* 555–560.

Committee on Quality, American Academy of Pediatrics. (1999). The diagnosis, treatment, and evaluation of the initial urinary tract infection in febrile infants and children. *Pediatrics, 103,* 843–852.

Dagan, R., Johnson, C. E., McLinn, S., Abughali, N., Feris, J., Leibovitz, E., Burch, D. J., & Jacobs, M. R. (2000). Bacteriologic and clinical efficacy of amoxicillin-clavulanate versus azithromycin in acute otitis media. *Pediatric Infectious Disease Journal, 19,* 95–104.

Deglin, J., & Vallerand, A. (1999). *Davis's drug guide for nurses* (6th ed.). Philadelphia: F. A. Davis.

Dowell, S. (1998). Principles of judicious use of antimicrobial agents for pediatric upper respiratory infections. *Pediatrics,* (Suppl.)*101,* 160–184.

Facts and Comparisons Staff. (1999). *Drug facts and comparisons.* St. Louis: Facts and Comparisons.

Fletcher, C. V., Kakudi, T. N., & Collier, A. C. (1999). Human immunodeficiency virus infection. In J. T. DiPito, R. L. Talbert,G. C. Yee, G. R. Matzke, B. G. Wells, & L. M. Posey (Eds), *Pharmacotherapy: A pathophysiologic approach* (4th ed., pp. 1930–1956). Stamford, CT: Appleton & Lange.

Gatifloxacin and moxifloxacin: Two new fluroquinolones. (2000). *Medical Letter on Drugs and Therapeutics, 42,* 15–17.

Gilbert, D. N., Moellering, R. C., Jr., & Sande, M. A. (1999). *The Sanford guide to antimicrobial therapy* (29th ed.). Hyde Park, VT: Antimicrobial Therapy.

Gleason, P., Kapoor, W., Stone, R., Lave, J., Obrosky, D., Schulz, R., Singer, D., Coley, C., Marrie, T., & Fine, M. (1997). Medical outcomes and antimicrobial costs with the use of the American Thoracic Society guideline for outpatients with community-acquired pneumonia. *Journal of the American Medical Association, 278*(1), 32–39.

Gonzales, R., Steiner, J. F., & Sande, M. (1997). Antibiotic prescribing for adults with colds, upper respiratory tract infections, and bronchitis by ambulatory care physicians. *Journal of the American Medical Association, 278,* 901–904.

Gooch, W. M., & Golantly, S. A. (2000). *A review of treatment guidelines in an era of drug-resistant pneumococcal pathogens: A review of the otitis media guidelines.* Laguna Niguel, CA: Institute for Medical Studies.

Groll, A. H., Piscitelli, S. C., & Walsh, T. J. (1998). Clinical pharmacology of systemic antifungal agents: A comprehensive review of agents in current clinical use, current investigational compounds, and putative targets for antifungal drug development. *Advances in Pharmacology, 44,* 343–501.

Gutierrez, K. (1999). Pharmacotherapeutics: Clinical decision-making in nursing. Philadelphia: Saunders.

Handbook of antimicrobial therapy. (2000). New Rochelle, NY: Medical Letter.

Hawkey, C., Tulassay, Z., Szczepanski, L., van Rensburg, C., Filipowicz-Sosnowska, A., Lanas, A., Wason, C., Peacock, R., & Gillon, K. (1998). Randomized controlled trial of *Heliobactoer pylori* eradication in patients on non-steroidal anti-inflammatory drugs: HELP NSAIDS study. *Heliobactoer* eradication for lesion prevention. *Lancet, 352*(9133), 1016–1021.

Helwig, H. (1997). Contemporary issues in the management of pediatric infections. *Pediatric Infectious Disease Journal* (Suppl.)*16,* S39– S41.

Hueston, W. J., & Mainous, A. G. (1998). Acute bronchitis. *American Family Physician, 57,* 1270–1279.

Jacobs, M. R. (1999). Activity of quinolones against mycobacteria. *Drugs,* (Suppl. 2)*58,* 19–22.

Kaplan, S. L. (1997). *Streptococcus pneumoniae:* Impact of antibiotic resistance in pediatrics. *Current Problems in Pediatrics, 27,* 187–195.

Kastrup, E. (Founding Editor). (1999). *Drug facts and comparisons.* St. Louis: Facts and Comparisons.

Katzung, B. (1998). *Basic and clinical pharmacology* (7th ed.). Stamford, CT: Appleton & Lange.

Klein, J. O. (1995). Antimicrobial therapy issues facing pediatricians. *Pediatric Infectious Disease Journal, 14,* 415–418.

Kolmos, H. J., & Little, P. (1999). Should general practitioners perform diagnostic tests on patients before prescribing antibiotics? *British Medical Journal, 318,* 799–803.

Kozyrskyj, A. L., Hildes-Ripstein, G. E., Longstaffe, S. E. A., Wincott, J. L., Sitar, D. S., Klassen, T. P., & Moffat, M. E. K. (1998). Treatment of acute otitis media with a shortened course of antibiotics: A meta-analysis. *Journal of the American Medical Association, 279,* 1736–1742.

Lampris, H. W., & Maddix, D. S. (1998). Clinical use of antimicrobial agents. In B. Katzung (Ed.), *Basic and clinical pharmacology* (7th ed., pp. 812–826). Stamford, CT: Appleton & Lange.

Levin, B. R., Lipsich, M., & Perrot, V. (1997). The population genetics of antimicrobial resistance. *Clinics in Infectious Disease,* (Suppl. 1)*24,* S9–S16.

Locksmith, G. J., Clark, P., & Duff, P. (1999). Maternal and neonatal infection rates with three different protocols for prevention of group B streptococcal disease. *American Journal of Obstetrics and Gynecology, 180,* 416–422.

Mangione-Smith, R., McGlynn, E. A., Elliott, M. N., Krogstad, P., & Brook, R. H. (1999). The relationship between perceived parental expectations and pediatrician antimicrobial prescribing behavior. *Pediatrics, 103,* 711–718.

Niederman, M. S., Skerett, S. J., Yamauchi, T., & Pinkowish, D. (1998). Antibiotics or not: Managing patients with respiratory infections. *Patient Care, 32,* 60–74.

Nyquist, A., Gonzales, R., Steiner, J. F., & Sande, M. A. (1998). Antibiotic prescribing for children with colds, upper respiratory tract infections, and bronchitis. *Journal of the American Medical Association, 279,* 875–877.

O'Dell, J. R. (1999). Is there a role for antibiotics in the treatment of patients with rheumatoid arthritis? *Drugs, 57,* 279–282.

Oeffinger, K. C., Snell, L. M., Foster, B. M., Panico, K. G., & Archer, R. K. (1998). Treatment of acute bronchitis in adults: A national survey of family physicians. *Journal of Family Practice, 46,* 469–475.

Ogle, J. W. (1999). Antimicrobial therapy for ambulatory pediatrics. *Annals of Pediatrics, 28,* 434–445.

Orenstein, R. (1999). Urinary tract infections in adults. *American Family Physician, 59,* 1225–1235.

Pichichero, M. E. (1997). Empiric antibiotic selection criteria for respiratory infections in pediatric practice. *Pediatric Infectious Disease Journal, 16,* S60–S64.

Pichichero, M. E., & Cohen, R. (1997). Shortened course of antibiotic therapy for otitis media, sinusitis, tonsillopharyngitis. *Pediatric Infectious Disease Journal, 16,* 680–695.

Piddock, L. J. V. (1999). Mechanisms of fluoroquinolone resistance: An update 1994–1998. *Drugs,* (Suppl. 2)*58,* 11–18.

Prevention of Bacterial Endocarditis [American Heart Association patient handout]. Based on standards published by same source in *JAMA 277,* 1794, 1997.

Rapid diagnostic tests for influenza. (1999). *Medical Letter on Drugs and Therapeutics, 41*(1068), 121–122.

Roman, R. S., Smith, J., Walker, M., Byrne, S., Ramotar, K., Dyck, B., Kabani, A., & Nicolle, L. E. (1997). Rapid geographical spread of a methicillin-resistant *Staphylococcus aureus* strain. *Clinics in Infectious Disease, 25,* 698–705.

Schaad, U. B. (1997). Toward an integrated program for patient care in pediatric infections. *Pediatric Infectious Disease Journal,* (Suppl.)*16,* S34–S38.

Schrag, S. J., Zywicki, S., Farley, M. M., Reingold, A. L., Harrison, L. H., Lefkowitz, L. B., Hadler, J. L., Danilia, R., Cieslak, P. R., & Schuchat, A. (2000). Group B streptococcal disease in the era of intrapartum antibiotic prophylaxis. *New England Journal of Medicine, 342,* 15–20.

Schussheim, A. E., & Fuster, V. (1999). Antibiotics for myocardial infarction: A possible role of infection in arthrogenesis and acute coronary syndromes. *Drugs, 57,* 283–291.

Schwartz, B., Mainous, A. G., & Marcy, S. M. (1998). Why do physicians prescribe antibiotics for children with upper respiratory tract infections? *Journal of the American Medical Association, 279,* 881–882.

Stahlmann, R., & Lode, H. (1999). Toxicity of quinolones. *Drugs,* (Suppl. 2)*58,* 37–42.

Steele, R. W., Thomas, M. P., Begue, R. E., & Despinasse, B. P. (1999). Selection of pediatric antibiotic suspensions: Taste and cost. *Infection Medicine, 16,* 197–200.

Talley, N. J., Vakil, N., Ballard, E. D., & Fennerty, M. B. (1999). Absence of benefit for eradicating *Helicobacter pylori* in patients with nonulcer dyspepsia. *New England Journal of Medicine, 341*(15), 1106–1111.

Thielman, N. M., & Neu, H. C. (1998). Principles of antimicrobial use. In T. M. Brody, J. Larner, & K. P. Minneman (Eds.), *Human pharmacology: Molecular to clinical* (3rd ed., pp. 641–654). St. Louis: Mosby.

Tiggs, B. B. (2000). Acute otitis media and pneumococcal resistance: Making judicious management decisions. *Nurse Practitioner: The American Journal of Primary Health Care, 25*(69), 73–80.

Turnbridge, J. (1999). Pharmacokinetics and pharmacodynamics of fluroquinolones. *Drugs, 58*(Suppl. 2), 29–36.

Two neuraminidase inhibitors for treatment of influenza. *Medical Letter on Drugs and Therapeutics, 41*(1063), 91–93.

United States Pharmacopeial Dispensing Information (USPDI). (1999). *Volume I: Drug information for the health care professional* (19th ed.). Englewood, CO: Micromedex Publishers.

VandeWaa, E. A., Henderson, J. D., White, G. L., & Nowatzke, T. J. (1998). Common helminthic infections: Treating wormlike parasites in primary care. *Clinician Reviews 8*(5), 75–77, 81–82, 85–90, 92.

CHAPTER 23

Drugs Used in Treating Inflammatory Processes

CHAPTER OUTLINE

Antigout and Uricosuric Agents

G out was the first form of arthritis to be recognized as crystal-induced. It is a syndrome caused by an alteration in purine metabolism, the end product of which is uric acid. This alteration results in hyperuricemia and in the deposition of urate crystals in various tissues. The key elements in treatment of this disorder are management of the acute pain and use of **antigout** and **uricosuric agents.** The drugs used to manage the pain are most often **nonsteroidal anti-inflammatory drugs (NSAIDs),** which are discussed later in the chapter. The two **antigout drugs, allopurinol (Zyloprim)** and **colchicine,** and the two **uricosuric agents, probenecid (Benemid)** and **sulfinpyrazone (Anturane)** are the focus of this section.

Pharmacodynamics

Antigout Drugs

Antigout drugs act to reduce the inflammatory process or to prevent the synthesis of uric acid. **Allopurinol** inhibits xanthine oxidase, the enzyme responsible for the conversion of hypoxanthine and xanthine to uric acid. This drug has a metabolite (alloxanthine), which is also an inhibitor of xanthine oxidase. **Allopurinol** acts directly on purine metabolism, reducing the production of

uric acid, without disrupting the biosynthesis of vital purines. **Allopurinol** is the only drug that acts directly on the pathophysiological cause of gout.

Administration of **allopurinol** generally leads to a fall in both serum and urinary uric acid in 2 to 3 days. The magnitude of this decrease is dose-dependent. A week or more of treatment may be necessary before the full effects of the drug can be seen.

Unlike **allopurinol, colchicine** does not affect purine metabolism. It binds to microtubular proteins to interfere with the function of the mitotic spindles and inhibit the migration of granulocytes to the inflamed area. It reduces lactic acid production by granulocytes, which decreases deposition of uric acid, and it interferes with kinin formation and reduces phagocytosis. Taken together, these actions decrease the inflammatory response to the deposited urate crystals.

Although it relieves pain in acute attacks, **colchicine** is not an **analgesic.** It is also not **uricosuric** and does not prevent gout from progressing to chronic gouty arthritis. Its prophylactic, suppressive effect helps reduce the incidence of acute attacks and relieves the patient's occasional residual pain and mild discomfort.

Uricosuric Drugs

Uricosuric drugs, unlike **antigout drugs,** increase the rate of uric acid secretion. Both **probenecid** and **sulfinpyrazone** inhibit renal tubular reabsorption of urate and thus increase the renal excretion of uric acid and decrease serum uric acid levels. Effective uricosuria reduces the miscible urate pool, retards urate deposition, and promotes reabsorption of urate deposits. **Sulfinpyrazone** also competitively inhibits platelet prostaglandin synthesis, which prevents platelet aggregation and gives the drug an antithrombotic effect. Both drugs lack anti-inflammatory activity. They are most useful for patients with reduced urinary excretion of uric acid. They are not intended for treatment of acute attacks.

Pharmacokinetics

Absorption and Distribution

All four drugs are well absorbed after oral administration (Table 23–1). **Allopurinol** is widely distributed to tissues. **Colchicine** concentrates mainly in white blood cells. **Probenecid** crosses the placenta without producing adverse effects in the fetus or infant. **Sulfinpyrazone** also crosses the placenta but may be hazardous to the fetus. Both **probenecid** and **sulfinpyrazone** are highly protein-bound and tend to displace other drugs that have a high affinity for the same binding sites.

Metabolism and Excretion

The liver metabolizes all four drugs. All have active metabolites. Both biliary and renal routes excrete **allopurinol** and **colchicine**. The other two drugs are excreted primarily in urine.

Pharmacotherapeutics

Precautions and Contraindications

All four drugs are associated with poor urate clearance in the presence of renal impairment. They should be used cautiously, and renal function tests should be performed regularly to determine appropriate dosage of the drug.

Allopurinol and **colchicine** are associated with hepatotoxicity. They are not recommended for patients with severe hepatic dysfunction. If patients taking these drugs develop anorexia, weight loss, or pruritus, evaluation of liver function should be part of the diagnostic workup. For milder hepatic disorders, close monitoring of liver function is required.

Colchicine, probenecid, and **sulfinpyrazone** are all used cautiously in the presence of peptic ulcer disease or spastic colon. Gastrointestinal (GI) adverse reactions from these drugs are likely to make these disorders worse. Because **probenecid** and **sulfinpyrazone** are sulfa-based drugs, patients with known or suspected **sulfa** allergies should not use them.

Pregnancy categories vary by drug. *Allopurinol* is **Pregnancy Category C, but there are no adequate, well-controlled studies in pregnant women. Use only when benefits clearly outweigh potential risks to the fetus.** *Colchicine* is **Pregnancy Category C when given orally, D when given parenterally. This drug can cause fetal harm when administered to pregnant women. Use only when benefits clearly outweigh risks to the fetus and other drugs are not effective.** *Probenecid* is **Pregnancy Category B. It crosses the placenta, but it has been used during pregnancy without producing harmful effects in the fetus.** *Sulfinpyrazone* is **Pregnancy Category D, but there are no adequate, well-controlled studies in pregnant women. Use only when its benefits clearly outweigh the potential risks to the fetus.**

Allopurinol has been found in breast milk. It is not known whether the other three drugs are excreted in breast milk. Exercise caution when prescribing these drugs for nursing women.

These drugs are generally not indicated for use in children except in rare disorders that a specialist would follow. No dosage schedules are published for children.

Table 23–1. Pharmacokinetics: Antigout and Uricosuric Agents

Drug	Onset	Peak (in plasma)	Duration	Protein Binding	Half-Life	Elimination
Allopurinol	2–3 d*	1.5 h allopurinol 4.5 h oxipurinol	1–2 wk*	NA	1–2 h allopurinol 15 h oxypurinol	20% in feces; remainder in urine
Colchicine	12 h†	0.5–2 h	Unknown	50%	10–60 min in plasma <46 h in leukocytes	10–20% in urine; remainder in bile and feces
Probenecid	30 min*	2–4 h	8 h	85–95%	5–8 h dose-dependent	In urine; primarily as metabolite
Sulfinpyrazone	NA	4 h	Unknown	98–99%	4 h	50% in urine; 90% as unchanged drug; 10% as metabolite

*Hypouricemic action.
†Anti-inflammatory action.

Adverse Drug Reactions

Urates tend to crystallize out in acid urine. Fluid intake of more than 3000 mL/day, along with sufficient sodium bicarbonate (3 to 7.5 g/day) or potassium citrate (7.5 g/d) maintains alkaline urine. Continue alkalization until the serum uric acid level returns to normal limits and the tophaceous deposits disappear.

Colchicine, probenecid, and **sulfinpyrazone** are associated with adverse reactions affecting the GI tract. Symptoms include nausea, vomiting, diarrhea, and abdominal pain. These symptoms are particularly troublesome for patients with active peptic ulcer disease or a history of it.

Probenecid and **sulfinpyrazone** are sulfa-based drugs. They have been associated with hypersensitivity reactions related to this base. Severe, anaphylactic reactions are rare and usually occur within several hours after administration of the first dose of a restart regimen, following prior use of the drug. The appearance of a hypersensitivity reaction requires immediate discontinuance of the drug.

Other adverse reactions are unique to specific drugs. **Allopurinol** is associated with a maculopapular skin rash that sometimes is scaly or exfoliative. The incidence of this adverse reaction is increased in the presence of renal disorders. Because skin reactions may be severe and sometimes fatal, the drug should be discontinued at the first sign of rash. The most severe reactions include fever, chills, arthralgia, cholestatic jaundice, eosinophilia, mild leukocytosis, or leukopenia.

Patients on standard therapy with **colchicine** who have elevated plasma levels because of renal function have developed myopathy and neuropathy that result in weakness. This problem is often unrecognized and misdiagnosed as polymyositis or uremic neuropathy. Proximal weakness and elevated serum creatine kinase are generally present. The condition resolves 3 to 4 weeks after drug withdrawal.

Colchicine also induces reversible malabsorption of vitamin B_{12}, perhaps because it alters the function of the ileal mucosa.

Drug Interactions

Colchicine has very few drug interactions. The other three drugs have many. **Probenecid** inhibits the tubular secretion of most **penicillins** and **cephalosporins** and usually increases plasma levels by any route these **antibiotics** are given. **Sulfinpyrazone** reduces renal tubular secretion of organic anions (e.g., **antimicrobials** and **sulfonamides**) and displaces other anions bound extensively to plasma proteins (e.g., **tolbutamide, warfarin**). **Salicylates** have a mutually antagonistic effect with both of these drugs.

Because these drugs, with the exception of **colchicine**, have many drug interactions, checking drug interactions before prescribing them is important. Table 23–2 lists the drug interactions.

Clinical Use and Dosing

GOUT. **Colchicine** given orally is the time-honored drug for treatment of acute gouty attacks, but its efficacy is limited by the adverse reactions that commonly occur with doses adequate to manage the symptoms. In addition, dosages must be adjusted for patients with impaired renal or hepatic function, and it must be administered with great caution to older adults. Oral **NSAIDs** or intra-articular injection of **corticosteroids** has largely replaced **colchicine** for this indication. When it is given, the usual regimen is an initial dose of 1 to 1.2 mg, followed by 0.5 to 1.2 mg every 1 to 2 hours, up to 16 doses, until relief is obtained or until adverse reactions (usually diarrhea, nausea, and vomiting) develop. Opiates may be needed to control the diarrhea. The total amount of drug needed to control pain and reduce inflammation during an acute attack is 4 to 8 mg. Articular pain and swelling usually abate within 12 hours and are usually gone in 24 to 48 hours.

All four drugs are used to prevent acute attacks or to manage gout between acute attacks. **Allopurinol,** the drug of choice for patients with a history of urinary calculi, renal insufficiency, chronic tophaceous gout, or high levels of serum urate, is given in doses of 200 to 300 mg/day for mild gout and 400 to 600 mg/day for moderately severe tophaceous gout. The minimum effective dose is 100 to 200 mg daily, and the maximum dose is 800 mg/day. Doses greater than 300 mg/day must be divided. Dosage adjustments for patients with renal insufficiency are based on creatinine clearance (CCr) values. These adjustments are depicted in Table 23–3.

For patients who have no more than one acute attack per year, the usual dose of **colchicine** is 0.5 to 0.6 mg/day for 3 or 4 days a week. For patients who have more than one acute attack per year, the dose is 0.5 to 0.6 mg every day. Serious cases may require 1 to 1.8 mg per day.

Probenecid is the **uricosuric** agent of choice because of its well-established safety and its relatively long duration of action. Therapy is not started until an acute gouty attack has subsided. Doses are 0.25 mg daily for 1 week and then 0.5 g twice daily thereafter. Gastric intolerance may indicate overdose, and decreasing the dosage may ease it. The dosage that maintains normal serum uric acid levels is continued for maintenance. When the patient has had no acute attacks for 6 months, the dose is decreased by 0.5 g every 6 months. Do not reduce the maintenance dose to the point where serum uric acid levels begin to rise.

In the presence of renal impairment, a once-daily dose of 1 g may be used. The daily dose may be increased in 0.5-mg increments every 4 weeks (usually to less than 2 mg/day) if symptoms are not controlled or the 24-hour

Table 23–2. Drug Interactions: Antigout and Uricosuric Agents

Drug	Interacting Drug	Possible Effect	Implications
Allopurinol	Angiotensin-converting enzyme inhibitors	Higher risk of hyper-sensitivity reaction	Avoid concurrent use
	Aluminum salts	Decreased effects of allopurinol	Separate administration
	Ampicillin	Rate of ampicillin-induced rash much higher	Warn patients
	Anticoagulants	Anticoagulant effect of some drugs enhanced; not warfarin	Use warfarin for anticoagulation; conflicting data
	Cyclophosphamide	Myelosuppressive effects enhanced; increased risk for bleeding	If must be used together, monitor for bleeding risk
	Theophylline	Theophylline clearance decreased with large doses of allopurinol; increased toxicity risk	Select different respiratory drug
	Thiazide diuretics	Increased incidence of hypersensitivity reactions	Avoid concurrent use or monitor for hypersensitivity
	Thiopurines	Clinically significant increases in pharmacological and toxic effect of thiopurines	Avoid concurrent use
	Uricosuric agents	Uricosuric agents that increase excretion of urate also likely to increase excretion of oxypurinol and lower degree of inhibition of xanthine oxidase; avoid concurrent use	Dosage adjustments may be needed if uricosuric added to treatment regimen
Colchicine	NSAIDs	Additive adverse GI effects	Avoid concurrent use; monitor for GI bleeding
Probenecid	Acyclovir	Decreased acyclovir renal clearance and increased bioavailability	Associated with IV use of drug; avoid this route
	Allopurinol	Increased blood levels for allopurinol	Beneficial effect; may be used therapeutically
	Barbiturates	Increased blood levels	Monitor central nervous system (CNS) effects
	Benzodiazepines (BDZs)	More rapid and prolonged BDZ effect	Monitor BDZ effects
	Clofibrate	Accumulation of clofibric acid; higher steady-state serum concentrations	Select different antilipidemic
	Dapsone	Possible accumulation of dapsone and its metabolites	Monitor for adverse effects or avoid concurrent use
	Dyphylline	Increased half-life, decreased clearance	May be used therapeutically to extend dyphylline dosing interval
	Methotrexate	Increased plasma level; therapeutic effects and toxicity increased	Avoid concurrent use
	NSAIDs	Increased plasma levels and toxicity	Avoid concurrent use
	Pantothenic acid	Renal transport inhibited; plasma levels increased	No specific action required
	Penicillamine	Effects of penicillamine attenuated	Avoid concurrent use

Continued on next page

Table 23–2. Drug Interactions: Antigout and Uricosuric Agents *(continued)*

Drug	Interacting Drug	Possible Effect	Implications
	Penicillins, cephalosporins	Inhibits tubular secretion of most penicillins and cephalosporins; usually increases plasma levels by any route these antibiotics are given	Monitor for adverse effects
	Salicylates	Mutually antagonistic	Avoid concurrent use
	Sulfonamides	Renal transport inhibited; plasma levels increase	Select different antimicrobial
	Sultonylureas	Half-life of sulfonylurea increased	Monitor blood glucose closely
	Zidovudine	Increased zidovudine bioavailability; cutaneous eruptions accompanied by malaise, myalgia, or fever have occurred	Avoid concurrent use
Sulfinpyrazone	Acetaminophen	Risk of hepatotoxicity may be increased	Conflicting data
	Anticoagulants, oral	Anticoagulant activity of warfarin enhanced: increased bleeding risk	Use probenecid if warfarin must be used
	Niacin	Reduce uricosuric activity of sulfinpyrazone	Avoid concurrent use
	Salicylates	Mutually antagonistic	Avoid concurrent use
	Theophylline	Increased theophylline clearance and decreased plasma levels	Avoid concurrent use or adjust dosage based on serum levels
	Tolbutamide	Decreased clearance and increased half-life of tolbutamide; hypoglycemia may result	Glyburide not affected; change hypoglycemic drug
	Verapamil	Increased clearance; decreased bioavailability	Select different calcium channel blocker

urate excretion is less than 700 mg. **Probenecid** is not effective in chronic renal failure if the glomerular filtration rate is 30 mL/minute or less.

Sulfinpyrazone is a potent **uricosuric** agent, but it must be given several times daily, is more likely than the other drugs to cause gastric adverse reactions, and can cause platelet dysfunction. For these reasons, it is prescribed only when **probenecid** and **allopurinol** are not tolerated. Initial dosage is 200 to 400 mg daily in two divided doses. Taking the drug with meals or milk reduces its adverse GI reactions. The dose is gradually increased to a maintenance dose of 400 mg daily in two divided doses. Doses can be as low as 200 mg/day or as high as 800 mg/day to control blood urate levels. Therapy is continued, even in the presence of acute exacerbations. This drug can be used concomitantly with **colchicine.** Patients previously controlled on **probenecid** may be transferred to **sulfinpyrazone** at the full maintenance dose.

MALIGNANCIES ASSOCIATED WITH HYPERURICEMIA. **Allopurinol** is approved for this indication. Doses of 600 to 800 mg daily for 2 or 3 days, with a high fluid intake, have proved effective. Similar consideration for dosage regulation as were given for other uses apply here.

Children age 6 to 10 with secondary hyperuricemia secondary to malignancy are given 300 mg daily. Younger children are generally given 150 mg/day. Another suggested dosing regimen is 1 mg/kg/day in four divided doses given every 6 hours to a maximum of 600 mg/day. After 48 hours of treatment, the dose is titrated according to uric acid levels.

RECURRENT CALCIUM OXALATE CALCULI. **Allopurinol** 200 to 300 mg/day in single or divided doses is given for this indication. The dose is adjusted up or down, based on 24-hour urinary urate determinations that measure the resultant control of hyperuricemia. Patients also benefit from dietary modifications such as increases in oral fluids and dietary fiber and from reductions in animal protein, sodium, refined sugars, oxalate-rich food, and excessive calcium intake.

UNLABELED USES. **Colchicine** also has several unla-

Table 23–3. Dosage Schedule: Antigout and Uricosuric Agents

Drug	Indication	Initial Dose	Maintenance Dose
Allopurinol	Management of gout	*Adults:* Mild disease: 200–300 mg/d Moderately severe, tophaceous: 400–600 mg/d	Minimum effective dose is 100–200 mg/d; maximum dose is 800 mg/d Doses >300 mg/d must be divided Dosage adjustments for renal insufficiency in adults: CCr 60 mL/min: 200 mg/d CCr 40 mL/min: 150 mg/d CCr 20 mL/min: 100 mg/d CCr 10 mL/min: 100 mg qod CCr <10 mL/min: 100 mg 3 times/wk
	Hyperuricemia associated with treatment of malignancy	*Adults:* 600–800 mg/d for 2–3 d with a high fluid intake *Children 6–10 y:* 300 mg/d (100 mg tid) *Children <6 y:* 150 mg/d (50 mg tid)	After 48 h titrate dose in all age groups according to serum uric acid levels Another recommended regimen for children: 1mg/kg/d in 4 divided doses given q6h; maximum dose 600 mg/d
	Recurrent calcium oxalate stones	*Adults:* 200–300 mg/d in single or divided doses	Dosage adjusted up or down based on control of hyper-uricemia according to 24-h urinary urate determinations
Colchicine	Acute gouty attacks	*Adults:* 1–1.2 mg followed by 0.5–1.2 mg every 1–2 h up to 16 doses	Total needed during acute attack is usually 4–8 mg
	Management of gout		Adults with <1 acute attack/y: 0.5–0.6 mg/d for 3–4 d/wk Adults with >1 acute attack/y: 0.5–0.5 mg/d Serious cases: 1–1.8 mg/d
Probenecid	Management of gout*	*Adults:* 0.25 mg qd for 1 wk	0.5 mg bid; if no acute attack in 6 mo, reduce dose by 0.5 mg/d every 6 mo
Sulfinpyrazone	Management of gout	*Adults:* 200–400 mg/d in 2 divided doses	400 mg/d in 2 divided doses; doses as low as 200 mg/d and as high as 800 mg/d have been used

*Probenecid is not effective for management of gout in the presence of chronic renal failure with CCr <30 mL/min.

beled uses. These purposes and the recommended doses follow:

1. Hepatic cirrhosis: 1 mg/day for 5 days each week
2. Primary biliary cirrhosis: 0.6 mg twice daily
3. Adjunctive therapy for amyloidosis: 0.5 mg daily in two divided doses
4. Refractory idiopathic thrombocytopenic purpura: 1.2 to 1.8 mg/day for 2 weeks or more
5. Skin manifestations of scleroderma: 1 mg/day

Rational Drug Selection

Specific disease processes for which each of these drugs is most appropriate have already been mentioned. Addi-

tional considerations in choosing the appropriate drug follow (Table 23–4).

RENAL INSUFFICIENCY. Because it blocks urate production, **allopurinol** is especially useful for patients with a history of urinary calculi, with renal insufficiency, or with excessive basal urinary uric acid excretion (>750 to 800 mg/24 hours). Serious adverse reactions occur in fewer than 2 percent of patients, typically within the first 2 months of therapy. Patients should be kept under close surveillance during this period. Toxicity seems more likely when **allopurinol** is given concomitantly with **thiazide diuretics.**

PEPTIC ULCER DISEASE. Intravenous (IV) **colchicine** rapidly provides a therapeutic plasma level and does not

Table 23–4. Available Dosage Forms: Antigout and Uricosuric Agents

Drug	Dosage Form	How Supplied
Allopurinol (Zyloprim)	Tablets: 100 mg	In bottles of 100 tablets
	Tablets: 300 mg	In bottles of 100, 500 tablets
(Generic)	Tablets: 100 mg, 300 mg	In bottles of 100, 500, 1000 tablets
Colchicine	Tablets: 0.5 mg, 0.6 mg	In bottles of 100 tablets
Probenecid (Benemid)	Tablets: 0.5 mg	In bottles of 100 tablets
(Generic)	Tablets: 0.5 mg	In bottles of 100, 1000 tablets
Sulfinpyrazone (Anturane)	Tablets: 100 mg	In bottles of 100 tablets
	Capsules: 200 mg	In bottles of 100 capsules
(Generic)	Tablets: 100 mg	In bottles of 100, 500 tablets
	Capsules: 200 mg	In bottles of 100, 500, 1000 capsules

cause GI adverse reactions. It is useful for patients who cannot take the drug orally, have peptic ulcer disease, or have contraindications to **NSAIDs.** Diluted in 20 mL of normal saline and given over 10 minutes, 2 mg usually provides relief within 6 to 8 hours. Care must be used to prevent extravasation because **colchicine** may cause tissue necrosis.

HIGH LEVELS OF SERUM URATE ASSOCIATED WITH SECONDARY GOUT. Allopurinol is the drug of choice because it is the only drug in this group that blocks urate production.

Monitoring

All patients receiving these drugs require serum uric acid level monitoring. A baseline assessment is done at initiation of therapy. Uric acid levels should be normal after 1 to 3 weeks of therapy, and serum levels should be drawn again then and periodically throughout therapy or in the presence of exacerbations. The upper limit of normal for men and postmenopausal women is 7 mg/dL; for premenopausal women, it is 6 mg/dL.

For **allopurinol,** liver and renal function must be assessed prior to initiation of therapy and periodically during the first few months of therapy, particularly for patients with preexisting liver disease. Perform blood urea nitrogen (BUN), serum creatinine, and CCr tests, and reassess dosages based on the results.

Probenecid and **sulfinpyrazone** both have blood dyscrasias (anemia, hemolytic anemia) as adverse reactions. Patients taking these drugs should have periodic complete blood counts (CBC).

Patients whose urine is being alkalinized to prevent crystallization of urates in the urine should have their acid-base balance monitored.

Patient Education

ADMINISTRATION. Each drug should be taken exactly as prescribed. A dose that is missed should be taken as soon as the patient remembers but without doubling doses. For **allopurinol,** if the dosing schedule is once daily, do not take it until the next day. If the dosing schedule is more than once a day, take up to 300 mg for the next dose. None of these drugs should be discontinued without first consulting the health care provider. Uric acid levels rise when the drug is stopped.

In the event of an acute attack during maintenance therapy, **allopurinol, probenecid,** and **sulfinpyrazone** should be continued while **colchicine** is added to the regimen to treat the acute attack. Dosage adjustments of the maintenance drugs may be necessary.

Allopurinol can be crushed and given with fluid or mixed with food for patients who have difficulty in swallowing.

Patients should avoid taking **aspirin** or **salicylates** while taking **probenecid** or **sulfinpyrazone.** These drugs are mutually antagonistic.

ADVERSE REACTIONS. The main adverse reaction for all these drugs is GI distress. Taking these drugs with food or milk may minimize gastric irritation.

Probenecid and **sulfinpyrazone** are sulfa-based drugs that have been associated with hypersensitivity reactions related to this base. Patients should be asked about **sulfa** allergies and taught the indications of a hypersensitivity reaction and the importance of reporting it. A hypersensitivity reaction requires immediate discontinuance of the drug. Other symptoms to report with these drugs include sore throat, fatigue, yellowing of the skin or eyes, and unusual bleeding or bruising. These drugs have been associated with blood dyscrasias and hepatotoxicity.

Allopurinol has been associated with a maculopapular rash that sometimes is scaly or exfoliative. Because this skin reaction can be severe or even fatal, patients should report to their health care provider the first indication of a rash. They should be seen to evaluate this rash, and discontinuance of the drug should be considered.

Drowsiness and dizziness have occasionally affected patients who are taking **allopurinol.** Caution patients to avoid driving or other activities requiring alertness until their response to the drug is known.

Patients taking standard doses of **colchicine** have developed proximal muscle weakness related to myopathy and neuropathy. Patients should be warned to report these symptoms to their health care provider. Stopping the drug usually reverses the symptoms within 3 to 4 weeks.

LIFESTYLE MANAGEMENT. To reduce available urates, an alkaline diet may be prescribed that includes reductions in animal protein, sodium, refined sugars, oxalate-rich food, and excessive calcium intake, as well as increases in oral fluids and dietary fiber. Fluid intake in excess of 3000 mL per day also reduces the risk for renal calculi. Because large amounts of **alcohol** increase uric acid concentrations and may decrease the effectiveness of medications, **alcohol** should be avoided or consumed in very small amounts.

Corticosteroids

Cortisol, the endogenous glucocorticoid in the body, is produced and secreted on the basis of feedback mechanisms of the hypothalamus-pituitary-adrenal (HPA) axis. The adrenal cortex synthesizes and secretes the steroid hormones that include mineralocorticoids and glucocorticoids and, to a lesser extent, androgens. Figure 23–1 depicts this feedback system. Exogenously administered **adrenal cortex hormones (corticosteroids)** affect this feedback mechanism.

Corticosteroids have a major role in the management of a variety of disease processes. In primary or secondary adrenal cortex insufficiency, they are used for replacement therapy. In rheumatic disorders, they may be short-term adjunctive therapy for acute episodes or exacerbation. These drugs are also used to treat collagen disease, dermatologic conditions, asthma, allergic rhinitis, neoplastic disorders, inflammatory bowel disease, and idiopathic thrombocytopenia purpura. The role of **inhaled corticosteroids** in management of respiratory disorders is covered in Chapter 15. **Topical corticosteroids** used to manage dermatologic conditions are covered in Chapter 21. This chapter focuses on the use of **systemic corticosteroids** to manage inflammatory conditions in primary care situations.

Pharmacodynamics

Glucocorticoids have metabolic, anti-inflammatory, and growth-suppressing effects. They also influence levels of awareness and sleep patterns. They increase blood glucose concentration by stimulating gluconeogenesis in the liver and by decreasing uptake of glucose into muscle, lymphatic, and adipose cells. In extrahepatic tissues, they stimulate protein catabolism and inhibit amino acid uptake and protein synthesis.

They inhibit the immune and inflammatory systems by their actions at several sites: depressing proliferation of T lymphocytes, including those that produce the antiviral protein interferon; decreasing natural killer cell activity; reversing macrophage activity; and suppressing the synthesis, secretion, and actions of chemical mediators involved in inflammatory and immune responses. These chemical mediators include interleukins, prostaglandins, leukotrienes, bradykinin, serotonin, and histamine.

Glucocorticoids also increase circulating erythrocytes, increase appetite, promote fat deposits in the face and cervical areas, increase uric acid excretion, and decrease serum calcium levels, possibly by inhibiting GI absorption of calcium. Their feedback activity on the HPA axis suppresses secretion and synthesis of adrenocorticotropic hormone (ACTH) and suppresses growth hormone secretion so that somatic growth is inhibited. Finally, they potentiate the effects of catecholamines, thyroid hormone, and growth hormone on adipose tissue.

Corticosteroids are synthetic **glucocorticoids** with the same multiple actions as the endogenous glucocorticoids, which may explain not only the variety of clinical uses for these drugs but also the wide range of adverse reactions.

Pharmacokinetics

Absorption and Distribution

Corticosteroids are all well absorbed from the upper jejunum (Table 23–5). Those with intramuscular (IM) formulations are well absorbed from IM sites. Injections of suspensions and esters produce greatly altered onset and duration times. Absorption is rapid for esters (sodium phosphates and sodium succinates) and relatively slow for other derivatives (acetates, acetonides, and tebutates). Absorption from local sites (e.g., intra-articular or intrasynovial) is slower than from IM sites. Because onset, peak, and duration of action vary, these drugs are classified into short-, intermediate-, and long-acting forms.

These drugs are reversibly bound to **corticosteroid**-binding proteins. **Corticosteroids** have significantly altered pharmacological effects on patients with altered protein-binding capacities.

All these drugs are widely distributed, cross the placenta, and probably enter breast milk.

Metabolism and Excretion

The liver metabolizes **hydrocortisone (Cortef)**, and this is the rate-limiting step in its clearance. The metabolism and excretion of other **corticosteroids** generally parallel those of **hydrocortisone**. Induction of hepatic enzymes increases the metabolic clearance of all **corticosteroids**.

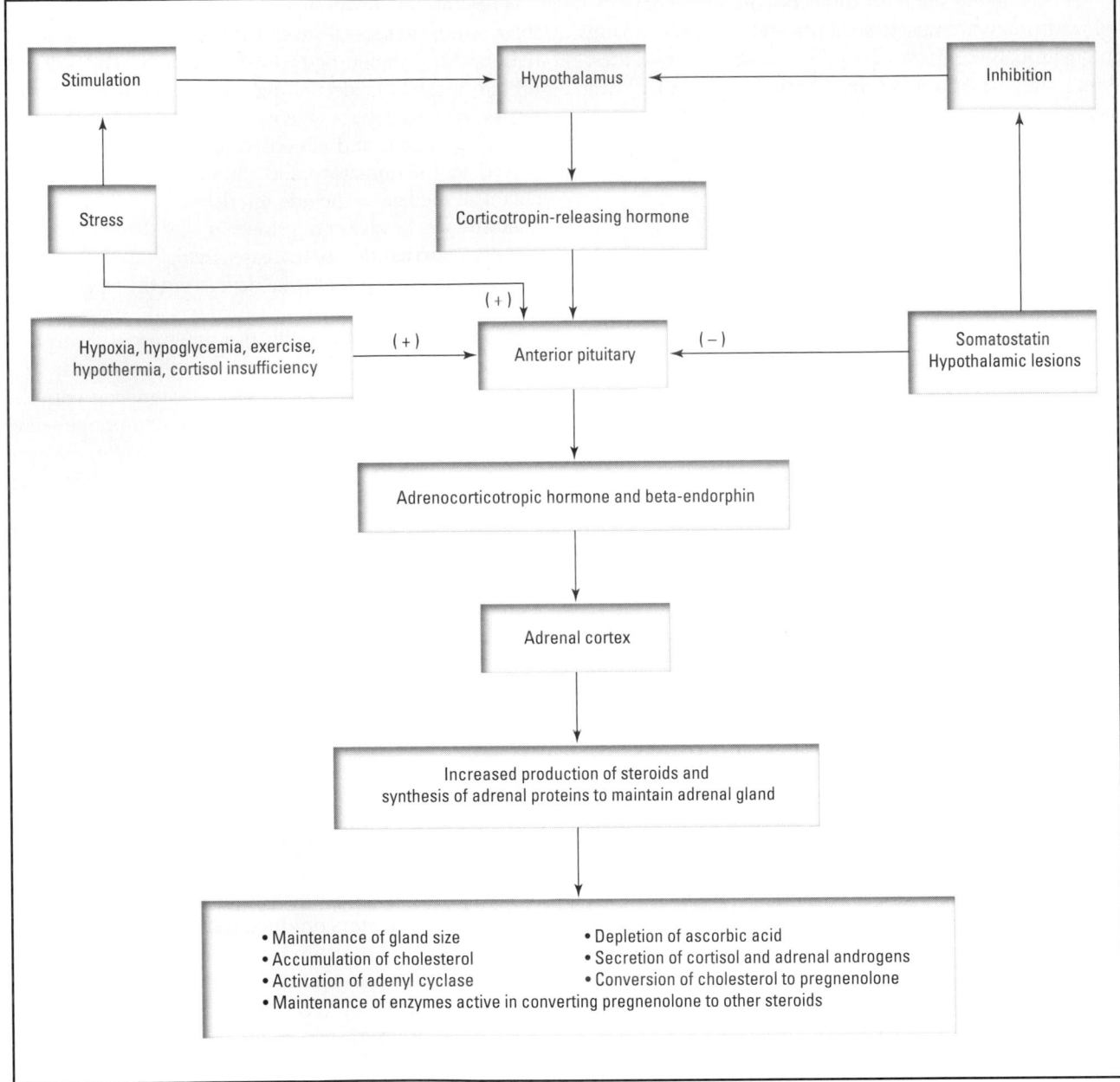

Figure 23–1. Hypothalamus-pituitary-adrenal axis and feedback loops.

The liver converts **cortisone (Cortone)** to **hydrocortisone**, and **prednisone (Deltasone)** is converted to **prednisolone (Delta-Crotef, Prelone)**. These metabolites are then clinically active and metabolized by the liver for clearance. Approximately 1 percent of the daily dose of the drug is excreted unchanged in urine. Renal clearance is increased when plasma levels are increased.

Pharmacotherapeutics

Precautions and Contraindications

The wide range of contraindications and warnings about cautious use associated with these drugs is a factor of their numerous actions. They are contraindicated in the presence of active untreated infections because they may mask the indications of infection, and new infections may appear during their use. A patient may also have decreased resistance, and the host defense mechanisms may be unable to prevent dissemination of the infection. **Corticosteroids** may exacerbate systemic fungal infections and activate latent amebiasis. Although they have been advocated for the treatment of chronic active hepatitis, they may be harmful in hepatitis positive for hepatitis B surface antigen.

For many disorders, these drugs should be used cautiously. Average and large doses of drugs with high relative mineralocorticoid potency (e.g., **cortisone** and **hy-**

Table 23–5. Pharmacokinetics: Selected Corticosteroids

Drug	Onset (hours)	Peak (hours)	Duration (days)	Protein Binding	Half-Life	RAP	RMP	Elimination
Cortisone* PO	Rapid	2	1.25–1.5	Very high	30 min P 8–12 h B	0.8	2	1% unchanged in urine
Cortisone* IM	Slow	20–48	1.25–1.5	Very high	—	0.8	2	1% unchanged in urine
Hydrocortisone* PO	Rapid	1	1.25–1.5	High	80–118 min P 8–12 h B	1	2	1% unchanged in urine
Hydrocortisone† IM	Slow	4–8	Varies	High	—	1	2	1% unchanged in urine
Methylprednisolone†	UK	1–2	1.25–1.5	High	78–188 min P 18–36 h B	5	0	1% unchanged in urine
Prednisolone†	1	1–2	1.25–1.5	High	115–211 min P 18–36 h B	4	1	1% unchanged in urine
Prednisone†	1	1–2	1.25–1.5	Very high	60 min P 18–36 h B	4	1	1% unchanged in urine
Triamcinolone†	UK	1–2	2.25	High	200+ min P 18–36 h B	5	0	1% unchanged in urine
Dexamethasone‡ PO	UK	1–2	2.75	High	110–210 min P 36–54 h B	20–30	0	1% unchanged in urine
Dexamethasone‡ IM	Rapid	8	6	High	—	20–30	0	1% unchanged in urine
Betamethasone‡ PO	UK	1–2	3.25	High	300+ min P 36–54 h B	20–30	0	1% unchanged in urine
Betamethasone‡ IM	1–3	UK	7	High	—	20–30	0	1% unchanged in urine

*Short-acting.
†Intermediate-acting.
‡Long-acting.
B = Biologic half-life.
P = Plasma half-life.
RAP = Relative anti-inflammatory potency.
RMP = Relative mineralocorticoid potency.
UK = Unknown.

drocortisone) can cause elevated blood pressure, salt and water retention, and increased excretion of potassium. These effects can be especially problematic for patients with hypertension and cardiovascular disorders (e.g., congestive heart failure [CHF]). Sodium restriction and potassium supplementation may be necessary. Edema can occur in the presence of renal disease with a fixed or decreased glomerular filtration rate (GFR). These drugs should be used with caution in renal insufficiency, acute glomerulonephritis, or chronic nephritis.

All **corticosteroids** increase calcium excretion, which creates problems for postmenopausal women and others at risk for osteoporosis.

Patients with diabetes mellitus may have difficulty maintaining glycemic control because **corticosteroids** alter the liver's glucose regulation. Patients with ulcerative colitis or peptic ulcer disease have an increased probability of impending perforation.

Some of these products contain tartrazine or sodium bisulfite, both of which can cause severe allergic reactions. Patients with these allergies should notify their health care provider, and the label of the drug should be read carefully for these inclusions.

Corticosteroids cross the placenta (*prednisone* has the least transport), and most are Pregnancy Category C. In animal studies, large doses resulted in cleft palate, stillborn fetuses, and decreased fetal size. Chronic ingestion during the first trimester in humans has shown a 1 percent incidence of cleft palate. In considering use of these drugs during pregnancy or in women with childbearing potential, the benefits must be carefully weighed against the potential risks to the fetus. Infants of mothers who have taken these drugs are observed closely for signs of hypoaldosteronism.

Corticosteroids appear in breast milk and could retard the nursing infant's growth, interfere with endogenous corticosteroid production, or cause other unwanted effects. Advise mothers taking these drugs not to nurse. However, several studies suggest that the amount excreted in breast milk is negligible with **prednisone** or **prednisolone** doses 20 mg or less per day and **methylprednisolone (Medrol)** doses 8 mg or less per day. For mothers who want to nurse, waiting 3 to 4 hours after taking the drug and using one of these drugs within these doses may be tried.

When given **corticosteroids**, children may experience altered growth and development, and they require careful monitoring if they must be on prolonged therapy. Some of these products contain benzyl alcohol, which has been associated with a fatal "gasping syndrome" in infants.

Older adults often have chronic disorders that are worsened by **corticosteroids**. Consider the risk-benefit factors of **steroid** use. Lower doses and careful monitoring of blood pressure, blood glucose, and electrolytes at least every 6 months is appropriate.

Adverse Drug Reactions

Adverse reactions can be discussed by the body system that is affected.

MUSCLE AND SKIN.   Common skin changes reported with **systemic corticosteroids** include atrophy and thinning of the skin, alopecia, acneiform eruptions, poor healing, purpura, striae, hirsutism, and desquamation. Myopathy is also seen, with marked muscle wasting. No relationship between dose or duration of therapy and these adverse reactions is apparent. Alteration in body fat is also noted, particularly in patients who take **corticosteroids** for more than 60 days, with the most common changes truncal obesity, buffalo hump, and moon facies.

SKELETAL TISSUES.   Osteoporosis develops in 11 to 20 percent of patients treated for more than 1 year. Skeletal fractures, many of the spine, ribs, and pelvis, may occur secondary to the reduced bone density.

OCULAR TISSUES.   Prolonged use may produce subcapsular cataracts, glaucoma with possible damage to the optic nerve, and increased risk for secondary ocular infections due to fungi or viruses.

GASTROINTESTINAL SYSTEM.   Corticisteroids have been implicated in the induction of peptic ulcer disease. Patients who appear to be at risk are those being treated for nephrotic syndrome or hepatic disease, are taking a total dose of **prednisone** exceeding 1 g, or have a history of ulcer disease, concomitant use of a known gastric irritant, or stress. Prophylaxis with **antacids** or **histamine$_2$ blockers** is suggested for patients with two or more of these risk factors (Lester, Knowles, & Shear, 1998). Patients also taking **NSAIDs** may require **misoprostol (Cytotec)**.

CARDIOVASCULAR SYSTEM.   Hypertension is the most common adverse reaction. This and other cardiovascular problems (e.g., fluid and electrolyte disturbances) are discussed in the Precautions and Contraindications section.

CENTRAL NERVOUS SYSTEM.   Delirium, agitation, insomnia, mood swings, and severe depression characterize **steroid** psychosis. The onset of symptoms is usually within 15 to 30 days. Predisposing factors include doses above 40 mg of **prednisone** or its equivalent dose in another drug, female gender, and a family history of psychiatric disorder. The incidence is correlated with dose. If the **steroid** cannot be stopped, **psychotropic drugs** are effective in relieving the symptoms.

ENDOCRINE SYSTEM.   Prolonged therapy may lead to adrenal suppression. The degree of suppression depends on dosage, relative **glucocorticoid** (anti-inflammatory) potency, biologic half-life, and duration of therapy. As a general rule, suppression occurs with doses above the physiological range that are given for more than 1 month. It can be minimized by using intermediate-acting agents on an alternate-day dosing schedule. Abrupt withdrawal after adrenal suppression has occurred may result in a withdrawal syndrome, with symptoms similar to those seen in adrenal insufficiency. To minimize this adverse reaction, the dose of **corticosteroids** used for prolonged therapy should be tapered. Recovery from HPA suppression can take up to 12 months.

The effect on glucose metabolism and regulation is discussed in the Precautions and Contraindications section. Amenorrhea, postmenopausal bleeding, and other menstrual irregularities have also been seen.

Drug Interactions

Additive hypokalemia may occur with drugs that also produce this adverse reaction. This hypokalemia increases the risk for toxicity in **digoxin**. Several drugs stimulate the metabolism of **corticosteroids**, and **oral contraceptives** decrease their metabolism. **NSAIDs** increase the risk for GI adverse reactions. Other specific drug interactions are presented in Table 23–6.

Clinical Use and Dosing

ADRENOCORTICAL INSUFFICIENCY.   For replacement of cortisol, under normal circumstances patients are given 15 to 20 mg of cortisol or its equivalent daily. Dosage

Table 23–6. Drug Interactions: Selected Corticosteroids

Drug	Interacting Drug	Possible Effect	Implications
Betamethasone, cortisone	Insulin, oral hypoglycemics	Decreased effectiveness, resulting in altered glycemic control	Monitor blood glucose levels more closely if drugs must be given concurrently
Hydrocortisone	Cholestyramine	Hydrocortisone area under the curve (AUC) decreased	Separate dose by 4 h and give hydrocortisone first
	Insulin, oral hypo-glycemics	Decreased effectiveness, resulting in altered glycemic control	Monitor blood glucose levels more closely if drugs must be given concurrently
Dexamethasone	Ephedrine	Decreased half-life and increased clearance of dexamethasone	Avoid concurrent administration
	Insulin, oral hypo-glycemics	Decreased effectiveness, resulting in altered glycemic control	Monitor blood glucose levels more closely if drugs must be given concurrently
Prednisone	NSAIDs, other GI irritants	Increased risk for GI bleed	Avoid concurrent use
	Insulin, oral hypo-glycemics	Decreased effectiveness, resulting in altered glycemic control	Monitor blood glucose levels more closely if drugs must be given concurrently
Methylprednisolone	Macrolide anti-microbials (e.g., erythromycin, clarithromycin)	Significant decrease in methylprednisolone clearance	Has been used therapeutically to decrease methylprednisolone dose
	Insulin, oral hypo-glycemics	Decreased effectiveness, resulting in altered glycemic control	Monitor blood glucose levels more closely if drugs must be given concurrently
All corticosteroids	Barbiturates	Decrease the pharmaco-logical effects of the corticosteroid	Avoid concurrent use
	Oral contraceptives	Corticosteroid half-life and concentration increased; clearance decreased	May require dosage adjustment
	Estrogens	Corticosteroid clearance decreased	May require dosage adjustment
	Hydantoins, rifampin	Corticosteroid clearance increased; reduced therapeutic effects	May require dosage adjustment
	Ketoconazole	Corticosteroid clearance decreased; AUC increased	Select different imidazole
	Digoxin	May increase risk of digitalis toxicity	Avoid coadminstration
	Isoniazid	Isoniazid serum concen-trations decreased	If must be used together, dosage adjustments may be needed; monitor therapy closely
	Potassium-depleting agents (e.g., thia-zide and loop diuretics, mez-locillin, piperacillin, ticarcillin)	Additive hypokalemia	Avoid concurrent use; monitor serum potassium levels
	Salicylates	Reduced serum salicylate levels; decreased thera-peutic effectiveness	Avoid concurrent use
	Somatrem	Inhibits growth-promoting effect of somatrem	Consult with endocrinologist for best action

schedules vary, but the simplest and least expensive in adults is **cortisone** 25 mg daily. **Hydrocortisone** 20 mg may also be used on the same schedule. To approach diurnal rhythms, the dose is given in the morning before 9 A.M. Equivalent doses of **prednisone** or another **corticosteroid** may be used but have no specific advantage. In addition, other **corticosteroids** have less relative mineralocorticoid potency, and an additional drug to provide mineralocorticoid activity might be required if they are used. **Cortisone** and **hydrocortisone** have intrinsic mineralocorticoid activity and require no additional drugs.

The response to any of these drugs is highly variable. Doses are highly individualized, and much higher doses given in divided doses may be needed. Specific doses and ranges for each of the **corticosteroids** for this indication, for both adults and children, is provided in Table 23–7.

INFLAMMATION. Any of the **corticosteroids** may be used to reduce or prevent inflammation. Because the need for mineralocorticoid activity is low to absent in this indication, drugs with more anti-inflammatory activity—**methylprednisolone**, **prednisone**, and **triamcinolone (Aristocort)**—are appropriate. **Betamethasone** also has only anti-inflammatory activity, but it is four to five times more potent than the other drugs, which increases the risk for adverse reactions. **Dexamethasone** is used most often in acute care to relieve the inflammation that causes intracranial pressure after closed head injury or cranial surgery. Doses are shown in Table 23–7.

IMMUNOSUPPRESSION. Although all **corticosteroids** have immunosuppressive capability, the most commonly used is **prednisone.** It has a short half-life, low cost, and negligible mineralocorticoid activity, and it is available in 5-mg and 20-mg tablets that make dosage changes simple for the patient to manage. Tapering doses can be complex, with different doses every day or every other day. When patients are being tapered from high doses (e.g., after organ rejection episodes), the tapering schedule may last for weeks. Patients can be instructed to take a specific number of tablets on day 1 and then reduce the dose by one tablet each day as a simple taper, without their having to keep track of the number of milligrams they are to take on any given day. **Prednisolone,** the active hepatic metabolite of **prednisone,** is useful in the presence of hepatic dysfunction. Other drugs in this class may also be used for this indication, and their dosing schedule is presented in Table 23–7.

Regardless of the disease process for which the drug is given, several overall dosing guidelines apply (Table 23–8). The following guidelines are adapted from *Drug Facts and Comparisons* (Kastrup 1998) and Goroll, May, and Mulley (1995):

1. The maximal activity of the adrenal cortex in producing cortisol is between 2 and 8 A.M. To best match this natural body rhythm, daily doses are best taken in the morning before 9 A.M.

2. The initial dose depends on the specific disease being treated. Maintain or adjust the dose until an acceptable response is achieved. Establish a time frame within which to expect this response. If such a response does not occur within that time frame, discontinue the **corticosteroid** and consult or refer the patient for other therapy.

3. After an acceptable response if achieved, determine the maintenance dose by decreasing the dosage in small amounts at intervals until the lowest dosage that maintains an adequate clinical response is reached. The lowest possible dose is always best, especially with long-term therapy, to avoid or reduce adverse reactions. In the presence of increased stress (e.g., trauma, surgery, or infection), a temporarily increased dosage may be needed.

4. If, after long-term therapy or because of spontaneous remission, the drug is to be stopped, withdraw it gradually to prevent an adrenal insufficiency crisis. Tapering is generally not necessary after short-term therapy (e.g., 1 to 2 weeks) because adrenal suppression has not occurred.

5. Most conditions that require chronic **corticosteroid** therapy can be well controlled on alternate-day therapy, although the therapy must usually be started with daily dosing. For alternate-day dosing, twice the daily dose is given every other morning before 9 A.M. It works best if the patient is taking an intermediate-acting drug but may be used with short-acting drugs as well. The purpose of this schedule is to provide the patient on long-term therapy the benefits of the drug while minimizing the HPA-axis suppression, withdrawal symptoms, and, for children, growth retardation. Long-acting agents may still produce HPA suppression, even with alternate-day dosing. The regimen is only for patients on long-term therapy who can be trusted to follow this schedule without needing the prompting of daily therapy. In the advent of a flare-up in the disease process, a return to daily dosing may be necessary, at least until the flare-up clears.

6. Unlike a tapering schedule, alternate-day scheduling retains the same total **steroid** dose. Switching is carried out by gradually increasing the dose on the first day and decreasing it on the second day until a double dose is taken every other day with no drug on the in-between days. A rough guideline for switching is to make changes in increments of 10 mg of **prednisone** (or its equivalent) when the daily dose is more than 40 mg, and in 5-mg increments when the daily dosage is 20 to 40 mg. Below 20 mg, the change is made in increments of 2.5 mg. The interval between changes varies from

Table 23–7. Dosage Schedule: Selected Corticosteroids

Drug	Indication	Dose	Notes
Betamethasone	Inflammation, immunosuppression	*Adults:* 0.6–7.2 mg/d PO as single or divided doses *Children:* 62.5–250 µg/kg/d PO in 3 divided doses	Long-acting. Suppresses HPA at doses >0.6 mg/d.
Cortisone	Adrenocortical insufficiency	*Adults:* 10–37 mg/d PO as single or divided doses *Children:* 0.7 mg/kg/d PO in divided doses	Has mineralocorticoid activity but may need additional drug; short-acting; suppresses HPA at doses >20 mg/d.
	Inflammation, immunosuppression	*Adults:* 25–300 mg/d PO in single or divided doses *Children:* 2.5–10 mg/kg/d PO as single or divided doses	Has mineralocorticoid activity but may need additional drug; short-acting; suppresses HPA at doses >20 mg/d.
Dexamethasone	Adrenocortical insufficiency	*Children:* 23.3 µg/kg/d PO in 3 divided doses	Not commonly used for this indication in adults; required addition of mineralocorticoid.
	Inflammation, immunosuppression	*Adults:* 0.5–9 mg/d PO in single or divided doses *Children:* 83.3–333.3 µg/kg/d PO in 3–4 divided doses	Long-acting. Suppresses HPA at doses >0.75 mg/d.
Hydrocortisone	Adrenocortical insufficiency	*Adults:* 15–25 mg/d PO in single or divided doses *Children:* 0.56 mg/kg/d PO in single or divided doses	Has mineralocorticoid activity; short-acting; suppresses HPA at doses >20 mg/d.
	Inflammation, immunosuppression	*Adults:* 20–240 mg/d PO in 1–4 divided doses *Children:* 2–8 mg/kg/d in single or divided doses	Has mineralocorticoid activity; short-acting; suppresses HPA at doses >20 mg/d.
	Inflammatory bowel disease	*Adults:* 100 mg nightly in retention enema for 21 d or until remission	Has mineralocorticoid activity; short-acting; suppresses HPA at doses >20 mg/d.
Methylprednisolone	Inflammation, immunosuppression	*Adults:* 4–48 mg/d PO in single or divided doses initially; up to 240 mg/d for maintenance *Children:* 0.117–1.67 mg/kg/d PO in 3–4 divided doses	Intermediate-acting; suppresses HPA at doses of 4 mg/d.
	Multiple sclerosis	*Adults:* 160 mg/d for 7 d; then 64 every other day for 1 mo	Intermediate-acting; suppresses HPA at doses of 4 mg/d.
Prednisolone	Adrenocortical insufficiency	*Adults:* 5–60 mg/d PO in single or divided doses *Children:* 0.14 mg/kg/d PO in 3 divided doses	Intermediate-acting; suppresses HPA at doses >5 mg/d.
	Inflammation, immunosuppression	*Adults:* 5–60 mg/d PO in single or divided doses *Children:* 0.5–2 mg/kg/d PO in 3–4 divided doses	Intermediate-acting; suppresses HPA at doses >5 mg/d.
	Multiple sclerosis	*Adults:* 200 mg/d for 7 d; then 80 mg every other day for 1 mo	Intermediate-acting; suppresses HPA at doses >5 mg/d.

Continued on next page

Table 23–7. Dosage Schedule: Selected Corticosteroids *(continued)*

Drug	Indication	Dose	Notes
Prednisone	Adrenocortical insufficiency	*Adults:* 5–60 mg/d PO in single or divided doses	Minimal mineralocorticoid activity; intermediate-acting; suppresses HPA at doses >5 mg.
	Inflammation, immunosuppression	*Adults:* 5–60 mg/d PO in single or divided doses *Children:* 0.14–2 mg/kg/d PO in 4 divided doses	Minimal mineralocorticoid activity; intermediate-acting; suppresses HPA at doses >5 mg.
	Nephrosis	*Children* >10 y: 20 mg qid PO *Children 4–10 y:* 15 mg qid PO *Children 18 mo-4 y:* 7.5–10 mg qid	Minimal mineralocorticoid activity; intermediate-acting; suppresses HPA at doses >5 mg.
Triamcinolone	Adrenocortical insufficiency	*Adults:* 4–12 mg/d PO in single or divided doses *Children:* 117 μg/kg/d in single or divided doses	No mineralocorticoid activity; requires addition of mineralocorticoid drug. Intermediate-acting; suppresses HPA at doses >4 mg/d.
	Rheumatic disorders	*Adults:* 8–12 mg/d PO	No mineralocorticoid activity; requires addition of mineralocorticoid drug. Intermediate-acting; suppresses HPA at doses >4 mg/d.
	Systemic lupus erythematosus	*Adults:* 20–32 mg/d PO	No mineralocorticoid activity; requires addition of mineralocorticoid drug. Intermediate-acting; suppresses HPA at doses >4 mg/d.
	Other inflammatory diseases or for immunosuppression	*Adults:* 4–48 mg/d PO in single or divided doses *Children:* 0.416–1.7 mg/kg/d PO in single or divided doses	No mineralocorticoid activity; requires addition of mineralocorticoid drug. Intermediate-acting; suppresses HPA at doses >4 mg/d.

For parenteral doses, see other sources.

1 day to several weeks and is empirically based on the clinical response.

7. The schedule for tapering and withdrawing is different. The goal is to reduce the drug to physiological levels or to eliminate the drug altogether. For doses above 40 mg, the dose is reduced by 10 mg of **prednisone** (or its equivalent) every 1 to 3 weeks. Doses below 40 mg require reductions of 5 mg every 1 to 3 weeks. Once the physiological dose is reached (5 to 7.5 mg/day), the patient can be switched to 1-mg tablets so that dosage reductions can be continued. Weekly or biweekly reductions can then be done 1 mg at a time.

Rational Drug Selection

LENGTH OF THERAPEUTIC ACTIVITY. **Corticosteroids** are classified according to their therapeutic effects into short-, intermediate-, and long-acting forms. Short-acting agents are less likely to produce HPA suppression, especially when taken only in the morning and in low doses on an alternate-day schedule. Long-acting agents are preferred if the effects of high doses must be sustained (e.g., increased intracranial pressure or organ transplant rejection).

RELATIVE POTENCY. Mineralocorticoid activity is desirable in adrenocortical insufficiency but not if the primary goal of therapy is anti-inflammatory or immunosuppressive. Drugs with higher relative mineralocorticoid potency (RMP) are selected for adrenal insufficiency. Drugs high in relative anti-inflammatory potency (RAP) are selected when the goal is to reduce inflammation or suppress the immune system.

Monitoring

Monitoring is based on the common adverse reactions associated with the use of **corticosteroids:** weight gain, edema, hypertension, and indications of excessive potassium loss and negative nitrogen balance associated with protein catabolism. Carefully monitor the growth and development of children on prolonged therapy.

Table 23–8. Available Dosage Forms: Selected Corticosteroids

Drug	Dosage Form	How Supplied
Betamethasone (Celestone)	Tablets: 0.6 mg Syrup: 0.6 mg/5 mL	In bottles of 100, 500 mg In 118 mL
Cortisone (Cortone)	Tablets: 25 mg	In bottles of 100 scored tablets
(Generic)	Tablets: 5 mg Tablets: 10 mg Tablets: 25 mg	In bottles of 50 scored tablets In bottles of 100 scored tablets In bottles of 100, 500 tablets
Dexamethasone (Decadron)	Tablets: 0.25 mg, 0.5 mg Tablets: 0.75 mg Tablets: 1.5 mg Tablets: 4 mg, 6 mg Elixir: 0.5 mg/5 mL	In bottles of 100 scored tablets In bottles of 12, 100 scored tablets In bottles of 50 scored tablets In bottles of 50 scored tablets In 100, 237 mL
(Generic)	Tablets: 0.25 mg, 0.5 mg Tablets: 0.75 mg Tablets: 1 mg Tablets: 1.5 mg Tablets: 2 mg Tablets: 4 mg, 6 mg Elixir: 0.5 mg/5 mL Oral solution: 0.5 mg/5 mL	In bottles of 100 tablets In bottles of 100, 1000 tablets In bottles of 100, 1000 scored tablets In bottles of 50, 100 tablets In bottles of 100 scored tablets In bottles of 50, 100 tablets In 100, 120, 240, 500 mL In 500 mL
Hydrocortisone (Cortef)	Tablets: 5 mg Tablets: 10 mg, 20 mg	In bottles of 50 scored tablets In bottles of 100 scored tablets
(Generic)	Tablets: 10 mg, 20 mg	In bottles of 100 tablets
Methylprednisolone (Medrol)	Tablets: 2 mg Tablets: 4 mg Tablets: 8 mg Tablets: 16 mg Tablets: 24 mg, 32 mg	In bottles of 100 scored tablets In bottles of 30, 100, 500 scored tablets In bottles of 25 scored tablets In bottles of 50 scored tablets In bottles of 25 scored tablets
(Generic)	Tablets: 4 mg Tablets: 10 mg	In bottles of 21, 100 tablets In bottles of 50 tablets
Prednisolone (Delta-Cortef, Generic)	Tablets: 5 mg	In bottles of 100, 500, 1000 tablets (Delta-Cortef tablets are scored)
(Prelone)	Syrup: 15 mg/5 mL	In 240 mL (cherry flavor)
Prednisone (Deltasone)	Tablets: 2.5 mg Tablets: 5 mg, 10 mg, 20 mg Tablets: 50 mg	In bottles of 100 scored tablets In bottles of 100, 500 scored tablets In bottles of 100 scored tablets
(Liquid Pred)	Syrup: 5 mg/5 mL	In 120, 240 mL
(Generic)	Tablets: 5 mg Tablets: 10 mg Tablets: 20 mg Tablets: 50 mg Oral solution: 5 mg/5 mL	In bottles of 100, 500, 1000, 5000 tablets In bottles of 100, 1000 tablets In bottles of 100, 500, 1000 tablets In bottles of 100 tablets In 500 mL

Continued on next page

Table 23–8. Available Dosage Forms: Selected Corticosteroids *(continued)*

Drug	Dosage Form	How Supplied
Triamcinolone (Aristocort)	Tablets: 1 mg Tablets: 2 mg Tablets: 4 mg Tablets: 8 mg	In bottles of 50 scored tablets In bottles of 100 scored tablets In bottles of 30, 1000 scored tablets In bottles of 50 scored tablets
(Kenacort)	Tablets: 8 mg Syrup: 4 mg/5 mL	In bottles of 50 tablets In 120 mL
(Generic)	Tablets: 4 mg	In bottles of 100, 500 tablets

Parenteral formulations are not presented here.

Laboratory monitoring begins with an initial assessment of serum electrolytes, glucose, and CBC. For patients on long-term therapy or high doses, annual monitoring of these parameters, as well as guaiac testing of stools and serum lipid analysis, is appropriate. For patients at risk for or with indications of GI adverse reactions, upper GI x-rays are desirable.

Systemic corticosteroids may produce subcapsular cataracts in as many as 30 percent of patients, and patients who have or are at risk for increased intraocular pressure (IOP) may experience increases in IOP while on these drugs. A slit-lamp examination is recommended every 6 to 12 months for patients on long-term **corticosteroid** therapy.

Patient Education

ADMINISTRATION. Instruct the patient to take the drug exactly as prescribed. Missed doses should be taken as soon as the patient remembers, unless it is almost time for the next dose. Doses should not be doubled. If the patient is being switched from daily to alternate-day therapy or is on a tapering or withdrawal protocol, make the changes as simple as possible and provide written instructions.

Corticosteroids should not be discontinued or the dosage changed without first consulting the health care provider. Adrenal insufficiency (anorexia, nausea, weakness, fatigue, dyspnea, hypotension, and hypoglycemia) may result when the drug is stopped suddenly. If these signs appear, the health care provider should be notified immediately. Adrenal insufficiency can be life-threatening.

In the event of an acute attack during maintenance therapy, the drug should be continued and the health care provider notified. Dosage or schedule adjustments of the maintenance drugs or the addition of another drug may be necessary. Determining the cause for the exacerbation is important because removal of that cause may be the main treatment chosen.

ADVERSE REACTIONS. Corticosteroids cause immunosuppression and may mask symptoms of infection. Instruct the patient to avoid people with known contagious illnesses and to report possible infections immediately. Patients should avoid vaccinations without first consulting their health care provider.

Review the probable adverse reactions with the patient. Patients should immediately report severe abdominal pain or tarry stools to their health care provider. They should also report unusual swelling, weight gain, tiredness, bone pain, nonhealing sores, visual disturbances, and behavioral or mood changes.

Discuss possible changes in body image, and explore coping mechanisms for them.

Advise patients to wear medical identification that describes their disease process and drug regimen in the event of a medical emergency that prevents patients from relating their medical history. They should also inform any health care professional who provides care that they are taking **corticosteroids.**

LIFESTYLE MANAGEMENT. A diet high in protein, potassium, and calcium and low in sodium and carbohydrates can counteract some of the adverse reactions associated with **corticosteroids.** Multivitamins with minerals are appropriate. Caloric management to prevent obesity should also be implemented. **Alcohol** should be avoided during therapy. Osteoporosis risk can be reduced not only with calcium intake but also with regular exercise. Because stress can be a source of HPA stimulation, stress management techniques are used.

Nonsteroidal Anti-Inflammatory Drugs

Inflammation, pain, and fever are common manifestations of many diseases. **NSAIDs** offer the advantage of having activity in all three areas, which allows a less complex and less costly regimen. They also reduce the need for **opioid analgesics,** which are associated with chemical dependency and addiction. These advantages have resulted in **NSAIDs** becoming the most widely used prescription and over-the-counter (OTC) drugs in use today.

Aspirin and other **salicylates** that are members of this class are discussed in the next section. **Acetaminophen (Tylenol)**, although not an **anti-inflammatory** drug by chemistry, is often used to treat pain and fever and so is included in this section.

Pharmacodynamics

The inflammatory response is the same, regardless of the injury. Destruction of cell membranes results in release of chemical mediators, including histamine, prostaglandins, leukotrienes, cytokines, oxygen radicals, and enzymes. The cascade of events is depicted in Figure 23–2. Two major enzymes, lipo-oxygenase and cyclo-oxygenase, are required to produce these mediators.

Although the exact mode of action of **NSAIDs** is not known, the major mechanism is thought to be inhibition of cyclo-oxygenase activity and prostaglandin synthesis. Inhibition of lipo-oxygenase, leukotriene synthesis, lyso-somal enzyme release, neutrophil aggregation, and various cell membrane functions may also occur. These agents may also suppress rheumatoid factor.

The **NSAIDs** are primarily used for their anti-inflammatory activity, but they are effective **analgesics** that are useful for the relief of mild to moderate pain. They also have antipyretic properties. Because the mechanism of antiplatelet activity is reversible binding to thromboxane, antiplatelet activity exists only while the **NSAID** is in the blood. For this reason, **NSAIDs** are not used for antiplatelet therapy.

Acetaminophen is an **analgesic** and **antipyretic** with no anti-inflammatory activity. Although its mechanism of action is not known, it is thought to act by inhibiting central and peripheral prostaglandin synthesis. The central inhibition is almost as potent as **aspirin,** but its peripheral action is minimal. It reduces fever by direct actions on the hypothalamic heat-regulating centers, which increase dissipation of body heat via vasodilation and sweating. It has the advantages of minimal GI irritation and of not affecting bleeding times, uric acid levels, or respiration.

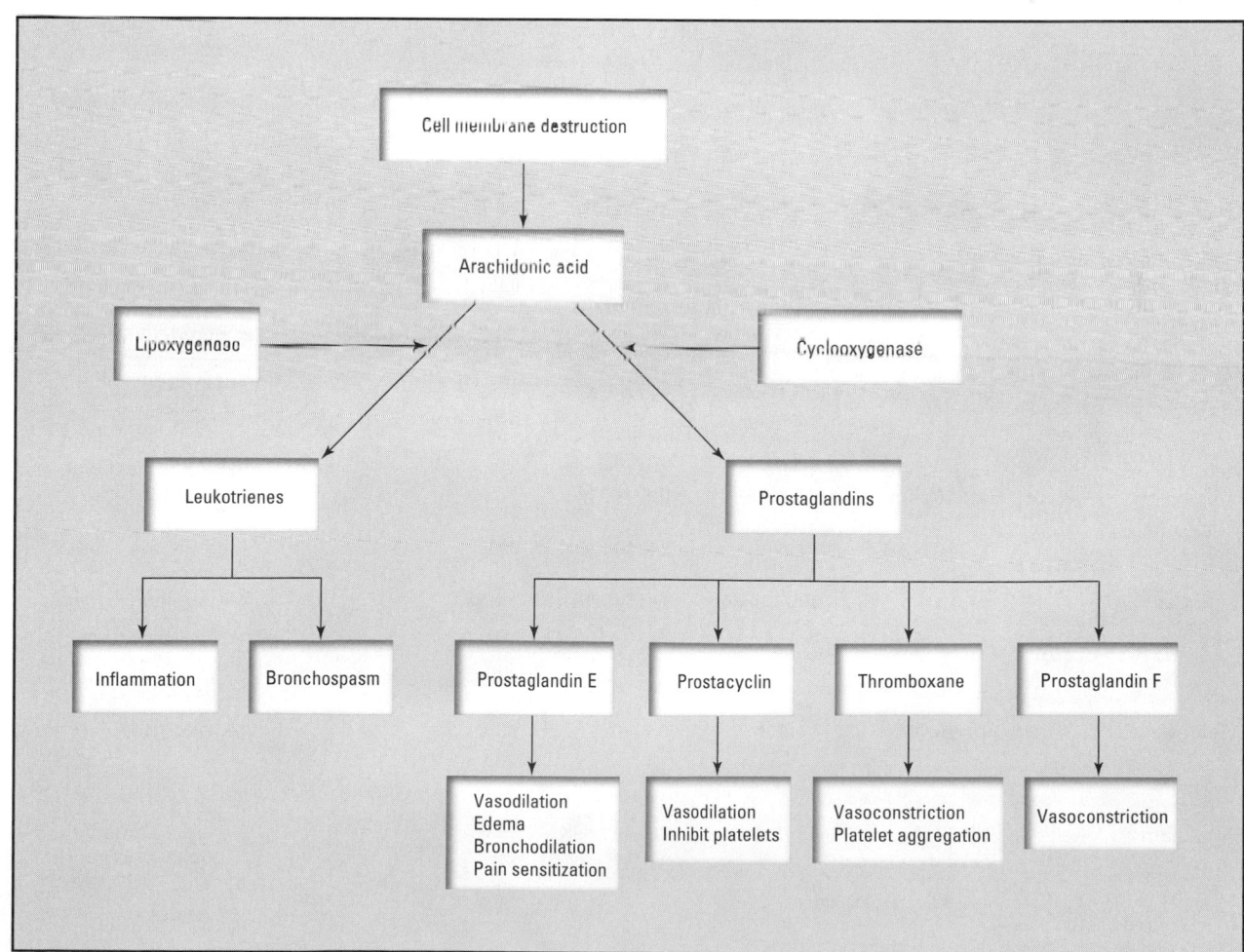

Figure 23–2. Sequence of events in inflammatory response. The sequence of events is the same, regardless of the source of injury.

Pharmacokinetics

Absorption and Distribution

After oral administration, **NSAIDs** are rapidly and almost completely absorbed (Table 23–9). **Naproxen sodium (Naprosyn)** is used as an **analgesic** because it is more rapidly absorbed. In general, food delays absorption but does not affect the total amount absorbed. Administration with food reduces GI adverse reactions. **Ketorolac (Toradol)** is the only drug in the class with an IM route of absorption.

All **NSAIDs** are more than 90 percent protein-bound. They are widely distributed in tissues, cross the placenta, and enter breast milk in low concentrations.

Acetaminophen is also rapidly and almost completely absorbed after oral administration. Rectal absorption is variable.

Serum protein binding is low at therapeutic concentrations but varies from 20 to 50 percent with toxic concentrations. It is relatively uniformly distributed in body tissues, crosses the placenta, and enters breast milk.

Metabolism and Excretion

The **NSAIDs** are all metabolized by the liver and excreted by the kidney, primarily as metabolites. **Sulindac (Clinoril)** and **nabumetone (Relafen)** are inactive prodrugs converted by the liver to active metabolites.

Table 23–9. Pharmacokinetics: Selected NSAIDs and Acetaminophen

Drug	Onset Anal./AntiR	Peak Anal./AntiR	Duration Anal./AntiR	Protein Binding	Half-Life	Elimination
Propionic Acid Group						
Ibuprofen	0.5 h/7 d	1–2 h/1–2 wk	4–6 h/UK	90 99%	1.8–2.5 h	10% unchanged in urine
Ketoprofen	0.5 h/NA	0.5–2 h/NA	4–8 h/NA	99%	2–4 h	60% metabolized by liver, some renal excretion
Naproxen	1 h/14 d	2–4 h/2–4 wk	7–12 h/UK	99%	12–15 h	Metabolites in urine
Naproxen sodium	1 h/14d	1–2 h/2–4 wk	7–12 h/UK	99%	10–20 h	Metabolites in urine
Oxaprozin	1 h/7 d	3–5 h/UK	24–48 h/UK	>99%	42–50 h	Metabolites in urine
Acetic Acid Group						
Diclofenac	1 h/1 wk	2–3 h/2 wk	4–8 h/UK	99%	1–2 h	>50% on first pass through liver; metabolites in urine
Indomethacin	0.5–2 h/7 d	1–2 h /1–2 wk SR: 2–4 h/—	4–6 h/UK	99% SR: 4.5–6 h	4.5 h	Metabolites in urine
Ketorolac	Varies /NA IM: 10 min	2–3 /NA IM: 0.5–1	4–6 h/NA IM: 4–6 h	99%	2.4–8.6 h*	92% in urine; 6% in feces
Nabumetone	1–2 h/1–2 d	5 h/2 wk	24–48 h/UK	99%	22.5–30 h*	Metabolites in urine
Sulindac	1 h/7 d	2–4 h/2–3 wk	7–16 h/UK	93–98%	7.8–16 h	Metabolites in urine
Fenamic Acid Group						
Meclofenamate	1 h/few days	0.5–1 h/2–3 wk	4–6 h/UK	>99%	40 min–2 h	Metabolites in urine
Mefenamic acid	Varies/NA	2–4 h/NA	6 h/NA	90%	2–4 h*	Metabolites in urine
Oxicams						
Piroxicam	15–30 min/ 7–12 d	3–5 h/2–3 wk	48–72 h/UK	99%	30–86 h	Minimal amounts unchanged in urine

*Prolonged in older adults and impaired renal function.
Anal. = Analgesic action.
AntiR = Antirheumatic action.
NA = No action; not used for this indication.
UK = Unknown.

Acetaminophen is extensively metabolized by the liver and excreted by the kidney primarily as inactive metabolites. When it is taken regularly or in large doses, the stores of one hepatic conjugate (glutathione) become depleted, and hepatic necrosis may occur. Half-life is prolonged in neonates, and severe hepatic dysfunction is related to its dependence on a liver function for metabolism.

Pharmacotherapeutics

Precautions and Contraindications

The only relative contraindications are for **ketorolac, mefenamic acid (Ponstel)**, and **nabumetone** in the presence of preexisting renal impairment. Because **NSAID** metabolites are excreted primarily by the kidneys, all others should be used with caution in the presence of renal function impairment. Renal function should be assessed prior to initiation of therapy and during therapy.

The liver extensively metabolizes **NSAIDs. Naproxen** may exhibit an increase in unbound fraction and reduced clearance of free drug in cirrhotic patients. A reduced dose may be necessary. The area under the curve (AUC) of **sulindac** may be increased in patients with cirrhosis because of alterations in sulfide formation and metabolism. Because the effects of hepatic disease on other **NSAIDs** are not known, they should be used cautiously in patients with hepatic impairment.

The liver also extensively metabolizes **acetaminophen.** High doses or long-term use and chronic alcoholism have been associated with hepatotoxicity. Avoid high doses or long-term use. For patients with chronic alcoholism, no safe dose has been determined. It should not be used for these patients.

GI adverse reactions are the most common reasons for cautious use. Serious GI bleeding, ulceration, and perforation can occur at any time without warning symptoms. Studies have not identified any subset of patients not at risk for these problems. A history of serious GI events, alcoholism, and smoking are the only specific factors associated with increased risk. Based on these data, active or chronic inflammation or ulceration of the GI tract relatively contraindicates use of all **NSAIDs**, especially **indomethacin (Indocin)** and **sulindac.** Other **NSAIDs** are sometimes used concurrently with a **cytoprotective agent** such as **sucralfate (Carafate)** or **misoprostol (Cytotec). Diclofenac** is produced in a combination with **misoprostol** under the brand name **Arthrotec. Cytoprotective agents** are discussed in Chapter 18. Wherever possible, however, these patients should be treated with nonulcerogenic drugs.

Indomethacin may aggravate depression or other psychiatric disturbances. A different **NSAID** should be chosen in this situation.

Age appears to increase the risk for adverse reactions to **NSAIDs.** The risk for serious ulcer disease is greater in adults over age 65. This risk appears to be dose-dependent, and reduced dosages may be necessary. **Ketorolac** is cleared more slowly in older adults. **Nabumetone** shows no difference in overall efficacy and safety between older adults and younger patients.

The *NSAIDs* are Pregnancy Category B (*ketoprofen [Orudis], naproxen, diclofenac, ibuprofen [Advil, Motrin], indomethacin, meclofenamate [Meclofen], piroxicam [Feldene], sulindac*) or Pregnancy Category C (*etodolac [Lodine], ketorolac, mefenamic acid, nabumetone, oxaprozin [Daypro]*). **There are no adequate and well-controlled studies in pregnant women, so use during pregnancy must be carefully weighed in terms of risks and benefits. Agents that inhibit prostaglandin synthesis may cause closure of the ductus arteriosus and other untoward effects in the fetus. Use in the first trimester is less troublesome;** *NSAIDs* **should be avoided during the last trimester.**

Acetaminophen **is Pregnancy Category B. Although it crosses the placenta, it has been routinely used during all stages of pregnancy. At therapeutic doses, it appears safe for short-term use.**

Most **NSAIDs** are excreted in breast milk. In studies, **ibuprofen** was not detected in breast milk, **naproxen** was detected at 1 percent of maternal concentration, and **ketorolac** was detected at a maximum milk:plasma ratio of 0.037. In general, nursing mothers should not use **NSAIDs** because of their potential effect on the infant's cardiovascular system. If they are used, select **ibuprofen, naproxen, or ketorolac.**

Acetaminophen is excreted in breast milk in low concentrations with reported milk:plasma ratios of 0.91 to 1.42 at 1 and 12 hours, respectively. No adverse effects on nursing infants were reported.

Mefenamic acid and **meclofenamate** are not recommended for children under age 14. Children under age 14 should not take **indomethacin** except in circumstances that clearly warrant the risk. Closely monitor the liver function of children between ages 2 and 14 who take it. Cases of hepatotoxicity, including fatalities, have been reported in children with juvenile rheumatoid arthritis. Other **NSAIDs** may be used to treat children, and pediatric doses are published for these drugs. **Acetaminophen** is also safe for children.

Adverse Drug Reactions

The most common adverse reactions with **NSAIDs** are GI disturbances, in particular nausea, vomiting, constipation, and diarrhea. Taking the drug with food can reduce these reactions. GI bleeding and ulceration were discussed in the Precautions and Contraindications section.

Acute renal insufficiency has occurred in patients

with preexisting renal disease or compromised renal perfusion. Patients at greatest risk are older adults, premature infants, those taking diuretics, and those with heart failure, systemic lupus erythematosus, or chronic glomerulonephritis. Stopping the drug usually brings recovery. Interstitial nephritis has occurred with increasing frequency in patients who take **NSAIDs,** and it may be due to altered prostaglandin metabolism.

Hematologic effects are less common but can be related to the actions of the drugs. **NSAIDs** inhibit platelet aggregation and may increase bleeding time. Decreased hemoglobin and hematocrit levels have occurred rarely. Patients with initial values below 10 g/dL who are to receive long-term therapy should have these values regularly monitored.

Fluid retention and peripheral edema are not severe but can be problematic for patients with compromised cardiovascular function. Patients with severe heart failure may have significant deterioration in hemodynamic function, presumably related to inhibition of prostaglandin-dependent compensatory mechanisms.

Cholestatic hepatitis, jaundice, and abnormal liver function tests have occurred rarely. Pancreatitis has developed in patients who take **sulindac.**

Adverse reactions associated with **acetaminophen** are few; however, those that do exist are significant. Acute hepatic necrosis occurs with doses of 10 to 15 g. Doses above 25 g are usually fatal. Children appear less susceptible to toxicity than adults because they have less capacity for glucuronidation, the metabolic pathway for **acetaminophen.** Acute poisoning is manifested by nausea, vomiting, drowsiness, confusion, liver tenderness, and renal failure, which occur within the first 24 hours and may persist for more than 1 week. Acute renal failure may also occur.

ACETAMINOPHEN POISONING. The course of **acetaminophen** poisoning is divided into four stages:

1. (12 to 24 hours): Nausea, vomiting, diaphoresis, and anorexia
2. (24 to 48 hours): Clinically improved; AST, ALT, bilirubin, and prothrombin levels begin to rise
3. (72 to 96 hours): Peak hepatotoxicity; AST of 20,000 not unusual
4. (7 to 8 days): Death or recovery

Acute **acetaminophen** poisoning should be referred to a poison control center hospital. If this is not possible, the following treatment regimen may be followed. If the acute ingestion is more than 150 mg/kg or the dose cannot be determined, obtain a serum **acetaminophen** assay 4 hours after ingestion. If the level is more than 300 mg/mL, hepatic damage has occurred in 90 percent of patients. Minimal hepatic damage results from a level below 120 mg/mL. Treatment is by gastric lavage in all cases, preferably within 4 hours of ingestion. Oral *N*-acetylcysteine is a specific antidote for **acetaminophen**

toxicity. Contact a poison control center for correct dosing of the antidote.

Anemia, neutropenia, pancytopenia, and thrombocytopenia also occur but are not severe. The skin eruptions and urticarial skin reactions that may develop are also transient and not severe.

Drug Interactions

Both **NSAIDs** and **acetaminophen** have many drug interactions. **NSAIDs** decrease the effectiveness of **antihypertensive drugs** because of their tendency to cause fluid retention and increased extracellular fluid volume. Coadministration with **anticoagulants** may prolong prothrombin time because both drugs affect platelet aggregation. Drugs that have adverse reactions associated with increased risk for GI bleeding or ulceration have an even higher risk if taken with **NSAIDs.** Drugs that require glucuronidation for metabolism may affect the metabolism of **acetaminophen** by competing for metabolic sites. These and other interactions are listed in Table 23–10.

Clinical Use and Dosing

RHEUMATOID ARTHRITIS. For patients with mild forms of rheumatoid arthritis and minimal joint involvement, an **NSAID** is appropriate first-line therapy. Although most **NSAIDs** have been used for this indication, those with a labeled indication for treatment of rheumatoid arthritis are **diclofenac, ibuprofen, indomethacin SR, ketoprofen, meclofenamate, nabumetone, naproxen, oxaprozin, piroxicam,** and **sulindac.** Doses of each of these drugs are presented in Table 23–11. These drugs do not significantly differ in their efficacy. Choice is determined by adverse reactions, cost, duration of action, and patient preference.

Age appears to increase the risk for adverse reactions to **NSAIDs,** except **nabumetone,** which shows no difference in overall efficacy and safety between older adults and younger patients. For women of childbearing age, Pregnancy Category may affect choice. **Nabumetone, piroxicam,** and **oxaprozin** have longer durations of action than the other drugs commonly used. **Ibuprofen** is the least expensive and is available OTC. **Diclofenac** comes in a combination with a **cytoprotective agent (misoprostol)** to reduce the risk for GI bleeding and ulceration, but this combination is quite expensive.

If a good clinical response occurs without signs of inflammation, the treatment regimen is continued. More advanced disease or patients with partial or poor response to **NSAIDs** require a change of drug therapy.

OSTEOARTHRITIS. The patient's pain and disability provide the guidelines for management of osteoarthritis. Initially, **acetaminophen** in doses up to 1 g qid are given to manage joint pain. If this drug fails to control pain,

Table 23–10. Drug Interactions: Selected NSAIDs and Acetaminophen

Drug	Interacting Drug	Possible Effect	Implications
Acetaminophen	Alcohol	Increased risk for hepatotoxicity	Avoid alcohol intake
	Anticholinergics	Delayed onset of action of acetaminophen; ultimate pharmacological effects not altered	No action required
	Beta-adrenergic blockers	Propranolol inhibits the enzyme systems responsible for glucuronidation and oxidation of acetaminophen, resulting in increased pharmacological effects	Select different beta-adrenergic blocker
	Contraceptives, oral	Increased glucuronidation, resulting in increased plasma clearance and decreased half-life of acetaminophen	Select NSAID for treatment if long-term therapy; not a problem with single dose
	Probenecid	Increases the therapeutic effectiveness of acetamino-phen	Used therapeutically
	Loop diuretics	Decreased effectiveness of diuretic because acetamino-phen may decrease renal prostaglandin excretion and decrease plasma renin activity	Avoid concurrent use
	Zidovudine	Decreased pharmacological effects of zidovudine related to enhanced nonhepatic or renal clearance of zidovudine	Avoid concurrent use; select NSAID for long-term use
All NSAIDs	Anticoagulants	May prolong prothrombin time (PT)	Avoid coadministration; monitor PT and patients closely; instruct patients to watch for indications of bleeding
	Beta adrenergic blockers	Antihypertensive effect impaired; sulindac and naproxen do not affect atenolol	Select appropriate drug match
	Hydantoins	Serum levels of phenytoin increased, resulting in increased pharmacological and toxic effects of phenytoin	If they must be used together, monitor serum levels and adjust dose accordingly
	Lithium	Serum lithium levels increased; sulindac has no effect or decreases levels	Avoid concurrent use or select sulindac; monitor serum levels
	Loop diuretics	Decreased effects of loop diuretics	Avoid concurrent use for long-term therapy or select different diuretic
	Probenecid	Probenecid may increase concentrations and toxicity risk of NSAIDs	Avoid concurrent use
	Salicylates	Decreased plasma concentra-tions of NSAIDs	Avoid concurrent use; offers no therapeutic advantage and significantly increases incidence of GI adverse reactions

Continued on next page

Table 23–10. Drug Interactions: Selected NSAIDs and Acetaminophen *(continued)*

Drug	Interacting Drug	Possible Effect	Implications
Indomethacin	Digoxin	May decrease digoxin serum levels; ibuprofen has similar effect	Select different NSAID
	Phenylpropanolamine	Increased blood pressure	Avoid coadministration
	Dipyridamole	Additive fluid retention	Select different NSAID
Indomethacin, naproxen	Thiazide diuretics	Decreased antihypertensive and diuretic action; sulindac may enhance effects	Avoid concurrent use; select sulindac if enhanced effect is desired

NSAIDs are prescribed. Although **NSAIDs** have both analgesic and anti-inflammatory actions, they do not alter the course of the disease or prevent joint destruction. All **NSAIDs** except **ketorolac** and **mefenamic acid** have an indication for treatment of osteoarthritis. Doses are presented in Table 23–11. As with rheumatoid arthritis, choice of **NSAID** is determined by adverse reactions, cost, duration of action, and patient preference. There is no significant difference in efficacy, and patient response is variable. For patients who experience adverse effects on the GI tract, adjunctive administration of **histamine₂ blockers** or **cytoprotective agents** may be needed. Both of these drug classes are discussed in Chapter 18.

MILD TO MODERATE PAIN. Almost every individual at some time experiences an episode of mild to moderate pain. Regardless of the source of the pain, **nonopioid analgesia** is the primary choice for management, especially if inflammation accompanies or is the cause of the pain. Although any **NSAID** may be used for this indication, several have been routinely used and proved effective. **Ibuprofen** is the most commonly used because it is inexpensive, available OTC, and short-acting so that acute pain can be managed without long-term effects and adverse reactions. For women of childbearing age, it is Pregnancy Category B, and for nursing women it is not detected in breast milk. **Naproxen sodium** is used as an **analgesic** because it reaches its peak more rapidly. Other drugs used for this indication include **ketoprofen, ketorolac, meclofenamate,** and **mefenamic acid.** When an injectable **NSAID** is needed, only **ketorolac** has such a formulation.

As with other indications, there is no clear difference in efficacy. Taking the drug around the clock, rather than as necessary, is more effective. Choice is based on adverse reactions, cost, duration of action, and patient preference. Health care providers often choose one short-acting drug (**ibuprofen, diclofenac, ketoprofen, ketorolac, meclofenamate**), an intermediate-acting one (**naproxen**), and a long-acting drug (**ketoprofen ER**) and use the same drugs repeatedly. Experience with a limited number of drugs provides more clinical knowledge, and there is no clear benefit to using more than a few. Because different patients seem to respond better to different **NSAIDs**, if one drug does not produce the desired effect, another one can be tried.

Acetaminophen is useful in treating mild to moderate pain that is not accompanied by or caused by inflammation. It is not intended for pain management for more than 5 days in children or 10 days in adults because of the increased risk for hepatic adverse reactions. For adults, 325 to 650 mg every 4 to 6 hours usually suffices. Children's doses are based on age, with doses published from 3 months to 14 years. After age 14, the adult dose is used. These doses are shown in Table 23–11.

PRIMARY DYSMENORRHEA. Ibuprofen, ketoprofen, mefenamic acid, and **naproxen** are the drugs used for this indication. Doses are shown in Table 23–11.

TENDINITIS AND BURSITIS. Indomethacin SR, naproxen, and **sulindac** are used for this indication. **Naproxen** and **sulindac** both are intermediate acting and provide longer duration of action than **indomethacin,** even in its sustained-release form. They also have fewer drug interactions. **Naproxen** is less likely to produce GI adverse reactions. These same three drugs are used to manage the pain in gout because it is associated with inflammation. Treatment choices are determined on the same basis.

FEVER. Ibuprofen is the **NSAID** of choice for fever. Doses are published for both adults and children. **Acetaminophen** may also be used for this purpose, but not for longer than 3 days. It is best used in those patients with **aspirin** allergy, blood coagulation disorders, upper GI disease, and the fever that accompanies the common cold, "flu," and other viral illnesses in children. It has also been used to prevent the fever and injection site pain from **DPT vaccinations.** A dose immediately following vaccination and every 4 to 6 hours thereafter for 48 to 72 hours is suggested.

Rational Drug Selection

There is no clear difference in efficacy between **NSAIDs.** The rationale for choices is provided in the discussion of

Table 23–11. Dosage Schedule: Selected NSAIDs and Acetaminophen

Drug	Indication	Dosage Schedule	Notes
Acetaminophen	Mild to moderate pain and/or fever	*Oral Doses* *Adults and children >14 y:* 325–650 mg every 4–6 h *or* 1 g tid or qid	Not to exceed 4 g/d
		Children 0–3 mo: 40 mg every 4 h *Children 4–11 mo:* 80 mg every 4 h *Children 1–<2 y:* 120 mg every 4 h *Children 2–3 y:* 160 mg every 4 h *Children 4–5 y:* 240 mg every 4 h *Children 6–8 y:* 320 mg every 4 h *Children 9–10 y:* 400 mg every 4 h *Children 11 y:* 480 mg every 4 h	For all ages of children, doses not to exceed 5 doses in 24 h
		Children 12–14 y: 640 mg every 4 h	Not to exceed 4 g/d
		Suppositories *Adults and children >12 y:* 650 mg every 4–6 h	Not to exceed 720 mg/d
		Children 3–11 mo: 80 mg up to every 6 h	Not to exceed 2.6 g/d
		Children 1–3 y: 80 mg up to every 4 h *Children 3–6 y:* 120–125 every 4–6 h *Children 6–12 y:* 325 mg every 4–6 h	
Etodolac	Osteoarthritis	*Adults:* 800–1200 mg/d in divided doses, followed by dosage adjustments within the range of 600–1200 mg/d in divided doses	Not to exceed 1200 mg/d; for patients ≤60 kg, do not exceed 20 mg/kg
	Analgesia	*Adults:* 200–400 mg every 6–8 h as needed	Not to exceed 1200 mg/d; for patients ≤60 kg, do not exceed 20 mg/kg
Diclofenac	Rheumatoid arthritis	*Adults:* 100–200 mg/d in divided doses (50 mg tid–qid *or* 75 mg bid) Chronic therapy with extended-release tablets: 100 mg/d	Doses above 225 mg/d not recommended
	Osteoarthritis	*Adults:* 100–200 mg/d in divided doses (50 mg tid–tid *or* 75 mg bid) Chronic therapy with extended-release tablets: 100 mg/d	Doses above 200 mg/d are not recommended
	Ankylosing spondylitis	*Adults:* 100–125 mg/d delayed-release tablets (25 mg qid with an extra dose at bedtime if needed)	Doses above 125 mg not recommended
	Analgesia, primary dysmenorrhea	*Adults:* 50 mg tid; some patients may need 100 mg tid initially, followed by 50 mg tid	After first day, maximum dose 200 mg; doses generally should not exceed 150 mg
Ibuprofen	Rheumatoid arthritis, osteoarthritis	*Adults:* 1.2–3.2 g/d (300 mg qid *or* 400, 600, or 800 mg tid–qid)	Not to exceed 3.2 g/d; higher doses usually needed for rheumatoid arthritis
	Juvenile arthritis	*Children:* 30–70 mg/kg/d in 3–4 divided doses; 20 mg/kg/d may be adequate in milder disease	
	Mild to moderate pain	*Adults:* 400 mg every 4–6 h as needed	Not to exceed 1200 mg/d
	Muscle sprain, strain (anti-inflammatory, analgesic)	*Adults:* 600 mg qid or 800 mg tid for 5 d	Not to exceed 3600 mg/d
		Children: 20–40 mg/k/d in divided doses	Not to exceed 50 mg/kg/d
	Primary dysmenorrhea	*Adults and children >12 y:* 400 mg every 4 h as needed	Not to exceed 1200 mg/d

Continued on next page

Table 23–11. Dosage Schedule: Selected NSAIDs and Acetaminophen *(continued)*

Drug	Indication	Dosage Schedule	Notes
	Fever reduction	*Adults:* 200–400 mg every 4–6 h *Children 6 mo–12 y:* 5 mg/kg for temperature <39.1°C (102.5°F) or 10 mg/kg for higher temperatures; may be repeated every 4–6 h	Not to exceed 1200 mg/d Not to exceed 40 mg/kg/d
	OTC use for pain and/or fever	*Adults:* 200 mg every 4–6 h while symptoms persist; if response is not adequate, may use 400 mg *Children 32–44 kg/11 y:* 300 mg every 6–8 h *Children 27–32 kg/9–10 y:* 250 mg every 6–8 h *Children 22–26 kg/6–8 y:* 200 mg every 6–8 h *Children 16–21 kg/4–5 y:* 150 mg every 6–8 h *Children 11–15 kg/2–3 y:* 100 mg every 6–8 h *Children 8–10 kg/12–23 mo:* 67 mg every 6–8 h *Children 5.5–7.9 kg/6–11 mo:* 50 mg every 6–8 h	Not to exceed 1200 mg/d; do not take for >10 d for pain or >3 d for fever
Indomethacin	Moderate to severe rheumatoid arthritis, ankylosing spondylitis, and osteoarthritis	*Adults and children >14 y:* 25 mg bid–tid initially; increase dose by 25–50 mg at weekly intervals until satisfactory response Sustained release: 75 mg can be taken daily as alternative to 25 mg tid or bid as alternative to 50 mg tid	Not to exceed 200 mg/d; for patients with persistent night pain or morning stiffness, give larger portion of dose at bedtime (up to 100 mg)
	Acute painful shoulder (bursitis or tendinitis)	*Adults and children >14 y:* 75–100 mg/d in 3–4 divided doses for 7–14 d	
	Acute gouty arthritis	*Adults:* 50 mg tid; taper to eliminate drug as soon as pain is relieved	Do not use sustained-release form
Ketoprofen	Rheumatoid arthritis, osteoarthritis	*Adults:* 75 mg tid *or* 50 mg qid initially Maintenance dose is 150–300 mg/d in 3–4 divided doses Extended release: 200 mg once daily	Reduce dose by 1/2–1/3 for older adults and those with renal impairment; not to exceed 300 mg/d
	Mild to moderate pain, primary dysmenorrhea	*Adults:* 25–50 mg every 6–8 h as needed	Doses >50 mg have not increased efficacy; not to exceed 300 mg/d
	OTC use for pain	*Adults and children >16 y:* 12.5 mg with full glass of liquid every 4–6 h; if pain or fever persists after 1 h, follow with 12.5 mg	Not to exceed 25 mg in a 4–6 h period or 75 mg/24 h
Ketorolac	Acute, moderately severe pain	*Adults <65 y:* 60 mg IM single dose or 30 mg every 6 h (not to exceed 120 mg/d); then 20 mg PO initially, followed by 10 mg every 4–6 h as needed (not to exceed 40 mg/d) *Adults >65 y* or *<50 kg* or *with renal impairment:* 30 mg IM single dose or 15 mg every 6 h (not to exceed 60 mg/d); then 10 mg PO every 4–6 h as needed (not to exceed 40 mg/d)	Not intended for >5 d combined IM and PO, or for minor or chronic pain; oral therapy is intended only as continuation from IM therapy

Continued on next page

Table 23–11. Dosage Schedule: Selected NSAIDs and Acetaminophen *(continued)*

Drug	Indication	Dosage Schedule	Notes
Meclofenamate	Rheumatoid arthritis, osteoarthritis	*Adults:* 200–400 mg/d in 3–4 equally divided doses	Not to exceed 400 mg/d
	Mild to moderate pain	*Adults and children >14 y:* 50–100 mg every 4–6 h	Not to exceed 400 mg/d
	Excessive menstrual bleeding, dysmenorrhea	*Adults and children >14 y:* 100 mg tid for up to 6 d, starting with first day of menstrual flow	Not to exceed 400 mg/d
Mefenamic acid	Acute pain	*Adults and children >14 y:* 500 mg, then 250 mg every 6 h as needed	Not to exceed 1 wk
	Primary dysmenorrhea	*Adults and children >14 y:* 500 mg, then 250 mg every 6 h as needed starting at onset of bleeding or symptoms	Should not be necessary for more than 2–3 d
Nabumetone	Rheumatoid arthritis, osteoarthritis	*Adults:* 1000 mg daily; may increase to 1500–2000 mg/d	Not to exceed 2000 mg/d
Naproxen	Rheumatoid arthritis, osteoarthritis, ankylosing spondylitis	*Adults:* 250–500 mg bid; may increase to 1.5 g/d for limited periods Delayed release: 375–500 mg bid Controlled release: 750–1000 mg once daily Naproxen sodium: 275–550 mg bid; may increase to 1.65 mg for limited periods	Morning and evening doses do not need to be equal; more than twice-daily dosing does not improve efficacy
	Juvenile arthritis	*Children:* 10 mg/kg/d in 2 divided doses Suspension: 13-kg child = 2.5 mL bid; 25-kg child = 5 mL; 38-kg child = 7.5 mL	
	Acute gout	*Adults:* 750 mg, then 250 mg every 8 h until attack subsides Controlled release: 1000–1500 mg once daily on first day, then 1000 mg once daily until the attack subsides Naproxen sodium: 825 mg, then 275 mg every 8 h until attack subsides	
	Mild to moderate pain, dysmenorrhea, acute tendinitis or bursitis	*Adults:* 500 mg, then 250 mg every 6–8 h as needed Controlled release: 1000 mg once daily; 1500 mg/d may be used for limited period	Not to exceed 1.25 g/d
		Naproxen sodium: 550 mg, then 275 mg every 6–8 h as needed *Children:* Naproxen suspension, 5 mg/kg/d in 2 divided doses	Not to exceed 1.375 g/d
	OTC use for pain	*Adults:* 200 mg with full glass of liquid every 8–12 h while symptoms persist; dose of 400 mg initially, then 200-mg doses, may be necessary *Adults >65 y:* Do not take >200 mg every 12 h *Children:* Do not give to children <12 y except under advice/ supervision of HCP	Not to exceed 600 mg/d

Continued on next page

Table 23–11. Dosage Schedule: Selected NSAIDs and Acetaminophen *(continued)*

Drug	Indication	Dosage Schedule	Notes
Oxaprozin	Rheumatoid arthritis, osteoarthritis	*Adults:* 1200 mg once daily; patients with low body weight or milder disease may use 600 mg once daily	Not to exceed 1800 mg/d or 26 mg/kg, whichever is lower; doses >1200 mg/d should be divided
Piroxicam	Rheumatoid arthritis, osteoarthritis	*Adults:* 20 mg once daily; may divide dose *Adults >65 y:* 10 mg once daily initially	
	Dysmenorrhea	*Adults:* 40 mg first day, then 20 mg/d	
Sulindac	Rheumatoid arthritis, osteoarthritis, ankylosing spondylitis	*Adults:* 150 mg bid	
	Acute gout, painful shoulder (tendinitis, bursitis)	*Adults:* 200 mg bid	Therapy usually not longer than 7 d

clinical use and dosing. **Acetaminophen** is used only for fever and for mild to moderate pain not associated with inflammation.

Monitoring

Monitoring is required only for long-term therapy. Because these drugs may produce acute renal insufficiency, assess renal function (serum creatinine) before initiation of therapy and annually throughout long-term therapy. A CBC prior to initiation of therapy and annually thereafter is appropriate because of the risk for GI bleeding. Any other monitoring is related to the disease being treated.

Patient Education

ADMINISTRATION. Take the drug exactly as prescribed (Table 23–12). A missed dose should be taken as soon as the patient remembers unless it is almost time for the next dose. For drugs taken more than once daily, ideally take the missed dose within 1 to 2 hours of the time it was scheduled. Do not double doses. Taking higher doses than those prescribed does not increase efficacy and may increase adverse reactions.

For some **NSAIDs,** there is a proscribed length of time beyond which the drug may not be taken. Patients should be informed of this time limitation. Taking the drug with food or a full glass of fluid and remaining in an upright position for 15 to 30 minutes may reduce GI discomfort and adverse reactions. Remind them to avoid **aspirin, alcohol,** or other GI irritants while taking these drugs.

ADVERSE REACTIONS. Advise patients about probable adverse reactions and what to do if they occur. The most common adverse reaction is GI bleeding. They should contact their health care provider if they experience coffee-ground emesis or black, tarry stools. The provider should also be notified of skin rash, itching, visual disturbances, weight gain, edema, or persistent headache. With **meclofenamate** and **mefenamic acid,** if rash, diarrhea, or other digestive problems occur, patients should discontinue the drug and contact their health care provider.

These drugs may cause drowsiness. Patients should avoid activities requiring mental alertness until their response to the drug is known.

LIFESTYLE MANAGEMENT. Lifestyle modifications are only those related to the disease being treated.

Aspirin and Nonacetylated Salicylates

Aspirin is the prototype drug for this class, which makes it one of the most used drug classes for the treatment and prevention of a wide variety of disorders. Although **salicylates** are prescribed for conditions similar to those the **NSAIDs** are used for, in addition to the analgesic, antiinflammatory, and antipyretic properties common to the **NSAIDs,** the **salicylates** also possess antiplatelet properties to varying degrees. This latter property accounts for some of their adverse reactions but also for the increased breadth of their use beyond those for which **NSAIDs** are prescribed. The ability of **aspirin** to reduce platelet aggregation has given it a role in managing rheumatic fever, transient ischemic attacks (TIAs), coronary artery disease, and deep vein thrombosis. The antiplatelet role of **aspirin** is discussed in Chapter 16. Its nonspecific antiinflammatory effect is invaluable in reducing cardiac workload for patients with severe carditis and heart failure. **Aspirin** has been shown to reduce the incidence of myocardial infarction (MI) in men and the incidence of death in all patients with unstable angina. **Salicylates** are

Table 23–12. Available Dosage Forms: Selected NSAIDs and Acetaminophen

Drug	Dosage Form	How Supplied
Acetaminophen (Tylenol)	Tablets: 325 mg, 500 mg	In bottles of 10, 24, 50, 100, 200 tablets
	Tablets: 500 mg extra strength	In bottles of 100 tablets
	Chewable tablets: 80 mg	In bottles of 30, 48, 96 (bubble gum and cherry-flavored chewables)
	Chewable tablets: 160 mg	In bottles of 24 grape and fruit-flavored chewable tablets
	Caplets: 325 mg	In bottles of 24, 50, 100 caplets
	Caplets: 650 mg extended relief	In bottles of 100 caplets
	Gelcaps: 500 mg extra strength	In bottles of 24, 50, 100 gelcaps
	Elixir: 160 mg/5 mL	In 60 and 120 mL (grape and cherry flavors)
	Liquid: 500 mg/15 mL	In 240 mL; with dosing cup
	Infant drops: 100 mg/mL	In 7.5, 30 mL; with 0.8-mL dropper
(Generic)	Tablets: 325 mg	In bottles of 50, 100, 1000 tablets
	Tablets: 500 mg	In bottles of 100, 1000 tablets
	Tablets: 650 mg	In bottles of 1000 tablets
	Chewable tablets: 80 mg	In bottles of 30, 100 chewable tablets
	Capsules: 500 mg	In bottles of 50, 100, 1000 capsules
	Elixir: 160 mg/5 mL	In 118 and 120 mL, pint and gallon
	Liquid: 160 mg/5 mL	In 120 and 500 mL
	Liquid: 500 mg/15 mL	In 237 mL
	Solution: 100 mg/mL	In 15 mL
	Suppository: 120 mg, 300 mg, 325 mg, 650 mg	In 12 individually foil-wrapped suppositories
Diclofenac (Voltaren)	Delayed release: 25 mg	In bottles of 60, 100 tablets
	Delayed release: 50 mg, 75 mg	In bottles of 60, 100, 1000 tablets
	Extended release: 100 mg	In bottles of 100 tablets
(Generic)	Delayed release: 25 mg, 50 mg, 75 mg	In bottles of 60, 100, 1000 tablets
Etodolac (Lodine)	Capsules: 200 mg, 300 mg	In bottles of 100 capsules
Ibuprofen (Advil)	Tablets: 200 mg	In bottles of 4, 8, 24, 50, 100, 165, 250 tablets
	Caplets: 200 mg	In bottles of 24, 50, 100, 154, 250 caplets
	Suspension: 100 mg/5mL	In 119 and 473 mL, fruit-flavored
(Motrin)	Tablets: 100 mg	In 100 scored, film-coated tablets
	Tablets: 200 mg	In bottles of 24, 50, 100, 130, 165
	Tablets: 300 mg, 500 mg, 600 mg, 800 mg	In bottles of 500 tablets
	Chewable tablets: 50 mg, 100 mg	In bottles of 100 citrus-flavored chewable tablets
	Caplets: 200 mg	In bottles of 24, 50, 100, 130, 165 caplets
	Gelcaps: 200 mg	In bottles of 24, 50 gelcaps
	Suspension: 100 mg/5 mL	In 60, 120, 480 mL, berry flavor
	Oral drops: 40 mg/mL	In 15 mL, berry flavor
(Generic)	Tablets: 200 mg	In bottles of 50, 100, 500 tablets
	Tablets: 300 mg, 400 mg, 600 mg	In bottles of 50, 100, 250 tablets
	Tablets: 800 mg	In bottles of 12, 15, 21, 30, 40, 50, 60, 100, 360, 500 tablets
Indomethacin (Indocin)	Capsules: 25 mg	In bottles of 100, 1000 capsules
	Capsules: 50 mg	In bottles of 100 capsules
	Suspension: 25 mg/5 mL	In 237 mL, pineapple-coconut-mint flavor
	Suppository: 50 mg	In 30 individually foil-wrapped suppositories
(Generic)	Capsules: 25 mg	In bottles of 60, 100, 500, 1000 capsules
	Capsules: 50 mg	In bottles of 23, 72, 100, 250, 500 capsules
	Sustained release: 75 mg	In bottles of 60, 100 capsules
	Suspension: 25 mg/5 mL	In 500 mL, fruit-flavored

Continued on next page

Table 23–12. Available Dosage Forms: Selected NSAIDs and Acetaminophen *(continued)*

Drug	Dosage Form	How Supplied
Ketoprofen (Orudis)	Tablets: 12.5 mg Capsules: 25 mg, 50 mg Capsules: 75 mg	In bottles of 24, 50 tablets In bottles of 100 tablets In bottles of 100, 500 tablets
(Oruvail)	Extended release:100 mg, 150 mg, 200 mg	In bottles of 100 capsules
(Generic)	Capsules: 25 mg, 50 mg Capsules: 75 mg	In bottles of 100 capsules In bottles of 100, 500 capsules
Ketorolac (Toradol)	Tablets: 10 mg Injection: 15 mg/mL Injection: 30 mg/mL	In bottles of 100 film-coated tablets In 1-mL Tubex syringes In 1- and 2-mL Tubex syringes
Meclofenamate (Meclofen)	Capsules: 50 mg, 100 mg	In bottles of 100 tablets
(Generic)	Capsules: 50 mg, 100 mg	In bottles of 100, 250, 500 capsules
Mefenamic acid (Ponstel)	Capsules: 250 mg	In bottles of 100 capsules
Nabumetone (Relafen)	Tablets: 500 mg, 750 mg	In bottles of 100, 500 film-coated tablets
Naproxen (Aleve)	Tablets: 200 mg	In bottles of 24, 50, 100 tablets
(Naprelan)	Controlled release: 375 mg Controlled release: 500 mg	In bottles of 100 tablets In bottles of 75 tablets
(Naprosyn)	Tablets: 250 mg, 375 mg, 500 mg Enteric coated: 375 mg, 500 mg Suspension: 125 mg/5mL	In bottles of 100, 500 tablets In bottles of 100 enteric-coated tablets In 474 mL, pineapple-orange flavor
(Naproxen)	Tablets: 250 mg, 375 mg, 500 mg Suspension: 125 mg/5 mL	In bottles of 100, 500, 1000 tablets In 5 and 500 mL, pineapple-orange flavor
(Naproxen sodium)	Tablets: 275 mg, 550 mg	In bottles of 100, 500, 1000 tablets
Oxaprozin (Daypro)	Caplets: 600 mg	In bottles of 100, 500 film-coated caplets
Piroxicam (Feldene)	Capsules: 10 mg Capsules: 20 mg	In bottles of 100 tablets In bottles of 100, 500 tablets
(Generic)	Capsules: 10 mg, 20 mg	In bottles of 100, 500, 1000 capsules
Sulindac (Clinoril)	Tablets: 150 mg, 200 mg	In bottles of 100 tablets
(Generic)	Tablets: 150 mg, 200 mg	In bottles of 60, 100, 500 tablets

There are many brand names for several of these drugs. Only the most commonly used are presented here.

also used topically as **keratolytic agents** and **counterirritants.** This role is discussed in Chapters 21 and 30.

Pharmacodynamics

All **salicylates** have analgesic, anti-inflammatory, antipyretic, and antiplatelet actions. The pharmacological effects are qualitatively similar. **Salicylates** lower body temperature through vasodilation of peripheral vessels, thus enhancing dissipation of heat. The anti-inflammatory and analgesic activities are mediated through inhibition of prostaglandin synthesis in the same manner as **NSAIDs.** However, **aspirin** more potently inhibits prostaglandin synthesis and has greater anti-inflammatory activity than the **NSAIDs.** The acetyl group of the **aspirin** molecule is thought to be responsible for these differences. **Aspirin** acetylates the cyclo-oxygenase enzyme in the prostaglandin biosynthesis pathway.

Aspirin also irreversibly inhibits platelet aggregation. Single analgesic-level doses prolong bleeding time. Acetylation of platelet cyclo-oxygenase prevents synthesis of thromboxane A, which is a potent vasoconstrictor and inducer of platelet aggregation for the life of the platelet (7 to 10 days). This drug has shown some success as an antiplatelet agent for patients with thromboembolic disease. For this indication, low doses appear to be more effective than higher ones. Further discussion is in Chapter 16.

The **nonacetylated salicylates (salsalate [Disalcid], choline magnesium trisalicylate [Trilisate],** and **choline salicylate [Arthropan]**) and **diflunisal (Dolobid),** which is a salicylic acid derivative not metabolized to salicylic acid, are not as potent as **aspirin** and do not possess the same degree of antiplatelet activity.

Pharmacokinetics

Absorption and Distribution

Salicylates are rapidly and completely absorbed after oral administration (Table 23–13). Bioavailability depends on the dosage form, gastric emptying time, gastric pH, presence of **antacids** or **buffering agents,** and particle size. The bioavailability of enteric-coated products may be erratic. The presence of food in the gut slows absorption, and absorption from rectal suppositories is also slower, resulting in lower salicylate levels.

Aspirin is partially hydrolyzed to salicylic acid during absorption and is distributed to all body tissues and fluids, including fetal tissue, breast milk, and the central nervous system (CNS). The highest concentrations are in plasma, the liver, the renal cortex, the heart, and lung tissues.

Protein binding of **salicylates** is concentration-dependent. At low concentrations (100 µg/mL), 90 percent is bound; at higher concentrations (400 mg/mL), only 76 percent is bound.

Diflunisal is also rapidly and completely absorbed after oral administration. It crosses the placenta and enters breast milk. The first dose tends to have slower onset of pain relief than other drugs but achieves comparable peak effects. More than 99 percent is bound to plasma proteins.

Metabolism and Excretion

Salicylic acid is eliminated by renal excretion of salicylic acid and by oxidation and conjugation of metabolites by the liver. The amount excreted depends on urine pH. As urine pH increases from 5 to 8, renal clearance of free ionized salicylate increases from 2 to 3 percent to more than 80 percent. Alteration of urine pH is used in the treatment of salicylate poisoning to increase excretion.

Aspirin has a half-life of 15 to 20 minutes. Salicylic acid's half-life is 2 to 3 hours at low doses; at higher doses, it ranges from 6 to 12 hours. Plasma levels increase disproportionately as **salicylate** doses increase.

Difunisal has a long half-life and nonlinear pharmacokinetics so that time to steady state is 3 to 4 days with 125 mg bid and 7 to 9 days with 500 mg bid. A loading dose shortens the time to steady state. Because 90 percent of each dose is eliminated by the kidneys, the half-life increases with renal impairment.

Pharmacotherapeutics

Precautions and Contraindications

Taking **salicylates,** especially **aspirin,** by children or adolescents with influenza or chickenpox has been associated with the development of Reye's syndrome, a rare

Table 23–13. Pharmacokinetics: Salicylates

Drug	Onset	Peak	Duration	Protein Binding	Half-Life	Elimination
Acetylsalicylic acid	15–20 min	1–3 h	3–6 h	90–91%; 25–76%*	15–20 min; 2–3 h; 15–30 h*	In urine and by liver*
Choline salicylate	5–30 min	1–3 h	3–6 h	90–91%; 25–76%*	15–20 min; 2–3 h; 15–30 h*	In urine and by liver*
Choline magnesium salicylate	5–30 min	1–3 h	3–6 h	90–91%; 25–76%*	15–20 min; 2–3 h; 15–30 h*	In urine and by liver*
Salsalate	5–30 min	1–3 h	3–6 h	90–91%; 25–76%*	15–20 min; 2–3 h; 15–30 h*	In urine and by liver*
Diflunisal	1 h	2–3 h	8–12 h	>99%	8–12 h	90% in urine; <5% in feces

*See discussion in text.

but life-threatening condition characterized by vomiting, lethargy, and eventually delirium and coma. The mortality rate is 20 to 30 percent, and permanent brain damage has been reported in survivors. Children or adolescents with influenza or chickenpox should not take **salicylates**. **Salicylates** probably should not be taken by anyone with any viral upper respiratory infection (URI).

Aspirin should be avoided for 1 week before any surgery because of the increased risk for postoperative bleeding on account of its antiplatelet effects. For similar reasons, **salicylates** in general are contraindicated for patients with active peptic ulcer disease or other GI bleeding–related disorders or a history of such disorders. **Salsalate** and **choline salicylate** may cause less GI irritation and bleeding than **aspirin**. The antiplatelet effects contraindicate **salicylate** use for patients who are taking **anticoagulants** or who have anemia or a history of blood coagulation defects.

Salicylates should be used cautiously for patients with hepatic impairment. Reversible hepatic encephalopathy has occurred after even therapeutic doses for rheumatoid arthritis. Cautious use is also required for patients with renal insufficiency because **salicylates** may cause a transient decrease in renal function and aggravate chronic kidney diseases. **Magnesium salicylates** are contraindicated in the presence of renal insufficiency because the kidney cannot eliminate the magnesium, and hypermagnesemia results.

Salicylates affect uric acid accumulation. In low doses (less than 2 g/day), they decrease urate excretion and raise serum uric acid levels. At high doses (3 to 5 g/day) they have a uricosuric effect; however, they are rarely tolerated at this high a dose. They should be used with caution in the presence of gout.

Aspirin is Pregnancy Category D; *salsalate* and *magnesium salicylate* are Pregnancy Category C. **Ingestion during pregnancy may produce anemia in the mother and increase the risk for postpartum hemorrhage. Inhibition of prostaglandin synthesis may cause constriction of the ductus arteriosus and other possible untoward effects in the fetus. Avoid use in pregnancy, especially during the third trimester.** *Diflunisal* **is Pregnancy Category C. Although its safety during pregnancy has not been established, it should not be used, especially during the last trimester.**

Salicylates are excreted in breast milk in low concentrations. Adverse effects on nursing infants have not been reported. **Diflunisal** is excreted in breast milk in concentrations of 2 to 7 percent of the maternal plasma. Because of potential adverse effects, discontinuing either this drug or nursing is recommended.

The safety and efficacy of **magnesium salicylate** and **salsalate** have not been established in children. **Aspirin** should not be used in children with acute febrile illness. Children with dehydration appear more at risk for **salicylate** toxicity.

Adverse Drug Reactions

The most common adverse reaction to **salicylates** is GI irritation and bleeding. Although fecal blood loss is lower with enteric-coated products, these drugs have erratic absorption and still must be used cautiously by patients with GI disorders. The amount of blood lost from GI bleeding secondary to **salicylate** use is usually clinically insignificant, but with prolonged use it can result in iron-deficiency anemia. Patients who have developed peptic ulcers while taking **salicylates** have healed these ulcers with the use of **histamine$_2$ blockers** and **antacids**, despite continued **salicylate** use. Only 20 to 25 percent of patients on chronic **aspirin** therapy for rheumatoid arthritis develop mucosal injury.

Hypersensitivity reactions have occurred with **salicylates**. Hypersensitivity to **salicylates** or **NSAIDs** contraindicates **aspirin** use and requires extremely cautious use of the other **salicylates**. Cross-sensitivity exists between **aspirin** and **NSAIDs** and between **aspirin** and tartrazine dye. This cross-sensitivity does not appear to occur with **choline salicylate**. **Aspirin** sensitivity is more prevalent in patients with asthma, nasal polyps, or chronic urticaria.

Salicylates are ototoxic at increased blood levels. They should be discontinued if dizziness, tinnitus, or impaired hearing develops. Temporary hearing loss disappears gradually when the drug is stopped.

TOXICITY. The acute lethal dose of **salicylates** in adults is 10 to 30 g, and in children it is 4 g. Chronic **salicylate** toxicity can occur when more than 100 mg/kg is ingested daily for 2 or more days. Signs of **salicylate** poisoning appear at serum levels of 200 μg/mL. Severe toxicity may occur at levels of 400 μg/mL. Respiratory alkalosis is seen initially. Hyperpnea and tachypnea occur as a result of increased CO_2 production and a direct stimulatory effect of the **salicylate** on the respiratory center in the brain. Other symptoms include nausea, vomiting, hypokalemia, tinnitus, disorientation, irritability, seizures, dehydration, hyperthermia, thrombocytopenia, and other hematologic disorders.

Treatment for **salicylate** toxicity includes induction of emesis or gastric lavage to remove any unabsorbed drug from the stomach. Activated charcoal diminishes **salicylate** absorption if it is given within 2 hours of ingestion. **Salicylate** levels and acid-base, fluid, and electrolyte balances are carefully monitored. The rest of therapy is supportive. Forced alkaline diuresis increases **salicylate** excretion. Hemodialysis is reserved for those patients with severe poisoning.

Drug Interactions

Aspirin may potentiate the anticoagulant action of **heparin, warfarin,** or **thrombolytic agents** (Table 23–14).

Table 23–14. Drug Interactions: Salicylates

Drug	Interacting Drug	Possible Effect	Implications
Acetylsalicylic acid	Angiotensin-converting enzyme inhibitors, beta-adrenergic blockers	Decreased antihypertensive effect because of prostaglandin inhibition	Consider discontinuing salicylate or selecting different antihypertensive
	Heparin, warfarin	Prolonged bleeding time, impaired platelet function	Avoid concurrent use
	Nitroglycerin	Unexpected hypotensive effects	Reduce nitroglycerin dose
	NSAIDs	Aspirin may decrease serum concentrations	Avoid concomitant use; no therapeutic advantage and may increase risk for GI bleed
All salicylates	Alcohol, cefamandole, cefoperazone, cefotetan, valproic acid, plicamycin	Increased risk for GI bleeding	Avoid alcohol while taking salicylates; select different antimicrobial or avoid use of salicylate
	Loop diuretics, aminoglycosides, bumetanide, ethacrynic acid	May increase risk for ototoxicity	Avoid concurrent use or monitor for tinnitus, hearing loss
	Probenecid, sulfinpyrazone	Salicylates antagonize uricosuric effects	Avoid concurrent use
	Spironolactone	Salicylates inhibit diuretic effects	Avoid concurrent use
	Sulfonylureas	Salicylates in doses >2 g/d have hypoglycemic effect; potentiate glucose-lowering effect	Select different drug combination
	Penicillins, phenytoin, methotrexate, valproic acid, sulfonamide	May enhance effects of these drugs	Monitor for potential dosage adjustments
	Foods that acidify urine*	Decreases renal excretion and increases serum levels of salicylates	May increase risk for toxicity
	Foods that alkalinize urine*	Increases renal excretion and decreases serum levels of salicylates	May be used therapeutically to treat overdose
Diflunisal	Acetaminophen	Concurrent administration may result in 50% increase in acetaminophen levels	Increased risk for hepatotoxicity; avoid concurrent use
	Heparin, warfarin	Competitively displaces warfarin from protein-binding sites; increased risk for bleeding	Avoid concurrent use; monitor PT/INR closely
	Hydrochlorothiazide (HCTZ)	Significantly decreased HCTZ plasma levels	Avoid concurrent use
	Aspirin, NSAIDs, colchicine, glucocorticoids, alcohol	Additive risk for GI bleeding	Avoid concurrent use
	Lithium	May increase serum lithium levels	Select different salicylate
	Probenecid	Increased risk of diflunisal toxicity	Avoid concurrent use or monitor closely for indications of toxicity
	Antacids	Concurrent administration decreases absorption of diflunisal	Separate administration by at least 1 h
	Indomethacin	Decreased renal clearance and significantly increased indomethacin serum levels	Avoid concurrent use
	Sulindac	Increased renal clearance and significantly decreased sulindac serum levels	Avoid concurrent use

*Foods that alkalinize urine: all fruits except cranberries, prunes, plums; all vegetables; milk. Foods that acidify urine: cheeses, cranberries, eggs, fish, grains, meats, plums, poultry, and prunes.

INR = international normalized ratio; PT = prothrombin time.

It may increase the risk for bleeding with **cefamandole, cefoperazone, cefotetan, valproic acid,** or **plicamycin.**

All **salicylates** may enhance the activity of **penicillins, phenytoin, methotrexate, valproic acid, sulfonylureas,** and **sulfonamides.** They may antagonize the beneficial effects of **probenecid** or **sulfinpyrazone** and blunt the therapeutic response to **diuretics, antihypertensives,** and some **NSAIDs. Glucocorticoids** decrease serum salicylate levels.

There is an increased risk for GI bleeding when aspirin is taken with any other drug with a similar adverse reaction. The risk for ototoxicity is increased when it is taken with any other drug with this adverse reaction (e.g., **aminoglycosides**).

Some foods contain **salicylate.** Foods and spices high in **salicylate** include curry, paprika, licorice, Benedictine liqueur, prunes, raisins, tea, and gherkins. Foods that acidify the urine may increase serum salicylate levels, and those that alkalinize the urine may have the opposite effect.

Clinical Use and Dosing

FEVER. Aspirin is the **salicylate** of choice for reduction of fever in adults. It is contraindicated for use with pregnant patients, however. To be used with children, the cause of the fever must first be determined. It is contraindicated in children and adolescents if the cause of the fever is influenza or chickenpox. While not clearly stated in the literature, this warning may extend to other viral URIs. Many providers do not use it as an **antipyretic** for any children since there are other drugs that do not carry the concern about Reye's syndrome. **Acetaminophen** or **ibuprofen** is probably better for fever management in children. Adult's and children's doses of **aspirin** are shown in Table 23–15.

Diflunisal is not recommended as an **antipyretic.** In single doses, it reduces fever in some patients but not in a clinically significant amount.

MILD TO MODERATE PAIN. Pain associated with inflammation is especially well managed with **salicylates** or **NSAIDs. Aspirin, choline salicylate, choline magnesium salicylate,** and **diflunisal** are all approved for this indication. **Aspirin** is the gold standard against which others are judged. It is inexpensive, available OTC, the most potent **analgesic** in the class, and short-acting, so that acute pain can be managed without long-term effects and adverse reactions. It is has limitations, however. **It is Pregnancy Category D, especially in the third trimester,** and contraindicated in children with influenza or chickenpox, as previously discussed.

Diflusinal offers the advantage of analgesia comparable to **aspirin** with longer-lasting responses. Like the other drugs in this group, it can be used for this indication, but all four are more often used to treat arthritic conditions.

RHEUMATOID ARTHRITIS. Salicylates or **NSAIDs** can be used to treat rheumatoid arthritis. Once again, **aspirin** is the gold standard. Serum levels can easily be measured to determine adherence and therapeutic efficacy, and it is the least expensive **salicylate. Nonacetylated salicylates** are less potent **anti-inflammatory agents,** but they have fewer adverse reactions than **aspirin.** The main disadvantages of **aspirin** are the high incidence of GI intolerance (take with food or use enteric-coated tablets), the inconvenience of taking four or five doses daily, and the relatively long interval (4 to 7 days) before a full anti-inflammatory effect is reached. A trial of therapy of 3 to 4 g per day for 4 to 6 days is recommended because 70 to 80 percent of patients who will respond will do so within this time frame. Older adults are predictably less tolerant to the adverse GI reactions, and their trial dose should be 2 to 3 g per day. If the response is inadequate and adherence has been good, a **salicylate** level should be drawn before changing drugs. If the drug level is within therapeutic parameters (20 to 25 mg/dL in adults; 15 to 20 mg/dL in older adults) without adequate response, or if the drug is not tolerated, another drug should be tried. If the **salicylate** level is too low, but the patient has been adherent and tolerates the **aspirin,** the dose should be increased by 325 to 650 mg/day until the desired anti-inflammatory level of the drug is reached.

The margin is narrow between a good therapeutic level and toxicity in treating patients with rheumatoid arthritis because the dose is higher than that used for fever or analgesia. The earliest manifestation of toxicity is tinnitus or mild deafness. **Aspirin** should be stopped immediately if these symptoms occur. Once they abate, it may be restarted at a lower dose, or an **NSAID** may be chosen. Toxicity is discussed in the adverse reactions section.

For patients whose main reason for discontinuing **aspirin** is GI intolerance, **salsalate** is a good alternative. It can be given in twice-daily dosing and has a much lower incidence of GI bleeding. **Choline salicylate** and **choline magnesium salicylate** can also be used and may be given in bid to qid dosing.

OSTEOARTHRITIS. Patients with osteoarthritis may present occasionally with acute or subacute painful episodes in which the underlying problem is inflammation. No drugs have proven efficacy in altering the course of osteoarthritis, but both **salicylates** and **NSAIDs** are used successfully to treat the pain associated with these exacerbations. **Aspirin** is an effective **analgesic** and **anti-inflammatory** that is usually well tolerated in divided doses of 1.2 to 2.4 g/day. **NSAIDs** tend to have more adverse reactions with no better pain relief when given at anti-inflammatory doses over more than a few days. **Acetaminophen** is helpful for analgesia but has no anti-inflammatory effects.

The **nonacetylated salicylates** are also effective and

Table 23–15. Dosage Schedule: Salicylates

Drug	Indication	Dose	Notes
Acetylsalicylic acid	Fever, pain, headache, dysmenorrhea	*Adults:* 325–650 mg every 4 h; with extra strength may use 500 mg every 3 h *or* 1 g every 6 h; not to exceed 4 g/d *Children 2–11 y:* 65 mg/kg/d in 4–6 divided doses*	
	Rheumatoid arthritis, osteoarthritis Juvenile rheumatoid arthritis	*Adults:* 3.2–6 g/d in divided doses *Children <25 kg:* 60–110 mg/kg/d in divided doses (every 6–8 h); start with 60 mg/kg/d and increase by 20 mg/kg/d after 5–7 d, then increase by 10 mg/kg/d after another 5–7 d *Children >25 kg:* 50–60 mg/kg/d with a similar dosing increase schedule	Toxicity risk increased at this dose Maintain a serum salicylate level of 15–30 mg/mL for anti-inflammatory effects
	Acute rheumatic fever	*Adults:* 5–8 g/d initially in 3–4 divided doses; increase dose to reach serum salicylate level of 15–30 mg/mL; not to exceed 8 g/d *Children:* 100 mg/kg/d for 2 wk, then decrease to 75 mg/kg/d for 4–6 wk; not to exceed 130 mg/kg/d	
	Transient ischemic attacks in men	*Adults:* 1300 mg/d in divided doses (650 mg bid or 325 mg qid)	Doses as low as 300 mg/d may be effective in some patients
	Myocardial infarction prophylaxis	*Adults:* 300–325 mg/d	81 mg/d doses may be used for patients who have fecal blood loss with higher doses, but once every 15 d must take one 325-mg dose
Choline salicylate	Fever, pain	*Adults and children >12 y:* 870 mg every 3–4 h; maximum 6 times/d	Has fewer adverse reactions than aspirin
	Rheumatoid arthritis	*Adults:* 870–1740 mg up to qid	
Choline magnesium salicylate	Fever, pain, rheumatoid arthritis	*Adults:* 2–3 g/d in divided doses or 150 mg bid *Children >37 kg:* 2.2 g/d in 2 divided doses* *Children <37 kg:* 50 mg/d in 2 divided doses*	
Salsalate	Rheumatic conditions	*Adults:* 1500 mg bid *or* 750 mg qid; not to exceed 4 g/d	
Diflunisal	Mild to moderate pain	*Adults:* 1 g initially, followed by 500 mg every 8–12 h	Half this dose initially and following may be effective
	Osteoarthritis	*Adults:* 500 mg–1 g/d in 2 divided doses; not to exceed 1.5 g/d	

*Dosing schedules are published for analgesia and fever reduction. Use cautiously. Not recommended for children with influenza or chickenpox because of risk for Reye's syndrome.

have fewer GI adverse reactions than **aspirin. Diflunisal** has the advantage of bid dosing but may take up to 2 weeks to achieve full anti-inflammatory effects. Although it is more expensive than **aspirin,** the cost may approach that of many of the **NSAIDs.** Discussion of **NSAIDs** is in the section preceding this one.

JUVENILE RHEUMATOID ARTHRITIS. Juvenile rheumatoid arthritis is an autoimmune disease that occurs in four different forms, all of which are characterized by joint inflammation. Pediatric specialists generally follow children with the disorder and determine their treatment protocol. **Salicylates** and **NSAIDs** are commonly part of this protocol.

Aspirin is prescribed in daily doses of 60 to 110 mg/kg for children. **NSAIDs** are prescribed if the child does not respond to or cannot tolerate **aspirin** therapy. **Nonacetylated salicylates** are not indicated for treatment of juvenile forms of rheumatoid arthritis.

ACUTE RHEUMATIC FEVER. After almost disappearing in the United States and Western Europe in the 1960s, rheumatic fever began a resurgence in the 1980s. Usually a sequela of group A beta-hemolytic streptococcal infection, the infection is treated with **antimicrobials,** but the inflammatory manifestations are treated with **aspirin.** Although this disorder is more common in children, it can also occur in adults. Dosage schedules for both are presented in Table 23–15.

MYOCARDIAL INFARCTION PROPHYLAXIS. Daily treatment of 300 to 325 mg **aspirin** in patients with MI has been associated with a 20 percent reduction in risk of subsequent and nonfatal reinfarction. In the International Study of Infarct Survival (ISIS-II) (Kastrup, 1998), patients who received a combination of **aspirin** 160 mg/day and **streptokinase** after the onset of a suspected MI had significantly fewer reinfarctions, strokes, and deaths than those who received placebo. The combination was also better than either drug alone. This result has led to the recommendation that, at the first sign of an MI (chest pain and other symptoms), patients should take one 325-mg **aspirin** tablet.

Prophylaxis protocols suggest 300 to 325 mg/day of **aspirin.** Doses of 81 mg/day may be used for patients who experience fecal blood loss or are intolerant to other GI adverse reactions from higher doses. To be effective, however, once every 15 days (the lifespan of platelets) a single dose of 300 to 325 mg should be taken to ensure adequate antiplatelet activity. **Nonacetylated salicylates** do not have adequate antiplatelet activity for this indication and have not been subjected to research to support their use.

TRANSIENT ISCHEMIC ATTACKS. **Aspirin** and **ticlopidine** have been used to prevent TIAs. The studies have been done with male patients, so use for female patients is based on extrapolation from these studies. Doses of at least 1500 mg/day appear to be needed for most patients, but a few studies have reported efficacy with doses as low as 300 mg/day. **Ticlopidine** is discussed in Chapter 16.

Dosing schedules for all of these drugs for each indication are presented in Table 23–15.

Rational Drug Selection

Rational drug selection is based largely on indication, cost, and convenience of therapy (Table 23–16). All of these are discussed in the Clinical Use and Dosing section.

Monitoring

A random **salicylate** level should be drawn 7 to 10 days after initiation of therapy. Periodic **salicylate** levels should be drawn during long-term management to check maintenance of therapeutic levels and monitor for toxic manifestations.

Because all of these drugs are eliminated by the kidney and dosage adjustments may be required based on renal function, serum creatinine levels should be assessed before therapy is begun and annually throughout long-term therapy. Urinary pH should also be monitored regularly. Sudden acidification of the urine can more than double the plasma **salicylate** level, resulting in toxicity.

Salicylates interfere with homeostasis. A CBC should be drawn prior to initiating therapy and at least annually throughout long-term therapy. A CBC should also be drawn and fecal occult blood studies should be done as well if there is any indication of GI bleeding.

Monitor hepatic function prior to antirheumatic therapy and if symptoms of hepatotoxicity occur. These problems are more likely in patients with rheumatic fever, juvenile rheumatoid arthritis, or preexisting hepatic diseases, especially children.

Ophthalmic effects have been reported in patients taking **diflunisal.** Ophthalmic studies are appropriate for patients who develop eye complaints during therapy.

Patient Education

ADMINISTRATION. Instruct the patient to take **salicylates** exactly as prescribed. Taking with food or a full glass of water and remaining in an upright position for 15 to 30 minutes after administration can reduce GI irritation. Food slows absorption but does not alter the total amount absorbed.

Remind patients not to crush or chew enteric-coated tablets or take **antacids** within 1 hour of enteric-coated tablets. Chewable tablets may be chewed, dissolved in liquid, or swallowed whole. Tablets with a vinegar-like odor (acetic acid) should be discarded.

Instruct patients not to increase the dose beyond that

Table 23–16. Available Dosage Forms: Salicylates

Drug	Dosage Form	How Supplied
Acetylsalicylic acid (Bayer Aspirin*)	Tablets: 325 mg Chewable tablets: 81 mg Enteric-coated tablets: 325 mg Timed-release tablets: 650 mg Caplets: 325 mg Caplets: 500 mg	In bottles of 12, 24, 50, 100, 200, 300 tablets In bottles of 36 In bottles of 50, 100 tablets In bottles of 30, 72, 125 tablets In bottles of 500, 100, 200 caplets In bottles of 30, 60 caplets
(Generic)	Tablets: 325 mg Tablets: 500 mg Enteric-coated tablets: 325 mg Enteric-coated tablets: 650 mg Enteric-coated tablets: 975 mg Suppository: 120 mg, 200 mg, 300 mg, 600 mg	In bottles of 100, 200, 250, 500, 1000 tablets In bottles of 100 tablets In bottles of 30, 60, 90, 100, 1000 tablets In bottles of 100, 1000 tablets In bottles of 100 tablets; prescription only In 12 individually foil-wrapped suppositories
Choline salicylate (Arthropan)	Liquid: 870 mg/5 mL	In 240 and 480 mL (mint-flavored)
Choline magnesium salicylate (Trilisate)	Tablets: 500 mg, 750 mg Tablets: 1 g Liquid: 500 mg/5 mL	In bottles of 100 scored tablets In bottles of 60 scored tablets In 237 mL (cherry-flavored)
Salsalate (Disalcid)	Capsules: 500 mg Tablets: 500 mg, 750 mg	In bottles of 100 capsules In bottles of 100, 500 tablets
(Generic)	Tablets: 500 mg, 750 mg	In bottles of 100, 500 tablets
Diflunisal (Dolobid)	Tablets: 250 mg, 500 mg	In bottles of 60 tablets

*There are many different brands of aspirin. Bayer was selected because it has several different forms.

prescribed. Increased doses increase the risk for **salicylate** poisoning. For patients taking **aspirin** for MI or TIA prophylaxis, increasing the dose has not proved to provide additional benefits but does increase the risk for adverse reactions.

ADVERSE REACTIONS. The most common adverse reactions are ototoxicity and GI irritation and bleeding. Advise patients to report tinnitus; unusual bleeding from the gums; bruising, black, tarry stools; or fever lasting longer than 3 days. Patients who are taking **salicylates** should not use **alcohol** or other substances that increase GI irritation.

The Centers for Disease Control and Prevention (CDC) warns against giving **aspirin** to children or adolescents with influenza, influenza-like syndromes, or chickenpox (varicella) because of a possible association with Reye's syndrome. Parents should be given this information.

LIFESTYLE MANAGEMENT. Rest, heat, exercise, and other lifestyle modifications are part of the management of arthritic conditions. The modifications are as important as the pharmacological management and should be stressed.

REFERENCES

Burns, C., Barber, N., Brady, M., & Dunn, A. (1996) *Pediatric primary care.* Philadelphia: Saunders.

Davis, A. (1996). Primary care management of chronic musculoskeletal pain. *Nurse Practitioner, 21*(8), 72–82.

Deglin, J., & Vallerand, A. (1998). *Davis's drug guide for nurses* (6th ed.). Philadelphia: F. A. Davis.

Ellershaw, J., & Kelly, M. (1994). Corticosteroids and peptic ulceration. *Palliative Medicine, 8,* 313–319.

Goroll, A., May, L., & Mulley, A. (1995). *Primary care medicine* (3rd ed.). Philadelphia: Lippincott.

Gutierrez, K. (1999). *Pharmacotherapeutics: Clinical decision-making in nursing.* Philadelphia: Saunders.

Jones, A. (1997). Primary care management of acute low back pain. *Nurse Practitioner, 22*(7), 50–68.

Kastrup, E. (Founding Ed.). (1998). *Drug facts and comparisons.* St. Louis: Facts and Comparisons.

Lester, R., Knowles, S., & Shear, N. (1998). The risk of systemic corticosteroid use. *Dermatologic Clinics, 16*(2), 277–288.

Ross, C. (1997). A comparison of osteoarthritis and rheumatoid arthritis: Diagnosis and treatment. *Nurse Practitioner, 22*(9), 20–41.

Smith, T. (1998). Cyclooxygenases as the principal targets for the actions of NSAIDs. *Rheumatic Disease Clinics of North America, 24*(3), 501–523.

CHAPTER 24

· · · · · · ·

Drugs Used in Treating Eye and Ear Disorders

CHAPTER OUTLINE

*T*his chapter discusses the medications used to treat eye and ear disorders, including the common **anti-infective agents** for conjunctivitis, the medications used for allergic conjunctivitis, and common **anti-inflammatory agents** used for ocular inflammation. Although primary care providers may not prescribe some of the glaucoma medications, many drugs interact with these ophthalmic medications, and therefore a basic understanding of these agents is necessary and included. **Eye lubricants** and **vasoconstrictors** are discussed here. The use of **fluorescein**, a diagnostic agent commonly used in primary care, is addressed in this chapter. The ear medications that are discussed in this chapter include the **anti-infectives, analgesics,** and **ceruminolytics.**

Drugs Used in Treating Eye Disorders

Ophthalmic Anti-infectives

Common eye infections that are treated by primary care providers include bacterial conjunctivitis, viral conjunctivitis, blepharitis, and hordeolum. Acute conjunctivitis is the most common disorder of the eye seen by the primary care provider (Wald, 1997). The commonly used **antibacterial agents** for conjunctivitis are **sulfacetamide sodium (Bleph-10)**, **erythromycin (Ilotycin)**, **tobramycin (Tobrex)**, **gentamicin (Garamycin)**, and the **fluoroquinolones norfloxacin (Noroxin)**, **ciprofloxacin (Ciloxan)**, and **ofloxacin (Ocuflox)**. The combination drugs **Polytrim** and **Polysporin Ophthalmic** may also be used and are discussed here. **Chloramphenicol (Chloroptic)** is rarely used in primary care because of its adverse effects. More serious infectious eye disorders such as herpesvirus infection, keratitis, and corneal ulcers are treated by ophthalmologists and therefore are not discussed at great length in this chapter, although the **antiviral agents** that may be used to treat viral eye infections are briefly discussed.

Pharmacodynamics

Ophthalmic antibiotics may be bacteriostatic or bactericidal.

Bacitracin is bacteriostatic and inhibits the incorporation of amino acids and nucleotides into the cell. It is active against many gram-positive (staphylococci, streptococci, clostridia, corynebacteria, and anaerobic cocci) and gram-negative (gonococci, meningococci, and fusobacteria) organisms.

Erythromycin is a bacteriostatic **macrolide antibiotic** that is active against a wide range of organisms. It binds to the 50 S ribosomal subunit, inhibiting bacterial protein synthesis. The gram-positive organisms that are susceptible to **erythromycin** include *Staphylococcus aureus*, *Streptococcus pyogenes*, *Streptococcus pneumoniae*, *Streptococcus viridans* group, and *Corynebacterium diphtheriae*. **Erythromycin** has limited gram-negative coverage. It is also active against *Chlamydia trachomatis*.

Sulfacetamide is a synthetic **sulfonamide** that inhibits bacterial dihydrofolate synthetase. It is active against the following susceptible organisms: streptococci, staphylococci, *Escherichia coli*, *Klebsiella pneumoniae*, *Pseudomonas pyocyanea*, *Neisseria gonorrhoeae*, and *C. trachomatis*.

Tobramycin is a broad-spectrum **aminoglycoside**. The exact mechanism by which it is bactericidal is unknown. It is active against staphylococci, streptococci, *Corynebacterium* species, *K. pneumoniae*, *Moraxella* species, *Proteus* species, beta-hemolytic streptococci, and *Haemophilus influenzae*. **Tobramycin** ophthalmic is not active against *N. gonorrhoeae* or *C. trachomatis*.

Gentamicin is a broad-spectrum **antibiotic** that is active against a wide range of gram-positive and gram-negative organisms. It is unclear how **gentamicin** causes cell death. It is active against staphylococci, *S. pneumoniae*, beta-hemolytic streptococci, *E. coli*, *H. influenzae*, *N. gonorrhoeae*, and *Enterobacter* species.

The **fluoroquinolones ciprofloxacin**, **norfloxacin**, and **ofloxacin** are bactericidal via inhibition of DNA gyrase. It is unclear how inhibition of DNA gyrase leads to cell death. The **fluoroquinolones** are active against staphylococci, *S. pneumoniae*, *H. influenzae*, *K. pneumoniae*, *Proteus* species, *Enterobacter* species, and *Pseudomonas aeruginosa*.

Polytrim is an **ophthalmic antibacterial** preparation that combines **polymyxin B** and **trimethoprim**. **Polymyxin B** binds to cell membranes with high affinity, specifically the phospholipids in the cell wall. This causes increased cellular permeability. **Polymyxin B** is generally active against gram-negative bacteria (*E. coli*, *P. aeruginosa*, *H. influenzae*). **Trimethoprim** inhibits bacterial dihydrofolate reductase. **Trimethoprim** has both gram-positive and gram-negative activity. **Trimethoprim** is active against *S. aureus*, *S. pneumoniae*, and *S. pyogenes*.

Polysporin Ophthalmic contains **polymyxin B** and **bacitracin**. This combination provides activity against gram-positive and gram-negative bacterial organisms, as discussed previously.

Two **antiviral ophthalmic agents** that may be prescribed by an ophthalmologist are **vidarabine (Vira-A)** and **trifluridine (Viroptic)**. **Vidarabine** inhibits viral DNA replication, although the exact mechanism of action is not known. **Vidarabine** has antiviral activity against herpes simplex virus (HSV) types 1 and 2, varicella-zoster virus, cytomegalovirus, vaccinia, and hepatitis B. The exact mechanism of action of **trifluridine** is not known, although it is thought to interfere with DNA synthesis. **Trifluridine** is active against HSV-1 and HSV-2, adenovirus, and vaccinia virus.

Pharmacokinetics

Ophthalmic antibiotic and **antiviral preparations** generally penetrate only the ocular fluid and tissues. Systemic absorption is minimal, although there may be enough absorption for sensitization to occur, specifically with **sulfacetamide**. There is no information regarding the metabolism and excretion of **ophthalmic anti-infectives**.

Pharmacotherapeutics

PRECAUTIONS AND CONTRAINDICATIONS. Hypersensitivity to any component of the preparation is a contraindication to its use. There may be cross-sensitivity between the individual **aminoglycosides (tobramycin** and **gentamicin)**. The same is found with the **fluoroquinolones**.

The vehicles used in ophthalmic ointments may retard corneal healing after ocular trauma or ocular surgery. Improvements in ophthalmic ointment vehicles have improved this situation, but manufacturers still warn that many preparations may retard corneal healing.

Purulent exudates that contain para-aminobenzoic acid may inactivate **sulfacetamide** antibacterial activity.

Antibacterial agents are not effective against fungal infection, viral infection, or all types of bacterial infection.

If the patient is not responding to therapy, reevaluation, including appropriate cultures, is indicated.

Erythromycin and *tobramycin* ophthalmic preparations are Pregnancy Category B. *Gentamicin, ciprofloxacin, norfloxacin, ofloxacin, polymyxin B,* and *sulfacetamide* are Pregnancy Category C. The *antiviral ophthalmic agents vidarabine* and *trifluridine* are both Pregnancy Category C. Safety for use during pregnancy has not been determined.

The use of the **sulfacetamide** and the **fluoroquinolones ciprofloxacin, norfloxacin,** and **ofloxacin** should be avoided during lactation because they are harmful to the infant and breast milk excretion is unknown.

Erythromycin and **tobramycin** are safe and effective in children. The safety of the **fluoroquinolones** (**ciprofloxacin, norfloxacin,** and **ofloxacin**) in children under age 1 year has not been established. **Sulfacetamide** and **polymyxin B–bacitracin** should not be prescribed to infants younger than 2 months old.

ADVERSE DRUG REACTIONS. All of the **ophthalmic anti-infective preparations** may cause local irritation, which is usually transient. Irritation may include burning, itching, and inflammation. Superinfection may occur with prolonged or repeated use of **ophthalmic anti-infectives.**

Bacitracin may cause blurred vision, which usually lasts only a few minutes.

Sulfacetamide ophthalmic preparations may cause a hypersensitivity reaction in patients who have previously exhibited sensitivity to **sulfonamides.** Stevens-Johnson syndrome is a rare adverse reaction that has been reported with **sulfacetamide** ophthalmic ointment use. Fever, bone marrow depression, and lupus erythematosus may rarely occur with **sulfonamides,** including topical preparations. There may be intense burning and stinging, especially with the 30% **sulfacetamide sodium** solution (**Sulamyd 30%**).

Aminoglycosides may cause localized ocular toxicity and hypersensitivity.

The **fluoroquinolones** may cause a white crystalline precipitate to form in the superficial portion of the cornea. This was observed in about 17 percent of the patients on **ciprofloxacin.** Lid margin crusting, crystals, scales, and the sensation of a foreign body in the eye are also reported with **ophthalmic fluoroquinolones.** Patients also report a bitter or bad taste in the mouth, specifically with **ciprofloxacin** solution. **Fluoroquinolones** may also cause photophobia, tearing, nausea, decreased vision, conjunctival hyperemia, and corneal staining.

The **ophthalmic antiviral preparations** may cause burning and irritation upon instillation into the eye. **Vidarabine** may also cause photophobia, pruritus, erythema, ocular pain, and, less commonly, increased lacrimation. Patients who are using **ophthalmic vidarabine** may develop superficial punctate keratitis after exposure to UV light, and they should wear sunglasses to protect their eyes when exposed to bright light. **Trifluridine** has adverse reactions similar to those of **vidarabine,** with the addition of reported increases in intraocular pressure.

DRUG INTERACTIONS. There are no drug interactions reported for ophthalmic preparations of **bacitracin, gentamicin, tobramycin, polymyxin B, bacitracin,** and **erythromycin.**

Sulfacetamide is incompatible with silver-containing preparations and should not be used in conjunction with ophthalmic products containing **silver salts,** including **silver nitrate.** Concomitant use of **ophthalmic sulfacetamide** with **zinc sulfate** causes a precipitate to form. Ester-type **local anesthetics** including **benzocaine, chloroprocaine, cocaine, procaine, propoxycaine,** and **tetracaine** should not be used concurrently with **sulfacetamide** because they can antagonize the therapeutic actions of the **sulfonamide.**

The **fluoroquinolones** (**ciprofloxacin, norfloxacin,** and **ofloxacin**) may increase **theophylline** levels and potentiate **oral anticoagulants.** These interactions are theoretical with ophthalmic use of **fluoroquinolones,** in that little is known regarding the amount of medication that is systemically absorbed, and whether enough is absorbed to cause a drug interaction. Table 24–1 presents drug interactions with **ophthalmic anti-infectives.**

CLINICAL USE AND DOSING

Conjunctivitis. The common organisms that are associated with bacterial conjunctivitis vary with the age of the patient. Newborns should be evaluated for ophthalmia neonatorum. Preschool children most commonly have bacterial conjunctivitis, with viral etiology (adenovirus) more likely in schoolchildren. *N. gonorrhoeae* conjunctivitis should be excluded in sexually active adolescents and adults. Adults may have viral or bacterial conjunctivitis. *Chlamydia* is seen in the neonate and sexually active teen and adult. Table 24–2 presents the clinical and laboratory features of conjunctivitis.

Ophthalmia Neonatorum. Any infant less than 1 month of age who presents with conjunctivitis should have Gram's stain, antigen detection tests, and cultures of the eye discharge to rule out gonococcal, chlamydial, or HSV origin. Gonococcal conjunctivitis in the newborn requires intramuscular (IM) **ceftriaxone** (50 mg/kg, maximum 125 mg). If there are extraocular manifestations, then a 7-day course of IM or intravenous (IV) **ceftriaxone** is warranted. Chlamydial conjunctivitis in the newborn requires treatment with systemic **erythromycin** (30 to 50 mg/kg/day) for 2 to 3 weeks. To prevent ophthalmia neonatorum, the Centers for Disease Control (CDC, 1989) recommends prophylactic administration of **antibiotic** eye medication within 1 hour of delivery. The recommended **antibiotics** are **erythromycin** 0.5% (1/4 to 1/2 inch to each eye), **tetracycline** 1% (1/4 to 1/2 inch to each eye), or **silver nitrate** 1% solution (2 drops to each eye).

Table 24–1. Drug Interactions: Ophthalmic Anti-infectives

Drug	Interacting Drug	Possible Effect	Implications
Sulfacetamide sodium	Silver preparations	Incompatibility	Do not use concurrently
Erythromycin	None reported		
Tobramycin	None reported		
Gentamicin	None reported		
Norfloxacin	Warfarin, theophylline, cyclosporine	May raise levels of these systemic drugs	Monitor theophylline level and PT/PTT times
Ciprofloxacin	Warfarin, theophylline, cyclosporine	May raise levels of these systemic drugs; may increase renal toxicity from cyclosporine	Monitor theophylline level
Ofloxacin	Warfarin, theophylline, caffeine, cyclosporine	May raise levels of these systemic drugs; may increase renal toxicity from cyclosporine	Monitor PT/INR levels closely
Polymyxin B–trimethoprim	None reported		
Polymyxin B–bacitracin ophthalmic	None reported		

PT = prothrombin time; PTT = partial thromboplastin time.
INR = international normalized ratio

Table 24–2. Clinical and Laboratory Features of Conjunctivitis

Type of Conjunctivitis	Common Patient Groups	Common Pathogens	Clinical Features
Ophthalmia neonatorum	Infants <1 mo	N. gonorrhoeae Chlamydia	Erythema, purulent exudate, chemosis
Bacterial conjunctivitis	Most common in children between 3 mo and 8 y; can happen at any age	H. influenzae S. aureus S. pneumoniae	Erythema, purulent discharge, itching, burning, matted eyelashes
Conjunctivitis-otitis syndrome	Predominantly in children <6 y	H. influenzae (~73% of patients)	Bacterial conjunctivitis accompanied by otitis media
Gonococcal conjunctivitis	Newborns, sexually promiscuous teens and adults	N. gonorrhoeae	Eye is markedly inflamed, with copious discharge and swollen lids
Blepharitis	Any age group	May be infected with S. aureus	Chronic or acute inflammation of the eyelash follicles
Hordeolum	Any age group	S. aureus	Tender, swollen red furuncle along eyelid margin
Viral conjunctivitis	Any age group, most common in children	Adenovirus Herpes simplex virus	Redness, chemosis, photophobia

Bacterial Conjunctivitis. Children between ages 3 months and 8 years are most likely to have staphylococcal, streptococcal, or *Haemophilus* conjunctivitis. Nontypable *H. influenzae* is seen more in warmer climates between May and October. *S. pneumoniae* is seen in colder climates and during the winter. *S. aureus* shows no geographic or seasonal pattern. In studies of children with acute bacterial conjunctivitis, *H. influenzae* is the most common organism (Wald, 1997).

Although bacterial conjunctivitis is considered a self-limited disease (unless caused by gonorrhea), patients who receive **topical antibiotic** therapy have faster clinical improvement. When conjunctivitis prevents the patient from going to school or work, **antibiotics** can speed the recovery. Most schools require treatment for the child to return to school.

Uncomplicated conjunctivitis may be treated with **sulfacetamide** 10% ophthalmic solution or ointment, **erythromycin** ointment, **trimethoprim–polymyxin B (Polytrim)**, or **bacitracin–polymyxin B (Polysporin)**. **Sulfacetamide** has no coverage against *H. influenzae*, a fact that should be considered in choosing an **antibiotic**. Gram's stain or culture can further guide the choice of **antibiotic**.

The second-line choices for uncomplicated bacterial conjunctivitis include **tobramycin, gentamicin,** or any of the **fluoroquinolones**. See Table 24–3 for dosing information.

Bacterial conjunctivitis caused by dacryostenosis may be treated with **erythromycin** ointment (Yetman & Coody, 1997).

Conjunctivitis-Otitis Syndrome. The syndrome of conjunctivitis accompanied by otitis media predominantly occurs in children younger than 6 years old. *H. influenzae* is the causative organism in the majority (73%) of patients with conjunctivitis-otitis syndrome (Wald, 1997). Treatment is **systemic antibiotics** that are effective against *H. influenzae*. **Amoxicillin** dosed at 75 to 90 mg/kg a day is the first-line drug of choice. If **systemic antibiotics** are prescribed, **topical ophthalmic** treatment is usually not needed. See Chapter 44 for management of otitis media.

Gonococcal Conjunctivitis. Purulent bacterial conjunctivitis usually responds to **topical antibiotic** therapy. An exception is hyperpurulent gonococcal conjunctivitis, which is usually found in the newborn and in sexually promiscuous teenagers and adults. The eye discharge should be Gram's-stained and cultured to confirm the diagnosis. Treatment consists of **parenteral antibiotics** and sterile saline irrigations to clear the exudate. Use of a beta-lactamase–resistant **cephalosporin** such as **ceftriaxone** is warranted. Because untreated gonococcal infection can penetrate the intact eye, treatment should begin as soon as the diagnosis is suspected.

Blepharitis. Blepharitis is an acute or chronic inflammation of the eyelash follicles and meibomian glands of the eyelids. Treatment consists of scrubbing the eyelashes with gentle, no-tears shampoo and applying **sulfacetamide sodium** 10% solution (1 or 2 drops twice a day) or **erythromycin** 0.5% ophthalmic ointment (1/4-inch ribbon to each eye twice a day) until the symptoms clear and then for an additional 7 days. The patient should not wear contact lenses during treatment, and the contacts should be sterilized before reinserting. Eye makeup should be discarded to prevent reinfection. (MacDonald, 1996).

Hordeolum. Hordeolum, commonly called a *sty,* is an infection of the sebaceous gland of the eyelash or eyelid. The causative organism is *S. aureus.* Treatment consists of warm, moist compresses four times a day for 15 minutes each time. **Antibiotic** eyedrops (**sulfacetamide** 10%) or ointment (**erythromycin** 0.5%) should be applied four times a day until the symptoms subside and then for an additional 2 to 3 days. The hordeolum usually spontaneously ruptures; if it does not, the patient should be referred to an ophthalmologist.

Viral Conjunctivitis. Viral conjunctivitis is usually caused by an adenovirus, HSV, or herpes zoster. Simple viral conjunctivitis caused by adenovirus is treated with **sulfacetamide** 10% solution or ointment four times a day or a broad-spectrum **antibiotic** such as **tobramycin,** to prevent secondary bacterial infection. The course of the conjunctivitis runs 12 to 15 days. Herpes keratitis is a potentially serious consequence of infection with herpes simplex. If herpes keratitis is suspected, a referral to an ophthalmologist for diagnosis and treatment is indicated. Two commonly used **antiviral agents** are **trifluridine** and **vidarabine.** Table 24–3 presents the dosage schedule of **ophthalmic anti-infectives.**

RATIONAL DRUG SELECTION

Efficacy. A determination of the suspected organism guides the choice of an **ophthalmic antibiotic.** If *H. influenzae* is high on the list of suspected organisms, then **sulfacetamide** should not be the first choice for treatment because it has poor coverage for *H. influenzae.* A combination product such as **Polysporin** or **Polytrim** provides good coverage for the common organisms that cause bacterial conjunctivitis. In infants, **erythromycin** is usually the drug of choice because of its good coverage, and ointment is more easily administered than drops (Table 24–4).

Cost. The least expensive **ophthalmic** is generally generic **erythromycin, bacitracin,** or **sulfacetamide** 10%. Broad-spectrum or newer formulas (**fluoroquinolones**) are more expensive.

MONITORING. There is no laboratory monitoring necessary with **ophthalmic anti-infectives.**

Table 24–3. Dosage Schedule: Ophthalmic Anti-infectives

Drug	Indication	Dose	Notes
Sulfacetamide sodium	Conjunctivitis Trachoma	Solution: 1–2 drops q2–3h during the day, less often at night Ointment: Small amount tid–qid and qhs Trachoma: 2 drops q2h with systemic therapy	Not recommended for children under 2 mo
Erythromycin	Conjunctivitis and flare-ups of chronic blepharitis Prophylaxis of ophthalmia neonatorum	Ointment: ¼- to ½-inch ribbon 2–3 times/d Ointment: ½-inch ribbon of ointment in each conjunctival sac no later than 1 h after birth	Safe in infants Use a new tube in each infant
Gentamicin	Conjunctivitis	Severe infections: 2 drops q1h or ½-inch ointment q3–4h; may prolong interval as infection improves Mild/moderate infections: ½ drop q4h *or* ½ inch of ointment bid–tid	May be used in children
Tobramycin	Susceptible infections of conjunctiva and cornea	Severe infections: 2 drops q1h or ½-inch ointment q3–4h; may prolong interval as infection improves Mild to moderate infections: 1–2 drops q4h *or* ½ inch of ointment bid–tid	Safe and effective in children >1 mo
Norfloxacin	Susceptible infections of conjunctiva and cornea	1–2 drops qid for up to 7 d; may administer q2h while awake on day 1	Not recommended for <1 y
Ciprofloxacin	Susceptible infections of conjunctiva and corneal ulcer	Solution: Corneal ulcer: day 1, 2 drops q15min, then 2 drops q30min; day 2, 2 drops q1h; days 3 to 14, 2 drops q4h; treat for 14 d or until corneal epithelialization occurs Conjunctivitis: 1–2 drops q2h while awake × 2 d; then 1–2 drops q4h while awake for next 5 d Ointment: For conjunctivitis: ½ inch tid × 2 d, then bid × 5 d	Solution not recommended for <1 y Ointment not recommended for <2 y
Ofloxacin	Susceptible infections of conjunctiva and corneal ulcer	Corneal ulcer: days 1 and 2, 1–2 drops q20min while awake and 4 and 6 h after retiring; days 3 to 9, 1–2 drops q1h while awake; thereafter, 1–2 drops qid	Not recommended for <1 y

Continued on next page

Table 24–3. Dosage Schedule: Ophthalmic Anti-infectives *(continued)*

Drug	Indication	Dose	Notes
		Conjunctivitis: 1–2 drops q2–4h while awake × 2 d, then 1–2 drops qid while awake for next 5 d	
Polymyxin-trimethoprim	Susceptible infections of conjunctiva and cornea	1 drop q3h for 7–10 d, up to 6 doses/d	Not recommended for <2 mo Contraindicated in ophthalmia neonatorum
Polymyxin B–bacitracin ophthalmic	Susceptible infections of conjunctiva and cornea	Ointment: Apply ½-inch ribbon q 3–4 h	May be used safely in children

Table 24–4. Available Dosage Forms: Ophthalmic Anti-infectives

Drug	Dosage Form	How Supplied
Sulfacetamide sodium		
Bleph-10	10% solution	In 2.5, 5, and 10 mL
	10% ointment	In 3.5 g
Sodium Sulamyd	10% solution	In 5 and 15 mL
	30% solution	In 15 mL
	10% ointment	In 3.5 g
Generic	10% solution	In 5 and 15 mL
	30% solution	In 15 mL
	10% ointment	In 3.5 g
Erythromycin		
Ilotycin, Generic	Ointment: 5 mg/g	In 3.5 g
Tobramycin		
Tobrex	Solution: 0.3%	In 5-mL dropper bottle
	Ointment: 3 mg/g	In 3.5 g
Generic	Solution: 0.3%	In 5-mL dropper bottle
Gentamicin		
Garamycin, Genoptic	Solution: 3 mg/mL	In 5-mL dropper bottle
	Ointment: 3 mg/g	In 3.5 g
	Solution: 3 mg/mL	In 5- and 15-mL dropper bottle
Generic	Ointment: 3 mg/g	In 3.5 g
Norfloxacin		
Chibroxin	Solution: 3 mg/mL	In 5-mL Ocumeters
Ciprofloxacin		
Ciloxan	Solution: 3 mg/mL	In 2.5- and 5-mL dropper bottles
Ofloxacin		
Ocuflox	Solution: 3 mg/mL	In 1- and 5-mL dropper bottles
Polymyxin B–trimethoprim		
Polytrim Ophthalmic	Solution: polymyxin B 10,000 U/g, trimethoprim 1 g/mL	In 10 mL
Polymyxin B–bacitracin ophthalmic		
Polysporin Ophthalmic, Generic	Ointment: polymyxin B 10,000 U/g, bacitracin 500 U/g	In 3.5 g

Clinical Pearl

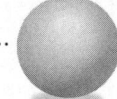

PROPER INSTILLATION OF EYE MEDICATIONS

Proper Instillation of Eyedrops
- Wash hands before administering eyedrops.
- Tilt head back or lie on back.
- Gently pull down lower eyelid to form a "pocket" to place the drop of medication into.
- Squeeze the medication onto the eye without touching eye with dropper.
- Close eye. Do not rub. Try not to blink.
- To prevent cross-contamination, do not use medication labeled for another patient.
- Wait at least 5 minutes between administration if administering more than one eye medication.

Proper Instillation of Eye Ointment
- Wash hands prior to administering eye medications.
- Warm the ointment by holding it in the hand for 1 to 2 minutes.
- With first use of a new tube, squeeze out and discard the first 1/4 inch of medication.
- Angle head back or lie on back.
- Gently pull down lower eyelid to form a "pocket" to place the drop of medication into.
- Squeeze 1/4 to 1/2 inch of medication onto the eye without touching eye with tip of tube.
- Close eye for 1 to 2 minutes. Do not rub.
- Wipe excess medication from around the eye with a tissue.
- To prevent cross-contamination, do not use medication labeled for another patient.
- Wait at least 10 minutes between administrations if administering more than one eye medication.
- Temporary blurred vision after administration of ophthalmic ointment.

PATIENT EDUCATION

Administration. Administration of ophthalmic medications can be challenging for patients. The patient should be instructed in the importance of keeping the tip of the dropper or tube from touching the eye, fingertips, or any other surface, to prevent contamination. Hands should be washed before and after instillation of eye medications. Eye medications should not be shared.

Ophthalmic ointment should be transferred from the tube onto a moistened cotton swab, then rolled into each conjunctival sac. Use one swab for each eye to prevent contamination.

Eyedrops are self-administered by holding the bottle of solution in the dominant hand and using the pointer finger of the other hand to gently pull down the lower eyelid to form a "pocket" for the solution to be dropped into. The patient can use this method for both eyes.

For children who may resist the "bull's-eye" method of instilling eyedrops, one of three methods may be used. School-age children can assist with the instillation by pulling down their own lower eyelid, while the parent or care provider instills the eyedrop into the pocket formed. If this method doesn't work, children can lie down on their backs and close their eyes, keeping the head still. After the eyedrops are placed on the internal canthus, children slowly open their eyes without moving the head. The eyedrops roll into the eyes. Younger children require immobilization to instill eyedrops or ophthalmic ointment. This can be accomplished by two people, one to hold the child and the other to administer the medication.

Adverse Reactions. The patient should be instructed that there might be transient burning or stinging with most of the **ophthalmic anti-infective agents.** If burning is severe or prolonged, the patient should contact the provider. Other adverse effects should be discussed with the patient, with instructions to report any unusual symptoms.

Lifestyle Management. The most important nonpharmacological measure is for the patient and family members to wash their hands thoroughly whenever the infected eyes are touched and before instilling medication. Handwashing will decrease spread of the infection to other contacts.

The patient with an eye infection should not share hand towels with the rest of the family. The patient with an eye infection should use a separate towel or paper towels to prevent the spread of infection to family members.

Eye makeup needs to be thrown away after an eye infection because mascara and other makeup can harbor bacteria or viruses, and the patient can become reinfected.

Clinical Pearl

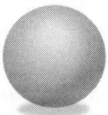

....

TIPS FOR ADMINISTERING EYE MEDICATIONS TO A CHILD

If only one adult is available to administer eyedrops, then the adult can sit on the floor with the child between his or her legs, with the child's legs in the same direction as the adult's. The child's head can be immobilized between the adult's thighs and the arms held firmly down under the adult's thighs. This leaves the adult's hands free to instill the medication. The child may kick, but this will not affect the administration of the medication. Although this method may sound drastic, trying to administer eye medication to a squirming toddler or preschooler can be almost impossible, and with this method the eyedrops can be effectively administered in less than 1 minute.

....

Purulent discharge can be removed with cotton balls moistened with warm water. The cotton ball is wiped gently from the interior canthus to the external canthus to remove discharge. A clean cotton ball should be used for each wipe and for each eye.

Antiglaucoma Agents

Glaucoma is a group of disorders in which elevated intraocular pressure (IOP) damages the optic nerve. In the United States, glaucoma is the leading cause of blindness in African-Americans and the third leading cause in whites (Moroi & Lichter, 1996). The patient may have open-angle glaucoma, in which a block at the level of the trabecular meshwork impairs aqueous humor reabsorption, or the patient may have angle-closure glaucoma, which develops when the normal path of the aqueous flow is interrupted in an eye with a shallow anterior chamber. Current medical therapies are aimed at decreasing the production of aqueous humor at the ciliary body and at increasing the outflow of this fluid from the angle structures. Glaucoma or the suspicion of glaucoma requires evaluation and treatment by an ophthalmologist. Primary care providers need to be aware of the medications that are prescribed, the drug interactions that may occur, and the adverse effects of the prescribed medications.

Pharmacodynamics

The **antiglaucoma agents** can be roughly divided into the following categories: **beta blockers, adrenergic agonists, miotics, carbonic anhydrase (CA) inhibitors, sympathomimetics,** and the **prostaglandin agonist latanoprost (Xalatan).**

BETA BLOCKERS. Beta-adrenergic antagonists, also known as **beta blockers**, reduce IOP by interference with the cAMP-induced production of aqueous humor by the ciliary processes in the eye, although the exact mechanism of action is not known. IOP is reduced in patients with either elevated or normal IOP. Visual acuity, pupil size, and accommodation do not appear to be affected by **ophthalmic beta blockers.**

MIOTICS, CHOLINESTERASE INHIBITORS. Echothiophate iodide (Phospholine) is an indirect-acting agent that inhibits the cholinesterase enzyme. Topical application to the eye causes intense miosis and muscle contraction. The IOP is reduced by a decreased resistance to aqueous outflow.

MIOTICS, DIRECT-ACTING. The direct-acting **miotics** are **parasympathomimetic (cholinergic) drugs** with muscarinic effects. When applied topically, these drugs produce pupillary constriction, stimulate the ciliary muscles, and increase aqueous humor outflow. They also reduce outflow resistance by contraction of the iris sphincter. IOP is decreased with the increase in outflow.

CARBONIC ANHYDRASE INHIBITORS. CA is an enzyme found in many tissues of the body, including the eye. Inhibition of CA in the ciliary processes of the eye decreases aqueous humor secretion, presumably by slowing the formation of bicarbonate ions, with subsequent reduction in sodium and fluid transport. Decreased aqueous humor secretion leads to decreased IOP.

SYMPATHOMIMETICS. It is believed that **sympathomimetics** reduce IOP by reducing the production of aqueous humor and by increasing aqueous humor outflow.

ALPHA-ADRENERGIC AGONISTS. Alpha-adrenergic agonists reduce IOP by reducing the production of aqueous humor and by increasing uveoscleral outflow.

PROSTAGLANDIN AGONIST. Latanoprost is a selective agonist of a prostaglandin receptor known as the FP receptor. **Latanoprost** increases the outflow of aqueous humor by acting on the FP receptor. This leads to decreased IOP.

Pharmacokinetics

Little is known about the specific pharmacokinetic parameters of the **beta blockers**. Duration of action is noted in Table 24–5. What is known is determined by clinical observation of pharmacodynamic responses. An unknown amount of absorption occurs, but systemic absorption is known to occur because both cardiac and pulmonary signs of beta-blocker activity can occur. **Beta blockers** are metabolized in the liver and excreted in the urine and feces.

The pharmacokinetics of **cholinesterase inhibitors** and the direct-acting **miotics** are not known. Duration of action is noted in Table 24–5.

Following topical administration into the eye, **brinzolamide (Azopt)** is absorbed systemically, although plasma concentrations remain low and generally below the level of detection. It is widely distributed, including into the breast milk in animal studies. It may cross the placenta. **Brinzolamide** is metabolized to *N*-desthyl brinzolamide and excreted primarily in the urine.

Dorzolamide (Trusopt), when applied topically to the eye, has some systemic absorption, although no free drug is measured in the plasma. **Dorzolamide** is excreted primarily unchanged in the urine.

Methazolamide (Neptazane) is an oral **CA inhibitor**. It is well absorbed from the GI tract. **Methazolamide** is distributed throughout the body including the plasma, cerebrospinal fluid, aqueous humor of the eye, red blood cells, bile, and extracellular fluid. Its exact metabolism is not described. Excretion is primarily renal, with 25 percent of the drug excreted unchanged in the urine.

The pharmacokinetics of the **sympathomimetics** is not known.

Following ophthalmic administration of **brimonidine (Alphagan)**, peak serum levels occur in 1 to 4 hours. **Brimonidine** is extensively metabolized in the liver and eliminated in the urine.

Latanoprost is absorbed through the cornea, where it is hydrolyzed to become biologically active. Plasma levels of **latanoprost** can be measured. Distribution is unknown. It is not known whether **latanoprost** crosses the placenta, although in animal studies adverse fetal effects were found. It is not known whether **latanoprost** is excreted in breast milk. **Latanoprost** is metabolized via fatty-acid beta oxidation in the liver. The metabolites are excreted primarily in the urine (88%). Table 24–5 presents the pharmacokinetics of **antiglaucoma agents**.

Table 24–5. Pharmacokinetics: Antiglaucoma Agents

Drug	Duration
Beta blockers	
Betaxolol, carteolol	12 h
Levobunolol, metipranolol, timolol	12–24 h
Miotics	
Carbachol	6–8 h
Pilocarpine	4–8 h
Echothiophate	Days/weeks
Carbonic anhydrase inhibitors	
Acetazolamide	8–12 h
Brinzolamide	N/A
Dorzolamide	About 8 h
Methazolamide	10–18 h
Sympathomimetics	
Epinephrine, dipivefrin	12 h
Alpha-adrenergic agonists	
Apraclonidine	7–12 h
Brimonidine	12 h
Prostaglandin agonists	
Latanoprost	24 h

Pharmacotherapeutics

PRECAUTIONS AND CONTRAINDICATIONS. Although primary care providers do not prescribe **ophthalmic antiglaucoma agents**, the medications are absorbed and systemic levels reached in great enough amounts to cause complications of chronic conditions. Coordination of care with the ophthalmologist will ensure the optimum care for the patient's glaucoma and other medical problems.

The **beta-blocker ophthalmic medications** are contraindicated in patients with asthma, a history of asthma, chronic obstructive pulmonary disease (COPD), or other pulmonary disease. There may be bronchospasm associated with the use of **topical beta blockers,** which may prove fatal to patients with respiratory disease.

Beta Blockers. **Beta blockers** suppress conduction through the AV node; therefore, **topical beta blockers** are contraindicated in patients with bradycardia or advanced atrioventricular (AV) block. **Beta blockers** should not be used in patients with compromised ventricular dysfunction, patients in cardiogenic shock, or patients with systolic congestive heart failure. Discontinue **topical beta blockers** at the first sign of cardiac failure. **Beta blockers** are contraindicated for patients with hypotension (standing blood pressure [SBP] less than 100 mm Hg).

Beta blockers should be used with caution in patients with poorly controlled diabetes mellitus because **beta blockers** can prolong or enhance hypoglycemia by interfering with glycogenolysis. **Beta blockers** may also mask the signs and symptoms of acute hypoglycemia. Because they may mask the clinical signs of hypothyroidism, **beta blockers** should be used with caution in patients with hyperthyroidism.

Patients using **beta blockers** during surgery should be monitored closely for signs of cardiac failure. Severe, protracted hypotension and difficulty in restarting the heart have been reported. **Beta blockers** may need to be withdrawn before surgery, with the last dose 2 days prior to surgery.

Beta blockers are contraindicated in patients with Raynaud's disease or peripheral vascular or cerebrovascular disease because decreased cardiac output can exacerbate symptoms.

Ophthalmic beta blockers are Pregnancy Category C. Fetal anomalies and fetotoxicity have been observed in animal studies. Most of the *ophthalmic beta blockers* are **excreted in breast milk and are contraindicated in breastfeeding.** *Ophthalmic beta-blocker agents* are used **in children, but they must be monitored closely.**

Miotics. The **miotics** are contraindicated when active inflammation of the eye is present. They are also contraindicated when constriction is not wanted, for example, in iritis, uveitis, and some forms of secondary glaucoma.

The *miotics* are Pregnancy Category C, with *demecarium (Humorsol)* given the classification of Pregnancy Category X. Use with caution in lactating women. Use with extreme caution in children.

Carbonic Anhydrase Inhibitors. **Dorzolamide** and **brinzolamide** contain **sulfonamide** and are absorbed in amounts great enough to cause hypersensitivity reactions in patients with **sulfonamide** sensitivity. *Dorzolamide* **and** *brinzolamide* **are Pregnancy Category C. They are contraindicated in lactation, and their safety for use in children is not known.**

Methazolamide is contraindicated in patients with hyponatremia, hypokalemia, renal disease, liver disease, suprarenal gland failure, hyperchloremic acidosis, adrenocortical insufficiency, and severe pulmonary obstruction. **It is Pregnancy Category C and not recommended for use in children.**

Sympathomimetics. **Apraclonidine (Iopidine)** is contraindicated in patients with **clonidine** hypersensitivity. **Dipivefrin (AKPro, Propine)** is contraindicated in patients with narrow-angle glaucoma and aphakic patients. *Apraclonidine* **is Pregnancy Category C, and** *dipivefrin* **is Pregnancy Category B. They are not recommended for use by nursing mothers or by children.**

Alpha-Adrenergic Agonists. **Brimonidine** is contraindicated in patients taking **monoamine oxidase inhibitors (MAIOs)**. **Brimonidine** should be used with caution in patients with cardiac, renal, or liver disease. **Brimonidine** should not be instilled with contact lenses in place. The patient should wait 15 minutes after instilling **brimoni-**dine before replacing contacts. *Brimonidine* **is Pregnancy Category B.** *Brimonidine* **should be avoided in children and lactating women.**

Prostaglandin Agonists. **Latanoprost** should not be administered while the patient is wearing contact lenses. **Latanoprost** should be used with caution in patients with intraocular inflammation (iritis) and aphakic patients. **It is Pregnancy Category C. It is not recommended for use during lactation or by children.**

ADVERSE DRUG REACTIONS. All of the **antiglaucoma medications** may cause transient discomfort or tearing. Blurred vision, photophobia, and hyperemia may also occur. Allergic conjunctivitis may occur with any of the **topical ophthalmic medications.**

Headaches and dizziness may occur with the use of **beta blockers.** Patients may exhibit systemic beta-blocker effects with the use of ophthalmic preparations. Symptoms include bradycardia, hypotension, bronchospasm, and, rarely, AV block.

Miotics may cause corneal clouding, ciliary spasm, headache, induced myopia, and retinal detachment. Patients may have systemic anticholinergic effects if excessive absorption occurs. These symptoms include headache, hypertension, salivation, sweating, nausea, and vomiting. Iris cysts may be seen with **cholinesterase inhibitors.**

Many patients (about 25%) report dysgeusia, or bitter taste in the mouth, after ocular administration of **CA inhibitors.** Superficial punctate keratitis is reported in 10 to 15 percent of patients using ophthalmic preparations.

Systemic CA inhibitors (methazolamide) may cause melena and GI upset, such as anorexia, nausea, and vomiting. Glycosuria and urinary frequency have been reported. Weakness, malaise, fatigue, bone marrow depression, thrombocytopenia, leukopenia, and hemolytic anemia have been reported with use of **methazolamide.** Renal calculi and nephrotoxicity have also been reported. Fever is a rare adverse effect of **methazolamide.**

The local effects of the **sympathomimetics** include conjunctival or corneal pigmentation. Systemic effects of **topical sympathomimetic** use include headache, hypertension, tachycardia, and cardiac arrhythmias (with excessive absorption).

The local effects of **alpha agonists** that occur in 10 to 30 percent of patients include the sensation of a foreign body in the eye and ocular pain. Systemic adverse effects include dry mouth, drowsiness, and headache. Corneal staining may occur.

The local adverse effects reported in 5 to 15 percent of patients taking **prostaglandin agonists** include foreign body sensations, keratopathy, and iridal discoloration. The iridal discoloration may be gradual (many months) and is caused by an increase in the amount of brown pigmentation in the iris because of an increased number of melanosomes in melanocytes. The color change may be permanent.

DRUG INTERACTIONS

Beta Blockers. The use of **ophthalmic beta blockers** with **systemic beta blockers** may cause additive beta-blockade effects. Coadministration of **ophthalmic timolol** has caused bradycardia and asystole.

Miotics. **Carbachol** and **pilocarpine** solution have no reported drug interactions. **Pilocarpine** ocular sustained-release inserts (**Ocusert Pilo**) potentiate the absorption of **epinephrine**. **Echothiophate** may potentiate the effects of **succinylcholine**, leading to respiratory and possibly cardiovascular collapse. **Echothiophate** may have additive effects when used with **systemic anticholinesterases** used in the treatment of myasthenia gravis. There is additive toxicity (increased parasympathomimetic effects) if organic pesticides or **carbamate** is absorbed by someone using **ophthalmic echothiophate**.

Carbonic Anhydrase Inhibitors. Concurrent use of **CA inhibitors (topical brinzolamide, dorzolamide,** and **systemic methazolamide)** and high-dose **salicylates** may lead to metabolic acidosis and **salicylate** toxicity, which allow greater penetration of **salicylate** into the central nervous system (**CNS**). This interaction is theoretical with the **topical CA inhibitors**. **CA inhibitors** may inhibit excretion of basic drugs and promote excretion of acidic drugs. The concurrent use of **oral** and **topical CA inhibitors** is not recommended.

Sympathomimetics. There are no known drug interactions with **ophthalmic dipivefrin**. **Apraclonidine** may interact with cardiovascular drugs. **Apraclonidine** should not be used by patients who are using **MAOIs** because concurrent use may cause a hypertensive crisis.

Alpha-Adrenergic Agonists The **alpha-adrenergic agonists** are contraindicated with the use of **MAOIs**. There may be additive CNS depression if **topical alpha-adrenergic agonists** are used concurrently with **CNS depressants**. **Tricyclic antidepressants** can affect the metabolism and uptake of circulating amines. Medications that may cause bradycardia (**beta blockers, antihypertensives,** and **cardiac glycosides**) may have additive depression of pulse and blood pressure if used concurrently with **alpha-adrenergic agonists**.

Prostaglandin Agonists. The only reported drug interaction noted with **latanoprost** is **thimerosal**, which can cause precipitation if administered concurrently. Advise the patient to wait at least 5 minutes between administration of the two ophthalmic medications.

Table 25–6 presents drug interactions with **antiglaucoma agents**.

CLINICAL USE AND DOSING

Glaucoma. **Antiglaucoma medications** are prescribed by ophthalmologists. Dosage is determined by the clinical condition of the patient.

RATIONAL DRUG SELECTION. The ophthalmologist determines what medication should be used, based on the patient's glaucoma type and underlying medical conditions.

MONITORING. The patient who is prescribed **antiglaucoma medications** may require monitoring of blood pressure and cardiovascular status. IOP is measured and monitored by the ophthalmologist. No laboratory monitoring is necessary.

PATIENT EDUCATION

Administration. The patient should be instructed to administer the medication exactly as the ophthalmologist has prescribed (Table 24–7). Abruptly stopping the medication can increase adverse effects.

Adverse Reactions. The patient should have been instructed by the ophthalmologist regarding the adverse effects of the medication. Reinforcement may be necessary. If the patient is experiencing adverse effects from the medication, the primary care provider can facilitate a referral back to the ophthalmologist.

Ocular Antiallergic and Anti-inflammatory Agents

There are a variety of **ocular antiallergic** and **anti-inflammatory drugs**. The **antiallergic** medications include the **mast cell stabilizers lodoxamide (Alomide)** and **cromolyn sodium (Crolom)**. **Levocabastine (Livostin), antazoline (Vasocon-A, Antazoline-V), ketotifen (Zaditor), pheniramine (Naphcon-A),** and **emedastine (Emadine)** are **antihistamines**. The nonsteroidal anti-inflammatory drugs (NSAIDs) are **flurbiprofen (Ocufen), suprofen (Profenal), diclofenac (Voltaren ophthalmic solution),** and **ketorolac (Acular)**. **Corticosteroid ophthalmic agents** are used as anti-inflammatories, although they are rarely used in primary care because of the serious adverse effects. **Anti-inflammatory agents** are found in single formula or in combination with **antibiotics**.

Pharmacodynamics

OPHTHALMIC ANTIALLERGIC AGENTS. The **mast cell stabilizers** limit hypersensitivity reactions by inhibiting the degranulation of sensitized mast cells that occur after exposure to specific antigens. They also inhibit the release of histamine and SRS-A (slow-reacting substance of anaphylaxis). They have no intrinsic antihistamine activity.

Ocular antihistamines are selective for the H_1 histamine receptor. They block the H_1 histamine receptors and inhibit histamine-stimulated vascular permeability in the conjunctiva. This relieves ocular pruritus associated with allergic conjunctivitis.

OCULAR ANTI-INFLAMMATORY AGENTS. The **ocular NSAIDs** have analgesic, antipyretic, and anti-inflammatory

Table 24–6. Drug Interactions: Antiglaucoma Agents

Drug	Interacting Drug	Possible Effect	Implications
Beta blockers Betaxolol, carteolol, metipranolol	Oral beta blockers	Additive effects, excessive hypotension, increased reduction of IOP	Use with caution
	Antihypertensive agents	Additive antihypertensive effects	Monitor blood pressure (BP)
	Antiarrhythmics (diltiazem, verapamil, amiodarone, digoxin)	Additive effects; may cause significant effects on AV node conduction; may cause complete heart block	Use with caution, monitor closely
	Beta-agonist bronchodilators (albuterol, Alupent, salmeterol)	Beta blocker may antagonize the effects of beta agonists	Use with caution; avoid concurrent use if possible
Levobunolol	Oral beta blockers	Additive effects, excessive hypotension, increased reduction of IOP	Use with caution
	Cimetidine	Interferes with hepatic metabolism of levobunolol, potentially increasing its effects	Avoid concurrent use
	Sympathomimetics, including inhaled beta agonists	Antagonism of desired therapeutic effects	Avoid concurrent use
Timolol	Oral beta blockers	Additive effects, excessive hypotension, increased reduction of IOP	Use with caution
	Antihypertensive agents	Additive antihypertensive effects	Monitor BP
	Antiarrhythmics (diltiazem, verapamil, amiodarone, digoxin)	Additive effects; may cause significant effects on AV node conduction; may cause complete heart block	Use with caution; monitor closely
	Verapamil	Coadministration of ophthalmic timolol has caused bradycardia and asystole	Do not use concurrently
	Beta-agonist bronchodilators (albuterol, Alupent, salmeterol)	Timolol may antagonize the effects of beta agonists	Use with caution; avoid concurrent use if possible
	Quinidine	Quinidine can potentiate timolol-induced bradycardia	Use with caution; monitor closely
Miotics Carbachol, pilocarpine	No significant interactions		
Echothiophate	Succinylcholine (anesthetic)	May potentiate succinylcholine, leading to possible respiratory and cardiovascular collapse	Do not use concurrently; consider stopping echothiophate before surgery
	Systemic anticholinesterases	Additive effects	Coadminister cautiously

Continued on next page

Table 24–6. Drug Interactions: Antiglaucoma Agents *(continued)*

Drug	Interacting Drug	Possible Effect	Implications
	Carbamate or organo-phosphate insecticides and pesticides	Increased parasympatho-mimetic effects	Warn patients who are gardeners or workers who may be exposed to these chemicals to protect themselves with masks, frequent washing of skin, and clothing changes
Carbonic anhydrase inhibitors Acetazolamide	Barbiturates, aspirin, lithium	Excretion decreased	May lead to decreased effectiveness of inter-acting drugs
	Amphetamines, quinidine, procainamide, tricyclic antidepressants	Excretion decreased	May result in toxicity to interacting drugs
Brinzolamide	No known drug interactions		
Dorzolamide	Oral CA inhibitors	Potential additive effects	Concurrent use not recommended
Methazolamide	Diflunisal Salicylates	Significant decrease in IOP Accumulation of metha-zolamide, resulting in CNS depression and metabolic acidosis	Avoid concurrent use Avoid concurrent use
	Topiramate	Increased risk of renal stone formation	Avoid concurrent use
	Basic pH drugs	Inhibited renal excretion of basic drugs	
	Acidic pH drugs	Promotes excretion of acidic drugs	Monitor potassium
	Corticosteroids, potassium-depleting diuretics	Hypokalemia	Monitor potassium
Sympathomimetics Epinephrine	Anesthetics (cyclopro-pane, halogenated hydrocarbons)	May cause cardiac arrhythmias	Discontinue epinephrine prior to surgery
Dipivefrin	No significant interactions		
Alpha-adrenergic agonists Apraclonidine	Cardiovascular agents: antihypertensives, cardiac glycosides, beta blockers MAOIs	Apraclonidine may reduce pulse and BP	If using concurrently, monitor pulse and BP frequently Concurrent use contraindicated
Brimonidine	CNS depressants: alcohol, barbiturates, opiates, sedatives, or anesthetics Beta blockers, anti-hypertensives Tricyclic antidepressants MAOIs	Additive CNS depression Brimonidine may reduce pulse pressure and BP Tricyclic antidepressants can lower circulating amines	Use with caution Use with caution; monitor cardiac status Monitor IOP closely if necessary to admin-ister concurrently Use contraindicated
Prostaglandin agonists Latanoprost	Thimerosal	Precipitation of latanoprost occurs when used concurrently	Administer at least 5–10 min apart

Table 24–7. Available Dosage Forms: Antiglaucoma Agents

Drug	Dosage Form	How Supplied
BETA BLOCKERS		
Betaxolol		
Betoptic*	Solution: 5.6 mg/mL	In 2.5, 5, 10, and 15 mL
Betoptic S*	Suspension: 2.8 mg/mL	In 2.5, 5, 10, and 15 mL
Carteolol		
Ocupress	1% solution	In 5- and 10-mL dropper bottles
Levobunolol		
Betagan	0.25% solution	In 5- and 10-mL bottles
	0.5% solution	In 2-, 5-, 10-, and 15-mL bottles
AKBeta, Generic	0.25% solution	In 5- and 10-mL bottles
	0.5% solution	In 5-, 10-, and 15-mL bottles
Metipranolol		
OptiPranolol	0.3% solution	In 5- and 10-mL dropper bottle
Timolol		
Timoptic	0.25%, 0.5% solution	In 2.5-, 5-, 10-, and 15-mL bottles
		In 2.5 and 5 mL
Timoptic-XE	0.25%, 0.5% gel	In 5-, 10-, and 15-mL bottles
Generic	0.25%, 0.5% solution	
MIOTICS		
Carbachol		
Isopto Carbachol	0.75% solution, 1.5% solution	In 15- and 30-mL dropper bottles
	2.25% solution	In 15-mL bottles
	3% solution	In 15- and 30 mL-dropper bottles
Carboptic	3% solution	In 15-mL bottle
Pilocarpine		
Isopto Carpine	Solution: 0.25%, 0.5%, 1%, 2%, 3%, 4%, 5%, 6%, 10%	In 15- and 30-mL dropper bottles
		In 15- and 30-mL dropper bottles
Pilocar	Solution: 0.5%, 1%, 2%, 3%, 4%, 6%	In 3.5 g
		In 15- and 30-mL dropper bottles
Pilopine HS	Gel: 4%	
Generic	Solution: 0.5%, 1%, 2%, 4%, 6%, 8%	
Echothiophate		
Phospholine Iodide	Powder for solution: 0.03%, 0.06%, 0.125%, 0.25%	In 5 mL diluent
CARBONIC ANHYDRASE INHIBITORS		
Acetazolamide		
Diamox	Tablets: 125 mg, 250 mg	In 100s
Brinzolamide		
Azopt*	1% suspension	In 2.5, 5, 10, and 15 mL
Dorzolamide		
Trusopt*	2% solution	In 5 and 10 mL

Continued on next page

Table 24–7. Available Dosage Forms: Antiglaucoma Agents *(continued)*

Drug	Dosage Form	How Supplied
Methazolamide Neptazane	Tablets: 25 mg, 50 mg	In 100s
SYMPATHOMIMETICS		
Epinephrine Epifrin*†	0.5% solution 1% solution 2% solution	In 15-mL dropper bottle In 10-mL dropper bottle In 15-mL dropper bottle
Glaucon*†	1% solution, 2% solution	In 10-mL dropper bottle
Dipivefrin Propine, generic	0.1% solution	In 5-, 10-, and 15-mL bottles
ALPHA-ADRENERGIC AGONISTS		
Apraclonidine Iopidine	1% solution 0.5% solution	In 0.25-mL dispenser In 5-mL drop-tainer
Brimonidine Alphagen*	0.2% solution	In 5- or 10-mL dropper bottle
Latanoprost Xalatan*	0.005% solution	In 2.5 mL

*Contains benzalkonium chloride, which cannot be administered with soft contact lenses in place.
†Contains sulfites.

activity. The ophthalmic **NSAIDs** reduce prostaglandin E₂ in aqueous humor by inhibition of prostaglandin biosynthesis. It is thought to be through the inhibition of cyclo-oxygenase enzyme, which is essential to the synthesis of prostaglandins.

Topical steroids exert an anti-inflammatory action. The exact mechanism of action for **ocular corticosteroids** is not known. They are thought to act by the induction of phospholipase A₂ inhibitory proteins. These proteins control the mediators of inflammation, such as prostaglandins and leukotrienes. **Corticosteroids** can increase IOP; the mechanism is not clear.

Pharmacokinetics

Limited systemic absorption occurs with the use of **ophthalmic anti-inflammatory** and **antiallergic agents.**

The metabolism and excretion of **ophthalmic antiallergic** and **anti-inflammatory agents** are unknown.

Pharmacotherapeutics

PRECAUTIONS AND CONTRAINDICATIONS. Hypersensitivity to any component of the product is a contraindication of any of the ophthalmic medications. Use caution with patients with known sensitivity to **acetylsalicylic**

acid when prescribing **NSAIDs** because cross-sensitivity may occur.

Ophthalmic Antiallergic Agents. Patients should not wear soft contact lenses while inserting any ophthalmic product that contains benzalkonium chloride (**cromolyn sodium, lodoxamide, ketotifen, emedastine, levocabastine**). Wear can be resumed within a few hours of discontinuing **cromolyn, levocabastine,** and **lodoxamide.** Patients who are using **ketotifen** and **emedastine** may wear their soft contacts if they wait at least 10 minutes after instilling the eyedrops to insert their contacts.

Emedastine, cromolyn sodium, and *lodoxamide* are Pregnancy Category B. *Antazoline, ketotifen,* and *levocabastine* are Pregnancy Category C, although no studies have been done in pregnant women. Safe use in lactation has not been established, although such minimal amounts are absorbed that use during lactation is probably safe.

Lodoxamide is safe in children as young as age 2 years. **Cromolyn sodium ophthalmic** can be prescribed to children older than age 4 years. The safety of **emedastine** and **ketotifen** in children younger than age 3 has not been established.

Ocular Anti-inflammatory Agents. Referral to an ophthalmologist is warranted for patients who appear to need corticosteroid therapy. They require slit-lamp examination to rule out herpes keratitis prior to initiating therapy.

Corticosteroid eye medications should not be administered to patients with acute, untreated purulent bacterial, viral, or fungal ocular infection. Prescribing **ophthalmic corticosteroids** to a patient with herpes keratitis can lead to serious complications, including blindness. This may also occur with **ocular NSAIDs**; therefore, a referral is indicated before treatment.

The *ocular NSAIDs* are Pregnancy Category C, and the *ocular corticosteroids* are also Pregnancy Category C. **Safety in children has not been established.**

ADVERSE DRUG REACTIONS. All **ophthalmic antiallergic** and **anti-inflammatory medications** may cause transient discomfort or tearing. Blurred vision, photophobia, and hyperemia may also develop. Allergic conjunctivitis may occur with any of the topical ophthalmic medications.

Other adverse reactions reported (1 to 5%) with the use of the **mast cell stabilizer lodoxamide** include dry eye, foreign body sensation, ocular itching and pruritus, and crystalline deposits. **Cromolyn sodium** may also cause itchy eyes, eye dryness and puffiness, and styes.

The most frequent adverse reaction reported with the use of **ocular H$_1$-histamine blockers** is headache. Conjunctival injection and rhinitis are reported in 10 to 25 percent of patients treated. The adverse reactions that occur in fewer than 5 percent of patients include asthenia, blurred vision, corneal staining, dysgeusia, hyperemia, keratitis, pruritus, rhinitis, and sinusitis.

Naphazoline may precipitate narrow-angle glaucoma. It may also cause mydriasis, increased IOP, and allergic dermatitis. Systemic adrenergic or antihistamine effects may occur with excessive use.

The **ocular NSAIDs** may cause minor ocular irritation upon instillation (up to 40% incidence). The other reported adverse reactions noted in 1 to 10 percent of patients using **ocular NSAIDs** include superficial ocular infection, superficial keratitis, ocular inflammation, corneal edema, and iritis. Reactions reported less frequently include corneal infiltrates, corneal ulcer, keratitis, and mydriasis.

The severe adverse reactions that can occur with the use of **ocular corticosteroids** include glaucoma (elevated IOP) with optic nerve damage, loss of visual acuity and field defects, cataract formation, secondary infection of the eye, exacerbation of existing infections, and perforation of the globe. Systemic side effects may develop with extensive use.

DRUG INTERACTIONS. There are no drug interactions noted with any of the **ocular antiallergic medications**.

Ocular NSAIDs may potentiate **oral anticoagulants**; the patient should be monitored for prolonged bleeding times if the drugs are used concurrently.

Ophthalmic steroids have no known drug interactions.

CLINICAL USE AND DOSING

Allergic or Vernal Conjunctivitis. Allergic conjunctivitis can occur in response to a variety of allergens; vernal conjunctivitis refers to conjunctivitis that occurs primarily in the spring, usually because of an allergen. The **mast cell stabilizers (lodoxamide, cromolyn sodium)** may be used to treat vernal conjunctivitis. They may be used safely for up to 3 months.

The **ophthalmic H$_1$ blocker ketotifen** can be prescribed for allergic conjunctivitis and ocular pruritus. The dose used in adults and children over age 3 years is 1 drop in the affected eye every 8 to 12 hours. The dosage for **levocabastine**, another prescription **ophthalmic H$_1$ blocker**, is 1 drop in the affected eye four times a day.

The OTC products available to treat allergic conjunctivitis combine a **decongestant** with an **antihistamine**. Products that combine **antazoline** and **naphazoline (Vasocon-A)** or **naphazoline** and **pheniramine (Opcon-A, Naphcon-A)** are used for temporary relief of the minor eye symptoms of itching and redness caused by pollen and other allergens such as animal hair. Patients may self-prescribe these products; therefore, the primary care provider needs to monitor the patient for proper use and the adverse effects associated with the use of these medications.

Ocular Inflammation. Consultation with an ophthalmologist is indicated in the treatment of ocular inflammation. The patient requires a slit-lamp examination to rule out herpes keratitis or other infectious disease before beginning therapy with **ocular anti-inflammatory agents**. The dosing of these agents may be found in Table 24–8.

RATIONAL DRUG SELECTION

Safety. The **ophthalmic mast cell stabilizers** are quite safe to use, even in children and in pregnant patients. The **ocular antihistamines** are safe and can be used in children as young as 2 years old **(lodoxamide)**. The **ophthalmic H$_1$ blockers** are safe for use in adults, with **ketotifen** safe for use in children as young as 3 years.

The **ocular NSAIDs** are safe for treating a clear case of vernal conjunctivitis. If the diagnosis is unclear, an ophthalmologic consult is indicated before prescribing to clarify the diagnosis and rule out herpes keratitis.

The **ophthalmic corticosteroid** preparations have serious adverse effects. They should be prescribed only by an ophthalmologist.

MONITORING. The primary care provider needs to monitor the patient for effectiveness of therapy. There is no specific laboratory monitoring necessary with these medications. IOP should be periodically monitored by a trained eye professional if using medications that may increase IOP, **ocular corticosteroids**, and **naphazoline**.

PATIENT EDUCATION

Administration. The patient should be instructed to use

Table 24–8. Dosage Schedule: Selected Ocular Antiallergic
and Anti-inflammatory Agents

Drug	Indication	Dose	Notes
Mast cell stabilizers			
Cromolyn sodium	Allergic or vernal conjunctivitis	Adults and children ≥4 y: 1–2 drops each eye 4–6 times daily	Safety in children <4 y is not known Advise the patient not to wear soft contact lenses while using ophthalmic cromolyn sodium
Lodoxamide	Vernal conjunctivitis, keratoconjunctivitis, vernal keratitis	Over age 2 y: 1–2 drops qid for up to 3 mo	Not recommended in children <2 y
Antihistamines			
Antazoline/naphazoline	Allergic conjunctivitis	Adults: 1–3 drops into eyes q3–4h	OTC; use for temporary relief of allergic conjunctivitis symptoms
Emedastine	Allergic conjunctivitis	Adults and children ≥3 y: 1 drop qid	Not recommended in children <3 y Soft contact wearers may reinsert lens 10 min after administration of emedastine
Ketotifen	Temporary prevention of ocular itching due to allergic conjunctivitis	Adults and children ≥3 y: 1–2 drops q8–12h	Not recommended in children <3 y Soft contact wearers may reinsert lens 10 min after administration of ketotifen
Levocabastine	Seasonal allergic conjunctivitis	Adults and children ≥12 y: 1 drop into affected eye qid for up to 2 wk	Not recommended for use in children
Pheniramine/naphazoline	Allergic conjunctivitis	Adults: Instill 1–2 drops q3–4h	OTC; use for temporary relief of allergic conjunctivitis symptoms
Olopatadine	Temporary prevention of ocular itching due to allergic conjunctivitis	Adults and children ≥3 y: 1–2 drops bid, at least 6–8 h interval	Not recommended in children <3 y Soft contact wearers may reinsert lens 10 min after administration of olopatadine
Nonsteroidal anti-inflammatory drugs			
Diclofenac	Postop inflammation after cataract surgery	After surgery, instill 1 drop into affected eye qid for 2 wk, beginning 24 h after surgery	Prescribed by ophthalmologists
Flurbiprofen	Postop inflammation after cataract surgery	On day of surgery, instill 1 drop into eye every 30 min, beginning 2 h prior to surgery	Prescribed by ophthalmologists
Ketorolac	Seasonal allergic conjunctivitis	Adults and children ≥12 y: 1 drop in affected eye(s) qid	Patients wearing hydrogel soft contact lenses may experience ocular irritation when using concurrently Advise patients not to wear contacts while using this drug
Suprofen	Postop inflammation after cataract surgery	On day of surgery, instill 2 drops into eye at 3, 2, and 1 h prior to surgery; after surgery, instill 2 drops into affected eye q4h for 1 d	Prescribed by ophthalmologists

Table 24–9. Available Dosage Forms: Ocular Antiallergic and Anti-inflammatory Agents

Drug	Dosage Form	How Supplied
Mast cell stabilizers		
Cromolyn sodium		
Crolom*, Opticrom*	4% solution	In 10 mL
Lodoxamide		
Alomide	0.1% solution	In 10 mL
Antihistamines		
Antazoline-naphazoline		
Vasocon-A*	Solution: antazoline 0.5%, naphazoline 0.027%	In 5 and 15 mL
Generic	Solution: antazoline 0.5%, naphazoline 0.027%	In 15 mL
Emedastine		
Emadine*	0.05% solution	In 5 mL
Ketotifen		
Zaditor*	0.025% solution	In 5 mL
Levocabastine		
Livostin	0.05% suspension	In 2.5 mL, 5 mL, 10 mL
Pheniramine-naphazoline		
Naphcon-A*, Naphazoline Plus*, Generic	Solution: 0.3% pheniramine, 0.025% naphazoline	In 15 mL
Olopatadine		
Patanol*	0.1% solution	In 5 mL
Nonsteroidal anti-inflammatory drugs		
Diclofenac		
Voltaren	0.1% solution	In 2.5 mL and 5 mL
Flurbiprofen		
Ocufen[†]	0.03%	In 2.5 mL
Ketorolac		
Acular*	0.5% solution	In 3 mL, 5 mL, 10 mL
Acular PF	0.5% solution, preservative free	Single-use vials: 12 × 0.4 mL
Suprofen		
Profenal[†]	1% solution	In 2.5 mL

*Contains benzalkonium chloride, which cannot be administered with soft contact lenses in place.
[†]Contains thimerosal.

the medication exactly as prescribed (Table 24–9). Overuse or underuse can adversely affect the outcome of the clinical condition. Advise the patient to avoid touching the dropper to the eye or other surface, which may contaminate the medication. To prevent cross-contamination, neither prescription nor OTC products should be shared with another person.

Adverse Reactions. Alert the patient to the adverse reaction of transient stinging and burning that may occur with the use of ocular medications. If the burning or stinging is intense or prolonged or if there is any other adverse reaction, the patient should contact the primary care provider.

Ocular Lubricants

Ocular lubricants offer tearlike lubrication for the relief of dry eyes and eye irritation. **Ocular lubricants** are also referred to as **artificial tears**. An **artificial tear** insert consisting of **hydroxypropyl cellulose (Lacrisert)**, which may be prescribed by an ophthalmologist or optometrist, is not discussed in this chapter.

Pharmacodynamics

Ocular lubricants contain a balanced solution of salts to maintain ocular tonicity, buffers to adjust pH, viscosity to prolong eye contact time, and preservatives.

Pharmacokinetics

Ocular lubricants are not absorbed in measurable amounts.

Pharmacotherapeutics

PRECAUTIONS AND CONTRAINDICATIONS. There are no true contraindications to the use of **ocular lubricants.**

Products that contain **benzalkonium chloride (Teargen, Akwa Tears, Puralube Tears, Comfort Tears, Dry Eyes, HypoTears, Ultra Tears, Isopto Plain, Isopto Tears, Just Tears, LubriTears, Moisture Drops, Murine, Nature's Tears, Nu-Tears, Nu-Tears II, Tearisol,** **OcuCoat, Tears Naturale, Tears Renewed)** should not be used with soft contacts.

ADVERSE DRUG REACTIONS. The **ocular lubricants** may cause mild stinging and temporary blurred vision.

DRUG INTERACTIONS. There are no significant drug interactions with the **ocular lubricants.**

CLINICAL USE AND DOSING
Dry Eye Syndrome. **Ocular lubricants** or **artificial tears** are used as needed to provide relief of dry eyes and ocular irritation. They can also be used as lubricants for artificial eyes. The patient should be instructed to instill 1 or 2 drops into the eye(s) three to four times a day as needed. Table 24–10 presents the dosing schedule.

Table 24–10. Dosage Schedule: Miscellaneous Ophthalmic Products

Drug	Indication	Dose	Notes
Ocular lubricants Artificial tears	Ocular irritation, xerophthalmia	*Adults and children:* Instill 1–2 drops into affected eye(s) 3–4 times/d as needed	
Ophthalmic vasoconstrictors Naphazoline	Relief of eye redness	Instill 1–2 drops qid as needed	Treatment should not continue for longer than 3 to 4 d without the supervision of an ophthalmologist
Oxymetazoline	Relief of eye redness	*Adults and children:* 1–2 drops in affected eye(s) bid–qid but no more frequently than every 6 h	OTC
Tetrahydrozoline	Relief of eye redness	*Adults:* Instill 1–2 drops into the affected eye(s) up to 4 times/d	OTC
Ophthalmic diagnostic products Fluorescein	Detection of corneal abrasion or defect	2% solution: Instill 1–2 drops into the eye; use Wood's lamp to detect staining of defect Strips: Moisten strip with sterile water and place at fornix in the lower cul-de-sac; the patient should close lid tightly and blink several times; use Wood's lamp to detect defect	After examination, excess stain can be removed with sterile saline solution Soft contact lenses can be reinserted 1 h after the eyes are flushed with saline to remove fluorescein

MONITORING. There is no laboratory monitoring needed with the use of **artificial tears.**

PATIENT EDUCATION

Administration. Advise the patient to avoid touching the dropper to the eye or another surface, which may contaminate the medication.

Adverse Reactions. Advise the patient that transient mild stinging and blurred vision may occur. The patient should contact the primary care provider if headache, eye pain, vision changes, prolonged redness, or discharge occurs.

Ophthalmic Vasoconstrictors

Ophthalmic vasoconstrictors are used in primary care to provide temporary relief of redness of the eye due to minor eye irritants. There are **ophthalmic vasoconstrictors** that are used by eye care specialists to dilate the pupil (**hydroxyamphetamine Hbr, 2.5 and 10% phenylephrine**) They are not covered in this chapter.

Pharmacodynamics

The **ophthalmic vasoconstrictors** are **sympathomimetic** agents that act by constricting the conjunctival blood vessels. The products used for eye redness are generally weak **sympathomimetic** solutions.

Pharmacokinetics

Information regarding the pharmacokinetics of the **ophthalmic vasoconstrictors** is not available, other than duration of action. The duration of action of **naphazoline** is 3 to 4 hours. Oxymetazoline's duration of action is 4 to 6 hours, and **tetrahydrozoline's** duration action of action is 1 to 4 hours.

Pharmacotherapeutics

PRECAUTIONS AND CONTRAINDICATIONS. The **ophthalmic vasoconstrictors** are contraindicated if the patient is sensitive to any of the components of the product. They are also contraindicated in any patient who has narrow-angle glaucoma.

The *ophthalmic vasoconstrictors* are Pregnancy Category C; the safety of their use in pregnancy has not been established.

ADVERSE DRUG REACTIONS. The patient may experience transient stinging or burning upon instillation. Blurring of vision may occur and is temporary, passing within minutes. Patients may experience mydriasis. Increased lacrimation, irritation, and discomfort may occur.

The most serious adverse reaction that may occur is increased IOP.

Rebound congestion or redness can develop with frequent or extended use of **ophthalmic vasoconstrictors.**

DRUG INTERACTIONS. There are no significant drug interactions with the use of **oxymetazoline** or **tetrahydrozoline.**

Tricyclic antidepressants and **maprotiline (Ludiomil)** may potentiate the pressor effects of **naphazoline.** If **MAOIs** are used with **ophthalmic sympathomimetics,** exaggerated adrenergic effects may result. Do not use **MAOIs** within 21 days of the **ophthalmic sympathomimetics.**

Systemic adverse effects may more easily occur if **ophthalmic sympathomimetics** are used with **beta blockers.**

CLINICAL USE AND DOSING

Relief of Eye Redness. **Ophthalmic vasoconstrictors** that are used for relief of eye redness due to irritation or allergic conjunctivitis include **tetrahydrozoline, oxymetazoline, naphazoline,** and **phenylephrine.** The usual adult dose is 1 or 2 drops instilled in the eyes four times a day. Use in children is not recommended.

RATIONAL DRUG SELECTION. Tetrahydrozoline, oxymetazoline, naphazoline (0.012%, 0.02%, 0.03%), and **phenylephrine 0.12%** are available OTC (Table 24–11). **Naphazoline 0.1%** is available only by prescription. **Phenylephrine 2.5 and 10%** are used only for pupil dilation and are instilled by eye care specialists.

MONITORING. There is no laboratory monitoring necessary with the use of **ophthalmic vasoconstrictors.**

PATIENT EDUCATION

Administration. Advise the patient to avoid touching the dropper to the eye or another surface, which may contaminate the medication. The patient should avoid prolonged or excessive use of **ocular vasoconstrictors** because rebound congestion or redness may occur.

Adverse Reactions. Advise the patient that transient mild stinging and blurred vision may occur.

Ophthalmic Diagnostic Products

The **ophthalmic diagnostic** that is used in primary care is **topical fluorescein sodium.** It is used to detect corneal epithelial defects or abrasions. The injectable form of **fluorescein** is used by ophthalmologists as a diagnostic aid in ophthalmic angiography. Only the topical form is discussed in this chapter.

Pharmacodynamics

Fluorescein is a yellow, water-soluble dibasic acid xanthine dye. It produces an intense fluorescent green color in alkaline (pH >5) solution. **Fluorescein** detects de-

Table 24–11. Available Dosage Forms: Miscellaneous Ophthalmic Products

Drug	Dosage Form	How Supplied
OCULAR LUBRICANTS		
Artificial tears (many available)		
Bion Tears	Preservative-free solution: dextran, hydroxypropyl methylcellulose	Single-use containers—28
Duratears Naturale	Ointment: lanolin, mineral oil	In 3.5 g
Hypotears	Solution: polyvinyl alcohol	In 15, 30 mL
	Preservative-free ointment: light mineral oil, white petrolatum	In 3.5 g
Lacri-Lube	Ointment: petrolatum, mineral oil	In 3.5, 7 g
Muro 128	Solution: sodium chloride	In 2, 15 mL
OPHTHALMIC VASOCONSTRICTORS		
Naphazoline		
Bausch & Lomb Allergy Drops	0.012% solution	In 15 mL
Bausch & Lomb Maximum Strength Allergy Drops	0.03% solution	In 15 mL
Clear Eyes	0.012% solution	In 15 mL
Comfort Eye Drops	0.03% solution	In 15 mL
Naphcon	0.012% solution	In 15 mL
Naphcon Forte	0.1% solution	In 15 mL
Vasocon Regular	0.1% solution	In 15 mL
Vasoclear	0.02% solution	In 15 mL
Oxymetazoline		
OcuClear	0.025% solution	In 30 mL
Visine LR	0.025% solution	In 15, 30 mL
Tetrahydrozoline		
Visine	0.05% solution	In 15, 22.5, 30 mL
Murine Plus, Generic	0.05% solution	In 15, 30 mL
OPHTHALMIC DIAGNOSTIC PRODUCTS		
Fluorescein	2% solution	In 1, 2, 15 mL
	Strips: 0.6, 1, 9 mg	In 100s, 300s

fects in the corneal epithelium. A corneal abrasion or corneal epithelial defects appears bright green. **Fluorescein** does not stain the intact cornea.

Pharmacokinetics

When used for the detection of corneal abrasion, **topical fluorescein** is not absorbed.

Pharmacotherapeutics

PRECAUTIONS AND CONTRAINDICATIONS. Hypersensitivity to **fluorescein** is a contraindication to its use.

Do not use **fluorescein** with soft contact lenses, which become stained. Lenses can be reinserted after the eyes are flushed with sterile saline and the patient waits an hour.

Fluorescein is Pregnancy Category C, although there are no reports of fetal complications or anomalies.

ADVERSE DRUG REACTIONS. There are no adverse drug reactions reported with **topical fluorescein** use, other than staining of soft contact lenses.

DRUG INTERACTIONS. There are no drug interactions with the use of **topical fluorescein.**

CLINICAL USE AND DOSING

Detection of Corneal Epithelial Defects. If a corneal abrasion or foreign body is suspected, the provider instills 1 or 2 drops of **fluorescein 2% solution** into the eye. After a few seconds, epithelial defects will stain. The use of a Wood's lamp enhances detection of defects. **Fluorescein strips** may be used. The strip is moistened with sterile water and placed at the fornix in the lower cul-de-sac close to the punctum. The patient should close the lid tightly over the strip until the desired amount of staining occurs. Have the patient blink several times to distribute the stain. After examination, excess stain can be removed with sterile saline solution.

MONITORING. There is no specific laboratory monitoring necessary with the use of **topical fluorescein.**

PATIENT EDUCATION

Administration. Advise the patient that the staining of the cornea is temporary and will resolve within a few hours. The patient should not be wearing soft contact lenses during the examination. Advise the patient to wait at least 1 hour before reinserting the contact lenses.

Drugs Used in Treating Ear Disorders

Otic Anti-infectives

Otitis externa (OE) is an acute, painful inflammatory condition of the external auditory canal. Commonly known as swimmer's ear, OE affects people of all ages, and it is the most common cause of visits for ear pain. It can easily be treated by a primary care provider, yet it can have serious, even life-threatening complications, especially in diabetic or immunocompromised patients.

OE occurs when there is a breakdown in a number of protective mechanisms. The normally acidic environment creates a hostile climate for bacterial growth. Cerumen is bacteriostatic and provides a protective layer that protects the epithelium against hyperhydration. Factors that alter these defenses and contribute to OE include an abrasion in the ear canal, water in the ear canal, and maceration of the skin from heat and moisture. With OE, the acidic environment in the ear canal is changed to neutral or basic, usually by retained moisture. Itching and a sense of fullness develop from damage to the epithelium caused by hyperhydration. Organisms invade wet intact skin, as well as damaged epithelium.

Pharmacodynamics

The medications used in the treatment of OE include combination products (**Cortisporin, Pediotic**) that contain a **corticosteroid (hydrocortisone)** and **antibiotic(s) (neomycin, polymyxin B, ciprofloxacin)**, **antibiotic** alone (**gentamycin, ofloxacin**), and acid or alcohol drops (**Otic Domeboro, Burow's Otic, VoSol, VoSol HC**) (Tables 24–12 and 24–13).

Hydrocortisone reduces the inflammation caused by OE. The exact mechanism of action for **topical corticosteroids** is not known. They are thought to act by the induction of phospholipase A_2 inhibitory proteins. These proteins control the mediators of inflammation, such as prostaglandins and leukotrienes.

Neomycin is active against *S. aureus* and *Proteus* and *Enterobacter* species. **Polymyxin B** is generally active against gram-negative bacteria (*P. aeruginosa, E. coli, H. influenzae*). **Gentamicin** is a broad-spectrum **aminoglycoside** that is active against *P. aeruginosa*, staphylococci, *S. pneumoniae*, beta-hemolytic streptococci, and *Enterobacter* species. The **fluoroquinolones (ciprofloxacin, ofloxacin)** are active against staphylococci, *S. pneumoniae, Proteus* and *Enterobacter* species, and *P. aeruginosa*.

Acid and alcohol solutions such as **Otic Domeboro** and **Burow's Otic** contain 2% acetic acid in aluminum acetate solution. Another acid solution, **VoSol Otic**, contains 2% acetic acid solution and 3% propylene glycol. These solutions reduce inflammation and are **antibacterial** and **antifungal**.

Pharmacokinetics

Information regarding the pharmacokinetics of otic preparations is not available.

Pharmacotherapeutics

PRECAUTIONS AND CONTRAINDICATIONS. Hypersensitivity to any component of the product is a contraindication to its use.

Ciprofloxacin is contraindicated if the tympanic membrane (TM) is perforated. **Cortisporin otic solution** is contraindicated if the TM is perforated. **Cortisporin otic suspension** may be used.

Prolonged use of **topical antibiotics** may lead to superinfection and overgrowth of nonsusceptible organisms and fungi.

ADVERSE DRUG REACTIONS. Local reactions, such as contact dermatitis, may occur with any of the otic preparations. Superinfection may develop with prolonged use. **Ofloxacin otic** may cause taste alteration. Dizziness, vertigo, and paresthesias have also been reported with otic **ofloxacin** use. Ototoxicity may occur with prolonged use of **Pediotic** and **Cortisporin otic solution.**

DRUG INTERACTIONS. There are no known drug interactions for the topical otic preparations.

CLINICAL USE AND DOSING

Acute Otitis Externa (Swimmer's Ear). Upon presentation of OE, the canal is swollen and full of discharge. The organisms found in OE (swimmer's ear) are usually gram-negative rods, *P. aeruginosa, Enterobacter* species, and *Proteus mirabilis. Pseudomonas* is the most common organism found in OE. Mycotic OE is less common, usually caused by *Aspergillus, Trichophyton,* or *Candida.* Occasionally, a furunculosis (small abscess) of the external canal may be caused by *S. aureus* or *S. pyogenes* carried there by dirty fingers.

Table 24–12. Dosage Schedule: Drugs Used in Treating Ear Disorders

Drug	Indication	Dose	Notes
Otic anti-infectives			
Gentamicin	Otitis externa	Use ophthalmic drops: 4 drops in affected ear qid for 7–10 d	Broad-spectrum coverage
Ofloxacin	Otitis externa Chronic suppurative otitis media with perforated tympanic membrane Otitis media in children with tympanostomy tubes	Age 1–12 y: 5 drops in affected ear bid for 10 d Age ≥12 y: 10 drops in affected ear for 10 d	To prevent dizziness, warm bottle in hand for 1–2 min prior to administering Not recommended for use in children <1 y
Otic anti-infective–steroid combination			
Hydrocortisone-neomycin–polymyxin B	Otitis externa Chronic suppurative otitis media with perforated tympanic membrane	Children: 3 drops of suspension in affected ear 3–4 times/d Adults: 4 drops of suspension in affected ear 3–4 times/d	Suspension is less ototoxic than solution; solution is contraindicated if TM is perforated
Hydrocortisone-ciprofloxacin	Acute otitis externa	Age ≥1 y: 3 drops in affected ear bid for 7 d	To prevent dizziness, warm bottle in hand for 1–2 min prior to administering Not recommended for use in children <1 y
Hydrocortisone-neomycin-colistin	Otitis externa	4 drops of suspension in affected ear 3–4 times/d	Contraindicated if TM perforated
Acid-alcohol solutions			
Acetic acid–aluminum acetate	Otitis externa	Clean ear canal; instill 4 drops 3–4 times/d for 7–10 d If canal swollen: Insert wick saturated with solution; instill 4–6 drops q2–3h; keep moist for 24 h	Contraindicated if TM perforated
Acetic acid–propylene glycol	Otitis externa	Clean ear canal; instill 5 drops 3–4 times/d for 7–10 d If canal swollen: Insert wick saturated with solution; instill 4–6 drops q2–3h; after 24 h, remove wick and instill 5 drops qid	Contraindicated if TM perforated Not recommended in children ≤3 y
Acetic acid–propylene glycol–hydrocortisone	Otitis externa	Clean ear canal, and instill 5 drops 3–4 times daily for 7–10 d May use cotton wick for first 24 h	Contraindicated if TM perforated Not recommended in children ≤3 y
Isopropyl alcohol–glycerine	Drying solution for ear canal	Instill 4–6 drops in each ear after swimming or bathing	

Continued on next page

Table 24–12. Dosage Schedule: Drugs Used in Treating Ear Disorders *(continued)*

Drug	Indication	Dose	Notes
Isopropyl alcohol–propylene glycol	Drying solution for ear canal	Instill 6–8 drops in each ear after swimming or bathing or bid	
Otic analgesics Benzocaine-antipyrine-glycerin	Analgesia in acute otitis media Adjunct in cerumen removal	Otitis media: Fill affected canal and insert cotton plug; may repeat every 1–2 h if needed Cerumen removal: Fill ear canal tid for 2–3 d	Contraindicated if TM perforated
Benzocaine-antipyrine–propylene glycol	Analgesia in acute otitis media	Fill ear canal and insert cotton plug; repeat q2–4h as needed	Contraindicated if TM perforated
Ceruminolytics Carbamide peroxide	Cerumen removal	Instill 5–10 drops in ear canal, keep drops in for several minutes, and repeat bid for up to 4 d	Contraindicated if TM perforated Not recommended in young children
Triethanolamine	Cerumen removal	Fill ear canal, insert cotton plug, allow to remain for 15–30 min, and flush ear	Contraindicated if TM perforated

Once it has been determined that the TM is intact, the canal can be gently cleaned with warm saline or with 3% hydrogen peroxide. If the TM cannot be visualized, irrigation should not be performed.

Topical medication is the treatment of choice.

A **steroid-antibiotic** drop that combines **hydrocortisone** with **neomycin** and **polymyxin B (Cortisporin Otic, Pediotic)**, **colistin (Coly-Mycin S Otic)**, or a **hydrocortisone-ciprofloxacin (Ciloxan HC)** suspension is instilled in the affected ear four times a day. The usual dose is 4 drops, and treatment should continue for 7 to 10 days. **Gentamicin** and **ofloxacin** provide good coverage for the common organisms, but the combination products decrease inflammation faster. **Ciprofloxacin** cannot be used if the TM is perforated.

A topical acid or alcohol solution (**Otic Domeboro, Burow's Otic, VoSol**) can be instilled into the ear four times a day if the TM is intact. A 1:1 mixture of vinegar and rubbing alcohol is just as effective, but it can be painful to administer. If excessive inflammation is present, a combination of acid with **hydrocortisone (VoSol HC)** may be effective.

If the canal is too swollen to allow the drops to be instilled, a wick of 0.25-inch gauze or cotton may be inserted into the swollen external canal for 24 to 36 hours. The medication can be dropped onto the wick.

Chronic Otitis Externa. Chronic EO can be inflammatory or infectious. Psoriasis, eczema, or seborrhea can cause inflammatory chronic OE. Chronic infectious OE may be caused by infected sinus tracts, cysts, or fungi.

The treatment for inflammatory chronic OE is determined by the severity of presentation. If the patient is complaining of chronic itching, accompanied by dry skin elsewhere on the body, the treatment consists of placing 2 or 3 drops of baby oil or mineral oil in the canal daily. If the patient has psoriasis in the external canal, it can be treated with **steroid** cream or lotion (see Chapter 30). Seborrhea can cause a scaly inflammation in the external auditory canal and behind the ears, usually accompanied by seborrhea of the forehead, eyelids, and face. Treatment is the use of **selenium sulfide** shampoo and **topical corticosteroids** (see Chapter 30).

If the ear canal is greatly inflamed, treatment includes cleansing the external canal of debris and using a **steroid otic** solution (**Decadron**) two or three times a day until the swelling decreases. If needed to relieve the inflammation, a wick can be placed and **Otic Domeboro** or **Burow's Otic** dropped onto the wick for 24 to 48 hours.

Malignant Otitis Externa. Malignant OE is a rare but potentially lethal infection caused by *P. aeruginosa*. Malignant OE occurs mainly in older patients with diabetes

Table 24–13. Available Dosage Forms: Drugs Used in Treating Ear Disorders

Drug	Dosage Form	How Supplied
Otic anti-infectives		
Gentamicin ophthalmic		
Garamycin, Genoptic	Solution: 3 mg/mL	In 5-mL dropper bottle
Generic	Solution: 3 mg/mL	In 5- and 15-mL dropper bottles
Ofloxacin		
Floxin	0.3% solution	In 5 mL
Otic anti-infective–steroid combination		
Hydrocortisone-neomycin-polymyxin B	Suspension: hydrocortisone 1%, neomycin 5 mg/mL, polymyxin B 10,000 U/mL	In 10 mL
Cortisporin Otic, Generic	Solution: hydrocortisone 1%, neomycin 5 mg/mL, polymyxin B 10,000 U/mL	In 10 mL
Pediotic	Suspension: hydrocortisone 1%, neomycin 5 mg/mL, polymyxin B 10,000 U/mL	In 10 mL
Hydrocortisone-ciprofloxacin	Suspension: hydrocortisone 10 mg/mL, ciprofloxacin 2 mg/mL	In 10 mL
Cipro HC Otic		
Hydrocortisone-neomycin-colistin	Suspension: hydrocortisone 1%, neomycin 5 mg/mL, colistin 3 mg/mL	In 10 mL
Coly-Mycin S Otic		
Acid-alcohol solutions		
Acetic acid–aluminum acetate	Solution	In 60 mL
Otic Domeboro, Burow's Otic		
Acetic acid–propylene glycol	Solution	In 15 mL and 30 mL
VoSol Otic		
Acetic acid–propylene glycol–hydrocortisone	Solution	In 15 and 30 mL
VoSol HC Otic		
Isopropyl alcohol–glycerin		
Swim-Ear	Liquid: 95% isopropyl alcohol, 5% anhydrous glycerin	In 30 mL
Isopropyl alcohol–propylene glycol		
EarSol	Drops: 44% isopropyl alcohol, propylene glycol	In 50 mL
Otic analgesics		
Benzocaine-antipyrine-glycerin	Solution	In 10 mL with dropper
Auralgan	Solution	In 15 mL with dropper
Generic		
Benzocaine-antipyrine–propylene glycol	Solution	In 13 mL with dropper
Tympagesic		
Ceruminolytics		
Carbamide peroxide		
Debrox	6.5% drops	In 30 mL with dropper
Murine Ear	6.5% drops	In 15 mL with dropper
Auro Ear Drops	6.5% drops	In 15 mL
Triethanolamine		
Cerumenex Drops	10% solution	In 6 and 12 mL with dropper

(90%). It develops when OE extends and invades the surrounding tissues, causing osteomyelitis of the base of the skull and purulent meningitis, accompanied by multiple cranial nerve palsies. Standard treatment includes **parenteral antibiotics** with an **aminoglycoside** and **carbenicillin** for 4 to 6 weeks, plus surgical debridement.

Prevention of Swimmer's Ear.   Most cases of acute OE (swimmer's ear) can be prevented by instilling isopropyl ear drops (**Swim-Ear, FarSol**) or 1 or 2 drops of rubbing alcohol into the ear canal to dry the ear after swimming. The commercial preparations have the advantage of less stinging with application if the skin is slightly macerated.

Table 24–12 presents the dosage schedule of drugs used in treating ear disorders.

MONITORING.   There is no laboratory monitoring necessary with these medications. The patient with a severely inflamed external canal requiring a wick should be reassessed 48 hours after treatment is begun and at the end of treatment to determine clinical cure. Patients with chronic EO need cleansing of the canal and reassessment every 2 to 3 weeks and may require alterations in topical medications, depending on clinical status.

PATIENT EDUCATION

Administration.   Advise the patient to hold the bottle of medication in the hand for a few minutes to warm the medication before instilling. The patient should lie on her or his side with the affected ear up, instill the drops, and keep the ear up for 2 minutes or insert a soft cotton plug to prevent the medication from draining out.

Adverse Reactions.   Advise patients to notify their primary care provider if adverse effects occur.

Otic Analgesics

Topical anesthetics are used in the ear to treat pain associated with otitis media. The **local anesthetic benzocaine** is used to provide pain relief until **systemic antibiotics** can take effect. **Benzocaine** is combined with **glycerin**, a hygroscopic agent, in **Auralgan Otic**. **Analgesic** eardrops are instilled into the affected ear three to four times daily or up to once every 1 to 2 hours as needed for pain.

Ceruminolytics

Some patients have an excessive accumulation of cerumen, which can lead to conductive hearing loss, impaction, and an environment for OE to develop. Patients who use cotton-tipped applicators (Q-Tips) to try to remove the cerumen actually push the cerumen farther into the canal. The cerumen often forms a hard plug that is painful to remove. Treatment includes instillation of mineral oil, which softens the wax, or the use of carbamide peroxide, which softens and emulsifies the wax. Once the cerumen is softened, the ear canal can be irrigated with *warm* water or saline. If the canal is excoriated, application of **antibiotic** or **steroid** eardrops for 7 to 10 days will prevent the development of OE.

REFERENCES

Centers for Disease Control. (1989). STD treatment guidelines. *Morbidity and Mortality Weekly Report, 8,*287.

Facts and Comparisons Staff. (1999). *Drug facts and comparisons.* St. Louis: Facts and Comparisons.

Gitinger, J. W. (1996). Eye diseases. In J.C. Bennett, & F. Plum, (Eds.), *Cecil textbook of medicine* (20th ed., pp. 2174–2183). Philadelphia: Saunders.

LaRosa, S. (1998). Primary care management of otitis externa. *Nurse Practitioner, 23*(6), 125–128, 131–133.

MacDonald, M. (1996). Eye problems. In C. E. Burns, N. Barber, A. M. Brady, & A. M. Dunn (Eds.), *Pediatric primary care: A handbook for nurse practitioners* (pp. 573–591). Philadelphia: Saunders.

Moroi, S. E., & Lichter, P. R. (1996). Ocular pharmacology. In J. G. Hardman & L. E. Limbard (Eds.), *Goodman & Gilman's the pharmacological basis of therapeutics* (9th ed., pp. 1619–1645). New York: McGraw-Hill.

Murphy, J. L. (Ed.). (1999). *Nurse practitioner prescribing reference.* New York: Prescribing Reference.

Nard, J. A. (2000). Otitis externa. In M. R. Dambro & J. A. Griffith (Eds.), *Griffith's 5 minute clinical consultant* (8th ed.). Baltimore: Williams & Wilkins.

Petersen-Smith, A. M. (1996). Ear disorders. In C. E. Burns, N. Barber, A. M. Brady, & A. M. Dunn (Eds.). *Pediatric primary care: A handbook for nurse practitioners* (pp. 593–607). Philadelphia: Saunders.

Rosenfield, J. A., & Clarity, G. (1998). The ear, nose and throat. In *Family medicine principles and practice* (5th ed.). New York: Springer.

Wald, E. R. (1997). Conjunctivitis in infants and young children. *Pediatric Infectious Disease Journal, 16*(2), S17–S20.

Yetman, R. J., & Coody, D. K. (1997). Conjunctivitis: A practice guideline. *Journal of Pediatric Health Care, 11*(5), 238–241.

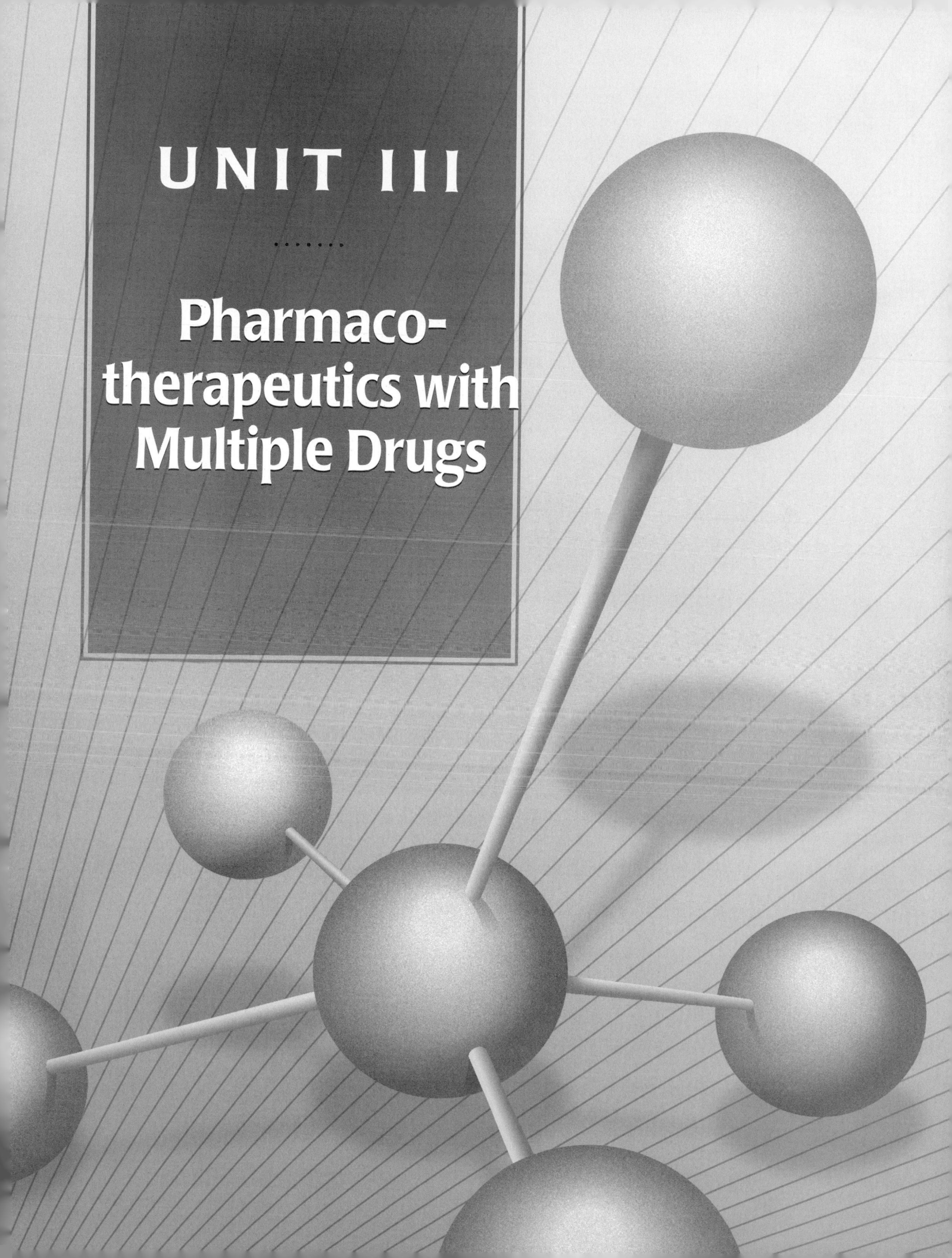

UNIT III

Pharmaco-therapeutics with Multiple Drugs

CHAPTER 25

·······

Anemia

CHAPTER OUTLINE

Anemias are extremely common in primary care practice. Of the three main forms of anemia, iron-deficiency anemia is the most common; approximately 20 percent of women, 50 percent of pregnant women, and 3 percent of men are iron-deficient. Infants and teenage girls are also at high risk for this disorder, and it is common in older adults. Anemia of chronic disease is the second most common form, as well as the most common in hematologic disorders in the older adult population. The third major form of ane-

mia is sickle cell disease, which affects more than 72,000 Americans, mainly of African ancestry. Approximately 1 in every 500 African-Americans and 1 in every 1000 Hispanics have sickle cell disease; about 2 million Americans or 1 of every 12 African-Americans carry the sickle cell trait.

The average American diet normally supplies adequate iron to prevent anemia, lack of energy, and related symptoms, but age-related growth and development needs and concomitant disease processes may interfere with the intake, metabolism, or utilization of dietary iron. For sickle cell anemia, iron intake and utilization are not the issue, but lack of energy is a central problem, with the alteration in oxygen transport and adenosine triphosphate (ATP) generation that is associated with this disorder.

Diagnosis and treatment of the various forms of anemia entail interpretation of blood studies and peripheral smears, prescription of lifestyle modifications in the form of diet and energy conservation, and prescription of drugs specific to each disorder. The focus of this chapter is the lifestyle modifications and drugs used to treat each disorder. The history, physical examination, and laboratory tests to diagnose specific anemias are not within the scope of this book.

Pathophysiology

The underlying pathophysiology in all types of anemia is a decrease in the oxygen-carrying capacity of the blood. *Iron-deficiency anemia* (IDA) decreases oxygen-carrying capacity because of a low hemoglobin concentration that is due to reduced red blood cell (RBC) production (lack of adequate iron intake, poor absorption of iron by the body, or lead poisoning) or acute or chronic blood loss. This produces a microcytic-hypochromic anemia that develops slowly after the normal stores of iron have been depleted in the body and particularly the bone marrow. *Folic acid–deficiency anemia* (FDA) decreases oxygen-carrying capacity because of a low hemoglobin concentration. Folic acid is necessary for the normal maturation and functioning of RBCs. FDA produces a macrocytic-normochromic anemia within 3 months of the start of an inadequate diet, more rapidly than pernicious anemia because folate stores are more rapidly depleted. *Pernicious anemia* (PA) also has a low hemoglobin concentration. Vitamin B_{12} is necessary for maturation and DNA synthesis in RBCs. PA produces a macrocytic-normochromic anemia that develops slowly, often over years, and it is frequently severe before it is diagnosed. Concomitant symptoms include glossitis and neuropathy; the latter is often used to clinically differentiate between FDA and PA. *Anemia of chronic disease* (ACD) is also associated with low hemoglobin, but it is caused by destruction of RBCs by a hyperactive reticuloendothelial system, decreased production of RBCs by hypoactive bone marrow, or altered iron metabolism, with defective transfer of iron from stores to the plasma. This produces a normocytic-normochromic anemia that also develops slowly and is often mild or asymptomatic. Patients with *sickle cell anemia* (SCA) have a normal amount of hemoglobin (normocytic-normochromic), but their RBCs contain an abnormal type of hemoglobin, hemoglobin S (HgbS). Sickle cell disease is actually a group of genetic disorders characterized by the predominance of this hemoglobin. These disorders include SCA, beta thalassemia syndromes, and hemoglobinopathies in which HgbS is associated with another abnormal hemoglobin. These disorders are found in people of African, Mediterranean, Indian, and Middle Eastern heritage. Sickle cell trait is not a disease and not a cause for abnormalities in the blood count, and it does not produce vaso-occlusive symptoms under physiological conditions.

There are two cardinal pathophysiological features of sickle cell disease: chronic hemolytic anemia and vaso-occlusion, which results in ischemic tissue injury. Low oxygen tensions in the blood from ischemia or decreased partial pressures of oxygen in the air cause HgbS to crystallize, which distorts the RBCs into a sickle shape and makes them fragile and easily destroyed. Hemolytic anemia may be related to repeated cycles of sickling and unsickling. Tissue injury is usually produced by hypoxia secondary to the obstruction of blood vessels by sickled erythrocytes. The sickled cells are unable to squeeze through the smaller blood vessels, and tissues supplied by these blood vessels undergo ischemia. The organs at greatest risk for damage are those with venous sinuses where blood flow is low and oxygen tension and pH are low (spleen and bone marrow) and those with a limited terminal arterial blood supply (eye and head of the femur and humerus). The kidney is also at risk, especially as the patient ages.

Regardless of the disease process, the decreased oxygen transport to tissues carries the same results. Decreased mitochondrial oxygenation at the cellular level leads to decreased ATP production and reliance on the glycolytic process, resulting in poor energy generation and the formation of lactic acid, which affects the body's acid-base balance. It also affects the functioning of the body's largest energy consumer, the sodium-potassium-ATPase pump. As this pump works less efficiently, fluid and electrolyte shifts occur. Activation of the renin-angiotensin-aldosterone system augments the fluid shifts, with resultant sodium and water retention.

A reduction in the number of circulating RBCs affects the consistency and volume of blood. The less viscous blood flows faster and more turbulently and may cause ventricular dysfunction, cardiac dilation, and heart valve insufficiency. Increased venous return to the heart stimulates the heart to pump harder and faster, resulting in tachycardia and the risk of heart failure. To better oxygenate the reduced number of RBCs, the respiratory rate and depth increase. If the anemia is severe enough to overcome the usual compensatory mechanisms, the patient experiences shortness of breath, a rapid pounding pulse, dizziness, and fatigue, even at rest.

Other body systems are also affected. Figure 26–1 in Chapter 26 depicts the pathophysiological changes associated with the decreased oxygen transport. These are the same changes that are seen in the patient with anemia, because the underlying pathology is the same.

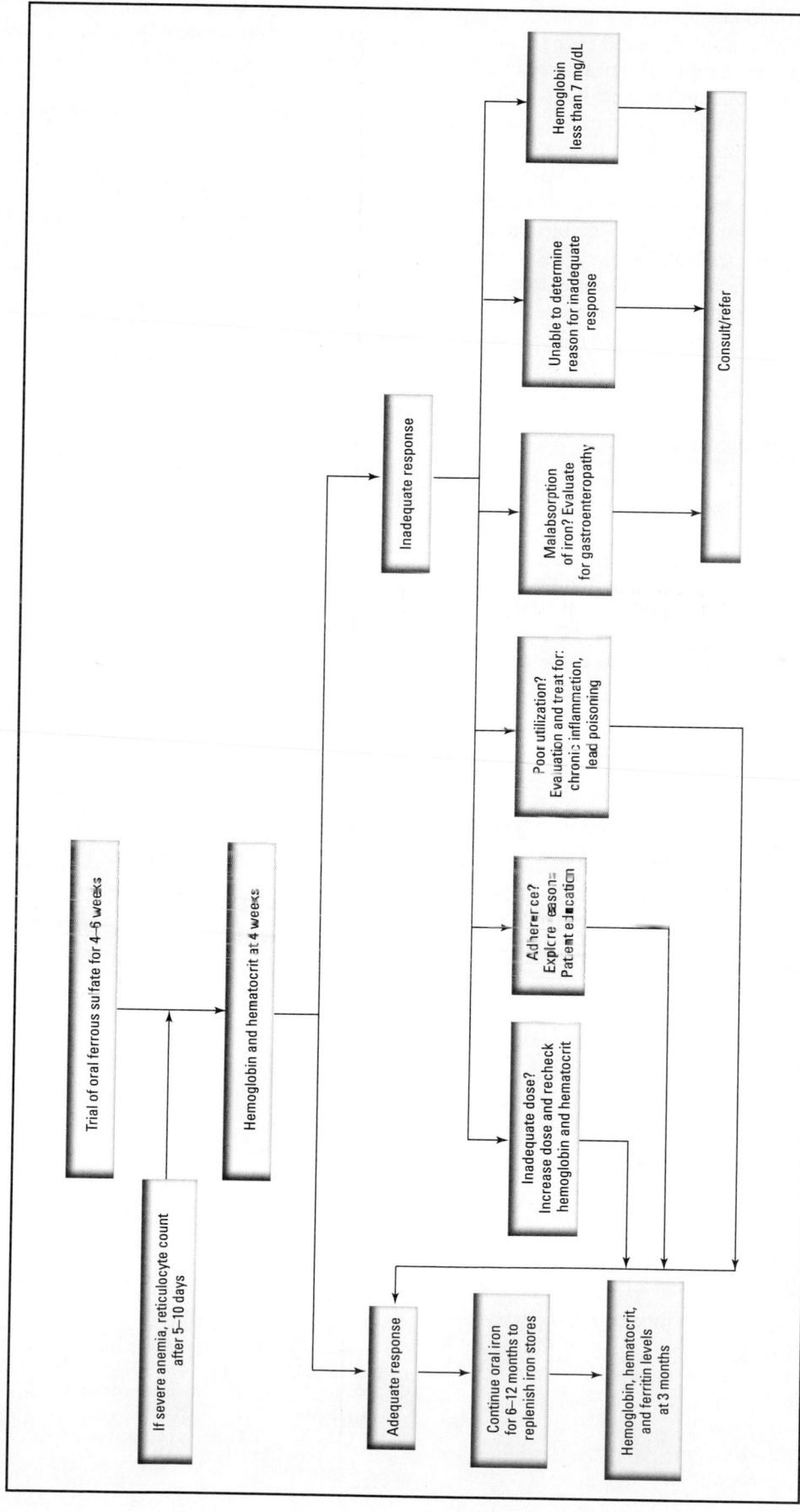

Figure 25–1. Drug treatment algorithm for iron-deficiency anemia.

Goals of Treatment

The ultimate goal of treatment for all types of anemia is to provide adequate oxygen transport to body tissues. For patients with IDA, FDA, and PA, this may be seen in a return to normal in the number and character of RBCs and to normal hemoglobin values. ACD is normocytic and normochromic, so the goal is a return to the normal number of RBCs and to normal hemoglobin values. Table 25–1 shows the normal blood indices for each age and sex grouping. The goal of treatment for SCA is prevention of the morbidity and mortality associated with this disease and reduction in the percentage of HgbS in the blood.

Rational Drug Selection

Iron-Deficiency Anemia

Risk Stratification and Screening

Growth and development and gender factors play important roles in risk stratification. The fetus stores iron during the last trimester, providing the infant with stores that usually last about 6 months. Preterm infants may have only 3 months of iron stores, and they grow at a more rapid rate, compounding the problem of poor iron stores. Although 95 percent of all iron from old RBCs is recycled, the diet is the major source of replacement iron. For infants, 50 percent of the iron in breast milk is absorbed, as opposed to 10 percent from cow's milk. Breastfeeding reduces the risk for IDA. The early addition of solid foods to the infant's diet may impair the ability to absorb iron, and solid foods should be introduced slowly, with conscious inclusion of foods high in iron. Consider iron supplementation for infants fed on formula. Infants should be screened with hemoglobin and hematocrit tests at age 9 to 12 months, when iron stores may be depleted and the possibility of anemia exists.

Iron needs increase during periods of rapid growth. Teenage girls are in a high-risk group because of their growth spurt and the onset of menstruation. National surveys suggest that teenage girls do not ingest adequate iron in their diets. This risk group should be screened with hemoglobin and hematocrit tests at age 12 to14 years, based on their onset of menstruation.

Children between age 1 and 2 years are particularly prone to IDA, according to the Centers for Disease

Table 25–1. Normal Anemia-Related Blood Values by Age and Gender

Age/Gender	Hemoglobin (g/100 cc)	Hematocrit	RBC Count (million/mm³)	Mean Corpuscle Volume (μm³) Concentration (pg/cell)	Mean Corpuscle Hemoglobin Concentration (pg/cell)	RBC Distribution Width
Infants 9–12 mo	11.4–14.1	32–41%	2.7–4.9	78	30–33	
Children 1–9 y	11–14.5	32–41%	3.7–5.3	77–81	31–34	
Children 9–12 y	12–15	34–43%	4.0–5.2	83–86	31–34	
Adolescents 12–14 y Male Female	12–16 11.5–15	35–45% 34–44%	4.5–5.3 4.1–5.1	78–88 78–90	31–34	
Adolescents 15–17 y Male Female	12.3–16.6 11.7–15.3	37–48% 34–44%	4.5–5.3 4.1–5.1	Adult levels Adult levels	31–34	
Adults 18+ y Male Female	13.2–17.3 11.7–15.5	40–54% 35–47%	4.2–5.4 3.6–5.0	Both genders: Microcytic = <87 Normocytic = 87–103 Macrocytic = >103	Both genders: Hypochromic = <32 Normochromic = 32–36 Hyperchromic = >36	Both genders: 11.5–14.5% CU

CU=conventional units.

Control and Prevention. Typically, they consume large quantities of milk, which is poor in iron, at a time when they need iron the most because of their growth. If they exhibit signs and symptoms consistent with anemia, they should be screened with hemoglobin and hematocrit tests. Lead poisoning can also contribute to IDA in young children. At-risk children should be screened for blood lead levels between age 12 and 72 months.

Although anemia is common in older adults, that is older men and postmenopausal women, in this population it is usually due to gastrointestinal (GI) blood loss associated with ulcers, the use of **aspirin** or **nonsteroidal anti-inflammatory drugs (NSAIDs),** or chronic disease rather than to iron deficiency. A study of carefully selected older adults (screened for health status, socioeconomic status, race, nutritional status, and altitude of residence) revealed that no older women had hemoglobin values of less than 12 g/dL, and only 2.3 percent of older men had values below 14 g/dL (Daly, 1989). Another study of healthy, very old people revealed little fluctuation in hemoglobin values, even into the ninth decade (Daly, 1989). With the exception of older adults with lower socioeconomic status, African-Americans, and patients with concomitant diseases that place them at risk, screening for IDA is not appropriate in the elderly (Daly, 1989).

Women generally have smaller stores of iron than men and have increased loss through menstruation, and their balance between intake and loss of iron is precarious. IDA occurs frequently in nonpregnant women of childbearing age because of menstruation, and it occurs to some extent in virtually all pregnant women because their iron stores have to serve the increased blood volume of the mother and be a source of hemoglobin for the growing fetus. Women in general should be screened for IDA at annual physical exams, and pregnant women should have this screening included as part of their regular prenatal care.

Table 25–2 displays common laboratory values associated with various anemias. The hemoglobin and hematocrit are used for screening; the other values are used to differentiate the type of anemia.

Algorithm

Treatment of IDA begins with prevention, but iron deficiency cannot be overcome with increased dietary intake alone. **Iron** supplements are always required.

Lifestyle Modification

The primary goal of management for IDA is prevention. The key to prevention of IDA not due to a disease process is adequate nutrition. Prevention starts with breastfeeding for infants. Because breast milk does not contain enough iron to allow the maximal growth of an infant who is more than 4 months old, breast-fed infants should receive supplemental **iron** drops, beginning at that age. Formula-fed infants should use an iron-fortified formula. Children and adults need to eat sufficient amounts of iron-rich foods. Foods rich in iron that the body can readily absorb include raisins, meats, fish, poultry, eggs, legumes, potatoes, and rice. The iron in many vegetables is poorly absorbed, so vegetarians must pay special attention to their intake of legumes and rice. Chapter 8 includes a more detailed discussion of nutrition. Table 25–3 presents iron intake recommendations for the prevention and treatment of IDA.

Table 25–2. Laboratory Findings in Selected Anemias

Test	Iron-Deficiency Anemia	Folic Acid–Deficiency Anemia	Pernicious Anemia	Anemia of Chronic Disease	Sickle Cell Anemia
Hemoglobin	Low	Low	Low	Low	Low (5–11 g/dL)
Hematocrit	Low	Low	Low	Low	Low (about 20%)
Reticulocyte count	Normal	Low	Low	Normal	Low (5–20%)
Plasma iron	Low	High	High	Normal or low	Normal
Total iron-binding capacity	High	Normal	Normal	Normal or low	Normal
Ferritin	Low	High	High	Normal	Normal
Transferrin	Low	Slightly high	Slightly high	Slightly low	Normal

Table 25–3. Iron Intake Recommendations for the Prevention and Treatment of Iron-Deficiency Anemia

Risk Group	Prevention	Treatment
Infants (age 6–12 mo)	• Breastfeeding for first y • Iron supplement after age 4 mo: 4–6 mo: 1 mg/kg/d 6–12 mo: 10 mg/d • Non-breast-fed infants need 1 mg/kg/d of iron from birth to 6 mo; 10 mg/d from 6–12 mo • Preterm infants may start on 2–4 mg/kg of iron at age 2 mo in anticipation of small iron stores • Begin iron-rich cereals at age 6 mo	Up to 6 mg/kg/d of elemental iron in 3–4 divided doses
Children 1–12 y: 12–21 y: Male: Female:	10 mg/d of iron 12–5 mg/d of iron 15–30 mg/d of iron Diet should include iron-rich foods	1–2 y: 6 mg/kg/d of elemental iron in 3–4 divided doses 2–12 y: 3 mg/kg/d of elemental iron in 3–4 divided doses 12–21 y: 150–250 mg of elemental iron/d Ferrous sulfate is best choice for oral iron Absorption enhanced by taking it on an empty stomach or with vitamin C and E; milk, antacids, tea, and food interfere with absorption
Adults Male: Female:	 12–15 mg/d of iron 15–30 mg/d or iron Diet should be high in iron-rich foods	150–250 mg of elemental iron/d (e.g., ferrous sulfate 300–325 mg tid or qid)
Pregnant and lactating women	30–60 mg of elemental iron daily during last two trimesters and while lactating	Ferrous sulfate 300–325 mg/d

Learning energy conservation techniques, such as planning rest periods, pacing activities, keeping objects within reach when performing tasks, and sitting down when doing chores are other important lifestyle modifications for the patient with IDA.

Drug Therapy

Once the decision is made to begin drug therapy, the choice of drug is based on age and gender variables. Figure 25–1 delineates the drug treatment algorithm for IDA. See Table 25–3 for the dosages of **iron** recommended for infants, children, adolescents, adults, and during pregnancy and lactation. Chapter 16 has a more detailed discussion of **iron** formulations, including their cost. Although Chapter 16 includes **ferrous sulfate, gluconate,** and **fumarate** formulations, **ferrous sulfate** is the least expensive and best absorbed. Slow-release and enteric-coated compounds have been advertised to re-

duce GI distress, and they require only once-daily dosing. However, they dissolve slowly and can bypass the proximal small bowel, where most absorption of iron takes place. They are also significantly more expensive. GI upset can be reduced by adjusting the dosage and by taking the drug with food. There is no evidence to suggest that these formulations are worth the extra cost.

Monitoring

The response to **iron** therapy is apparent within 10 days of initiating therapy. The first change noted in blood values is an increase in the reticulocyte count, followed by a rise in hemoglobin concentration of 0.1 to 0.2 g/100 cc per day. If the anemia is severe (hemoglobin less than 8 g/dL), a reticulocyte count can be obtained 5 to 10 days after initiating therapy. If the anemia is not severe, the hemoglobin and hematocrit levels are checked at 4 weeks, and the ferritin level is also assessed at 3 months.

Outcome Evaluation

Several weeks of therapy are required to bring hemoglobin levels back into the normal range, and replenishing iron stores may take months. Speed is not the issue, however, unless there is rapid blood loss. In that case, consultation or referral to a physician is appropriate. Hemoglobin, hematocrit, and RBC indices should be evaluated at 4 weeks, 3 months, and annually.

If the hemoglobin level does not return to normal limits within 6 weeks, the inadequate response should be evaluated. If the dose is inadequate, it may be increased. Starting with a lower dose and gradually increasing it reduces the likelihood of adverse reactions that may hamper adherence to the treatment regimen. Persistent, unrecognized blood loss should be sought with stool specimens for occult blood and for ova and parasites. Referral to a gastroenterologist for x-rays and endoscopy may be necessary. The source of the blood loss should then be treated. If there is a history of poor weight gain, diarrhea and other GI symptoms, or surgery on the GI tract, malabsorption syndromes should be ruled out. Poor iron utilization can result from chronic inflammation, lead poisoning, or sideroblastic anemia. Chronic inflammation can be demonstrated with elevated sedimentation rates, elevated iron and total iron-binding capacity levels, low percentage of iron saturation, and high ferritin levels. Lead poisoning is demonstrated with increased serum lead levels and basophilic stippling on RBC morphology. Sideroblastic anemia is usually found in infancy. Laboratory values reveal high ferritin levels, normal or high iron and total iron binding capacity levels, and elevated bone marrow stores of iron. Each of these disorders must be treated before iron therapy can be successful. When the history, physical examination, and standard laboratory analyses do not lead to a determination of the cause of the inadequate response, or the initial hemoglobin level is less than 7 g/dL, consultation with or referral to a hematology specialist is appropriate.

Patient Education

Patient education related to IDA should focus on:

1. Understanding the pathophysiology of IDA and its potential long-term effects
2. Recognizing the importance of prevention and the role of diet and energy conservation
3. The importance of adherence to the treatment regimen
4. The need for follow-up visits with the primary care provider because IDA can recur

Prevention of iron deficiency is discussed in some detail in Chapter 16. Stress to the patient that a diet with sufficient amounts of iron-rich foods may avoid the need for supplemental **iron** therapy, but only after the IDA has been resolved.

When diet alone is inadequate or when iron needs are very high, as in pregnancy, drug therapy is initiated. Patient education specific to drug therapy includes:

1. The reason for taking **iron**
2. Doses and schedules for the drug
3. Potential drug interactions and the need to inform other providers that they are taking **iron**
4. Possible adverse reactions and ways to reduce them. The most common adverse reactions that lead to nonadherence are GI problems such as nausea and constipation. Taking **iron** with food reduces the total amount absorbed but can also reduce the nausea. Adequate fluids and fiber can prevent constipation.

Additional patient education related to **iron** therapy is presented in Chapter 16.

Folic Acid–Deficiency Anemia

Risk Groups

Several patient populations, including age-based, gender-based, and concomitant disease based groups, are at risk for folic acid deficiency. Certain drugs are also associated with effects on dihydrofolate reductase, an enzyme critical to folate synthesis.

Infants who are fed powdered milk products or goat's milk develop this deficiency because these products are deficient in both folic acid and vitamin B_{12}. Older children who are exclusively vegetarian or who have severe nutritional deficiencies, absorption problems, or tapeworm infestations are also at risk. Prolonged cooking of vegetables destroys folates and can result in deficiency if such foods are the only source of this vitamin. Older adults whose diets lack vegetables, eggs, and meat often develop folic acid deficiency.

Women are not especially at risk unless they become pregnant. Pregnant women have increased folate requirements and may become deficient, especially if their diets were already marginal. Evidence suggests that maternal folic acid deficiency is associated with increased risk for neural tube defects in the fetus.

Disease states associated with folic acid deficiency caused by impaired absorption include sprue, heavy giardial infections, and short bowel syndrome. Disease states that result in deficiency because of increased demand include hyperthyroidism, hemolytic anemia, malignancy, and other chronic debilitating disorders. Alcoholics and patients with liver disease develop deficiency because of poor diet and reduced hepatic storage of folates. There is also evidence that **alcohol** interferes with the absorption and metabolism of folates. Patients undergoing renal dialysis lose folates from the plasma during dialysis, and that results in deficiency.

Drugs that interfere with folate absorption or metabolism include **phenytoin (Dilantin)** and some other **anticonvulsants, methotrexate (Folex), oral contraceptives, isoniazid (INH), triamterene (Dyrenium), trimethoprim (Trimpex),** and **pyrimethamine (Daraprim).** Patients who take these drugs, especially on a long-term basis, should be monitored for folate deficiency.

Drug Therapy

Oral **folic acid** is well absorbed, and doses of 1 to 2 mg/day result in correction of the deficiency in 4 to 5 weeks. Hemoglobin levels begin to rise within the first week, and the anemia is completely corrected in 1 to 2 months. Because of the potential teratogenic effects of folate deficiency in pregnant women, women of childbearing age should take prophylactic doses of 0.1 to 0.4 mg/day and continue this dose throughout any pregnancy. **Folic acid** supplementation to prevent deficiency should also be considered in the other high-risk patients mentioned previously. Detailed discussion of clinical use and dosing of **folic acid** is provided in Chapter 16.

Monitoring

The only monitoring required is to follow hemoglobin and hematocrit levels at regular intervals. The timing of such assessment is based on the acute versus chronic nature of the cause of the deficiency.

Patient Education

Patient education focuses on prevention as well as treatment. Diet and appropriate cooking methods are central to prevention, especially for strict vegetarians. Women of childbearing age should have the need for **folic acid** supplementation discussed during health care provider encounters for any reason. Alcoholics require special attention and help in correcting this addiction. When diet alone is inadequate or folate needs are very high, as in pregnancy, drug therapy is initiated. Patient education specific to drug therapy includes:

1. The reason for taking **folic acid**
2. The doses and schedule for the drug
3. The fact that some drugs may potentially interfere with folate metabolism
4. The need to inform their providers that they are taking supplemental **folic acid.** More specific discussion of patient education is found in Chapter 16.

Pernicious Anemia

Risk Groups

The underlying disorder in PA is usually defective secretion of gastric intrinsic factor, which is necessary for vitamin B_{12} absorption. It is most common in northern Europeans and older adults, but can occur in any age or ethnic group. Partial or total gastrectomy and small bowel resection are the two most common iatrogenic causes of this problem. The former surgery removes the parietal cell–containing portion of the stomach that secretes intrinsic factor, and the latter surgery removes a portion of the bowel that absorbs the vitamin B_{12}–intrinsic factor complex. Diseases of the terminal ileum, fish tapeworm, thyroid diseases, and bacterial overgrowth in the small bowel from stasis can also cause PA. Nutritional deficiency is rare but may be seen in strict vegetarians after several years without meat, eggs, or dairy products.

Screen for PA any of these risk groups and other patients who present with the neurological symptoms of peripheral neuropathy, symmetrical paresthesias in the hands and feet progressing to ataxia from loss of vibratory and position sense, memory loss, depression, agitation, personality change or central visual scotomata. This is especially true for older adults, in which some of these changes may be confused with senile dementia.

Drug Therapy

Because the underlying problem in almost all cases of pernicious anemia is malabsorption, parenteral therapy with **vitamin B_{12}** is required. With the exception of the correctable disease processes in the risk groups previously mentioned, the injections must be taken for the remainder of the patient's life. Correctable conditions require treatment of the underlying problem, and parenteral therapy continues temporarily. **Oral vitamin B_{12}** is useful only for the rare case of nutritional deficit and for patients who cannot take the parenteral form. Parenteral doses begin at 100 µg; oral doses up to 1000 µg may result in enough absorption to correct the problem in some cases.

The hematologic response to parenteral **vitamin B_{12}** is rapid. The bone marrow usually returns to normal within 48 hours. Reticulocytosis begins on the second or third day and is usually maximal by the fifth to tenth day. Hemoglobin and hematocrit levels should return to normal within 1 to 2 months. Sudden drops in serum potassium levels have been reported with **vitamin B_{12}** therapy. Serum potassium levels should be monitored and supplemental **oral potassium** given if needed.

Chapter 16 has a detailed discussion of rational drug selection and dosing for **vitamin B_{12}**. Although it is not urgent to treat most cases of PA, the reversibility of neurological deficits is, to some extent, dependent upon their duration. Patients with neurological symptoms should have this disorder promptly diagnosed and treated. When neurological symptoms are present, twice-monthly dosing is recommended for 6 months prior to beginning the usual monthly dose.

Monitoring

Reticulocyte counts, hemoglobin and hematocrit, iron, folic acid, and vitamin B$_{12}$ serum levels are obtained prior to treatment, between the fifth and seventh day of therapy, and then frequently until the hemoglobin and hematocrit are normal. Relapse of symptoms is not uncommon in the presence of continuing therapy. Blood counts should continue at regular intervals throughout the patient's lifetime, based on individual response to therapy. Because of the potential for sudden drops in serum potassium levels, these should also be monitored at the same time as hemoglobin and hematocrit levels are drawn. The Schilling test is used for diagnosis but not as a monitoring tool.

Patient Education

Patient education related to PA should focus on:

1. Understanding the pathophysiology of PA and its potential long-term effects
2. The importance of adherence to the treatment regimen
3. The need for follow-up visits with the primary care provider in that PA and its symptoms can recur, even with continuing therapy

Patient education specific to the drug therapy includes:

1. The reason for taking the **vitamin B$_{12}$**
2. The fact that the **oral vitamin B$_{12}$** found in multivitamin tablets or the higher doses found in health food stores are not appropriate to treat the problem
3. The doses and schedule for the drug
4. The fact that patients need to take the drug for the remainder of their lives

Anemia of Chronic Disease

Risk Stratification and Screening

This form of anemia is the most common form in older adults and is associated with several specific chronic diseases, including chronic renal failure, osteomyelitis, tuberculosis, rheumatoid diseases, hepatitis, carcinoma, myeloma, lymphoma, and leukemia. Older adults with any chronic illness and patients of any age with these illnesses should be evaluated for the presence of anemia. ACD is usually mild and asymptomatic, but some patients may present with fatigue, shortness of breath, loss of appetite, weight loss, or light-headedness after mild activity. Because these symptoms may be the same as those seen with the underlying chronic illness, it is important to include evaluation for anemia in the workup for these disorders.

Algorithm

There is no effective therapy directed specifically at ACD. Treatment of the underlying chronic disease is necessary to resolve the anemia. Sometimes patients have a concomitant IDA that is amenable to treatment with **iron,** but otherwise oral **iron** is not necessary. When ACD is caused by chronic renal failure, the cause is probably associated in part with decreased production of erythropoietin by the kidney. In this case, administration of **epoetin alfa (Epogen)** may lead to an increase of 6 to 10 percent in the hematocrit within 6 weeks. The malignant diseases causing ACD may also require the use of this drug, which is discussed in Chapter 16. The main focus of therapy for ACD, besides treatment of the underlying disease, is energy conservation.

Sickle Cell Anemia

This chapter does not discuss the total management of sickle cell disease. The reader is referred to National Institutes of Health publication 95–2117 for a complete discussion and guidelines for management of common problems, such as pain and infection. This chapter focuses on management of the anemia and precipitants of sickling and the resultant ischemia.

Prevention

Prevention of the morbidity and mortality associated with the hemolytic anemia of sickle cell disease is focused on avoidance of the precipitants of a sickling crisis. Serious bacterial infections, especially those due to *Streptococcus pneumoniae, Haemophilus influenzae,* and *Mycoplasma pneumoniae,* are a major cause of sickling. Patients and their parents need to be taught early recognition of signs and symptoms of these infections, and early aggressive treatment is critical. Children with sickle cell disease should also receive pneumococcal and influenza **vaccines** and all other childhood immunizations. Dehydration is another precipitant. Adequate hydration (2 quarts/day or more in children and adults) should be stressed, especially during periods of elevated environmental temperature and physical activity. Exposure to cold, with its resultant vasoconstriction, can precipitate a sickling event and should be avoided. Although strenuous exercise may precipitate a sickling event, there is no evidence that most exercise is harmful, and the beneficial effects of exercise are well known. Children with sickle cell disease are encouraged to participate in physical activities and set their own limits. Exercise capacity is reduced by as much as 50 percent in adults with sickle cell disease. Participation in noncompetitive recreational activities that do not involve strenuous exercise should be encouraged. Any activity that results in exhaustion, whether recreation or employment, should be discouraged. Exercise under adverse conditions, such as cold weather, high altitude, or cold water exposure, should also be avoided.

Dietary Counseling

Dietary counseling is an important part of patient care. Mothers should be encouraged to breast-feed their infants, although iron-fortified formulas are an acceptable alternative. Foods high in iron should be encouraged in children and adults. Chapter 6 has more information on foods high in iron.

Drug Therapy

Patients with SCA do not usually have concurrent IDA. **Supplemental *iron* should not be prescribed unless the patient is documented to have reduced iron stores by specific assessments of the serum ferritin level or measurement of serum iron and iron-binding capacity.** Children with SCA are often microcytic in the absence of iron deficiency. The incidence of alpha thalassemia trait is also quite high in African-Americans and may produce microcytosis in the absence of iron deficiency. Routine administration of supplemental **folic acid** is also not necessary unless the diet history reveals inadequate folate intake, for example, low intake of green leafy vegetables. Most patients eat poorly during painful crises, and daily supplements of 1 mg of **folic acid** should be prescribed during those times. Other reasons for **folate** supplementation are discussed in Chapter 8. The danger of masking a vitamin B_{12} deficiency is small, but African-American patients are at risk. There is no evidence that any other form of vitamin supplementation is of value in sickle cell disease.

Infections also enhance susceptibility to vaso-occlusive events and their subsequent ischemia. Prophylactic **penicillin** is so effective in reducing the number of life-threatening episodes of pneumococcal sepsis in children under age 5 that most states screen newborns for sickle cell disease so they can be placed on the drug by age 2 to 3 months. Oral **penicillin VK** 125 mg bid is given until age 3 years, then 250 mg bid is given until age 5 years. Prophylaxis in older children has not been shown to be beneficial and may be unnecessary after pneumococcal immunizations are complete and antibody titers are protective. **Penicillin** is discussed in more detail in Chapter 22.

Although there is no drug to cure sickle cell disease, **hydroxyurea (Hydrea)** has been shown to reduce the frequency of sickle cell crisis in adults by as much as 50 percent. The Multicenter Study of Hydroxyurea (MSH) in Sickle Cell Anemia (Bonds, 1995) did not enroll children. The dosing schedule in the MSH trial was 15 mg/kg initially, with the dose increased by 5 mg/kg every 12 weeks

until the maximum dose of 35 mg/kg/day was reached unless toxicity was observed. If toxicity occurred, treatment was stopped until the bone marrow recovered and then was restarted at a dose 2.5 mg/kg less than the previous dose. If no toxicity occurred after 12 weeks on the lower dose, the subsequent dose was increased by 2.5 mg/kg/day. Toxicity was defined as absolute neutrophil counts lower than 2000/mm^3, absolute reticulocyte counts lower than 80,000/mm^3, platelet counts lower than 80,000/mm^3, or a fall in hemoglobin from greater than or equal to 7 g/dL to 4.5 to 5 g/dL if reticulocytes were lower than 320,000 or hemoglobin lower than 4.5 g/dL.

Hydroxyurea may not be appropriate for all patients and should not be used for patients likely to become pregnant or those unwilling or unable to follow instructions regarding treatment. This drug is a cytotoxic agent and has the potential to cause life-threatening cytopenia. The onset of leukopenia and thrombocytopenia may occur within 10 days of beginning therapy. White blood cell and platelet counts should be monitored prior to and periodically during therapy. Because it attacks rapidly growing cells, stomatitis, anorexia, nausea, vomiting, and diarrhea may occur. Good oral hygiene and monitoring of nutritional status are important. If the decision is made to try this drug, referral to or consultation with a hematologist is suggested.

Experimental drug therapy is being tried with **erythropoietin** to determine its capability in augmenting the production of hemoglobin F (HgbF) (fetal). HgbF interferes with the polymerization of HgbS in solution and with the sickling of HgbS RBCs. **Butyrate,** a simple fatty acid widely used as a food additive, is also being investigated as an agent that may increase HgbF production. Their role in therapy, alone or in combination with **hydroxyurea,** is still unclear. **Erythropoietin** is discussed in Chapter 16. **Clotrimazole (Mycelex),** commonly used to treat fungal infections, is under investigation to prevent the loss of water from RBCs that contributes to sickling. Antifungal agents are presented in Chapter 22.

Transfusions

With the mild to moderate anemia common to sickle cell disease, body systems except the eye and the spleen adapt fairly well to the reduced oxygen-carrying capacity of the blood. Most patients with sickle cell disease are relatively asymptomatic from their anemia and do not require transfusions to improve oxygen-carrying capacity. Transfusions may be used for specific indications when the anemia is severe or to prevent chronic complications. According the National Heart, Lung, and Blood Institute (NHLBI, 1995), indications for RBC transfusions include:

1. In severely anemic patients, simple transfusions without exchange when:

a. Patients are so anemic that they have physiological derangement that is manifested by impending or overt high-output cardiac failure, dyspnea, postural hypotension, angina, or cerebral dysfunction.

b. Patients have had a sudden diminution in hemoglobin concentration, particularly patients who are having an acute splenic or hepatic sequestration crisis, manifested by rapid spleen or liver enlargement and rapidly falling hematocrit.

c. Patients exhibit fatigue and dyspnea, usually at hemoglobin levels lower than 5 g/dL and a hematocrit less than 15 percent.

2. When there is a need to improve microvascular perfusion by decreasing the proportion of erythrocytes containing HgbS, an exchange transfusion is indicated unless the patient is severely anemic and has good cardiac function. Conditions for exchange transfusion include:

a. Acute or suspected cerebrovascular accident (CVA) or transient ischemic attack (TIA)

b. Multiorgan failure syndrome, including fat embolization

c. Acute chest syndrome or other acute lung disease, when arterial oxygen cannot be maintained at near-normal levels or when the process progresses despite **antibiotic** and other indicated therapy

d. Acute priapism unresponsive to therapy

e. Surgery on the posterior segment of the eye, even if done under local **anesthesia** or preparation for general **anesthesia**

3. Chronic transfusion programs, usually initiated by exchange transfusion, when:

a. Children have had CVA, to prevent further complications.

b. Chronic congestive heart failure exists in conjunction with other treatment.

In any case, the goal is a percentage of hemoglobin A (HgbA) greater than 50 to 70 percent. This usually requires repeated transfusion every 3 to 4 weeks. Maintaining this percentage has reduced the rate of cerebral infarction in children by 90 percent. When indications for transfusion exist, referral to or consultation with a physician is required. These serious conditions often require hospitalization.

Conditions that are not indications or are contraindications for transfusion therapy include: chronic steady-state anemia, uncomplicated acute painful crises, infections, minor surgery not requiring prolonged general **anesthesia** (e.g., myringotomy), aseptic necrosis of the hip or shoulder not requiring surgery, and uncomplicated pregnancy.

Transfusions are not without complications. Volume overload may require administration of **furosemide (Lasix)**, especially if the patient has cardiac dysfunction or minimal cardiac reserve. Iron overload can occur with chronic transfusions, usually after 1 to 3 years of therapy. Serum ferritin levels should be measured periodically. If the level is above 2000 ng/mL and transfusions are still required, chronic chelation therapy using nightly subcutaneous injections of **deferoxamine (Desferal)** 5 nights each week over several months is recommended by the NHLBI. Complications of this therapy include ototoxicity, ophthalmic toxicity, allergic reactions, growth failure, unusual infections, and pulmonary hypersensitivity. Annual visits to ophthalmological and audiological specialists for early detection of possible adverse reactions should be arranged. Ongoing education and support are usually necessary to maintain adherence to therapy. **Deferoxamine** should be discontinued during acute bacterial infections.

Bone Marrow Transplantation

Successful bone marrow transplantation can cure SCA. These transplants should be considered for severely affected children. According to Jones (1998), bone marrow transplantation has been successful for some children but has not been successful for adults. There appears to be a narrow window of opportunity when transplantation may be advantageous. Referral to a physician in a major medical center is usually required, and these transplants are still considered experimental.

Monitoring

Hemoglobin, hematocrit, reticulocyte counts, platelet counts, and white blood cell counts should be done frequently during the first year of life to establish the patient's baseline. After the first year, hemoglobin and hematocrit are relatively stable and need to be checked only once or twice a year in stable patients. Stable patients also require annual urinalysis, blood urea nitrogen (BUN), creatinine, and liver enzyme studies to monitor for evidence of organ damage. Before administration of transfusions, RBC antigens are needed. Patients with sickle cell disease are often difficult to crossmatch.

Most adults with sickle cell disease should have regular medical evaluations every 3 to 6 months. Blood counts, urinalysis, and routine chemistry tests should be done annually. With advancing age, complications such as chronic organ failure often require more frequent visits and more extensive laboratory evaluations. Attention focuses primarily on abnormalities in renal function and complications such as gallstones, aseptic necrosis, leg ulcers, and priapism.

Outcome Evaluation

The overall goal of therapy is the reduction in the number of sickling crises and prevention of organ damage. Hemoglobin level goals are 9 g/dL or greater, but levels of at least 7 g/dL may be acceptable in asymptomatic patients. The goal for percentage of HgbS is 30 percent or less. Outcomes for chronic transfusion therapy were presented previously.

Patient Education

Patient and parental information related to SCA should focus on:

1. Understanding the pathophysiology of sickle cell disease and the organs commonly damaged
2. Recognizing the importance of prevention, especially the central role of prevention of infection and avoidance of precipitants of sickling
3. Learning how to administer prophylactic **antibiotics** and other drugs
4. The importance of adherence to the treatment regimen
5. The need for regular follow-up visits with a primary care provider to manage this chronic disease
6. The role of genetic counseling

Prevention requires the parents and the patient to learn specific assessment skills. Any sign of illness in a child with sickle cell disease can be serious. Table 25–4 describes indications for seeking immediate medical help for infants, children, and adults. Patient education related to the administration of **penicillin** is discussed in Chapter 22. Measures to minimize the risk of vaso-occlusive events beyond prevention of infection were discussed previously. The hazards of cigarette smoking and excessive **alcohol** intake and the benefits of a well-planned exercise program should be included.

Although IDA is not common for patients with sickle cell disease, prevention of IDA with a diet that includes sufficient amounts of iron-rich foods should be discussed. When **iron** is required, follow the patient education instructions for IDA.

Patient education specific to the use of **hydroxyurea** includes:

1. Take the drug exactly as prescribed, even if nausea, vomiting, or diarrhea occurs.
2. If a dose is missed, do not take it at all; do not double doses.
3. Notify the health care provider of fever, chills, sore throat, loss of appetite, nausea, vomiting, diarrhea, bleeding gums, bruising, petechiae, or blood in the urine, stool, or emesis.
4. Avoid alcoholic beverages, **aspirin**, and **NSAIDs**, which may increase risk of bleeding.
5. Inspect oral mucosa for erythema and ulceration. If it occurs, use a sponge brush and rinse mouth with water after eating and drinking. If mouth pain interferes with eating, contact the health care provider for lidocaine-based mouthwash.

Table 25–4. Indications for Seeking Immediate Medical Attention for Infants, Children, and Adults with Sickle Cell Disease

Infants and Children
Rapid breathing or a breathing problem
Coughing frequently
Cranky and crying more than usual
Screaming when touched
Very tired or little energy; very weak
Vomiting, diarrhea
Does not want to eat
Has fewer wet diapers
Has pain or swelling in the abdomen
Has swollen hands or feet
Has pale blue or gray lips or skin
Adolescents and Adults
High fever
Productive cough
Sudden dyspnea
Weakness
Dizziness or postural hypotension
Angina
Very tired or little energy
Swollen hands or feet
Cloudy or foul-smelling urine; hematuria
Vomiting
Diarrhea
Acute priapism

6. Encourage fluid intake of 2000 to 3000 cc of non-caffeinated fluid daily.
7. Review need for contraception during therapy because of the teratogenic potential of this drug.

Patient education related to the other drugs used in treatment of sickle cell disease and its complications is presented in the Unit II chapters that include these drugs. Patient education related to the other complications of

Anemia

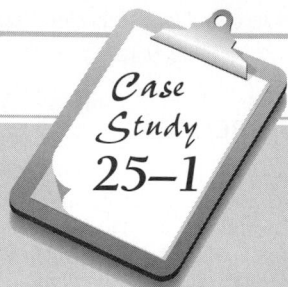

Complaint

Fatigue, tachycardia, and shortness of breath

History

Margaret is a 16-year-old female who presents at the clinic with fatigue, tachycardia, and shortness of breath during exercise in gym class. Her history includes onset of menses at age 12 with regular cycles, 5 days in length. She does not take any vitamin supplements. Her high school permits the students to leave the campus for lunch, and her lunch choices consist largely of fast foods. She does not eat breakfast. A specific question about iron-rich food indicated a low intake. Her weight is appropriate for her height. She is satisfied with her weight but does not want to gain any weight.

Assessment

Her laboratory values show hemoglobin at 9 g/dL, hematocrit at 32 percent, an RBC count of 3.8, a low mean corpuscular volume (MCV), and a reticulocyte count that is 0.4 percent of total RBCs. Suspecting IDA, her health care provider orders further laboratory studies that include low serum iron and ferritin levels and an increased total iron-binding capacity. Her physical examination has no findings outside normal parameters for her age and gender except slightly pale skin and conjunctiva.

Initial Management Plan

Margaret is diagnosed with mild to moderate IDA.

Initial therapy will include dietary measures, but because IDA cannot be corrected by diet alone, drug therapy will also be included. Her management plan is:

1. Start on generic ferrous sulfate tablets at 300 mg tid. Ferrous sulfate in this form is the least expensive and best absorbed of the ferrous compounds. Instruct her to take the drug on an empty stomach or with citrus juice. If she has GI problems, she may take the drug with food. This reduces absorption, but her anemia is mild to moderate, and an increased dose will not be required.
2. After assessing her knowledge base about dietary iron, begin teaching about food high in iron and place her on an iron-rich diet. Because eggs and whole-grain cereals are good sources of iron, begin by having her eat breakfast. Handy snacks such as raisins should be included. Margaret does not do the cooking at home, and her parents are included in the discussion of diet.
3. Keep her on the oral iron supplement for 4 weeks.
4. Have her keep a diet diary for these 4 weeks.

Follow-up Visit

At her follow-up visit in 4 weeks, she reported that she is now able to participate in gym class without tachycardia or shortness of breath. Hemoglobin and hematocrit levels are drawn. Because her anemia was not severe, a reticulocyte count was not drawn after 1 week of therapy. Her laboratory studies at this visit are minimally within the normal range for her age. A review of her diet diary shows that she has improved her intake of iron, although it could still be better, and she is eating breakfast. She did experience GI upset and began taking her tablets with her meals. She had forgotten about taking them with citrus juice.

Modifications to Management Plan

Based on this information, her management plan now includes:

1. Continue ferrous sulfate for 6 more months. Treatment for this length of time is required to correct the anemia and replenish iron stores.
2. Reinforce the need for iron-rich foods in her diet and negotiate ways to fit these foods into her diet.
3. Have her return to the clinic in 3 months for hemoglobin, hematocrit, and ferritin levels. If these are acceptable, keep her on supplemental iron for another 6 months and then determine need for further therapy.

Continuing Care

At the next visit, Margaret's laboratory results were within normal limits. Although she was inconsistent in her dietary changes, this is to be expected in adolescents. She was praised for her successes and encouraged to continue doing her best with the diet. Because adolescent females are a high-risk group for IDA, daily supplementation with ferrous sulfate 300 mg was continued.

sickle cell disease is detailed in the NIH publications in the reference list.

REFERENCES

Bonds, D. (January 30, 1995). *Clinical alert: Drug treatment for sickle cell anemia.* Rockville, MD.: National Institutes of Health, National Heart, Lung, and Blood Institute.

Burns, C., Barber, N., Brady, M., & Dunn, A. (1996). *Pediatric primary care.* Philadelphia: Saunders.

Daly, M. (1989). Anemia in the elderly. *American Family Physician, 39*(3), 129–136.

Goroll, A., May, L., & Mulley, A. (1995). *Primary care medicine* (3rd ed.). Philadelphia: Lippincott.

Haliotis, F., & Papanastasiou, D. (1998). Comparative study of tolerability and efficacy of iron protein succinylate versus iron hydroxide polymaltose complex in the treatment of iron deficiency in children. *International Journal of Clinical Pharmacology and Therapeutics, 36*(6), 320–325.

Jones, L. (1998). Sickle cell anemia in adults: Avoiding crises, organ damage. *Annals of Internal Medicine, 128*(12), 1055–1056.

National Heart, Lung, and Blood Institute. (1996). *Facts about sickle cell anemia* (National Institutes of Health publ. 96–4057). Rockville, MD.: NIH.

National Heart, Lung, and Blood Institute. (1995). *Management and therapy of sickle cell disease* (National Institutes of Health publ. 95–2117). Rockville, MD.: NIH.

Richer, S. (1997). A practical guide for differentiating between iron deficiency anemia and anemia of chronic disease in children and adults. *Nurse Practitioner, 22*(4), 82–103.

Use of folic acid–containing supplements among women of childbearing age—United States, 1997. *Morbidity and Mortality Weekly Report, 47,* 131–134.

CHAPTER 26

·······

Chronic Stable Angina and Low-Risk Unstable Angina

CHAPTER OUTLINE

A ngina is a clinical syndrome typically characterized by deep, poorly localized chest or arm discomfort that is reproducibly associated with physical exertion or emotional stress and promptly relieved by rest or **nitroglycerin**. The pathophysiology behind it is an imbalance between myocardial oxygen supply and demand (ischemia) associated with coronary artery disease (CAD). Several million Americans suffer from ischemic heart disease, and more than 600,000 die each year from this disorder or its complications. Chronic stable angina is the form most commonly seen in primary care, but even these patients have a mortality risk of 2 to 12 percent annually.

Treatment includes both pharmacological and surgical interventions. Pharmacological management includes the use of **nitrates, beta-adrenergic blockers, calcium channel blockers,** and **aspirin.** These drugs are discussed in detail in Chapters 12, 14, and 16. Concomitant disorders often include diabetes mellitus, hyperlipidemia, and hypertension, so that the treatment regimen can be quite complex; Chapters 31, 37, and 38, respectively, discuss management of these specific disorders. The focus of this chapter is the long-term management of chronic stable angina and low-risk unstable angina that is usually done by primary care providers.

Pathophysiology

The coronary arteries supply oxygen to the myocardium. Oxygen extraction from these vessels is at maximum efficiency at all times, and there is no oxygen reserve during periods of increased oxygen demand. Ischemia occurs when demand exceeds supply. The only mechanism available to increase oxygen supply is to dilate the arteries and bring more blood flow to the myocardium.

Imbalances between myocardial supply and demand can result from a variety of conditions. Supply is reduced by (1) hemodynamic factors such as increased resistance in coronary vessels, hypotension, and decreased blood volume; (2) cardiac factors such as decreases in diastolic filling time, increases in heart rate, and valvular incompetence; (3) hematologic factors such as the oxygen content of the blood, the acid-base status of the blood, and anemia; and (4) systemic disorders, such as shock, that reduce blood flow or the availability of oxygen. Demand is increased by (1) high systolic blood pressure; (2) increased ventricular volume; (3) increased thickness of the myocardium (ventricular hypertrophy); (4) increased heart rate resulting from exercise, stress, hyperthyroidism, fever, anemia, or hyperviscosity of the blood, and (5) conditions that heighten the myocardium's contractile response.

Another leading cause of imbalance between supply and demand is the decreased blood flow associated with atherosclerosis. Plaque formation results in narrowing or occlusion of the artery. Narrowing of a major coronary artery by more than 50 percent impairs blood flow sufficiently to hamper cellular metabolism under conditions of increased demand. Thrombus formation can also result from ulceration of atherosclerotic plaque. Platelet aggregation releases prostaglandin thromboxane A_2, a potent vasoconstrictor capable of causing vasospasms. Thromboxane A_2 also promotes platelet aggregation, resulting in a vicious circle of vasoconstriction and platelet buildup in the arterial walls.

Ischemia with pain is angina. There are three types of angina: chronic stable angina, unstable angina, and Prinzmetal's angina. Chronic stable angina (exertional angina) is caused by narrowing of the arterial lumen and hardening of the arterial walls, so that the affected vessels cannot dilate in response to the increased myocardial oxygen demand associated with physical exertion or emotional stress. Research indicates that up to 90 percent of ischemia is asymptomatic (silent ischemia). Diabetes mellitus and hypertension are associated with an increased prevalence of silent ischemia. Ischemia with or without pain has the same prognosis. In both cases, the myocardium is at risk.

On the cellular level, the myocardium becomes cyanotic within the first 10 seconds of impaired oxygen supply, and electrocardiographic (ECG) changes occur. Deprived of oxygen, the myocardial cells convert to anaerobic metabolism, and lactic acid accumulates. Myocardial nerve fibers are irritated by this lactic acid and transmit a pain message to the cardiac nerves and upper thoracic posterior nerve roots. Under ischemic conditions, cardiac cells are viable for about 20 minutes. The supply-demand imbalance must be resolved during this time to prevent permanent damage.

Pharmacodynamics

Nitrates affect the supply-demand equation on both sides. Dilating peripheral blood vessels results in decreased systemic vascular resistance (afterload), venous pooling, and decreased venous return to the heart. Myocardial oxygen demand is reduced by the reduced cardiac workload. The decreased venous return to the heart also decreases left ventricular end-diastolic pressure (preload), resulting in decreased wall tension and an increased transmyocardial gradient. This increased gradient improves perfusion between the coronary arteries on the outside of the heart and the subendocardium on the inside of the heart and increases oxygen supply to the myocardium. **Nitrates** also dilate coronary arteries to some extent, but doing so is difficult in severe atherosclerotic arteries, and this effect is now thought to be only a small part of their action in relieving ischemia.

Beta-adrenergic blockers affect the supply-demand equation on the demand side. Both **beta$_1$ selective agents** and **nonselective beta-adrenergic blockers** decrease the force of myocardial contractility and decrease heart rate and conduction velocity. **Nonselective beta-adrenergic blockers** also decrease systemic vascular resistance and blood pressure (afterload). All of these reduce myocardial oxygen demand.

Calcium channel blockers affect the supply-demand equation on both sides of the equation. Inhibition of calcium entry into cells reduces smooth muscle contraction, which results in peripheral vasodilation that leads to decreased venous return to the heart (preload) and then to decreased oxygen demand. **Calcium channel blockers** also decrease coronary artery spasm and relax coronary artery smooth muscle, causing dilation and improved myocardial oxygen supply. **Verapamil** and **diltiazem** also significantly reduce myocardial contractility and slow conduction through calcium-dependent fibers in the sinoatrial (SA) and atrioventricular (AV) nodes, resulting in decreased heart rate. These two actions decrease myocardial oxygen demand. The **dihydropyridines** do not have this action.

Aspirin inhibits the synthesis of thromboxane A_2 in the production of platelets. This action reduces platelet aggregation to stop the cycle of vasoconstriction and platelet buildup. Research has clearly demonstrated a role for this drug in primary prevention of myocardial infarction (MI) as an adjunct to risk factor management.

Goals of Treatment

The more immediate goals are to control symptoms and restore an optimal level of exercise capacity. The ultimate goals of therapy are to reduce the risks of MI and death. Although the clinical course of some patients may extend for 15 or 20 years, most patients with chronic stable angina are still at increased risk for cardiovascular morbidity and mortality. Their prognosis is strongly affected by the number and locations of coronary artery stenosis, the severity of the ischemia, and the presence of other CAD risk factors, such as smoking, hypertension, hyperlipidemia, low high-density lipid (HDL) cholesterol, diabetes mellitus, and age and gender considerations. Achievement of these goals is through improving oxygen supply and decreasing oxygen demand.

Rational Drug Selection

Angina is associated with MI and sudden cardiac death in the mind of provider and public alike. This presents a two-edged sword in therapeutic management: recognition of the potential complications, leading to consistent adherence to the treatment regimen, versus denial of the seriousness of the disorder, leading to lack of adherence to the treatment regimen. The health care provider can improve adherence by placing angina in a realistic perspective and tailoring treatment options to each patient's needs. For effective management, the choice of treatment should be low cost, limited in complexity, and with the fewest possible adverse reactions. To achieve this treatment protocol, lifestyle modifications and pharmacological therapy are chosen based on risk stratification, grade of angina, and specific patient variables. For each of these variables, the therapy discussed includes lifestyle modifications, initial monotherapy, and two- and three-drug therapy.

Risk Stratification

Major Risk Factors

The major risk factors for CAD are age, family history, smoking, hypertension, hypercholesterolemia, low HDL cholesterol, and diabetes mellitus (discussed in Chapter 37 and shown in Table 37–1). In addition, conditions discussed here that decrease oxygen supply and increase oxygen demand are also major risk factors for ischemic heart disease. These include heart failure (see Chapter 34), anemia (see Chapter 25), hyperthyroidism (see Chapter 39), valvular heart disease, and morbid obesity.

Patients with angina only on exertion, a normal resting ECG, and symptoms that can be controlled by rest and intermittent **nitroglycerin** should be started on lifestyle modifications and have any concurrent aggravating factors or disease processes treated. For example, hypertension itself can cause angina, and elevated cholesterol contributes to the continued development of atherosclerosis. Their treatment is critical. Patients with known CAD, age 60 and older, with ECG changes on exertion, and with diabetes are considered high risk for unstable angina and should be started on both lifestyle modifications and drug therapy.

Classification System for Grading Angina

The New York Heart Association and the Canadian Cardiovascular Society have devised a classification system for grading the severity of angina (Table 26–1). The lower the class, the more likely the patient's angina can be controlled by lifestyle modification and intermittent **nitroglycerin** (Table 26–2). The higher the class, the more likely the patient is to require multiple drug therapy.

Treatment Algorithms

It is not within the scope of this book to discuss the testing involved in the diagnosis and grading of angina. The treatment protocol discussed assumes accurate diagnosis of angina with the appropriate diagnostic tools, including laboratory testing, chest x ray, ECG, and exercise testing. Once the diagnosis is made, protocols are based on the grade or class of angina and the risk profile. Table 26–3 shows the protocol, including drug therapy and surgical interventions, based on the grade or class of angina and the risk profile.

Lifestyle Modification

Fundamental to the management of all types and grades of angina is the reduction of risk factors through lifestyle modification. Lifestyle modifications may prevent the development of complications commonly associated with myocardial ischemia and have little cost. Even when they cannot control angina alone, they may reduce the number and dosage of drugs required for angina management and prevent the need for surgical intervention. All patients should be advised to stop smoking, maintain appropriate levels of blood pressure and cholesterol, follow the Step 1 diet for cholesterol management (see Chapter 37), and achieve to the extent possi-

Table 26–1. Grading of Angina by the New York Heart Association and the Canadian Cardiovascular Society

Class	New York Heart Association	Canadian Cardiovascular Society
Class I	Proven coronary artery disease without symptoms	Ordinary physical activity, such as walking or climbing stairs, does not cause angina. Angina occurs with strenuous, rapid, or prolonged exertion at work or recreation.
Class II	Angina only with unusually strenuous physical exertion	Slight limitation of ordinary activity. Angina occurs on walking or climbing stairs rapidly; walking uphill; walking or stair climbing after meals; in cold wind; under emotional stress; or only during the few hours after awakening. Walking more than two blocks on the level and climbing more than one flight of ordinary stairs at a normal pace and in normal conditions does not cause angina.
Class III	Angina during routine physical activity	Marked limitations of ordinary activity. Angina occurs on walking one to two blocks on the level and climbing one flight of stairs in normal conditions and at a normal pace.
Class IV	Angina during minimal activity or rest	Inability to carry on any physical activity without discomfort. Angina may occur at rest.

Table 26–2. Risk Profiles Associated with Angina

Risk	Lifestyle Risk	Physiological Risk
Low	• Nonsmoker • Normotensive • Low cholesterol • Negative family history	• Mild stable angina (class I–II) • Good exercise tolerance tests • Normal ventricular function on echocardiography
High	• Smoker • Hypertensive • Hypercholesterolemia • Positive family history	• Severe angina (class III–IV) • Unstable angina • Poor exercise test performance • Impaired ventricular function
Uncertain	• Obesity • Sedentary lifestyle • Type A personality • Emotional stress	Silent ischemia

Table 26–3. Treatment Protocol Based on Grade/Class and Risk Profile

Grade/Class	Risk Profile	Treatment Protocol
Class I–II	Low risk	• Lifestyle modification • Intermittent nitroglycerin • Initial monotherapy
Class I–II	High risk	• Bypass surgery or • Lifestyle modification and initial drug therapy; drug therapy may progress
Class III–IV	High risk	Angioplasty or bypass surgery with lifestyle modification postoperatively
Unstable angina	Low risk	Lifestyle modification and initial drug therapy; drug therapy may progress

ble their ideal body weight. Table 26–4 discusses the main lifestyle modifications appropriate for patients with angina. They are similar to those appropriate for patients with hypertension and hypercholesterolemia.

Concurrent with lifestyle modifications, patients with angina should have any concomitant diseases—such as hypertension, hypercholesterolemia, severe anemia, hyperthyroidism, hypoxic lung disorders, diabetes mellitus, and critical valvular stenosis—treated and brought under control. These patients should also be placed on daily doses of **aspirin**. Although **aspirin** has not been demonstrated in randomized clinical trials to prevent the onset of angina, it has been extensively studied in the treatment and prevention of acute MI (Gruppo Italiano, 1990; ISIS-2, 1988; Juul-Moller, et al., 1992; Steering Committee, 1989; Third International Study, 1992). In these studies, it was associated with preventing reinfarction and significantly reduced recurrent ischemic events. In another trial (Garcia-Dorado, et al., 1995), the use of **aspirin** was associated with a significant reduction in admissions to the hospital for unstable angina.

Although **aspirin** is not a symptomatic treatment for the patient with stable or unstable angina, **aspirin** is beneficial in decreasing the risk for MI, a risk that is higher in the angina population. All patients should be given 81 to 325 mg of **aspirin** daily as an **antithrombotic agent**. Data indicate that 81 mg per day is effective for patients who cannot tolerate the higher doses because of their history of gastrointestinal (GI) bleeding disorders or cancer. This low dose, however, must be augmented by doses of 325 mg on at least 2 days each month (e.g., the 1st and the 15th days of the month). Enteric-coated tablets may also decrease risks for GI bleeding, but bioavailability concerns have been raised.

When these initial therapies have not resulted in improved exercise tolerance or decreased episodes of angina, or when the patient is class III or class IV on the grading scale or high risk, initial drug therapy is begun. Figure 26–1 delineates the drug treatment protocol for chronic stable angina and low-risk unstable angina.

Drug Therapy

Initial Monotherapy

Nitrates, beta-adrenergic blockers, and **calcium channel blockers** are the mainstays of initial drug therapy for angina. Each has a group of patients for whom they are

Table 26–4. Lifestyle Modifications

Attain Ideal Body Weight.
Excess weight increases cardiac workload and increases oxygen demand. It is also associated with hypertension, and loss of as little as 10 lb can significantly reduce blood pressure.

Increase Aerobic Physical Activity Within the Limitations of Angina.
The overall goal of anginal therapy is to restore optimal exercise capacity. The presence of angina, however, indicates an imbalance in oxygen supply and demand and denotes possible damage to the myocardium. Start with a level of activity that does not produce pain, and gradually increase the activity level by 1 min each day as long as there is no angina. Even limited activity is preferred to no activity. Daily activity is preferred to intermittent activity.

Reduce Sodium Intake to No More Than 2400 mg of Sodium or 6 g of Sodium Chloride.
Sodium helps the body retain water, which increases the amount of blood volume. This increases cardiac workload and increases oxygen demand. It is also associated with hypertension. Reduced intake of this level can often be achieved by not adding salt during cooking or on the table and by watching hidden sources of salt, such as canned foods.

Maintain Adequate Intake of Dietary Potassium (approximately 60 mEq/d).
The heart is heavily dependent on potassium for contractility.

Reduce Intake of Dietary Saturated Fats and Cholesterol.
Cholesterol and saturated fats are implicated in the development of atherosclerosis, which narrows coronary arteries and makes angina worse. The level of reduction depends upon serum cholesterol levels. Hypercholesterolemia requires lower levels than those required for patients with normal cholesterol levels. Start with the American Heart Association Step 1 diet.

Stop Smoking.
Nicotine is implicated in several ways in making angina worse. Absorbed nicotine increases blood pressure and heart rate, thus increasing myocardial oxygen demand. Nicotine also causes vasospasm, and the rise in carboxyhemoglobin from smoke inhalation reduces oxygen supply. Even passive smoke inhalation can reduce exercise tolerance in patients with angina. The low doses of nicotine found in nicotine replacement therapy (NRT) do not significantly elevate blood pressure or heart rate, and NRT may be used to aid in smoking cessation.

Limit Alcohol Intake.
For men and heavier patients, alcohol intake should be no more than 1 oz (30 cc) of ethanol (e.g., 24 oz beer, 10 oz wine, 2 oz 100-proof whiskey)/d. For women and lighter-weight patients, the intake should be no more than 1/2 oz/d.

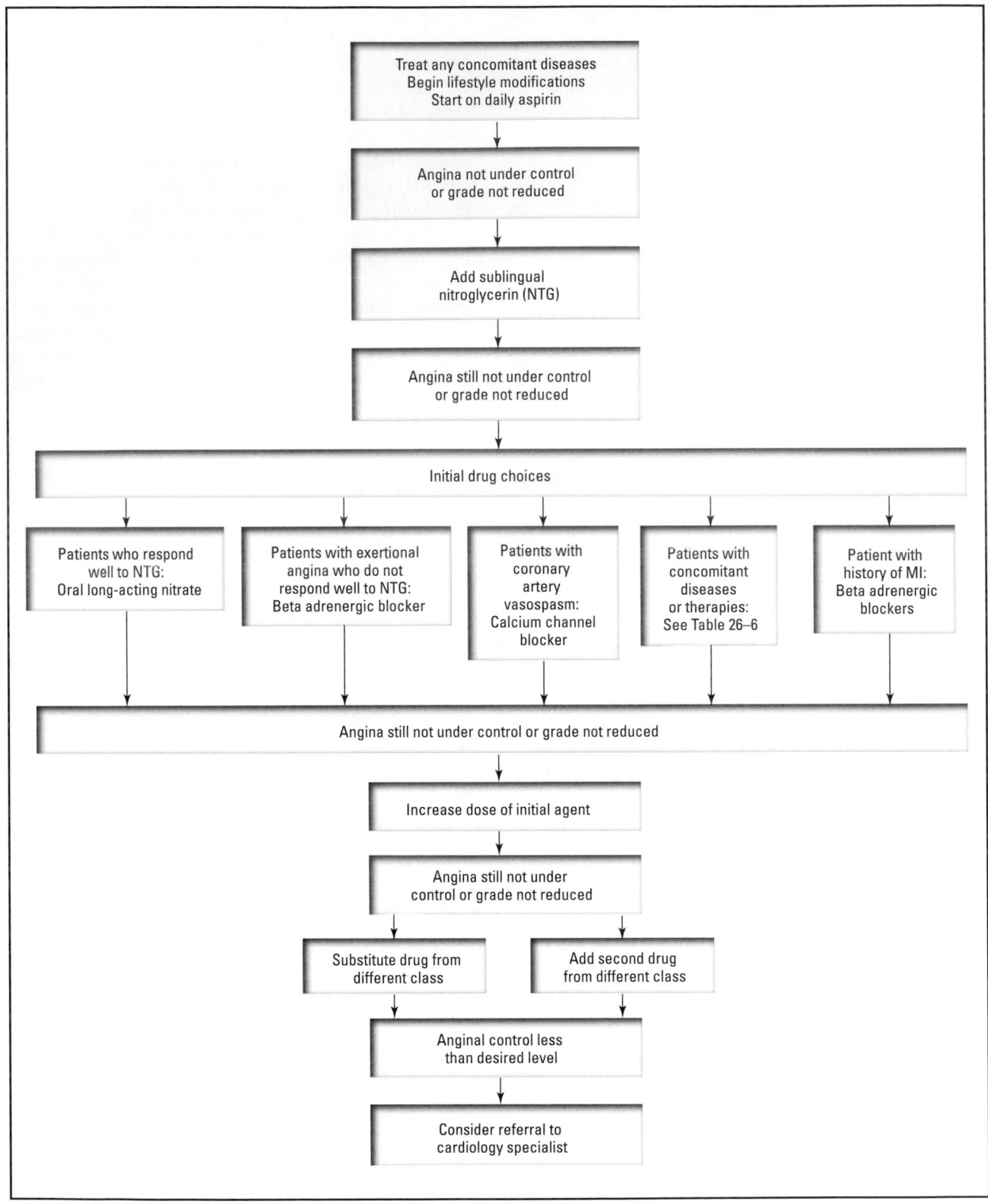

Figure 26–1. Drug treatment protocol for chronic stable angina and low-risk unstable angina.

best suited and a group for whom they are contraindicated. Detailed discussions of each of these classes of drugs are given in Chapters 12 and 14. The focus here is on their role in angina management.

Nitrates are the preferred treatment for most angina

patients. They are the oldest and best studied of the **antianginals,** are useful for all types of angina, effectively treat some of the complications (congestive heart failure) and aggravating conditions (hypertension) associated with angina, are cost-effective, and have a variety of routes of administration that allow flexibility for the patient. They are more effective than **beta-adrenergic blockers** in relieving and preventing anginal episodes in patients with vasospastic angina.

Initially, **nitroglycerin** 0.3 to 0.4 mg sublingual tablets or translingual spray is used for immediate symptom relief. All patients with angina should carry some form of rapid-acting **nitrate** with them at all times. They should be instructed to use this medication at the first sign of angina, even if they are uncertain if the symptoms are angina. If symptoms persist after three doses of this drug taken at 5-minute intervals, they should go to the hospital for medical attention. Chapter 14 has specific information on the treatment protocol and storage of **nitroglycerin** in its various forms.

For patients who respond well to sublingual or translingual **nitroglycerin** and who experience angina episodes more than "rarely," long-acting oral or transdermal **nitrates** are generally indicated. Among the available drugs, the most cost-effective is **isosorbide dinitrate (Isordil)** given bid or tid, with a 10- to 12-hour **nitrate**-free interval to compensate for **nitrate** tolerance. The timing of the **nitrate**-free interval should coincide with the time of

fewest episodes of angina. The schedule that seems most effective is 7 A.M. and 2 P.M. daily. Headache is the most common adverse reaction, but tachyphylaxis to this problem develops, and the headaches resolve. Starting with low doses and slowly increasing the dose reduces the incidence of headache.

Beta-adrenergic blockers decrease myocardial oxygen demand and are the drugs of choice for exertional angina. Because they do not improve myocardial oxygen supply and **propranolol (Inderal)** has been reported to increase the risk for coronary artery vasospasm in some patients, their main roles are in treating patients who do not respond well to **nitrates** and in preventing recurrence of MIs in patients with CAD. They are especially useful for patients with exertional angina whose lifestyle involves frequent vigorous activity, patients with resting tachycardia (e.g., hyperthyroidism), and for patients who have concomitant diseases that might benefit from beta-adrenergic blockade. Table 26–5 shows these concomitant diseases. **Beta-adrenergic blockers** are contraindicated for patients with overt heart failure, reactive airway diseases, and vasospastic angina. The most cost-effective and convenient **beta-adrenergic blocker** is

Table 26–5. Drug Choice Based on Concomitant Disease States

Drug Choice	EFFECT ON CONCOMITANT DISEASE STATES	
	Favorable Effects	**Unfavorable Effects**
Nitrates	Heart failure Hypertension	Migraine headaches MI
Beta-adrenergic blockers	Arrhythmias, atrial tachycardia Hypertension "Stage fright" Migraine headaches Hyperthyroidism Post MI	Heart failure Advanced AV block Reactive airway disease Claudication/Raynaud's syndrome (can use beta-1 selective drug) Diabetes mellitus (may try beta-1 selective drug) Depression Hypercholesterolemia
Calcium Channel Blockers Dihydropyridines	Hypertension, isolated systolic hypertension Systolic heart failure Raynaud's syndrome, peripheral vascular disease	Peripheral edema
Verapamil	Atrial trachycardias Hypertension Migraine headache MI	Advanced AV block Constipation Heart failure Concurrent use with beta blockers may cause additive bradycardia
Diltiazem	Atrial tachycardia Diabetes mellitus MI	Advanced AV block Heart failure
Amlodipine	Atherosclerosis Heart failure	

atenolol (Tenormin), with its once-daily dosing, low adverse reactions profile, and beta-1 selectivity. **Beta-adrenergic blockers** are discussed in more detail in Chapter 12.

Calcium channel blockers, like the nitrates, improve myocardial oxygen supply and decrease oxygen demand. They are the initial drugs of choice when coronary artery vasospasm is suspected to be a contributing mechanism to the angina. They are also effective for patients with exertional angina who have fixed atherosclerotic CAD; when **beta-adrenergic blockers** or **nitrates** are ineffective, contraindicated, or poorly tolerated; and when a concomitant disease might benefit from the use of a **calcium channel blocker**. Table 26–5 shows these concomitant diseases. Studies have also shown one **calcium channel blocker, amlodipine (Norvasc),** to be effective in inhibiting vascular smooth-muscle cell proliferation in atherosclerosis, and it may have a protective mechanism in preventing or retarding the progression of atherosclerosis. It also has the advantage of a long half-life that allows once-daily dosing without resorting to a sustained-release form.

There have been concerns raised about the potential for **calcium channel blockers** to negatively affect long-term survival in patients post-MI. Studies have shown that this problem is specific to the dramatic lowering of blood pressure associated with the use of short-acting **nifedipine (Adalat),** and other studies did not support an association between long-acting forms of **nifedipine** or other **calcium channel blockers** and long-term survival in this population; one study (Reicher-Reiss et al., 1998) found that low-dose, short-acting **nifedipine** therapy used in a randomized clinical trial for 1 year was not associated with increased mortality during a 5-year follow-up.

When initial monotherapy with low to moderate doses is not adequate to control angina or to reduce the grade from a higher class (III–IV) to a lower one (I–II), two choices are possible. One is to increase the dose of the monotherapy drug. This is always done with considerations for the potential adverse reactions associated with that drug. In some cases, the addition of a second drug to minimize the adverse reactions and provide an additive effect to maximize benefits may be more appropriate than significant increases in the initial drug. The second option is to substitute a drug from a different class. **Nitrates** and **calcium channel blockers** are both effective, for example, in vasospastic angina, but not all patients respond well to **nitrates.** Table 26–6 presents selected drugs in each class and their indications in specific types of angina.

Two-Drug Therapy

Combinations of **beta-adrenergic blockers** and **calcium channel blockers** have been shown to be more effective than the individual drugs used alone. Their effects on reducing myocardial oxygen demand are complementary, making it possible to use lower doses of both drugs, and many of their adverse reactions cancel out. Lower doses also reduce the risk of hypotension. Patients not adequately controlled by either drug alone tend to benefit from the addition of the second drug. Patients adequately controlled by monotherapy with either of these drugs do not seem to benefit from addition of the second drug. They are a questionable combination for patients with left ventricular (LV) dysfunction because they may induce heart failure or bradycardia in these patients. **Verapamil** should be avoided in this combination.

Combinations of a **long-acting nitrate** and a **beta blocker** are also safe, effective, and low in cost. Their effects are additive, permitting lower doses of both drugs, and their adverse reactions often cancel out. The **beta-adrenergic blocker** slows any reflex tachycardia caused by the **nitrate,** which helps to reduce myocardial oxygen demand. **Nitrates** decrease preload and minimize increases in LV end-diastolic volume that may be caused by the **beta-adrenergic blocker.**

Combinations of **long-acting nitrates** and **calcium channel blockers** are rarely used because of the high risk for hypotension and because their adverse reaction profiles are additive. This combination is usually reserved for refractory cases of vasospastic angina.

Table 26–6. Selected Drug Choices Based on Type of Angina

Drug Choice	Chronic Stable Angina	Exertional Angina	Vasospastic Angina	Unstable Angina
Amlodipine	X	X	X	
Atenolol	X	X		
Diltiazem	X	X	X	
Isosorbide dinitrate	X	X	X	
Nifedipine	X	X	X	
Verapamil				X

When the addition of a second drug greatly improves angina, it is worthwhile to attempt gradual reduction of prior drug doses over time. For example, if the addition of a **beta-adrenergic blocker** to high-dose **nitrate** therapy greatly improves angina, gradual reduction in the **nitrate** doses can be tried.

Once a combination of two drugs has been initiated, if the response is still not adequate, similar choices are possible as with monotherapy. One is to increase the dose of one or both of the drugs in the combination. The other is to add a third drug to the regimen.

Three-Drug Therapy

Patients with severe (class III–IV) angina who are refractory to two-drug regimens may be tried on a combination of three drug classes. The addition of a **calcium channel blocker** to a combination of a **nitrate** and a **beta-adrenergic blocker** is the usual sequence. When this level of regimen is required, referral to a cardiologist is appropriate.

Table 26–7 presents the drugs commonly used to treat angina, whether alone or in combination with other drugs.

Additional Patient Variables

Older Adults

The treatment protocol for angina is the same for older adults as it is for other adults, with consideration for the usual changes in pharmacokinetics in this age group. Lifestyle modifications are always first-line therapy because of their safety and cost. When drugs are chosen, consideration should be given to the risks for CAD and MI, which are higher in older adults. Older adults, however, may have chronic airway diseases, and **nonselective beta-adrenergic blockers** are contraindicated with this concomitant disease. Congestive heart failure is also common and particularly lethal in older patients. **Nitrates** have an important role in this disease process, whereas the negative inotropic effects of some **calcium channel blockers** may make this disorder worse. Hypertension and hypercholesterolemia are also more common in older adults. Table 26–5 shows the appropriate drug class selection for each of these disease processes.

Women

Postmenopausal women not on **hormone replacement** therapy are at the same risk as age-cohort men for the development of atherosclerosis and CAD. Research has consistently shown a marked decrease in the risk of major CAD and the symptoms of angina associated with it among women who take **estrogen** or **estrogen plus progestin** as compared with women who do not use **hormone replacement** after menopause (Grodstein et al., 1996; Postmenopausal writing group, 1995; Stampfer et al., 1991). Given this risk profile, women with angina should be assessed for use of **estrogen** as a central part of their therapy. Women of all ages are at higher risk for silent myocardial ischemia. Studies that have included significant percentages of female patients have found

Table 26–7. Drugs Commonly Used: Angina

Drug	Brand Name
Beta-adrenergic blockers	
Atenolol	(Tenormin)
Propranolol	(Inderal)
Calcium channel blockers	
Amlodipine	(Norvasc)
Diltiazem	(Cardizem)
Felodipine	(Plendil)
Nifedipine sustained release	(Procardia XL)
Nitrates	
Isosorbide dinitrate	(Isordil)
Isosorbide mononitrate	(Imdur)
Nitroglycerin (sublingual)	(Nitrostat)

that taking **aspirin** produced the same lowering of all-cause mortality and lower incidence of nonfatal MI and stroke as found in men (Harpaz, et al., 1996). There is no gender-based difference in the treatment protocol for angina. There may be differences based on concomitant disease states such as hypertension and hypercholesterolemia (discussed in Chapters 37 and 38). Premenopausal women are at higher risk for anemia that may affect myocardial oxygen supply. Treatment for anemia is discussed in Chapter 25.

Concomitant Diseases

Drugs used to treat angina may improve the management of some diseases and worsen others. Selection of an angina drug that treats a concomitant disease can simplify the overall therapeutic regimen, reduce cost, and increase the likelihood of adherence. It is not within the scope of this book to discuss all possible concomitant disease states, but those most common in patients with angina that might benefit from appropriate drug selection to treat the angina are discussed here.

MYOCARDIAL INFARCTION. Angina is usually associated with CAD, the major underlying mechanism behind MI. Both **aspirin** (Kromholz, et al., 1996) and **beta-adrenergic blockers** have been associated with MI prophylaxis. **Diltiazem (Cardizem)** in its long-acting form has been shown to decrease mortality for patients with non–Q wave MIs. **Calcium channel blockers** should be avoided after MI for patients with poor ejection fractions (less than 40%) because of their negative inotropic effects. **Nitrates** tend to cause reflex tachycardia. The increased myocardial oxygen demand associated with this tachycardia cannot be adjusted for with coronary arteries that are unable to effectively dilate or are blocked. They should be used with caution. **Angiotensin-converting enzyme (ACE) inhibitors** are useful after MI to prevent heart failure and mortality. Although they are not drugs of choice to treat angina, they do have antiatherogenic effects, diminish myocardial oxygen demand, and increase nitric oxide through their action on the bradykinin system. Post-MI patients who are given **ACE inhibitors** may also benefit from reduced angina.

HEART FAILURE. Heart failure is commonly associated with higher grades of angina. Several drugs used to treat angina also reduce blood pressure and improve myocardial function to reduce the risk for development of heart failure. **Isosorbide dinitrate,** combined with the vasodilator **hydralazine,** reduces both preload and afterload for patients with heart failure. This combination is the only one besides **ACE inhibitors** to be associated with decreased morbidity and mortality from heart failure. The **dihydropyridines amlodipine** and **felodipine (Plendil)** are the only **calcium channel blockers**

demonstrated to be safe in treating angina with concomitant heart failure caused by advanced LV dysfunction. The negative inotropic effects of **beta-adrenergic blockers** can make heart failure worse, and these drugs should be avoided. Lifestyle modifications are also central to heart failure prevention and management (discussed in Chapter 34).

HYPERTENSION. Lifestyle modifications are the first approach to treatment of both hypertension and angina. Emphasis is placed on control of weight; reduced intake of sodium, saturated fat, cholesterol, and **alcohol;** and increased physical activity for both disease processes. All drug classes used to treat angina are helpful in the treatment of hypertension. **Beta-adrenergic blockers** are preferred because of cost and MI prophylaxis. **Calcium channel blockers** are also acceptable for patients with hypertension. **Nitrates** are best reserved for normotensive patients. Chapter 38 discusses the concomitant use of these drugs in more detail.

HYPERCHOLESTEROLEMIA. As with hypertension, lifestyle modifications are the first approach to treatment. The only class of **antianginal drugs** that negatively affects hypercholesterolemia is **beta-adrenergic blockers.** They increase triglycerides and cholesterol transiently and reduce the level of HDL. Because this alteration in lipid levels is transient, these drugs should not be avoided when there are other compelling reasons for the use of a **beta-adrenergic blocker,** such as MI prophylaxis.

PERIPHERAL VASCULAR DISEASES. The vasoconstrictive effects of **beta-adrenergic blockers** have an adverse effect on peripheral blood flow that contraindicates their use for patients with concomitant peripheral vascular disease (PVD). The peripheral vasodilating effects of the **dihydropyridine group** of calcium channel blockers have resulted in their having an "unlabeled" use in the treatment of Raynaud's syndrome. They are the drugs of choice for patients with concomitant PVD.

DIABETES MELLITUS. Calcium channel blockers are preferred because of their lower effects on glucose metabolism. They have also been shown to have some degree of renal protection. **Beta-adrenergic blockers** decrease insulin secretion and may mask the signs of hypoglycemia. The one sign of hypoglycemia that is not masked is diaphoresis, and patients with diabetes who are taking these drugs should be taught to test their blood glucose levels in the event of a diaphoretic episode. If a **beta-adrenergic blocker** must be used to treat angina for compelling reasons, these adverse reactions are associated with $beta_2$ blockade, and use of a $beta_1$ selective drug reduces but does not eliminate these problems.

ASTHMA AND CHRONIC AIRWAY DISEASES. Beta-adrenergic blockers in both oral and topical ophthalmic forms may exacerbate asthma and other chronic airway diseases. They should be avoided unless the reasons for their use are compelling.

Other disease processes that are affected positively or negatively by the drugs commonly used to treat angina are shown in Table 26–5.

Cost

The cost of **antianginal** drug therapy should be considered in drug selection, especially because patients are often on multiple drugs and a significant proportion of patients who are older may be on fixed incomes. In general, generic formulations are acceptable and cheaper than brand-name drugs.

Nitrates are the cheapest of the **antianginals**. Among the **nitrates, nitroglycerin** sublingual is significantly cheaper than the translingual spray. The spray, however, has a much longer shelf life and may actually be closer in price if the patient uses the drug rarely. **Isosorbide dinitrate** comes in a generic form that is almost 10 times less expensive than **isosorbide mononitrate**. Despite bioavailability differences between the two drugs, there appears to be no clear advantage to the more expensive **mononitrate**.

The **beta-adrenergic blockers** are in the middle in cost. An older drug, **propranolol (Inderal)**, is relatively inexpensive, but its lipid solubility increases the adverse reactions profile, and it must be taken 2 to 4 times each day. It is also a **nonselective beta-adrenergic blocker**, along with **labetalol, nadolol, and timolol**. Lack of selectivity results in more adverse reactions. The drug of choice is **atenolol**. It is the least expensive, is $beta_1$ se-

---

PATIENT EDUCATION

Angina

Related to the Overall Treatment Plan/Disease Process

☐ Pathophysiology of angina and its prognosis

☐ Role of lifestyle modifications in improving prognosis and keeping down the number and cost of required drugs

☐ Importance of adherence to the treatment regimen

☐ Indications of complications that need to be reported and the need for regular follow-up visits with the primary care provider

Specific to the Drug Therapy

☐ Reason for taking the drug(s) and the anticipated action of the drug(s) on the disease process

☐ Doses and schedules for taking the drugs

☐ Possible adverse reactions and what to do when they occur

☐ Interactions between lifestyle modification and these drugs

Reasons for Taking the Drug(s)

Patient education about specific drugs used to treat angina is provided in Chapters 14 and 16. Specific information related to angina includes: Reasons for the drugs being given. Antianginal drugs are given to reduce cardiovascular morbidity (especially myocardial infarction) and mortality. Some drugs do both of these things; most do one or the other. The expectation should be clear about what these drugs can and cannot do. Stable angina is a chronic condition that requires lifelong treatment, and so the regimen should be incorporated into the daily life of the patient. Even well-managed angina can become unstable and may require urgent management. Knowledge of when and how to use sublingual or translingual nitroglycerin is important.

Continued on next page

PATIENT EDUCATION

Angina (continued)

Drugs as Part of the Total Treatment Regimen

Angina therapy is based on lifestyle modification. These modifications are not always easy to maintain, but they are equally as important as drugs in successful control of symptoms and prevention of complications. Among the lifestyle modifications is sodium restriction to reduce extracellular fluid volume, decrease afterload, and reduce myocardial oxygen demand. Care should be taken not to reduce salt and fluid too quickly, which may result in fluid volume deficit, leading to hypotension and a reduction in myocardial oxygen supply. Patients should be taught signs and symptoms of fluid volume deficit to report. None of the antianginal drugs directly reduces fluid volume, but all except aspirin have vasodilating actions that may make fluid volume deficit worse. Sodium reduction may also lead some patients to seek salt substitutes that have potassium as part of their contents. Changes in potassium levels can significantly affect myocardial functioning, so these substitutes should be used sparingly. Nonsalt herbal seasoning is encouraged.

Another central lifestyle modification is regular aerobic exercise, such as walking or cycling. The amount and type of exercise must be carefully monitored and targeted to anginal symptoms. Patients can be referred to a cardiac rehabilitation program at the start of their exercise program so that their response can be monitored. Later, they can monitor their own response and determine the pace and amount of exercise that works for them. The key is gradually increasing, regular aerobic exercise. Several of the antianginal drugs, especially the nitrates, have the potential to cause orthostatic hypotension. Exercise should be timed to avoid this adverse reaction, and adequate fluids should be taken while exercising.

---

lective, has a long half-life so that it can be taken only once daily, and has low lipid solubility and a low adverse reactions profile.

Calcium channel blockers are the most expensive **antianginals.** Short-acting forms are less expensive but must be taken several times each day, and some research suggests an increased mortality risk for short-acting **nifedipine.** It should be prescribed only in its long-acting form. **Diltiazem** in its short-acting form is among the least expensive; its sustained-release form is significantly more expensive. **Verapamil** is the least expensive, but it has limited use, and almost 100 percent of patients who take it develop constipation. This constipation usually requires an additional medication (stool softener) to treat the problem, and by the time the cost of the second drug is added in, all cost savings are lost. **Amlodipine,** because it is a newer formulation, is not inexpensive. The expense needs to be weighed against its range of uses, once-daily dosing, reduced peripheral edema, decreased incidence of reflex tachycardia, and antiatherogenic properties.

Aspirin brands do not appear to have significant advantages over generics. Enteric coating makes this drug more expensive, and there have been recent questions about inconsistent bioavailability with enteric coating.

Monitoring

The most important monitoring parameters are the presence, characteristics, and timing of angina episodes. Precipitating factors such as exercise, effort that involves use of the arms above the head, cold environment, walking after a meal, emotional stress, anger or anxiety, or coitus need to be reviewed. Some of these may be corrected by lifestyle modifications. For class I–II, low-risk angina patients, initial diagnostic tests may involve exercise treadmill testing and exercise echocardiography. After laboratory data and other monitoring parameters specific to the drugs they are taking, an annual 12-lead ECG, complete blood count (CBC), and blood chemistry are probably enough. For class III–IV or high-risk angina patients, monitoring parameters should be determined in collaboration with a cardiology specialist.

Outcome Evaluation

Figure 26–1 shows the drug treatment protocol for angina management. Evaluation for angina control occurs throughout the protocol. The main indication for

Angina

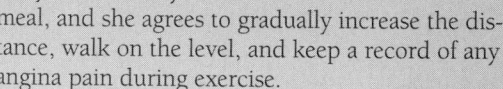

Complaint

Recurrent chest pain

History

Mary is a 61-year-old white woman who is a non-insulin-dependent diabetic being managed on Glucophage. She is 5 ft 7 in tall and weighs 188 lb. In addition to her weight and the presence of diabetes, other cardiovascular risk factors include a history of high-normal hypertension (134/86 mm Hg) and borderline high cholesterol (210 mg/dL). Her younger brother died suddenly last year from a myocardial infarction. She does not smoke or drink alcohol. Other pertinent medical problems include estrogen deficiency syndrome (postmenopausal) being managed on estrogen (Premarin) 0.625 mg daily.

She comes to the clinic today asking for advice about recurrent chest pain. For the past 6 months, she has experienced episodic chest pains almost daily. She describes her pain as "catching me around the heart [she points to the left submammary area] and sometimes inside my breast bone [she points to the lower sternum]. Sometimes it feels like I am getting stabbed, but usually it just aches. Sometimes it gives me indigestion." The indigestion is described as " a kind of heavy feeling that goes away if I stop what I am doing and try to get up the gas." The symptoms usually last only a minute or two and are relieved by rest. The pain is associated with exertion such as vacuuming the house or walking quickly. She can walk two blocks on the level without symptoms if she takes her time.

Assessment

After a cardiac workup, Mary is diagnosed with class II exertional angina. Her cardiac risk history places her at high risk.

Initial Management Plan

Mary's initial management plan is:

1. Start on aspirin 325 mg daily. Mary is started on this dose because she has no history of GI disease and, with her high-risk cardiac status, she needs full antithrombotic activity.
2. Integrate Step 1 American Heart Association diet with her American Diabetes Association (ADA) diet. This is not difficult because the goals of both diets are very similar. She has been inconsistent in her adherence to her ADA diet, however, so she receives a referral to a dietitian and a support group. Lifestyle modifications are more likely to be adhered to with concurrent social support. The long-term goal is to achieve a weight of 140 lb. To achieve this goal, a weekly weight loss goal of 1 to 2 lb is planned.
3. Begin daily aerobic exercise. Mary already tries to walk short distances every evening after dinner. The timing of her exercise is changed to avoid activity after a heavy meal, and she agrees to gradually increase the distance, walk on the level, and keep a record of any angina pain during exercise.
4. After assessing her knowledge base about the diagnosis and its management, begin appropriate teaching. This will include when and how to use sublingual nitroglycerin and angina literature from the American Heart Association.
5. Management of her diabetes is coordinated with her diabetic specialist.

Follow-up Visit

At her follow-up visit in 1 month, Mary reports that she is taking her aspirin and that her appointment with the dietitian gave her some good ideas about the diet. She has lost 4 lb. She is now walking 3 to 4 blocks in the morning before breakfast and has had no episodes of chest pain during these morning walks. She does continue to experience "indigestion" when she is doing heavy housework or when she is "stressed" at work. This indigestion is now described as substernal discomfort and heaviness, and it is unrelated to meals. Her sublingual nitroglycerin relieves this discomfort within 2 minutes. Rest alone relieves it in about 5 minutes. On several occasions, she took nitroglycerin before doing some heavy housework, and she experienced no indigestion or chest pain. Her blood pressure today is 126/00 mm Hg.

Modifications to Management Plan

Mary's treatment plan includes continuance of her aspirin and sublingual nitroglycerin. Her diet is not changed, and her exercise regimen now has a goal of walking 1/2 to 1 mile daily. Modifications to her treatment plan include:

1. Obtain an ECG. Her ECG today is normal. This is important because it helps to rule out left ventricular dysfunction. Left ventricular dysfunction would suggest referral for additional, possibly invasive, cardiac testing and would influence the choice of drugs.
2. Start diltiazem 30 mg q8h. Mary has responded well to nitroglycerin and might be started on an oral long-acting nitrate, but calcium channel blockers are preferred with diabetics because of their limited effect on glucose metabolism. Calcium channel blockers also have demonstrated some degree of renal protection, and Mary is not on an ACE inhibitor for her hypertension, so this renal protection is important. A formulation that allowed once-

continued

Angina (continued)

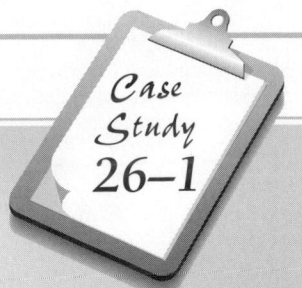

Case Study 26–1

daily dosing would simplify her treatment regimen, but cost is a factor for Mary, and the sustained-release forms are significantly more expensive.

3. Obtain appropriate laboratory tests, including a lipid profile. With her Step 1 diet, her weight loss, and her exercise, her cholesterol level is now 196 mg/dL, her LDL cholesterol is less than 120 mg/dL, and her HDL cholesterol is above 40 mg/dL. No new treatment beyond continuing the diet and exercise is required.
4. Schedule a follow-up visit in 2 months unless her symptoms worsen.

Continuing Care

At her follow-up visit, Mary is delighted that her weight is down another 6 lb, her blood pressure is 120/80 mm Hg, and she reports only one episode of chest pain, which was associated with the need to run a short distance to catch a bus. One month later, she is still doing well, and she will be followed on an annual basis. She continues to be seen regularly by her diabetes specialist and has an "open" referral to the dietitian if she needs more help with her diet.

---

substitution of a drug from a different class or the addition of more drugs is inadequate control of angina or failure to reduce the grade or class to a lower grade or class of angina.

There are situations in which to worry about treating an angina patient and times when referral to a specialist is appropriate:

1. When chronic stable angina becomes unstable—Unstable angina means that it is new or accelerating or has become unpredictable in its characteristics or precipitating factors. It is important to rule out the possibility that it is still stable angina but that changes in lifestyle or the onset of a concomitant illness is causing changes in the anginal symptoms. However, the time taken to rule this out should be very short, especially if ECG changes are noted. In general, patients with new-onset unstable angina should be referred to a specialist for urgent workup.
2. When the patient has "ominous" findings on an exercise tolerance test—These tests are usually administered by a specialist, who would probably be the one to first notice the findings.
3. When a post-MI patient develops new-onset angina, especially with ECG changes—The more recent the MI, the higher the risk. Urgent referral is required.
4. When an MI is suspected, based on anginal and other symptoms—Obtain an ECG, draw appropriate laboratory studies, and obtain a consult with a physician.
5. When standard therapy is not successful in improving exercise tolerance and reducing the incidence of angina symptoms, when a secondary cause of the angina that may require surgical intervention is suspected, or when the patient has complex concomitant disease processes—Consul-

tation is appropriate. This may result in a referral, but it is generally not urgent.

Patient Education

Patient education should include a discussion of information related to the overall treatment plan as well as that specific to the drug therapy, reasons for taking the drug, drugs as part of the total treatment regimen, and adherence issues.

REFERENCES

Barron, H., Viskin, S., Lundstrom, R., Swain, E., Truman, A., Wong, C. & Selby, J. (1998). Beta blocker dosages and mortality after myocardial infarction: Data from a large health maintenance organization. *Archives of Internal Medicine, 158*(5), 449–453.

Behar, S. (1998). Treatment of angina pectoris with calcium antagonists: Long-term follow-up. *Cardiovascular Drugs and Therapy, 12,* 119–124.

Camargo, C., Stamfer, M., Glynn, R., Grodstein, F., Gaziano, J., Manson, J., Buring, J., & Hennekens, C. (1997). Moderate alcohol consumption and risk for angina pectoris or myocardial infarction in U.S. male physicians. *Annals of Internal Medicine, 126*(5), 372–375.

Garcia-Dorado, D., Theroux, P., Toronos, P., Sambola, A., Oliveras, J., Santos, M., & Soler Soler, J. (1995). Previous aspirin use may attenuate the severity of manifestations of acute ischemic syndromes. *Circulation, 92*(7), 1743–1748.

Goroll, A., May, L., & Mulley, A. (1995). *Primary care medicine* (3rd ed.) Philadelphia: Lippincott.

Grodstein, F., Stampfer, M., Manson, J., Coldits, G., Willett, W., Rosner, B., Speizer, F., & Hennekens, C. (1996). Postmenopausal estrogen and progestin use and the risk of cardiovascular disease. *New England Journal of Medicine, 335*(7), 453–461.

Gutstein, D., & Fuster, V. (1997). Management of stable coronary artery disease. *American Family Physician, 56*(1), 99–105.

Haim, M., Shotan, A., Boyko, V., Reicher-Reiss, H., Benderly, M., Goldbourt, U., & Behar, S. (1998). Effect of beta-blocker therapy in patients with coronary artery disease in New York Heart Association classes II and III. *American Journal of Cardiology, 81,* 1455–1460.

Harpaz, D., Benderly, M., Goldbourt, U., Kishon, Y., & Behar, S. (1996). Effect of aspirin on mortality in women with symptomatic or silent myocardial ischemia. *American Journal of Cardiology, 78*(11), 1215–1219.

ISIS-2 Collaborative Group. (1988). Randomized trial of intravenous streptokinase, oral aspirin, both or neither among 17,187 cases of suspected acute myocardial infarction: ISIS-2. *Lancet, 332,* 349—360.

Italiano Per Lo Studio Della Sopravivenza Nell Infarcto Miocardiso. (1990). GISSI-2: A factorial randomized trial of alteplase versus streptokinase and heparin versus no heparin among 12,490 patients with acute myocardial infarction. *Lancet, 336,* 65–71.

Juul-Moller, S., Edvardsson, N., Jahnmatz, B., Rosen, A., Sorensen, S., & Omblus, R. (1992). Double-blind trial of aspirin in primary prevention of myocardial infarction in patients with stable chronic angina pectoris: The Swedish angina pectoris aspirin trial (SAPAT) group. *Lancet, 340*(8833), 1421–1425.

Katzung, B. (1998). *Basic and clinical pharmacology.* (7th ed.) Stamford, CT: Appleton & Lange.

Krumholz, H., Radford, M., Ellerbeck, E., Hennen, J., Meehan, T., Petrillo, M., Wang, Y., & Jencks, S. (1996). Aspirin for secondary prevention after acute myocardial infarction in the elderly: Prescribed use and outcomes. *Archives of Internal Medicine, 124*(3), 292–298.

Madjlessi-Simon, T., Mary-Krause, M., Fillette, F., Lechat, P., & Jaillon, P. (1996). Persistent transient myocardial ischemia despite beta adrenergic blockade predicts a higher risk of adverse cardiac events in patients with coronary artery disease. *Journal of American College of Cardiology, 27,* 1586–1591.

Parmley, W. (1998). Optimum treatment of stable angina pectoris. *Cardiovascular Drugs and Therapy, 12,* 105–110.

Postmenopausal Estrogen/Progestin Interventions Trial writing group. (1995). Effects of estrogen or estrogen/progestin regimens on heart disease risk factors in postmenopausal women. *Journal of the American Medical Association, 273,* 199–208.

Reicher-Reiss, H., Behar, S., Boyko, V., Mandelzweig, L, Kaplinsky, E., & Goldbourt, U. (1998). Long-term mortality follow-up of hospital survivors of a myocardial infarction randomized to nifedipine in the SPRINT study. *Cardiovascular Drugs and Therapy, 12,* 171–176.

Savonitto, S. (1998). Selection of drug therapy in stable angina pectoris. *Cardiovascular Drugs and Therapy, 12,* 197–210.

Stampfer, M., Colditz, G., Willett, W., Manson, J., Speizer, F., & Hennekens, C. (1991). Postmenopausal estrogen therapy and cardiovascular disease: Ten-year follow-up from the Nurses' Health Study. *New England Journal of Medicine, 325*(11), 756–762.

Steering Committee of the Physicians' Health Study Research Group. (1989). Final report on the aspirin component of the ongoing physician's health study. *New England Journal of Medicine, 321,* 129–135.

Stepien, O., Gogusev, J., Zhu, D., Iouzalen, L., Herembert, T., Drueke, T., & Marche, P. (1998). Amlodipine inhibition of serum-, thrombin-, or fibroblast growth factor-induced vascular smooth-muscle cell proliferation. *Journal of Cardiovascular Pharmacology, 31,* 786–793.

Third International Study of Infarct Survival Collaboration Group. (1992). ISIS-3: A randomized comparison of streptokinase versus tissue plasminogen activator versus anistreplase and of aspirin plus heparin versus aspirin alone among 41,299 cases of suspected acute myocardial infarction. *Lancet, 339,* 753–770.

CHAPTER 27

....

Anxiety and Depression

CHAPTER OUTLINE

rimary care providers are often the first health care professionals patients consult when they are struggling with symptoms of anxiety and depression. They may not clearly state the problem as such but rather present a combination of physical, emotional, and social symptoms intertwined with a request for health care evaluation and treatment. Physiological causes for these symptoms are ruled out in making a diagnosis of anxiety or depression.

Mind and body work together and can affect functioning physically, cognitively, emotionally, behaviorally, and socially. Psychosocial stressors can deplete serotonin and norepinephrine neurotransmitter resources. With fewer of these neurotransmitters available in the brain, physiological symptoms occur, depending on the location of the reduction in the brain. For example, with decreased serotonin in the frontal cortex and in the hypothalamus, the most common symptoms are poor concentration and decision making, decreased appetite, decreased libido, and difficulty in sleeping. Consequently, the patient might not be able to perform as well at work, might have difficulty maintaining sexual intimacy, and feel fatigue and decreased self-esteem. Medications can treat only physiologically based symptoms, and the primary care provider needs to know how to rationally prescribe for mental health problems.

Using a single mode of treatment for major depressive or anxiety disorders (i.e., only medications or only psychotherapy) is much less effective than using a multimodal approach (American Psychiatric Association, 1996; Gabbard, 1996). The primary care provider can best serve the patient by explaining how medications can help with the physiological aspects of the symptoms and how therapy or counseling can assist in learning new skills in handling stress. This chapter describes the pathophysiology of anxiety and depression and the physiological, psychological, and behavioral manifestations. It is not within the scope of this book to discuss the diagnosis of these disorders in any depth. For further discussion of the diagnostic process, see management texts and the *Diagnostic and Statistical Manual* (DSM IV-R; American Psychiatric Association, 1994) for diagnostic criteria. The treatment protocol presented here assumes appropriate diagnosis of anxiety or depression.

Pathophysiology

Anxiety and depressive symptoms result from an interaction of the central nervous, peripheral nervous, and endocrine systems, as well as the generalized stress response. Usually the generalized stress response is mediated by the immune system in producing cortisol to activate the fight, flight, or freeze response, which is a function of the peripheral nervous system. For review of the various functions of the brain and their anatomic locations, see a basic physiology text They are summarized briefly next.

Nervous System

The main structures of the brain involved in the anxiety and mood symptoms include the frontal cortex, the diencephalon, the brainstem and cerebellum, and the limbic system. The frontal lobe is responsible for higher integrative functions such as executive control, personality traits, expression of emotionality, problem solving, decision making, and conceptualization. The diencephalon acts as a relay center for sensory input and motor output between the cerebral cortex and deeper areas of the brain. The hypothalamus maintains the internal milieu, such as appetite, sleeping and wakefulness, sex drive, body temperature, and endocrine functions through the hypothalamic-pituitary-endocrine axes. The vegetative symptoms of depression, such as poor appetite, difficulty in sleeping (including insomnia and hypersomnia), and low sex drive, arise from inadequate functioning of the hypothalamus.

The brainstem contains the three nuclei where essential neurotransmitters are produced: the locus ceruleus for serotonin, the raphe nucleus for norepinephrine, and the substantia nigra for dopamine. Also within the brainstem lies the reticular activating system, which maintains attentiveness. Interconnecting all these structures is the limbic system, a network of neuronal fibers connecting the basal ganglia, thalamus, hypothalamus, cingulate gyrus, hippocampus, amygdala, and eventually the frontal cortex. The hippocampus and amygdala store memories, especially those with intense emotional overtones, and are responsible for learning and formation of emotions. The limbic system, therefore, serves to connect most of the major structures involved in emotion, perception, learning, cognition, and behavior. Clearly, it is of vital importance in understanding and intervening in mental health problems. The endocrine system becomes involved in mental health symptoms by virtue of activation of the hypothalamic-pituitary-endocrine axes. These axes are discussed in more detail in Chapter 19.

Neurotransmitters

Neurotransmitters (NTs) are biochemicals that permit neurons to communicate with each other for a whole-body response. The primary NTs involved in most behavioral symptoms, including anxiety and depression, are serotonin (5HT), norepinephrine (NE), dopamine (DA), gamma-aminobutyric acid (GABA), and acetylcholine (ACh). There are other NTs involved in psychiatric symptoms, but their mechanisms are still exploratory and are not discussed in this chapter. Each NT has a specific neuroreceptor to which it can bind. The receptors may have several subtypes. For example, 5HT has at least 15 receptor subtypes to which binding of $5HT_2$ may contribute to improved appetite but diminished sexual response (Tollefson, 1998). Blocking $5HT_2$ postsynaptic receptors and blocking 5HT reuptake presynaptically will result in improved depressive symptoms without interfering with sexual response. Table 27–1 depicts the various receptors and the effects of receptor activity.

Serotonin and norepinephrine follow very similar pathways; however, NE acts more as an arousing or activating agent, and 5HT acts on mood or the general tenor of emotion (Cooper, Bloom, & Roth, 1996; Kaplan & Sadock, 1998). Epinephrine and NE activity are discussed in more detail in Chapter 12.

GABA is a different kind of NT in that it acts on the chloride channel of the neural membrane to produce an extended hyperpolarization of the neuron, thereby inhibiting additional impulses momentarily. The highest concentration of GABA receptors is found in the amygdala. GABA has two types of receptors: GABA-A, coupled with the chloride channels, and GABA-B, associ-

Table 27–1. Effects of Neurotransmitter Receptor Activation

Receptor Activity	Effects of Receptor Activity
Acetylcholine blockade	• Second most potent action of cyclic antidepressants • Potentiation of effects of drugs with anticholinergic properties, including OTC cold medications • Adverse reactions: dry mouth, blurred vision, constipation, urinary retention, sinus tachycardia, lengthening of QT interval, memory disturbances
Alpha$_1$ adrenergic blockade	• Potentiation of antihypertensives acting by way of alpha$_1$ blockade • Adverse reactions: postural hypotension, dizziness, reflex tachycardia, sedation
Alpha$_2$ adrenergic blockade	• Antagonism of antihypertensives acting as alpha$_2$ stimulants (e.g., clonidine, methyldopa) • Adverse reactions: sexual dysfunction
Dopamine reuptake blockade	• Antidepressant, antiparkinsonian effect • Adverse reactions: psychomotor activation, aggravation of psychosis
Dopamine$_1$ blockade	• May mediate antipsychotic effect
Dopamine$_2$ blockade	• In mesolimbic area, antipsychotic effect correlates with clinical efficacy in controlling positive symptoms of schizophrenia; an inverse relationship exists between dopamine$_2$ blockade and therapeutic antipsychotic dosage • In nigrostriatal tract, contributes to extrapyramidal adverse reactions (rigidity, tremor) • In hypothalmus-pituitary area, contributes to endocrine adverse reactions (galactorrhea, gynecomastia) and sexual dysfunction in men
Dopamine$_3$ blockade	• May mediate antipsychotic effect on negative symptoms of schizophrenia
Dopamine$_4$ blockade	• May mediate antipsychotic effect on positive symptoms of schizophrenia
Histamine$_1$ blockade	• Most potent action of cyclic antidepressants and mirtazapine • Potentiation of effects of other CNS drugs • Adverse reactions: sedation, drowsiness, postural hypotension, weight gain
Norepinephrine reuptake blockade	• Antidepressant effect • Potentiation of pressor effects of norepinephrine • Interaction with guanethidine (interferes with antihypertensive effect) • Adverse reactions: tremors, tachycardia, sweating, insomnia, erectile and ejaculation problems
Serotonin reuptake blockade	• Antidepressant, antiobsessive effect • Can increase or decrease anxiety, depending on dose • Potentiation of drugs with serotonergic properties (e.g., L-tryptophan, phentermine); watch for serotonin syndrome
Serotonin$_1$ blockade	• Antidepressant, anxiolytic, and antiaggressive action
Serotonin$_2$ blockade	• Anxiolytic, antidepressant, antipsychotic, antimigraine effect • May correlate with clinical efficacy in decreasing negative symptoms of schizophrenia; may compensate for (decrease) extrapyramidal effects caused by dopamine$_2$ blockade • Adverse reactions: hypotension, ejaculatory problems, sedation

ated with the second messenger system. The GABA receptor is very complex, with several subunits permitting many different binding sites. **Benzodiazepines,** for example, bind to and enhance the action of the GABA-A receptors and indirectly modulate the chloride ion channel of the GABA receptor. As neuroscience continues to evolve, much more knowledge is forthcoming about the complexity of the GABA receptor, and new drugs will likely have remarkably different pharmacodynamics.

Neuroconduction-Neurotransmission Cascade

Communication between neurons is accomplished through a cascade of electrical and neurochemical events. Initially, there is a wave of depolarization of the neural covering down the axon into the nerve terminal. This depolarization is caused by voltage-sensitive calcium entering the cell and changing the charge momentarily from positive to negative. The calcium influx causes the vesicles containing the NTs to migrate down the neuron to the terminal neuronal membrane. The vesicle fuses with the membrane and releases the NT into the synaptic cleft between two neurons. The NT can then bind with a postsynaptic neuroreceptor, causing another change in ionic conductance of the second cell and activating intracellular processes in the receptive cell. Once the NT is bound to a neuroreceptor, the G-protein transforms it, and second messengers (inositol and cyclic adenosine monophosphatase) act on it to permit the DNA in the cell nucleus to replicate the message and implant it into another vesicle for further transport. If the NT does not bind to a postsynaptic receptor, the action of the NT is terminated by diffusing back into the presynaptic cell, or an active transport system carries it back into the presynaptic cell, where it is enzymatically degraded by monoamine oxidase. The neuroconduction-neurotransmission cascade in depicted in Figure 27–1.

Pharmacodynamics

All the current psychoactive drugs act on this neuroconduction-neurotransmission cascade in some way. Drugs may inhibit the uptake or transport into the presynaptic cell, thereby making more of the NT available for eventual binding to a receptor. This, in turn, places a demand on the postsynaptic cells to produce or reduce receptors on the cell membrane and improve receptor binding. Another mechanism interferes with the ionic action of conduction through blocking the calcium or sodium channels, thereby slowing down or speeding up conduction and movement of the vesicle to the cell membrane. Neuroscientists are already beginning to develop drugs that act on the second messenger system, thereby influencing actual message replication.

There are eight classes of drugs used for anxiety and depression: **nonselective norepinephrine-serotonin reuptake inhibitors (tricyclics** and **heterocyclics), serotonin-selective reuptake inhibitors (SSRIs), serotonin-norepinephrine reuptake inhibitors (SNRIs), norepinephrine-dopamine agonists, serotonin agonist reuptake inhibitors, norepinephrine-selective reuptake inhibitors (NRIs), monoamine oxidase inhibitors (MAOIs),** and **benzodiazepines (BDZs).** Each class acts on NTs in a different way.

Nonselective Norepinephrine-Serotonin Reuptake Inhibitors

Nonselective norepinephrine-serotonin reuptake inhibitors (imipramine [Tofranil], desipramine [Norpramin], amitriptyline [Elavil], nortriptyline [Pamelor], and doxepin [Sinequan] were previously referred to as **tricylic antidepressants.** They affect the NE, 5HT, ACh, and histamine receptors to increase availability of NE and 5HT to bind to postsynaptic receptors. They do this by inhibiting their transport back into the presynaptic neuron when the postsynaptic receptors have failed to pick up the NT in the synaptic cleft.

Serotonin-Selective Reuptake Inhibitors

Serotinin-selective reuptake inhibitors (fluoxetine [Prozac], paroxetine [Paxil], sertraline [Zoloft], fluvoxamine [Luvox], and citalopram [Celexa]) act by blocking the transport mechanism that returns unhound 5HT left in the synaptic cleft into the presynaptic neuron, thereby terminating the transmission of the message carried by that receptor. When the transport mechanism is blocked, more serotonin is available to bind to the postsynaptic 5HT receptor.

Serotonin-Norepinephrine Reuptake Inhibitors

Serotonin-norepinephrine reuptake inhibitors (nefazodone [Serzone], trazodone [Desyrel], and venlafaxine [Effexor]) block the reuptake mechanism of NE and 5HT that ultimately serves to block $5HT_2$ postsynaptic receptors and permit serotonin to easily bind to $5HT_{1A}$. Because $5HT_{1A}$ receptors densely populate the limbic system, increasing 5HT binding here probably accounts for modulating emotions such as sadness, aggression, and anxiety.

Norepinephrine-Dopamine Agonists

Norepinephrine-dopamine agonists consist of only one drug, **bupropion (Wellbutrin.) Bupropion** affects the frontal cortex, the limbic system, the caudate, and the brainstem. In the limbic system, it affects the ventral medial hypothalamus (Kaplan & Sadock, 1998) by increasing NE and DA and the reticular activating system that extends from the brainstem upward through the hypothalamus and the thalamus and then to the cerebral frontal cortex. Also important is what it does not affect. It does not block 5HT reuptake or inhibit monoamine oxidase. It does provide a mild degree of DA reuptake

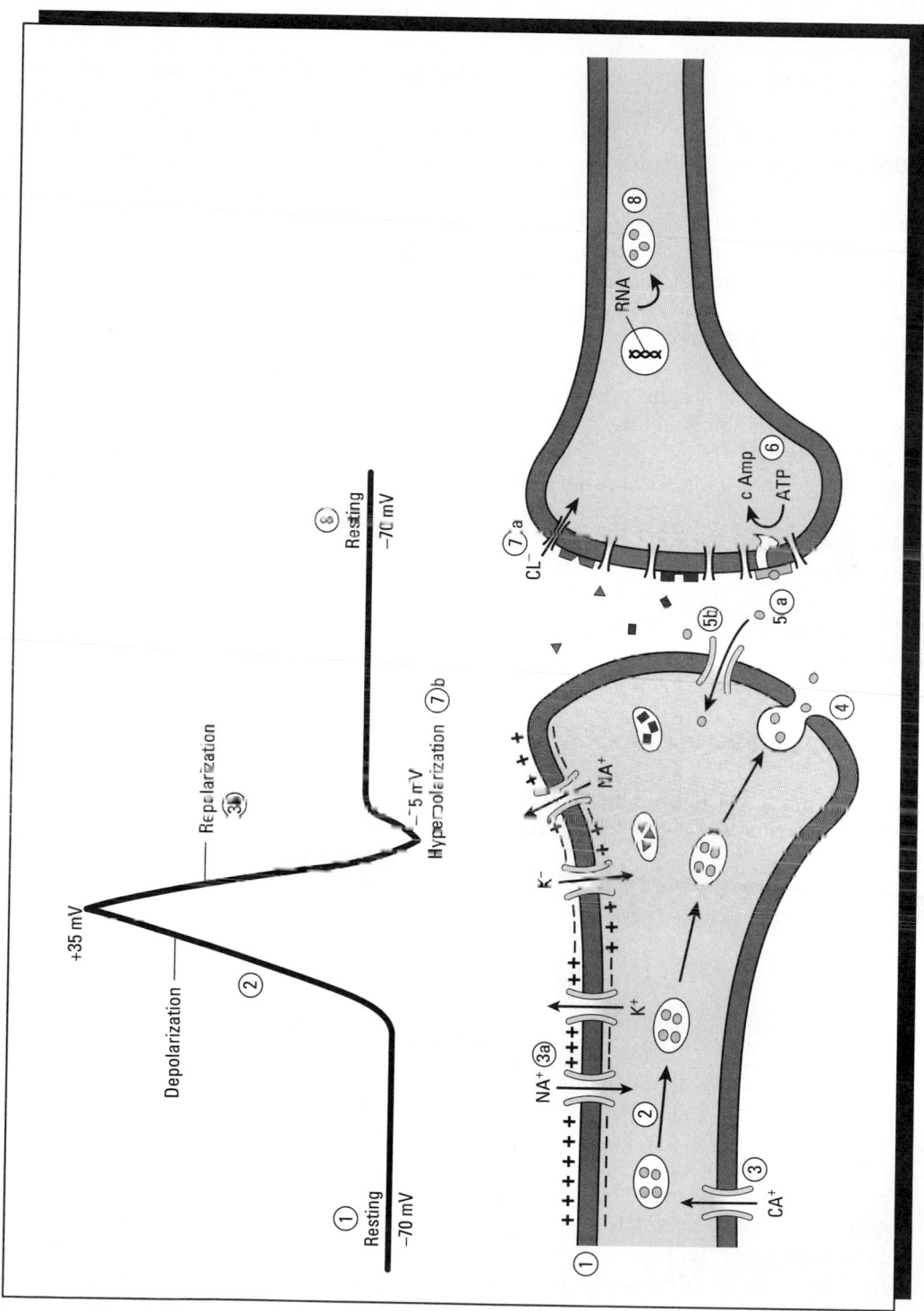

Figure 27–1. Neuroconduction-neurotransmission cascade.

blockade; more important, however, the active metabolites of **bupropion** block the reuptake of NE (Kaplan & Sadock, 1998). It is likely that the NE reuptake blockade, especially in the frontal cortex, serves to activate and calm at the same time. **Bupropion** possibly acts on the serotonergic neurons indirectly through the DA blockade and therefore creates a compensatory increase in 5HT release in the synaptic space.

Serotonin Agonist Reuptake Inhibitor

Mirtazepine (Remeron) is a recent addition to the **psychotropics** used to treat anxiety and depression. It is a **serotonin agonist reuptake inhibitor** that blocks the reuptake of NE and the dendritic reuptake of 5HT, resulting in an increase in 5HT available for release from the presynaptic neuron and more NE available in the synaptic cleft. Additionally, it blocks the postsynaptic $5HT_2$ and $5HT_3$ receptors, leaving all the 5HT available to bind with the $5HT_1$ receptors.

Norepinephrine-Specific Reuptake Inhibitors

Reboxetine is a soon-to-be-released **norepinephrine-specific reuptake inhibitor.**

Monoamine Oxidase Inhibitors

Monoamine oxidase inhibitors (phenelzine [Nardil] and **tranylcypromine [Parnate])** inhibit monoamine oxidase, the enzyme that contributes to degradation of the monoamines (DA, 5HT, and NE), thereby allowing more availability of these NTs for postsynaptic binding.

Benzodiazepines

The last class of **psychotropics** used to treat anxiety and depression is the **BDZs.** They are divided into the short-acting agents (**alprazolam [Xanax], clonazepam [Klonopin], lorazepam [Ativan], oxazepam [Serax],** and **temazepam [Restoril]**) and long-acting agents (**chlordiazepoxide [Librium], clorazepate [Tranxene], diazepam [Valium], prazepam [Centrex],** and **quazepam [Dormalin]**). **BDZs** act on the chloride ion channel of GABA-A receptors when they are bound to their adjacent **BDZ** receptor. In doing so, they enhance GABA neurotransmission, which then lengthens hyperpolarization of the impulse, thus slowing down responses to successive impulses. The net effect is to decrease reactivity of the brain. **BDZs** have four main effects: anxiolytic, anticonvulsant, muscle relaxation, and sedation.

Buspirone is a **nonbenzodiazepine GABA agonist** that also is used to treat anxiety. It does not act directly on the GABA receptor but seems to act as an agonist to the $5HT_{1A}$ and the DA_2 receptors. The effect of DA is not yet understood, but the action on 5HT occurs primarily in the hippocampus and, to a lesser extent, the frontal cortex. This unusual combination of actions places it in a class of its own. By its main action on the limbic system, it reduces anxiety, and its lesser effect on the frontal cortex prevents cognitive impairment.

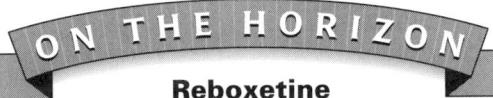

Reboxetine

Reboxetine, an **NRI,** (soon to be released), selectively blocks the reuptake of NE without affecting DA, 5HT, or histamine and with only weak ACL blockade. With this higher NE release and binding, studies show greater activation, drive, and motivation in patients with severe melancholic depression manifested by psychomotor retardation and hypersomnia. This would likely bring a much greater response and recovery rate of clients in a severe and debilitating depression without significant side effects or drug-drug interactions. **Reboxetine** may replace the difficult-to-manage **MAOIs** in the treatment of vegetative and melancholic depressive symptoms. **Reboxetine** has a relatively short half-life, requiring twice-daily dosing. It is rapidly absorbed through the gastrointestinal tract and has a peak plasma time of 2 hours. It has no inhibitory effects on the CYP-450 system and therefore will have few drug-drug interactions (Dostert, Benedetti, & Poggesi, 1997).

Goals of Treatment

The goals for treatment of anxiety disorders are resolution of symptoms and prevention of relapse. To meet these goals requires lifestyle modifications through counseling as well as drug therapy. The goals of treatment are very similar for depression: relief of symptoms, stabilization of mood, and prevention of relapse. Specific expected outcomes related to work with the therapist are individualized to the patient but may include (1) practicing relaxation exercises for 20 minutes for 5 of 7 days, (2) participating with friends in both entertainment and support, (3) exercising for at least 15 minutes daily for 5 of 7 days, (4) using affirmation to replace negative thinking, and (5) identifying contributing events in the past and present and working with the therapist to reach some peaceful balance and resolution.

Rational Drug Selection

Anxiety

Anxiety is a normal emotion in response to threat or anticipation of harm. The total body responds to threat through the autonomic system by preparing the body to flee the situation, remain and fight, or remain and freeze. The central nervous system (CNS) activates the frontal lobe to enable problem solving and thinking about the situation, as well as the memory centers to consider previous situations and responses. Finally, the rest of the cortex reacts interactively to enable the person to ask for help from others and use environmental resources to deal with the situation. Clearly, anxiety serves an adaptive purpose, and to automatically medicate anxiety may be countertherapeutic. When a patient maladaptively responds to stress, the provider should consider medication. In deciding to prescribe medication, first identify the target symptoms and then determine if they meet the criteria for a diagnosis. Many managed health care insurers do not cover medications without a diagnosis establishing medical necessity. DSM IV-R describes specific categories of anxiety disorders, with criteria for each diagnosis. If the client's symptoms do not fully meet the criteria or present a mixed picture, it is advisable to refer the client to an advanced practice psychiatric–mental health practitioner or other mental health professional. Figure 27–2 presents the algorithm for treatment of anxiety.

The primary neural pathways involved in anxiety include 5HT, NE, and GABA. Therefore, pharmacological intervention can use **nonselective norepinephrine-serotonin reuptake inhibitors, SRIs,** and/or **SNRIs. BDZs** and **beta-adrenergic blockers** have minor roles. **Beta-adrenergic blockers** are discussed in Chapter 12.

Nonselective norepinephrine-serotonin reuptake inhibitors can be used for these anxiety symptoms as well as for panic attacks and chronic pain. They usually take 2 to 4 weeks to produce the full therapeutic effect, with gradual improvement beginning with the vegetative symptoms, then arousal symptoms, before relief of mood symptoms. Unfortunately, these drugs have many adverse reactions because of their action on the cholinergic and histamine receptors, and a patient can easily overdose on these drugs and die from cardiac consequences. They are not first-line therapy; there are better and safer drugs.

Serotonin-selective reuptake inhibitors can be used for these symptoms as well as for obsessive-compulsive disorders and panic attacks. They also usually take 2 to 4 weeks to provide the full therapeutic effect, with gradual improvement beginning with the vegetative symptoms, then arousal symptoms, before relief of mood symptoms. They have fewer adverse reactions than the **nonselective** drugs and are often first-line therapy.

Serotonin-norepinephrine reuptake inhibitors affect both of these NTs. The complementary blocking of 5HT and NE permits targeting symptoms of both mood and arousal, therefore, they are useful for treating depression, sleep-pain disorders, and anxiety disorders such as obsessive-compulsive disorder, panic, and social phobia, as well as attention deficit disorders and eating disorders (Kaplan & Sadock, 1998). **Venlafaxine** demonstrates some unique effects on the G-coupling mechanism after postsynaptic receptor binding, which may decrease the time needed to reach full therapeutic effect; therefore, it has an earlier onset of action.

In the past, **GABA agonists** and **BDZs** have been used to treat anxiety; however, they have potential for cognitive impairment, tolerance, and dependence. Because the **SRIs** and **SNRIs** have not been found to be addicting, they can be given with less serious consequences.

Psychiatrists and advanced practice psychiatric–mental health nurses prescribe **BDZs** least often, and many of the clinical specialties and primary care providers prescribe them the most often. This is probably because the **BDZs** provide relatively immediate relief of anxiety symptoms. Over time, however, patients need a higher dosage to bring about the same effect, and when they abruptly stop taking them, they experience symptoms of anxiety and even panic. **Long-acting BDZs** are much less likely to produce tolerance and are prescribed initially while introducing an **SRI** for long-term management.

Other drugs that can be advantageous in anxiety are those that affect the ion channels of neurons, such as **beta-adrenergic blockers (propranolol [Inderal]** and **atenolol [Tenormin])** and the **nonbenzodiazepine GABA agonists** (e.g., **buspirone [BuSpar], valproate [Depakote],**

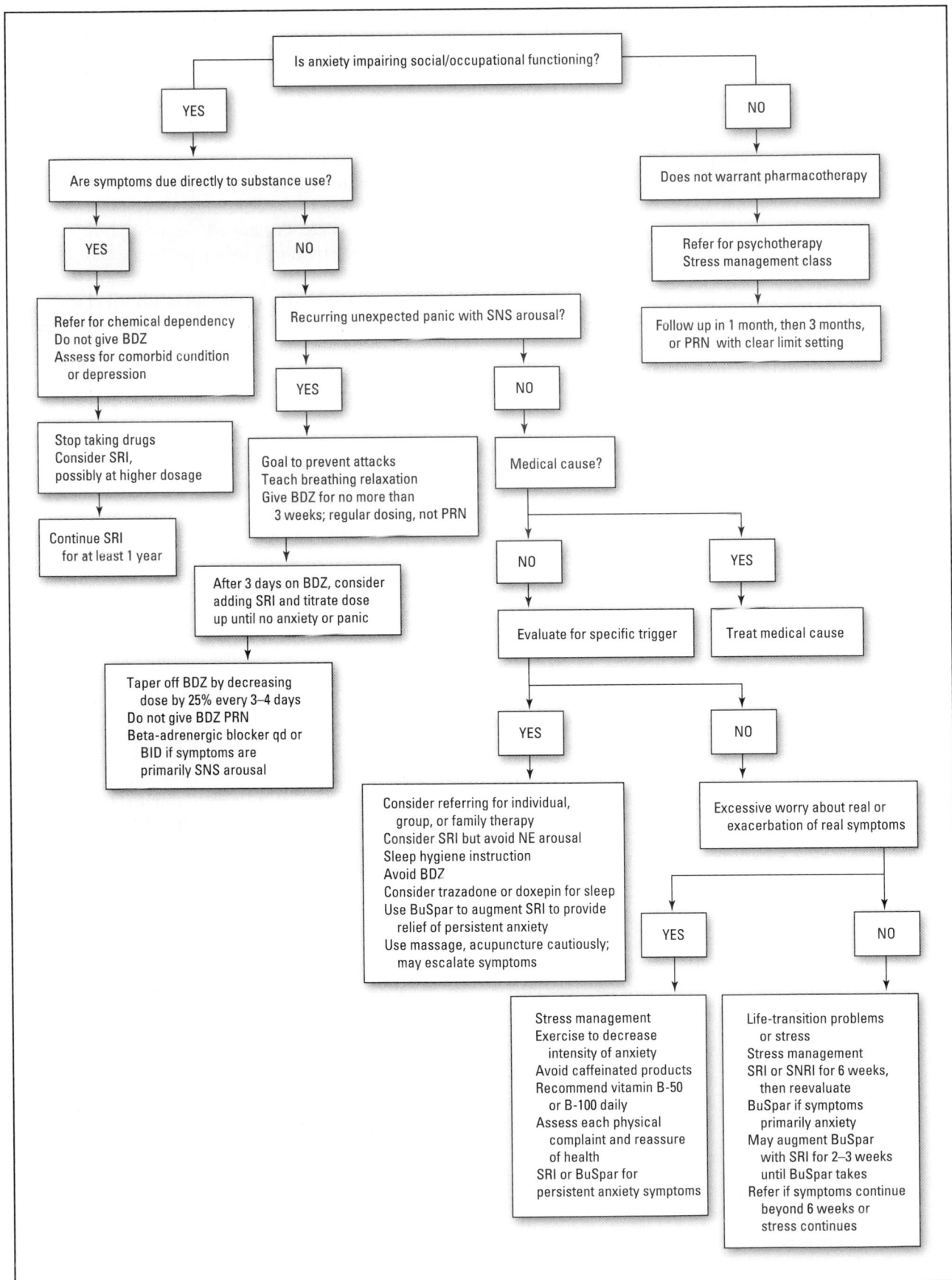

Figure 27–2. Treatment algorithm for anxiety.

and **lamotrigine [Lamictal]**). **Beta-adrenergic blockers** are particularly effective with panic disorders, especially if primarily associated with sympathetic nervous system (SNS) arousal.

Buspirone does not produce tolerance or dependency. It requires about 2 weeks to reach full therapeutic level. It cannot be taken as needed and must be taken on a regular basis and usually more than once a day. **Buspirone** seems to be especially effective with patients who have generalized anxiety disorder but is not at all effective with panic or anxiety attacks. **Buspirone** also is helpful in augmenting the **SRIs** and **SNRIs** and in treating patients with agitated or anxious depression. Because there seems to be no cross-tolerance, **buspirone** is a helpful drug to use with clients in alcohol or drug recovery. The drug must be taken every day to be effective and cannot be used to relieve immediate anxiety.

Panic and Adjustment Disorders

Long-acting BDZs are the first-line drugs of choice for panic disorder because the anxiety is so acute that the patient seeks relief in whatever way possible. Taking the medication when the panic is occurring inadvertently conveys to the client that the panic is inevitable and can be relieved only with the medication. Instead, it is best to identify any particular patterns to the panic (e.g., nighttime panic or situationally determined panic) and prescribe anticipatory to the event. In this way, the severe anxiety is prevented rather than treated after the fact by an as-needed dose. The drug is prescribed at bedtime if the panic is nighttime or at lunch time if the panic is midday. After a week on the **BDZs**, if the symptoms are adequately relieved and there are no panic attacks, the prescriber can introduce an **SRI**, such as **paroxetine (Paxil)**, at an ordinary initial dosage and titrated upward as the **BDZ** is titrated downward. In this case, tapering off the **BDZ** is more for symptom coverage while the **SRI** is being introduced than for prevention of withdrawal symptoms. For many patients, this is an effective way of treating panic or adjustment disorder with anxiety or mixed anxiety and depression. The **BDZ** may need to be reinstated if breakthrough panic symptoms occur. The drug should be short-term with patients with adjustment disorder, but patients with panic disorder may need to stay on some medication plan for up to a year. The patient with adjustment disorder is likely to spontaneously get better within 6 weeks or when the situation is resolved and not need a referral for psychotherapy. The patient with panic disorder may benefit from a referral for psychotherapy to learn stress management strategies.

Depression

Depression is an interesting phenomenon among Americans in that there is an implicit stigmatizing notion that people who are depressed have weak characters and, therefore, depression needs to be denied. Yet the English language has many terms and idioms to describe the gamut of severity of depression such as *the blues, having a funky day, down in the dumps, doldrums, low, sad, gloomy, despairing, disheartened,* and *despondent*. In fact, the rate for diagnosed depression has steadily increased since World War II, with an impressive peak between 1960 and 1975 (Klerman & Weisman, 1989). Until recently, depression was seen as a disorder of adults, but recent studies indicate that it is important to recognize and treat childhood and teenage depression as a protection against future more severe and more frequent bouts (Hughs et al.,1990). A genetic predisposition is implied because the risk for depression among first-degree relatives is 2 to 10 times higher than among unrelated or distantly related people (Kaplan & Sadock, 1998).

There are different kinds and degrees of depression severity. DSM IV-R identifies major depressive disorder as the acute form (onset symptoms for at least 2 weeks) and dysthymia (symptom duration longer than 2 years) as the chronic form. The spectrum of depression may also be considered from the degree of severity of symptoms ranging from mild, through moderate, to severe and with psychotic features. Although the predominant symptoms include depressed mood, diminished interest, fatigue and loss of energy, diminished concentration, and feelings of worthlessness and hopelessness, another presentation includes irritability, sensitivity to rejection, agitation, hostility, and anxiety in the atypical depression.

Instead of or in addition to emotional and behavioral symptoms of depression, patients may present with a myriad of somatic symptoms. Prepubertal children complain of gastrointestinal symptoms or may say they are sick to avoid going to school. Adults, especially those older than 65, commonly express depression through cardiovascular, gastrointestinal, and genitourinary systems and low back pain or other muscular pain. Especially in older adults, cognitive deficits may predominate to falsely lead the clinician to diagnose dementia.

A frustrating problem for primary care providers is the relative frequency with which depression accompanies other mental disorders (Fogelson, Bystritsky, & Sussman, 1988; Preskorn & Fast, 1993). Patients with panic attacks are often also depressed. Studies show they have a higher lifetime risk for suicide than those without any mental disorder. These patients often experience marriage and family conflicts, occupational difficulties and unemployment, financial strain, and drug and **alcohol** abuse (Kaplan & Sadock, 1998). With friends becoming burned out and greater constriction in social support due to fear and embarrassment about having repeat panic attacks, the person begins to experience symptoms of major depressive disorder.

People with personality disorders, especially borderline, avoidant, and dependent disorders, have associated intermittent depression. Those with borderline personality disorder may fear rejection and abandonment by friends and family; when they do experience inevitable disappointment, they feel it much more strongly than others would. In trying to cope with the perceived loss, they feel an abandonment type of depression. Similarly, those with dependent personality disorder may have exhausted their social resources and respond with depression and immobility. These patients often unconsciously turn to their primary care providers for nurturing. They may use outpatient and even emergency care excessively with what may be seen by the primary care provider as minor problems. The primary care provider should recognize the behavior as a clumsy or misguided attempt to have someone care for them instead of interpreting the behaviors as manipulative or malingering. In this case, the primary care provider would have better results by treating the problems as a masked depression.

Medical disorders may underlie depressive symptoms and confuse both the mental health nurse practitioner and the primary care nurse practitioner. Because the symptoms of depression overlap extensively with hypothyroidism, ruling out thyroid dysfunction with appropriate laboratory studies is essential. Additionally, unrecognized malignancies (including brain tumors) may be disguised as depression. Other conditions include chronic renal failure, autoimmune disorders, and biochemical lesions in the midbrain and brainstem such as parkinsonism and Huntington's disease. Similarly, some medical treatments may induce depression, most notably **antihypertensive** medications that antagonize the biogenic NTs. Figure 27–3 presents the algorithm for depression.

Keeping in mind the basic neurophysiological mechanisms that contribute to the target symptoms of depression and anxiety, providers can more accurately and deliberatively assess and treat the condition. Conceptually, both anxiety and depression can be medicated with the same groups of drugs. Additional classes of drugs that are commonly used to treat depression include **norepinephrine-dopamine agonists, serotonin agonist reuptake inhibitors,** and **MAOIs.**

Bupropion is currently the only **norepinephrine-dopamine agonist.** Because it affects the frontal cortex, limbic system, caudate, and brainstem, it has many uses in treating target symptoms of depression, attention deficit disorder, and social phobia, as well as disturbances in satiety such as eating disturbances, substance abuse, and nicotine dependency. In fact, **bupropion** is being increasingly used to help with smoking cessation, weight loss, depression, and postopioid addiction because of its activity in the hypothalamus at the reward and satiety center.

Because of the slow onset of therapeutic effects, it sometimes helps to start a client on low doses of an **SRI,** add the **bupropion** 3 or 4 days later, gradually increase the **bupropion** dose until therapeutic effects become evident, and then taper off the **SRI.** Additionally, **bupropion** is an early choice of medications to augment the effects of **SRIs** in patients with refractory depression.

Mirtazapine, the only **serotonin agonist reuptake inhibitor,** is very effective in reducing anxiety and depressive symptoms without contributing to $5HT_2$ and $5HT_3$ receptor activity resulting in anxiety, insomnia, sexual dysfunction, or gastrointestinal effects. Two major problems with **mirtazapine** include weight gain and drowsiness due to significant histamine blockade. Oddly enough, more adverse reactions occur at the lower or higher doses. The best outcomes result when patients take a middle range of doses from 30 to 45 mg, and drowsiness occurs most often in the 7.5- to 15-mg range.

The **MAOIs** have been available since the early 1960s and have only recently fallen out of use because of the newer and safer drugs available. **MAOIs** block monoamine oxidase by binding to the enzyme and permanently inactivating it. Synthesis of replacement monoamine oxidase requires about 2 weeks. This allows for levels of the catecholamines (DA and NE) and 5HT to rise, but it also decreases monoamine oxidase availability for two other amines found in human diets, tyramine and phenylethylamine. Monoamine oxidase is a natural rate-limiting substance that is needed to detoxify tyramine in the human body before it causes such severe events as a sudden rise in pulse and blood pressure. Therefore, use of the **MAOIs** requires dietary restrictions of tyramine-containing foods such as any aged meats and cheeses and fermented products (e.g., wine, beer, sauerkraut, soy sauce).

Although studies show the **MAOIs** to be particularly effective with atypical depression, mixed anxiety and depression, panic disorder, eating disorders, and depression accompanying borderline personality disorder, they can also be very difficult to manage with a potentially suicidal person. It is safest and most prudent for the advanced practice nurse to avoid using **MAOIs** and consider the **SRIs** and the **SNRIs** as the first-line drugs to treat depression and anxiety.

Lifestyle Modifications

If the patient is also highly self-critical, has low self-esteem, and lacks assertiveness, medication will not directly improve these symptoms, but improved thinking and reduced sensitivity through medication and therapy will improve the psychological symptoms.

Drug Therapy

Lifestyle modifications brought about through counseling alone are rarely enough to treat anxiety or depres-

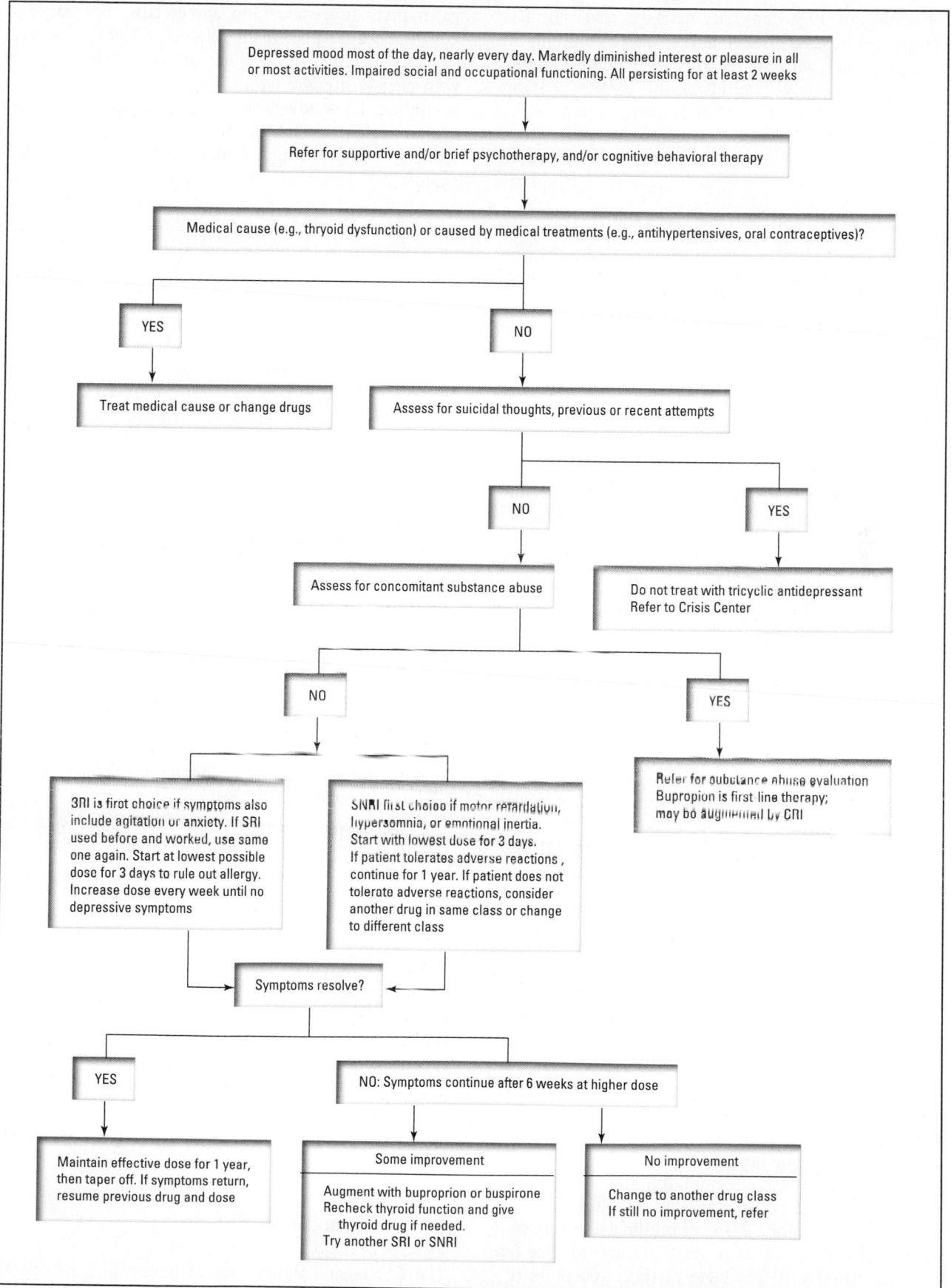

Figure 27–3. Treatment algorithm for depression.

sion. Selection of appropriate drugs is also central to therapy and is based on several variables. Symptoms improve gradually, with full responsiveness taking about 2 to 4 weeks at steady-state dosage if the primary symptoms are depression. Anticipate relief of anxiety within the first 2 to 3 days; then expect appetite and concentration to improve within the first 1 to 2 weeks. The last symptoms to improve are sleep and then dysphoric mood and consequential behaviors.

Treatment algorithms that include lifestyle modifications and drug therapy are presented in Figures 27–2 for anxiety and 27–3 for depression. Understanding the biochemistry of the brain and how drugs act on it permits clinicians to prescribe in a deliberate and thoughtful manner instead of simply following a protocol. Because the terms *antidepressant* and *anxiolytic* do not distinctively describe the NT action of these drugs, it helps to consider what NTs are involved in order to predict response and adverse drug reactions. The focus of prescribing then becomes clear identification of the target symptoms that are distressing, determining if those symptoms are amenable to biologic therapy, and selecting a drug that is specific to the putative mechanism of the symptoms. Knowing the regions of the brain and tissue interaction that mediate symptoms also aids in selecting appropriate pharmacotherapy. If symptoms are predominantly cognitive (e.g., indecisiveness, poor motivation) and vegetative (e.g., poor appetite, difficulty sleeping, low libido), the frontal cortex and hypothalamus are involved, and probably there is some dysfunction in the NE and 5HT systems. Drugs that increase the levels of these two NTs are most appropriate. The treatment algorithms assist the provider in beginning to think through the treatment process. Patients often do not follow these algorithms as nicely as we would like.

Adverse Drug Reactions

The **SRIs** are not specific for the receptor subtype to which 5HT binds. Instead, all the available **SRIs** can bind with any 5HT receptor subtype. The binding of 5HT to the $5HT_2$ receptor may be implicated in the sexual adverse reactions of the **SRIs**. With $5HT_2$ antagonists (e.g., **nefazodone** and **trazodone**) and the $5HT_{14}$ agonist **buspirone (BuSpar)**, however, the sexual dysfunction effects are minimal (Schatzberg, Cole, & DeBattista, 1997). **Buspirone** also does not produce cognitive or memory impairment or disinhibition euphoria like the **benzodiazepines** and does not interact with **alcohol** (Janicak et al., 1997). Because the **SRIs** have minimal to no effects on NE, DA, histamine, or ACh, there are few adverse reactions associated with blockade of these receptors (e.g., anxiety, restlessness, drowsiness, constipation, and orthostasis). Reduced sexual desire, delayed or absent or-

gasm, premature ejaculation, and erectile disturbance occur in about 35 percent of patients. Clinical experience suggests that men have fewer sexual adverse reactions with **paroxetine** and women have fewer problems with **sertraline**. These adverse reactions usually do not become evident for about a month, which may be due simply to relief of depression and therefore recognition of sexual dysfunction. It is important to advise patients of these adverse reactions and ask them to report these problems, which can be corrected. The most direct correction is lowering the dose or changing to another **SRI** or **SNRI**. If the patient does not want to try a different medication and the lowered dose does not help, other strategies might include adding **bupropion** or considering a **serotonin antagonist** (e.g., **amantadine [Symmetrel]** or **cyproheptadine [Periactin]**) prior to anticipated symptoms. Another option might be drug holidays with **paroxetine** or **sertraline**, but this is not possible with **fluoxetine** on account of its long half-life. **Citalopram (Celexa)** may have fewer sexual dysfunction adverse reactions and would be the first choice of change, or consider **nefazodone or venlafaxine**. It is fairly easy to change within the **SSRI** class by substituting the equivalent dosage at the next dose time.

Table 27–2 lists the dose equivalents for all **antidepressants**, including **SSRIs**. In changing from an **SSRI** to **bupropion**, it is advisable to first add the **buspirone** and then titrate off the **SSRI**. Changing from an **SSRI** to an **SNRI** can be the same direct change to the equivalent dose, but there may be NE-mediated adverse reactions, especially restlessness and anxiety. Dosage schedules for each of these drugs is presented in Chapter 13.

Bupropion has a dose-dependent increased risk for seizures in patients with bulimia (Schatzberg, Cole, & DeBattista, 1997; Kaplan & Sadock, 1998); therefore, it should not be given in single doses over 150 mg. The lowered seizure threshold and relatively short half-life require **bupropion** to be administered in two or three daily doses. A new slow-release preparation helps with a more even distribution, but, because of the seizure potential, it still requires multiple daily dosing. It has a benign adverse reaction profile because it does not affect the cholinergic pathways and has even been used to reverse the sexual dysfunction adverse reactions of **SSRIs** because it seems to block $5HT_2$ receptors.

Serotonin-norepinephrine reuptake inhibitors have adverse reactions similar to those of **SSRIs**, including insomnia, somnolence, and nausea. Like the **SSRIs**, drugs in this class could contribute to sexual dysfunction.

Drug Interactions

The **SSRIs** are highly protein-bound and inhibit the CYP-450 isoenzyme system to varying extents. They interact with many other drugs to a significant degree. Pa-

Table 27–2. Dose Equivalents for Antidepressants

Generic Drug Name	Equivalent Dose
Amitriptyline	100
Bupropion	150
Citalopram	20
Desipramine	150
Doxepin	150
Fluoxetine	20
Imipramine	150
Maprotiline	75
Mirtazapine	30
Nefazodone	150
Nortriptyline	50
Paroxetine	20
Protriptyline	20
Sertraline	50
Trazodone	150
Trimipramine	100
Venlafaxine	100

tients who are taking several other drugs may benefit from a drug choice that has fewer drug interactions. **SNRIs** show less protein binding than the **SSRIs**, are weak inhibitors of the CYP-450 2D6 isoenzyme system, and have fewer drug-drug interactions (Schatzberg, Cole, & DeBattista, 1997). **MAOIs** can have dangerous interactions with over-the-counter medications and herbal remedies that contain **ephedrine.**

The CYP-450 enzymes are responsible for the metabolism of many **psychotropic drugs** and have drug interactions based on this metabolism. Table 27–3 summarizes the major drug interactions based on CYP-450.

Convenience

Nefazadone and **venlafaxine** have short half-lives, necessitating two to three daily doses. **Venlafaxine** is available in an extended-release form, permitting more continuous blood levels and thereby reducing the occurrence of restlessness and anxiety when the blood level drops prior to the second dose. Frequently, patients who already have an anxiety disorder or agitation associated with depression cannot tolerate the anxiety caused by missed doses and refuse to continue taking the medication. With the **Effexor XR,** however, patients tolerate this drug much better. Other dosing schedules are discussed in Chapter 13. Adherence is improved with drugs that can be taken once daily.

Drug Dependency

Patients who abuse other substances, especially **alcohol,** are more likely to develop tolerance and dependency to all **psychotropics,** especially **BDZs.** When the clinician identifies that the patient has developed a tolerance to the **BDZ,** it is time to consider a withdrawal plan. Of special notice should be the patient who is taking very large doses of medication, such as 60 to 120 mg of **diazepam** a day. If the patient is taking a **short-acting BDZ** (e.g., **alprazolam**), a long-acting drug (e.g., **clonazepam [Klonopin]**) can be substituted at a comparable dosage before beginning the taper. Usually, tapering by 25 percent a week adequately prevents withdrawal symptoms and rebound anxiety (Kaplan & Sadock, 1996; Maxmen & Ward, 1995). A patient who has difficulty with the taper should be referred to a drug treatment program, a psychiatrist, or an advanced psychiatric–mental health nurse for discontinuance.

Monitoring

Patients need to know the provider is concerned and does not think they are "weak" or "bad" for having symptoms. It is important to follow up on the recommendations within the first week after initiation of therapy, which can usually be handled by a telephone consultation. Once the patient has good response and adverse reactions are tolerable, progress should be monitored in 6 months and again in 1 year. After 1 year, tapering the drug for possible discontinuance is tried. If symptoms return within 3 weeks, drug therapy is again initiated at the effective dose for another 6 months.

Outcome Evaluation

Outcome evaluation and appropriate referral points are presented in the algorithms.

Advance practice primary care nurses are likely to see patients with depressive and anxiety symptoms in their practice, whether or not the patients directly identify their concerns as depression or anxiety. Therefore, it is important to assess possible explanations for multiple somatic symptoms, especially those that involve the au-

Table 27–3. Four Cytochrome P-450 Isoenzymes and Potential Drug Interactions

Isoenzyme	Substrates	Inhibitors	Comments
1A2	Acetaminophen, caffeine, theophylline, trimipramine, doxepin, clomipramine, amitriptyline, tacrine, propranolol, clozapine, phenacetin, trazodone, mirtazapine, alprazolam	Citalopram, fluoxetine, fluvoxamine, nefazodone, moclobemide, fluoroquinolones, grapefruit juice	
2D6	Fluoxetine, sertraline, amitriptyline, clomipramine, desipramine, imipramine, nortriptyline, trimipramine, maprotiline, venlafaxine, nefazodone, trazodone, paroxetine, bupropion, flurazepam, type I antiarrhythmics, dextromethorphan, oxycodone, codeine, haloperidol, perphenazine, risperidone, thioridazine, propranolol, alprenolol, timolol, metoprolol, indoramin	Citalopram, fluoxetine, fluvoxamine, paroxetine, sertraline, nefazodone, trazodone, venlafaxine, amitriptyline, clomipramine, quinidine, fluphenazine, haloperidol, perphenazine, thioridazine, methadone	Not the most abundant isoenzyme but important for metabolism of many psychotropic medications 7–10% of whites have limited or absent capacity ("poor metabolizers") to metabolize
2C19	Citalopram, moclobemide, clomipramine, nortriptyline, desipramine, trimipramine, diazepam, hexobarbital, omeprazole, phenytoin, fluoxetine, venlafaxine, phenelzine	Citalopram, fluvoxamine, fluoxetine, paroxetine, sertraline, venlafaxine, mirtazapine, imipramine, moclobemide, tranylcypromine, diazepam, cimetidine, felbamate, omeprazole	All 2C subfamily comprises 20% of P-450 system Significant polymorphism in 18% Japanese, 19% African-Americans, 8% Africans, and 3–5% whites
3A4	Astemizole, loratadine, alprazolam, clonazepam, diazepam, midazolam, triazolam, estazolam, flurazepam, carbamazepine, ethosuximide, amitriptyline, imipramine, clomipramine, bupropion, nefazodone, sertraline, trazodone, venlafaxine, citalopram, calcium channel blockers, amiodarone, disopyramide, lidocaine, propafenone, quinidine, erythromycin, acetaminophen, alfentanil, codeine, androgens, dexamethasone, estrogens	Fluvoxamine, fluoxetine, paroxetine, sertraline, nefazodone, venlafaxine, mirtazapine, diltiazem, verapamil, clarithromycin, itraconazole, ketoconazole, cimetidine, dexamethasone, grapefruit juice	Potentially dangerous arrhythmias for those taking antihistamines, tricyclic antidepressants Accounts for 30% of all P-450 isoenzymes

tonomic system (e.g., increase in heart and respiratory rate, constipation, diarrhea, dizziness, blurred vision), poor concentration, insomnia or hypersomnia, loss of appetite and libido, fatigue, restlessness, irritability, and increased or absent emotionality. Because many medical problems may mimic depression and anxiety as well as the reverse, a thorough examination including laboratory studies can help the practitioner narrow the clinical options and therefore treat appropriately.

Medications target physiological symptoms only; and all the **psychotropic** medications act specifically on neural pathways in different parts of the brain. The psychological and social symptoms, such as low self-esteem, social withdrawal, and poor communication, can be better treated with psychotherapy. Because the physiological, psychological, and social symptoms occur together in depression and anxiety, the advanced practice primary care nurse would serve the patient best by not only prescribing medications but also discussing psychotherapy and referring the patient to a therapist to learn some new ways of coping with stress.

The choice of medication in treating depression and anxiety depends on the prominent symptoms the patient presents, comorbid conditions, other medications the patient is taking, and their tolerance of adverse reactions. Additionally, because mental disorders are often familial, it helps to know if anyone else in the family has similar symptoms and what medications have worked for them. When several choices are reasonable, select the medication that other blood relatives have had success with because they are likely to affect the patient the same.

Clinical guidelines recommend that symptoms of depression and anxiety are best treated with a combination of medications and psychotherapy (AHCPR, 1995; American Psychiatric Association, 1996). The primary care advanced practice nurse is in a pivotal position in initiating pharmacological treatment and in assisting the patient to find a mental health therapist for behavioral treatments. It is important, therefore, to have readily available a list of therapists and their areas of expertise. When recommending therapy, the primary care nurse should provide two to three names of therapists. Discussing with the patient features of a therapist the patient would feel most comfortable with (e.g., gender, discipline, geographical area, or ethnicity) invites the patient to follow up on the referral. It is also helpful to tell the patient a little about each referral specific to therapeutic style (e.g., interactive, good listener), theoretical orientation (e.g., cognitive-behavioral, interpersonal), and special interests (e.g., family conflicts, developmental transitions, sexual orientation). Of course, this requires the nurse to know something about the therapists, and that information is acquired through networking and collaboration.

Frequently, the primary care provider takes on the prescribing and medication management role while the patient is in therapy and after therapy is concluded. Maintaining an open line of communication with the patient's signed authorization for the release of information reduces confusion in treatment direction.

Working with the patient who is depressed and/or anxious is challenging and hard work. Respectful and collaborative consulting with mental health professionals yields rewarding outcomes for both patient and provider. Probably the greatest reward is seeing and hearing about the improvement the patient is making. It is tempting for both patient and mental health professional to attribute success to the medications, but to do so invalidates the power and capacity of patients. Medications can only help the brain return to its normal functioning. It is the whole person who makes the changes necessary for recovery to mental health.

Patient Education

Patient education is critical in attaining the patient's cooperation and participation in taking the medications. Compliance is least likely to be an issue with well-informed patients who understand the biology of their symptoms as well as the biology of how the medication works. The various pharmaceutical companies that produce **psychotropic** medications have informative patient education material that can supplement the clinician's teaching.

One of the most frequent errors in treating depression is ending medication treatment prematurely. When patients begin to feel better, they believe they no longer need the medication. However, the medications focus on correcting the brain's functioning, and the brain's resumption of proper function may take up to a year or longer, depending on how long the patient has been depressed. Undertreatment of depression leaves the patient vulnerable to future depressive episodes that are more severe than previous episodes. Patients need to know that they will be taking the medication for at least a year and then will need to taper off the medication to see if the symptoms resume. Another error in prescribing **psychotropic** medications is maintaining a dose insufficient to adequately treat the symptoms. The goal is complete resolution of the target symptoms, not just improvement. In most cases, this goal is reasonable and attainable if the dosage is raised to completely treat the symptoms. Because all the medications that are now available for depression and anxiety have a 2- to 4-week lag time for complete remission of symptoms, the trial of any medication requires 4 to 6 weeks before deciding it is ineffective unless the patient cannot tolerate adverse reactions of the drug. It helps to tell the patient that some symptoms remit earlier than others; usually anxiety with or without depression is the first to remit, whereas improvements of mood and sleep disturbance are likely to happen later.

Last, remember that prescribing for patients who have anxiety and depressive symptoms hinges on how the provider relates to the patient. A caring relationship in which the patient feels heard, believed, and taken seriously allows complete assessment, accurate medication decisions, and effective medication monitoring in collaboration with the patient. The placebo effect of **psychotropic** medication is about 35 percent, which means that the patient's belief that the medication will help is a powerful tool in having the medication work. Therefore, the provider should tell the patient that this medication will help, explain what to look for as the improvement occurs, and ask that the prescriber is kept informed of how the medication affects the patient, both positively and negatively.

REFERENCES

Agency for Health Care Policy and Research. (1995). *Depression in primary care: Vol. 2. Treatment of major depression.* Rockville, MD: U.S. Department of Health and Human Services.

American Psychiatric Association. (1994). *Diagnostic and statistical manual of mental disorders* (4th ed. Revised). Washington, DC: American Psychiatric Association.

American Psychiatric Association. (1996). *Practice guidelines.* Washington, DC: American Psychiatric Association.

Burgess, A. W., Hartman, C. R., & Clements, P. T. (1995). Biology of memory and childhood trauma. *Journal of Psychosocial Nursing, 33,* 16–26.

Cooper, J. R., Bloom, F. E., & Roth, B. H. (1996). *The biochemical basis of neuropharmacology* (7th ed.). New York: Oxford University Press.

Dostert, P., Benedetti, M. S., & Poggesi, I. (1997). Review of the pharmacokinetics and metabolism of reboxetine, a selective noradrenaline reuptake inhibitor. *European Neuropsychopharmacology, 7* (Suppl. 1), S23–S35.

Fogelson, D. L., Bystritsky, A., & Sussman, N. (1988). Interrelationships between major depression and the anxiety disorders: Clinical relevance. *Psychiatric Annals, 18,* 158–167.

Gabbard, G. O., & Atkinson, S. D. (1996). *Synopsis of treatments of psychiatric disorders* (2nd ed.). Washington, DC: APA Press, Inc.

Hughs, C., Preskorn, S. H., Tucker, S., Hassanein, R., & Wrona, M. (1990). Follow-up of adolescents initially treated for prepubertal onset of major depressive disorder with imipramine. *Psychopharmacology Bulletin, 26*(2), 244–256.

Janicak, P. G., Davis, J. M., Preskorn, S. H., & Ayd, F. J. (1997). *Principles and practice of psychopharmacotherapy* (2nd ed.). Baltimore: Williams & Wilkins.

Kaplan, H. I., & Sadock, B. J. (1996). *Pocket handbook of psychiatric drug treatment.* Baltimore: Williams & Wilkins.

Kaplan, H. I., & Sadock, B. J. (1998). *Synopsis of psychiatry* (8th ed.). Baltimore: Williams & Wilkins.

Kessler, R. C., McGonagle, K. A., Zhao, S., Nelson, C. B., Hughes, C. B., Eschelman, S., Wittchen, H. U., & Kendler, K. S. (1994) Lifetime and 12-month prevalence of DSM-III-R psychiatric disorders in the United States: Results from the national co-morbidity survey. *Archives of general psychiatry, 56,* 8.

Klerman, G. L., & Weisman, M. M. (1989). Increasing rates of depression. *Journal of the American Medical Association, 261,* 2229–2235.

Maxmen, J. S., & Ward, N. G. (1995). *Psychotropic drugs fast facts* (2nd ed.). New York: W. W. Norton.

Preskorn, S. H., & Fast, G. (1993). Beyond signs and symptoms: The case against a mixed anxiety and depression category. *Journal of Clinical Psychiatry, 54*(Suppl.), 9–15.

Restak, R. M. (1995). *Brainscapes.* New York: Hyperion.

Schatzberg, A. F., Cole, J. O., & DeBattista, C. (1997). *Manual of clinical psychopharmacology* (3rd ed.). Washington, DC: American Psychiatric Press.

Tollefson, G. D. (1998). Selective serotonin reuptake inhibitors. In A. F. Schatzberg & C. B. Nemeroff (Eds.), *The American Psychiatric Press textbook of psychopharmacology* (2nd ed.). Washington, DC: American Psychiatric Press.

Van der Kolk, B. A. (1998). The psychology and psychobiology of developmental trauma. In A. Stoudemire (Ed.), *Human behavior: An introduction for medical students.* New York: Lippincott-Raven.

CHAPTER 28

·······

Asthma and Chronic Obstructive Pulmonary Disease

CHAPTER OUTLINE

Asthma

According to the National Heart, Lung, and Blood Institute (NHLBI) and the World Health Organization (WHO), asthma affects more than 100 million people worldwide. The American Medical Association (1997) reports that asthma affects 14 to 15 million Americans. This chapter focuses on the pharmacological management of asthma according to the current guidelines established by the NHLBI-WHO Study Group on the Global Strategy for Asthma Management and Prevention (1995) and the National Asthma Education and Prevention Program (1997). The chapter briefly discusses the pathophysiology of asthma to help explain the rationale for selecting appropriate medications. Monitoring and outcome evaluations are essential in asthma therapy, as adjustments can have a significant impact on a patient's activity level, and patient education is the key to having patients with asthma feel that they have control over a chronic illness. The overall goal of the asthma portion of the chapter is to enable the health care provider to render optimum care for patients with asthma.

Pathophysiology

In the past, asthma was seen as episodic bronchospasm occurring in response to specific and nonspecific stimuli. It is now known that asthma is a chronic inflammatory disorder of the airways. The airway inflammation is present even between flare-ups and can significantly alter lung function. Based on this information, the National Asthma Education and Prevention Program (NAEPP) defines *asthma* as "a chronic inflammatory disorder of the airways in particular, mast cells, eosinophils, T lymphocytes, macrophages, neutrophils, and epithelial cells. In susceptible individuals, this inflammation causes recurrent episodes of wheezing, breathlessness, chest tightness, and coughing, particularly at night or early morning. These episodes are usually associated with widespread, but variable airflow obstruction that is often reversible either spontaneously or with treatment. The inflammation also causes an associated increase in the existing bronchial hyperresponsiveness to a variety of stimuli" (1997). When asthma therapy is adequate, inflammation can be decreased over the long term, thereby preventing most asthma-related problems.

Chronic Inflammation

The lungs of patients who have died from asthma are visually noted to be overinflated. Both large and small airways are plugged with mucus and a mixture of cell de-

bris, inflammatory cells, and serum proteins. Microscopic examination reveals extensive infiltration of the airway lumen and wall with eosinophils, mononuclear cells accompanied by vasodilatation, evidence of microvascular leakage, and epithelial disruption (NHLBI, 1995). The airway smooth muscle is often hypertrophied, with new vessel formation, increased numbers of epithelial goblet cells, and deposition of interstitial collagen beneath the epithelium. These changes further support the theory of chronic inflammation in asthma.

New insight into asthma has been gained with the use of fiberoptic bronchoscopy with lavage. This technique allows for the study of the cellular changes in asthma that lead to inflammation and altered lung function. Through a series of interrelated cellular mechanisms, mast cells, eosinophils, epithelial cells, macrophages, and activated T cells have been shown to affect lung function (Fig. 28–1). These cells can influence airway function by a number of routes. The release of histamine and leukotrienes can lead directly to bronchoconstriction. The release of proinflammatory cytokines from the mast cells, macrophages, and T cells activates the neutrophils, eosinophils, and macrophages, and this activation leads to the chronic inflammation associated with asthma. Cytokines can also cause the changes found on autopsy: smooth muscle hypertrophy, increased vascular permeability, and mucus secretion.

Airway Hyperresponsiveness

Airway hyperresponsiveness is a hallmark of asthma, leading to the clinical symptoms of wheezing, chest tightness, and dyspnea after exposure to stimuli such as allergens, environmental irritants, viral infections, exercise, and cold air. The inclination of airways to narrow too easily and too much is a major aspect of asthma, along with the chronic inflammation noted previously. Until recently, treatment of asthma focused on treating acute attacks with bronchodilator therapy. It is now known that the underlying inflammation influences the airway in such a way as to cause airway hyperresponsiveness. An allergen may trigger the release of a multitude of cellular mediators, cytokines, and chemokines, which result in increased smooth-muscle responsiveness. Therefore, treating only the bronchoconstriction without treating the underlying inflammation leads to treatment failure if inflammation is present. Treatment of asthma and decreasing airway inflammation not only reduces symptoms but also decreases airway hyperresponsiveness.

Airflow Obstruction

Airflow obstruction is caused by a variety of changes in the airway. Acute bronchoconstriction and airway edema are two causes already discussed. Chronic mucus

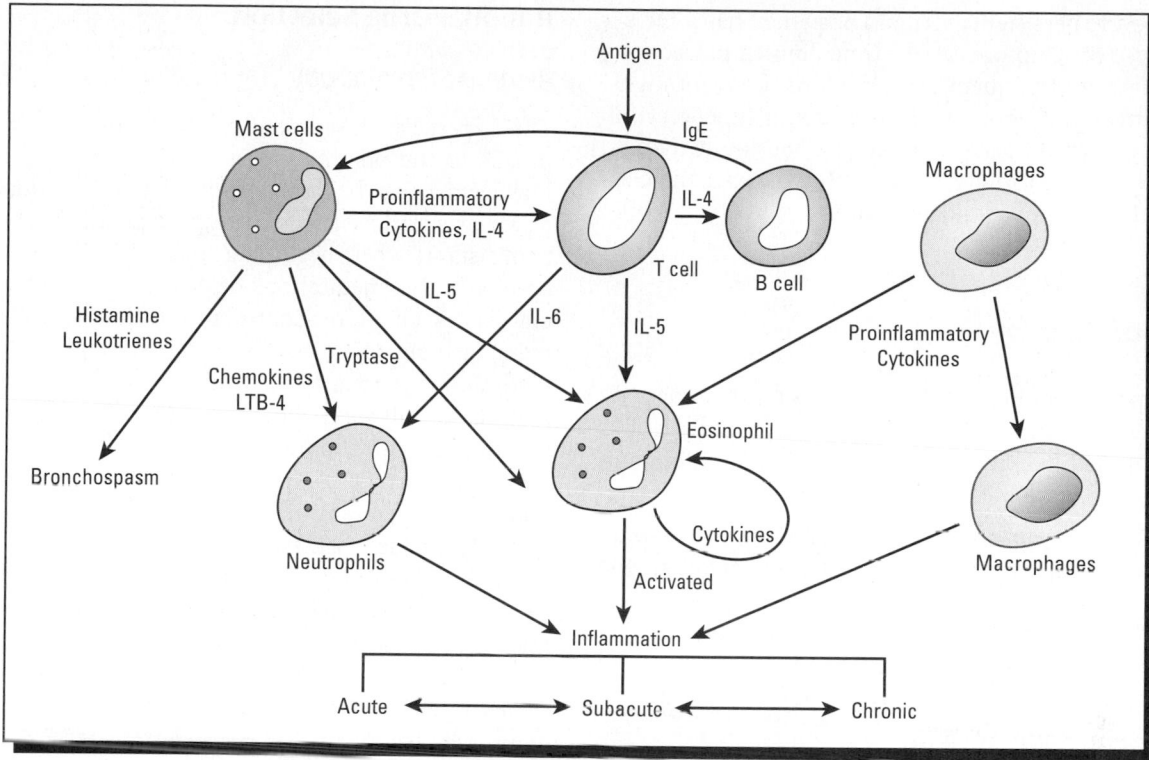

Figure 28–1. Cellular mechanisms involved in airway inflammation. (From National Asthma Education and Prevention Program, [1997]. *The Expert Panel report II: Guidelines for the diagnosis and management of asthma.* NIH Pub. No. 97–4051. Bethesda, MD: National Heart, Lung, and Blood Institute, National Institutes of Health.)

plug formation caused by increased mucus secretion can also influence airflow. It is now known that in some patients airway changes are only partially reversible. Chronic inflammation leads to airway remodeling. Histological evidence indicates that there is an alteration in the amount and composition of the extracellular matrix in the airway wall. This change is not fully understood but suggests a rationale for early, aggressive treatment with **anti-inflammatory** therapy.

Understanding the role of inflammation and the cellular mechanisms involved has led to new treatment strategies. Understanding the multiple mechanisms involved in airway inflammation has led to treatment aimed at either multiple components (**inhaled corticosteroids**) or specific mediators of inflammation. Recent development of **leukotriene modifiers** has shown that treatment aimed at specific mediators can be successful. Leukotrienes are responsible, in part, for increased mucus production, bronchoconstriction, and eosinophil infiltration. **Leukotriene modifiers,** as described in Chapter 15, are either **leukotriene receptor antagonists (zafirlukast** and **montelukast)** or **leukotriene synthesis inhibitors (zileuton).** Research continues to develop a better understanding of the pathology of asthma and treatment targeted at controlling the cellular changes that occur in acute and chronic asthma.

Classification of Asthma

Asthma severity is determined by clinical features before treatment. There are four classifications of severity, based on need for medication to relieve symptoms, nighttime symptoms, and lung function:

1. Mild intermittent asthma: Symptoms occur less often than twice a week and the patient is asymptomatic between exacerbations, nighttime symptoms are less than twice a month, and peak expiratory flow (PEF) is greater than 80 percent predicted.

2. Mild persistent asthma: Symptoms occur more often than twice a week but less often than once a day and exacerbations may affect activity, nighttime symptoms occur more often than twice a month and less than once a week, and PEF is greater than 80 percent predicted, with 20 to 30 percent variability.

3. Moderate persistent asthma: The patient is having daily symptoms, requires daily use of a **beta agonist,** exacerbations occur more often than twice a week and affect activity, nighttime symptoms occur more often than once a week, and PEF is greater than 60 percent to less than 80 percent, with more than 30 percent variability.

4. Severe persistent asthma: The patient has some degree of symptoms all the time, limited physical activity and frequent exacerbations, frequent nighttime symptoms, and decreased lung function (PEF less than 60 percent predicted, with more than 30 percent variability). Table 28–1 outlines the classifications of asthma severity.

Goals of Therapy

The Expert Panel Report II: Guidelines for the Diagnosis and Management of Asthma, developed by the NHLBI's National Asthma Education and Prevention Program (1997), clearly defines the goals of asthma therapy:

1. Prevent chronic and troublesome symptoms (e.g., coughing or breathlessness in the night, in the early morning, or after exertion).
2. Maintain (near) "normal" pulmonary function.
3. Prevent recurrent exacerbations of asthma and minimize the need for emergency department visits or hospitalizations.
4. Provide optimal pharmacotherapy with minimal or no adverse effects.
5. Meet patients' and families' expectations of and satisfaction with asthma care.

Rational Drug Selection

Asthma Step Therapy

The Expert Panel Report II recommends a stepwise approach to the pharmacological management of asthma. Management can begin at a higher level and gradually step down or start low and move up, depending on the patient's status when beginning treatment. The panel recommends that medications be categorized into two general classes: long-term-control medications to achieve and maintain control of persistent asthma and quick-relief medications to treat acute symptoms and exacerbations. Asthma severity determines the amount and frequency of medication, with suppression of airway inflammation the goal. One essential component of asthma treatment is the patient's cooperation in keeping a log of asthma symptoms. This patient self-assessment enables the provider to track the effectiveness of therapy and make treatment decisions based on medication use, nighttime symptoms, and PEF. Although step therapy is a helpful framework, the clinician must individualize therapy based on a patient's individual circumstances and response to therapy.

Initiating Control of Asthma

The Expert Panel II prefers an aggressive approach of gaining quick control with a higher level of therapy and

Table 28–1. Classification of Asthma Severity

Step	Symptoms	Nighttime Symptoms	Lung Function
Step 4 Severe persistent	• Continual symptoms • Limited physical activity • Frequent exacerbations	Frequent	• FEV_1 or PEF: ≤60% predicted • PEF variability: >30%
Step 3 Moderate persistent	• Daily symptoms • Daily use of inhaled short-acting beta$_2$ agonist • Exacerbations affect activity • Exacerbations ≥twice a week; may last days	>Once a week	• FEV_1 or PEF: >60 to <80% predicted • PEF variability: >30%
Step 2 Mild persistent	• Symptoms >twice a week but <once a day • Exacerbations may affect activity	>Twice a month	• FEV_1 or PEF: ≥80% predicted • PEF variability: 20–30%
Step 1 Mild intermittent	• Symptoms ≤twice a week • Asymptomatic and normal PEF between exacerbations • Exacerbations brief (from a few hours to a few days); intensity may vary	≤Twice a month	• FEV_1 or PEF: >80% predicted • PEF variability: <20%

Source: National Asthma Education and Prevention Program. (1997). *The Expert Panel report II: Guidelines for the diagnosis and management of asthma.* NIH Pub. No. 97–4051. Bethesda, MD: National Heart, Lung, and Blood Institute, National Institutes of Health.
Clinical features before treatment: The presence of one of the features of severity is sufficient to place a patient in that category. An individual should be assigned to the most severe grade in which any feature occurs.

then stepping down the care (NAEPP, 1997). A treatment algorithm for asthma is shown in Figure 28–2. Drugs commonly used to treat asthma are shown in Table 28–2.

MILD INTERMITTENT ASTHMA. Treatment for mild intermittent asthma symptoms consists of using short-acting **inhaled beta$_2$ agonists** as needed for symptoms. Patients with mild intermittent asthma have asthma symptoms only when exposed to their asthma triggers (e.g., allergens, viral respiratory illness, chemical inhalants), people who have only exercise-induced asthma, and infants and children who wheeze with viral upper respiratory infections (NHLBI, 1995.) Using short-acting **beta$_2$ agonists** more than twice a week may indicate a need to step up to step 2 therapy or to initiate long-term-control therapy. Education at this step is introducing the patient and family to the use of medication and teaching them about asthma, proper inhaler technique if appropriate, care during exacerbation of symptoms, and environmental controls to known allergens.

Drazen et al. (1996) conducted a comparison study of 255 patients with mild asthma in which patients followed for 16 weeks were to administer their inhaled **albuterol** either on a regular schedule (126 patients) or as needed (129 patients). The study concluded that there were no significant differences between the study groups' peak flow variability, forced expiratory volume (FEV), the number of puffs of supplemental **albuterol** needed, asthma symptoms, asthma quality-of life score, or airway responsiveness to **methacholine.** This study underscores the expert panel recommendation that patients with mild asthma use their **albuterol** inhaler on an as-needed basis, which enables patients to feel that they have some control over their asthma. Mild intermittent asthma is not inconsequential, as attacks can be severe, and it varies from patient to patient.

MILD PERSISTENT ASTHMA. The recommended treatment for patients with mild persistent asthma is one long-term-control medication daily. The primary treatment is **inhaled anti-inflammatory** medication. Treatment is started with inhaled low-dose **corticosteroids, cromolyn (Intal), or nedocromil (Tilade).** Children are usually started on a trial of **cromolyn** or **nedocromil.** The suggested beginning dose of inhaled **steroids** is 200 to 500 µg per day of **beclomethasone dipropionate (Beclovent, Vanceril)** or **budesonide (Pulmicort Turbuhaler)** or the equivalent. Sustained-release **theophylline** to serum concentrations of 5 to 15 µg/mL is an alternative therapy, but it should be used with caution and with close monitoring of serum **theophylline** levels. **Zileuton (Zyflo)** or **zafirlukast (Accolate)** may also be considered for patients over age 12, although their place in therapy is yet to be fully established because of their relative newness. The **leukotriene-receptor antagonist montelukast (Singulair)** has been approved for use in children as young as 6, but there is little research as to the effectiveness or safety of long-term use of this medication in children. Inhaled

short-acting **beta$_2$ agonists** are used as needed to relieve symptoms. If symptoms persist, inhaled **corticosteroids** should be increased to 750 to 800 µg per day of **beclomethasone dipropionate** or the equivalent. If a patient is requiring daily use of inhaled **beta$_2$ agonists** and is using the medications correctly, then step 3 therapy is indicated. Patient education at this step is teaching self-monitoring and developing and reviewing the self-management plan.

MODERATE PERSISTENT ASTHMA. Patients with moderate persistent asthma require long-term preventive medication to maintain control of their asthma. The dose of **inhaled corticosteroids** should be 800 to 2000 µg of **beclomethasone dipropionate** (12 to 20 puffs/day at 42 µg/puff) or the equivalent. **Long-acting bronchodilators** in addition to inhaled **corticosteroids** may also be considered, especially for nighttime symptoms. Quick relief of symptoms is obtained with short-acting inhaled **beta$_2$ agonists.** A more severe exacerbation may require **oral corticosteroids.** If control of symptoms is not achieved and the patient is adhering to the asthma plan, including correct inhaler technique, then increasing the treatment to step 4 is indicated. Having patients record their medication use and symptoms is essential at all steps but critical at step 3 because documentation is helpful in determining whether referral to an asthma specialist is indicated if the patient needs step 4 therapy.

SEVERE PERSISTENT ASTHMA. Treatment for patients with severe persistent asthma symptoms requires daily **inhaled** high-dose **corticosteroids,** daily **long-acting bronchodilators,** and frequent use of **oral corticosteroids.** The **inhaled corticosteroid** dose should be in the high range, which is 800 to 2000 µg of **beclomethasone dipropionate** (more than 20 puffs/day at 42 µg/puff) or the equivalent. Patients need approximately 48 puffs per day of 42 µg/puff **beclomethasone** to achieve the 2000-µg dose or 24 puffs per day of 84 µg/puff strength. Long-acting **bronchodilators** can be either inhaled **beta$_2$ agonists,** sustained-release **theophylline,** or long-acting **beta$_2$ agonist** tablets. In addition, patients may require a once-a-day dose of inhaled short-acting **beta$_2$ agonist,** such as upon rising. If long-term **oral corticosteroids** are required, the lowest dose possible to achieve results should be used and on an alternate-day schedule if possible. **Inhaled corticosteroids** are preferable to **systemic corticosteroids,** and the maximum dose should be used before long-term systemic therapy is initiated. Exacerbations require short bursts of high-dose **systemic corticosteroids.** All patients who require step 4 treatment need referral to an asthma specialist.

Monitoring Control

Once control is achieved, patients need to be monitored every 1 to 6 months to determine if a step up or step

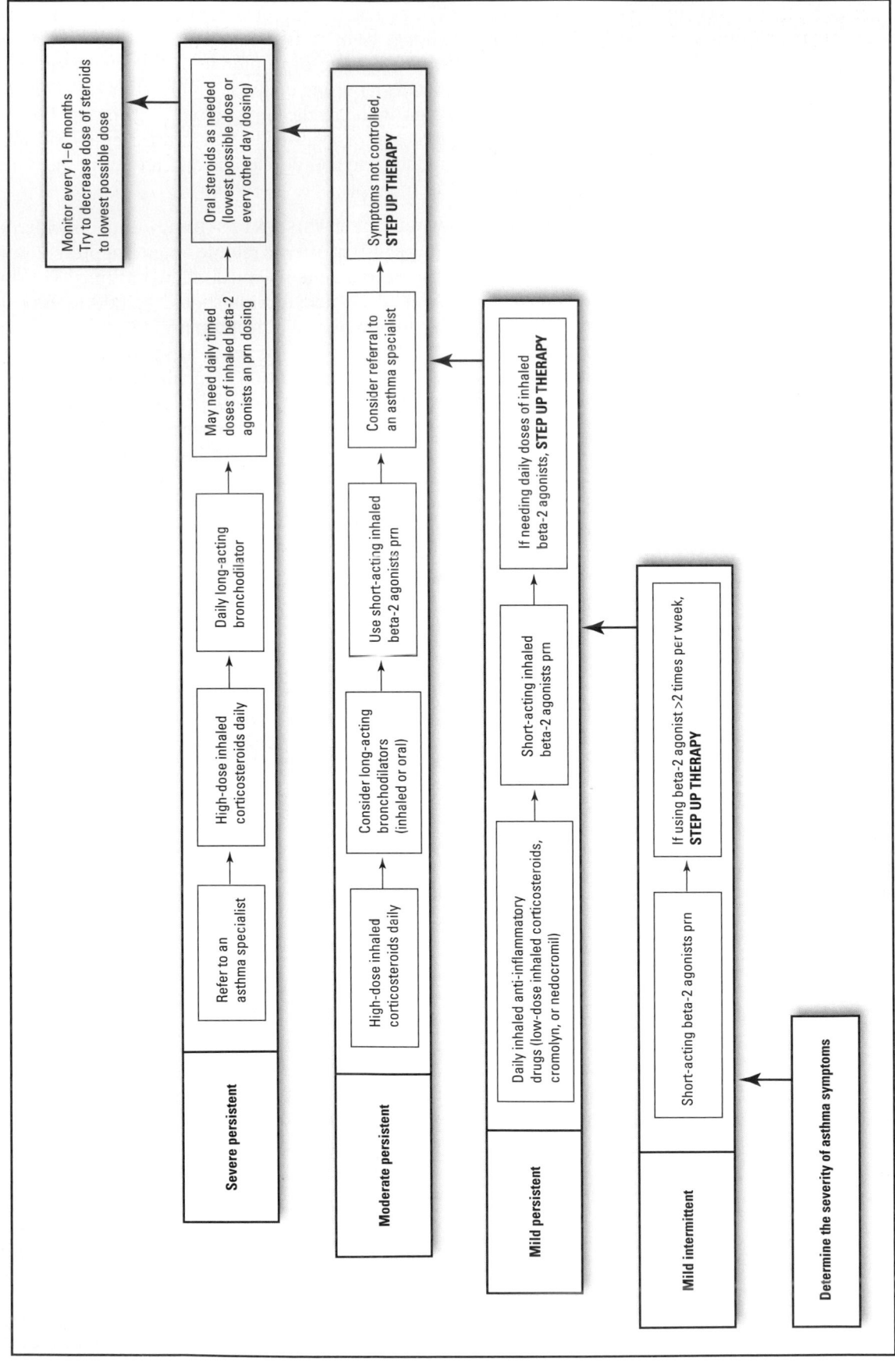

Figure 28–2. Treatment algorithm for asthma.

Table 28–2. Drugs Commonly Used: Asthma and COPD

Drug	Dosage	Special Notes	How Supplied
Short-Acting Bronchodilators Albuterol (Ventolin, Proventil)	**Inhaled** 2 puffs q4–6h 2 puffs 5 min prior to exercise **Nebulizer** (run over 10 to 15 min) *Adults:* Dilute 0.5 mL of 0.5% solution in 3-mL normal saline *or* give 1 unit dose *Children:* 0.01–0.03 mL/kg of 0.5% solution diluted in 2-mL normal saline **Oral** *Adults:* 2–4 mg tid or qid up to a max of 32 mg/d *Children 6–12 y:* 2 mg tid or qid *Children <6 y:* 0.1 mg/kg divided tid	• May repeat dose in 5–10 min during exacerbations. • Check proper inhaler technique with every clinic visit.	**Metered Dose Inhaler** 90 µg/puff **Solution for Nebulizer** 0.5% (5 mg/mL) 0.083 in unit-dose vial **Oral** Tablets: 2 mg, 4 mg Extended-release tabs: 4 mg, 8 mg Syrup: 2 mg/5 mL
Terbutaline (Brethine)	**Inhaled** 2 puffs every 4–6h; do not repeat more often than every 4–6h **Oral** *Adults and children >15 y:* 5 mg tid; maximum 15 mg/24 h *Children 12 to 15 y:* 2.5 mg tid; maximum 7.5 mg/24 h **Parenteral** *Adults:* 0.5 mg SC in the lateral deltoid; may repeat in 15–30 min; maximum dose 0.5 mg in 4 h	• Not recommended for children younger than 12 y. • Terbutaline is used to control premature contractions in pregnant women; use with care in the patient in the third trimester nearing her expected date of confinement (EDC), as it may affect labor.	**Inhaler** 0.2 mg/puff **Oral** Tablets: 2.5 mg, 5 mg **Parenteral** 1 mg/mL
Bitolterol (Tornalate)	**Inhaled** *Adults and children >12 y:* For bronchospasm: 2 puffs 1–3 min apart, followed by a third puff if needed For prevention of bronchospasm: 2 puffs every 8 h	Not recommended for children younger than 12 y.	**Inhaler** 0.37 mg/puff
Pirbuterol (Maxair inhaler)	**Inhaled** *Adults and children >12 y:* 1–2 puffs every 4–6 h; maximum 12 puffs/d	Not recommended for children younger than 12 y.	**Inhaler** 0.2 mg/puff
Long-Acting Bronchodilator Salmeterol Inhaler (Serevent)	**Inhaled** *Adults and children >12 y:* For asthma and control of bronchospasm: 2 puffs bid For exercise-induced asthma: 2 puffs 30–60 min prior to exercise	Not to be used for short-term relief. Patients need to have a short-acting bronchodilator also prescribed for short-term relief	**Inhaler** 25 µg/puff

Continued on next page

Table 28–2. Drugs Commonly Used: Asthma and COPD *(continued)*

Drug	Dosage	Special Notes	How Supplied
		and told not to use drug for acute exacerbations. If using salmeterol twice a day, do not use another dose for exercise-induced asthma; a short-acting bronchodilator or cromolyn should be used.	
Anticholinergic Agents Ipratropium bromide (Atrovent)	**Inhaler** *Adults and children >12 y:* 2 puffs qid; maximum 12 puffs/24 h **Nebulizer** 1 unit dose	• Can be mixed with albuterol 0.5% solution for nebulizer use if used within 1 h. • Contraindicated in patients with soybean or peanut allergy.	**Inhaler** 18 µg/puff **Solution for Nebulizer** 500 µg per unit-dose vial
Combination Inhaled Medications Albuterol/ipratropium bromide (Combivent)	**Inhaled** *Adults:* 2 puffs qid	• Primarily used for COPD patients. • Simplifies medication regimen by combining two commonly prescribed medications. • Not recommended for children.	**Inhaler** Ipratropium 18 µg/puff combined with albuterol 90 µg/puff
Systemic Corticosteroids Prednisone	*Adults:* "Burst" therapy 40–60 mg/d in 1 or 2 doses *Children:* "Burst" 1–2 mg/kg/d in 1–2 doses; maximum of 40–50 mg/d	If given in short "bursts" of 3–10 days, dose does not have to be tapered.	**Tablets** 5 mg, 10 mg, 20 mg
Prednisolone (Prelone, Pediapred syrup)	*Children:* "Burst" 1–2 mg/kg/d in 1–2 doses; maximum of 40–50 mg/d	Same as for prednisone.	**Syrup** Pediapred 5 mg/5 mL Prelone 15 mg/5 mL

Inhaled Anti-inflammatory Agents
Cromolyn (Intal)
	Inhaled
	Adults and children >5 y:
	  4 puffs qid initially, wean down to 2 puffs bid–tid; may use 2 puffs prior to exercise or allergen exposure
	Nebulizer
	Adults and children >2 y:
	  1 unit dose qid, weaning down to bid
		• Must be used continuously for 3–4 wk before maximum effect is achieved.
		• Very safe to use in children, with fewer adverse reactions than inhaled steroids.
			Inhaler
			0.8 mg/puff
			Solution for Nebulizer
			20 mg/2-mL ampule

Continued on next page

Table 28–2. Drugs Commonly Used: Asthma and COPD *(continued)*

Drug	Dosage	Special Notes	How Supplied
Nedocromil (Tilade)	**Inhaled** *Adults and children >6 y:* 2–4 puffs bid–qid **Nebulizer** *Adults and children >2 y:* 1 ampule via nebulizer qid		**Inhaler** 1.75 mg/puff **Solution for Nebulizer** 11 mg/2.2-mL ampule
Inhaled Corticosteroids Beclomethasone dipropionate (Beclovent, Vanceril)	**Adult** *Low dose:* 168–504 µg daily in divided doses either bid, tid, or qid (4–12 puffs of 42 µg) *Medium dose:* 504–840 µg daily in divided doses (12– 20 puffs of 42 µg) *High dose:* >840 µg daily in divided doses (>20 puffs of 42 µg) **Children** *Low dose:* 84–336 µg daily in divided doses (2–8 puffs of 42 µg) *Medium dose:* 336–672 µg daily in divided doses (8– 16 puffs/d of 42 µg) *High dose:* >672 µg daily in divided doses (>16 puffs/d of 42 µg)		**Inhaler** 42 µg/puff 84 µg/puff
Budesonide (Pulmicort Turbuhaler)	**Adult** *Low dose:* 200–400 µg daily (1 or 2 inhalations daily) *Medium dose:* 400–600 µg daily (2–3 inhalations daily) *High dose:* >600 µg daily (>3 inhalations daily) **Children** *Low dose:* 200 µg daily (1 inhalation daily) *Medium dose:* 200–400 µg daily (2–3 inhalations daily) *High dose:* >400 µg/d (>2 inhalations daily)	Not recommended for children younger than 6 y.	**Turbuhaler** 200 µg/dose
Flunisolide (Aerobid)	**Adult** *Low dose:* 500–1000 µg daily (2–4 puffs daily divided in bid dose) *Medium dose:* 1000–2000 µg daily (4–8 puffs divided bid) *High dose:* >2000 µg daily (>8 puffs divided bid)	Rinse mouth after use.	**Inhaler** 250 µg/puff

Continued on next page

Table 28–2. Drugs Commonly Used: Asthma and COPD *(continued)*

Drug	Dosage	Special Notes	How Supplied
	Children *Low dose:* 500–750 μg (2–3 puffs daily) *Medium dose:* 1000–1250 μg daily (4–5 puffs daily divided bid) *High dose:* >1250 μg daily (>5 puffs divided bid)		
Fluticasone (Flovent)	**Adult** *Low dose:* 88–264 μg daily (2–6 puffs of 44 μg divided bid) *Medium dose:* 264–660 μg daily (2–6 puffs of 110 μg daily divided bid) *High dose:* >660 μg (>6 puffs 110 μg *or* >3 puffs 220 μg) **Children** *Low dose:* 88–176 μg daily (2–4 puffs of 44 μg divided bid) *Medium dose:* 176–440 μg daily (2–4 puffs 110 μg divided bid) *High dose:* >440 μg (>4 puffs 110 μg *or* >2 puffs 220 μg)		**Inhaler** 44 μg/puff 110 μg/puff 220 μg/puff
Triamcinolone Acetonide (Azmacort)	**Adults** *Low dose:* 400–1000 μg daily divided in bid, tid, or qid doses (4–10 puffs) *Medium dose:* 1000–2000 μg daily in divided doses (10–20 puffs) *High dose:* >200 μg daily in divided doses (>20 puffs) **Children** *Low dose:* 400–800 μg per day in divided doses (4–8 puffs daily) *Medium dose:* 800–1200 μg daily in divided doses (8–12 puffs) *High dose:* >1200 μg daily in divided doses (>12 puffs)		**Inhaler** 100 μg/puff
Leukotriene Modifiers Zafirlukast (Accolate)	**Adults** 20 mg bid	• Not recommended for children. • Must be taken on an empty stomach.	**Oral** 20-mg tablets
Montelukast (Singulair)	**Adults** 10 mg once daily in the P.M. **Children 6–14 y** 5 mg once daily in the P.M.	Not recommended for children younger than 6 y.	**Oral** 10-mg tablets 5-mg chewable tablets

Continued on next page

Table 28–2. Drugs Commonly Used: Asthma and COPD *(continued)*

Drug	Dosage	Special Notes	How Supplied
Zileutin (Zyflo)	**Adults** 600 mg qid	• Not recommended for children. • Evaluate liver function prior to initiating therapy and routinely during therapy; contraindicated in acute liver disease.	*Oral* 600-mg tablets

down in therapy is indicated. Step therapy is meant to be a dynamic program of therapy in which changes in a patient's symptoms require movement up or down. For appropriate treatment decisions to be made, it is essential that patients be monitored frequently and that they maintain a self-assessment record. The Expert Panel II is of the opinion that the dose of inhaled **corticosteroids** may be reduced about 25 percent every 2 to 3 months to the lowest dose possible to maintain asthma control (NAEPP, 1997). Most patients with persistent asthma require daily medication to suppress underlying airway inflammation, and they may relapse if inhaled **corticosteroids** are withdrawn completely.

If at any time control of asthma symptoms is not achieved and sustained, the health care provider has a number of actions to take. First and most important, the provider must review and observe the patient's medication administration. Improper inhaler technique can create havoc in management of asthma, as the patient is not getting relief at increasing "doses" of medication. This problem can lead to unnecessary changes in therapy. The patient's inhaler technique should be reviewed at every visit because research has shown that technique deteriorates between visits. The provider needs to be aware that the prescribed regimen may not be followed at home, and intensive education may be needed to ensure compliance.

Managing Exacerbations

A temporary increase in **anti-inflammatory** therapy may be needed to reestablish control or treat exacerbations. The need for **oral steroids** is characterized by increased need for **short-acting bronchodilators** or decreased PEF (20% or greater), reduced tolerance to activity, and increased nocturnal symptoms. A short "burst" of **oral prednisone** is often effective. The appropriate dose is 40 to 60 mg per day as a single or divided (twice a day) dose (1 to 2 mg/kg in children to a maximum of 60 g/day) for 3 to 10 days. If the **steroid** burst is successful (the PEF returns to normal and symptoms improve), then no other treatment is necessary. If the **prednisone** burst

does not control symptoms, then a step up to a higher level is indicated. If frequent bursts of **steroids** are required, then higher-level care is needed.

Maintaining Control of Asthma

Factors that influence maintaining control of asthma include exposure to allergens, barriers to care (e.g., financial), and self-management issues. Allergy testing and referral to an allergy specialist may be necessary to maintain effective control of asthma symptoms. Families in crisis have difficulty in maintaining a complex medication regimen, and every effort should be made to simplify the treatment for all patients regardless of their resources.

Home Management of Exacerbations of Asthma

Home management of asthma exacerbations is an integral part of asthma management. Patients need to be educated to recognize early symptoms of decreasing lung function and to adjust their medications accordingly. The Expert Panel II (NAEPP, 1997) recommends the following home pharmacological therapy, which is described in detail in Figure 28–3:

1. Increase frequency of inhaled **beta$_2$ agonists.**
2. Initiate or increase **corticosteroid** treatment under certain circumstances. For mild exacerbations in patients who are already using **inhaled corticosteroids**, double the dose until the PEF returns to the patient's predicted normal range. For moderate to severe exacerbations, a course of **oral steroids** is required. **Systemic steroids** may also be necessary for patients who continue to have persistent decreased lung function in spite of doubling **inhaled corticosteroid** dose. Patients who are able to self-manage their asthma should have **oral prednisone** tablets or syrup at home with a management plan so they can begin therapy immediately.
3. Patients need to continue more intensive therapy (step up in care) for several days until the PEF returns to normal.

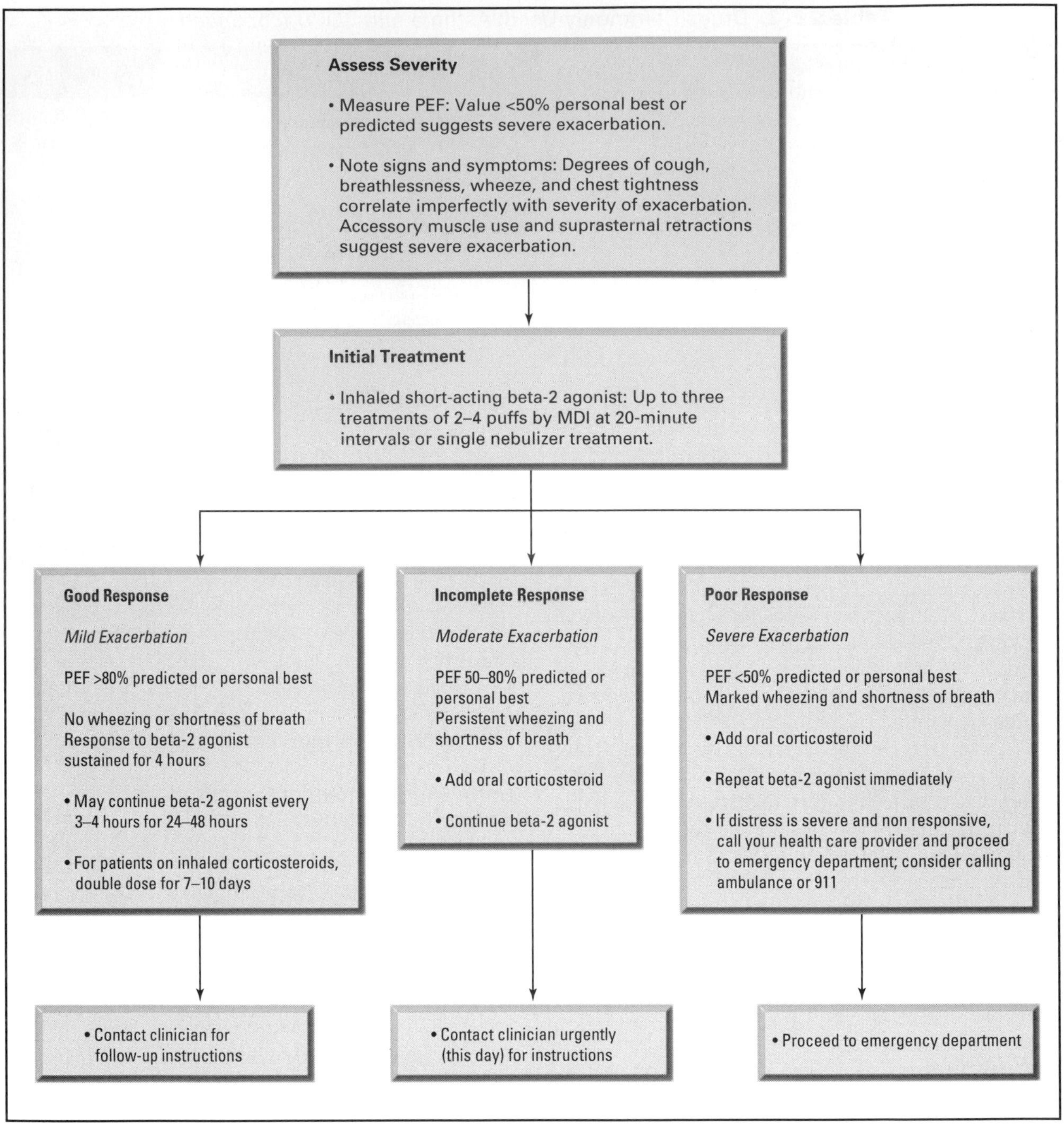

Assess Severity

• Measure PEF: Value <50% personal best or predicted suggests severe exacerbation.

• Note signs and symptoms: Degrees of cough, breathlessness, wheeze, and chest tightness correlate imperfectly with severity of exacerbation. Accessory muscle use and suprasternal retractions suggest severe exacerbation.

Initial Treatment

• Inhaled short-acting beta-2 agonist: Up to three treatments of 2–4 puffs by MDI at 20-minute intervals or single nebulizer treatment.

Good Response

Mild Exacerbation

PEF >80% predicted or personal best

No wheezing or shortness of breath
Response to beta-2 agonist sustained for 4 hours

• May continue beta-2 agonist every 3–4 hours for 24–48 hours

• For patients on inhaled corticosteroids, double dose for 7–10 days

Incomplete Response

Moderate Exacerbation

PEF 50–80% predicted or personal best
Persistent wheezing and shortness of breath

• Add oral corticosteroid

• Continue beta-2 agonist

Poor Response

Severe Exacerbation

PEF <50% predicted or personal best
Marked wheezing and shortness of breath

• Add oral corticosteroid

• Repeat beta-2 agonist immediately

• If distress is severe and non responsive, call your health care provider and proceed to emergency department; consider calling ambulance or 911

• Contact clinician for follow-up instructions

• Contact clinician urgently (this day) for instructions

• Proceed to emergency department

Figure 28–3. Management of asthma exacerbations: Home treatment. (From National Asthma Education and Prevention Program. (1997). *The Expert Panel report II: Guidelines for the diagnosis and management of asthma.* NIH Pub. No. 97–4051. Bethesda, MD: National Heart, Lung, and Blood Institute, National Institutes of Health.)

4. Patients should contact their health care provider any time they begin **oral steroids** or increase their **inhaled corticosteroid** dose, if the attack is severe, or if emergent treatment is necessary.

Patient Variables

PREGNANCY. Pregnant women with asthma need to be monitored closely for changes in lung function. Adequate oxygenation is essential for the fetus to develop normally. Poorly controlled asthma can lead to low birth weight, increased perinatal morbidity, and prematurity. In general, asthma therapy is the same for pregnant women as for other patients with asthma. They need to be educated and monitor their PEF throughout the pregnancy. Any changes in PEF require prompt treatment and modification in pharmacological therapy. Wendel et al.'s (1996) randomized controlled study of 105 pregnant women with asthma concluded that asthma should be managed aggressively in pregnancy and that **inhaled cortico-steroids** should be used to treat airway inflammation. They concluded that use of **intravenous aminophylline** in hospitalized patients did not improve outcomes over the use of inhaled **beta$_2$ agonists**. Most medications used to treat asthma are **Pregnancy Class C**, as noted in Chapter 15. Oral forms of **beta$_2$ agonists** should be used selectively in patients who are in labor, as **terbutaline** is a tocolytic (unlabeled use). Inhaled forms of **beta$_2$ agonists** are less likely to affect uterine contractions (*Drug Facts and Comparisons*, 1998).

PEDIATRIC PATIENTS.   Pediatric patients under age 5 require special management strategies. First, diagnosing asthma in infants and young children is difficult. Asthma is often underdiagnosed and undertreated in this age group because objective measures of lung function are difficult to obtain and treatment decisions are made on clinical assessment. Some health care providers are reluctant to label children as having asthma, and often the child is given a label of chronic bronchitis, wheezy bronchitis, "happy wheezer," or the like and therefore does not receive adequate treatment. Note that not all wheezing and coughing are asthma, and the patient may have less common conditions such as cystic fibrosis, vascular ring, tracheomalacia, congenital heart disease, foreign body aspiration, and primary immunodeficiency.

Among children younger than 5, the most common cause of asthma symptoms is viral respiratory infection. As most infants and toddlers get repeated viral respiratory infections, susceptible children may have repeated episodes of asthma symptoms. Parents are often frightened and frustrated with these repeated exacerbations. Parental stress associated with frequent health care visits, uncertain diagnosis, missed work because of the child's illness, or guilt about needing to work when they want to be at home with the child can make working with these families a challenge for the provider. Ladebauche suggests that "development of a partnership with parents of an infant with asthma should begin as soon as the diagnosis is established. Open communication between health care provider and parents should be used to clearly define roles and expectations of care" (1997). Partnering with parents and establishing an asthma management plan will often enable parents to feel as if they have control and that they have a clearly defined plan of action for exacerbations. Lieu et al. (1997) found that having a written asthma management plan and starting medications at the onset of cold or flu lowered the odds of an emergency department visit in a case-control study of children up to age 14 with asthma in a large regional health management organization. Parents can be taught how to identify and anticipate asthma symptoms, such as the beginning of a child's upper respiratory infection symptoms. Parents can learn to identify objective parameters of concern, such as respiratory rate or use of accessory muscles for breathing. Asthma education must be written and frequently repeated to stressed and often fatigued parents. It is best to provide in-depth teaching when the child is well so the parents can be at their optimum and not distracted by the child's condition.

The Expert Panel II recommends that all children with asthma symptoms be given a therapeutic trial of **bronchodilators**, specifically **beta$_2$ agonists** by inhaled route or oral syrup. The NIH Expert Panel developed a step-wise approach for managing infants and young children with asthma symptoms (Table 28–3). Use of **bronchodilators** more than twice a week is an indication of the need for daily **anti-inflammatory** medication. Daily long-term therapy should begin with **cromolyn** or **nedocromil**. They are considered safer for children and are without the potential but small risk of delayed growth that inhaled **corticosteroids** present. If the child's asthma is severe enough to require daily inhaled **corticosteroids**, the dose range is 100 to 400 µg/day of **beclomethasone** (2 to 10 puffs per day at 42 µg/puff). If step 3 therapy is required, the Expert Panel II opinion is that control should be established quickly with higher doses of inhaled **corticosteroids** and that therapy should be stepped down after 2 to 3 months to the lowest dose required to maintain control. Referral to an asthma specialist is essential for all children who require step 3 or 4 care. Poor control at step 2 may also be a reason to consider referral. Exacerbations caused by viral upper respiratory infections can be quite severe, and **systemic corticosteroids** may be needed often in this age group because of the number of viral upper respiratory infections that children get in infancy.

Delivery of medication to infants and young children can be a challenge. There are several delivery devices available, but the dose of medication received can vary considerably among devices and age groups. Nebulizer therapy is preferred for children younger than 2 years to deliver **cromolyn** and **beta$_2$ agonists.** Nebulizers may be used in older children who are unable to use metered-dose inhalers (MDIs) well enough to get therapeutic effects. MDIs with either a spacer or a face mask can be used. An MDI and spacer with face mask is an alternative strategy in infants if there is a need for portable treatment, such as for traveling or daycare. It is also a good choice if the family is financially stressed and the cost of a nebulizer and **albuterol** inhalation solution is prohibitive. Prior to changing or stepping up therapy, patients and parents must be assessed for proper use of delivery devices.

Older children and adolescents often have to manage symptoms at school or otherwise away from parents, and they must be included in the asthma management plan. They are developmentally interested in learning and mastering new skills. Including school-age children in decisions regarding their care and allowing them to

Table 28–3. Stepwise Approach for Managing Infants and Young Children (Age 5 Years and Younger) with Acute or Chronic Asthma Symptoms

Step 4 Severe persistent	• Daily anti-inflammatory medication • High-dose inhaled corticosteroid with spacer/holding chamber and face mask • If needed, add systemic corticosteroids 2 mg/kg/d and reduce to lowest daily or alternate-day dose that stabilizes symptoms	Bronchodilator as needed for symptoms (see step 1) up to 3 times a day
Step 3 Moderate persistent	• Daily anti-inflammatory medication *Either:* • Medium-dose inhaled corticosteroid with spacer/holding chamber and face mask, *or* • Once control is established, medium-dose inhaled corticosteroid and nedocromil *or* • Medium-dose inhaled corticosteroid and long-acting bronchodilator (theophylline)	Bronchodilator as needed for symptoms (see step 1) up to 3 times a day
Step 2 Mild persistent	• Daily anti-inflammatory medication, either cromolyn (nebulizer is preferred or MDI) *or* nedocromil (MDI only) • Infants and young children usually begin with a trial of cromolyn or nedocromil *or* • Low-dose inhaled corticosteroid with spacer/holding chamber and face mask	Bronchodilator as needed for symptoms (see step 1)
Step 1 Mild intermittent	No daily medication needed Step down: Review treatment every 1–6 mo; if control is sustained for at least 3 mo, a gradual stepwise reduction in treatment may be possible	Bronchodilator as needed for symptoms ≤twice a week Intensity of treatment will depend on severity of exacerbation. *Either:* • Inhaled short-acting $beta_2$ agonist by nebulizer or face mask and spacer/holding chamber *or* • Oral $beta_2$ agonist for symptoms With viral respiratory infection • Bronchodilator q4–6h up to 24 h (longer with physician consult) but, in general, repeat no more than once every 6 wk Consider systemic corticosteroid if • Current exacerbation is severe *or* • Patient has history of previous severe exacerbations Step up: If control is not achieved, consider step up; first, review patient's medication technique, adherence, and environmental control (avoidance of allergens or other precipitant factors)

Source: National Asthma Education and Prevention Program. (1997). *The Expert Panel report II: Guidelines for the diagnosis and management of asthma.* NIH Pub. No. 97–4051. Bethesda, MD: National Heart, Lung, and Blood Institute, National Institutes of Health.

accept responsibility for their asthma management can increase their sense of accomplishment and self-confidence (Ladebauche, 1997). School-age and adolescent children need to be able to effectively administer inhaled medications. Therefore, as children with asthma get older and gain independence, the provider needs to observe the child's inhaler technique and make adjustments as necessary. The health care provider needs to provide a written asthma management plan for the school, with clearly defined instructions for handling exacerbations and exercise-induced asthma, if appropriate. Many schools do not allow students to carry and self-administer medications. If possible, a plan that allows children to self-administer asthma medication at school is ideal. This plan has to be worked out between the parent, the school, and the health care provider.

Sports and physical activities are essential to a healthy lifestyle for children. Every attempt should be made to control asthma symptoms so that children can participate in physical activities. Treatment just prior to activity often prevents the cough and wheeze some children experience with exercise. Poor exercise tolerance is an indication of poorly controlled asthma and the need to modify the asthma management plan. Adding a long-term-control medication such as **cromolyn** or **beclomethasone** usually improves exercise tolerance. Guidance from the health care provider can assist parents and children in choosing appropriate sports. Often, children allergic to pollens cannot play outdoor sports such as baseball or soccer yet can participate in swimming, basketball, and gymnastics without problems. Restricting physical activity should be a last resort.

OLDER ADULTS. Older adults with asthma symptoms often present with a variety of other disease processes. The provider must first determine how much of the airflow obstruction is reversible and how much is due to other obstructive lung disease (chronic bronchitis, emphysema). Often a trial of 2 to 3 weeks of **systemic corticosteroids** is necessary to determine the extent of reversibility of airway disease. Inhaled long-term-control medications can then be introduced if indicated.

The medications used to treat asthma have increased adverse effects in the older patient. Those with preexisting ischemic heart disease may also be more sensitive to **beta$_2$ agonist** adverse effects, including tremor and tachycardia. Concomitant use of **anticholinergics** and **beta$_2$ agonists** may be beneficial in the older patient. **Theophylline** clearance is reduced, causing increased serum **theophylline** levels. Frequent monitoring of blood levels is necessary if **theophylline** is used for the older patient. **Systemic corticosteroids** can cause confusion, agitation, and changes in glucose metabolism. There is also a dose-dependent reduction in bone mineral content that may be associated with **inhaled corticosteroid** use. Low to medium doses appear to have no major effect on bone density. Older patients may be at more risk because of preexisting osteoporosis, lower estrogen levels (in women), and a sedentary lifestyle. The Expert Panel II (NAEPP, 1997) recommends concurrent treatment with **calcium** and **vitamin D** supplements and, as appropriate, **estrogen** replacement for older patients on high-dose **inhaled corticosteroid** therapy.

Another concern in older patients is that the medications used to treat other chronic diseases may cause asthma exacerbations or require medication adjustments. Patients who are taking **theophylline** need to be assessed for medications that affect **theophylline** clear-

ance. The **nonselective beta blockers,** including some **beta blockers** in eyedrops used to treat glaucoma, can result in mutual inhibition of therapeutic effects if used with **beta$_2$ agonists. Nonsteroidal anti-inflammatory drugs (NSAIDs)** used to treat arthritis may cause asthma exacerbation. At each visit for asthma-related symptoms, it is essential to assess the patient's complete history, including all medications the patient takes.

Special Situations

SEASONAL ASTHMA. Seasonal asthma is identified when patients appear to have asthma symptoms only in relationship to certain pollens and molds. Seasonal asthma is managed in the same stepwise approach to long-term management of asthma that was previously discussed. If the patient has predictable seasonal asthma—each spring, for example—long-term **anti-inflammatory** treatment should be initiated approximately 1 month before the anticipated onset of symptoms and continued through the season. **Cromolyn,** a **mast cell stabilizer,** is a good choice for initial treatment of seasonal asthma.

COUGH VARIANT ASTHMA. Cough variant asthma is seen especially in young children. Cough variant asthma is diagnosed when cough, usually at night, is the principal symptom. Daytime examination may be normal, thereby often delaying or confusing the diagnosis. A therapeutic trial of **bronchodilator** medication is often diagnostic of cough variant asthma. Monitoring PEF changes between morning and evening readings may also assist in the diagnosis. Management is according to the stepwise approach to long-term management of asthma.

EXERCISE-INDUCED BRONCHOSPASM. Exercise-induced bronchospasm (EIB) should be anticipated in all patients with asthma, although some patients exhibit asthma symptoms only when exercising. Bronchospasm is due to hyperventilation of air that is cooler and dryer than that of the respiratory system, which causes loss of heat and water from the lungs. The diagnosis of EIB is made first by history of cough, shortness of breath, chest pain or tightness, or wheezing during or right after exercise. Formal diagnosis can be made in a laboratory or by having patients exercise strenuously enough to increase their heart rate to 80 percent of maximum for 4 to 6 minutes. Otherwise healthy patients can run in the hallway or stairway of the clinic if appropriate. The PEF measurements are taken before and at 5-minute intervals for 20 to 30 minutes. A 15 percent decrease in PEF is compatible with EIB.

The goal of EIB therapy is for patients to be able to participate in any activity they choose without asthma symptoms. Teachers and coaches need to be notified that a child or an athlete has EIB. The Expert Panel II (NAEPP, 1997) recommends the following treatment strategies:

1. Short-acting **beta$_2$ agonists** used just prior to exercise prevent EIB in 80 percent of patients for 2

to 3 hours. **Salmeterol** has been shown to prevent EIB for 10 to 12 hours.

2. **Cromolyn** and **nedocromil** inhaled shortly before exercise is also effective in preventing EIB.

3. A lengthy warm-up before exercise may decrease the need for repeated medications if the patient can tolerate continuous exercise without symptoms.

4. Long-term-control therapy with **inhaled anti-inflammatory** medication may be indicated and helpful in reducing airway responsiveness and therefore decreasing EIB.

SURGERY. Surgery places patients with asthma at risk for complications during and after surgery. These complications include acute bronchoconstriction triggered by intubation, hypoxemia and possible hypercapnia, impaired cough effectiveness, atelectasis, and respiratory infections. The more severe the patient's asthma prior to surgery, the higher the likelihood of complications. Prior to surgery, the asthmatic patient should have an evaluation that includes symptoms, review of medications, and pulmonary function testing. If possible, patients ought to be at their personal best PEF. A short burst of **systemic corticosteroids** may be necessary to reach ideal lung function. Patients who have received **systemic corticosteroids** in the past 6 months require **intravenous hydrocortisone** during the surgical period.

Monitoring

Monitoring patients with asthma is a continuous process, beginning with the initial diagnosis. The Expert Panel II recommends ongoing monitoring of the following six areas: signs and symptoms, pulmonary function, quality of life and functional status, history of asthma exacerbations, pharmacotherapy, and patient-provider communication and patient satisfaction.

Monitoring Signs and Symptoms of Asthma

All patients should be taught to monitor and recognize their asthma symptoms. Recording symptoms and PEF on a self-assessment diary enables the patient and the provider to track asthma symptoms and determine if there is adequate control. Clinical signs of asthma should be assessed at each visit through physical examination and appropriate questioning of the patient. Questions should be asked about the recent past (example: In the past 2 weeks, how many times have you had nighttime symptoms?). Questions about longer periods give a more generalized response (example: Have your symptoms been better or worse since your last visit?). Assessment of symptoms should differentiate between daytime symptoms, nighttime symptoms, and symptoms that occur in the early morning and that do not improve after inhaling a short-acting **beta$_2$ agonist**.

Monitoring Pulmonary Function

Monitoring lung function is essential to diagnosis and management of asthma. Lung function can be monitored by spirometry and peak flow monitoring. The Expert Panel II (NAEPP, 1997) recommends that spirometry tests be done at the time of initial assessment, after treatment is initiated and PEF has stabilized to determine "normal" airway function for the individual patient, and then every 1 to 2 years to assess the maintenance of airway function. Spirometry may also be needed to check the accuracy of PEF readings before making major treatment decisions if there is a question about the reliability of the PEF. Peak flow meters are used for ongoing monitoring, not diagnosis, of asthma. Patients who have frequent exacerbations or require long-term therapy need to have a peak flow meter at home and be comfortable with its use. Monitoring PEF is essential to management of moderate to severe asthma in order to determine the severity of exacerbations and to guide treatment decisions. Daily PEF readings help to detect early changes in asthma status, help to evaluate response to changes in medication therapy, and provide a quantitative measure of airflow obstruction. The Expert Panel II does not recommend long-term daily peak flow monitoring of patients with mild intermittent or mild persistent asthma, although PEF may be helpful during exacerbations. Patients should be given in-depth teaching regarding peak flow meter use, which may require more than one visit or referral to a nurse clinician who can teach proper peak flow meter use. Patients need to establish their personal best PEF and use that reading as the basis of their action plan. The patient should use the same brand of peak flow meter or reestablish personal best PEF if changing brands because there is no universal normative value for peak flow meters and the PEF may vary between brands. Peak flow meters are usually covered by insurance if the provider writes a prescription for the item.

Monitoring Quality of Life and Functional Status

Monitoring quality of life and functional status is essential to determine if the goals of asthma therapy are being met. The Expert Panel II recommends that the following areas of quality of life be periodically assessed:

1. Missed work or school because of asthma
2. Reduction in usual activities
3. Any disturbances in sleep due to asthma
4. Any change in caregiver activities due to child's asthma (for caregivers of children with asthma)

Monitoring History of Asthma Exacerbations

Monitoring the history of asthma exacerbation is essential at every visit. The provider must question the patient and evaluate self-monitoring records to determine exacerbation, both self-treated and those treated by other health care providers (e.g., emergency department visit, hospitalization). Changes in drug treatment are based on the exacerbation history.

Monitoring Pharmacotherapy

Monitoring the effectiveness of pharmacological therapy is key to successful asthma treatment. The following should be monitored: patient adherence to the regimen, inhaler technique, level of usage of as-needed **inhaled short-acting beta$_2$ agonist,** frequency of **oral corticosteroid** "burst" therapy, and changes in dosages of **inhaled anti-inflammatory** or other long-term-control medication. The provider must also determine if the patient is at the appropriate level of step therapy and if changes need to be made. At each visit, an up-to-date asthma action plan has to be reviewed and revised as appropriate.

Monitoring Patient-Provider Communication and Patient Satisfaction

Patient satisfaction and patient-provider communication should be assessed routinely. Two aspects of patient satisfaction should be assessed and addressed as appropriate: satisfaction with asthma control and satisfaction with quality of care (NAEPP, 1997).

Outcome Evaluation

Evaluating the effectiveness of asthma therapy is an ongoing process, as described in the Monitoring section. The best outcome for asthma patients is being able to accomplish their activities of daily living, whatever their lifestyle, with minimal asthma symptoms.

The Expert Panel II recommends that referral to an asthma specialist be made if there are difficulties in achieving or maintaining control, if immunosuppressive therapy is being considered, or if a patient requires step 4 (step 3 if patient is an infant or young child) care.

Patient Education

Patient education should include a discussion of information related to the overall treatment plan as well as that specific to the drug therapy, reasons for taking the drug, drugs as part of the total treatment regimen, and adherence issues.

The key to asthma patient education is to establish and maintain a partnership between the patient, family, and the health care team. Patients and families are being asked to manage complex medical regimens, detect and self-treat most exacerbations (unless severe), and communicate appropriately with the team. Asthma educa-

tion is cost-effective and can reduce morbidity for both adults and children.

Chronic Obstructive Pulmonary Disease

Chronic obstructive pulmonary disease (COPD) is the term commonly used to refer to conditions of chronic airflow limitation. Other terms used include chronic obstructive airway disease and chronic obstructive lung disease. It is the fifth leading cause of death in the United States, affecting more than 15 million people. The primary risk factor is cigarette smoking (85% caused by smoking), although occupational exposure (grain, coal, asbestos) and air pollution are also known factors.

COPD is a heterogeneous disorder that includes primarily chronic bronchitis and emphysema but also includes peripheral airway disease and asthmatic bronchitis. The diagnosis of obstructive lung disease is determined by spirometry tests of lung function. A positive diagnosis of COPD is made when the forced expiratory volume in 1 second (FEV$_1$) and the ratio to the forced vital capacity (FVC) is less than 75 percent. There are clear differences between the clinical presentations of emphysema and chronic bronchitis. Patients with emphysema are older at diagnosis and often thinner than patients with chronic bronchitis (Table 28–4). The primary symptom seen in emphysema is dyspnea, whereas cough with copious sputum production is often the presenting symptom in chronic bronchitis. Laboratory values differ in that patients with emphysema are typically barrel-breasted and breathe through pursed lips ("pink-puffers"), whereas patients with chronic bronchitis are typically obese and suffer from significant hypoxemia, cyanosis, and carbon dioxide retention ("blue-bloaters").

Pathophysiology

The pathophysiology of COPD is characterized by both acute and chronic inflammation. There are also changes in cellular proliferation, leading to tissue destruction, loss of structural ciliated columnar cells, squamous and goblet cell metaplasia, glandular and smooth-muscle hypertrophy, and scarring. Clinically, these changes lead to worsened obstruction, hyperinflation of the lungs, increased sputum production, recurrent respiratory infections, and altered gas exchange. As the disease progresses, the patient experiences respiratory muscle fatigue, ventilatory disorders, cardiovascular compromise, and poor quality of life.

Emphysema

Emphysema is closely linked to cigarette smoking and the damage to the respiratory tract from the chronic cellular changes smoking produces. The chronic, progressive destruction of the alveolar structures found in emphysema is thought to be caused by an imbalance between proteases and antiproteases in the lower respiratory tract. Proteases, specifically polymorphonuclear neutrophil (PMN) elastase and pulmonary alveolar macrophage (PAM) elastase, work unchecked to destroy alveolar structures and their elastin network. Cigarette smokers have increased numbers of PMNs and PAMs in their lungs, which results in the loss of elastic recoil and structural support found in the lungs of smokers with emphysema. These findings are also found in patients with genetic alpha$_1$ antitrypsin deficency, which accounts for 2 percent of patients with emphysema. Alpha$_1$ antitrypisn functions as an antiprotease in the lung to inhibit neutrophil elastase. Therefore, the same structural changes occur in these patients as occur in smokers with emphysema.

Chronic Bronchitis

Cigarette smoking is also the major contributor to the development of chronic bronchitis. Other inhaled irritants are also known to cause chronic bronchitis, among them dust, grain dust, fumes, and asbestos. There are three direct effects of inhaling bronchial irritants that contribute to the development of chronic bronchitis: (1) stimulation of mucus secretion in the airways, (2) impaired mucus clearance due in part to interference with ciliary activity, and (3) decreased resistance to bronchopulmonary infection because of altered alveolar macrophage function. Clinically, the patient presents with a chronic cough that is due to accumulation of the secretions. Airflow obstruction is due to inflammation of the airways and the thick secretions. The increased mucus is an excellent medium for recurrent bronchial infections, which cause further damage to the airways.

PATIENT EDUCATION

Asthma

Related to the Overall Treatment Plan and Disease Process

☐ Basic facts about asthma. Use a variety of teaching methods such as illustrations, video, written pamphlets or books, and models. Repeat key facts at every visit until the patient and/or family demonstrates an understanding of asthma. An example would to be to show the patient a drawing of a normal airway and an airway affected by asthma. The provider can then demonstrate how different medications act on different components of asthma (bronchodilator relaxes smooth muscle, anti-inflammatory decreases inflammation, etc.). This information can be repeated when reviewing medications at each visit until a clear understanding is demonstrated.

☐ Medication skills. This includes proper inhaler use, spacer use if appropriate, when to take quick-relief medications, and nebulizer use if appropriate.

☐ Self-monitoring skills. This includes self-assessment of symptoms, peak flow monitoring, and how to record symptoms and PEF on self-assessment diary. Recognizing early signs of declining lung function is essential knowledge for the patient and family.

☐ Environmental control and avoidance strategies will enable the patient and family to avoid possible asthma triggers. Discussion of how environmental exposure to allergens and irritants can worsen asthma symptoms and how to avoid triggers at home, work, and school will assist patients in learning self-management.

Specific to the Drug Therapy

☐ Reason for the drug being given and its anticipated action in the disease process.
☐ Doses and schedules for taking the drug.
☐ Coping mechanisms for complex and costly drug regimens.
☐ Interactions between other treatment modalities and these drugs.

continued

PATIENT EDUCATION

Asthma (*continued*)

Reasons for the Drug(s) Being Taken

Patient education about specific drugs is provided in Chapter 15.

Drugs as Part of the Total Treatment Regimen

Information should be provided concerning drugs as part of the total treatment regimen and individualized to the patient's age and asthma severity.

Many educational resources are available, the best of which are from the NIH and WHO. These documents include the following:

☐ The Expert Panel Report 2: Guidelines for Management of Asthma. National Education Prevention Program. NIH Publication No. 97–4051 (1997).

☐ Global Initiative for Asthma. Asthma Management and Prevention. A Practical Guide for Public Health Officials and Health Care Professionals (1995).

☐ Global Initiative for Asthma. Asthma Prevention Program. A Pocket Guide for Physicians and Nurses (1995).

What You and Your Family Can Do about Asthma

These documents are published on the Internet. The Expert Panel Report 2 can be found at *www.nhlbi.nih.gov/nhlbi/nhlbi.htm* and the NIH/WHO Global Initiative for Asthma documents can be found at *www.ginasthma.com*

Other resources include the following:

☐ National Asthma Education and Prevention Program. NHLBI Information Center, PO Box 30105, Bethesda, MD 20824-0105, (301) 251–1222, *www.nhlbi.nih.gov/nhlbi/nhlbi.htm*

☐ Allergy and Asthma Network, Mothers of Asthmatics, Inc., 3554 Chain Bridge Road, Suite 200, Fairfax, VA 22030 2709, (703) 385–4403, *www.pdoi.com/healht/aanma* (Also a booklet: What Everyone Needs to Know about Asthma)

☐ Asthma and Allergy Foundation of America, 1123 15th Street NW, Suite 502, Washington, DC 20005, (800) 7AS-THMA

☐ American Academy of Allergy, Asthma, and Immunology, 611 East Wells Street, Milwaukee, WI 53202, (800) 822–2762, *www.aaaai.org*

Adherence Issues

☐ Health care providers should be aware of the potential problem of nonadherence with the treatment regimen and should discuss the importance of adherence with the patient and family members.

Goals of Therapy

The major goals of treatment for patients with COPD are to slow the disease process and maintain quality of life. Although medications such as **antibiotics, bronchodilators,** and **corticosteriods** are part of the treatment, other nonpharmacological measures have just as much impact. Most important, the patient must quit smoking. Nutrition and infection protection are key in maintaining optimum health. Exercise and pulmonary rehabilitation improve function and quality of life for the patient with COPD. A well-managed regimen of medication and non-

Pediatric Patient with Asthma

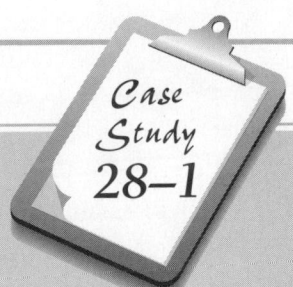

Complaint

"My son has been coughing and wheezing for the past 24 hours."

History

Zack, age 6, presents to the office with symptoms of worsening cough and wheeze for the past 24 hours. He is accompanied by his mother, who is a good historian. She reports that her son started having symptoms of a viral upper respiratory infection (URI) 2 to 3 days ago, beginning with a runny nose, low-grade fever of 100.5°F orally, and loose cough. Wheezing started on the day before the visit, so Zack's mother started administering albuterol MDI 2 puffs before bed and then 2 puffs at around 2 A.M. The cough and wheezing appear worse today, according to the mother. Zack had difficulty taking deep-enough breaths to inhale this morning's dose of albuterol, even using the spacer.

Zack has been a patient at the clinic since birth and is up to date on his immunizations. His growth and development have been normal, and he has been generally healthy except for mild intermittent asthma. His asthma is usually precipitated by a viral URI. He has required oral prednisone an average of two or three times per year for the past 3 years. He has an albuterol MDI at home with a spacer, which his parents are comfortable using. He is in first grade. This is the first asthma exacerbation of the school year, and his mother expresses a concern about sending him to school with an inhaler.

Assessment

Zack is afebrile with a respiratory rate of 36 and a tight cough every 1 or 2 minutes. He weighs 45 lb. The examination is all within normal limits except for his breath sounds. He has diffuse expiratory wheezes and mild retractions. Pulse oximeter readings indicate oxygen saturation of 93%.

Initial Management Plan

Zack's initial management plan is as follows:

1. In the clinic: Zack is given a nebulizer treatment of albuterol inhalation solution 2.5 mg in 2 cc saline. His lungs have better aeration after the treatment, with scattered wheezes. The tight cough has subsided. Pulse oximeter reading is now 98%.
2. Teaching: Once Zack has better aeration and decreased cough, the practitioner will use a placebo MDI to check his inhaler technique. He is able to use the MDI with spacer fairly well without assistance.
3. Exacerbation plan: Zack is given a prescription for prednisone 20 mg PO bid for 3 to 5 days. His mother is instructed to begin the prednisone immediately upon filling the prescription and to give two doses today. She is also instructed to have Zack use his inhaler every 4 to 6 hours until the cough and wheeze have been gone for 24 hours. Zack may return to school the next day if the cough and wheeze improve. A school asthma management plan is written out for the mother to take to the school, and a prescription is given for a second albuterol MDI and spacer for school use.
4. Follow-up and asthma teaching: The mother is instructed to return to the clinic in 1 to 2 weeks for follow-up and to develop a written asthma treatment plan.

Follow-up Visit

At his follow-up visit 10 days later, Zack is much improved. Zack and his parents are taught how to use a peak flow meter, and an asthma treatment plan is developed.

Modifications to Management Plan

The asthma treatment plan now includes the use of the peak flow meter to track PEF and to detect exacerbations earlier in the course of a viral illness. The plan also includes a small emergency supply of oral prednisone at home for use in exacerbations, following clear written guidelines of when to start the medication. The parents are to contact their primary care practitioner if they start the prednisone.

Principles Demonstrated

Zack's case demonstrates the use of steroid burst therapy for mild intermittent asthma, as well as establishment of a written plan for further exacerbations. It also illustrates the beginning independence that children with asthma must learn in order to manage their illness at school. A written asthma treatment plan for home and school is essential for successful treatment. A home emergency supply of prednisone can be given to patients if clear guidelines are given as to its use and appropriate education given.

Adult Patient with Asthma

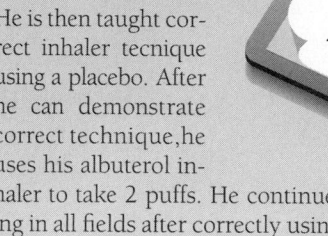

Case
Study
28–2

Complaint

"I need a refill for my inhaler."

History

Rick, age 25, is being seen in your clinic for the first time. He recently moved to the area and is establishing with you as a primary provider. His chief complaint is that he needs a refill for his asthma inhalers and is hoping you "know more about asthma than the last provider" because his asthma has "never" been under control in spite of trying many different inhalers. He has never seen an asthma specialist and has never had a written asthma treatment plan.

Rick reports having asthma "all his life," beginning in early childhood. As a child, he remembers being hospitalized a couple of times for asthma. He reports the mainstay of his treatment has been to use an albuterol inhaler the past few years. He remembers being on oral medicine before but cannot remember the name. He has no other health problems except that he smokes one pack of cigarettes per day. Upon further exploration, he reports that he used the different inhalers for only a short time, because "they didn't work."

Assessment

Rick's examination is normal except for soft expiratory wheezes and a loose cough. He did have his albuterol inhaler with him, and when asked to demonstrate the use of his inhaler, he demonstrated such poor technique that he probably did not inhale any medication at all.

Initial Management Plan

Rick's initial management plan is as follows:

1. Get old records regarding previous asthma treatment.
2. In the clinic today: Rick is given a brief overview of the pathophysiology of asthma, using a diagram of a normal airway and an asthma-affected airway to demonstrate the different components of asthma.

He is then taught correct inhaler tecnique using a placebo. After he can demonstrate correct technique, he uses his albuterol inhaler to take 2 puffs. He continues to have wheezing in all fields after correctly using the inhaler. The practitioner decides to take an aggressive approach to management and so decides to prescribe prednisone 40 mg daily for 7 days, a triamcinolone inhaler 4 puffs 4 times a day, and albuterol 2 puffs prn symptoms. A written asthma management plan is given to Rick. He is to return in 1week for follow-up and to begin asthma education.

Follow-up Visit

Rick is scheduled with the practitioner for a medium-length visit to review how the treatment plan is going. He is then scheduled with the nurse educator for extensive asthma education and reinforcement of the asthma management plan. Smoking cessation is discussed during the follow-up visit. He is also scheduled for spirometry testing. Peak flow meter use is taught.

Continuing Care

Rick is asked to record medication use and PEF. Rick will need to be seen regularly until his asthma is controlled at the lowest-possible inhaled corticosteroid dose.

With each visit, Rick's inhaler technique will be checked. Always check inhaler technique before making any treatment decisions. Do not assume that a patient who has asthma for many years understands the pathophysiology of the disease. These patients can benefit from asthma teaching just as much as newly diagnosed patients. Rick's case also demonstrated a decision to use step 4 therapy and then to wean down to the lowest dose of inhaled corticosteroid. Smoking cessation should be encouraged in all patients with asthma.

pharmacological therapies enhances the outcome for patients with COPD.

Rational Drug Selection

The medication regimen for the COPD patient often includes different medications, each treating a different aspect of the disease. Drugs commonly used to treat COPD are shown in Table 28–2.

Bronchodilators

Bronchodilators are the mainstay of pharmacological therapy for COPD patients. They treat the reversible component of COPD and maximize airflow. Inhaled **beta$_2$ agonists** are the first-line choice for COPD therapy. They can be administered by MDI, by nebulizer, or orally. They are effective and much safer than **theophylline,** which historically was used to treat COPD patients. Patients who have been stable on **theophylline** for years can continue, as long as serum **theophylline** levels are monitored. **An-**

Table 28–4. Clinical Features of Emphysema and Chronic Bronchitis

Characteristic	Chronic Bronchitis	Emphysema
Age at onset of symptoms	40–50 y	50–60 y
Primary symptoms	Cough	Dyspnea
Sputum	Copious, usually purulent	Scant, usually mucoid
Chest x-ray	Peribronchial thickening, often evidence of old inflammatory disease	Hyperlucent, overinflated lung, flattened diaphragm
Weight	Frequently obese	Thin, often marked weight loss
Total lung capacity	Normal or slightly decreased	Increased
Chest examination	Noisy chest, slight hyperinflation	Clear, may have slight end-expiratory wheeze, marked hyperinflation
Cor pulmonale with heart failure	Common	Infrequent until end stages of disease

ticholinergic agents such as **ipratropium bromide (Atrovent)** reduce the volume of sputum without changing the viscosity, which, in addition to their bronchodilation effects, may make them the drug of choice in COPD. One caution is that **ipratropium bromide** is not effective for immediate relief of bronchospasm on account of its slow onset of action; therefore, regular dosing is necessary. Two studies concluded that the combination of a **beta$_2$ agonist** and **ipratropium bromide**, administered by nebulizer, provided higher FEV$_1$ readings and greater symptomatic relief than the **beta$_2$ agonists** alone (Colice, 1996; Tashkin et al., 1996). New MDIs with combined **albuterol** and **ipratropium bromide (Combivent)** may be more convenient and economical for patients with COPD who require both medications.

Corticosteroids

Corticosteroids are most useful in the short-term treatment of acute COPD exacerbation because of their anti-inflammatory effects (Johannsen, 1994). If, in spite of maximal therapy with **bronchodilators,** the patient continues to have significant airway obstruction, a course of **systemic corticosteriods** is indicated. **Prednisone** is given as a dose of 40 to 60 mg daily for 10 to 14 days. At that time, the patient should have a 20 to 30 percent increase in pulmonary function (FEV$_1$). Some patients respond to a 10-day burst of **corticosteroids,** and the medications can be discontinued. Other patients require a taper of medication to the lowest **prednisone** level required to prevent recurrent attacks and relieve bronchospasm. The **prednisone** dose is tapered over 1 to 2 weeks and then to 5 mg over 5 days. Tapering may lead to recurrence of symptoms, and patients should be educated regarding monitoring their symptoms and PEF

during tapering. Adverse effects are minimal at dosages of 10 mg per day or 15 to 20 mg every other day. Alternate-day dosages should be used if possible.

Once patients are stable and bronchospasms are relieved, the patient should be started on an **inhaled corticosteroid** such as **beclomethasone.** Adding **inhaled steroids** allows a reduced **systemic corticosteroid** dose. In general, **inhaled steroids** can replace 7.5 to 10 mg per day of **oral prednisone** (Matthay & Arroliga, 1996). Education about the slow onset of **inhaled corticosteroids** is necessary so patients are aware of the need to continue and slowly taper the **prednisone** over many weeks as the **inhaled steroids** are introduced. Patients need to be cautioned to rinse their mouths after inhaled **steroid** use to prevent oral candidiasis, an adverse effect of **inhaled steroids.**

Oxygen

In some patients, home **oxygen** therapy is necessary. **Oxygen** therapy can be used short-term during acute exacerbations or long-term in chronically hypoxemic patients. The goals of supplemental **oxygen** therapy are to correct arterial hypoxemia and prevent secondary organ damage; ideally, oxygen saturation should be greater than 90 percent. In patients experiencing an acute exacerbation of COPD, a drop in partial pressure of oxygen in arterial blood (PaO$_2$) to below 55 mm Hg is an indication for short-term supplemental **oxygen.** These patients should be monitored to determine when **oxygen** therapy can be discontinued. For the chronically hypoxemic COPD patient, continuous home **oxygen** therapy is associated with increased survival rate. The mortality is closely correlated with number of hours per day the patient receives supplemental **oxygen.** Survival is highest in patients receiv-

Clinical Pearl

OXYGEN THERAPY

One note of caution in providing **oxygen** therapy to some patients with COPD who have poor ventilatory capacity: These patients, known as "carbon dioxide retainers," no longer rely on rises in $PaCO_2$ as the primary drive to breathe. If these patients receive too much **oxygen,** raising their PaO_2 above their normal baseline, hypoventilation may occur. This results in CO_2 retention and the somnolence, lethargy, and coma that occur with carbon dioxide narcosis. Monitoring arterial blood gases is essential in all patients receiving **oxygen** therapy.

ing 12 hours per day or less of **oxygen.** Patients should be started on continuous **oxygen** therapy if they demonstrate persistent hypoxemia at rest (PaO_2 less than 55 mg Hg and less than 88% oxygen saturation). Patients with cor pulmonale or polycythemia with PaO_2 less than 59 mm Hg and less than 89 percent oxygen saturation require supplemental **oxygen.** Patients on continuous **oxygen** therapy require arterial blood gas studies after 1, 3, and 6 months of therapy. Supplemental **oxygen** improves exercise tolerance, neuropsychological function, and quality of life, all key factors in the patient's emotional health in learning to live with this chronic disease.

Antibiotics

Because patients with COPD have an excess of thick pulmonary mucus and decreased ciliary clearance of secretions, they are susceptible to repeated bronchial infections. Infection is considered present when the patient is producing a purulent sputum. The common organisms found in the sputum of patients with COPD patients are *Haemophilus influenzae, Streptococcus pneumoniae, Mycoplasma pneumoniae,* and *Moraxella catarrhalis.* The most common organism is *S. pneumoniae.* Antibiotic choices have to cover these organisms until sputum cultures are available to determine sensitivity. **Amoxicillin-clavulanic acid, erythromycin,** and double-strength **sulfamethoxazole-trimethoprim** are all appropriate first-line choices. Resistant organisms require a change

in **antibiotic** therapy after drug susceptibility studies are completed. Length of treatment is 7 to 14 days.

Immunizations

Infection prevention is essential in management of patients with COPD, and vaccination against respiratory infections is an integral component in preventing illness in these patients. Protection against influenza virus is recommended annually. Optimally, the **influenza vaccine** should be administered between October and January, the earlier in the influenza season the better, to allow adequate antibody response. Patients with COPD also require a **pneumococcal vaccine** every 6 years regardless of age. Patients should be taught the importance of these **vaccines,** so they remember to get them.

Smoking Cessation

Smoking is a major contributor to COPD. Cigarette smoking results in severe destruction of lung tissue, and the damage is largely irreversible. To halt the progression of COPD, the patient must stop smoking. The benefits of smoking cessation include an eventual return to a nearly normal age-related rate of ventilatory function.

There are many new medications that can help the patient stop smoking. Smoking cessation is discussed in depth in Chapter 41.

Clinical Pearl

INFLUENZA VACCINE REMINDERS

The health care provider should keep a tickler file of chronic respiratory patients (those with asthma and COPD), so they can be reminded by phone or mail each fall to get their **influenza vaccine.**

Chronic Obstructive Pulmonary Disease

Related to the Overall Treatment Plan and Disease Process

The patient needs to be taught the following areas of self-management:

☐ Smoking cessation. This is a difficult area of education because of the physical and psychological addiction to cigarettes. Many patients have attempted to quit smoking previously and need to be encouraged to try again, using some of the pharmacological interventions available to aid in tobacco cessation.

☐ Pathophysiology of COPD. A basic understanding of the changes in the pulmonary system that occur with COPD will assist the patient in understanding the role that the different medications play in the treatment regimen.

☐ Medication skills. Patients with COPD often have other chronic illnesses that require routine medications. Administering a complex regimen of multiple medications can be overwhelming, especially to older patients. Written schedules (in large print) and divided pill boxes are two strategies for medication management. Providing the patient with the generic and trade names of medications will decrease medication confusion. Having the patient bring all medications in for review will prevent medication errors. Often the patient may be seeing other providers, including specialists who may also be prescribing medications. It is the role of the primary care provider to coordinate between specialty providers and monitor medications the patient is taking. Encourage patients to use a magnifying glass to read the generic names on the MDI canisters, as the canister color may change with different brands of the same medication.

Specific to the Drug Therapy

☐ Reason for the drug being given and its anticipated action in the disease process
☐ Doses and schedules for taking the drug
☐ Coping mechanisms for complex and costly drug regimens
☐ Interactions between other treatment modalities and these drugs

Reasons for the Drug(s) Being Taken

Patient education about specific drugs is provided in Chapter 15.

Drugs as Part of the Total Treatment Regimen

The total treatment regimen also includes teaching self-monitoring skills, including, if indicated, proper use of a peak flow meter.

Infection control measures are also taught. Patients with COPD are at high risk for respiratory infections. They need to be taught the importance of annual influenza vaccine and the need for a pneumococcal pneumonia vaccine every 6 years. They need to avoid crowds and people, especially children, with respiratory infections.

Adherence Issues

Health care providers should be aware of the potential problem of nonadherence with the treatment regimen and should discuss the importance of adherence with the patient and family members.

Chronic Obstructive Pulmonary Disease

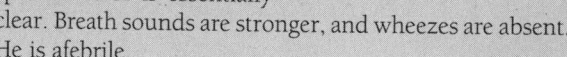

Case Study 28–3

Complaint

"I've had a cough and fever for 2 days."

History

A 62-year-old white man, Mr. Thompson, presents to the clinic for a worsening cough and fever for 2 days. His grandchildren recently visited, and he thinks that he may have caught his grandson's cold. He has been using his inhaler with minimal relief. He also notes that his sputum is dark green, and there seems to be an increased amount.

Mr. Thompson was diagnosed with COPD 6 years ago. His normal medications include Combivent (albuterol and ipratropium bromide) MDI 2 puffs four times a day and hydrochlorothiazide 12.5 mg daily for his blood pressure. He smokes half a pack of cigarettes per day, a decrease from his previous two-pack-a-day 45-year habit. He has not had any shots since he was in the military, many years ago. He has been hospitalized once in the past with pneumonia. Except during the hospitalization, he has never required oxygen therapy.

Assessment

In general, Mr. Thompson is slightly breathless and barrel-chested. His vital signs are: BP 145/88, pulse 94, respiration 20, and temperature 99.8°F. Breath sounds are diminished and bronchial in quality; there are scattered expiratory wheezes, no crackles. Heart sounds are distant, no murmur, and best heard beneath the ziphoid. No cyanosis or clubbing is evident, and there is trace edema of both ankles. His chest x-ray shows hyperinflation of the lungs, flattened hemidiaphragm of the lungs, and no infiltrate.

His CBC is as follows: WBC 10,500, Hct 44%, Segs 70%, and Bands 8%. Pulse oximetry is 91% on room air. Sputum Gram's stain is as follows: 4+ PMNs, 2+ pleomorphic gram-negative rods, and few epithelial cells.

Initial Management Plan

Mr. Thompson's initial management plan is as follows:

1. Review records to determine past treatment of exacerbations.
2. In the clinic today: Mr. Thompson is prescribed Septra DS 1 bid for 7 days, prednisone 40 mg daily for 7 days, and guaifenesin with codeine 5 to 10 cc q4h prn cough. He is asked to demonstrate the use of his inhaler and is noted to be using his inhaler correctly. He is to continue to use the Combivent qid. The patient is to return in 2 weeks for follow-up, sooner if his respiratory status worsens.

Follow-up Visit

At this follow-up visit in 2 weeks, Mr. Thompson's breathing is a lot easier, but he still has a cough. The sputum color is essentially clear. Breath sounds are stronger, and wheezes are absent. He is afebrile.

Modifications to Management Plan

Pulmonary function tests are ordered. Pneumococcal vaccine is given, and Mr. Thompson is advised to get his influenza vaccine every fall. He is also instructed to continue using the Combivent qid and to make an appointment to be seen after the pulmonary function tests are completed to discuss the results.

Continuing Care

Mr. Thompson's pulmonary function tests reveal FVC 75% predicted for his age and height; FEV_1 is 62% predicted for his age and height and improves by 19% after the use of a bronchodilator. His ABGs are pH 7.39, pCO_2 45, and pO_2 94.

When Mr. Thompson returns to discuss his pulmonary function tests, the practitioner discusses smoking cessation at length with him and refers him to a local American Lung Association program for smoking cessation. He is to stop using the Combivent inhaler. New prescriptions for ipratropium (Atrovent) 4 puffs tid on a scheduled basis and an albuterol MDI, which he is to use 2 puffs prn wheezing, are given to him. He is also instructed to contact his health care provider if he has increased cough, especially if he is febrile and if his sputum color changes to green or yellow. The health care provider discusses with the patient and his wife his wishes in the future if he experiences respiratory failure, specifically his wishes regarding mechanical ventilation.

Mr. Thompson's case demonstrates the care of a patient with COPD during an acute exacerbation, using bronchodilators, steroid burst therapy, and antibiotics. At the follow-up visit, smoking cessation and immunizations, key components in the treatment of patients with COPD, are addressed. Modification of the treatment regimen based on pulmonary function tests creates a treatment plan based on the patient's pulmonary function when he is well. Addressing the patient's wishes regarding aggressive end-of-life care is fundamental and best done when the patient is well and at least one other family member is present.

Monitoring

Monitoring patients with COPD has four aspects related to pulmonary function and quality of life: signs and symptoms of COPD, pulmonary function, pharmacotherapy, and quality of life.

All patients should be taught how to monitor their symptoms for worsening pulmonary function. Patients with chronic bronchitis need to monitor their sputum for changes in color from their baseline to more purulent. Any symptoms of respiratory infection must be reported to their health care provider so that appropriate **antibiotic** therapy can be started. During times of poor outdoor air quality, these patients need to remain indoors and report any signs of respiratory distress to their health care provider. Patients with COPD may require increased use of **bronchodilators** or **oxygen** during these times.

Monitoring pulmonary function is done by spirometry, peak flow meter, oxygen saturation (pulse oximetry), and arterial blood gases. Patients can be taught to use a peak flow meter to monitor lung function at home and determine their need for changes in their medication regimen in times of illness or poor air quality. All patients with COPD need objective monitoring of lung function on a regular basis to identify worsening of function and therefore need for a change in their treatment regimen.

Patients should bring their medications to every visit to the health care provider. MDI use should be reviewed and technique monitored with each visit. Patients who use more than the recommended amounts of **beta$_2$ agonists** need to be assessed closely to determine the reason for the increased use. Is the patient using the inhaler incorrectly, or is the disease progressing? Increased use of **inhaled bronchodilators** is an indication for reevaluation of the medication regimen and a possible need for systemic steroids. Patients on supplemental **oxygen** therapy require arterial blood gases, as previously mentioned, at 1, 3, and 6 months after beginning therapy. Any change in respiratory status is an indication for repeat arterial blood gas determination. All patients require a written medication management plan that is reviewed at every visit.

Monitoring quality of life at every visit can determine if the treatment regimen is successful. Is the patient able to tolerate activities of daily living without assistance? Exercise tolerance, activity level, and nutrition all need to be evaluated. The financial burden of a chronic illness such as COPD is significant, and referral to a social worker may be necessary to help the patient pay for prescribed treatment.

Outcome Evaluation

Successful management of patients with COPD includes their self-assessment of quality of life, as well as physical parameters of optimal treatment. As COPD is chronic and for the most part irreversible, outcome evaluation is based on the patient's having the best quality of life for the disease state. The successfully managed patient with COPD has optimal activity tolerance, which varies for each patient. Pharmacological management is aimed at decreasing bronchospasm and secondary infections. Therefore, the amount of bronchospasm and the number of infections determine if treatment is successful.

Patient Education

Patient education should include a discussion of information related to the overall treatment plan as well as that specific to the drug therapy, reasons for taking the drug, drugs as part of the total treatment regimen, and adherence issues.

Patient education for the COPD patient centers on maintaining optimum pulmonary function and quality of life. Teaching self-management is the basis of successful treatment.

REFERENCES

American Medical Association (1997). *Managing asthma today: Integrating new concepts.* Chicago, IL: American Medical Association.

Autio, L., & Rosenow, D. (1999). Effectively managing asthma in young and middle adulthood. *Nurse Practitioner, 24*(1), 100–111.

Colice, G. L. (1996). Nebulized bronchodilators for outpatient management of stable chronic obstructive pulmonary disease. *American Journal of Medicine, 100*(Suppl. 1A), 1A-11S–1A-18S.

Drazen, J. M., Israel, E., Boushey, H. A., Chinchilli, V. M., Fahy, J. V., Fish, J. E., Lazarus, S. C., Lemanske, R. F., Martin, R. J., Peters, S. P., Sorkness, C., & Szefler, S. J. (1996). Comparison of regularly scheduled with as-needed use of albuterol in mild asthma. *New England Journal of Medicine, 335*(12),841–847.

Drombrowski, M., Thom, E., & McNellis, D. (1999). Maternal-fetal medicine units (MFMU) studies of inhaled corticosteroids during pregnancy. *Journal of Allergy and Clinical Immunology, 103*(2, part 2), S356–S359.

Facts and Comparisons Staff. (1998). *Drug facts and comparisons.* St. Louis: Facts and Comparisons.

Georgitis, J. W. (1999). The 1997 asthma management guidelines and therapeutic issues relating to the treatment of asthma. *Chest, 115*(1), 210–217.

Johannsen, J. M. (1994). Chronic obstructive pulmonary disease: Current comprehensive care for emphysema and bronchitis. *Nurse Practitioner, 10*(1), 59–67.

Konig, P., & Shaffer, J. (1996). The effect of drug therapy on long-term outcome of childhood asthma: A possible preview of the international guidelines. *Journal of Allergy and Clinical Immunology, 98*(6), 1103–1111.

Ladebauche, P. (1997). Managing asthma: A growth and developmental approach. *Pediatric Nursing, 23*(1), 37–44.

Lieu, T. A., Quesenberry, C. P., Capra, A. M., Sorel, M. E., Martin, K. E., & Mendoza, G. R. (1997). Outpatient management practices associated with reduced risk of pediatric asthma hospitalization and emergency department visits. *Pediatrics, 100*(3), 334–341.

Luskin, A. T. (1999). An overview of the recommendation of the working group on asthma and pregnancy. *Journal of Allergy and Clinical Immunology, 103*(2), S350–S353.

Matthay, R. A., & Arroliga, A. C. (1996). Chronic airways diseases. In J. C. Bennett & F. Plum (Eds.), *Cecil textbook of medicine* (20th ed.). Philadelphia: Saunders.

National Asthma Education and Prevention Program. (1997). *The Expert Panel report II: Guidelines for the diagnosis and management of asthma.* NIH Pub. No. 97–4051. Bethesda, MD: National Heart, Lung, and Blood Institute, National Institutes of Health.

National Heart, Lung, and Blood Institute. (1995). *Global strategy for asthma management and prevention NHLBI/WHO report.* NIH Pub. No. 95–3659. Bethesda, MD:882 National Institutes of Health.

Simmons, M. S., Nides, M. A., Rand, C. S., Wise, R. A., & Tashkin, D. P. (1996). Trends in compliance with bronchodilator inhaler use between follow-up visits in a clinical trial. *Chest, 109*(4), 963–968.

Tashkin, D. P., Bleecker, E. Braun, S. Campbell, S., DeGraff, A. C.,

Hudgel, D. W., Boyars, M. C., & Sahn, S. (1996). Results of a multicenter study of nebulized inhalant bronchodilator solutions. *American Journal of Medicine, 100*(Suppl. 1A), 1A-62S–1A-69S.

VanAndel, A. E., Reisner, C., Menjoge, S. S., & Witek, T. J. (1999). Analysis of inhaled corticosteroid and oral theophylline use among patients with stable COPD from 1987 to 1995. *Chest, 115*(3), 703–707.

Wendel, P. J., Ramin, S. M., Barnett-Hamm, C., Rowe, T. F., & Cunningham, F. G. (1996). Asthma treatment in pregnancy: A randomized controlled study. *American Journal of Obstetrics and Gynecology, 175*(1), 150–154.

Williams, D. M. (1995). Chronic obstructive airways disease. In L. Y. Young & M. A. Koda-Kimble (Eds.), *Applied therapeutics.* Vancouver: Applied Therapeutics.

CHAPTER 29

·······

Contraception

CHAPTER OUTLINE

C hoosing a method of contraception (birth control) is an intimate process and one in which patients, male and female, often seek advice from their health care provider. Considerations that must be addressed include the age of the patient, frequency of sexual relations, safety of the method chosen, safe sex practices, the health and medical conditions of the patient, and cost.

There are many contraceptive options available to patients, including abstinence. These options are presented in Table 29–1. This chapter focuses on the pharmacological methods, which are usually considered the most effective.

Pharmacological methods include **oral contraceptives,** subdermal implants, **depot medroxyprogesterone acetate** injection, and intrauterine devices.

Oral contraceptives (OCs) contain **estrogen** or **progesterone,** or both. These preparations vary with the type of **progestins** but have many properties in common. They are well absorbed. Combination products are taken daily for 3 weeks with 1 pill-free week interval. Continuous **progestins** are taken daily throughout the cycle.

Levonorgestrel (Norplant) is the only currently available subdermal implant. It is composed of six silicone capsules, each containing 36 mg of **levonorgestrel,** which is released daily over 5 years.

Depot medroxyprogesterone acetate (DMPA), which has 150 mg of active ingredient, is given deep intramuscularly (IM) in large doses every 3 months.

Intrauterine devices include **CU T 380A (Paragard)** and **progesterone T (Progestasert).** CU T 380A is made of polyethylene, with fine copper wire wound around each vertical stem of the **T** portion of the device. The vertical stem is impregnated with barium sulfate so that the device can be seen under x-ray. Ninety percent of the women worldwide who use an intrauterine device use this device. It has been approved for 10-year usage.

Table 29–1. Contraceptive Options

Type	Advantages	Disadvantages	Effectiveness
Pharmacological Methods			
Oral contraceptive	Continuous contraceptive protection Reversible Some noncontraceptive health benefits	Must remember to take daily Increases risk of blood clots, heart attack, stroke, esp in smokers >35 y Common adverse effects include nausea, vomiting, weight gain, irregular bleeding	99% or greater
Subdermal implant	Continuous contraception protection up to 5 y Reversible No need to remember to take daily	Office minor surgical procedure with local anesthetic Adverse effects include irregular bleeding, headache, nausea, removal difficulties, depression, dizziness	99% or greater
Depot medroxyprogesterone acetate (DMPA)	Continuous contraception for 3 mo No need to remember to take daily	Medical visits for quarterly injection Delayed return to fertility (up to 18 months) Some adverse effects, such as weight gain, menstrual bleeding irregularities	99% or greater
Intrauterine device (formulated with copper or progestin)	Continuous contraception No need to remember to take daily	May be expelled or perforate uterus May increase pelvic inflammatory disease risk for some women	99% or greater
Barrier Methods			
Male condom (alone)	Easily obtained Best protection method from sexually transmitted diseases Good results when used with spermicide	May reduce sensation Less sexual spontaneity Breakage possible Provided by male partner	88–98%
Female condom	*Less breakage *Made from polyurethane, not latex *Not provided by male	More expensive than male condoms *Requires anticipation, less spontaneous *Requires some education for proper use	88–98%
Diaphragm (with spermicide)	Insertion up to 8 h before intercourse	Reapplication of spermicide necessary for repeated intercourse Comfort level with insertion important Increases risk of urinary tract, bladder infections Requires anticipation and planning	82–94%
Cervical cap	Insertion 1/2 h to 48 h before	Increased risk of changes in cervical cells (only in first 4 mo) May have vaginal odor and discharge Requires practice for proper insertion	82–94%

Continued on next page

Table 29–1. Contraceptive Options *(continued)*

Type	Advantages	Disadvantages	Effectiveness
Spermicide (alone)	Easily obtained Good results when used with barrier methods	Insertion necessary at least ½ h before intercourse Reapplication necessary for repeated intercourse May be messy May increase risk of urinary tract infections, especially when used with diaphragm	79–97%
Surgical Methods Tubal ligation (female sterilization)	Continuous contraception No need to remember to use daily	Permanent method Surgical procedure	99% or greater
Vasectomy (male sterilization)	Continuous contraception No need to remember to use daily	Provided by the male partner Permanent method Surgical procedure has less risk for complications	99% or greater
Behavioral Methods Periodic abstinence (part of natural family planning)	Inexpensive	Requires careful planning and motivation Prohibits intercourse for up to half the menstrual cycle Not for women with irregular cycles	80–99%
Withdrawal	Inexpensive	Provided by male partner Leakage of sperm often occurs before ejaculation	72%

Progesterone T releases 65 µg of **progesterone** daily. The T consists of ethylene vinyl acetate copolymer. The copolymer contains 38 mg of **progesterone** and the barium sulfate for x-ray visibility.

Pathophysiology

Estrogens are primarily responsible for the development of the secondary sexual characteristics of the developing female. Estrogens and progestins cause proliferation of the vaginal and uterine mucosa, increased secretion of the cervix, and fullness in the breasts. Control of estrogen and progesterone secretion is by the hypothalamus through the pituitary gland. Gonadotropin-releasing hormone (GnRH) from the hypothalamus controls follicle-stimulating hormone (FSH) and luteinizing hormone (LH) from the anterior pituitary. The FSH and LH stimulate follicular development in the ovary; LH stimulates androgen production, and FSH stimulates the androgen conversion into estrogen in the granulosa cells of the ovarian parenchyma. In the presence of adequate estrogen, LH surge is responsible for ovulation. Without fertilization of the ovum, the progesterone-rich corpus luteum degenerates. It is the cessation of progesterone secretion that causes the menstrual flow.

Naturally occurring estrogens have the following effects on the reproductive tract:

ON THE HORIZON

Contraceptive Patch

Soon to be released by Ortho Pharmaceuticals is the "contraceptive patch." It contains the same active ingredients as **Ortho-Cyclen.** It will be dosed as one patch per week and will especially be useful for those patients who forgot to take their pill.

1. Suppression of FSH and LH. During the first 2 weeks of the menstrual cycle, high levels of estrogens suppress the pituitary gland.
2. Secretions within the uterus and the cells lining the uterus are altered.
3. Ovum transport is accelerated.
4. High levels of estrogens cause the corpus luteum to degenerate.

Naturally occurring progestins are precursors to estrogens, androgens, and adrenocortical steroids, which is why progestins can be both positive and negative in their estrogenic effects. Progesterone is produced in the ovary by the corpus luteum after successful ovulation. The progestin-dominant or luteal phase causes the following:

1. Suppression of LH, which partially inhibits ovulation
2. Thickened cervical mucus, which inhibits transportation of sperm
3. Inhibition of enzymes that allow the sperm to fertilize the ovum
4. Slowed ovum transport and changed fallopian tube secretions
5. Atrophy of endometrial cells, which prevents implantation (Hatcher et al., 1998)

Endogenous estrogens are produced in the ovary and transformed in the liver to estradiol, estrone, and estriol. Fat tissue, hair follicles, and muscle convert androgens to estrogens, but not the most potent form, estradiol.

Pharmacodynamics

The primary synthetic **estrogen** in oral contraception is **ethynyl estradiol.** Synthetic **estrogens** and **progestins** were developed to improve oral absorption. Synthetic **progestins** developed for oral contraception have been derived from progesterone or testosterone. The significant clinical difference is their androgenic effects. The more androgenic **progestins** cause increased hyperlipidemia, reduced glucose tolerance, acne, and increased cardiovascular disease. **First-** and **second-generation progestins** norethindrone (Ortho-Novum 1/35, Norinyl 1 + 35, Micronor), di-norgestrel (Lo/Ovral), and **levonorgestrel (Triphasil, Tri-Levlen, Nordette),** are the most common members in current use. The **third-generation progestins** desogestrel (Ortho-Cept, Desogen) and **norgestimate (Ortho-Cyclen, Ortho Tri-Cyclen)** have fewer reported androgenic effects than older **progestins** (Katzung, 1998). There have been no properly controlled studies to compare **levonorgestrel** to **norgestimate** and **desogestrel.** What is known is that members of all three generations of **progestins** are safe and effective when used with 35 mcg or less of **ethinyl estradiol** (Katzung, 1998; Dickey, 1994; Speroff & Darney, 1996).

Other systems and functions of the body are affected by hormone administration. The nervous system seems to be activated by **estrogen** and depressed by **progesterone,** causing elation at midcycle and moodiness prior to menstruation. Hormone administration may also change vitamin and mineral absorption (Dickey, 1994). For example, serum blood or plasma levels of vitamin A, copper, and iron may increase with the administration of **OCs,** and serum blood or plasma levels of thiamine (vitamin B_1), riboflavin (vitamin B_2), pyridoxine (vitamin B_6), cobalamin (vitamin B_{12}), ascorbic acid (vitamin C), folacin (folic acid), magnesium, and zinc may decrease.

Endocrine functions affected by hormone administration include increased levels of corticosteroid-binding globulin, yet the rate of secretion of cortisol is not altered. Plasma renin and aldosterone are both increased. Thyroxine-binding globulin is increased, but the free thyroxine remains normal. Stimulation of sex hormone–binding globulin (SHBG) causes reduced levels of androgens. At higher levels of **estrogen,** androgens can be suppressed. Contraceptive hormones effect changes in blood coagulation similar to those seen during pregnancy. There is an increase in factors VII, VIII, IX, and X and a decrease in antithrombin III. Women taking **OCs** need larger amounts of **warfarin (Coumadin)** to prolong their prothrombin time. They also have higher iron and total iron-binding capacity, similar to patients with hepatitis. Alterations in liver function range from mild, as in protein synthesis, to more severe, as in altered drug excretion and metabolism. Changes in bile clearance and composition increase the incidence of gallstone formation. Lipid metabolism is dramatically affected by 100-μg oral contraceptives, but the formulations with less than 50 μg have minimal effects. **OC** use also causes reduced carbohydrate absorption from the gastrointestinal tract, and **progestin** increases insulin levels. **Estrogens** increase cardiac output, blood pressure, and heart rate mildly in most women, but some have a marked response and require close monitoring. Although acne is improved on **OCs,** increased pigmentation can also occur and require consistent use of sun blocks. Darker-pigmented females are more subject to this effect (Katzung, 1998).

Goals of Treatment

Treatment goals of pharmacological contraception are to use the safest, best-tolerated, and most effective method that the patient desires. The best method for patients may require knowledge about their religion, culture, and education and the approval of their sex partner or parent.

Clinical Pearl

BREAST CANCER RISK

The risk for breast cancer is calculated based on early menarche (<12 years), single marital status, late age at birth of first child (>30 years), nulliparity and lower parity, family history of breast cancer (more than one first-degree relative who was diagnosed before menopause), and late menopause (>50 years) (DMPA, 1995).

Safety

A weak association has been established between the development of liver cancer and women using **OCs** longer than 8 years. Breast cancer risk determination is controversial because research suggests that women who start **OC** use before age 18 have a slightly higher relative risk of cancers before age 46. Oral contraception for longer than 10 years demonstrates a slightly higher trend in breast cancer. For these women, (age 46 to 54 at the time of diagnosis), the increased relative risk occurred with recent use and use longer than 12 years (WHO, 1995).

More reassuring news comes from case-controlled studies in New Zealand, Kenya, Mexico, and Thailand that disprove tumorigenesis with **DMPA** (DMPA, 1995). Analysis of this pooled data indicates that **DMPA** does not promote tumor formation, but rather it could accelerate the growth of preexisting early tumors. This hypothesis is not new. It has been used to understand the effects estrogen and progesterone have on breast tissue. Patients need to know what their absolute risks are before using any hormonal contraception.

Cardiovascular disease risk related to lipid metabolism is difficult to quantify because so many other risk factors are involved. Formulations lower than 50 μg seem to have no detrimental effects. In general, the cardiovascular risk factors other than **OC** use play the predominant role in the occurrence of ischemic stroke and myocardial infarction (Lewis, 1998). Patients who smoke share an increased risk for heart attack, stroke, and thromboembolic phenomena (deep venous thrombosis and pulmonary embolism) as they approach age 35. At that time, the risks for morbidity and mortality far outweigh the benefits (Hatcher et al., 1998).

Tolerance

Thirty years of experience in prescribing **OC** have provided much data with which to knowledgeably help patients decide which **OC** they should choose. Current **OCs** have less **estrogen**; therefore, they cause fewer of the pregnancy-like symptoms that had earlier been so distressing. The **third-** and **fourth-generation progestins** show fewer weight changes, improved complexion, and reduced mood swings. Improved packaging has also improved compliance.

Effectiveness

The theoretical effectiveness is 99 percent or greater with most hormonal therapies. Patients have lower discontinuation rates and therefore fewer unwanted pregnancies if they are well educated about emergency hormonal contraception and use a backup method such as spermicide and condoms. Commonly used **OCs** are presented in Table 29–2.

Clinical Pearl

ESTROGEN

Although many forms and doses of **estrogen** are available, the adverse effects and precautions are the same for all of them.

Table 29–2. Drugs Commonly Used: Pharmacological Contraception

Monophasic	Estrogens (mg)	Progestins (mg)	
Alesse	Ethinyl estradiol 0.02	Levonorgestrel 0.1	
Loestrin 21 1.5/30	Ethinyl estradiol 0.03	Norethindrone 1.5	
Loestrin 21 1/20	Ethinyl estradiol 0.02	Norethindrone 1.0	
Desogen	Ethinyl estradiol 0.03	Desogestrel 0.3	
Lo-Ovral	Ethinyl estradiol 0.03	Norgestrel 0.3	
Nordette	Ethinyl estradiol 0.03	Levonorgestrel 0.15	
Ortho-Cyclen	Ethinyl estradiol 0.03	Norgestimate 0.25	
Ortho-Cept	Ethinyl estradiol 0.03	Desogestrel 0.3	
Levlen	Ethinyl estradiol 0.03	Levonorgestrel 0.15	
Brevicon, Modicon	Ethinyl estradiol 0.035	Norethindrone 0.5	
Demulen 1/35	Ethinyl estradiol 0.035	Ethynodiol diacetate 1.0	
Genora 1/35 Ortho-Novum 1/35 Norinyl 1+35 Nelova 1/35	Ethinyl estradiol 0.035	Norethindrone 1.0	
Ovcon 35	Ethinyl estradiol 0.035	Norethindrone 0.4	
*Genora 1/50 Ortho-Novum 1/50 Norinyl 1+50 Nelova 1/50	Mestranol 0.05	Norethindrone 1.0	
*Ovcon 50	Ethinyl estradiol 0.05	Norethindrone 1.0	
*Demulen 1/50	Ethinyl estradiol 0.05	Ethynodiol diacetate 1.0	
*Ovral	Ethinyl estradiol 0.05	Norgestrel 0.5	
Biphasic Jenest-28	**Phase 1 (mg)** Ethinyl estradiol 0.035 Norethindrone 0.5	**Phase 2 (mg)** Ethinyl estradiol 0.035 Norethindrone 1.0	
Nelova	Ethinyl estradiol 0.035 Norethindrone 0.5	Ethinyl estradiol 0.035 Norethindrone 1.05	
Ortho-Novum 10/11	Ethinyl estradiol 0.035 Norethindrone 0.5	Ethinyl estradiol 0.035 Norethindrone 1.05	
Triphasic Triphasil, Tri-Levlen	**Phase 1 (mg)** Ethinyl estradiol 0.03 Levonorgestrel 0.05	**Phase 2 (mg)** Ethinyl estradiol 0.04 Levonorgestrel 0.075	**Phase 3 (mg)** Ethinyl estradiol 0.03 Levonorgestrel 0.125
Ortho-Novum 7/7/7	Ethinyl estradiol 0.035 Norethindrone 0.5	Ethinyl estradiol 0.035 Norethindrone 0.75	Ethinyl estradiol 0.035 Norethindrone 1.0
Tri-Norinyl	Ethinyl estradiol 0.035 Norethindrone 0.5	Ethinyl estradiol 0.035 Norethindrone 1.0	Ethinyl estradiol 0.035 Norethindrone 0.5

Continued on next page

Table 29–2. Drugs Commonly Used: Pharmacological Contraception *(continued)*

Monophasic	Estrogens (mg)	Progestins (mg)	
Ortho Tri-Cyclen	Ethinyl estradiol 0.035 Norgestimate 0.18	Ethinyl estradiol 0.035 Norgestimate 0.215	Ethinyl estradiol 0.035 Norgestimate 0.25
Continuous Micronor Nor-QD	**Compound and Dosage** Norethindrone 0.35 mg		
Ovrette	Norgestrel 0.075 mg		
Parenteral Progestin Norplant	**Compound and Dosage** Levonorgestrel 36 mg per capsule (kit with 6 capsules and other items)		
DMPA	Medroxyprogesterone acetate 150 mg IM		

This dosage is not recommended in primary care.
Adapted from *Drug Facts and Comparisons,* 1999.

Rational Drug Selection

Guidelines

There are more than two dozen formulations of **OCs**, as well as injectable and implantable contraceptives. If they are all similar in effectiveness and well tolerated, choosing among them may seem difficult. Over the years, investigators have studied the relative potency of the estrogens and progestins. These statements tend to be based on hormonal effects on one or two organ systems or biochemical changes, not on all the functions affected by the hormone. Many systems are involved within a body, and each woman herself may have more or less endogenous hormone; therefore, this relative potency debate may be oversimplified. Practitioners should use information about the patient's age, menstrual activity, personal habits, and present state of health to make choices for first-time OC users (Speroff and Darney, 1996) (Table 29–3).

Cost

Most contraceptives are priced so that the cost per year is the same for all products. For example, the cost of the intrauterine device is similar to the cost of an OC spread out over the life of the intrauterine device. The variable

Clinical Pearl

....

EMERGENCY CONTRACEPTION

Emergency contraception is the use of 2 tablets of **norgestrel** 0.5 mg, **ethinyl estradiol** 50 mg **(Ovral)** 12 h apart, within 72 h of unprotected intercourse.

The alternative is 4 tablets of **norgestrel** 0.3 mg, **ethinyl estradiol** 30 mg **(Lo/Ovral)**, **levonorgestrel** 0.15 mg, **ethinyl estradiol** 30 mg **(Nordette, Levlen)**; or **levonorgestrel** 0.05, 0.075, 0.125 mg, **ethinyl estradiol** 30, 40, 30 mg **(Triphasil** or **Tri-Levlen)**, yellow pills only, 12 h apart (Hatcher et al., 1998).

Levonorgestrel (Plan B) has been released as emergency contraception. It is two pills spaced 12 hours apart within 72 hours of unprotected intercourse. This method uses **progestin** (each pill = 20 **Ovrette**) only and is more effective and with less nausea than multiple **OCs** (Hatcher, 1999).

....

Table 29–3. Guidelines for Choice of Oral Contraception for First-Time Users

First-Time User	Continuous Progestin*	Combination 1st and 2nd Generation†	Combination 3rd Generation‡	Ethinyl Estradiol 30–35 µg	Ethinyl Estradiol 20 µg
Nonsmoker Adolescent	–	+	+	+	–
Postpartum under age 35 breastfeeding	+	–	–	–	–
Perimenopausal	+	–	–	–	+
Smoker Adolescent	–	+	+	+	–
Postpartum under age 35 breastfeeding	+	–	–	–	–
Perimenopausal	–	–	–	–	–
Menstrual flow (patients under age 35) Heavy flow	+	+	+	+	–
Regular to light flow	–	+	+	+	+

Examples:
*Norethindrone 0.35 mg (Micronor).
†Ethinyl estradiol 35 µg, norethindrone 1 mg (Ortho-Novum 1/35); ethinyl estradiol 30 µg, norgestrel 0.3 mg (Lo/Ovral).
‡Ethinyl estradiol 35 µg, norgestimate 0.25 mg (Ortho-Cyclen); ethinyl estradiol 30 µg, desogestrel 0 15 µg (Desogen, Ortho-Cept).

factor is whether your patient's health insurance pays for an **OC** or if the program pays only for an inserted device. Most communities have county or private not-for-profit contraceptive centers with a sliding-scale fee schedule to assist women in need. Several of the first **OCs** are now available in generic formulations, with the result of cost savings and no evident loss of efficacy. Although the cost has escalated over the past three decades, the benefits of fewer unwanted pregnancies, less blood loss, and fewer days of work lost on account of cyclic illness far improve the quality of life for most women.

Patient Variables

Differences in a woman's physiological and psychological response to **estrogens** and **progestins** make choosing **OCs** more of an art than a science. Yet taking a thorough history, performing a complete physical examination, and obtaining a baseline laboratory profile rule out potential patients for whom **OCs** should not be prescribed. Patient variables that require withholding **OCs** or monitoring more closely are listed in Table 29–4.

Patients may also choose **OCs** for their noncontraceptive benefits. Indications for choosing an **OC** include the following:

1. Women with endometriosis who are not ready to get pregnant

2. Need for short- or long-term birth control
3. Acne improvement
4. Heavy, painful, or unpredictable menses
5. Forty percent reduction in risk for ovarian cancer
6. Recurrent ovarian cysts
7. Forty percent lower risk of endometrial cancer
8. Fifty to seventy-five percent fewer surgical cases of benign breast disease (Hatcher et al., 1998)

Drug Variables

Providers and patients have been concerned about reduced OC effectiveness while the patients take **antibiotics**. Yet a review of the literature has validated this problem in only two classes of drugs: **rifampin (Rifadin, Rimactane)**, used to treat tuberculosis, and **griseofulvin (Gris-PEG, Fulvicin, Grisactin)**, used to treat fungal infections. The mechanism of action is thought to be induction of liver enzymes. **Antibiotics** currently available are not liver-enzyme inducers. There is a potential risk of reduced absorption with **penicillin (Pen Vee K)** and broad-spectrum **tetracycline (many generics, Achromycin V, Panmycin)** (Cottet, 1996).

Another area of concern has been the effect of **OCs** on laboratory values. Previous thyroid test methods were affected by protein binding, but the new TSH is not (Katzung, 1998). Lipid levels (cholesterol, triglycerides, and high-density lipoprotein cholesterol) may be af-

Table 29–4. Contraindications: Contraceptive Hormones

Absolute contraindications	Thromboembolic disorder or history
	Cerebrovascular accident or history
	Coronary artery disease or history
	Known or suspected breast cancer
	Known or suspected dependent neoplasia
	Pregnancy
	Benign or malignant liver tumor
	Impaired liver function (at present)
	Previous cholestasis during pregnancy
	Classic migraine headache
Strong contraindications	Common migraine headache (if prescribed, use lowest estrogen formulation)
	Hypertension (diastolic BP >90 mm Hg; systolic BP >140 mm Hg on three or more separate visits)
	Mononucleosis (only during acute phase)
	Major surgery within the next 4 wk
	Long leg cast or major lower leg injury
	Over age 40 (if patient also has a second risk factor for cardiovascular disease such as hypertension or diabetes)
	Over age 35 (if patient is a heavy smoker, e.g., >15 cigarettes/d)
	Abnormal genital bleeding (may not be easily defined)
	Systemic lupus erythematosus (may exacerbate the disease)
Possible contraindications	Hyperlipidemia (if triglycerides are not high and if vascular disease is absent)
	Seizure disorder (possibility of reduced effectiveness because of enzyme induction)
May consider prescribing	Smoker (only if 1 y has passed since quitting: the 20-μg formulation has no clotting or platelet impact)
	Depression (low dose should be tolerated)
	Benign breast disease (may even help after 2 y of therapy)
	Sickle cell disease (benefits outweigh the risks, but use lowest estrogen formulations)
	Diabetes mellitus/gestational diabetes (if under age 35 and a nonsmoker with no vascular complications/no contraindications)
	Hemorrhagic disorders (not contraindicated)

fected by **OCs**. A baseline lipid profile and an assessment of the family history of lipid disease rule out falsely elevated lipid tests.

Dosing Regimens

Oral contraceptives are recommended to be dosed uniformly, one pill a day. The Food and Drug Administration (FDA) has standardized package inserts so that patients are not confused by conflicting instructions. Formulations of 35 μg or less are recommended to reduce undesirable adverse effects and morbidity. Each packet contains 3 weeks of active ingredients and 1 week of seven inert pills.

During the week of no medication, women menstruate. The package insert has information for common concerns and questions that should be referred to because some women may be using **OCs** for medical or gynecological problems rather than birth control.

Progestin-only OCs are dosed daily beginning with day 1 of the menstrual cycle and taken continuously with no week of inert tablets.

Monitoring

The initial history and physical examination with baseline laboratory tests, which include Pap smear, complete

Clinical Pearl

LMP NOTATION

Last menstrual period (LMP) should be considered a vital notation to be displayed at the top of each chart note in a patient's medical record, because every woman is pregnant until proved otherwise.

blood count, glucose, and lipid profile, serve as a point of reference for future measurements.

Monitoring for the adverse effects of **OCs** should be done initially, at 3 months, and then annually. Serious effects that could be caused by **OCs** include abnormal vaginal bleeding; hypertension; amenorrhea; unilateral numbness, weakness, or tingling, indicating possible cerebral spasm or occlusion; breast pain or mass; leg pain; chest pain; sudden loss of vision from possible thromboembolic phenomena; and jaundice (Hatcher et al., 1998).

In addition to screening for adverse drug effects, use these "well-patient" visits to screen for asymptomatic sexually transmitted diseases and reinforce barrier protection for those at risk for disease. Use of tobacco and alcohol are the two most common lifestyle habits that contribute to morbidity and mortality at all ages. Both have interaction effects on the organ systems of patients who use an **OC**. Patients with a chronic disease such as diabetes, seizure disorder, or migraine headache require more frequent monitoring visits based on their individual conditions.

Oral Contraceptives

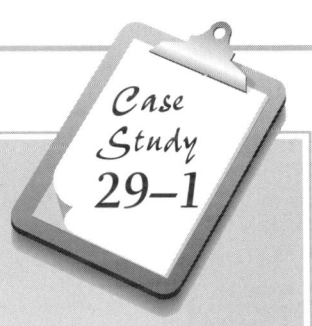

Case Study 29–1

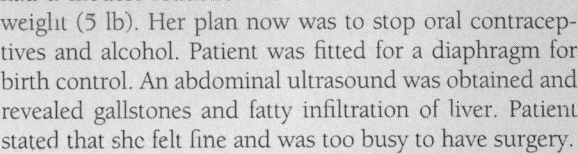

Complaint

"I've gained weight since starting my birth control pills."

History

Anita, age 29, a white female, presented for her wellness examination. Family history was positive for hyperlipidemia and hypertension.

Assessment

Physical examination revealed height 5′ 3″, weight 170, BP 120/70, pulse 80. HEENT: demonstrated no funduscopic evidence of hypertension, no thyroid gland mass or enlargement. Breasts: no dominant mass, nipple discharge, or lymphadenopathy, breast self-examination taught. Cardiovascular: normal sinus rhythm without murmur. Lungs: clear to auscultation. Abdomen: obese, normal bowel tones, no palpable mass or organomegaly. Pelvic: normal Pap smear. Laboratory values: total cholesterol 241, triglycerides 171, LDL 161, and HDL 46, uric acid 7.0 and liver function GGT 107.

Initial Management Plan

Anita was found to have abnormal liver function and lipid abnormalities since instituting oral contraception 2 years earlier. She had also gained 55 pounds in that same time interval.

Her initial treatment plan was to:

1. Reduce dietary fats
2. Begin exercising

Follow-up Visit

At Anita's 1-month follow-up visit, there was no improvement in weight or laboratory abnormalities. She stated that although she has tried to diet, she eats out a lot and travels weekly.

Modifications to Management Plan

Anita was to continue the original plan and return in 3 months.

Continuing Care

At Anita's 3-month follow-up visit, there were no improvements in her laboratory values, although she had a modest reduction in weight (5 lb). Her plan now was to stop oral contraceptives and alcohol. Patient was fitted for a diaphragm for birth control. An abdominal ultrasound was obtained and revealed gallstones and fatty infiltration of liver. Patient stated that she felt fine and was too busy to have surgery.

At her 4-month follow-up visit, there was no improvement in laboratory tests, and she had regained the weight she had lost. She used no alcohol. An internist was consulted regarding her treatment plan. Patient was asymptomatic and did not want surgery because of high job demands and possible divorce. Consultant reinforced my plan and recommended continued monitoring.

At a 10-month follow-up visit, mild improvement in liver function test and lipids was seen and Anita stated that she "felt fine."

At a 17-month follow-up visit, there were no changes from her 10-month follow-up, except that she was now divorced.

Anita did not return for 3 years. At that time, she presented with general malaise. She was afebrile and had back pain. Her blood pressure was normal. Urinalysis showed a trace of blood and elevated bilirubin. Physical exam revealed icteric conjunctiva. Laboratory values reveal elevated amylase, white blood cells, and liver function tests. Anita was referred to a surgeon for obstruction of the common bile duct with gallstones and pancreatitis, secondary to the obstruction. She was hospitalized 3 months later and found to have chronic liver disease. She is being monitored by a gastroenterologist and may need liver transplantation if cirrhosis progresses.

This case indicates that patients need monitoring when on oral contraceptives. High-risk patients (family history of hyperlipidemia) who experience weight gain and use OCs may develop gallstones. With laparoscopic cholecystectomy, patients miss very little time from work, and recovery is usually uneventful.

Clinical Pearl

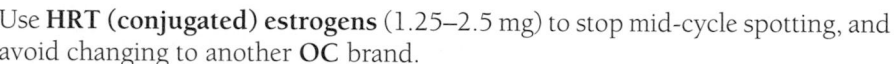

NEW-USER SPOTTING

Use **HRT (conjugated) estrogens** (1.25–2.5 mg) to stop mid-cycle spotting, and avoid changing to another **OC** brand.

Outcome Evaluation

Adverse effects require immediate consultation and discontinuation of **OCs** until the cause of the adverse symptom rules out OC etiology. Exceptions that can be handled less urgently are abnormal vaginal bleeding, amenorrhea, and blood pressure elevation. Breakthrough bleeding frequently occurs in the initial cycles of use of any **OC** formulation. If the patient has not missed any doses, reassure her that break-through bleeding has not been associated with reduced efficacy. It is not necessary to stop the dosing regimen while resolving the problem. The endometrium breaks down because of the low estrogen component of the **OC**. Use 1.25 mg **conjugated estrogens** or 2 mg **estradiol** for 7 days no matter where in the cycle spotting occurs (Speroff and Darney, 1996). If this treatment is not effective, schedule an examination to rule out infection and pregnancy. Amenorrhea is a common concern that may result after several months or years of **OC** use. **Progestins** atrophy the endometrium, and some women welcome scanty or no menses. For others, no monthly cycle produces anxiety, which is usually relieved by a negative pregnancy test. Amenorrhea caused by **DMPA** may be a result of low estrogen levels (less than 30 picograms). Giving exogenous **estrogen** should correct lower estrogen levels. Patients at risk for osteoporosis (smokers, fair skin, small frame, and positive family history) should have estrogen levels measured annually (Hatcher et al., 1998).

Hypertension may be **OC**-induced, especially in women with a positive family history. Persistent blood pressure elevation is frequently the reason for reducing the **estrogen** component in the **OC**, switching to a **progestin-only OC**, or choosing another method of birth control. Also, consider other birth control options to prevent unplanned pregnancy while monitoring blood pressure elevations. Nausea and breast pain experienced throughout the cycle would warrant switching **OCs**. Either **estrogen** or **progestin** could cause these symptoms. Try using a totally different **OC**. World Health Organization (WHO) data have caused concern that secondary amenorrhea produced by long-term DMPA use may lead to osteoporosis (McGee, 1997). If patients choose to stay on the injectable contraceptive, then **calcium** and **vitamin D** supplementation should be offered. In addition, patients may need bone density measurements if there is any suspicion of fracture. Weight gain has been more frequently reported with the use of injectable or implantable contraceptives (Hatcher et al., 1998).

Patient Education

Patient education should include a discussion of information related to the overall treatment plan, as well as that specific to the drug therapy, reasons for taking the drug, drugs as part of the total treatment regimen, and adherence issues.

Frequently, there is much to discuss and not enough time during the office visit; therefore, provide the patient with literature packets that can be reviewed at home with family or friends on topics like sexually transmitted disease prevention, why have Pap smears, how to quit smoking, and a self-test for possible **alco-**

Clinical Pearl

OC USE AND WEIGHT

Return of fertility may be sooner in women of lower body mass index (BMI).

Women with BMI greater than 27 will probably gain even more weight on **depot medroxyprogesterone.**

Clinical Pearl

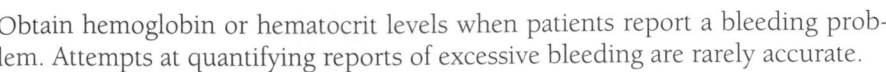

REPORT OF BLEEDING

Obtain hemoglobin or hematocrit levels when patients report a bleeding problem. Attempts at quantifying reports of excessive bleeding are rarely accurate.

PATIENT EDUCATION

Pharmacological Contraception Related to the Overall Treatment Plan/Disease Process

- ☐ Normal physiology of the menstrual cycle and how the oral contraceptives affect ovulation through suppression of the hypothalamic-ovarian axis
- ☐ Safety issues
- ☐ Need for regular follow-up visits with the primary care provider (every 6 months for patients age 15 to 24, every 3 years after three normal Pap smears for patients age 25 to 45)
- ☐ How to say no when choosing to abstain
- ☐ Importance of adhering to treatment plan (dosing schedule), including what to do if an error in treatment plan occurs, such as missed pills or condom breakage (emergency contraception works for all birth control methods)
- ☐ Self-monitoring of symptoms of adverse effects that need immediate attention
- ☐ Safe-sex practices, including use of OC and protection with female or male condoms for sexually transmitted diseases

Specific to the Drug Therapy

- ☐ Reason for the drug's being given and its anticipated action.
- ☐ Doses and schedules for taking the drug. For example, combination oral contraceptives are taken for 3 weeks with 1 week of inert or placebo pills, whereas progestin-only pills are taken day 1 of the menstrual period continually with no disruption. Progestin intrauterine devices need to be replaced annually, whereas Paragard may be left in place 10 years unless complications such as pain, bleeding, or menstrual disruption occurs.
- ☐ Possible adverse effects and what to do if they occur. For example, barrier methods may cause irritation or allergy (latex and nonoxyl-9), depot preparations may cause amenorrhea or spotting and desired fertility may take up to 18 months; if the patient has implanted progestin, it needs to be removed surgically and warn the patient to expect that fertility is immediate.
- ☐ Interactions between other treatment modalities and these drugs. For example, emphasize the dangers of smoking and OCs at any age. Also advise the patient to stop OCs 4 weeks before and 2 weeks after major surgery to prevent thrombus formation.

continued

PATIENT EDUCATION

Pharmacological Contraception Related to the Overall Treatment Plan/Disease Process (*continued*)

Reasons for Taking the Drug(s)

Hormonal contraception has highest efficacy at a time in a woman's life when she is very fertile (age 15 to 35). Progestin-only contraception is preferred while breast-feeding to maintain good milk production and avoid infant exposure to high-dose estrogen.

Drugs As Part of the Total Treatment Regimen

As a method of birth control, hormonal contraception is safe, efficacious, and immediately reversible. Studies have followed millions of women over 30 years with noncontraceptive benefits such as reduced uterine and ovarian cancer (Dickey, 1994; Hatcher et al., 1998; and Speroff & Darney, 1996). There is also less blood loss anemia with hormonal contraceptives.

Adherence Issues

Abnormal vaginal bleeding is the commonest cause of discontinuing the OC (Rosenberg & Waugh, 1998).

Education about emergency contraception is necessary because it works for couples using any birth control method. This prescription is not an abortifacient. Prevention of pregnancy before implantation is contraception (done within 72 hours). Implantation takes place at least 7 days after ovulation (Glasier, 1997). Remind older, nonsmoking women that low-dose oral contraception (30 and 20 µg) may be continued until menopause (Speroff and Darney, 1996).

---

hol abuse. When contacting the patient with the results of physical examinations and laboratory data, use this opportunity to provide reinforcement of any health teaching. Also, be available by phone for urgent questions. A 5-minute phone consultation may prevent discontinuance of the OC and an unplanned pregnancy.

REFERENCES

Cottet, C. (1996). Do antibiotics decrease the effectiveness of oral contraceptives? *Oregon Nurse, 61*(3), 3–5.

Dickey, R. (1994). *Managing contraceptive pill patients* (8th ed.). Durant, OK: CIP.

DMPA and breast cancer: A largely reassuring analysis. (1995). *WHO Drug Information, 9*(1), 20–22.

Glasier, A. (1997). Emergency postcoital contraception. *New England Journal of Medicine, 337*(15), 1058–1064.

Hatcher, R. (1999). *Proceedings of regional CME: Oral contraceptives for the millennium.* Portland, OR: Oregon Nurses Association.

Hatcher, R., Stewart, F., Trussell, J., Kowal, D., Guest, F., Stewart, G., & Cates, W. (1998). *Contraceptive technology* (16th ed.). New York: Irvington.

Kastrup, E. (Ed.) (1998). *Drug facts and comparisons.* St. Louis: Facts and Comparisons.

Katzung, B. (1998). *Basic and clinical pharmacology* (7th ed.). Norwalk, CT: Appleton & Lange.

Kimble-Haas, S. (1998). The intrauterine device: Dispelling the myths. *The Nurse Practitioner, 23*(11), 58–73.

Lewis, M. (1998). Myocardial infarction and stroke in young women: What is the impact of oral contraceptives? *American Journal of Obstetrics and Gynecology, 179*(3), S68–S77.

McGee, C. (1997). Secondary amenorrhea leading to osteoporosis: Incidence and prevention. *American Journal of Primary Health Care, 22*(5), 38, 41–42, 44–45.

Mendelsohn, M., & Karas, R. (1999). *New England Journal of Medicine, 340*(23), 1801–1811.

Oral contraceptives and breast cancer: More insight into a complex association. (1995). *WHO Drug Information, 9*(1), 18–20.

Rosenberg, M., & Waugh, M. (1998). Oral contraceptive discontinuation: A prospective evaluation of frequency and reasons, *American Journal of Obstetrics and Gynecology, 179*(3), 577–582.

Speroff, L., & Darney, P. (1996). *A clinical guide for contraception* (2nd ed.). Baltimore: Williams & Wilkins.

Winkler, U. (1998). Effects of hemostatic variables of desogestrel and gestodene containing oral contraceptives in comparison with levonorgestrel containing contraceptive: A review. *American Journal of Obstetrics and Gynecology, 179*(3):S51-S61.

CHAPTER 30

· · · · · · ·

Dermatologic Conditions

CHAPTER OUTLINE

he skin is the body's largest organ, and it is uniquely accessible for diagnosis and treatment. Primary care providers see patients with dermatologic problems on a daily basis, with skin-related problems accounting for 9 percent of clinic visits.

The most common dermatologic diagnosis in adult primary care is dermatitis (15.8%), with bacterial skin infections the second most common (14% of visits) (Feldman et al., 1998.). This chapter addresses the pharmacological management of common dermatologic conditions seen in primary care. Accurate diagnosis of the condition is assumed.

Dermatitis

Eczema (atopic dermatitis), contact dermatitis, diaper dermatitis, and seborrheic dermatitis are four common forms of dermatitis seen in primary care.

Eczema is a chronic skin disorder that affects all ages. It often begins in infancy and affects 10 to 15 percent of chil-

dren. It may resolve during puberty, only to recur in adolescence or adulthood. The pattern of rash with eczema varies with age. Infants have the rash on the face, scalp, trunk, and the extensor surface of the extremities. In infants, the rash is usually acute or subacute, red, and vesicular. Eczema in adolescents and adults is usually chronic, with scaling, dryness, and lichenification on the flexure surfaces of the extremities, face, neck, hands, and upper chest. Eczema tends to worsen during the winter months.

Contact dermatitis is an acute inflammatory reaction of the skin to an irritant or allergen. It can be differentiated from eczema because it is generally not chronic or recurring and is usually distributed on exposed skin.

Diaper dermatitis (diaper rash) can occur in any patient who is incontinent and uses an occlusive barrier type of garment or diaper; however, it is most commonly seen in infants and toddlers.

Seborrheic dermatitis is a common inflammatory dermatitis characterized by erythematous, eczematous patches with yellow, greasy scale. It is usually localized to hairy areas and to areas with high concentrations of sebaceous glands. It can be found on the forehead, eyebrows, nasolabial folds, ear canals, neck, chest, intertriginous areas, the diaper or groin area, and intergluteal fold. In infants under age 6 months, the scaling seen on the scalp without inflammation is commonly called *cradle cap*, and in adolescents and adults it is called *dandruff*.

Pathophysiology

Eczema

The exact etiology of eczema is unknown. Patients with eczema have high IgE antibody levels, but an exact immune cause has not been proved. A predisposition to pruritus and a reduced threshold of irritant responsiveness are believed to be key elements. Pruritus leads to increased scratching, which increases skin trauma, leading to increased itching (itch-scratch-itch cycle). Stroking the skin causes an abnormal reaction of dermatographism, a white line.

There is a high correlation between eczema and other atopic diseases, with 50 to 80 percent of children with eczema later developing asthma, allergic rhinitis, or hay fever. There is often a positive family history for allergic disorders or asthma.

Contact Dermatitis

There are two types of contact dermatitis, irritant and allergic. Both are usually confined to the point of contact with the irritant or allergen. This contact usually produces erythema, papules, and/or vesicles.

Irritant contact dermatitis is caused by contact of the skin with an irritating substance. The effect may be mild to severe. Irritating substances can be acid or alkali, solvents, or detergents. There is no immunologic response as part of the inflammatory response in irritant contact dermatitis.

Allergic contact dermatitis is a delayed hypersensitivity response to an allergen. The allergen can be a variety of items in the environment, usually a small-molecular-weight substance that binds to the proteinaceous components of the skin to form a sensitizing antigen. Sensitization to the substance or allergen takes 10 to 14 days to develop after the first exposure. Dermatitis occurs within 1 to 7 days of subsequent exposure to the allergen. The most common allergens causing allergic contact dermatitis are certain plants (poison oak, ivy, and sumac), metals (especially in snaps, zippers, and jewelry), clothing (wool), cosmetics (fragrance or preservatives), topical medications (neomycin, anesthetics such as benzocaine, topical antihistamine), hair dyes, and soaps. Avoidance usually prevents the allergic response.

Diaper Dermatitis

Diaper dermatitis is an inflammatory disorder of the skin caused by a breakdown of the skin's natural barrier in the perineal or "diaper" area. The rash is often striking for its clear borders that coincide with the borders of the diaper or protective undergarment.

Forms of diaper dermatitis include irritant dermatitis, caused by chemical or mechanical irritation. Chemical irritation is caused by contact with urine and feces. Mechanical irritation is due to chafing of the diaper or undergarment on the skin folds. If the irritant dermatitis becomes chronic, the skin may appear dry. The rash may become more generalized and inflammatory, involving the creases and all the area that the diaper covers. The skin can become ulcerated or eroded with chronic irritation.

Infectious dermatitis may be caused by *Candida albicans* (candidiasis) and is usually a superinfection that can occur after a patient has had irritant dermatitis in the diaper area for 3 to 5 days. Candidiasis is suspected when there is a beefy red confluent rash with satellite lesions that are either red papules or pustules.

Other forms of diaper dermatitis include seborrheic dermatitis, psoriasiform napkin dermatitis, and atopic dermatitis. These disorders in the diaper area are treated the same as dermatitis on other parts of the body.

Seborrheic Dermatitis

The exact cause of seborrheic dermatitis is unknown. It is possibly related to increased production of sebum or an abnormal lipid composition of sebum. Seborrheic dermatitis is rare in children over age 6 to 12 months and in those who are prepubertal because the sebaceous glands are involuted and dormant during this time and become active again with puberty.

Goals of Treatment

With all forms of dermatitis, the primary goals are to decrease the inflammation and discomfort caused by the dermatitis.

Rational Drug Selection

With all forms of dermatitis, rational drug selection is based first on decreasing the symptoms of an acute exacerbation and then on preventing, decreasing, and/or controlling the frequency and severity of further exacerbations.

Eczema

ACUTE EXACERBATIONS

Topical corticosteroids. **Topical corticosteroids** are adrenocorticosteroid derivatives incorporated into a vehicle suitable for application to the skin. The anti-inflammatory effect of **topical steroids** is nonspecific and acts against most causes of inflammation. At the cellular level, they appear to inhibit the formation, release, and activity of the endogenous mediations of inflammation. When applied to inflamed skin, **steroids** inhibit the migration of macrophages and leukocytes into the area by reversing vascular dilation and permeability. This decreases edema, erythema, and pruritus.

Variable amounts of the drug are absorbed through the skin, depending on the drug used, the vehicle used, the amount of skin surface area the medication is applied to, and the condition of the skin. Absorption is enhanced by increased skin temperature, hydration, and application to denuded areas, intertriginous areas, or skin surfaces with thin stratum corneum layer (face or scrotum). Occlusive dressings enhance skin penetration and therefore increase drug absorption. Infants and children have a higher proportion of body surface area to body weight, and therefore they absorb proportionally more medication. Following topical administration, **corticosteroids** enter the bloodstream and are metabolized and excreted the same as **systemic steroids.** Therefore, in infants and young children, the lowest effective strength of **topical steroid** is used to prevent systemic corticosteroid effects. *Topical corticosteroids* **are Pregnancy Category C. In pregnant patients, do not use** *corticosteroids* **extensively, for long periods, or in large amounts.**

The penetration of the **topical steroid** varies with the medication's vehicle. Ointments are more occlusive and therefore more potent, and they are good for scaly areas. Creams are less occlusive and usually less potent. Lotions are usually the least potent. Table 30–1 presents the common **topical steroids** used for eczema. The potency of any **steroid** can be increased approximately tenfold by occlusion with plastic wrap. Therefore, to increase the effects of a **steroid,** apply an occlusive dressing over the area. Do not use occlusive dressings more than 12 hours per day, or systemic steroid effects may occur. In young children, occlusive dressings are rarely used. A diaper is very occlusive, and **steroid** use should be avoided in the diaper area unless a low-strength **steroid** is needed for short periods (e.g., 2 days). Higher-strength **steroid** creams can be mixed with a moisturizer to enhance the effects.

There are many **topical steroid** preparations available, and it is impossible for any practitioner to be familiar with all of them. Familiarity with one or two agents in each category is reasonable. The most commonly used low-potency **topical steroid** is **1% hydrocortisone.** Moderate-potency **topical steroids** include **hydrocortisone valerate 0.2% (Westcort)** and **triamcinolone acetonide 0.1% (Aristocort, Kenalog).** High-potency **steroids** include **betamethasone dipropionate, augmented 0.05% (Diprolene),** and **triamcinolone acetonide 0.5% (Aristocort, Kenalog).** Each provider needs to know what medications are allowed from each category in the formulary they are using.

Oral corticosteroids. **Oral corticosteroids** are occasionally used to treat severe eczema. Patients with eczema who receive **oral corticosteroids** for another disease, such as asthma, see a striking improvement in their skin. Improvement in acute exacerbations is often dramatic, a mixed blessing in the treatment of this chronic illness. Patients often feel so good that they may have the false impression that the **steroids** "cured" their eczema. Given the major adverse effects observed with prolonged or frequently repeated **corticosteroid** therapy, routine use of **oral steroids** for eczema is contraindicated. If **oral steroid** therapy for severe eczema is considered, consultation with a physician is indicated. A patient who is using **oral steroids** must understand that the effects are short-term and that **oral steroid** preparations cannot be used frequently. When the oral preparation is started, patients must be started on a comprehensive prevention routine to prevent severe exacerbations. They need to be warned that their eczema will return after the **steroids** wear off.

Antipruritics. **Antipruritics** are used to control the itching associated with eczema and to break the itch-scratch-itch cycle. Commonly used oral agents are the **antihistamines diphenhydramine (Benadryl) and hydroxyzine (Atarax).** These drugs have antipruritic and sedative actions. Pruritus can disrupt sleep; therefore, mild sedation can be helpful to prevent nocturnal itching, especially in children. **Cetirizine (Zyrtec),** a metabolite of **hydroxyzine** without its sedative effects, can be used during the day to achieve an antipruritic effect without sedation. Another **antipruritic** is the tricyclic compound **doxepin (Sinequan),** which has potent histamine$_1$ and histamine$_2$ blocking action.

Topical antipruritics can be used and should be considered if severe pruritus is present. **Doxepin cream (Zonalon)** can be used for moderate to severe pruritus associated with eczema. Care should be taken when prescribing **doxepin** for topical use because significant amounts can be absorbed systemically if it is used over 10 percent of the body surface area or if used for a long time. Drowsiness occurs in more than 20 percent of patients using **doxepin** cream, especially if it is used on more than 10 percent of body surface area.

Available **topical antipruritics** that are safer to use than **doxepin** are **Aveeno** cream (colloidal oatmeal–based) and **Moisturel** emollient cream or lotion (petrolatum, glycerine based). These over-the-counter (OTC) agents can be used liberally on large surface areas with no harmful effects.

Emollients. **Emollients** play a key role in both acute exacerbations of eczema and in long-term therapy. Their use is discussed in the long-term therapy section.

Table 30–1. Drugs Commonly Used: Dermatitis and Psoriasis

Drug	Indication	Strengths Available	Dose	Notes
TOPICAL CORTICOSTEROIDS				
Low-Potency Hydrocortisone (Hytone, Cortisporin, Cortaid)	Dermatitis	Cream, lotion, ointment: 1%, 2.5%	Apply a thin layer 2–4 times/d until healed	Available OTC
Triamcinolone acetonide (Aristocort, Aristocort A, Kenalog)	Dermatitis	Cream, lotion, ointment: 0.025%	Apply a thin layer 3–4 times/d until healed	Prescription required
Intermediate-Potency Hydrocortisone valerate (Westcort)	Dermatitis	Cream, ointment: 0.2%	Apply a thin layer 2–3 times/d until healed	Should be used with caution on the face; choose lower potency on face
Triamcinolone acetonide (Aristocort, Kenalog)	Dermatitis	Cream, lotion, ointment: 0.1%	Apply a thin layer 3–4 times/d until healed	Should be used with caution on the face; choose lower potency on face
High-Potency Betamethasone dipropionate, augmented (Diprolene)	Dermatitis	Emollient cream, lotion: 0.05%	Apply a thin film 1–2 times/d until healed; maximum of 45 g of cream or 50 mL of lotion/wk	Avoid abrupt cessation if used for chronic conditions; not recommended in children
Triamcinolone acetonide (Aristocort, Kenalog)	Dermatitis	Cream: 0.5%	Apply sparingly to affected area 2–3 times daily until healed	Avoid abrupt cessation if used for chronic conditions; use with caution and sparingly in children
ORAL CORTICOSTEROIDS				
Prednisone	Contact dermatitis (severe or if large skin surface area is involved)		*Adults:* 0.5–1 mg/kg/d (40–60 mg/d; maximum 60 mg/d *Children:* 1 mg/kg/d; maximum 40 mg/d	Dose is usually tapered after the first 10–14 d, with tapering taking 1–2 wk Severe cases may need a 2- to 3-wk course; 2 wk is the minimum length of treatment for severe poison oak or ivy dermatitis

Continued on next page

Table 30–1. Drugs Commonly Used: Dermatitis and Psoriasis *(continued)*

Drug	Indication	Strengths Available	Dose	Notes
Methylprednisolone (Medrol Dosepak)	Contact dermatitis (severe or if large skin surface area is involved)		Premeasured dose pack; dose is preset at 24 mg on day 1, tapering 4 mg/d to a dose of 4 mg on day 6	Allows for easy tapering over 6 d 6-d course may not be long enough for some patients
ANTIPRURITIC AGENTS				
Diphenhydramine (Benadryl)	Pruritus associated with dermatitis	Elixir: 12.5 mg/5 mL Chewable tablets: 12.5 mg Tablets: 25 mg	*Adults:* 25–50 mg every 4–6 h *Children age 2–6:* 6.25 mg; maximum 37.5 mg/ 24 h *Children age 6–12:* 12.5–25 mg q4–6h; maximum 150 mg/24 h	May cause drowsiness
Hydroxyzine (Atarax)	Pruritus associated with dermatitis	Syrup: 10 mg/5 mL Tablets: 10, 25, 50, 100 mg	*Adults:* 25 mg 3–4 times/d *Children <age 6:* 12.5 mg 3–4 times/d; maximum 50 mg/ 24 h *Children age 6 and older:* 12.5– 25 mg 3–4 times/ d; maximum 50–100 mg/24 h	May cause drowsiness
Cetirizine (Zyrtec)	Pruritus associated with dermatitis	Syrup: 1 mg/mL Tablets: 5, 10 mg *Children age 2–5:*	*Adults:* 5–10 mg once daily mines 2.5 mg initially; can increase dose to 5 mg/d either as one 5-mg dose or 2.5 mg q12h *Children age 6 and older:* 5– 10 mg once daily	Less sedation than other antihista- Should not be used concurrently with alcohol or other CNS depressants as it may poten- tiate the depres- sant effect
Doxepin (systemic: Sinequan)	Pruritus associated with dermatitis	Capsules: 10, 25, 50, 75, 100, 150 mg	Dose range is 25– 150 mg/d in single or divided doses; suggested start- ing dose is 75 mg/d, then titrate up or down as indicated Use dose that achieves effect with fewest adverse effects	Not recommended in children Do not use within 14 d of monoamine oxidase inhibitors (MAOIs) Contraindicated in patients with acute myocardial infarc- tion (MI), urinary re- tention, or glucoma Pregnancy Category C; not recommended during pregnancy

Continued on next page

Table 30–1. Drugs Commonly Used: Dermatitis and Psoriasis *(continued)*

Drug	Indication	Strengths Available	Dose	Notes
Doxepin (topical: Zonalon)	Moderate to severe pruritus associated with atopic dermatitis (eczema)	Cream: 5%	Apply a thin film to affected areas 4 times/d in 3- to 4-h intervals	Interacts adversely with alcohol, cimetidine, and MAOIs; avoid these drugs during therapy Contraindicated in children Pregnancy Category B Patients with untreated narrow-angle glaucoma and urinary retention should not use PO or topical form
SHAMPOOS FOR SEBORRHEIC DERMATITIS				
Ketoconazole shampoo (OTC: Nizoral)	Seborrheic dermatitis	2% shampoo	Apply to wet scalp, massage for 1 min, rinse, and repeat; leave on scalp for 3 min, then rinse well	See package Pregnancy Category C
Selenium sulfide shampoo (Selsun Blue, Head & Shoulders Intensive Treatment, Excel)	Seborrheic dermatitis	OTC: 1% shampoo Rx: 2.5% shampoo	Apply to wet hair and massage in for 2–3 min before rinsing completely; apply twice a wk until control is achieved, then weekly thereafter For cradle cap: Apply 1% shampoo to scalp, avoiding eyes; rinse thoroughly	See package Advise patient that the shampoo will loosen crusted scales and that these scales may appear loose in the hair after the first few shampoos; brush to remove the scales from the hair; this will resolve after a few treatments
Coal tar shampoo (OTC: Zetar, Neutrogena T/Gel, Tegrin Medicated, Denorex, Theraplex T, Ional T Plus)	Seborrheic dermatitis	1%: Zetar, Theraplex T 2%: Ionol T Plus, Neutrogena T/Gel 5%: Tegrin Medicated 7% Tegrin Medicated Extra conditioning 9% Denorex 12.5%: Extra Strength Denorex	Rub into wet hair and scalp and then rinse; repeat and leave shampoo in for 5 min, rinse well; may be used daily– weekly; follow package directions	See package Do not use if there are open infected lesions Use with caution in children under age 2 May cause sun sensitivity for 24 h after application

Continued on next page

Table 30–1. Drugs Commonly Used: Dermatitis and Psoriasis *(continued)*

Drug	Indication	Strengths Available	Dose	Notes
Pyrithione zinc (OTC: Head & Shoulders shampoo, Zincon, Danex, DHS, Sebulon, ZNP Bar)	Seborrheic dermatitis	1% shampoo: Head & Shoulders, Zincon, Danex 2% shampoo: DHS Zinc, Sebulon 2% soap: ZNP Bar	Shampoo: apply, lather, rinse, and repeat; use once or twice weekly Soap: wet skin, lather, rinse, and repeat; use once or twice a wk	See package
Sulfur and salicylic acid shampoo (Fostex, Sebex, Sebulex)	Seborrheic dermatitis	5% sulfur and 3% salicylic acid: Maximum Strength Meted 3% salicylic acid and 5% colloidal sulfur: MG400 2% sulfur and 2% salicylic acid: Fostex Medicated Cleansing, Sebex, Sebulex	Follow package directions	See package
TOPICAL ANTIPSORIATICS				
Coal tar (OTC: Zetar, Medotar, Taraphilic, MG217 Medicated, MG217 Dual Treatment, Fototar, Tegrin for Psoriasis, Oxipor VHC)	Psoriasis	Emulsion: 30% (Zetar) Ointment: 1% (Medotar, Taraphilic), 2% (MG217 Medicated) Cream: 2% (Fototar) Lotion: 5% (MG217 Dual Treatment, Tegrin for Psoriasis); 48.5% (Oxipor VHC) Various generics: 20%	Follow package directions Rinse well after use	May cause staining Contraindicated if patient is taking tetracycline, psoralins, and topical retinoids May cause contact irritant dermatitis Pregnancy Category C
Anthralin (Dithrocreme, Lansan, Anthra-Derm, Dithro-Scalp)	Psoriasis	Cream: 0.1%, 0.25%, 0.5%, 1% Scalp cream: 0.25%, 0.5%	Begin with a low concentration (0.1%); apply a small amount to affected areas; rub in gently, avoiding healthy surrounding skin; leave on for 10 min, then wash off; after 1 wk, may increase to 15–20 min	May stain skin and clothes Pregnancy Category C; safety in young children unknown May alternate with other therapies (retinoids, topical steroids, UV light)

Continued on next page

Antibiotics. **Antibiotics** may be necessary to treat secondary infections of *Staphylococcus aureus*, beta-hemolytic streptococci, a virus, or a fungus. If a bacterial infection is suspected, treat for 10 days with an **antibiotic** that is effective against *S. aureus* and streptococci. **Cephalexin** (**Keflex**), **amoxicillin/clavulanate** (**Augmentin**), and **cefprozil** (**Cefzil**) are all effective. **Erythromycin** may be used, depending on the resistance level of the staphylococci. **Azithromycin** (**Zithromax**) can be used for **penicillin**- and **cephalosporin**-allergic patients. If there is re-

Table 30–1. Drugs Commonly Used: Dermatitis and Psoriasis *(continued)*

Drug	Indication	Strengths Available	Dose	Notes
			Increase strength in incremental steps until lesions are healed and skin looks and feels normal Scalp cream: begin with low concentration (0.25%); apply to scalp after combing hair to remove scales; leave on for 10–20 min; use daily for at least 1 wk; increase strength if needed	
Calcipotriene (Dovonex)	Psoriasis	Ointment, solution, cream: 0.0005%	Apply twice daily to affected area; rub in gently and completely Treat for 6–8 wk; improvement usually noted after 1–2 wk	Pregnancy Category C; should not be used during pregnancy or in children Older patients have a higher incidence of adverse skin reactions Rare reports of rapid onset of hypercalcemia

current bacterial infection, a 3-week course of treatment is necessary.

LONG-TERM THERAPY. Eczema is a chronic disorder, and the patient often cycles between mild to moderate dry skin and exacerbations that can be mild to severe. Once an exacerbation quiets, patients must continue to care for their skin to prevent further exacerbations. The keys to long-term therapy are adequate hydration of the skin and avoidance of agents that cause exacerbations.

Emollients. **Moisturizers, lubricants,** and **emollients** help retain water in the skin. They are composed of petrolatum, lanolin, or other agents such as colloidal oatmeal in an emulsion. The **emollient** is applied after patients bathe one to four times per day. They pat their skin dry and then apply the lotion or cream liberally to all affected areas. This procedure traps the moisture in the skin. Ointments provide the most occlusive barrier; creams are the next best. Lotions offer the convenience of easy application over large areas of skin but are not as occlusive as ointments and creams. Patients often decrease their use of **emollients** between exacerbations,

and a review and reinforcement of their use during each clinic visit will increase compliance.

Of all the **emollient** products available, many are eliminated because they have additives such as perfumes or other chemicals, to which many patients with eczema are sensitive. Commonly used **emollients** are **Aveeno** cream or lotion, **Eucerin** cream or lotion, **Lubriderm** lotion, and **Moisturel** lotion. **White petrolatum (Vaseline)** or **vegetable shortening (Crisco)** can be used in severe cases. If the patient uses a lotion, make sure it does not contain **alcohol,** which is drying and irritating. Occasionally, patients are sensitive to the lanolin in **Eucerin,** which is a natural product derived from sheep's wool. Because large amounts are needed to be effective, expense can play a role in choosing an **emollient. White petrolatum** is inexpensive and a good treatment choice for patients with limited resources.

NONPHARMACOLOGICAL MEASURES. Nonpharmacological measures include hydrating baths and avoiding skin irritation and offending agents that cause exacerbations. Patients should be told to wear rubber or plastic gloves when

Clinical Pearl

DERMATITIS

- For eczema, combine one 30-g tube of medium-potency **corticosteroid** cream (**Elocon** or **Westcort**) with 16 oz of **moisturizer** lotion (**Lubriderm, Aquaphor**) to enhance the effect of the **steroid.** To mix, have the family or patient pour the lotion into a clean bowl, add the cream, and use a wire whisk to mix. Pour the mixture back into the lotion bottle and label appropriately. This can be safely applied up to four times a day to large surface areas.
- Occluding the surface with plastic wrap will increase penetration of the **topical corticosteroid.** Do not do this in children, as it will increase the systemic absorption of the **steroid.**
- For contact dermatitis, caution the patient using bath oils against slipping in the tub. Children should be supervised at all times when using bath dermatologics, which can all cause the tub to be slippery. Older adults should also be monitored.
- For the patient with hand dermatitis, wearing cotton gloves overnight after applying a thick layer of **emollient** will increase absorption, and the patient will often see a significant improvement overnight.

their hands may be exposed to harsh chemicals or detergents. They should avoid irritating fabrics such as wool. Soft cotton clothing allows the skin to breathe. Careful avoidance of perfumed lotions and soaps prevents flare-ups related to the additives in these products. Some patients have food sensitivities that exacerbate their eczema.

Baths are used to hydrate the skin. The patient should take a warm—not hot—bath for 20 minutes. The skin is patted dry, and **emollients** are applied immediately to maintain the skin's hydration. The patient should use a mild soap for cleansing the groin and axillae, not harsh deodorant soaps. After a bath is also a good time to apply **corticosteroid** creams or ointments, if needed.

Contact Dermatitis

The treatment for both types of contact dermatitis is the same. If a small area of skin is affected, a **topical corticosteroid** cream is usually effective. If more than 10 percent of the skin surface must be treated or if the allergic contact dermatitis is severe, then **oral corticosteroids** are used. Wet dressings or baths are soothing to the inflamed skin. **Oral antihistamines** may help control pruritus.

TOPICAL CORTICOSTEROIDS. Topical corticosteroid creams or ointments are effective in treating mild to moderate contact dermatitis. A low-potency (**hydrocortisone** 1% or 2.5% cream) or intermediate-potency (**hydrocortisone valerate** 0.2% or **triamcinolone acetonide** 0.1%) cream can be used. (See Table 30–1 for prescribing information.) The patient should begin to experience relief in 2 to 3 days, with complete healing in 2 to 3 weeks.

ORAL CORTICOSTEROIDS. Oral corticosteroids (**prednisone** or **methylprednisolone**) are used if the contact

dermatitis is severe or if a large skin surface area is involved. A 2- to 3-week course of therapy may be needed for severe cases, with 2 weeks usually the minimum length of therapy required for severe poison oak or ivy dermatitis. See Table 30–1 for prescribing information.

WET DRESSINGS OR BATHS. Wet dressings or baths provide comfort. **Aluminum acetate solution (Burow's, Domeboro)** is an astringent wet dressing applied for 30 minutes four times a day for relief of inflammation associated with contact dermatitis. **Emollient** baths that contain colloidal oatmeal solids (**Aveeno**) or oils (**Alpha Keri Bath Oil, Lubriderm Bath Oil**) can be used to provide relief from pruritus associated with contact dermatitis. Baths may be used as needed for comfort.

Diaper Dermatitis

Drug therapy in the treatment of diaper dermatitis is aimed at protecting the skin, decreasing inflammation, and treating *Candida* infection. Nonpharmacological interventions are also used to prevent irritant diaper dermatitis.

BARRIER MEDICATIONS. Barrier medications are used to protect the skin from the irritant effects of contact with urine and feces. Plain **white petrolatum** is an effective and inexpensive barrier agent. Vitamins A and D are added to petrolatum to create a barrier OTC medication, **A&D Ointment. Zinc oxide** is a commonly used barrier that has a drying effect as well. It is combined with a variety of other agents such as **petrolatum** (**Diprotex, Diaparene, Bottom Better**), **cod liver oil and talc (Desitin)**, and **balsam of Peru (Balmex)**, which is thought to promote wound healing. Plain **zinc**

oxide is an effective barrier that is less expensive than the many diaper rash products. Barrier medications should be used at the first sign of irritation.

ANTI-INFLAMMATORY MEDICATIONS. Anti-inflammatory medications are used to decrease the inflammation associated with diaper dermatitis. Because of the occlusive nature of diapers and undergarments, a low-dose **hydrocortisone** (0.5% or 1%) should be used for a brief period. Low-dose **hydrocortisone** can be used for 2 to 3 days in the diaper area safely if it is applied sparingly (pea-sized amount) and used two to three times a day. Stronger **corticosteroid** preparations or combination medications containing midpotency **steroids** with an **antifungal** should not be used in the diaper area.

ANTIFUNGAL MEDICATIONS. Candidiasis is treated with a topical antifungal agent that is effective against *C. albicans*. Commonly used medications are **nystatin (Mycostatin)**, **miconazole (Monistat-Derm)**, and **clotrimazole (Lotrimin)**. All of these medications are applied twice daily until the *Candida* infection is clear. **Miconazole** and **clotrimazole** are available OTC and are usually not covered by insurance plans. **Nystatin** is available by prescription only and is usually covered by insurance. If a patient does not respond to the OTC products, a trial of **nystatin** is warranted.

WET SOAKS. Wet soaks or sitz baths are used to decrease inflammation and provide comfort. **Burow's solution** soaks or compresses can be used if the rash is weepy. Commercial diaper wipes often contain **alcohol**, which stings, and they should be avoided during diaper dermatitis. A spray bottle of clean water allows adequate cleansing without further irritating the area.

NONPHARMACOLOGICAL MANAGEMENT. Nonpharmacological management includes exposure to air, frequent diaper changes, and changing the diaper or protective garment brand. Expose the affected area to air by leaving the diaper off, or blow-dry the area with a hair dryer on low heat held several inches away from the skin two to three times a day.

Seborrheic Dermatitis

The mainstay of treatment for seborrheic dermatitis is topical **antiseborrheic** shampoos. **Topical corticosteroids** may also be used for nonhairy areas such as the face.

ANTISEBORRHEIC SHAMPOOS. Antiseborrheic shampoos should be used as prescribed to control dandruff. A variety of preparations are available to treat scalp seborrhea or dandruff. **Selenium sulfide**, one of the most commonly prescribed shampoos for seborrhea, is available OTC (**Selsun Blue, Head & Shoulders Intensive**) as 1% **selenium sulfide**; prescription formulas (**Exsel,**

Selun) contain 2.5% **selenium sulfide**. **Coal tar** shampoos are available OTC and range in strength from 0.5% (**DHS Tar**) to 12% (**Extra Strength Denorex**) **coal tar**. **Pyrithione zinc**, the active ingredient in OTC shampoos such as **Head & Shoulders**, may also be used to treat seborrheic dermatitis. Bar soap containing **pyrithione zinc** is available for use on body areas with seborrheic dermatitis (**ZNP Bar**). Shampoos that combine **sulfur** and **salicylic acid** can also be used (**Sebulex, Fostex**). For treating cradle cap, low-strength **selenium sulfide** (1%) is generally recommended, and care should be taken to keep the shampoo out of the infant's eyes and to rinse the hair well. Table 30–1 presents prescribing information.

TOPICAL CORTICOSTEROIDS. Topical corticosteroids are used for inflammatory seborrhea that does not respond to medicated shampoo. Low-potency **steroid** lotion or gel is applied two to three times daily to affected areas. Ongoing use of **topical steroids** may be needed when seborrheic dermatitis recurs. Table 30–1 presents prescribing information.

Monitoring

Monitoring for all forms of dermatitis includes assessing the patient for effectiveness of therapy and determining if the patient has experienced any adverse effects or developed a secondary infection.

Outcome Evaluation

For all forms of dermatitis, effective management controls exacerbations and provides comfort measures to decrease pruritus or other symptoms. If the initial therapy has not controlled the exacerbation, increasing the potency of the initial medication or switching to another medication may be indicated. However, before switching to another medication, the provider should observe the patient's medication administration technique, which may be the problem. Secondary skin infections, if they occur, should be treated promptly. Referral to a dermatologist may be necessary if therapy is not managing the dermatitis, if high-potency **topical corticosteroids** are indicated, or if the patient has an unusual presentation.

Patient Education

Patient education should include a discussion of information related to the overall treatment plan as well as that specific to the drug therapy, reasons for taking the

PATIENT EDUCATION

Dermatitis

Related to the Overall Treatment Plan/Disease Process

☐ Pathophysiology
☐ Role of preventive and nonpharmacological measures if appropriate
☐ Importance of adherence to the treatment regimen
☐ Self-monitoring of symptoms
☐ What to do when symptoms worsen
☐ Need for follow-up visits with the primary care provider

Specific to the Drug Therapy

☐ Reason for taking the drug and its anticipated action on the disease process
☐ Doses and schedules for taking the drug
☐ Possible adverse effects and what to do if they occur
☐ Interactions between other treatment modalities and these drugs

Reasons for taking the Drug(s)

Patient education about specific drugs is provided in the appropriate chapter.

Specifically for Eczema

☐ Pathophysiology of eczema, that it is a chronic disorder requiring ongoing care, and that there is an itch-scratch-itch cycle that needs to be addressed, but that it is a recurring disease that can be controlled.
☐ Avoidance of offending agents that cause exacerbations.
☐ Appropriate use of topical corticosteroids should be demonstrated. With a sample, the provider can demonstrate how far a pea-sized amount of topical medication can be spread. The patient or caregiver applying the medication should be aware of the adverse effects of overuse of topical corticosteroids.
☐ Avoidance of irritants or agents that cause exacerbation of the eczema should be taught, with a written list of common irritants provided to the patient.
☐ Long-term therapy (skin hydration and emollient use) versus acute therapy.

Specifically for Contact Dermatitis

☐ Pathophysiology
☐ The appropriate application of topical corticosteroids should be demonstrated.
☐ Appropriate use of antipruritic medication.

Specifically for Diaper Dermatitis

☐ The parent or patient should be educated about the underlying pathophysiology of diaper dermatitis, in that it is usually an irritant dermatitis caused by chemical irritation from urine or feces, complicated by mechanical irritation of the diaper or undergarment rubbing and chafing the skin.

continued

PATIENT EDUCATION

Dermatitis *(continued)*

☐ Describing the characteristics of a secondary infection with *Candida* will assist with early identification and treatment of this common complication in diaper dermatitis.

☐ Nonpharmacological management such as sitz baths, air drying, and frequent diaper changes should be discussed.

☐ If properly treated, the skin should return to normal in the area in 3 to 4 days. If the patient is not responding to treatment in 48 hours, then a reevaluation is necessary.

Specifically for Seborrheic Dermatitis

☐ The patient should know that seborrheic dermatitis cannot be cured and can only be controlled and that treatment will probably need to be continued long-term in adolescents and adults. In infants with cradle cap, it will usually resolve around age 6 months.

☐ Signs and symptoms of secondary infection so that the patient can contact the health care provider if symptoms of a secondary infection occur.

Drugs as Part of the Total Treatment Regimen

The total treatment regimen includes pharmacological and nonpharmacological measures. Be sure the patient and/or family members are aware of the specific measures to be taken.

Adherence Issues

Health care providers should be aware of the potential problem of nonadherence and should discuss the importance of completing the entire treatment regimen with the patient and/or family members.

drug, drugs as part of the total treatment regimen, and adherence issues.

Psoriasis

Psoriasis is a chronic skin condition that affects 1 to 3 percent of the population worldwide. It is characterized by sharply defined, symmetrical, erythematous patches with a distinctive silver scale. There are two peak ages of onset: from age 16 to 22 and from age 57 to 60. However, it may occur at any age. Men and women are equally affected, but it is more common in whites than in darker-skinned people. There is a positive family history for the disease in 30 percent of patients. The disease may remain localized to a few areas, or it may become generalized. The condition is lifelong and may occur in an intermittent or a continuous pattern.

Pathophysiology

The exact pathogenesis of psoriasis is unclear. There is a significant decrease in the amount of time that it takes for a psoriatic epidermal cell to travel to the skin surface and be cast off. A normal skin cell travels to the surface in 26 to 28 days; with psoriasis, the cells take only 3 to 4 days. This decreased time does not allow normal cell maturation to take place.

Lesions of active psoriasis can develop in areas of epidermal trauma. Surgery, a sunburn, or scratch marks can all heal, leaving psoriatic lesions in their place (Koebner's phenomenon). Exacerbations may be triggered by beta-hemolytic streptococcal infections, as well as by some medications (e.g., **lithium, beta-adrenergic antagonists, angiotensin-converting enzyme inhibitors, antimalarial drugs,** and **indomethacin**).

Extensor surfaces are affected more commonly, with other common sites being the intergluteal fold, the eyebrows, and around the ears. Nails may develop pits and ridges, may be thick and discolored, and have splinter hemorrhages.

Goals of Treatment

Although psoriasis is a chronic, lifelong, recurrent disease, the goal of therapy should be complete control of symptoms and clearing of psoriatic lesions. It should be emphasized to the patient that psoriasis is a treatable disease and that control is possible with continued, conscientious use of medication.

Rational Drug Selection

The management of psoriasis consists of topical medication and phototherapy for mild to moderate psoriasis (less than 20% of the body involved) and the addition of systemic medications for severe psoriasis (more than 20% of the body involved). Patients with severe disease are usually referred to a dermatologist; therefore, systemic treatment is covered only briefly in this chapter.

Topical Therapy

Topical therapy for psoriasis consists of **topical steroids, coal tar** or **keratolytic shampoos** for scalp involvement, **keratolytic agents** for thick plaques, **anthralin,** and **calcipotriene.**

TOPICAL STEROIDS. Topical steroids are used to treat psoriasis because of their anti-inflammatory effects on the plaques. Moderate- to high-potency **steroids** are used because the lesions are generally **steroid**-resistant. (See Table 30–1.) Occlusion with plastic may be necessary for best results. The **steroid** cream or ointment is applied two to three times per day. Chronic **topical corticosteroid** use can cause tachyphylaxis and may have adverse effects such as atrophy and telangiectasia. Intermittent or "pulse" therapy minimizes some of these effects and has the best long-term outcome. If **topical corticosteroids** are used in the intertriginous areas or on the face, a low-dose medication should be chosen. Regardless of the **topical steroid** used, 3 weeks of continuous use is the limit. Patients should be discouraged from using **steroids** for longer periods. **Topical corticosteroids** should be reserved for psoriasis flare, and another medication used for ongoing therapy.

COAL TAR. Coal tar (**Zetar, Medotar, Tegrin for Psoriasis**) affects psoriasis by enzyme inhibition and antimitotic action. **Tar** preparations include creams, shampoos, ointments, lotions, gels, and oils. They range in strength from 1 to 20 percent. They have few adverse effects and are safer to use than **topical steroids** and **anthralin.** The major problem is that they are messy and can stain the skin and clothes. The **tar** preparation is applied to the affected areas once or twice daily. If using **coal tar** shampoo or bath emulsion, the patient should be instructed to rinse well after use. **Tar** preparations make the patient photosensitive; therefore, the patient should be instructed to avoid sunlight and ultraviolet light. (See Table 30–1.)

ANTHRALIN. Anthralin (**Dithrocreme**) is an antimitotic agent that is used for chronic psoriasis. It has an antiproliferative effect. Although it is effective, **anthralin** has the disadvantages of being irritating and of staining skin and clothing. Careful instructions for use increase the likelihood of a successful outcome with this difficult-to-administer medication. Table 30–1 presents prescribing information.

CALCIPOTRIENE. Calcipotriene (**Dovonex**) is a vitamin D_3 derivative that regulates cell differentiation and proliferation and suppresses lymphocyte activity. **Calcipotriene** is available in a cream, ointment, or solution preparation. It is effective and safe for short- or long-term treatment. Table 30–1 presents prescribing information.

Phototherapy

Patients with psoriasis respond very well to phototherapy. Phototherapy with ultraviolet-B (UVB) light is effective in managing psoriasis by reducing DNA synthesis of epidermal cells. UVB light treatment is easy for the patient to use and can produce long-lasting remissions of 2 to 4 months. A newer therapy consisting of narrowband UVB light is currently under investigation. UVB therapy is usually prescribed by a dermatologist. The use of commercial tanning beds is not recommended.

Systemic Medications

Systemic medications used for psoriasis are **methotrexate, oral retinoids,** and **cyclosporine.** All have serious adverse effects and therefore should be prescribed only by a dermatologist and only if the patient meets criteria determined by the American Academy of Dermatology. To try to decrease the adverse effects, the medications may be prescribed intermittently or on a rotational basis. Patients should be advised to avoid pregnancy before, during, and for a period of time after taking these drugs. The primary care provider will need to consult with the dermatologist and observe the patient for adverse effects if any of these medications are prescribed.

Monitoring

The patient who is being treated for psoriasis should be monitored for effectiveness of therapy and for adverse effects of the medication.

Outcome Evaluation

Psoriasis lesions should eventually clear, with the skin returning to the patient's normal look and feel. If the patient is using the medication correctly and there is unsatisfactory clinical response, or if skin irritation occurs, then either the medication needs to be changed or the strength increased. Skin irritation is a common adverse effect of psoriasis medications, especially if the patient gets the medication on the surrounding skin. Review proper administration technique prior to changing the therapy.

Patient Education

Successful treatment of psoriasis requires educating the patient on the following key points:

1. The patient should understand the pathophysiology of psoriasis, that it is a chronic disease but that remission is possible if adequately treated.
2. Proper application of topical medications will not only optimize treatment but also decrease adverse effects of the medications.
3. Many of the medications stain the skin and clothing. The patient should be aware of this problem and instructed on how to minimize the staining.
4. Some medications cause photosensitivity; therefore, the patient needs to understand the hazards of sun exposure and use protective clothing and sunscreen.

Acne and Acne Rosacea

Acne affects an estimated 17 to 28 million Americans, accounting for 4.4 percent of internist visits. It is the number one condition seen by dermatologists, accounting for 18 percent of visits (Feldman, 1998). Approximately 85 percent of adolescents have acne to some degree, although acne can also occur in patients in their twenties to forties. Adolescent acne is more common in boys than in girls; however, adult acne is more common in women than in men. Males have a higher incidence of severe acne at all ages (Landow, 1997).

Although acne may be a minor problem from a medical standpoint, multiple studies have determined that acne has a significant impact on the patient's quality of life (Lasek & Chren, 1998; Mallon et al., 1999). The adolescent is stereotyped as being the most concerned about acne, but studies have indicated that the older the patient, the more the impact acne has on quality-of-life scores, regardless of severity (Lasek & Chren, 1998). Acne patients reported levels of social, psychological, and emotional problems that were as great as those reported by patients with chronic disabling asthma, epilepsy, diabetes, back pain, or arthritis (Mallon et al., 1999). The practitioner needs to address the patient's concerns about acne with this in mind.

Pathophysiology

The underlying cause of acne is multifactorial. A genetic susceptibility appears to predispose some people to acne. Acne begins below the skin surface in the pilosebaceous unit of the sebaceous glands. In acne, the sebaceous glands are enlarged and sebum production is increased, probably because of adrenogenic hormones. In patients with acne, there is an alteration in the keratinization process in the follicular infrainfundibulum. This causes the extra sebum to occlude the hair follicle and produce microcomedones. These may enlarge with time and form closed comedones (whiteheads) or open comedones (blackheads). *Propionibacterium acnes* organisms colonize the follicles and convert the triglycerides in the sebum into free fatty acids. Free fatty acids are a factor in the synthesis of chemoattractants that draw inflammatory elements, leading to the inflammation associated with acne. The patient may have superficial papules and/or pustules or deeper nodules, depending on the intensity of the inflammatory process.

Goals of Treatment

At this time, there is no cure for acne. The goal is to control the acne and keep visible lesions and medication adverse effects to a minimum. Management goals that will control acne are (1) to control the inflammatory process associated with acne by altering the bacterial flora and (2) to decrease the obstruction of the sebaceous ducts.

Rational Drug Selection

Acne treatment should be approached in a stepwise manner. If the acne is mild or moderate, a beginning therapy might include **topical retinoids** and **topical antibiotics.** If after 6 to 8 weeks this is not completely effective, an **oral**

antibiotic might be added or a change in topical therapy initiated. For moderate to somewhat severe acne, the patient is usually started on an **oral antibiotic** and topical preparations combined. For severe, recalcitrant, nodular acne, the patient is prescribed **isotretinoin (Accutane).** Figure 30–1 presents an algorithm of the pharmacological management of acne.

Topical Agents

The topical agents used for acne can be divided into two categories: **topical retinoids** and **topical antibiotics.**

TOPICAL RETINOIDS. Topical retinoids (tretinoin [Retin-A]) or retinoid-like compounds (**adapalene [Differin]**) are used to treat inflammatory and noninflammatory acne. They act to alter the abnormal keratinization process of acne that leads to microcomedo formation. Additionally, they stimulate mitotic activity and increase the turnover of follicular epithelial cells, causing extrusion of the comedones. Clinically, this causes an initial worsening of acne, as comedones that were previously under the skin are extruded. This worsening is not a reason for discontinuation of treatment. Patients should be reassured that their faces will clear after approximately 6 to 8 weeks of treatment.

Both preparations can cause some skin irritation, especially in fair-skinned patients or patients with sensitive skin. Atopic people can be quite sensitive to these products. The patient should not use any harsh toners, astringents, scrubs, or cleansers while on **topical retinoid** therapy because these increase irritation. The patient's skin is more photosensitive when **topical retinoids** are used, and patients should be advised to use noncomedogenic sunscreen for any sun exposure.

The patient should avoid the eyes and mucous membranes when applying these products. There may be transient stinging, burning, or pruritus immediately after applying **topical retinoids.** Redness and peeling may occur with excessive application. There is no improved response to **topical retinoids** if they are used more than recommended, but there is a dramatic increase in skin irritation. Table 30–2 presents the drugs commonly used to treat acne.

TOPICAL ANTIBIOTICS. **Topical antibiotics** are thought to act to control acne by their bacteriostatic or bactericidal activity against *P. acnes*. They control the inflammatory process, probably by decreasing the free fatty acids that *P. acnes* produces. Applied topically, **antibiotics** have an uneven, erratic penetration into the follicles. Therefore, they are usually used in mild acne, for maintenance after a course of **oral antibiotics,** or in conjunction with **topical retinoids.** There is a concern that resistant *P. acnes* may develop if **topical antibiotics** are overused. The **topical antibiotics** that are approved for use include **benzoyl peroxide,** available by prescription (**Benzac, Desquam-X, Desquam-E**) or OTC (**Dryox, Fostex, Neutrogena**

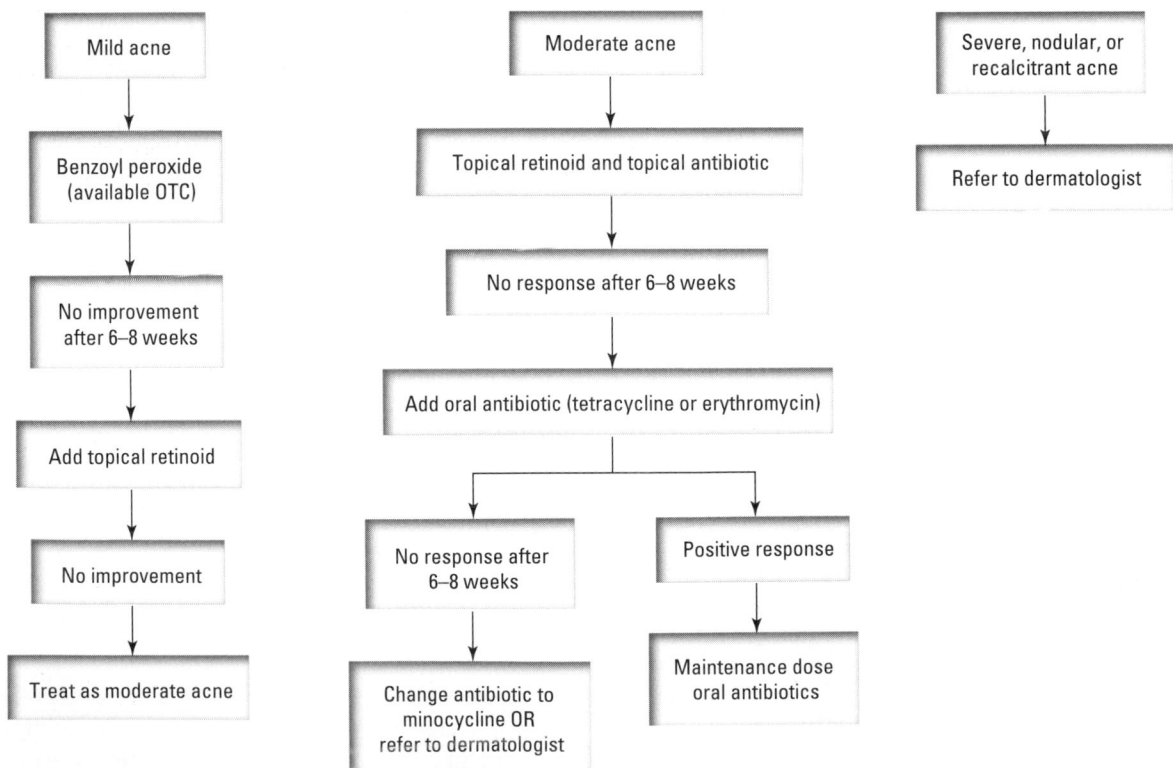

Figure 30–1. Algorithm: pharmacological management of acne.

Table 30–2. Drugs Commonly Used: Acne

Drug	Indication	Strengths Available	Dose	Notes
Topical Retinoids				
Tretinoin (Retin-A)	Acne	Cream: 0.025%, 0.05%, 0.1% Gel: 0.025%, 0.01% Liquid: 0.05%	Apply to affected areas once daily after washing face with a mild cleanser; begin with 0.025% cream and increase strength or to bid if needed Sensitive-skin patients may need to dose every other night	Wash hands after application Normal use of cosmetics is permissible, but instruct patient to use noncomedogenic products Pregnancy Category C; pregnant women should be switched to another product
Adapalene (Differin)	Acne	Gel: 0.1% (alcohol-free) Lotion: 0.1% (30% alcohol)	Apply to affected areas once daily (HS) after washing with a gentle cleanser; avoid eyes, lips, and mucous membranes	Avoid harsh soaps, cleansers, or alcohol-containing products, which increase skin irritation while using adapalene Pregnancy Category C May be used in children over age 12
Topical Antibiotics				
Benzoyl peroxide (Rx: Benzac, Desquam-X, Desquam-E) (OTC: Dryox, Fostex, Neutrogena Acne Mask, Clearasil)	Acne	Liquid wash: 2.5%, 5%, 10% Bar: 5%, 10% Mask: 5% Lotion: 5%, 5.5%, 10% Cream: 5%, 10% Gel: 2.5%, 4%, 5%, 10%, 20%	For cleansers, wash once or twice daily; rinse well and pat dry For other formu: apply once daily; gradually increase to 2–3 times daily if needed; apply after cleansing skin	Has a drying action, causes comedolysis, and has a mild desquamation effect (irritating to the skin) Pregnancy Category C; topical application during pregnancy is generally considered safe May be used in children >12 Bleaches fabrics Inactivates tretinoin and cannot be applied simultaneously
Erythromycin (Staticin, Akne-Mycin, A/T/S, Eryderm, Erymax, Ery-Sol, T-Stat, Erygel)	Acne	Solution: 1%, 2% Gel: 2% Ointment: 2%	Apply to affected areas bid after washing face with a mild cleanser	Pregnancy Category B Do not use concurrently with clindamycin

Continued on next page

Table 30–2. Drugs Commonly Used: Acne *(continued)*

Drug	Indication	Strengths Available	Dose	Notes
Benzoyl peroxide/ erythromycin (Benzamycin)	Acne	Gel	Apply to affected areas once or twice/d (gel dries to a crusty white appearance; therefore, patient may prefer evening application; patient may use plain benzoyl peroxide in the morning if this is a concern)	Pregnancy Category C Bleaches fabrics Must be kept refrigerated; stable for only 3 mo after mixed Adverse effects include skin irritation and sun sensitivity
Clindamycin (Cleocin, Clinda-Derm, C/T/S)	Acne	Gel, lotion, topical solution	Apply thin layer to affected areas bid	Use with caution in patients with eczema Although rare, there are reports of colitis with topical administration If patient develops diarrhea, stop medication and investigate cause Pregnancy Category B Do not use in children under age 12 Adverse effects include skin dryness and irritation, burning, and peeling
Tetracycline (Topicycline)	Acne	Topical solution: 2.2 g/mL	Apply to affected areas bid; apply until skin is thoroughly wet (stinging and burning may occur but subside after a few minutes)	Pregnancy Category B May be staining to clothes; yellowing of skin may be removed by washing Assess patient for sulfite sensitivity Topicycline contains sodium bisulfite
Metronidazole **(Metro-Gel, Noritate)**	Acne rosacea	Gel: 0.75% Emollient cream: 1%	Apply a thin film bid to entire affected area after washing	Improvement should be noted within 3 wk, but there may be continued improvement through 9 wk of treatment Pregnancy Category B Some mild skin irritation may be noted

Continued on next page

Table 30–2. Drugs Commonly Used: Acne *(continued)*

Drug	Indication	Strengths Available	Dose	Notes
Oral Antibiotics Tetracycline (Achromycin)	Acne (long-term treatment)	Capsules: 250, 500 mg Tablets: 250, 500 mg	Initially, 500 mg bid for 1–2 mo After control is achieved, dose may be lowered to 500 mg qd for 1–2 mo; then determine maintenance dose of 125–500 mg daily	Must be taken on an empty stomach; poorly absorbed if taken with calcium-containing foods, milk, or antacids Pregnancy Category D; do not prescribe to lactating women or children under age 8 (may cause staining of teeth)
Erythromycin base (E-Mycin, Ery-Tab), erythromycin estolate (Ilosone), erythromycin ethylsuccinate (EryPed, E.E.S.)	Acne (long-term treatment)	Erythromycin base: capsules: 250, 333, 500 mg Erythromycin estolate: tablets: 250, 500 mg; suspension 125 mg/5 mL, 250 mg/5 mL Erythromycin ethylsuccinate: chewable tablets: 200 mg; tablets: 400 mg; suspension: 200 mg/5 mL, 400 mg/5 mL	Initially, 1000 mg/d in divided doses (usually qid) After control is achieved, dose can be decreased to 250–500 mg/d	Some dermatologists prescribe a "burst" of 750 mg for 7–10 d if acne is cyclical such as menstrual-associated acne Inexpensive Pregnancy Category B May cause gastrointestinal (GI) upset; take with food or milk
Minocycline (Minocin)	Acne (acne resistant to tetracycline and erythromycin)	Capsules: 50, 100 mg Tablets: 50, 100 mg	Initially, 100 mg bid, then wean to 50 mg qd after control is achieved	Expensive Must be taken on an empty stomach Pregnancy Category D; do not prescribe to lactating women or children <8 y

Acne Mask, Clearasil); erythromycin (Staticin, Akne-Mycin, A/T/S, Eryderm, Erymax, Ery-Sol, T-Stat, Erygel), clindamycin (Cleocin, Clinda-Derm, C/T/S), and tetracycline (Topicycline). A combination product of **benxoyl peroxide** and **erythromycin (Benzamycin)** is superior to either agent alone. Prescribing information is given in Table 30–2.

Oral Agents

Oral agents used for acne are divided into three categories: **oral antibiotics**, hormonal therapy, and **isotretinoin** (an **oral retinoid**). **Oral antibiotics** are prescribed for moderate to severe acne and are within the scope of practice of primary care providers. **Isotretinoin** is prescribed for severe nodulocystic acne but only by dermatologists because of its adverse effects.

ORAL ANTIBIOTICS. Oral antibiotics are active against *P. acnes*, which helps transform comedones into inflam-

matory pustules and papules. **Oral antibiotics** do not affect existing lesions, but they prevent future lesions by decreasing sebaceous fatty acids by decreasing *P. acnes* colonization. They may also have an anti-inflammatory effect independent of their action against *P. acnes*. No one **antibiotic** is considered superior, but **tetracycline** is often used because it has been studied the most extensively and is inexpensive. Table 30–2 presents prescribing information for **tetracycline (Achromycin V)**, **erythromycin (erythromycin base [E-Mycin, Ery-Tab], erythromycin estolate [Ilosone], erythromycin ethylsuccinate [EryPed, E.E.S.], and minocycline [Minocin]).**

HORMONAL THERAPY. Hormonal therapy can be prescribed to women who require birth control who also have mild to moderate acne. Two **oral contraceptives** currently have Food and Drug Administration (FDA) approval for use in acne: **Ortho Tri-Cyclen** and **Ortho-Cyclen**. The **oral contraceptives** appear to control the inflammatory

Clinical Pearl

ACNE

Tell patients who are using **benzoyl peroxide** or **Benzamycin** that it can bleach clothes and towels. Advise them to use an old or white pillowcase on their bed and an old or white towel to dry their hands after using these agents.

---

component of acne. The patient is prescribed a premeasured dose pack and takes one pill daily. Effects on acne are seen in 3 to 6 months of continued use. For full prescribing information, see the chapter on **oral contraceptives.**

ISOTRETINOIN. Isotretinoin (Accutane) is the most potent agent for treating acne. It is reserved for severe recalcitrant cystic acne. Its exact mechanism of action is unknown but thought to be related to decreased sebum production (by 90%) and **isotretinoin's** ability to decrease abnormal keratinization. **Isotretinoin** is prescribed for a period of 15 to 20 weeks and may need to be repeated. The toxicity profile and its ability to cause fetal malformations require that the prescriber provide extensive education and close monitoring throughout therapy. The adverse effects of dry skin, cheilitis, and pruritus are seen in almost all patients taking the drug. The major concern is the use of the drug in women who may become pregnant; therefore, there are very stringent requirements and consent that must be met before the drug is prescribed. For female patients, a pregnancy test needs to be performed before beginning therapy and then monthly throughout therapy. Liver enzyme and lipid levels should also be obtained before beginning therapy and monitored throughout therapy. *Isotretinoin* is **Pregnancy Category X.** It should not be prescribed to teenagers who have not completed their linear growth. Because of the toxic effects of **isotretinoin,** it is rarely prescribed by a primary care provider and is usually prescribed only by a dermatologist.

Acne Rosacea

Acne rosacea, commonly referred to as *rosacea,* is a skin condition that usually affects middle-aged patients. It is a chronic inflammatory disorder that affects the blood vessels and pilosebaceous glands of the face. The patient often has a characteristic red-colored nose. An important hallmark characteristic is easy flushing and blushing of the face associated with the ingestion of **alcohol,** spicy foods, or caffeine-containing beverages.

Patients with acne rosacea have papules and pustules superimposed on diffuse erythema and telangiectasia over the central portion of the face. Hyperplasia of the sebaceous glands, connective tissue, and vascular bed can lead to a large bulbous red nose, called *rhinophyma.* The patient may also have ocular involvement that may require the care of an ophthalmologist.

Topical metronidazole (Metro-Gel, Noritate) is used to treat acne rosacea. The mechanism by which **metronidazole** works to improve the inflammation of rosacea is unknown but is probably related to its antibacterial effect. Rosacea usually responds well to **metronidazole,** but the **antibiotic** must be continued for life, as the rosacea will recur if the medication is discontinued. Table 30–2 presents prescribing information.

Monitoring

The patient needs to be monitored for effectiveness and adverse effects of the acne medication.

Laboratory testing before and during therapy may be indicated for some patients. The primary care provider may be involved in obtaining and monitoring these tests. For female patients, especially those taking **tetracycline, minocycline,** and **isotretinoin,** pregnancy testing is recommended prior to beginning treatment and as indicated throughout therapy.

Outcome Evaluation

The patient needs to use an acne medication for at least 6 to 8 weeks before effectiveness can be determined. If there is no response after that time, then a change in therapy can be considered, either adding another medication or changing the regimen completely. Before determining the medication is not effective, review administration of the medication with the patient. The adverse effects associated with topical acne treatments include skin irritation and some redness and peeling. Mild symptoms usually improve if the frequency of administration is decreased slightly. If possible, the strength of the topical medication can be decreased if there is mild to moderate irritation. Severe skin irritation warrants discontinuing the medication and switching to another.

PATIENT EDUCATION

Acne

Related to the Overall Treatment Plan/Disease Process

☐ Pathophysiology

☐ Role of preventive and nonpharmacological measures if appropriate

☐ Importance of adherence to the treatment regimen

☐ Self-monitoring of symptoms

☐ What to do when symptoms worsen

☐ Need for follow-up visits with the primary care provider

Specific to the Drug Therapy

☐ Reason for the drug's being given and its anticipated action on the disease process

☐ Doses and schedules for taking the drug

☐ Possible adverse effects and what to do if they occur

☐ Interactions between other treatment modalities and these drugs

Reasons for Taking the Drug(s)

Patient education about specific drugs is provided in the appropriate chapter.

Specifically for Acne

☐ The patient should understand that it will take at least 6 weeks to determine if treatment is effective. Tying this into the explanation of normal skin growth will help the patient understand why it takes so long for the medication to work.

☐ Whatever level of treatment the patient is started on, the patient needs to understand what alternatives there are if the chosen treatment is not effective.

Drugs as Part of the Total Treatment Regimen

The total treatment regimen includes pharmacological and nonpharmacological measures. Be sure the patient and/or family members are aware of the specific measures to be taken.

Adherence Issues

Health care providers should be aware of the potential problem of nonadherence and should discuss the importance of completing the entire treatment regimen with the patient and/or family members.

Patient Education

Patient education should include a discussion of information related to the overall treatment plan as well as that specific to the drug therapy, reasons for taking the drug, drugs as part of the total treatment regimen, and adherence issues.

Skin Infections

Skin infections commonly seen in primary care include bacterial, viral, and fungal skin infections.

Bacterial skin infections are common and seen in any age patient. The skin infections seen in primary care include impetigo, a furuncle (boil or abscess), perianal streptococcal infection, and cellulitis. All require prompt treatment with the appropriate **antibiotic.**

Many viral skin infections can affect the skin, often causing rashes. Herpes simplex virus infection, herpes zoster (shingles), and varicella (chickenpox) are the common viral infections seen in primary care.

Fungal skin infections can be divided into two types: *Candida* infections and dermatophyte infections. Dermatophyte or tinea infections include tinea of the scalp (tinea capitis or ringworm of the scalp), tinea of the skin (tinea corporis or ringworm), tinea cruris ("jock itch"), tinea of the feet (tinea pedis or athlete's feet), and tinea versicolor. Onychomycosis, a fungal infection of the nails, is another type of fungal skin infection.

Pathophysiology

Bacterial Skin Infections

The most common bacterial organisms found in skin infections are *S. aureus* and *Streptococcus pyogenes*. The organism usually enters the skin through a break in the skin. The bacteria cause an inflammatory infectious process to begin.

Viral Skin Infections

Viral skin infections include herpes viral infections, varicella, and herpes zoster.

Herpes viral infections are spread by intimate contact between a person shedding the virus and a susceptible host. With inoculation into the skin or mucous membrane, herpes simplex virus (HSV) begins to replicate. The incubation period is 4 to 6 days. As replication continues, local inflammation and cell lysis lead to the distinctive vesicle with an erythematous region. The virus generally ascends the peripheral sensory nerves to the dorsal root ganglia. HSV replicates in the dorsal root ganglia and then enters an inactive or latent stage. The herpesvirus is unique in that it establishes latency for varying periods of time. HSV can be reactivated and enter a replication cycle at any time. There are two HSV infections, HSV-1 and HSV-2, with HSV-1 generally associated with nongenital infection and HSV-2 associated with genital infection.

Varicella (chickenpox) is a highly contagious disease caused by the varicella-zoster virus, a herpesvirus. It is spread by direct contact, in droplets, and by airborne transmission. The virus infects individuals by the conjunctivae or respiratory tract, replicating in the nasopharynx and upper respiratory tract. It spreads systemically to cause a viremia, resulting in a disseminated vesicular rash after an incubation period of 10 to 14 days. The patient is contagious for 1 to 2 days prior to the rash eruption and until all the lesions are dry. After the rash clears, the virus enters a latent phase and remains inactive in the dorsal root ganglia.

Herpes zoster (shingles) is caused by reactivation of latent varicella-zoster virus. The reason for the reactivation is unknown, although stress seems to have some impact. The incidence of the disease increases with age and immunosuppression. The patient usually experiences burning and pain along the dermatome prior to the vesicles erupting. The lesions are generally unilateral and appear along a dermatome, although there may occasionally be scattered lesions. The diagnosis is confirmed with Tzanck smear or viral culture.

Fungal Skin Infections

Candida infections are caused by *C. albicans,* which is commonly found on the skin and mucosal tissues in the oral, intestinal, and vaginal areas. Considered a normal flora in these areas, an overgrowth can lead to infection and erythema, ulceration, and characteristic white plaques. In the mouth, oral candidiasis is known as *thrush*. In women, a vaginal *Candida* infection is known as a *yeast* infection (see Chapter 42.) *Candida* is diagnosed by examination of scrapings from the area, using potassium hydroxide (KOH) preparation.

Dermatophytes are a group of fungi that live on the keratin of the stratum corneum, nails, and hair. Symptoms of dermatophyte infection include pruritus, scaling, occasional vesicles, and, in tinea corporis, characteristic annular lesions with raised edges and clearing in the center. Tinea versicolor can have clinical findings of multiple scaling, discrete macules that can be hypopigmented or hyperpigmented.

Onychomycosis is a fungal infection of the fingernails or toenails.

Goals of Treatment

The goals of treatment for skin infections are to decrease the severity of the infection or eradicate it (as appropriate), alleviate symptoms, and heal the skin area and return it to normal (as appropriate).

Rational Drug Selection

Bacterial Skin Infections

IMPETIGO.   Impetigo is a bacterial infection (*S. aureus* or *S. pyogenes*) of the superficial layers of the skin, which begins as vesicles that rupture, leaving a hallmark golden or honey-colored crust. **Topical mupirocin ointment (Bactroban)** is used if the impetigo is mild (up to five singular lesions). **Topical mupirocin** is considered the most effective **topical antibiotic;** however, it is available only by prescription and is expensive. The OTC ointments **bacitracin**

Table 30–3. Drugs Commonly Used: Skin Infections

Drug	Indication	Strengths Available	Dose	Notes
Topical Antibiotics Mupirocin (Bactroban)	Bacterial skin infections	2% ointment (15, 30 g) (available Rx only)	Apply to affected area tid until healed	Pregnancy Category B Safe in children
Polymyxin B/neomycin/ bacitracin (Polysporin, Neosporin, Triple Antibiotic Ointment)	Bacterial skin infections	Triple antibiotic combination (available OTC)	Apply a small amount to affected area 1–3 times/d until healed	Do not use if the patient has a neomycin sensitivity Topical use is safe in pregnancy and in young children
Bacitracin (Bacitracin, Baciguent)	Bacterial skin infections	Bacitracin only ointment (available OTC)	Apply to affected area 1–3 times/d until healed	May use in patients with neomycin sensitivity Safe during pregnancy and in young children
Systemic Oral Antibiotics Cephalexin (Keflex)	Bacterial skin infections	Capsules: 250, 500 mg Suspension: 125 mg/5 mL, 250 mg/5 mL	*Adults:* 500 mg every 12 h for 7–10 d *Children:* 25–50 mg/kg/d divided qid or tid; treat for 7–10 d	Inexpensive Pregnancy Category B Safe in children Well tolerated
Amoxicillin/clavulanate (Augmentin)	Bacterial skin infections	Tablets: 250 mg amoxicillin with 125 mg clavulanate; 500 mg with 125 mg Chewable tablets: 125 mg amoxicillin with 31.25 mg clavulanate; 200 mg with 28.5 mg; 250 mg with 62.5 mg; 400 mg with 57 mg; 125 mg with 31.25 mg/ 5 mL; 200 mg with 28.5/5 mL; 250 mg with 62.5 mg/ 5 mL; 400 mg with 57 mg/5 mL	*Adults:* 500 mg of amoxicillin every 12 h *or* 250 mg every 8 h for 7–10 d *Children > 3 mo:* 25–45 mg/kg/d of amoxicillin divided every 12 h (use 200 mg/5 mL or 400 mg/5 mL strength suspension) *or* 20–40 mg/kg/d of amoxicillin if using 125 mg/5 mL or 250 mg/5 mL strength suspension; treat for 7–10 d; use higher amounts with more severe infections	Broad-spectrum coverage Moderately expensive Pregnancy Category B May cause gastro-intestinal (GI) upset, especially at higher doses Children's dose is based on amoxicillin content Due to clavula-nate content, two 250-mg tablets are not the same as one 500-mg tablet; suspen-sion doses are also not equivalent

Continued on next page

Table 30–3. Drugs Commonly Used: Skin Infections *(continued)*

Drug	Indication	Strengths Available	Dose	Notes
				Children should not be given the 250-mg tablet until they weigh >40 kg
Cefadroxil (Duricef)	Bacterial skin infections	Tablets: 1 g Capsules: 500 mg Suspension: 125 mg/5 mL, 250 mg/5 mL, 500 mg/5 mL	*Adults:* 1 g once/d for 10 d *Children:* 30 mg/kg/d divided into 2 doses every 12 h	Pregnancy Category B First-generation cephalosporin Convenient dosing
Cefprozil (Cefzil)	Bacterial skin infections	Tablets: 250, 500 mg Suspension: 125 mg/5 mL, 250 mg/5 mL	*Adults and children age 12 and older:* 250–500 mg every 12 h for 7–10 d *Children 2–12:* 20 mg/kg/d divided into 2 doses 12 h apart for 7–10 d	Broad-spectrum coverage Expensive Pregnancy Category B
Erythromycin base (E-Mycin, Ery-Tab) erythromycin estolate (Ilosone), erythromycin ethylsuccinate (EryPed, E.E.S.)	Mild to moderate bacterial skin infections	Erythromycin base: 250, 333, 500 mg capsules Erythromycin estolate: 250-, 500-mg tablets; 125 mg/5 mL, 250 mg/5 mL suspension Erythromycin ethylsuccinate: 200-mg chewable tablets; 400-mg tablets; 200 mg/5 mL, 400 mg/5 mL suspension	*Adults:* 250–500 mg qid for 10 d *Children:* 20–50 mg/kg/d qid for 10 d	Inexpensive Pregnancy Category B May cause GI upset; take with food or milk
Azithromycin (Zithromax)	Bacterial skin infections	Capsules: 250 mg; Z-pak (6, 250-mg tablets with instructions for daily dosing) Suspension: 100 mg/5 mL; 200 mg/5 mL	*Adults:* 500 mg single dose the first d followed by 250 mg daily for days 2–5 *Children:* 10 mg/kg as one single dose on the first day, then 5 mg/kg/d on days 2–5; do not exceed adult dose	Convenient dosing; 5-day course of treatment Broad spectrum Pregnancy Category B
Antivirals Acyclovir (Zovirax), topical	HSV infection, herpes zoster, varicella	3% ointment (3, 15 g)	Apply to lesion every 3 h 6 times/d for 7 d	Pregnancy Category C Use a finger cot or glove when applying ointment to prevent spread of virus

Continued on next page

Table 30–3. Drugs Commonly Used: Skin Infections *(continued)*

Drug	Indication	Strengths Available	Dose	Notes
Acyclovir (Zovirax), oral	HSV infection, herpes zoster, varicella	Tablets: 400, 800 mg Suspension: 200 mg/5 mL	*Adults:* Genital herpes: Initial: 200 mg every 4 h 5 times/d for 10 d Chronic: 400 mg bid or 200 mg 3–5 times/d for up to 12 mo Intermittent: 200 mg q4h 5 times/d for 5 d; begin at first sign of occurrence Herpes zoster: 800 mg q4h 5 times/d for 7–10 d Varicella: 20 mg/kg 4 times/d for 5 d; maximum 800 mg/dose; begin within 24 h of first lesion *Children age 2 and older:* Varicella: 20 mg/kg 4 times/d for 5 d; maximum 800 mg/dose; begin within 24 h of first lesion	Pregnancy Category C Decrease dose in renal patients
Famciclovir (Famvir)	HSV infection, herpes zoster	Tablet: 125, 250, 500 mg	Genital herpes: Initial episode: 125 mg q12h for 5 d; begin as soon as symptoms appear Recurrent episodes: 125 mg q12h for 5 d Suppression therapy: 250 mg q12h for up to 12 mo Herpes zoster: 500 mg q8h for 7 d; begin within 72 h of lesions appearing	Not recommended in patients <18 Decrease dose in renal patients Pregnancy Category B Register pregnant patients exposed by famciclovir by calling 800-366-8900 ext 5231
Valacyclovir (Valtrex)	HSV infection, herpes zoster	Caplet: 500 mg, 1 g	Genital herpes: Initial episode: 1 g daily for 10 d Recurrent episodes: 500 mg q12h for 5 d, started within 24 h of first symptom of outbreak	Not recommended in children Decrease dose in renal patients Pregnancy Category B Register pregnant patients exposed by

Continued on next page

Table 30–3. Drugs Commonly Used: Skin Infections *(continued)*

Drug	Indication	Strengths Available	Dose	Notes
			Herpes zoster: 1g q8h for 7 d; begin within 48–72 h of first lesions appearing	valacyclovir by calling 800-722-9292 ext 39437
Antifungals Nystatin (Mycostatin, Nilstat)	Oral *Candida* infection	Suspension: 100,000 U/mL Pastilles: 200,000 U each	*Adults and children:* 2–3 mg in each inner cheek qid (total dose 4–6 mL); have patient hold medication in mouth as long as possible before swallowing; treat for 48 h after clinical cure to prevent relapse *Infants:* 1 mL each cheek qid (2 mL per dose total) until 48 h after clinical cure; may apply medication to inner cheeks and tongue with cotton swab prior to administering the 1-mL dose via dropper	Safe in pregnancy and in young children and even in debilitated infants Well tolerated, even with prolonged administration
Nystatin (Mycostatin, Nilstat, Nystex)	Cutaneous *Candida* infection	Cream, ointment, powder	Apply to affected areas 2–3 times/d until healed	Safe in pregnancy and in children
Clotrimazole (Mycelex)	Oral *Candida* infection	Troches: 10 mg	*Adults and children >3:* 1 troche 5 times/d for 14 d; dissolve slowly in mouth	Not recommended in children Pregnancy Category C; not recommended for use in pregnancy May cause elevated liver function tests
Clotrimazole (Lotrimin, Mycelex)	Dermatophyte infections of the skin	1% cream (Rx and OTC); 1% solution (Rx and OTC); 1% lotion (Rx)	Apply to affected area bid for 2 wk Tinea pedis: treat for 4 wk	Pregnancy Category B Safe in children

Continued on next page

Table 30–3. Drugs Commonly Used: Skin Infections *(continued)*

Drug	Indication	Strengths Available	Dose	Notes
Gentian violet	Oral *Candida* infection	Solution: 1%, 2% (available OTC)	Apply with cotton swab to entire inner surface of the mouth 2 times/d until healed	Stains everything it touches purple; warn patient/parents about staining of mouth; stain resolves within a couple of days of discontinuing therapy
Fluconazole (Diflucan)	Oral *Candida* infection	Tablets: 50, 100, 150, 200 mg Suspension: 10 mg/mL, 40 mg/mL	*Adults:* 200 mg first d, then 100 mg daily for 2 wk minimum *Infants and children:* 6 mg/kg on the first d, then 3 mg/kg daily for 2 wk minimum	Pregnancy Category C Interacts with cimetidine, hydrochlorothiazide, rifampin, cyclosporine, phenytoin, and theophylline; monitor closely if patient is taking one of these medications with fluconazole
Miconazole (Micatin, Monistat-Derm, Micatin)	Dermatophyte infections of the skin	2% cream (Micatin, Monistat-Derm); 2% powder (Micatin); 2% spray (Micatin Liquid) (available OTC)	Apply to affected area 2–3 times/d for 2 wk Tinea pedis: treat for 4 wk	Topical use safe in pregnancy and in children
Tolnaftate (Tinactin, Ting, Aftate, Absorbine)	Dermatophyte infections of the skin	1% cream, solution, gel, powder, spray powder, spray liquid (available OTC)	Apply to affected area bid for 2–3 wk; if skin is thickened, treatment may take 4–6 wk	Safe for topical use in pregnancy Not recommended for use in children <2 y
Terbinafine (Lamisil)	Dermatophyte infections of the skin	Cream	Apply to affected and immediate surrounding areas 1–2 times/d until symptoms are significantly improved (usually 1–4 wk) Tinea pedis: apply to affected and immediate surrounding areas until symptoms are significantly improved	Pregnancy Category B; safety in children <12 has not been established Clinical improvement may continue for 2–4 wk after therapy is stopped

Continued on next page

Table 30–3. Drugs Commonly Used: Skin Infections *(continued)*

Drug	Indication	Strengths Available	Dose	Notes
Sulconazole (Exelderm)	Dermatophyte infections of the skin	1% cream; 1% solution (Rx required)	Massage medication into affected area 2 times/d for 2 wk For tinea pedis, apply for 4 wk	Pregnancy Category C; use only if clearly needed
Ciclopirox (Loprox)	Dermatophyte infections of the skin	1% cream; 1% lotion (Rx required)	Massage medication into affected area 1–2 times/d for 3 wk For tinea pedis, apply bid for 4 wk	Pregnancy Category C; safety in children <10 has not been established
Ketoconazole (Nizoral)	Dermatophyte infections of the skin	2% cream	Massage medication into affected area once/d for 2 wk For tinea pedis, apply for 6 wk	Pregnancy Category C May be used to treat cutaneous *Candida* infections
Econazole (Spectazole)	Dermatophyte infections of the skin	1% cream (Rx required)	Massage medication into affected area once/d for 2 wk minimum For tinea pedis, apply for 4-wk minimum	Pregnancy Category C; do not use in first trimester; use in second and third trimesters only if clearly needed
Oxiconazole (Oxistat)	Dermatophyte infections of the skin	1% cream; 1% lotion (Rx required)	Massage medication into affected area 1–2 times/d for 2 wk For tinea pedis, apply for 4 wk	Pregnancy Category B; use only if clearly needed
Griseofulvin Microsize (Fulvicin U/F, Grifulvin V, Grisactin)	Tinea capitis, onychomycosis	Tablets: 250, 500 mg Capsules: 125, 250 mg Suspension: 125 mg/5 mL	Tinea capitis: *Adults:* 500 mg daily for 4–6 wk *Children:* 11 mg/kg/d for 4–6 wk Onychomycosis: *Adults:* 750–1000 mg daily in divided doses; treat fingernail infection for 4 mo; toenail infection for 6 mo *Children:* 11 mg/kg/d; treat fingernail infection for 4 mo; toenail infection for 6 mo	Pregnancy Category C; safe in children >2 y Renal, liver, and hematopoietic function tests need to be drawn and monitored every 8 wk if on prolonged therapy Best absorbed if taken with a high-fat meal

Continued on next page

Table 30–3. Drugs Commonly Used: Skin Infections *(continued)*

Drug	Indication	Strengths Available	Dose	Notes
Griseofulvin Ultramicro-size (Fulvicin P/G, Grisactin Ultra, Gris-PEG)	Tinea capitis, onychomycosis	Tablets: 125, 165, 250, 330 mg	Tinea capitis: *Adults:* 330–375 mg daily for 4–6 wk *Children:* 7.3 mg/kg/d for 4–6 wk Onychomycosis: *Adults:* 660–750 mg daily in divided doses; treat fingernail infection for 4 mo; toenail infection for 6 mo *Children:* 7.3 mg/kg/d; treat fingernail infection for 4 mo; toenail infection for 6 mo	Pregnancy Category C; safe in children >2 y Renal, liver, and hematopoietic function tests need to be drawn and monitored every 8 wk if on prolonged therapy Best absorbed if taken with a high-fat meal
Ketoconazole (Nizoral)	Tinea capitis, onychomycosis	Tablets: 200 mg	*Adults:* 200 mg daily; may increase to 400 mg daily if inadequate clinical response; minimum length of treatment is 4 wk *Children 2 y and older:* 3.3–6.6 mg/kg/d	Monitor hepatic function prior to initiating therapy and monthly during therapy Pregnancy Category C; may be prescribed to children age 2 and older Not first-line treatment for onychomycosis because of possible hepatotoxicity Use with caution if patient is taking medications that are primarily metabolized by the liver Coadministration with astemizole is absolutely contraindicated because of secondary cardiotoxic effects

Continued on next page

Table 30–3. Drugs Commonly Used: Skin Infections *(continued)*

Drug	Indication	Strengths Available	Dose	Notes
Itraconazole (Sporanox)	Onychomycosis	Capsules: 100 mg	*Adults:* Daily dosing schedule: toenails: 200 mg daily for 12 wk Pulse schedule: toenails: 400 mg daily for 1 wk/ mo for 3–4 mo; for fingernails: 200 mg bid for 7 d, then 3 wk without medication, then 200 mg bid for 7 more d *Children:* Pulse schedule: 5 mg/kg/d for 1 wk/mo for 3–4 consecutive mo	If used for more than 8 consecutive wk, liver enzymes and electrolytes should be drawn prior to and every 8 wk during treatment Pregnancy Category C; do not administer to pregnant women or women considering pregnancy In children, use griseofulvin as first-line therapy Coadministration with astemizole is absolutely contraindicated because of secondary cardiotoxic effects Coadministration with cisapride, midazolam, triazolam, simvastatin, and lovastatin is also contraindicated
Terbinafine (Lamisil)	Onychomycosis	Tablets: 250 mg	Fingernail infection: 250 mg daily for 6 wk Toenail infection: 250 mg daily for 12 wk	Not recommended for use in children; safety not established Liver enzymes and complete blood count (CBC) should be monitored every 6 wk Pregnancy Category B; delay treatment until after pregnancy

and combinations of **bacitracin, polymyxin B sulfate,** and **neomycin (Polysporin, Neosporin,** and **Triple Antibiotic Ointment)** may be used if there are one or two lesions and the patient is not **neomycin**-sensitive.

Oral antibiotics, such as **cephalexin (Keflex)** or **amoxicillin-clavulanate (Augmentin),** or **erythromycin** or **azithromycin (Zithromax)** if the patient is **penicillin**-allergic, are indicated if the patient has more than five lesions or if the lesions continue to worsen after 2 to 3 days of topical therapy.

Table 30–3 presents prescribing information.

FURUNCLE.   Treatment of a small furuncle, which is usually caused by *S. aureus,* may include warm packs and **systemic antibiotics.** A larger boil or abscess may require incision and drainage, as well as **systemic antibiotics.** Gram's stain and culture of the drainage will determine if the organism will be sensitive to the **antibiotic** of choice.

PERIANAL STREPTOCOCCAL INFECTION.   Perianal streptococcal infection, a localized infection of the perianal area, usually occurs in children. The rash is caused by group A beta-hemolytic streptococci. The diagnosis is confirmed by a perianal swab and culture. The treatment of choice is **penicillin,** with **erythromycin** prescribed to **penicillin**-allergic patients.

CELLULITIS.   Cellulitis is a painful, erythematous, spreading bacterial infection involving the soft tissue. The patient can become quite ill if untreated, including developing sepsis. The causative organisms are most commonly *Streptococcus pneumoniae, S. aureus,* or, in children, *Haemophilus influenzae.* Treatment is with **systemic antibiotics** that are effective against these organisms. If the clinical assessment warrants it, an initial dose of an **intramuscular antibiotic (ceftriaxone)** can be given, followed by **oral antibiotic** treatment. **Oral antibiotic** treatment with a broad-spectrum **antibiotic** such as **amoxicillin-clavulanate** or a **cephalosporin** is indicated. Blood and tissue aspirate cultures will guide the practitioner in determining if the organism is sensitive to the **antibiotic** of choice. Close follow-up, usually within 24 hours, is indicated to determine if the clinical status is improving or worsening. **Parenteral antibiotics** may be needed.

Viral Skin Infections

HSV INFECTIONS, VARICELLA, AND HERPES ZOSTER.   The treatment of HSV infections, varicella, and herpes zoster includes the use of **acyclovir (Zovirax),** which can be used topically or systemically. **Acyclovir** has inhibitory action against HSV-1, HSV-2, and varicella-zoster virus. It decreases the duration of acute infections in HSV-2 infections and, when used to treat herpes zoster, shortens the time to lesion scabbing and decreases the length of viral shedding. When prescribed for patients with varicella, **acyclovir** decreases the number of vesicular lesions, shortens the time to healing, and decreases fever by the second day.

Other antiviral agents that may be prescribed include **famciclovir (Famvir)** and **valacyclovir (Valtrex),** which are the drugs of choice for recurrent outbreaks of HSV infection. **Famciclovir** can also be used for treatment of herpes zoster. It decreases the healing time by shortening the time to crusting and healing and decreases the length of viral shedding. **Valacyclovir** is a hydrochloride salt of L-valyl ester of acyclovir, is rapidly converted to acyclovir, and is active against HSV infections, varicella, and herpes zoster.

Comfort measures with **antipruritics,** such as **antihistamines,** and wet soaks are also part of the treatment plan.

Table 30–3 presents prescribing information.

Fungal Skin Infections

ORAL CANDIDIASIS.   Oral candidiasis (thrush) is commonly found in infants and immunocompromised patients. Prompt treatment is essential to maintain adequate nutrition and for patient comfort. The treatment of choice is a topical application of an **antifungal** agent, such as **nystatin (Mycostatin), clotrimazole (Mycelex),** or **gentian violet,** or oral administration of the **systemic antifungal**

Clinical Pearl

THRUSH

Infants (and some older or very ill patients) are unable to hold **nystatin** suspension in their mouth. To achieve better results with **nystatin** administration, instruct the parents or caregivers to dip a clean cotton-tipped applicator into the **nystatin** solution, then rub the medication into the areas of thrush on the inner cheeks. Use a clean swab for each side and do not redip the applicator into the **nystatin.** After swabbing on the **nystatin,** the parent or caregiver can then administer 1 to 2 mL to each cheek.

fluconazole (**Diflucan**). Table 30–3 presents prescribing information.

TINEA CAPITIS. With tinea capitis (ringworm of the scalp), the patient presents with a characteristic bald patch, with crusting or scaling. *Microsporum* species usually present with broken hairs and a fine gray scale. *Trichophyton tonsurans* (black dot tinea) presents with tiny black dots that are the remains of broken hair shafts.

Treatment of tinea capitis consists of **oral antifungal** therapy with **griseofulvin (Grifulvin V, Grisactin)** and biweekly shampooing with a **sporicidal** shampoo (**selenium sulfide or ketoconazole**). Tinea capitis should always be treated with a **systemic antifungal**, never a topical agent. Children should be kept out of school for the first 2 to 3 days of treatment to avoid spreading the infection. Treatment should continue for 6 to 8 weeks or until 2 weeks after KOH or culture is negative. Close contacts should be empirically treated with **sporicidal** shampoo twice a week. Resistant cases can be treated with **terbinafine, fluconazole,** or **itraconazole,** based on the sensitivity as determined by culture. Table 30–3 presents prescribing information.

TINEA CORPORIS AND TINEA CRURIS. Tinea corporis (ringworm) is commonly caused by *Microsporum canis, T. tonsurans,* or *Epidermophyton floccosum.* The classic presentation is an annular lesion with raised borders and a clear center. There may be scaling and usually some erythema. The infection spreads by direct contact with an infected person or animal, with household pets a common source of infection.

Tinea cruris ("jock itch") affects the skin of the groin, upper thighs, and intertriginous folds. It is more common in males and rarely occurs before adolescence. It is caused by the dermatophytes *E. floccosum, T. rubrum, Trichophyton mentagrophytes,* and *C. albicans.* Tinea cruris is worse in hot, humid weather. The lesions are scaly with a raised border, erythematous, and slightly brown in color. Treatment for both tinea corporis and tinea cruris is **topical antifungal** cream, with **miconazole (Micatin, Monistat-Derm), tolnaftate (Tinactin),** and **clotrimazole (Lotrimin, Mycelex)** the least expensive and most commonly prescribed. Other **topical antifungals** that may be used include **terbinafine (Lamisil), sulconazole (Exelderm), ciclopirox (Loprox), ketoconazole (Nizoral), econazole (Spectazole),** and **oxiconazole (Oxistat).** Table 30–3 presents prescribing information.

TINEA PEDIS. Tinea pedis (athlete's foot) is caused by the dermatophytes *E. floccosum, T. rubrum, T. mentagrophytes,* and *C. albicans.* It is more common in males and rarely presents before puberty. It can present in three forms: interdigital maceration, scaling, and fissuring; a "moccasin" distribution of persistent dry scale with minimal inflammation; or scattered pustules and vesicles on the sole and lateral aspects of the feet. The nonpharmacological management includes measures to keep the feet dry and well aired such as wearing sandals whenever possible, wearing clean cotton socks, and drying the feet carefully after bathing. Pharmacological management is with **topical antifungals**, similar to those used for tinea corporis: **miconazole, clotrimazole, tolnaftate, terbinafine, sulconazole, ciclopirox, ketoconazole, econazole,** and **oxiconazole.** However, the length of treatment is usually longer. Table 30–3 presents prescribing information.

TINEA VERSICOLOR. Tinea versicolor (pityriasis versicolor) is caused by *Pityrosporum orbiculare* (formerly called *Malassezia furfur*). Clinically, the infection appears as multiple scaling, discrete, oval-shaped macules that may be hypopigmented or hyperpigmented. The color of the macules ranges from salmon to brown, and they are usually seen on the trunk, neck, and shoulders. The infection is associated with warm, humid weather. Treatment consists of topical application of **selenium sulfide** shampoo (**Selsun**) or a **topical antifungal**, commonly one of the **imidazoles (miconazole, clotrimazole, econazole).** The patient should be educated to observe for recurrence, which up to 50 percent of patients experience. The shampoo is applied to the affected area and left on for 10 to 15 minutes every day for 1 week. It may also be used prophylactically once a month. The **topical antifungal** is used for 2 to 4 weeks and is rubbed into the affected area twice a day.

ONYCHOMYCOSIS. Onychomycosis is a fungal infection of the nail, either fingernail or toenail. The common dermatophyte that is found in onychomycosis is tinea unguium, with *Candida* infections also a cause. Effective treatment usually involves months of a **systemic antifungal** medication, commonly **griseofulvin, ketoconazole, itraconazole,** or **terbinafine.** Topical treatment is usually not effective. Table 30–3 presents prescribing information.

Monitoring

For all skin infections, the patient should be monitored to determine the effectiveness of the medication in treating the infection, compliance with the prescribed therapy, adverse effects, and the development of secondary infection.

Outcome Evaluation

For skin infections, improvement should be noted, usually within 24 to 48 hours. If not, a change in therapy may be indicated, with resistance suspected. Secondary

Skin Infections

Related to the Overall Treatment Plan/Disease Process

- ☐ Pathophysiology
- ☐ Role of preventive and nonpharmacological measures if appropriate
- ☐ Importance of adherence to the treatment regimen
- ☐ Self-monitoring of symptoms
- ☐ What to do when symptoms worsen
- ☐ Need for follow-up visits with the primary care provider

Specific to the Drug Therapy

- ☐ Reason for taking the drug and its anticipated action on the disease process
- ☐ Doses and schedules for taking the drug
- ☐ Possible adverse effects and what to do if they occur
- ☐ Interactions between other treatment modalities and these drugs

Reasons for Taking the Drug(s)

Patient education about specific drugs is provided in the appropriate chapter.

Specifically for Bacterial Skin Infections

- ☐ Explanation regarding the suspected cause of the infection and the rationale for the antibiotic treatment chosen
- ☐ Handwashing should be stressed to prevent spread of the skin infection to the patient or others
- ☐ Clear guidelines regarding notifying the practitioner if the infection is getting worse
- ☐ Improvement should be noted in 24 to 48 hours; if not, a change in therapy may be indicated

Specifically for Viral Infections

- ☐ Expectations of the medication. The healthy patient will have resolution of the vesicular lesions even without pharmacological intervention. Effective antiviral therapy decreases the time to scabbing and healing of lesions and decreases viral shedding time. In immunocompromised patients, the medication will help decrease the severity of the outbreak.
- ☐ How the virus can become dormant and recur at a later time, even many years later.
- ☐ Patients using topical acyclovir need to be instructed to use a glove or finger cot to apply the ointment to prevent getting the virus on their hands and spreading it; also, the patient may experience a transient burning when the medication is applied.

continued

PATIENT EDUCATION

Skin Infections *(continued)*

☐ It should be stressed to the patient and/or family members that the patient is contagious until the lesions are healed or scabbed over, even if antiviral agents are being taken; the patient should avoid contact with immunocompromised individuals and avoid sexual intercourse if the patient has genital herpes lesions.

Specifically for Fungal Infections

☐ The patient and/or family members should understand how the fungal infection is spread and how contagious the infection is.
☐ Family members and pets should be checked for signs of infection and treated if indicated.
☐ The provider should stress the possibility of relapse if the medication regimen is not followed correctly and for the full treatment time.

Drugs as Part of the Total Treatment Regimen

The total treatment regimen includes pharmacological and nonpharmacological measures. Be sure the patient and/or family members are aware of the specific measures to be taken.

Adherence Issues

Health care providers should be aware of the potential problem of nonadherence and should discuss the importance of completing the entire treatment regimen with the patient and/or family members.

---

skin infections, if they occur, should be treated promptly. Referral to a dermatologist may be necessary if therapy is not managing the infection.

Patient Education

Patient education should include a discussion of information related to the overall treatment plan as well as that specific to the drug therapy, reasons for taking the drug, drugs as part of the total treatment regimen, and adherence issues.

Skin Infestations

Skin and hair infestation with arthropods, most commonly lice and scabies, is a frequently seen problem in primary care. Head lice infestation is at epidemic levels in school-age children, with 6 to 12 million people in the United States affected each year. Scabies is common at all ages and is more common when poor hygiene or crowded living conditions are present.

Pathophysiology

Lice

Pediculosis is infestation of the body with lice. The affected body area helps to determine what arthropod is present. The skin signs seen with pediculosis are pruritus, excoriation from scratching, adenopathy (occasionally) in the affected region, and the presence of lice or nits.

The common name for infestation with *Pediculus humanus capitis* is head lice (pediculosis capitis). The mite of head lice is usually visible, and the nits or eggs are visualized attached to the hair shaft. The female louse lays approximately four eggs per day and has a lifespan of 2 to 4 weeks. Head lice are spread by direct contact with another infected person or by indirect contact with a hairbrush, hat, or article of clothing that the lice or nits have been transferred to. Outbreaks in schools are seen when children share hats or hairbrushes. When outer garments are hung in a close group, which is often the case in school, the lice can travel from coat to coat and spread to an unsuspecting new household. Diagnosis is made by observing mites or nits.

Body lice (pediculosis corporis), the common name for infestation with *Pediculus humanus corporis,* are uncommon. They usually are not seen on the body but on the seams of clothing and undergarments. They come onto the body to feed and leave hemorrhagic pinpoint macules where they extract blood. There is often excoriation from scratching. The common sites for body lice are the belt line, collar, and underwear areas. Diagnosis is made by examining the clothing and underwear for the presence of mites and nits.

Infestation with *Phthirus pubis* is commonly called *pubic lice* (pediculosis pubis). Patients often refer to it as *crabs.* The mites are quite small and may need to be examined under a handheld magnifying glass, as they may be mistaken for a freckle. The mites and nits are found on the pubic hair and the hair of the perianal region. They may extend up to the hair on the abdomen and to the hair on the upper thighs. The eyelashes and axillary hair may also be involved. Pubic lice are never seen before pubertal hair development. They are often sexually transmitted. Diagnosis is made by observing the mite or nits in the pubic hair.

Scabies

Scabies is a highly contagious infestation with *Sarcoptes scabiei.* The female scabies mite burrows under the skin and lays eggs as she tunnels. The eggs hatch in about 2 weeks. The surface of the skin has characteristic curving burrows and excoriated papules. The burrows are in the horny layer of the skin and are seen most frequently on the sides of the fingers, the interdigital webs, flexor surfaces of the wrists, elbows, axillae, and genitalia. In infants, the scabies mite can often be found on the entire body, including the trunk and face. There may be a secondary infection present.

The incubation period is 1 to 2 months after contact with another infested person or with unwashed clothing recently worn by an infected person. Bed partners can be infected even if there is no body contact. Often the first sign of infestation with scabies is intense pruritus, which occurs 2 to 6 weeks after the first exposure to the mite. The itching is caused by sensitization to the mite feces. Definitive diagnosis is made by scraping a burrow that reveals mites or eggs.

Goal of Treatment

The goals of treatment are to completely eradicate the arthropods and to educate the patient and family about the disease and how to prevent further infestations.

Rational Drug Selection

Pharmacological management of lice and scabies consists of the use of **ectoparacides.** The specific medication used varies by the type of infestation and the age of the patient. For head lice, there is a choice of OTC products and, in the case of resistance to OTC products, prescription **lindane** or a variety of nonpharmacological remedies. For body lice, the treatment of choice is **lindane** and washing infested clothing and bedding. Pubic lice are treated with **lindane** shampoo. Scabies is treated with **permethrin** or **lindane.** Nonpharmacological, environmental measures are a key part of the treatment of any infestation because patients can reinfect themselves or other family members and restart the infestation cycle.

Head Lice

Head lice can cause great distress to the family. It is important to treat head lice aggressively and completely to prevent recurrence. Unfortunately, resistance to some **pediculicides** has made treating head lice at times a clinical challenge. The OTC products available for treating head lice include **pyrethrins** and **permethrin. Lindane,** a prescription drug, is used as a second-line agent for resistant head lice.

Although all of the head lice treatments are relatively safe, they are classified as neurotoxic agents, and they should be used exactly as directed on the package. To limit exposure, the medication should be washed off at a sink, rather than in a shower. Cool or lukewarm water should be used to minimize absorption caused by vasodilation (Chesney & Burgess, 1998). After treatment, the hair should be combed to remove all the nits. There are special combs available for this, or slow, patient combing can be effective. Advise parents to comb hair a minimum of 20 minutes, dividing hair in sections (Clore & Longyear, 1993). Treat only family members who are actively infested. Do not treat head lice prophylactically.

PYRETHRINS. Pyrethrins are combined with **piperonyl butoxide (RID, Pronto, A-200)** and are available OTC. Pyrethrins are 100 percent insecticidal and 70 to 80 percent ovicidal. The shampoo is applied to dry hair and left on for 10 to 20 minutes, with the time varying by brand. It is important for the product to be applied to dry hair to enable the **pediculicide** to enter the insect's body better. The patient should be retreated in 1 week regardless of whether there is evidence of infestation. Pyrethrins have no residual activity and can be used in young children and pregnant women if used as directed.

PERMETHRIN. Permethrin is a synthetic compound related to **pyrethrins.** It is available OTC in 1% cream (**Nix**) or prescription strength 5% cream (**Elimite**). Only **Nix** has FDA approval for use on head lice. **Nix** is 97 percent insecticidal and 70 to 80 percent ovicidal. **Permethrin** is a cream rinse that is applied after shampooing. It is important that the shampoo not have any conditioner in the formula, which makes the **permethrin** less effective. The cream rinse is left in the hair for 10 minutes before rinsing off. Treatment should be repeated in 1 week, regardless of whether signs of infestation are present. **Permethrin** cream rinse has residual activity against lice for up to 10 days.

LINDANE. **Lindane** is a prescription product used as a second-line agent for head lice. The popular brand of **lindane, Kwell,** is no longer on the market, but multiple generic brands of the product are available. **Lindane** is 67 percent insecticidal and 45 to 70 percent ovicidal. **Lindane** is neurotoxic and should not be used in pregnant women or in infants. **Lindane** is applied to dry hair, working in small quantities of water to create a good lather. The shampoo is left on for 4 minutes. The amount of shampoo prescribed for short hair is 1 oz; for long hair, 2 oz. The shampoo should be rinsed well. **Lindane** has no residual activity against head lice.

NONPHARMACOLOGICAL TREATMENTS. With the growing problem of resistance and concern over exposing children to repeated doses of **pediculicides**, there are growing anecdotal reports about the success of various nonmedicated therapies. Popular and safe remedies are mayonnaise (full-fat variety), olive oil, and petroleum jelly. It is thought that they asphyxiate the lice by blocking their breathing apparatus or immobilize them and affect their ability to feed. A patient who would like to try these treatments should apply a thick layer of the product and cover with a shower cap. The product is left on from 1 hour to overnight, then shampooed out.

The provider may be asked by a frustrated parent about other nonpharmacological remedies. It is important to give the parent clear guidelines regarding the use of unproven and possibly dangerous interventions, such as using lamp oil or other flammable liquid. Products developed for animals, such as dog lice shampoo, are also not advised.

Body Lice

The treatment for body lice is **topical pediculicides, lindane** and **permethrin.** Body lice live on clothing and underwear and come to the skin only to feed, so it is important to instruct the patient to wash all clothing and bedding in hot water to kill lice and nits that are on the clothing.

LINDANE. **Lindane** is applied to the total body as a cream or lotion and left on for 8 to 12 hours (overnight). The amount needed for an adult is 2 oz. **Lindane** should not be used in infants. **It is Pregnancy Category B but should not be used as a first-line medication in pregnant patients because there have been no adequate studies in pregnant patients. If it is prescribed during pregnancy, then it should not be used more than twice during a pregnancy.**

PERMETHRIN. **Permethrin** 5% (Elimite) may be used for body lice. It is slightly safer in pregnant patients and

can be used in children as young as 2 months. **Permethrin** is applied from head to toe and left on for 8 hours (overnight), then showered off.

Pubic Lice

LINDANE. Pubic lice are treated with an application of **lindane** 1% cream, lotion, or shampoo. A thin layer of cream or lotion is applied to the hair and skin surrounding the pubic area and left on for 12 hours. If **lindane** shampoo is used, the shampoo is massaged into dry pubic hair and left on for 5 to 10 minutes. If axillary or thigh hair is also infested, then use the cream or lotion. Reapply in 7 days if there is evidence of live lice. Sexual partners should also be treated concurrently. Bedding and clothes should be washed.

Scabies

When treating scabies, the provider may choose between **permethrin** and **lindane.** The provider may choose the drug based on patient age and toxicity of the agent. All family members should receive treatment, even if asymptomatic. Family members may be in the incubation period, and so all members of the household need treatment to prevent recurrence. Although one treatment is curative, the inflamed burrows and pruritus may last for up to 3 weeks after treatment with a **scabicide.** Families need to be educated regarding this prolonged healing phase. Patients should not be re-treated unless living mites are observed.

PERMETHRIN. **Permethrin 5% cream (Elimite, Acticin)** is the drug of choice for the treatment of scabies in young children and pregnant women. It is 90 percent effective against the scabies mite and can be used in infants as young as 2 months old and in pregnant women. The cream is massaged into the skin from the neck to the soles of feet. It should be left on for 8 to 14 hours and then washed off in the shower. Infants require special application of **permethrin** to the scalp, temple, forehead, hands, and feet. One to two oz of **permethrin** per family member is prescribed.

LINDANE. **Lindane** 1% lotion or cream is used for scabies in children over 6 months of age and in nonpregnant adult patients. It is applied in a thin layer from the neck down to the soles of the feet and left on for 8 to 12 hours (overnight) and then washed off thoroughly. If there are crusted lesions present, a tepid bath should be taken prior to application to soften the lesions. The patient should dry the skin thoroughly before applying **lindane.** Two oz of **lindane** per family member are prescribed.

TOPICAL CORTICOSTEROIDS. **Topical corticosteroids** are used after scabies treatment to treat pruritus and inflammation associated with the scabies mite. **Hydrocortisone** 1% or 2.5% or a stronger **corticosteroid,** if indicated, is applied to affected areas twice a day until lesions are healed.

Monitoring

Patients and families need to be monitored for appropriate use of the medication and for effectiveness of treatment. The patient should be monitored for sensitivity to the medication prescribed. If medications are used appropriately, there is rarely an adverse reaction from them, although skin irritation or sensitivity may occur.

Outcome Evaluation

If effective treatment has been implemented, then the lice or scabies should be eradicated. Before resistance is assumed, the provider should review how the patient or family used the medication and if environmental measures were adequate.

Patient Education

Patient and family education is the key to effective eradication of lice and scabies. In prescribing treatment for lice or scabies, the following are key areas of education that need to be covered:

1. Explanation of how the patient was most likely infected with the lice or scabies and how they can be passed on to other family members or, in the case of pubic lice, sexual partners. The incubation period and early symptoms should be discussed to identify other contacts that may be infected, such as school contacts.
2. Proper use of the prescribed medication and environmental measures that may be taken. Written instructions should also be provided. Environmental measures that should be taken for lice and scabies include washing sheets, towels, clothing, and headgear worn recently in hot water and laundry soap. They need to be in a hot dryer for at least 20 minutes to kill any remaining nits or scabies that may be on the clothing. Clothing that cannot be put in a hot water wash must be dry-cleaned or pressed with a hot iron. Remind parents to wash coats and car seat covers if indicated. Items that cannot be washed or dry-cleaned, such as stuffed animals, should be placed in a plastic bag for 3 to 4 weeks; for scabies, only 4 days is needed. Brushes and combs should be washed in hot water and soaked for 1 hour in disinfectant such as Lysol or rubbing alcohol and then rinsed with hot water. Vacuum-

ing play areas, floors, rugs, and furniture will pick up any nits or lice that may have been transferred to these areas. Parents should be told that insecticidal sprays or bombs are not necessary.

Alopecia Androgenetica (Male Pattern Baldness)

Alopecia androgenetica (male pattern baldness) affects men and some women. It involves hair loss from the frontal, vertex, and occipital regions of the scalp in men and thinning of the hair in the frontoparietal area or diffuse hair loss in women.

Pathophysiology

Common male pattern baldness is genetically determined. The process can begin at any time after puberty. There is not actual hair loss, but a conversion of thick hair to fine, unpigmented vellus hairs, which are poorly seen.

The process is androgen-dependent. A male who has a disorder that lowers testosterone production will never go bald, regardless of genetics; a woman who has a masculinizing disorder that raises androgen levels will develop classic male pattern baldness.

Goals of Treatment

A realistic goal is to achieve moderate to dense hair growth with continued use of **topical minoxidil (Rogaine)** for at least 4 months. If treating with **finasteride (Propecia),** a realistic goal would be increased hair growth after 3 months of continued treatment.

Rational Drug Selection

Alopecia androgenetica can be treated topically with **minoxidil** or systemically with **finasteride.** Choosing between the two medications can often be a simple task based on the patient profile. If the patient is also being treated for benign prostatic hypertrophy (BPH), then **finasteride** is the drug of choice. For a female patient, **minoxidil** is the only choice available.

Minoxidil

Minoxidil, the first drug approved by the FDA to treat male pattern baldness, is available OTC. The patient may be seeking a recommendation from the prescriber or self-prescribing and seeking information regarding its use. It is important to note that **minoxidil** does not treat balding of the frontoparietal areas in men, only in women. **Minoxidil** is effective in treating balding on the vertex of the scalp in men.

Minoxidil 2% topical solution is applied to the scalp twice daily for the entire length of treatment. The patient applies 1 mL directly to the affected area of the scalp (vertex area in men and frontoparietal area in women). The medication should be applied to a dry scalp. Patients should be instructed to wash their hands after using their fingers to rub the medication into the scalp. Twice-daily application for at least 4 months may be needed to obtain observable hair growth. If the medication is discontinued, the hair in the treated area will shed in 3 to 4 months.

Minoxidil **should not be used by pregnant patients (Pregnancy Category C) or by children under age 18.** **Minoxidil** is generally well tolerated. The topical solution contains **alcohol** and therefore may be irritating upon application. Patients may be sensitive to **minoxidil** and develop contact dermatitis. **Minoxidil** topical solution used as directed has minimal cardiac effects, but if large amounts are applied there is a potential for cardiac adverse effects.

Finasteride

Finasteride is a type II 5-alpha reductase–specific inhibitor that inhibits the conversion of testosterone into 5-alpha dihydrotestosterone (DHT). Development of alopecia androgenetica is dependent upon DHT, as is the prostate gland. **Finasteride** is also used in treatment of BPH. **Finasteride** is effective in treating vertex and anterior midscalp baldness in men. Hair regrowth is noted after 3 months of daily treatment, with full treatment effect achieved after 6 to 12 months of use.

The dose of **finasteride** is 1 mg once daily with or without food. Continued use is necessary to have continued benefit. If treatment is stopped, hair will return to untreated levels within 12 months.

Finasteride should be prescribed with caution in patients with hepatic dysfunction because the drug is metabolized extensively in the liver. It causes a decrease in serum prostate specific antigen (PSA) levels, even in the presence of prostate cancer. **It is Pregnancy Category X.** *Finasteride* **exposure during pregnancy, even in small quantities, may produce abnormalities of the external genitalia in male offspring. Pregnant women or a woman planning a pregnancy should not handle crushed tablets.** *Finasteride* **may be potentially absorbed from the semen. When a male patient's sexual partner is pregnant or may become pregnant, the patient should either avoid exposing his partner to his semen or discontinue** *finasteride.* **There is a small possibility (3% or less) of developing decreased libido, erectile dysfunction, or ejaculation disorder while taking** *finasteride.*

Monitoring

The patient being treated for male pattern baldness needs to be monitored for effectiveness of treatment and adverse effects of the medication. The major adverse effect seen with **minoxidil** is dermatitis or sensitivity to the topical solution, which is treated by discontinuing the medication. **Topical steroids** should not be used concurrently with **minoxidil**. The patient should also be observed for possible cardiac adverse effects. **Finasteride** is generally well tolerated, and adverse effects are usually mild. If the patient experiences sexual dysfunction, then the drug should be discontinued. The patient should be monitored for prostate cancer with a digital rectal examination and PSA levels because **finasteride** causes a low PSA level, even in the presence of prostate cancer. If the patient's sexual partner is of childbearing age, he should be warned about the severe effects that **finasteride** can have on the developing fetus. Monitoring for use of birth control, with condoms used to prevent semen exposure, is necessary if there is a possibility of the patient's partner becoming pregnant.

Outcome Evaluation

It may take 3 to 4 months to determine if **minoxidil** or **finasteride** is effective. The provider should schedule a follow-up appointment with the patient for 3 to 4 months after beginning therapy to determine effectiveness.

Patient Education

In treating a patient with alopecia androgenetica, the following key points should be covered in patient education:

1. The pathophysiology and cause of male pattern baldness.
2. Realistic expectations of therapy, including what type of hair loss the drug treats; how long therapy takes until effects are noticed; that if treatment is stopped, hair shedding will occur; and that the new hair initially may be fine and almost colorless, but with continued treatment the hair should develop the same color and texture as the rest of the hair on the scalp.
3. Caution that the patient should take the medication exactly as prescribed or as indicated by the instructions if taking OTC **minoxidil**.
4. Adverse effects of the medications, especially the hazards to women from **finasteride** exposure.

REFERENCES

Burns, C. E., Barber, N, Brady, A. M., & Dunn, A. M. (1996). *Pediatric primary care: A handbook for nurse practitioners.* Philadelphia: Saunders.

Chesney, R. J., & Burgess, I. F. (1998). Lice: Resistance and treatment. *Contemporary Pediatrics, 15*(11), 180–190.

Clore, E. R., & Longyear, L. A. (1993). A comparative study of seven pediculicides and their nit removal combs. *Journal of Pediatric Health Care, 7*(2), 55–60.

Cooper, K. D., Menter, A., Ritchlin, C. T., Taylor, J. R., & Zanolli, M.D. (1999). Psoriasis: New clues to causation, new ways to treat. *Patient Care for the Nurse Practitioner, 2*(5), 42–50.

Drug Facts and Comparisons. (1999). *Drug facts and comparisons.* St. Louis: Facts and Comparisons.

Feldman, S. R., Fleischer, A. B. Jr., & McConnell, R. C. (1998). Most common dermatologic problems identified by internists, 1990–1994. *Archives of Internal Medicine, 158*(7), 726–730.

Guzzo, C., Lazarus, G. S., & Werth, V. P. (1996). Dermatological pharmacology. In J. G. Hardman & L. E. Limbird (Eds.). *Goodman and Gilman's the pharmacological basis of therapeutics* (9th ed.). New York: McGraw-Hill.

Hansen, R. C., Krafchik, B. R., Lane, A. T., Odio, M. R., & Schachner, L. A. (1998). Dealing with diaper dermatitis. *Contemporary Pediatrics, 5*(May Suppl.), 5–10.

Landow, K. (1997). Dispelling myths about acne. *Postgraduate Medicine, 102*(2), 94–99, 103–104, 110–112.

Lasek, R. J., & Chren, M. M. (1998). Acne vulgaris and the quality of life of adult dermatology patients. *Archives of Dermatology, 134*(4), 454–458.

Mallon, E., Newton, J. N., Klassen, A., Stewart-Brown, S. L., Ryan, T. J., & Finlay, A. Y. (1999). The quality of life in acne: A comparison with general medical conditions using generic questionnaires. *British Journal of Dermatology, 140*(4), 672–676.

Murphy, J. L. (Ed.). (1999). *Nurse practitioner prescribing reference.* New York: Prescribing References.

Parker, F. (1996). Skin diseases. In J. C. Bennett & F. Plum (Eds.). *Cecil textbook of medicine* (20th ed.). Philadelphia: Saunders.

Resnick, S. D. (1998). Principles of topical therapy. *Pediatric Annual, 27*(3), 171–176.

Suarez, S., & Friedlander, S. F. (1998). Antifungal therapy in children: An update. *Pediatric Annual, 27*(3), 177–184.

CHAPTER 31

·······

Diabetes Mellitus

CHAPTER OUTLINE

D iabetes mellitus, in one of its forms, occurs in almost 6 percent of the population of the United States, and recently there has been a disturbing increase in its incidence. It is more prevalent in several ethnic groups; African-Americans, Hispanics, Native Americans, and Asian-Americans have a two to five times higher rate of diabetes than the rest of the population.

The annual cost of diabetes care is estimated to be $91.8 billion, with $46.7 billion of that the direct costs of care. It is the leading cause of blindness and end-stage renal disease, and it accounts for approximately 67,000 lower extremity amputations annually (DiPiro et al., 1999).

Diabetes mellitus is actually a heterogeneous group of complex metabolic disorders that share common alterations in glucose metabolism. They differ in age at onset, genetic predisposition, treatment options, and the complications developed. Table 31–1 provides a brief comparison of these differences. It is not within the scope of this book to discuss all the permutations of diabetes in any detail. For that discussion, readers are referred to pathophysiology and management-related texts. This chapter focuses on the pharmacological management of type 1 and type 2 diabetes mellitus. Gestational diabetes, which

requires consultation with the obstetrical provider, is not discussed here.

Pathophysiology

Type 1 Diabetes Mellitus

Several pathogenic processes are involved in the development of diabetes mellitus. Type 1 diabetes, which ac-

Table 31–1. Comparison of Type 1 and Type 2 Diabetes Mellitus

Characteristic	Type 1	Type 2
Age at onset	Usually during childhood or adolescence, but can occur at any age, even in eighth and ninth decades	Usually after age 40, and risk for it increases with age, obesity, and lack of physical activity
Type of onset	Signs and symptoms abrupt, but disease process may be present for years	Insidious and gradual
Genetic susceptibility	HLA-DR3 and DR4 and others; 50% concordance in monozygotic twins	Frequent genetic background, but no relation to HLA; almost 100% concordance in monozygotic twins
Environmental factors	Viruses, toxins	Obesity, nutrition; more common in women with prior gestational diabetes and in patients with hypertension or hyperlipidemia
Etiology	Unknown; postulated causes include heredity, autoimmune disease, and viral infections	Unknown; heredity is highly associated
Islet cell antibody and pancreatic cell–mediated immunity	Present at onset	Absent
Endogenous insulin	Secretion is markedly diminished early in disease; may be totally absent later	Levels may be low (insulin deficiency), normal, or high (insulin resistance)
Nutritional status	Thin, catabolic state	Obesity is common
Symptoms	Polydipsia, polyphagia, polyuria, fatigue, and weight loss	May be asymptomatic; polydipsia or polyuria may be present
Ketosis	Prone at onset or during insulin deficiency	Resistant except during infection or stress
Control of diabetes	Often difficult with wide glucose fluctuations	Variable
Dietary management	Essential	Essential; sometimes controlled with diet and exercise
Insulin	Insulin therapy is mandatory	Required for 30–40% of patients as disease progresses
Sulfonylureas and other oral agents	Not efficacious	Efficacious
Complications	Occur in a majority of patients after >5 y, but reduced incidence for those with tight control	Frequent, but reduced incidence for those with tight control

counts for 10 percent of total diabetes, results from an autoimmune destruction of the beta cells of the pancreas and islet cells, which leads to insulin deficiency. Tyrosine phosphatases IA-2 and IA-2 beta autoantibodies are seen in 85 to 90 percent of patients with type 1 diabetes. The remainder of patients with type 1 diabetes have no known etiology (idiopathic). Most patients with idiopathic type 1 diabetes are African- or Asian-Americans.

There is a strong genetic connection to the DQA and B genes and to certain human leukocyte antigens (HLA). Five groups of HLA have been recognized: A, B, C, D, and DR. Type 1 diabetes susceptibility has been linked to HLA-DR3 and DR4 loci. Because twin studies have shown only 50 percent concordance, environmental factors, chemical agents, and dietary agents are likely contributing factors. Genetic counseling for parents is based on statistical risk. If one child has type 1 diabetes, other siblings have a 5 to 10 percent chance of developing type 1 diabetes. The risk is 45 percent if the sibling is an identical twin. The offspring of a father with type 1 diabetes has a 4 to 6 percent risk, and the offspring of a mother with type 1 diabetes has a 2 to 3 percent risk. Theoretically, when a person with the appropriate genetic characteristics is exposed to a viral infection, the beta cells are destroyed directly, or an autoimmune process is triggered, which in turn destroys the beta cells. The onset and progression of hyperglycemic symptoms are usually rapid and acute in type 1 diabetes. Some patients, particularly children and adolescents, may present with ketoacidosis as the first manifestation of the disease. Adults with type 1 diabetes may retain residual beta cell function sufficient to prevent ketoacidosis for many years.

Successful treatment requires **insulin** replacement. If the disease progresses without treatment, diabetic ketoacidosis (DKA), weight loss, and muscle wasting may develop. Once treatment is initiated, the patient may go into temporary remission, despite the continued destruction of beta cells ("honeymoon phase"). Eventually, the destruction reaches a point where hyperglycemia occurs again, and **insulin** therapy is required throughout the rest of the disease process.

Type 2 Diabetes Mellitus

Type 2 diabetes pathogenesis is complex, and manifestations vary greatly across patients. There is a strong genetic influence, but no HLA type has been found. For type 2 diabetes, genetic counseling is based on known higher familial risk. The siblings of a person with type 2 diabetes are at a 7 to 14 percent risk for developing type 2 diabetes. The offspring of parents who both have type 2 diabetes have a 15 to 45 percent chance of developing it. Children and young adults with type 2 diabetes have a 50 percent chance of transmitting the disease to their offspring.

Plasma insulin levels in type 2 diabetes may by low, normal, or high. Although the specific etiology of this form of diabetes is not known, autoimmune destruction of beta cells does not occur. The metabolic defects associated with this disorder are (1) impaired basal and stimulated insulin secretion, (2) an increased rate of endogenous hepatic glucose production, and (3) decreased tissue responsiveness to insulin as a result of receptor or postreceptor defects. Most patients with this form of diabetes are obese, and obesity plays a major role in type 2 diabetes by downregulating insulin receptors in skeletal muscle and fat cells. The gradual onset and progression of type 2 diabetes allows patients to adapt to the symptoms without realizing that the disease process is producing them.

Because there is sufficient endogenous insulin supply to inhibit the development of DKA, **insulin** is not mandatory, although it may be used later in the disease process or during acute illness or stress. Patients can, however, develop hyperglycemic, hyperosmolar nonketosis (HHNK). **Oral hypoglycemic agents** and other **oral antidiabetic agents** are effective in addressing one or more of the metabolic defects in type 2 diabetes.

Complications

Long-term complications of both types of diabetes are based on target organ damage. The organs most commonly involved are the eyes, heart, kidneys, and nervous system. Retinopathy with potential loss of vision; nephropathy leading to renal failure; peripheral neuropathy with risk of foot ulcers, amputation, and Charcot's joint; and autonomic neuropathy with gastrointestinal, genitourinary, and cardiovascular symptoms and sexual dysfunction may occur. Patients with diabetes have an increased incidence of atherosclerotic cardiovascular, peripheral vascular, and cerebrovascular diseases. They are at increased risk for hypertension, abnormalities of lipid metabolism, and periodontal disease (American Diabetes Association, 1998).

Diagnosis

In 1998, the American Diabetes Association (ADA) modified the diagnostic criteria for diabetes mellitus. The revised criteria are shown in Table 31–2. Three ways to diagnose diabetes are possible, and each must be confirmed on a subsequent day by a different one of the three methods. For example, one instance of symptoms with a casual plasma glucose of 200 mg/dL or more, confirmed on a subsequent day by a fasting plasma glucose of 126 mg/dL or more, warrants the diagnosis of diabetes. An intermediate group of patients whose glucose levels, although not meeting the criteria for diabetes, are nevertheless too high to be considered

Table 31–2. Diagnostic Criteria for Diabetes Mellitus, Impaired Glucose Tolerance, and Impaired Fasting Glucose

Diagnostic Category	Diagnostic Criteria
Diabetes mellitus	Symptoms of diabetes plus casual plasma glucose concentration ≥200 mg/dL. Casual is defined as any time of day without regard to time since last meal. The classic symptoms of diabetes are polyuria, polydipsia, and unexplained weight loss. OR Fasting plasma glucose ≥126 mg/dL. Fasting is defined as no caloric intake for at least 8 h. OR 2-h postload plasma glucose in an oral glucose tolerance test ≥200 mg/dL. The test should be performed as described by the World Health Organization, using a glucose load containing the equivalent of 75 g anhydrous glucose dissolved in water.
Impaired glucose tolerance	Random or 2-h postprandial plasma glucose ≥140 mg/dL and <200 mg/dL.
Impaired fasting glucose	Fasting plasma glucose ≥110 mg/dL and <126 mg/dL.

normal is also recognized. These patients are said to have impaired glucose tolerance (IGT) or impaired fasting glucose (IFG). Patients with these two disorders are at risk for diabetes and cardiovascular disease and probably have insulin-resistance syndrome. Although approximately 25 percent of them will go on to develop diabetes, it is important not to label them as patients with diabetes until a definite diagnosis is made because of social, insurance, and job limitations that may occur. Further discussion of the diagnosis of diabetes is found in the ADA Clinical Practice Recommendations (1998). The material in this chapter assumes an appropriate diagnosis of diabetes.

Pharmacodynamics

Insulin

Insulin is used in the management of both types of diabetes. Naturally occurring insulin promotes the storage of fat as well as glucose and influences cell growth and metabolic functions in a wide variety of tissues. Its action on glucose transporters is discussed in detail in Chapter 19. In summary, these receptors "open the gate" to allow glucose to enter the cell. The total number of insulin receptors can be downregulated by such factors as obesity and long-standing hyperglycemia, which may explain why weight loss can be a significant factor in diabetes management.

Insulin acts on the liver to increase storage of glucose as glycogen and resets the liver after food intake by reversing the amount of catabolic activity. It also decreases urea production, protein catabolism, and cAMP in the liver; promotes triglyceride synthesis; and increases potassium and phosphate uptake by the liver.

Insulin promotes protein synthesis by increasing amino acid transport and by stimulating ribosomal activity. It also promotes glycogen synthesis to replace glycogen stores used during muscle activity.

Finally, insulin reduces the circulation of free fatty acids and promotes the storage of triglycerides in adipose tissue. This process is accomplished, in part, by suppression of cAMP production and dephosphorylation of the lipases in fat cells.

Administration of the drug **insulin** produces the same effect as the naturally occurring hormone. Although it is given largely to control blood glucose in patients with diabetes, that is not its only effect on the body.

Oral Antihyperglycemic Agents

Sulfonylureas

Oral agents are efficacious for only type 2 diabetes, and most drugs act on different aspects of the metabolic defects. **Sulfonylureas** increase endogenous insulin secretion by the beta cells and may improve the binding between insulin and insulin receptors or increase the number of receptors. Hypoglycemic effects appear to be due to increased endogenous insulin production and to improved beta-cell sensitivity to blood glucose levels or suppression of glucose release by the liver.

Biguanides

Biguanides are **oral antihyperglycemic drugs.** Their pharmacology and chemistry are different from the **sulfonylureas. Metformin (Glucophage)** was first released in the United States in September 1995 and to date is the only drug in this class used clinically. **Metformin** increases peripheral glucose uptake and utilization, improves hepatic response to blood glucose levels so that the liver produces appropriate amounts of glucose, and decreases intestinal absorption of glucose. Together, these actions improve glucose tolerance and lower both basal and postprandial plasma glucose levels. Unlike the **sulfonylureas, metformin** does not stimulate insulin release from the pancreatic beta cells.

Alpha-Glucosidase Inhibitors

Alpha-glucosidase inhibitors are also **oral antihyperglycemic drugs,** but their pharmacodynamics are different from the **sulfonylureas** and the **biguanides. Acarbose (Precose)** was first released in January 1996. **Miglitol (Glyset)** was approved in 1998 and released to the public in 1999. **Alpha-glucosidase inhibitors** do not act directly on any of the defects in metabolism seen in type 2 diabetes mellitus. They competitively inhibit and delay the absorption of complex carbohydrates (CHO) from the small bowel. **Alpha-glucosidase inhibitors** have no inhibitory activity against lactase and do not induce lactose intolerance. They lower blood glucose levels after meals. Unlike the **sulfonylureas,** they do not enhance pancreatic beta-cell secretion of insulin. Like **metformin,** they are not associated with weight gain and diminish the weight-increasing effects of **sulfonylureas** when given in combination with them. Their activity is effective on any CHO food intake, including liquid diets taken via a nasogastric tube.

Thiazolidinediones

Another class of drugs used to treat type 2 diabetes mellitus is the **thiazolidinediones.** They are **oral antihyperglycemic drugs. Troglitazone (Rezulin)** was first released in March 1997. It was removed from the market in 1999 because of the adverse reactions associated with liver damage. **Pioglitazone (Actos) and rosiglitazone (Avandia)** are newer drugs in this class. They have been associated with less risk of liver damage. **Thiazolidinediones** activate a nuclear receptor that regulates gene transcription, resulting in expression of proteins that improve insulin action in the cell. This action leads to increased utilization of available insulin by the liver and muscle cells and also in adipose tissue. In addition, these drugs reduce hepatic glucose production so that the liver produces appropriate amounts of glucose. Taken together, these actions improve glucose tolerance and lower both basal and postprandial plasma glucose levels. Unlike the **sulfonylureas, thiazolidinediones** do not produce hypoglycemia in diabetic or nondiabetic patients, except in special situations, and do not cause hyperinsulinemia because they do not stimulate insulin release from the pancreatic beta cells. Like **metformin,** they have a modest impact on lipids because of their actions in the liver.

Meglitinides

The last class of drugs, the **meglitinides,** has a different mechanism of action than any of the other drugs used to treat type 2 diabetes. They are short-acting insulin secretagogues. **Repaglinide (Prandin)** was first released in April 1998 and to date is the only drug in this class used clinically. **Repaglinide** closes ATP-dependent potassium channels in the beta-cell membrane by binding at specific receptor sites. This potassium channel blockade depolarizes the beta cell and leads to an opening of calcium channels. The resultant influx of calcium increases the secretion of insulin. Because its time in the plasma is less than 2 hours, the effect is very short. The end result of **repaglinide** stimulation of insulin secretion is a lowering in postprandial blood glucose levels. It does not directly affect fasting blood glucose levels or any of the other defects in metabolism seen in type 2 diabetes.

Each of these drug classes is discussed in detail in Chapter 19.

Goals of Treatment

The overall goals for the treatment of diabetes are (1) near normalization of blood glucose (tight glycemic control), (2) prevention of acute complications such as hypoglycemia, (3) prevention of progression of the disease to target organ damage, and (4) appropriate patient-oriented self-management. The overall goals of treatment of diabetes have not changed, but the results of the Diabetes Control and Complications Trial (DCCT) (American Diabetes Association, 1993) have altered the glycemic targets. These new targets are depicted in Table 31–3. This trial conclusively demonstrated that in patients with type 1 diabetes, the risk for development or progression of retinopathy, nephropathy, and neuropathy is reduced 50 to 75 percent by intensive treatment regimens when compared with conventional regimens. This implies that complete normalization of glycemic levels may prevent complications (American Diabetes Association, 1998). A similar trial currently in progress is testing patients with type 2 diabetes. Without waiting for data from the second trial, both types of diabetes are highly likely to benefit from tight glycemic control.

Rational Drug Selection

Diabetes is a lifelong disease that may be asymptomatic until target organ damage occurs. For this reason, providers often find themselves prescribing lifestyle modifications or drugs to treat a problem that patients have no clear evidence that they have and when they do not feel acutely ill. For effective management, the choice of treat-

Table 31–3. American Diabetes Association Glycemic Control Targets

Biochemical Index	Nondiabetic Value	Goal for Patient with Diabetes	Additional Action Suggested
Fasting blood glucose	<110 mg/dL	80–120 mg/dL	<80 mg/dL or >140 mg/dL
Bedtime blood glucose	<120 mg/dL	100–140 mg/dL	<100 mg/dL or >160 mg/dL
HbA$_{1c}$	<6%	<7%	>8%

HbA$_{1c}$ = Glycosylated hemoglobin. The values shown are for the general population. Patients with comorbid disease and the very young may require different targets. The targets for older adults are generally 10 percent higher. Additional action suggested may include enhanced self-management education, comanagement with a diabetes team, referral to an endocrinologist, change in drug therapy, or more frequent contact with the patient.
Adapted from American Diabetes Association, 1998.

ment should be low cost, limited in complexity, and with the fewest possible adverse reactions. This is especially important because diabetes is a largely self-managed disease. To achieve this treatment protocol, management is chosen based on the type of diabetes, the desired glycemic target, the severity of hyperglycemia, and specific patient variables. These management variables are discussed here in terms of stepped therapy, including lifestyle modification, initial monotherapy, and stepping up to multiple drugs.

Algorithms

Type 1 Diabetes

Patients with type 1 diabetes have an absolute lack of insulin and must be given exogenous **insulin** to sustain life and prevent DKA. The algorithm for type 1 diabetes begins simultaneously with lifestyle modifications and the administration of **insulin.** Patterns of administration and adjustments in dosage are based on blood glucose levels and assessment of glycosylated hemoglobin (HbA$_{1c}$) testing every 3 months initially and then every 6 months. Monitoring is discussed later. Figure 31–1 shows the algorithm for management of type 1 diabetes.

Type 2 Diabetes

Type 2 diabetes is a more complex disease, and some endogenous insulin is present. The algorithm for type 2 diabetes begins with lifestyle modifications. If glycemic targets are not met with diet, exercise, and, if appropriate, weight loss, drug therapy is initiated with a single drug. Based on glycemic control, the single drug is continued, or other drugs are added to the regimen. Monitoring with HbA$_{1c}$ is similar for both types of diabetes. Figure 31–2 shows the algorithm for management of type 2 diabetes.

Lifestyle Modifications

Nutrition therapy, including consultation with a nutritionist; exercise; and, if appropriate, weight loss con-

tinue to be the cornerstones of diabetes management. Patients using **insulin** are encouraged to eat at consistent times synchronized with the action of the **insulin** preparation. Patients on intensive therapy may make adjustments in short-acting **insulin** dosages based on the carbohydrate content of their meals and snacks and for deviations from usual eating patterns. Adequate nutritional knowledge to make these adjustments is required. The benefits of other lifestyle modifications in type 1 diabetes have not been supported by evidence (Berger & Muhlhauser, 1999). The prescription of regular exercise is beneficial in general and may help with weight loss and positive feelings of health, but it does not appear to directly affect the progression of type 1 diabetes. It is important, however, for the patient with diabetes to understand the effect exercise has on glucose uptake by skeletal muscle and the resultant alteration in plasma glucose levels. Exercise may also be prescribed because of comorbid conditions.

Lifestyle modifications do appear to make a difference with type 2 diabetes (Table 31–4). Some patients (approximately 10%) achieve glycemic targets with lifestyle modifications alone (Campbell, 1998). Nutritional goals for patients with type 2 diabetes include achieving and maintaining not only glycemic control but also appropriate lipid levels and blood pressure. Calories, protein, total fat, saturated fat and cholesterol, carbohydrates, sweeteners, fiber, sodium, and **alcohol** are all included in specific recommendations. Exercise prescriptions for patients with type 2 diabetes are 50 to 80 percent of maximal heart rate, three to four times per week. Exercise is not recommended if the patient is in poor glycemic control. Specific recommendations related to nutrition and exercise are found in the ADA clinical practice recommendations (1998).

Drug Therapy

Drug therapy is first-line therapy in type 1 diabetes and second-line therapy in type 2 diabetes. The choice of drug and the decision of monotherapy versus combination therapy are based on the type of diabetes, the

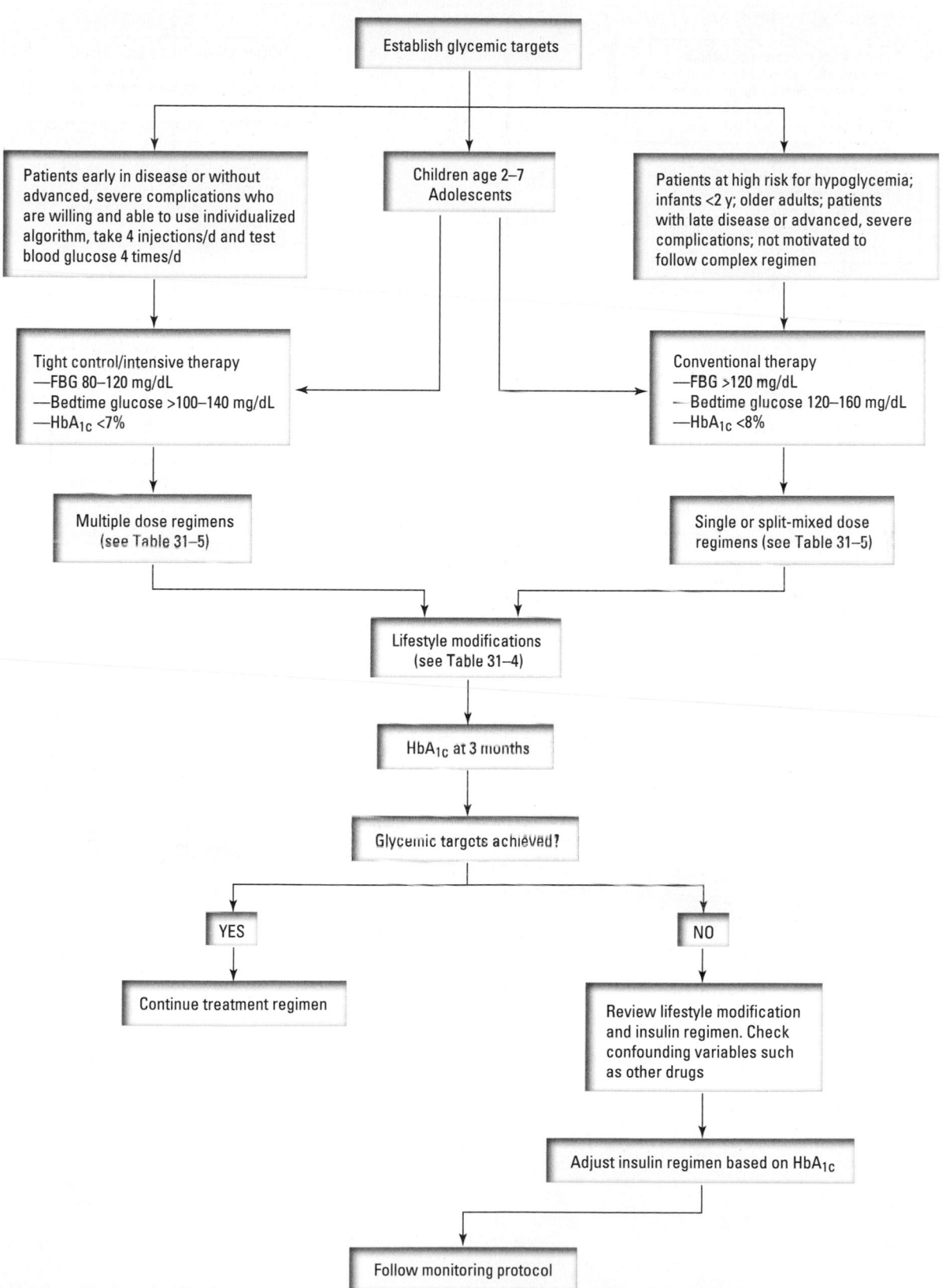

Figure 31–1. Treatment algorithm for type 1 diabetes.

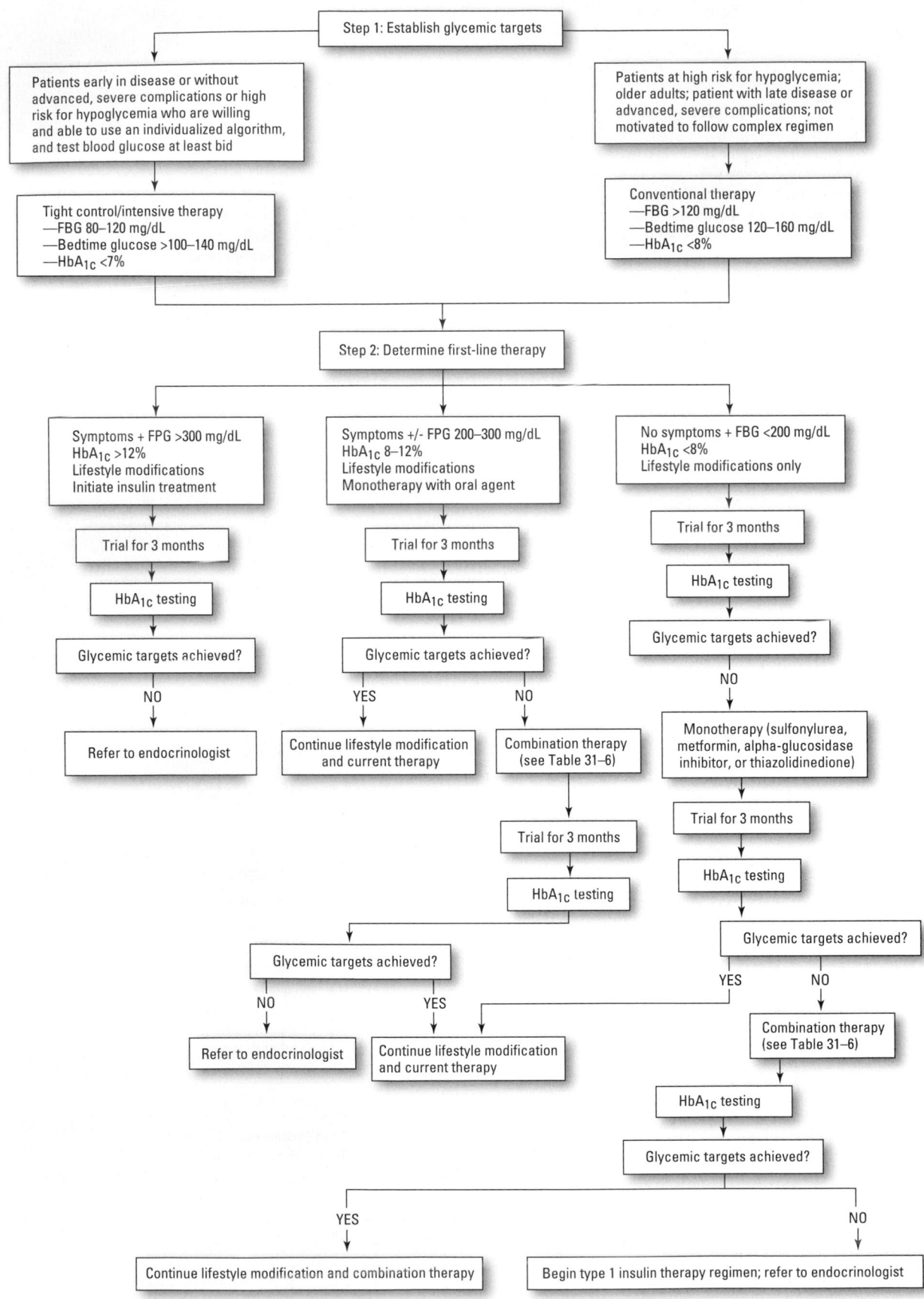

Figure 31–2. Treatment algorithm for type 2 diabetes.

Table 31–4. Lifestyle Modifications for Patients with Diabetes

Nutrition	
Type 1	• Eat at consistent times synchronized with the action of the insulin preparation.
Type 1 and type 2	• Moderate caloric restriction. • Space meals, spreading nutrient intake, especially carbohydrates, throughout the day. • 10–20% of daily caloric intake derived from both animal and vegetable proteins. • In the presence of nephropathy, total protein intake may be restricted to 0.7–0.8 g/kg/d. • <10% of calories from saturated fats and <10% from polyunsaturated fats. • 60–70% of total calories from monounsaturated fats and carbohydrates. In the presence of lipid abnormalities, saturated fat may be reduced to 7% of total calories. • <200 mg of cholesterol/d. • Total carbohydrate content is more important than type of carbohydrate. Fruits and milk have a lower glycemic response than most starches, and sucrose produces a glycemic response similar to bread, rice, and potatoes. Sucrose should be substituted 1:1 for other carbohydrates and not added to the meal plan. • Fiber recommendations are the same as for persons without diabetes. • Sodium restriction, if any, is related to any concomitant hypertension. • Abstention from alcohol is advised. If consumed, it is best done with meals and no more than 2 drinks of alcohol/d for men and no more than 1/d for women (1 alcoholic beverage = 12 oz beer, 5 oz wine, or 1.5 oz distilled spirits).
Exercise	
Type 1 and type 2	• Exercise affects uptake of glucose by muscle and fat tissue; it can affect plasma glucose levels. Time the exercise to coincide with caloric intake. Carbohydrate-based food should be readily available during and after exercise. • Increase aerobic physical activity to 60–80% of maximal heart rate for 20–30 min 3–4 d/wk. Obese or low-activity patients may need to start with as little as 3 min of activity/d and increase the activity by 1 min/d until the desired 20–30 min is achieved. • Do not exercise if your fasting plasma glucose is >250 mg/dL, casual plasma glucose is >300 mg/dL, or ketones are present. • Monitor blood glucose before and after exercise. • Learn the glycemic response to different exercise conditions.
Weight Loss	
Type 1 and type 2	• Moderate caloric restriction (250–500 calories less than average daily intake as calculated from a food history). • Moderate weight loss (5–9 kg or 10–20 lb), irrespective of starting weight, has been shown to affect insulin sensitivity.

glycemic control desired, patient variables, and concomitant disease processes.

Monotherapy

Type of Diabetes

TYPE 1 DIABETES. Patients with type 1 diabetes require **insulin.** Combinations of short-acting, intermediate-acting, and long-acting agents may be used. The pattern of administration of **insulin** is based on the patient's blood glucose, dietary, and exercise patterns. Patients in the DCCT study on tight control used combinations of short-acting and intermediate-acting **insulins** given three to four times per day. Those on very tight control used long-acting **insulin** at night with short-acting **insulin** before each meal or more frequently, based on self-monitored glucose measurements. A third group used an **insulin** pump. Patients who are intelligent, motivated,

and reliable can be taught to regulate their blood sugar with this degree of control. Less capable patients risk hypoglycemic reactions on this regimen and might not be appropriate candidates or might need higher fasting blood sugar targets than the more capable patients. Table 31–5 lists the commonly used **insulin** regimens.

TYPE 2 DIABETES. Patients with type 2 diabetes can have a variety of oral agents tailored to their specific disease process. Lean patients are less likely to be insulin-resistant and more likely to benefit from a **sulfonylurea.** Obese patients are more likely to benefit from a **biguanide** that acts more on glucose utilization and hepatic glucose storage and production. Patients with high risk for hypoglycemia benefit from drugs that are less likely to produce that effect. Patients with high postprandial blood glucose levels may benefit from an **alpha-glucosidase inhibitor.** At some point in their disease, many patients with type 2 diabetes may require the addition of **insulin.** These drugs are discussed in more detail in Chapter 19.

Table 31–5. Commonly Used Insulin Regimens

Regimen	Types of Insulin	Schedule	Advantages	Disadvantages
Single dose	Intermediate-acting	Given at 7 A.M.	• One injection covers noon and evening meals • Reduced risk for hypoglycemia during sleep	No fasting, breakfast, or nighttime coverage
Split-mixed dose (20/30 premix)	Intermediate- and short-acting	Both given at 7 A.M. and 5 P.M.	• Two injections provide 24-h coverage	Two injections are required Patient must adhere to set meal pattern
Split-mixed dose	Intermediate- and short-acting	Both at 7 A.M.; short-acting at 6 P.M.; intermediate at 9 P.M.	• Three injections provide coverage for 24 h • Risk for 3 A.M. hypoglycemia reduced	Three injections required
Multiple doses	Intermediate- and short-acting	Intermediate at 9 P.M.; short-acting before each meal	• More flexibility at mealtimes for amount of food intake	Four injections required and premeal glucose checks Requires highly individualized algorithm
Multiple doses	Short- and long-acting	Long-acting at 7 A.M. and 7 P.M.; short-acting before each meal	• Pattern more closely simulates normal endogenous insulin pattern • Some flexibility allowed in food intake	Requires 3–4 injections and premeal and bedtime blood glucose checks Requires highly individualized algorithm

Age

Approximately three-quarters of all newly diagnosed cases of type 1 diabetes occur in patients under age 18 years. Care of these patients requires integration of diabetes management with the growth and development needs of children, adolescents, and their families. Young patients with diabetes are best cared for by a team that can deal with these special needs. Glycemic targets may need to be modified to take into account that children younger than age 7 lack hypoglycemic awareness because they lack the cognitive capacity to recognize and respond to hypoglycemic signals. Tight control also should be undertaken with extreme caution in children age 2 to 7 years because hypoglycemia may impair normal brain development, which is not complete until age 7. Overly aggressive dietary manipulation can contribute

to lack of adherence, especially in adolescents. Schools and daycare settings must be involved in the treatment of the diabetes, often participating in administration of drugs. Treatment regimens must take all of these needs into account.

Older adults are more likely to have type 2 diabetes and use oral agents to treat their disease. They may suffer severe consequences from a hypoglycemic episode, especially patients with significant atherosclerosis who may be vulnerable to permanent injury (American Diabetes Association, 1998). Glycemic targets for older adults are generally 10 percent higher than those for younger patients. All **sulfonylureas** may produce severe hypoglycemia. Second-generation drugs are less likely than first-generation drugs to have this adverse reaction. **Glimepiride (Amaryl),** a third-generation **sulfonyl-**

urea, is least likely to cause this adverse reaction. The risk for hypoglycemia with **repaglinide** is about the same as with second-generation **sulfonylureas**. Drugs that are less likely to produce hypoglycemia include **metformin, alpha-glucosidase inhibitors,** and **thiazolidinediones. Metformin** is especially appropriate for older adults who also need to lose weight because it also has been associated with overall reductions in diabetes-related mortality (O'Conner, Spann, & Woolf, 1998; Peterson & Spann, 1998; Zimmerman & Hagen, 1998). **Alpha-glucosidase inhibitors** are well tolerated in older adults and have a good safety profile in this population (Rabasa-Lhoret & Chiasson, 1998). **Thiazolidinediones** have been associated with liver dysfunction and are not first-line drugs in older adults.

Race

Arslanian and Danadian (1998) report "convincing evidence" that African-American children have higher insulin secretion both before and during puberty and lower insulin sensitivity during adolescence. If we extrapolate that African-American adults may continue this lower insulin sensitivity, then it is appropriate to select drugs that improve insulin sensitivity to treat type 2 diabetes in African-Americans of all ages. Drugs with this characteristic include **metformin** and the **thiazolidinediones.**

Obesity

Obesity contributes to diabetes by downregulating insulin receptors, and it also contributes to many of the complications associated with diabetes. Weight loss alone improves short-term glycemic levels and has the potential to improve long-term metabolic control (American Diabetes Association, 1998). **Metformin** is the oral agent most associated with fostering weight loss (Zimmerman & Hagen, 1998) and is the first-line treatment choice for patients with central obesity (Peterson & Spann, 1998). The lack of weight gain associated with **alpha-glucosidase inhibitors** suggests that they might also be helpful to patients with diabetes who are obese. **Sulfonylureas** have been associated with weight gain in most studies; weight gain has been reported with **thiazolidinediones** in some studies.

Concomitant disease processes also affect drug choice. Often these disease processes reflect target organ damage from diabetes. The pathophysiological changes associated with the disease process and/or the drugs commonly used to treat it contribute to determining the best drug therapy, especially for patients with type 2 diabetes.

Coronary Artery Disease and Heart Failure

Atherosclerosis occurs earlier in patients with diabetes than it does in those without elevated glucose levels. This significantly increases the risk for cardiovascular disease, which is a leading cause of death in patients with diabetes. The DCCT trial demonstrated no increased risk for patients with type 1 diabetes on intensive therapy, and there are some observational studies showing fewer cardiovascular events and less mortality in better-controlled type 2 diabetes. Daily intake of **aspirin** has also been shown to reduce cardiovascular events in patients with diabetes (American Diabetes Association, 1998).

Metformin has been associated with improving cardiovascular risk through its action in improving lipid levels. There has been an increased frequency of lactic acidosis, however, in patients with congestive heart failure who take **metformin,** and it is now not recommended for patients requiring pharmacological therapy for congestive heart failure (Zimmerman & Hagen, 1998). **Insulin** may be required for these patients.

A bolded warning appears in all **sulfonylurea** material stating that the administration of **oral hypoglycemic drugs** has been reported to be associated with increased cardiovascular mortality as compared with treatment by diet alone or diet plus **insulin.** Although the research that resulted in the warning was for only one drug in this class, the warning has been extended to all. Some recent studies have suggested that this warning may need to be rethought.

Sulfonylureas are the drugs among the oral agents most associated with risk for hypoglycemia. Hypoglycemia may be difficult to recognize in patients who are concurrently taking **beta-adrenergic blockers** because these drugs mask the signs and symptoms of hypoglycemia, with the exception of diaphoresis. Patients with coronary artery disease, heart failure, or hypertension are commonly treated with **beta-adrenergic blockers.** If **sulfonylureas** must be given concurrently with **beta-adrenergic blockers, glimepiride** is less likely to cause hypoglycemia than other drugs in the class.

Clinical studies have presented conflicting evidence on the ability of **thiazolidinediones** to modify cardiovascular risk. They are not recommended for treating patients with diabetes who also have cardiovascular disease or risks for it (Umland & Romanelli, 1999).

Angiotensin-converting enzyme (ACE) inhibitors are central to the management of heart failure and hypertension. These drugs also have been shown to significantly reduce the incidence of diabetic nephropathy. They are the drugs of choice for patients with diabetes who also have these cardiovascular disorders. **Calcium channel blockers** in combination with **ACE inhibitors** also are a rational choice in coexisting cardiovascular diseases and diabetes (Parving, 1998). **Calcium channel blockers** have limited effects on glucose metabolism, and the **non-dihydropyridine type** have been shown to have some degree of renal protection.

Coronary artery disease is further discussed in Chapter 26, and heart failure is discussed in Chapter 34.

Hyperlipidemia

Having diabetes is now considered equivalent in cardiovascular risk to having established cardiovascular disease, and a major reason for this risk is the incidence of hyperlipidemia in patients with diabetes. The NCEP and the ADA both recommend aggressive lipid-lowering in patients with diabetes, and the ADA urges that these patients be placed in the same risk category as patients without diabetes but with established coronary heart disease (CHD). The ADA also recommends that low-density lipoprotien (LDL) cholesterol levels in patients with type 2 diabetes should be below 130 mg/dL and, if they also have CHD, below 100 mg/dL. Triglyceride levels should be lower than 200 mg/dL.

Diabetes, particularly type 2, can cause a lipid abnormality with a high level of very low density lipoprotein (VLDL) and a low level of high-density lipoprotein (HDL). This is seen clinically as high triglyceride levels (200 to 400 mg/dL) and low HDL levels (<35 mg/dL). Diabetic control by itself seldom normalizes lipid abnormalities, even with tight glycemic control. A significant number of these patients need direct lipid management (Carmena, 1998). Two classes of **antihyperlipidemic drugs** are first-line therapy for patients with diabetes. **Reductase inhibitors** have consistently demonstrated ability to reduce cardiovascular risk and are first-line therapy when the main goal is reduction of LDL cholesterol. Their action is less prominent in reduction of VLDL and triglycerides, but they also have this action. **Fibric acid derivatives** act more directly on VLDL and triglycerides. They may be used alone or in conjunction with **reductase inhibitors** (Gotto, Pasternak, & Weart, 1999). **Nicotinic acid (niacin)** also effectively lowers triglycerides; however, it is associated with increased uric acid levels, which also occur in some patients with diabetes. It may also increase insulin resistance. **Colestipol (Colestid)** and **cholestyramine (Questran)** may improve lipid levels, but they may pose problems for patients with diabetic gastropathy. Discussion of **antihyperlipidemic drugs**, including dosing schedules, is included in Chapters 14 and 37.

Metformin has a modestly favorable impact on lipids because of its actions in the liver (Zimmerman & Hagen, 1998). In clinical studies, **metformin** alone or in combination with a **sulfonylurea** lowered mean fasting serum triglycerides, total cholesterol, and LDL and had no adverse effect on HDL (Bailey & Turner, 1996). It is an appropriate oral agent for patients with diabetes who also have lipid abnormalities. The combination of **gemfibrozil (Lopid)**, a **fibric acid derivative**, with **metformin** and a Step 2 lipid-control diet is the most efficacious in both controlling lipid and lowering blood glucose levels.

Acarbose (Precose), an **alpha-glucosidase inhibitor**, has also shown beneficial effects for patients with hypertriglyceridemias. It acts on the pathogenesis of these disorders, lowering production of endogenous triglycerides (Malaguarnera et al., 1998).

Troglitazone, a **thiazolidinedione**, lowers triglyceride and free fatty acid levels and increases HDL cholesterol levels (Zimmerman & Hagen, 1998). It is also appropriate therapy for patients with concurrent hypertriglyceridemia. The required frequent monitoring of liver function based on reports of severe hepatotoxicity, however, has increased its cost, so that it is not the first choice.

Further discussion of hyperlipidemia occurs in Chapter 37.

Hypertension

Hypertension (HTN) is a common comorbid condition in patients with diabetes. Of the 25 million people with diabetes worldwide, approximately 50 percent are also hypertensive (MacLeod & McLay, 1998). In type 1 diabetes, HTN is often a manifestation of diabetic nephropathy. In type 2 diabetes, it is often part of a syndrome that includes glucose intolerance, insulin resistance, obesity, hyperlipidemia, and coronary artery disease. In both types of diabetes, the presence of HTN is associated with increased cardiovascular risk, especially for stroke and ischemic heart disease. Control of HTN has been demonstrated to reduce the rate of progression of diabetic nephropathy and hypertensive cerebrovascular disease. This control is more important than glycemic control in reducing the risk for cardiovascular disease.

Some drugs used to treat HTN also address other complications of diabetes. ACE inhibitors, as mentioned before, reduce the risk for diabetic nephropathy through their reduction of intraglomerular pressure and a reduction in glomerulosclerosis. They have a unique, specific, and beneficial effect on the kidneys of both normotensive and hypertensive patients with diabetes. The ADA and the National Kidney Foundation, along with others, agree on the use of **ACE inhibitors** for all patients with diabetes, even those who are normotensive (Aiello, 1998; American Diabetes Association, 1998). Although they have not yet been approved for this use, **angiotensin II receptor antagonists** show a great deal of promise regarding their effects on diabetic nephropathy, and three multicenter, randomized, double-blind clinical trials are currently assessing their efficacy (Makrilakis & Bakris, 1998). **Alpha-adrenergic blockers** are recognized to improve insulin sensitivity and have a neutral or mildly beneficial effect on the lipid profile. They do not appear to have a beneficial effect on diabetic nephropathy. **Non-dihydropyridine calcium channel blockers** have a neutral effect on glucose metabolism and have been shown to decrease proteinuria. **Dihydropyridines** have never been shown to consistently reduce urinary protein excretion or to prevent glomerulosclerosis (Makrilakis & Bakris, 1998).

Other drugs used to treat HTN, however, can have adverse effects on glycemic control. In very low doses, diuretics may safely be used for patients with diabetes (Black, Cohen, & Davis, 1993; O'Conner et al., 1998), but at moderate to high doses they adversely affect glucose metabolism. They may also potentiate orthostatic hypotensive changes in patients with diabetic neuropathy. **Thiazide diuretics** have been shown to increase peripheral insulin resistance and hepatic glucose release. Both of these actions interfere with glycemic control. In one study, they were associated with a fourfold excess mortality in patients receiving **diuretics** versus those who were not (MacLeod & McLay, 1998). **Thiazide diuretics** have demonstrated a slowed progression of nephropathy (Makrilakis & Bakris, 1998).

Beta-adrenergic blockers may precipitate diabetes among hypertensive obese patients because of their increase in insulin resistance. **Beta$_1$ selective adrenergic blockers,** by contrast, sometimes increase insulin levels. Clearly, if this class of drugs must be used for patients with diabetes (e.g., for myocardial infarction prevention), the choice should be one with beta$_1$ selectivity. The lack of hypoglycemic awareness with this class of drugs has been discussed previously.

HTN is discussed in more detail in Chapter 38.

Nephropathy

Microalbuminuria (30 to 300 mg/24 hours) has been shown to be the earliest stage of diabetic nephropathy. Patients with microalbuminuria are likely to progress to clinical albuminuria and a decreased glomerular filtration rate over a period of years. Once albuminuria occurs, the risk for end-stage renal disease is high in patients with type 1 diabetes and significant for those with type 2 (American Diabetes Association, 1998). Aiello (1998) discusses in detail the pathophysiology, risk factors, diagnostic testing, and management of diabetic nephropathy. Intensive diabetic management and maintenance of blood pressure below 130/85 mm Hg have been effective in reducing the rate of progression to end stage. **ACE inhibitors** have also been demonstrated to significantly delay the progression of diabetic nephropathy.

Patients with significant renal disease should not use **metformin** because of the risk for lactic acidosis. Caution should be exercised with **sulfonylureas** or **alpha-glucosidase inhibitors.**

Neuropathy

Diabetic neuropathy (DN) is the earliest and most common complication of diabetes. Its onset is often insidious. The role of tight glycemic control in preventing or delaying the onset of this complication is clear.

Peripheral diabetic neuropathy may result in pain, loss of sensation, and muscle weakness, and it is a major risk factor for development of ulceration and lower extremity amputations. In addition to maintaining HbA$_{1c}$ concentrations of 7 percent or less, therapies are also directed at other factors in DN. Neuropathic pain is often severe and intractable. Treatment is based on trial and error. No one method is superior to others for an individual patient. **Tricyclic antidepressants** have been used for their effect on the intrinsic pain-suppressing pathways. **Nortriptyline (Aventyl, Pamelor)** and **desipramine (Norpramin)** are more useful when the patient also experiences orthostatic hypotension because they are less likely to exacerbate it. **Gabapentin (Neurontin),** an **anticonvulsant,** acts by stabilizing neuronal membranes. Therapy is begun at low doses, followed by gradual titration. These drugs are discussed in more detail in Chapter 13.

Autonomic involvement can affect gastrointestinal, cardiovascular, and genitourinary function. **Metoclopramide (Reglan),** a **prokinetic agent,** is the most commonly used drug to treat gastroparesis; however, it has a relatively high incidence of adverse reactions, especially in children and older adults. This increased risk for adverse reactions is significant because gastric emptying problems are more common in older adults (Valentine, 1998). **Cisapride (Propulsid)** may also be used to enhance antral contractility and increase gastric emptying. It has the added benefit of acting on lower esophageal sphincter tone to reduce gastroesophageal reflux (Koch, 1998).

Genitourinary dysfunction includes reduced bladder contraction force, resulting in urinary stasis, increased risk for bladder infections, and impotence. Bladder contraction force can be enhanced by the use of a **cholinergic agonist** such as **bethanechol (Urecholine).** Impotence has been successfully treated with **alpha-adrenergic blockers** that increase vascular blood flow. **Sildenafil (Viagra)** is being advertised for treatment of impotence.

ON THE HORIZON

Recombinant Human Nerve Growth Factor

A new type of drug used to treat the underlying mechanism of DN is currently in phase III trials. **Recombinant human nerve growth factor** shows promise in improving neurological function and preventing the development of DN.

Retinopathy

Diabetic retinopathy (DR) is a highly specific vascular complication of both type 1 and type 2 diabetes. After 20 years of diabetes, nearly all patients with type 1 and more than 60 percent of patients with type 2 diabetes have some degree of retinopathy. It is the most frequent cause of blindness among adults age 20 to 74. The DCCT study clearly demonstrated that tight glycemic control reduced or prevented the development of retinopathy by 27 percent as compared with conventional therapy and reduced the progression by 34 to 76 percent. Aside from the appropriate use of **insulin** or **oral antidiabetic agents** to maintain HbA_{1c} at 7 percent or less, there are no pharmacological therapies available to treat this disorder.

Combination Therapy

When monotherapy does not achieve glycemic targets, the treatment regimen is stepped up to combination therapy. There is no evidence that switching drugs within a specific class improves glycemic control. A common mistake is to stop one class of drug and start another. A more rational approach is to add a second drug. Table 31–6 shows the most common combination regimens and the types of patients for whom they are appropriate.

If the initial drug was a **sulfonylurea,** addition of **metformin,** an **alpha-glucosidase inhibitor,** or a **thiazolidinedione** is the next logical step. Individual characteristics such as obesity (**metformin** induces weight loss), renal function (**thiazolidinediones** are hepatically eliminated), and time of day for lack of glycemic control (**alpha-glucosidase inhibitors** are especially good for postprandial hyperglycemia) help in making the choice. Second-generation **sulfonylureas** are best for patients who are taking multiple medications to minimize potential drug interactions and because they have the advantage of being given once daily, thereby reducing the complexity of the drug regimen and improving adherence. Among this group of drugs, **glimepiride** binds to different insulin receptors more than other **sulfonylureas** and may be effective when others are not. It is also associated with a lower incidence of hypoglycemic reactions.

Depending on the classes used, addition of a different drug follows different steps. If the drug to be added is **metformin,** the dose of the **sulfonylurea** must first be reduced, usually by half, before adding the **metformin** because these drugs tend to potentiate each other, and adverse reactions are more likely without dosage adjustments.

Table 31–6. Commonly Used Drug Combinations

Drug Combinations (Frequently Used and Well-Studied)	Appropriate Patients
Sulfonylurea + metformin	Obese patients or those who experience weight gain with sulfonylurea. Have synergistic effect so doses of both can be reduced. Metformin associated with weight loss. Also useful for patients with high triglyceride levels and increased fasting blood glucose despite sulfonylurea.
Sulfonylurea + insulin	Patients whose main defect is insufficient secretion of insulin by beta cells. Also useful for patients with fasting hyperglycemia in the morning.
Sulfonylurea + thiazolidinedione	Patients with high triglyceride levels. Sulfonylurea stimulates insulin secretion; thiazolidinediones decrease hepatic production and triglyceride levels. Also useful for patients with impaired renal function. Better with thin patients.
Sulfonylurea + alpha-glucosidase inhibitor	Patients with hyperinsulinemia, often seen in obese. Sulfonylurea stimulates insulin secretion and may produce hyperinsulinemia and induce weight gain. Alpha-glucosidase inhibitor reduces hyperinsulinemia and counteracts the weight gain that sulfonylurea may cause. Also useful for patients with postprandial hyperglycemia despite sulfonylurea.
Metformin + repaglinide	Patients with postprandial hyperglycemia despite metformin who want tight control. Repaglinide is short-acting insulin secretagogue. Useful for patients with postprandial hyperglycemia.
Metformin + insulin	Patients desiring tight control. Metformin does not stimulate insulin secretion.
Alpha-glucosidase inhibitor + insulin	Patients desiring tight control. Alpha-glucosidase inhibitor does not stimulate insulin secretion.

Additional regimens infrequently used, not well studied, and not FDA-approved include (1) sulfonylurea + metformin + insulin and (2) metformin + alpha-glucosidase inhibitor.

The same steps related to reduction in the **sulfonylurea** dose arise when an **alpha-glucosidase inhibitor** is added to the regimen. Because of their mechanism of action, **alpha-glucosidase inhibitors** alone do not cause hypoglycemia, but they may do so in combination with **sulfonylureas**. Treatment of this hypoglycemia cannot be accomplished with the usual ingestion of sucrose (hard candy or soft drinks), fructose, or starches because they are disaccharides and **alpha-glucosidase inhibitors** delay their absorption. Because there is no inhibitory activity against lactase or monosaccharides, milk, lactose, and glucose can be used to treat the hypoglycemia.

Thiazolidinediones and **sulfonylureas** taken together have additive effects on each other's actions, so the initial dose of the **sulfonylurea** does not need to be reduced. Reduction may occur later. Both fasting and postprandial blood glucose levels of patients decrease. It is important to monitor these levels closely when **thiazolidinediones** are added to the treatment regimen to avoid hypoglycemia. While blood glucose levels dropped, in one study weight went up, with gains of 5.8 to 13 lb. Other studies have not replicated this finding, so the use of this combination for obese patients with diabetes is based on the experience of the provider.

Repaglinide dosing, when added to **metformin,** has an additive effect. **Metformin** can also be added to **repaglinide** therapy if there is inadequate control with **repaglinide** alone, with no change in dosing of either drug.

Insulin may also be added to the regimen. When it is combined with a **sulfonylurea,** the **insulin** is initially given at bedtime and the **sulfonylurea** in the morning (bedtime **insulin,** daytime **sulfonylurea** [BIDS] or suppertime mixed **insulin,** daytime **sulfonylurea** [SMIDS]). This regimen takes advantage of the increased insulin secretion produced by the **sulfonylurea** while the bedtime **insulin** suppresses hepatic glucose production during the early morning hours. This combination is especially useful for patients with elevated fasting blood glucose levels.

When **insulin** is added to the treatment regimen, close monitoring of blood glucose levels is also critical. Significant drops in blood glucose, with risk for hypoglycemic reactions, have occurred.

Each of these drug combinations is discussed in more detail, including specific dosing schedules, in Chapter 19.

Monitoring

The ADA has recommendations for laboratory evaluation of patients with diabetes at the initial visit and as part of continuing care. Laboratory evaluation at the initial visit includes the following:

1. Fasting plasma glucose. A random plasma glucose test may be performed in an undiagnosed symptomatic patient for diagnostic purposes.

2. HbA_{1c}. This test is to provide baseline data because it will be the test used for ongoing evaluation of glycemic control.

3. Fasting lipid profile. Hyperlipidemias are common in patients with diabetes and contribute significantly to cardiovascular risk.

4. Serum creatinine. This test is given to all adults but to children only if proteinuria is present. Diabetic nephropathy is a frequent complication of diabetes. Early intervention is necessary to prevent the development of end-stage renal disease.

5. Urinalysis. Urinalysis includes tests for glucose, ketones, protein, and sediment. Increased urine glucose indicates that the renal threshold for glucose has been exceeded. Ketones are associated with DKA. Protein is an early indicator of impaired renal function. Sediment evaluation may indicate urinary tract infection.

6. Tests for microalbuminuria. Tests are given for microalbuminuria to pubertal and prepubertal patients with type 1 diabetes for at least 5 years and to all patients with type 2 diabetes. Microalbuminuria is the earliest indicator of impaired renal function.

7. Urine culture. Culture urine if sediment is abnormal or symptoms of urinary tract infection are present.

8. Thyroid function tests. The presence of thyroid disorders may cloud the diagnosis and complicate the treatment of diabetes.

9. Electrocardiogram in adults. Cardiovascular disease is a complication of diabetes, and this study serves as a baseline. Taken alone, electrocardiograms are not sufficient to diagnose most cardiac conditions, but they are part of the diagnostic testing for these disorders.

Laboratory evaluation of continuing care includes the following:

1. HbA_{1c} should be performed to document the degree of glycemic control. Because HbA_{1c} reflects mean glycemia over the preceding 2 to 3 months, it should be measured every 3 months initially and then every 6 months in patients who are meeting treatment goals and who have stable glycemic control. See Table 31–3 for glycemic targets.

2. Adult patients should be tested annually for lipid disorders with fasting cholesterol, triglyceride, HDL, and calculated LDL measurements. The targets for management are LDL below 100 mg/dL, HDL above 45 mg/dL, and triglycerides below 200 mg/dL. Tests resulting in higher values should be repeated for confirmation, and then management should be instituted according to the NCEP guidelines.

3. Children older than age 2 should have a lipid profile after the diagnosis of diabetes and when glucose control has been established. If values fall within

PATIENT EDUCATION

Diabetes Mellitus

Related to the Overall Treatment Plan/Disease Process

☐ Pathophysiology of diabetes and the long-term effects of inadequate management on target organs

☐ Role of lifestyle modification, especially dietary therapy, in improving outcomes and keeping the number and cost of required drugs down

☐ Importance of adherence to the treatment regimen

☐ Need for regular follow-up visits with the primary care provider and other specialists

Specific to the Drug Therapy

☐ Reason for taking the drug(s) and the anticipated action of the drug(s) on the disease process

☐ Doses and schedules for taking the drugs

☐ Possible adverse reactions (especially hypoglycemia, DKA, and HHNK), how to prevent them, and what to do if they occur

☐ Interactions between lifestyle modifications and these drugs

Reasons for Taking the Drug(s)

Patient education about specific drugs is provided in Chapter 19. More specific information related to diabetes includes the following: Tight glycemic control and management of hypertension and hyperlipidemia are central to reducing morbidity and mortality from the leading cause of death in the United States, which is cardiovascular disease, and to preventing retinopathy and end-stage renal disease. The risks of these complications must be discussed while maintaining the potential for good quality of life with appropriate treatment.

Drugs as Part of the Total Treatment Regimen

The expectations should be clear about what the drugs can and cannot do. Dietary and other lifestyle modifications complement drug therapy and are equally important. Diabetes is a chronic condition. Self-management requires incorporation of drugs, diet, exercise, and glucose self-monitoring into the everyday life of the patient with diabetes.

Adherence Issues

Nonadherence to the treatment regimen may result in increased risk for complications and reduced life expectancy. Health care providers should be aware of potential problems with nonadherence, discuss the importance of adherence at each follow-up visit, and assist patients in removing barriers to adherence such as lack of social support and cost of the treatment regimen. A team approach with the patient as an active partner should be maximized. Patient education booklets are available from the American Diabetes Association, which can be accessed on the Internet at *www.ada.org*.

Diabetes Mellitus

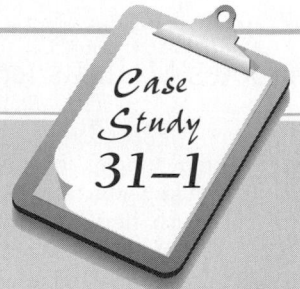

Case Study 31–1

Complaint

"I've been urinating a lot."

History

Marion is a 45-year-old overweight patient who presents at the urgency care clinic with frequency, urgency, and burning on urination. She has had urinary tract infections before, and the symptoms are similar. The triage nurse orders a urinalysis, and the results are consistent with a urinary tract infection. However, the urinalysis also shows protein in the urine and a high glucose level. A casual plasma glucose level is drawn and shows 420 mg/dL. Her blood pressure is 150/90. When these values are reported to her, she states that she is not surprised. Her mother and her aunt both have type 2 diabetes, and she has used her mother's glucose monitor to check her own blood glucose levels in the past. When they are high, she adjusts her diet. Because this is an urgency care setting, her urinary tract infection is treated; a fasting chemistry panel, lipid profile, glycosylated hemoglobin, and thyroid function tests are ordered, and she is referred to her primary care provider for workup of probable type 2 diabetes. Screening for microalbuminuria is postponed until her urinary tract infection is cured because urinary tract infections can cause transient elevations in urinary albumin excretion.

Assessment

Marion's primary care provider reviews her laboratory findings. They include the following:

1. Fasting plasma glucose 300 mg/dL
2. Triglycerides 350 mg/dl
3. HDL cholesterol 35mg/dL
4. HbA$_{1c}$ 10%
5. Serum creatinine 1.2
6. Thyroid function studies within normal limits

Measurement of the albumin to creatinine ratio in a spot collection is also performed, resulting in a finding of 30 mg/g. Although this is consistent with microalbuminuria, there is marked day-to-day variability in albumin excretion, so at least two of three tests done in a 3- to 6-month period should show elevated levels before a patient is designated as having microalbuminuria.

Initial Management Plan

Because Marion has now satisfied the criteria for a diagnosis of diabetes and has concurrent hypertension, hyperlipidemia, and probable microalbuminuria, her initial treatment plan is as follows:

1. Begin a diet with calories reduced 300 kcal/day below her usual intake to facilitate weight loss. Weight loss alone will improve insulin uptake by upregulating insulin receptors. Protein is restricted to 0.7g/kg/day to retard the rate of fall in glomerular filtration rate. Recommendations vary from 0.8 g/kg/day for patients without overt nephropathy to 0.6 g/kg/day for those who demonstrate elevated serum creatinine levels. Total fat intake should be <10 percent of calories, with increased use of monounsaturated fats as the fat source, and dietary cholesterol <200 mg/day (Step 2 NCEP diet). Increased use of monounsaturated fats is helpful in treating elevated triglycerides. Sodium is restricted to 2000 mg/day to treat her hypertension in the likely presence of early nephropathy.

2. Start an exercise program.

3. Initiate drug therapy with glimepiride (Amaryl) Sulfonylureas as monotherapy are effective in achieving adequate blood glucose control in 50 percent of newly diagnosed patients with diabetes. Glimepiride is the least expensive of the branded drugs in this group, has coverage for once-daily dosing, and is the least likely to produce hypoglycemia. Because she will be taking drugs for her hypertension and perhaps for her hyperlipidemia, her regimen will be complex, and anything that can reduce this complexity will be helpful in increasing adherence. Unfortunately, it may also produce weight gain, but metformin, another possible choice that assists in weight loss and improves the lipid profile, is risky for patients with impaired renal function. If it is added later to the regimen, it will be done in very low doses.

4. Diet and exercise may control her hypertension, but ACE inhibitors are recommended for all patients with type 2 diabetes to prevent the progression of nephropathy, so it is appropriate to add one to her treatment regimen. Lisinopril (Zestril) 5 mg daily is chosen because it is available in scored 10-mg tablets that can be halved to keep the cost down and make it possible to increase the dose if needed without a new prescription.

5. Some patients can correct their hyperlipidemia with diet and exercise. She is being placed on a Step 2 NCEP diet. To refrain from making her regimen

continued

Diabetes Mellitus (*continued*)

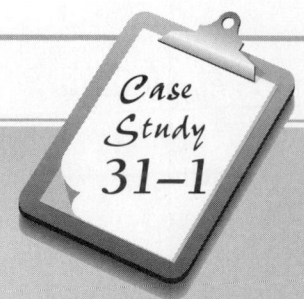

too complex initially, no antihyperlipidemic drug will be prescribed at this first visit.

6. Teach her self-monitoring of glucose, including how to keep a log of diet, exercise, fingerstick glucose levels, and drugs taken.

7. Schedule follow-up visits weekly until her blood glucose level is <140 mg/dL and she is competent to conduct the treatment protocol.

Follow-up Visit

Marion is seen weekly for 3 weeks. She begins to lose weight at a rate of 2 lb/week, and her blood glucose level is <140 mg/dL, which meets the interim target but is still

not at the final target of <120 mg/dL. Because she has seen family members manage their diabetes, she learns quickly with their support. A repeat HbA_{1c} has dropped to 8.2 percent, but it, too, is still not at target. She expresses some difficulty with her dietary changes but is "working on it."

Modifications to Management Plan

She will be seen every 3 months for the next year, with monitoring of her HbA_{1c} and review of her diabetic log.

accepted risk levels, the test should be repeated every 5 years. Tests resulting in abnormal values require institution of therapy according to NCEP guidelines.

4. Routine urinalysis should be performed yearly in adults. If the urinalysis is positive for protein, a quantitative measure is helpful in determining a treatment plan. If it is negative for protein, the urine should be tested for microalbuminuria. Screening for microalbuminuria in patients with type 1 diabetes should begin with puberty and after 5 years' duration of diabetes. Because of the difficulty in establishing a precise date when type 2 diabetes began, screening for patients with type 2 diabetes should begin at the time of diagnosis.

Outcome Evaluation

Outcome evaluation is against glycemic targets and prevention or development of the common complications of diabetes. The ADA has published a position statement on the standards of care for patients with diabetes, including outcome evaluation. These standards include joint establishment of treatment goals and glycemic targets with the patient. Because diabetes requires a considerable amount of self-management, treatment goals and glycemic targets should take into account patient characteristics, such as the patient's capacity to understand and carry out the treatment regimen, the risk for severe hypoglycemia, and other factors that may increase risk or decrease benefit (e.g., very young or very old, end-stage renal disease, advanced cardiovascular or cerebrovascular disease, or other concomitant diseases that will materially shorten life expectancy). In addition,

children with diabetes require integration of factors associated with growth and development into their treatment regimen.

To provide this standard of care, a team effort is required, especially when children are the patients. Consultation between diabetic specialists, diabetic educators, nutritionists, and the primary care provider is critical throughout treatment. If this consultation is ongoing, times when treatment requires more input from a specific member of the team (e.g., intercurrent illness, DKA, HHNK, or recurrent hypoglycemia) will be defined by the team, and interactions between patients and their various providers will be seamless.

Patient Education

Patient education related to diabetes includes management of the disease process, counseling about the risk for development of diabetes, prevention of complications, and the role of the patient in self-management. It is not within the scope of this book to discuss all the patient education required. For that information, the reader is referred to the ADA Clinical Practice Recommendations (1998). The focus of patient education here is the part that is related to pharmacological management.

Because diabetes requires self-management by the patient as an active member of the treatment team, it must take top priority in a patient's consciousness.

To facilitate adherence to the treatment regimen, patient education should focus on understanding the pathophysiology of diabetes and the long-term effects of inadequate management on target organs; the role of lifestyle modification, especially dietary therapy, in improving outcomes and keeping the number and cost of required drugs down; the importance of adherence to the treatment regimen; and the need for regular follow-up visits with the primary care provider and other specialists.

REFERENCES

Aiello, J. (1998). Preventing diabetic nephropathy: The role of primary care. *Nurse Practitioner, 23*(2), 12–31.

American Diabetes Association. (1993). Implications of the diabetes control and complications trial. *Diabetes Care, 16*(11), 1517–1520.

American Diabetes Association. (1998). Clinical practice recommendations, 1998. *Diabetes Care, 21*(1), S5–S97.

Arslanian, S., & Danadian, K. (1998). Insulin secretion, insulin sensitivity and diabetes in black children. *Trends in Endocrinology and Metabolism, 9*(5), 194–199.

Bailey, C., & Turner, R. (1996). Drug therapy: Metformin. *New England Journal of Medicine, 334*(9), 574–579.

Berger, M., & Muhlhauser, I. (1999). Diabetes care and patient-orientated outcomes. *Journal of the American Medical Association, 281*(18), 1676–1678.

Bernstein, G. (1998). The diabetic patient in your practice. *Emergency Medicine, 30*(7), 66–75.

Black, H., Cohen, J., & Davis, B. (1993). Influence of long-term, low-dose, diuretic based hypertensive therapy on glucose, lipid and mortality. *Hypertension, 21,* 335–343.

Boden, G., Chen, X., & Iqbal, N. (1998). Acute lowering of plasma fatty acids lowers basal insulin secretion in diabetes and nondiabetic subjects. *Diabetes, 47*(10), 1609–1612.

Cabanas, E. (1998). Maturity-onset diabetes of the young: Recent findings indicate insulin resistance/obesity are not factors. *Diabetes Educator, 24*(4), 477–480

Campbell, R. (1998). Glimepiride: Role of a new sulfonylurea in the treatment of type 2 diabetes mellitus. *Annals of Pharmacotherapy, 32*(10), 1044–1052.

Carmena, R. (1998). Requirements for claims of favorable effects on serum lipids by oral antidiabetic agents. *American Journal of Cardiology, 81*(8), 56F–57F.

DiPiro, J., Talbert, R., Yee, G., Matzke, G., Wells, B., & Posey, L. (1999). *Pharmacotherapy: A pathophysiological approach.* Stamford, CT: Appleton and Lange

Estacio, R., & Schrier, R. (1998). Antihypertensive therapy in type 2 diabetes: Implications of the appropriate blood pressure control in diabetes (ABCD) trial. *American Journal of Cardiology, 82,* 9R–14R.

Flick, M., & Schumann, L. (1997). Non-insulin-dependent diabetes mellitus. *Journal of the Academy of Nurse Practitioners, 9*(7), 337–344.

Fossum, E., Hoieggen, A., Moan, A., Rostrup, M., & Kjeldsen, S. (1999). Insulin sensitivity is related to physical fitness and exercise blood pressure to structural vascular properties in young men. *Hypertension, 33*(3), 781–786.

Fried, R. (1998). Infections in diabetes mellitus. *Emergency Medicine, 30*(7), 84–87.

Gavin, J., & Peters, A. (1999). Syndrome X: Implications for cardiovascular risk. *Patient Care for the Nurse Practitioner,* February, 14–18.

Genuth, S., Palmer, J., & Zimmerman, B. (1999). New diagnostic criteria for diabetes. *Patient Care for the Nurse Practitioner,* February, 2–6.

Giacca, A., Groenewoud, Y., Tsui, E., McClean, P., & Zinman, B. (1998). Glucose production, utilization, and cycling in response to moderate exercise in obese subjects with type 2 diabetes and mild hyperglycemia. *Diabetes, 47*(11), 1763–1770.

Goodpaster, B., Keeley, D., Wing, R., Meier, A., & Thaete, F. (1999). Effects of weight loss on regional fat distribution and insulin sensitivity in obesity. *Diabetes, 48*(4), 839–847.

Gotto, A., Pasternak, R., & Weart, C. (1999). Statins: New uses to improve outcomes. *Patient Care for the Nurse Practitioner, 2*(7), 16–32.

Koch, K. (1998). Diabetic gastropathy: A clinical overview. *Patient Care Nurse Practitioner,* May, 1–10.

Lombardo, R. (1998). Gastrointestinal complications in diabetes. *Emergency Medicine, 30*(7), 76–83.

MacLeod, M., & McLay, J. (1998). Drug treatment of hypertension complicating diabetes mellitus. *Drugs, 56*(2), 189–202.

Makrilakis, K., & Bakris, G. (1998). Diabetic hypertensive patients: Improving their prognosis. *Journal of Cardiovascular Pharmacology, 31*(Suppl. 2), A34–S40.

Malaguarnera, M., Giugno, I., Panebianco, M., & Pistone, G. (1998). Beneficial effects of acarbose on familial hypertriglyceridemias. *International Journal of Clinical Pharmacology and Therapeutics, 36*(8), 441–445.

Marre, M., Bouhanick, B., Gilles, B., Glaaois, Y., LeJeune, J., Chatellier, J., & Alhenc-Gelas, F. (1999). Renal changes on hyperglycemia and angiotensin-converting enzyme in type 1 diabetes. *Hypertension, 33*(3), 775–780.

Mattock, M., Barnes, D., Viberti, G., Keen, H., Burt, D., Hughes, J., Fitzgerald, A., Sandu, B., & Jackson, P. (1998). Microalbuminuria and coronary health disease in NIDDM. *Diabetes, 47*(11), 1786–1792.

Mogensen, C. (1998). Natural history of cardiovascular and renal disease in patients with type 2 diabetes: Effect of therapeutic interventions and risk modification. *American Journal of Cardiology, 82,* 4R–8R.

Murtaugh, M., Ferris, A., Capacchione, C., & Reece, A. (1998). Energy intake and glycemia in lactating women with type 1 diabetes. *Journal of the American Dietetic Association, 98*(6), 642–648.

O'Conner, P., Spann, S., & Woolf, S. (1998). Care of adults with type 2 diabetes mellitus: A review of the evidence. *Journal of Family Practice, 47*(5), S13–S22.

Parving, H. (1998). Calcium antagonists and cardiovascular risks in diabetes. *American Journal of Cardiology, 82,* 42R–44R.

Peterson, K., & Spann, S. (1998). Primary care for patients with type 2 diabetes: Moving beyond hyperglycemia. *Journal of Family Practice, 47*(5), S63–S64.

Plosker, G., & Faulds, D. (1999). Troglitazone: A review of its use in the management of type 2 diabetes mellitus. *Drugs, 57*(3), 409–438.

Rabasa-Lhoret, R., & Chiasson, J. (1998). Potential of alpha-glucosidase inhibitors in elderly patients with diabetes mellitus and impaired glucose tolerance. *Drugs and Aging, 13*(2), 131–143.

Testa, M., & Simonson, D. (1998). Health economic benefits and quality of life during improved glycemic control in patients with type 2 diabetes mellitus: A randomized, controlled, double-blind trial. *Journal of the American Medical Association, 280*(17), 1490–1496.

Umland, E., & Romanelli, A. (1999). Cardiovascular effects of troglitazone. *Annals of Pharmacotherapy, 33*(2), 229–232.

Valentine, V. (1998). Diabetic gastropathy in the elderly. *Patient Care Nurse Practitioner,* May, 17–21.

Westerbacka, J., Vehkavaara, S., Bergholm, R., Wilkinson, I., Cockcroft, J., & Yki-Jarvinen, H. (1999). Marked resistance of the ability of insulin to decrease arterial stiffness characterizes human obesity. *Diabetes, 48*(4), 821–827.

Zimmerman, B., & Hagen, M. (1998). An evaluation of new agents in the treatment of type 2 diabetes. *Journal of Family Practice, 47*(5), S37–S43.

CHAPTER OUTLINE

Gastroesophageal Reflux Disease

astroesophageal reflux disease (GERD) is a common problem in primary care. Approximately 10 percent of Americans suffer from daily heartburn, and up to 50 percent have monthly symptoms (Tucker & Schumann, 1999). The severity of the disease varies from occasional postprandial discomfort to severe esophageal inflammation, stricture, bleeding, and even esophageal carcinoma.

Evaluation and management of GERD is best carried out in a stepwise fashion. In most cases, the primary care provider can manage diagnosis and treatment. Ten to 15 percent of patients with GERD require referral to a gastroenterologist. Although the focus of this chapter is drug therapy, lifestyle modification is central to successful management of GERD and is also discussed.

Pathophysiology

GERD results from the reflux of chyme from the stomach into the esophagus. The physiological action of the lower esophageal sphincter (LES) is critical to maintaining a pressure barrier between the stomach and the esophagus. In patients with GERD, the resting tone of the LES tends to be less than normal, permitting transient relaxation of the LES 1 to 2 hours after eating. This relaxation allows gastric contents to regurgitate into the esophagus. The acid is usually neutralized and cleared from the esophagus by peristaltic action within 1 to 3 minutes and sphincter tone is restored, but the LES is a complicated region of smooth muscle and many factors can contribute to poor functioning.

The function of the LES is regulated by the interaction of hormonal, neural, and dietary factors. The hormone gastrin increases resting tone, whereas estrogen, progesterone, glucagon, secretin, and cholecystokinin all decrease sphincter tone. The vagus nerve and alpha-adrenergic stimulation help to maintain resting tone. Tobacco, **alcohol,** peppermint, chocolate, and foods with high concentrations of fat or carbohydrate all decrease LES tone.

Drugs also contribute to LES tone (Table 32–1). Those that increase tone include **bethanechol (Urecholine), metoclopramide (Reglan), pentobarbital (Nembutal), histamine,** and **antacids. Anticholinergics, theophylline, meperidine (Demerol),** and **calcium channel blockers** are among the drugs that decrease LES tone. Some of these drugs are used to treat GERD.

Factors that increase intra-abdominal pressure can also contribute to GERD by affecting the pressure gradient. Vomiting, coughing, and bending all increase intra-abdominal pressure. Increased abdominal pressure during pregnancy may contribute to GERD, but the underlying cause is the increased circulating estrogen and progesterone.

Transient relaxation of LES tone is not the only factor in GERD. Decreased secondary peristalsis and defective mucosal resistance to caustic liquids have also been implicated. These factors are also targets of treatments for GERD.

The severity of the esophagitis that results from GERD depends on the composition of the gastric contents, the length of time they are in contact with the esophageal mucosa, and the epithelial resistance to acid. If the chyme is highly acidic or contains bile salts and pancreatic enzymes, reflux esophagitis can be severe. Patients with decreased esophageal peristalsis have longer exposure times between the chyme and the esophageal mucosa. Delayed gastric emptying contributes to reflux esophagitis by lengthening the period during which reflux is possible and by increasing the acid content of chyme.

Signs and Symptoms

Most patients complain of burning substernal pain that radiates upward, often aggravated by meals and by lying down and relieved by sitting up. The burning substernal pain can be confused with the chest pain associated with angina or myocardial infarction and cause considerable patient distress. Nocturnal aspiration of reflux contents can cause recurrent pneumonia, bronchospasm, and cough.

Sore throat, hoarseness, and halitosis are associated with reflux into the back of the throat. A reflex salivary hypersecretion is sometimes described, especially in children.

Dysphagia usually suggests long-standing GERD with acute inflammation or stricture, or both. Solid food may stick in the distal esophagus; repeated swallows and significant amounts of liquid may be required to ensure passage into the stomach.

Older adults, who may have decreased gastric acidity or decreased pain perception, may not report these symptoms despite significant disease. They are also more likely to self-treat.

Diagnosis

Diagnosis involves radiographic and endoscopic evaluation of the upper gastrointestinal (GI) tract. These procedures are determined in consultation with or by referral to a gastroenterologist. For further discussion of the diagnostic process associated with GERD, the reader is referred to management texts. The treatment protocol presented here assumes appropriate diagnosis of GERD.

Table 32–1. Foods and Drugs That Influence GERD

Foods and Drugs	Action on LES Tone
Foods Chocolate, spearmint, peppermint, decaffeinated coffee, high-fat or high-carbohydrate meals, alcohol	Decrease LES tone
Acid foods, citrus fruit and juices, caffeine	Increase gastric acid secretion
Fatty foods	Delay gastric emptying
Drugs Tobacco	Decreases LES tone and increases gastric acid secretion
Anticholinergics, theophylline, meperidine, calcium channel blockers	Decrease LES tone
Bethanechol, cisapride, metoclopramide, pentobarbital, histamine, antacids	Increase LES tone

Pharmacodynamics

Each of the contributing factors to the development of GERD is a target for pharmacological management. Drugs can be used to increase LES tone, to reduce the amount of acid in the chyme, to improve peristalsis and thereby decrease the time chyme is available to produce reflux, and to decrease the exposure of the mucosa to highly acid material. The classes of drugs with these actions include antacids, histamine$_2$ blockers, cytoprotective agents, prokinetics, and proton pump inhibitors. Figure 32–1 depicts the site of action of each of these classes of drugs.

Drugs to Improve Lower Esophageal Sphincter Tone

Metoclopramide and **bethanechol** serve a dual purpose in the management of GERD; they improve LES tone and

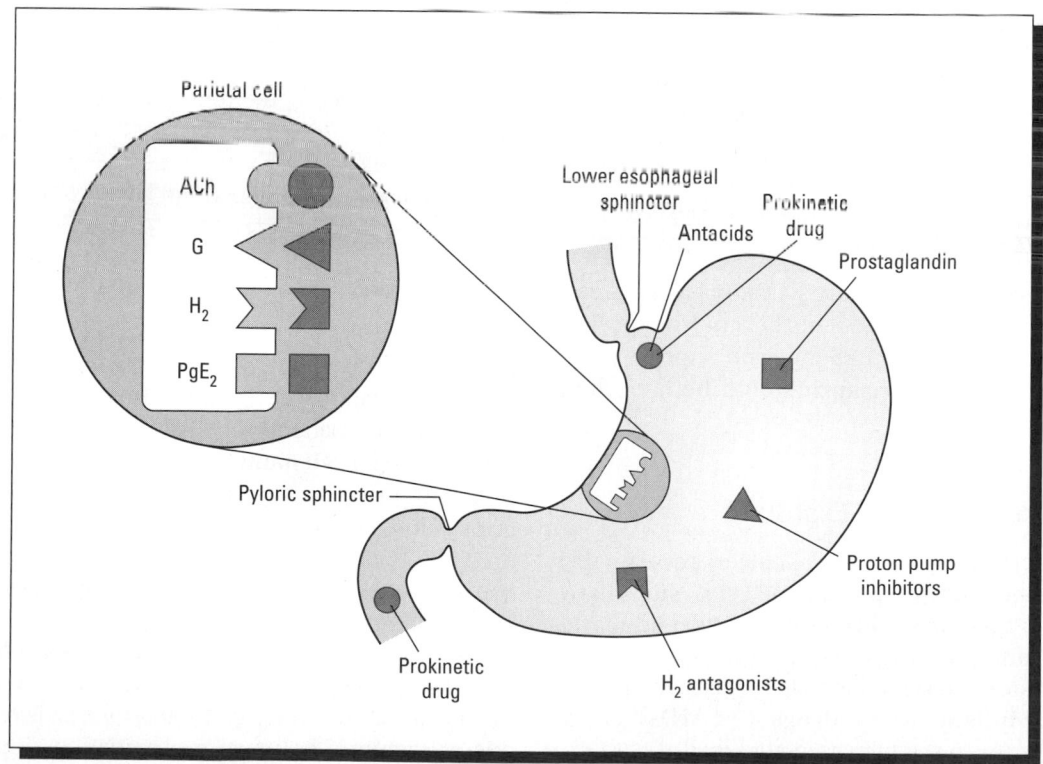

Figure 32–1. Sites of action of drugs used to treat GERD and PUD.

have a prokinetic function. They are most useful for patients who have reflux without burning pain and for those with gastroparesis. **Metoclopramide** and **bethanechol**, however, have not consistently demonstrated significant healing of esophageal lesions.

Antacids also serve a dual purpose; they improve LES tone and increase gastric pH. They are first-line drug therapy, along with lifestyle modifications.

Drugs to Reduce the Amount of Acid

Two main classes of drugs are used to reduce acid secretion. **Histamine₂ blockers** act on the parietal cells to decrease the amount of acid produced. They are added to **antacid** therapy or used to replace high-dose **antacid** therapy, providing better symptom relief and increasing esophageal healing to about 50 percent (Chiba et al., 1997).

Proton pump inhibitors act one step earlier in the production of acid and decrease almost 100 percent of acid secretion. Patients with symptoms refractory to lifestyle modification and **histamine₂ blocker** therapy and those with erosive esophagitis are candidates for therapy with this class of drugs. They improve esophageal healing to about 80 percent (Chiba et al., 1997).

Time required for healing is as important as the amount of healing. Study data (Chiba et al., 1997) suggest that healing demonstrated by endoscopy at 8 weeks is significantly higher (83.6%) for **proton pump inhibitors** than for **histamine₂ blockers** (51.9%). Note, however, that the length of therapy with **proton pump inhibitors** is limited to no more than 12 weeks without a break in therapy.

Drugs to Improve Peristalsis

A few patients continue to report symptoms despite reduced acid secretion. These patients benefit from **prokinetics,** which both improve LES tone and improve peristalsis. **Metoclopramide, cisapride,** and **bethanechol** were discussed previously.

Drugs to Decrease Mucosal Exposure

Two **cytoprotective** agents are available to decrease the exposure of the gastric mucosa to acid: **sucralfate (Carafate)** and **misoprostol (Cytotec).** Older adults or those taking multiple drugs may benefit from **sucralfate. Misoprostol** is reserved largely for use when **nonsteroidal anti-inflammatory drugs (NSAIDs)** are a contributing factor to the increased acid load.

The pharmacokinetics and pharmacodynamics of each of these categories of drugs are discussed in more detail in Chapter 18.

Goals of Treatment

There are four goals of therapy for patients with GERD: (1) reduce or eliminate the symptoms; (2) heal any esophageal lesions; (3) manage or prevent complications such as stricture, Barrett's esophagus, or esophageal carcinoma; and (4) prevent relapse. To meet these goals requires both lifestyle modification and drug therapy.

Rational Drug Selection

Algorithm

For most patients, GERD is treated with stepped therapy. The steps are based on symptom relief and degree of esophageal damage.

Step 1 involves lifestyle modifications and over-the-counter (OTC) **antacids.** Most patients have tried some step 1 interventions before they seek health care. This step alone may be sufficient for patients with mild disease and only occasional symptoms. If progression to other steps is required, step 1 interventions are continued throughout the other steps. Figure 32–2 depicts the stepped algorithm for GERD.

Lifestyle Modifications

Antireflux maneuvers, dietary changes, and cessation of smoking are central to the management of GERD regardless of the step. Antireflux maneuvers reduce back pressure on the LES from intra-abdominal contents. Dietary changes reduce the total volume and acid content of the stomach. Smoking is a factor in reducing LES tone and increasing gastric acid secretion. Table 32–2 lists appropriate lifestyle modifications.

Drug Therapy

Antacids are also appropriate for step 1. Chapter 18 discusses the various drugs in this class and provides suggestions for rational drug choice from among them.

Step 2 is for patients who fail to achieve symptom relief with step 1. **Histamine₂ blockers** are added at this step, with or without **prokinetic** agents. Doses of **histamine₂ blockers** for GERD are generally about twice those used for peptic ulcer disease (PUD). There is no evidence that once-daily or nocturnal dosing is effective for acute treatment or maintenance therapy, and they must be taken at least twice a day. Endoscopy is probably warranted at this step to assess the degree of esophageal damage. Consultation with a gastroenterologist is required for this procedure. The practice of initiating empiric treatment without diagnostic tests is questionable because of the risks associated with Barrett's esophagus and the difficulty in distinguishing GERD symptoms from *Heli-*

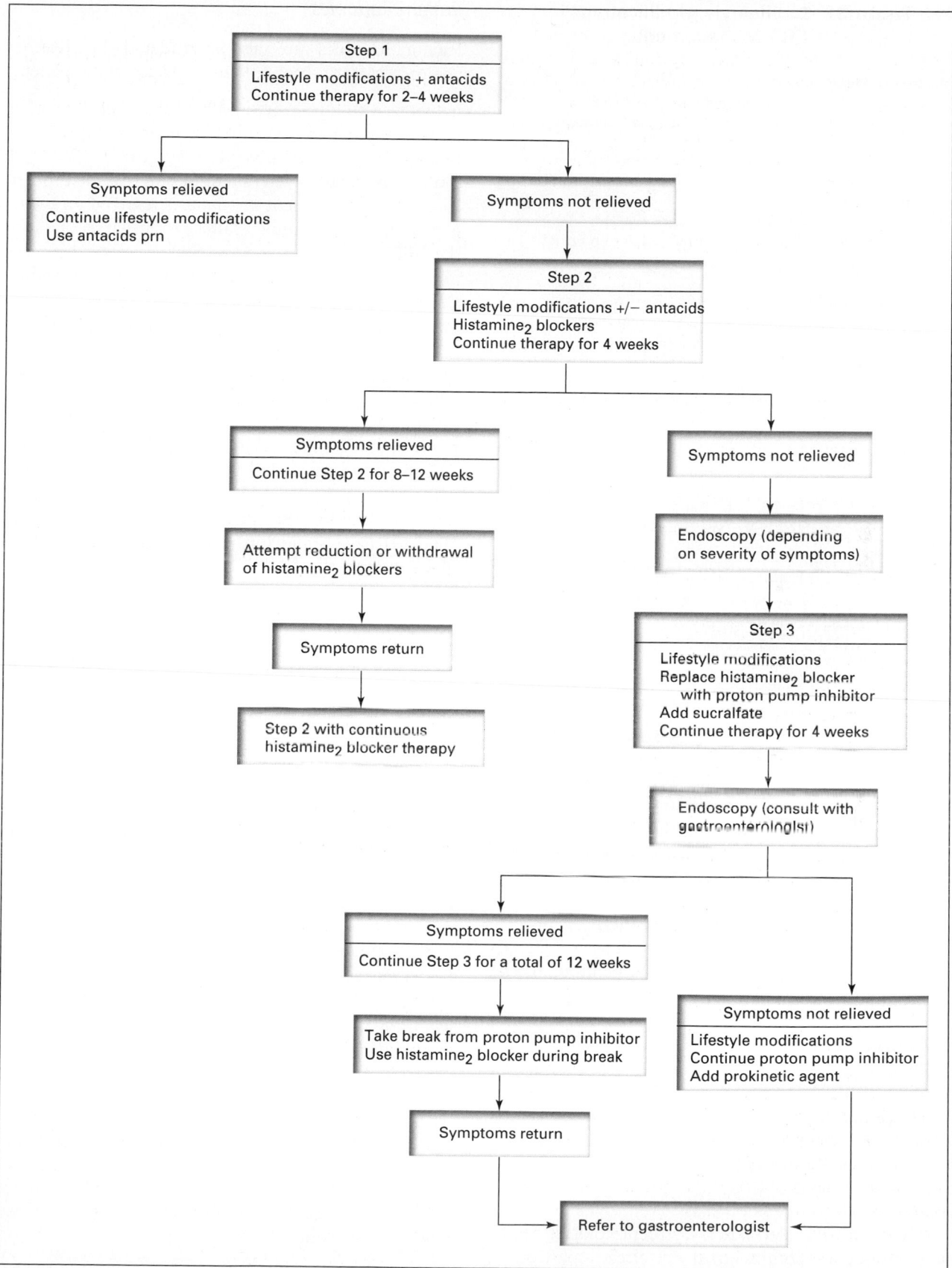

Figure 32–2. Stepped-approach algorithm for management of GERD.

Table 32–2. Lifestyle Modifications in GERD Management

Antireflux Maneuvers
- Sleep with the head of the bed elevated 6 to 8 inches with bed blocks or wedges or by using a hospital bed.
- Avoid the recumbent position within 3 hours after eating.
- Avoid bending over within 3 hours after eating.
- Avoid exercise, especially strenuous exercise, within 3 hours after eating.
- Attain and maintain appropriate body weight.
- For infants, in addition to the above, maintain upright position during and for at least 20 minutes after eating.

Dietary Considerations
- Avoid spicy, acidic, tomato-based, or fatty foods.
- Avoid chocolate, peppermint, onions, and citrus fruits and juices.
- Limit your intake of coffee, tea, alcohol, and colas.
- Eat moderate amounts of food at each meal. Do not gorge yourself.
- Avoid eating meals or bedtime snacks within 3 hours of going to bed.
- Reserve fluid intake for after or between meals.
- For infants, in addition to the above, thicken feedings with 1 tablespoon of rice cereal per ounce of formula.

Smoking Cessation
- Stop smoking. Smoking both lowers LES tone and increases the secretion of gastric acid.
- Smoking cessation is a high priority.

cobacter pylori–associated disease. Both disorders require additional specific diagnostic and treatment intervention. The American College of Gastroenterology's algorithm for the diagnosis and management of GERD suggests diagnostic testing fairly early in the process of management. None of these diagnostic procedures is inexpensive, but the long-term cost of failure to appropriately diagnose the problem can be significantly higher. Tucker and Schumann (1999) discuss these issues in their article.

Histamine₂ blockers are appropriate if there is no erosive disease. For older adults, **prokinetic** agents present some problems (discussed later). The addition of **sucralfate** 1 g before each meal and at bedtime instead of a **prokinetic** may be preferable for this age group. Rational drug choice among **histamine₂ blockers** and between **prokinetics** is discussed in Chapter 18.

Step 3 is initiated if symptoms are refractory after 4 weeks of step 2 therapy or if endoscopy shows evidence of erosive disease. **Proton pump inhibitors** are central to management at this step. They replace the **histamine₂ blocker.** **Sucralfate** is added for mucosal protection for patients of all ages. This is the last phase that is appropriately managed by the primary care provider.

Step 4 requires referral to a gastroenterologist. Step 3 interventions are continued. If not already part of the regimen, a **prokinetic** agent is added and surgery is considered.

Patient Variables

Patient variables are also considered in treatment choices. Primary among them is the age of the patient.

INFANTS AND CHILDREN. Forty-seven percent of infants younger than 2 months old regurgitate gastric contents at least twice daily. Most outgrow GERD by 10 months to 1 year. Given that most outgrow the problem, aggressive management in infants is reserved for the few experiencing concomitant failure to thrive secondary to the GERD.

Lifestyle modifications are similar to those for adults. Despite the limited number of research studies on the use of GERD-related drugs for children, they are being used for this indication.

Antacids are considered safe for pediatric use. Along with dietary adjustments, they are first-line therapy.

Clinical research supports the efficacy and safety of **histamine₂ blockers** in children as well (Glassman, George, & Grill, 1995; Hart, 1996; Hyman, 1994). Those with twice-daily dosing schedules are more likely to foster adherence in children. **Ranitidine (Zantac)** and **famotidine (Pepcid)** have liquid formulations that make pediatric dosing easier.

Cisapride is the preferred **prokinetic** agent for children. It has minimal adverse reactions in this age group. **Metoclopramide** commonly has adverse reactions in children, including restlessness, insomnia, somnolence, dystonia, and extrapyramidal symptoms. Some of the drug's antidopaminergic adverse reactions do not resolve with drug withdrawal. It is not recommended for children.

There is little published research on the use of **proton pump inhibitors** for children. Because the long-term effects of their use in children are not known, they are recommended only for cases refractory to all other measures and reserved for the final step in therapy.

There is no children's dosing schedule for **sucralfate.** It has been used but does not have Food and Drug Administration (FDA) approval for children.

In summary, infants over 2 months of age with mild GI symptoms, who are gaining weight and demonstrating age-appropriate development, can be treated empirically with lifestyle modifications and short-term (2 to 4 weeks) use of **antacids** (step 1) and **histamine₂ blockers** (step 2). When this treatment is not successful, step 3 with **cisapride** can be tried. If this therapy fails after 2 weeks, referral is required.

For children, lifestyle modification should be given a carefully monitored trial of at least 4 weeks before drug therapy is instituted. Family members and the school nurse should be involved in the therapy so that consistency can be maintained.

OLDER ADULTS. **Antacids** are generally safe in older adults, but those with constipation as an adverse reaction may be more problematic for older adults. In addition, many **antacids** have high sodium content, and some older adults are on low- to moderate-sodium diets.

Among the **histamine₂ blockers, famotidine (Pepcid)** is generally safe in the older population but should be used with caution in cases of renal insufficiency. **Nizatidine (Axid)** may cause asymptomatic ventricular tachycardia and carries a risk of hepatocellular injury. **Ranitidine (Zantac)** and **cimetidine (Tagamet)** carry risks for confusional states and toxicity in older adults. Because older adults are often taking several prescription and OTC drugs, the increased number of drug interactions associated with **cimetidine** also makes it a less attractive choice.

Among the **prokinetics, metoclopramide** has a risk for central nervous system (CNS) toxicity. In addition, it is contraindicated in congestive heart failure, renal failure, and hypokalemia, all of which are more common in older adults. **Metoclopramide** requires careful thought and monitoring in older adults.

Monitoring

Endoscopy to demonstrate the presence of lesions and their healing is the gold standard. It is usually reserved for patients who required at least step 3 therapy. For patients requiring ongoing step 3 or 4 therapy, some specialists recommend an annual endoscopy. Given its cost, others suggest endoscopy every 2 to 3 years because Barrett's esophagus is not reversible.

Esophagitis is the cause of 5 to 10 percent of all cases of upper GI bleeding. Monitoring by complete blood count at annual exams is appropriate. The remainder of monitoring is clinical evaluation of symptoms.

Outcome Evaluation

Figure 32–2 shows the treatment algorithm for GERD. Outcome evaluation targets relief of symptoms. Evaluation also includes the other goals for therapy: healing of lesions, prevention of complications, and prevention of relapse.

Relapse rates are high for patients with GERD. Lifestyle modifications and some drug therapy are commonly required for life. **Histamine₂ blocker** therapy may be required chronically but at reduced doses. Return of symptoms for a patient who has been pain-free and is adherent to the treatment regimen suggests that the provider should increase the dosage of the current drug or move the patient to the next step in the algorithm and arrange for endoscopy evaluation.

Referral to a pediatric specialist is warranted for any infant younger than 2 months old who presents with vomiting or other symptoms of GERD. Children and infants over age 2 months who are unresponsive to short-term (2 to 4 weeks at each step) empiric treatment or have suspected or demonstrated complications also require referral.

Patients who have mild or typical symptoms and who respond to conservative treatment (step 1 or 2) can be managed by the primary care provider. Patients who do not respond to 4 weeks of step 2 therapy should have endoscopy, which means at least consultation with a gastroenterologist. Patients with erosive disease or who do not respond to step 3 therapy require referral to a specialist. These patients are at high risk for Barrett's esophagus, which carries with it a 30-fold greater risk for developing esophageal cancer than the general population.

Patient Education

Patient education should include a discussion of information related to the overall treatment plan as well as that specific to the drug therapy, reasons for the drug being taken, drugs as part of the total treatment regimen, and adherence issues.

Peptic Ulcer Disease

PUD is a common clinical problem estimated to have a lifetime incidence of 5 to 10 percent. Between 1 and 2 percent of the population has an ulcer at any point in time, and approximately 200,000 to 400,000 new cases are seen in the United States each year. The rate of hospital admission for uncomplicated ulcer has decreased significantly, but the incidence has not decreased, making this largely a disease that is treated in the primary care setting. The peak incidence is in the fifth decade for men and the sixth decade for women. *H. pylori* infection has been firmly established as a major cause of PUD, but the "best" treatment option for this infection is still evolving. Reduction of stress and other factors that increase gastric acid secretion are still included in disease management.

Pathophysiology

PUD is a chronic inflammatory condition of the stomach and duodenum. It is the result of increased acid and pepsin secretion; impaired mucosal cytoprotection; use of NSAIDs; *H. pylori*; personal factors such as genetics, smoking, and stress; or a combination of these causes.

PATIENT EDUCATION

Gastroesophageal Reflux Disease

Related to the Overall Treatment Plan/Disease Process

☐ Pathophysiology of gastroesophageal reflux and its long-term risks for permanent esophageal damage and cancer of the esophagus

☐ Central role of lifestyle modifications in improving prognosis and keeping the number and cost of required drugs down

☐ Importance of adherence to the treatment regimen

☐ Need for follow-up visits with the primary care provider if the symptoms do not resolve or recur

Specific to the Drug Therapy

☐ Reason for the drug(s) being given and the anticipated action of the drug(s) on the disease process

☐ Doses and schedules for taking the drug(s)

☐ Possible adverse reactions and what to do when they occur

☐ Coping mechanisms for complex and costly drug regimens

☐ Interaction between lifestyle modifications and these drugs

Reasons for Taking the Drug(s)

Patient education about specific drugs is provided in Chapter 18. More specific information related to GERD: Drugs used to treat GERD are given to reduce symptoms, heal any esophageal ulcers, reduce the risk for permanent esophageal damage or cancer, and prevent relapse of symptoms. Different drugs have different roles with each of these. The expectations should be clear about what the drugs can and cannot do. Drugs alone will not correct the disorder.

Drugs as Part of the Total Treatment Regimen

Lifestyle modification is equally important in disease management. GERD is a chronic condition. Patients with GERD must understand the lifelong nature of the disorder and the need to incorporate the treatment regimen into their everyday lives.

Adherence Issues

Any disease process where lifestyle modifications are central to management is prone to problems with adherence. Health care providers should be aware of the potential problem of nonadherence, discuss the importance of adherence at each follow-up visit, and assist patients in removing barriers to adherence such as the complexity and cost of the treatment regimen and the presence of adverse reactions.

The incidence of gastric ulcers differs from that of duodenal ulcers. Gastric ulcer disease is about one-fourth as common as duodenal ulcer disease. The pathophysiology of the disorders also varies. Table 32–3 compares the incidence, pathophysiology, and signs and symptoms of the two disorders.

Gastric Ulcer Disease

Gastric ulcers tend to develop in the antral region, adjacent to the acid-secreting mucosa of the body. Although the pathogenesis of gastric ulcer disease is unclear, it is generally thought that the underlying defect is the

Gastroesophageal Reflux Disease

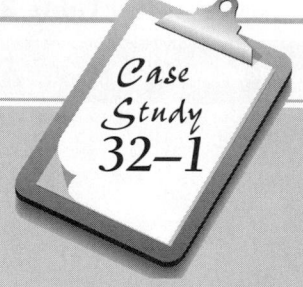

Case Study 32–1

Complaint

"My heartburn has been waking me up at night."

History

Greg is a 47-year-old man who presents at the clinic with complaints of intermittent nocturnal gastroesophageal reflux. History reveals that he awakens experiencing burning pain substernally and in the back of his throat. This results in "my larynx closing down" and his being "almost unable to breathe." As soon as he can breathe effectively, he swallows "a lot" of antacid and flushes it down with water. The entire episode is very frightening, and he is often afraid to go back to sleep. Because he already has a problem with mild sleep apnea, he is becoming increasingly tired and unable to function at work related to lack of sleep. He now sleeps only in his recliner. He is also concerned about the substernal pain because his father had a myocardial infarction at age 49 and required coronary artery bypass surgery. He is 5 feet 9 inches tall and weighs 178 pounds, with much of his excess weight carried in his abdomen. He is not a smoker, "occasionally" has three or four beers with friends, and "often" has pizza or submarine sandwiches for lunch with a "diet cola." He takes no drugs other than the antacid after a reflux episode.

Assessment

A chest x-ray and ECG are negative for cardiopulmonary disease, and Greg is diagnosed by history with GERD.

Initial Management Plan

Greg's initial management plan includes the following:

1. Discuss lifestyle modifications with a focus on weight loss, antireflux maneuvers, and dietary changes. Approximating ideal body weight will reduce intra-abdominal pressure. Antireflux maneuvers and dietary changes will reduce total volume and acid content of the stomach. With nocturnal GERD, taking food and fluids no closer than 3 hours before bedtime can significantly reduce symptoms.
2. Begin ranitidine 150 mg bid. Greg is already using antacids on a prn basis to reduce acid load. He can continue to take an antacid at bedtime. The addition of a histamine$_2$ blocker will help to reduce gastric acid secretion.
3. Draw a CBC for a baseline to assess for any potential future GI bleeding.
4. Schedule a follow-up visit in 1 month to see how things are going.

Follow-up Visit

At his follow-up visit, Greg states that the number of episodes is much lower and they are less severe, but he has still had two episodes. Careful history taking reveals that both of these episodes related to "lapses" in following the lifestyle modification. In both cases, he had friends visit, and they had consumed "three or four" beers each about 1 hour before he went to bed. He still sleeps in his recliner because "I don't want to have that feeling of not being able to breathe again." He continues to report that he does not feel rested upon awakening in the morning. He has lost 4 pounds.

Modifications to Management Plan

Greg's treatment plan now is as follows:

1. Stress the importance of lifestyle modifications while acknowledging that they are sometimes difficult to consistently maintain.
2. Leave the drug regimen in place for an additional 4 weeks. The episodes are less severe and fewer, so a full trial of 8 weeks is appropriate.
3. Follow-up visit in 1 month.

His episodes are consistently nocturnal and not postprandial so he is not tested for *H. pylori*. He has few episodes, so the risk for esophageal damage is mild to moderate at this time. Endoscopy is postponed.

Continuing Care

One month later, Greg's condition is the same. He has lost another 4 pounds, has followed the lifestyle modifications faithfully, and yet has had two nocturnal episodes of GERD. The decision is made to move him to step 3 therapy.

1. Discontinue the ranitidine.
2. Prescribe omeprazole 20 mg each morning. Proton pump inhibitors reduce a greater percentage of stomach acid, can be given once daily so that adherence is good, and have a higher healing rate for any esophageal lesions.
3. If he continues to have episodes of GERD after 4 weeks of omeprazole, consultation with a gastroenterologist will be done.

Four weeks later, Greg is symptom-free. He is sleeping in his bed and feeling more rested. His treatment plan at this time is as follows:

1. Continue the omeprazole for 4 more weeks, then discontinue it. Treatment can last as long as 12 weeks, but healing is generally accomplished in 8 weeks.
2. Return to the ranitidine bid regimen with prn antacids.
3. If symptoms recur, repeat 8-week regimen of omeprazole, send Greg for endoscopy, and consult with a gastroenterologist.

Table 32–3. Comparison of Gastric and Duodenal Ulcer Disease

Characteristic	Gastric Ulcer	Duodenal Ulcer
Age at onset	Age 50–70 years	Age 20–50 years
Gender	Equal in men and women	Most common in men
Cancer risk	Increased	Not increased
Pathophysiology Parietal cell mass	Normal or decreased	Increased
Acid production	Normal or decreased	Increased
Serum gastrin	Increased	Normal
Serum pepsinogen	Normal	Increased
Associated gastritis	More common	Usually not present
Helicobacter pylori	Present in 60–80% of cases	Present in 95–100% of cases
Clinical manifestations: pain	Located in upper abdomen Intermittent Pain>antacid>relief pattern Food>pain pattern	Located in upper abdomen Intermittent Pain>antacid or food>relief pattern Nocturnal pain common
Clinical course	Chronic ulcer without pattern of exacerbation and remission	Pattern of exacerbation and remission for years*

*This pattern is significantly affected by eradication of *H. pylori*.

disruption of the gastric mucosal barrier. A variety of substances can disrupt this barrier. They are summarized in Table 32–4. Another suggested contributing factor is increased duodenal gastric reflux of bile across an incompetent pyloric sphincter. An increased concentration of bile salts disrupts the gastric mucosa and decreases the electrical potential across the gastric mucosal membrane. This altered electrical potential permits the diffusion of hydrogen ions into the mucosa, where they disrupt permeability and cellular structure. Once the barrier is broken, the damaged submucosal areas exposed to hydrogen ions release histamine, which stimulates an increase in acid and pepsinogen production, causes local vasodilation, and increases capillary permeability. The pepsinogen produces mucosal erosion, resulting in the formation of ulcers. The disrupted mucosa becomes edematous and loses plasma proteins. Destruction of small blood vessels results in bleeding.

Pyloric stenosis has also been given as a possible cause of gastric ulcer formation. With pyloric deformity, there is poor gastric emptying, resulting in stasis and antral distention. This distention leads to increased gastrin release and gastric acid production.

Chronic gastritis has also been associated with the development of gastric ulcers. It may precipitate ulcer formation by limiting the ability of the mucosa to secrete a protective layer of mucus. Decreased mucosal synthesis

Table 32–4. Substances That Can Disrupt the Gastric Mucosal Barrier

Drugs Alcohol
Aspirin
Caffeine*
Corticosteroids
NSAIDs
Tobacco
Other Causes Bile and pancreatic secretions
Physiological and psychological stress
Salmonella
Spicy, irritating foods*
Staphylococcus organisms
Uremia associated with renal failure

*See discussion in Lifestyle Modifications section.

of prostaglandin (e.g., NSAIDs) may also create an ulcerogenic environment.

Duodenal Ulcer Disease

Infection with *H. pylori* is the major cause of duodenal ulcers. With the exception of patients taking **NSAIDs,** 95 to 100 percent of patients with duodenal ulcer are infected with this organism. It is a spiral-shaped bacterium that lives attached to or just above the gastric mucosa. Once *H. pylori* is acquired, colonization continues for life unless the organism is eliminated by **antimicrobial** treatment or the usually late-in-life development of atrophic gastritis. Essentially everyone who carries the organism in the gastric mucosal layer has evidence of some tissue reaction (e.g., an inflammatory response and chronic active gastritis), yet most colonized patients remain asymptomatic for life. The strain of *H. pylori* with which an individual is colonized (spiral shape, flagella, and specific ability to attach to Lewis B antigens in persons with type O blood) affects risk for disease.

Once attached to the mucosal layer, *H. pylori* releases toxins, proteases, and phospholipase enzymes that promote inflammation and impair the integrity of the mucosal layer. The inflammatory process includes the release of histamine, which acts the same on the duodenal mucosa and on the gastric mucosa. The end result is ulceration.

There is one caveat in the rush to eradicate *H. pylori*. It appears that, like many other bacteria (e.g., *Escherichia coli*), *H. pylori* may serve a useful function in our bodies and only occasionally cause disease. A cofactor may need to be present for duodenal ulcers to form. Hypersecretion of acid and pepsin, inadequate secretion of bicarbonate by the duodenal mucosa, a greater-than-usual number of parietal cells in the gastric mucosa, serum gastrin levels that remain high longer than normal after eating, failure of a feedback mechanism whereby acid in the gastric antrum inhibits gastrin release, and rapid gastric emptying that overwhelms the buffering capacity of the bicarbonate-rich pancreatic secretion may all contribute to ulcer formation.

Because colonization with *H. pylori* appears to increase the risk for duodenal ulcers but seems to decrease the risk for certain other diseases (e.g., esophageal diseases), an important question for providers is which patients should be treated. Because there is little evidence of improvement in symptoms of nonulcer dyspepsia by eradication of *H. pylori,* patients with this disorder probably should not be treated. Nevertheless, eradication of *H. pylori* is associated with reduced development of chronic atrophic gastritis, a precursor to one form of gastric cancer. Patients with risk factors for gastric cancer probably should be treated. Blaser (1999) discusses these issues and recommends that providers search for and treat *H. pylori* only in those patients with PUD and gastric mucosal–associated lymphoid tissue (MALT)

lymphomas. In such patients, the benefits outweigh the risks.

Diagnosis

Diagnosis involves radiographic and endoscopic evaluation of the upper GI tract and testing for *H. pylori* colonization. Patients who have previously diagnosed duodenal ulcers or who no have history of ingestion of **NSAIDs,** no evidence of a hypersecretory state, and no history of treatment with an **antimicrobial** that might have cured *H. pylori* are so likely to have *H. pylori* infection that a diagnostic test adds little information but does add cost.

Diagnostic procedures are determined in consultation with or by referral to a gastroenterologist. For further discussion of the diagnostic process associated with PUD, the reader is referred to management texts. The treatment protocol presented here assumes appropriate diagnosis of PUD.

Pharmacodynamics

The same drugs that are used to treat GERD are used to treat gastric and duodenal ulcers that are not caused by *H. pylori*. Reduction of acid secretion is accomplished with **histamine$_2$ blocker** or **proton pump inhibitor** therapy with a trial of 6 weeks. **Sucralfate** may be used to protect the gastric mucosa. **Antacids** may provide some symptom relief but do little to heal ulcers. These drugs were previously discussed here and in Chapter 18, which also presents the dosing schedule for treatment of PUD.

When eradication of *H. pylori* is desired, treatment includes a 2-week course of **antimicrobial** therapy. Antimicrobial agents used include **clarithromycin, tetracycline, amoxicillin,** and **metronidazole**. They are given in double or triple drug regimens with **histamine$_2$ blockers, proton pump inhibitors,** or **bismuth subsalicylate.** Acid suppression by the **histamine$_2$ blocker** or **proton pump inhibitor** in conjunction with the **antimicrobial** helps alleviate the ulcer-related symptoms, heals gastric mucosal inflammation, and may enhance the efficacy of the **antimicrobial** agent against *H. pylori* at the mucosal surface. **Antimicrobials** are discussed in more detail in Chapter 22.

Goals of Treatment

Goals of treatment for PUD are similar to those for GERD: (1) reduce or eliminate the symptoms, (2) heal any ulcers, (3) manage or prevent complications such as GI bleeding or the development of gastric carcinoma, and (4) prevent relapse. To meet these goals requires both lifestyle modification and drug therapy, but lifestyle modification is less important in PUD than in GERD.

Rational Drug Selection

Algorithm

The treatment algorithm is slightly different for patients with gastric disease as compared with those who have duodenal disease. Both are treated with a stepped approach. The steps are based on symptom relief, presence of complications, and likelihood of *H. pylori* infection. Ulcers that are associated with **NSAID** use are discussed in Chapter 23.

As with GERD, step 1 involves lifestyle modifications and OTC **antacids**. Most patients have tried some step 1 interventions before they seek health care. This step alone may be sufficient for patients with mild disease and only occasional symptoms, but this step alone is not likely to heal any ulcers. Progression to step 2 is usually required, especially for duodenal ulcers and for those that are a result of *H. pylori* infection. Figure 32–3 depicts the stepped algorithm for gastric ulcer disease, and Figure 32–4, that for duodenal ulcer disease.

Step 2 for patients with uncomplicated gastric ulcers and typical histories is the addition of **histamine₂ blockers** twice a day and **sucralfate** 1 g four times a day before meals and at bedtime. This regimen reduces gastric acid secretion and provides mucosal protection. It will heal most gastric ulcers, but a longer duration of treatment than that used to heal duodenal ulcers is commonly needed with this regimen to heal gastric ulcers because the average ulcer size is larger and healing does not correlate as well with gastric acid secretion. **Proton pump inhibitors** may be used instead of **histamine₂ blockers**. Although they are more expensive, they heal a higher percentage of ulcers but are intended for no more than 12 weeks of therapy. Maintenance therapy with an **antisecretory** agent, usually a **histamine₂ blocker**, at the full healing doses is necessary. Prevention of recurrence usually lasts only as long as maintenance therapy is continued, and up to 90 percent of ulcers recur once maintenance therapy is stopped.

Ulcers complicated by bleeding require endoscopy for diagnosis of the lesion. Healing should also be documented by endoscopy after 8 weeks of **antisecretory therapy**. There is inconsistent support for the use of **proton pump inhibitors** versus other drugs for healing ulcers associated with bleeding.

For duodenal ulcers, step 2 involves testing for *H. pylori* except when diagnostic testing adds cost but little additional information as previously discussed. Noninvasive testing includes serologic tests and breath tests. These tests do not determine if an ulcer is present but indicate if the patient is infected with *H. pylori*. Invasive tests include endoscopy, during which biopsy specimens are obtained. These tests diagnose both ulcers and infection. Table 32–5 depicts the sensitivity, specificity, and relative cost of these tests. Serologic testing is the least expensive and appropriate for most patients because, in a population with a high prevalence of *H. pylori* infection, the positive predictive value of this test is 95 percent for patients with active infection (Speicher, 1998). Patients with evidence of active bleeding or in a population where prevalence of *H. pylori* colonization is not high may need invasive testing.

Patients without *H. pylori* infection are treated in the same manner as gastric ulcer patients. Conventional treatment with a **histamine₂ blocker** and **sucralfate** heals 70 to 90 percent of duodenal ulcers with 8 weeks of treatment. Replacing the **histamine₂ blocker** with a **proton pump inhibitor** shortens healing time to about 4 weeks.

Patients with *H. pylori* infection have one of the drug protocols for eradication of that organism instituted at step 2. Table 32–6 shows the various drug protocols. Treatment with one of these protocols heals up to 90 percent of duodenal ulcers in 6 to 8 weeks. In addition, many clinical treatment trials have demonstrated that curing infection is associated with a marked reduction in ulcer recurrence rates. Duodenal and gastric ulcers recur in up to 80 percent of patients treated with drugs to reduce gastric acid but not treated for eradication of *H. pylori* infection. By comparison, 6 to 15 percent of patients have recurrent ulcers when their *H. pylori* infection is cured.

In 1994, the National Institutes of Health (NIH) expert panel in the area of GI and infectious disease recommended that patients with ulcers who are infected with *H. pylori* undergo **antimicrobial** therapy to eradicate that infection. Economic analysis demonstrates that curing an ulcer takes less time and costs substantially less than the cost of treating ulcer symptoms over a patient's lifetime. The most extreme treatment, vagotomy or ulcer surgery, costs approximately $17,000. Maintenance with **antisecretory agents** costs approximately $11,000 over 15 years. In comparison, the drug protocol for eradication of *H. pylori* costs less than $1000 and takes 14 to 17 days (Gold, 1999).

Maintenance therapy with an **antisecretory** agent is not generally required after eradication of *H. pylori*. However, it is prudent to prescribe maintenance therapy for certain high-risk groups: smokers; patients over age 60; patients with chronic obstructive pulmonary disease, coronary artery disease, or renal failure; patients with a history of bleeding or perforated ulcer; patients with persistent symptoms; and those who must take **NSAIDs** or other ulcerogenic drugs.

Step 3 for patients with gastric or duodenal ulcers is for those who fail to become symptom-free or who develop complications such as GI bleeding while on **antisecretory therapy**. This step requires referral to a gastroenterologist. Surgery is contemplated at this step for gastric ulcer patients.

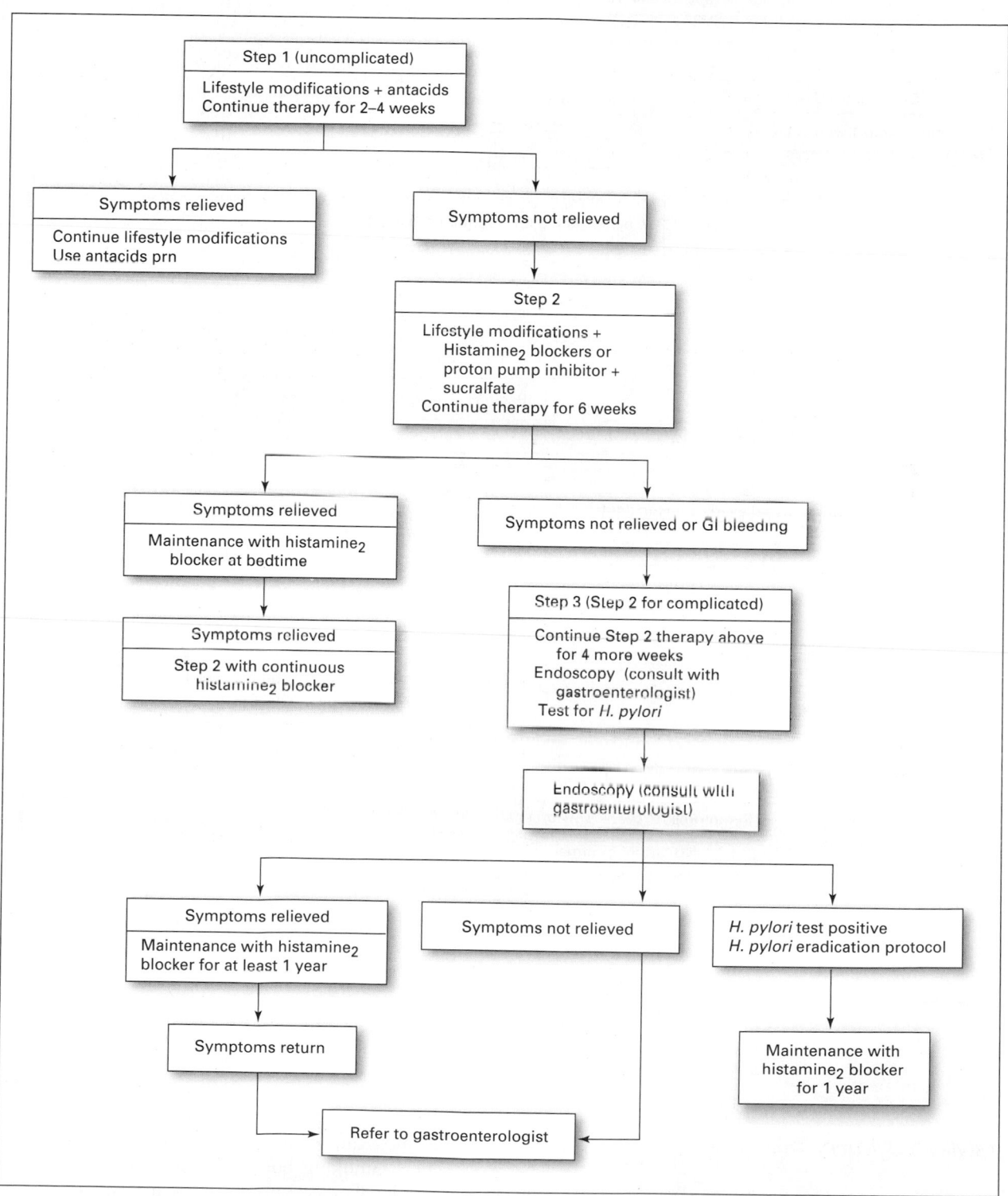

Figure 32–3. Algorithm for gastric ulcer disease.

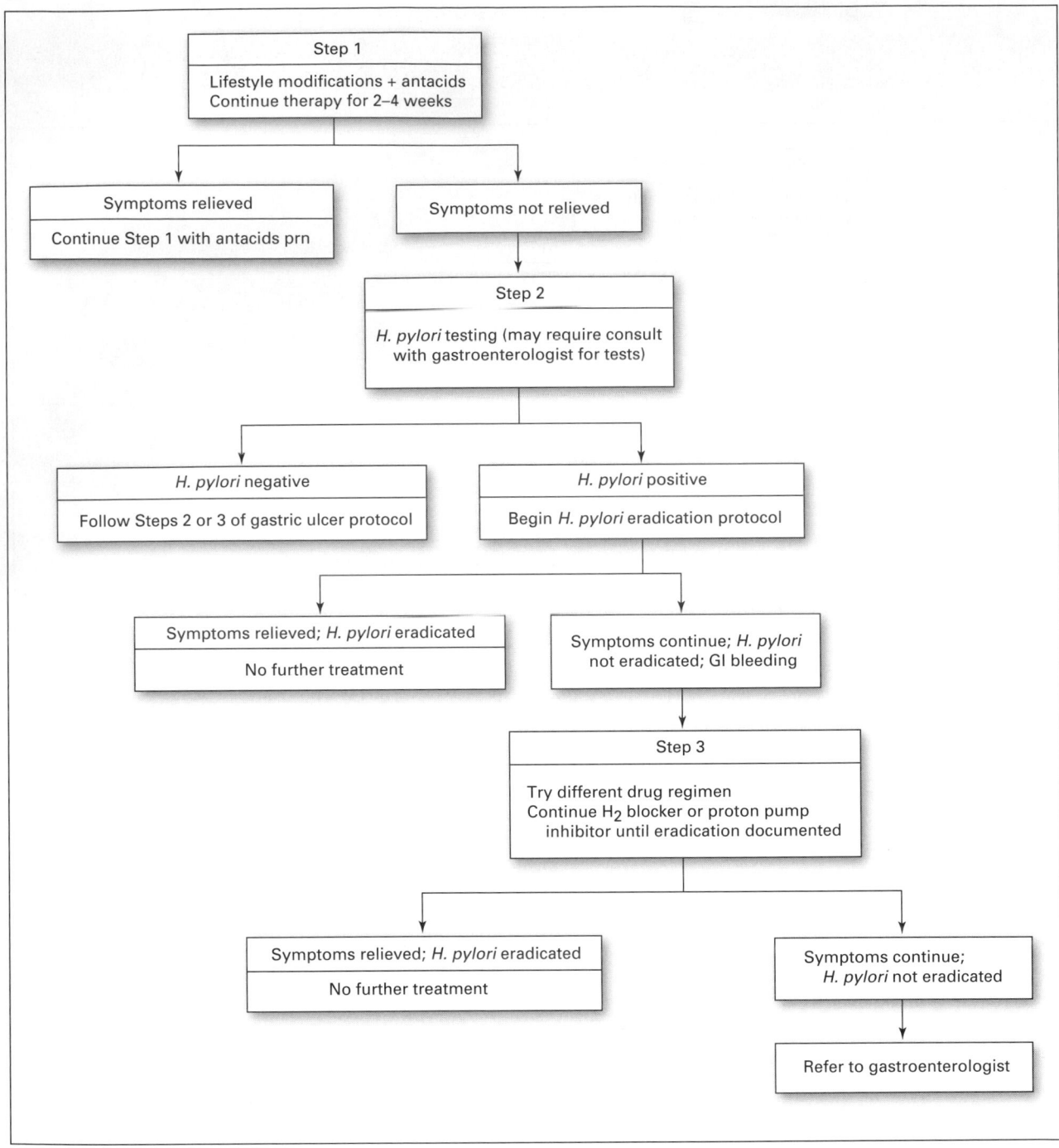

Figure 32–4. Algorithm for duodenal ulcer disease.

Lifestyle Modifications

There is no evidence that dietary modifications affect the course of PUD. Frequent small meals and decreased consumption of spices, **alcohol,** caffeine, and fruit juices have never been demonstrated to effect healing. Dietary changes should be directed at those substances that cause symptoms in each particular patient.

The most important lifestyle modification is smoking cessation. Smoking both increases the risk for gastric and duodenal ulcers and delays their healing.

Aspirin and **NSAIDs** are known to be ulcerogenic. Their use should be discouraged. One study (Chan et al., 1997), however, found that eradication of *H. pylori* infection prior to beginning **NSAID** therapy decreased the risk for ulcer formation in patients taking **NSAIDs.**

Table 32–5. Invasive and Noninvasive Diagnostic Tests for *H. pylori*

Test	Sensitivity	Specificity	Relative Cost*
Noninvasive			
Serologic evaluation	88–99%	85–95%	1
Urea breath test	90–98%	90–100%	2
Invasive			
Biopsy urease test	89–98%	95–100%	4
Culture of biopsy specimen	72–92%	100%	5
Histologic evaluation	93–99%	95–99%	5

*Relative cost is calculated against the cost of serologic evaluation, which is given a relative value of 1.

Drug Therapy

Currently, the FDA approves eight treatment regimens; however, several other combinations have been used successfully. Regimens include double or triple drug therapy with a variety of drugs. The FDA-approved treatment options (as of July 1998) and other regimens with reported success rates above 90 percent are presented in Table 32–6.

Antimicrobial resistance and lack of adherence to a complex regimen for 2 weeks are the two main reasons for treatment failure. To overcome these problems, reducing the regimen to 7 days has been tried. The results have not been favorable. Laine and colleagues (1998) conducted a multicenter trial of dual and triple therapies, all but one of which were 7-day regimens. Conclusions drawn from their data are:

1. Dual therapy seems to be inadequate for the eradication of *H. pylori*.
2. Eradication rates were 57 to 59 percent with these regimens.
3. Regimens that include **metronidazole** seem to be less effective, presumably because there is more resistance to this agent. DiPiro and colleagues (1999) report a resistance rate as high as 50 percent.
4. Even the best triple-therapy regimen may not be adequate if given for only 7 days. Eradication rates were 67 to 82 percent.
5. The best regimens seem to be those that are at least 10 days long and include two **antimicrobials** and an **antisecretory** agent.

DiPiro and colleagues (1999) state that when **amoxicillin** is substituted for **tetracycline,** eradication rates decline to 75 percent from 90 percent. Increasing the length of therapy to up to 1 month did not seem to improve on this lower rate. The Centers for Disease Control and Prevention (CDC) fact sheet (1999) recommends that **amoxicillin** be reserved for patients who cannot take **tetracycline.** The computer link to this fact sheet is shown in the reference list.

Selection among the protocols is based on cost, convenience, ability to tolerate the adverse drug reactions of the total regimen, **antimicrobial** resistance, patient variables, and eradication rates. Eradication rates, shown in Table 32–6, were discussed previously related to length of regimen and dual versus triple therapy.

Dual-drug regimens, those that do not contain a **proton pump inhibitor** (they are expensive), and those that contain **amoxicillin** (which is less expensive), may be lower in cost and more convenient, but eradication data suggest that they are not the most likely to be efficacious. For each patient, assess the likelihood of adherence and use the most cost-effective but simplest drug regimen that will get the job done.

Adverse Drug Reactions for the Total Regimen

Adverse drug reactions have been reported in up to 70 percent of patients taking bismuth-based four-drug regimens. These reactions are lower (30 percent) for patients taking **proton pump inhibitor**–based regimens. They are lowest for two-drug regimens (15%), but these regimens are equally low in efficacy. **Metronidazole**-based regimens have increased adverse reactions (DiPiro, 1999). Overall, the best regimen for tolerability appears to be **proton pump inhibitor**–based three-drug regimens. Happily, these regimens also are highly efficacious.

Antimicrobial Resistance

There is increasing concern about **antimicrobial** resistance, regardless of the disease process for which these drugs are being used. Chapter 22 discusses resistance to the various **antimicrobials.** Resistance associated with *H. pylori* eradication has been linked to the length and complexity of the treatment regimen and the tolerability of adverse reactions. Resistance to **metronidazole** is most common and higher in women, probably because of its use to treat genital infections. Resistance to **clarithromycin** is low (10%), as is resistance to **amoxicillin**

Table 32–6. Drug Treatment Protocols for *H. pylori* Eradication

Drug 1	Drug 2	Drug 3	Comments	Eradication Rate
Omeprazole 40 mg qd	Clarithromycin 500 mg tid		× 14 d + omeprazole 20 qd × 14 d*	70%
Omeprazole 20 mg bid	Clarithromycin 500 mg bid	Amoxicillin 1g bid	× 10 d*	>90%
Omeprazole 20 mg bid	Clarithromycin 250 mg bid	Metronidazole 500 mg bid	× 14 d	>90%
Lansoprazole 30 mg tid	Amoxicillin 1g tid		× 14 d*	<60%
Lansoprazole 30 mg bid	Amoxicillin 1g bid	Clarithromycin 500 mg tid	× 10 d*	NA
Lansoprazole 30 mg bid	Amoxicillin 1g bid	Clarithromycin 500 mg bid	× 10 d*	NA
Tetracycline 500 mg qid	Metronidazole 250 mg qid	Bismuth subsalicylate 2 tabs qid	× 14 d + histamine₂ blocker for 4 wk*	>90%
Tetracycline 500 mg qid	Clarithromycin 500 mg tid	Bismuth subsalicylate 2 tabs qid	× 14 days + antisecretory drug	>90%
Amoxicillin 500 mg qid	Clarithromycin 500 mg tid	Bismuth subsalicylate 2 tabs qid	× 14 d + antisecretory drug	>90%
Amoxicillin 500 mg qid	Metronidazole 250 mg tid	Bismuth subsalicylate 2 tabs qid	× 14 d + antisecretory drug	>90%
Amoxicillin 750 mg tid	Clarithromycin 500 mg tid		× 14 d + antisecretory drug	>90%
Amoxicillin 750 mg tid	Metronidazole 500 mg tid		× 14 d + antisecretory drug	>85%
Ranitidine bismuth citrate (RBC) 400 mg bid	Clarithromycin 500 mg tid		× 14 d + RBC for 14 d*	<60%
RBC 400 mg bid	Clarithromycin 500 mg bid		× 14 d + RBC for 14 d*	<60%

All regimens are taken with meals.
*These treatment protocols are FDA-approved.

and **tetracycline.** Acquired resistance occurs in up to two-thirds of treatment failures. Changing drugs and trying a different treatment regimen may be useful in these instances.

Patient Variables

Several patient variables need to be considered. Patients with allergies to any of the drugs in a treatment regimen require a different regimen. Women of childbearing age require careful consideration before they are prescribed

tetracycline because of the risk for fetal harm. Each of the drugs in these regimens has potential drug interactions. Other drugs the patient may be taking must be taken into account.

Given all these parameters, the treatment regimen with good to excellent eradication rates, a low to medium adverse reactions profile, likelihood of adherence based on complexity of the regimen and moderate cost, and limited **antimicrobial** resistance appears to be **clarithromycin** plus **amoxicillin** plus **omeprazole**, all taken twice a day for 14 days.

PATIENT EDUCATION

Peptic Ulcer Disease

Related to the Overall Treatment Plan/Disease Process

☐ Understanding the pathophysiology of ulcer formation and its long-term risks for bleeding and cancer of the stomach

☐ Role of lifestyle modifications in total treatment regimen

☐ Importance of adherence to the treatment regimen, especially in light of antimicrobial resistance

☐ Need for follow-up visits with the primary care provider if the symptoms recur or do not resolve

Specific to the Drug Therapy

☐ Reason for the drug(s) being given and the anticipated action of the drug(s) on the disease process

☐ Doses and schedules for taking the drug(s)

☐ Possible adverse reactions and what to do when they occur

☐ Coping mechanisms for complex and costly drug regimens

☐ Interactions between lifestyle modifications and these drugs

Reasons for Taking the Drug(s)

Patient education about specific drugs is provided in Chapters 18 and 22. More specific information related to PUD includes: Drugs used to treat PUD are given to reduce symptoms, heal any ulcers, reduce the risk for complications, and prevent relapse of symptoms. Different drugs have different roles with each of these. The expectations should be clear about what the drugs can and cannot do.

Drugs as Part of the Total Treatment Regimen

Lifestyle modification is important in disease management. PUD is often a chronic condition, requiring lifelong maintenance therapy.

Adherence Issues

Any disease process where lifestyle modifications are required or where a complex regimen of three or four drugs over a period of weeks is required is likely to have problems with adherence. Health care providers should be aware of the potential problem of nonadherence, discuss the importance of adherence, and assist patients in removing barriers to adherence, such as the complexity and cost of the treatment regimen and the presence of adverse reactions.

Monitoring

Monitoring parameters for each of the drugs in these treatment regimens are presented in Chapters 18 and 22. Documentation of ulcer healing by endoscopy 4 to 8 weeks after the end of therapy is the gold standard. Cost considerations suggest reserving it for patients who are at high risk for complications, patients with recurrence, and those who will be on long-term therapy. The urea breath test can be used to screen symptomatic patients who are suspected of having recurrent ulcers associated with *H. pylori* infection. Documentation by endoscopy is optional for low-risk patients.

Outcome Evaluation

Figures 32–3 and 32–4 show the treatment algorithms for PUD. Outcome evaluation targets relief of symptoms. Evaluation also includes the other goals for therapy: healing of lesions, prevention of complications, and prevention of relapse. Relapse rates are high for patients with PUD but can be significantly reduced with appropriate maintenance therapy or eradication of *H. pylori* infection.

Patients with PUD who remain symptom-free without drugs or on maintenance therapy require no more frequent follow-up than with their annual physical examination.

Patients with PUD not associated with *H. pylori* infection who are not responsive to therapy or who develop complications such as bleeding require consultation with or referral to a gastroenterologist. Patients with *H. pylori* infection–associated ulcers that do not respond to the first course of antimicrobial therapy should have a second course of therapy with a different drug combination. If they still have symptoms and eradication fails, referral to a gastroenterologist is appropriate. Other causes, such as Zollinger-Ellison syndrome, may be present.

Patient Education

Patient education should include a discussion of information related to the overall treatment plan as well as that specific to the drug therapy, reasons for the drug being taken, drugs as part of the total treatment regimen, and adherence issues.

REFERENCES

Ault, D., & Schmidt, D. (1998). Diagnosis and management of gastroesophageal reflux in infants and children. *Nurse Practitioner, 23* (60), 78–100.

Bazaldua, O., & Schneider, F. (1999). Evaluation and management of dyspepsia. *American Family Physician, 60*(6), 1773–1784, 1787–1788.

Blaser, M. (1999). In the world of black and white, *Helicobacter pylori* is gray. *Annals of Internal Medicine, 130*(8), 695–697.

Centers for Disease Control and Prevention. (1999). *Heliobacter pylori:* Fact sheet for health care providers. *www.cdc.gov/ncidod/dbmd/hpylori.htm.*

Chan, F., Sung, J., Chung, C., To, K., Yung, M., Leung, V., Lee, Y., Chan, C., Li, E., & Woo, J. (1997). Randomized trial of eradication of *Helicobacter pylori* before non-steroidal anti-inflammatory drug therapy to prevent peptic ulcers. *Lancet, 350,* 975–979.

Chiba, N., DeGara, C., Wilkinson, J., & Hunt, R. (1997). Speed of healing and symptoms relief in grade II to IV gastroesophageal reflux disease: A meta-analysis. *Gastroenterology, 112,* 1798–1810.

Deglin, J., & Vallerand, A. (1998). *Davis's drug guide for nurses* (6th ed.). Philadelphia: F. A. Davis.

DiPiro, J., Talbert, R, Yee, G., Matzke, G., Wells, B., & Posey, L. (1999). *Pharmacotherapy: A pathophysiological approach* (4th ed.). Stamford, CT: Appleton & Lange.

Drewitz, D., Sampliner, R., & Garewal, H. (1997). The incidence of adenocarcinoma in Barrett's esophagus: A prospective study of 170 patients followed 4.8 years. *American Journal of Gastroenterology, 92,* 212–215.

Earnest, D., & Robinson, M. (1999). Treatment advances in acid secretory disorders: The promise of rapid symptom relief with disease resolution. *American Journal of Gastroenterology, 94*(11, Suppl.), S17–S24.

Glassman, M., George, D., & Grill, B. (1995). Gastroesophageal reflux in children: Clinical manifestation, diagnosis and therapy. *Gastroenterology Clinics of North America, 24,* 71–98.

Gold, B. (1999). *H. pylori:* The key to cure for most ulcer patients. Atlanta: Division of Bacterial and Mycotic Diseases, National Center for Infectious Diseases, Centers for Disease Control and Prevention.

Hart, J. (1996). Pediatric gastroesophageal reflux. *American Family Physician, 54*(8), 2463–2471.

Hyman, P. (1994). Gastroesophageal reflux: One reason why baby won't eat. *Journal of Pediatrics, 125*(6) S103–S109.

Kastrup, E. (1998). *Drug facts and comparisons.* St. Louis: Facts and Comparisons.

Khuroo, M., Yattoo, G., Javid, G., Khan, B., Shah, A., Gulzar, G., & Sodi, J. (1997). A comparison of omeprazole and placebo for bleeding peptic ulcer. *New England Journal of Medicine, 336,* 1054–1058.

Laine, L., Estrada, R., Trujillo, M., Knigge, K., & Fennerty, M. (1998). Effect of proton-pump inhibitor therapy on diagnostic testing for *Helicobacter pylori. Annals of Internal Medicine, 129*(7), 547–550.

Laine, L., Franz, J. Baker, A., & Neil, G. (1997). A United States multicenter trial of dual and proton pump inhibitor-based triple therapies for *Helicobacter pylori. Alimentary Pharmacologic Therapy, 11,* 913–917.

Middlemiss, C. (1997). Gastroesophageal reflux disease: A common condition in the elderly. *Nurse Practitioner, 22*(11), 51–59.

National Institutes of Health Consensus Development Conference. (1994). *Helicobacter pylori* in peptic ulcer disease. *Journal of the American Medical Association, 272,* 65–69.

Navuluri, R., & Yue, S. (1999). Understanding peptic ulcer disease pharmacotherapeutics. *Nurse Practitioner, 24*(3), 128–132.

Nefesoglu, F., Ayanoglu-Dulger, G., Ulusoy, N., & Imeryuz, N. (1998). Interaction of omeprazole with enteric-coated salicylate tablets. *International Journal of Clinical Pharmacology and Therapeutics, 36*(10), 549–553.

Schmidt, B. (1999). *Instructions for pediatric patients* (2nd ed.). Philadelphia: Saunders.

Speicher, C. (1998). *The right test* (3rd ed.). Philadelphia: Saunders.

Sung, J., Chan, F., Wu, J., Leung, W., Suen, R., Ling, T., Lee, Y., Cheng, A., & Chung, S. (1999). One-week ranitidine bismuth citrate in combination with metronidazole, amoxicillin and clarithromycin in the treatment of *Helicobacter pylori* infection: The RBC-MACH study. *Alimentary Pharmacology and Therapeutics, 13*(8), 1079–1084.

Tucker, K., & Schumann, L. (1999). Gastroesophageal reflux disease. *Clinical Advisor, 2*(4), (April), 52–58.

Van der Hulst, R., Rauws, E., Koycu, B., Keller, J., Bruno, M., Tijssen, J., & Tytgat, G. (1997). Prevention of ulcer recurrence after eradication of *Helicobacter pylori:* A prospective long-term follow-up study. *Gastroenterology, 113,* 1082–1086.

Yamamoto, T., Takano, K., Sanaka, M., Kuyama, Y., Yamanaka, M., Koike, Y., & Mineshita, S. (1998). Pharmacokinetic characteristics of cisapride in elderly patients. *International Journal of Clinical Pharmacology and Therapeutics, 36*(8), 432–434.

CHAPTER 33

·······

Headaches

CHAPTER OUTLINE

eadaches are a common presenting complaint in primary care, accounting for 18 million outpatient visits per year in the United States. This makes headaches the seventh leading chief complaint in ambulatory clinics. More than 80 percent of adult Americans report that they experience recurrent headache, with 35 to 50 percent labeling their headache severe enough to disrupt their activities of daily living (Marin, 1998; Smith, 1998). The cost of direct medical care for migraine is $1 billion, and the cost to American employers, $13 billion annually because of missed work days and impaired work function (Hu, 1999). Successful pharmacological management of headache can improve the quality of life for millions of Americans.

Headaches affect all age groups, from preverbal children to the older patient. When asked, 20 to 40 percent of school-age children report having had headaches. The onset of migraine usually occurs between the ages of 15 and 25, although younger children may experience migraine. The peak incidence of headache is in young adulthood (age 25 to 34), with the incidence waning as the patient population gets older. Onset of headache after age 50 or headaches increasing in frequency or severity should lead to the investigation of underlying neurological disease.

The most common types of headaches can be classified as migraine, tension-type, and chronic daily headache, which may present as a mixed form of tension type and migraine, or transformed migraine. Drug-rebound headache is also identified as a cause of chronic daily headache. Cluster headaches are rare but severely debilitating. The pharmacological management of these common types of headaches is discussed in this chapter. Pathological headaches, caused by space-occupying lesions, alterations in intracranial pressure, or other pathology, are not discussed here, other than to note when the differential should lead to pathology rather than to common headaches.

Migraine

Migraine headaches are a complex multifactorial condition, which may be classified into three categories: migraine with aura (classic migraine), migraine without aura (common migraine), and complicated migraine. Classification of migraine, although important for accurate diagnosis, does not affect the pharmacological management. This chapter discusses acute or abortive therapy and preventive therapy, as well as nonpharmacological therapy for treating migraine.

Pathophysiology

There are several theories regarding the pathogenesis of migraine headache. The vascular theory proposes that the aura preceding migraine is caused by vasoconstriction of intracranial vessels, and vasodilation of the affected vessels results in the typical vascular headache pain that throbs in unison with the pulse. The vascular theory has been disputed because not all migraine sufferers have a pulsatile quality to their headache pain.

Considerable evidence associates migraine with changes in serotonin activity that result in release of vasoactive neurotransmitters (substance P, bradykinin, neurokinin A, and calcitonin gene-related peptides). This produces an inflammatory response around the blood vessels of the dura mater and pia mater and is accompanied by dilation of cerebral blood vessels. Specific excitatory serotonin receptors ($5-HT_2$), when activated, can lead to migraine. Many of the abortive agents used for migraine appear to stimulate inhibitory serotonin receptors ($5-HT_1$ and $5-HT_{1D}$) or block $5-HT_2$ receptors.

There is a strong familial component to migraine, with 20 to 60 percent of patients reporting a family history of migraine. Migraine is two to three times more prevalent in women than in men. Women with migraines may have increased headaches around the time of their menstrual periods and if they are taking estrogen-containing medications, such as oral contraceptives. Other known triggers of migraine include **alcohol,** strong light, noxious odors, extreme fatigue, and certain foods. Table 33–1 lists common triggers that may precipitate a migraine headache in patients prone to migraine.

Goals of Treatment

The overall goal of therapy is to minimize the impact of migraine headaches on patients' quality of life, social functioning, and ability to work. A second goal is prevention of migraine by avoiding each patient's identified triggers and prophylaxis for frequent migraine sufferers. Minimiz-

Table 33–1. Common Migraine Triggers

Factor	Triggers
Environmental factors	Noxious smells and fumes Bright light or glare Tobacco smoke
Foods	Caffeine (coffee, tea, caffeine-containing medications or beverages) Nuts, peanut butter, pea pods, lima or navy beans Alcohol (red wine, beer, liquor) Aged cheese MSG (in Chinese food, seasoning salt, processed foods, soups) Chocolate (sweets, foods, drinks) Nitrites and nitrates (processed meats, hot dogs) Onions Avocados Dairy products (ice cream, yogurt, cheese, sour cream, milk, cream) Pickled or smoked foods (pickled herring, smoked fish) Citrus fruits, bananas, figs, raisins Aspartame (in many foods and drinks labeled "sugar-free") Sulfites Yeast products (in bread, donuts)
Lifestyle	Hunger/fasting Oversleeping Inadequate sleep Stress Lack of exercise Prolonged sitting in an uncomfortable position Extended computer usage
Hormonal	Menses Menopause Oral contraceptives Hormonal replacement therapy
Medications	Nitroglycerin Oral contraceptives Antihypertensives Theophylline Antibiotics (TMP-SMZ, griseofulvin) Histamine$_2$ blockers (cimetidine, ranitidine) Analgesic or ergotamine overuse Indomethacin

ing adverse effects of pharmacotherapy and avoidance of medication overuse/abuse that can lead to drug-rebound headache should also be goals of both the provider and the patient.

Rational Drug Selection

Pharmacological management of migraine is divided into two major components: acute or abortive therapy and preventive or prophylactic therapy. Most patients with migraine need only abortive therapy for their headaches. If migraine frequency is greater than twice a month and/or severely debilitating or if abortive agents are ineffective, the health care provider should consider prescribing daily preventive therapy.

Acute Therapy

Acute or abortive therapy is aimed at reversing, aborting, or reducing pain and accompanying symptoms of an attack that is in progress or is anticipated. Acute therapy for migraines can range from simple over-the-counter (OTC) **analgesics** to intramuscular (IM) **dihydroergotamine** that needs to be administered in a clinic or emergency room setting. Oral (PO) therapy may not be effective in patients with associated nausea or vomiting. The stepwise approach to selecting migraine medications for acute treatment is helpful, based on the severity of the pain and associated symptoms. Figure 33–1 is an algorithm that addresses the steps in acute migraine therapy. Although this section discusses pharmacological treatment, nonpharmacological therapy—specifically applying ice to the head and/or lying down in a darkened room—must accompany the medication. The patient must be advised not to try to "work through" a migraine by just taking medication.

SIMPLE ANALGESICS. Simple **analgesics** such as **aspirin (ASA)** and **acetaminophen (APAP)** or **nonsteroidal anti-inflammatory drugs (NSAIDs)** are the first step in the acute treatment of mild to moderate migraine that is not associated with severe nausea or vomiting. Patients often self-medicate with OTC **analgesics,** relying on advertising messages to choose a medication (Sheftell, 1997). The health care provider needs to be aware that most patients have already self-medicated to treat their migraines and that they are often seeking care because their treatment is no longer effective. If the provider decides to begin treatment with an OTC product, educating the patient about the rationale for starting with an OTC product will increase compliance.

Clinical experience and population-based studies have demonstrated the effectiveness of OTC **analgesics** in treating migraine, especially if taken early. The mechanism of action for the various OTC preparations is not completely understood. **ASA** is thought to have antiprostaglandin and antiplatelet activity that might deliver relief from migraine attack. Recent evidence is that **ASA** may also act centrally and has serotoninergic activity (Sheftell, 1997). **APAP** is thought to act centrally and inhibit prostaglandin synthesis. **NSAIDs** also inhibit prostaglandin syntheseis and have a central analgesic mechanism of action. Their anti-inflammatory and antipyretic activity may also contribute to migraine relief. **Caffeine** is an ingredient in many OTC "headache" preparations (Table 33–2) and plays a role as an **analgesic** adjuvant when added to **ASA** or in combination with **APAP.** Currently, only one OTC preparation is Food and Drug Administration (FDA) –approved to be labeled specifically for migraine pain, and that is a combination of **ASA, APAP,** and **caffeine (Excedrin Migraine).**

The dosing of **ASA** or **APAP** should be limited to a 1000-mg dose (10 to 15 mg/kg for children) at the beginning of migraine symptoms or aura, with a maximum of 4000 mg per day. Rebound headaches are possible if **ASA** or **APAP** is used more than 3 days per week.

The **NSAIDs** have been found to diminish the severity and duration of migraine attacks. Although no **NSAID** has been found to be better than another in clinical trials, there is a variable response to the different agents that differs from patient to patient. The use of **NSAIDs** can involve trying multiple medications before an effective agent is found. **Naproxen sodium (Anaprox, Aleve)** is often a first choice for migraine, as it is quickly absorbed and well tolerated. The initial starting dose of **naproxen sodium** is 550 mg, followed by 550 mg twice a day or 275 mg every 6 to 8 hours. The dose of **naproxen sodium** for children is 10 to 20 mg/kg/day divided in twice-daily dosing. Although the majority of **NSAIDs** are given PO, **indomethacin (Indocin)** is also available in suppository form, which may be helpful if the patient is nauseated or vomiting. **Ketorolac (Toradol)** is the only **NSAID** available in an injectable form, which can also be used if the patient is vomiting. Table 33–2 shows the dosing for commonly used **NSAIDs.**

MIDRANGE ANALGESICS. Midrange **analgesics** are commonly prescribed to treat both migraine and tension-type headaches. Combination products that combine either **butalbital** with **ASA** or **APAP (Fiorinal** or **Fioricet)** or **isometheptene** with **acetaminophen** and **dichloralphenazone (Midrin)** are effective in treating mild to moderate migraine. These products should be used cautiously because rebound headaches can occur if they are taken in greater than recommended dosages or more than 2 days per week. Drug-rebound headache is discussed later in this chapter.

HIGH-RANGE ANALGESICS. High-range **analgesics** include the commonly used **opioids,** which act centrally to treat the pain of migraine. Although **opioids** are controversial in the treatment of migraine, there are patients for whom an **opioid** is the drug of choice. An **opioid** can be prescribed if the patient is pregnant, if vasoconstrictor medications are contraindicated, or if the migraine is not responsive to **ergotamine** or **serotonin agonists** (discussed later).

Codeine either alone or in combination with **ASA (Aspirin** with **codeine #3)** or **APAP (Tylenol** with **codeine #3)** is the **opioid** most commonly used to treat migraine. The dose of **codeine** should be 30 to 60 mg, with the lowest effective dose used. **Meperidine (Demerol)** can be given IM if the patient is unable to take oral medications because of nausea and/or vomiting. The maximum initial dose is 150 mg in an adult, and a dose of 50 to 100 mg can be repeated every 3 to 4 hours. Intranasal **butorphanol (Stadol)** can be tried in patients who fail **nonopioid therapy** or who have contraindications to other migraine medications. The dose of one spray in one nostril has a rapid onset (less than 15 minutes) and can be repeated in 1 hour if needed. Adverse effects include orthostasis and sedation. The patient should limit its use to no more than twice a week. Other **opioids** that are prescribed for migraine, even though there is little clinical information to support their effectiveness over newer **nonnarcotic agents,** include **oxycodone** and **hydrocodone. Opioids** must be prescribed carefully because of their potential for physical dependence, tolerance, and addiction. Therefore, they should be limited to patients with severe but infrequent headaches or the oc-

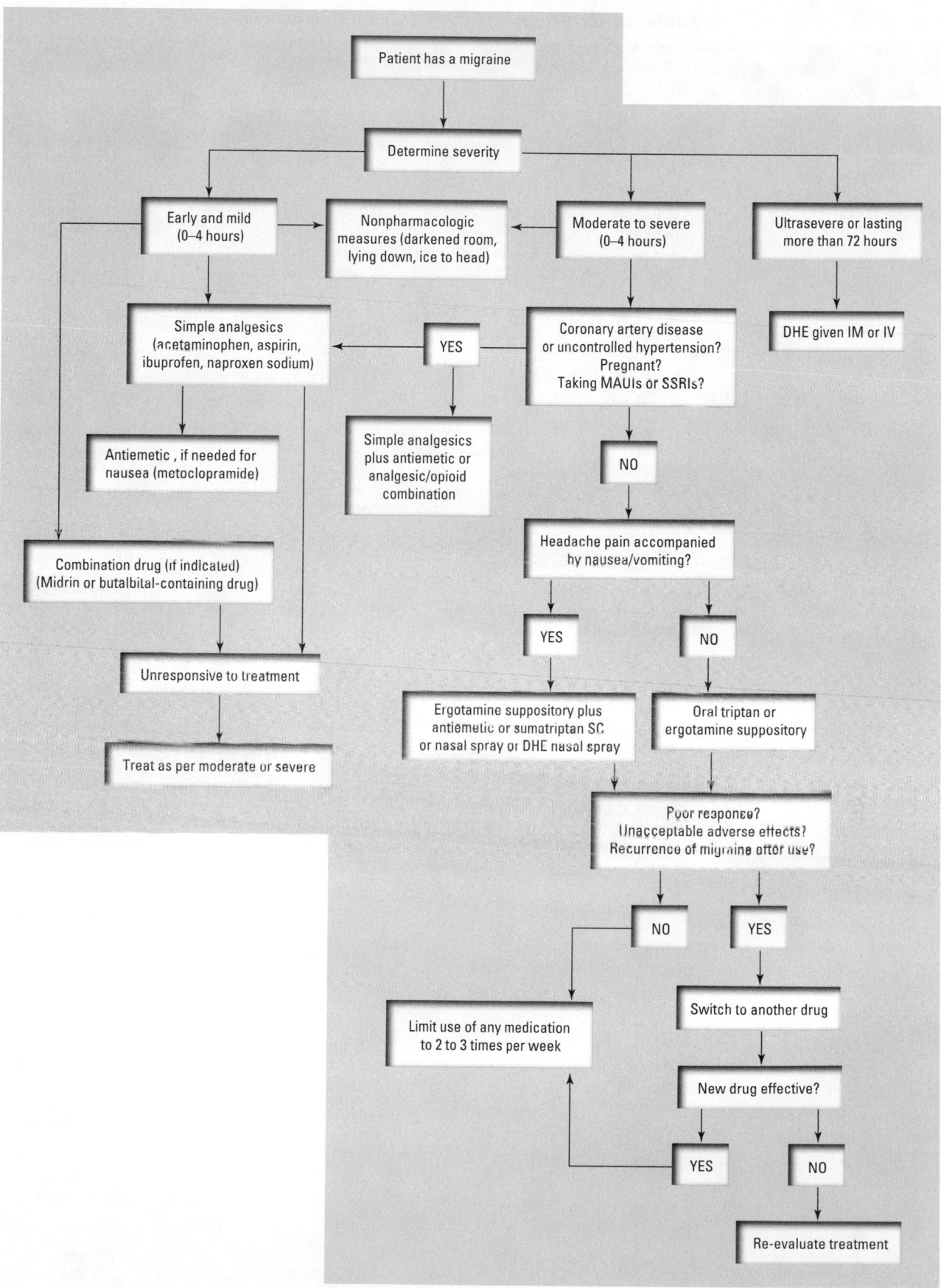

Figure 33–1. Treatment algorithm for acute migraine headache.

Table 33–2. Drugs Commonly Used: Headaches

Drug	Initial Dose	Maximum Dose	Strengths Available	Rebound Potential	Comments
		ACUTE THERAPY			
Nonnarcotic Analgesics Acetaminophen (OTC: Tylenol)	*Adults:* 650–1000 mg at onset and every 4–6 h *Children:* 10–15 mg/kg/dose	*Adults:* 4000 mg/day 2–3 d/wk 30 dosages/mo *Children:* 5 doses in 24 h	*Tablets:* 160, 325, 500, 650 mg *Liquid:* 80 mg/0.8 mL 160 mg/5mL *Chewable:* 80, 160 mg *Suppositories:* 80, 120, 325, 650 mg	Yes	Safe in pregnancy, lactation, and in most patients
Aspirin (OTC: Bayer, Bufferin, Ecotrin)	*Adults:* 650–1000 mg at onset and every 4–6 h *Children:* Not recommended for use in children	*Adults:* 4000 mg/d 2–3 d/ wk 30 dosages/mo	*Tablets:* 325, 500, 650, 975 mg *Suppositories:* 300, 600 mg	Yes	Contraindicated in pregnancy (Category D) Avoid use within 1 wk of surgery
Ibuprofen (OTC: Motrin IB, Advil, Nuprin; Rx: Motrin)	*Adults:* 200–800 mg at onset, then every 6 h *Children:* 5–10 mg/kg initially; may repeat every 6–8 h	*Adults:* 2400 mg/d *Children:* 40 mg/kg/d	*OTC tablets:* 100, 200 mg *Rx tablets:* 400, 600, 800 mg *Suspension:* 100 mg/5 mL *Chewable:* 50, 100 mg	Unlikely	Contraindicated in third trimester of pregnancy; safe during lactation Use with caution in kidney disease, ulcer disease, gastritis
Naproxen (Rx: Naprosyn)	*Adults:* 500 mg at onset, then 250 mg every 6–8 h *Children:* 2.5–5 mg/kg initially and may repeat every 12 h	*Adults:* 1000 mg/d *Children:* 15 mg/kg/d	*Tablets:* 250, 375, 500 mg *Suspension:* 125 mg/mL	Unlikely	Contraindicated in third trimester of pregnancy; safe during lactation Absorbed more slowly than naproxen sodium Use with caution in kidney disease, ulcer disease, gastritis
Naproxen sodium (OTC: Aleve; Rx: Anaprox)	*Adults:* 825 mg at onset, then 200–550 mg in 3–4 h *Children:* Use suspension form of naproxen	*Adults:* 1375 mg/d	*OTC tablets:* 200 mg *Rx tablets:* 275, 550 mg	Unlikely	Contraindicated in third trimester of pregnancy; safe during lactation Naproxen sodium absorbed more quickly than naproxen, reaches peak levels in half the time Use with caution in kidney disease, ulcer disease, gastritis

Continued on next page

Table 33–2. Drugs Commonly Used: Headaches *(continued)*

Drug	Initial Dose	Maximum Dose	Strengths Available	Rebound Potential	Comments
Ketorolac (Rx: Toradol)	*Adults:* 30–60 mg initially, may repeat 30–60 mg every 6 h *Children:* Not recommended in children <16 y old	*Adults:* 120 mg/d	*Injection:* 15 mg/mL, 30 mg/mL for IM injection	Unlikely, but frequent use should be avoided	Use for emergency treatment of severe migraine in patients who cannot use other medications Contraindicated in pregnancy, lactation, kidney disease, ulcer disease, gastritis
Aspirin/acetaminophen/ caffeine combination (OTC: Excedrin, Vanquish)	*Adults:* 2 tablets every 6 h	*Adults:* 8 tablets/d, 2 d/wk	*Excedrin:* APAP 250 mg, ASA 250 mg, caffeine 65 mg *Vanquish:* APAP 165 mg, ASA 227 mg, caffeine 33 mg	Yes	Same precautions as for ASA and APAP
Combination Analgesics Butalbital compounds (Rx: Fiorinal, Fioricet, Esgic Plus)	*Adults:* 2 tablets at onset, then 1 tablet every 4–6 h *Children:* Not recommended	*Adults:* 6 tablets per attack 2 d/wk 30 tablets	*Fiorinal:* Butalbital 50 mg, ASA 325 mg, caffeine 40 mg *Fioricet:* Butalbital 50 mg, APAP 325 mg, caffeine 40 mg *Esgic Plus:* Butalbital 50 mg, APAP 500 mg, caffeine 40 mg	Yes	Same as for ASA and APAP
Isometheptene compound (Rx: Midrin, Isocom)	*Adults:* *Migraine:* 2 capsules at onset, then 1 capsule every h if needed for relief *Tension headache:* 1 or 2 capsules at onset, followed by one capsule every 4 h *Children:* Not recommended	*Migraine:* 5 per 12 h, 2 d/wk 20 per mo *Tension headache:* 8 per 24 h, 2 d/wk 20 per mo	*Midrin, Isocom:* Isometheptene 65 mg, dichloral-phenazone 100mg, APAP 325 mg	Yes	Adverse interaction with monoamine oxidase inhibitors (MAOIs) Contraindicated in uncontrolled hypertension, coronary artery disease (CAD), peripheral vascular disease (PVD)

Continued on next page

Table 33–2. Drugs Commonly Used: Headaches *(continued)*

Drug	Initial Dose	Maximum Dose	Strengths Available	Rebound Potential	Comments
Narcotic Analgesics Codeine-containing compounds (Rx: Tylenol #3, Empirin #3)	*Adults:* 1 or 2 tablets at onset of attack, then 1 every 4–6 h *Children:* Aspirin-containing preparations contraindicated	*Adults:* 6 tablets per attack, 2 d/wk 10–15 doses/mo	*Tylenol #3:* APAP 300 mg with codeine 30 mg *APAP with codeine liquid:* Codeine 12 mg and APAP 120 mg/5 mL *Empirin #3:* ASA 325 mg with codeine 30 mg	Yes and habit forming	Relatively safe during pregnancy Should not be considered first-line therapy Monitor use carefully; if patient is needing more than 15 tablets/mo, reevaluate treatment Contraindicated in substance abuse patients Should not be prescribed for chronic daily headache
Meperidine (Rx: Demerol)	*Adults:* Maximum initial dose 150 mg, can repeat 50–100 mg every 3–4 h if needed		*IM injection:* 25 mg/mL, 50 mg/mL, 75 mg/mL, 100 mg/mL	Yes	May be used in pregnancy Patients must have someone to drive them home after receiving medication Use only as "rescue" medication Use sparingly and infrequently when other treatments have been ineffective
Butorphanol (Rx: Stadol NS)	*Adults:* 1 spray to one nostril; may be repeated in 1 h *Children:* Not recommended	*Adults:* 2 sprays (2 mg) per attack, 2 d/wk	*Stadol NS:* Nasal spray 1 mg/spray	Probably	Can be used as a "rescue" medication Effective for nocturnal headaches Side effects of orthostasis and sedation May be used with caution in pregnancy
Ergot Derivatives Ergotamine tablets (Rx: Ergostat, Ergomar)	*Adults:* One tablet sublingual at onset of attack; may repeat every 30 min; max 3 tablets per attack *Children:* Not safe in children	*Adults:* 3 tablets/d, 2 d/wk and 10 mg/wk	Sublingual 2-mg tablets	Yes	Contraindicated in pregnancy (Category X) and lactation Contraindicated in CAD and PVD May cause severe nausea and vomiting

Continued on next page

Table 33–2. Drugs Commonly Used: Headaches *(continued)*

Drug	Initial Dose	Maximum Dose	Strengths Available	Rebound Potential	Comments
Ergotamine and caffeine combination (Rx: Cafergot, Wigraine)	*Adults:* *Tablets:* 2 tablets at onset, then 1 tablet every 30 min if needed, up to 6 tablets per attack *Suppositories:* 1/3–1 suppository at onset; may repeat 1 suppository in 1 h, if needed *Children:* Not recommended	*Adults:* 6 tablets or 2 suppositories per attack, 2 d/wk, 10 mg/wk	*Cafergot & Wigraine tablets:* Ergotamine 1 mg, caffeine 100 mg *Cafergot & Wigraine suppositories:* Ergotamine 2 mg, caffeine 100 mg	Yes	Pregnancy Category X; contraindicated in lactation, CAD, PVD May cause nausea and vomiting Suppository form better absorbed May premedicate with an antiemetic
Dihydroergotamine (Rx: DHE 45, Migranal)	*Adults:* *Injection:* 1 mg IV/IM at onset; may repeat 1-mg dose hourly for total maximum of 3 mg IM or 2 mg IV *Intranasal:* 1 spray each nostril at onset; may repeat in 15 min *Children:* Not recommended	*Adults:* IM: 3 mg/attack IV: 2 mg/attack IM/IV: 6 mg/wk IM home use: 18 doses/mo *Intranasal:* 6 sprays/24 h, 8 sprays/wk	*DHE 45 injection:* 1 mg/mL *Migranal:* 0.5 mg/spray	Unlikely	Contraindicated in pregnancy, lactation, CAD, PVD, and hypertension Premedicate with antiemetic metoclopramide for greater effectiveness
Serotonin Receptor Agonists Sumatriptan (Rx: Imitrex)	*Adults:* *Oral:* 25–100 mg initially; may be repeated every 2 h for up to 24 h *SC injection:* 6 mg; may repeat ×1 in 1 h *Intranasal:* 5, 10, or 20 mg; may repeat once after 2 h if needed *Children >10 y:* Consult with physician or pediatric neurologist *Oral:* poor and erratic absorption in children *SC injection:* 0.1 mg/kg/dose; may repeat once after 2 h *Nasal spray:* works well in children; consult for dosing *Children <10 y:* Not recommended	*Adults:* *Oral:* 300 mg/d, 4 headaches per mo *SC injection:* 2 injections/d, 4 headaches per mo *Intranasal:* 40 mg/d, 4 headaches per mo	*Tablets:* 25, 50 mg *SC injection:* 6 mg/mL single dose vial *Nasal spray:* 5 mg/spray, 20 mg/spray	Likely	Contraindicated in pregnancy, ischemic heart disease, CAD, and uncontrolled hypertension None of the triptans can be used within 24 h of ergotamine-containing medications or other triptans Concurrent use of a triptan or use within 2 wk of MAOIs is contraindicated All the triptans interact with selective serotonin reuptake inhibitors (SSRIs), causing serotonin syndrome

Continued on next page

Table 33–2. Drugs Commonly Used: Headaches *(continued)*

Drug	Initial Dose	Maximum Dose	Strengths Available	Rebound Potential	Comments
Naratriptan (Rx: Amerge)	*Adults* : One 1 mg or 2.5 mg tablet at onset of migraine; may repeat dose in 4 h, if needed *Children 12–17:* Adult doses are used *Children <12 y:* Safety has not been established	*Adults:* 5 mg/24 h, 4 headaches per mo	*Tablets:* 1 mg, 2.5 mg	Likely	Same contraindications as for sumatriptan Longer half-life than other triptans, less likely to cause rebound headache Interacts with oral contraceptives
Rizatriptan (Rx: Maxalt, Maxalt-MLT)	*Adults* (either form): Take 5–10 mg at onset of migraine; may repeat in 2 h, if needed *Children:* Not recommended in patients <18 y	*Adults:* 30 mg/24 h, 4 headaches per mo *Propranolol patients:* use 5-mg dose, up to 3 doses in 24 h	*Maxalt tablets:* 5, 10 mg *Maxalt-MLT orally disintegrating tablets:* 5, 10 mg	Likely	Same contraindications as for sumatriptan Use with caution in patient concurrently taking propranolol
Zolmitriptan (Rx: Zomig)	*Adults:* 2.5 mg or less initially (may break 2.5-mg tablet in half); repeat if headache returns after 2 h *Children:* Safety not established	*Adults:* 10 mg/24 h, 4 headaches per mo	*Tablets:* 2.5 mg, 5 mg	Likely	Same contraindications as for sumatriptan Use with caution in patients with hepatic dysfunction (<2.5-mg dose) Interacts with oral contraceptives and cimetidine
Antiemetics Metoclopramide (Rx: Reglan)	*Adults:* 10 mg either orally or IV either before ergotamine derivative or concurrently with analgesic *Children:* Not recommended	*Adults:* 40 mg/d	*Tablets:* 5 mg, 10 mg *Injection:* 5 mg/mL	N/A	Interacts with cimetidine, digoxin, MAOIs, and cyclosporine Safe in pregnancy (Category B)
PREVENTIVE THERAPY					
Beta Blockers Propranolol (Rx: Inderal)	*Adults:* Start with 60–80 mg/d, and increase every 3–7 d *Children:* 0.5–1 mg/kg/d divided bid and increased every 3–4 d	*Adults:* 240–320 mg/d (monitor blood pressure (BP) and heart rate (HR): systolic BP should be >100 mm Hg and HR >50 bpm) *Children:* 2–4 mg/kg/d	*Tablets:* 10, 20, 40, 60, 80 mg	N/A	Contraindicated in chronic heart failure (CHF), asthma, chronic obstructive pulomonary disease (COPD), PVD, diabetes mellitus, depression, Wolff-Parkinson-White syndrome

Continued on next page

Table 33–2. Drugs Commonly Used: Headaches *(continued)*

Drug	Initial Dose	Maximum Dose	Strengths Available	Rebound Potential	Comments
					Pregnancy Category C but safer than some other preventive agents Start with a trial of 3 mo; as response improves over time, it needs to be tapered slowly (over a week) if discontinued Interacts with many drugs including cimetidine, oral contraceptives, calcium channel blockers
Timolol (Rx: Blocadren)	*Adults:* Start at 20 mg/d; increase slowly *Children:* Not recommended	*Adults:* 60 mg/d	*Tablets:* 5, 10, 20 mg	N/A	Pregnancy Category C Contraindications and drug interactions similar to propranolol
Metoprolol (Rx: Lopressor)	*Adults:* Start at 100 mg/d; increase slowly *Children:* Not recommended	*Adults:* 250 mg/d	*Tablets:* 50, 100 mg	N/A	Pregnancy Category C Contraindications include bradycardia, second- or third-degree heart block, overt heart failure Interacts with many drugs, including calcium channel blockers, digoxin, clonidine, and oral contraceptives
Atenolol (Rx: Tenormin)	*Adults:* 100 mg/d *Children:* Not recommended	*Adults:* 200 mg/d	*Tablets:* 25, 50, 100 mg	N/A	Pregnancy Category D Contraindications include bradycardia, second- or third-degree heart block, overt heart failure Interacts with many drugs, including calcium channel blockers, digoxin, clonidine, and oral contraceptives
Tricyclic Antidepressants Amitriptyline (Rx: Elavil)	*Adults:* Start with 10 mg qHS and increase every 2	*Adults:* 150 mg/d	*Tablets:* 10, 25, 50, 75 100 mg	N/A	Contraindicated in patient with narrow-angle glaucoma,

Continued on next page

Table 33–2. Drugs Commonly Used: Headaches *(continued)*

Drug	Initial Dose	Maximum Dose	Strengths Available	Rebound Potential	Comments
	wk to a total daily dose of 20–50 mg *Children:* Not recommended for children <12 y				urinary retention, pregnancy, breastfeeding, concurrent use of MAOIs cannot use (within 14 d of each other), and in suicidal patients
Anticonvulsants Divalproex (Rx: Depakote)	*Adults:* Initial dose is 125–250 mg bid; may increase 125 mg weekly *Children:* Safety and effectiveness for migraine prevention has not been studied in children <16 y	*Adults:* 1000 mg/d	*Tablets:* 125, 250, 500 mg	N/A	Requires baseline assessment of liver function, platelet count, and bleeding time, as hepatic failure and thrombocytopenia are rare adverse effects Monitor liver function tests (LFTs) and complete blood count (CBC) every 2 wk ×3 Pregnancy Category D
NSAIDs Naproxen sodium (OTC: Aleve; Rx: Anaprox)	*Adults:* 550 mg bid	*Adults:* 1375 mg/d	*OTC tablets:* 200 mg *Rx tablets:* 275, 550 mg	Unlikely	Contraindicated in third trimester of pregnancy; safe during lactation Use with caution in kidney disease, ulcer disease, gastritis
Calcium Channel Blockers Verapamil (Rx: Calan, Isoptin)	*Adults:* Start with 40 mg bid and slowly increase *Children:* Not recommended	*Adults:* 480 mg/d	*Tablets:* 40, 80, 120 mg	N/A	Contraindicated in pregnancy (Category C), Parkinson's disease, and depression May be first-line choice in patients with hypertension who cannot take beta blockers
Serotonin Antagonist Methysergide (Rx: Sansert)	*Adults:* Start with 2 mg bid; increase slowly *Children:* Not recommended	*Adults:* 8–14 mg/d	*Tablets:* 2 mg	N/A	Most serious side effect is retroperitoneal fibrosis or related conditions with prolonged therapy Patient should have a drug-free period of 3–4 wk after every 6 mo of treatment Contraindicated in pregnancy, CAD, PVD, impaired renal or liver function, and hypertension

casional headache that is unresponsive to nonnarcotic agents.

ERGOT DERIVATIVES. **Ergot derivatives** have been used for many years to treat migraine. **Ergotamine** and **dihydroergotamine (DHE)** act as vasoconstrictors that lead to a decline in the amplitude of pulsation in the extracranial arteries and decreased hyperperfusion of the basilar artery area, without decreasing cerebral hemispheric blood flow. **Ergotamine** controls up to 70 percent of acute migraine attacks, but its adverse effects of nausea and vomiting and its unpredictable oral absorption limit routine use. Pretreatment with an **antiemetic** decreases the nausea and vomiting associated with ergotamine use. **Ergotamine suppositories (Wigraine, Cafergot)** are better absorbed than PO preparations and can be quite effective if administered at the beginning of migraine symptoms. Misuse of **ergotamine** may lead to drug-rebound headaches, and use should be limited to two doses, twice a week or less (total weekly dose of 10 mg maximum), up to 12 doses per month. Another caution with **ergotamine** is that the vasoconstriction can have serious effects on patients with peripheral vascular disease, coronary heart disease, hypertension, and impaired hepatic or renal function. Exceeding recommended amounts of **ergotamine** can lead to vasospastic adverse effects. *Ergotamine* derivatives are **contraindicated in pregnancy because they can produce prolonged uterine contractions that can result in abortion. Thus all forms of *ergotamine* are Pregnancy Category X.** *Ergotamine* is not recommended for children.

DHE, although chemically similar to **ergotamine,** does not cause the same peripheral vasoconstrictor effects, making it safer to use. It also causes less nausea than **ergotamine** and does not require pretreatment with an **antiemetic.** DHE is effective even well into the course of a headache, unlike **ergotamine,** which must be taken at the beginning of migraine symptoms. **DHE** can be administered IM **(D.H.E. 45)** or intranasally **(Migranal).** **DHE** has a longer duration of action than **sumatriptan,** and so headache recurrence rates are lower. The dosage of **DHE 45** is 1 mg (or 1 mL) IM or intravenously (IV) initially and can be repeated at 1-hour intervals to a maximum of 3 mg IM or 2 mg IV. IM **DHE** can be prescribed for home use if the patient has proper instructions regarding administration. Monthly limits for IM **DHE** is 18 ampules or 12 headache events. The dose of intranasal **DHE** is 1 spray (0.5 mg) in each nostril, repeated after 15 minutes, for a dose of 2 mg. Maximum dose is 6 sprays in a 24-hour period and 8 sprays per week. Although intranasal **DHE** is easier to administer, the patient should be warned that it has a slow onset of action. Precautions for **DHE** are the same as for **ergotamine;** it is contraindicated in pregnancy, coronary artery disease, peripheral vascular disease, and hypertension. **DHE** is not recommended for children.

SEROTONIN RECEPTOR AGONISTS. **Serotonin receptor agonists** act selectively as 5-HT_1 **receptor agonists,** causing vasoconstriction and apparently blocking release of vasoactive substances that lead to migraine. **Sumatriptan (Imitrex)** was the first **selective serotonin receptor agonist** developed specifically to treat migraine; newer agents include **naratriptan (Amerge), rizatriptan (Maxalt),** and **zolmitriptan (Zomig).** As they differ slightly in pharmacokinetics and individual response, trial of a different **serotonin receptor agonist** is warranted if one is not effective.

Sumatriptan is effective in decreasing the severity of headache in 54 to 80 percent of patients. It is also effective in relieving the nausea, photophobia, and phonophobia that can accompany migraine. **Sumatriptan** should be taken after the aura of migraine passes, as it is found to be effective only after the headache symptoms appear. **Sumatriptan** is available in PO, subcutaneous (SC), and intranasal forms. The dose for PO **sumatriptan** is 25 to 100 mg initially and may be repeated every 2 hours for up to 24 hours (maximum 300 mg in 24 hours). Although an initial dose of 25 mg should be tried with a patient who has never had **sumatriptan,** research has shown that an initial dose of 50 to 100 mg is superior in relieving migraine symptoms (Pfaffenrath et al., 1998.) The initial SC dose of **sumatriptan** is 6 mg, and 82 percent of patients report relief in 20 minutes. The dose may be repeated in 1 hour if there is no relief, for a maximum of two 6-mg doses in 24 hours. Intranasal **sumatriptan** has a slower onset than SC (2 hours versus 20 minutes) and is less effective in relieving headache (62 percent at 2 hours), yet intranasal dosing may be more appealing for children and for patients who fear self-administration of

Clinical Pearl

ERGOTAMINE SUPPOSITORIES

Ergotamine suppositories can provide relief if taken at the beginning of a migraine attack. For patients who have not used **ergotamine** before, instruct them to use one-third of a 2-mg suppository initially and repeat in 30 to 60 minutes. Refrigeration makes the suppository easier to slice.

Clinical Pearl

SEVERE MIGRAINE HEADACHE

First-line treatment for a severe migraine should be **DHE** given IM, IV, or intranasally or sumatriptan given PO or SC. For ultrasevere attacks or relief of status migrainosus (migraine lasting >72 hours), **DHE** is considered the drug of choice, with doses repeated every 8 hours for 24 hours or more, preceded by **metoclopramide** to prevent nausea.

injectable medication. After a dose of **sumatriptan**, up to 40 percent of headaches recur within 10 to 14 hours, and a second dose may be necessary. Do not repeat the dose of **sumatriptan** if the patient does not respond initially to the first dose.

Naratriptan is similar to **sumatriptan** in its mechanism of action but differs in its pharmacokinetics. **Naratriptan** has a higher PO bioavailability (about 70%) and a longer half-life (6 hours) than **sumatriptan**. This might lead to a lower rate of headache recurrence, with only 17 to 28 percent of patients reporting recurrence (Mathew, 1997). These differences may lead the practitioner to choose **naratriptan** as the first-line **triptan**. **Naratriptan** has been studied in adolescents (age 12 to 17), and the reported adverse events do not differ from the adult studies. One factor that may prevent the use of **naratriptan** is that its half-life and plasma levels are increased with concurrent use of **oral contraceptives**, and the dose should be lowered.

Rizatriptan, also a **5-HT$_1$ serotonin receptor agonist**, has oral bioavailability that is better than **sumatriptan** (about 45% versus 15%) but not as good as **naratriptan**. Because its half-life is similar to **sumatriptan** (both 2 to 3 hours), cost and PO absorption may be factors when choosing between **rizatriptan** and **sumatriptan**. **Rizatriptan** is available in PO tablet or PO disintegrating tablet, which may be preferred for some patients with nausea as a major symptom of migraine. One caution with **rizatriptan** is that plasma levels of **rizatriptan** are increased significantly when taken with **propranolol**, and concurrent use should be avoided.

Zolmitriptan has a higher PO bioavailability than **sumatriptan** and **rizatriptan** (60 percent in females, 38 percent in males) and a similar half-life. **Zolmitriptan** is the only **triptan** that interacts with **cimetidine** (doubles the half-life and plasma levels of **zolmitriptan**), and this may be a factor in prescribing. **Zolmitriptan's** half-life and clearance are also affected by **oral contraceptives**.

All **triptans** are contraindicated in patients with coronary artery disease or uncontrolled hypertension because of their potential to constrict coronary artery vessels. The **triptans** are contraindicated in pregnancy. None of the **triptans** can be used if **ergotamine derivatives** have been used in the prior 24 hours on account of increased vasospastic reactions; their effects may be additive. The **triptans sumatriptan, zolmitriptan,** and **rizatriptan** interact with **monoamine oxidase inhibitors (MAOIs)**, and should not be used concurrently or within 2 weeks of discontinuing the **MAOI**. All of the **triptans** interact with **selective serotonin reuptake inhibitors (SSRIs)**, causing serotonin syndrome. **Sumatriptan** can be used in children, but consultation with a pediatric neurologist is advisable.

ANTIEMETICS. **Antiemetics** are an integral part of migraine management. Gastric emptying and oral absorption of medications are decreased in migraine patients, especially those patients with nausea and vomiting as a component of their migraine. A dose of **metoclopramide (Reglan)** is often recommended as part of migraine therapy. Some think that **metoclopramide** should be a first-line therapeutic agent in patients with nausea as a significant component of migraine (Peroutka, 1998). Other commonly used **antiemetics** are the **phenothiazine**

Clinical Pearl

TRIPTANS

It is advisable to administer the first dose of any of the **triptans** under direct supervision. The patient should receive the first dose in the clinic (or urgent care center) and be monitored for any adverse cardiovascular effects.

antiemetics, perphenazine (Trilafon), prochlorperazine (Compazine), and **chlorpromazine (Thorazine)**.

Preventive Therapy

Preventive therapy should be considered for any patient who experiences severely incapacitating or frequent severe migraines (more than two per month) and patients who cannot tolerate abortive medications because of either chronic illness (coronary artery disease or hypertension) or the adverse effects of abortive medications. Preventive medication is also recommended if the patient is taking abortive medication more than twice a week. The primary goal of preventive therapy is to use the least amount of medication with the fewest side effects to decrease migraine symptoms. If drug-rebound headache is suspected, it must be treated first before starting the patient on preventive therapy; this topic is covered later in this chapter.

Patients must understand that preventive therapy will not completely eliminate migraine and that a 50 percent reduction in migraine attacks is considered a success. Fewer than 10 percent of patients become headache-free with preventive therapy. The patient must also be aware that it may take 4 weeks before preventive therapy begins to be effective and that there is an increase in effectiveness for 3 months. It is common for patients to discontinue preventive therapy after only a couple of weeks and label it as ineffective. Education is the key to success for preventive therapy. Another component to preventive therapy is a headache diary that is initiated prior to preventive therapy and then maintained to determine the frequency, severity, and duration of migraine. This tool enables the provider to assess the effectiveness of preventive therapy.

Because preventive therapy cannot completely eliminate migraines, the patient should also have acute or abortive medications to take for migraine. The provider should recognize interactions between preventive and acute therapies and prescribe accordingly (see Table 33–2). The significance of avoiding migraine triggers, which cannot be overlooked in migraine prevention, is discussed later in the chapter.

BETA BLOCKERS. Beta blockers are one of the first-line choices for migraine preventive therapy, with up to 44 percent reduction in migraine reported. The mechanism of action in migraine prevention is not clear, but it is thought that they may affect the central catecholaminergic system and brain serotonin (5-HT$_2$) receptors. They also block beta receptors in vascular smooth muscle to prevent arterial dilatation. **Propranolol (Inderal)** and **timolol (Blocadren)** are the only beta blockers that have been FDA-approved for migraine preventive therapy, although **nadolol (Corgard)**, **metoprolol (Lopressor)**, and **atenolol (Tenormin)** have also been shown to be effective.

Propranolol is typically started at a dose of 60 to 80 mg a day and slowly increased every third or fourth day to a maximum of 240 mg per day in adults. Twice-daily dosing has the highest compliance rate. Individual response varies, and the patient should be monitored closely. A pulse below 50 or a systolic blood pressure below 100 mm Hg in the adult suggests that the maximum dosage has been reached. The dose in children is 0.5 to 1 mg/kg a day, divided into two doses and titrated every 3 to 4 days, to a maximum of 2 to 4 mg/kg/day. Pediatric patients should be monitored closely, and consultation with a pediatric neurologist before initiating and during therapy is advisable. A trial of 3 months in both adult and pediatric patients is necessary as the response improves over time. Treatment should be reassessed every 6 months, and it may be discontinued. **Propranolol** needs to be tapered slowly (over a week) to prevent drug withdrawal headache. Adverse effects of **propranolol** include fatigue, lethargy, and depression, and it should not be the first-line drug in depressed patients. It is also not well tolerated by athletes. **Propranolol** is contraindicated in patients with congestive heart failure, asthma, chronic obstructive pulmonary disease, peripheral vascular disease, diabetes mellitus, or Wolff Parkinson-White syndrome. *Propranolol is Pregnancy Category C but safer than some of the other preventive agents.*

If **propranolol** is not effective or not well tolerated, one of the other **beta blockers** can be tried; failure to respond to one **beta blocker** does not predict response to another. If a patient has asthma or other respiratory disorders, **metoprolol** and **atenolol** may be used because they are cardioselective. See Table 33–2 for dosing of these agents.

TRICYCLIC ANTIDEPRESSANTS. Tricyclic antidepressants, specifically **amitriptyline (Elavil)**, are effective in reducing the frequency, severity, and duration of migraine attacks. **Amitriptyline** modulates neurotransmitters and appears to affect the central serotonin receptor function. Its antimigraine effect is unrelated to its antidepressant effect, and the antimigraine effect can often be achieved at lower doses than are required to treat depression. The patient should be started on 10 mg a day taken before bed and increased every 2 weeks to a total daily dose of 20 to 50 mg. Adverse effects that should be monitored include drowsiness (most common), dry mouth, weight gain, constipation, and orthostatic hypotension. **Amitriptyline** is contraindicated in patients with narrow-angle glaucoma, urinary retention, pregnancy, breastfeeding, and concurrent use of MAOIs. Other **tricyclic antidepressants** that may be used include **nortriptyline (Pamelor, Aventyl)**, which causes less drowsiness and anticholinergic effect than **amitriptyline**.

DIVALPROEX. **Divalproex (Depakote)** recently received FDA labeling as a preventive treatment for migraine.

Divalproex reduces the number of migraine attacks and also reduces the duration and intensity. It is notably appropriate to use in the patient with coexisting seizure disorder. The initial dose for migraine preventive therapy is 125 to 250 mg twice daily. The dosage can be increased by 125 or 250 mg weekly, to a maximum dose of 1000 mg per day. Patients who are started on **divalproex** require baseline assessment of liver function, platelet count, and bleeding time, as hepatic failure and thrombocytopenia are rare adverse effects. Clinical monitoring of symptoms for liver failure or bleeding disorders is more indicative of potential problems than routine laboratory monitoring. **Divalproex** serum concentrations should be monitored during therapy if poor compliance, toxicity, or drug reactions are suspected. *Divalproex* is Pregnancy Category D.

NONSTEROIDAL ANTI-INFLAMMATORY DRUGS. NSAIDs may also be used for migraine preventive therapy. The most commonly used NSAID is **naproxen sodium,** dosed at 550 mg twice a day. **NSAIDs** are particularly effective in treating menstrual migraines if daily dosing is started the week before menses and continued for a week after. In older patients, **NSAIDs** may pose a higher risk of causing nephrotoxicity or gastrointestinal problems.

CALCIUM CHANNEL BLOCKERS. Calcium channel blockers are also commonly used for migraine preventive therapy, although their effectiveness has had mixed results, and they should not be a first-line choice. **Calcium channel blockers** are thought to prevent migraine by inhibiting vasospasm of the cerebral arteries and by preventing cerebral hypoxia during migraine attacks. **Verapamil (Calan, Isoptin)** is the most commonly used for migraine prevention. **Nifedipine** and **diltiazem** are not as effective in controlling migraines and probably should not be prescribed for this use. **Calcium channel blockers** may be the first-line choice for patients with hypertension who cannot take **beta blockers.** Dosing of **verapamil** is shown in Table 33–2. Adverse effects include sedation, weight gain, depression, and extrapyramidal symptoms. **Calcium channel blockers** are contraindicated in pregnancy, Parkinson's disease, and depression.

METHYSERGIDE. Methysergide (Sansert) is an **ergot derivative** that is a **5-HT$_2$ receptor agonist** that inhibits or blocks the effects of serotonin. **Methysergide** is not commonly used because of its potential for adverse effects (reported in 30 to 50% of patients). The most serious adverse effect is retroperitoneal fibrosis or related conditions with prolonged therapy. If **methysergide** is prescribed, the patient should have a drug-free period of 3 to 4 weeks after every 6 months of treatment. **Methysergide** is contraindicated in pregnancy. **Ergot derivatives** should be avoided in patients with coronary artery disease, peripheral vascular disease, impaired renal or liver function, or hypertension.

Nonpharmacological Management of Migraine

Nonpharmacological management of migraine includes a variety of interventions and alternative therapies. The first and most important is migraine trigger identification and avoidance. Alternative therapies, including nontraditional health care, should be addressed; up to 70 percent of patients who seek alternative therapy never discuss it with their health care provider. Lifestyle issues such as stress and work environment can be modified to decrease migraine attacks or make them more manageable.

IDENTIFYING TRIGGERS. Identifying and avoiding triggers can significantly decrease migraines. Many patients identify certain foods, odors, or medications that may cause headache. Table 33–1 lists common migraine triggers. Patients need to be encouraged to use their headache diary to determine if something is a trigger. Common foods like chocolate, yogurt, or the food additive aspartame can trigger a migraine, and patients are often not aware that something is provoking their headaches. Smoking cessation and sleep regulation may also prove helpful in headache prevention.

ALTERNATIVE THERAPIES. Alternative therapies that may assist in the treatment of migraine vary considerably. A naturopath may prescribe herbal medicine to treat migraines. Other alternative therapies that may be beneficial

---

ON THE HORIZON

New Medications for Migraine Headaches

New medications are being developed for the treatment of migraine headaches. Four new **triptans** are under development: **eletriptan (Relpax), frovatriptan (Miguard), almotriptan,** and **alniditan. Ganaxolone** is a synthetic form of neuroactive **steroid** produced by humans, and it appears to decrease inflammation of the brain lining. **Dotarizine,** which is in clinical trials, may have use as a prophylactic agent. **S-fluoxetine** is being developed and may be used for headache preventive therapy.

include acupuncture, aromatherapy, chiropractic manipulation, hypnosis, and reflexology. Patients can try massage therapy, relaxation therapy, and yoga, which all appear to reduce the tension and stress that may lead to migraine. The health care provider should have access to local health education classes that teach yoga and relaxation classes or a local massage therapist for referral. A simple technique of applying ice to the head can often decrease the severity of pain associated with migraine; patients can be encouraged to try this simple technique as an adjunct to or a substitute for their medication.

BIOFEEDBACK. Biofeedback techniques are helpful for many patients. Biofeedback is thought to change vascular dilatation. Although the exact mechanism is unclear, some patients do report improvement in their migraine symptoms. Biofeedback is often combined with other relaxation therapies and may give the patient a feeling of control and mastery over the migraine symptoms.

Monitoring

Patients with migraine headaches should keep a headache diary, especially when a new treatment is begun or if modifications are made in the therapy. The health care provider can use the diary to determine if the treatment is decreasing the frequency, duration, or severity of the migraine. The diary can also track adverse side effects of the medication prescribed. Overuse of medication can be determined, and an alternative plan developed. Patients should also have their blood pressure monitored for hypertension if they are on a **triptan, ergotamine derivative, beta blocker,** or **calcium channel blocker**. Patients on **divalproex** should have their liver function and complete blood count (CBC) tested every 2 weeks for a total of 6 weeks.

Outcome Evaluation

The goal of migraine treatment is to minimize the impact of migraine headaches on patients' quality of life, social functioning, and ability to work. It is evaluated by discussing with patients how their migraine is affecting their quality of life and by having them record in their headache diary when their headaches adversely affect their quality of life and ability to work. Modification of the treatment plan multiple times until the optimal treatment is found is important in achieving the goal of minimal impact from migraine on quality of life.

Avoidance of patients' identified migraine triggers often decreases the frequency of headache. It is evaluated by having patients record in their headache diaries any headache associated with a specific trigger. If patients are unable to determine if a specific item is a trigger, an elimination diet may be tried. Patients eliminate one item from the common triggers list for 2 weeks and then reintroduce it into their diet. This process may take weeks or months, but the reward of identifying a trigger is worth the perceived inconvenience.

Before beginning preventive therapy for frequent migraine sufferers, patients must be clear that the final goal is to reduce the frequency of migraine by 50 percent and that total elimination of migraine is not a realistic goal. Evaluating the success of preventive therapy by use of the headache diary and by demonstrating a decrease in frequency to the patient will assist in clarifying the true success of treatment. It is essential to treat patients for an adequate amount of time (2 to 3 months) before a change in treatment.

Patient Education

Patient education should include a discussion of information related to the overall treatment plan as well as that specific to the drug therapy, reasons for taking the drug, drugs as part of the total treatment regimen, and adherence issues.

Patient education is the key to successful migraine treatment. Patient education related to migraine should focus on the following:

1. An understanding of the diagnosis and nature of migraines.
2. The nonpharmacological measures to prevent and treat migraines, such as trigger identification and avoidance and the use of relaxation, massage, or ice to counter pain.
3. Education about the medication that is prescribed. Specifically expected side effects, adverse side effects, interactions with other medications, and maximum dosages. Drug-rebound headache should be addressed at the beginning of treatment.
4. The patient as an integral part of the treatment plan. Therapy is less effective if the patient does not keep a headache diary or uses the medication in a way other than how it was prescribed.
5. Realistic expectations of treatment. The patient will probably not be migraine-free, but the goal is to decrease the severity and frequency of migraines. Acute treatment should provide relief within an hour or two, or a change in therapy may be indicated.
6. Caution the patient about using OTC medications to treat the headache unless they are part of the treatment plan.

Education resources available for both the patient and the provider on the Internet and in print enable better understanding of the pathology and treatment of migraine and other headaches. The patient needs to be directed to reliable information. There are numerous patient-health

PATIENT EDUCATION

Headaches

Related to the Overall Treatment Plan/Disease Process

☐ Pathophysiology of headache

☐ Role of lifestyle modifications

☐ Importance of adherence to the treatment regimen

☐ Self-monitoring of symptoms and associated symptoms

☐ What to do when symptoms and associated symptoms worsen

☐ Need for regular follow-up visits with the primary care provider

Specific to the Drug Therapy

☐ Reason for taking the drug and its anticipated action in the disease process

☐ Doses (including maximum dosage) and schedules for taking the drug

☐ Possible adverse effects and what to do if they occur

☐ Interactions between other treatment modalities and these drugs

Reasons for Taking the Drug(s)

Patient education about specific drugs is provided in the appropriate chapters. Specific reasons for taking the drug(s) should be discussed on an individual basis, depending on the diagnosis and nature of the headache. Drug-rebound headache should also be discussed at the beginning of treatment.

Drugs as Part of the Total Treatment Regimen

The total treatment regimen includes pharmacological and nonpharmacological measures, as well as the headache diary. A realistic expectation and goals of the individualized treatment plan should be presented.

Adherence Issues

Nonadherence with the treatment regimen may affect functional status. Health care providers should be aware of the potential problem of nonadherence and discuss the importance of adherence with the patient and family.

organizations, pharmaceutical manufacturers, online support groups, and even Websites that are maintained by private individuals. Table 33–3 provides a short list of the patient-health sites and provider information sites that are considered reliable, comprehensive, and trustworthy and that may be helpful for the health care provider who cares for patients with headaches.

Tension-type Headaches

Up to 90 percent of all headaches could be classified as tension-type headache. At least 15 percent of patients

have experienced their first tension headache by age 10. Tension-type headaches can occur daily and may become persistent and intractable. Like migraine, 75 percent of patients with chronic tension-type headaches are women. Patients may suffer from both tension-type and migraine headaches.

The patient usually describes a bandlike pressure that is persistent dull pain. The pain is usually bilateral in location and nonpulsating. The headache may change in intensity and last from 30 minutes to 7 days. Unlike migraine, tension-type headaches are not worsened by physical activity. The patient may have mild nausea or photophobia, but severe nausea, vomiting, and aura are

Table 33–3. Headache Resources for Patients and Health Care Providers

American Association for the Study of Headache
www.aash.org
19 Mantua Rd.
Mount Royal, NJ
(609) 423-0082
This Website for the AASH has an excellent "Headache FAQs" section, listing the most frequently asked questions about headache, that can be printed up for patients.

JAMA Migraine Information Center
www.ama-assn.org/special/migraine
Extensive information for the health care provider who is caring for migraine patients, including pharmacological and nonpharmacological treatment.

American Council for Headache Education
www.achenet.org
19 Mantua Rd.
Mount Royal, NJ
(609) 423-0082
This site is geared for patients and is connected with the AASH. There is patient information on headaches in general, migraines, and prevention and treatment of headaches, as well as a discussion forum for patients.

National Headache Foundation
www.headaches.org
428 W. Saint James Pl., 2nd floor
Chicago, IL 60614
(800) 843-2256

absent. Tension headaches may increase in frequency and severity in times of stress or emotional upheaval. Chronic tension-type headache is diagnosed when the headache is present for more than 15 days per month.

Pathophysiology

The pathology of tension-type headaches is poorly understood. It was thought that muscle contraction was the primary cause of tension headache, and it was previously called muscle contraction headache. The patient may exhibit tenderness of the extracranial soft tissue and of the cervical or masseter muscles. The muscle pain and tenderness in tension headaches may resemble fibromyalgia. Prolonged stress, eyestrain, and sitting for long periods, such as when using a computer, may lead to increased tension headaches. There is little agreement currently about the cause of tension headaches.

Goals of Therapy

The primary goal of tension-type headache treatment is to decrease the frequency and severity of headache and to provide acute relief of headache once it begins. Although total eradication of headache may not be possible, a combination of relaxation therapy and preventive medication when necessary usually decreases the frequency of headache.

Rational Drug Selection

The pharmacological management of tension-type headaches, like migraine, focuses on acute or abortive treatment and preventive therapy. A key distinction between tension headache and migraine treatment is that tension headaches do not respond to **ergotamine derivatives** or **triptans.**

Acute Therapy

Acute therapy in the treatment of tension-type headaches includes a combination of pharmacological and nonpharmacological therapy.

MILD ANALGESICS. For mild to moderate tension headaches, OTC **analgesics** are quite effective. **ASA, APAP,** or one of the **NSAIDs (ibuprofen** or **naproxen),** taken at the beginning of a tension headache, can be effective in relieving headache pain. The dosing is the same as for migraine. Patients should be cautioned not to use OTC **analgesics** for headache more than two to three times per week because they can cause drug-rebound headache. Patients often self-medicate with OTC products prior to seeking care for their headaches, and therefore a history of what the patient has taken for headache relief and in what amounts is necessary. This history assists the health care provider in determining if the headache has received adequate amounts of **analgesic** or if the tension headache is complicated by drug-rebound headache.

COMBINATION MEDICATIONS. Combination medications are commonly prescribed to treat both migraine and tension-type headaches. Products that combine either **butalbital** with **ASA** or **APAP** or **isometheptene** with **APAP** and **dichloralphenazone** are effective in treating tension headache. These products should be used cautiously because rebound headaches can occur if dosages are higher than recommended or if they are taken more than 2 days per week. The provider should distribute a maximum of 30 tablets of either of these medications per month to make sure the patient is not overusing them.

NONPHARMACOLOGICAL MEASURES. Nonpharmacological measures should be an integral part of acute tension headache treatment. Topical heat or cold packs should be applied. Massage therapy and relaxation therapy help to relax the muscle tension that can aggravate tension headaches.

Preventive Therapy

Preventive therapy should be considered if the patient is having more than one to two headaches per week. Used more than twice a week, the medications used for acute tension headache therapy all have the potential for causing drug-rebound headaches. A trial of preventive medication is likely to be helpful and should be considered early in treatment.

BETA BLOCKERS. **Beta blockers** can be used for prophylactic treatment of tension headache. The dosing and contraindications are the same as for migraine preventive therapy.

TRICYCLIC ANTIDEPRESSANTS. **Tricyclic antidepressants** are successful in reducing tension headaches in patients who are depressed and in those who are not. They appear to enhance the endogenous pain-suppressing systems in the brain. **Amitriptyline** and **nortriptyline** are used in same dosages as for migraine (see Table 33–2). Patients with tension-type headaches may also have depression, and dosing for depression may be successful if a lower dose is not effective.

NONPHARMACOLOGICAL THERAPY. Nonpharmacological therapy is central in the preventive treatment of tension-type headaches. Stress management, biofeedback, and regular exercise can help to reduce medication use for tension headaches. Alternative therapies such as acupuncture and herbal medicine prescribed by a naturopath may improve headache symptoms. Referral to a psychologist or psychiatrist may assist in identifying and treating underlying anxiety that may be contributing to the tension headaches.

Monitoring

Monitoring for effectiveness of acute or preventive medication prescribed for tension headache should be done frequently (every 1 to 2 months) at the beginning of treatment. The patient must keep a headache diary to assist in determining if treatment is successful. Once a patient is stable on an acute or preventive medication, the patient can be seen less frequently. The provider should continue to monitor the use of combination drugs (**butalbital** and **isometheptene** compounds) to safeguard against potential drug-rebound headaches developing from overuse.

Outcome Evaluation

Evaluating the success of tension-type headache therapy is achieved by monitoring the patient's headache diary to determine if there is a decrease in the frequency or severity of headaches. If the patient develops new skills, such as stress reduction or relaxation, or begins exercising regularly, these efforts ought to be acknowledged by the health care provider. As tension-type headaches often last off and on for many years, reevaluation and reworking the treatment regimen may happen multiple times.

Patient Education

Patient education should include a discussion of information related to the overall treatment plan as well as that specific to the drug therapy, reasons for taking the drug, drugs as part of the total treatment plan, and adherence issues. For general patient education information, see the previous Patient Education display.

Patient education information specific to treating tension-type headaches should focus on the following principles:

1. Patients need to know what tension-type headaches are and how they differ from migraines or pathological headaches.
2. Medication education ensures that the acute or preventive medications are taken appropriately. Prevention of drug-rebound headache should be addressed early in the treatment.
3. Nonpharmacological therapies should be encouraged and the patient given local resources available, such as yoga classes, relaxation tapes, and massage therapists.
4. The importance of the patient's participation by keeping a headache diary needs to be stressed. Because most treatment decisions are based on response to therapy, the headache diary is invaluable to the successful management of headaches.

Chronic Daily Headaches

Approximately 35 to 45 percent of patients who seek treatment at headache centers suffer from daily or near daily headaches (Mathew, 1997). Chronic daily headaches (CDH) can be classified as chronic tension-type headache, transformed migraine, hemicrania continua, drug-rebound headache, or new daily persistent headache. Chronic tension-type headaches have already been addressed. Drug-rebound headache is addressed later in this chapter. New persistent daily headache (NPDH) is uncommon, the onset is usually abrupt (patients can often pinpoint the date), and it is usually self-limiting. The cause is thought to be Epstein-Barr virus–induced immune changes. Treatment of NPDH is not discussed in this chapter because little information is available; these patients should be referred to a neurologist for care.

Pathophysiology

The pathology of CDH is often unclear and of mixed origin. There is a clear difference between transformed migraine and hemicrania continua. The boundary between chronic tension-type headache and transformed migraine is less clear and may require a neurology referral for treatment.

Transformed migraine refers to CDH that starts as episodic migraine headache with onset in adolescence. The initial migraines have the pathogenesis of migraine discussed earlier. In transformed migraine, the overuse of **analgesics** appears to alter platelet membrane transduction, affecting circulating serotonin levels. Other abnormalities in blood biochemistry, such as low intracellular levels of magnesium, may also play a role in transformed migraine (Mendizabal, 1998). There is also a higher incidence of coexisting psychopathology, with a strong association between migraine and depression, anxiety disorders, panic disorders, and neuroticism.

Hemicrania continua, also known as chronic paroxysmal hemicrania, is a rare headache syndrome, and the pathogenesis is unknown. The patient, most often a woman, suffers from multiple (10 to 20) and short-lived (less than 20 minutes) episodes of severe unilateral, excruciating pain in the area of the eye, forehead, and temple.

Goals of Treatment

The first goal of treatment for CDH is to break the pattern of daily headache. The patient is then stabilized on prophylactic or preventive therapy.

Rational Drug Selection

Transformed Migraine

In most patients with transformed migraine, the daily headache cycle can be broken by using repeated doses of IV **DHE**. Approximately 70 to 80 percent of patients respond to **DHE**. The patient is given a test dose of 0.33 mL of **DHE** with 5 mg of **metoclopramide** or 10 mg of **prochlorperazine (Compazine)**, followed by 0.5 mL of **DHE** and one of the **antinausea medications** every 6 hours for 48 to 72 hours. This treatment usually requires inpatient treatment. **DHE** is contraindicated in coronary and peripheral vascular disease.

Alternatives to **DHE** include **chlorpromazine (Thorazine)** and **prochlorperazine.** If the patient has drug-rebound headache due to misuse of **analgesics, ergots,** or combination medications, the patient has to be detoxified, which is discussed later in this chapter. Treatment of transformed migraine may require consultation with a neurologist.

Preventive pharmacotherapy can be started after the headache cycle is broken. The patient usually responds to migraine-preventive medications such as **propranolol, divalproex,** or a **tricyclic antidepressant. Amitriptyline** is a good choice if the patient is also depressed. **Fluoxetine (Prozac)** may also be used as a preventive medication; the dose is 40 mg daily. The patient is on preventive medication until the headache days are reduced by 50 percent, and then an additional 3 to 4 weeks, for a total of 6 to 12 weeks.

The patient should also receive alternative therapy to treat CDH. Behavioral counseling, biofeedback therapy, relaxation therapy, physical exercise, and acupuncture are all valid alternative therapies for treatment of CDH.

Hemicrania Continua

Hemicrania continua or chronic paroxysmal hemicrania is a rare disorder that responds completely to **indomethacin** and to nothing else. **Indomethacin (Indocin)** 75 to 150 mg is given daily. Referral to a neurologist is recommended.

Monitoring

Monitoring of patients with CDH who are on preventive therapy requires the patient to keep a diary of headache and medication use. Patients' blood pressure should be monitored if they are on a **beta blocker,** and liver function monitored if on **divalproex,** as per migraine therapy monitoring. Ongoing monitoring of headache is necessary, as 31 percent may have recurrence of headache in spite of preventive medication.

Outcome Evaluation

Patients with CDH are difficult to treat. Treatment success is determined by how effective it has been in breaking the cycle of daily headaches and how effective the preventive treatment is. The patient's headache diary is key in the evaluation of the success of treatment.

Patient Education

Patient education should include a discussion of information related to the overall treatment plan as well as

that specific to the drug therapy, reasons for taking the drug, drugs as part of the total treatment plan, and adherence issues. For general patient education information, see the previous Patient Education display.

Patient education information specific to treating CDH should focus on the following principles:

1. Education about the nature of the disorder, particularly that it is biologic in origin, with neurochemical changes producing the headache.
2. Overuse of **analgesics**, leading to drug-rebound headache, must be emphasized.
3. The influence of stress, anxiety, depression, and inability to relax should be discussed, and the patient encouraged to use nonpharmacological therapies to decrease headache.

Cluster Headaches

Cluster headaches are characterized by intense pain lasting for 15 minutes to 2 hours; they occur in "clusters" of several weeks or months, with the headache subsiding for months at a time, often to recur. The patient can experience one to three attacks a day, usually at the same time of day. They occur most frequently at night, awakening the patient from sleep. Men are affected more than women, with onset in their late twenties. The pain of a cluster headache is unique in that it occurs behind or around one eye, with tearing, conjunctival injection, and drooping of the eyelid common symptoms. There may be nasal congestion, facial flushing, and sweating. The pain is so severe that the patient is unable to lie down or sit still, often pacing the floor in pain.

Pathophysiology

There is no clear etiology for cluster headaches. It is most likely a neuronal disorder originating in the hypothalamus. The clockworklike timing of cluster headaches suggests that the circadian pacemaker or biologic "clock" is dysfunctional.

Goals of Treatment

Relieving the pain of an acute cluster headache and decreasing the length of time of the cluster are the goals of cluster headache management.

Rational Drug Therapy

Most patients with cluster headaches require acute and preventive therapy. The acute attacks are severe and last only a short time; therefore, the intervention must be fast-acting. The patient usually requires both acute and preventive medications to manage the headache.

Acute Therapy

Oxygen therapy administered via a 100 percent nonrebreather mask for 15 to 30 minutes often provides immediate relief of cluster headache.

Ergotamine derivatives are also effective for acute cluster headaches, although the PO forms are poorly absorbed. **Ergotamine suppositories** or **DHE** intranasally or IM has a more rapid onset and is preferred (see Table 33–2 for dosing). **Ergotamine** may also be administered in a 2-mg dose given before bed if nocturnal attacks occur frequently.

Intranasal lidocaine is thought to be effective in treating cluster headache. The patient lies supine, hyperextends the head 45 degrees, and rotates it 30 degrees to the side of the headache. The **lidocaine nasal solution** is then dripped into the nostril on the affected side over 30 seconds. The onset is approximately 5 minutes.

Sumatriptan, if administered SC, may provide relief of acute cluster headaches, although it is not considered a first-line drug. Intranasal **sumatriptan** may also be effective.

Preventive Therapy

Ergotamine administered in a 2-mg dose before bed can prevent nocturnal cluster headaches. **Ergotamine** 1 mg given four times a day may also prevent cluster headaches. **Ergotamine** should be withdrawn every seventh day to prevent ergotism and to determine if the cluster has ceased.

Verapamil can prevent cluster headaches in some patients. **Calcium channel blockers** are thought to prevent cluster headache by inhibiting vasospasm of the cerebral arteries. Dosing of **verapamil** is given in Table 33–2. Cluster headaches appear to need dosing in the high range to achieve headache reduction.

Divalproex can be effective in preventing cluster headaches. The dosing is the same as for migraine prophylaxis (see Table 33–2).

Lithium appears to have some effect on cluster headaches in some patients, and a trial of **lithium** is warranted if the patient does not respond to other preventive medications. The dose for cluster headache prevention is 300 mg daily to a maximum of 300 mg three times a day. The patient needs careful monitoring for adverse effects, including electrocardiogram (ECG), electrolytes, thyroid function, creatinine, and CBC studies.

Nonpharmacological therapies include avoidance of all **alcohol** during the clustering of headaches because **alcohol** often precipitates a headache. Patients often are able to drink **alcohol** between headache clusters without adverse effects. Tobacco, stress, anger, and vigorous physical activity should be avoided. The patient needs to maintain a normal sleep pattern, if possible. Cluster headaches do not appear to respond to self-care measures such as massage and relaxation.

Monitoring

Cluster headaches can be severely disabling, and the intense pain and loss of sleep can significantly affect the patient's quality of life. The health care provider needs to monitor the patient for suicidal thoughts during the headache. The headache diary helps to monitor the effectiveness of acute and preventive medications. A patient treated with **lithium** requires careful monitoring of ECG and chemistries throughout treatment.

Outcome Evaluation

Cluster headaches by definition are self-limiting and will eventually stop, regardless of treatment. The focus of care is to provide measures that shorten or prevent cluster headaches during the cluster. Evaluation of the effectiveness of acute and preventive therapy is accomplished by self-report with a headache diary. Modifications in pharmacological management of cluster headaches should be based on the headache diary.

Patient Education

Patient education should include a discussion of information related to the overall treatment plan as well as that specific to the drug therapy, reasons for taking the drug, drugs as part of the total treatment plan, and adherence issues. For general patient education information, see the previous Patient Education display.

Patient education information specific to treating cluster headaches should focus on the following principles:

1. Educating the family about cluster headache, particularly the fact that it is a benign condition, in spite of the severe pain experienced during attacks.
2. Self-management of acute medications. The headache is usually brief, and therefore the patient must be able to self-medicate to provide relief. The pain may be gone by the time the patient can get transportation to a medical clinic.
3. Avoidance of **alcohol** is crucial during clusters of headaches.

Drug-Rebound Headaches

Drug-rebound headache should be considered in any patient who reports daily use of **analgesics**, combina-

tion medications such as **butalbital** or **ergotamine derivatives** or one of the **triptans. Caffeine** can also cause withdrawal headache when abruptly discontinued. The headache recurs as the medication wears off, compelling the patient to take another dose of medication, which causes a cycle of medication overuse and rebound. The patient may never have complete relief of pain. A careful history of all the medications, including OTC **analgesics,** that the patient takes on a daily basis can help to determine if drug rebound is the issue or if a patient has CDH.

The health care provider needs to be aware of the clinical features of drug-rebound headaches. The following clinical characteristics are found in drug-rebound headache (Mathew, 1997):

1. Headaches are daily or near daily, occurring most frequently in the early morning (2 A.M. to 5 A.M.).
2. The headaches occur in patients who have a headache disorder and use more **analgesics** than the recommended amounts.
3. The headaches worsen as the **analgesic** wears off, causing the patient to take more medication.
4. The slightest physical or mental exertion brings on a headache.

Pathophysiology

Dependence on either **ergotamine** or the OTC **analgesics** is thought to have physical and psychological elements. The overuse of simple **analgesics** (ASA or **APAP**), either alone or in combination with **butalbital** or **caffeine,** has a high potential for causing drug-rebound headache. Although the exact process is unclear, it is thought to suppress or alter the central pain-control mechanism. **Ergotamine** causes a clear pharmacological dependence and subsequent withdrawal. When a patient has **analgesic**-rebound headache, other headache therapies used for acute or preventive therapy may be resistant to treatment. The patient must be detoxified before preventive therapy can be started.

Goals of Therapy

The goal of treating drug-rebound headache is that the patient will no longer be taking daily doses of **analgesics** or **ergotamine** and will be stabilized on preventive medication. The goal during the withdrawal period should be minimizing the intensity of the withdrawal headache.

Rational Drug Therapy

Anticipating withdrawal from daily or near-daily use of **analgesics, butalbital**-containing drugs, or **ergotamine** can make the patient anxious. The provider needs to adequately prepare the patient prior to the detoxification process, as discussed in the Patient Education section. Preventive therapy can be started when the withdrawal process is started or 2 to 3 weeks before or after the withdrawal process. Preventive therapy for migraine and tension-type headache has already been discussed. The advantage of starting preventive therapy either before or after the withdrawal process begins is that the patient may interpret withdrawal symptoms as adverse effects of preventive therapy (Moore & Noble, 1997). The practitioner should consult with a neurologist prior to embarking on detoxification of a patient with drug-rebound headache.

Withdrawal from the simple **analgesics, ASA** and **APAP** or **caffeine**-containing medications, is usually done on an outpatient basis. The patient stops taking the **analgesic** and is started on **Midrin** for 1 week and **cyproheptadine (Periactin)**. Another regimen involves a different class of **analgesic (naproxen), intranasal DHE**, and **antiemetics**.

Butalbital-containing drugs (**Fiorinal, Fioricet**) may need to be tapered slowly because severe problems can develop with abrupt cessation. Serious withdrawal symptoms, such as delirium and seizures, can appear without warning. **Butalbital** use of less than 8 pills (400 mg) per day can be treated on an outpatient basis. Suggested regimens include **Midrin** *plus* **clonazepam (Klonopin)** for 1 week and then taper *or* **phenobarbital** for 1 week *plus* **promethazine (Phenergan)** for 1 to 2 weeks. If the patient is using more than 8 pills per day, then inpatient drug detoxification is necessary, using IV **DHE, metoclopramide**, and IV fluids.

Ergotamine overuse can lead to ergotism as well as CDH. If the patient is taking 0.5 to 1 mg of **ergotamine** (either PO or rectally), the patient can be treated as an outpatient. One treatment is to give **naproxen** daily for 1 to 3 weeks *plus* **methylergonovine (Methergine)** *plus* **promethazine** for 1 to 2 weeks (Moore & Noble, 1997). If the patient is taking more than 1 mg per day of **ergotamine**, then inpatient treatment will probably be needed to provide supportive care. The withdrawal headache from **ergotamine** takes up to 72 hours to appear and lasts 72 hours or more.

Monitoring

Monitoring begins with the provider's regulating the number of doses of acute relief medication the patient is allowed to have each month. If OTC **analgesic** overuse is suspected, then the provider needs to determine the number of doses the patient is taking in a day or a week. During the withdrawal period, the patient's symptoms need to be monitored. If the patient requires IV medica-

tion or fluid intervention, the patient may need to be hospitalized. After the patient has been successfully detoxified from the medication, the provider needs to monitor the effectiveness of the preventive medication in preventing headaches. Effective preventive medication decreases the need for acute therapy. Ongoing assessment of **analgesic** and **ergotamine** use will determine if the patient is overusing again.

Outcome Evaluation

The successful outcome in drug-rebound headache is a patient who is detoxified from the offending medication and is somewhat headache-free. The patient may still have an occasional headache and need acute or preventive therapy. Up to 31 percent of patients have recurrence of CDH and often get back into the pattern of overuse of acute therapy medications (Mathew, 1997).

Patient Education

Patient education should include a discussion of information related to the overall treatment plan as well as that specific to the drug therapy, reasons for taking the drug, drugs as part of the total treatment plan, and adherence issues. For general patient education information, see the previous Patient Education display.

When discussing drug-rebound headache with the patient, the provider must be careful to avoid terms like "drug abuse." Patients with drug-rebound headache began with a primary headache disorder and fell into a pattern of overuse, and to label them as "abuser" can be devastating. Before and during the detoxification period, the provider should explain the plan of care and establish patients' trust. They are about to embark on a process that will surely cause moderate to severe headache, which they have been trying to avoid.

The following principles regarding drug-rebound headache and the withdrawal process need to be discussed with the patient:

1. A clear description of drug-rebound headache and how it develops should be given to the patient.
2. After stopping the medication, the headache will get worse within 24 hours (72 hours for **ergotamine**) and may last from days to weeks.
3. Patients must be assured that interventions will be taken to make them comfortable and to decrease the severity of headache, including hospitalization, if needed.
4. It may take 1 to 3 months for the patient to have a normal response to acute therapy.

Migraine Headache

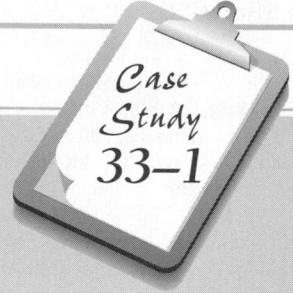

Case Study 33–1

Complaint

"My migraine headaches won't go away."

History

Susan is a 32-year-old white woman who presents to the clinic with recurrent migraine. She reports that she has a moderate to severe migraine once a week, on average. She uses SC Imitrex (sumatriptan), and most of the time the headache resolves with one dose. She was told to return for a checkup if she had to use the Imitrex more than two or three times a month.

Susan is married and has four children. She experienced her first migraine at age 18 and has no other health problems. Initially, her migraines were managed with Cafergot (ergotamine and caffeine), but when Imitrex was introduced a few years ago, she switched and has had good results. She is otherwise healthy. She reports a two- to four-cup-a-day intake of coffee; usually, one of those "cups" is a double latte. She occasionally uses Anacin for relief of mild headache—she thinks only once or twice a week. She has never been hospitalized overnight for her migraines but has gone to the emergency room for "pain medicine" before she switched to Imitrex.

Assessment

Afebrile, vital signs all WNL, weight 135 lb (stable). The physical examination is completely within normal limits. Her neurological exam is unremarkable.

Initial Management Plan

As Susan is not acutely experiencing a migraine, she is asked to keep a headache diary for 3 to 4 weeks. She is to record the day and time of the headache; its severity; if Imitrex, Anacin, or other medication was taken; and how effective the treatment was. The provider also discusses migraine triggers and gives her a handout of common migraine triggers. She is asked to record on her headache diary the amount of caffeine-containing drinks she consumes and to note if she can identify any other stressors.

Upon further discussion, the provider discovers that Susan reports that her stress level has increased recently. The provider discusses stress reduction and relaxation exercises or classes to help Susan manage her stress. She states that she does not have time for classes, so the provider encourages Susan to take a daily short walk (without her children). Susan is concerned at first that the provider did not prescribe a new medication for her migraines and does not know why she needs to keep a headache diary. After reassurance that the headache diary is necessary to determine the appropriate course of treatment, she states that she is willing to "try" to keep a headache diary and will return in 4 weeks.

Follow-up Visit

When Susan returned to the clinic, she brought a fairly complete headache diary for the 4 intervening weeks. She stated that at first she was unsure that it made any difference, but she did discover a couple of triggers to her migraines that she was unaware of. She discovered that on certain days when her children had a before-school class, she often had less sleep the previous night because she had to get up early to get everyone ready. She also would skip breakfast those days and plan on grabbing something later. Susan discovered the combination of decreased sleep, no breakfast, and the stress of getting everyone ready and to class on time often triggered a migraine by early afternoon on those days. She also stated that she probably underestimated her caffeine intake on the previous visit and routinely had 4 to 5 caffeine-containing beverages. She was not aware that the soda that was her favorite cold beverage contained caffeine. The headache diary also revealed that Susan was taking Anacin twice a week for headaches, Imitrex five times over the 4 weeks, and occasional doses of Tylenol, averaging twice a week. The health care provider reviewed the headache diary and medication use with Susan and addressed the concern of developing drug-rebound headache with more frequent use of analgesics.

Modifications to Management Plan

A plan is developed between the provider and Susan to start her on a preventive medication, propranolol 40 mg bid. She is to continue to keep the headache diary, and she agreed to gradually decrease her caffeine intake and analgesic use.

Continuing Care

Susan is seen again in 1 month and 2 months after preventive therapy is started. After 1 month of propranolol, her dose is increased to 60 mg bid because she was still having three migraines per month. Her headache diary indicated that she had decreased her caffeine intake by approximately half and was not using any Anacin. After 2 months of propranolol, her migraines have decreased in frequency to once a month, and she is not reporting any adverse effects of the beta blocker at a dose of 60 mg bid. She still has Imitrex to use as acute therapy for her migraines. Susan began a program of walking daily with a friend and is now walking approximately 2 to 3 miles at least 4 days a week. She is proud of her accomplishment and states that she hasn't felt this well in many years. The provider encourages her to continue to monitor her use of acute medications, including OTC medications for headaches. She is to return for care in 6 months or if her headaches increase in frequency or severity before that time.

REFERENCES

American Association for the Study of Headache. (1999). Headache: Frequently asked questions. *www.aash.org/faqs.*

Biondi, D. M., Elkind, A. H., & Silberstein, S. D. (1998). Emerging migraine treatments. *Patient Care Nurse Practitioner, 1*(7), 10–26.

Genzen, J. R. (1998). The Internet and migraine: Headache resources for patients and physicians. *Headache, 38,* 312–314.

Hu, X. H. (1999). Burden of migraine in the United States: Disability and economic costs. *Archives of Internal Medicine, 159,* 813–818.

Journal of the American Medical Association. (1999). Managing migraine today (II): Pharmacological and nonpharmacological treatment. JAMA Migraine Information Center. *www.ama-assn.org/special/migraine/treatmnt/treatmnt.htm.*

Mannix, L. K., Frame, J. R., & Solomon, G. D. (1997). Alcohol, smoking and caffeine use among headache patients. *Headache, 37,* 572–576.

Marin, P. A. (1998). Pharmacology update: Pharmacologic management of migraine. *Journal of the American Academy of Nurse Practitioners, 10*(9), 407–412.

Mathew, N. T. (1997). Transformed migraine, analgesic rebound and other chronic daily headaches. *Neurologic Clinics, 15*(1), 167–186.

Mendizabal, J. E. (1998). The clinical challenge of chronic daily headaches. *Patient Care Nurse Practitioner, 1*(5), 41–46.

Mertens, R., Muilenburg, N, Rasmussen, D., Grazer, R., Kleinman, M., Dow, B., Wallace, P., Lee, N., & Brown, B. (1998). Clinical guidelines: Headache in primary care. Kaiser Permanente Northwest Intranet.

Moore, K. L., & Noble, S. L. (1997). Drug treatment of migraine: Part I. Acute therapy and drug-rebound headache. *American Family Physician, 56*(8), 2039–2048.

Noble, S. L., & Moore, K. L. (1997). Drug treatment of migraine: Part II. Preventive therapy. *American Family Physician, 56*(9), 2279–2286.

Peroutka, S. J. (1998). Beyond monotherapy: Rational polytherapy in migraine. *Headache, 38,* 18–22.

Pfaffenrath, V., Cunin, G., Sjonell, G., & Prendergast, S. (1998). Efficacy and safety of sumatriptan tablets (25 mg, 50 mg and 100 mg) in the acute treatment of migraine: Defining the optimum doses of oral sumatriptan. *Headache, 38,* 184–190.

Pryse-Phillips, W. E. M., Dodick, D. W., Edmeads, J. G., Gawel, M. J., Nelson, R. F., Purdy, A., Robinson, G., Stirling, D., & Worthington, I. (1997). Guidelines for the diagnosis and management of migraine in clinical practice. *CMAJ, 156,* 1273–1287.

Sheftell, F. D. (1997). Role and impact of over-the-counter medication in the management of headache. *Neurologic Clinics, 15*(1), 187–198.

Smith, C. M. (1998). Differential diagnosis of headache. *Journal of the American Academy of Nurse Practitioners, 10*(11), 519–524.

Tfelt-Hansen, P. (1997). Prophylactic pharmacotherapy of migraine. *Neurologic Clinics, 15*(1), 153–165.

Ziegler, D. K. (1997). Opioids in headache treatment: Is there a role? *Neurologic Clinics, 15*(1), 199–207.

CHAPTER 34

·······

Heart Failure

CHAPTER OUTLINE

Heart failure is a major health problem that the National Heart, Lung, and Blood Institute estimates affects more than 2 million Americans annually and causes the deaths of 200,000 of them each year. Despite aggressive investigation into treatment options, until very recently the 5-year mortality rate was 50 percent. Of particular importance in its management is the design of a treatment program targeted at the patient's underlying pathophysiology. Such a carefully designed program maximizes outcomes and prevents such treatment complications as prerenal azotemia and dehydration. Because multidrug regimens are often necessary, patient education is essential to limit complications and hospitalizations that result from poor adherence to the treatment regimen.

Pathophysiology

Heart failure is a clinical syndrome that occurs when the cardiac output is inadequate to satisfy the oxygen demands of the body. The primary deficit is a defect in the excitation-contraction coupling mechanism. Contractility of heart muscle is a function of the interaction of calcium with the actin-troponin-tropomyosin system. Activator calcium released from the sarcoplasmic reticulum facilitates the interaction of actin with myosin to create the cross-bridging that produces contraction. The amount of calcium released depends on the amount in stores and the amount that enters the cell during the plateau phase of the action potential. In heart failure, the sarcomeres of the muscle cells are altered in length so that limited numbers of cross-bridges can form and function appropriately, and contractile force degenerates. The reduced force at systole causes the ventricles to supply inadequate blood volume to the body, and blood pressure drops, even though the ventricle is very full and over-stretched. This triggers counterregulatory mechanisms in the rest of the body, activating the sympathetic nervous system (SNS) and the renin-angiotensin-aldosterone (R-A-A) system (Fig. 34–1). The SNS increases heart rate, tries to increase contractile force, and increases venous tone. The R-A-A system triggers the retention of sodium and water to increase blood volume and venous return (increased afterload). Initially, this brings more venous return to the heart and increases the amount of blood available to the body. In the long-term, these adaptive mechanisms actually create more failure. The ventricle

that is already full and stretched is required to deal with more volume (increased preload), and the stressed myocardium begins to undergo structural changes. The cells generated during these changes (remodeling) are often abnormal and include a proliferation of connective tissue cells as well. These cells utilize energy inefficiently and have little contractile ability. The problem is compounded by the denial of adequate oxygen as the increased heart rate shortens the diastolic filling time and the coronary arteries have less time to fill. The heart itself demands more oxygen supply and has less.

Types of Heart Failure

Three main forms of heart failure can occur. Systolic dysfunction typically occurs acutely and often follows a

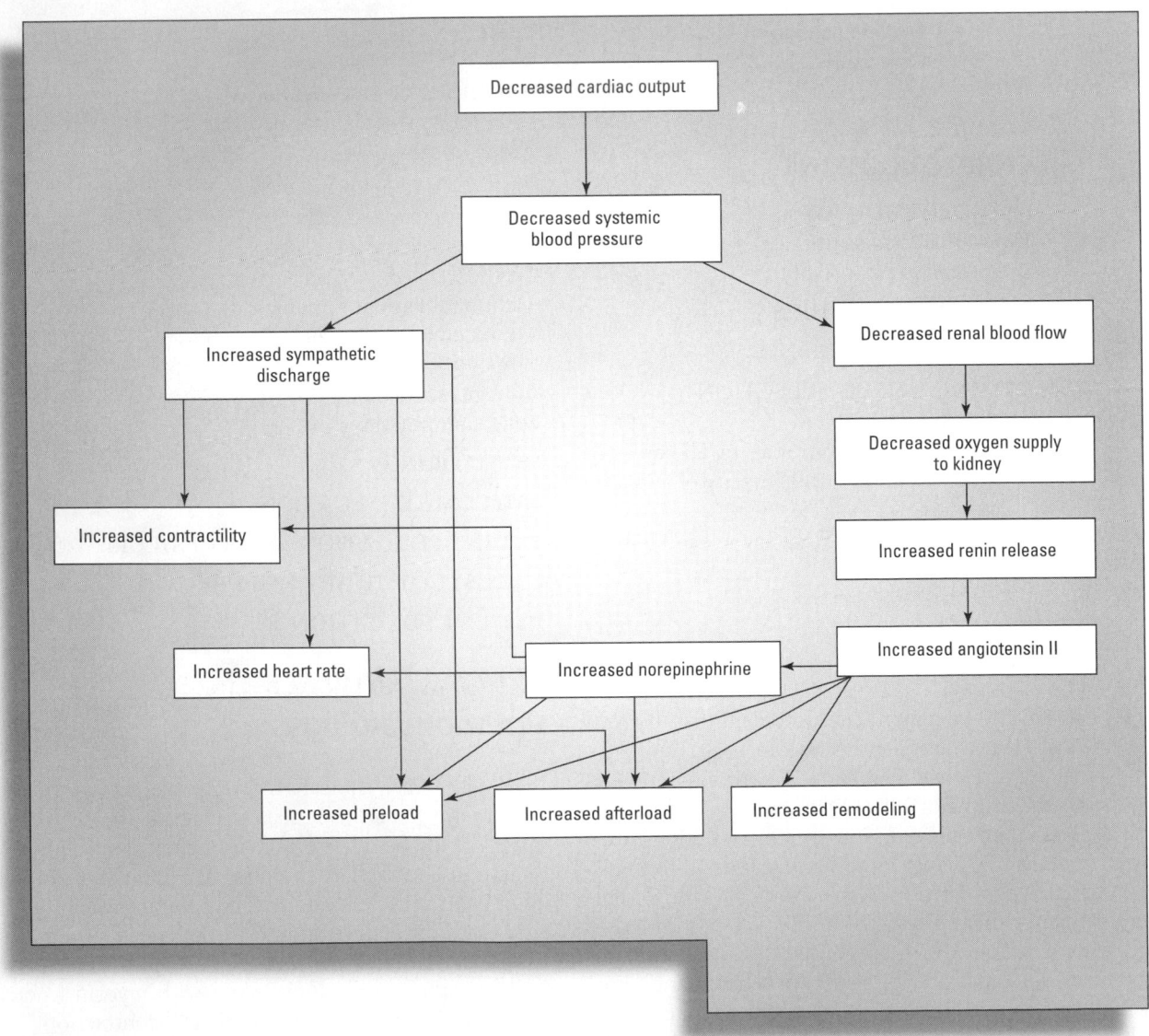

Figure 34–1. Compensatory responses in heart failure.

myocardial infarction (MI). Other potential causes include nonischemic cardiomyopathy, use of **alcohol** and other drugs that depress the myocardium, and conditions that lead to volume overload. The problem is inadequate force generated to eject blood from the ventricles, resulting in decreased cardiac output and ejection fractions of less than 45 percent. Up to 50 percent of patients with heart failure have this form.

Diastolic dysfunction results from inadequate relaxation to permit normal filling. Although cardiac output is reduced, ejection fractions may remain within normal limits. Potential causes include valvular dysfunction, hypertrophic and ischemic cardiomyopathy, uncontrolled hypertension, and hypothyroidism. Up to 40 percent of patients with heart failure have this form. Coronary artery disease (CAD) and atherosclerosis are significant contributing factors for combined systolic-diastolic dysfunction. Framingham data suggest that 76 percent of patients with heart failure have hypertension or CAD alone or in combination as the cause. Treatment of these underlying disorders often improves the performance of the heart muscle.

"High-output" failure is a fairly rare form that takes place when the demands of the body are so great that even increased cardiac output is insufficient. Causative factors include hyperthyroidism, anemia, and arteriovenous shunts. Treatment for this form is directed at the underlying pathology and is not discussed here.

Symptoms of Heart Failure

Symptoms have been described as depending on whether the left or the right ventricle is affected. Lung-focused symptoms (often referred to as "congestion") are associated with left-sided failure, and body-focused symptoms, such as edema, are associated with right-sided failure. With the exception of cor pulmonale, which is clearly right-sided in nature, progression of the disease usually involves both ventricles, and the terminology of left versus right failure is less useful clinically. In older adults, the peripheral edema thought to be associated with right heart failure is actually more often related to venous insufficiency. Peripheral venous disease should be considered as a causative or contributing factor to symptoms in older adults. Regardless of which ventricle is more involved, initial symptoms and those found in mild cases include fatigue, dyspnea on exertion, and unexplained weight gain. Chest x-ray reveals redistribution of pulmonary blood flow to the upper lung fields and/or cardiomegaly. Later in the disease progression and in moderate cases, the fatigue increases; orthopnea develops and may include paroxysmal nocturnal dyspnea. Chest x-ray shows pulmonary edema. In later and more severe cases, a third heart sound (S3) can be heard, the murmur of mitral regurgitation is common, and the chest x-ray shows

pleural effusions. The clinical course of the disease depends in large part on the point at which the patient is diagnosed and treatment is started, the appropriate targeting of that treatment, and the underlying pathology.

Pharmacodynamics

Only a small number of heart failure cases are attributable to specific disorders that can be treated with or improved by surgery. The mainstay of heart failure therapy is drug treatment targeted to altering the physiological mechanisms that create or arise from heart failure. Five main categories of drugs are used to treat heart failure. **Diuretics** reduce preload by decreasing extracellular fluid volume and can be used to decrease hypertension that increases afterload. **Angiotensin-converting enzyme (ACE) inhibitors** act on the R-A-A system to decrease preload and afterload. They also affect heart tissue remodeling so that fewer abnormal myocardial cells are generated. **Digoxin**, a **cardiac glycoside**, improves myocardial contractility and cardiac output. **Beta-adrenergic blockers** affect the SNS counterregulatory mechanism of heart failure. **Nitrates** improve systolic and diastolic ventricular function by improving oxygen transport to the myocardium.

Goals of Treatment

There are three goals of therapy used to determine treatment options: improvement of symptoms, reduction in morbidity, and reduction in mortality. Specific drug therapies have research support documenting their efficacy in attaining one or more of these goals. Physiological goals are to decrease overload (preload and/or afterload), improve contractility, and decrease heart rate. Rational drug selection can be based on these goals, on the mechanism behind the dysfunction, and on the symptom severity of the disease process.

Rational Drug Selection

Guidelines

The Agency for Health Care Policy and Research (AHCPR; see USDHHS, 1994) has produced a clinical practice guideline for the management of patients with left-ventricular dysfunction. This guideline includes steps in accurate diagnosis, pharmacological and nonpharmacological therapies, counseling, and patient education.

Initial treatment for heart failure is focused on reversing underlying pathologies if possible and treating precipitating factors. Lifestyle modification is the first step and includes limitation of activity, reduction in weight as appropriate, limitation of sodium intake to about 2400 mg per day, cessation of smoking, limitation of **alcohol** intake, and a "heart healthy" diet low in cholesterol and saturated fat. These modifications can reduce the demands on the heart, decrease the risk for or facilitate the treatment of hypertension and CAD, and remove a drug that directly depresses the myocardium. Lifestyle modification is appropriate in all stages of heart failure and is an adjunct to successful drug therapy. Table 38–2 in the chapter on hypertension delineates lifestyle modifications that are used in hypertension management, which are also appropriate with heart failure.

Pharmacological therapy is instituted for all patients with heart failure. Pharmacodynamic, pharmacokinetic, and pharmacotherapeutic considerations related to the main drug categories used to treat heart failure are presented in Chapter 14. In determining initial therapy, the presence or absence of fluid overload is considered first. In the presence of fluid overload, a **diuretic** is the initial drug of choice. Next, variables for use of a specific category of drug are considered. Each of the classes of drugs used to treat heart failure addresses the goals of therapy, the severity of the disease, and the underlying pathophysiology in different ways. Concomitant diseases, age, and pregnancy also must be factored into decision making in drug selection. Although it is possible to recommend an approach to drug selection, each of these variables must be considered to facilitate individualizing drug choice. Figures 34–2 and 34–3 show drug algorithms for patients with heart failure.

Drug Choice Based on Goals of Therapy, Pathophysiology, and Severity of Disease

Diuretics

Diuretics improve symptoms and reduce morbidity (Table 34–1). There is no evidence that they affect mortality. Their main function is reducing preload associated with volume overload. **Thiazide diuretics** have long been and remain the drugs of choice early in the disease process and for patients with mild disease. **Loop diuretics** are effective as add-on therapy late in the disease and for patients with more significant heart failure. **Potassium-sparing diuretics** are too weak to be of benefit as monotherapy. They can be useful as concurrent therapy with **thiazide** or **loop diuretics** to counterbalance the potassium loss common to these latter two groups of drugs.

The AHCPR guideline states that **diuretics** should be started immediately when patients present with symptoms or signs of volume overload. In appropriate dosage, preload can be reduced without causing clinically significant decreases in cardiac output. For mild to moderate disease, start therapy with 50 mg **hydrochlorothiazide (HCTZ)**. If the heart failure is more severe, use a **loop di-**uretic such as **furosemide (Lasix)** 20 to 40 mg bid. **Loop diuretics** can cause marked diuresis. Before starting them, discontinue the **thiazide diuretic.** For **loop diuretics,** divide the daily dose to prevent great diuresis at one time. If the patient does not respond adequately to the divided dose, try giving the entire daily dose in the morning before increasing the dose. The goal with **diuretics** is to give the lowest-possible dose that achieves the desired effect. Single daily doses are effective, but during times of increased pathology, oral absorption may be compromised, and the intravenous (IV) route or high doses of oral formulations may be needed. Dosing schedules are given in Chapter 14. Monitor weight gain, changes in dyspnea on exertion, and electrolytes. Diuretic resistance may occur in the presence of decreased renal perfusion or renal stenotic or obstructive pathologies, or with the concurrent administration of **nonsteroidal anti-inflammatory drugs (NSAIDs).** If symptoms seem resistant to the standard doses of the diuretic, check creatinine clearance. **Thiazide diuretics** cannot be used with creatinine clearances that are lower than 25 mL/minute. **Loop diuretics** and **indapamide (Lozol)** can be used with these low creatinine clearances.

Although **diuretics** may be used as monotherapy, they are commonly given with other drugs. Concurrent administration of **vasodilator** therapy may be instituted to improve renal blood flow. Patients may also benefit from the addition of **metolazone (Zaroxolyn)** for its synergistic action on diuresis. Although initiation of **diuretic therapy** is important for patients who have heart failure with volume overload, it is also important to avoid excessive diuresis, especially for patients who are also on sodium restrictions. Volume depletion can lead to hypotension and prerenal azotemia. For patients concurrently taking **ACE inhibitors**, renal insufficiency can be induced. **Diuretics** may be stopped, if necessary, to allow rehydration before starting an **ACE inhibitor.** They can be reintroduced after the dose of the **ACE inhibitor** has been stabilized. **ACE inhibitors** augment the effectiveness of **thiazide** and **loop diuretics** because they decrease glomerular filtration fractions and increase the delivery of solute and water to the distal nephron segments that are responsive to the action of these diuretics.

Long-term use of **diuretics** can stimulate increased R-A-A activity and sodium retention, which are both counterproductive in treating heart failure. This result is less likely with low doses. In addition to the potential for fluid volume changes, **thiazide** and **loop diuretics** present risks for acid-base and electrolyte disturbances that can be proarrhythmic. Monitoring for these problems is discussed in detail in Chapter 14. The most common electrolyte problem is hypokalemia. Any **potassium** supplementation must be based on serum levels because not all patients become hypokalemic or require supplementation beyond dietary changes. **Potassium** supple-

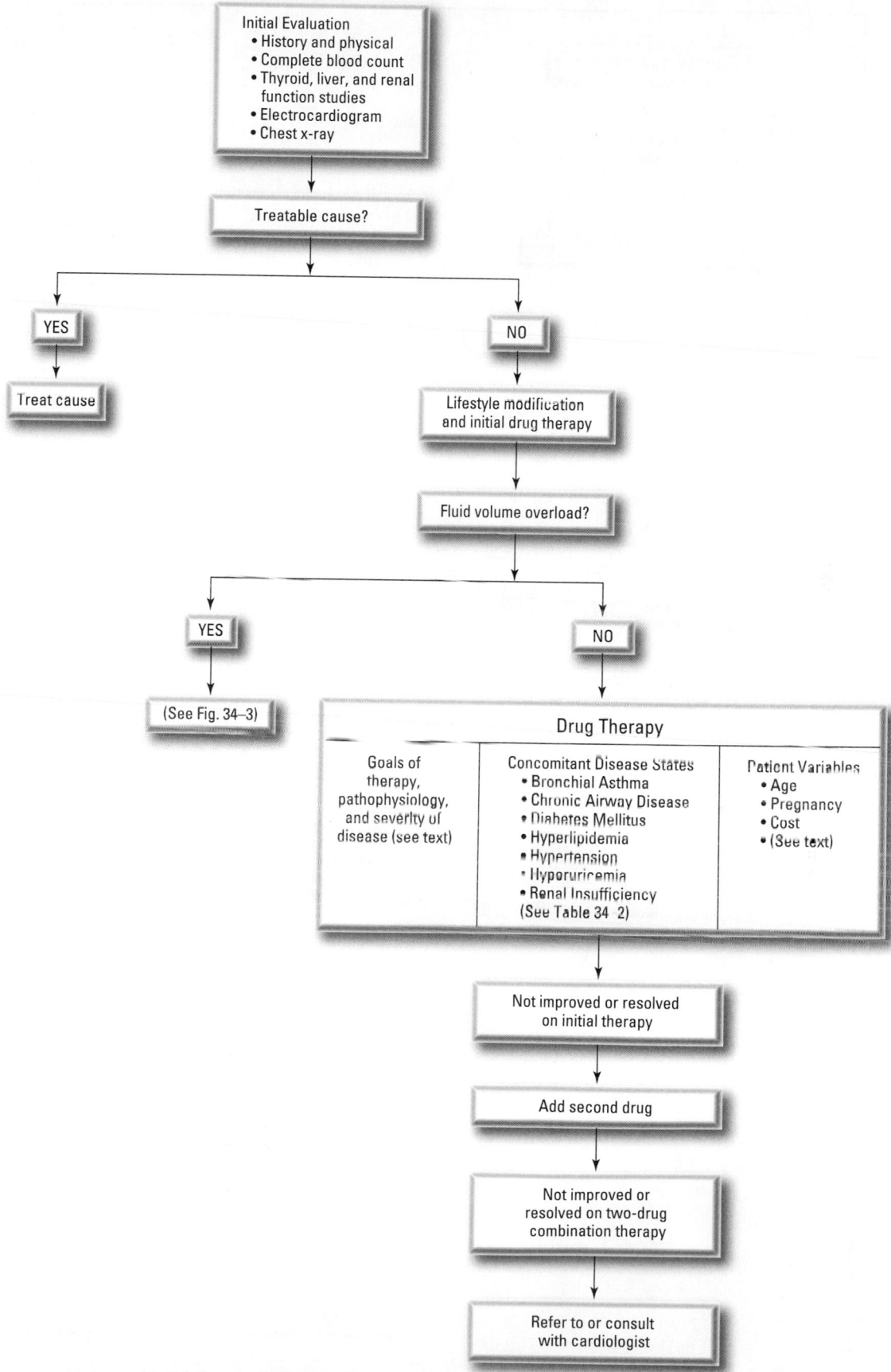

Figure 34–2. Drug treatment algorithm based on treatment and patient variables.

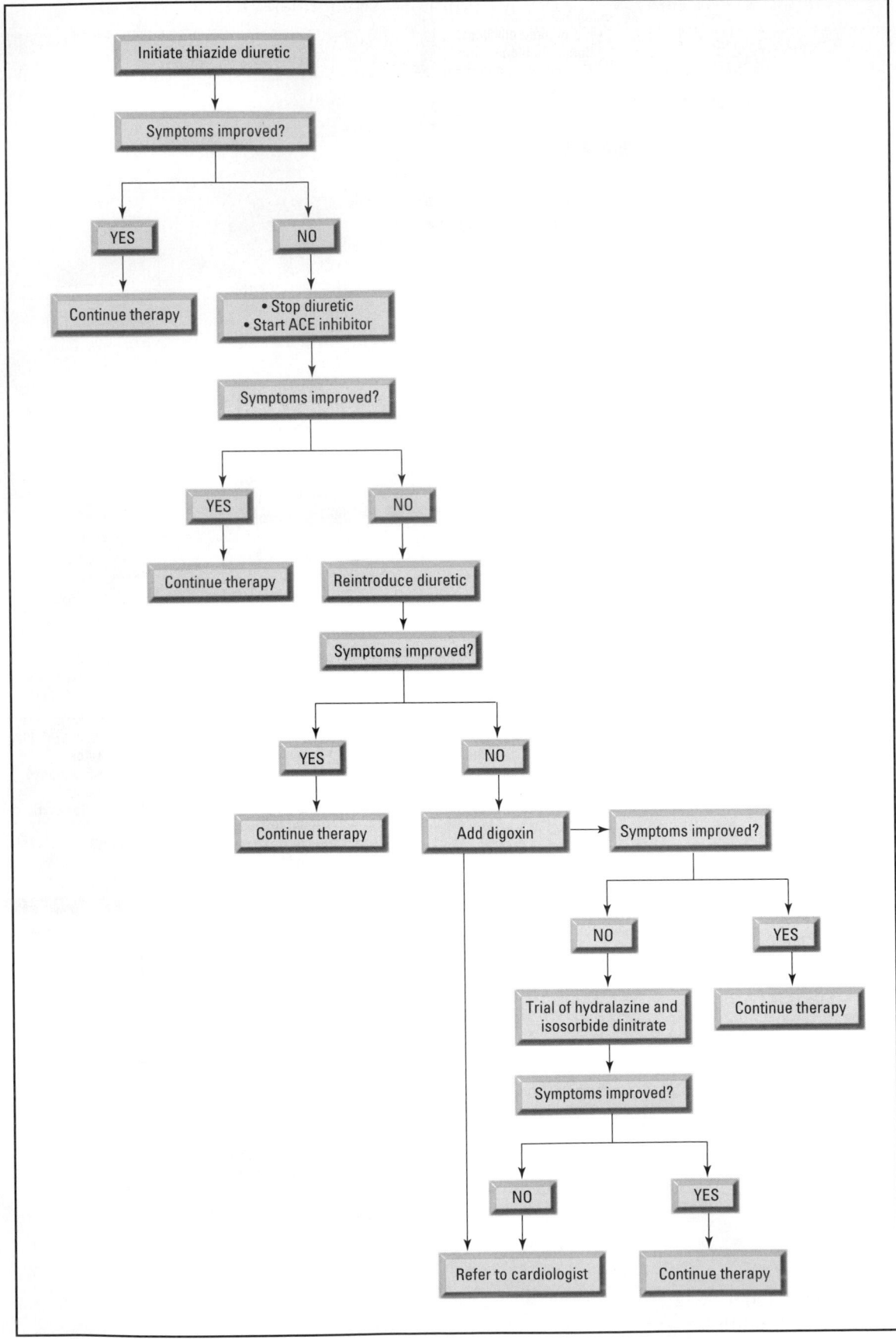

Figure 34–3. Drug treatment algorithm based on fluid volume status: Patient with fluid volume overload.

Table 34–1. Drugs Commonly Used: Heart Failure

Drug	Indication	Initial Dose	Target Dose	Maximum Dose	Special Notes
Thiazide diuretics*: Hydrochlorothiazide	Initial therapy for volume overload.	25 mg qd	As needed	50 mg qd	Cost[†] $1.04 (generic)
Loop diuretics*: Furosemide, bumetanide, torsemide	Added therapy when resistant to standard therapy or for decompensation. Furosemide is first choice. Torsemide is best when high doses of furosemide are required.	10–40 mg qd 0.5–1 mg qd 5 mg qd	As needed As needed As needed	240 mg qd 10 mg qd 20 mg qd	Cost[†] $1.73 (generic)
ACE inhibitors: Captopril, enlapril, lisinopril, quinapril	All subsets of patients. Initial therapy or if symptoms not relieved by diuretic. Drug of choice for patients with diabetes.	6.25 mg tid 2.5 mg bid 5 mg qd 5 mg bid	50 mg tid 10 mg bid 20 mg qd 20 mg bid	100 mg tid 20 mg bid 40 mg qd 20 mg bid	Cost[†] $19.35 $21.53 $23.59
Angiotensin II receptor antagonist: Losartan	Patients intolerant to ACE inhibitors.	25 mg qd	50 mg qd	100 qd	
Digoxin*	If symptoms unrelieved by ACE inhibitor and diuretic.	0.125 mg qd	As needed	As needed	
Hydralazine	With Isosorbide dinitrate for intolerance to ACE inhibitor.	10–25 mg tid	75 mg tid	100 tid	
Isosorbide dinitrate	With hydralazine for intolerance to ACE inhibitor.	10 mg tid	40 mg tid	80 mg tid	
Beta blockers: Labetalol, carvedilol	Patients with diastolic dysfunction or cardiomyopathy in whom reduced heart rate can improve cardiac output.	100 mg bid 3.125 mg bid	400–800 mg 6.25–25 mg bid	1.2 g/d 25 mg bid	

*Dosage for infants and children are given in Chapter 14.
[†]Cost in 1998 dollars to pharmacist for 30-day prescription at lowest recommended dose.

ments must be used cautiously, if at all, for patients concurrently taking **ACE inhibitors,** which cause elevated potassium. Oral **potassium** supplements should provide **chloride** as well to prevent diuretic-induced hypo-

kalemic alkalosis. Hypomagnesemia is also common and may impair potassium repletion. **Diuretics** also contribute to abnormal glucose and lipid metabolism. Care must be taken and diagnostic tests frequently monitored when **diuretics** must be used for patients with diabetes or lipid abnormalities.

Angiotensin-Converting Enzyme Inhibitors

Angiotensin-converting enzyme (ACE) inhibitors have been shown to improve symptoms, decrease morbidity, and decrease mortality. They affect both preload and afterload through their vasodilating effects, decrease the incidence of remodeling by reducing the local generation and action of angiotensin II in heart muscle, and prevent neurohormonal counterregulatory mechanisms that worsen heart failure through their action on the R-A-A system. Patients taking **ACE inhibitors** show moderate increases in ejection fraction, decreased left ventricular end-diastolic filling pressures, and improved myocardial energy metabolism. Because they are the only drugs that address all of the pathological mechanisms that produce heart failure, they are appropriate for all subsets of patients unless these patients are pregnant or have bilateral renal artery stenosis, serum potassium levels above 5.5 mEq, or a history of angioedema. They are also useful for preventing the development of heart failure in patients with ventricular dysfunction but no overt symptoms. A significant reduction in the development of symptomatic heart failure and death due to any cause has been demonstrated in these patients. As monotherapy or in combinations, **ACE inhibitors** are superior to all other drugs and drug combinations used to treat heart failure.

Although these drugs are most effective with systolic dysfunction, it is often difficult to ascertain if the patient has systolic or diastolic dysfunction at the time of the initial examination. However, 90 percent of patients with heart failure have some left ventricular dysfunction (LVD). **ACE inhibitors** are the drugs of choice for LVD and create few ill effects for patients with diastolic dysfunction, even though they are less efficacious with diastolic dysfunction. These drugs are safe to start before it is clear which of the two types of dysfunction exists.

Therapy should be started immediately if **diuretic** monotherapy does not improve exercise tolerance and reduce symptoms, especially for patients with mild to moderate congestive heart failure and absence of an S3. There is no need to wait until the disease has progressed. **ACE inhibitors** are also commonly used as primary therapy, with **diuretics** added if symptoms persist or if volume overload develops at a later time. This is consistent with the AHCPR guidelines. Start with a low dose to prevent risks of hypotension and hypoperfusion, especially of the kidneys. Beginning with 6.25 mg **captopril (Capoten)**, the only short-acting **ACE inhibitor**, permits discontinuance with rapid clearance of the drug should a renal problem occur. Gradually increase **ACE inhibitor** therapy to improve exercise tolerance and relieve symptoms, while monitoring blood pressure and renal function. Blood pressure monitoring is critical not only to assure renal perfusion but also to prevent dizziness and falls. Many patients with heart failure are older adults at high risk for falls with even a limited decrease in cerebral perfusion. Renal function must also be closely watched with blood urea nitrogen (BUN), creatinine, and urinalysis. Any deterioration in renal function may require dosage reductions. Because **ACE inhibitors** alter aldosterone function, potassium levels may rise. Regular monitoring of serum electrolytes is important. Use of **potassium-wasting diuretics** as concurrent therapy may be helpful. **Potassium-sparing diuretics** are not used.

Debate continues on the choice of the best **ACE inhibitor** for long-term therapy. In randomized, controlled studies, both short-acting and long-acting formulations were equally effective. The long-acting formulations demonstrate some greater risk of prolonged hypotension and impairment of renal function, but only at high doses. However, long-acting forms provide a higher affinity for the ACE receptors and more stable drug levels. They also provide a less complex treatment regimen that is more likely to result in adherence because all **ACE inhibitors** except **captopril** have once-daily dosing. The dosing schedule for different **ACE inhibitors** and the process for changing to a long-acting form is discussed in Chapter 14.

A dry, "tickle" cough occurs in up to 15 percent of patients and is the leading reason patients give for choosing to discontinue therapy. This adverse effect appears to be related to the action of **ACE inhibitors** on the bradykinin system. Because they do not affect this system, **angiotensin II receptor antagonists (ATRA)** have actions similar to **ACE inhibitors** but do not produce the cough. Although it has not been officially approved for treatment of heart failure, in a recent trial (Pitt et al., 1997), **losartan (Cozaar)** reduced mortality more than **captopril** did in older adults with heart failure. Further trials are needed to determine if other drugs in this class have a similar effect and to support the use of **ATRAs** in heart failure. **Losartan** is being used clinically because of its actions on the R-A-A system. To date, **losartan** should be reserved for patients for whom **ACE inhibitors** are indicated, but who are unable to tolerate them.

Cardiac Glycosides

Digitalis was once the only effective drug to treat heart failure. Its ability to increase contractility by increasing intracellular calcium and inhibiting the sodium-potassium-ATPase pump deals directly with the primary deficit in heart failure. Unfortunately, clinical research demonstrates that therapy directed at noncardiac targets, such as fluid volume and counterregulatory mechanisms, is more effective in treating heart failure than are the **inotropes**. Although **digoxin** increases the force of contraction, thereby improving functioning and symptoms and reducing hospitalizations, it has little if any effect on mortality. The development of **ACE inhibitors,** combined with the risks of toxicity and multiple drug interactions associated with the **cardiac glycosides (CGs),** has moved **digoxin** to a second-line drug except for selected cases. It remains the drug of choice for heart failure secondary to atrial fibrillation with a rapid ventricular response (it slows heart rate) and uncontrolled hypertension. **Digoxin** also remains a cornerstone of treatment for heart failure in patients with severe systolic dysfunction (ejection fractions less than 40 percent and an audible S3). In fact, the presence of S3 is a potent predictor of response to **CG** therapy. **Digoxin** is less beneficial with ejection fractions of more than 40 percent or in heart failure secondary to hypertrophic cardiomyopathies. Patients with severe aortic stenosis or poorly compliant, hypertrophied ventricles often require elevated end-diastolic filling pressures to support forward stroke volume. Excessive reduction of preload may markedly decrease cardiac output in these patients, so **diuretics** cannot be used. **Digoxin** is the drug of choice here, although it is not a substitute for valve surgery. **Digoxin** is not useful in heart failure associated with idiopathic hypertrophic subaortic stenosis (which it actually worsens), recurrent transient ischemia, or mitral stenosis (unless the patient also has atrial fibrillation).

For stable patients, therapy can be started with an oral maintenance dose without resorting to a loading dose. Using a daily dose of 0.25 mg, a therapeutic blood level can be achieved in 5 to 7 days. Check the serum level in 1 week and make any needed adjustments on the basis of clinical response and serum level. Less stable patients require hospitalization for loading doses. Monitor patients on **digoxin** by following heart rate and rhythm, potassium levels, and renal function. Routine monitoring of serum **digoxin** levels is generally overdone. Monitoring should occur in addition to clinical judgment rather than as a substitute for it. Chapter 14 has detailed discussion of the reasons for and process of monitoring associated with the use of **digoxin,** as well as the process of initiating and maintaining **digoxin** therapy.

The decision to begin **digoxin** therapy should not be made lightly. It should not be used unless there is clear evidence of chronic systolic dysfunction or one of the disease processes just mentioned. **Digitalis** toxicity occurs in as many as 25 percent of patients, and the mortality rate from this toxicity averages 22 percent. The AHCPR guidelines suggest that patients with mild to moderate heart failure often become asymptomatic on optimal doses of **ACE inhibitors** and **diuretics** and do not require **digoxin. Digoxin** should be added for those patients whose symptoms persist despite optimal doses of these two drugs. For patients already on **digoxin,** research evidence supports symptom deterioration when it is suddenly withdrawn. For these patients, **digoxin** should not be withdrawn unless a reversible cause of

heart failure has been fully corrected or there is no basis for using the drug in the first place.

Nitrates

Nitrates are effective for a subset of patients whose primary pathology is increased preload. They are relatively selective to epicardial vasculature and improve systolic and diastolic ventricular function by increasing coronary blood flow. They are also effective after MI and for those with CAD as the primary cause of their heart failure. They reduce symptoms and have some effect on mortality when used as monotherapy in the acute setting. Improvement in mortality in primary care has been demonstrated only when **isosorbide dinitrate** is combined with **hydralazine,** a peripheral vasodilator. This combination is usually reserved for patients who are intolerant of **ACE inhibitors.** Problems with **nitrate** tolerance require special timing of doses, with **nitrate**-free intervals daily. Chapter 14 includes discussion of this problem. The dosage of **isosorbide dinitrate** that produces the most sustained hemodynamic effects and minimizes the development of tolerance appears to be 40 mg q8h. The dosage of **hydralazine** is up to 800 mg q8h to reduce afterload. This is not a long-term management solution.

Beta-Adrenergic Blockers

Beta-adrenergic blockers are used for a subset of patients with diastolic dysfunction or cardiomyopathies for whom decreased heart rate could improve cardiac output. **Beta-adrenergic blockers** are also important for MI prophylaxis for patients who develop heart failure secondary to an acute MI. Care must be taken in prescribing these drugs because they may precipitate acute decompensation. Very low doses are used, and several months are required to show improvement. **Labetalol (Normodyne)** appears to be promising for this use. **Labetalol** is a **nonselective beta-adrenergic blocker** with some alpha-receptor blockade. This combination of actions results in no significant change in cardiac output or heart rate so that the benefits of beta blockade on MI prophylaxis can exist with reduced risk for acute decompensation. It can also be used safely with **digoxin** because it does not abolish this drug's inotropic action. **Carvedilol (Coreg),** another **alpha-beta–adrenergic blocker,** is also being used to treat patients with severe heart failure not resolved by other drugs used in combination. A major drawback for this drug is its expense. Both of these drugs can be used in combination with **ACE inhibitors** to improve left ventricular function.

Calcium Channel Blockers

With the exception of **amlodipine (Norvasc), calcium channel blockers** have not been shown to improve symptoms and may actually worsen them. **Calcium channel**

blockers find rare use for patients with diastolic dysfunction only, and few patients have isolated diastolic dysfunction. Generally, their use with heart failure should be avoided. **Amlodipine** has been demonstrated to be safe for treating angina and hypertension in patients with advanced LVD when used in addition to **ACE inhibitors, diuretics,** or **digoxin**. The safety appears related to its long half-life; calcium channel blockade is maintained at a consistent level and does not have the peaks and troughs associated with most calcium channel dosing, even of sustained-release forms.

Cost

The drugs used to treat heart failure vary in cost from minimal to quite expensive. **Diuretics** are among the least expensive, but they vary from **indapamide (Lozol)** ($25 per month) to generic **HCTZ** ($1.04 per month). The latter is the drug of choice for a variety of reasons, and cost certainly also makes it desirable. None of the **ACE inhibitors** is inexpensive, but **captopril** is now available as a generic formulation, making it less expensive even when it must be administered three times daily. Because **digitalis** has been used for so long, it is among the least expensive. The best choice of **digitalis** formulation is **digoxin**. Despite a slightly higher cost, the Glaxo Wellcome brand (**Lanoxin**) is preferred because of the variable absorption of many other brands. Table 34–1 includes a cost index for many of the drugs commonly used to treat heart failure.

Additional Patient Variables

Concomitant Diseases

Hypertension (HTN) is a common concurrent disorder with heart failure and may contribute to its etiology (Table 34–2). Initial therapy for HTN is monotherapy with **diuretics,** especially for sodium-sensitive patients such as African-Americans, older adults, those who are obese, and those with renal insufficiency. The most effective **diuretics** for both HTN and heart failure are the thiazides. **Loop diuretics** are less effective for HTN but have some use there, and they are helpful for subsets of patients with severe heart failure. **ACE inhibitors** are drugs of choice for treating HTN in young and white patients. The dose for treating HTN, however, is double the dose used to treat heart failure, and the lower dose is required for patients who have both disorders. In patients with low ejection fractions (less than 40 percent), the vasodilating effects of **ACE inhibitors** provide adequate perfusion, even with systolic blood pressure (SBP) at or below 90 mm Hg.

Patients with diabetes may experience increased glucose levels with **diuretics. Thiazide diuretics** in low doses are the least likely to cause this adverse response, followed by **loop diuretics.** Because of their demonstrated effect in reducing diabetic nephropathy, **ACE inhibitors** are clearly the drugs of choice to treat heart failure in patients with diabetes. **Angiotensin II receptor blockers** may also reduce diabetic nephropathy, but this effect has yet to be demonstrated by longitudinal studies. **Calcium channel blockers** have also been shown to have some renal protection. **Angiotensin II receptor antagonists** and **calcium channel blockers** are also acceptable drugs for patients with diabetes because of their limited effects on glucose metabolism, lipid profiles, and renal function. **Beta-adrenergic blockers** are generally avoided for patients with diabetes because they have an adverse effect on peripheral blood flow, prolong hypoglycemia, and mask most hypoglycemic symptoms. Patients with diabetes who need MI prophylaxis and have concurrent heart failure, however, may be placed on low doses of **beta-adrenergic blockers** and taught to monitor their blood glucose more closely and to recognize diaphoresis as their main indicator of hypoglycemia.

Hyperlipidemia leading to atherosclerotic changes is also a common concurrent disorder that may contribute to the etiology of heart failure. **Diuretics** have been associated with transient elevation in lipid levels. Although they are not the first choice for these patients, this transient problem does not rule them out. **ACE inhibitors, angiotensin II receptor blockers, calcium channel blockers,** and **digoxin** do not affect lipid levels and may

ON THE HORIZON

CGP 48506

Drugs targeted at the sensitivity of the actin-troponin-tropomyosin system to calcium have been tried in the past. The action of **phosphodiesterase inhibitors,** such as **theophylline,** is in this area. In general, these drugs have produced little improvement. **CGP 48506** is an investigational drug targeted at calcium sensitivity. It is still undergoing development.

Table 34–2. Drug Choice Based on Concomitant Disease States

Disease State	Preferred	Second Choice	Avoid	Comments
Asthma and chronic airway disease	• ACE inhibitors	• Angiotensin II receptor antagonists (if cough with ACE inhibitor)	• Beta-adrenergic blockers • Alpha-beta–adrenergic blockers	Beta- and alpha-beta–adrenergic blockers may be used if MI prophylaxis is critical.
Diabetes	• ACE inhibitors	• Thiazide diuretics • Angiotensin II • Calcium channel blockers	• Beta-adrenergic blockers • Alpha-beta–adrenergic blockers	Beta- and alpha-beta–adrenergic blockers may be used if MI prophylaxis is critical. Calcium channel blockers only in selected subsets of patients.
Renal insufficiency	• Thiazide diuretics • Loop diuretics	• Digoxin	• ACE inhibitors	ACE inhibitors may be used for patients with diabetes with renal insufficiency with careful monitoring.
Hyperlipidemia	• ACE inhibitors, • Angiotensin II receptor antagonists • Digoxin	• Thiazide diuretics • Loop diuretics	• Beta-adrenergic blockers • Alpha-beta–adrenergic blockers	Beta- and alpha-beta–adrenergic blockers may be used if MI prophylaxis is critical.
Hypertension	• Thiazide diuretics • Loop diuretics • ACE inhibitors	• Beta-adrenergic blockers • Alpha-beta–adrenergic blockers	• Calcium channel blockers	Calcium channel blockers only in selected subsets of patients.
Hyperuricemia	• Digoxin	• ACE inhibitors	• Thiazide diuretics • Loop diuretics	Diuretics may be used and combined with drug to reduce uric acid if they are critical to heart failure management.

be used for patients with hyperlipidemia. **Beta-adrenergic blockers** increase triglycerides transiently and reduce levels of high-density lipids.

Hyperuricemia can be a problem for patients with gout. **Diuretics** can produce this adverse effect. The least likely to do so are the **thiazides**, followed by the **loop diuretics. ACE inhibitors** do not affect uric acid levels directly but can influence renal function, which may indirectly affect uric acid metabolism. **Digoxin** does not affect uric acid metabolism.

Bronchial asthma or chronic airway disease may occur with heart failure, especially in older adults. Chronic airway obstruction is the underlying cause of cor pulmonale, right-sided heart failure. Bronchial activity is unchanged by **ACE inhibitors.** In the 10 to 15 percent of patients taking these drugs who experience a cough, **angiotensin II receptor antagonists** are an alternative. **Alpha-beta–adrenergic blocker** and **beta-adrenergic blockers** are contraindicated in bronchospastic disorders.

Impaired renal function and electrolyte disturbances also influence drug selection. Because **digoxin** is excreted essentially unchanged by the kidney, renal impairment suggests cautious use and close monitoring of serum drug levels. Renal impairment is also associated with increased potassium levels, and the administration of **potassium-wasting diuretics** often results in decreased potassium levels. Both of these situations increase the risk for **digitalis** toxicity. Dosage adjustments of **digoxin** are required for patients with decreased renal function, especially older adults. Renal clearance is a factor in the choice of **diuretic**, as previously discussed. **Thiazide** and **loop diuretics** may cause hypokalemia. **ACE inhibitors** are contraindicated in bilateral renal artery stenosis, and careful monitoring of renal function is required with their use.

Age

Digoxin has a long history of use in infants and children. **Thiazides** and **loop diuretics** are approved for use with pediatric patients. Both of these drug groups have specific pediatric formulations. Safety has not been established in pediatric patients for **ACE inhibitors**. Older adults have a higher risk for **digitalis** toxicity, and the indications of toxicity are different in children and older adults than they are in most adults. **Digitalis** toxicity is discussed in Chapter 14.

Pregnancy

ACE inhibitors are contraindicated in pregnancy. **Digoxin** has been used, but blood levels must be monitored closely to avoid toxicity. **Diuretics** decrease plasma volume and may decrease plasma placental perfusion. They are used only when benefits clearly outweigh risks. Jaundice and thrombocytopenia have been seen in neonates after use in the mother. **Beta-adrenergic blockers** are considered safe in the latter part of pregnancy. A general rule of thumb sometimes proposed is that drugs safe to be used in infants are safe for use in pregnancy, but it is important to remember that consideration must be given to the maternal-fetal drug concentration ratio. Some drugs develop much higher levels of concentration in the fetus than they do in the maternal circulation, and the dose that is therapeutic for the mother may be too high for the neonate. It is best to avoid any drug during pregnancy unless the benefits clearly outweigh the risk to the fetus.

Drug Combinations

Adherence to a treatment regimen is less likely as the regimen becomes more complex. Drug combinations can increase that complexity. They should be reserved for situations in which monotherapy is ineffectual.

Common combinations include **diuretics** and **ACE inhibitors.** When using this combination, withholding or decreasing the dose of the **diuretic** to permit rehydration prior to initiating the **ACE inhibitor** reduces the chances of renal dysfunction and hypotension. The **diuretic** may be reintroduced later with positive effects because the **ACE inhibitor** improves the action of the **diuretic** on the renal tubule. With this combination,

monitor blood pressure, potassium, BUN, and creatinine levels, and decrease the **diuretic** dose if blood pressure falls or prerenal azotemia develops.

Diuretics are also commonly used with **digoxin** for patients with systolic dysfunction. The **diuretics** reduce afterload, and **digoxin** improves contractility. Care must be taken with this combination concerning serum potassium levels, as was previously discussed.

For patients who remain symptomatic on a combination of an **ACE inhibitor** and a **diuretic**, **digoxin** may be added. With this combination, fluid status and serum potassium levels must be carefully monitored. For patients with persistent dyspnea after optimal doses of **diuretics**, **ACE inhibitors**, and **digoxin**, a trial of **hydralazine** and **isosorbide dinitrate** may be given. The addition of a vasodilator to an **ACE inhibitor** may relieve symptoms, particularly for patients with hypertension or evidence of severe mitral regurgitation.

Whenever drug combinations involving more than two drugs are required or patients remain symptomatic on standard one- or two-drug therapy, referral to a cardiologist is essential. Consultation with a cardiologist may be appropriate for all patients with more than mild heart failure.

Monitoring

Monitoring to assess effectiveness in treating the pathology includes daily weights and symptom assessment. Monitoring specific to each drug class is presented in Chapter 14. Renal function assessment is common to all of the drug classes. Serum drug level monitoring is important for **digoxin**. Serum potassium levels are also monitored in all patients with heart failure. Hypokalemia, which may result from **diuretic** therapy, enhances sensitivity to the toxic effects of **digoxin** and is proarrhythmic in all patients with heart failure. Hypomagnesemia may impair the effectiveness of **potassium** replacement therapy and should be assessed for patients with refractory hypokalemia. The Heart Failure Guideline Panel recommends against the use of other tests (e.g., echocardiography, exercise testing) for monitoring the response to treatment of patients with heart failure. No data exist to suggest that monitoring these endpoints contributes information beyond that obtained from a careful history and physical examination (USDHHS, 1994). Repeated testing may be useful for patients with a new heart murmur or sudden deterioration, even though they are adherent to the treatment regimen.

Outcome Evaluation

A careful history and physical examination should be the mainstay in determining outcomes and directing ther-

PATIENT EDUCATION

Heart Failure

Related to the Overall Treatment Plan and Disease Process

☐ Pathophysiology of heart failure, its prognosis, and its long-term effects on other organs of the body besides the heart

☐ Role of lifestyle modifications, including dietary and activity modifications, in improving prognosis and keeping the number and cost of required drugs down

☐ Importance of adherence to the treatment regimen

☐ Self-monitoring of symptoms of worsening failure, including daily weights

☐ What to do when symptoms worsen

☐ Need for regular follow-up visits with the primary care provider

Specific to the Drug Therapy

☐ Reason for the drug's being given and its anticipated action in the disease process

☐ Doses and schedules for taking the drug

☐ Possible adverse effects and what to do if they occur

☐ Coping mechanisms for complex and costly drug regimens

☐ Interactions between other treatment modalities and these drugs

Reasons for Taking the Drug(s)

Patient education about specific drugs is provided in Chapter 14. Specifically for heart failure, additional information includes the following: These drugs are given to reduce mortality, reduce symptoms, and improve functional status. Some drugs do all of these (ACE inhibitors); most do only one. The expectations should be clear about what the drugs can and cannot do. Heart failure is a chronic condition that rarely occurs in a short space of time, and it is not likely to be corrected in a short space of time, if at all. Patients with heart failure must understand the seriousness of this diagnosis, including the 5-year mortality rate of 50 percent and the potential need for surgeries such as heart transplant. All of this must be done while maintaining hope and emphasizing that good quality of life is possible.

Drugs as Part of the Total Treatment Regimen

The total treatment regimen includes sodium restriction and avoidance of excessive fluid intake. Diuretics reduce fluid volume and may interact with dietary restrictions, resulting in orthostatic hypotension. Care should be taken not to reduce fluid volume too quickly, which exacerbates the problem of decreased cardiac output and may lead to hypotension or renal insufficiency. Patients should report symptoms of fluid volume deficit. They should be told to rise slowly from a supine to a standing position to permit the body to redistribute body fluids. Sodium restriction may lead some patients to seek salt substitutes that have a potassium salt as part of their contents. For patients taking ACE inhibitors, this can result in excessively high potassium levels. Such salt substitutes should be avoided. Nonsalt herbal seasoning is more appropriate.

continued

PATIENT EDUCATION

Heart Failure *(continued)*

Regular aerobic exercise such as walking or cycling may improve functional status and decrease symptoms. Regular, gradually increased exercise may lead to enough improvement, in some cases, to reduce the drugs needed. Timing of exercise with the peak action of drugs is important. Patients are often able to predict the timing of voiding after taking a diuretic or times when other drugs are more likely to produce dizziness. Exercise timing should take these into consideration.

Adherence Issues

Nonadherence with the treatment regimen in heart failure may reduce life expectancy and certainly affects functional status. Health care providers should be aware of the potential problem of nonadherence, discuss the importance of adherence at each follow-up visit, and assist patients in removing barriers to adherence (e.g., cost, adverse effects, or complexity of the regimen).

Heart Failure

Case Study 34–1

Complaint

"I'm feeling tired and bloated."

History

David, a 32-year-old white man, came to the office for follow-up 1 week after hospitalization for severe chest pain and arrhythmias consistent with left ventricular dysfunction. He was diagnosed during hospitalization with cardiomyopathy and heart failure with an ejection fraction of 40 percent by cardiac catheterization.

His chief complaint today is fatigue and feeling slightly "bloated," despite 1 week on hydrochlorothiazide (HCTZ) 50 mg daily. His family and personal history is unremarkable except for a congenital renal pelvic junction stricture repaired at age 16. There is no further history of renal impairment, and his creatinine today is 0.8 mg/dL. He had one episode of chest pain last night that was "not enough to go to the hospital." He denies syncope and is not a smoker. He has a sedentary, "high-stress" job and rarely exercises except on an occasional weekend. His diet includes excess salt and cholesterol.

Assessment

Physical examination is remarkable for a blood pressure of 150/90 mm Hg, a pulse of 85, and respiratory rate of 24. Heart sounds do not include an S3, but his lungs exhibit bibasilar crackles that do not clear on coughing. Peripheral pulses are 2+/4+ throughout with 1+ pedal edema in the ankles and mild facial edema. His height is 75 inches and his weight is 220 lb.

Initial Management Plan

In addition to his medical diagnosis of heart failure, nursing diagnoses include activity intolerance, fluid volume excess, and knowledge deficit about his disease and its management. His management plan is as follows:

1. Discontinue the HCTZ so that an ACE inhibitor can be started. Usually this would be stopped for 2 days to permit rehydration before starting the ACE inhibitor. His continued edema and bibasilar crackles, however, indicate fluid volume excess, so hydration is not a concern. The HCTZ will be stopped today, and the ACE inhibitor started immediately.

2. Prescribe captopril 6.25 mg orally twice daily for 7 days. He has no contraindications to ACE inhibitors, the drugs of choice for this type of heart failure. His serum creatinine today is 0.8 mg/dL, providing a baseline for renal assessment. A complete blood count and serum electrolytes are drawn today to provide additional baselines.

3. After assessment of his knowledge base about the diagnosis and its management (with special emphasis on lifestyle and ACE inhibitors), teaching is begun for David and his family.

4. His next follow-up visit for evaluation of therapy and a serum creatinine level will be in 1 week.

continued

Heart Failure (*continued*)

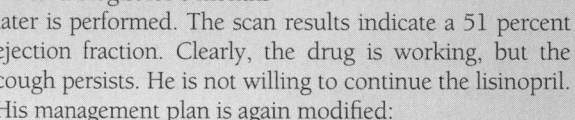

Follow-up Visit

At his follow-up visit 1 week later, David's serum creatinine is 1.5 mg/dL. This is an acceptable increase, based on the action of the ACE inhibitor on the renal system. His edema is decreased, and he has had no further episodes of chest pain. His weight is 213 lb, indicating improved cardiac output that has resulted in improved renal function.

Modifications to Management Plan

His new management plan is as follows:

1. Change his ACE inhibitor to lisinopril (Zestril) 5 mg daily. This is a long-acting ACE inhibitor that can be given once daily. In addition, it comes in a scored capsule so that it can be dispensed as 10 mg and halved. This improves cost because both strengths cost the same.
2. Increase the dose to 10 mg in 2 weeks if permitted by continued renal assessment. This is a stable dose for heart failure. Ordering the 10-mg tablets as the base means only one prescription need be filled, and dosage changes can be made as needed using the existing drug.
3. Assess for adverse effects and adherence, and continue patient and family teaching.

Continuing Care

David's only adverse response is a persistent "tickle" cough that interrupts his sleep to the extent that he requires encouragement from his family to remain on the drug. He agrees to do so until a multiple gated acquisition (MUGA) scan scheduled by his cardiologist for 6 months later is performed. The scan results indicate a 51 percent ejection fraction. Clearly, the drug is working, but the cough persists. He is not willing to continue the lisinopril. His management plan is again modified:

1. Change his drug to an angiotensin II receptor antagonist: losartan (Cozaar) 50 mg daily. Although angiotensin II receptor antagonists have research evidence for their use only in older adults, they provide the R-A-A activity inhibition desired in David's type of failure. They do not, however, affect the kinin system, and the importance of this system's action in resolving heart failure is not yet known.
2. Evaluate cardiac function by physical exam and symptoms in 2 weeks. If cardiac status deteriorates, choose a different drug.
3. Discuss evaluation of cardiac status with cardiologist.

Two years later, David has altered his diet to reduce sodium and trans–fatty acid intake, and he now engages in regular exercise. He has a new job that is less stressful. He remains on losartan 50 mg daily. He has experienced no more chest pain or rhythm disturbances. His weight is stable at 195 lb, and he has no edema. In the absence of symptoms indicating worsening failure, he will be followed every 6 months to assess cardiac function.

---

apy. The history includes questions about physical functioning, appetite, mental health, sleep disturbances, sexual functioning, cognitive function, and ability to perform the usual activities of daily living, including occupational and social activities. Specific questions are asked about the presence of weight gain, orthopnea, paroxysmal nocturnal dyspnea, edema, and dyspnea on exertion. The patient should report weight increases greater than 2 lb in any single day, increased pulmonary symptoms, and ankle edema. A worsening of any of these parameters requires evaluation of the treatment regimen and may indicate the need to adjust the therapy, especially **diuretic** dosage.

Heart failure is generally a chronic condition that can be adequately managed in primary care. Consultation or referral to a cardiologist is appropriate when any of the following occurs:

1. Symptoms markedly worsen or the patient becomes excessively hypotensive.
2. The patient is refractory to standard therapy.
3. There is evidence of renal failure or **digitalis** toxicity.
4. Adequate support is not present in the home to permit the patient to be treated in that situation.

Patients who remain symptomatic on a combination of an **ACE inhibitor,** a **diuretic**, and **digoxin** should be seen by a cardiologist at least once. Persistent volume overload despite standard pharmacological management may require more aggressive administration of the current **diuretic**, more potent **diuretics** via the IV route, or a combination of **diuretics.** Additional testing beyond the usual monitoring may demonstrate evidence of concurrent disorders that may be the source of the resistance to therapy. These disorders may be amenable to other therapies. Surgical intervention may be needed, and hospitalization may be appropriate.

As with all chronic conditions, lack of adherence to a therapeutic regimen is unfortunately common. Several factors in the management of heart failure foster this nonadherence. Lifestyle management is central to the treatment regimen for all stages and types of heart failure, and difficulty in achieving and maintaining lifestyle changes is well documented. Adverse drug reactions and drug costs are also factors. Table 38–9 in the chapter on hypertension details some activities that can improve adherence, and Chapter 6 has additional material to improve positive outcomes.

Patient Education

Patient education should include a discussion of information related to the overall treatment plan as well as that specific to the drug therapy, reasons for the drug being taken, drugs as part of the total treatment regimen, and adherence issues.

REFERENCES

Aronow, W. (1998). The ELITE study: What are its implications for the drug treatment of heart failure? *Drugs & Aging, 12*(6), 423–428.

Cauffield, J., Gums, J., & Grauer, K. (1997). The serum digoxin concentration: Ten questions to ask. *American Family Physician, 56*(2), 495–503.

CONSENSUS Trial Study Group. (1987). Effect of enalapril on mortality in severe congestive heart failure. *New England Journal of Medicine, 316,* 1429–1435.

The Digitalis Investigation Group. (1997). The effect of digoxin on mortality and morbidity in patients with heart failure. *New England Journal of Medicine, 336,* 525–533.

Goroll, A., May, L., & Mulley, A. (1995). *Primary care medicine* (3rd ed.). Philadelphia: Lippincott.

Hardman, J., Limbird, L., Molinoff, P., & Ruddon, R. (Eds.). (1996). *Goodman and Gilman's the pharmacological basis of therapeutics* (9th ed.). New York: McGraw-Hill.

Katzung, B. (1998). *Basic and clinical pharmacology* (7th ed.). Stamford, CT: Appleton & Lange.

Packer, M. (1997). Effects of beta-adrenergic blockade on survival of patients with chronic heart failure. *American Journal of Cardiology, 80*(11), 46L-54L.

Packer, M., Bristow, M., Cohn, J., Colucci,W., Fowler, M., Gilbert, E., & Shusterman, N. (1996). The effect of carvedilol on morbidity and mortality in patients with chronic heart failure. *New England Journal of Medicine, 334,* 1349–1355.

Packer, M., Gheorghiade, M., Young, J., Constantini, P., Adams, K., Cody, R., Smith, L., Van Voorhees, L., Gurley, L., & Joily, M. (1993). Withdrawal of digoxin from patients with chronic heart failure treated with angiotensin-converting enzyme inhibitors. RADIANCE study. *New England Journal of Medicine, 329,* 1–7.

Pfeffer, M., Braunwald E., Moye, L., Basta, L., Brown, E., Jr., Cuddy, T., Davis, B., Geltman, E., Goldman, S., Flaker, G., Klein, M., Lamas, G., Packer, M., Rouleau, J., Rouleau, J. L., Rutherford, J., Wertheimer, J., & Hawkins, C. (1992). Effect of captopril on mortality and morbidity in patients with left ventricular dysfunction after myocardial infarction. *New England Journal of Medicine, 327*(10), 669–677.

Pitt, B., Segal, R., Martinez, F., Meurers, G., Cowley, A., Thomas, I., Deedwania, P., Ney, D., Snavely, D., & Chang, P. (1997). Randomized trial of losartan versus captopril in patients over 65 with heart failure (Evaluation of Losartan in the Elderly Study, ELITE). *Lancet, 349,* (9054), 747–752.

Riaz, K., & Forker, A. (1998). Digoxin use in congestive heart failure. *Drugs, 55*(6), 747–758.

The SOLVD Investigators. (1991). Effect of enalapril on survival of patients with reduced left ventricular ejection fraction and congestive heart failure. *New England Journal of Medicine, 325,* 293.

The SOLVD Investigators. (1992). Effect of enalapril on mortality and development of heart failure in asymptomatic patients with reduced left ventricular ejection fractions. *New England Journal of Medicine, 327,* 685.

Uretsky, B., Young, J., Shahidi, F., Yellen, L., Harrison, M., & Joily, M. (1993). Randomized study assessing the effect of digoxin withdrawal in patients with mild to moderate chronic congestive heart failure: Results of the PROVED trial. *Journal of American College of Cardiology, 22,* 955–962.

U.S. Department of Health and Human Services. (1994). Heart failure: Management of patients with left-ventricular systolic dysfunction. (AHCPR Publication No. 94–0613). Rockville, MD: U.S. Department of Health and Human Services.

CHAPTER 35

....

Human Immunodeficiency Virus Disease and Acquired Immunodeficiency Syndrome

CHAPTER OUTLINE

uman immunodeficiency virus (HIV) disease and its sequel, acquired immunodeficiency syndrome (AIDS), are currently the most important infectious diseases in the United States, with more than 665,000 cases of AIDS reported to the Centers for Disease Control and Prevention (CDC) through June 1998. More than 400,000 deaths have been due to AIDS since the beginning of the epidemic. Since 1995, the natural history of HIV disease has been altered because of increasingly effective **antiviral** therapy. A growing list of potent medications, used in increasingly complex combinations, has slowed the progression of HIV disease leading to AIDS and has dramatically reduced the death rates for people living with HIV. One consequence of this dramatic improvement in outcome is that the older case definition of AIDS no longer accurately reflects the epidemiology of the disease and is much less useful in predicting the needs for prevention and treatment services. In response, 31 states currently have HIV case reporting, resulting in an additional 17,311 new cases of HIV infection reported from July 1997 through June 1998. Although the numbers are not known precisely, it is estimated that at least 700,000 people are living with HIV in the United States and that only 50 percent of them know they are HIV-infected and are receiving ongoing health care.

Pathophysiology

AIDS is a clinical syndrome characterized by progressive immune system suppression, resulting in the development of opportunistic diseases. It is caused by chronic HIV infection. The first reported cases were described in 1981, the causative agent of AIDS was identified as HIV in late 1983, a serologic test for HIV infection was available in 1985, and the first therapy was licensed in 1987. HIV is a member of a family of viruses known as retroviruses, so named because they are able to create DNA copies of their RNA genome, thus reversing (*retro*) the usual flow of genetic information. HIV is a lentivirus, a type of virus that characteristically produces diseases with a long incubation period leading to cancer, severe immune suppression, or both. The basic pathology in AIDS is a loss of CD4-positive T lymphocytes, cells critical to maintaining cell-mediated immune function. This damage results in progressively severe immune dysfunction.

Transmission

There are three principal means of HIV transmission that have been identified: blood, sexual contact, and mother-to-child transmission. The frequency of transmission is influenced by the amount of infectious virus present in the body fluid and the extent of contact an individual has with the body fluids.

Stages

The natural history of HIV disease progresses through several stages. After viral transmission, a symptomatic primary HIV infection, often called *acute retroviral syndrome,* occurs in 50 to 90 percent of the people infected. The onset of symptoms is usually 2 to 4 weeks following infection, but the incubation may be as long as several months in rare cases. Typically, a flulike viral syndrome develops, with fever, lymphadenopathy, pharyngitis, rash, and myalgias or arthralgias. Diarrhea, headaches, and nausea and vomiting are also common. At this stage, serologic tests are not helpful because seroconversion to a positive HIV antibody test usually occurs at 4 to 12 weeks after exposure and infection. Therefore, diagnosis of acute retroviral syndrome must be confirmed by tests for HIV mRNA (viral load). Generally, 95 percent or more of patients seroconvert within 6 months after HIV transmission.

The period from infection to 6 months following HIV transmission is known as *early HIV disease*. At around 6 months after infection, HIV establishes a "set point," representing a stable balance between immune suppression of the virus and ongoing viral replication. In any individual patient, this steady-state set point seems to be relatively stable over a period of years in the absence of **antiretroviral therapy (ART)**. One possible effect of early therapy is to alter this set point to a level associated with longer survival.

The next stage is asymptomatic infection. During this period, the patient is clinically asymptomatic and generally has no abnormal findings on physical examination except enlarged lymph nodes. Symptomatic HIV infection is marked by the development of common infections and other conditions that are more severe and persistent in the presence of HIV infections but by themselves do not define AIDS. Examples of the conditions include thrush, oral hairy leukoplakia, peripheral neuropathy, cervical dysplasia, constitutional symptoms, and recurrent herpes zoster.

Advanced HIV disease is the development of AIDS as defined by the 1993 CDC case definition. This definition includes a list of conditions indicative of severe immunosuppression, as well as the inclusion of all patients with a CD4+ count below 200 cells per mm^3.

Goals of Treatment

The overall goal of **ART** is to achieve maximal and sustained suppression of HIV replication. Such suppression is important in preventing further immune damage and reducing the possibility of the emergence of drug-resistant viral variants. Currently, the most effective intervention in altering the course of HIV disease is proper use of **ART**. Highly active **antiretroviral drugs** are intended to improve survival, reduce or eliminate symptoms, regain immune function, and block the evolution of drug-resistant strains of HIV. In addition, prophylaxis medications can, to a great extent, prevent the development of certain opportunistic infections when the immune system becomes markedly compromised.

Rational Drug Selection

The clinical management of HIV-infected individuals has become increasingly complex as new drug combinations have been evaluated and found effective. In addition, practical strategies must be identified so that virologic suppression can be attained with therapy plans that patients can adhere to consistently. The treatment of HIV disease is a dynamic, rapidly changing arena, as newer drugs are developed and different combinations evaluated.

Principles of Therapy

The Public Health Service has identified certain principles of therapy of HIV infection. First, ongoing HIV replication leads to immune system damage and progression to AIDS. HIV infection is always harmful, and long-term survival free of clinically significant immune dysfunction is unusual. The extent of HIV replication and its rate of CD4+ T-cell destruction are indicated by plasma HIV RNA levels. The extent of HIV-induced immune damage that has already occurred is indicated by the CD4+ T-cell counts. Therefore, plasma HIV RNA and CD4+ T-cell levels must be regularly measured to determine the risk for disease progression in an HIV-infected person and to identify when to initiate or modify antiretroviral treatment regimens. Treatment decisions should be individualized based on the risk of disease progression as indicated by plasma HIV RNA levels and CD4+ measurements. The goal of therapy should be the maximum achievable suppression of HIV replication. The use of potent combination **ART** to suppress HIV replication to below the levels of detection of sensitive viral-load assays limits the potential for selection of **antiretroviral**-resistant HIV variants.

The most effective way to achieve sustained suppression of HIV replication is the concomitant initiation of combinations of effective anti-HIV drugs that the patient has not taken before and that are not cross-resistant with **antiretroviral agents** with which the patient has been treated previously. Each **antiretroviral** drug used in combination therapy should be used according to optimal schedules and dosages. Because the currently available effective **antiretroviral drugs** are limited in number and mechanism of action, and cross-resistance between specific drugs has been shown, remember that any change in **ART** increases future therapeutic limitations.

These principles should be applied to HIV-infected children, adolescents, and adults. However, the treatment of HIV-infected children involves unique pharmacological, virologic, and immunologic considerations. Women should receive optimal **ART** even if they are pregnant. In fact, **antiviral** therapy of the pregnant woman with **AZT** alone or with standard three-drug combinations has dramatically reduced the rates of vertical transmission from mother to child. Additionally, persons with acute primary HIV infection should be treated with combination **ART** to suppress viral replication to undetectable plasma HIV RNA levels. Finally, even those with undetectable viral loads should be considered infectious and counseled to avoid behaviors that are associated with transmission or acquisition of HIV.

In view of these principles, a key question becomes when to start **antiretroviral drug** therapy. There are certain times when most experts agree that the initiation of **ART** is warranted. If a person has symptomatic HIV disease, decreasing CD4+ T-cell counts, high viral load, or primary HIV infection, initiation of therapy is indicated.

However, the potential benefits of early intervention must be weighed against the risks of early therapy. One major factor is nonadherence for patients who are not yet ready to commit to a complex drug regimen and potential adverse effects that may decrease their quality of life. Therefore, the clinician and the patient need to have an indepth discussion of the potential toxicities and the complexities of the **antiretroviral** regimen. Table 35–1 presents these risks and benefits.

In patients with primary infection, the period between infection and the time of emergence of an antibody response and establishment of a steady-state set point of HIV RNA in the blood, combination therapy results in dramatic and sustained viral suppression. If therapy is initiated early enough, the dissemination of HIV within the body is in theory blunted, and the result is decreased viral reservoirs. It may not be possible to eradicate the virus, but early treatment of primary infection may have important long-term

Table 35–1. Risks and Benefits of Early Initiation of Antiretroviral Therapy in the Asymptomatic HIV-Infected Patient

Potential Benefits
- Control of viral replication and mutation; reduction of viral burden
- Prevention of progressive immunodeficiency; potential maintenance or reconstruction of a normal immune system
- Delayed progression to AIDS and prolongation of life
- Decreased risk of selection of resistant virus
- Decreased risk of drug toxicity
- Possible decreased risk of viral transmission

Potential Risks
- Reduction in quality of life from adverse drug effects and inconvenience of current maximally suppressive regimens
- Earlier development of drug resistance
- Transmission of drug-resistant virus
- Limitation in future choices of antiretroviral agents due to development of resistance
- Unknown long-term toxicity of antiretroviral drugs
- Unknown duration of effectiveness of current antiretroviral therapies

Source: U.S. Department of Health and Human Services. (1999). Report of the NIH panel to define principles of therapy of HIV infection and guidelines for the use of antiretroviral agents in HIV-infected adults and adolescents. *Morbidity and Mortality Weekly Report, 47* (4/24/98; revis. 5/99), RR-5.

benefits. Newly infected people tend to have a relatively homogeneous swarm of viruses, and early treatment may minimize viral diversification. Other arguments for treating primary infection include the idea that the set point could possibly be lowered, with a subsequent slowing of disease progression. Also, it may also reverse much of the immune system damage that occurs during this early infection period.

Early initiation of potent **ART** is supported by recent data. Theoretically, the earlier the therapy is initiated, the less damage occurs. However, there has been no long-term experience with early therapy. Also, it is possible that if therapy is started too early or not managed well, future treatment options may be compromised. These considerations need to be balanced with the patient's wishes and ability to adhere to a treatment regimen. **Highly active antiretroviral therapy (HAART)** refers to a combination of **antiretroviral drugs** that are capable of suppressing HIV replication to undetectable levels and sustaining an undetectable level for a prolonged period.

Treatment of asymptomatic patients with established HIV infection and early disease with high CD4+ T-cell counts and low viral load is controversial. Arguments against early treatment include (1) the increased potential for adherence failures with longer-duration therapy, (2) the risk of longer exposure to unknown long-term adverse effects of medication, (3) the impact on quality of life caused by unpleasant adverse effects and the need to adhere to a regimen, and (4) the possible earlier selection of drug-resistant HIV strains. There are also potentially decreased future options for changing medication if resistance develops and possible exhaustion of benefit from current therapy because the duration of efficacy of suppression is not known. Finally, there is the increased cost of early initiation of therapy. The reasons for starting therapy in asymptomatic patients are similar to those for treating primary infection. Some clinicians believe that a patient with a detectable viral load should be offered **ART**.

Nucleoside Reverse Transcriptase Inhibitors

There are currently six **nucleoside reverse transcriptase inhibitors (NRTIs)** approved in the United States: **AZT** (1987), **ddI** (1991), **ddC** (1992), **d4T** (1994), **3TC** in combination with **AZT** (1995), the **Combivir** combined formulation of **AZT** and **3TC (1997)**, and **abacavir** (1998). These drugs mimic natural nucleotides, which are molecules that are the building blocks of DNA and RNA. The **NRTIs** compete with the natural nucleotides for incorporation by HIV's reverse transcriptase enzyme into newly synthesized viral DNA chains, resulting in chain termination. The **nucleoside**

analogues remain a key component of combination **antiretroviral** regimens.

Zidovudine (Retrovir; formerly **AZT)** was the first **nucleoside analogue** approved by the Food and Drug Administration (FDA). It is indicated for the treatment of HIV disease when **ART** is warranted. **Zidovudine** is supplied in 100-mg capsules and 300-mg tablets. The recommended total oral daily dose of **zidovudine** is 600 mg per day in divided doses in combination with other **antiretroviral** agents and 500 mg or 600 mg per day in divided doses for monotherapy. The major dose-limiting toxicity of **zidovudine** is reversible bone marrow toxicity manifested as anemia or leukopenia. Fatigue, rashes, severe muscle pain, muscle inflammation, nausea, insomnia, and headaches are also associated with **zidovudine** therapy.

Lamivudine (Epivir; formerly **3TC)**, a synthetic **nucleoside analogue** with activity against HIV, is indicated in combination with **zidovudine** for the treatment of HIV infection. Supplied in 150-mg tablets, the recommended dose of **lamivudine** for adults and adolescents is 150 mg twice daily. Adverse events that have been reported include headache, nausea, malaise, fatigue, nasal signs and symptoms, diarrhea, neuropathy, neutropenia, and anemia. Some patients with HIV infection who have chronic liver disease due to hepatitis B virus (HBV) infection experienced clinical or laboratory evidence of recurrent hepatitis upon discontinuation of **lamivudine.** Therefore, caution is warranted when considering stopping **lamivudine** in those also infected with HBV.

Lamivudine and **zidovudine** are also available in combination **Combivir** tablets containing 150 mg of **lamivudine** and 300 mg of **zidovudine.** The recommended dosage of **Combivir** for adults and adolescents is 1 tablet twice daily. In controlled trials of **lamivudine** 300 mg per day plus **zidovudine** 600 mg per day, adverse events that were reported included anorexia, abdominal pain and cramps, dyspepsia, neuropathy, insomnia, dizziness, depressive disorders, nasal signs and symptoms, cough, skin rashes, myalgias, arthralgias, and musculoskeletal pain.

Didanosine (Videx; formerly **ddI)** is indicated for the treatment of HIV. It is supplied in chewable/dispersible buffered tablets in strengths of 25, 50, 100, and 150 mg. The dosing interval for **didanosine** should be 12 hours. All **didanosine** formulations should be taken on an empty stomach, at least 30 minutes before or 2 hours after eating. Adults should take 2 tablets at each dose so that adequate buffering is provided to prevent gastric acid degradation of **didanosine.** The recommended dose for patients weighing 60 kg or more is 200 mg twice a day or 400 mg once daily. For patients weighing less than 60 mg, the recommended dosage is 125 mg twice a day or 400 mg once daily. The major toxicity of **didanosine** is pancreatitis. Other adverse events include lactic acidosis, severe hepatomegaly with steatosis, and retinal and visual changes.

Zalcitabine (Hivid; formerly ddC) in combination with **zidovudine** is indicated for the treatment of HIV infection in patients with limited prior exposure to **zidovudine**. **Zalcitabine** is also indicated in combination with **protease inhibitor**s for the treatment of HIV disease. In patients with advanced HIV disease who are intolerant to or who have disease progression while receiving **ART, zalcitabine** monotherapy is indicated for the treatment of HIV infection. **Zalcitabine** is supplied as 0.375-mg and 0.75-mg tablets, and the recommended monotherapy dose is 0.75 mg orally every 8 hours. The recommended combination regimen is 0.75 mg **zalcitabine** and 200 mg **zidovudine** every 8 hours. Reported toxicities include fatigue, headache, fever, abdominal pain, oral lesions, vomiting, nausea, diarrhea, abnormal hepatic function, peripheral neuropathy, convulsions, and rash.

Stavudine (Zerit; also known as d4T) is approved by the FDA for adults and children with HIV infection. It is most effective when used in combination with other **antiretrovirals. Stavudine** is supplied in 15-, 20-, 30-, and 40-mg capsules and as an oral solution. **Stavudine** doses should be given 12 hours apart, and the recommended dosages are based on weight. For those weighing 60 kg or more, the dose is 20 mg twice daily, and for those weighing less than 60 kg, the recommended dose is 15 mg twice daily. Peripheral neuropathy is the most frequently observed toxicity of **stavudine.** Other reported adverse events at the dose of 40 mg twice daily include headache, chills, fever, diarrhea, rash, nausea, vomiting, abdominal pain, myalgias, insomnia, and anorexia.

The most recently approved **nucleoside analogue** is **abacavir** (Ziagen), which was approved in December 1998 to treat HIV-1 in adults and children. **Abacavir** is supplied as 300-mg tablets or an oral suspension. The recommended dosage for adults is 300 mg twice daily in combination with other **antiretroviral agents.** Fatal hypersensitivity reactions have been associated with **abacavir** therapy. Therapy with **abacavir** should *not* be restarted following a hypersensitivity reaction because more severe symptoms will recur within hours and may include life-threatening hypotension and death. Hypersensitivity reactions have been reported in approximately 5 percent of patients taking **abacavir.** The reaction is characterized by symptoms indicating involvement of multiple organs or body systems. Symptoms usually appear within the first 6 weeks of treatment, although these reactions may occur at any time during therapy. Frequently observed signs and symptoms include fever, skin rash, fatigue, and gastrointestinal (GI) problems such as nausea, vomiting, diarrhea, or abdominal pain. Other signs and symptoms include malaise, lethargy, myalgia, arthralgia, edema, shortness of breath, and paresthesias. Physical findings include lymphadenopathy, mucous membrane lesions, and rash. The rash usually is maculopapular or urticarial but may be variable in appearance.

Hypersensitivity reactions have occurred without rash. Laboratory abnormalities include elevated liver function tests, increased creatine phosphokinase or creatinine, and lymphopenia. Anaphylaxis, liver failure, hypotension, and death have occurred in association with hypersensitivity reactions. Symptoms worsen with continued therapy but often resolve when therapy is discontinued.

Nonnucleoside Reverse Transcriptase Inhibitors

The FDA has approved three **nonnucleoside reverse transcriptase inhibitors (NNRTIs): delavirdine** (1997), **nevirapine** (1996), and **efavirenz** (1998). This group of medications is structurally diverse, but all bind near the catalytic site of HIV-1 reverse transcriptase and are very specific. As noncompetitive inhibitors of reverse transcriptase, their antiviral activity is additive or synergistic with most other **antiretrovirals.** However, drug interactions dictate dosage adjustments with **protease inhibitors.**

As a class of medications, the **NNRTIs** may cause mild to moderate skin rash that can be managed with **antihistamines.** Occasionally, the skin eruption is more severe, and rare cases of Stevens-Johnson syndrome have been observed.

Delavirdine (Rescriptor) is indicated for the treatment of HIV-1 infection in combination with other appropriate **antiretroviral agents.** It is supplied as a 100-mg tablet, and the recommended dosage is 400 mg three times daily (a total of 12 tablets per day). The tablets may be dispersed in water prior to taking. **Delavirdine** may be taken with or without food. The most significant side effect of **delavirdine** is rash, which occurs in about 18 percent of people who take the drug. Adverse events of moderate or severe intensity that occurred in patients taking **delavirdine** in combination included headache, fatigue, nausea, diarrhea, vomiting, increased alanine aminotransferase (ALT) and aspartate aminotransferase (AST), rash, and itching. Because of possible effects of **delavirdine** on the hepatic metabolism of certain drugs, coadministration of **delavirdine** with certain nonsedating **antihistamines, sedative hypnotics, antiarrhythmics, calcium channel blockers, ergot alkaloid preparations, amphetamines,** and **cisapride** may result in serious or life-threatening adverse events. Resistance to **delavirdine** emerges rapidly in vitro and when this drug was tested as a monotherapy; therefore it should never be given alone for any length of time.

Nevirapine (Viramune), the second **NNRTI** released, has been approved for use in combination with approved **nucleoside analogues** for the treatment of HIV-1 infection. Approval was based on surrogate endpoint data, but subsequent studies demonstrated clinical benefit in combination regimens. Supplied in 200-mg white tablets, the recommended dose is one 200-mg tablet daily for the first 14 days, followed by one 200-mg tablet twice daily in combination with **antiretroviral agents.** The initial lower dose has been found to decrease the occurrence of skin rash. **Nevirapine** may be taken with or without food. The most frequently reported adverse events are skin rash, fever, nausea, headache, and abnormal liver function tests. Rashes are usually mild to moderate maculopapular, erythematous, cutaneous eruptions, with or without pruritus, located on the trunk, face, and extremities. Most severe rashes occurred within the first 28 days of treatment. **Nevirapine** therapy should be discontinued if patients experience severe rash or a rash accompanied by constitutional findings. Resistance to **nevirapine** emerges rapidly when **nevirapine** is used as a monotherapy or in suboptimal combinations.

The newest **NNRTI** to be approved is **efavirenz (Sustiva)**. **Efavirenz** is indicated in combination with other antiretroviral agents and is supplied in 50-, 100-, and 200-mg capsules. The recommended dosage of **efavirenz** is 600 mg orally once a day in combination with a **protease inhibitor** and/or two **NRTIs**. **Efavirenz** may be taken with or without food; however, a high-fat meal may increase the absorption of **efavirenz,** resulting in more side effects. The most significant adverse events associated with **efavirenz** are nervous system symptoms and rash. Fifty-two percent of patients receiving **efavirenz** reported central nervous system and psychiatric symptoms, including dizziness, somnolence, insomnia, abnormal dreaming, confusion, abnormal thinking, impaired concentration, amnesia, agitation, depersonalization, hallucinations, and euphoria. **Efavirenz** should be taken at bedtime to improve the tolerability of the nervous system side effects. Because of the rapid emergence of resistance to **NNRTIs** given as monotherapy, **efavirenz** must be given in combination with other **antiretrovirals.**

Protease Inhibitors

In 1996, at the International Conference on AIDS in Vancouver, a new era in the treatment of HIV disease was introduced. **HAART** involves the use of a **protease inhibitor (PI)** combined with two **nucleoside analogues.** This strategy provides a major advancement in moving toward HIV as a clinically manageable condition.

There are currently five **PIs** approved for use in the United States: **indinavir** (1996), **nelfinavir** (1997), **ritonavir** (1996), **saquinavir** (1995), and **amprenavir** (1999). The mechanism of action for the **PIs** targets a later stage of the viral replication cycle than do the **reverse transcriptase inhibitors.** A **PI** binds within the catalytic site of the viral protease enzyme. The viral protease enzyme plays a crucial role in the maturation of the virus as it buds off from an infected cell by cutting free the viral enzyme's reverse transcriptase and integrase

from large precursor polyproteins and allowing the virus's structural elements to assemble properly. The virus can become infectious only if the protease enzyme is successful. The development of resistance-conferring mutations has been associated with failure of **PIs** to suppress viral load and subsequent clinical progression.

The common toxicities associated with **PIs** are generally different from those seen with the **nucleoside analogues.** GI adverse effects, especially diarrhea, are among the first that patients experience. These drugs have also been known to induce hepatitis or to exacerbate preexisting viral hepatitis secondary to the metabolism of **PIs** by the liver.

As the use of **PIs** becomes more commonplace and patients have been on these drugs for longer periods, certain adverse events are beginning to emerge. Abnormal fat distribution in the absence of weight gain in patients taking **PIs** has been reported in increasing numbers. The lipodystrophy can present as loss of fat from the face and limbs, an increased abdominal girth (protease paunch), or development of a "buffalo hump" (pads of fat behind the neck or on the back). New-onset diabetes and exacerbation of existing diabetes have been observed with the use of **PIs.** The incidence of new or worsening diabetes on **PIs** has been low. Recently, it has also been reported that premature coronary artery disease has rarely occurred in patients on **PIs.**

Recently, more research has looked at dual **PIs** therapy. The rationale for this approach is that the coadministration of two **PIs** together slows their clearance and dramatically improves the pharmacokinetic profile. Examples of the combinations studied include **indinavir-nelfinavir, indinavir-ritonavir, nelfinavir-ritonavir, nelfinavir-saquinavir,** and **ritonavir- saquinavir.**

Table 35–2 presents the drugs commonly used in HIV disease.

Indinavir (Crixivan) is a peptidomimetic **PIs** approved for the treatment of HIV-infected adults "when antiretroviral therapy is warranted." The approval was based primarily on surrogate marker data including viral load and CD4+ counts. **Indinavir** is supplied in capsule form and is available in 200-mg and 400-mg strengths. The recommended dosage of **indinavir** is 800 mg orally every 8 hours. For optimal absorption, it should be taken without food but with water 1 hour before or 2 hours after a meal. However, this can be difficult for a patient to tolerate. Alternatively, it may be taken with other liquids such as skim milk, juice, coffee, or tea or with a light meal (e.g., dry toast with jelly or corn flakes with skim milk and sugar). It should not be taken with meals high in calories, fat, and protein. Adequate hydration must be maintained, and it is recommended that the patient drink at least 1.5 L of liquids during the course of 24 hours. Nephrolithiasis has been reported in approximately 4 percent of patients receiv-

Table 35–2. Drugs Commonly Used: HIV Disease

Drug	Dosing Recommendations	Form	Adverse Reactions	Notes
Protease Inhibitors Indinavir (Crixivan)	800 mg q8h; separate dosing with didanosine by 1 h	200-, 400-mg capsules	Nephrolithiasis, GI intolerance, nausea, increased indirect bilirubinemia, headache, asthenia, blurred vision, dizziness, rash, metallic taste, thrombocytopenia, hyperglycemia, fat redistribution and lipid abnormalities, possible increased bleeding episodes in patients with hemophilia	Take 1 h before or 2 h after meals; may take with skim milk or low-fat meal; levels decrease by 77% Store at room temperature
Ritonavir (Norvir)	600 mg q12h; separate dosing with didanosine by 2 h	100-mg capsules, 600-mg/7.5 mL PO solution	GI intolerance, nausea, diarrhea, vomiting, paresthesias (circum-oral and extremities), hepatitis, asthenia, taste perversion, triglycerides increase >200%, transaminase elevation, elevated creatine phosphokinase (CPK) and uric acid, hyperglycemia, fat redistribution and lipid abnormalities, possible increased bleeding episodes in patients with hemophilia	Take with food if possible, which may improve tolerability; levels increase 15% Refrigerate capsules; oral solution should not be refrigerated
Saquinavir (Invirase)	400 mg bid with ritonavir	200 mg capsules	GI intolerance, nausea, diarrhea, headache, elevated transaminase enzymes, hyperglycemia, fat redistribution and lipid abnormalities, possible increased bleeding episodes in patients with hemophilia	No food effect when taken with ritonavir Store at room temperature
Saquinavir (Fortovase)	1200 mg tid	200-mg capsules	GI intolerance, nausea, diarrhea, abdominal pain, dyspepsia, headache, elevated transaminase enzymes, hyperglycemia, fat redistri-	Take with large meal; levels increase 6-fold Refrigerate or store at room temperature (up to 3 mo)

Continued on next page

Table 35–2. Drugs Commonly Used: HIV Disease *(continued)*

Drug	Dosing Recommendations	Form	Adverse Reactions	Notes
			bution and lipid abnormalities, possible increased bleeding episodes in patients with hemophilia	
Nelfinavir (Viracept)	750 mg tid	250-mg tablets, 50-mg/g oral powder	Diarrhea, hyperglycemia, fat redistribution and lipid abnormalities, possible increased bleeding episodes in patients with hemophilia	Take with meal or snack; levels Increase 2- or 3-fold Store at room temperature
Nucleoside Reverse Transcriptase Inhibitors Zidovudine (AZT, ZDV) (Retrovir)	200 mg tid *or* 300 mg bid *or* with 3TC as Combivir, 1 bid	100-mg capsules, 300-mg tablets, 10-mg/mL IV solution, 10-mg/mL oral solution	Bone marrow suppression, anemia, neutropenia, GI intolerance, headache, insomnia, asthenia, lactic acidosis	Take without regard to meals
Didanosine (ddI) (Videx)	Tablets: >60 kg: 200 mg bid <60 kg: 125 mg bid	25-, 50-, 100-, 150-mg tablets; 167-, 250-mg sachets	Pancreatitis, peripheral neuropathy, nausea, diarrhea, lactic acidosis	Take 30 min before or 1 h after meal; levels decrease 55%
Zalcitabine (ddC) (Hivid)	0.75 mg tid	0.375-, 0.75-mg tablets	Peripheral neuropathy, stomatitis, lactic acidosis	Take without regard to meals
Stavudine (d4T) (Zerit)	>60 kg: 40 mg bid <60 kg: 30 mg bid	15-, 20-, 30-, 40-mg capsules	Peripheral neuropathy, lactic acidosis	Take without regard to meals
Lamivudine (3TC) (Epivir)	150 mg bid <50 kg: 2 mg/kg bid *or* with ZDV as Combivir 1 bid	150-mg tablets, 10-mg/mL oral solution	Minimal toxicity, lactic acidosis	Take without regard to meals
Abacavir (ABC) (Ziagen)	300 mg bid	300-mg tablets, 20-mg/mL oral solution	Hypersensitivity reaction, fever, rash, nausea, vomiting, malaise, fatigue, loss of appetite, lactic acidosis	Take without regard to meals
Nonnucleoside Reverse Transcriptase Inhibitors Nevirapine (Viramune)	200 mg PO qd × 14 d, then 200 mg PO bid	200-mg tablets	Rash, increased transaminase levels, hepatitis	Take without regard to meals

Continued on next page

Table 35–2. Drugs Commonly Used: HIV Disease *(continued)*

Drug	Dosing Recommendations	Form	Adverse Reactions	Notes
Delavirdine (Rescriptor)	400 mg PO tid, *or* 4 100-mg tablets in 3 oz or more water to produce slurry; separate dosing with didanoside or antacids by 1 h	100-mg tablets	Rash, increased transaminase levels, headaches	Take without regard to meals
Efavirenz (Sustiva)	600 mg PO qHS	50-, 100-, 200-mg capsules	Rash, increased transaminase levels, CNS symptoms, false-positive cannabinoid test	Avoid taking after high-fat meals; levels increase 50%

Source: Adapted from U.S. Department of Health and Human Services. (1999). Report of the NIH panel to define principles of therapy of HIV infection and guidelines for the use of antiretroviral agents in HIV-infected adults and adolescents *Morbidity and Mortality Weekly Report, 47* (4/24/98; revis. 5/99), RR-5.

ing **indinavir** in clinical trials. Other drug-related clinical adverse experiences of moderate or severe intensity in more than 2 percent of patients treated with **indinavir** alone or in combinations with **zidovudine** include abdominal pain, asthenia, fatigue, flank pain, malaise, nausea, diarrhea, vomiting, acid regurgitation, anorexia, dry mouth, back pain, headache, insomnia, dizziness, somnolence, and taste perversion. A dose reduction of **rifabutin** to half the standard dose is recommended if it is given with **indinavir**. If **ketoconazole** is administered concurrently, a dose reduction of **indinavir** to 600 mg every 8 hours should be considered. Also, if **indinavir** and **didanosine** are administered together, they should be given at least 1 hour apart on an empty stomach. If a patient has mild to moderate hepatic insufficiency because of cirrhosis, the dosage of **indinavir** should be reduced to 600 mg every 8 hours.

Nelfinavir (Viracept) is indicated for the treatment of HIV infection when **ART** is warranted. The indication is based on surrogate marker changes in patients who received **nelfinavir** in combination with **nucleoside analogues** or alone for up to 24 weeks. **Nelfinavir** is supplied as a light blue, capsule-shaped tablet in a 250-mg strength. **Nelfinavir** is an inhibitor of the HIV-1 protease and results in the production of immature, noninfectious HIV. The recommended dose is 750 mg (three 250-mg tablets) three times daily. **Nelfinavir** should be taken with a meal or light snack. Antiviral activity is enhanced when **nelfinavir** is administered in combination with **nucleoside analogues**. Therefore, it is recommended that **nelfinavir** be used in combination with **nucleoside analogues**. Drug-related adverse experiences of moderate or severe intensity include diarrhea, nausea, flatulence, abdominal pain, asthenia, and rash. **Nelfinavir** should not be administered concurrently with **astemizole, triazolam, midazolam, ergot derivatives,** **amiodarone,** or **quinidine** because **nelfinavir** may affect the hepatic metabolism of these drugs and create the potential for serious or life-threatening adverse events.

Ritonavir (Norvir) is also a peptidomimetic **PI** of both HIV-1 and HIV-2 proteases. **Ritonavir** is FDA-approved for use alone or in combination with **nucleoside analogues** in patients with HIV infection when therapy is warranted. The drug is supplied as an oral solution (80 mg/mL) and as a 100-mg soft-gelatin capsule (released in July 1999). The soft-gelatin capsules should be stored in a refrigerator when possible. However, refrigeration is not required if the capsules are used within 30 days and stored below 77°F. Common adverse reactions include fatigue, vomiting, diarrhea, loss of appetite, abdominal pain, taste disturbance, peripheral neuropathy, headache, and dizziness. **Ritonavir** is metabolized principally by the liver, and administering the drug to patients with impaired hepatic function requires caution. **Ritonavir** should not be used with certain medications including some **nonsedating antihistamines, sedative hypnotics, antiarrhythmics,** or **ergot alkaloid preparations.** Drugs that must not be coadministered with **ritonavir** include **amiodarone, astemizole, bepridil, bupropion, clozapine, encainide, flecainide, meperidine, piroxicam, propafenone, propoxyphene, quinidine, rifabutin, alprazolam, clorazepate, diazepam, estazolam, flurazepam, midazolam, triazolam,** and **zolpidem.** The dose of **clarithromycin** should be reduced in patients with renal failure. Coadministration of **ritonavir** with **desipramine** increases plasma concentrations of **desipramine;** therefore, the dose of **desipramine** should be reduced. **Ritonavir** also reduces plasma concentrations of **ethinyl estradiol,** so that an increased hormone dosage of **oral contraceptives** should be used or alternative contraception methods should be considered. When given with **saquinavir,** the plasma concentration of **saquinavir** is dramatically increased. The plasma concentration of **theophylline** is decreased when given with **ritonavir.**

Saquinavir (Fortovase, Invirase) is also a peptidomimetic **PI.** It is indicated for the treatment of HIV infection based on changes in surrogate markers. **Saquinavir** is approved for use in adults in combination with other **antiretrovirals.** The drug was first approved with a hard-gel capsule formulation **(Invirase)** that was poorly absorbed when given orally. More recently, a soft-gel formulation **(Fortovase)** with increased bioavailability was approved. The recommended dosage of **Invirase** is 600 mg three times daily taken with a full meal. The dose of **Fortovase** is 1200 mg three times daily. Food aids the absorption of **Fortovase.** Adverse events include diarrhea, abdominal discomfort, nausea, dyspepsia, abdominal pain, headache, paresthesias, extremity numbness, asthenia, and myalgias. **Saquinavir** should not be coadministered with **rifampin, triazolam, midazolam,** or **ergot derivatives.**

Amprenavir (Agenerase) is an HIV **PI** approved to treat HIV-1 in adults and children in April 1999. This drug is supplied in 150-mg capsules. The recommended dosage is 1200 mg twice daily. Absorption from the soft-gel capsule appears unaffected by the presence of food. Because of the low capsule strength, the dosing regimen requires taking 16 tablets daily. The predominant route of elimination is biliary excretion, and **agenerase** undergoes limited hepatic metabolism. Reported toxicities include headache, diarrhea, and skin rash.

Other Drug Strategies

An interesting medication occasionally used in the treatment of HIV infection is **hydroxyurea.** Although it has no direct anti-HIV activity, it functions in concert with the **NRTIs** through its inhibition of ribonucleotide reductase. This decreases the intracellular production of natural deoxyribonucleotide triphosphates (dNTPs) and increases the effectiveness of the **NRTI analogues.** In short-term clinical trials, **hydroxyurea** has been shown to increase the anti-HIV activity of **didanosine.** The effect of **hydroxyurea** on the antiviral activity of other **NRTIs** is less well understood. The current dosage for **hydroxyurea** is 500 mg twice daily. The drug is generally well tolerated in patients with CD4 counts above 200 cells per mm^3; however, mild to moderate anemia and/or neutropenia may occur.

Initiation of Antiretroviral Therapy

Much controversy has surrounded the attempt to establish guidelines for when **ART** should be initiated. A consensus has emerged that **ART** should be initiated relatively early in the infection. Current U.S. guidelines recommend therapy as the CD4 decreases to 350 to 500 cells per mm^3 or the viral load increases to above 10,000 to 20,000 copies per mL. Therapy is also recommended for all symptomatic patients, regardless of viral load or CD4 T-cell count. The risks must be weighed against the potential benefits of early intervention, including nonadherence for patients not ready to commit to a complex regimen. Table 35–3 presents indications for the initiation of **ART** in the chronically HIV-infected patient.

Once the decision to begin therapy has been made, the next decision is which drugs should be used as initial therapy. Generally, three agents are superior to two agents in suppressing viral replication. Which combination to use as initial therapy remains unclear and depends on a variety of factors. The drug combination potency, expected

Table 35–3. Indications for the Initiation of Antiretroviral Therapy in the Chronically HIV-Infected Patient

Clinical Category	CD4* T-Cell Count and HIV RNA	Recommendation
Symptomatic	Any value	Treat
Asymptomatic	CD4 T cells <500/mm³ *or* HIV RNA >10,000 (bDNA) or >20,000 (RT-PCR)	Treatment should be offered. Strength or recommendation is based on prognosis for disease-free survival and willingness of the patient to accept therapy.
Asymptomatic	CD4 T cells >500/mm³ *and* HIV RNA <10,000 (bDNA) or <20,000 (RT-PCR)	Many experts would delay therapy and observe; however, some experts would treat.

*Some experts would observe patients with CD4 T-cell counts between 350 and 500/mm³ and HIV RNA levels <10,000 (bDNA) or <20,000 (RT-PCR).
Source: Adapted from U.S. Department of Health and Human Services. (1999). Report of the NIH panel to define principles of therapy of HIV infection and guidelines for the use of antiretroviral agents in HIV-infected adults and adolescents. *Morbidity and Mortality Weekly Report, 47* (4/24/98; revis. 5/99), RR-5.

duration of benefit, development of resistance, toxicity, potential interactions with other medications, ease of use, and cost must all be considered in making a selection. Initial therapy should include two **nucleoside analogues** in combination with a **PI** or **NNRTI.** Table 35–4 presents a listing of the preferred recommendations. See the CDC guidelines for detailed criteria.

Because the overall goal of **ART** is to maintain viral suppression for as long as possible, it becomes necessary to change therapies in the face of virologic failure. The modification of therapy is complicated and depends on the goal of therapy and the options still available for the patient. Some guiding principles can be helpful. First, the reason for failure of the current regimen should be established. For example, if the patient was unwilling or unable to comply with the regimen, a second regimen may fail. A second key factor is cross-resistance within drugs in a specific **antiretroviral** class. Once the decision is made to switch therapy, all drugs should be switched simultaneously, and the switch should occur as soon as possible. Table 35–5 presents guidelines for changing an **antiretroviral** regimen.

Even in the face of persistent virologic failure, a CD4 count and clinical benefit are usually observed. Therefore, continued therapy is typically indicated, even if all other options have been tried. However, there are times when therapy may be discontinued if patients develop advanced debilitating disease and request that **antiretroviral drugs** be stopped, or if there is no effective viral load or CD4 count effect with combination therapy and discontinuation may be a reasonable option. If therapy is stopped on account of intolerance, all **antiretroviral medications** should reasonably be stopped simultaneously and a new combination restarted at a later date.

ART is an increasingly complex, rapidly evolving area of medicine. Given the development of resistance and the patterns of cross-resistance within each drug classification, as well as the complicated picture of toxicities that emerge with the use of **antiretroviral** medications, it is clear that patients should be cared for by clinicians with experience and expertise in HIV medicine. Therefore, early consultation with an HIV specialist is imperative in designing an **ART** regimen.

Prevention of Opportunistic Infections

A second area of therapy that must be considered in treating HIV-infection is the prevention of opportunistic infections in patients infected with HIV. The CDC with the U.S. Department of Health and Human Services has released the 1999 "USPHS/IDSA Guidelines for the Prevention of Opportunistic Infections," with clear recommendations for the prevention of certain common opportunistic infections. *Pneumocystis carinii* pneumonia prevention should be pursued whenever the CD4+ count is below 200 cells or oropharyngeal candidiasis is present. *Mycobacterium tuberculosis* prophylaxis is indicated in any person with a tuberculin skin test (TST) reaction 5 mm or more or prior positive TST result without treatment or contact with a case of active tuberculosis. *Toxoplasma gondii* prophylaxis should be initiated if IgG antibody testing for *Toxoplasma* is positive and the CD4+ count is below 100 cells. The fourth strongly recommended prevention is for *Mycobacterium avium* complex (MAC) in persons with a CD4+ count below 50. Table 35–6 presents selected prophylaxis recommendations.

There are also several opportunistic diseases for which prophylaxis is generally recommended. **Pneumococcal vaccination** is recommended for all patients. For all patients who test anti-HBc negative, **hepatitis B vaccine** in three doses is also recommended. All patients should receive the **influenza vaccine** annually as well. Finally, any patient who is anti-HAV negative and has chronic hepatitis C should receive the **hepatitis A vaccine.**

One question that has come to light in the wake of successful **HAART** is whether primary prophylaxis may be discontinued when the patient displays a marked increase in CD4+ cell count above the limits used to indicate that prevention is recommended. See the current CDC guidelines for the detailed criteria for discontinuing and restarting opportunistic infection prophylaxis.

Table 35–4. Preferred Antiretroviral Agents

One choice each from column A and column B. Drugs are listed in random, not priority, order.	
Column A	**Column B**
Indinavir	ZDV + ddI
Nelfinavir	d4T + ddI
Ritonavir	ZDV + ddC
Saquinavir-SGC	ZDV + 3TC
Ritonavir + Saquinavir SGC or HGC	d4T + 3TC
Efavirenz	ddI + 3TC

Source: Adapted from U.S. Department of Health and Human Services. (1999). Report of the NIH panel to define principles of therapy of HIV infection and guidelines for the use of antiretroviral agents in HIV-infected adults and adolescents. *Morbidity and Mortality Weekly Report, 47* (4/24/98; revis. 5/99), RR-5.

Cost

With the advent of effective, long-term combination therapy to treat HIV and AIDS, the cost of prescriptions has become a significant factor. The choice of medications and the complexity of the regimen dramatically affect the

Table 35–5. Guidelines for Changing an Antiretroviral Regimen for Suspected Drug Failure

Criteria for changing therapy include a suboptimal reduction in plasma viremia after initiation of therapy, reappearance of viremia after suppression to undetectable, significant increases in plasma viremia from the nadir of suppression, and declining CD4 T-cell numbers.

When the decision to change therapy is based on viral-load determination, it is preferable to confirm with a second viral-load test.

Distinguish between the need to change a regimen because of drug intolerance or inability to comply with the regimen versus failure to achieve the goal of sustained viral suppression; single agents can be changed or dose reduced in the event of drug intolerance.

In general, do not change a single drug or add a single drug to a failing regimen; it is important to use at least two new drugs and preferably to use an entirely new regimen with at least three new drugs.

Many patients have limited options for new regimens of desired potency; in some of these cases, it is rational to continue the prior regimen if partial viral suppression was achieved.

In some cases, regimens identified as suboptimal for initial therapy are rational because of limitations imposed by toxicity, intolerance, or nonadherence. This especially applies in late-stage disease. For patients with no rational alternative options who have virologic failure with return of viral load to baseline (pretreatment levels) and declining CD4 T-cell count, there should be consideration for discontinuation of antiretroviral therapy.

Experience is limited with regimens using combinations of two protease inhibitors or combinations of protease inhibitors with nevirapine or delavirdine; for patients with limited options due to drug intolerance or suspected resistance, these regimens provide possible alternative treatment options.

There is limited information about the value of restarting a drug that the patient has previously received. The experience with zidovudine is that resistant strains are often replaced with "wild-type" zidovudine-sensitive strains when zidovudine treatment is stopped, but resistance recurs rapidly if zidovudine is restarted. Although there is preliminary evidence that this occurs with indinavir, it is not known if similar problems apply to other nucleoside analogues, protease inhibitors, or NNRTIs, but a conservative stance is that they probably do.

Avoid changing from ritonavir to indinavir, or vice versa, for drug failure because high-level cross-resistance is likely.

Avoid changing between nevirapine, delavirdine, and efavirenz, or vice versa, for drug failure because high-level cross-resistance is likely.

The decision to change therapy and the choice of a new regimen require the clinician to have considerable expertise in the care of people living with HIV. Physicians who are less experienced in the care of persons with HIV infection are strongly encouraged to obtain assistance through consultation with or referral to a clinician with considerable expertise in the care of HIV-infected patients.

Source: U.S. Department of Health and Human Services. (1999). Report of the NIH panel to define principles of therapy of HIV infection and guidelines for the use of antiretroviral agents in HIV-infected adults and adolescents. *Morbidity and Mortality Weekly Report, 47* (4/24/98; revis. 5/99), RR-5.

cost to the patient. Table 35–7 gives some indication of the expense involved in the treatment of this disease.

Adherence to the Medication Regimen

An increasingly significant area affecting the outcome of long-term **ART** is the patient's adherence to the medication regimen. Medication adherence in general has been studied frequently over the past 30 years. The medical literature suggests that adherence is almost universally less than 100 percent, with most estimates falling in the range of 30 to 60 percent. Successful adherence has been defined as more than 80 percent of doses taken. However, there have been no studies to show that 80 percent or better adherence is therapeutically effective for combination **ART**. In addition, several clinical reports have demonstrated that resistance can develop when patients miss a few days or even a few doses of medication.

Certain trends emerge regarding patient characteristics as predictors of adherence. Generally, sociodemographic characteristics are poor predictors of adherence. Patients' beliefs, knowledge, and expectations strongly influence medical decision making and willingness to begin and then adhere to therapy. If a person understands the purpose of medications, believes the treatment will be helpful, and perceives the need for treatment, then adherence is greater. It is therefore imperative that the health care provider and the patient discuss combination therapy early in treatment so that later therapy can be successful.

Table 35–6. Selected Opportunistic Disease Prophylaxis in Adults and Adolescents Infected with Human Immunodeficiency Virus

Pathogen	Indication	First Choice	Alternative
Pneumocystis carinii	CD4+ count <200 cells µL *or* oropharyngeal candidiasis	• Trimethoprim-sulfamethoxazole (TMP-SMZ), 1 DS PO qd TMP-SMZ, 1 SS PO qd	• Dapsone 50 mg PO bid *or* 100 mg PO qd • Dapsone 50 mg PO qd *plus* pyrimethamine 50 mg PO qw *plus* leucovorin 25 mg PO qw • Dapsone 200 mg PO *plus* pyrimethamine 75 mg PO *plus* leucovorin 25 mg PO qw • Aerosolized pentamidine 300 mg qm via Respirgard II nebulizer • Atovaquone 1500 mg PO qd TMP-SMZ 1 DS PO tiw
Mycobacterium tuberculosis —Isoniazid-sensitive	TST reaction 5 mm or more *or* prior positive TST result without treatment *or* contact with case of active tuberculosis (TB)	• Isoniazid 300 mg PO *plus* pyridoxine 50 mg PO qd × 9 mo *or* • Isoniazid 900 mg PO *plus* pyridoxine 100 mg PO biw × 9 mo • Rifampin 600 mg *plus* pyrazinamide 20 mg/kg PO qd × 2 mo	• Rifabutin 300 mg PO qd *plus* pyrazinamide 20 mg/kg PO qd × 2 mo • Rifampin 600 mg PO qd × 4 mo
—Isoniazid-resistant	Same; high probability of exposure to isoniazid-resistant TB	• Rifampin 600 mg *plus* pyrazinamide 20 mg/kg PO qd × 2 mo	• Rifabutin 300 mg PO qd *plus* pyrazinamide 20 mg/kg PO qd × 2 mo • Rifampin 600 mg PO qd × 4 mo • Rifabutin 300 mg PO qd × 4 mo
—Multidrug-resistant	Same; high probability of exposure to multidrug-resistant TB	• Choice of drug requires consultation with public health authorities	• None
Toxoplasma gondii	IgG antibody to *Toxoplasma* and CD4+ count <100 cells µL	• TMP-SMZ 1 DS PO qd	• TMP-SMZ 1 SS PO qd • Dapsone 50 mg PO qd *plus* pyrimethamine 50 mg PO qw *plus* leucovorin 25 mg PO qw • Atovaquone 1500 mg PO qd with or without pyrimethamine 25 mg PO qd *plus* leucovorin 10 mg PO qd
Mycobacterium avium complex	CD4+ count <50 cells µL	• Azithromycin 1200 mg PO qw *or* clarithromycin 500 mg PO bid	• Rifabutin 300 mg PO qd • Azithromycin 1200 mg PO qw *plus* rifabutin 300 mg PO qd

Source: Adapted from U.S. Department of Health and Human Services. (1999). USPHS/IDSA guidelines for the prevention of opportunistic infections in persons infected with human immunodeficiency virus. *Morbidity and Mortality Weekly Report, 48*, RR-10.

Active substance abuse is likely to affect adherence to combination therapy, although it is not an absolute. Consider issues such as the drugs used, available drug treatment resources, and support systems. A second potential barrier to adherence is neurocognitive impair-

ment. Problems with memory to frank dementia can occur in HIV patients.

Critical elements to establishing and maintaining adherence to a treatment regimen include the complexity of the regimen and how it blends into the patient's personal

Table 35–7. Medication Costs per Month as Reported by a Local Outpatient Pharmacy

Medication	Strength/Number	Cost per Month
Retrovir	300 mg/ #60	$314.75
Epivir	150 mg/ #60	$270.10
Combivir	#60	$579.75
Videx	100 mg/ #120	$226.05
Hivid	0.375 mg/ #90	$177.60
Hivid	0.75 mg/ #90	$221.35
Zerit	20 mg/ #60	$262.00
Zerit	40 mg/ #60	$283.05
Ziagen	300 mg/ #60	$361.20
Viramune	200 mg/ #60	$265.00
Rescriptor	100 mg/ #360	$249.60
Sustiva	200 mg/ #90	$337.90
Invirase	200 mg/ #270	$603.10
Fortovase	200 mg/ #480	$538.00
Norvir	100 mg/ #360	$686.20
Crixivan	400 mg/ #180	$477.80
Viracept	250 mg/ #270	$599.90

life circumstances. The combination therapy regimen must fit into the daily routine. A key variable is the two-way provider-patient communication. Patients have to believe that the therapy will have a profound effect on their health so that the benefits outweigh the burdens of the medication regimen.

Before the patient begins **ART,** it is helpful to address anticipated problems or barriers to adherence. This can potentially include rehearsal with a week's worth of jellybeans to see what areas of the person's life are problematic to the prescribed schedule. Other techniques that may be helpful are writing a treatment plan, keeping a medication log, linking taking medications to certain daily activities in the person's life, and using a pillbox to prepare the medication doses for a week at a time. Social assistance can also make a major difference, especially at the beginning of the regimen. Still, there is a lot more to be learned about the issues affecting adherence to a complex **antiretroviral** regimen.

Monitoring

Decisions about initiating or changing **ART** should be guided by monitoring the viral load and CD4+ T-cell count and by assessing the patient's clinical condition. The viral load and CD4+ T-cell count should be measured when therapy is initiated, 4 weeks after therapy is started, and every 3 to 4 months thereafter. Two baseline viral RNA tests are recommended before starting therapy. Along with these surrogate markers, the patient should be clinically assessed for early signs of toxicity or intolerance to any of the medications, as well as for the development of opportunistic infections or malignancies.

Outcome Evaluation

As stated early in this chapter, the key goals of therapy are to suppress the viral load to undetectable levels for as long as possible and to prevent opportunistic infections. Therefore, the outcome evaluation for **ART** must be based on viral load, CD4+ cell counts, and clinical assessment of the patient.

There is another important way to look at outcomes of **ART.** In a recent observational study, 1255 patients, each of whom had at least one CD4+ count below 100 cells per mm^3, were followed from January 1994 through June 1997. In this group, the mortality rates declined from 29.4 per 100 person-years in 1995 to 8.8 per 100 person-years in the second quarter of 1997. These reductions occurred regardless of gender, race, age, and risk factors for HIV transmission. In addition, the incidence of any of three major opportunistic infections (*P. carinii* pneumonia, MAC disease, and cytomegalovirus retinitis) declined from 21.9 per 100 person-years in 1994 to 3.7 per 100 person-years by mid-1997. Stepwise reductions in morbidity and mortality were associated with increases in the intensity of **ART** (classified as none, monotherapy, combination therapy without any **PI,** and combination therapy with a **PI**). The most benefit was seen with combination **ART,** and the inclusion of **PIs** in the regimens conferred additional benefit. The results of this study illustrate that the recent declines in morbidity and mortality are attributable to the use of more intensive **antiretroviral** regimens. Therefore, effective **ART** is imperative in the treatment of HIV disease.

Patient Education

The complexity of the medication regimens used to treat HIV infection make patient education imperative but difficult. Specific guidelines for how to take medications

HIV Disease

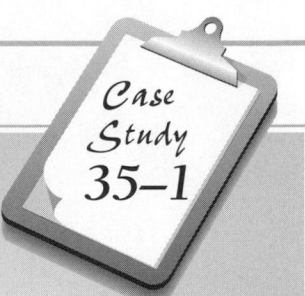

Case Study 35–1

Complaint

"I'm HIV positive."

History and Assessment

Ben, a 45-year-old white man, was found to be HIV positive in June 1995. At that time, his CD4+ cell count was 685 cells per mm³, and his viral load was undetectable. Ben chose to postpone therapy and be monitored every 3 to 6 months.

In March 1999, his CD4+ cell count had declined to 514 cells per mm³, and the viral load was now 41,520. Because of the measurable viral load and the decreasing CD4+ cell count, Ben was advised to begin therapy. In counseling sessions, Ben expressed some fear about starting therapy because it represented a long-term commitment and would force him to acknowledge his illness on a daily basis.

Initial Management Plan

After much discussion concerning the risks and benefits of beginning therapy, Ben was given prescriptions for Combivir and indinavir. The side effects of each were reviewed, and the medication instructions were provided in writing.

Follow-up and Modifications to Management Plan

A 1-week follow-up call to the patient revealed that Ben had not started the medications, but he stated that he intended to start in the next 3 days. The reasons given for the delay were that he wanted to start the medications on a Friday in case he experienced any side effects, but he was still hesitant to begin therapy.

After another discussion with the health care provider, Ben began therapy. He experienced some nausea when taking the indinavir but no other side effects. He was instructed to take indinavir with a small, low-fat meal. Within 1 week, Ben was experiencing no side effects.

Continuing Care

After 4 weeks of therapy, another viral load was drawn. The viral load had dropped to 191, which was a significant motivator for Ben to continue the medications as ordered. At 4 months of therapy, the viral load was undetectable, and Ben continues to be free of side effects.

---

and what adverse reactions should be reported to the health care provider are determined by which drug regimen has been selected. It is important to work with patients to design a regimen that will fit their lifestyle and establish strategies for incorporating the regimen into daily activities.

There is no cure for HIV infection, so patient education must include safe sex practices and transmission information. Patients should always use a latex condom during every act of sexual intercourse. Sexual practices that might result in oral exposure to feces should be avoided to reduce the risk for intestinal infections. Injection drug users should be counseled to never reuse or share syringes, needles, water, or drug preparation equipment. HIV-positive women in the United States are instructed to use infant formula as an alternative to breastfeeding to decrease the incidence of vertical transmission.

REFERENCES

Abrams, C., Cotton, D., Markowitz, M., & Mayer, K. (1998). *AIDS/HIV treatment directory*. New York: AmFAR.

Bartlett, J. G. (1998). *1998 Medical management of HIV infection*. Baltimore: Johns Hopkins University.

Centers for Disease Control and Prevention. (1998). *HIV/AIDS Surveillance Report, 10*(1).

Cohen, P. T., Sande, M. A., & Volberding, P. A. (Eds.). (1999). *The AIDS knowledge base* (3rd ed. HIV InSite version). *http://hivinsite.ucsf.edu//akb/1997/.*

Levy, J. A. (1998). *HIV and the pathogenesis of AIDS*. Washington, DC: ASM Press.

Liming, J. (February 1999). Personal communication.

Palella, F. J., Delaney, K. M., Moorman, A. C., Loveless, M. D., Fuhrer, J., Satler, G. A., Aschman, D. J., & Holmberg, S. D. (1998). Declining morbidity and mortality among patients with advanced human immunodeficiency virus infection. *New England Journal of Medicine, 338,* 13.

Sande, M. A., & Volberding, P. A. (1999). *The medical management of AIDS*. (6th ed.). Philadelphia: Saunders.

U.S. Department of Health and Human Services. (1998). Report of the NIH panel to define principles of therapy of HIV infection and guidelines for the use of antiretroviral agents in HIV-infected adults and adolescents. *Morbidity and Mortality Weekly Report, 47,* RR-5.

U.S. Department of Health and Human Services. (1999). Report of the NIH panel to define principles of therapy of HIV infection and guidelines for the use of antiretroviral agents in HIV-infected adults and adolescents. *Morbidity and Mortality Weekly Report, 47*(April 24, 1998; revis. May 1999), RR-5.

U.S. Department of Health and Human Services. (1999). USPHS/IDSA guidelines for the prevention of opportunistic infections in persons infected with human immunodeficiency virus. *Morbidity and Mortality Weekly Report, 48,* RR-10.

U.S. Food and Drug Administration. Approved drugs for HIV/AIDS or AIDS-related conditions. *http://www.fda.gov/oashi/aids/stat_app.html.*

CHAPTER 36

....

Hormone Replacement Therapy and Osteoporosis

Hormone Replacement Therapy

*L*iterature about **hormone replacement therapy (HRT)** is abundant in popular magazines as well as in professional journals. Nurse practitioners (NPs) need to evaluate this literature with their clients. Menopausal **hormone therapy** is indicated for three conditions: vasomotor instability (hot flashes), urogenital atrophy, and osteoporosis. In the early 1970s, women were told to take **estrogens** until the day they died. Then a 1977 study showed that unopposed **estrogen therapy** caused adenomatous hyperplasia of the uterus, a precancerous condition. However, what was soon realized was that use of **progesterone** to oppose the **estrogen** effect on the uterine lining was the necessary treatment, and cyclic postmenopausal therapy was reestablished.

Cancer risks and adverse effects of **conjugated estrogens** were erroneously compared with data of the first, very potent **ethinyl estradiol estrogen** used in the **oral contraceptive** preparations of the 1960s. The potency ratio at that time was approximately 1:20, with **conjugated estrogens** the less potent. This type of data extrapolation contributed to persistent fears that postmenopausal **estrogens** cause cancer, heart attack, deep venous thromboembolism, and stroke. See Chapter 29 for a discussion of **estrogen** and **progesterone** adverse effects when they are used as **contraceptives.**

In the 1980s, postmenopausal **estrogen therapy** was prescribed for another indication. Data from the Framingham studies suggested that women using **estrogen** whose families had had coronary artery disease (CAD) may develop clinical disease later than their counterparts without **hormone therapy.** The Postmenopausal Estrogen/Progestin Interventions (PEPI) Trial and the Nurses Collaborative Study validated this thesis. At the same time, other researchers asked if the risk of cancer to the uterus and breast cancels the benefit of the improved lipid profile. Many more women die of early CAD than of breast and uterine cancer. It may be that for those patients the small but real risk of later cancer is one they will take. The decade of the 1990s saw a dramatic rise in health care costs. Health maintenance organizations sprouted as the health care industry attempted to slow down rising costs by demanding cost-effective therapies. The Heart and Estrogen/Progestin Replacement Study (HERS) was the first large randomized trial that looked at reduction in mortality by using menopausal **estrogens.** The results were unexpected. Women with CAD did not live longer. In fact, these women died earlier in the first year of therapy. Those women without cardiovascular disease benefited but not until the fourth and fifth years of therapy (Grodstein et al., 1997).

Pathophysiology

Between the ages of 42 and 56, most women experience a decline in ovarian hormone function, with the resultant natural cessation of menses. At menarche, the ovary starts production of three steroids: progestin, androgen, and estrogen. These three steroids have a dramatic effect on the brain, hypothalamus, pituitary, and the ovary itself. Sex hormones play an important role in the dynamic process of the formation and remodeling of neuronal circuits and neurotransmitters (Paganini-Hill, 1998). The target organs of ovarian steroids are the uterine epithelium, the uterine tubes, the breasts, and the vagina. Ovulation decreases a few years prior to menopause. The ovary ages as a result of exhaustion of follicles. Lack of ovarian function may also be the result of surgical castration or ovarian disease. If left intact, the postmenopausal ovary continues to produce androgens. These androgens, as well as those from the adrenal gland, are then converted in fatty tissues and hair follicles into less potent estrogens, estrone and estriol. This peripheral conversion of androgens may vary greatly, so that some women pass through menopause without seeking therapy and others are miserable and seek treatment. Initially, women experience hot flashes, insomnia, vaginal atrophy, and depression. Later on (2 to 5 years), insidious changes occur, such as loss of bone mass

and changes in cholesterol and lipoprotein ratios. Osteoporosis is treated separately later in this chapter. The incidence of atherosclerotic diseases is low in premenopausal women, rises in postmenopausal women, and is reduced again in postmenopausal women who take **estrogens.** The direct effects of estrogen on blood vessels promote vasodilatation and delay the development of atherosclerosis. It is possible that the negative effects on hepatic coagulation factors and fibrinogen offset the beneficial effect on lipids. The route of administration (transdermal or vaginal) of **estrogens** also reduces the hepatic problem, as well as some of the lipid benefit. Coadministration of **progestin** blunts part of the beneficial effects on lipids. The possible clinical effects of estrogen metabolites, phytoestrogens, and peripheral conversion of testosterone to estradiol need to be explored (Mendelsohn & Karas, 1999). Replacement by exogenous **estrogen** is aimed at relieving signs and symptoms of estrogen deficiency, such as hot flashes, insomnia, genital-urinary atrophy, and emotional lability. Staying on **hormonal therapy** indefinitely may be necessary to sustain the benefit on bone mass and blood vessel disease.

Goals of Treatment

Goals of **HRT** are safe, well-tolerated, and effective therapy. Treatment of menopausal symptoms with prescription medications has risks that require careful selection and screening of patients. To prevent endometrial hyperplasia in women with intact uteri, the addition of a **progestin** is necessary. Breast cancer risk has been studied with conflicting results. No increased association of cancer in **HRT** has been shown unless treatment extends beyond 10 years. In those women who did develop breast cancer, the diagnosis was the more unusual types that have low malignant potential (Colditz et al., 1995).

Relief of menopausal symptoms can be dramatic after the initiation of **hormonal therapy.** Women feel more in control of their bodily functions and emotional stability, and reestablish more restful sleep patterns. Relief from dyspareunia due to vaginal atrophy improves sexual relations. **Estrogen** treatment of the urethral mucosa often relieves urinary urgency. Although most patients have a beneficial effect from **HRT,** a small percentage describe a flare of headaches, fluid retention, breast tenderness, and change or resumption of erratic menses. Weight gain at midlife occurs because basal metabolism reduces 10 percent each decade, not because of **estrogen** therapy. In a 15-year prospective and cross-sectional study of 671 women age 65 to 94, no differences in body mass index (BMI) between baseline and follow-up were found in women who used **hormone therapy** and controls (Kritz-Silverstein & Barrett-Connor, 1996).

Treatment of postmenopausal women with **estrogen** causes a delayed increase in risk of cardiovascular disease as a result of improved serum lipid levels (Anonymous, 1997 Clinical Reviews, 1996). Reduction in colon and rectal cancers was correlated with postmenopausal **estrogen** use (Grodstein et al., 1997; Newcomb & Storer, 1995). These two studies demonstrated that **HRT** use statistically reduces the risk of colon cancer. Colon cancer is the second most common cancer in women. **Estrogen replacement therapy (ERT)** influences several neurotransmitter systems, including those using acetylcholine. Acetylcholine levels in patients with Alzheimer's disease are found to be reduced by 90 percent. In addition, **ERT** enhances cerebral blood flow and facilitates glucose transport into brain cells. Therapeutic doses of **estrogens** show changes in brain organization for memory in postmenopausal women (Shaywitz et al., 1999).

Rational Drug Selection

Estrogen Therapy

To make a rational drug selection, the questions to ask are: "What are the risks versus benefits to me? Am I concerned about pure scientific reasons to take or reject therapy, or are there quality of life issues that are more important?" Risks and benefits and quality of life issues need to be considered each year when prescriptions are renewed for menopausal and postmenopausal **hormone therapy.** In addition, nonpharmacological behaviors such as weight loss, smoking cessation, reduced **alcohol** intake, regular exercise, and healthy dietary habits need to be encouraged at all office visits. There is information available to consider when choosing **estrogen** as therapy for the short- and long-range complications of estrogen deficit.

The absolute contraindications to **estrogen** that are listed in Table 29-3 are similar to those for **hormonal contraception.** The exceptions are smoking and hypertension. The morbidity and mortality associated with **ethinyl estradiol** and smoking in women age 35 or older do not exist with the use of the less potent forms of **estrogen.** In addition, **conjugated estrogens** as well as **estradiol** do not have the ability to stimulate renin substrate the way **ethinyl estradiol** does, so hypertension is not a contraindication (August, 1998).

The first menopausal **estrogens** were **conjugated equine estrogen** derived from stallion urine, greater in es-

trogen content than of a pregnant mare or even the pregnant human. Next, synthetic formulations of **estradiol** were manufactured, but those have had wider use in Europe. Most recently **estropipate** has been derived from plant sources so that patient preferences may be respected.

Combinations of **estrogen** and **progesterone (Premarin, Estrace,** and **Ogen)** are used when the uterus is intact. Women who have had a hysterectomy take only **estrogen.** There are several safe combinations of therapies for use in menopause. Low-dose **vaginal estrogens** (with the ring or cream) do not increase the risk of endometrial hyperplasia as do the oral forms (Weiderpass et al., 1999). In addition, use of the **estradiol**-releasing vaginal ring has a positive effect on urethral and vaginal atrophy symptoms without causing adverse effects (Eriksen, 1999).

If the uterus is present, the following may be prescribed:

1. **Estrogen** (0.625 mg) plus **medroxyprogesterone acetate** (MPA) 2.5 mg daily **(Prempro)**
2. **Estrogen** (0.625 mg) plus **micronized progesterone** 100 mg daily
3. **Estrogen** (0.625 mg) daily plus **MPA** 10 mg for 10 to 12 days
4. **Estrogen** (0.625 mg) daily plus **MPA** 5 mg for 14 days **(Premphase)**
5. **Estrogen** (0.625 mg) daily plus **micronized progesterone** 200 mg for 12 days (Writing Group for the PEPI Trial, 1996)
6. **Estrogen** (0.625 for days 1 to 25 plus **MPA** 10 days 16 to 25 (the first regimen used, which has the disadvantage of more hot flashes)
7. **Estrogen** (0.625 mg) plus **progestin** Monday through Friday (may experience more hot flashes)

If the uterus is not present, the following are commonly prescribed: **Estrogen** (0.625 mg) for 5 days each week, or 25 days each month, or daily all month.

When initiating therapy in older women, begin with low doses (0.3 mg) of **conjugated estrogens** every other day for 2 months. Next, increase the **estrogens** to daily use for another 2 months. Add **MPA** 2.5 mg daily if patient has a uterus. If symptoms such as bleeding or breast pain do not occur, increase **estrogen** up to 0.625 mg daily. Some women may need only the lower **estrogen** dosages as long as they have adequate diet, **calcium** intake of 1500 mg, and 800 IU of **vitamin D** (Recker et al., 1999).

Clinical Pearl

....

REDUCING BREAST PAIN AS AN ADVERSE EFFECT OF ESTROGEN

For the **estrogen** adverse effects of breast pain, reduce the dose of patch hormone by securing a small bandage to the center of the side that touches the skin.

....

Progesterone Therapy

Use of **progestins** for the treatment of postmenopausal symptoms and in conjunction with **estrogen** to prevent hyperplasia of the endometrium is considered "unlabeled" use. **Progesterone (Provera, Aygestin, Prometrium)** use has been validated by numerous research studies in postmenopausal therapies. It is not cost-effective for pharmaceutical companies to petition the Food and Drug Administration (FDA) for more indications when **MPA** has gone off patent.

Use **progesterone** early in therapy to alleviate symptoms and counter the **estrogen** effect on the uterine endometrium. Delay use of **estrogen** in obese patients (BMI more than 27) because of their higher endogenous **estrogen** levels. Obesity itself is a risk factor for endometrial cancer. Some women may show vasoconstriction (Raynaud's phenomenon) with **estrogen.** This effect was not present when women took **estrogen** in combination with **progesterone** (Fraenkel et al., 1998).

Natural **progesterone** has fewer adverse effects than synthetic agents such as **MPA.** Natural **progesterone** is indicated for women with hypertension and abnormal lipid profiles. Some researchers favor exclusive use of **progesterone.** More research is necessary concerning its use for affective disorders and allergic symptoms (Murray, 1998).

Progesterone dosing regimens include the following:
1. **Norethindrone acetate (Aygestin)** 2.5 to 5.0 mg, which is equivalent to
2. **Medroxyprogesterone acetate (Provera)** 5 to 10 mg, which is equivalent to
3. **Micronized progesterone (Prometrium)** 100 to 200 mg

Some women cannot tolerate daily or monthly **progestin** because of emotional lability. Quarterly **progestin** therapy has been shown to be as safe as monthly cyclic therapy in a Kaiser-Permanente Study (Ettinger et al., 1994).

Testosterone Therapy

When traditional **HRT/ERT** is not successful in suppressing hot flashes and improving sex drive, **estrogen** in combination with **testosterone** has been used empirically. Peripheral conversion of androgens may augment **ERT** and reduce hot flashers. Masculinizing adverse effects such as lower voice and increased facial and body hair can occur when **testosterone** is used alone. These adverse effects may not regress after **testosterone** is withdrawn. Traditionally, **testosterone** has been used topically (2%) in aquaphor or petrolatum for vulvar "dystrophies." See Chapter 42 for newer treatments for vulvovaginitis.

Formulations available are the following:
1. **Esterified estrogen** 0.625 mg plus **testosterone** 1.25 mg
2. **Esterified estrogen** 1.25 mg plus **testosterone** 2.5 mg (this higher **estrogen** is used in post-oophorectomy patients younger than 49)
3. **Conjugated estrogens** 0.625 mg plus **testosterone** 5 mg
4. **Conjugated estrogens** 1.25 mg plus **testosterone** 10 mg

Available transdermal formulations with and without **progestin** are the following:
1. **Estradiol** comes in 0.05 mg and 0.1 mg **(Estraderm)** and 0.03 mg, 0.05 mg, and 1 mg **(Vivelle).**
2. **Estradiol** and **norethindrone (Combipatch)** comes in 0.1 mg/0.5 mg or 0.05 mg/0.25 mg.

Once women are through the early phase of menopause and have stopped erratic bleeding, a convenient combination pill or patch may be prescribed.

Figure 36–1 presents a treatment algorithm for **HRT/ERT.**

Monitoring

Women taking **hormonal therapy** for menopausal symptoms have similar adverse effects and precautions no matter what the **estrogen** source and the route of administration. Schedule a complete history, physical examination, and mammogram annually. Liver function tests need to be done at baseline, along with a lipid profile, and repeated annually if abnormal. All women over age 45 need to be screened for adult-onset diabetes mellitus (Scharbo-Dehann, 1996). Some sources recommend endometrial biopsies at baseline and every year or two. Most authorities agree that abnormal bleeding and all postmenopausal bleeding require uterine sampling.

Outcome Evaluation

Women may present for treatment complaining of heavy menses. When the bleeding problem is serious enough to cause a drop of 2 g of hemoglobin within one menstrual cycle, management usually requires specialty care. The patient may need a dilatation and curettage. It is not uncommon for fibroids and hyperplasia to cause this degree of bleeding. Both conditions may require referral and surgery.

Postmenopausal bleeding—that is, bleeding of any degree after 12 or more months of amenorrhea—needs an evaluation that includes history, physical, pelvic examination, mammogram, pelvic ultrasound, and endometrial biopsy. Laboratory tests are necessary to rule out bleeding disorders and endocrine disease. If all of the workup demonstrates no disease, then referral for an inpatient dilatation and curettage is indicated.

Frequently, older women present with symptoms of urinary incontinence or chronic bladder infections.

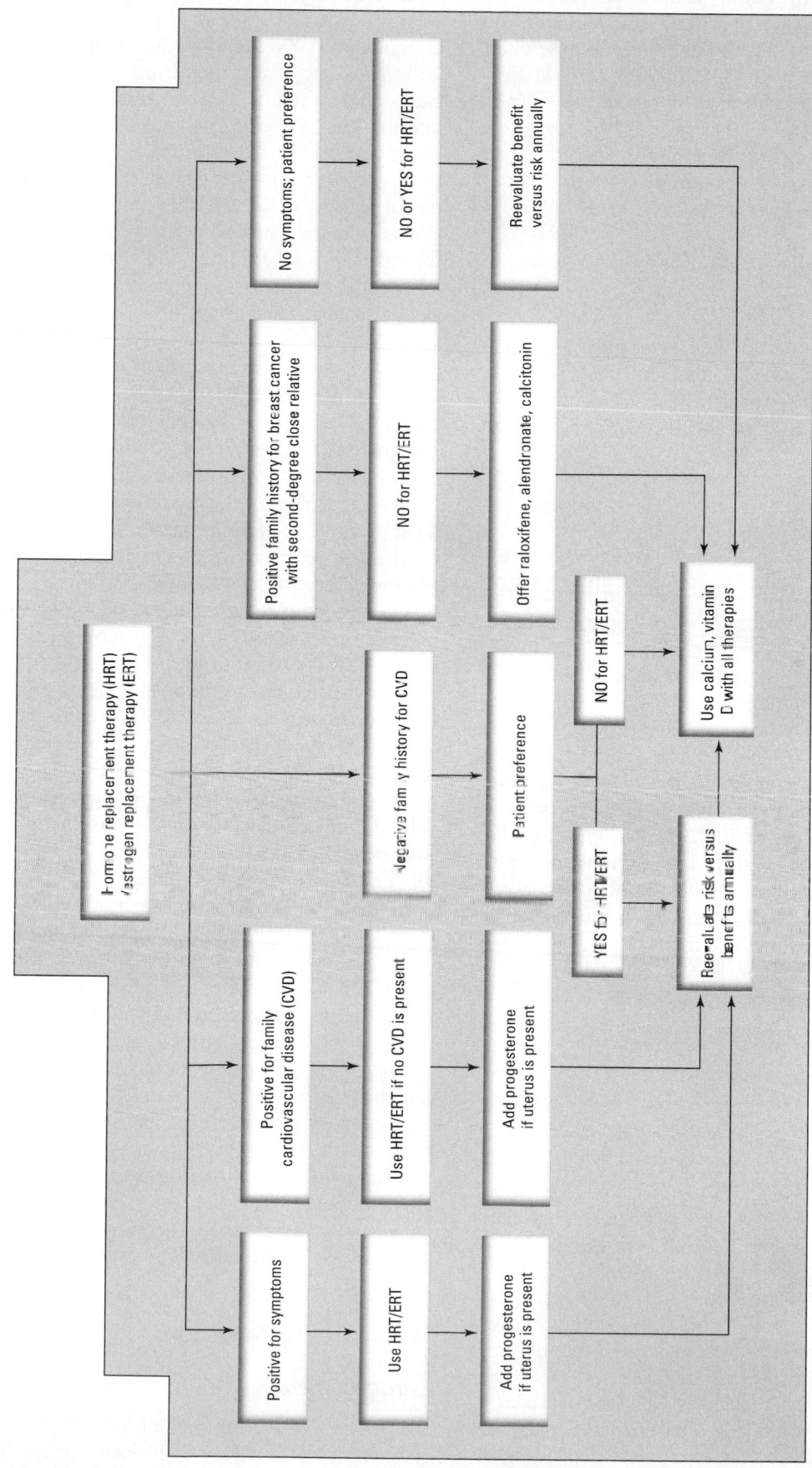

Figure 36–1. Treatment algorithm: Hormone replacement therapy/estrogen replacement therapy.

If there is blood and the culture is negative (even as few as 8 to 10 red blood cells per high-powered field), the patient will need a urological evaluation. Because older women who have not been on **HRT** have cervical atrophy, performing an endometrial biopsy in the office is too painful. Other areas of concern in the older woman are pigmented vulvar lesions, ulcerations, and thickened white patches, all of which require biopsies to rule out cancer.

Patient Education

Patient education should include a discussion of information related to the overall treatment plan as well as that specific to the drug therapy, reasons for taking the drug, drugs as part of the total treatment regimen, and adherence issues.

Osteoporosis

Estrogen therapy has long been the gold standard for both prevention and treatment of osteoporosis. Estrogens reduce the bone-resorbing action of parathyroid hormone (PTH). Estrogen receptors have been found in bone, which validates the hypothesis that estrogen may have direct effects on bone remodeling (Katzung, 1998). Both the PEPI and CHART studies observed that 20 percent of white women over age 50 are vulnerable to mortality from hip and spine fractures. In those who survive, 50 percent require nursing home care. Men also suffer from osteoporosis, but at a later age and more gradually than women. There are several well-known risk factors for osteoporosis such as family history, women of slight build and fair complexion (Scandinavian), age, and diets low in calcium and vitamin D. See Table 36–1 for the risk factors of osteoporosis.

Pathophysiology

Besides immediate physical problems, there are also more serious, longer-lasting effects of estrogen deficiency. Osteoporosis is a generalized metabolic disease characterized by decreased bone mass as a result of an imbalance in the bone-remodeling process. The bone resorbers (osteoclasts) exceed the bone formers (osteoblasts). With the acceleration of bone loss, back, hip, and wrist fractures occur. The bones of the body contain 98 percent of body calcium. Calcium enters the body through the intestine. PTH and vitamin D principally regulate calcium homeostasis. Other hormones such as calcitonin, prolactin, growth hormone, insulin, thyroid, glucocorticoids, and sex hormones are secondary regulators, depending on specific physiological circumstances.

Pharmacodynamics

Of the 600 to1000 mg of calcium consumed daily, only 100 to 250 mg is absorbed from the gut. In the steady state, renal excretion of calcium and phosphate balances intestinal absorption. The movement of calcium and phosphate across the intestinal lining is closely regulated. Intestinal diseases can disrupt this balance. Hormonal regulation of calcium, mentioned earlier, greatly affects calcium metabolism. Ions such as sodium and fluoride also have an impact on calcium balance. Drugs taken for other diseases, such as **thiazides** for hypertension, also affect calcium metabolism.

Goals of Treatment

The goals of treatment for osteoporosis are that the pharmacological therapy be inexpensive, safe, and effective. Nonpharmacological therapy (and prevention) includes an appropriate exercise program.

The best treatment for osteoporosis is prevention. Developing a healthy lifestyle while building bone mass is the most cost-effective strategy. Excessive dieting and exercise or fad diets that are deficient in essential nutrients contribute to reduced bone mass. **Calcium** is the least expensive drug used in osteoporosis therapy. Generic **calcium carbonate (Tums)** costs pennies a day.

Patients have benefited from research focused on osteoporosis treatment. Several new therapies have been developed such as the **bisphosphonates (alendronate), raloxifene,** and **calcitonin. Calcitonin** provides relief from bone pain and builds bone mass without any harmful effects on the breast or uterus.

Research indicates that postmenopausal women need some additional drug therapy besides a healthy lifestyle to prevent and treat osteoporosis. Newer drugs such as **calcitonin, alendronate,** and **raloxifene** have not had as wide usage as **estrogen,** and so they are recommended at this time only if the patient has contraindications to **HRT.**

Prevention of osteoporosis includes a high-impact aerobic exercise program; however, excessive exercise is not good because stress fractures may result. For treatment of osteoporosis, weight-bearing activity like brisk walking (20 minutes three to four times per week) is ideal. Resistance training (lifting weights or using strength-training machines) is a slow process, so programs should start low and work up over a period of months.

Rational Drug Selection

Estrogen Therapy

See the prescribing information presented earlier in the chapter for **HRT.** Dosing is the same for osteoporosis as the recommendations for **HRT/ERT.**

PATIENT EDUCATION

Hormone Replacement Therapy

Related to the Overall Treatment Plan/Disease Process

- ☐ Pathophysiology of the changes that take place in the female physiology at menopause that make a woman vulnerable to atrophy of the genital organs, vasomotor instability, and emotional lability, and when lower estrogen levels cause undesirable lipid patterns.
- ☐ Role of lifestyle modifications and the various treatment protocols and medications available
- ☐ Importance of adherence to the treatment regimen
- ☐ Need for regular follow-up visits with the primary care provider, including annual screening tests such as mammography

Specific to the Drug Therapy

- ☐ Reasons for the drug's being given
- ☐ Doses and schedules for taking the drug
- ☐ Possible adverse effects and what to do if they occur, especially if uterine bleeding occurs
- ☐ Interactions between other treatment modalities and these drugs

Reasons for Taking the Drug(s)

Specifically, additional information includes the following: Quality-of-life issues such as relief of hot flashes, target organ atrophy prevention; and treatment of osteoporosis; prevention of early heart disease, which may be more successful, especially in families who have a hereditary tendency for cardiac disease; and the preliminary data on retention of cognition, which seems promising.

Drugs as Part of the Total Treatment Regimen

The total treatment regimen includes the following: Therapy with alternative herbs and healthier lifestyle, which may relieve symptoms but have not proved to bestow reduced morbidity, as has drug therapy; hormonal therapy is indicated for vaginal atrophy and bladder outlet syndrome; and referral to an appropriate specialist to provide the appropriate care when adverse effects occur as a result of estrogen therapy.

Adherence Issues

Nonadherence to the treatment regimen may be a result of various causes. Nonadherence due to the possible risk of cancer should be discussed, and the absolute risk of cancer rather than relative risk of cancer should be calculated annually. The possibility of minor discomforts, such as breast tenderness, bloating, fluid retention, and the need for follow-up visits, should be discussed prior to therapy. If irregular or unexpected bleeding occurs, patients should be advised to contact their health care provider for modifications to the treatment regimen rather than stop therapy on their own.

Hormone Replacement Therapy

Complaint

"I think I might be pregnant."

History

Maria Gonzales, age 45, presents complaining of hot flashes and fatigue. She reports (through an interpreter) that her last menstrual period was 2 months ago and that she wonders if she is pregnant. She states that her husband "takes care" of birth control.

Mrs. Gonzales works for a local plant nursery and is physically active but has gained 15 lb since her last examination at age 42. Menarche was at age 9 years and she has delivered six children. One child died at birth from prolapsed umbilical cord. Her children range in age from 25, 23, stillborn, 19, 12, and 7. Family history is significant for father deceased at age 56 of coronary artery disease. Mother and two siblings in Mexico have diabetes. She thinks that their diabetes is controlled on "pills." Four other siblings live nearby.

Assessment

Vital signs are blood pressure 140/90, pulse 88, height 4'10", and weight 150 pounds. Physical examination reveals a Hispanic female appearing her stated age. Abnormal findings are "benign cellular change" on Pap smear. BMI is 32. Cholesterol level is 230 mg/dL, and HDL is 40 mg/dL. Legs indicate venous disease with a trace of pitting edema in both ankles. Urine pregnancy test was negative, with specific gravity 1.020. Mammograms are described as early involutional changes.

Initial Management Plan

Based on her assessment data, she is diagnosed as perimenopausal. Mrs. Gonzales's management plan is as follows:

1. MPA 10 mg daily the first 10 days each month.
2. Change in diet. Diet analysis reveals traditional Mexican food of rice or toast and coffee for breakfast. Lunch at work is a taco or burrito and fruit juice. Supper is meat, vegetables, beans (refried), and several tortillas. Most days Mrs. Gonzales eats four to eight tortillas, and most are fried in oil. A realistic change in diet is to use spray oil instead of deep-frying and eat four tortillas each day instead of eight. Switch to pinto beans, and substitute brown rice served with milk at breakfast.
3. Dietary supplementation. Work keeps Mrs. Gonzales outdoors (vitamin D) most of the year, but supplements of calcium are needed, to include 800 additional mg of calcium carbonate. Expected weight loss would be 3 to 5 lb each month, with a goal of 20 lb loss in total.
4. Follow-up visit. Return to clinic in 1 month (12 hours fasting) for full lipid panel.

Follow-up Visit

At her follow-up visit, Mrs. Gonzales's vital signs are BP 142/88, weight 148. She feels "a little better." She is sleeping without as many hot flashes but has lost only 2 lb. After the first 10 days of MPA 10 mg daily, she had a withdrawal bleed of just a trace. Fasting lipids levels today reveal total cholesterol 225 mg/dL, triglycerides 250 mg/dL, LDL 140 mg/dL, and HDL 40 mg/dL.

Modifications to Management Plan

Mrs. Gonzales's new management plan is as follows:

1. After 3 to 6 months of cyclic progesterone, plan conjugated estrogens 0.3 mg and 5–10 mg of MPA daily. If the progestin causes mood changes, consider micronized progesterone 200 mg 10 to 14 days each month. According to Andersen et al. (1999), benefits in cardiovascular risk factors such as lowering the fibrinogen level are not affected by cyclic or continuous estrogen/progestin administration.
2. After elevated triglycerides of 250 mg/dL (desirable <100 mg/dL), elevated LDL 140 mg/dL (optimal <100 mg/dL), and elevated total cholesterol 225 mg/dL (optimal being <200 mg/dL) were discovered, Mrs. Gonzales was prescribed a cholesterol-lowering drug (pravastatin) 10 mg qd. Mrs. Gonzales has a strong family history of diabetes and coronary artery disease, as well as borderline blood pressure readings, obesity, abnormal lipids, and menopause (six risk factors for cardiovascular disease).
3. Return to clinic in 1 month to monitor liver function tests and to see how the HRT and pravastatin affect Mrs. Gonzales's lipid levels

Calcium Therapy

The typical American diet provides 600 to 1000 mg calcium. The best calcium sources are dairy products and certain vegetables such as broccoli. Yogurt has more than 400 mg per 8-oz serving, and broccoli has 150 mg.

Calcium supplementation, up to 1200 mg, is frequently necessary during childhood growth, pregnancy, and lactation. Calcium as a part of a daily diet is found in plentiful and cheap sources. Buying **calcium** supplementa-

Table 36–1. Osteoporosis: Risk Factors

Modifiable Risk Factors	Unmodifiable (Internal) Risk Factors
• Depression	Female gender
• Low-calcium diet	Blue eyes
• Eating disorders (anorexia or bulimia)	Small, thin body frame
• Use of medications such as steroids, anticonvulsants, excessive thyroid hormone, some cancer medications	Age 50 and older
• Sedentary lifestyle	White, Asian, or Native American
• Cigarette smoking	Family history of osteoporosis
• Excessive alcohol intake	Early menopause
	Abnormal absence of menstruation (polycystic ovary [PCO] disease)
	Low testosterone levels (men)
	Difficulty in absorbing calcium from the gut

tion is also economical. Table 36–2 presents information on available **calcium** preparations.

When increased demand after menopause exceeds the typical dietary intake (1500 mg), **calcium** alone as a supplement is not enough to prevent or treat osteoporosis. Patients need pharmacotherapy, used in conjunction with **vitamin D**, exercise, and avoidance of certain lifestyle behaviors. Optimum response is when **estrogen** is added to the regimen.

Some patients complain of constipation with **calcium** in combination with **carbonate**, and other formulations need to be substituted. The presence of milk allergy and lactose intolerance can also greatly affect the amount of calcium in the diet and make supplementation mandatory.

Calcium is always ingested in combination with other ions. Depending on which ion, the dose may need to be given away from mealtimes to avoid reduced absorption.

Most **calcium supplement**s in combination are only 40 to 50 percent active, so the practitioner needs to calculate the number of tablets depending on the size of tablet. A 600-mg **Tums** tablet has 240 mg of active calcium, and six **Tums** tablets fulfill the requirements for a postmenopausal woman.

Alendronate Therapy

Alendronate (Fosamax), a third-generation drug in the family of **biphosphonate compounds,** has been used in clinical trials for years, but FDA approval of earlier compounds restricted their use to specialists because of the adverse effects and complicated dosing regimen. **Alendronate** is indicated for prevention as well as treatment of women with diagnosed osteoporosis who cannot or will not take **estrogen.** Osteoporosis must be diagnosed

by fracture or bone mass density (BMD). Table 36–3 presents methods used for measuring bone density.

Before treatment can be initiated, secondary causes of osteoporosis must be ruled out. Malignancies, anemias, Paget's disease, hyperthyroidism, hyperparathyroidism, nutritional deficiencies, osteomalacia, renal disease, sarcoidosis, Cushing's syndrome, pituitary disease, and hypogonadism are the most common causes. A complete history and physical examination and certain screening blood and urine chemistries can rule out these diseases.

Bone resorption is inhibited with the resulting asymptomatic reduction in calcium and phosphate concentrations. The decrease in serum phosphate by **alendronate** may reflect the positive bone mineral balance as well as a decrease in renal phosphate reabsorption. Most information about improvement in calcium metabolism is from the benefits shown in Paget's disease and the hypercalcemia of malignancies.

Alendronate is approximately $50 per month as compared with $30 per month for **estrogen** and **estrogen-progestin** therapies. This cost is pennies compared with the costs of surgery, hospitalization, and rehabilitation for fracture care once bone thinning has progressed. Table 36–4 presents the approximate yearly costs of various therapies for the treatment of osteoporosis.

Patients with a history of gastrointestinal (GI) bleeding, peptic ulcer disease, and gastroesophageal reflux disease (GERD) may not be the best candidates for **alendronate** because of the esophageal irritation common with this drug.

Adequate supplementation with **calcium** and **vitamin D** is necessary before initiating therapy. No dosage adjustment is necessary as long as renal function remains between 35 and 60 mL/minute. At this time, **alendronate** cannot be used with **estrogen.**

Table 36–2. Calcium Preparations

Drug	Active Calcium	How Supplied
Calcium acetate	25%	1000 mg in 180 and 1000 tablets per bottle (250 mg calcium)
Calcium carbonate	40%	650 mg in 1000 tablets per bottle (260 mg calcium)
Calcium citrate	21%	950 and 2376 mg in 100 and 300 tablets per bottle (200 mg and 500 mg calcium)
Calcium glubionate	6.5%	1.8 g per 5 mL in 480 mL with sweetener choices of saccharin, sorbitol, or sucrose (115 mg calcium)
Calcium gluconate	9.3%	500-mg, 650-mg, 975-mg, and 1-g tablets in 500 and 1000 tablets per bottle (45, 58.5, 87.75, and 90 mg of calcium)
Calcium lactate	13%	325 mg and 650 mg in 1000 tablets per bottle (42.5 mg and 84.5 mg of calcium)
Tricalcium phosphate	39%	1565.2 mg in 60 tablets per bottle (600 mg calcium)

Adapted from Kastrup, E. (Ed.). (1998). *Drug facts and comparisons.* St. Louis: Drug Facts and Comparisons.

Table 36–3. Methods for Bone Density Measurements

Test	Sites Measured	Approximate Cost	Comments
Dual energy x-ray absorptiometry (DXA)	Spine, hip, total body	$150–$200	Limitations: misdiagnoses low bone mass in patients with arthritis Available: yes, but not in all cities
Peripheral dual energy x-ray absorptiometry (P-DXA)	Wrist, finger	$50	Limitations: for older adults Available: yes
Quantitative computed tomography (QCT)	Spine	$100–$150	Limitations: machine must be recalibrated between uses Available: yes
Peripheral QCT (pQCT)	Forearm, wrist	$40–$60	Limitations: better for younger patients needing multiple sites Available: yes
Radiographic absorptiometry (RA)	Hand	$60	Limitations: Requires normal baseline; not available for patients with arthritis who have no baseline Available: yes
Single photon absorptiometry (SXA)	Wrist	$50	Limitations: older adults Available: yes
Single energy x-ray absorptiometry (SXA)	Wrist, heel	$35–$120	Limitations: older adults Available: yes
Ultrasound	Heel, tibia, finger	$30–$50	Limitations: new, younger, no x-ray Available: yes
Peripheral instant x-ray imaging (PIXI)	Wrist, heel	$50	Limitations: older adult or young Available: European approval only

Adapted from American Academy of Family Physicians. (1997). *Osteoporosis: Diagnosis and patient management monograph* (pp. 1–20). Leawood, KS: American Academy of Family Physicians.

Table 36–4. Therapies for Osteoporosis: Approximate Cost per Year

Therapy	Approximate Cost per Year
Alendronate (Fosamax) 5 mg PO qd (prevention); 10 mg PO qd (treatment)	$640
Conjugated estrogen (Premarin) 0.625 mg PO qd	$166
Conjugated estrogen (CE) with medroxyprogesterone (MPA) (generic Provera) 0.625 mg CE and 5 mg MPA PO qd	$238
Micronized estradiol (generic Estrace) 1mg PO qd	$105
Transdermal estradiol (Estraderm, Climara, Vivelle) 0.05 mg TD (to apply 1–2 times/wk)	$126–$561
Esterified estrogen (Estratab, Menest) 0.625 mg PO qd	$159
Raloxifene (Evista) 60 mg PO qd	$659
Salmon calcitonin (Miacalcin) 200 IU intranasally qd	$837

Adapted from Koder, M. (1999). Prevention strategies for postmenopausal osteoporosis. *Oregon Drug Use Review Board,* *7*(1), 6–7.

Alendronate 10 mg is taken with a full glass of water in the morning 30 minutes before any other food or drugs. Patients should remain upright to reduce the chance of esophageal irritation. Administer milk or **antacids** to bind **alendronate** in case of accidental overdosage.

Calcitonin Therapy

When given by the intranasal route, **calcitonin** increases spinal bone mass in postmenopausal women with established osteoporosis. **Calcitonin** cannot prevent bone loss in the early postmenopausal woman. This drug is indicated only for women who have severe disease and cannot take **estrogen.** It also has an unexplained analgesic effect on osteoporotic fracture pain.

Single injections of **calcitonin** transiently inhibit bone resorption and osteoclasts. Low serum calcium levels increase the secretion of endogenous **calcitonin,** with a resulting small decrease in serum calcium. **Calcitonin** is administered intranasally (200 IU per day). Currently, this therapy has been shown to be more effective in spinal fractures, rather than in hip and wrist fractures. Use the nasal route of administration for patients with established bone loss. This drug is not for prevention in early menopause. Rhinitis and nasal irritation are the commonest complaints. Examine the nasal mucosa carefully.

Calcitonin should be refrigerated before opening and then kept at room temperature once opened. Dosing with **calcitonin** 200 IU intranasally requires alternating nostrils every other day to reduce mucosal irritation. Other adverse effects are fatigue and flulike symptoms.

Calcitonin therapy is the most costly per month but has its place for pain relief in osteoporosis and for those patients unable to use **estrogen.**

Raloxifene Therapy

Raloxifene (Evista) is a **selective estrogen receptor modulator (SERM)** that has estrogen-like effects on bone (increases BMD) and on lipid (decreases total and low-density lipoprotein [LDL] cholesterol) metabolism. Unlike **estrogen,** it does not stimulate breast and uterine tissues. This drug is an improvement over **tamoxifen** and may well prove to be a breast cancer antagonist after further clinical trials. It is indicated for prevention and treatment of osteoporosis in women who do not want to or are unable to take **estrogen** therapy. It shares with **estrogen** the precaution to avoid use in women who have previously had deep vein thrombus or embolism. It cannot be used in combination with **estrogen** because the receptors affected are different in the presence of **estrogen.**

Raloxifene therapy suppresses bone resorption and bone formation, as reflected by serum and urine markers of bone turnover. In addition, it decreases total and LDL cholesterol and fibrinogen, which are effects formerly attributed only to **ERT.** When compared with **estrogen** and **progesterone, raloxifene's** adverse reactions were in the areas of more hot flashes, genital and urinary infection, and chest pain. **HRT,** by contrast, demonstrated more vaginal bleeding, breast pain, and flatulence (Kastrup, 1998).

A previous history of venous thromboembolic events such as deep vein thrombosis, pulmonary embolism, and retinal artery embolism is a contraindication for use. Patients with multiple risk factors for osteoporosis should receive bone density measurements (BDMs) to assess their need for this drug.

Patients need to be warned that the drug should be discontinued 72 hours prior to prolonged bed rest and to avoid inactivity while traveling by car or plane. Women need to know that this medication will not stop hot flashes; in fact, it could trigger hot flashes at the beginning of therapy.

The dose of **raloxifene** is 60 mg daily without regard to meals. Make sure patients consume or supplement 1500 mg of **calcium** and 800 IU of **vitamin D** daily.

Figure 36–2 present a treatment algorithm for osteoporosis.

Monitoring

Estrogen requires the same monitoring when prescribed for osteoporosis as when it is used for **HRT.** Obtain annual renal function tests on all patients over age 65 and on those with potentially reduced renal function, such as patients with diabetes.

The use of **calcium** alone for supplementation rarely needs blood test follow-up, but treatment of conditions with **vitamin D** and **high-dose calcium** can induce high levels in serum and then in the kidney. The monitoring interval between tests for BDMs has not been standardized but will probably be in 1 to 2 years.

Monitoring of **alendronate** is aimed at electrolyte measurement, renal function, and GI symptoms of patients over age 65 and of those with multiple medical conditions. Known drug-drug interactions are with **ranitidine,** **calcium supplements, antacids,** and **aspirin.**

Use of **calcitonin** presents the possibility of allergy because circulating antibodies have been detected in 2 to 18 months of therapy. **Calcitonin** is derived from mammal thyroid glands.

Drug interactions have been observed in **raloxifene** with **cholestyramine** and **warfarin,** so coadministration should be avoided. Evaluation of this therapy can be done every 2 years with bone densitometers, but beneficial effects may be demonstrated as early as 1 year after therapy (Kastrup, 1998).

Outcome Evaluation

Osteoporosis is expected to begin 2 to 5 years after menopause in women not using **HRT.** Assess patients who have had fractures, unusual bone pain, high-risk physical characteristics, or a history of systemic **cortisone** use. The NP can begin this evaluation with a history and physical examination and then consult before obtaining laboratory tests or imaging studies. If any of these tests or imaging studies indicate pathology, then referral for specialty care is indicated.

Patients who have other medical conditions and multiple medications to manage are candidates for consultation or referral. Consider referral if more than one consultation is made with the specialist over medication choices. After therapy is established and the patient is not having adverse drug effects, most primary care providers handle routine monitoring.

Patient Education

Patient education should include a discussion of information related to the overall treatment plan as well as that specific to the drug therapy, reasons for taking the drug, drugs as part of the total treatment regimen, and adherence issues.

ON THE HORIZON

Sodium Fluoride

As a treatment for osteoporosis, **sodium fluoride (Slow Fluoride)** is a new formulation of an old drug that has been used for more than 30 years in Europe. The FDA has found that its adverse effects of gastritis, bone pain, and stress fractures far outweigh its benefits of increased bone density and has not approved it for general use. If approved, it will be used with **calcium citrate** and delivered in cycles of 12 months on and 2 months off therapy (Kessenich, 1996).

Ongoing research may prove that **SERMs** will prevent fractures in patients with osteoporosis, as do **estrogen, alendronate,** and **calcitonin.**

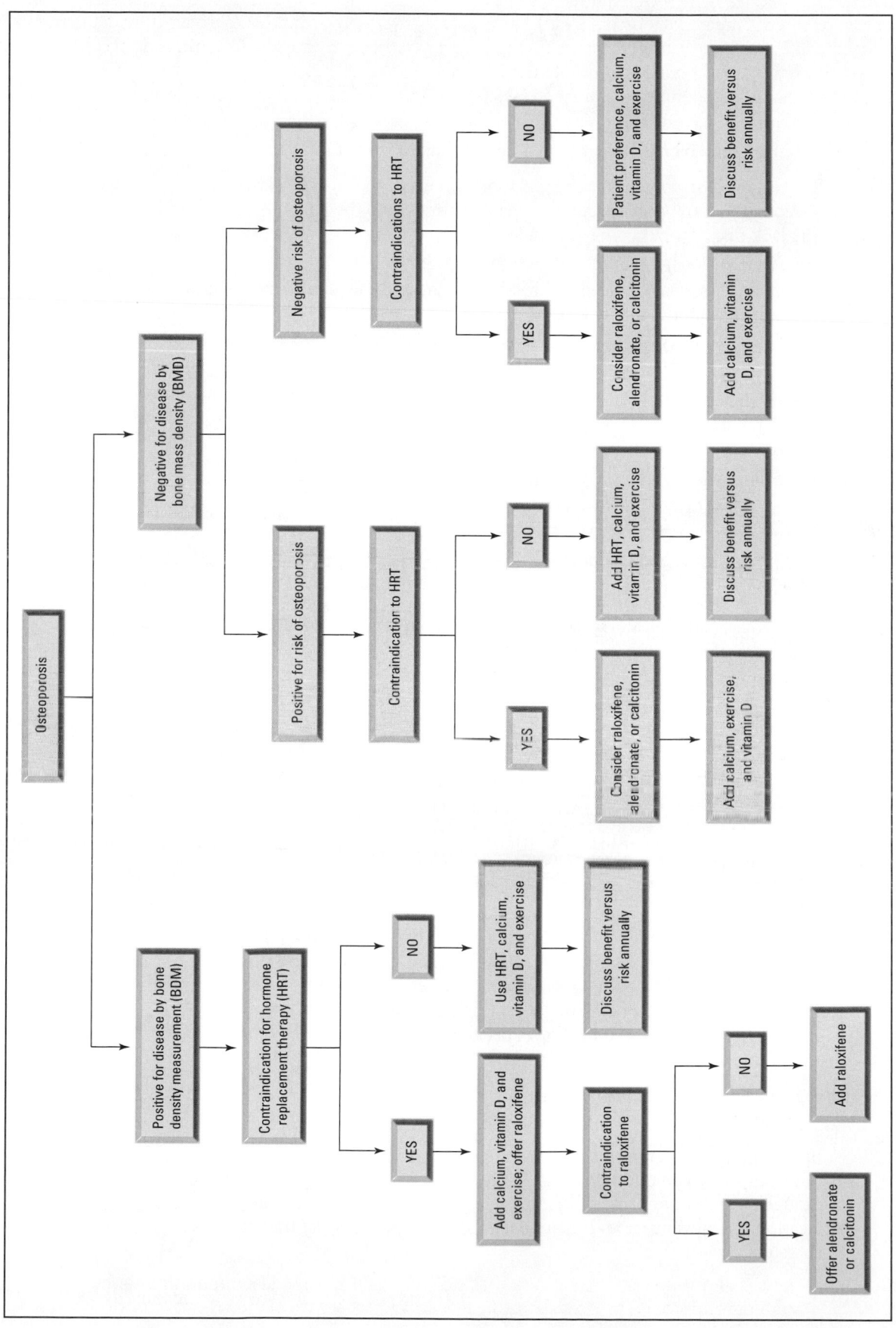

Figure 36–2. Treatment algorithm: Osteoporosis.

Osteoporosis

Related to the Overall Treatment Plan/Disease Process

☐ Pathophysiology of the dynamic relationship between the osteoclasts and osteoblasts in the process of bone metabolism to help the patient understand how the lack of estrogen begins a cascade of events ending with the increased risk of osteoporosis in the early years after cessation of menses

☐ Role of excessive alcohol, nicotine, and caffeine and low intakes of calcium and vitamin D as modifiable risks for osteoporosis

☐ Role of nondrug treatments such as diets high in calcium and vitamin D, exercise, and avoidance of the high-risk lifestyles

☐ An understanding of how knowledge of family history, ethnicity, and genetic characteristics help to identify patients with unmodifiable risk factors for osteoporosis

☐ Importance of adherence to the treatment regimen

☐ Importance of supplementing the diet with additional calcium (up to 1600 mg) and vitamin D (800 mg) to the osteoporosis therapy

☐ Self-monitoring of symptoms

☐ What to do when symptoms worsen

☐ Need for regular follow-up visits with the primary care provider and for screening tests such as bone mineral densities (BMDs) every 2 years

Specific to the Drug Therapy

☐ Reason for the drug to be taken and its anticipated action in the disease process

☐ Doses and schedules for taking the drug

☐ Possible adverse effects and what to do if they occur

☐ Interactions between other treatment modalities and these drugs

Reasons for Taking the Drug(s)

Patient education specifically for osteoporosis should include the following: that prevention of osteoporosis is more successful, especially in those who have a hereditary tendency for bone loss disease; treatment of fractures is far more expensive than drug therapy; and postmenopausal fractures are associated with early loss of independent living and reduced life expectancy.

Drugs as Part of the Total Treatment Regimen

The total treatment regimen includes lifestyle modification: healthy diet, dietary supplements, and exercise. However, these lifestyle modifications may not be enough, especially in older patients. Some form of drug therapy is usually necessary. Although several nonhormone therapies are available, estrogen therapy has the best indication for prevention and treatment of spine, hip, and wrist fractures associated with osteoporosis.

continued

PATIENT EDUCATION

Osteoporosis *(continued)*

Adherence Issues

Adherence issues include the following:

☐ Media reports about disease and drug therapies have an increasing impact on patients and primary care practices.

☐ Membership in health maintenance organizations may affect the choice of drugs patients will receive.

☐ Patients' fears or issues about drug therapy may not be based on facts.

☐ Drug therapy educational handouts should be available to patients and their families.

☐ Monitoring appointments are problematic if patients are homebound or transportation is difficult.

Osteoporosis

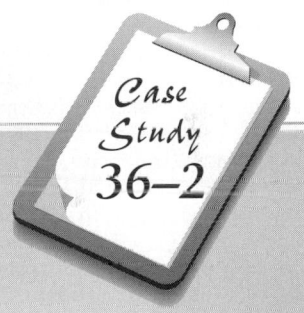

Case Study 36–2

Complaint

"I want to be checked for osteoporosis."

History

Mrs. Miller, a 67-year-old white woman, presents with concerns about possible osteoporosis. She has used no estrogen therapy in the last 20 years since menopause and has been an insulin-dependent diabetic for more than 16 years.

Mrs. Miller has a hereditary group of diseases called syndrome X, which includes diabetes, hyperuricemia, hypertension, hypothyroidism, and hyperlipidemia. At ages 45 and 51, she had breast biopsies. One of these biopsies showed a benign hyperplasia, which causes increased cancer risk. Estrogen may increase cancer risk in patients with mammary hyperplasia. In her thirties, Mrs. Miller had conization of the cervix, which revealed carcinoma in situ. Family history included hypertension in both parents and a maternal aunt with osteoporosis. Current medications include levothyroxine 125 mcg, metformin 500 mg bid, glyburide 5 mg bid, lisinopril 10 mg bid, diltiazem 240 mg XL, ASA two tabs daily, pravastatin 20 mg daily, and calcium and garlic pills, strength unknown.

Assessment

Mrs. Miller's vital signs are 140/86, height 64", and weight 149.5 lb. Physical examination reveals a woman who appears her stated age. Abnormal findings include decreased arterial-to-venous ratio in right eye; chloasma around eyes; grade 1/6 diastolic murmur heard loudest in the right second intercostal space; dense, nodular breasts (characteristic of mammary dysplasia); and severe vulvar and vaginal atrophy. Abnormal laboratory tests include Pap smear with atrophic changes, total cholesterol 239, triglycerides 236, HDL 26, and LDL 166. Her Hgb A_{1c} is 7.3 (indicating good blood sugar control over the past 3 months). Bone mineral density revealed bone mass less than 2 standard deviations from normal (osteoporosis).

Initial Management Plan

Based on her assessment data, Mrs. Miller is diagnosed with osteoporosis. Her management plan is as follows:

1. Maintain all previous medications, and add raloxifene 60 mg.
2. Make sure that the calcium supplement is sufficient, and calculate the dietary intake from foods to equal 1600 mg, as well as 800 mg of vitamin D.
3. Follow-up visit. Return to clinic in 1–2 months after starting new medication like raloxifene.

Follow-Up Visit:

At her follow-up visit (actually at 6 months), Mrs. Miller's vital signs are BP 140/88 and weight 152 lb. Laboratory tests demonstrate cholesterol 218 mg/dL, triglycerides 200 mg/dL, HDL 26 mg/dL, and LDL 158 mg/dL.

Modifications to Management Plan

Consider increasing metformin to 500 mg tid for high triglycerides, and substitute atorvastatin if cholesterol is not less than 200mg/dL on subsequent visits. Patients with diabetes need to have lower blood pressure, lower serum lipids, and lower Hgb A_{1c} measurements than patients without diabetes on account of the increased risk of heart disease in all types of diabetes mellitus.

REFERENCES

Adkins, C. (1997). Bone mass and the risk of breast cancer. *New England Journal of Medicine, 337*(3), 199.

Andersen, L., Gram, J., Skouby, S., & Jespersen, J. (1999). Effects of hormone replacement therapy on hemostatic cardiovascular risk factors. *American Journal of Obstetrics and Gynecology, 180*(2, Pt. 1), 283–289.

August, P. (1998). Sex, hormones, and hypertension: What is—and is not—known. *Women's Health in Primary Care, 1*(10), 21–28.

Baker, V., & Jaffe, R. (1995). Clinical uses of anti-estrogen. *Obstetrical and Gynecological Survey, 51*(1), 45–59.

Berga, S. (1996). The physician as a guardian of bone health. *Internal Medicine Alert,* (2).

Buring, J. (1998). *Women's health study update* (Harvard Medical School and Brigham and Women's Hospital), 8(1), 4.

Colditz, M., Hankinson, S., Hunter, D., Willet, W., Manson, J., Stampfer, M., Hennekens, C., Rosner, B., & Speizer, F. (1995). The use of estrogens and progestins and the risk of breast cancer in postmenopausal women. *New England Journal of Medicine, 332*(24), 1589–1593.

Don't be swayed into taking boron for your bones. (1999). *Tufts University Health & Nutrition Letter, 8,* 3.

Eriksen, B. (1999). A randomized, open, parallel-group study on the preventive effect of an estradiol-releasing vaginal ring (Estring) on recurrent urinary tract infections in postmenopausal women. *American Journal of Obstetrics and Gynecology, 180*(5), 1072–1079.

Ettinger, B., & Grady, D. (1993). The waning effect of postmenopausal estrogen therapy on osteoporosis, *New England Journal of Medicine, 329*(16), 1192–1193.

Ettinger, B., Selby, J., Citron, J., Vangessel, A., Ettinger, V., & Hendrickson, M. (1994). Cyclic hormone replacement therapy using quarterly progestin. *Obstetrics and Gynecology, 83*(5), 693–700.

Fraenkel, L., Zhang, Y., Chaisson, C., Evans, S., Wilson, P., & Felson, D. (1998). *Annals of Internal Medicine, 129*(3), 208–211.

Grodstein, F., Stampfer, M., Colditz, G., Willet, W., Manson, J., Joffe, M., Rosner, B., Fuchs, C., Hankinson, S., Hunter, D., Hennekens, C., & Speizer, F. (1997). Postmenopausal hormone therapy and mortality. *New England Journal of Medicine, 336,* 1769–1775.

Harvard Medical School. (1997). Does HRT increase vein clots? *Harvard Heart Letter, 7*(9), 6.

Kastrup, E. (Ed.). (1998). *Drug facts and comparisons.* St. Louis: Facts and Comparisons.

Katz, W. (1998). Osteoporosis: The role of exercise in optimal management. *Physician and Sports Medicine, 26*(2), 33–35, 39–43.

Katzung, B. (1998). *Basic and clinical pharmacology* (7th ed.). Norwalk, CT: Appleton & Lange.

Kessenich, C. (1996). Update on pharmacotherapeutics for osteoporosis. *Nurse-Practitioner, 21*(8), 19–24.

Koder, M. (1999). Prevention strategies for postmenopausal osteoporosis. *Oregon Drug Use Review Board, 7*(1), 6–7.

Kritz-Silverstein, D., & Barrett-Connor, E. (1996). Long-term postmenopausal hormone use, obesity, and fat distribution in older women. *Journal of the American Medical Association, 275*(1), 46–49.

Liu, J. (1998). Natural progesterone. *Health News (New England Journal of Medicine), 4*(4), 3.

McClung, M. (1998). Latest management of osteoporosis. Proceedings of Regional CME. Ashland, OR: Oregon Nurses Association.

Mendelsohn, M., & Karas, R. (1999). The protective effects of estrogen on the cardiovascular system. *NEJM 340*(23), 1801–1811.

Murray, J. (1998). Natural progesterone: What role in women's health care? *Women's Health in Primary Care, 8,* 671–674, 677–680, 686–687.

Newcomb, P., & Storer, B. (1995). Postmenopausal hormone use and risk of large-bowel cancer. *Journal of the National Cancer Institute 87*(14), 1067–1071.

Paganini-Hill, A. (1998). Alzheimer's disease in women. *Female Patient, 23,* 12–18.

Recker, R., Davies, K., Dowd, R., & Heaney, R. (1999). The effect of low-dose continuous estrogen and progesterone therapy with calcium and vitamin D on bone in elderly women. *Annals of Internal Medicine, 130*(11), 897–904.

Scharbo-Dehann, M. (1996). Hormone replacement therapy, *Nurse Practitioner, 21*(12), 1–13.

School of Public Health. (1998). A consumer's guide to replacement hormones. *University of California at Berkeley Wellness Letter 13*(12), 4–5.

Shaywitz, S., Shaywitz, B., Pugh, K., Fullbright, R., Skudlarski, P., Mencl, W., Constable, R., Naftolin, F., Palter, S., Marchione, K., Katz, L., Shankweiler, D., Fletcher, J., Lacadie, C., Keltz, M., & Gore, J. (1999). Effect of estrogen on brain activation patterns in postmenopausal women during working memory tasks. *Journal of the American Medical Association, 281*(13), 1197–1202.

Weiderpass, E., Baron, J., Adami, H., Magnusson, C., Lindgren, A., Bergstrom, R., Correia, N., & Persson, I. (1999). Low-potency oestrogen and risk of endometrial cancer: A case-control study. *Lancet, 353*(9167), 1824–1828.

Writing Group for the PEPI Trial. (1996). Effects of hormone replacement therapy on endometrial histology in postmenopausal women. *Journal of the American Medical Association, 275*(5), 370–375

CHAPTER 37

· · · · · · ·

Hyperlipidemia

CHAPTER OUTLINE

Cardiovascular diseases are the major cause of death in the United States. Almost 500,000 people die each year from heart attacks, most commonly related to coronary artery disease (CAD). Atherosclerosis is the major cause of CAD. It is characterized by deposits of cholesterol and other lipoproteins on the walls of arteries. Elevated serum lipoprotein levels are one of the four best-established risk factors for CAD. More specifically, the risk for CAD is associated with serum cholesterol levels greater than 200 mg/dL, fasting triglyceride levels greater than 150 mg/dL, and low-density lipoprotein (LDL) levels greater than 130 mg/dL. Lifestyle and pharmacological therapies are directed toward bringing elevated levels of these lipoproteins down to specific levels

associated with reduced cardiovascular disease risk. In the Framingham study, a 10 percent decrease in cholesterol level was associated with a 2 percent decrease in the incidence of CAD morbidity and mortality. Drugs that affect lipid levels differentially affect LDLs, high-density lipoproteins (HDLs), very low density lipoproteins (VLDLs), and triglyceride levels. The choice of drug is based on how that drug affects each of these.

This chapter focuses on the relationship of hyperlipidemia to atherosclerosis and the management of hyperlipidemia based on the National Cholesterol Education Program (NCEP) guidelines. Chapter 14 provides specific information for each of the drugs used to lower plasma lipid levels.

Pathophysiology

Serum fat and cholesterol are carried in the circulation in complexes of lipids and proteins called lipoproteins. Fat is transported as triglycerides and phospholipids, and cholesterol is transported in free and esterified forms. Most of the cholesterol in plasma is carried in LDLs. High concentrations of LDLs are associated with an increased risk of CAD. Serum lipoproteins are formed via two pathways: dietary, or exogenous, and liver synthesis, or endogenous.

Exogenous Pathway

After a meal, fat and cholesterol are absorbed, esterified into triglycerides and cholesterol in the intestinal cells, and then packed into chylomicrons. The chylomicrons are transported via the lymphatic system to the thoracic duct and enter the venous circulation. Activated endothelial lipoprotein lipase then hydrolyzes the triglycerides into free fatty acids and glycerol, which are removed from the circulation by fat and muscle cells. Surface cholesterol is transferred to HDL. The chylomicrons shrink during this process and become remnants, which are removed from the circulation by apolipoprotein E after it binds to a liver receptor.

This pathway is central to the lifestyle modifications that are the core of hyperlipidemia therapy. Drugs that affect absorption of fat and cholesterol in the intestine (**bile acid–binding resins**) and drugs that increase lipolysis of triglycerides via lipoprotein lipase (**fibric acid derivatives**) also have some of their mechanism of action through this pathway.

Endogenous Pathway

VLDLs are synthesized and secreted by the liver into the circulation. They are triglyceride-rich with some cholesterol present. VLDL interacts with lipoprotein lipase in the capillary endothelium to hydrolyze triglycerides into free fatty acids and glycerol, which are then absorbed by fat and muscle cells. About 50 percent of the VLDL remnants are taken up by apolipoprotein B and E receptors in the liver, and the other 50 percent stay in the circulation and become intermediate-density lipoproteins (IDLs). IDLs are then enriched with cholesterol by hepatic triglyceride lipase to become LDLs, which carry about 75 percent of the circulating cholesterol. LDL circulates for about 2 to 3 days and is removed for use by all tissue types.

LDL receptors in the liver are downregulated by the presence of LDL; therefore, one mechanism for lowering LDL is drug therapy that increases the number of LDL receptors in the liver (**bile acid–binding resins, HMG-CoA reductase inhibitors**). Drugs that inhibit VLDL synthesis in the liver (**niacin, fibric acid derivatives**) also reduce LDL via the endogenous pathway.

Atherogenesis

There are four main types of lipoproteins: VLDLs, IDLs, LDLs, and HDLs. The lipoproteins that contain apolipoprotein B100 have been identified as the vehicles that facilitate transport of cholesterol into the arterial wall, leading to atherogenesis. LDLs are the major culprits in this process. LDL levels are increased in those who consume large amounts of saturated fats and/or cholesterol, who have defects in the LDL receptor (familial hypercholesterolemia), or have a polygenic form of increased LDL. When serum LDL levels exceed a threshold of 130 mg/dL, they cross the arterial wall and become embedded in the arterial lumen. Here they undergo oxidation and are taken up by macrophages. Atherosclerotic plaque is made up of foam cells, which are, in turn, made up of transformed macrophages and smooth muscle cells that have been filled with cholesterol. Glycation of lipoproteins in poorly controlled diabetes contributes to foam cell generation. Arterial hypertension also accelerates the process.

HDLs are thought to function as acceptors of free cholesterol as it passively diffuses out of cells. This reverse transport is the mechanism by which cholesterol may be removed from atherosclerotic plaques. Figure 37–1 shows the relationship of lipid metabolism to atherosclerotic plaque formation. Apolipoprotein A-I is the major apoprotein in HDL, and the level of this apoprotein and the level of HDL are both associated with decreased CAD risk and decreased atherogenesis. Women have higher HDL levels than men do, in part because of their higher estrogen levels, and the administration of **estrogen** to postmenopausal women can be a part of hyperlipidemia therapy. Exercise increases HDL; obesity and smoking decrease it. Although LDLs are most commonly the lipoprotein toward which therapy is directed, the ratio of total cholesterol to HDL is actually the most powerful predictor of atherosclerotic CAD risk. Table 37–1 shows the positive and negative risk factors for CAD.

Goals of Treatment

The positive relationship between elevated cholesterol levels, atherosclerosis, and CAD is well established. The overarching goal for management of hyperlipidemia is to reduce morbidity and mortality from CAD by reducing atherogenesis. Multiple patient variables based on risk profiles are considered in setting individual lipoprotein level goals. CAD risk is the main guide to the type and intensity of cholesterol-lowering ther-

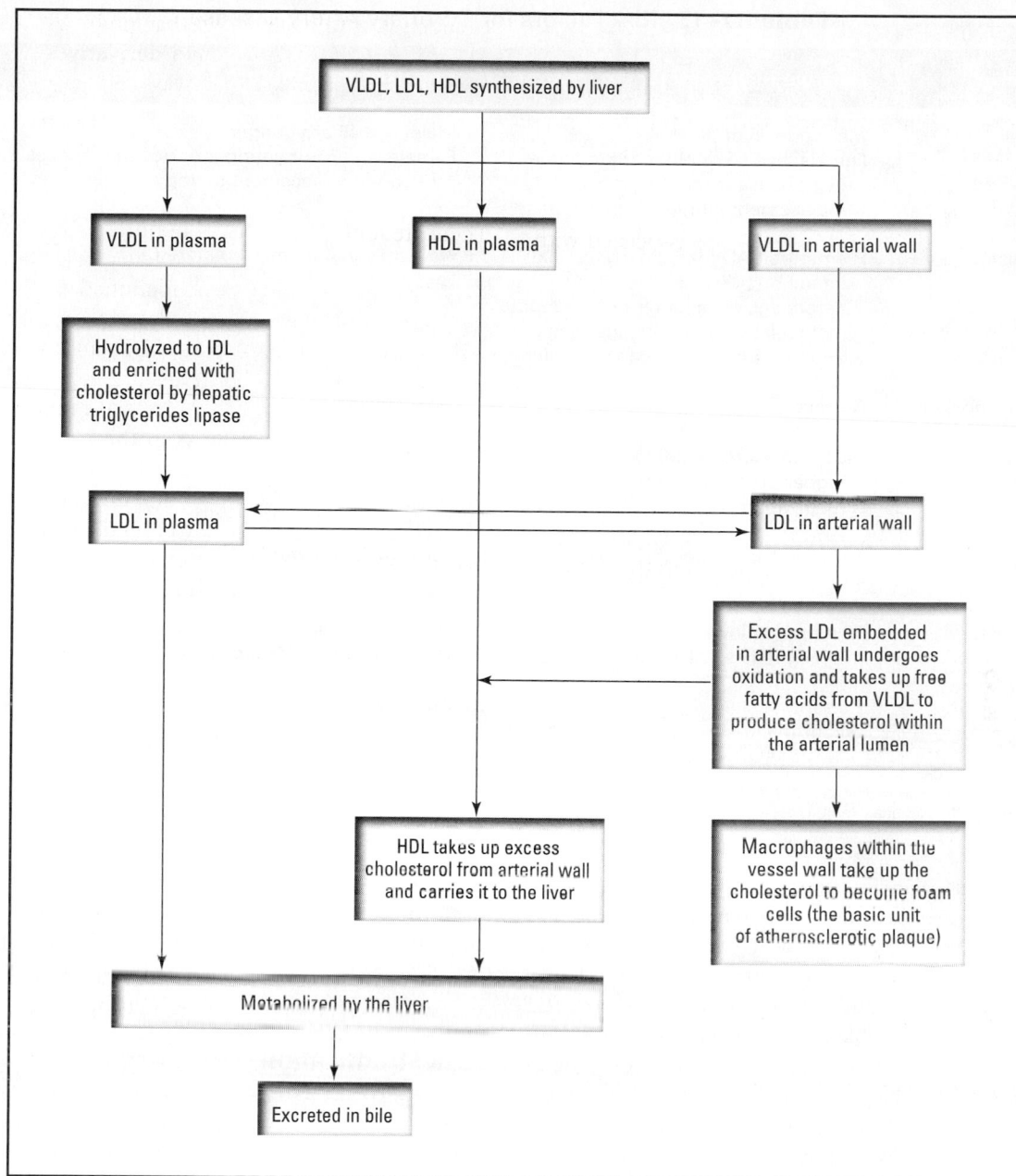

Figure 37–1. Relationship of lipid metabolism to atherosclerotic plaque formation. Excess LDL embedded in the arterial wall undergoes oxidation and takes up free fatty acids from VLDL to produce cholesterol within the arterial lumen. If the excess cholesterol is not taken up by HDL and carried to the liver, macrophages within the vessel wall create atherosclerotic plaque from this excess cholesterol.

apy. Those at high risk for CAD receive more aggressive therapy and have lower target cholesterol and LDL levels than those with less risk. For individuals free of CAD risk, total cholesterol levels below 200 mg/dL and HDL levels above 35 mg/dL are considered acceptable. For those with existing CAD, total cholesterol levels are less important, and the goal becomes LDL levels below 100 mg/dL and HDL levels above 60 mg/dL. Table 37–2 presents the treatment goals for LDL cholesterol levels based on the presence or absence of CAD and risk factors. The Second Report of the NCEP Expert Panel on Detection, Evaluation, and Treatment of High Blood Cholesterol (NCEP, 1993) presents algorithms for treatment based on risk stratification. The discussion in this chapter is taken from or consistent with those algorithms.

Rational Drug Selection

Hyperlipidemia presents a problem in therapeutic management because it is usually asymptomatic until damage

Table 37–1. Risk Factors for Coronary Artery Disease

Risk Factor	Positive Risk Factors	Negative Risk Factors
Age	Male: age 45 or older Female: age 55 or older or premature menopause without estrogen replacement therapy	Male: age 45 or younger Female: age 55 or younger or postmenopausal on estrogen replacement therapy
Family history	Premature CAD (definite myocardial infarction [MI] or sudden death before age 55 in father or first-degree male relative or before age 65 in mother or first-degree female relative)	No family history of premature CAD
Cigarette smoking	Current	Nonsmoking
Hypertension	Blood pressure 140/90 mm Hg or higher or taking antihypertensive medication	Normotensive
LDL cholesterol	160 mg/dL or higher (high risk) 130–159 mg/dL (borderline high risk)	130 mg/dL or lower (low risk)
HDL cholesterol	35 mg/dL or lower (major positive risk factor)	60 mg/dL or higher (major negative risk factor)
Diabetes mellitus	Presence, especially if poorly controlled	Absence

From the National Cholesterol Education Program (1993). *Second report of the Expert Panel on Detection, Evaluation, and Treatment of High Blood Cholesterol in Adults (adult treatment panel II)*. NIH Publ. No. 93-3095). Rockville, MD: National Institutes of Health. National Heart, Lung and Blood Institute.

to the cardiovascular system occurs. In addition, the central aspects of treatment are lifestyle modifications, especially dietary, which include the reduction of substances in the diet that are often perceived as making food taste good. Finally, patients often want a prescription for a drug that will "cure" the problem, and the drugs that are prescribed for hyperlipidemia are considered last-resort treatments because they have potentially serious adverse reactions. For effective management, the treatment protocol must be palatable, low cost, and with the fewest possible adverse reactions. To achieve this treatment protocol, management is based on presence or absence of CAD and

Table 37–2. Low-Density Lipoprotein Goal Based on Coronary Artery Disease

Patient Category	LDL Goal
Without CAD and <2 risk factors	<160 mg/dL
Without CAD and with >2 risk factors	<130 mg/dL
With CAD	<100 mg/dL

From the National Cholesterol Education Program (1993). *Second report of the Expert Panel on Detection, Evaluation, and Treatment of High Blood Cholesterol in Adults (adult treatment panel II)* NIH Publ. No. 93-3095). Rockville, MD: National Institutes of Health. National Heart, Lung and Blood Institute.

associated risk factors and specific patient variables. For each of these variables, lifestyle management, initial monotherapy, and stepping up to multiple drug therapy are discussed.

Risk Stratification

A gradient potential of CAD risk, taking into account lipid levels and the presence of other CAD risk factors, has been delineated by the NCEP expert panel. Table 37–1 presents the CAD risk factors delineated by the NCEP expert panel: age greater than 45 in men and 55 in women, family history of premature CAD, smoking, hypertension, cholesterol levels, and diabetes mellitus. Age, gender, and diabetes are discussed later in a section about additional patient variables.

CAD tends to cluster in families, and a positive family history of clinical CAD or sudden death in first-degree male relatives before age 55 or first-degree female relatives before age 65 is an important risk factor. The family history should include the presence or absence of high cholesterol levels and nonlipid risk factors and the age of onset of each risk factor. This provides data to assess for inherited lipoprotein disorders.

The NCEP expert panel does not list race as a risk factor for CAD. However, CAD death rates are 3 to 70 percent higher among blacks than among whites in the same age groups through age 74, and the current decline in age-adjusted CAD death rates in the United States is less striking in blacks than in whites. Reasons for these differences are not clear, but the prevalence of hypertension among blacks may be a significant factor. No separate algorithm for lipid management based on race is recommended.

High Risk

Patients at high risk for CAD are those with LDL cholesterol levels above 160 mg/dL, HDL cholesterol levels below 35mg/dL, and clinical evidence of CAD or other atherosclerotic disease, such as peripheral arterial insufficiency or symptomatic artery disease. Also at high risk, but slightly less so, are those with the same lipid levels and two or more CAD risk factors in addition to hyperlipidemia but no clinical evidence of current CAD. Patients in this risk group require both lifestyle modification and drug therapy, often with more than one drug.

Moderate Risk

Patients at moderate risk for CAD are those with LDL cholesterol levels of 130 to 159 mg/dL, HDL cholesterol levels above 35 mg/dL but below 60 mg/dL, no clinical evidence of CAD, and fewer than two other CAD risk factors in addition to hyperlipidemia. Patients in this group require lifestyle modification and may require drug therapy but often with only one drug.

Low Risk

It should be noted that this group still has a risk, although the risk is low. Patients at low risk for CAD are those with LDL cholesterol below 130 mg/dL, HDL cholesterol levels above 60 mg/dL, total cholesterol-to-HDL ratio below 4.5, VLDL cholesterol levels 50 to 100 mg/dL or fasting triglycerides 250 to 500 mg/dL, no clinical evidence of CAD, and fewer than two CAD risk factors. Patients in this group require information about diet, physical activity, and risk factor reduction.

Treatment Algorithms

Lifestyle Modifications

Lifestyle modifications are the core of treatment for hyperlipidemia. Clinical trials have demonstrated that lowering serum cholesterol reduces new CAD events in patients with existing CAD and reduces CAD mortality in primary prevention for patients without CAD. Some analysis of drug trials, however, has raised the possibility of increases in non-CAD mortality resulting from drug therapy. Dietary therapy has not been found to be associated with increased non-CAD mortality. Therefore, evidence that cholesterol lowering will reduce CAD morbidity and mortality supports efforts to use dietary therapy in primary prevention and as first-line therapy in secondary prevention and to reserve drug therapy for high-risk patients in whom the benefits outweigh the risks of potential adverse reactions.

The general aim of dietary therapy is to lower cholesterol to target levels while still maintaining a nutritionally adequate eating pattern. Such therapy involves two steps.

The Step 1 diet emphasizes the choice of fruits, vegetables, grains, cereals, and legumes, as well as poultry, fish, lean meats, and low-fat dairy products. It involves an intake of saturated fat of 8 to 10 percent of total calories, no more than 30 percent of total calories from all fats, and less than 300 mg of cholesterol per day. Concerning acceptable fats, recent evidence suggests that monounsaturated fats, such as olive oil, canola oil, and high-oleic forms of sunflower seed and safflower oil, may cause almost as much of a decrease in LDL cholesterol levels as the polyunsaturated oils. The Step 1 diet does not require a dramatic alteration in the diet of most patients and is generally well tolerated. Total cholesterol and LDL cholesterol levels usually fall by 5 to 15 percent on this diet.

Patients without CAD on the Step 1 diet should have their total cholesterol level measured and their adherence to the diet assessed at 4 to 6 weeks and at 3 months. Although the goal is to lower LDL levels, this group of patients is at lower risk, and most can be managed during dietary therapy on the basis of total cholesterol levels, thus avoiding the additional cost and inconvenience of obtaining a fasting blood sample, required for LDL estimation. For low-risk patients, the dietary therapy should be given at least a 6-month trial. Further discussion related to monitoring patients on this regimen follows later.

If the cholesterol goal has not been achieved with the Step 1 diet, the patient is generally referred to a dietitian. With the aid of the dietitian, the patient progresses to Step 2. The Step 2 diet reduces intake of saturated fat to less than 7 percent of calories and reduces the intake of cholesterol to less than 200 mg per day. This diet requires careful attention to the whole diet to reduce intake of saturated fat and cholesterol to the specified levels and still maintain an acceptable and nutritious diet. Total cholesterol and dietary adherence are assessed at 4 to 6 weeks and at 3 months. If the desired goal is reached, long-term monitoring can begin. Only if total cholesterol remains substantially above the target goal should drug therapy be considered. A minimum of 6 months of intensive diet therapy and counseling should be done in primary prevention before drug therapy is initiated. Figures 37–2 and 37–3 delineate the algorithm for primary prevention in adults without evidence of CAD, including target goals for total cholesterol and HDL levels.

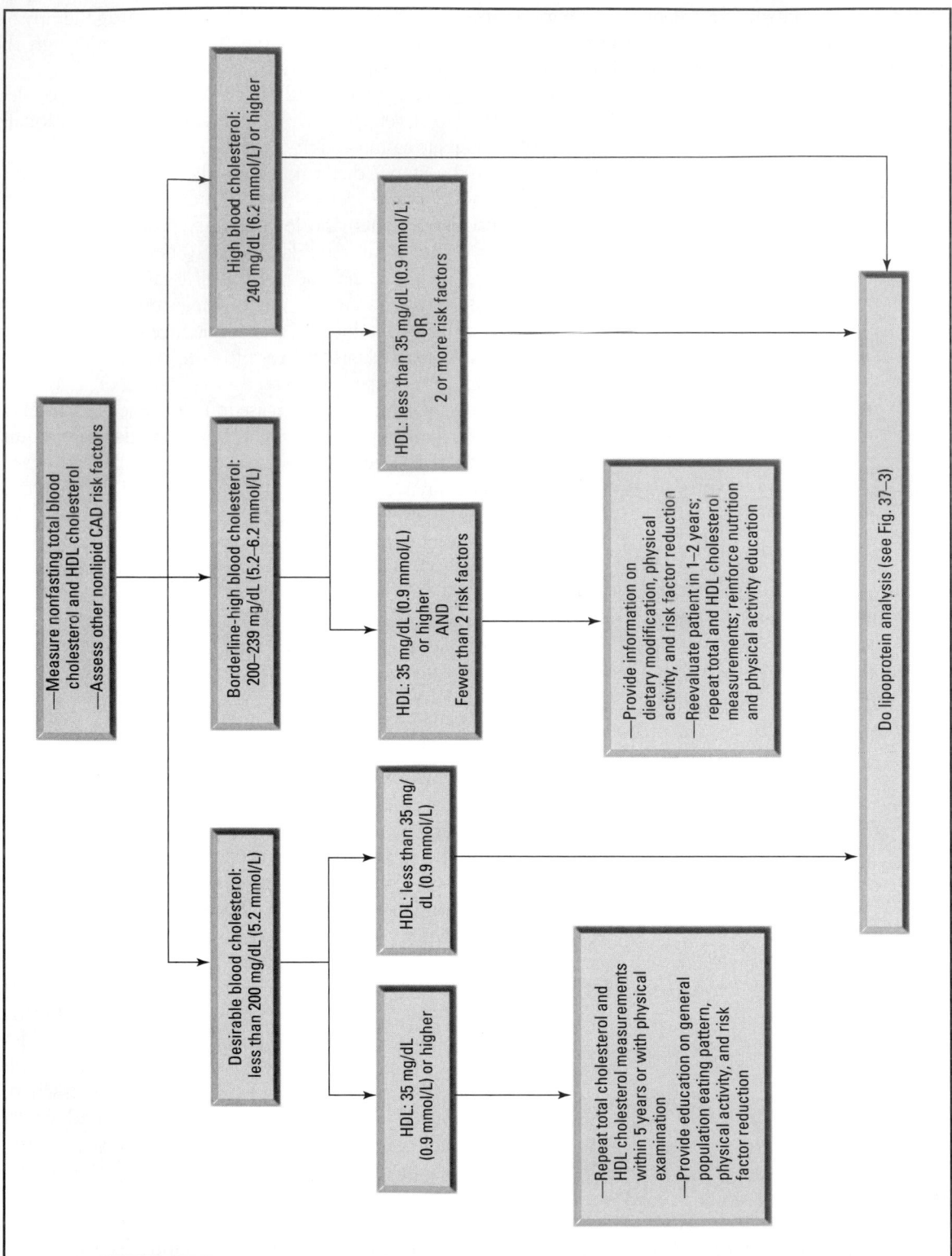

Figure 37–2. Primary prevention in adults without evidence of CAD. (From the National Cholesterol Education Program [1993]. *Second report of the Expert Panel on Detection, Evaluation, and Treatment of High Blood Cholesterol in Adults [adult treatment panel II].* [National Institutes of Health. National Heart, Lung and Blood Institute. NIH Publ. No. 93–3095]. Rockville, MD: NIH.)

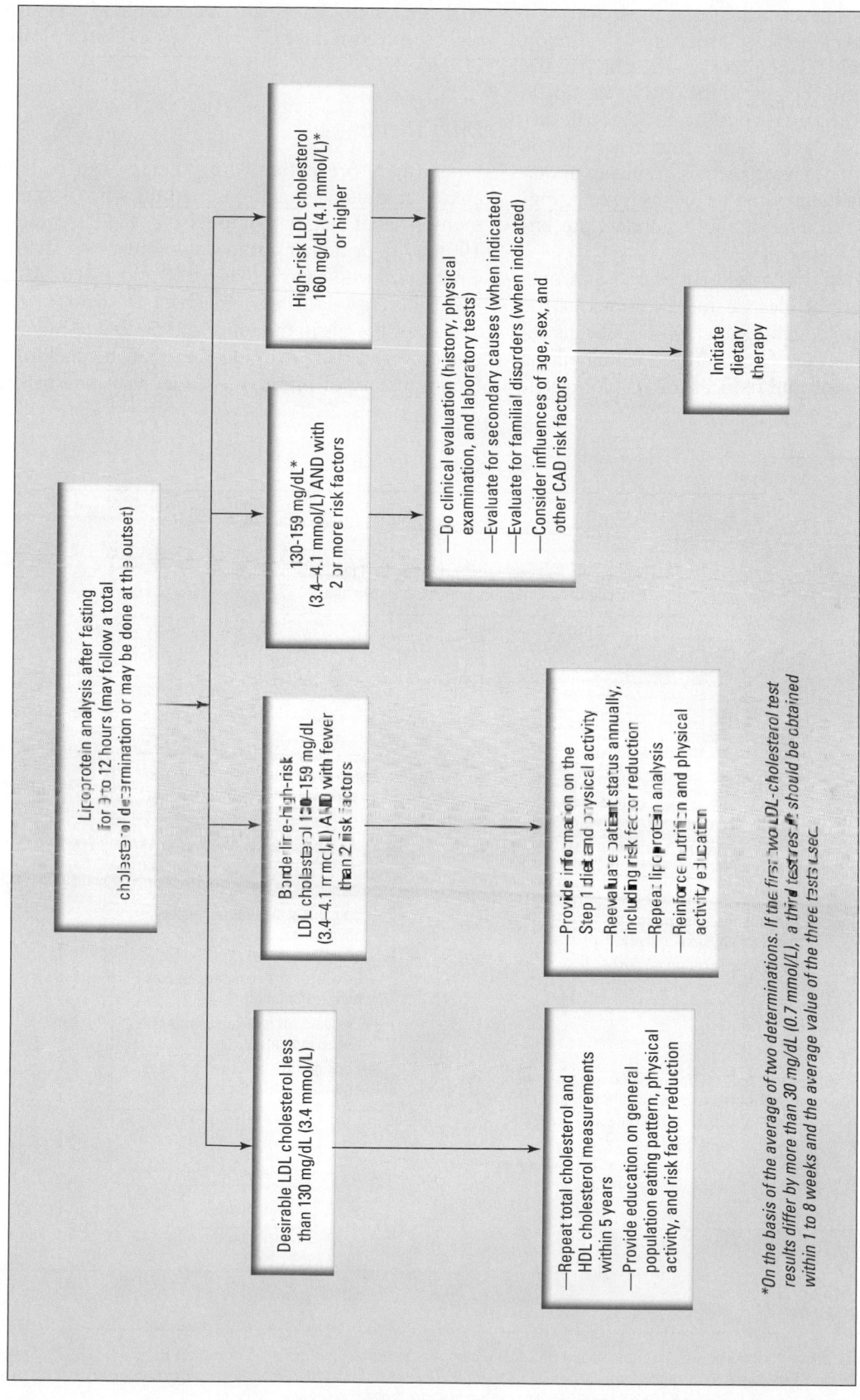

Figure 37-3. Primary prevention in adults without evidence of CAD based on lipoprotein analysis. (From the National Cholesterol Education Program [1993]. *Second report of the Expert Panel on Detection, Evaluation, and Treatment of High Blood Cholesterol in Adults [adult treatment panel II]*. [National Institutes of Health. National Heart, Lung and Blood Institute. NIH Publ. No. 93–3095]. Rockville, MD: NIH.)

Patients with established CAD or other atherosclerotic disease should begin immediately on the Step 2 diet. LDL cholesterol levels and dietary adherence are assessed at 4 to 6 weeks. If the goal of therapy for secondary prevention (LDL cholesterol level 100 mg/dL or less) is achieved, the patient remains on this therapy. If the goal of therapy is not achieved, drug therapy is considered. Although diet therapy is essential for these patients, their risk profile is higher, and the period for assessment of results from diet before initiating drug therapy can be relatively short. Figure 37–4 delineates the algorithm for secondary prevention in adults with evidence of CAD.

Weight reduction in overweight patients and aerobic exercise are also central lifestyle modifications in the treatment of hyperlipidemia (Table 37–3). Weight reduction enhances the LDL cholesterol-lowering effects of diet and drug therapy and reduces the risk for developing diabetes. Exercise promotes lowering of LDL cholesterol levels and also reduces triglyceride levels, raises HDL cholesterol levels, and reduces blood pressure. All of these effects reduce CAD risk beyond simply lowering LDL levels.

Drug Therapy

For primary prevention, drug therapy can be considered in middle-aged and older adults who, despite a 6-month trial of dietary therapy, have (1) LDL cholesterol 190 mg/dL or higher without two other risk factors for CAD or (2) who have between 160 and 190 mg/dL with two other risk factors. Some patients who have LDL cholesterol levels in the range of 160 to 220 mg/dL and one powerful risk factor, such as diabetes mellitus or a family history of premature CAD, also may be candi-

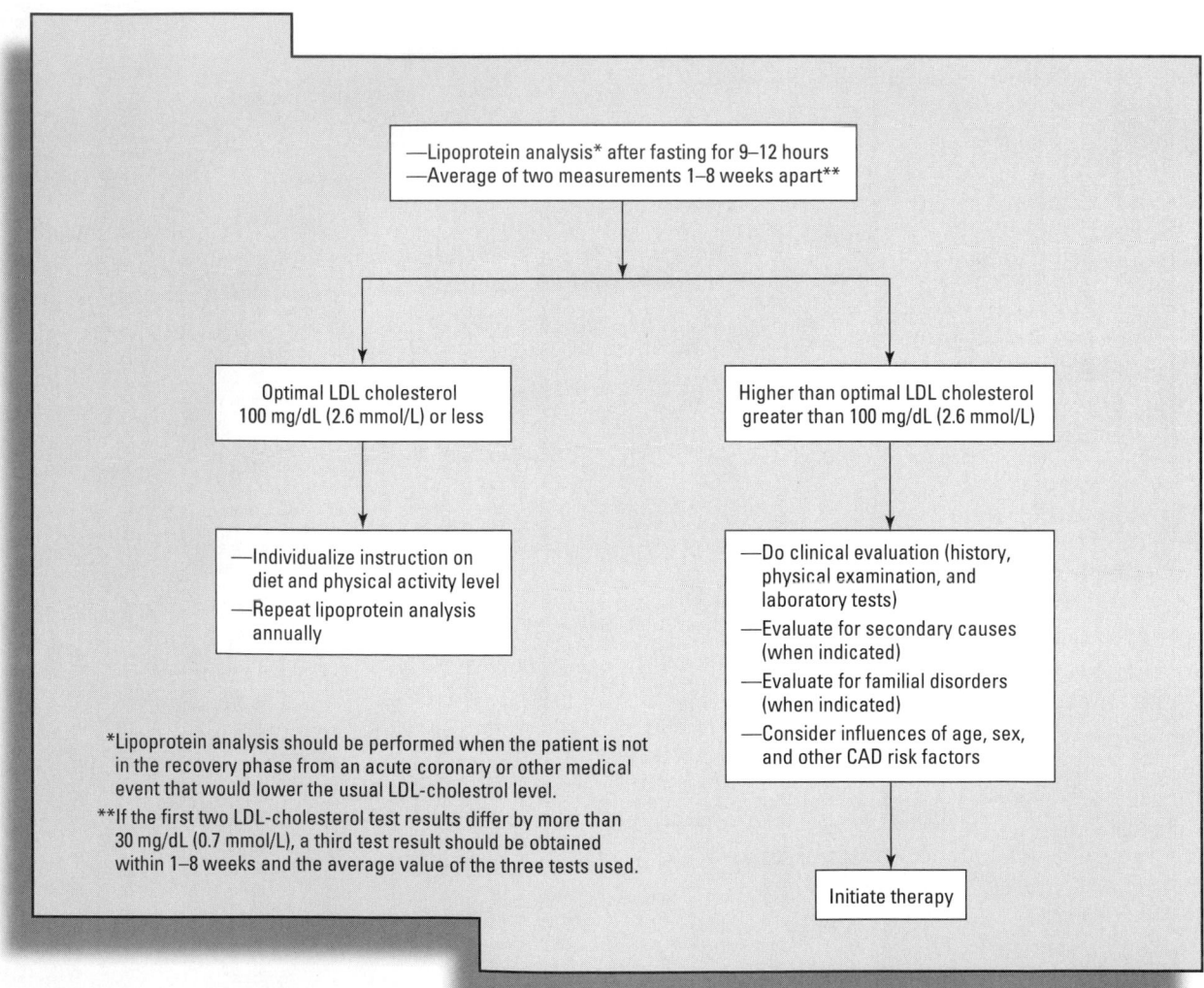

Figure 37–4. Secondary prevention in adults with evidence of CAD. (From the National Cholesterol Education Program [1993]. *Second report of the Expert Panel on Detection, Evaluation, and Treatment of High Blood Cholesterol in Adults [adult treatment panel II].* [National Institutes of Health. National Heart, Lung and Blood Institute. NIH Publ. No. 93–3095]. Rockville, MD: NIH.)

Table 37-3. Lifestyle Modifications

Reduce Intake of Saturated Fats
- Saturated fat intake should be 8–10% of total calorie intake; 7% for Step 2 diets. Monounsaturated fats are the best choice for fat intake.

- Total fat intake should be 30% or less of total calorie intake.

- Visible fat (cream, butter, margarine, salad dressing) is restricted to 1 tsp/meal.

- Foods high in fat content (nonlean meat, olives, nuts) are avoided.

- Cooking methods are steaming, baking, broiling, grilling, or stir-frying with small amounts of fat.

Reduce Cholesterol Intake
- Total cholesterol intake should be less than 300 mg per day; 200 mg per day for Step 2 diet.

- No more than 3 egg yolks per week; 1 egg yolk for Step 2 diets. Egg whites or egg substitutes may be used as desired.

- Organ meats and shrimp are restricted because they are high in cholesterol although low in fat.

- Red meat and milk products are major sources of fat and cholesterol. Severely limit red meat. Skim milk is highly recommended.

Eat a Well-Balanced Diet
- A diet rich in fruits and vegetables, high in fiber, and moderate in protein is recommended.

Lose Weight
- As little as 10 lb of weight loss can significantly affect CAD risk.

Limit Alcohol Intake
- Especially if triglycerides are high, alcohol intake should be limited to no more than 1 oz (30 mL) of ethanol (e.g., 24 oz beer, 10 oz wine, 2 oz 100-proof whiskey) per day or 1/2 oz (15 mL) ethanol per day for women and lighter-weight people.

Increase Aerobic Activity
- 30–45 min most days of the week is recommended. Obese and low-activity patients may need to start with as little as 3 min of activity per day and increase by 1 min each day until the desired 30–45 min is achieved.

Stop Smoking

---

dates for drug therapy. The goals of therapy are the same as those for diet therapy: LDL cholesterol levels below 160 mg/dL for those without risk factors and below 130 mg/dL for those with risk factors. These are minimal goals, and lower levels are more desirable. Exceptions are made for young adult men (under age 35) and premenopausal women. Their treatment is discussed later in this chapter.

Clinical judgment beyond the usual algorithm is required for patients who do not meet the criteria for drug therapy but have not achieved the treatment targets on lifestyle modifications alone. Examples include those without two risk factors whose LDL remains in the range of 160 to 190 mg/dL, young adults in the range of 190 to 220 mg/dL, and those with two risk factors with LDL levels in the range of 130 to 160 mg/dL. In general, maximal efforts should be made to achieve lower cholesterol levels by nonpharmacological means first, and then low doses of **bile acid–binding resins** may be used for these patients, especially for men.

The use of drugs as primary prevention for men and women with average cholesterol levels (patients who do not meet NCEP criteria for elevated lipid levels) is controversial. The NCEP document states that this practice has not yet been demonstrated to affect mortality and morbidity outcomes from cardiovascular disease. A study published in the May 1998 *Journal of the American Medical Association* (Downs et al., 1998), however, reports reduced risk for first acute major coronary events in men and women with average total cholesterol and LDL levels and below-average HDL levels. These findings support the inclusion of the HDL levels in risk-factor assessment that is part of the current NCEP guidelines but also suggest the need for reassessment of the guidelines regarding pharmacological intervention for this group of patients.

Although the AFCAPS/TexCAPS study (Downs et al., 1998) used **lovastatin**, a **reductase inhibitor**, if the goal is to increase HDL levels as well as lower LDL levels, **nicotinic acid** would seem to be another excellent choice for this purpose. Studies need to test this drug and determine its effectiveness, especially in light of the introduction of a slow-release form that is effective without significant adverse reactions.

For secondary prevention, drug therapy generally is indicated for patients with established CAD or other atherosclerotic disease if the LDL cholesterol level is above 130 mg/dL. If the level is in the range of 100 to 129 mg/dL, clinical judgment must weigh the potential benefit, the risk of adverse reactions to the drugs, and the cost of the drugs to make a clinical decision on drug therapy. The goal of this therapy is an LDL level no higher than 100 mg/dL. If the goal of therapy is not attained after 3 months with a single drug, consideration should be given to adding a second drug. Combination therapy should be undertaken only after counseling the patient about potential benefits and risks. Such therapy is costlier, requires regular supervision by the health care provider, and exposes the patient to a greater array of potential adverse reactions. Some of the drawbacks of combination therapy may be avoided by using low doses of each drug.

The choice of which drug to use is based largely on the elevated lipoprotein involved (Table 37–4). Detailed discussion of each drug class is provided in Chapter 14. In general:

1. **Nicotinic acid (niacin)** is effective in lowering total cholesterol and triglyceride levels and raising HDL levels. There is evidence that it reduces total mortality in secondary prevention trials. It has several adverse reactions, however, that are difficult to overcome and increase the likelihood of nonadherence. To keep the dose low enough to reduce these adverse reactions and still effectively control VLDL and LDL levels, **nicotinic acid** may be combined with a **bile acid–binding resin.** Slow-release nicotinic acid (Niaspan) has been studied as another way to reduce adverse effects. Based on these studies, a 2-g/day dose proved advantageous in reducing lipid levels without causing any significant adverse reactions. **Nicotinic acid** is best for treating patients who have elevated total cholesterol and triglycerides, low HDL levels, or both. Because **nicotinic acid** is a vitamin and sold over the counter (OTC), the Food and Drug Administration (FDA) issued a statement on the OTC use of any cholesterol-lowering drugs, including **nicotinic acid.** The FDA concluded that the nature of hypercholesterolemia and its potential sequelae are such that OTC use of these

Table 37–4. Commonly Used: Hyperlipidemia

Drug	Initial Dose	Target Dose	Maximum Dose	Special Notes
Bile acid–binding resins Cholestyramine (Questran)	16 g/day	10–16 g/day	24 g/day	Cost: $91.20
Colestipol (Colestid)	20 g/day	10–20 g/day	24 g/day	Cost: $79.31
Fibric acid derivatives Fenofibrate (Tricor)	67 mg/day	67–134 mg/day	201 mg/day	
Gemfibrozil (Lopid)	1200 mg/day	1200–2400 mg/day	2400 mg/day	Cost: $60.20
HMG-CoA reductase inhibitors Atorvastatin (Lipitor)	10 mg/day	5–40 mg/day	80 mg/day	
Fluvastatin (Lescol)	20 mg/day	40 mg/day	40 mg/day	
Lovastatin (Mevacor)	20 mg/day	10–40 mg/day	80 mg/day	Cost: $59.90
Pravastatin (Pravachol)	20 mg/day	20 mg/day	40 mg/day	Cost: $53.99
Simvastatin (Zocor)	10 mg/day	20 mg/day	40 mg/day	Cost: $54.02
Nicotinic acid (niacin) Generic	1 g tid	1.5–3.5 g/day	8 g/day	Cost: $6.44
Nicotinic Acid (regular release) (Niacor, Nicolar)	1 g tid	1.5–3.5 g/day	8 g/day	Cost: $23.04 (Niacor); $88.13 (Nicolar)
Nicotinic acid (slow- or extended-release) (Niaspan)	375 mg/day	500–750 mg/day	1 g/day	

* Cost in 1998 dollars to the pharmacist for 30 days of treatment based on average wholesale price listings and usual dose.

drugs is not a safe and effective means for treating this condition.

2. **Bile acid–binding resins** have a strong record of efficacy and safety. They are most useful for patients with moderately elevated LDL levels, those with a low CAD risk profile who are unable to reduce their LDL by diet alone, and young adult men and premenopausal women. Low doses can be effective for patients whose LDL cholesterol is close to their target goal and who just need a little extra help. They are also useful, together with **fibric acid derivatives,** to treat patients with familial combined hyperlipidemia who are intolerant to niacin. Their main drawback is their GI adverse reaction profile. They are contraindicated for patients with high triglyceride levels.

3. **HMG-CoA reductase inhibitors** are highly effective at lowering LDL. A modest decrease in triglycerides and increase in HDL may also occur. Recent long-term studies have shown them to be safe and to reduce risk for CAD when used alone or in combination. They are especially useful for severe forms of hypercholesterolemia and for maximal lowering of LDL levels in secondary prevention. For high-risk CAD patients, this class of drugs should be tried first. If patient response is not adequate after 4 months, the patients should be switched to a different drug or given a trial on a combination of drugs. Combinations of **reductase inhibitors** with low-dose **niacin** have shown promise for the highest-risk patients and are the most efficacious and practical combination for treatment of familial combined hyperlipidemia. For treating this disorder, **reductase inhibitors** also have a highly synergistic action with **bile acid–binding resins.** To assure absorption, the **reductase inhibitor** should be given at least 1 hour before or 4 hours after the **bile acid–binding resin.**

4. **Fibric acid derivatives** are effective triglyceride-lowering drugs that may modestly lower LDL and raise HDL for some patients. Elevated triglycerides are not an independent risk factor for CAD and because these drugs usually do not produce substantial reductions in LDL cholesterol, they are not appropriate for maximal lowering of LDL levels in secondary prevention. They are valuable for patients with very high triglyceride levels, for diabetic patients with elevated triglycerides, and for patients with familial dysbetalipoproteinemia.

5. Drug combinations are commonly used for patients with more than one lipoprotein abnormality. For elevated LDL and triglycerides below 200 mg/dL, the main goal is to lower LDL levels because hypertriglyceridemia does not carry the same risk for CAD as elevated LDL cholesterol levels. Combinations of **reductase inhibitors** with low-dose **nico-**tinic acid are used for high-risk patients; **bile acid–binding resins** combined with low-dose **nicotinic acid** are best for younger adults and patients without high CAD risk. If the triglyceride level is 200 to 400 mg/dL, **nicotinic acid** may be combined with **fibric acid derivatives.**

Additional Patient Variables

Children and Adolescents

Atherosclerosis can begin in childhood, and fatty streaks have been seen in children as young as 10 years old. Up to 25 percent of children and adolescents have cholesterol levels above 200 mg/dL. Genetic disorders of lipid metabolism occur in 0.5 to 1 percent of the population. These children often have total cholesterol levels 1.5 to 3 times higher than normal. Approximately 80 percent of these children will experience symptomatic CAD prior to age 20. The remaining percentage of elevated cholesterol is related to the same environmental factors that result in adult hyperlipidemia. These children are assessed for the same CAD risk factors as adults.

Acceptable cholesterol levels in children are slightly lower than in adults. Total cholesterol should be below 170 mg/dL (LDL below 110 mg/dL). Borderline cholesterol levels are 170 to 199 mg/dL, and high cholesterol levels are 200 mg/dL or above. Figure 37–5 shows the treatment algorithm for children.

As with adults, the goal is primary prevention. Lifestyle modifications include aerobic exercise; weight control; and a diet that includes breastfeeding, late introduction of solid foods, control of salt intake, and reduced saturated fat and cholesterol intake. Reduction in other risk factors, such as smoking and excess weight, and appropriate management of hypertension and diabetes are essential. These changes should always be tried first, with at least a 6-month trial before drugs are considered.

When drug therapy is considered, the child should be referred to a pediatrician with experience in lipid disorders. Among the available **antihyperlipidemics, nicotinic acid** is the only one with established safety in children under age 18. Use of **HMG-CoA reductase inhibitors** is restricted to children with heterozygous or homozygous familial hyperlipidemia with some residual receptor activity. Adolescent females are considered of childbearing age and should follow the guidelines for women of childbearing age given later in this chapter.

Young Adult Men

Young adult men (age less than 35) experience increased risk of developing CAD related to elevated cholesterol levels, but those with moderately high LDL cholesterol (160 to 220 mg/dL) are at relatively low risk for

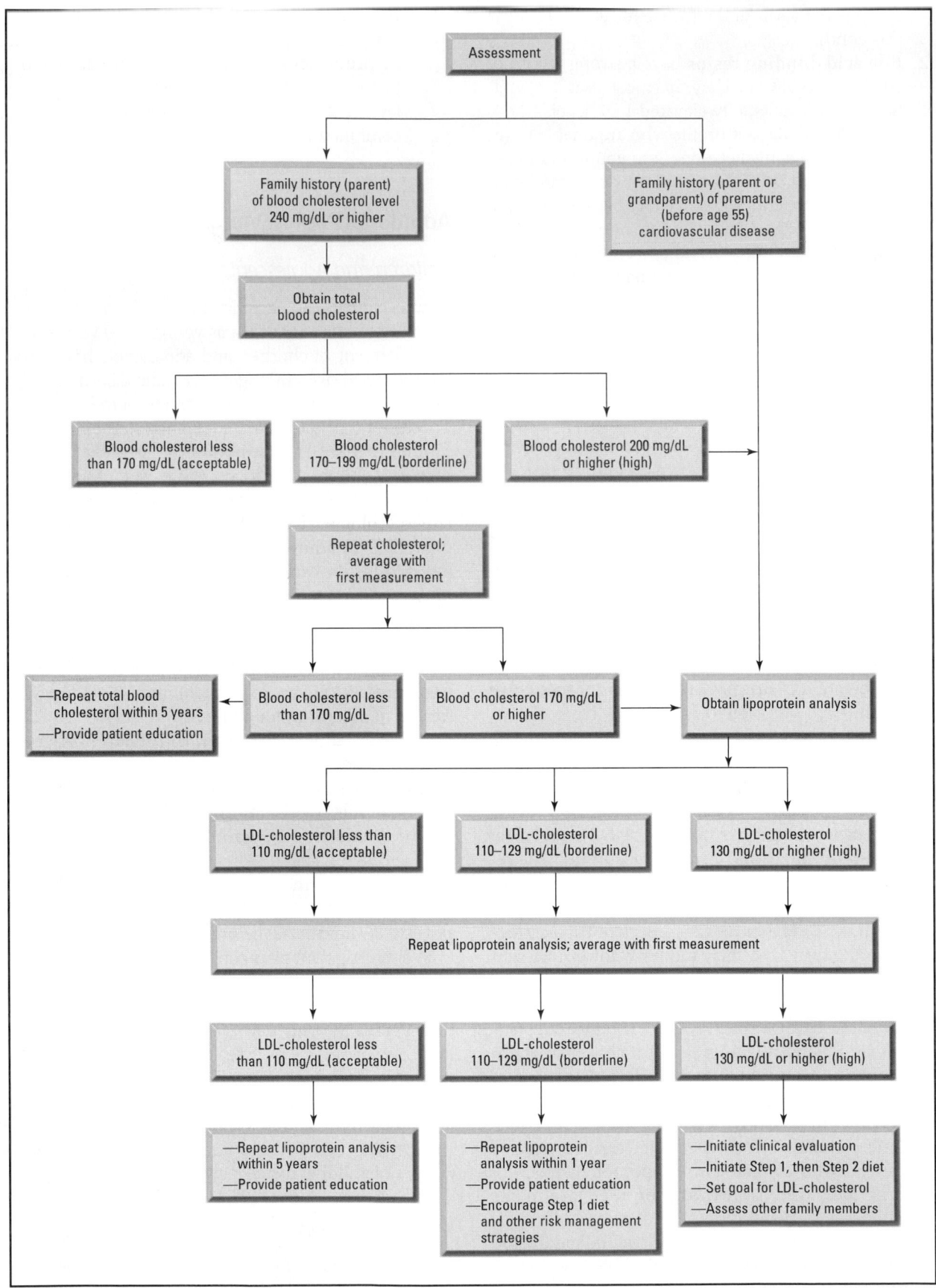

Figure 37–5. Management of blood cholesterol in children.

developing CAD in the near future unless they have additional risk factors. They are generally classified as low risk, and the focus of cholesterol-lowering therapy should be diet and exercise. For those without other risk factors, drug therapy should be delayed when LDL levels are in the range of 190 to 220 mg/dL. In general, drug therapy is considered only when LDL levels reach 220 mg/dL or multiple other risk factors are present. When drugs are chosen, **bile acid–binding resins** in low doses are first line, followed by **HMG-CoA reductase inhibitors.**

Older Adults

Despite the fact that the relative risk of CAD related to elevated cholesterol is weaker in older adults than in young and middle-aged adults, a high cholesterol level leads to more CAD events in older people. Lowering CAD risk by reducing total cholesterol, and specifically LDL levels, is critical in this population. Angiographic studies have shown that even advanced coronary atherosclerosis may respond to reductions in cholesterol. Some older adults, however, are not candidates for aggressive cholesterol lowering. They include those with severe concurrent illnesses such as congestive heart failure, dementia, advanced cerebrovascular disease, or active malignancy. Older adults who are otherwise healthy should have cholesterol-lowering therapy.

How aggressive the therapy is depends, as it does in younger patients, on the degree of CAD risk. The same algorithm based on CAD risk can be used. The Second Report of the NCEP, (NCEP 1993) added age as an independent risk variable for CAD so that older adults are more likely to exhibit two risk factors than are younger patients, which may alter their placement on treatment algorithms. In addition, older adults are less likely to achieve the LDL goal with diet therapy alone and are more likely to require some drug therapy. **HMG-CoA reductase inhibitors** are the first-line drugs in this age group. They are well tolerated, with only minor diarrhea and occasional sleep pattern disturbance the most common problems. Most can be taken once daily so they do not add much complexity to an existing treatment regimen. **Niacin** is also effective, but its adverse reactions are not well tolerated. It may also trigger hypotension that can be dangerous, especially in older patients, who may also be on other drugs that can produce orthostatic changes. **Bile acid–binding resins** have risks for impaction and constipation and so are not a good choice for older people.

Women

Elevated cholesterol levels confer CAD risk on women as well as men, but the correlation is lower before age 55. Until that age, women are at lower risk for CAD than their male counterparts, in part because of their higher estrogen levels. After age 55, the most common cause of death in both men and women is cardiovascular disease.

Premenopausal women are in the lowest risk group, but risk increases progressively after menopause. For premenopausal women, diet, exercise, and weight loss for overweight patients are the treatment of choice. If patients are without other CAD risk factors, drug therapy should be delayed when LDL levels are in range of 190 to 220 mg/dL. Drug therapy is considered only when LDL levels are at least 220 mg/dL or multiple other risk factors are present. For postmenopausal women, **estrogen** replacement therapy has been significantly correlated with reduced CAD morbidity and mortality and may obviate the need for therapy beyond lifestyle modification. If postmenopausal women have very high LDL levels or multiple other risk factors, they should be treated with the drugs discussed in the section on older adults.

Nicotinic acid and *fibric acid derivatives* are **Pregnancy Category C. Risks and benefits should be carefully weighed before giving these drugs to pregnant women. All** *HMG-CoA reductase inhibitors* are **Pregnancy Category X and should not be given to women who have the potential to become pregnant. No pregnancy category has been assigned to the** *bile acid–binding resins.* **Women of childbearing age with elevated cholesterol levels are best managed with lifestyle modifications. If drug therapy is required and they are not on a well-established birth control program, they may be placed on** *bile acid–binding resins.* **If this is not effective, they should probably be referred to a lipid specialist. All** *antilipidemics* **should be avoided during breastfeeding.**

Concomitant Disease States

Drugs used to treat hyperlipidemia may improve the management of some diseases and worsen others. It is not within the scope of this book to discuss all possible diseases that may coexist with hyperlipidemia, but the most common diseases that benefit from appropriate selection of a drug to treat the hyperlipidemia are discussed here.

DIABETES MELLITUS. Diabetes mellitus, particularly type 2 (non-insulin-dependent diabetes mellitus [NIDDM]), can cause a high-VLDL, low-HDL lipid abnormality. This is seen clinically as high triglyceride levels (200 to 400 mg/dL) and low HDL levels (less than 35 mg/dL). The therapy combination that works best is **gemfibrozil (a fibric acid derivative)**, Step 1 or 2 diet therapy, **glucophage (Metformin)**, and weight loss. **Nicotinic acid** also effectively lowers triglycerides and may be substituted for the **gemfibrozil.**

HYPOTHYROIDISM. Hypothyroidism often presents with hypercholesterolemia. This is seen clinically as elevated cholesterol, high LDL, and mild VLDL elevation.

Every patient with elevated cholesterol should be screened for hypothyroidism because the best treatment for the lipid disorder is to treat the primary problem: hypothyroidism.

HYPERTENSION. Hypertension and hyperlipidemia commonly occur together. Patients with concomitant hypertension and hypercholesterolemia should have both treated aggressively because CAD risk is synergistically increased. Lifestyle modifications are the first approach to treatment of both. When drug therapy is chosen, drug effects on both disorders are considered. **Nicotinic acid** can cause orthostatic hypotension and should be used with caution for patients who are being treated with **antihypertensives** that have this same adverse reaction potential. None of the other classes of drugs used to treat hyperlipidemia has direct effects on blood pressure. Drugs used to treat hypertension sometimes have effects on cholesterol levels. This interaction is discussed in detail in Chapter 38. For example, **thiazide diuretics** and **beta-adrenergic blockers**, considered first-line therapy in treating hypertension, can cause short-term increases in cholesterol levels. Efficacy, safety, cost, and prevention of myocardial infarction (MI), however, mean that they still may be safely used. Drugs that affect lipid levels should not be avoided if their use means less than optimal blood pressure control. If an **antihypertensive** induces a rise in serum cholesterol that moves a patient into a group where lipid-lowering drug therapy becomes necessary, and a different **antihypertensive** proves equally efficacious in treating the hypertension but has less effect on lipid levels, substitution of the latter **antihypertensive** probably would be appropriate.

Cost

In today's health care environment, cost effectiveness of therapy is always an issue. The aggregate cost of CAD in the United States is a staggering $50 to $100 billion per year for medication, treatment, and lost wages. Prevention of CAD could greatly reduce this economic burden, and the management of cholesterol levels is one way to prevent CAD. Patients in high-risk categories for CAD related to elevated cholesterol levels have the greatest likelihood of significant benefit from cholesterol reduction. For example, in men age 35 to 64 and women age 35 to 54 with established CAD, intervention with standard doses of **HMG-CoA reductase inhibitors** has been estimated to save significant amounts of money otherwise spent on CAD events in untreated patients. In older men and women, the cost-benefit ratios are even better. From a public health standpoint, therefore, the cost of cholesterol treatment is clearly justified for this group of patients. Patients at lower risk have a less favorable cost-benefit ratio, but it is still relatively acceptable. For this group, the ratio depends to some extent on the drug chosen. On an individual basis, even low-risk patients may have justification for cholesterol reduction therapy.

Obviously, dietary management and reduction of major risk factors, such as smoking and limited physical activity, have the best cost-benefit ratio and are justified from the standpoint of both public health and the individual patient. When drug therapy is chosen, the cost includes laboratory assessment and monitoring as well as the price of individual drugs. The largest component of expense, however, is the cholesterol-lowering drug itself. Drug cost can be a significant issue, especially for older adults who are on fixed incomes. Table 37–4 shows the monthly cost of selected drugs used to treat hyperlipidemia. **Nicotinic acid** in its generic form is clearly the least expensive, and even the slow-release form is less expensive than other **antilipidemic drugs.** The most commonly used drugs, the **HMG-CoA reductase inhibitors,** are midrange in cost. Chapter 14 has a detailed discussion of the cost of all of the **antilipidemics.**

Monitoring

Monitoring for effectiveness of dietary therapy is discussed in that section. Drug therapy is not usually initiated until a 6-month trial of dietary therapy has been completed. Determination of the drug to treat the lipid disorder is based on a minimum of two lipoprotein determinations during maximum dietary therapy. This provides a baseline for future determination of drug efficacy.

With good drug adherence, maximum lowering of the LDL cholesterol is achieved within 4 to 6 weeks of initiating therapy. The first follow-up of LDL cholesterol levels should be made 6 to 8 weeks after initiating therapy. **Nicotinic acid** is the exception to this rule, with repeat measurements made when the dose has been stable for 4 to 6 weeks. A second measurement of LDL cholesterol levels is done 6 weeks after the first measurement. A minimum of two measurements is essential for evaluating the efficacy of the drug. After the target LDL cholesterol level is reached, patients should be followed at 8- to 12-week intervals for 1 year. After 1 year of therapy, during which the response has been established and there is no evidence of toxicity, patients should be followed at 4- to 6-month intervals. Additional laboratory studies specific to each drug class beyond the lipoprotein determinations are discussed in Chapter 14.

Outcome Evaluation

Discontinuation of treatment is quickly followed by a return of the cholesterol to pretreatment levels. Long-term

Hyperlipidemia

Related to the Overall Treatment Plan and Disease Process

☐ Pathophysiology of lipid disorders and their long-term effects on cardiovascular morbidity and mortality

☐ Role of lifestyle modification, especially dietary therapy, in improving outcomes and keeping the number and cost of required drugs down

☐ Importance of adherence to the treatment regimen

☐ Need for regular follow-up visits with the primary care provider

Specific to the Drug Therapy

☐ Reason for the drug(s) being given and the anticipated action of the drug(s) on the disease process

☐ Doses and schedules for taking the drug(s)

☐ Possible adverse reactions, how to prevent them, and what to do if they occur

☐ Interaction between lifestyle modifications and the drug(s)

Reasons for Taking the Drug(s)

Patient education about specific drugs is provided in Chapter 14. More specific information related to hyperlipidemia includes the reasons for drug(s) being taken: Antilipidemics are given to reduce morbidity and mortality from the leading cause of death in the United States—cardiovascular disease. Discuss the risk of cardiovascular disease with the patient while maintaining the potential for good quality of life with adequate treatment.

Drugs as Part of the Total Treatment Regimen

The expectations should be clear about what the drugs can and cannot do. Drugs are supplements to dietary and other lifestyle modifications, not substitutes for them. Lipid disorders are chronic conditions. Lifestyle modifications and drug regimens need to be incorporated into patients' everyday lives. Discontinuation of treatment will result in return of lipids to pretreatment levels.

Adherence Issues

Nonadherence to the treatment regimen may increase patients' risk for cardiovascular morbidity and reduce their life expectancy. Health care providers should be aware of potential problems with nonadherence, discuss the importance of adherence at each follow-up visit, and assist patients in removing barriers to adherence, such as lack of social support and cost of the treatment regimen. Utilization of other health team members, especially the dietitian, should be maximized. Patient education booklets available from the American Heart Association and the National Cholesterol Education Program may supplement dietary instruction.

Hyperlipidemia: Anne

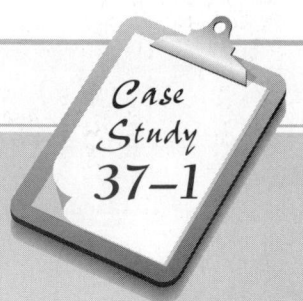

Case Study 37–1

Complaint

Annual physical examination.

History

Anne is a 57-year-old white woman with a family history of elevated cholesterol levels and coronary artery disease. Her father had an MI at age 52, and her mother required bypass surgery for coronary artery occlusion at age 71. Her mother's total cholesterol level was greater than 300 mg/dL before she was placed on therapy after her bypass, and her mother's blood pressure requires treatment with diuretics to maintain an acceptable level. Anne has no personal history or family history of diabetes. She is 67 inches tall and weighs 188 lb. She underwent surgical menopause at age 40 and is currently on estrogen replacement therapy. Assessment of her dietary patterns indicates an unacceptably high intake of saturated fat and cholesterol.

Assessment

Anne's physical examination is essentially normal, with no abnormal heart sounds and a blood pressure of 130/70 mm Hg. Her annual labs, including a thyroid screen and ECG, are also normal. Her lipid profile is total cholesterol 253, triglycerides 129, LDL cholesterol 160, HDL cholesterol 60, and cholesterol:HDL ratio 4.2. She has the following positive CAD risk factors: male first-degree relative with MI before age 55, an elevated cholesterol level, and a borderline high LDL level. Negative risk factors include being female over age 55 but on estrogen replacement therapy, nonsmoking, no hypertension, no diabetes, and an HDL level 60 mg/dL or higher.

Initial Management Plan

Based on her assessment data, Anne is diagnosed with mild hyperlipidemia without CAD risk factors. (The negative risk factors replace the positive risk factors.) Her management plan is as follows:

1. Begin dietary therapy at Step 1. This diet is generally tolerated well by most patients, and her lipoprotein elevations are not severe. According to the NCEP guidelines, diet modification is first-line therapy for patients without CAD and with fewer than two risk factors. The goal is to reduce her LDL level to 130 mg/dL or less. Pamphlets from the American Heart Association on the Step 1 diet were given and discussed.

2. Discuss physical exercise and weight loss. Anne's exercise is limited to the walking associated with her work as a staff nurse. She recently bought a treadmill with the goal of beginning to exercise. The goal is to start walking on the treadmill for 5 minutes each day for 1 week and then increase by 1 minute each day until she reaches 30 minutes a day. Patients who are essentially sedentary need to start low and go slow with exercise, or they will have sore muscles, become quickly discouraged, and quit exercising. This goal gives her a chance to be successful. Weight loss goals are 1 lb per week, with a terminal goal of a weight of 140 lb. Adherence to a Step 1 diet usually results in this pace of weight loss.

3. Return to the clinic in 4 weeks to assess progress and draw new lipid levels.

Follow-up Visit

Anne was able to follow her treatment plan and showed improvement in her lipid levels at each follow-up visit during the next year. One year later, her weight was 146 lb, and her lipid levels were total cholesterol 204, triglycerides 120, LDL cholesterol 120, HDL cholesterol 68, and cholesterol:HDL ratio 3.0.

Modifications to Management Plan and Continuing Care

Anne will be followed with her annual physical examination and will have her total cholesterol and HDL cholesterol levels measured at the time of this exam.

---

cholesterol control means lifelong adherence to the treatment regimen. Achieving long-term clinical control of high blood cholesterol requires the same interest and attention from the patient and the primary care provider as was given to the initial evaluation and treatment decisions. Effective use of follow-up visits and skillful employment of adherence-enhancing techniques are required, including nurturing the patient-provider relationship. The primary care provider can manage hyperlipidemia in most patients. Severe forms of hypercholesterolemia are often the result of a genetic disorder of lipoprotein metabolism. Consultation with a lipid specialist is needed only for patients with these severe, complex forms of lipid disorders or patients who do not respond to standard therapy.

Patient Education

Patient education should include a discussion of information related to the overall treatment plan as well as

Hyperlipidemia: Anne's Mother

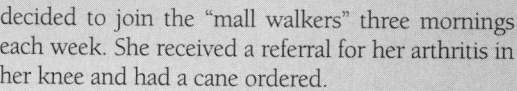

Case Study 37–2

History and Assessment

Anne's mother was a different story. At age 71, she experienced an MI and had subsequent bypass surgery. Her total cholesterol level at that time was 300 mg/dL, her LDL level was greater than 160, and her HDL was less than 35 mg/dL. She was postmenopausal but not on estrogen replacement because of a history of breast cancer. Her blood pressure was 160/94 mm Hg. She was 63 inches tall and weighed 250 lb. She was married and had a strong social support system of friends and family.

Initial Management Plan

Anne's mother's management plan at that time was as follows:

1. Begin diet therapy at Step 2. Patients with CAD and severely elevated lipoprotein levels begin immediately with Step 2. Because this change in diet required significant modifications, she was referred to a dietitian. Her MI had been quite serious, and she was very motivated to engage in diet therapy, but it was initially very difficult because both she and her husband had a history of a diet quite high in saturated fat and cholesterol. Family support, especially from her daughter, was central to her success.

2. Discuss exercise and weight loss. She had "struggled" with her weight most of her life and was not optimistic about any chance of losing weight. Weight loss is also difficult in older adults because of slower metabolism rates. A limited goal was set to lose half a pound per week. She was essentially sedentary because of arthritis in her right knee but was totally independent in her activities of daily living. She decided to purchase an exercise bike and try riding it for short periods each day. In addition, both she and her husband decided to join the "mall walkers" three mornings each week. She received a referral for her arthritis in her knee and had a cane ordered.

3. In addition to medications for her hypertension (a loop diuretic and potassium) and for her heart (digoxin), begin therapy with a lipid-lowering drug. The drug chosen was lovastatin (Mevacor). HMG-CoA reductase inhibitors are generally well tolerated by older adults, and once-daily dosing added little to her complex drug treatment regimen.

Follow-up Visit and Continuing Care

Anne's mother was followed up in 4 weeks and is much improved. In addition to the drugs just listed, she is also on an ACE inhibitor. Much to her surprise, she has lost 49 lb, has been able to incorporate the Step 2 diet into her life with only occasional "slips," and can work for about 2 hours in her garden daily. She has been unusually adherent to her drug regimen and has each drug carefully scheduled throughout the day. Her blood pressure is now 130/70, and there is discussion about reducing her diuretic to a low-dose thiazide that will not require potassium supplementation. Her total cholesterol level is now 186 mg/dL, with an LDL of 100 mg/dL. Her HDL is now above 35 mg/dL. Last week, she, Anne, and the rest of the family celebrated her 75th birthday.

that specific to the drug therapy, reasons for the drug being taken, drugs as part of the total treatment regimen, and adherence issues.

REFERENCES

Andrews, T., Raby, K., Barry, J., Naimi, C., Allred, E., Ganz, P., & Selwyn, A. (1997). Effect of cholesterol reduction on myocardial ischemia in patients with coronary disease. *Circulation, 95*(2), 324–328.

Ballantyne, C. (1998). Low-density lipoproteins and risk for coronary artery disease. *American Journal of Cardiology, 82*(9A), 3Q–12Q.

Blankenhorn, D. (1991). Angiographic trials testing the efficacy of cholesterol lowering in reducing progression or inducing regression of coronary atherosclerosis. *Coronary Artery Disease, 1*(2), 875–879.

Burns, C., Barber, N., Brady, M., & Dunn, A. (1996). *Pediatric primary care: A handbook for nurse practitioners*. Philadelphia: Saunders.

Choinowska-Jezierska, J., & Adamska-Dyniewska, H. (1998). Efficacy and safety of one-year treatment with slow-release nicotinic acid. Monitoring of drug concentration in serum. *International Journal of Clinical Pharmacology and Therapeutics, 36*(6), 326–332.

Davidson, M. (1998). What kind of data should be available to probe the effects of nutrients, food supplements or vitamins on serum lipoprotein levels and/or atherosclerosis? *The American Journal of Cardiology, 81*(8), 80F–83F.

Downs, J., Clearfield, M., Weis, S., Whitney, E., Shapiro, D., Beere, P., Langendorfer, A., Stein, E., Kruyer, W., & Gotto, A. (1998). Primary prevention of acute coronary events with lovastatin in men and women with average cholesterol levels. *Journal of the American Medical Association, 279*(20), 1615–1622.

Frye, R. (1997). Clinical reality of lowering total and LDL cholesterol. *Circulation, 95*(2), 306–307.

Goroll, A., May, L., & Mulley, A. (1995). *Primary care medicine* (3rd ed.). Philadelphia: Lippincott.

Gotto, A. (1998). Triglyceride as a risk factor for coronary artery disease. *American Journal of Cardiology, 82*(9A), 22Q–25Q.

Herd, J. (1998). Relation of clinical benefit to metabolic effects in lipid-lowering therapy. *American Journal of Cardiology, 82*(6A), 22M–25M.

Jukema, J., van Boven, A., Zwinderman, A., Van der Laarse, A., & Bruschke, A. (1998). Proposed synergistic effect of calcium channel blockers with lipid-lowering therapy in retarding progression of coronary atherosclerosis. *Cardiovascular Drugs and Therapy, 12,* 111–118.

Katzung, B. (1998). *Basic and clinical pharmacology* (7th ed.). Stamford, CT: Appleton & Lange.

Klag, M., Ford, D., Mead, L., He, J., Whelton, P., Liang, K., & Levine, D. (1993). Serum cholesterol in young men and subsequent cardiovascular disease. *New England Journal of Medicine, 328(5),* 313–318.

Kwiterovich, P. (1998). The antiatherogenic role of high-density lipoprotein cholesterol. *American Journal of Cardiology, 82(9A),* 13Q–21Q.

Lewis, S., Collier, I., & Heitkemper, M. (1996). *Medical surgical nursing: Assessment and management of clinical problems* (4th ed.). St. Louis: Mosby.

Manolio, T., Ettinger, W., Tracy, R., Kuller, L., Borhani, N., Lynch, J., & Fried, L. (1993). Epidemiology of low cholesterol levels in older adults: The Cardiovascular Health Study. *Circulation, 87(3),* 1033–1036.

McCarron, D., Oparil, S., Chait, A., Haynes, R., Kris-Etherton, P., Stern, J., Resnik, L., Clark, S., Morris, C., Hatton, D., Metz, J., McMahon, M., Holcomb, S., Snyder, G., & Pi-Sunyer, F. (1997). Nutritional management of cardiovascular risk factors. *Archives of Internal Medicine, 157,* 169–177.

National Cholesterol Education Program. (1992). Report of the expert panel on blood cholesterol levels in children and adolescents. *Pediatrics, 89,* 525–584.

National Cholesterol Education Program. (1993). *Second report of the Expert Panel on Detection, Evaluation, and Treatment of High Blood Cholesterol in Adults (adult treatment panel II).* NIH Publ. No. 93–3095. Rockville, MD: National Institutes of Health, National Heart, Lung and Blood Institute.

Neaton, J., Blackburn, H., Jacobs, D., Kuller, L., Lee, D., Sherwen, R., Shih, J., Stamler, J., & Wentworth, D. (1992). Serum cholesterol level and mortality findings for men screened in the Multiple Risk Factor Intervention Trial. *Archives of Internal Medicine, 152(7),* 1490–1500.

Orloff, D. (1998). Update on the U.S. Food and Drug Administration regulatory approach to over-the-counter cholesterol-lowering drugs. *American Journal of Cardiology, 81(8),* 79–80.

Ornish, D., Brown, S., Scherwitz, L., Billings, J., Armstrong, W., Ports, T., McLanahan, S., Kirkeeide, R., Brand, R., & Gould, K. (1990). Can lifestyle changes reverse coronary heart disease? The Lifestyle Heart Trial. *Lancet, 336(8708),* 129–133.

Ornish, D., & Denke, M. (1994). Dietary treatment of hyperlipidemia. *Journal of Cardiovascular Risk, 1(4),* 283–286.

Ornish, D., Scherwitz, L., Billings, J., Brown, S., Gould, K., Merritt, T., Sparler, S., Armstrong, W., Ports, T., Kirkeeide, R., Hogeboom, C., & Brand, R. (1998). Intensive lifestyle changes for reversal of coronary heart disease. *Journal of the American Medical Association, 280(3),* 2001–2007.

Pearson, T. (1998). Lipid-lowering therapy in low-risk patients. *Journal of the American Medical Association, 279(20),* 1659–1661.

Rosenson, R., & Tangney, C. (1998). Antiatherothrombotic properties of statins: Implications for cardiovascular event reduction. *Journal of the American Medical Association, 269(20),* 1643–1650.

Strychar, I., Champagne, F., Ghadirian, P., Bonin, A., Jenicek, M., & Lasater, T. (1998). Impact of receiving blood cholesterol test results on dietary change. *American Journal of Preventive Medicine, 14(2),* 103–110.

Tzivoni, D., & Klein, J. (1998). Effect of lipid-lowering therapy on myocardial ischemia. *Cardiovascular Drugs and Therapy, 12,* 135–139.

Weintraub, M. (1998). Guidance for industry: Over-the-counter treatment of hypercholesterolemia. *American Journal of Cardiology, 81(8),* 78F–79F.

Wong, N., Wilson, P., & Kannel, W. (1991). Serum cholesterol as a prognostic factor after myocardial infarction: The Framingham Study. *Archives of Internal Medicine, 115,* 687–693.

CHAPTER 38

· · · · · · ·

Hypertension

CHAPTER OUTLINE

Hypertension is the most common cardiovascular disease in America. According to the sixth report of the Joint National Committee (JNC) on Prevention, Detection, Evaluation, and Treatment of High Blood Pressure (NHBPEP, 1997), approximately 50 million adult Americans have hypertension, and the disorder is also found in children. Sustained arterial hypertension re-

sults in end-organ damage to the eyes and brain and is a leading cause of renal failure and cardiac disease. The JNC report (NHBPEP, 1997) states, "If the U.S. population retained the average blood pressure levels of young adults, there would be less cardiovascular disease" (p. 8). Such a goal is attainable for a large percentage of patients with hypertension with current treatment regimens. Unfortunately, "Nearly three-fourths of adult Americans with hypertension are not controlling their blood pressure to below 140/90 mm Hg" (NHBPEP, 1997, p. 8). A factor in this lack of control is nonadherence to the treatment regimen. Chapter 6 focuses on issues related to nonadherence. This chapter discusses treatment regimens that can enable people to control their blood pressure. The diagnosis and clinical evaluation of hypertension are discussed in some detail in the JNC report, and the reader is encouraged to obtain and use that information. Specific recommendations in this chapter are taken from or consistent with the information in that report.

Pathophysiology

Systemic arterial pressure is a function of stroke volume, heart rate, and total peripheral resistance. Alterations in any of these factors result in changes in blood pressure. The major organs involved in regulation of blood pressure are the heart (heart rate and stroke volume), the sympathetic nervous system (SNS) (total peripheral resistance), and the kidney (extracellular fluid volume). Disease processes that may affect stroke volume and heart rate include any that increase extracellular fluid volume, the activity of the SNS, or plasma epinephrine levels and those that produce cardiac rhythm disturbances. Disease processes that affect total peripheral resistance include any that narrow the arteriolar radius or increase blood viscosity. Figure 38–1 shows the relationship of these factors to blood pressure control. In both normotensive and hypertensive patients, blood pressure is maintained by moment-to-moment adjustments in this system.

Categories of Hypertension

Blood pressure is categorized into six levels, ranging from optimal to stage 3 hypertension. Table 38–1 shows the blood pressure readings that fall into each of these categories and the recommended follow-up for each category.

Pharmacodynamics

Only a small percentage of cases of hypertension are attributable to identifiable causes. These causes are often treated with surgery. The bulk of cases (approximately 90 to 95%) are diagnosed as essential hypertension. Because these cases have no identifiable cause, the treatment necessarily depends on interfering with normal physiological mechanisms that regulate blood pressure. Four main classes of drugs lower blood pressure through this interference. **Diuretics** lower blood pressure by depleting the body of sodium and reducing extracellular fluid volume. **Beta-adrenergic blockers** and other drugs acting on the SNS lower blood pressure by reducing peripheral vascular resistance, inhibiting cardiac contractility, and increasing venous pooling in capacitance vessels. Direct **vasodilators** reduce pressure by relaxing vascular smooth muscle, thereby dilating resistance vessels and increasing the area over which blood must flow. Finally, agents that act in the renin-angiotensin-aldosterone (R-A-A) system reduce pressure by decreasing sodium and water retention (aldosterone action), by decreasing vasoconstriction (angiotensin direct action), and by increasing vasodilation (bradykinin action). More detailed pharmacokinetics and pharmacodynamics of each of these categories of drugs are discussed in Chapters 12 and 14.

Goals of Treatment

The positive relationship between hypertension and cardiovascular risk has been long established. "This relationship is strong, continuous, graded, consistent, independent, predictive and etiologically significant for those with or without coronary artery disease" (NHBPEP, 1997, p. 11). The first goal of hypertension management is reduction in cardiovascular risk. A positive relationship has also been shown between hypertension and end-organ damage to the eyes, brain, and kidneys. The second goal is prevention of this end-organ damage. To meet these two goals, it is necessary to do the following:

1. Prevent the rise of blood pressure with age.
2. Improve control of hypertension to below 140/90 mm Hg.
3. Increase recognition of the importance of controlling isolated systolic hypertension.
4. Improve recognition of the importance of high-normal blood pressure on the development of hypertension.
5. Reduce ethnic, socioeconomic, and regional variations in hypertension.
6. Improve opportunities for well-tolerated, affordable treatment options, including lifestyle modifications and pharmacological treatment.

Rational Drug Selection

Hypertension presents a unique problem in therapeutic management. It is usually a lifelong disease but is asymptomatic until end-organ damage occurs. For this reason, providers often find themselves prescribing lifestyle modifications or drugs that have disturbing adverse reactions to treat a problem that does not make the patient feel ill. For effective management, the choice of treatment should be low in cost, limited in complexity, and with the fewest possible adverse reactions. To achieve

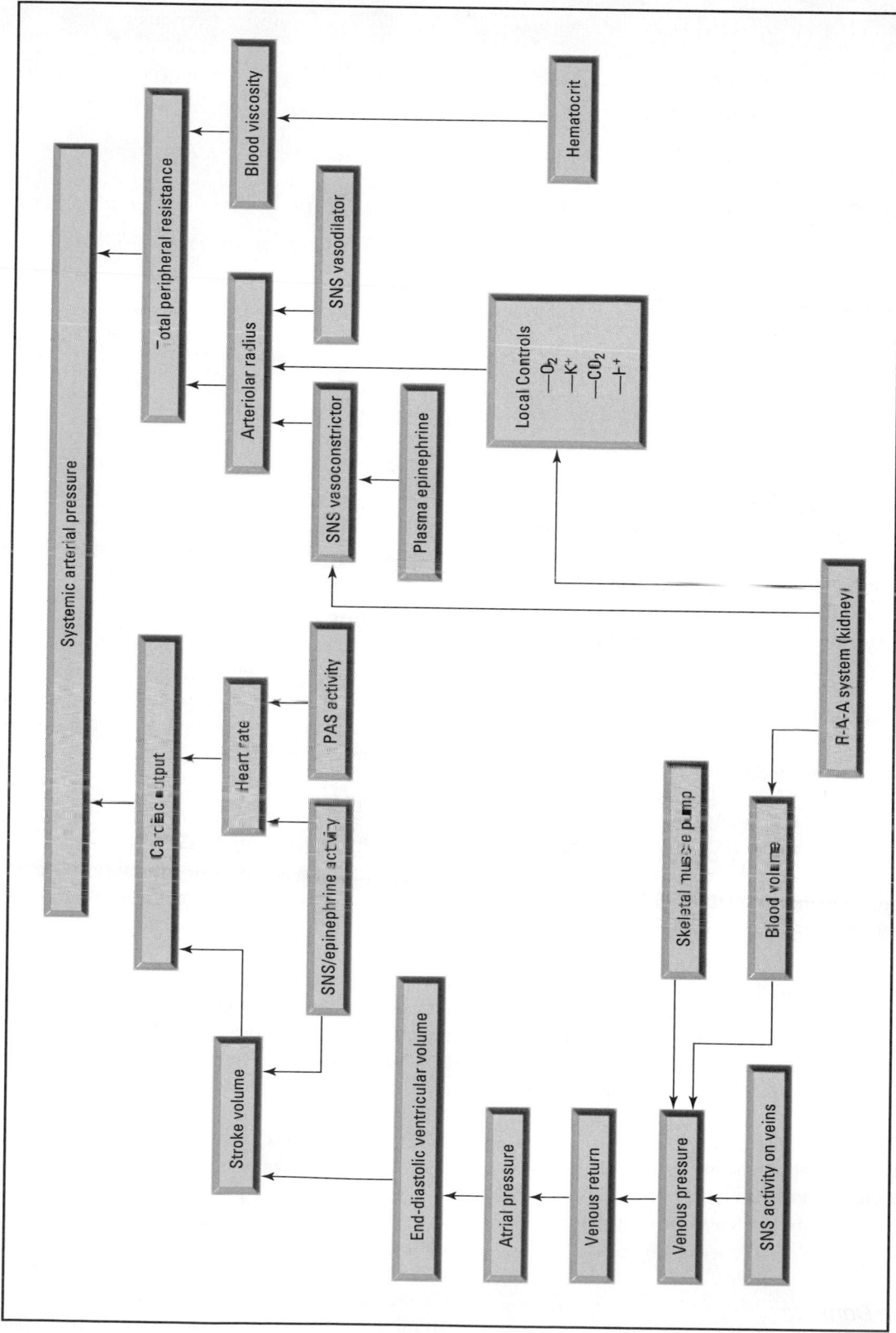

Figure 38–1. Regulation of blood pressure. Systemic arterial pressure is determined by cardiac output and total peripheral resistance. Increases in cardiac output or total peripheral resistance increase systemic arterial pressure, and decreases in these factors decrease systemic arterial pressure. Antihypertensive drugs act at one or more of these anatomical sites of blood pressure control.

Table 38–1. Categories of Hypertension and Their Follow-up

Category	Systolic Blood Pressure (mm Hg)	Diastolic Blood Pressure (mm Hg)	Follow-up
Optimal	Less than 120 *and*	Less than 80	None
Normal	Less than 130 and	Less than 85	Recheck in 2 y
High normal	130–139 *or*	85–89	Recheck in 1 y
Hypertension stage 1	140–159 *or*	90–99	Confirm within 2 mo
Hypertension stage 2	160–170 *or*	100–109	Evaluate or refer to source of care within 1 mo
Hypertension stage 3	180 or higher *or*	110 or higher	Evaluate or refer to source of care immediately or within 1 wk, depending on clinical situation

From the National High Blood Pressure Education Program (1997). *The sixth report of the Joint National Committee on Prevention, Detection, Evaluation, and Treatment of High Blood Pressure* (NIH Publ. No. 98-4080). Rockville, MD: National Institutes of Health, National Heart, Lung and Blood Institute.

this treatment protocol, management is based on category of hypertension, risk stratification, and specific patient variables. For each of these management variables, this chapter discusses stepped therapy, including lifestyle management, initial monotherapy, stepping up to multiple drugs, and stepping down when possible.

Risk Stratification

The risk of cardiovascular disease in patients with hypertension is determined by the level of blood pressure, the presence or absence of major risk factors, and the presence or absence of target organ damage. These factors independently modify the risk for cardiovascular disease secondary to hypertension and should be assessed for during the routine evaluation of all patients.

Major Risk Factors

Major risk factors for the development of hypertension include smoking, dyslipidemia, diabetes mellitus, age older than 60, male gender or postmenopausal female, and family history of cardiovascular disease in female family members under age 65 and in male family members under age 55. Obesity and physical activity are also predictors of cardiovascular risk and interact with the other risk factors but are less important in the selection of **antihypertensive drugs.**

Target Organ Damage

Disease processes that are associated with hypertension include left ventricular hypertrophy, angina or myocardial infarction (MI), prior coronary revascularization, heart failure, stroke or transient ischemic attack, nephropathy,

peripheral arterial disease, and retinopathy. Patients with these diseases should be screened for hypertension because these are often indications of target organ damage.

Risk Groups

Based on the category of blood pressure, major risk factors, and target organ damage, an empiric stratification of patients into risk groups has been established to facilitate therapeutic decisions.

Risk Group A

Patients with high-normal blood pressure or stages 1 to 3 hypertension who do not have clinical cardiovascular disease, major risk factors, or target organ damage are in risk group A. Patients in this group with stage 1 hypertension are candidates for a trial of up to 1 year of vigorous lifestyle modification with vigilant blood pressure monitoring. Lifestyle modifications may prevent the development of hypertension, can reduce cardiovascular risk factors, and cost little or nothing. Even when they cannot control hypertension alone, they may reduce the number and dosage of drugs required to manage hypertension. Table 38–2 details lifestyle modifications that have proved effective in hypertension management. Excess body weight (more than 27 body mass index), for example, is correlated closely with hypertension. Deposition of body fat in the upper part of the body, as evidenced by a waist circumference of more than 34 inches in women or more than 39 inches in men, is associated with risk for dyslipidemia, diabetes, and coronary heart disease mortality, as well as hypertension.

If the blood pressure goal is not achieved by lifestyle modifications alone, drug therapy should be added (Table 38–3). For those with stage 2 or 3 hypertension, drug therapy is essential.

Table 38–2. Lifestyle Modifications

- Lose weight. Loss of as little as 10 lb may significantly reduce blood pressure.

- Limit alcohol intake to no more than 1 oz (30 mL) ethanol (e.g., 24 oz beer, 10 oz wine, 2 oz 100-proof whiskey) per day or 1/2 oz (15 mL) ethanol per day for women and lighter-weight people.

- Increase aerobic physical activity to 30–45 min most days of the week. Obese or low-activity patients may need to start with as little as 3 min of activity per day and increase the activity by 1 min each day until the desired 30–45 min is achieved.

- Reduce sodium intake to no more than 100 mmol (2400 mg of sodium or 6 g of sodium chloride) per day. This can often be achieved by not adding salt during cooking or on the table and by watching hidden sources of salt such as canned foods.

- Maintain adequate intake of dietary potassium (approximately 90 mmol per day).

- Maintain adequate intake of dietary calcium and magnesium for general health.

- Stop smoking. The low doses of nicotine found in nicotine replacement therapy (NRT) do not significantly affect blood pressure, and NRT may be used as needed to aid in smoking cessation.

- Reduce intake of dietary saturated fat and cholesterol for overall cardiovascular health.

Adapted from the National High Blood Pressure Education Program (1997). *The sixth report of the Joint National Committee on Prevention, Detection, Evaluation, and Treatment of High Blood Pressure* (NIH Publ. No. 98-4080). Rockville, MD: National Institutes of Health, National Heart, Lung and Blood Institute.

Risk Group B

Risk group B includes patients with hypertension who do not have clinical cardiovascular disease, target organ damage, or diabetes mellitus but do have one or more major risk factors. Most patients with hypertension are in this group. For those with stage 1 hypertension and only one risk factor, lifestyle modification for up to 6 months with vigilant blood pressure monitoring is appropriate. If more than one risk factor is present, initial management is with drug therapy. Lifestyle modification and management of reversible risk factors are also strongly recommended for this latter group.

Risk Group C

Risk group C patients have hypertension and clinically manifested cardiovascular disease or target organ damage. This group includes all patients with diabetes, with or without other risk factors. Initial management is with drug therapy: "It is the clinical opinion of the JNC VI executive committee that some patients who have high-normal blood pressure as well as renal insufficiency, heart failure or diabetes mellitus should be considered for prompt pharmacologic therapy" (NHBPEP, 1997, p. 17).

Although lifestyle modifications are appropriate for all risk groups, implementation of these modifications

Table 38–3. Treatment Protocol by Blood Pressure Stage and Risk

Blood Pressure Stage	Risk Group A (No Risk Factors, No Target Organ Damage, No Clinical Cardiovascular Disease)	Risk Group B (At Least 1 Risk Factor, Not Including Diabetes, No Target Organ Damage, No Clinical Cardiovascular Disease	Risk Group C (Target Organ Damage, Clinical Cardiovascular Disease and/or Diabetes with or without Other Risk Factors)
High normal (130–139/85–89)	Lifestyle modification	Lifestyle modification	Drug therapy
Hypertension stage 1 (140–159/90–99)	Lifestyle modification	Lifestyle modification	Drug therapy
Hypertension stages 2 and 3 (160 or greater/100 or greater)	Drug therapy	Drug therapy	Drug therapy

Adapted from the National High Blood Pressure Education Program (1997). *The sixth report of the Joint National Committee on Prevention, Detection, Evaluation, and Treatment of High Blood Pressure* (NIH Publ. No. 98-4080). Rockville, MD: National Institutes of Health, National Heart, Lung and Blood Institute.

should not delay the start of an effective **antihypertensive drug** regimen for patients in higher risk groups.

Stepped Therapy

Once the decision is made to begin drug therapy, initial drug choices are based on the presence or absence of complications, specific indications of specific drugs, and compelling indications from concurrent disease processes. Figure 38–2 shows this decision-making protocol.

Initial Drug Therapy

For most patients, the lowest dose of the initial drug should be used to prevent adverse reactions and too much or too abrupt a reduction in blood pressure. The dose is then slowly titrated upward, based on patient response. If blood pressure remains uncontrolled after 1 to 2 months, the next dosage level should be prescribed. The ideal drug should provide 24 hours of efficacy with at least 50 percent of the peak effect remaining at the end of the 24 hours. Long-acting formulations are preferred over short-acting because (1) adherence is better with once-daily dosing; (2) for many agents, fewer tablets mean lower cost; (3) control of hypertension is smoother; and (4) the risk of sudden death, heart attack, and stroke on account of abrupt changes in blood pressure is lessened.

When the decision is made to begin drug therapy and there are no clear indications for another type of drug, a **diuretic** or a **beta-adrenergic blocker** should be chosen because they have been shown to reduce morbidity and mortality in numerous randomized controlled trials (RCTs). As shown in Figure 38–2, there are compelling indications for specific other agents, also based on RCTs. **Angiotensin-converting enzyme (ACE) inhibitors**, for example, are drugs of choice in diabetes mellitus, heart failure, and MI. Other concomitant diseases that may affect the choice of drugs are discussed later.

Monotherapy is best when it controls hypertension because adherence is likely to be better, cost is lower, and adverse reactions are apt to be fewer. Moderate to severe hypertension, however, commonly requires a combination of two or more drugs from different classes, acting by different mechanisms. Newly developed formulations that include such combinations may permit the best of both worlds; the patient takes just one pill or capsule yet receives the benefit of two drugs.

Some **antihypertensive drugs** are not well suited for monotherapy because they cause troublesome adverse reactions in almost all patients who take them. These drugs include **direct-acting smooth-muscle vasodilators, central alpha$_2$ agonists,** and **peripheral adrenergic antagonists.** These drugs can be used effectively when combined with other drugs that address these adverse reactions.

Stepping Up to Multiple Drugs

If the initial monotherapy drug choice is inadequate at that drug's full dose, two options are considered: addition of another drug or substitution by a different drug. If the patient is tolerating the first choice well, a second drug may be added from another class. The choice of the second drug is influenced by how it might affect the adverse reaction profile of the first drug or by how well these drugs have been shown to work together in clinical studies. An adequate dose of **hydralazine** results in compensatory tachycardia and salt and water retention. The addition of a **beta-adrenergic blocker** prevents the tachycardia, and the addition of a **diuretic** prevents salt and water retention. An **ACE inhibitor** and a **nondihydropyridine calcium channel blocker** may reduce proteinuria in a patient with diabetes better than either drug alone.

If a **diuretic** was not chosen as the first drug, it is usually indicated as the second-step drug because its addition will enhance the effects of most other agents. If the second drug controls the hypertension satisfactorily, an attempt may be made to withdraw the first drug and return to monotherapy. If the patient is having significant adverse reactions or no response from the initial drug, an agent from another class is substituted. For example, a persistent cough may be annoying enough that a patient will not continue to take an **ACE inhibitor.** Because they do not affect the kallikrein system, **angiotensin II receptor antagonists (ATRAs)** do not produce this cough, nor do they have the problem with angioedema that is a contraindication to the use of an **ACE inhibitor.** Because the hemodynamic effects are similar, an **ATRA** may be substituted for the **ACE inhibitor.** Documentation of equal long-term cardiac and renal protection for patients with systolic dysfunction and diabetic nephropathy is only recently coming forward, however, and to date **ATRAs** should be reserved for patients for whom **ACE inhibitors** are indicated but who are unable to tolerate them.

Modification of this protocol may be needed for patients with stage 3 hypertension, those in risk group C, or those at especially high risk for a coronary event or stroke. For these patients, single-drug therapy initially may not be adequate. The intervals between the addition of a second or third drug should be decreased, and the maximum dose of some drugs may be increased. Patients with average systolic blood pressure (SBP) of 200 mm Hg or higher and average diastolic blood pressure (DBP) of 120 mm Hg or more require immediate drug treatment and, if symptomatic target organ damage is present, may require hospitalization.

Stepping Down

Although hypertension is generally accepted to be a lifelong disease, after it has been controlled effectively for at least 1 year, a decrease in the dosage and number of **antihypertensive drugs** should be considered. The reduction

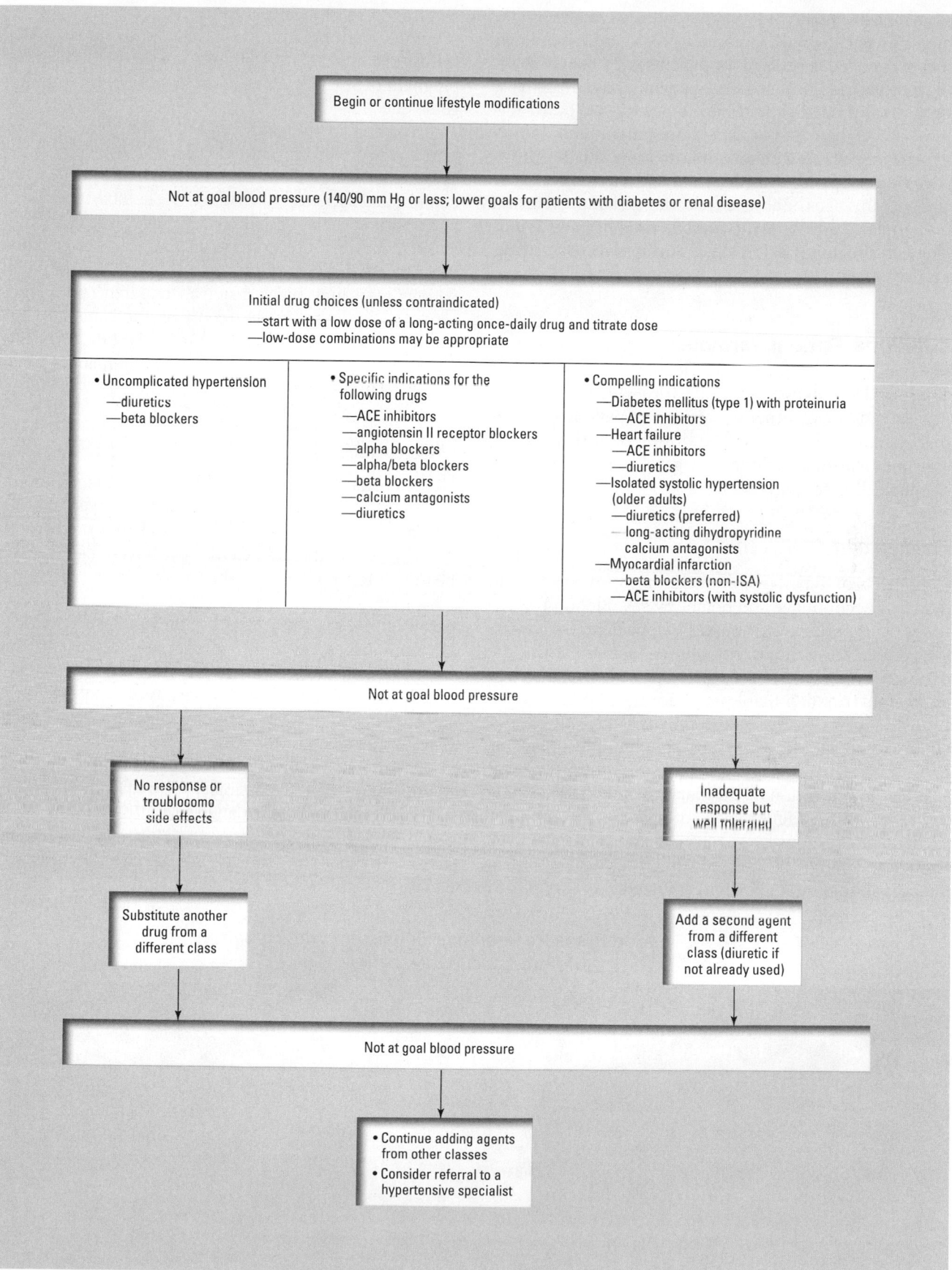

Figure 38–2. Treatment protocol for hypertension management.

should be deliberate, slow, and progressive and accompanied by vigilant blood pressure monitoring. Step-down therapy is often successful for patients who also are making lifestyle modifications. Any patient whose drugs have been discontinued should have regularly scheduled follow-up visits because blood pressure usually rises again to hypertensive levels within months to years after the drugs have been stopped. This return of hypertension is especially common in the absence of continued improvements in lifestyle. If adherence to lifestyle modifications is not likely, maintaining a low-dose **antihypertensive drug** may be preferable to complete discontinuance of all drugs.

Additional Patient Variables

The prevalence of hypertension varies with age, race, education, and many other variables. The patient variables that affect the clinical use and dosing of **antihypertensive medications** include age, gender, race, and concomitant diseases and therapies.

Children and Adolescents

Definitions of hypertension in children and adolescents take into account age and height by sex. Blood pressure in the 95th percentile or higher is considered hypertension. Table 38–4 shows the values consistent with a diagnosis of hypertension for girls and boys based on age and height. An identifiable cause for the hypertension is more likely in younger children than it is in adults, and such causes should always be sought. The treatment protocol is similar to that used for risk group A adults. Lifestyle modifications are initially used, with drug therapy reserved for higher levels of blood pressure or for inadequate response to lifestyle modifications. Although the choice of drugs is similar to that for adults, dosages should be smaller and adjusted very carefully in

children. The clinical use and dosing sections for the drugs in Chapters 12 and 14 have children's doses. **ACE inhibitors** and **ATRAs** should not be prescribed for pregnant or sexually active girls because of their teratogenic effects.

According to the sixth report of the Joint National Committee on the Prevention, Detection, Evaluation, and Treatment of High Blood Pressure (NHBPEP, 1997), uncomplicated hypertension alone is not sufficient reason to restrict asymptomatic children from participating in physical activities because exercise may actually lower blood pressure and prevent hypertension. Detailed recommendations regarding hypertension in children and adolescents can be found in the report by the National High Blood Pressure Education Program (NHBPEP) Working Group of Hypertension Control in Children and Adolescents. (NHBPEP, 1997) .

Older Adults

Hypertension is very common in older adults, occurring in 60 to 71 percent of the population over age 60. Among older adults, SBP pressure is a better predictor of coronary heart disease (CHD), cardiovascular disease, heart failure, end-stage renal disease, and all-cause mortality than is DBP. An even better predictor is pulse pressure (SBP minus DBP), which indicates reduced vascular compliance in large arteries. Evidence of this increased risk has led to recognition of the importance of treating isolated systolic hypertension in older adults rather than accepting increased blood pressure as a "normal" part of aging.

Measurement of blood pressure in older adults requires consideration of the possibility of pseudohypertension caused by excessive vascular stiffness. In addition, older adults are more likely to experience orthostatic changes, and their blood pressure should always be measured standing as well as in the lying position.

Table 38–4. Blood Pressure Readings Consistent with Hypertension in Children and Adolescents

Age (Years)	Girls (50th Percentile for Height)	Girls (75th Percentile for Height)	Boys (50th Percentile for Height)	Boys (75th Percentile for Height)
1	104/58	105/59	102/57	104/58
6	111/73	112/73	114/74	115/75
12	123/80	124/81	123/81	125/82
17	129/84	130/85	136/87	138/88

Adapted from the report by the NHBPEP Working Group on Hypertension Control in Children and Adolescents. From the National High Blood Pressure Education Program (1997). *The sixth report of the Joint National Committee on Prevention, Detection, Evaluation, and Treatment of High Blood Pressure* (NIH Publ. No. 98-4080). Rockville, MD: National Institutes of Health, National Heart, Lung and Blood Institute.

Large RCTs have shown that **antihypertensive drug** therapy reduces risk for stroke, CHD, cardiovascular disease, and mortality in patients over age 60 with any form of hypertension, but especially with isolated systolic hypertension. The Systolic Hypertension in the Elderly Program (SHEP, 1991) demonstrated that drug therapy directed at isolated systolic hypertension in adults over age 60 decreased the 5-year incidence of cardiovascular events by 32 percent, with a 27 percent decrease in nonfatal MI and in the rate of coronary events.

As in younger patients, therapy should begin with lifestyle modifications. Older adults respond especially well to reduced salt intake and weight loss because they are prone to sodium retention and volume excess. Dietary sodium intake should be reduced to less than 2300 mg per day. If these measures do not achieve the blood pressure goal, drug therapy should begin. In general, the initial dose should be about half that used in younger patients. **Thiazide diuretics** and **beta-adrenergic blockers** in combination with **diuretics** are recommended because they have been shown in RCTs to reduce morbidity and mortality and because they are less expensive for patients who are often on fixed incomes. When compared with each other, **diuretics** are more effective than **beta-adrenergic blockers** and "are preferred because they have significantly reduced multiple endpoint events" (NHBPEP, 1997, p. 45). **Thiazide diuretics** are particularly useful for isolated systolic hypertension because of their greater effects on SBP than on DBP. Morbidity and mortality are both improved in older adults when SBP is reduced while DBP is held stable at between 85 and 90 mm Hg. It is important to monitor potassium levels with the drugs, especially if the patient is also on **digitalis.** Even mild hypokalemia may be problematic for older adults with coronary artery disease (CAD). Drug combinations that include both a **thiazide diuretic** and a **potassium-sparing diuretic** are useful for patients who have repeated episodes of hypokalemia. Long-acting **dihydropyridine calcium channel blockers** are appropriate alternatives, but they are more expensive. Drugs that have high risk for orthostatic changes **(peripheral adrenergic blockers, alpha-adrenergic blockers,** and high doses of **diuretics)** and those that can affect cognitive function **(central alpha$_2$ agonists)** should be avoided or, if there is a compelling reason for their use, used with extreme caution.

The blood pressure goal for older adults is the same as it is for younger patients, below 140/90 mm Hg. An interim goal of less than 160 SBP may be acceptable for patients with marked systolic hypertension. Any reduction in blood pressure has some benefit, and the closer to the ideal goal, the better. Additional recommendations can be found in the report by the NHBPEP Working Group on Hypertension in the Elderly.

Women

Although there are no demonstrated clinical differences between men and women related to blood pressure outcomes or responses to therapy, women do have some unique variables related to hypertension: use of **oral contraceptives** and **hormone replacements** and pregnancy. Women taking **oral contraceptives** have a small but detectable increase in both SBP and DBP, but these are usually within the normal range. Hypertension is two to three times more common in women taking these drugs, especially if they are also obese. A strong correlation has also been found in hypertension risk for women who smoke and take **oral contraceptives.** Women over age 35 who smoke should be discouraged from using **oral contraceptives** and highly encouraged to stop smoking. If hypertension develops in women taking **oral contraceptives,** the drugs should be discontinued. Blood pressure usually returns to normal in a few months. If hypertension continues, therapy for hypertension should be begun. **Oral contraceptives** are often prescribed on a yearly basis, but a more prudent approach may be to prescribe them semiannually so that blood pressure can be checked every 6 months.

The presence of hypertension is not a contraindication to postmenopausal **estrogen replacement** therapy. Blood pressure does not increase significantly with **hormone replacement therapy (HRT).** In most women with or without hypertension, **HRT** has shown clear benefit on cardiovascular risk factor profiles. A few women may experience a rise in blood pressure attributable to **HRT,** however, so all women receiving **HRT** should have their blood pressure monitored more frequently after the therapy is initiated.

Hypertension that is present and observable before pregnancy or diagnosed before the 20th week of pregnancy is chronic hypertension, not pregnancy-induced hypertension. The goal of hypertension management for chronic hypertension in pregnant women is to minimize short-term risks while avoiding therapy that compromises the fetus (Table 38–5). **Methyldopa (Aldomet)** has been studied the most and is recommended for women whose chronic hypertension is first diagnosed in pregnancy. **Beta-adrenergic blockers** are equally effective and are safe during the second and third trimesters, but their use in the first trimester has been associated with growth retardation in the fetus. If the hypertension is diagnosed before the pregnancy, **diuretics** and many other **antihypertensives** may be continued. Chapters 12 and 14 delineate safety issues in pregnancy for various drugs used to treat hypertension. **ACE inhibitors** and **ATRAs** should never be used in pregnancy because of their teratogenic effects. Women with hypertension who become pregnant while on these drugs should have a different class of **antihypertensive drugs** substituted for them.

Table 38–5. Antihypertensives Recommended in Pregnancy

The report of the NHBPEP Working Group on High Blood Pressure in Pregnancy permits continuation of drug therapy in women with chronic hypertension (except for ACE inhibitors). In addition, angiotensin II receptor blockers should not be used during pregnancy. In women with chronic hypertension with diastolic levels of 100 mm Hg or greater (lower when end-organ damage or underlying renal disease is present) and in women with acute hypertension when levels are 105 mm Hg or greater, the following drugs are recommended:

Recommended Drug	Comments
Beta blockers	Atenolol (C) and metoprolol (C) appear to be safe and effective in late pregnancy; labetalol (C) also appears to be effective.
Calcium antagonists	Potential synergism with magnesium sulfate may lead to precipitous hypotension (C).
Central alpha agonists	Methyldopa (C) is the recommended drug of choice.
Direct vasodilators	Hydralazine (C) is the parenteral drug of choice, based on its long history of safety and efficacy.
Diuretics	Diuretics (C) are recommended for chronic hypertension if prescribed before gestation or if patients apper to be salt-sensitive; they are not recommended in preeclampsia.

ACE inhibitors (D) and angiotensin II receptor blockers (D) may result in fetal abnormalities including death; these drugs should not be used in pregnancy.
Pregnancy Category C = adverse effects in animals; no controlled trials in humans; use if risk appears justified. Pregnancy Category D = positive evidence of fetal risk.
From the National High Blood Pressure Education Program (1997). *The sixth report of the Joint National Committee on Prevention, Detection, Evaluation, and Treatment of High Blood Pressure* (NIH Publ. No. 98-4080). Rockville, MD: National Institutes of Health. National Heart, Lung and Blood Institute.

Pregnancy-induced hypertension (PIH) is a pregnancy-specific condition. It occurs primarily during the first pregnancy and after 20 weeks of gestation. It may be superimposed on existing chronic hypertension. A detailed summary of hypertension in pregnancy was published in a report by the NHBPEP Working Group on High Blood Pressure in Pregnancy (NHBPEP, 1997).

Racial and Ethnic Minorities

The prevalence of hypertension among different racial and ethnic groups varies. Native Americans have the same or slightly higher prevalence rates than the white population. Hispanics have the same to slightly lower prevalence rates, despite their increased incidence of obesity and type 2 diabetes mellitus. South Asians have about the same prevalence and appear to be more responsive to **antihypertensive drugs** that are whites. The prevalence of hypertension in African-Americans is among the highest in the world. Hypertension develops at younger ages than in whites, and the average blood pressure is much higher than in the white population. They also have a higher rate of stage 3 hypertension and more end-organ damage from their hypertension. Their stroke rate is 80 percent higher; their heart disease mortality is 50 percent higher; and their hypertension-related end-stage renal disease is 320 percent higher than that of the general population.

The underlying pathology associated with hypertension in African-Americans is thought to be salt sensitivity. In general, this population has low renin activity, and so the R-A-A system is thought not to play a major role. This increased sensitivity to salt, along with the high prevalence in this population of obesity, cigarette smoking, and type 2 diabetes mellitus, means that lifestyle modifications are especially efficacious. Salt intake should be reduced to less than 6 g per day, and weight should be reduced, if necessary, to approach ideal body weight. If these modifications do not result in achievement of the blood pressure goal, **diuretics** have been proved in RCTs to reduce morbidity and mortality and are the first agents of choice unless there are compelling reasons to choose another drug class. **Calcium channel blockers** and **alpha-beta adrenergic blockers** are also effective in this population. Monotherapy with **ACE inhibitors** is less effective because of the low renin activity. In the presence of diabetes mellitus, however, **ACE inhibitors** may be used in combination with a **diuretic.** Monotherapy with **beta-adrenergic blockers** is also less effective but may be used in combination with a **diuretic** for post-MI patients.

The high prevalence of stage 3 hypertension in the African-American population means that they frequently require multidrug therapy, which may result in a higher prevalence of adverse reactions. For the proportion of African-Americans who do not trust the white-dominated medical system, these adverse effects—related to drugs that treat a disease that exists for them only because a medical device (the blood pressure cuff) tells them they have it—increase their distrust, especially when these adverse effects include such personal problems as impotence. All possible steps should be taken to deal with adherence issues in this population, with consideration for cultural ramifications.

Concomitant Diseases and Therapies

Antihypertensive drugs may improve the management of some diseases and worsen that of others (Table 38–6). Selection of an **antihypertensive** that also treats a concomitant disease can simplify the overall therapeutic regimen, reduce cost, and increase the likelihood of adherence. It is not within the scope of this book to discuss all possible diseases that may coexist with hypertension, but the most common diseases that benefit from appropriate selection of an **antihypertensive** are discussed here.

CEREBROVASCULAR DISEASE. Clinically evident cerebrovascular disease is an indication for hypertensive therapy. Treatment is initially withheld until the patient is stable, and then treatment is instituted with a goal to reduce blood pressure gradually. To avoid orthostatic hypotension, drugs that have high risk for orthostatic changes (**peripheral adrenergic blockers, alpha-adrenergic blockers,** and high doses of **diuretics**) should not be chosen.

CORONARY ARTERY DISEASE. Coexisting CAD and hypertension place patients at especially high risk for cardiovascular morbidity and mortality. **Antihypertensive therapy** is essential, and its benefits well established. Blood pressure should be reduced to a goal of 140/90 mm Hg, with lower blood pressure desirable in patients with angina. Excessively rapid lowering of blood pressure, however, may result in reflex tachycardia and sympathetic stimulation and should be avoided. **Antihypertensive drugs** that have reflex tachycardia and sympathetic stimulation as adverse reactions (**alpha-adrenergic blockers, nitrates,** and **peripheral vasodilators**) should also be avoided. **Long-acting calcium channel blockers** and **beta-adrenergic blockers** are especially helpful to patients with concomitant angina. **Short-acting calcium channel blockers** should not be used. After MI, **beta-adrenergic blockers** with intrinsic sympathomimetic activity are the drugs of choice because they reduce the risk of subsequent MI or sudden cardiac death. **ACE inhibitors** and **ATRAs** are also useful after MI, especially with concomitant left ventricular dysfunction, to prevent heart failure and mortality. Chapter 35 further discusses this management protocol.

LEFT VENTRICULAR HYPERTROPHY. Left ventricular hypertrophy (LVH) is a cardiac adaptation to the increased afterload generated by persistent hypertension. LVH is a major independent risk factor for sudden cardiac death, MI, stroke, and other cardiovascular events. In addition to lifestyle modification with salt reduction and weight loss, **antihypertensive drugs** (except **direct vasodilators** such as **hydralazine** and **minoxidil**) are capable of reducing left ventricular mass and wall thickness and reducing cardiovascular risks. The combination of an **ACE inhibitor** and a **diuretic** has proved to be more effective than any other class or combination of classes in regressing LVH and reducing cardiovascular risks.

HEART FAILURE. Hypertension is the major cause of left ventricular failure in the United States. Control of blood pressure with lifestyle modifications and drug therapy improves myocardial function and reduces the risk for heart failure and cardiovascular mortality. **ACE inhibitors** alone or in conjunction with **diuretics** or **digoxin** are the most effective drugs for this purpose. When **ACE inhibitors** are not well tolerated, studies dating from late 1997 have shown that the **ATRA losartan (Cozaar)** may be equally effective alone or in the same combinations. When **ACE inhibitors** are contraindicated (renal artery stenosis, angioedema, or pregnancy), the vasodilator combination of **hydralazine** and **isosorbide dinitrate** is also effective. The **alpha-beta–adrenergic blocker carvedilol (Coreg)** has also been shown to be beneficial when combined with an **ACE inhibitor,** but **carvedilol** is quite expensive. The **dihydropyridines** amlodipine (Norvasc) and **felodipine (Plendil)** have been demonstrated to be safe for treating angina and hypertension in patients with advanced left ventricular dysfunction when they are used in addition to **ACE inhibitors, diuretics,** or **digoxin,** but other **calcium channel blockers** are not recommended for these patients. Chapter 34 discusses the treatment of heart failure in more detail.

RENAL PARENCHYMAL DISEASE. Hypertension may result from any form of renal disease that reduces the number of functioning nephrons, leading to salt and water retention and then to increased extracellular fluid (ECF) volume. Evaluation of renal function in hypertensive patients should include serum creatinine levels (even small elevations reflect large losses in glomerular filtration rate) and urinalysis to detect proteinuria or hematuria. Reversible causes of renal failure should always be sought and treated. Blood pressure goals for patients with proteinuria in excess of 1 g per 24 hours should be 125/75 mm Hg or less, with whatever **antihypertensive therapy** is necessary. Sodium restriction is recommended to a level lower than that recommended for uncomplicated hypertension, and dietary restriction of potassium and phosphorus is recommended when creatinine clearance is below 30 cc per minute.

All classes of **antihypertensive drugs** are effective, and multiple drugs may be needed. **ACE inhibitors** have been the most effective in patients with diabetic nephropathy, proteinuria of 1 g or more per 24 hours, and renal insufficiency. **ACE inhibitors** are the drug class of choice to control hypertension and slow progression of renal failure for all patients who have hypertension and renal insufficiency

Table 38–6. Drug Choice Based on Concomitant Disease States

Disease State	Drug Choice
Compelling Indications Unless Contraindicated Diabetes mellitus (type 1) with proteinuria	ACE inhibitors
Heart failure	ACE inhibitors Diuretics
Isolated systolic hypertension (older adults)	Diuretics (preferred) CA (long-acting DHP)
Myocardial infarction	Beta blockers (non-ISA) ACE inhibitors (with systolic dysfunction)
May Have Favorable Effects on Comorbid Conditions Angina	Beta blockers CA
Atrial tachycardia and fibrillation CA (non-DHP)	Beta blockers CA (non-DHP)
Cyclosporine-induced hypertension (caution with the dose of cyclosporine)	CA
Diabetes mellitus (types 1 and 2) with proteinuria	ACE inhibitors (preferred) CA
Diabetes mellitus (type 2)	Diuretics (low dose)
Dyslipidemia	Alpha blockers
Essential tremor	Beta blockers (non-CS)
Heart failure	Carvedilol Losartan potassium
Hyperthyroidism	Beta blockers
Migraine	Beta blockers (non-CS) CA (non-DHP)
Myocardial infarction	Diltiazem hydrochloride Verapamil hydrochloride
Osteoporosis	Thiazides
Preoperative hypertension	Beta blockers
Prostatism (BPH)	Alpha blockers
Renal insufficiency (caution in renovascular hypertension and creatinine 265.2 mmol/L or higher [3 mg/dL])	ACE inhibitors
May Have Unfavorable Effects on Comorbid Conditions ***(May Be Used with Special Monitoring Unless Contraindicated)*** Bronchospastic disease	Beta blockers
Depression	Beta blockers Central alpha agonists Reserpine (contraindicated)
Diabetes mellitus (types 1 and 2)	Beta blockers Diuretics (high dose)

Continued on next page

Table 38–6. Drug Choice Based on Concomitant Disease States *(continued)*

Disease State	Drug Choice
Dyslipidemia	Beta blockers (non-ISA) Diuretics (high dose)
Gout	Diuretics
Heart block (second and third degree)	Beta blockers (contraindicated) CA (non-DHP) (contraindicated)
Heart failure	Beta blockers (except carvedilol) CA (except amlodipine besylate, felodipine)
Liver disease	Labetalol hydrochloride Methyldopa (contraindicated)
Peripheral vascular disease	Beta blockers
Pregnancy	ACE inhibitors (contraindicated) Angiotensin II receptor blockers (contraindicated)
Renal insufficiency	Potassium-sparing agents
Renovascular disease	ACE inhibitors Angiotensin II receptor blockers

CA = calcium channel blocker; CS = cardiac specific; DHP = dihydropyridine; non-ISA = non-intrinsic sympathomimetic action.
From the National High Blood Pressure Education Program (1997). *The sixth report of the Joint National Committee on Prevention, Detection, Evaluation, and Treatment of High Blood Pressure* (NIH Publ. No. 98-4080). Rockville, MD: National Institutes of Health. National Heart, Lung and Blood Institute.

unless they are specifically contraindicated. In patients with serum creatinine levels of 3 mg/dL or more, ACE inhibitors should be used with caution. Chapter 14 provides more detailed discussion of this treatment protocol. Thiazide diuretics are not effective with renal insufficiency manifested by serum creatinine levels 2.5 mg/dL or more, and loop diuretics such as furosemide (Lasix) are needed, often at relatively large doses. Potassium-sparing diuretics should be avoided in renal insufficiency. Chapter 14 also discusses the use of diuretics in more detail.

RENOVASCULAR DISEASE. Clinical clues to renovascular disease associated with hypertension include (1) onset of hypertension before age 30, especially without a family history, or recent onset of significant hypertension after age 55; (2) accelerated or persistent hypertension; and (3) acute renal failure precipitated by antihypertensive therapy, especially with ACE inhibitors or ATRAs. Treatment of this disease process is best done surgically, and no specific antihypertensive medications are recommended.

DIABETES MELLITUS. Antihypertensive drug therapy should be initiated, along with lifestyle modifications (especially weight loss), to reach a blood pressure goal of below 130/85 mm Hg for all patients with diabetes mellitus. ACE inhibitors, ATRAs, alpha-adrenergic blockers, calcium channel blockers, and diuretics in low doses are preferred because of their lower effects on glucose metabolism, lipid profiles, and renal function. Of this group, ACE inhibitors are considered best because of their demonstrated reduction in risk for diabetic nephropathy. If they are not well tolerated, ATRAs may be considered. Calcium channel blockers have also been shown to have some degree of renal protection.

Beta-adrenergic blockers have an adverse effect on peripheral blood flow, prolong hypoglycemia, and mask most hypoglycemic symptoms. If there is a compelling reason for a patient with diabetes to use them, they should be combined with a diuretic. The patient should be taught that beta-adrenergic blockers do not mask diaphoresis as a symptom of hypoglycemia; this symptom should be carefully watched for and lead to immediate blood glucose monitoring. Chapter 12 discusses this treatment protocol in more detail.

DYSLIPIDEMIA. Lifestyle modifications are the first approach to treatment of both dyslipidemia and hypertension. Emphasis is placed on control of weight; reduced intake of sodium, saturated fat, cholesterol, and alcohol; and increased physical activity. When drug therapy is chosen, drug effects on lipid metabolism are the primary consideration. Alpha-adrenergic blockers may decrease serum cholesterol to a limited degree and increase HDL.

ACE inhibitors, ATRAs, **calcium channel blockers,** and **central adrenergic agonists** have neutral effects on lipids. **Beta-adrenergic blockers** increase triglycerides transiently and reduce levels of high-density lipids (HDLs). They are chosen mainly for patients with previous MIs who need their protective effects against sudden cardiac death and recurrent MI. In high doses, **thiazide** and **loop diuretics** can cause at least short-term increases in levels of cholesterol, triglycerides, and low-density lipids (LDLs). Dietary modifications can reduce these effects. Low doses of **thiazide diuretics** do not produce these effects and can be safely used. According to the NHBPEP (1997, p. 50) document, "In the Systolic Hypertension in the Elderly Program and the Hypertension Detection and Follow-up Program, both of which used **diuretics** as initial monotherapy or in combination, the risks for cerebrovascular and coronary events were reduced equally in persons with normal lipid levels and those with elevated lipid levels."

Lowering lipid levels also reduces cardiovascular risks that are shared in common with hypertension. Selection of appropriate cholesterol-lowering drugs is discussed in the guidelines from the National Cholesterol Education Program (1993).

BRONCHIAL ASTHMA OR CHRONIC AIRWAY DISEASES. Hypertension is relatively common in acute asthma and may be related to treatment with **beta agonists** or **systemic corticosteroids.** Bronchial reactivity is unchanged by **ACE inhibitors,** which are safe for most patients with asthma. If the patient is one of the 10 to 15 percent who experience the adverse effect of a cough, **ATRAs** are an alternative. **Beta-adrenergic blockers** and **alpha-beta–adrenergic blockers** may exacerbate asthma and should not be used unless there are compelling reasons for doing so. The topical ophthalmic **beta-adrenergic blockers** such as **timolol (Timoptic)** may also worsen asthma.

Many over-the-counter drugs used as **decongestants** and cold and asthma remedies contain a sympathomimetic drug that can raise blood pressure. They are generally safe when taken in limited doses by patients who are on **antihypertensive therapy. Cromolyn sodium, ipratropium bromide,** or **corticosteroids** by inhalation can be used safely for nasal congestion by patients with hypertension.

Cost

The cost of **antihypertensive drug therapy** should be considered in drug selection, especially for patients who require multiple drugs (Table 38–7). In most cases, generic formulations are acceptable and cheaper. Nongeneric newer agents are usually more expensive than **diuretics** or **beta-adrenergic blockers,** especially in that both of these classes come in generic formulations. If the newer agent is equally effective and there are no compelling reasons for its use, cost should be a major factor in choosing the initial therapy. If the newer agent is more effective or there is a compelling reason for its use, cost should be a secondary consideration. Using combinations can also reduce drug cost. Table 38–8 lists some of the more common drugs found in combination tablets.

Shopping at different sources to check prices is often worthwhile. Some drugs have the same cost for a higher-dose as for a lower-dose tablet, and the tablet can be divided to reduce cost. These cost-saving measures are discussed in more detail in Chapters 12 and 14.

Treatment costs include not only the price of the drug but also the price of any routine or special laboratory tests, supplemental therapies, clinic visits, and time lost from work for clinic visits. Maintaining contact with a patient and regularly checking blood pressure are important factors in adherence, but they can also add cost. Teaching the patient how to do home blood pressure monitoring and use of telecommunication or e-mail to maintain contact can reduce these costs.

In an era of managed care, the cost of treating hypertension is always under scrutiny. Managed care agencies can be reminded, however, that the cost of hypertension management that results in good control is lower than the cost that may be avoided by reducing hypertension-associated heart disease, stroke, and renal failure, which may result in expensive hospitalizations. RCTs have shown that these reductions occur in a relatively short period of time and are sustained for years.

Monitoring

The single-most important monitoring parameter is blood pressure measurement. Home or clinic blood pressure measurement in the early morning before the patient has taken the **antihypertensive** drug(s) provides data about the adequacy of management related to the surge in blood pressure after arising. Measurement in the late afternoon or evening helps to monitor control across the day. Because the stress of a clinic visit may result in higher blood pressure readings in the clinic, blood pressure goals based on home monitoring should be lower than those based on clinic monitoring.

Laboratory data and other monitoring parameters related to specific drugs are discussed in Chapters 12 and 14 for each drug class. Annual evaluations for target organ damage should include a 12-lead electrocardiogram (ECG), urinalysis, complete blood count (CBC), blood chemistry (potassium, sodium, creatinine, fasting glucose, total cholesterol), and HDL levels. Optional tests include creatinine clearance, 24-hour urine protein, LDL levels, thyroid-stimulating hormone levels, and limited

Table 38–7. Selected Antihypertensive Drugs and Their Cost

Drug	Dosage (mg/day)	Cost*
ACE Inhibitors		
Benazepril	10–40	$19.09
Captopril	12.5–150	$19.35
Enalapril	2.5–40	$21.53
Lisinopril	5–40	$23.59
Alpha₁-Adrenergic Blockers		
Prazosin	1–20	$7.72 (generic)
Terazosin	1–20	$36.67
Angiotensin II Receptor Antagonist		
Losartan	25–100	
Beta-Adrenergic Blockers		
Atenolol	25–100	$20.26 (generic)
Metoprolol	50–200	$13.53 (generic)
Propranolol	40–240	$4.10 (generic)
Propranolol extended-release	80–240	$23.10 (generic)
Calcium Channel Blockers		
Amlodipine	2.5–10	$35.36
Diltiazem CD	120–360	$31.32
Diltiazem SR	120–360	$48.00
Diuretics		
Furosemide	20–320	$1.73 (generic)
Hydrochlorothiazide	12.5–50	$1.04 (generic)
Indapamide	2.5–5	$26.42
Spironolactone	25–100	$2.51 (generic)
Triamterine	50–150	$9.77

*Cost in 1998 dollars to pharmacist for 30-day prescription at lowest recommended dosage.

echocardiography. For patients with diabetes, microalbuminuria and glycosylated hemoglobin studies are essential. Physical examination includes funduscopic examination, neurological examination, and assessment of heart and lung sounds, peripheral pulses, and bruits.

Outcome Evaluation

Figure 38–2 shows the treatment protocol for hypertension management. Evaluation against specific blood pressure goals occurs throughout the protocol. The main indications for substitution of a drug from a different class are no response and troublesome adverse reactions to initial drug therapy. Specific drugs to substitute were previously discussed. When this substitution does not result in achievement of the goal blood pressure, drugs from other classes are continually added until the goal is reached.

When standard therapy is not successful in achieving goal blood pressure (refractory hypertension), when a secondary cause of the hypertension is suspected, when the patient has complex concomitant conditions, or

Table 38–8. Common Combinations of Antihypertensive Drugs

Drug Combination	Brand Name
Beta-Adrenergic Blockers and Diuretics Atenolol 50 or 100 mg/chlorthalidone 25 mg	Tenoretic
Metoprolol 50 or 100 mg/hydrochlorothiazide 25 or 50 mg	Lopressor HCT
Propranolol 40–80 mg/hydrochlorothiazide 25 mg	Inderide
ACE Inhibitors and Diuretics Benazepril 5, 10, or 20 mg/hydrochlorothiazide 6.25, 12.5, or 25 mg	Lotensin HCT
Captopril 25 or 50 mg/hydrochlorothiazide 15 or 25 mg	Capozide
Enalapril 5 or 10 mg/hydrochlorothiazide 12.5 or 25 mg	Vaseretic
Lisinopril 10 or 20 mg/hydrochlorothiazide 12.5 or 25 mg	Zestoretic
Angiotensin II Receptor Antagonists and Diuretics Losartan 50 mg/hydrochlorothiazide 12.5 mg	Hyzaar
Calcium Channel Blockers and ACE Inhibitors Amlodipine 2.5 or 5 mg/benazepril 10 or 20 mg	Lotrel
Diltiazem 180 mg/enalapril 5 mg	Teczem
Felodipine 5 mg/enalapril 5 mg	Lexxel
Other Combinations Triamterene 37.5, 50, or 75 mg/hydrochlorothiazide 25 or 50 mg	Dyazide, Maxzide
Spironolactone 25 or 50 mg/hydrochlorothiazide 25 or 50 mg	Aldactazide
Hydralazine 25, 50, or 100 mg/hydrochlorothiazide 25 or 50 mg	Apresazide
Methyldopa 250 or 500 mg/hydrochlorothiazide 15, 25, 30, or 50 mg	Aldoril
Prazosin 1, 2, or 5 mg/polythiazide 0.5 mg	Minizide

when renal failure worsens even with adequate control, referral to a hypertension specialist is appropriate. Referral to a physician for immediate hospitalization is indicated with evidence of malignant hypertension (greater than 130 mm Hg diastolic reading, retinal hemorrhages, bulging disks, mental status changes, or new-onset heart failure).

Adherence Issues

Lack of adherence to a therapeutic regimen to control blood pressure is unfortunately very common. Several factors in hypertension management foster this nonadherence. Lifestyle modification is a foundation of hypertension management, and difficulty in achieving and maintaining lifestyle changes is well documented. Adverse drug reactions and drug costs are also factors in non-

adherence. Sexual dysfunction, fatigue, and depression are common adverse reactions to several classes of **antihypertensive drugs.** A systematic team approach that utilizes health professionals and community resources can assist in providing the necessary education, support, and follow-up to improve adherence. Table 38–9 details some activities that can improve adherence. Chapter 6 has additional material to improve positive outcomes.

Patient Education

Patient education should include a discussion of information related to the overall treatment plan as well as that specific to the drug therapy, reasons for the drug's being taken, drugs as part of the total treatment regimen, and adherence issues.

Table 38–9. Factors to Improve Adherence to Therapy

- Be aware of signs of patient nonadherence to antihypertensive therapy and monitor for them.

- Establish the goal of therapy jointly with the patient: to reduce blood pressure to nonhypertensive levels with minimal or no adverse effects.

- Educate patients about the disease and involve them and their families in its treatment; have them measure blood pressure at home.

- Maintain regular contact with patients; consider telecommunication.

- Keep treatment regimen as inexpensive and simple as possible.

- Encourage lifestyle modifications and provide support for them.

- Integrate drug regimen into routine activities of daily living.

- Prescribe drugs according to pharmacological principles, favoring long-acting formulations.

- Be willing to stop unsuccessful therapy and try a different approach.

- Anticipate adverse reactions and adjust therapy to prevent, minimize, or ameliorate them.

- Continue to add effective and tolerated drugs, stepwise, in sufficient doses to achieve the goals of therapy while reducing the likelihood of adverse reactions.

- Encourage a positive attitude about achieving therapeutic goals.

- Use nurse case management and a team approach.

Adapted from the National High Blood Pressure Education Program (1997). *The sixth report of the Joint National Committee on Prevention, Detection, Evaluation, and Treatment of High Blood Pressure* (NIH Publ. No. 98-4080). Rockville, MD. National Institutes of Health, National Heart, Lung and Blood Institute.

PATIENT EDUCATION

Hypertension

Related to the Overall Treatment Plan and Disease Process

☐ Pathophysiology of hypertension and its long-term effects on target organs

☐ Role of lifestyle modifications in improving prognosis and keeping the number and cost of required drugs down

☐ Importance of adherence to the treatment regimen

☐ Self-monitoring of blood pressure

☐ Indications of target organ damage

☐ Need for regular follow-up visits with the primary care provider

Specific to the Drug Therapy

☐ Reason for taking the drug(s) and the anticipated action of the drug(s) on the disease process

☐ Doses and schedules for taking the drug(s)

☐ Possible adverse reactions and what to do when they occur

☐ Coping mechanisms for complex and costly drug regimens

☐ Interaction between lifestyle modifications and these drugs

continued

PATIENT EDUCATION

Hypertension *(continued)*

Reasons for Taking the Drug(s)

Patient education about specific drugs is provided in Chapters 12 and 14. More specific information related to hypertension includes the reasons for taking the drug(s): Antihypertensive drugs are given to reduce mortality and decrease target organ damage. Some drugs do both; most do one or the other. The expectations should be clear about what the drugs can and cannot do. Hypertension is a chronic condition that rarely develops in a short space of time and is not likely to be corrected in a short space of time, if at all. Patients with hypertension must understand the lifelong nature of the disorder and the need to incorporate the treatment regimen into their everyday lives. The risk of target organ damage must be discussed, but hope must be maintained, and the potential for good quality of life with adequate treatment must be emphasized.

Drugs as Part of the Total Treatment Regimen

The total treatment regimen includes salt reduction and avoidance of excessive fluid intake. Diuretics reduce fluid volume and may interact with dietary sodium reduction, resulting in orthostatic hypotension. Care should be taken not to reduce salt and fluid too quickly. Patients should be taught to report signs and symptoms of fluid volume deficit. Sodium reduction may lead some patients to seek salt substitutes that have potassium as part of their contents. For patients taking ACE inhibitiors or ATRAs, this choice can result in excessively high potassium levels. Such salt substitutes should be avoided. Nonsalt herbal seasoning is more appropriate.

Vasodilators can produce orthostatic hypotension. Tell patients to rise slowly from a supine position to permit the body to redistribute body fluids.

Regular aerobic exercise such as walking or cycling can improve blood pressure control. Gradually increased, regular exercise may lead to improvement in blood pressure level and reduce the drug(s) needed.

Adherence Issues

Nonadherence with the treatment regimen may reduce life expectancy and affect the functioning of target organs. Health care providers should be aware of the potential problem of nonadherence, discuss the importance of adherence at each follow-up visit, and assist patients in removing barriers to adherence, such as the complexity and cost of the treatment regimen and the presence of adverse reactions.

Hypertension: Ray

Complaint

Physical examination.

History

Ray is a 49-year-old African-American man with a strong family history of hypertension. His father and brother both died at early ages from cardiac disease related to hypertension. He has no personal or family history of diabetes. He has not seen a health care provider or had his blood pressure evaluated for several years.

Assessment

His physical examination and lab work were both negative except for grade 1 retinopathy and a blood pressure of 164/104. His height is 71 inches, and his weight is 196 lb.

Initial Management Plan

Ray is diagnosed with essential hypertension after three consecutive blood pressure readings in the same range. A patient with a blood pressure of 164/104, target organ damage (grade 1 retinopathy), and another major risk factor (family history of cardiovascular disease) is classified as stage 2, risk group B. Initial therapy for Ray will be drug therapy with lifestyle modifications as adjunct therapy. His management plan is as follows:

1. Start him on low-dose diuretic therapy with hydrochlorothiazide 25 mg q A.M. African-American patients respond best to diuretic therapy as initial therapy. Starting with a low dose reduces the likelihood of adverse effects.
2. Place Ray on a low-sodium diet (2500 mg sodium). African-Americans are salt-sensitive, and even small reductions in sodium levels often decrease their blood pressure.
3. After assessment of his knowledge base about the diagnosis and its management, begin teaching for Ray and his family.
4. Draw appropriate labs (see Monitoring section of this chapter).
5. Obtain 12-lead ECG.
6. Target blood pressure is less than 140/90 mm Hg.

Follow-up Visit

At his follow-up visit 1 week later, his blood pressure was taken (150/84), and his ECG and labs were reviewed. His ECG showed mild LVH, his urinalysis had trace protein, and his serum creatinine was 1.2 mg /dL. All other data were within normal limits, and he had no abnormal heart or lung sounds. The diuretic was reducing his blood pressure but not to the target level, and new evidence was present of beginning renal target organ damage. He stated that he had experienced no significant adverse effects from the diuretics, but his diet diary indicated that he still needed more information about the low-sodium diet, as his sodium intake was more than 4 g/day.

Modifications to Management Plan

Based on the new evidence, Ray's new management plan included the following:

1. Refer Ray and his wife to a dietitian.
2. Increase his hydrochlorothiazide to 50 mg per day.
3. Teach home blood pressure monitoring.
4. Schedule follow-up visit in 4 weeks.

Continuing Care

After a 6-month trial of diet, aerobic exercise, weight loss, and hydrochlorothiazide, Ray's blood pressure was still not quite at target (146/85). A second drug had to be added. Several different classes are good choices. Beta-adrenergic blockers have cardioprotective qualities, and he has a family history of cardiovascular disease, but African-Americans respond less well to this class than do other ethnic groups. ACE inhibitors have both cardiac and renal protective qualities. Ray also has an indication of early hypertensive renal damage. African-Americans generally are low in renin genetically and do not benefit as much as other ethnic groups from ACE inhibitors. Calcium channel blockers work quite well with African-Americans, have some helpful cardiac effects in the absence of heart failure, and also have some renal protective effects. Unfortunately, a long-acting formulation must be used, the best one (diltiazem) is quite expensive in its long-acting form, his health insurance has no prescription coverage, and his financial status is such that the cost is likely to result in nonadherence. To keep his treatment regimen as simple as possible and to keep down the cost, the following plan is developed:

1. Change his once-daily drug to a combination tablet of metoprolol 50 mg (a beta blocker) and hydrochlorothiazide 50 mg (a diuretic) that must be taken bid but has a fairly low cost. In addition, metoprolol is beta$_1$ selective, so the number of adverse effects is lower.
2. Assess for adverse effects and adherence, and continue patient and family teaching.
3. Schedule a 6-month follow-up visit to review blood pressure diary, diet, and therapy.

At the next visit, Ray had achieved the target blood pressure but was still struggling to keep his sodium below 3 g per day. Recognizing that lifestyle modifications are not easy to make and that 3 g per day was significantly better than the 5 to 6 g he had been eating, he and his wife were praised for their progress and put in contact with a support group of other hypertensive patients.

REFERENCES

Aellig, W. (1998). Adverse reactions in antihypertensive therapy. *Cardiovascular Drugs and Therapy, 12,* 189–196.

Andersen, P., Seljeflot, I., Herzog, A., Arnesen, H., Hyermann, I., & Holme, I. (1998). Effects of doxazocin and atenolol on atherothrombogenic risk profile in hypertensive middle-aged men. *Journal of Cardiovascular Pharmacology, 31*(5), 677–683.

Barker, W., Mullooly, J., & Linton, K. (1998). Trends in hypertension prevalence, treatment, and control in a well-defined older population. *Hypertension, 31*(2), 552–559.

Brogden, R., & Wiseman, L. (1998). Moexipril: A review of its use in the management of essential hypertension. *Drugs, 55*(6), 845–860.

Higashi, Y., Oshima, T., Sasaki, S., Nakano, Y., Kambe, M., Matsuura, H., & Kajiyama, G. (1998). Angiotensin-converting enzyme inhibition, but not calcium antagonism, improves a response of the renal vasculature to L-arginine in patients with essential hypertension. *Hypertension, 32*(1), 16–24.

Katzung, B. (1998). *Basic and clinical pharmacology* (7th ed.). Stamford, CT: Appleton & Lange.

Mancia, G., Failla, M., Grazappiolo, A., & Giannattasio, C. (1998). Present and future role of combination treatment in hypertension. *Journal of Cardiovascular Pharmacology, 31*(Suppl. 2), S41–S44.

Messerli, F., Grossman, E., & Goldbourt, U. (1998). Are beta-blockers efficacious as first-line therapy for hypertension in the elderly? *Journal of the American Medical Association, 279*(23), 1903–1907.

Mourad, J., Girerd, X., Boutouyrie, P., Safar, M., & Laurent, S. (1998). Opposite effects of remodeling and hypertrophy on arterial compliance in hypertension. *Hypertension, 31*(2), 529–533.

National Cholesterol Education Program. (1993). *Second report of the expert panel on detection, evaluation, and treatment of high blood cholesterol in adults (Adult Treatment Panel II).* NIH Publ. No. 93-3095. Rockville, MD: National Institutes of Health, National Heart, Lung, and Blood Institute.

National High Blood Pressure Education Program. (1997). The sixth report of the Joint National Committee on Prevention, Detection, Evaluation, and Treatment of High Blood Pressure (NIH Publ. No. 98–4080). Rockville, MD: National Institutes of Health, National Heart, Lung, and Blood Institute.

Papademetrious, V., Prisant, L., Neutel, J., & Weit, M. (1998). Efficacy of low-dose combination of bisoprolol/hydrochlorothiazide compared with amlodipine and enalapril in men and women with essential hypertension. *American Journal of Cardiology, 81,* 1363–1365.

Parati, G., Ulian, L., Santucciu, C., Omboni, S., & Mancia, G. (1998). Difference between clinic and daytime blood pressure is not a measure of the white coat effect. *Hypertension, 31*(5), 1185–1189.

Sadowski, A., & Redeker, N. (1996). The hypertensive elder: A review for the primary care provider. *Nurse Practitioner, 21*(5), 99–112.

Sever, P. (1998). The heterogeneity of hypertension: Why doesn't every patient respond to every hypertensive drug? *Journal of Cardiovascular Pharmacology, 31*(Suppl. 2), S1–S4.

Systolic Hypertension in the Elderly Cooperative Research Group. (1991). Prevention of stroke by antihypertensive drug treatment in older persons with isolated systolic hypertension. *Journal of the American Medical Association, 265,* 3255.

Thrift, A., McNeil, J. Forbes, A., & Donnan, G. (1998). Three important subgroups of hypertensive persons at greater risk of intracerebral hemorrhage. *Hypertension, 31,* 1223–1229.

Weir, M., Chrysant, S., McCarron, D., Canossa-Terris, M., Cohen, J., Gunter, P., Lewin, A., Mennella, R., Kirkegaard, L., Hamilton, J., Weinberger, M., & Weder, A. (1998). Influence of race and dietary salt on the antihypertensive efficacy of an angiotensin-converting enzyme inhibitor or a calcium channel antagonist in salt-sensitive hypertensives. *Hypertension, 31,* 1088–1096.

Weir, M., Gray, J., Paster, R., & Saunders, E. (1995). Differing mechanisms of action of angiotensin converting enzyme inhibition in black and white hypertensive patients. *Hypertension, 26*(1), 124–130.

CHAPTER 39

·······

Hyperthyroidism and Hypothyroidism

T hyroid disorders are among the most common disease processes seen in primary care. Untreated clinical or subclinical thyroid disease can result in long-term complications in every body system, especially the cardiovascular system.

In children, hyperthyroidism can produce car-diomegaly and heart failure. In adolescents, it can interfere with normal growth, and in older adults it is associated with heart failure and osteoporosis. Untreated hyperthyroidism in pregnancy increases the risk for first-trimester spontaneous abortion, stillbirths, and neonatal mortality. Hyperthyroidism is seen in 2 percent of all women and in one-tenth as many men. It is most common in ages 20 to 40.

In children, hypothyroidism can result in decreased mental and physical growth. In adults, it increases the risk for heart disease related to altered lipoprotein metabolism. Hypothyroidism is also more common in women, with a prevalence of 6 per 1000, but its prevalence increases with aging. Approximately 5 percent of older adults manifest evidence of hypothyroidism. Although there are many other thyroid disorders, these two are the most prevalent and are the focus of this chapter.

Treatment for these two disorders includes lifestyle management and drug therapy. Pharmacological management includes **synthetic thyroid hormones, antithyroid agents** such as **propylthiouracil (PTU), methimazole (Tapazole),** and **radioactive iodine (I 131).** These drugs are discussed in detail in Chapter 19. Symptom management may also include other drugs, such as **beta-adrenergic blockers,** which are discussed in Chapter 12. This chapter discusses the management of hyperthyroidism and hypothyroidism that is usually done by primary care providers.

Thyroid Hormone Synthesis

The synthesis of thyroid hormones is dependent on the functioning of the hypothalamic-pituitary-thyroid axis. Synthesis begins with the secretion of thyrotropin-releasing hormone (TRH) by the hypothalamus in response to cold, stress, and decreased levels of thyroxine (T_4). TRH stimulates the synthesis and release of thyroid-stimulating hormone (TSH) by the anterior pituitary. TSH, in turn, stimulates the production of thyroid hormones. Thyroid hormones (T_4 and T_3) are synthesized from iodine and tyrosine molecules by follicular cells in the thyroid gland. T_4 can be converted to T_3 peripherally when additional thyroid hormone is needed. In fact, 80 percent of circulating T_3 is the result of peripheral conversion from T_4. Conversion of T_4 to T_3 is stimulated by cold temperatures and stress. Conversion is inhibited by acute and chronic illness, starvation, and some drugs. Table 39–1 shows drugs that have clinically significant effects on thyroid function. T_4 and T_3 in plasma are reversibly bound to protein, mainly thyroxine-binding globulin. Only a small portion (0.04% of total T_4 and 0.4% of total T_3) exists in a free form, and only this free form is clinically active. The amount of active thyroid hormone in the plasma produces a feedback loop that inhibits or further stimulates TRH and TSH secretion to decrease or increase thyroid hormone production. This mechanism is depicted in Chapter 19.

Thyroid Function Tests

Several thyroid function tests can be used to evaluate thyroid function. These tests and their normal values are

Table 39–1. Drug Effects on Thyroid Function

Drug	Effect on Thyroid Function
Amiodarone	• Releases iodine as drug is metabolized • Inhibits peripheral conversion of T_4 to T_3 • Can produce thyrotoxicosis
Carbamazepine	Increases metabolism of T_4, resulting in decreased total T_4
Estrogen	Increases thyroid-binding globulin levels
Glucocorticoids	Impair basal and TRH-stimulated TSH concentration
Levodopa	Chronic administration displaces thyroid hormone from thyroid-binding globulin, resulting in suppressed TSH response
Lithium	Blocks iodine uptake by thyroid gland, resulting in decreased hormone production
Phenytoin	• Decreases TSH response to TRG by 50% • Enhances cellular uptake and metabolism of T_4, resulting in decreased total T_4
Propranolol	Inhibits peripheral conversion of T_4 to T_3
Salicylates (in doses > 4 g/d)	Suppress TSH response by inhibiting binding of T_4 and T_3 to thyroid-binding globulin
Theophylline	Beta-adrenergic stimulation of hypothalamus results in increased TSH response

Table 39–2. Thyroid Function Tests

Test	Normal Value	Values in Hyperthyroidism	Values in Hypothyroidism
Free thyroxine index (FT$_4$I)	1.3–4.2	High	Low
Free triiodothyronine index (FT$_3$I)	22–56	High	Normal or low
Free T$_4$ (FT$_4$)	0.7–1.86 ng/dL (9–24 pmol/L)	High	Low
Free T$_3$ (FT$_3$)	0.2–0.52 ng/dL (3–8 pmol/L)	High	Low
Thyrotropin-stimulating hormone (TSH)	0.3–5 mU/mL	Low	High
Thyrotropin-releasing hormone (TRH)	>6 µU/mL in serum TSH 45 min after injection; blunted TSH response (<2 µU/mL) in patients >age 40	No response	Exaggerated rise

listed in Table 39–2. The most commonly used tests in primary care are TSH and free T$_4$ values. The sensitive or ultrasensitive forms of the TSH test should be used to avoid missing subclinical conditions.

Hyperthyroidism

Pathophysiology

Hyperthyroidism, also known as *thyrotoxicosis*, occurs when there is a breakdown in the feedback loop and the body's tissues are exposed to excessive levels of thyroid hormone. The cause of this excessive secretion may be a hyperfunctioning thyroid nodule, anterior pituitary disorders, toxic multinodular goiter, or thyroiditis, including postpartum thyroiditis (McDermott, 1998; Schilling, 1997). By far the most common etiology is Graves' disease, which accounts for 60 to 90 percent of all hyperthyroidism. Graves' disease is an autoimmune disorder characterized by abnormal IgG autoantibodies that bind to TSH receptors and activate excessive glandular growth and hormone production.

Regardless of the etiology of hyperthyroidism, the clinical features are attributable to the metabolic effects of increased circulating levels of thyroid hormone. These effects include heat intolerance and increased sensitivity to stimulation by the sympathetic division of the autonomic nervous system. Table 39–3 shows the most common systemic effects of hyperthyroidism.

Pharmacodynamics

Antithyroid drugs reduce the production of thyroid hormones. **PTU** and **methimazole** inhibit the synthesis of new thyroid hormone by the thyroid gland but do not inactivate existing or stored hormone. **PTU** also inhibits the peripheral conversion of T$_4$ to T$_3$. Neither of these drugs treats the underlying pathophysiology of hyperthyroidism. A treatment trial of at least 1 year is required, but only 20 percent of patients treated with at least 1 year of therapy go into spontaneous remission. Dosing schedules for these two drugs are provided in Chapter 19. Both drugs are inexpensive and relatively free of adverse reactions.

Beta-adrenergic blockers address the symptoms of hyperthyroidism by decreasing the sympathetic stimulation from the autonomic nervous system. The most commonly prescribed drugs in this class are **propranolol**, because of its short half-life, and **atenolol**, because of its once-daily dosing. **Propranolol** is the less expensive of the two, but neither is very expensive. The drugs are gradually withdrawn as the patient becomes euthyroid. Dosing schedules for this indication are discussed later in this chapter.

Iodides block peripheral conversion of T$_4$ to T$_3$ and inhibit hormone release. **Potassium iodide** was the earliest of the **iodides** to be used for this purpose. It is mainly restricted to preoperative preparation before thyroid surgery. Doses are discussed later in this chapter.

Goals of Treatment

The goal of therapy for patients with hyperthyroidism is correction of the hypermetabolic state, with a minimum of adverse reactions and with the smallest incidence of hypothyroidism. This means symptom relief and normalization of TSH and free T$_4$ levels. **Beta-adrenergic blockers** can produce this effect in the short term, but definitive therapy usually requires at least the addition of **antithyroid agents**.

Table 39–3. Systemic Effects of Hyperthyroidism

Body System	Clinical Manifestation	Underlying Mechanism
Cardiovascular	Increased cardiac output, decreased peripheral vascular resistance, tachycardia at rest, arrhythmias	Increased metabolism and need to dissipate heat
Respiratory	Dyspnea and reduced vital capacity	Weakness of respiratory muscles
Gastrointestinal	• Increased appetite with concurrent weight loss • Diarrhea, nausea, vomiting, abdominal pain • Decreased serum lipid levels • Decreased tissue stores of glucose, protein, and vitamins	Increased utilization of carbohydrates, proteins, and fats to support rapid metabolism Increased peristalsis and cholesterol conversion salts Malabsorption of fat, fat stores depleted for energy, increased excretion of cholesterol in feces Increased glucose utilization, use of protein as energy source, and impaired conversion of B vitamins to their coenzymes, causing an increased need for water- and fat-soluble vitamins
Integumentary	• Excessive sweating, flushing, warm skin • Temporary hair loss; hair fine, soft, and straight; nails grow away from nail beds	Need to dissipate heat Hyperdynamic circulatory state
Reproductive	Oligomenorrhea or amenorrhea in women; impotence or decreased libido in men	Hypothalamic or pituitary disturbances; increased production of sex hormone–binding globulin
Neurological	• Restlessness, short attention span, fatigue, insomnia, emotional lability • Ocular manifestations, including decreased blinking and fine tremor of the lid	Alteration in cerebral metabolism Hyperactivity of sympathetic nervous system
Musculoskeletal	• Hypercalcemia • Loss of muscle mass	Excessive bone resorption Excessive protein catabolism
Endocrine	• Enlarged gland; systolic or continuous bruit of thyroid gland • Diminished sensitivity to exogenous insulin	Hyperactivity of the gland and increased circulation to support that hyperactivity Increased insulin degradation

Rational Drug Selection

It is not within the scope of this book to discuss the testing involved in the diagnosis of hyperthyroidism. The treatment protocol discussed here assumes appropriate diagnostic tools, including laboratory data, and accurate diagnosis of the disorder. Once the diagnosis has been made, treatment regimens are determined.

Three main avenues of treatment are used for patients with hyperthyroidism: (1) **antithyroid drugs,** (2) **radioactive iodine,** and (3) surgery. Because **radioactive iodine** and surgery are usually the province of physicians, this chapter discusses **antithyroid drugs** and **beta-adrenergic blockers. Iodides** are sometimes useful as supplemental drugs and are discussed in this minor role.

Lifestyle Management

Lifestyle management is diet-related. The thyroid gland requires adequate amounts of iodine to produce thyroid hormones. In a hyperthyroid state, iodine is especially important, and patients should be taught how to include adequate iodine in their diets. Additionally, the potential for nutritional deficits is high, related to the hypermetabolic state. A high-calorie (4000 to 5000 kcal/day) may be necessary to satisfy hunger and prevent tissue breakdown. To provide this number of calories, six meals a day may be required, as well as snacks that are high in protein, carbohydrates, minerals, and vitamins, particularly vitamins A, B_6, and ascorbic acid. Caffeinated fluids and highly seasoned food should be avoided because they augment the symptoms of hyperthyroidism.

Drug Therapy

Choices in drug therapy are based on patient variables (severity of the disease, duration of the disease, age of the patient, pregnancy, and the likelihood of patient adherence to the treatment regimen) and on drug-related variables (cost and adverse reactions). Figure 39–1 depicts drug choices based on these variables.

Patient Variables

SEVERITY OF DISEASE. **Antithyroid drugs** are prescribed with the intent of achieving spontaneous remission of the disease. Patients most likely to achieve remission are those with mild disease and small goiters. Because these drugs do not inhibit the action of existing or stored thyroid hormone, clinical response typically takes 4 to 8 weeks. **PTU** is available in 50-mg tablets, and the dose varies from 150 to 300 mg daily. Because of its short half-life, the dose is divided and taken three times daily. **Methimazole** comes in 5- and 10-mg tablets, and dosing is usually started at 15 mg daily. Its longer half-life means that once-daily dosing may be tried. **Beta-adrenergic blockers** may be added temporarily to reduce symptoms while the patient is awaiting clinical response to the **antithyroid drugs**. Adequate doses of these drugs are determined by measuring resting and exercising heart rates and degree of symptom relief.

DURATION OF DISEASE. Beta-adrenergic blockers provide excellent symptomatic relief for transient disorders such as thyroiditis because spontaneous remission is the rule. **Aspirin, nonsteroidal anti-inflammatory drugs (NSAIDs)**, and **corticosteroids** may also be used in subacute thyroiditis to control inflammatory symptoms. These drugs are equally useful for postpartum thyroiditis, when they are given for 3 months. Dosage is based on symptom relief.

Graves' disease is of longer duration. Endocrinologists do not agree on the best treatment for Graves' disease, except in the case of older adults and cardiac patients, for whom **radioactive iodine** is the treatment of choice. For younger or middle-aged patients, an initial 1-year trial of **antithyroid drugs** is considered a reasonable starting point for treatment. Both drugs are equally useful. **PTU** has some peripheral activity, but this effect does not appear to be clinically significant except at high doses, where it is especially useful for severe hyperthyroidism and thyroid storm. **PTU** is initiated at 300 mg daily in three equally divided doses given 8 hours apart. Patients with severe disease may require 400 mg daily. Maintenance doses are 100 to 150 mg daily. **Methimazole** is commonly initiated at 20 to 30 mg daily. One advantage to **methimazole** is that doses may be divided and given every 8 hours, or once-daily dosing may be tried. Once-daily dosing reduces the complexity of the

treatment regimen. Once control of symptoms and appropriate levels of thyroid hormone production are achieved, the doses of both drugs can be tapered to the lowest amount needed to maintain a euthyroid state. Treatment is continued for 12 to 24 months and then stopped to see if a relapse occurs. Relapse is more common for patients treated less than 12 months. Patients who fail to achieve control of symptoms with **antithyroid drugs,** who are unable to tolerate the therapy, or who experience a relapse after completion of therapy are candidates for **radioactive iodine** or surgery.

The treatment regimen often includes supplementation with **beta blockers** for symptom relief. The common dose for **atenolol** is 50 mg/day, and for **propranolol** it is 20 to 40 mg qid. **Atenolol** offers the advantages of fewer adverse reactions, based on its beta$_1$ selectivity, and once-daily dosing for patients who are less adherent if the regimen is too complex. **Propranolol** is less expensive and offers the advantage of peripheral blockage of conversion of T$_4$ to T$_3$.

AGE OF PATIENT. Older adults are treated with **radioactive iodine.** They may be pretreated with **antithyroid drugs** to bring them closer to euthyroid status before **radioactive iodine** therapy is initiated. Younger and middle-aged patients are discussed in the previous section.

Some endocrinologists prefer **antithyroid drug** therapy in childhood Graves' disease (AACE, 1995). There are children's doses for both drugs, but the preferred drug is **PTU**. Dosage schedules for both **methimazole** and **PTU** are shown in Chapter 19. Treatment lasts 6 to 18 months; most patients are treated for at least 1 year. As with adults, relapse is less likely with the longer duration of therapy.

PREGNANCY. *Radioactive iodine is contraindicated during pregnancy because it crosses the placenta. Antithyroid drugs are the treatment of choice, even though both cross the placenta and they are listed as Pregnancy Category D. Because the amount of drug that crosses the placenta is low with PTU, it is clearly preferred over methimazole. The lowest-possible dose of PTU is used to keep the mother's thyroid function at the upper limit of normal. Pregnancy itself has an ameliorating effect on Graves' disease, so that the dose of drug required usually decreases as the pregnancy progresses. In some cases, the drug can be withdrawn 2 to 3 weeks before delivery.*

Pregnant women with Graves' disease may transfer large amounts of thyroid-stimulating antibody to the fetus and induce fetal thyrotoxicosis. The infant's thyroid function should be tested at birth.

Postpartum patients who are receiving **antithyroid drugs** should consult their provider before choosing to nurse their infants. Breast milk can transfer **antithyroid drugs;** however, the amount is small, especially with **PTU,** and unlikely to induce significant hypothyroidism.

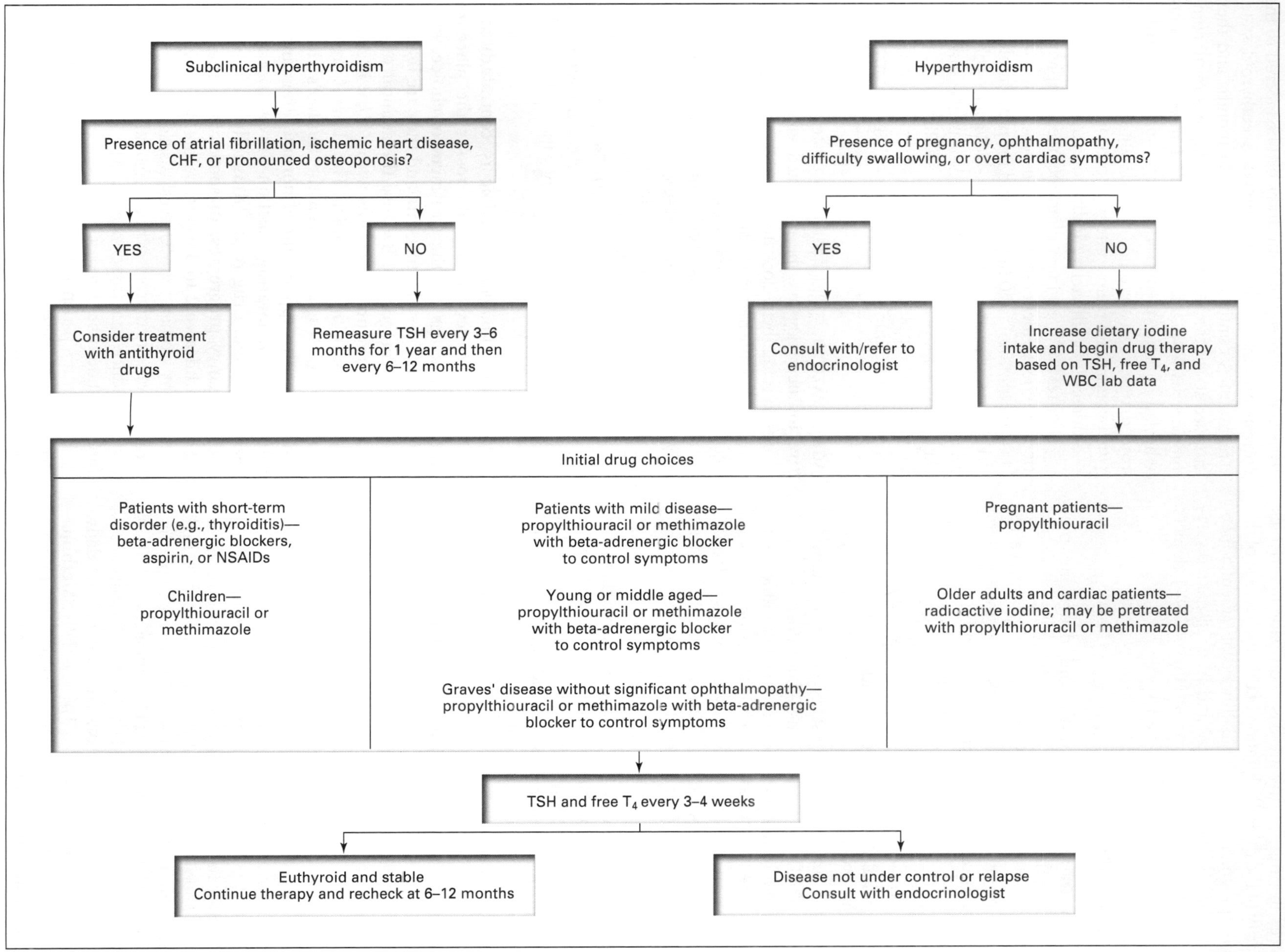

Hyperthyroidism

Presence of pregnancy, ophthalmopathy, difficulty swallowing, or overt cardiac symptoms?

NO

YES

Increase dietary iodine intake and begin drug therapy based on TSH, free T$_4$, and WBC lab data

Consult with/refer to endocrinologist

Initial drug choices

Pregnant patients—propylthiouracil

Older adults and cardiac patients—radicactive iodine; may be pretreated with propylthioruracil or methimazole

Patients with mild disease—propylthiouracil or methimazole with beta-adrenergic blocker to control symptoms

Young or middle aged—propylthiouracil or methimazole with beta-adrenergic blocker to control symptoms

Graves' disease without significant ophthalmopathy—propylthiouracil or methimazole with beta-adrenergic blocker to control symptoms

TSH and free T$_4$ every 3–4 weeks

Disease not under control or relapse Consult with endocrinologist

Euthyroid and stable Continue therapy and recheck at 6–12 months

Subclinical hyperthyroidism

Presence of atrial fibrillation, ischemic heart disease, CHF, or pronounced osteoporosis?

NO

YES

Remeasure TSH every 3–6 months for 1 year and then every 6–12 months

Consider treatment with antithyroid drugs

Patients with short-term disorder (e.g., thyroiditis)—beta-adrenergic blockers, aspirin, or NSAIDs

Children—propylthiouracil or methimazole

Figure 39–1. Drug therapy algorithm: Hyperthyroidism.

The potential risk should be discussed, and careful monitoring of mother and infant is important.

ADHERENCE.   Drug treatment is effective only if the drugs are taken as prescribed. Adherence to a treatment regimen is less likely if it is complex or leads to significant adverse reactions. **Antithyroid drugs** have limited adverse reactions but may need to be taken three times daily, making the treatment regimen complex. This complexity is especially problematic if the treatment regimen also involves a **beta-adrenergic blocker** that has significant adverse reactions and must also be taken three times daily but on a different schedule. To facilitate adherence, **methimazole** and **atenolol** both can be given once daily, and both have fewer adverse reactions than other drugs in their classes.

Drug-Related Variables

COST.   According to Goroll, May, and Mulley (1995), at doses up to 30 mg/day, **methimazole** is about 30 percent less expensive than a comparable dose of **PTU**. Other sources (Kastrup, 1998) rate **methimazole** as more expensive than **PTU**. Cost appears to be a significant variable, but the prices must be assessed at local pharmacies to determine which is less expensive.

ADVERSE REACTIONS.   A rare (0.3 to 0.6%) but potentially fatal complication of **antithyroid drug** therapy is agranulocytosis. The risk for this adverse reaction increases with age, beginning at about age 40, and is dose-independent for **PTU** and dose-dependent for **methimazole**. Patients taking less than 30 mg/day of **methimazole** have not experienced this adverse reaction, making it the safer of the two drugs.

In summary, properly monitored, either **PTU** or **methimazole** is a reasonable choice for therapy. **PTU** is preferred for specific indications, and **methimazole** is preferred on the basis of hematologic adverse reactions and ease of administration.

Preoperative Preparation

In addition to consideration of selected variables, all of these drugs can be used in preparation for thyroid surgery. Preoperative administration of **antithyroid drugs** is required to avoid precipitating thyroid storm. Doses are similar to those used to treat the disease. Six to 8 weeks of preoperative treatment is required. **Beta-adrenergic blockers** may also be prescribed and have the advantage that only 1 to 2 weeks of preoperative therapy is required. **Atenolol,** with its more sustained half-life, is particularly useful. The addition of **potassium iodide** to **beta-blocker** therapy produces more rapid and greater preoperative control. This combination is especially use-ful for patients who must undergo surgery fairly quickly and for those who fail to achieve control (resting pulse of less than 90 beats per minute) on **beta blockers** alone. The **iodide** dose is 2 to 6 drops of solution mixed in a full glass of fruit juice, water, broth, or milk tid for 10 days before surgery. Administration with meals minimizes gastrointestinal irritation.

Ophthalmopathy

Although ophthalmopathy is caused by a different mechanism from that which causes hyperthyroidism, it is a common concurrent problem for patients with Graves' disease. Approximately 20 percent of patients with eye involvement that predates the treatment of their hyperthyroidism experience an exacerbation after treatment is initiated (Goroll, May, & Mulley, 1995). Successful treatment of hyperthyroidism does not appear to make the eye condition worse, but treatment-induced hypothyroidism seems to increase the risk for worsening the eye disorder. **Radioactive iodine** has the highest risk for post-treatment hypothyroidism, with up to 50 percent of patients becoming hypothyroid (McDermott, 1998). **Antithyroid drugs** are much less likely to result in post-treatment hypothyroidism and are often chosen in preference to other therapies for patients with ophthalmopathy.

Monitoring

Monitoring therapy includes attention to clinical status and thyroid function test results. Clinical status is assessed by watching weight, degree of heat tolerance, appetite, anxiety level, energy level, resting heart rate, and skin texture and temperature. For patients with ophthalmopathy, assessment also includes this symptom. The same tests that are used to diagnose hyperthyroidism are used to monitor the effectiveness of treatment. The amount of circulating thyroid hormone is monitored by changes in TSH and free T_4. TSH is the best outcome measure because the goal is normalization of TSH. It also provides the earliest evidence of overtreatment or development of hypothyroidism.

Initially, patients are seen every 3 to 4 weeks, and TSH and free T_4 levels are drawn at these times until they are euthyroid. Once the patient is stable and euthyroid, the frequency of visits and thyroid testing is extended to 6 months and then annually, based on symptom relief.

Pregnant patients are usually monitored by an endocrinologist. When a primary care provider is monitoring them, thyroid function tests must be done at each monthly visit because the progression of pregnancy is associated with decreased thyroid hormone production, and dosage adjustments are commonly required. Pregnant patients with Graves' disease may have thyroid-stimulating antibodies in their circulation that can cross the placenta and affect the fetus. Measurement of maternal thyroid-stimulating antibody may be useful to assess potential fetal risk (American Association of Clinical Endocrinologists, 1995).

Close monitoring of white blood cell (WBC) counts is important during the first 4 months of therapy. Mild leukopenia is common, occurring in up to 10 percent of patients. Although it does not require discontinuance of the drug, leukocyte counts below 1500 mm^3 are indications for stopping therapy (Goroll, May, & Mulley, 1995). Agranulocytosis, a rare but potentially fatal adverse reaction, usually occurs within 2 months and rarely beyond 4 months after initiation of therapy with **antithyroid drugs.** Monitoring the leukocyte count is not very helpful in relation to this disorder because onset is rapid. It is prudent, however, to obtain a baseline WBC count before initiating therapy.

Outcome Evaluation

Figure 39–1 shows the drug treatment protocol for hyperthyroidism. Evaluation is based on reduction of clinical symptoms and normalization of TSH and free T$_4$ levels. The main indications for substituting a different treatment modality (surgery) or a different drug (**radioactive iodine**) for **antithyroid drugs** are a patient's failure to achieve control of symptoms with **antithyroid drugs,** a patient's inability to tolerate the therapy, and relapse after completion of therapy with **antithyroid drugs.**

Consultation with or referral to an endocrinologist is sometimes appropriate:

1. Refer a patient who requires surgery or **radioactive iodine** therapy. These patients require hospitalization and a thyroid scan, and the endocrinologist can order these and work with the surgeon.
2. Hyperthyroidism during pregnancy presents special concerns and is best managed by a clinical endocrinologist (AACE, 1995) or in consultation with an endocrinologist. Lactating women also are best managed with at least consultation with an endocrinologist.
3. Patients with severe ophthalmopathy associated with Graves' disease also require consultation or referral, depending on the degree of symptoms. Visual impairment may require hospitalization and very high dose **corticosteroid** therapy or surgical decompression.
4. Referral is also considered when the patient has an obstruction to swallowing or desires cosmetic improvement that may require surgery.
5. "Prompt hospital admission is needed if heart failure, rapid atrial fibrillation or angina develops" (Goroll, May, & Mulley, 1995, p. 571).

Patient Education

Patient education should include discussion of information related to the overall treatment plan, as well as that specific to the drug therapy, reasons for taking the drug, drugs as part of the total treatment regimen, and adherence issues.

Hypothyroidism

Pathophysiology

The underlying mechanisms that cause hypothyroidism can be primary or secondary. Primary disorders are based on the hypothalamic-pituitary-thyroid gland feedback system and occur when the hypothalamus responds to a decreased thyroid hormone level with an increase in TRH, resulting in increased TSH secretion, which in turn stimulates thyroid gland enlargement, goiter formation, and preferential synthesis of T$_3$ over T$_4$. Of all patients with hypothyroidism, 95 percent have primary thyroid disease (Heitman & Irizarry, 1995). In secondary disorders, the TSH response is inadequate, so that the gland is normal or reduced in size, and both T$_3$ and T$_4$ synthesis are equally reduced.

Primary Disease

Hashimoto's thyroiditis is an immune-mediated disorder in which all components of the thyroid gland are injured, but especially the TSH receptors. Antibodies generated to attack glandular antigens impair TSH response, hormone synthesis, and hormone release. Most patients with this disorder have mild disease and may remain euthyroid. Approximately 70 percent go on to develop permanent hypothyroidism.

A common variant of this disorder is postpartum thyroiditis, which may affect up to 5 percent of postpartum women. Antibody production in this disorder peaks in 3 to 4 months after delivery and then declines. Symptoms resolve spontaneously, and most patients return to euthyroid states.

Congenital hypothyroidism occurs in infants as a result of absent thyroid tissue (thyroid dysgenesis) and hereditary defects in thyroid hormone synthesis. It is more common in female infants. Because thyroid hormone is essential for embryonic growth, especially of brain tissue, an infant with no T$_4$ during fetal life will be mentally retarded. This condition can largely be reversed with administration of T$_4$ immediately after birth. Capillary blood screening of all infants in the United States and Canada before discharge from the hospital or birthing center tests for this disorder. Infants suspected of the disorder are referred immediately to a pediatric endocrinologist.

PATIENT EDUCATION

Hyperthyroidism

Related to the Overall Treatment Plan and Disease Process

☐ Understanding the pathophysiology of hyperthyroidism and its prognosis
☐ Role of iodine intake in thyroid hormone production
☐ Importance of adherence to the treatment regimen
☐ Need to take the drug for at least 1 year
☐ Indications of relapse or complications that need to be reported
☐ Importance of discussing pregnancy or the potential for pregnancy with the primary care provider
☐ Need for regular follow-up visits with the primary care provider

Specific to the Drug Therapy

☐ Discussion of the reasons for taking the drug(s) and the anticipated action of the drug(s) on the disease process. It is especially important to inform the patient that antithyroid drugs take 4 to 8 weeks to have a noticeable effect.
☐ Doses and schedules for taking the drug(s).
☐ Possible adverse reactions and what to do when they occur.
☐ Patient education specific to antithyroid drugs is provided in Chapter 19.
☐ Patient education specific to beta-adrenergic blockers is provided in Chapter 12.

Endemic iodine deficiency has not been a problem in the United States since the early 1900s. The addition of iodine to table salt has largely eliminated this form of hypothyroidism.

Secondary Disease

Secondary hypothyroidism most commonly is a result of a pituitary disorder. The net result is inadequate TSH production, and the thyroid gland does not produce either thyroid hormone. Common disorders of the pituitary that are associated with secondary hypothyroidism include Cushing's syndrome, acromegaly, and pituitary adenomas.

Other secondary causes of hypothyroidism include the administration of drugs that reduce thyroid hormone production (see Table 39–1) and treatment or overtreatment of hyperthyroidism.

Regardless of the etiology of hypothyroidism, the clinical features are attributable to the metabolic effects of decreased circulating levels of thyroid hormone. These effects include decreased energy metabolism and heat production. The patient develops a low basal metabolic rate, cold intolerance, lethargy, and a slightly lowered body temperature. Table 39–4 shows the most common systemic effects of hypothyroidism.

Pharmacodynamics

For patients who are clinically hypothyroid, replacement therapy with thyroid hormones is indicated. Administration of **synthetic thyroid hormones (levothyroxine [T_4], liothyronine [T_3], and liotrix** [a 4:1 mixture of T_4 and T_3]) produces the same effects on body tissues as the body's own thyroid hormones, including the negative feedback required to reduce further secretion of TSH. Dosing schedules for these drugs are provided in Chapter 19. These drugs are inexpensive and relatively free of adverse reactions, but there are conditions (discussed later in this chapter) in which they are contraindicated or used with caution.

Goals of Treatment

The goal of therapy for patients with hypothyroidism is correction of the hypometabolic state with a minimum of adverse reactions. Adequate replacement should result in resolution of fatigue, loss of excess weight, improved functioning of all body systems, and prevention of complications, especially cardiovascular and neurological ones. This means normalization of TSH and free T_4 levels.

Hyperthyroidism

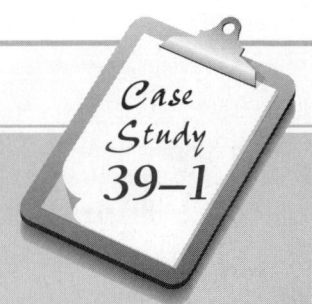

Complaint

"I've been feeling more fatigued and short of breath when I run."

History

Linda Allen is a 25-year-old married white woman. She is a buyer for a large department store. She recently moved to accept a significant promotion. Since moving, she noticed that she has become tense and irritable. She attributed this at first to the stress of her new job. She has also noticed sensitivity to heat and increased perspiration. She has recently lost 10 pounds and has occasional bouts of diarrhea. Linda noticed that she seems to have a fine tremor in both hands. Normally, she jogs 3 to 5 miles a day but has had to stop because of increasing fatigue and dyspnea. Sometimes her heart starts pounding and when she takes her pulse it is between 110 and140 bpm. These symptoms have caused her to come to the clinic. She belongs to an HMO and has regular physical exams and prophylactic medical and dental care. She has no children, but would like to become pregnant.

Assessment

Her physical examination reveals a regular pulse of 102 and respiratory rate of 18. Her blood pressure is 130/60. Her skin is smooth, moist, and slightly flushed. Her hair is fine and friable. Her thyroid gland is palpable and slightly enlarged. A grade II-III systolic murmur is heard over the aortic and pulmonic area. Her deep tendon reflexes are 3+/4+. She has no ophthalmopathy, and the rest of her physical examination is within normal limits.

Her laboratory data reveal a TSH of <0.1 mU/mL and a free T_4 of 5 ng/dL. Her WBC is 6000. Other laboratory values are within normal limits although her potassium is 3.5 mEq/L, her sodium is 135 mEq/L, and her calcium is 8.5 mg/dL.

Initial Management Plan

After a complete workup, Linda is diagnosed with hyperthyroidism. Because she has no ophthalmopathy and her disease state is of recent onset, drug therapy is chosen to manage her disease process. After consultation with an endocrinologist, her initial management plan is:

1. Start propylthiouracil 100 mg PO q8h. This drug is chosen because Linda is sexually active and has the potential to become pregnant. Pregnancy and the risk associated with treating hyperthyroidism while pregnant are discussed. She chooses to postpone trying to become pregnant at this time, but pregnancy can occur even with the best planning. Stress the need to take the drug consistently and that the length of treatment will be at least 1 year. She is to immediately report any sore throat or fever.

2. Start atenolol 50 mg daily. Atenolol is a beta$_1$ selective beta-adrenergic blocker that is useful in treating the symptoms until the propylthiouracil can exert full effect. It is chosen because of its once-daily dosing and because she has cardiac symptoms associated with her hyperthyroidism.

3. Discuss iodine intake and need for increased calories. Her goal is to gain back the 10 pounds she lost. To evaluate attainment of this goal, she is to weigh twice weekly. Daily weights are good assessments of fluid status, but nutritional weight gain usually takes more than 1 day.

4. Suggest daily multivitamin capsule with minerals. She drinks 2 to 3 cups of coffee a day. She is counseled to change to a caffeine-free beverage.

5. Over-the-counter antidiarrheals such as Pepto-Bismol may be used for the occasional bouts of diarrhea.

6. After assessment of her knowledge base about hyperthyroidism and its management, begin appropriate teaching.

Follow-up Visit

At her follow-up appointment in 3 weeks, Linda reports that her symptoms are improving. She has gained 2 pounds. Her TSH is now 0.2 mU/mL, her free T_4 is 3 ng/dL, and her WBC is 5500. Her thyroid function is improving, but she is still not euthyroid.

Modifications to the Treatment Plan

1. Begin a taper program for the atenolol with a goal to have her stop taking it in 3 weeks. (See Chapter 12 for an appropriate taper.)

2. Continue her propylthiouracil at the same dose.

3. Draw serum electrolyte labs. Her potassium at this visit is 3.8 mEq/L. That is an improvement but still requires monitoring.

4. Schedule a follow-up visit in 4 weeks. Have Linda contact the clinic if symptoms return as she reduces the atenolol.

Continuing Care

Four weeks later, lab values are euthyroid and she is asymptomatic. Her dose of propylthiouracil is decreased to 50 mg q8h which will be continued for the next 12 months. She will continue to come to the clinic for TSH and WBC counts every 4 weeks for the next 2 months and will be seen at 6 months and 12 months from initiation of therapy and then annually. Decisions regarding stopping therapy at 12 months to assess for possible remission will be made at that time

Table 39–4. Systemic Effects of Hypothyroidism

Body System	Clinical Manifestation	Underlying Mechanism
Cardiovascular	Reduced stroke volume and heart rate (reduced cardiac output); increased peripheral vascular resistance to maintain blood pressure; decreased blood flow to tissue; sinus bradycardia; ECG changes	Decreased metabolic demands and loss of regulatory and rate-setting effects of thyroid hormone.
Hematologic	Decreased red blood cell mass (normocytic/ normochromic anemia); macrocytic anemia associated with B_{12} deficiency and inadequate folate or iron absorption	Decreased basal metabolic rate and oxygen requirements, decreased production of erythropoietin. Possible association between thyroid hormone and hematologic response to B_{12}.
Respiratory	Dyspnea, hypoventilation, CO_2 retention	Myxedematous changes in respiratory muscles.
Gastrointestinal	Decreased appetite, constipation, weight gain, fluid retention; decreased protein metabolism (lightly positive nitrogen balance); decreased glucose absorption; elevated serum lipid levels	Decreased metabolic demand; reduced peristaltic activity; increased capillary permeability to proteins; depressed insulin degradation; depressed lipid synthesis and degradation.
Renal	Increased total body water; reduced erythropoietin production; dilutional hyponatremia	Reduced blood flow and glomerular filtration rate, leading to decreased excretion of water.
Integumentary	Dry, flaky skin; dry, brittle hair; reduced growth of nails and hair; slow wound healing; myxedema; cool skin	Reduced sweat and sebaceous gland secretion; increased hyaluronic acid binds water and causes a puffy appearance; decreased circulation to skin; reduced tissue regeneration.
Reproductive	Anovulation, decreased libido, high incidence of spontaneous abortion in women; decreased libido and oligospermia in men	Increased estriol formation in women; decreased androgen secretion in men; decreased levels of sex hormone–binding globulin in both genders.
Neurological	Confusion, slow speech and thinking; memory loss; hearing loss; night blindness; slow, clumsy movements; cerebellar ataxia	Decreased cerebral blood flow, resulting in cerebral hypoxia.
Musculoskeletal	Muscle and joint aching and stiffness; reduced deep tendon reflexes; increased bone density	Decreased innervation of muscles; decreased bone formation and resorption.
Endocrine	Increased TSH production; decreased cortisol turnover rate but normal serum cortisol levels	Impaired thyroid hormone synthesis; decreased deactivation of cortisol.

Rational Drug Selection

The testing involved in the diagnosis of hypothyroidism is not within the scope of this book. The treatment protocol discussed here assumes appropriate diagnostic tools, including laboratory data, and accurate diagnosis of the disorder. Once a diagnosis has been made, a treatment regimen is determined.

Thyroid hormones were originally ground-up thyroid glands of animals, and such preparations are still available today. Because the pharmacokinetics of such drugs and the concentration of thyroid hormone within them are highly variable, they have been replaced in practice with synthetic formulations. Patients may purchase the "natural" forms in health food stores, and complementary health care providers may prescribe them. It is important to ask in the history about this possibility. The focus of this chapter is **synthetic thyroid hormones.**

Drug Therapy

Patients develop the symptoms of hypothyroidism slowly and are often quite low in thyroid hormone before they are diagnosed. These patients have adapted to this low level of hormone and are very sensitive to the effects of synthetic **thyroid hormone** replacement. Treatment of mild to moderate hypothyroidism should be gradual.

According to Goroll, May, and Mulley (1995), with adequate therapy the first signs of clinical response to therapy are a modest weight loss, an increase in pulse rate, and resolution of constipation. Other symptoms, such as myxedema, cardiovascular problems, and elevated creatine kinase levels, take more time to improve. Most patients feel better in about 2 weeks and clinical resolution usually occurs in about 3 months.

All of the synthetic forms of **thyroid hormone** have been successfully used to treat hypothyroidism. Drug choice is based on patient and drug variables. Figure 19–2 depicts the treatment algorithm based on these variables.

Patient Variables

AGE AND GENDER. Women older than 50 with markedly elevated TSH levels (10 mU/mL or higher) found by screening exam have the highest risk for complications from hypothyroidism, such as cardiac conditions associated with altered lipid metabolism. Research evidence is not sufficient to recommend or discourage treatment, but the best option seems to be to treat patients who have symptoms that may be caused by hypothyroidism and follow them closely to see if symptoms improve. Some providers choose to treat these patients even if they are asymptomatic (Helfand & Redfern, 1998).

Men, younger women, and patients with a mildly elevated TSH level (6 to 9 mU/mL) found at screening have a lower risk for complications. No strong evidence supports treatment, especially if patients are asymptomatic (Helfand & Redfern, 1998). These patients should have TSH levels drawn every 2 to 5 years to see if the disease progresses to the point where treatment is appropriate. Symptomatic patients probably should be treated.

PREGNANCY. *Thyroid hormones are Pregnancy Category A. They may be given during pregnancy, and therapy begun before pregnancy should not be stopped. The increased metabolic rate common to pregnancy often requires higher doses. Increasing a patient's maintenance dose by 25 percent usually provides adequate coverage. TSH levels should then be checked in 4 weeks to determine the need for any further dosage adjustment.*

CONCOMITANT DISEASES. **Thyroid hormone** replacement is generally contraindicated after recent myocardial infarction. If hypothyroidism is a complicating or causative factor of the cardiac problem, judicious use of small doses may be called for. Coronary artery disease may worsen when **thyroid hormones** are given because the increased heart rate increases oxygen demand by the heart muscle and decreases the oxygen supply by decreasing the diastolic filling time. If **thyroid hormones** are required, the lowest-possible dose is used, with careful monitoring for indications of worsening cardiovascular disease. Although both **levothyroxine** and **liothyronine** have content stability, **liothyronine** is three to four times more active than **levothyroxine**, making it more likely to produce cardiotoxicity. For patients with concomitant cardiac disorders, **levothyroxine** should be used. In patients with angina, the administration of **thyroid hormone** replacement may precipitate unstable angina. **Beta-adrenergic blockers** may be concurrently administered to decrease this risk.

Long-term use of **levothyroxine** therapy in women has been associated with decreased bone density in the hip and spine. Women with osteoporosis and those who are postmenopausal and not on **estrogen** replacement require low doses and frequent monitoring. Data are not available on whether other **thyroid hormones** present the same problem.

Approximately 10 percent of patients with type 1 diabetes mellitus develop chronic thyroiditis, with an insidious onset of subclinical hypothyroidism. Women with this disorder are also more likely to develop postpartum thyroiditis. Sensitive TSH levels should be drawn at regular intervals on patients with type 1 diabetes, and hypothyroidism treated with **levothyroxine.**

Some patients with infertility and menstrual irregularities have underlying chronic thyroiditis with subclinical hypothyroidism. If these patients have elevated TSH levels, **levothyroxine** replacement therapy may normalize the menstrual cycle and restore fertility.

A few patients who are diagnosed with depression have primary hypothyroidism. The workup for depression should include TSH measurement and treatment of any hypothyroidism with appropriate doses of **levothyroxine.**

Levothyroxine is the drug of choice for treating congenital hypothyroidism. Tablets may be crushed and added to infant formula. This process is discussed in Chapter 19. Congenital hypothyroidism requires referral to an endocrinologist.

Drug-Related Variables

PHARMACOKINETICS. **Levothyroxine** has a longer half-life than the other two drugs, and it can be safely withheld for up to 2 weeks, if necessary, without altering the patient's thyroid status. AACE (1995) advocates the use of a high-quality brand of **levothyroxine**, and that brand should be continued throughout treatment.

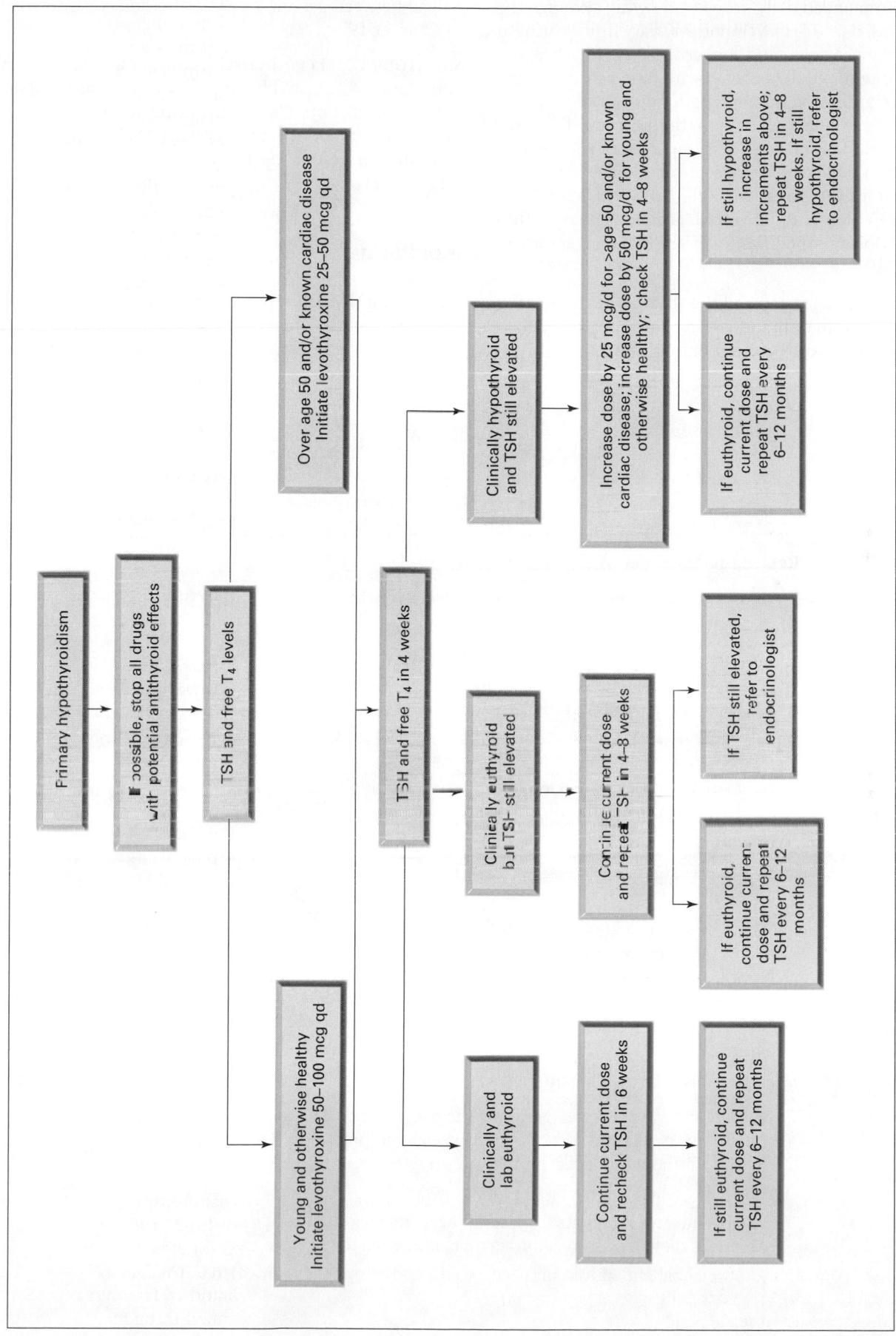

Figure 39-2. Drug therapy algorithm: Hypothyroidism.

The recommended daily dose is 1.6 µg/kg, although the dose is based on TSH levels and will vary from patient to patient. Lower doses and longer intervals for changing doses are required for patients who have cardiovascular disorders or long-standing hypothyroidism. If there is a need to rapidly correct a hypothyroid state, **liothyronine** is preferable because of its rapid onset and dissipation of action. The advantages of rapid onset and dissipation, however, must be weighed against the wide swings in T_3 levels and possible cardiotoxicity of **liothyronine.** Dosing schedules for both drugs are shown in Chapter 19.

COST.   Generic forms of all the **thyroid hormones** are less expensive than brand names; however, bioequivalence does not exist between brands and cannot be as-

sumed between generic forms. A cost index is provided in Chapter 19.

MONITORING.   **Levothyroxine** is the easiest to monitor with standard TSH and free T_4 laboratory measurements of thyroid function. Monitoring **liothyronine** therapy is more difficult, and it is best used for TSH suppression.

Liotrix offers no clear benefit over either of these other drugs on any of these parameters.

Monitoring

Monitoring **thyroid replacement** therapy has three parameters: clinical symptoms, TSH, and free T_4. Despite some controversy, clinical symptoms alone are generally

---

PATIENT EDUCATION

Hypothyroidism

Related to the Overall Treatment Plan and Disease Process

☐ Understanding the pathophysiology of hypothyroidism and its prognosis.

☐ Role of iodine intake in thyroid hormone production.

☐ Importance of adherence to the treatment regimen.

☐ Length of time the drug will need to be taken. For those with thyroiditis, this may be less than 12 months. For many with primary hypothyroidism, the treatment will be lifelong. The patient should be informed not to stop taking the drug without first consulting the health care provider.

☐ Indications of relapse or complications that need to be reported.

☐ Importance of discussing pregnancy or the potential for pregnancy with the primary care provider.

☐ Need to wear a medical identification bracelet stating that they are taking thyroid hormone replacement and to inform any provider who sees them that this is the case. This is especially important if this provider prescribes any new drugs for the patient.

☐ Need for regular follow-up visits with the primary care provider, which will include laboratory monitoring of thyroid function to determine the status of the hypothyroidism and any needed dosage adjustments of the drug therapy.

Specific to the Drug Therapy

☐ Discussion of the reasons for taking the drug(s) and the anticipated action of the drug(s) on the disease process. It is especially important to inform the patient that thyroid hormone replacement may take 4 to 8 weeks to have a noticeable effect.

☐ Doses and schedules for taking the drug(s).

☐ Possible adverse reactions (e.g., rapid heart rate, cardiac arrhythmias, chest pain, insomnia, diarrhea, or heat intolerance) and what to do when they occur.

☐ Additional patient education specific to thyroid hormones is provided in Chapter 19.

Hypothyroidism

Complaint

"I can't sleep and I've gained 15 pounds over the last 6 months."

History

Juanita is a 45-year-old woman who presents at the clinic with difficulty sleeping, depression, lack of energy, and an unexplained weight gain of 15 pounds within the last 6 months. Her eyelids are puffy and she reports that her menstrual cycle has been erratic.

Assessment

Routine laboratory tests were within normal limits except for slightly low hemoglobin and hematocrit..

Initial Management Plan

Juanita was diagnosed with onset of menopause; hormone replacement therapy was begun. TSH and free T_4 levels were ordered and she was scheduled for a follow-up visit in 1 month.

Follow-up Visit

At the time of the follow-up, Juanita is increasingly fatigued, has increased facial swelling, and is having decreased ability to think clearly. Her physical examination reveals the following vital signs: temperature 97°F, pulse 60, respirations 20, and blood pressure 96/60. Her skin is cool, dry, and flaky. Her lungs are clear and her heart sounds are normal. Her thyroid is palpable and slightly enlarged, nontender, and without nodules or bruit. Her movements are slow and her gait is clumsy. Her laboratory data include the following: TSH 150 mU/mL, free T_4 0.1 ng/dL. Other laboratory data are within normal limits, except for the continued low hemoglobin and hematocrit, and a slightly elevated cholesterol level. Juanita is diagnosed with hypothyroidism.

Modifications to the Management Plan

1. Continue estrogen-progesterone replacement therapy.
2. Initiate thyroid hormone replacement with levo-thyroxine 100 µg each morning. Starting doses for this drug vary from 50 to 100 µg/day. The 100 µg/ day dose is chosen because she is less than 50 years old and otherwise healthy, and her TSH is quite high. If she had any indication of cardiac problems, the dose would have been 25 or 50 µg/day to start.
3. After assessment of her knowledge base about hypothyroidism and its management, begin appropriate teaching. Recognizing that she has difficulty concentrating at this time, the focus of the teaching is on how to take her drugs; written material including drug administration and other teaching about hypothyroidism is sent home with her.
4. Schedule a follow-up appointment in 4 weeks with repeat TSH, free T_4, and CBC at that time. A minimum of 4 weeks is needed for thyroid hormone status to stabilize after initiation of therapy. Although a longer time may be chosen between visits for assessment of the efficacy of the treatment, shorter times are better for initial assessment.

Continuing Care

At her follow-up appointment in 3 weeks, Juanita reports that her symptoms are improving. She has increased appetite and energy levels and has lost 5 pounds. She is more mentally alert and her facial puffiness is improving. Her TSH is now 6 mU/mL, her free T_4 is 0.7 ng/dL, and her CBC is within normal limits. Her cholesterol level is improved but still slightly high. Her thyroid function is improving, but she is still not euthyroid. Her treatment plan now includes:

1. Continue her levothyroxine 100 µg/day.
2. Schedule a follow-up visit with repeat TSH and lipid profile in 6 weeks.
3. Continue teaching related to hypothyroidism.

At her next follow-up appointment, her TSH is 3.5 mU/mL, and she is asymptomatic. Her lipid profile is now also within normal limits. She will be followed at 6 months and then anually.

---

not an effective monitoring parameter because they do not correlate well with laboratory findings. They are important in conjunction with laboratory data.

The most accurate monitoring parameter is a sensitive TSH test because it correlates most closely with physiological measurements of **thyroid hormone** effects. TSH is evaluated for diagnosis, at initiation of therapy, and every 4 to 8 weeks after therapy has begun until the pa-tient achieves stable euthyroid status. Normalized and stable TSH levels often take 6 to 12 months to achieve. TSH is also repeated 6 to 8 weeks after any dosage adjustment because it takes approximately this amount of time for the new dosage to stabilize, especially with the long half-life of **levothyroxine.** Once the patient is euthyroid and stable, TSH monitoring occurs every 12 months, depending on symptoms and stability.

If the TSH level falls below the lower limit of normal or becomes undetectable, the dose of **thyroid hormone** used for replacement is excessive. Measurement of free T_4 can help to determine how excessive the dose is. Free T_4 may correlate poorly with physiological status during the initial therapy period. It is more reliable once the patient is stable (e.g., after 12 months).

During pregnancy, elevated estrogen increases thyroid-binding globulin levels, which alters total T_4 values but not free T_4. During pregnancy, both TSH and free T_4 levels are evaluated to determine appropriate replacement dosage. Tests are done at 8 weeks and 6 months of gestation. The goal is to normalize TSH and maintain free T_4 at the upper limits of normal. Primary care providers should consult with an endocrinologist for management of pregnant patients.

Anemia is a frequent concomitant disease with hypothyroidism. A complete blood count (CBC) should be drawn at initiation of therapy. After a thorough workup of any anemia to assess for other possible causes (e.g., iron deficiency, blood loss, vitamin B_{12} or folic acid deficiency), hypothyroidism should be treated with standard **thyroid hormone** replacement. Management of anemia, including monitoring parameters, is discussed in Chapter 25.

Other common concomitant disorders with hypothyroidism that require monitoring include hypercholesterolemia and hypertension. Management of these disorders, including monitoring parameters, is discussed in Chapters 37 and 38.

Outcome Evaluation

Figure 19–2 shows the drug treatment protocol for hypothyroidism. Evaluation is based on reduction of clinical symptoms and normalization of TSH and free T_4 levels. Times when consultation with or referral to an endocrinologist is appropriate include:

1. Failure to achieve control of symptoms or normalized TSH within 12 months by standard doses despite patient adherence to the treatment regimen.
2. Relapse after a period of stability on a standard dose.
3. Pending surgery. Careful anesthesia planning is required because clearance of anesthetics is reduced.
4. Pregnancy. Hypothyroidism during pregnancy presents special concerns and is best managed by a clinical endocrinologist (AACE, 1995) or in consul-

tation with an endocrinologist. Lactating women also are best managed with at least consultation with an endocrinologist.
5. Congenital hypothyroidism. Infants with suspected congenital hypothyroidism should be seen without delay by a pediatric endocrinologist (Mitchell, 1995).

Patient Education

Patient education should discuss the overall treatment plan, as well as information specific to the drug therapy, reasons for taking the drug, drugs as part of the total treatment regimen, and adherence issues.

REFERENCES

American Association of Clinical Endocrinologists. (1995). AACE clinical practice guidelines for the evaluation and treatment of hyperthyroidism and hypothyroidism. *Endocrine Practice, 1,* 54–62.

Bringmann, I., van Leeuwen, B., Hennemann, G., Beckett, G., & Toft, A. (1999). Outcome of treatment of hyperthyroidism. *Journal of Endocrinology Investigation, 22*(4), 250–256.

Fantz, C., Dagogo-Jack, S., Landenson, J., & Gronowski, A. (1999). Thyroid function during pregnancy, *Clinical Chemistry, 45*(12), 2250–2258.

Goroll, A., May, L., & Mulley, A. (1995). *Primary care medicine* (3rd ed.). Philadelphia: Lippincott.

Heitman, B., & Irizarry, A. (1995). Hypothyroidism: Common complaints, perplexing diagnosis. *Nurse Practitioner, 20*(3), 54–60.

Helfand, M., & Redfern, C. (1998). Screening for thyroid diseases: An update. *Annals of Internal Medicine, 129,* 144–158.

Kastrup, E. (Founding Ed.). (1998). *Drug facts and comparisons.* St. Louis: Facts and Comparisons.

Leigh, S. (1999). Two hormones better for treating hypothyroidism. *Medical Tribune, 40*(6), 15.

McDermott, M. (July 1998). Thyroid disease. Presentation at the 23rd National Primary Care Nurse Practitioner Symposium, Keystone, CO.

Mitchell, M. (1995). Congenital hypothyroidism. *Advance for Nurse Practitioners 3*(4),(April), 13–16.

Norcross, W. (February 1997). Diagnosis and management of thyroid disorders. Nurse Practitioner Association for Continuing Education Conference, San Diego.

Roti, E., Gardini, E., Magotti, M., Pilla, S., Minelle, R., Salvi, M., Monica, C., Maestri, D., Cencetti, S., & Braverman, L. (1999). Are thyroid function tests too frequently and inappropriately requested? *Journal of Endocrinology Investigation, 22*(3), 184–190.

Schilling, J. (1997). Hyperthyroidism: Diagnosis and management of Graves' disease. *Nurse Practitioner, 22*(6), 72–90.

Woeber, K. (1999). The year in review: The thyroid. *Annals of Internal Medicine, 131*(12), 959–962

CHAPTER 40

Pneumonia

CHAPTER OUTLINE

Adult Patients with Pneumonia

Pneumonia affects more than 4 million people a year in the United States, making it one of the more commonly seen medical problems. The incidence rates average 12 per 1000, increasing with age to more than 30 per 1000 in patients over age 75. As in most bacterial illnesses, those of the extremes of age are most severely affected, with infants and older adults often requiring hospitalization and intravenous (IV) **antibiotics.**

Pathophysiology

Pneumonia develops when an organism invades the lung parenchyma and the host defenses are depressed. Bacterial pneumonia results when the lung's primary defense mechanisms are altered, either by a viral infection or by immunologic problems. Chronically ill patients of all ages are more prone to pneumonia, usually because of their underlying medical problem. There may be other origins of pneumonia besides bacterial organisms, such as viral, fungal, rickettsial, and parasitic organisms; inflammatory processes; and inhalation of toxic substances.

The predominant organism found in pneumonia depends on the age and health status of the patient. For all ages (except neonates), *Streptococcus pneumoniae* is the most commonly found organism in pneumonia. It is identified as the causative organism in 60 to 75 percent of adults with bacterial pneumonia. Table 40–1 lists the common pathological agents for community-acquired pneumonia (CAP) at different ages.

In the past, practitioners attempted to determine the most likely pathogen by the clinical presentation of the patient, using terms like *typical* and *atypical*. Typical infections were those caused by *S. pneumoniae, Haemophilus influenzae, Staphylococcus aureus,* or gram-negative bacteria. The presentation of typical pneumonia included fever, chills, yellow or green sputum, pleuritic chest pain, and lobar consolidation on chest x-rays; the presentation of atypical pneumonia included a gradual onset of cough, no or scant sputum, low-grade fever, myalgias, arthralgias, and lack of consolidation on x-rays. It was thought that patients with atypical pneumonia most likely had *Mycoplasma pneumoniae, Legionella pneumophila,* or a viral infection. In clinical practice, these classifications have little usefulness, as numerous studies have shown that few reliable clinical features distinguish between the different bacterial pathogens (ATS, 1993).

Goals of Treatment

The ultimate goal of treatment for all patients is return to their respiratory status before the illness. Initially, patients who are responding to empiric **antibiotic** therapy should show improved clinical condition in 48 to 72 hours. The patient's chest x-ray may actually deteriorate, however, and not return to baseline for weeks or months. In previously healthy adults younger than 50, 66 percent of patients with pneumonia return to baseline chest x-rays within 4 weeks. In older patients or those who have previously had respiratory or other chronic illness, only 26 percent of patients have normal chest x-rays by the fourth week of treatment (ATS, 1993). Children may require 6 to 8 weeks for the chest x-ray to return to normal (Kercsmar, 1998). Therefore, a clear chest x-ray may not be the best indicator of successful treatment initially. The best indicator of improvement in clinical status is that the overall clinical manifestations of pneumonia (e.g., fever and increased white blood cell [WBC] count) should improve.

Rational Drug Selection

Guidelines

In 1993, the American Thoracic Society (ATS) issued guidelines for the initial management of adults with CAP that discuss the diagnosis, assessment of severity, and initial **antimicrobial** therapy. These guidelines, similar to those used in Europe and Canada (Woodhead, 1998), break down the treatment into severely ill and not severely ill patients, patients who require hospitalization,

Table 40–1. Community-Acquired Pneumonia: Common Pathogens by Age

Age	Common Pathogens
Neonates	Coliform bacteria, cytomegalovirus, enterovirus, group B streptococci, herpesvirus, *Mycoplasma hominis, Ureaplasma urealyticum*
Infants age 4 to 16 weeks	Cytomegalovirus, influenza virus, parainfluenza virus, respiratory syncytial virus (RSV), *Chlamydia trachomatis, Haemophilus influenzae, Staphylococcus aureus, Streptococcus pneumoniae, U. urealyticum*
Children up to age 5 years	Adenovirus, group A streptococci, influenza virus, RSV, *H. influenzae, S. aureus, S. pneumoniae*
Children over 5 years through adolescence	Influenza virus, varicella, *Chlamydia pneumoniae, H. influenzae, Legionella pneumophila, Mycoplasma pneumoniae, S. pneumoniae*
Adults under age 60 years with no comorbidity	Respiratory viruses, *C. pneumoniae, H. influenzae, M. pneumoniae, S. pneumoniae;* other (1%): endemic fungi, *Legionella* spp., *Mycobacterium tuberculosis, S. aureus*
Adults over age 60 years or with comorbidity	Aerobic gram-negative bacilli, respiratory viruses, *H. influenzae, S. aureus, S. pneumoniae;* other (1%): endemic fungi, *Legionella* spp., *Moraxella catarrhalis, M. tuberculosis*

and those who require intensive care unit (ICU) hospitalization (ATS, 1993; Rodrigues & Fein, 1995). These categories are as follows:

1. CAP in patients no older than 60 who have no evidence of comorbidity and who can be treated in an outpatient setting
2. CAP in patients older than age 60 or with evidence of comorbidity who can be treated in an outpatient setting
3. CAP requiring hospitalization but not admission to an ICU
4. Severe CAP, generally requiring admission to an ICU

Basically, the practitioner needs to take into consideration the age of the patient, the severity of the illness at initial presentation, and the treatment setting (outpatient or hospital). Because most primary care practitioners are in the ambulatory setting, the first two categories, which outline the treatment of the outpatient, are discussed here.

The practitioner must first evaluate the patient for advanced age and coexisting illness, both of which can affect the clinical presentation of CAP and increase its morbidity and mortality. Patients older than 65 appear to have increased risk factors and a slightly different group of pathogens than younger patients. Existing illnesses that the ATS identifies as complicating factors in CAP include chronic obstructive airway disease, diabetes mellitus, and chronic renal failure. **Alcohol** abuse and malnutrition also contribute to complicating the outcome for patients with CAP. Patients who are older or who have existing illnesses are more likely to have aerobic gram-negative infections.

In selecting treatment, the practitioner must also decide whether to treat the patient on an outpatient basis or in a hospital. The presence of any one of the following warrants admission to a hospital: respiratory rate greater than 30, temperature above 101°F, a PaO_2 less than 60 mm Hg, or a $PaCO_2$ greater than 50 mm Hg on room air. Even in the absence of any of these complicating factors or findings, the severity of the overall clinical picture may warrant hospitalization.

If the patient can be treated on an outpatient basis, the practitioner, using the ATS guidelines, determines the appropriate treatment based on the age of the adult patient and the existence of a comorbidity. The treatment decision is based on the slightly different organism found in each group. Figure 40–1 is an outpatient treatment algorithm for adults with CAP.

Dosing Regimen

Initial empiric therapy for the patient younger than 60 without comorbidity is to treat with a **macrolide** or **tetracycline. Erythromycin** 500 mg given orally (PO) qid for 7 to 14 days is the least expensive, and it provides coverage against most of the common organisms in this age category. Patients may also be prescribed **erythromycin**

333 mg tid or 500 mg bid, although these forms are slightly more expensive. If patients have gastrointestinal (GI) upset from the **erythromycin** at a dose of 500 mg qid, they may respond to 250 mg of **erythromycin** given qid. Smokers or patients who cannot tolerate **erythromycin** should be started on PO **azithromycin (Zithromax)** 500 mg on day 1 and 250 mg daily for days 2 through 5. Some isolates of *S. pneumoniae* may be resistant to **tetracycline**, so it should be used only in patients who are allergic or intolerant to **macrolides**. Another option is to prescribe **amoxicillin (Amoxil)** 500 mg PO tid plus **doxycycline** PO bid for 7 to 14 days. The patient should begin to exhibit clinical response in 48 to 72 hours; therefore, unless the patient is deteriorating, treatment should not be altered for 72 hours (Rodrigues & Fein, 1995).

Patients who are over age 60 or have preexisting chronic illness can be treated on an outpatient basis if they are not severely ill. If the patient is mildly ill, the practitioner has a choice of oral medications from which to choose. The least expensive choice is **trimethoprim-sulfamethoxazole (Septra DS)** 1 tablet twice a day for 10 to 14 days. Another choice for treatment is a **second-generation cephalosporin** or **amoxicillin/clavulanate (Augmentin)** 875 mg PO bid for 10 to 14 days. **Erythromycin** or another **macrolide** should be prescribed if *Legionella* is suspected. If the patient is moderately ill but still able to take **oral antibiotics**, the practitioner may broaden the coverage and start with **amoxicillin/clavulanate** or **levofloxacin (Levaquin)** 500 mg PO daily for 10 to 14 days (expensive). The patient should begin to demonstrate clinical improvement in 48 to 72 hours.

If the patient is over age 60 or has comorbidities, is stable enough for home therapy, but oral intake is not assured, there is the option of home parenteral therapy. The drugs of choice for these patients are **ceftriaxone (Rocephin)** 1 g daily via IV or intramuscularly (IM) or **levofloxacin** 500 mg IV daily. Once clinical response is observed, the patient is switched to oral therapy, as described previously. Although parenteral therapy is expensive, it is still much more cost effective than a hospital stay.

Patient Variables

PATIENT WITH A NURSING HOME–ACQUIRED PNEUMONIA. Nursing home–acquired pneumonias are not categorized separately by the ATS guidelines because of lack of appropriate studies. The ATS document does identify certain pathogens that are more common in residents of long-term care facilities: **methicillin**-resistant *S. aureus, Mycobacterium tuberculosis,* and certain viral agents (adenovirus, respiratory syncytial virus [RSV] and influenza). These pathogens should be part of the differential for treating a patient who resides in a long-term care facility, yet the ATS recommends that nursing home patients should be initially treated in the same fashion as other patients over age 60.

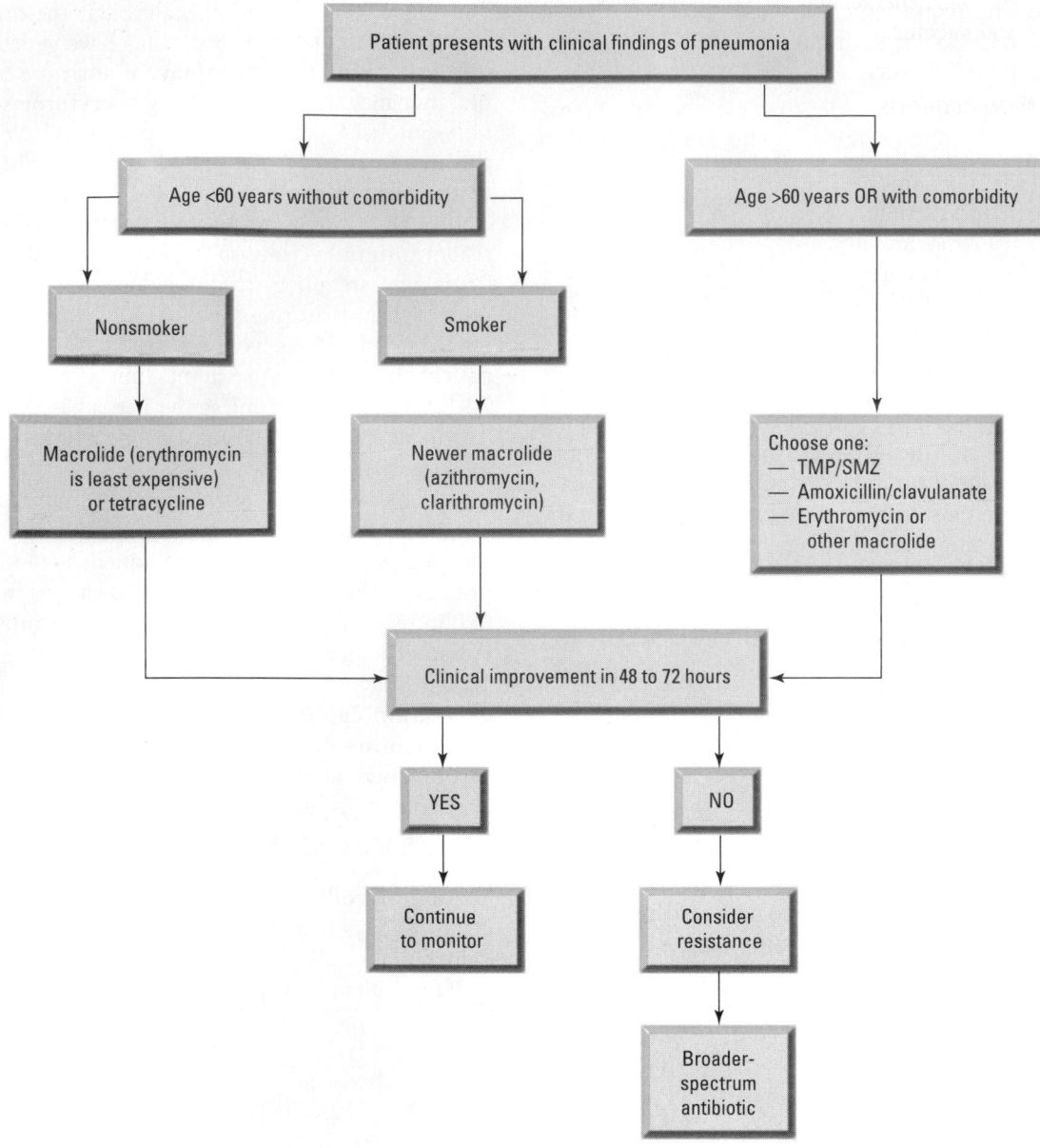

Figure 40–1. Treatment algorithm: Outpatient treatment of adults with community-aquired pneumonia.

PREGNANT PATIENT WITH PNEUMONIA. Pregnant women are at a slightly higher risk for infections than other women because of diminished lymphocyte function during pregnancy. There are risk factors that appear to be associated with antepartum pneumonia: anemia, prior lung disease, and illicit drug use. The pathogens found in CAP are also the predominant pathogens in antepartum patients with pneumonia. Viruses such as influenza (both type A and type B), varicella, and measles are associated with significant morbidity for pregnant women with pneumonia (Riley, 1997).

A review of the effects of pneumonia on pregnant patients suggests that maternal and fetal morbidity remain a concern. The complications found were maternal death, preterm labor, and fetal death. The most common complication is preterm labor (Riley, 1997).

Antibiotic therapy for the pregnant patient is similar to treatment of other adults with CAP: **erythromycin, trimethoprim-sulfamethoxazole,** or a **third-generation cephalosporin. Tetracycline** is not used during pregnancy because it may cause discoloration of deciduous teeth in neonates.

Prevention of viral causes of pneumonia is key to the health of the pregnant patient. The patient who has not previously had varicella should receive the **varicella vaccine** prior to planning a pregnancy. (It cannot be given during pregnancy.) The pregnant patient should receive an **influenza vaccine** in the fall of the year, and any patient with a chronic medical condition should receive a **pneumococcal vaccine.**

Lifestyle Modifications

Although the mainstay of treatment is **antibiotic** therapy, other measures improve outcome. Adequate hydration enables the patient to liquefy any secretions present. Also, patients who are ill with pneumonia often are anorectic and have decreased fluid intake, so education regarding "pushing" fluids is helpful. Rest is one aspect of therapy that younger working patients may have a hard time accepting. Encouraging patients to not work for a few days will speed the healing process. Tobacco smoke irritates the lungs and increases the coughing associated with the pneumonia. The patient and other household members should refrain from smoking.

Monitoring

The practitioner needs to monitor the patient's clinical status closely. Early identification of the need for hospitalization will enhance the outcome of the illness. The patient's fever, respiratory status, hydration, and activity tolerance all need to be monitored for early signs of either improvement or deterioration.

Outcome Evaluation

As previously mentioned, the patient needs to be monitored for response to empiric **antibiotic** therapy. The patient should become afebrile in 2 to 4 days. Leukocytosis most often resolves by the fourth day of treatment. Radiographic improvement usually requires more time and is not an indicator of improvement. If the chest x-ray worsens yet the patient shows clinical improvement, that is the natural progression of the disease. In severe CAP, if the radiographic findings worsen *and* the clinical picture worsens, then that is a predictor of increased morbidity and mortality (ATS, 1993; Rodrigues & Fein, 1995).

If there is no improvement in clinical status within 72 hours, the practitioner needs to consider that the pathogen is not being treated appropriately. There are two possibilities. One is that the **antibiotic** chosen is not treating the pathogen. An example would be using **amoxicillin** when the pathogen is *Mycoplasma*. Another consideration is that the pathogen is resistant to the **antibiotic** chosen. In an era of increasing **antibiotic** resistance, the practitioner is always choosing between the narrowest treatment spectrum and the shotgun approach to treatment. There are more powerful oral **antibiotics** available than those the ATS recommends for empiric therapy, but if all practitioners routinely overprescribe them, resistance will soon develop. Therefore, the prudent practice is to start with the recommendation and save the broader-spectrum **antibiotics** for true cases of resistance.

Patient Education

Patient education related to pneumonia should focus on the following:

1. Understanding that pneumonia may be bacterial, viral, or mycoplasmal and the expected course of improvement for each. The patient should know that the initial clinical picture may not clearly indicate what type of pathogen is causing the pneumonia. The response to treatment will help to clarify the pathogen.
2. Education about the **antibiotic** prescribed, including expected adverse reactions, drug interactions, and length of treatment.
3. Lifestyle modifications, such as increased hydration, smoking cessation, and rest, should all be discussed.
4. Symptoms of worsening status should be described and the patient told to notify the practitioner or seek urgent care if symptoms worsen rather than improve. Patients should be told to expect clinical improvement in 48 to 72 hours.

Patient education should also focus on prevention.

Pediatric Patients with Pneumonia

Pneumonia in the pediatric patient can cause the infant or child to become quite ill very rapidly. Specific pathogens

Clinical Pearl

Patients with chronic medical conditions who are at high risk for infections should get a **pneumococcal vaccine.** The **influenza vaccine** previously was advised for patients with chronic medical or respiratory infections (e.g., chronic obstructive pulmonary disease (COPD), asthma); now it is recommended for any patient who has significant contact with the public.

are more likely at certain ages. In children, treatment is determined by the organism most likely to be causing the pneumonia or by positive cultures for a specific organism. Children may be treated on an outpatient basis if their clinical condition is stable. Indications for hospitalization in children beyond early infancy include moderate to severe respiratory distress, failure to respond to oral **antibiotics,** lobar consolidation in more than one lobe, immunosuppression, empyema, abscess or pneumatocele, or underlying cardiopulmonary disease. This section focuses on the outpatient treatment of pneumonia in children. Neonates (children younger than 30 days old) with pneumonia require hospitalization, with few exceptions; therefore, this group is not discussed in this chapter.

Pathophysiology

The cause of pneumonia in more than 90 percent of children with bacterial pneumonia is *S. pneumoniae* (Goodman & Brady, 1996). In children, the most common organisms after *S. pneumoniae* vary according to age (see Table 40–1). *S. pneumoniae* is rarely found in neonates, whereas perinatal infection from group B streptococci is often the leading pathogen in this age group. *Chlamydia trachomatis,* another perinatal infection, can occur in 5 to 20 percent of 3- to 16-week-old infants whose mother has untreated disease at the time of birth. The clinical findings or age can often differentiate among the pathogens that cause pneumonia in children.

Goals of Treatment

The goals of treatment for pediatric patients with pneumonia are the same as the goals for adults with pneumonia.

Rational Drug Selection

Patient Variables

INFANTS WITH CHLAMYDIAL PNEUMONIA. Infants who are 3 to 16 weeks old and who present as afebrile, with a repetitive staccato cough and tachypnea, cervical adenopathy, crackles (wheezing is rare), and hyperinflation and bilateral diffuse infiltrates on chest x-ray, most likely have chlamydial pneumonia. Diagnosis is confirmed by detecting chlamydia-specific IgM in serum.

Drug Therapy. The standard treatment for infants with confirmed chlamydial pneumonia is **erythromycin (EryPed)** 50 mg/kg daily for 14 days. These infants can

usually be treated as outpatients if they are able to eat and maintain hydration.

CHILDREN WITH BACTERIAL PNEUMONIA. Bacterial pneumonia in children usually occurs as a secondary infection following a viral infection. Primary bacterial pneumonia is less common. The viral infection affects the lung defenses, setting the stage for secondary bacterial infection. The pathogen is *S. pneumoniae* in 90 percent of childhood cases of bacterial pneumonia. The clinical findings may include the following: fever (usually high), cough, shaking and chills, tachypnea, tachycardia, cyanosis, fine crackles (rales), decreased breath sounds, abdominal pain, and vomiting. The symptoms can worsen suddenly, and children can become quite ill. Definitive diagnosis of a bacterial infection includes an elevated WBC with a left shift (more than 15,000), a chest x-ray that demonstrates lobar consolidation, and positive blood or nasopharyngeal cultures. If pneumatoceles are seen on chest x-ray, suspect staphylococcal pneumonia.

Drug Therapy. If *S. pneumoniae* is the suspected organism, based on the clinical picture, then high-dose **penicillin** or **amoxicillin** (75 mg/kg daily divided in three doses) is the drug of choice (Schreiber & Jacobs, 1995). Some authors suggest giving one IM dose of **penicillin G** (100,000 U/kg daily), followed by PO **penicillin** or **amoxicillin** (Goodman & Brady, 1996). Another choice is **erythromycin** or **trimethoprim-sulfamethoxazole.** If highly resistant pneumococci are in the community, the practitioner may choose between IV or IM **ceftriaxone** (50 mg/kg in one daily dose, not to exceed 2 g/day) or inpatient treatment using **vancomycin** (Schreiber & Jacobs, 1995). Patients who are treated early in the course of the illness usually respond to high-dose **penicillin** or **amoxicillin.**

If *S. aureus* is the confirmed or highly suspected organism, the patient may be treated with IM or IV **ceftriaxone** (50 mg/kg in one dose daily) or hospitalized and given **methicillin.** Patients with *S. aureus* pneumonia are usually quite ill and require hospitalization for at least a few days. They may require a chest tube if there is significant empyema.

CHILDREN AND ADOLESCENTS WITH *MYCOPLASMA* PNEUMONIA. Mycoplasmal pneumonia is the most common type in children over age 5 years. The disease is usually mild. The typical history includes upper respiratory symptoms, fever, dry cough, malaise, sore throat, headache, and possibly chills. The patient may have been treated with **amoxicillin** for "bronchitis" without improvement. Chest x-ray reveals bronchovascular markings with areas of atelectasis. Confirmation of *M. pneumoniae* as the pathogen is determined by the presence of *Mycoplasma*-specific IgG or IgM in the serum (Kercsmar, 1998).

Table 40–2. Drugs Commonly Used: Community-Acquired Pneumonia

Drug	Dose	Length of Treatment	Strengths Available	Notes
Amoxicillin (Amoxil, Trimox)	*Adults:* 500 mg q8h *Children:* 40–50 mg/kg/day divided in three doses *or* high-dose therapy: 75/mg/kg/day in 3 doses	7–4 days	*Capsules:* 250 mg, 500 mg *Chewable tablets:* 125 mg, 250 mg *Powder for suspension:* 50 mg/mL, 125 mg/5 ml, 250 mg/5 mL	
Amoxicillin/clavulanate (Augmentin)	*Adults:* 875 mg q12h *Children* <3 mo: 30 mg/kg/day of amoxicillin divided q12h *Children* >3 mo: 45 mg/kg/day of amoxicillin divided q12h (use 200 mg/5 mL or 400 mg/5 mL strength suspension) *or* 30–40 mg/kg/day of amoxicillin if using 125 mg/5 mL or 250 mg/5 mL strength suspension	10–14 days for all patients	*Tablets:* 250 mg amoxicillin with 125 mg clavulanate, 500 mg amoxicillin with 125 mg clavulanate *Chewable tablets:* 125 mg amoxicillin with 31.25 mg clavulanate, 200 mg amoxicillin with 28.5 mg clavulanate, 250 mg amoxicillin with 62.5 mg clavulanate, 400 mg amoxicillin with 57 mg clavulanate *Suspension:* 125 mg amoxicillin with 31.25 mg clavulanate/5 mL, 200 mg amoxicillin with 28.5 mg clavulanate/5 mL, 250 mg amoxicillin with 62.5 mg clavulanate/5 mL, 400 mg amoxicillin with 57 mg clavulanate/5 mL, 400 mg amoxicillin with 57 mg clavulanate	Children's dose is based on amoxicillin content. Because of the clavulanate content, two 250-mg tablets are not the same as one 500-mg tablet. Because of the different clavulanate levels in the suspensions, it is not appropriate to dose the 125-mg/5-mL or the 250-mg/5-mL suspensions twice a day. Children should not be given the 250-mg tablet until they are >40 kg.
Azithromycin (Zithromax)	*Adults:* 500 mg on day 1, then 250 mg daily for days 2–5 *Children:* day 1, 10 mg/kg, followed by 5 mg/kg on days 2–5	5 days	*Capsules:* 250 mg *Z-pak:* six 250-mg tablets with instructions for daily dosing *Suspension:* 100 mg/5 mL, 200 mg/5 mL	Expensive. Good choice for smokers who cannot tolerate erythromycin.
Ceftriaxone (Rocephin)	*Adults:* 1 g daily *Children:* 50 mg/kg daily	Based on clinical response, switch to oral therapy when able	*Powder for injection:* 250 mg, 500 mg, 1 g	Broad spectrum. Expensive but less expensive than hospitalization.

Continued on next page

Table 40–2. Drugs Commonly Used: Community-Acquired Pneumonia *(continued)*

Drug	Dose	Length of Treatment	Strengths Available	Notes
Erythromycin base (E-Mycin, Ery-Tab)	*Adults:* 250–500 mg q6h *or* 333 mg q8h *or* 500 mg q12h *Children:* 30–50 mg/kg/day divided into tid dosing	*Adults:* 7–14 days *Children:* 10–14 days	*Tablets:* 250 mg, 333 mg, 500 mg	Should be taken with food to decrease GI upset.
Erythromycin estolate (Ilosone)	*Adults:* 250–500 mg q6h *or* 333 mg q8h *or* 500 mg q12h *Children:* 30–50 mg/kg/day divided into tid dosing	*Adults:* 7–14 days *Children:* 10–14 days	*Tablets:* 500 mg *Capsules:* 250 mg *Suspension:* 125 mg/5 mL, 250 mg/5 mL	Should be taken with food to decrease GI upset.
Erythromycin ethylsuccinate (E.E.S., EryPed)	*Adults:* 400 mg q6h *Children:* 30–50 mg/kg/day divided in q6h *or* q12h dosing	*Adults:* 7–14 days *Children:* 10–14 days	*Tablets:* 400 mg *Chewable tablets:* 200 mg *Drops:* 100 mg/2.5 mL *Suspension:* 200 mg/5 mL, 400 mg/5 mL	Should be taken with food to decrease GI upset.
Levofloxacin (Levaquin)	*Adults:* 500 mg once a day	7–14 days	*Tablets:* 250 mg, 500 mg *Injection:* 500 mg	Expensive.
Trimethoprim-sulfamethoxazole (TMP/SMZ, Septra, Bactrim)	*Adults:* 160 mg TMP, 800 mg SMZ q12h *Children* >2 mo: 8 mg/kg TMP, 40 mg/kg SMZ q12h	10–14 days for all patients	*Tablets:* 80 mg TMP/400 mg SMZ *Double-strength tablets:* 160 g TMP/800 mg SMZ *Oral suspension:* 40 mgTMP/200 mg SMZ per 5 mL	Cannot be used in infants <2 mo

Drug Therapy. The treatment of choice for mycoplasmal pneumonia is **erythromycin** (40 to 50 mg/kg daily given qid or tid or, for larger children, 333 mg PO tid for 10 days). This is inexpensive and provides good coverage for other atypical organisms. Another choice is **azithromycin** (10 mg/kg on day 1 and 5 mg/kg on days 2 through 5). **Azithromycin (Zithromax)** is packaged in a "Z-pak," a handy dose for older children; printed on the package are instructions to take two 250-mg capsules on day 1 and one capsule daily thereafter. **Clarithromycin (Biaxin)** may also be prescribed.

Monitoring

Patients with bacterial pneumonia need to be monitored closely for clinical improvement or deterioration. If the patient is being treated with the appropriate **antibiotic,** children often show rapid improvement, much faster than adults. Children can also deteriorate rapidly, and any infant who is not hospitalized needs to be seen in clinic the following day for reassessment.

Initial culture results are usually available in 24 hours, and the practitioner needs to determine (1) if the appropriate **antibiotic** has been chosen and (2) the level of resistance the organism has to the chosen **antibiotic.** If the patient is improving clinically, there is no need for repeat blood counts or cultures. If the patient is not improving or the clinical condition worsens, a repeat chest x-ray can determine if effusions or empyema is developing.

Patients with mycoplasmal pneumonia should be monitored for clinical improvement. The cough may last for weeks after the infection is treated. *M. pneumoniae* can spread to the blood, central nervous system, heart, skin,

Pneumonia

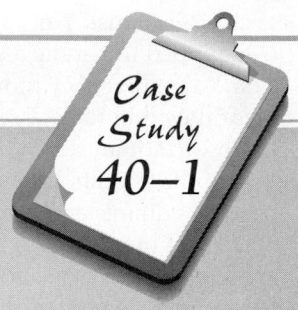

Complaint

"I've been coughing for 2 days."

History

George is a 48-year-old man who presents to the clinic with a 2-day history of fever and productive cough (sputum reported to be greenish). His history includes mild hypertension and a half-pack per day smoking habit. He reports that he used to smoke one pack per day, but has cut back. He is currently not taking medication for his high blood pressure because he didn't like the adverse reactions. No other family members are ill, but "something is going around" at work.

Assessment

On physical exam, George is pale and ill-appearing but able to ambulate into the exam room and onto the table without assistance. His oral temperature is 38.2°C, and his BP is 135/82. Breath sounds are positive for decreased breath sounds in the left lower lobe with scattered crackles. A chest x-ray reveals a consolidation in the left lower lobe.

Initial Management Plan

It is assumed that George has either *S. pneumoniae* or another bacterial pneumonia. Because he is a smoker, *H. influenzae* is also a possibility.

1. Begin oral antibotics. Azithromycin (Zithromax) is chosen for its broadened coverage for *H. influenzae*. George is prescribed a Z-pak to simplify administration.
2. He is also advised to take acetaminophen 650 mg PO every 4 hours for fever and discomfort.
3. Define signs of worsening respiratory status and parameters for returning to the clinic for reevaluation or seeking after-hours care.
4. Explain proper medication administration and maintenance of adequate hydration.
5. Suggest decreasing his smoking further to decrease the irritation to lung tissue. Be sure to congratulate him on having cut back.

Follow-up Visit

A follow-up telephone call found George to be improving. He was instructed to continue his antibiotics until he had taken all of them and to contact his health care provider if his symptoms worsened.

and joints, so monitoring for these complications is prudent. A child with sickle cell disease who develops mycoplasmal pneumonia develops a more severe pulmonary disease than the average child (Goodman & Brady, 1996).

All children with pneumonia need monitoring of their hydration status. Nutritional intake should also be assessed in infants who may be ill for a few days. The parents' ability to successfully administer medication and their ability to monitor their child's status are essential to the successful outpatient treatment of children with pneumonia.

Outcome Evaluation

Like the adult patient, the child with pneumonia must be monitored for response to the **antibiotic** therapy. The child should become afebrile in 2 to 4 days. There may be a residual cough for weeks, which should lessen with time. If the child's clinical status fails to improve in 48 to 72 hours, then the treatment plan must be reconsidered.

There may be bacterial resistance to the **antibiotic,** or the patient might have mycoplasmal pneumonia, which requires a **macrolide antibiotic.**

Patient Education

Patient education when a child has bacterial pneumonia focuses on the following:

1. How to assess the child's respiratory status and signs of respiratory deterioration. Clear instructions such as "If breathing over __ breaths per minute, call the practitioner" help parents monitor their child at home.
2. A clear plan of where the parents should take a child whose status worsens during the evening or night. Given the variable insurance rules regarding after-hours care, the practitioner needs to explain to parents how to access high-quality pediatric after-hours care in the event of deterioration in the

child's status. Not all urgent care clinics are equipped to handle a child in respiratory distress, and an emergency room is probably the best place for the child to be assessed.

3. How to administer medication appropriately. Make sure the parents have a medicine syringe to accurately administer the oral medications. Some medications must be taken on an empty stomach, and others must be taken with food, and the parents need to be reminded about any special instructions regarding the administration of the **antibiotic.**

4. The parents need to know how to assess hydration and what parameters are expected for urine output. Instructions that clearly define minimal output are the easiest to understand; for example, "Your infant should have a wet diaper every 6 to 8 hours at a minimum."

REFERENCES

American Thoracic Society. Pneumonia guidelines (adapted from Niederman et al.). Website: *www.thoracic.org.*

Goodman, M., & Brady, M. (1996). Respiratory disorders. In C. E. Burns, N. Barber, M. A. Brady, & A. M. Dunn (Eds.), *Pediatric primary care: A handbook for nurse practitioners.* Philadelphia: Saunders.

Johanson, W. G. (1996). Overview of pneumonia. In C. J. Bennett & F. Plum (Eds.), *Cecil textbook of medicine* (20th ed.). Philadelphia: Saunders.

Kercsmar, C. M. (1998). The respiratory system. In R. E. Behrman & R. M. Kliegman, *Nelson essentials of pediatrics* (3rd ed.). Philadelphia: Saunders.

Marrus, T. K., & Chan, C. K. (1998). Use of guidelines in treating community-acquired pneumonia. *Chest, 113,* 1689.

Niederman, M. S., Bass, J. B., Campbell, G. D., Fein, A. M., Grossman, R. F., Mandell, L. A., Marrie, T. J., Sarosi, G. A., Torres, A., & Yu, V. L. (1993). Guidelines for the initial management of adults with community-acquired pneumonia: Diagnosis, assessment of severity, and initial antimicrobial therapy. *American Review of Respiratory Disease, 148,* 1418. (This document has been adapted as the pneumonia guidelines by the ATS board and is located at the ATS Website: *www.thoracic.org.*)

Riley, L. (1997). Pneumonia and tuberculosis in pregnancy. *Infectious Disease Clinics of North America, 11,* 119.

Rodrigues, J. C., & Fein, A. M. (1995). Community-acquired pneumonia. *Emergency Medicine, 27*(3), 79–90.

Schreiber, J. R., & Jacobs, M. R. (1995). Antibiotic-resistant pneumococci. *Pediatric Clinics of North America, 42,* 519.

Woodhead, M. (1998). Community-acquired pneumonia guidelines: An international comparison. *Chest, 113,* 183S.

CHAPTER 41

....

Smoking Cessation

CHAPTER OUTLINE

D uring 1996, a random telephone survey of U.S. citizens in 49 states and the District of Columbia revealed that the mean prevalence of current smoking was 23.6 percent. Smoking is the leading cause of death in the United States, accounting for more than 430,000 deaths annually. Tobacco use contributes to the development of cancers, cerebrovascular disease, cardiovascular disease, dental disease, gastrointestinal (GI) disorders, and respiratory disease, making it the most preventable health problem in developed countries. Smokers who do not quit by age 35 have a 50 percent chance of dying from a tobacco-related disease. Patients' tobacco use needs to be addressed by all primary care providers, especially those who care for children, as 90 percent of smok-

ers begin smoking as teenagers. Secondhand or environmental exposure to tobacco smoke also poses a health hazard to nonsmokers, and the health care provider plays an important role in educating parents of young children about the effects of secondhand smoke. Education about secondhand smoke should be used as an opportunity to offer tobacco cessation to the smoking family member, thereby decreasing the health risks for the whole family.

A review of the physiological and psychological process of addiction will assist the health care provider in understanding the rationale for pharmacological intervention. Tobacco smoke contains many different chemicals, many of them known health hazards (ammonia, formaldehyde, carbon monoxide, benzene, arsenic, and lead). The addictive component in tobacco is nicotine. **Nicotine** has all the components of an addictive substance, similar to **heroin:** (1) production of transient mood alterations, (2) compulsive use despite damage to the individual and family members, (3) a reinforcing nature, (4) ability to produce dosage tolerance, (5) withdrawal symptoms upon cessation, and (6) a tendency to produce relapse behavior (Sheahan & Wilson, 1998).

The many forms of tobacco include cigarettes, pipes, cigars, smokeless tobacco, and snuff, and patients can be addicted to any of them. The health care provider needs to assess if the patient is using any form of tobacco and address cessation in the patient's plan of care. Although behavioral modification also plays an important part in quitting, it is discussed only briefly as a component of the treatment plan because this chapter focuses on pharmacological management.

Pathophysiology

Nicotine is a naturally occurring substance that is soluble in water and lipids. It is readily absorbed from many sites, including the lungs, mucosa, skin, and GI tract.

Nicotine Delivery

Nicotine is absorbed rapidly from tobacco smoke into the pulmonary circulation. It is then transported via the bloodstream to the brain, where it reaches the nicotine cholinergic receptors in 10 to 15 seconds after a puff. The mean time to peak concentration in the bloodstream is 7 to 8 minutes. Each puff contributes to maintaining the **nicotine** concentration. With each cigarette averaging 10 puffs, the pack-a-day smoker reinforces the blood **nicotine** level 200 times per day, with each puff providing distinct reinforcement of the habit. Smokeless tobacco is absorbed more slowly from the oral or nasal cavity.

Nicotinic Receptors

The neuronal nicotinic receptors appear to be complex, with the complexity contributing to the different responses to **nicotine agonists.** Chronic use of **nicotine** results in an increased number of brain nicotinic receptors, which appears to be an important factor in the development of tolerance of and dependence on **nicotine.**

Nicotine has both stimulant and depressant effects in the central nervous system (CNS). The stimulant effect is exerted mainly at the cortex, producing increased alertness and cognitive performance. **Nicotine** activates the nucleus accumbens "reward" system in the limbic system, causing increased extracellular fluid dopamine levels in the region. This increases the "reinforcing" quality of **nico-**

tine. Intravenous (IV) administration of **nicotine** activates neurohormonal pathways, releasing acetylcholine, norepinephrine, dopamine, serotonin, vasopressin, beta endorphins, growth hormone, and adrenocorticotropic hormone (ACTH).

Nicotine Withdrawal Syndrome

Nicotine withdrawal syndrome is characterized by craving, nervousness, irritability, impatience, hostility, labile mood, difficulty in concentrating, restlessness, and anxiety. Physical symptoms include decreased heart rate, increased appetite, and weight gain averaging 5 to 6 pounds. Somatic complaints such as myalgia, headache, constipation, and fatigue are common. The urge to smoke is closely related to low blood **nicotine** levels, which bring on early morning withdrawal symptoms. The smoker may not be smoking to achieve the effects of **nicotine** but rather to avoid withdrawal symptoms.

Goals of Treatment

The goal of tobacco cessation treatment is the complete discontinuation of tobacco. It can be achieved either "cold turkey" without pharmacological intervention or by using **nicotine replacement therapy,** which is then gradually reduced over time to zero. If **bupropion (Zyban)** is used, the goal is for the patient to be tobacco-free at the end of the 7 to 12 weeks of therapy.

Rational Drug Selection

The pharmacological management of tobacco cessation involves two different treatment modalities, **nicotine replacement therapy** and the **antidepressant bupropion.** The combination of **bupropion** and **nicotine replacement** via a **nicotine patch** provides higher long-term rates of smoking cessation (Jorenby et al., 1999).

Nicotine Replacement Therapy

Nicotine replacement therapy comes in four different forms: **gum, transdermal** or **patch, inhaler,** and **nasal spray.** The **gum** and **transdermal patch Nicotrol** are available over the counter (OTC); the **inhaler, spray,** and the **transdermal patch brands Prostep, Habitrol,** and **Nicoderm** are by prescription. Although the patient can self-treat with the OTC products, the health care provider should educate the patient regarding their proper use to ensure successful treatment. **Nicotine replacement** does not achieve the same peak levels of nicotine as smoking, but it does achieve a level high enough to suppress **nicotine** withdrawal symptoms. **Nicotine replacement ther-**

apy is recommended for patients who smoke more than 20 cigarettes per day (one pack), patients who smoke within 30 minutes of awakening in the morning, and patients who have tried to quit previously and have failed because of strong withdrawal symptoms and craving within the first week of quitting.

Nicotine polacrilex gum **is Pregnancy Category C, and** *transdermal nicotine* **is Pregnancy Category D, as** *nicotine* **is associated with decreased fetal breathing movements, probably caused by decreased placental perfusion.** *Nicotine replacement therapy* **is contraindicated immediately after myocardial infarction (MI) in patients with life-threatening arrhythmias and severe or worsening angina pectoris.**

Nicotine Gum

Nicotine gum improves smoking cessation rates of 40 to 60 percent compared with controls through 12 months of follow-up. The active ingredient in **nicotine gum** (Nicorette) is **nicotine polacrilex**, a **nicotine** resin complex. The **nicotine** is bound to an ion exchange resin that is released only during chewing. The medication is administered when the patient places a piece of gum in his or her mouth and chews slowly five to eight times, until a peppery taste appears. The patient then "parks" the gum in the buccal space. Intermittent chewing and parking the gum over 30 minutes promotes slow buccal absorption. Chewing too quickly causes an excess amount of **nicotine** to be released into the bloodstream, causing nausea, throat irritation, and hiccoughs. The patient should avoid smoking while chewing **nicotine gum**, as toxicity symptoms may occur (nausea, vomiting, and headache). **Nicotine gum** should not be the first-line choice for patients with temporal mandibular joint (TMJ) disease or peptic ulcer disease on account of adverse effects.

Nicotine polacrilex gum takes 30 minutes to reach its peak serum concentration. The patient who is just beginning a tobacco cessation program should chew one piece of 2-mg or 4-mg gum per hour. Abstinence rates appear to be higher when the patient chews the gum on a fixed schedule of every hour or every 2 hours. The patient who smokes more than 25 cigarettes per day should be started on the 4-mg dose initially and not exceed the maximum number of pieces per day of gum (30/day of 2 mg, 20/day of 4 mg). Acidic foods (coffee, soft drinks, juice) interfere with the buccal absorption of **nicotine** from **nicotine polacrilex** and should be avoided for 15 minutes before, during, and 15 minutes after chewing the gum.

After the patient has successfully quit smoking for 2 to 3 months, a gradual weaning of the gum dosage should begin; it should be complete 4 to 6 months from the beginning of treatment. Suggestions for a gradual withdrawal of treatment are as follows:

1. If the patient is on a 4-mg dose, decrease dose to 2 mg, and keep the timing the same.
2. Decrease the total number of pieces per day by one or more pieces every 4 to 7 days.
3. Substitute sugarless gum for one piece of **nicotine gum** every 4 to 7 days, gradually reducing the number of pieces of **nicotine gum** and increasing the number of pieces of sugarless gum.
4. Decrease the total time chewed from 30 minutes per piece to 15 minutes.

Treatment is stopped when the patient is chewing one to two pieces of **nicotine gum** per day. The use of **nicotine gum** past 6 months is not recommended.

Nicotine Transdermal System

The **transdermal nicotine system,** or **"patch,"** provides a slow, cutaneous absorption of **nicotine** over many hours. The **patch** is applied to clean, nonhairy skin on the upper body or upper arm when the patient wakes up. Peak **nicotine** levels occur in 2 to 6 hours (brand dependent) and then gradually decrease. Once the **patch** is removed, **nicotine** levels in the blood reach a nondetectable level in 10 to 12 hours in nonsmokers. There are different strengths of **patches** available and **patches** that are for 16-hour and for 24-hour use, allowing for dose regulation (Table 41–1). The 16-hour **patch** works well for the light to average smoker but is not effective for early morning withdrawal symptoms. The 24-hour **patch** provides a steady-state blood level of **nicotine,** with minimal peaks and troughs, and avoids morning withdrawal symptoms. The disadvantage of the 24-hour **patch** is that there are more adverse effects, including sleep disruption. Evaluat-

Clinical Pearl

NICOTINE GUM

Patients complain about the taste of the **nicotine gum.** Suggest that the patient try the mint-flavored variety, which patients seem to tolerate better.

Table 41–1. Drugs Commonly Used: Smoking Cessation

Drug	Strength Available	Dosage	Comments
Nicotine Gum Nicotine polacrilex (Nicorette)	2 mg 4 mg	If smoking <20–25 cigarettes/d: chew one 2-mg piece every 1–2 h (at least 9/d), max of 30/d. If smoking >20–25 cigarettes/d: chew one 4-mg piece every 1–2 h (at least 9/d), max of 20/d. After 6 wk decrease dose to one every 2–4 h for 3 wk, then one piece every 4–8 h for 3 wk, and then discontinue. Alternative: After 6 wk, gradually wean the dose by decreasing one piece of gum/d every 4–7 d.	Abstinence rates are higher if gum is chewed on a scheduled basis, rather than prn. Acidic foods and drinks interfere with absorption, so they should be avoided during and for 15 minutes before and after chewing nicotine gum. The use of nicotine gum for longer than 6 mo is not recommended.
Nicotine Transdermal Patch Habitrol (Rx)	21 mg/d 14 mg/d 7 mg/d	21 mg/d for first 6 wk, 14 mg/d for next 2 wk, and 7 mg/d for final 2 wk. *Low-dose regimen*:* 14 mg/d for 6 wk, then 7 mg/d for final 2 to 4 wk. *Length of treatment:* 8 to 12 wk.	24-h patch. Apply to clean, nonhairy area on upper body or upper arm upon waking.
Nicoderm CQ (OTC)	21 mg/d 14 mg/d 7 mg/d	21 mg/d for first 6 wk, 14 mg/d for next 2 wk, and 7 mg/d for final 2 wk. *Low-dose regimen*:* 14 mg/d for 6 wk then 7 mg/d for final 2–4 wk *Length of treatment:* 8–12 wk.	24-h patch. Apply to clean, nonhairy area on upper body or upper arm upon waking. May remove after 16–24 h.
Nicotrol transdermal (OTC)	15 mg/16 h 10 mg/16 h 5 mg/16 h	15 mg/16 h for first 4–12 wk, 10 mg/16 h for 2 wk, then 5 mg/16 h for final 2 wk. *Alternative:* Use 15 mg/16 h patch daily for 6 wk, then discontinue. *Length of treatment:* 14–20 wk.	16-h patch. Apply to clean, nonhairy area on upper body or upper arm upon waking. Remove after 16 h (before bed).
Prostep (Rx)	22 mg/d 11 mg/d	22 mg/d for 4–8 wk, then 11 mg/d for 2–4 wk. *Low-dose regimen*:* 11 mg/d for 4–8 wk. *Length of treatment:* 6–12 wk.	24-h patch. Apply to clean, nonhairy area on upper body or upper arm upon waking.
Nicotine Nasal Spray Nicotrol NS (Rx)	0.5 mg/spray One dose = 1 mg, or one spray in each nostril	Start with 1–2 doses (2–4 sprays)/h, Max of 5 sprays/h, 40 sprays/d. *Length of treatment:* 3 mo maximum.	Can be used ad lib. Advise patient not to sniff, inhale, or swallow the spray.

Continued on next page

Table 41–1. Drugs Commonly Used: Smoking Cessation *(continued)*

Drug	Strength Available	Dosage	Comments
Nicotine Inhaler Nicotrol inhaler (Rx)	10 mg/cartridge (4 mg nicotine delivered)	Patient puffs on mouthpiece frequently and continuously for 20 min. Initially, begins with at least 6 cartridges/d (max 16 cartridges/d) for the first 3–6 wk. Gradually decrease over 12 wk. *Length of treatment:* max 6 mo.	Provides oral stimulation similar to smoking.
Antidepressant Bupropion (Zyban) (Rx)	150-mg tablet	Begin 150 mg/d 1–2 wk prior to quit date. Increase dose to 150 mg bid (at least 8 h apart) after 3 d. *Length of treatment:* 7–12 wk.	May be combined with nicotine replacement. Avoid bedtime dosing, which may cause insomnia. Do not use with other forms of bupropion.

*Low-dose therapy is used for patients weighing less than 100 lb, patients with cardiovascular disease, and patients who smoke one-half pack per day or less.

ing the patient's smoking habit and determining if early morning withdrawal is an issue will enable the provider to prescribe the best transdermal system for the patient. **Transdermal nicotine** approximately doubles 6- to 12-month abstinence rates over those produced by placebo interventions.

The **transdermal nicotine system** has the advantage of delivering a steady-state level of **nicotine** that prevents **nicotine** withdrawal symptoms while allowing the smoker to work on the behavioral aspects of quitting. Unlike **nicotine gum**, the **patch** has the advantage of not reinforcing the oral aspects of smoking. Patients appreciate the ease of administration and once-daily dosing. Weaning off the **transdermal nicotine system** is accomplished by decreasing the dose of the **patch** on a scheduled basis. One disadvantage of the **nicotine patch** is that patients report that they are unable to self-regulate the dose if they are exhibiting withdrawal symptoms. This makes the **patch** less effective for highly dependent smokers, and a highly dependent smoker who is started on a **transdermal nicotine system** should be started on a high-dose 24-hour system to decrease withdrawal symptoms. The patient *must* refrain from smoking while using the **nicotine patch** because life-threatening dysrhythmias or MI may occur.

The most common adverse effect of the **nicotine patch** is skin irritation, with 35 to 47 percent of patients reporting some skin irritation during clinical trials. Advising the patient to change the site every day and not to reuse the site within a week can minimize this problem. The amount of skin irritation differs with the brand and dose used, so a change may alleviate the problem. If the patient exhibits symptoms of sleep disturbance or insomnia while using the **transdermal nicotine system**, first determine if the patient has signs of too high a dose or early morning withdrawal. Delayed onset of sleep is usually associated with too high a dose and early awakening associated with withdrawal symptoms. The provider can either switch the patient from the 24-hour to the 16-hour **patch** to decrease the dose or, if the patient is already using the 16-hour **patch**, decrease the dose. If withdrawal is the problem, then increase the **patch** from a 16-hour to a 24-hour or increase the dose of the **patch**. The patient needs to be aware that some adjustment of the dose may be necessary to provide effective relief of symptoms with minimal adverse effects. Advise the patient to report any adverse effects so that adjustments can be made.

Other adverse effects observed include symptoms of **nicotine** toxicity (headache, nausea, and vomiting) with higher-dose **patches** and with smoking while using a patch. If symptoms of toxicity occur, remove the **patch** and flush the skin area with water. *Do not use soap,* which increases **nicotine** absorption from the site. **Nicotine** will continue to be delivered into the bloodstream for a number of hours because there is a deposit of **nicotine** under the skin. Patients should report any symptoms of toxicity immediately to their health care provider.

Nicotine Nasal Spray

Nicotine nasal spray (Nicotrol NS) is a newer form of **nicotine replacement therapy.** The usual dose is 1 to 2 sprays in each nostril per hour, not to exceed 5 sprays per hour. The advantage to **nicotine nasal spray** is rapid achievement of peak blood levels, with peak levels

Clinical Pearl

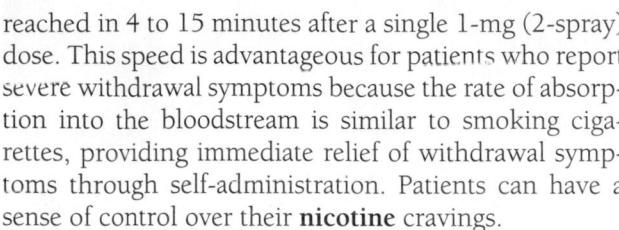

NICOTINE PATCH

Advise patients to dispose of used **nicotine patches** out of the reach of children. There is enough **nicotine** left in a *used* **patch** to lead to toxic levels in a child.

reached in 4 to 15 minutes after a single 1-mg (2-spray) dose. This speed is advantageous for patients who report severe withdrawal symptoms because the rate of absorption into the bloodstream is similar to smoking cigarettes, providing immediate relief of withdrawal symptoms through self-administration. Patients can have a sense of control over their **nicotine** cravings.

Patients need to be instructed *not to inhale, swallow, or sniff* the spray, unlike many other inhaled medications. The most common adverse effect is nasopharyngeal and ocular mucosa irritation. The use of **nicotine nasal spray** can cause serious arrhythmias and elevated blood pressure and should be avoided immediately after MI because it may cause angina.

With **nicotine nasal spray,** there is potential for abuse, as patients report a "head rush" and the sensation of feeling good, similar to cigarette smoking. Careful monitoring of the use of **nicotine spray** and advising patients of the potential for replacing their cigarette addiction with an addiction to the **nicotine spray** can help to avoid this problem. Three months is the recommended maximum length of treatment with **nicotine nasal spray.**

Nicotine Inhaler

The **nicotine (Nicotrol) inhaler** has recently become available to add to the delivery methods of **nicotine replacement therapy.** The **inhaler** consists of two parts, a cartridge containing 10 mg of **nicotine** (4 mg of delivered drug) and a mouthpiece. The patient puffs continuously on the inhaler for 20 minutes, providing the **nicotine** equivalent of two cigarettes. The patient should use at least 6 cartridges per day for 3 to 6 weeks. A maximum of 16 cartridges is used for the first week and then reduced gradually over 12 weeks. Adverse effects include coughing, mouth and throat irritation, and dyspepsia. In clinical studies, the **nicotine inhaler** group had an abstinence rate of 28 percent at 12 months (Hjalmarson et al., 1997).

Antidepressants

Antidepressants are thought to be helpful in smoking cessation because of the relationship between depressed mood and smoking behavior. During tobacco withdrawal, patients often exhibit depressed and anxious moods. Several **antidepressants** have been shown to be effective in smoking cessation, including **bupropion, doxepin,** and **nortriptyline.** This chapter discusses **bupropion (Zyban),** currently the only **antidepressant** approved by the Food and Drug Administration (FDA) for smoking cessation.

Bupropion

Bupropion is chemically unrelated to other **antidepressants,** and the mechanism by which it enhances the ability to abstain from smoking is unknown. It is presumed that **bupropion's** action as a weak inhibitor of neuronal uptake of dopamine accounts for its ability to assist in smoking cessation. **Bupropion** is started 1 to 2 weeks before the quit-smoking date. The patient begins taking 150 mg daily for 3 days and then increases the dose to 150 mg twice a day at least 8 hours apart, avoiding bedtime dosing. On the quit day the patient can quit cold turkey or use a **nicotine replacement therapy** along with the **bupropion. Bupropion** and the **nicotine patch** are a successful combination, more successful than the **nicotine patch** alone. Therapy continues for 7 to 12 weeks.

Bupropion is contraindicated in patients with seizure disorders, bulimia, and anorexia nervosa and within 14 days of the use of **monoamine oxidase inhibitors (MAOIs). Although it is Pregnancy Category B, it is not recommended during pregnancy** or for use in children under age 18. **Nondrug treatments should be tried first in pregnant patients.** If used with **nicotine replacement therapy,** the patient should be monitored for hypertension. **Bupropion** is the active ingredient in **Wellbutrin,** used to treat depression. The concurrent use of **bupropion (Zyban)** and **Wellbutrin** is contraindicated. The most frequent adverse effects of **bupropion** are insomnia (40%), dizziness (10%), and dry mouth (10%). Constipation is also a reported adverse effect, and the patient should be advised to increase fiber and fluid intake during treatment.

Nonpharmacological Treatment of Nicotine Addiction

The Agency for Health Care Policy and Research (AHCPR) has published *Smoking Cessation: Clinical Practice Guide-*

Clinical Pearl

CONSTIPATION AND TOBACCO CESSATION

Many patients experience constipation during tobacco cessation as the stimulating effects of **nicotine** on the GI system are decreased. Increased dietary fiber, increased fluids, and use of a bulk-producing **laxative (Metamucil** or **Citrucel)** will help with this problem.

lines (Fiore et al., 1996). These guidelines recommend a number of nonpharmacological interventions:

1. Smoking cessation interventions should include either individual or group counseling.
2. Smokers should be offered access to support through a telephone hot line or help line or online support group when feasible, as a self-help intervention.
3. Smoking cessation interventions should include problem solving, skills training, relapse prevention, and stress management to increase cessation success rates.

The cost effectiveness of the AHCPR smoking cessation guidelines has been evaluated, and the most cost-effective intervention involved intensive counseling and the **nicotine patch** (Cromwell et al., 1997).

Other nonpharmacological therapies include hypnosis, acupuncture, and massage. Self-massage of the ear or hand with circular or stroking motions decreases feelings of anxiety, depressed mood, withdrawal cravings, and craving intensity in smoking patients attempting to quit (Hernandez-Reif, Field, & Hart, 1999). Relaxation and exercise are also central to smoking cessation therapy to counter the anxiety that is associated with **nicotine** withdrawal and to decrease the amount of weight gained during cessation. The successful treatment of the smoker who desires to quit will include a variety of treatment modalities, both pharmacological and nonpharmacological.

Patient Variables

Pregnancy

A pregnant woman who smokes places herself and her fetus in danger. Smoking is associated with low birth weight and prematurity, as well as increased perinatal mortality. Smoking cessation during pregnancy is ideal for the developing fetus. Pregnant smokers are advised to quit smoking without the use of *nicotine replacement therapy.* **The benefits and risks of** *nicotine replacement therapy* **have not been studied on pregnant patients, but the risk of smoking is thought to outweigh the short-term risk of low-dose** *nicotine replacement.* **Therefore, the FDA has reclassi-**

fied *nicotine gum* **as a Pregnancy Category C medication; the** *transdermal patch* **and** *inhaled* **forms continue to be classified as Pregnancy Category D. The manufacturer of** *Nicorette gum* **continues to recommend that nonpharmacological measures be used first.** *Bupropion (Zyban)* **is not recommended during pregnancy. The number to register pregnant patients exposed to** *bupropion* **is (888) 825–5249, ext. 39441.**

Children

Children should never receive **nicotine replacement products** or **bupropion** for tobacco cessation. Their use is usually experimental, and they are rarely **nicotine**-addicted. Primary education about tobacco use is the appropriate method to be used with children who may be tempted to smoke. Toxic levels of **nicotine** are reached quickly in children, and all **nicotine** products should remain out of their reach.

Adolescents

Adolescent patients pose a challenge because most adult smokers began as teenage smokers. Physically and psychologically, they can be addicted to tobacco. The peer group norm can lead teens to use tobacco, even when they know it is illegal and a poor choice for them to make. Tobacco cessation programs in this age group need to be geared toward identifying the teen smoker early and providing support for quitting. Many teens report that their health care provider did not even ask if they used tobacco (Schubiner et al., 1998). The provider who identifies a teen smoker who is ready to quit can choose a variety of options. It is essential for the teen to have a peer support group of other teen nonsmokers. Many schools have drug and **alcohol** counselors on staff who organize support groups in the school. There has been little research in adolescents regarding **nicotine replacement therapy.** Because adolescent smokers report the same **nicotine** withdrawal and cravings as adults, a teenager who smokes 20 or more cigarettes per day warrants the trial use of **nicotine replacement. Transdermal nicotine replacement** has been studied in adolescent patients and may be the best choice for treatment. Buying tobacco products is illegal for adolescents under age 18. Writing a prescription for the product and having the parent purchase the product will allow the patient access to **nicotine replacement therapy.** The adolescent needs to have clear directions regarding not smoking while using **nicotine replacement** and regarding the symptoms of **nicotine** toxicity. Careful education and monitoring of the patient throughout therapy will decrease adverse outcomes.

Monitoring

The patient needs to be monitored closely during all phases of tobacco cessation. As patients begin therapy, they need to be monitored for signs of **nicotine** withdrawal or, in the case of **nicotine replacement, nicotine** toxicity. The dose of **nicotine replacement** can be adjusted up or down, based on a patient's clinical symptoms. As patients are weaned down on the dose of **nicotine replacement** (every 2 to 3 weeks), they need to be monitored for increasing withdrawal symptoms. After patients are weaned off **nicotine replacement,** they need to be continually assessed as to their abstinence from tobacco. It is not unusual for patients to relapse, and the health care provider needs to provide support for their repeated attempts to quit.

Smoking alters the metabolism of several medications, and patients taking them need to be monitored closely and the dosage of their medications adjusted accordingly as they successfully quit. Both smoking and **nicotine** can increase circulating cortisol and catecholamines. Patients taking **adrenergic agonists (isoproterenol, phenylephrine)** or **adrenergic blockers (beta blockers)** must be monitored closely as they decrease their **nicotine** dependence. Smoking may reduce the diuretic effects of **furosemide** and reduce cardiac output, and smoking cessation may reverse these actions. **Glutethimide (Doriden)** absorption may be decreased with smoking cessation. First-pass metabolism of **propoxyphene (Darvocet)** may be decreased with smoking cessation. Smoking cessation potentiates **theophylline, insulin, pentazocine, oxazepam, tricyclic antidepressants (e.g., imipramine), caffeine,** and **acetaminophen.** Careful assessment of medications that the patient is taking prior to

beginning a tobacco cessation program will decrease the adverse effects during cessation.

Outcome Evaluation

The goal of tobacco cessation is for the patient to be tobacco-free at the end of treatment. Understanding that **nicotine** is highly addictive and that there are behavioral patterns ingrained in a smoker's habit can help define successful treatment. The patient who quits smoking cold turkey and is successful over the long term clearly has a positive outcome. The patient who uses **nicotine replacement** or **bupropion** for a number of weeks and then is tobacco-free for a long period of time (more than 12 months) also has a positive outcome.

The reality of tobacco cessation treatment is that many patients relapse. Recognizing that many smokers quit for a while two or three times before successfully achieving long-term cessation will enable the patient and the provider to view any period of abstinence as one step closer to long-term success. By supporting patients during this process and assuring them that they are not failures if they begin smoking again, the health care provider preserves an environment where patients can again attempt quitting when they are ready.

Patient Education

Patient education should include a discussion of information related to the overall treatment plan as well as that specific to the drug therapy, reasons for the drug's being taken, drugs as part of the total treatment regimen, and adherence issues.

Educational Resources

Many resources pertaining to tobacco cessation are available for providers and patients. The American Lung Association (ALA) has local chapters that can provide posters, written educational materials to promote tobacco

---

ON THE HORIZON

Tobacco Cessation Therapies

The future looks promising for tobacco cessation therapies. There is currently a sublingual form of **nicotine replacement** available in Europe, which may gain FDA approval for use in the United States. Research continues on **antidepressants,** specifically **nortriptyline,** which may also be effective in the treatment of **nicotine** addiction.

Smoking Cessation

Related to the Overall Treatment Plan/Disease Process

☐ Education regarding the physical and psychological aspects of tobacco addiction

☐ Role of lifestyle modifications

☐ Importance of adherence to the treatment regimen

☐ Need for regular follow-up visits with the primary care provider

Specific to the Drug Therapy

☐ Doses and schedules for taking the drug

☐ Possible adverse effects and what to do if they occur

☐ Interactions between other treatment modalities and these drugs

Reasons for Taking the Drug(s)

These drugs are given to help a person stop smoking. The medications that are used for smoking cessation need to be used as prescribed; overuse or underuse will increase treatment failure or lead to adverse effects.

The patient needs to understand the danger of nicotine toxicity, know the symptoms, and have clear instructions to cease the medication and notify the health care provider. The patient must not smoke while using a nicotine replacement. Nicotine replacement products, even after they are used, can be toxic to children and to pets; therefore, all of the products need to be handled carefully and disposed of properly after use.

Drugs as Part of the Total Treatment Regimen

The total treatment regimen includes nonpharmacological strategies. Nonpharmacological strategies such as relaxation, massage, exercise, and group therapy should be discussed and patients encouraged to incorporate multiple strategies to help them be successful.

A weight gain of 5 to 8 lb is common during tobacco cessation. Patients need to avoid strict diets during tobacco cessation and increase exercise during cessation treatment. After they have been tobacco-free for a few months, they can then work on weight reduction. Encouraging exercise during treatment will decrease the amount of weight gained.

Adherence Issues

Patients should know that having quit before and resumed their habit does not predict that they cannot be successful and that patients often quit for a while and then lapse two or three times before they succeed.

Many patients need external motivation to be successful at tobacco cessation. Identifying each patient's motivation and reminding her or him of it at each visit will assist patients in refocusing their goals when they feel like giving up. Common motivators include the health of their children or spouse and their own health. Pointing out the cost savings of quitting smoking, which can add up to over $1000 a year for a pack-a-day smoker, can also help patients focus on their goal. Have them place a photo of what they will buy with their savings in a prominent place (the refrigerator or bathroom mirror) as a reminder.

Smoking Cessation

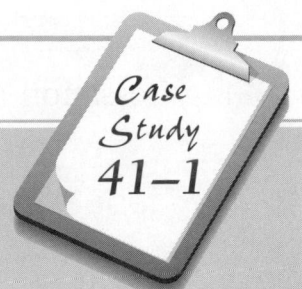

Complaint

"I think I want to quit smoking."

History

Ben, a 42-year-old white man, presents to the clinic for a blood pressure check. A nurse at a mall health screening had told him that his blood pressure was a little elevated. He denies any other physical complaints. He also mentions that the nurse told him that if he quits smoking, his blood pressure might go down.

Ben has been a patient at the clinic for 8 years but is seen on average every 18 months for minor acute problems, the last visit being 2 years ago (for bronchitis). He has never had an elevated BP in the clinic. The chart reveals that tobacco cessation has been addressed previously, but he was not ready to quit. Ben reports that he began smoking when he was 15 years old and became a regular 1.5-pack-per-day smoker when he was 19 or 20 (35-pack-year history). He at first denies any physical symptoms from smoking but does admit to a morning cough and shortness of breath during moderate exercise. He did try to quit cold turkey in his late twenties and again in his mid-thirties but was unsuccessful. He is interested in the "pill" that helps people stop smoking, and he also saw an ad on TV for "the patch." His wife is a nonsmoker, and he has two teenage children.

Assessment

Ben is well nourished and well developed. His BP is 132/90 at the beginning of the visit; when retaken at the end of the visit, it was 128/88. The rest of his vital signs are within normal limits (WNL).

Upon physical examination, he is noted to have a cough with deep inspiration and no clubbing or cyanosis noted. Breath sounds are clear. The rest of the examination is WNL. He denies any symptoms of depression.

Initial Management Plan

The provider assesses Ben's smoking habit and determines that he smokes the most before work in the morning (usually 3 to 4 cigarettes between arising and getting to work) and in the evening. Smoking is not allowed at work, and he gets only 30 minutes for lunch, allowing 1 or 2 cigarettes at lunch and 1 at each of his two breaks. After work, he begins smoking in the car on the way home and has an average of 2 to 3 cigarettes per hour until bed. Ben considers himself to be highly dependent on cigarettes and readily admits to nicotine withdrawal symptoms if he is not able to have his early morning cigarettes.

The provider discusses the different treatment options and decides to use a combination of bupropion (Zyban) and transdermal nicotine (Habitrol.) The initial management plan is as follows:

Ben is given a prescription for Zyban and told to take one 150-mg tablet for 3 days and then 1 tablet bid for the course of treatment, avoiding bedtime dosing. His blood pressure will need careful monitoring for hypertension during therapy. Ben sets a quit date of 10 days later and is given a prescription for Habitrol 21-mg/24-hour patches. He is told to return to the clinic a day or two after he quits smoking and begins the patch.

Follow-up Visit

Ben reports that he quit 2 days previously, on day 10 of the Zyban. He felt some cravings in the morning of the previous day but less so after the patch had been on for 24 hours. He reports that he had some trouble at work during lunch, as all the men he has lunch with smoke and he did not realize that he was used to smoking as a part of his work routine. His blood pressure is 136/88.

The provider encourages Ben and discusses strategies for dealing with situations where he previously smoked. He is encouraged to take a quick walk after eating his lunch to give him less time to sit with the smokers. He reports that his family is very supportive and his wife made a special meal to celebrate his quit day. The patient is instructed to stay on the same dose of Zyban (150 mg bid) and continue the Habitrol 21-mg patch for 6 weeks. He is to return in 1 week or sooner, if needed.

Three Days Later

Ben comes to the clinic with severe nausea. During lunch he had been offered a cigarette by a coworker and decided to smoke one. He became nauseated after a few minutes, but it is subsiding . Nicotine toxicity is discussed and the danger of smoking while using the nicotine transdermal patch is reviewed. The provider encourages Ben to not have lunch with the group of coworkers who smoke if he can. He is to return for his scheduled visit in 4 days.

Follow-up Visit One Week after Quit Date

Ben returns to the clinic feeling better and remains tobacco-free. His blood pressure is WNL, and he reports no withdrawal symptoms. He has been walking at lunch for the past 2 days with a coworker who quit 6 months previously by using the nicotine patch. He states that he now understands the necessity of having support outside his family for quitting. The walking makes his lunchtime go faster, and he has less time to be concerned about smoking. He is to return in 2 weeks.

continued

Smoking Cessation (*continued*)

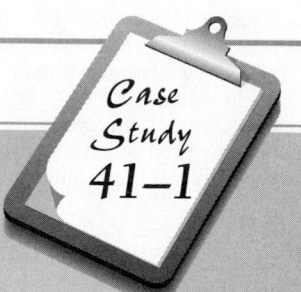

Case Study 41-1

Follow-up Visit Three Weeks after the Quit Date

Ben reports that he is feeling successful with his smoking cessation. He is now walking at lunch and also walks with his wife three or four nights a week. He is less short of breath when he walks, and his morning cough is decreasing. His blood pressure is WNL, and his weight is stable. He is instructed to continue on his current treatment regimen for 3 more weeks and then decrease the dose of his patch to 14 mg/day. He is to make an appointment for 1 to 2 days after decreasing the dose.

Follow-up Visit Six Weeks after the Quit Date

The morning after changing the dose, Ben reports some mild cravings, but they decreased. He is now walking nightly with his wife and at lunch. He reports that three men are now walking together at lunch, as another coworker is also quitting by using the nicotine patch. His BP remains WNL. He is instructed to stay on the 14-mg/day dose of Habitrol for 2 weeks and then decrease to 7 mg/day. He is to return to the clinic in 2 weeks.

Follow-up Visit Eight Weeks after the Quit Date

Ben has decreased his dose of Habitrol to 7 mg/day without problems. He continues to walk and is looking forward to being off the medication. His BP remains WNL, and his weight is stable. He is to continue the Habitrol 7-mg patch for 2 more weeks and then quit and return to the clinic in 3 to 4 weeks. He is to continue the Zyban for 4 more weeks.

Twelve Weeks after the Quit Date

Ben's family has planned a backpacking trip for the following week to celebrate his successful quitting. He has been off the Habitrol for 2 weeks and reports only mild cravings for the first couple of days after the last patch. He stopped the Zyban a week previously without problems. He states that he feels "really good." He is instructed to continue the physical activity and continue to avoid places where smoking is the norm. He is to return as needed and is told that the provider would be calling in 3 to 4 weeks to check on him.

Continuing Care

Telephone Follow-up Sixteen Weeks after the Quit Date

Ben reports that he remains tobacco-free. Walking with his wife nightly has improved the communication in his marriage. He found out that his family had been worrying about his health and that they are all proud of his accomplishment. He has made new friends based on common interests rather than on who is smoking at breaktime and at lunch. The provider reminds him that a relapse can still happen and to call if he has concerns.

One Year Later

Ben comes to the clinic for a routine physical. He has remained smoke-free. He has lost 6 lb over the last 6 months from the increased exercise, and his blood pressure is 122/84.

---

cessation, and materials for the Great American Smoke-out, an annual antismoking event. Both the American Cancer Society (ACS) and the American Heart Association (AHA) have local chapters that can also provide educational materials to health care providers. There are Websites devoted to tobacco cessation that health care providers can access. One helpful site is the Physician's Guide to the Internet, which summarizes the AHCPR recommendations and provides clinical guidelines for prescribing **nicotine replacement.** A full executive summary of the AHCPR *Clinical Guidelines* is available there, as well as an 8-page "Information for Patients" handout that can be downloaded and given to patients who are starting or considering **nicotine replacement therapy.** The Help Your Patient Stop Smoking Website is located at *www. physiciansguide.com/pgi/smoke1.html.* At the RxList Website, *www.rxlist.com,* the provider can type in a medication

and print extensive patient handouts on the medication. With the abundance of resources available to the health care provider, patient education should be easily incorporated into the care of the patient.

REFERENCES

Centers for Disease Control. (1997). State-specific prevalence of cigarette smoking among adults, children's and adolescents' exposure to environmental tobacco smoke—United States, 1996. *Morbidity and Mortality Weekly Report, 46,* 1038–1043.

Cromwell, J., Bartosch, W. J., Fiore, M. C., Hasselblad, V., & Baker, T. (1997). Cost effectiveness of the clinical practice recommendation in the AHCPR guidelines for smoking cessation. *Journal of the American Medical Association, 278,* 1759–1766.

Fiore, M. C., Bailey, W. C. Cohen, S. C., et al. (1996). *Smoking cessation: Clinical practice guidelines* (DHHS Pub. 96-0692). Rockville, MD: U.S. Department of Health and Human Services, Public Health Service, Agency for Health Care Policy and Research.

Heishman, S. J., Balfour, D. J. K., Benowitz, N. L., Hatsukami, D. K., Lindstrom, J. M., & Ockene, J. K. (1997). Society for research on nicotine and tobacco. *Addiction, 92*(5), 615–633.

Hernandez-Reif, M., Field, T., & Hare, S. (1999). Smoking cravings are reduced by self-massage. *Preventive Medicine, 28*(1), 28–32.

Hjalmarson, A., Nilsson, F., Sjöström, L., & Wiklund, O. (1997). The nicotine inhaler in smoking cessation. *Archives of Internal Medicine, 157,* 1721–1728.

Hurt, R. D., Offord, K. P., Croghan, I. T., Croghan, G. A., Gomez-Dahl, L. C., Wolter, T. D., Dale, L. C., & Moyer, T. P. (1998). Temporal effects of nicotine nasal spray and gum on nicotine withdrawal symptoms. *Psychopharmacology, 140,* 98–104.

Jimenez-Ruiz, C., Kunze, M., & Fagerstrom, K. O. (1998). Nicotine replacement: A new approach to reducing tobacco-related harm. *European Respiratory Journal, 11,* 473–479.

Jorenby, D. E., Leischow, S. J., Nides, M. A., Rennard, S. I., Johnston, J. A., Hughes, A. R., Smith, S. S., Muramoto, M. L., Daughton, D. M., Doan, K., Fiore, M. C., & Baker, T. B. (1999). A controlled trial of sustained-release bupropion, a nicotine patch, or both for smoking cessation. *New England Journal of Medicine, 340*(9), 685–691.

Krawiec, J. V., & Pohl, J. M. (1998). Smoking cessation and nicotine replacement therapy: A guide for primary care providers. *American Journal for Nurse Practitioners, 2*(1), 15–33.

Prochazka, A. V., Weaver, M. J., Keller, R. T., Fryer, G. E., Licari, P. A., & Lofaso, D. (1998). A randomized trial of nortriptyline for smoking cessation. *Archives of Internal Medicine, 158,* 2035–2039.

Schneider, N. G., Lunell, E., Olmstead, R. E., & Fagerström, K. (1996). Clinical pharmacokinetics of nasal nicotine delivery: A review and comparison to other nicotine systems. *Clinical Pharmacokinetics, 31*(1), 65–80.

Schubiner, H., Herrold, A., & Hurt, R. (1998). Tobacco cessation and youth: The feasibility of brief office interventions for adolescents. *Preventive Medicine, 27*(5), A47–A54.

Sheahan, S. L., & Wilson, S. M. (1998). Smoking cessation tips: Family system and addiction perspectives. *Journal of the American Academy of Nurse Practitioners, 10*(9), 393–401.

Smoking cessation. (1999). *Nurse Practitioners Prescribing Reference,* Summer, 237–240.

Thorndike, A. N., Rigotti, N. A., Stafford, R. S., & Singer, D. E. (1998). National patterns in the treatment of smokers by physicians. *Journal of the American Medical Association, 279*(8), 604–608.

CHAPTER 42

·······

Sexually Transmitted Diseases and Vaginitis

CHAPTER OUTLINE

Sexually Transmitted Diseases

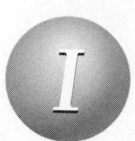 n the 1950s and 1960s, **penicillin** was the magic bullet for most sexually transmitted diseases (STDs). By 1995, **antibiotic** resistance threatened

control of bacterial infections such as syphilis, gonorrhea, and chlamydia. The number of patients requiring services for STDs has increased in proportion to those who are sexually active, and the number of patients with viral diseases has increased exponentially. The seroprevalence of herpes simplex virus type 2 (HSV-2) is now 20.8 percent. In the third National Health and Nutrition Examination Surveys

(NHANES III), seropositivity correlated with a higher lifetime number of sexual partners and with cocaine use, both of which are behavioral risk factors associated with the acquisition of human immunodeficiency virus (HIV) (Fleming et al., 1997). As many as 50 percent of those infected with HSV-2 are asymptomatic shedders of the virus. Because 20 percent of people now have HSV-2 infection, those who have unprotected sexual contact with multiple partners are virtually guaranteed to acquire HSV-2 (Arvin & Prober, 1997).

Scientific identification of the viral genotype of human papillomavirus (HPV) has enabled primary care providers to view cancer of the cervix as an STD. Although most HPV infection causes all Pap smears to appear atypical, genotypes 16, 18, 31, 33, and 35 have malignant potential, so that a seemingly innocuous wart could herald a potentially lethal disease.

Pathophysiology

With the onset of puberty, the vagina becomes estrogenized, and the glycogen content increases. Lactobacilli (Döderlein's bacilli) predominate and are responsible for the breakdown of glycogen to lactic acid. The pH of the normal vagina should be 3.5 to 4.1. Most women grow between three and eight types of bacteria. Usually a treatment such as **antibiotic therapy** or a behavior such as having multiple sex partners triggers a nonphysiological response, and the ecosystem of the vagina becomes disturbed enough to produce pathological symptoms. Beyond menopause, women may experience vulvovagi-

nal pain as a result of a thin, superficial epithelium. This reduced layer of epithelial cells can make the woman more vulnerable to infection and trauma. Infection can be from her own perineal bacterial flora, and the trauma can be a result of normal sexual relations. Other common irritants to the vaginal ecosystem are "forgotten" tampons, douches, contraceptive preparations, and even stress. Vaginal secretions consist of proteins, polysaccharides, amino acids, enzyme inhibitors, and immunoglobulins that are produced primarily from the cervix and to a lesser extent by Bartholin's and Skene's glands, endometrial and oviductal fluid, and transudate from vaginal squamous epithelium and exfoliated squamous cells. The peak times for production of these secretions are pregnancy and midcycle in a menstruating woman (Sorbel, 1997).

In women, STDs often present with discharge and vaginal irritation, but not all vaginitis is infectious. Differential diagnosis of vaginal discharge is presented in Table 42–1. Treatments for infectious vaginitis that may be acquired without sexual contact as well as noninfectious vaginitis are discussed later in this chapter.

Genital contact between people is required for transmission of most STDs, although fomite transmission (such as through vibrators, toilet seats, and bath towels) has occurred with hardier organisms. Women tend to experience more morbidity than men because of the secretions deposited during the sex act. Transmission from one partner to the other can be facilitated or impeded by alterations in vaginal pH, the presence of inflammation caused by **spermicides,** and the mucosal integrity of either partner. Bacteria and viruses can invade the mucosal

Table 42–1. Differential Diagnosis of Vaginal Discharge

Discharge Appearance	Symptoms	pH	Diagnostic Tests	Microscope Findings	Disease/ Syndrome
White, curdy	+ Burn, itch	<4.5	Culture/KOH	Budding yeast hyphae	Monilia Candidiasis
Mucopurulent, thick	+ Irritating	Normal	DNA/culture	WBCs>10/hpf	GC/Chlamydia
Thin, white, odor	+ Itch, odor a big issue	>4.5	+ Amine/ culture-change in vaginal flora	"Clue cells" (coccoid bacteria that obscure epithelial cell borders)	Bacterial vaginosis (BV)
Blood-tinged, purulent	+ Itch, dysuria, foul odor	<4.5	Wet mount = + Trichomonads	Trichomonads >10 WBCs/hpf	Trichomoniasis
Nonspecific, white	+ Pruritus, burn	3.5–4.5	Culture reports change in normal flora	4+ *Lactobacillus*	Cytologic
Scanty, may be white or yellow	+ Burn, sore, cracks	>5–7	Culture is negative	Several epithelial cells	Atrophic
White	None	3.8–4.2	Not necessary	1–2+ *Lactobacillus*	Normal

lining of the oral, genital, or anal tract. All bodily secretions, especially blood, can transmit infection from human to human.

Goals of Treatment

There is no dearth of literature to validate that STDs are preventable through safe sexual behavior. The first goal of therapy is to educate patients about those behaviors, especially those patients between ages 15 and 25, when the incidence of chlamydia infection is the highest. In a recent study of college-age females, the incidence of abnormal Pap smears associated with the presence of HPV was increasing at an alarming rate. Increased risk of acquiring HPV infection was significantly associated with younger age, Hispanic ethnicity, black race, an increased number of vaginal-sex partners, high frequencies of vaginal sex and alcohol consumption, anal sex, and partners who had an increased number of lifetime partners (Ho et al., 1998). Prevention of long-term sequelae of unsafe sex is the second goal of therapy. Four complications of STDs are tubal occlusion leading to infertility and ectopic pregnancy, neonatal morbidity and mortality caused by transmission during pregnancy and parturition, genital cancers, and possible exposure to HIV because of its association with other STDs. The third goal of therapy is to choose the most specific, cost-effective drug that has the best regimen for adherence, after verifying the diagnosis and assessment of pregnancy. The fourth goal of therapy is to reduce morbidity and provide comfort for those chronic viral and inflammatory conditions that are not curable.

Rational Drug Selection

Guidelines

Treatment for STDs is based on national guidelines recommended by the Centers for Disease Control and Prevention (CDC) because of the substantial impact on public health. The following recommendations are consistent with the *Guidelines for the Treatment of Sexually Transmitted Diseases* (U.S. Department of Health and Human Services, 1998) and are presented in Table 42–2. Chapter 18 has more information about the specific **antibiotics** and **antifungals.** Chapters 19 and 20 discuss drugs used for inflammatory disorders and for conditions of the integumentary system.

SYPHILIS. This systemic disease has been present in society for centuries. The increase of congenital cases (fourfold) since 1950 may be a result of illicit drug use. It is spread by direct contact of the mucosal tissue to infected lesions. Diagnostic symptoms may present as early as 5 days and as late as 90 days after exposure to the organism.

Primary infection presents with ulcer or chancre at the site of infection. Secondary infection has manifestations that include rash, mucocutaneous lesions, and adenopathy. Tertiary syphilis has cardiac, neurological, ophthalmic, auditory, or gummatous lesions. If syphilis is prevalent in the geographic area, screening should be repeated in the high-risk or pregnant patient at 28 weeks gestation to avoid possible neonatal transmission. The high-risk category for repeated screening is described as a person who has a history of multiple sex partners, a history of current or recent STDs, or a user of street drugs (Hatcher, 1998). Neurosyphilis may occur at any stage but is most common in late latent stage. During the late latent phase, the infected patient is not infectious, unless pregnant or through blood transmission. Misdiagnosis or delayed diagnosis is possible because of the low level of suspicion in many family practice settings. Vaginal "warts" are not all HPV viral disease. Anogenital condylomata lata are a common symptom of secondary syphilis, as well as a generalized papulosquamous eruption.

GONORRHEA. First isolated in 1879, this gram-negative intracellular diplococcus can be transmitted through the urethra, rectum, pharynx, vagina, or eye. The incubation can be 2 days to 2 weeks. The rate of transmission is 70 percent from male to unprotected female. Complications of infection are pelvic inflammation, salpingitis, or disseminated gonococcus (GC) infection characterized by pustular dermatitis. An infected pregnant woman is at risk for endometritis after procedures such as therapeutic abortions, chronic villus sampling, or dilatation and curettage. Between 30 and 50 percent of newborns of women with gonococcal cervicitis develop gonococcal conjunctivitis. In those who remain infected, the etiology is usually reinfection, not treatment failure (U.S. Department of Health and Human Services, 1998).

CHLAMYDIA. Chlamydia is a silent disease with serious sequelae such as pelvic inflammatory disease, ectopic pregnancy, and infertility. The recommendation to screen all patients plus early treatment can prevent the sequelae. The CDC data validate coinfection with gonorrhea; therefore, dual therapy is an accepted standard. Treatment of sex partners is important. Most practitioners treat the sex partner when diagnostic tests are positive because reinfection is common. Although the 7-day therapy is effective, if poor compliance is suspected, then the single 1-g dose of **azithromycin** is recommended. Alternative therapy with **erythromycin** is recommended for pregnant women, but adverse reactions and reduced effectiveness make it less desirable for nonpregnant women. Routine follow-up is not usually necessary, unless treatment is with **erythromycin.** It may be more beneficial to screen high-risk patients at 3- or 6-month intervals.

CHANCROID. This disease is endemic in some areas of this country. It has been found as a coinfection with HIV and, to a lesser extent, with syphilis and HSV. Diagnosis

Table 42–2. Drugs Commonly Used: Sexually Transmitted Diseases

Pathogen	First Choice	Alternative Choice
Bacterial Pathogens Syphilis, primary and secondary	Benzathine penicillin G Adults: 2.4 million units (IM) one dose Children: 50,000 units/kg in one dose	Pregnant patients allergic to penicillin should be desensitized Nonpregnant use doxycycline 100 mg bid for 2 wk *or* tetracycline 500 mg qid for 2 wk
Syphilis, early latent (tertiary)	Benzathine penicillin G Adults: 2.4 million units (IM) one dose	Same as above
Syphilis, late latent or unknown	3 weekly doses of benzathine penicillin G 2.4 million units	Same as above, only for 4 wk duration
Gonococcal infections (cervix, urethra, and rectum)	Cefixime 400 mg PO *plus* azithromycin 1 g PO in one dose	*Or* ceftriaxone 125 mg (IM) in one dose *or* ciprofloxacin 500 mg PO in one dose *or* ofloxacin 400 PO in one dose *or* doxycycline 100 mg bid for 7 d
Gonococcal infections (pharynx)	Same as above except for cefixime	Spectinomycin 2 g (IM) one dose
Chlamydia (adults and adolescents)	Azithromycin 1 g PO one dose *or* doxycycline 100 mg bid for 7 d	Erythromycin base 500 mg PO qid for 7 d *or* erythromycin ethylsuccinate 800 qid PO for 7 d *or* ofloxacin 300 PO bid for 7 d
Chlamydia (pregnancy)	Erythromycin base 500 mg PO qid for 7 d *or* amoxicillin 500 mg PO tid for 7 d	Erythromycin ethylsuccinate 800 mg PO qid for 7 d *or* erythromycin ethylsuccinate 400 mg PO qid for 14 d *or* erythromycin base 250 mg PO qid for 14 d
Chancroid	Azithromycin 1 g PO in one dose *or* ceftriaxone 250 mg (IM) in one dose *or* ciprofloxacin 500 mg PO bid for 3 d *or* erythromycin base 500 mg PO qid for 7 d	Ciprofloxacin is not for patients under age 18 years and those who are pregnant
Granuloma inguinale (donovanosis)	Trimethoprim-sulfamethoxazole one double-strength (DS) tablet PO bid for 3 wk *or* doxycycline 100 mg PO bid for 3 wk	Ciprofloxacin 750 PO bid for 3 wk *or* erythromycin base 500 mg PO qid for 3 wk
Lymphogranuloma venereum	Doxycycline 100 mg PO bid for 21 d	Erythromycin base 500 mg PO qid for 21 d
Bacterial vaginosis	Metronidazole 500 mg PO bid for 7 d *or* clindamycin cream 2% 5 g (one applicator) at bedtime for 7 d *or* metronidazole gel 0.75% 5 g (one applicator) at bedtime bid for 5 d	Metronidazole 2 g PO one dose *or* clindamycin 300 mg bid for 7 d
Viral Pathogens Herpes simplex types 1 and 2	**First Episode** Acyclovir 400 mg PO tid for 7–10 d *or* acyclovir 200 mg PO 5 times for 7–10 d *or* famciclovir 250 mg PO tid for 7–10 d *or* valacyclovir 1 g PO bid for 7–10 d	**Recurring Episodes** Same dosage as first episode except for 5 days of treatment Suppression daily is same dosage but given: acyclovir 400 bid; famciclovir 250 mg bid; valacyclovir 500 mg once daily; valacyclovir 1000 mg once daily
Human papillomavirus (HPV) (cervical)	Provider-applied (nonpregnant): needs specialized training to treat	Patient-applied (nonpregnant): needs colposcopy, biopsy prior to treatment Patient-applied (pregnant): needs specialist management

Continued on next page

Table 42–2. Drugs Commonly Used: Sexually Transmitted Diseases *(continued)*

Pathogen	First Choice	Alternative Choice
Human papillomavirus (HPV) (vaginal)	Provider-applied (nonpregnant): cryotherapy: apply every 2 wk; OK with pregnancy, *or* TCA or BCA 80–90% Apply every week; allow tissues to heal between applications; OK with pregnancy, *or* podophyllin resin 10–25%; apply, dry, wash off by 4 h; treat weekly *or* surgical removal by shave technique, curettage, or electrosurgery; *alternative therapies:* intralesional interferon, not with pregnancy, *or* laser surgery, not with pregnancy	Patient-applied (nonpregnant): Podofilox 0.05% solution or gel bid for 3 d, 4 d off, up to 4 cycles Imiquimod 5% cr: Apply 3 times a week at hs, wash off in A.M. Duration 8–16 wk Patient-applied (pregnant): not safe
Human papillomavirus (HPV) (urethral)	Provider-applied (nonpregnant): cryosurgery *or* podophyllin 10–25% as above	Patient-applied (nonpregnant): none Patient-applied (pregnant): none
Human papillomavirus (HPV) (anal, outside sphincter)	Provider-applied (nonpregnant): cryosurgery *or* TCA or BCA 80–90% as above *or* surgical removal	Patient-applied (nonpregnant): none Patient-applied (pregnant): none
Human papillomavirus (HPV) (oral)	Provider-applied (nonpregnant): cryosurgery *or* surgical removal	Patient-applied (nonpregnant): none Patient-applied (pregnant): none
Fungal Pathogen Candidiasis	*Intravaginal* Butoconazole 2% 5 g for 3 d Clotrimazole 1% 5 g for 7–14 d Clotrimazole 100-mg tablet 2 tabs for 3 d Clotrimazole 100-mg tab for 7 d Clotrimazole 500-mg tab given only once Miconazole 2% 5 g for 7 d Miconazole 200 mg supp for 3 d Miconazole 100-mg supp for 7 d Nystatin 100,000-unit tab for 14 d Tioconazole 6.5% oint 5 g in one dose Terconazole 0.4% cr 5 g for 7 d Terconazole 0.8% cr 5 g for 3 d Terconazole 80-mg supp for 3 d	*Oral* Fluconazole 150-mg tablet in one dose
Protozoan Pathogen Trichomoniasis	Metronidazole 2 g PO in one dose	Metronidazole 500 mg PO bid for 7 d
Ectoparasitic Pathogens Pubic lice	Permethrin 1% crème rinse to affected areas, wash off in 10 min *or* lindane 1% shampoo applied 4 min to the affected area and wash off *or* pyrethrins with piperonyl butoxide applied to affected areas, wash off in 10 min Permethrin 5 % cream: apply to all body, wash off 8–14 h	Not for pregnant women or children under age 2
Scabies		Lindane 1% apply to all body, wash off after 8 h *or* sulfur 6% ointment to all areas nightly for 3 nights; wash off 24 h after last dose

Adapted from U.S. Department of Health and Human Services. (1998). *Guidelines for treatment of sexually transmitted diseases.* Atlanta: Centers for Disease Control and Prevention.
TCA = trichloroacetic acid; BCA = bichloroacetic acid.

is difficult because of the lack of available and sensitive media. As a result, treatment is initiated when the following criteria are satisfied: one or more painful ulcers, negative tests for syphilis and HSV, and the appearance of ulcers with suppurative inguinal adenopathy. Although treatment is successful, there still may be significant scarring. In those men who are uncircumcised or have HIV disease, response may not be as good. Follow-up in this group is recommended because lack of response may indicate presence of HIV disease, and this person should be retested at 3-month intervals. If the lymphadenopathy is fluctuant, incision and drainage may be necessary to enhance healing.

GRANULOMA INGUINALE (DONOVANOSIS). Ulcers that are painless, without lymphadenopathy, and progress to large beefy lesions that are difficult to heal also characterize this disease. Most infections are endemic in tropical and developing areas of India, Papua New Guinea, central Australia, and southern Africa. Treatment is long, a minimum of 3 weeks, and relapse is common within 6 to 18 months despite the best therapy. Sex partners should have clinical signs and symptoms prior to initiation of therapy.

LYMPHOGRANULOMA VENEREUM. Lymphogranuloma venereum is another disease rarely seen in the United States, but it shares characteristics with chancroid, such as unilateral tender lymphadenopathy and self-limited genital ulcers. Homosexual men may present with proctocolitis and women with perianal inflammation, with the complication being strictures or fistulas. Local lesions (buboes) may require incision and drainage. Serum is required for diagnosis. These patients may need further testing to rule out the high rate of coexisting STDs.

BACTERIAL VAGINOSIS. Bacterial vaginosis (BV), the most prevalent of vaginal infections, may be caused by *Prevotella* spp., *Mobiluncus* spp., *Gardnerella vaginalis,* or *Mycoplasma hominis.* Although treatment of the sex partner has been recommended in recurrent cases, research has not validated its efficacy. BV has also caused endometritis and pelvic inflammatory disease after invasive procedures such as endometrial biopsy, intrauterine device insertion, cesarean delivery, hysterectomy, and therapeutic abortion. One preliminary study using **metronidazole** postabortion reduced infection substantially. Recent studies have proved BV to be a cause of preterm labor. Therefore, BV must be diagnosed once the diagnosis of pregnancy is made. The criteria during assessment must include three of the four following signs and symptoms: a homogeneous, white, *noninflammatory* discharge that smoothly coats the vaginal walls; vaginal pH of more than 4.5; positive Whiff test with 10% potassium hydroxide (KOH); and presence of "clue cells" (vaginal epithelial cell peppered with coccoid bacteria) under high-power microscopy. Treatment is recommended after the first trimester to avoid teratogenic potential. Systemic treatment is recommended because two randomized studies show increased preterm delivery in those treated with **clindamycin** vaginally. Theoretically, systemic therapy has better penetration of upper genital tract tissues.

VULVOVAGINAL CANDIDIASIS. Vulvovaginal candidiasis (VVC) may be caused by several yeast species, although *Candida albicans* or other *Candida* species are the most common. The **azoles** as a drug class are the most effective treatment. In 90 percent of infections, a single oral dose of **fluconazole** provides a cure. The patient with chronic recurrent disease is often diabetic. Women who control their blood sugar closely have fewer reported infections. Although this disease is often diagnosed when women are checked for STDs, it is not necessarily passed sexually, but sex partners may be treated simultaneously if they are symptomatic with penile *Candida.* **Azoles** do stimulate the P-450 enzyme system in the liver and have potential drug interactions with **calcium channel antagonists, cisapride, warfarin, oral hypoglycemic agents, phenytoin, protease inhibitors, theophylline,** and **rifampin.**

HERPES SIMPLEX VIRUS TYPE 1 AND HERPES SIMPLEX VIRUS TYPE 2. Genital herpes is recurrent and incurable. Two serotypes of herpes simplex virus (HSV) have been identified: herpes simplex virus type 1 (HSV-1) and herpes simplex virus type 2 (HSV-2). Most recurrences are a result of HSV-2. Medications are up to 75 percent effective for symptom relief and speed of healing ulcers. Suppressive therapy is recommended for patients who experience six or more episodes each year. The drugs listed in Table 42–2 are safe, but long-term therapy has been validated only for **acyclovir.** At present, 45 million people have serologically proven HSV-2 infection, and 50 percent of those shed virus without obvious symptoms. Systemic medication is recommended as superior to topical. Most patients experience fewer episodes after 1 year of suppressive therapy. Episodic therapy is effective in shortening the duration of outbreaks if started within the first 24 hours. Treatment of genital herpes in HIV-infected patients is controversial and should be deferred to a specialist's recommendations. Prenatal exposure to **antivirals** is too limited to predict pregnancy outcomes. Prenatal infection can be life-threatening, and protected sex is necessary if sex partners are infected. Transmission to the infant is common if the disease is acquired late in pregnancy. Cesarean delivery does not ensure protection from HSV-2 infection.

HUMAN PAPILLOMAVIRUS. Most HPV infections are asymptomatic or not visible. Reports indicate that more than 20 types are currently transmitted. Types 6 and 11 are visible "warts," but the other types (16,18, 31, 33, and 35) are associated with cervical dysplasia. Patients with visible warts may be infected with several types simultaneously. These lesions may be cervical, vaginal, or perianal. The removal of these warts should be based on symptoms because there is no proof that removal reduces infectivity or the development of cervical cancer. In practice, most patients want removal of any visible warts. Treatment regimens should be changed if warts do not resolve in three to six treatments. Treatment of these lesions may result in chronic pain syndromes of the vulva, but these are extremely rare.

TRICHOMONIASIS. *Trichomonas* spp. are protozoa, and protozoan infections require a different therapeutic approach. This infection requires treatment of sex partners. Men are rarely symptomatic but may harbor it in the prostate gland for years if left untreated. In women, the vaginal discharge is impressive, with a foul odor. Pregnancy complicates treatment until after the first trimester, but treatment is imperative because preterm labor and premature labor are possible complications. The diagnosis is often missed because wet mounts must be viewed quickly to capture the classic trichomonad movement. Urine sediment microscopy may frequently demonstrate this organism fortuitously.

GENITAL LICE. Genital lice, commonly called *crabs*, are an ectoparasitic infection that is treated differently based on where the lice are found (e.g., scalp, body, or the pubic area). The organism is genetically programmed to attach to hair of different diameters. Considerable resistance to medication for treatment of head lice has been seen, but pediculosis is still eradicated by the methods listed in Table 42–2. Decontamination of household and personal items with hot washing or dry-cleaning is usually adequate. Pubic lice cannot live away from the body for more than 72 hours, and fumigating the home is not necessary if the previous methods are observed.

SCABIES. With scabies, another ectoparasitic infection, the most common symptom is pruritus, but this takes 6 weeks to develop after exposure to *Sarcoptes scabiei*. Scabies is passed sexually in adults, but children may become infected by sleeping on infected sheets at a friend's house. Contrary to previous instructions, **lindane** should not be used immediately after bathing and by people with extensive dermatitis. This caution will prevent potential seizures. In addition, it should not be used during pregnancy and in children under age 2.

Special Treatment Situations

Delay in treatment can result in pelvic inflammatory disease. As a result, a woman who presents for care with signs of constitutional symptoms needs to be treated as if she has all types of infection. She may need an intravenous (IV) **antibiotic** if her temperature is high and if she cannot tolerate oral drugs. In addition, an assault victim, pregnant or nonpregnant, can present as a treatment dilemma. To prevent harm to the developing fetus, the assault victim needs to be treated urgently. Table 42–3 reviews special treatment situations.

HEPATITIS. Serologic testing is necessary for all suspected cases of hepatitis. It is easy to assume that IV drug

Table 42–3. Special Treatment Situations

SEXUAL ASSAULT
Pregnant
• Needs specialty consultation; may need hospitalization
Nonpregnant
• Hepatitis B vaccine (if not already immunized and empiric treatment) *and*
• Ceftriaxone 125 mg (IM) in one dose *and*
• Metronidazole 2 g PO in one dose *and*
• Azithromycin 1 g PO in one dose *or*
• Doxycycline 100 mg PO bid for 7 d
PELVIC INFLAMMATORY DISEASE (PID)
Pregnant
• Needs specialty consultation; may need hospitalization
Nonpregnant
Regimen A
• Ofloxacin 400 mg PO bid for 14 d *and*
• Metronidazole 500 mg PO bid for 14 d
Regimen B
• Ceftriaxone 250 mg (IM) once *or*
• Cefoxitin 2 g (IM) *plus* probenecid 1 g PO in a single concurrent dose *or*
• Other parenteral third-generation cephalosporin *plus*
• Doxycycline 100 mg PO bid for 14 d

users have hepatitis B or C, but, in fact, outbreaks of hepatitis A have been reported in drug users. Only 1.8 percent of patients die from liver disease as a result of hepatitis A, but there is considerable morbidity, well worth the cost and inconvenience of two injections. Hepatitis A and B are the only **vaccine**-preventable diseases that can be passed sexually.

Chronic infections of hepatitis B occur in 1 to 6 percent of infected adults but in 90 percent of infected newborns. Hepatitis B virus (HBV) is passed through vertical transmission. Prevention aimed at several groups is necessary. Prevention strategies include screening all pregnant women, vaccinating all newborns (started in 1992; new recommendations are being developed), vaccinating older children at high risk (e.g., Alaskan Natives, Pacific Islanders, and residents in households with first-generation immigrants from countries that have high levels of endemic disease), vaccinating children age 11 and 12 who do not fit into the preceding categories, and vaccinating teens and adults at high risk (sexual behaviors confer increased risk).

Monitoring

Drug sensitivity and patient intolerance frequently necessitate use of alternate drugs. In diseases such as syphilis, the importance of using **penicillin** is so crucial that the

ON THE HORIZON

Treatment of STDs

Clinical development and trials are in progress for **vaccines** against a number of STDs. Numerous **antiviral** agents have been investigated for the treatment of chronic HBV infections. Those agents that appear promising are **interferon alpha-2b** and **antiretroviral agents** such as **lamivudine.** The type of patient who responds the most favorably to these treatments usually has the following characteristics: (1) low pretherapy HBV DNA levels, (2) high pretherapy alanine aminotransferase levels, (3) short duration of infection, (4) acquisition of disease in adulthood, (5) active histology, and (6) female gender (U.S. Department of Health and Human Services, 1998).

Use of **azithromycin** in a single 1-g dose in pregnant patients found positive for chlamydia is an unlabeled use for this **antibiotic.** The female condom also appears to have a potential impact against STDs because of its superior strength, polyurethane construction, and increased protection to the vulva. Studies remain to be completed to validate efficacy of this nonlatex product.

patient needs to be orally desensitized. Because of the possibility of anaphylaxis, consultation with a physician expert in this process is necessary. Fortunately, most other STDs can be eradicated with a single oral or parenteral dose, and the therapy is of short duration. Although treatments are quite effective, follow-up is necessary to be sure all sexual partners are treated. Asymptomatic partners are frequently resistant to treatment and may require education and assistance from the local health department. Laboratories are required by law to report these diseases to the state, so patients need to know that they will be contacted for verification of treatment.

Outcome Evaluation

Infection in the genital tract with chlamydia or gonorrhea, if not treated in a timely manner, may ascend, invade the fallopian tubes, and cause life-threatening pelvic inflammatory disease and sepsis. A pregnant patient with an untreated STD may spontaneously abort and hemorrhage. Sepsis and bleeding require hospitalization and parenteral therapy. Consultation and referral to a gynecologist must be completed swiftly to prevent further complications. The specialist, in turn, will need information that only you may possess: the patient's full past medical history, laboratory findings, previous treatments, and drug allergies.

Patient Education

Patient education should include a discussion of information related to the overall treatment plan as well as that specific to the drug therapy, reasons for taking the drug, drugs as part of the total treatment regimen, and adherence issues.

Vaginitis

Treatment of female genital complaints across a woman's lifespan is common in primary care practice. Because of embarrassment, many young and old patients try to get treatment over the phone. Diagnosing vaginal discharge and vulvar conditions requires examination of the area affected and microscopic examination of vaginal secretions. Not all practitioners are adept at microscopy, but in this area the diagnosis may be elusive without prompt examination of vaginal discharge. This chapter earlier discussed the most common STDs and their treatment. Vaginal infections can be sexually transmitted, but some may also be acquired without sexual contact: vulvovaginal candidiasis, some types of bacterial vaginosis, cytolytic vaginosis, atrophic vaginitis with secondary bacterial infection, and some types of streptococcal infections. *Staphylococcus aureus,* found in toxic shock syndrome, is associated with foreign bodies (tampons) inadvertently left during menses. Treatment of vulvovaginal infections is discussed separately from those vulvovaginal conditions that present with vaginal burning, pruritus, and dyspareunia, yet are not infectious.

Pathophysiology

Normal vaginal discharge contains desquamated vaginal epithelial cells, cervical secretions, lactic acid, and bacteria that are both anaerobic and aerobic. Vaginal microflora, predominantly *Lactobacillus,* appear under the

PATIENT EDUCATION

Sexually Transmitted Diseases

Related to the Overall Treatment Plan/Disease Process

☐ Importance of Pap smears in women and testicular self-exams (TSE) in men
☐ Prevention of high-risk sexual behaviors

Specific to the Drug Therapy

☐ Many over-the-counter products are available to treat symptoms (see Table 42–2)
☐ Douching is no longer recommended because of the potential for pelvic infection and destroying the normal flora of *Lactobacillus*
☐ Bacterial vaginosis (BV) must be diagnosed and treated on the same day in patients suspected of being pregnant (BV may cause preterm labor)
☐ Importance of assessment of pregnancy status BEFORE prescribing

Reasons for Taking the Drug(s)

☐ Prevention of serious complications such as pelvic inflammatory disease and infertility
☐ Prevention of transmission of infection to the uninfected (public health issue)
☐ Prevention of dyspareunia, which affects normal sexual relations

Drugs as Part of the Total Treatment Regimen

☐ Importance of seeking treatment when symptoms appear
☐ Importance of culturing asymptomatic young persons (age 15–24) every 6 months

Adherence Issues

☐ Importance of following the labeled instructions to totally eradicate the infection
☐ Importance of contacting the health care provider if side effects or rash appears
☐ The potential for drug interactions (the macrolides with antifungal, systemic antifungals, and birth control pills)

microscope as unclumped rodlike organisms. Hormones, age influence, and infections may alter the delicate balance. The most common infections are due to bacteria, yeast, and parasites.

Conditions not covered earlier in the chapter are discussed here.

Cytolytic Vaginosis

In cytolytic vaginosis, an overgrowth of *Lactobacillus* occurs late in the menstrual cycle. It is frequently treated as a chronic yeast infection. Diagnosis is made by absence of *Trichomonas*, hyphae, clue cells, and white blood cells under microscopy. The pH may be as low as

3.5, and treatment is aimed at raising the pH rather than eradicating all bacteria. Treatments that involve douching of medications are discouraged. Instead, patients are encouraged to make vaginal suppositories from clear gelatin capsules (size "0") filled with sodium bicarbonate (baking soda) and dose twice weekly in the last week of the menstrual cycle.

Atrophic Vaginitis

Atrophic vaginitis with secondary infection occurs when thinned vaginal epithelium has reduced defenses against the common perineal bacteria. Culturing is necessary, as well as microscopy. See Table 42–2 for treatment once

Table 42–4. Treatment for Noninfectious Vulvovaginal Conditions

Condition	Drug Used	Nondrug Treatment
Chemical or other irritants spermicidals, douching solutions	Systemic steroid burst Medrol Dosepak	Avoid products with color and fragrance Always use sanitary pads Treat urinary incontinence with hygiene and disposable pads Referral to urology for surgical correction
Allergic, hypersensitivity, contact dermatitis, lichen simplex, foreign body	Steroid burst if severe reaction occurs Topical preferred over systemic	Avoidance and education about use of excessive hygiene measures Use of Crisco and avoidance of detergents in older women
Traumatic vaginitis (may be factitious)	Treat with short-term (2–4 wk) clobetasol 0.05% tid. May add hydroxyzine (Atarax) 10 mg prn	Education and counseling about breaking the scratch-itch cycle
Postpuerperal atrophic vaginitis	Vaginal application of conjugated or synthetic estrogen 1 g twice weekly	Water-soluble vaginal lubricant during intercourse—over a dozen effective lubricant choices
Desquamative inflammatory vaginitis (steroid responsive)	If short course is helpful, consult about length of therapy; need tissue diagnosis	Avoid harsh scrubbing, soaps, and other over-the-counter vaginal products
Erosive lichen planus	Steroids are usually necessary; need tissue diagnosis and consult or refer	Avoid excessive hygiene measures; there are "vulvar" specialists in gynecology
Collagen vascular disease, Behçet's and pemphigus syndromes	Refer aggressive and painful lesions for diagnosis and treatment May use low-dose (25–50 mg) tricyclic antidepressants for pain control	Support groups may be helpful for some patients
Hormonal Changes (normal responses) 1 Midcycle	None	If culture and microscopy clear, then educate and reassure patient
2 After intercourse	None	If culture and microscopy are clear, then educate and reassure
3 Atrophic	If culture and microscopy are clear, then vaginal estrogen or Estratest hs [in two dosages 1.25 mg or 0.625 mg (conjugated estrogen) with 2.5 mg or 1.25 (methyltestosterone)]	May require 3–6 mo of therapy for full therapeutic benefit
Epithelial disorders (previously called dystrophies), lichen sclerosis (white lesions)	Clobetasol ointment 0.05% bid for 4 wk, then once daily for 4 wk, then twice per wk for maintenance	Support group may be helpful for some patients

Adapted from Goroll (1995), Sorbel (1997), and Bornstein (1998).

the infecting organism is diagnosed and Table 42–4 for treatment of the underlying atrophic condition.

Toxic Shock Syndrome

S. aureus associated with toxic shock syndrome can be life-threatening. This patient requires immediate refer-

ral for hospitalization. Patients who are using tampons are the typical victims of this syndrome. Some women harbor *S. aureus* in their normal vaginal secretions but experience no symptoms until using tampons sets up an anaerobic climate. Criteria for making this diagnosis and treatment are based on CDC guidelines and include four of the following five diagnostic criteria: fever of

38.9°C (102°F) or higher, presence of a diffuse macular erythroderma, desquamation 1 to 2 weeks after onset of illness (palms and soles), hypotension (orthostatic changes of 15 mm Hg diastolic pressure or syncope), and involvement of three or more organ systems (GI, muscular, mucous membrane, renal, hepatic, hematologic, and central nervous system) (American Academy of Pediatrics, 1997).

Noninfectious Vaginal Conditions

Noninfectious vaginal conditions may result from the following:

1. Normal cyclic hormonal changes, which occur at midcycle under high estrogen levels and premenses, which is under progestin dominance. The volume changes concern some women, and microscopy may be necessary to reassure the patient.
2. Irritant or allergic products, such as those found in hygiene and contraceptive products (e.g., **spermicides** and latex).
3. Atrophic conditions, such as those associated with the postpartum period and breastfeeding and those associated with postmenopausal vaginal atrophy.

Other Conditions

Less common and more worrisome are inflammatory, collagen, and epidermal sclerosing conditions, which are commonly diagnosed in older women: inflammatory conditions related to trauma from excessive washing, wiping, and scratching; inflammatory conditions reflecting collagen-vascular disease; and inflammatory conditions associated with white or pigmented lesions that may be dysplastic or cancers.

Goals of Treatment

The goals of treatment are to treat the infection or inflammation, prevent reinfection, and prevent complications of the infection or inflammation.

The infection cannot be treated without an accurate diagnosis. Patients often call the office numerous times for prescriptions for yeast infections, yet frequently they do not have monilial vaginitis. This telephone diagnosis has a fifty-fifty chance of being correct. Patients end up spending money on medications that probably will not help their symptoms. For patients age 15 to 24, there is a good chance the problem is chlamydia, but for patients age 50 to 70, vaginal symptoms are more often related to atrophy of the genital tissues, vulvar presentation of collagen-vascular disease, or cancer.

Reinfection occurs when the etiology of the vaginal irritation is not known. If lack of estrogen is making the vaginal tissues thin and vulnerable to bleeding, then treatment with an **antibiotic** alone allows the infection to recur. Treatment with **vaginal estrogen** or the **vaginal ring** thickens the vaginal epithelium and permits natural defenses (intact mucous membranes) to prevail.

Complications of the infection can occur when symptoms of itching and irritation go untreated and the affected tissues thicken and lose elasticity (lichenification). When vulvar tissues become inflamed and heal, they often shrink in size so that the vagina will not allow sexual penetration. Early and aggressive treatment of conditions such as lichen sclerosus delays permanent hardening of the epidermis and dermal layers of the vulva.

Rational Drug Selection

Guidelines

Treatment of venereal infections is dictated by the CDC guidelines, but treatment for nuisance infections may vary according to the preference of the health care provider. Many women prefer the convenience of taking one pill (one dose that lasts a week) for yeast infection, but some authorities fear emergence of resistance of *C. albicans* with chronic oral medication (Sinofsky, 1999). The concept of keeping treatments specific is encouraged throughout medicine. Choice of a specific drug instead of a broad-spectrum drug reduces the problem of developing resistant organisms.

Cost

Many fungal infections are easily eradicated with **topical antifungals** such as **miconazole**, which is available over the counter.

Patient Variables

For most patients, wait to treat *Trichomonas* vaginal infections until after the first 12 weeks of pregnancy. Nevertheless, pregnant women need to have bacterial vaginosis treated early because preterm labor is possible with this seemingly minor infection. The presence of other medical conditions, such as diabetes, use of **progestin-containing contraceptives,** and tissue immunity factors, contribute to chronic monilial vaginitis.

Drug Variables

Many vulvovaginal conditions can be treated topically with as much efficacy as oral medication. Use of **intravaginal antibiotics** and **antifungals** does not affect the absorption of **oral contraceptives** or other medications that patients may be taking. **Topical steroids** can be used for longer periods without suppressing the adrenal gland and reducing total body immunity.

PATIENT EDUCATION

Vaginitis

Related to the Overall Treatment Plan/Disease Process

☐ Knowledge of many causes of vaginal irritation, ranging from allergy to inflammatory conditions associated with local and systemic disease

☐ Knowledge of the physiological changes in vaginal epithelium from age 12 to age 50

☐ Hygiene issues such as types of clothing for underwear, wiping correctly, and emptying bladder before and after intercourse

Specific to the Drug Therapy

☐ Many over-the-counter products that were previously under prescriptive authority are available to treat symptoms and are still efficacious

☐ Douching is no longer recommended because of the potential for pelvic infection and its destruction of the normal flora of *Lactobacillus*

Reasons for Taking the Drug(s)

☐ Prevention of dyspareunia, which affects normal sexual relations

☐ Control of miserable chronic conditions like lichen sclerosus

Drugs as Part of the Total Treatment Regimen

☐ Importance of seeking treatment when symptoms first appear to obtain the correct diagnosis

☐ Drug treatment early may prevent long-term morbidity (atrophy, sclerosis, and cancers)

Adherence Issues

☐ Importance of following the labeled instructions to totally eradicate the infection
☐ Importance of contacting the health care provider if side effects or rash appears
☐ Potential for drug interactions (the macrolides with antifungal, systemic antifungals, and birth control pills)

Monitoring

Episodic vaginal irritations that require topical treatment do not need to be monitored, but when patients become chronically infected or require oral medications, then pelvic examination and microscopy of vaginal discharge must be scheduled.

Outcome Evaluation

When a patient has a dermal condition that the practitioner has not seen before, a consultation is required. Consultation is also necessary when pigmented or white lesions are seen during examination. If patients remember that they were born with pigmented lesions (birthmarks), then biopsy is not necessary.

When patients do not respond to initial or follow-up treatments, consider referral. If the provider is not adept or comfortable with vulvar biopsies, then referral for specialty care is necessary. When conditions of the vulva appear in the very young (patients age 1 to 12), in older adults (patients age 60 and older), or in the pregnant patient, referral is recommended.

Patient Education

Patient education should include a discussion of information related to the overall treatment plan as well as

Vaginitis

Complaint

A 45-year-old woman, Mrs. Vee, complained of vaginal burning and itching after sexual relations with her husband of 25 years.

History

Vaginal smears for hormone effect demonstrated nonovulatory pattern so Mrs. Vee was prescribed progestin during the last 10 days of her menstrual cycle. The result was relief of irritability and mood swings. This response would be consistent with late luteal phase defect, common in perimenopausal women. The next year brought repeated cases of vaginal irritation, some with yeast and some a "shift in the normal flora" when cultured.

Assessment

BP 102/82, weight 130 lb, height 5′ 1″. Physical examination reveals that the Skene's, Bartholin's, and urethral glands are noninflamed; vaginal mucosa is mildly inflamed; scant discharge is present; cervix is parous; uterus is anterior, normal size, shape, and consistency; no adnexal mass is palpated; and rectal examination is negative for blood or mass.

Cervical cultures obtained grew 1+ *E. coli* and 3+ B-strep, not group A. Thyroid function is normal, urinalysis normal, blood sugar normal, and Pap smear obtained on day 11 demonstrated no cancer cells and moderate estrogen effect.

Initial Management Plan

Use metronidazole 500 mg bid for 5 to 7 days and amoxicillin 500 bid for same duration. Consider lubricated condoms until burning and irritation subside. If symptoms recur within 2 months, consider treating spouse.

Follow-up Visit

Six months later, Mrs. Vee complained of itching, vaginal burning, and odor. Cervical culture demonstrated "shift in the normal vaginal flora" without a specific pathogen. Menses have become scanty. Cyclic irritability is lasting longer than 2 weeks.

Modifications to Management Plan

Insert homemade suppository using size "0" clear gelatin capsules filled with boric acid vaginally at bedtime for three consecutive nights. Empiric trial of vaginal estrogen 1 g twice weekly and continue the 10 days of Provera premenstrually.

Continuing Care

Diagnosis: bacterial vaginosis secondary to atrophic vaginitis.

Vaginal symptoms greatly improved on empiric estrogen. Patient stopped coming in for vaginal burning and itch after intercourse. This woman presents with a common perimenopausal problem of vaginal atrophy that frequently looks like infection, then irritation, then possibly allergy, thinning of the vaginal epithelium, resulting in reduced tolerance to the trauma of sexual relations.

---

that specific to the drug therapy, reasons for taking the drug, drugs as part of the total treatment regimen, and adherence issues.

REFERENCES

American Academy of Pediatrics. (1997). *Red book: Report of the Committee on Infectious Disease* (24th ed.). Elk Grove Village, IL.: American Academy of Pediatrics.

Arvin, A., & Prober, C. (1997). Herpes simplex virus type 2: A persistent problem (editorial). *New England Journal of Medicine, 337*(16), 1158–1159.

Baggish, M. and Miklos, J. (1995). Vulvar pain syndrome: A review. *Obstetrical and Gynecological Survey, 50*(8), 618–627.

Bornstein, J., Heifetz, S., Kellner, Y., Stolar, Z., & Abramovici, H. (1998). Clobetasol dipropionate 0.05% versus testosterone proprionate 2% topical application for severe vulvar lichen sclerosus. *American Journal of Obstetrical Gynecology, 178*(1), Part 1, 80–83.

Daly, S., Doyle, M., English, J., Turner, M., Clinch, J., & Prendiville, W. (1998). Can the number of cigarettes smoked predict high-grade cervical intraepithelial neoplasia among women with mildly abnormal cervical smears? *American Journal of Obstetrical Gynecology, 179*(3), 399–402.

Diaz-Mitoma, F., Sibbald, G., Shafran, S., Boon, R., & Saltzman, R. (1998). Oral famciclovir for the suppression of recurrent genital herpes. *Journal of the American Medical Association, 280*(10), 887–892.

Eason, E., & Feldman, P. (1996). Contact dermatitis associated with the use of Always sanitary napkins. *Canadian Medical Association, 154*(8), 1173–1176.

Eisen, D. (1994). The vulvovaginal-gingival syndrome of lichen planus. *Archives of Dermatology, 130*(11), 1379–1382.

Fleming, D., McQuillan, G., Johnson, R., Nahmias, A., Aral, S., Lee, F., & St. Louis, M. (1997). Herpes simplex virus type 2 in the United States, 1976–1994. *New England Journal of Medicine, 377*(16), 1105–1111.

Fugate, K., & McCluskey, M. (1996). The impact of sexually transmitted diseases on fertility. *Obstetrical and Reproductive Clinics of North America, 7*(3), 521–534.

Goroll, A., May, L., & Mulley, A. (1995). *Primary care medicine,* (3rd ed.). Philadelphia: Lippincott.

Hall, D. (1996). Lichen sclerosus: Early diagnosis is the key to treatment. *Nurse Practitioner, 21*(12), 57–62.

Hatcher, R., Trussell, J., Stewart, F., Cates, W., Stewart, G., Guest, F., & Kowal, D. (1998). *Contraceptive technology* (17th ed.). New York: Ardent Media.

Ho, G., Bierman, R., Beardsley, L., Chang, C., & Burk, R. (1998). Natural history of cervicovaginal papillomavirus infection in young women. *NEJM 338*(7), 423–428.

Ivey, J. (1997). The adolescent with pelvic inflammatory disease: Assessment and management. *Nurse Practitioner, 22*(2), 57–62.

Janos, M., & White, G. (1997). The vestibulitis syndrome. *Journal of Reproductive Medicine, 42*(3), 145–152.

Kastrup, E., (Ed.) (1998). *Drug facts and comparisons.* St. Louis: Drug Facts and Comparisons.

Katzung, B. (1998). *Basic and clinical pharmacology* (7th ed.). Norwalk, CT: Appleton & Lange.

Kusseling, F., Shaperio, M., Greenberg, J., & Wenger, N. (1996). Understanding why heterosexual adults do not practice safer sex: A comparison of two samples. *AIDS Education and Prevention, 8*(3), 247–257.

Landers, D. (1996). Vaginitis/cervicitis: Diagnosis and treatment options in a limited resource environment. *Women's Health Issues, 6*(6), 342–348.

Mashburn, J., & Scharbo-DeHaan, M. (1997). A clinical guide to interpretation of the Pap smear. *Nurse Practitioner, 22*(4), 115–118, 124, 126–127.

Mott, A. (1998). Prevention and management of pelvic inflammatory disease by primary care provider. *American Journal for Nurse Practitioners, 2*(5), 7–9, 13–15.

National Cancer Institute Workshop. (1989). The 1988 Bethesda system for reporting cervical and vaginal cytological diagnoses. *Journal of the American Medical Association, 262*(12), 931–934.

O'Keefe, R., Scurry, J., Dennerstein, G., Sfameni, S., & Brenan, J. (1995). *British Journal of Obstetrics and Gynaecology, 102,* 780–786.

Orr, D., & Fortenberry, J. (1998). Editorial. *Journal of the American Medical Association, 280*(6), 564–565.

Raab, S., Steiner, A., & Hornberger, J. (1998). The cost-effectiveness of treating women with a cervical vaginal smear diagnosis of atypical squamous cells of undetermined significance. *American Journal of Obstetrical Gynecology, 179*(2), 411–412.

Rodriquez, M., Schiff, E., & Tzakis, A. (1998). Hepatitis A: Potentially serious disease. *Annals of Internal Medicine, 129*(6), 506.

Secor, R. (1997). Vaginal microscopy: Refining the nurse practitioner's technique. *Clinical Excellence for Nurse Practitioners, 1*(1), 29–34.

Sinofsky, F. (1999). Vulvovaginal candidasis: Topical versus oral therapy, *The Female Patient, 24*(5), 35–39.

Sorbel, J. (1996). Treating resistant vaginal infections. *Physician Assistant, 20*(4), 116–120.

Sorbel, J. (1997). Vaginitis. *New England Journal of Medicine, 337*(26), 1896–1903.

Spitzer, M. (1998). Cervical screening adjuncts: Recent advances. *American Journal of Obstetrical Gynecology, 179*(2), 544–556.

Talan, D., & Moran, G. (1998). CDC update: Tetanus among injection drug users. *Annals of Emergency Medicine, 32*(3), 385–386.

U.S. Department of Health and Human Services. (1998). *Guidelines for treatment of sexually transmitted diseases.* Atlanta: Centers for Disease Control and Prevention.

U. S. Preventive Services Task Force. (1996). *Guide to clinical preventive services* (2nd ed.). Baltimore: Williams & Wilkins.

Veljovich, D., Stoler, M., Andersen, W., Covell, J., & Rice, L. (1998). Atypical glandular cells of undetermined significance: A five-year retrospective histopathologic study. *American Journal of Obstetrcal Gynecology, 179*(2), 382–390.

Wendel, G., Stark, B., Jamison, R., Molina, R., & Sullivan, T. (1985). Penicillin allergy and desensitization in serious infections in pregnancy. *New England Journal of Medicine, 312,* 1229–1232.

CHAPTER 43

·······

Tuberculosis

CHAPTER OUTLINE

*T*uberculosis (TB) presents a serious threat to global health, with an estimated 8 to 10 million new cases worldwide each year and 3 million deaths annually. Nearly one-third of the world population is infected with *Mycobacterium tuberculosis* (about 1.7 billion persons). In 1993, the World Health Organization (WHO) declared a global emergency concerning TB.

In the United States, TB presents a significant health problem, even though it is preventable and curable.

Over the past decade, the number of people with TB in the United States has increased, in part because of an epidemic of people with human immunodeficiency virus (HIV) infection, immigration, declining living conditions for certain segments of the population, and decreased funding for federal and local health promotion programs aimed at preventing and treating TB.

Drug-resistant TB has been increasing since the mid-1980s. Federal funding for TB programs decreased in the

1970s, and states spent less money on TB prevention. Because of this and the growing HIV epidemic, the emergence of drug-resistant TB was inevitable. Congress has since increased funding for TB from nothing in 1976 to $9 million in 1986 and to $120 million in 1996 in response to the growing TB epidemic. The Centers for Disease Control and Prevention (CDC) has established three National Model TB Centers (San Francisco, Newark, and New York City) and a National Tuberculosis Surveillance Network.

Both primary and acquired drug resistance may occur. Acquired resistance stems from inadequate or inappropriate treatment regimens prescribed by providers or from noncompliance by patients. The dimensions of the problem can be staggering; New York City reportedly has a 30 percent incidence of multidrug-resistant TB. The problem is even more acute in less developed countries, with Nepal reporting resistance rates of 48 percent (Parsons et al., 1997).

The diagnosis and treatment of TB has become complex. Diagnostic criteria depend not only on the results of testing but also on the patient's immigration and immune status. Multidrug regimens that vary according to the patient's risk factors require the practitioner to be familiar with a wide variety of treatment regimens. Compliance with long treatment courses is an issue in the treatment of TB. Noncompliance has also led to the emergence of drug-resistant TB. This chapter addresses the treatment of TB and strategies to increase compliance with the treatment regimen, as well as the drug regimen used for TB prevention.

Pathophysiology

Tuberculosis is an infectious disease caused by *M. tuberculosis*. The organism is inhaled into the alveolus where it is ingested by the pulmonary macrophage. The bacilli multiply and spread to local pulmonary areas and to extrathoracic organs via the lymphatic system. The infected macrophage releases a substance that attracts T lymphocytes. The infected macrophage presents antigens from the phagocytosed bacilli to the lymphocytes, producing a series of committed immune effector cells (Iseman, 1996). This causes a delayed-type hypersensitivity and, combined with the newly activated macrophages, leads to intracellular killing of the bacilli and granuloma formation.

M. tuberculosis and most of the other mycobacteria grow quite slowly, with a doubling time of 18 hours. Thus skin test reactivity does not occur until 4 to 6 weeks after infection, with longer intervals noted. Colonies on culture media do not appear for 3 to 5 weeks, creating delays in culture confirmation and drug susceptibility testing.

Infection is spread almost exclusively by aerosolization of contaminated lung secretions. This organism affects primarily the pulmonary tissue, although extrapulmonary TB is not uncommon, especially in the immunocompromised patient. Patients with cavitary lung disease cough frequently and therefore are particularly infectious. The aerosolized droplets can remain suspended in room air for many hours. The skin and respiratory mucous membranes of a healthy, normally exposed person are resistant to invasion. The problem occurs with heavy or prolonged exposure to an infected or immunocompromised person. The very young and the very old or debilitated are also more susceptible because of decreased host defenses.

Pulmonary TB presents with the classic symptoms of TB: cough with productive, purulent secretions, often with blood streaks. Other symptoms include wide temperature variations, malaise, fatigue, wasting, chest pain, and dyspnea. Sweating, including night sweats, is common.

Extrapulmonary TB presents with a more problematic set of symptoms, often mimicking other diseases. Lymphatic TB may present initially as unilateral, painless cervical lymphadenopathy. TB bacilli can also settle in the genitourinary tract, bones or joints, meninges, gastrointestinal (GI) tract, and pericardium. When these extrapulmonary sites are infected, the symptoms are often vague and difficult to define. The suspicion of TB and intradermal testing as part of a workup for other diseases may lead to a quicker diagnosis. Also of concern is that the tuberculin skin test can be negative 20 to 25 percent of the time. Appropriate biopsy and culture of affected tissues or cerebrospinal fluid, which usually require consultation with a specialist in infectious diseases, increase the likelihood of an accurate diagnosis.

Goals of Treatment

The initial goal of treatment in TB is an accurate diagnosis. This requires a practitioner who understands the current guidelines for skin testing and puts TB high on the differential list for any pulmonary or other illness with vague presenting symptoms. A second goal is the patient's completion of the recommended therapy, as failure to complete therapy can lead to drug-resistant TB. Finally, the effectiveness of treatment must be evaluated.

Patients who have positive sputum cultures at the beginning of treatment should have monthly cultures, and the culture should convert to negative. A final chest x-ray is needed for documentation of baseline for future films, but the x-ray is not as important as the sputum examination. In patients with radiographic abnormalities consistent with TB, an effort should be made to establish a diagnosis via sputum culture. Bronchoscopy may be necessary to obtain an accurate diagnosis. If presumptive treatment is the only option, the key indicators for response to therapy are the chest x-ray findings. Improvement should be noted within the first 3 months of therapy. If there is no improvement, then either resistance or inaccurate diagnosis must be considered.

Rational Drug Selection

Risk Stratification

Although anyone may become infected with TB, some populations are identified as being at greater risk: children up to age 4 years, the infirm elderly, and immunocompromised patients, including those with HIV infection or acquired immunodeficiency syndrome (AIDS) and organ transplant recipients. Foreign-born people from high-prevalence countries are also at higher risk. The regions in the world where infection and disease are most prevalent include Latin America, Asia, and Africa. In the United States, certain populations are identified as being at higher risk, specifically medically underserved, low-income populations, including high-risk racial or ethnic minority populations (people who are homeless, blacks, Hispanics, and Native Americans). American nonwhite patients have a peak incidence of TB between ages 25 and 44, significantly younger than that of whites, which is over age 70. Residents of long-term care facilities (nursing homes, prisons, and mental institutions) are also at higher risk.

Screening

The decision to screen for TB is usually based on the patient's presenting with an identified risk factor. In some areas of the country, routine TB testing is part of all health maintenance visits because of an increased incidence of TB in the area. Many pediatric health care providers routinely screen all 12-month-old infants. Patients identified as being "at risk" are those with compromised immune systems (e.g., HIV-positive, immunosuppressive therapy, or prolonged **adrenocorticosteroid** therapy), close contacts of patients with newly diagnosed infectious TB, injection drug users known to be HIV-seronegative, foreign-born persons from high-prevalence countries, medically underserved low-income populations, and residents and staff of long-term care facilities. All health care providers should be screened routinely.

The most commonly used screening test and the test recommended for screening is an intradermal injection of tuberculosis protein antigens (such as **purified protein derivative [PPD]**). In 48 to 72 hours, an induration response is considered positive, based on the population being tested. For adults and children with HIV infection, close contacts of people with infectious TB, and patients with fibrotic lesions on chest x-ray (especially in upper lung regions), an induration of 5 mm or more is considered positive. A reaction of 10 mm or more is considered positive for other high-risk adults and children, including

infants and children under age 4. For people not considered at risk for TB infection, a reaction of 15 mm or more is considered positive.

Drug Therapy for Infectious Tuberculosis

Treatment of infectious TB requires the practitioner to apply three basic principles, as recommended by the American Thoracic Society (1994):

1. Treatment regimens must contain multiple drugs to which the organisms are susceptible.
2. The drugs must be taken regularly.
3. Drug therapy must continue for a sufficient period of time.

There are many possible combinations of drugs and rhythms of administration, but the initial phase of treatment is critical to prevent drug resistance and improve outcomes. This chapter discusses three treatment regimens that may be used. As newer medications are approved, these regimens may change, but the basic principles remain. Also, although short-term regimens rely heavily on expensive drugs, these regimens are generally more cost-effective than less expensive regimens. Therefore, drug cost should not affect the treatment protocol.

Six-Month Regimen

A 6-month regimen is recommended for patients with fully susceptible organisms who adhere to treatment. It consists of 2 months of four-drug therapy: **isoniazid (INH)**, **rifampin (RIF)**, **pyrazinamide (PYZ)**, and **ethambutol (ETH)**, followed by 4 months of **INH** and **RIF**. This four-drug therapy is effective even when the infecting organism is resistant to **INH**. Streptomycin is substituted for **ETH** in children too young to be monitored for visual acuity. This 6-month treatment can be used in patients who have HIV infection and in uninfected patients. Patients who have HIV infection should be monitored for treatment response, and their therapy should be prolonged if suboptimal response is found.

Nine-Month Regimen

A 9-month regimen of **INH** and **RIF** may be used for patients who cannot take **PYZ**. ETH (**streptomycin** in young children) should also be included in the treatment protocol until drug susceptibility studies are completed (for the first 2 months).

Twelve-Month Regimen

A 12-month course of treatment with **RIF** and **ETH** is necessary if the patient has a strain that is resistant to **INH**. Realistically, patients will usually be started on the four-drug regimen and then continued for the full 12 months of treatment with **RIF** and **ETH** because the initial cultures and sensitivity report may not be available for 6 to 8 weeks from the date of diagnosis.

Dosages for the drugs commonly used for treatment and prevention are shown in Table 43–1.

Drug Therapy for Drug-Resistant Tuberculosis

Drug-resistant TB has been increasing since the mid-1980s. Microbial resistance to antituberculosis drugs may be either initial or acquired. Initial resistance occurs in the patient who has never been treated for TB. Risk factors for initial resistance include exposure to a patient who has drug-resistant TB, immigration from a country with a high prevalence of drug resistance, and a greater than 4 percent incidence of resistance in the community. Acquired or secondary resistance occurs in the patient who has been previously treated for TB. Poorly or inadequately treated TB is the leading cause of secondary resistance. Poor treatment regimens allow resistant organisms to emerge.

For treatment of drug- or multidrug-resistant TB, the administration of at least two drugs to which there is demonstrated susceptibility is recommended. If there is isolated **INH** resistance, the 6-month, four-drug (**INH, RIF, ETH, PYZ**) protocol is effective.

If **INH** resistance is documented in a patient on the 9-month regimen (without **PYZ**), then the **INH** should be discontinued. If **ETH** was included in the initial regimen, then treatment with **RIF** and **ETH** should continue for a minimum of 12 months. If the initial treatment did not include **ETH**, then drug susceptibility should be repeated. **INH** needs to be discontinued, and two new drugs should be added. The regimen may need to be adjusted when drug susceptibility tests are final.

If the patient is resistant to multiple first-line drugs (**INH, RIF, ETH, PYZ**), then at least three new drugs that the organism is susceptible to should be administered. These second-line drugs include **capreomycin (Capastat), cycloserine (Seromycin), ethionamide (Trecator), kanamycin (Kantrex),** and **para-aminosalicylic acid (Sodium P.A.S.)** (see Table 43–1). This regimen should be followed until sputum cultures are clear; then the patient should have 12 months of two-drug therapy. Often, 24 months of therapy are given to patients who have TB that is resistant to multiple first-line drugs. Patients with resistant TB should have their medications administered via directly observed therapy (DOT) (see Table 43–2).

The role of newer **antibiotic agents** in the treatment of TB is unknown. The **quinolones** and newer **antibiotics** are commonly used, although clinical trials as to their effectiveness are still being done. Second-line treat-

ment usually requires injectable medications, which complicates the treatment regimen. Any patient who demonstrates resistance must be seen by an infectious disease specialist who treats patients with TB. As mentioned previously, inadequate treatment is one of the leading causes of secondary resistance.

Algorithm

Treatment of TB begins with an accurate diagnosis. Once a screening test for TB is considered positive, treatment begins, even if a definitive diagnosis of TB has not been made. Therapy may be altered, based on the patient's risk factors or on the sensitivity of the organisms to the medications being used. A treatment algorithm is presented in Figure 43–1.

Extrapulmonary Tuberculosis

Extrapulmonary TB is often difficult to diagnose. Once a bacteriologic examination has determined a diagnosis of TB, the treatment is basically the same as for pulmonary TB. Although there is not as much research regarding the effectiveness of shortened treatment for extrapulmonary TB, clinical experience indicates that 6 to 9 months of therapy is probably effective. Infants and children with miliary TB, bone or joint TB, and TB meningitis should receive 12 months of therapy.

Response to treatment is more difficult to monitor in patients with extrapulmonary TB and must often be determined based on clinical and radiographic improvement. Bacteriologic evaluation of extrapulmonary sites often requires invasive procedures to evaluate treatment. Referral to an infectious disease specialist is usually necessary to ensure optimal treatment.

Patient Variables

Pregnancy and Lactation

Tuberculosis infection during pregnancy presents like TB in nonpregnant patients. The clinical symptoms include cough, weight loss, fever, malaise and fatigue, and hemoptysis. Eighty-five percent of patients have upper lobe disease; extrapulmonary TB is rare in pregnant patients. TB screening during pregnancy is recommended for all patients. Positive results are the same as for nonpregnant patients. Patients who have active untreated TB at the time of delivery need to be placed in respiratory isolation and separated from their infants. This is motivation to treat TB prior to delivery.

The initial treatment regimen for pregnant women is **INH** and **RIF**. **ETH** should be included unless **INH** re-

Table 43–1. Drugs Commonly Used: Tuberculosis

Drug	Daily Dose	Twice-Weekly Dose	Route	Notes
First-line Agents Ethambutol (EMB)	*Adults:* 15–25 mg/kg *Children:* 15–25 mg/kg (maximum 2500 mg)	*Adults:* 50 mg/kg *Children:* 50 mg/kg/ dose (maximum 2500 mg)	PO	Ocular toxicity is a major adverse reaction (blurred vision, color blindness, optic neuritis). Regularly monitor visual acuity and color vision. Contraindicated in children too young to test for visual acuity (<6 y).
Isoniazid (INH)	*Adults:* 10–20 mg/kg up to a maximum of 300 mg daily *Children:* pretreatment dose: 10–15 mg/kg (maximum 300 mg); prevention dose: 10 mg/kg (maximum 300 mg)	*Adults:* 900 mg *Children:* 20–30 mg/kg/dose (maximum 900 mg)	PO, IM, IV	Monitor liver function monthly in high-risk patients. Patients require vitamin B supplements while taking drug. Significant interaction with phenytoin and antifungals (azoles).
Pyrazinamide (PYZ)	*Adults:* 25–30 mg/kg *Children:* 20–40 mg/kg (maximum 2000 mg)	*Adults:* 30–35 mg/kg *Children:* 50 mg/kg/dose (maximum 2000 mg)	PO	Urate levels always increase; do not stop drug unless severe gout develops.
Rifampin (RIF)	*Adults:* 600 mg *Children:* 10–20 mg/kg PO daily (maximum 600 mg)	*Adults:* 600 mg *Children:* 10–20 mg/kg/dose (maximum 600 mg)	PO, IV	Turns urine and other body fluids (tears) red. Major drug interactions with many drugs (oral contraceptives, anticoagulants, methadone, corticosteroids, estrogen replacement, calcium channel blockers, beta blockers, cyclosporine, antifungal azoles, phenytoin, theophylline, sulfonylureas, haloperidol, and others).
Streptomycin (SM)	*Adults:* 12–15 mg/kg *Children:* 15 mg/kg	*Adults:* 15 mg/kg up to 1 g *Children:* 20–40 mg/kg dose (maximum 1 g)	IM	Can be nephrotoxic and ototoxic; monitor renal function and decrease dose in patients with impaired renal function.
Second-Line Agents Capreomycin	*Adults:* 15–30 mg/kg up to 1 g *Children:* 15–30 mg/kg (maximum 1 g)		IM	May cause renal, auditory, and vestibular toxicity; monitor patients closely.
Cycloserine	*Adults:* 15–20 mg/kg up to 1 g *Children:* 15–20 mg/kg (maximum of 1 g)		PO	May cause psychosis, personality changes, convulsions, rash.

Continued on next page

Table 43–1. Drugs Commonly Used: Tuberculosis *(continued)*

Drug	Daily Dose	Twice-Weekly Dose	Route	Notes
Ethionamide	*Adults:* 15–20 mg/kg up to 1 g *Children:* 15–20 mg/kg (maximum 1 g)		PO	Hepatitis may be an adverse reaction; monitor liver function.
Kanamycin	*Adults:* 15–30 mg/kg up to 1 g *Children:* 15–30 mg/kg (maximum 1 g)		IM	May cause auditory, renal, and vestibular toxicity.
Para-aminosalicylic acid	*Adults:* 150 mg/kg up to 12 g *Children:* 150 mg/kg (maximum 12 g)		PO	May cause GI disturbances, hepatitis, sodium load, hypersensitivity.

sistance is unlikely. The length of therapy is 6 months. **Pyridoxine (vitamin B$_6$)** should be added to the regimen in pregnant patients to decrease the incidence of peripheral neuropathy associated with **INH** (Riley, 1997).

There is a 2.5-fold higher risk of **INH**-induced hepatitis in pregnant patients than in other patients (Riley, 1997). **RIF** may also be associated with maternal hepatitis. Monthly monitoring of liver function tests may prevent this adverse outcome.

Isoniazid, RIF, and **ETH** all cross the placenta, but these drugs have not been demonstrated to have teratogenic effects (American Thoracic Society, 1994). *Streptomycin* is contraindicated because of its harmful effects on the fetus, including congenital deafness and altered ear development. *Streptomycin* **is Pregnancy Category D.**

Breastfeeding is not contraindicated during treatment. There are small amounts of **INH** (0.75 to 2.3%) and **RIF** (0.05%) excreted into breast milk, but these amounts are well below the therapeutic dose. **ETH** and **PYZ** are both excreted in very small amounts as well. The risk of toxic reactions in the infant may be further minimized if the mother breast-feeds just prior to taking a dose of TB medication.

Pediatric Patients

PRIMARY PULMONARY TUBERCULOSIS. Older infants and children who present with primary pulmonary TB are often asymptomatic, with a positive skin test. Often the chest x-ray is normal or shows only minimal abnormalities (infiltrates with hilar adenopathy). Primary infection in older children and adolescents presents with an upper lobe infiltrate and cavitation without calcification. In infants and children under age 3 years with primary pulmonary infection, the disease may be progressive and merge with miliary TB or progressive central

nervous system (CNS) disease to produce TB meningitis (Prince, 1998). Eighty percent of infected children between ages 4 and puberty do not progress to disease (Goodman & Brady, 1996). Progressive disease does occur in immunocompromised children of all ages.

PROGRESSIVE PULMONARY TUBERCULOSIS. Progressive pulmonary TB in children occurs when the primary infection is not contained and produces bronchopneumonia or when the lesions involve a whole lobe (usually middle or lower) and cavitation develops. Weight loss, fever, night sweats, malaise, hemoptysis, and productive cough are common symptoms.

MILIARY TUBERCULOSIS. Infants and children under age 3 years frequently develop miliary TB, which is widespread dissemination with infection of multiple organs. The lesions are the size of millet seeds, thus the name *miliary* TB. The infant or child is quite ill, often with a sudden onset, and may have a high fever, weakness, malaise, anorexia, hepatosplenomegaly, and night sweats. The chest x-ray reveals diffuse miliary infiltrates. The tuberculin skin test **(PPD)** may be nonreactive as a result of anergy (Prince, 1998.) The child may need a liver or bone marrow biopsy to determine an accurate diagnosis.

TUBERCULOSIS MENINGITIS. TB meningitis is the most serious complication of TB. It usually occurs in young children (under age 5 years) and within 6 months of primary infection. There are three stages of the disease: prodromal (lasts 1 week), neurological involvement, and then increasing neurological involvement resulting from increasing intracranial pressure. The skin test **(PPD)** is positive in two-thirds of cases, but anergy may be present in very ill patients.

DRUG THERAPY. Drug therapy for pediatric patients depends on the infection or disease category, as noted in Table 43–3. The standard **anti-TB drugs INH** and **RIF** are used for asymptomatic infection and for 6 to 9

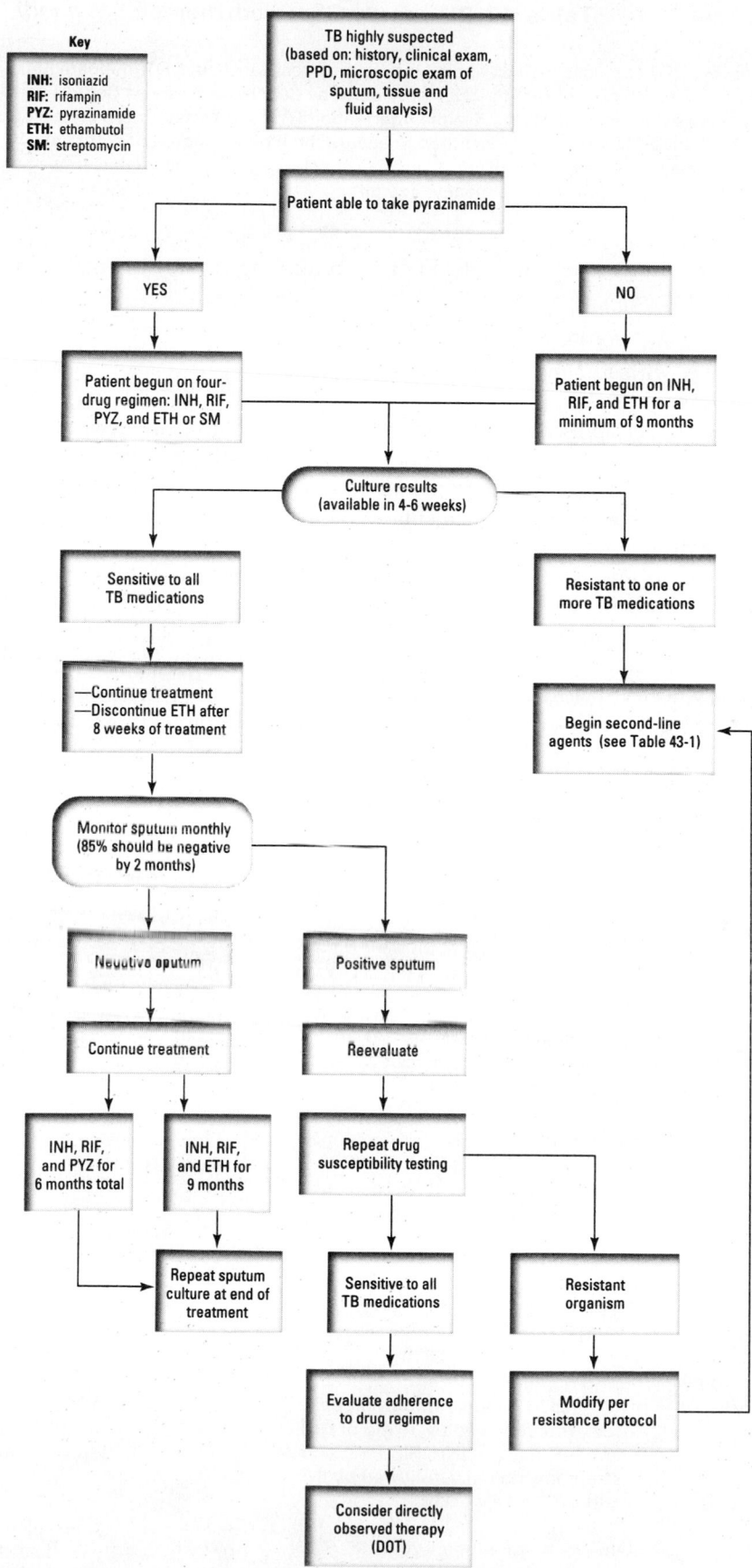

Figure 43–1. Treatment flowchart: Tuberculosis.

Table 43–2. Directly Observed Therapy

Directly observed therapy (DOT) reduces the risk of developing drug resistance. In DOT, the patient is required to take all of the medication in front of a health care or other service provider. The Centers for Disease Control and Prevention (CDC), the American Thoracic Society (ATS), and the World Health Organization (WHO) recommend the widespread or universal use of DOT in the treatment of TB. DOT has been demonstrated to ensure the highest degree of compliance with the medication regimen. There are many ways to increase compliance with DOT, including convenient clinic times and locations and incentives such as food, clothing, bus or carfare money, and gifts.

months. Multidrug regimens, as noted in Table 43–3, are used for progressive disease.

Adverse Reactions. **Rifampin** and **INH** can be administered to children safely, with minimal adverse reactions. Patients should be monitored for liver function alterations, especially if the patient presents with a flulike illness. Young children rarely have the **pyridoxine** deficiency associated with **INH** that can be prevented in adolescents and adults with **vitamin B₆** supplementation. **ETH** is an effective drug, but its main limitation is ocular toxicity, which causes optic neuritis, leading to blurred vision, color blindness, and visual field constriction. Although the visual changes associated with **ETH** are reversible, it should not be prescribed to children under age 6 years, whose visual changes cannot be accurately monitored. **Streptomycin** can be used in children in place of **ETH**, but it is used for only a short time (up to 12 weeks), and patients should be monitored for ototoxicity and nephrotoxicity. **PYZ** is used in

multidrug therapy in children and has few adverse reactions.

Newborn Infants

Management of the newborn infant whose mother (or other household contact) has TB is based on individual considerations. Approximately 50 percent of infants born to mothers with active disease will have TB in the first year of life (Prince, 1998). Unfortunately, in infants the skin test may not be positive until age 6 months.

If the mother has a positive **PPD** but no evidence of active disease, then the family and household contacts must be investigated. If no evidence of active disease is found in the mother or extended family, the infant needs to have a Mantoux (**5 TU PPD**) skin test at 4 to 6 weeks of age and at 3 to 4 months of age. If the TB status of household contacts cannot be evaluated, the infant may be started on **INH** (10 mg/kg per day).

Table 43–3. Treatment of Tuberculosis in Infants, Children, and Adolescents

Disease Category	Drug Therapy	Comments
Asymptomatic infection (positive skin test only)	*9-mo regimen:* INH-susceptible: INH daily INH-resistant: RIF daily	Twice-weekly therapy may be used if daily therapy is not feasible. Patients who are HIV-positive and children should be treated for 12 mo.
Pulmonary disease	*6-mo regimen:* INH, RIF, and PYZ daily for first 2 mo, followed by 4 mo of INH and RIF daily *or* INH, RIF, and PYZ daily for 2 mo, followed by 4 mo of INH and RIF twice weekly *9-mo regimen:* 9 mo of INH and RIF daily *or* 1 mo of INH and RIF daily, followed by 8 mo of INH and RIF twice weekly	If drug resistance is a concern, then a four-drug regimen is used (INH, RIF, PYZ, and ETH or streptomycin) for the first 2 mo.
Extrapulmonary TB (meningitis, miliary, bone, and joint)	*12-mo regimen:* INH, RIF, PYZ, and streptomycin daily for 2 mo, followed by 10 mo of INH and RIF daily *or* INH, RIF, PYZ, and streptomycin daily, followed by INH and RIF twice weekly	Four-drug therapy is used for the first 2 mo of treatment, until drug susceptibility is known.
Extrapulmonary TB (other than meningitis, miliary, bone, or joint)	Same as for pulmonary disease	

If the mother has newly diagnosed TB but is not contagious at delivery, the newborn infant requires a chest x-ray and Mantoux test at age 4 to 6 weeks. If these are negative, then the child is monitored at age 3 to 4 months and again at 6 months, with repeat Mantoux skin tests. **INH** is started at birth and discontinued at 3 to 4 months (some sources say 6 months) if the **PPD** is negative and there is no active disease in the family. The infant should receive **INH** even if the initial chest x-ray and **PPD** are negative because cell-mediated immunity of a degree sufficient to mount a significant reaction to skin testing can develop as late as age 6 months in an infant infected at birth. The mother may breast-feed. The infant should be examined carefully at monthly intervals. In cases of poor compliance, maternal positive sputum, or uncertain supervision, the infant may be given **BCG (bacille Calmette-Guérin) vaccine. BCG** does not prevent tuberculosis but may decrease the severity of the disease.

If the mother has active disease and is contagious at the time of delivery, the infant and mother should be separated until the mother is no longer contagious. The infant is managed the same as if the maternal disease were not contagious at the time of delivery.

If the mother has hematogenous spread of TB (bone, meningitis, or miliary TB), congenital TB is possible. If the infant is suspected of having congenital TB, **INH** is given for 6 months. If the **PPD** is positive at 6 months, then the **INH** is continued until age 9 months. Like any mother with active disease at delivery, a chest x-ray and Mantoux skin test should be done shortly after birth, and the infant should be monitored closely, with monthly assessments.

The HIV-Positive Patient

Worldwide, 8 to 10 percent of all cases of TB are associated with HIV infection. In the early stages of HIV infection, the clinical manifestations of TB are similar to those of a normal host. As the T-lymphocyte count decreases, changes occur:

1. There is a steady reduction in the percentage of patients who will have a positive TB skin test, decreasing to 10 to 20 percent of patients with advanced AIDS.
2. Extrapulmonary TB increases, with 60 to 80 percent of patients with CD4 counts below 50 demonstrating extrapulmonary infection.
3. Changing patterns of disease are noted on chest x-ray films (Iseman, 1996).

The treatment regimen for patients with HIV infection or AIDS as well as TB is altered to address the issue of decreased absorption of the **anti-TB medications** because of a variety of AIDS-associated enteropathies. This problem causes decreased serum levels of TB medications, leading to treatment failure. Direct measurement of drug serum levels should be undertaken early in the treatment course. There should also be close monitoring of the patient's response to treatment. The patient will probably require high-range drug dosing and a longer length of treatment.

Patients with HIV infection or AIDS are usually on multiple drugs besides the **anti-TB medication;** therefore, the patient should be monitored for interactions between the medications. **RIF** is known to alter the liver's metabolism of many drugs, leading to treatment failure or suboptimal response in the patient on multiple medications. There is also a complex drug interaction between **rifampin** and **protease inhibitors** that can create a therapeutic challenge, possibly leading to changes in the **antiretroviral** regimen. Providing an optimal outcome to a patient with HIV infection or AIDS with TB will most likely require referral to an infectious disease specialist.

Monitoring

Patients with positive pretreatment sputum for *M. tuberculosis* are best monitored by repeat sputum cultures monthly until sputum cultures are negative. After 2 months of treatment with **INH** and **rifampin,** more than 80 percent of patients who had positive sputum cultures at the beginning of treatment should have converted to negative. A patient who has a negative sputum culture no longer needs monthly evaluation but should have a sputum smear and culture at the end of the course of treatment.

Radiographic monitoring is not as important as sputum examination during the course of treatment. At the completion of treatment, a chest x-ray should be done to provide a baseline for comparison with any future films.

In patients with negative pretreatment sputum yet radiographic findings consistent with TB, an extensive effort to make a microbiologic diagnosis is necessary. These patients would most likely need medical evaluation by a pulmonologist. Bronchoscopy to perform biopsies and bronchoalveolar lavage should be considered to confirm the diagnosis of TB. If presumptive treatment is started without sputum cultures, then the chest x-rays should be repeated. Failure to show improvement of the lesions on the chest film after 3 months of therapy strongly suggests a misdiagnosis or a lesion that is an old TB lesion (not currently active).

Adverse Reactions to the Medications

Patients should also be monitored for adverse reactions to the medications used to treat TB by means of a baseline measurement of hepatic enzymes, bilirubin, serum creatinine, a complete blood count (CBC), and platelet count. Patients who are taking **PYZ** require a baseline serum uric acid. A baseline ophthalmology examination for visual acuity and a red-green color examination are required for patients on **ETH.** These baseline tests are used to determine any underlying abnormality that would affect the treatment regimen. Children generally do not require baseline laboratory tests, except visual acuity, unless there is some underlying medical condition that may complicate the treatment regimen.

Once treatment is begun, patients are monitored clinically for adverse reactions. There is usually no need for routine laboratory tests unless there were abnormalities to begin with. Patients should be made aware of the symptoms associated with the most common adverse reactions to the medications. They should report all flulike illness immediately and see their health care provider at least monthly during treatment. At the monthly visit, the provider should ask specific questions regarding adverse reactions to the medication and follow any positive answer with confirming laboratory tests.

Adult patients treated for TB are at risk for peripheral neuropathy associated with **INH** therapy; therefore, they also need **pyridoxine (vitamin B$_6$)** to decrease the likelihood of developing this serious but avoidable adverse reaction.

Outcome Evaluation

Because of the lengthy treatment time for TB and the increased incidence of resistant organisms found with inadequate treatment, include both the actual sputum culture evaluation and the patient's compliance with the medication regimen in judging the success of the treatment. Ideally, the patient will have TB-free sputum within the first 2 months of treatment and a clear sputum culture throughout the rest of the treatment. After treatment, no standard follow-up is required. If a patient is immunosuppressed, reevaluation is suggested 6 months after treatment is completed. Any relapse is most likely to occur within the first 2 years after treatment.

Patient Education

Extensive patient education is essential to successful TB treatment. The patient must understand the purpose for the long, multidrug treatment regimen and be a partner in the process. Compliance is a major issue in TB treatment; therefore, all teaching should have the underlying theme of taking all medication as scheduled. Research has found that patients who receive health education and counseling have higher compliance rates (Ailinger & Dear, 1998). The lengthy treatment requires that education be repeated and reviewed at the monthly visits. Because patients may be illiterate or understand little English, education should be presented in a variety of media,

such as videotapes in a patient's primary language. Peer health counselors may also be helpful in educating patients with TB.

Prevention of Tuberculosis

Most patients infected with the tubercle bacillus never develop active TB. The goal of preventive therapy is early identification of those patients who are at risk of developing active TB so that they can be treated with drugs to prevent their conversion to active disease. Patients at risk for developing active TB include those who have been newly exposed to persons with active TB and those who have dormant infections that are at risk for reactivation.

Skin testing with **PPD** or Mantoux is a necessary screening test to determine if the patient has been infected. Evaluation of the results of the skin test is based on the likelihood of infection and the risk of active TB if infection has occurred. If the patient is HIV-positive or has fibrotic lesions on chest x-ray, a reaction of 5 mm or more is considered positive. A reaction of 10 mm or more is considered positive in other at-risk patients, including infants and children. In patients who are not in any high-risk category or high-risk environment, a result of 15 mm or more is considered positive.

Patients are considered high risk if they have the following medical conditions: diabetes mellitus, prolonged therapy with **adrenocorticosteroids,** immunosuppressive therapy, hematologic or reticuloendothelial diseases such as leukemia or Hodgkin's disease, injection drug use by a patient known to be HIV-seronegative, end-stage renal disease, and any clinical presentation that consists of substantial rapid weight loss or chronic malnutrition. A person who is in a high-incidence group with a skin test reaction of 10 mm or more is a candidate for preventive therapy, even without any of these risk factors. High-incidence groups include foreign-born people from high-prevalence countries; medically underserved, low-income populations; and residents of long-term care facilities.

Pathophysiology

Most cases of TB in the United States occur from reactivation of latent infection acquired at an earlier time, months or years before, when the patient's immune system was able to mount a sufficient defense. The patient has no outward sign of ever having been infected by TB. All that remains to identify that the patient was exposed to TB is a positive tuberculin skin test. Reactivation, leading to active infection, occurs in patients who, for whatever reason, cannot muster a sufficient immune response.

PATIENT EDUCATION

Tuberculosis

Related to the Overall Treatment Plan and Disease Process

☐ A clear description of the pathophysiology and mode of transmission of TB: Patients need to understand that they can be infectious to their close contacts if they do not receive adequate treatment.

☐ A thorough outline of the complete treatment regimen, including an estimated length of time for treatment: Patients need to know up front that they will be receiving months and possibly more than a year of treatment.

☐ Importance of adherence to the treatment regimen.

☐ Importance of regularly scheduled follow-up appointments.

Specific to the Drug Therapy

☐ A written plan of the medication schedule is essential, especially with multidrug regimens.

☐ Possible adverse effects of the medications and importance of reporting immediately to the health care provider any vague, flulike symptoms.

Reasons for Taking the Drug(s)

These drugs are given to prevent or eliminate infection by *Mycobacterium tuberculosis*.

Drugs as Part of the Total Treatment Regimen

Tuberculosis medications are a part of the total treatment regimen, which also includes strict pulmonary care.

Adherence Issues

Extensive patient education is essential to successful treatment. The patient must understand the purpose for the long, multidrug treatment regimen and be a partner in the treatment. Compliance is a major issue; therefore, all teaching should have the underlying theme of taking all medication as scheduled. Research has found that patients who receive health education and counseling have higher compliance rates (Ailinger & Dear, 1998). The long period of treatment requires education that is repeated and reviewed at the monthly visits. To teach patients who may be illiterate or who understand only minimal English, education should be conducted in a variety of media, such as videos in the patient's primary language. Peer health counselors may also help to educate patients with TB. Directly observed therapy (DOT) may enhance compliance and adherence with therapy.

Drug Therapy

Drug therapy for TB prevention consists of **INH** alone. It is given in a single daily dose of 300 mg for adults and 10 to 15 mg/kg for children, not to exceed 300 mg. For many years, the standard length of preventive therapy has been 12 months. More recently, 6- and 9-month regimens have been used. Patients who are HIV-positive should receive 12 months of therapy. The American Academy of Pediatrics recommends 9 months of therapy for children. A recent recommendation from the CDC is a 2-month regimen of daily **RIF** and **PYZ** as an alternative to the 12-month therapy. This short-course preventive therapy regimen recommendation is based on the results of several randomized, controlled clinical trials in HIV-infected persons (CDC, 1998). This shortened

Tuberculosis

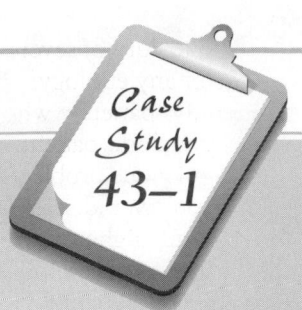
Case Study 43–1

Complaint

"I've had a cough for three weeks."

History

Maria is a 27-year-old Hispanic female who presents with a cough for 3 weeks. She has had a low-grade fever off and on during that time. A native of Mexico, Maria has lived in the United States for the past 13 years. Four months ago, she returned to Mexico for a 2-week visit with family members who live in a rural village. She is married and has four children. Other than the current cough, she has had no major acute or chronic illnesses. Her only hospitalizations have been when her children were born. She has had no known exposure to TB.

Assessment

Maria's vital signs are as follows: temperature 100.4°F, pulse rate 84, respiratory rate 24, and blood pressure 124/78 mm Hg. She weighs 126 lb, a 10-lb weight loss since her last visit.

Her physical exam is negative except for an occasional cough and decreased breath sounds in the upper left lung.

Diagnostic tests reveal the following: chest x-ray is positive for a 6-cm cavitary lesion in upper left lobe, PPD skin test is 12 mm of induration when read at 48 hours, sputum smear is positive for acid-fast bacilli (a culture is pending), and HIV testing is negative.

Initial Management Plan

Because of the high likelihood that Maria has TB, she is started on a four-drug regimen of antituberculosis medications: INH (300 mg daily), ETH (1 g daily), PYZ (2 g daily), and RIF (600 mg daily) for the first 2 months.

Four-drug therapy is recommended for the first 2 months of treatment (1) because drug susceptibility tests may take weeks and (2) to decrease the development of resistant TB strains from inadequately treated disease. Maria is also started on pyridoxine to prevent peripheral neuropathy associated with INH. A report is made to the public health department, and an investigation of household contacts is begun. Everyone in Maria's family needs to be tested.

Follow-up Visit

After 1 month of treatment, Maria reports that she is tolerating the medication well. Two of her children also had positive skin tests, with negative chest x-rays, and they are now on INH. Maria reports that her cough is better and the fever is gone. A repeat sputum culture is obtained, and a refill of medication for 1 month given. The initial sputum culture results indicated that Maria's TB strain is susceptible to all four drugs that she is taking. Maria is to be seen monthly for the 6 months of her treatment.

Modifications to Management Plan

None at this time.

Continuing Care

After 2 months of treatment, the ETH and PYZ are discontinued. Maria will continue on INH and RIF twice weekly for the remaining 4 months. She will have monthly sputum cultures until they are negative and at the end of treatment.

---

regimen may be useful in settings where longer courses of preventive therapy are difficult to administer or monitor (e.g., jail inmates or migrant workers).

The **INH** should be dispensed in monthly allotments, with the patient's compliance monitored at least monthly. For patients who may have questionable adherence, DOT is recommended. If resources prohibit daily DOT, then **INH** may be given twice a week at the dose of 15 mg/kg. Data on this treatment regimen are limited, but studies from the treatment of active disease indicate that intermittent therapy effectively prevents TB.

Prior to beginning drug therapy with **INH,** evaluate the patient as follows:

1. Exclude active TB, by both radiographic and bacteriologic tests. All patients with a positive skin test require a chest x-ray to rule out pulmonary TB. If the chest x-ray is consistent with pulmonary TB, then an extensive evaluation to rule out active disease is necessary. Bacteriologic studies of the sputum and comparisons with old x-rays are helpful in gaining a clear clinical picture of whether the patient has active disease. Because of the risk of developing **INH**-resistance when only **INH** is used for active disease, if there is any suspicion of active disease, then the patient should be started on multidrug therapy until the final diagnosis is clarified.

2. Determine if the patient has a history of adequate TB preventive therapy.

3. Find out if the patient has had prior **INH** therapy to determine if the patient has had adequate drug therapy.

4. Look for any contraindications to the administration of **INH** therapy: previous **INH**-induced hep-

atitis, history of severe **INH** reactions, or liver disease of any etiology.

5. Identify patients who require special cautions. They include patients over age 35, daily **alcohol** use, previous problems with **INH** therapy, current chronic liver disease, pregnancy, injection drug use, and higher-risk groups for developing fatal hepatitis (women, particularly black and Hispanic women). Hepatitis risk is also increased in the postpartum period.

Monitoring

As previously mentioned, patients receiving preventive TB therapy with **INH** should be monitored at least monthly. At the monthly visit, the health care provider carefully assesses the patient's compliance and asks the patient about symptoms of adverse effects of **INH**, specifically liver damage. A standardized form should be used to evaluate the patient for symptoms of liver damage, including unexplained anorexia; nausea; vomiting; dark urine; icterus; rash; persistent paresthesias of the hands and feet; persistent fatigue, weakness, or fever for more than 3 days' duration; and abdominal tenderness. If these or other signs or symptoms occur during preventive therapy, patients should contact their health care provider immediately.

Of those receiving **INH** therapy, 10 to 20 percent will have mildly abnormal liver enzymes, which usually resolve even if the **INH** is continued. Patients over age 35 have a higher frequency of hepatitis; therefore, a baseline transaminase should be obtained before therapy is begun for such patients, and the study should be repeated monthly during therapy. If values are greater than three to five times normal, then **INH** should be discontinued (American Thoracic Society, 1994). Other patients at risk for developing hepatitis are those who have chronic liver disease, injection drug users, and patients who use **alcohol** daily. Monthly liver function tests are not a substitute for monthly clinical evaluations of the patient on preventive therapy.

Outcome Evaluation

The success of preventive TB therapy is determined by the absence of active disease and by whether the patient has been compliant with the prescribed drug treatment. Because patients who are receiving preventive therapy often do not feel ill or have any overt symptoms, compliance with the long treatment regimen is even more difficult than for patients with active TB.

Patient Education

Education for patients receiving preventive TB therapy is similar to education for those receiving treatment for active TB. The key difference is stressing the need for months of treatment to a patient who often has no symptoms and feels well. Compliance with the treatment regimen is essential, and the health care team cannot emphasize it enough.

REFERENCES

Ailinger, R. L., & Dear, M. R. (1998). Adherence to tuberculosis preventive therapy among Latino immigrants. *Public Health Nursing*, 15(1), 19–24.

American Thoracic Society. (1994). Treatment of tuberculosis and tuberculosis infection in adults and children. *American Journal of Respiratory and Critical Care Medicine*, 149, 1359–1374.

Bradford, W. Z., & Daley, C. L. (1998). Multiple drug-resistant tuberculosis. *Infectious Disease Clinics of North America*, 12(1), 157–171.

Centers for Disease Control and Prevention. (1998). Prevention and treatment of tuberculosis among patients infected with human immunodeficiency virus: Principles of therapy and revised recommendations. *Morbidity and Mortality Weekly Report*, 47, 911–912 (no. RR-20).

Goodman, M. H., & Brady, M. A. (1996). Infectious diseases. In C. E. Burns, N. Barber, M. A. Brady, & A. M. Dunn (Eds.), *Pediatric primary care: A handbook for nurse practitioners* (pp. 481–485). Philadelphia: Saunders.

Heymann, J. S., Sell, R., & Brewer, T. F. (1998). The influence of program acceptability on the effectiveness of public health policy: A study of directly observed therapy for tuberculosis. *American Journal of Public Health*, 88(3), 442–445.

Hwang, M. Y. (1998). JAMA patient page: Fighting TB. *Journal of the American Medical Association*, 280(19), 1724.

Iseman, M. D. (1996). Tuberculosis. In J. C. Bennett & F. Plum (Eds.), *Cecil's textbook of medicine* (20th ed., pp. 1683–1689). Philadelphia: Saunders.

Parsons, L. M., Driscoll, J. R., Taber, H. W., & Salfinger, M. (1997). Drug resistance in tuberculosis. *Infectious Disease Clinics of North America*, 11(4), 905–927.

Prince, A. (1998). Infectious diseases. In R. E. Behrman & R. M. Kliegman (Eds.), *Nelson's essentials of pediatrics* (3rd ed., pp. 356–362). Philadelphia: Saunders.

Rey, E., Pons, G., Crémier, O., Van Zelle-Kervroëdan, F., Pariente-Khayat, A., d'Athis, P., Badonal, J., Olive, G., & Gendrel, D. (1998). Isoniazid dose adjustment in a pediatric population. *Therapeutic Drug Monitoring*, 20(1), 50–55.

Riley, L. (1997). Pneumonia and tuberculosis in pregnancy. *Infectious Disease Clinics of North America*, 11(1), 119–133.

Swanson, D. S., & Starke, J. R. (1995). Drug-resistant tuberculosis in pediatrics. *Pediatric Clinics of North America*, 42(3), 553–581.

CHAPTER 44

......

URI, Otitis Media, and Otitis Externa

CHAPTER OUTLINE

pper respiratory infections (URIs) are the most common minor acute illnesses seen in primary care. The most common secondary infections seen with viral URIs are sinusitis and, in children, otitis media. Practitioners encounter these illnesses countless times among their patients and should be aware of the pathogens commonly found and the pharmacological and nonpharmacological management of these illnesses. This chapter discusses the pharmacological management of these acute illnesses, as well as the management of otitis externa.

Viral Upper Respiratory Infection

Viral URIs, also known as common colds, are the most frequent disease seen in a primary care practice and also the number one cause of absenteeism from work and school. The frequency of viral URIs varies with age, with adults averaging 3 to 4 colds a year and children age 1 to 5 averaging 7 or 8. Infants have an average of 6 or 7 colds per year, but being in daycare increases their incidence of colds to 9 to 11 in the first year of life.

A viral URI usually starts with the symptoms of nasal congestion, rhinorrhea, malaise, and scratchy throat. The nasal discharge typically starts out thin and clear and then thickens and progresses to a green or yellow color. Generalized muscle aches may be present, but fever is usually absent in adults. Young children may have a low-grade fever for 2 or 3 days. Fever in adults or a high fever in children suggests influenza or a secondary infection, such as sinusitis or otitis media. URI symptoms are irritating but not severe. More severe symptoms should be investigated for secondary infection or other bacterial infection. Most patients are symptom-free in 7 to 10 days from the beginning of the illness.

Pathophysiology

The rhinovirus causes approximately 50 percent of all viral URIs. There are more than 100 serotypes of rhinovirus; therefore, even though immunity is produced by rhinoviral infections, the patient can quickly become infected with another strain of rhinovirus. The common story heard in the clinic is that a person just got over a cold and now has it back. Other viruses found with the common cold include, but are not limited to, adenovirus, respiratory syncytial virus, parainfluenza virus, and influenza viral strains. These viruses are transmitted between people by airborne droplets or by direct transmission of the virus in secretions via hand contact.

Goals of Treatment

Viral URIs are self-limiting and require no treatment other than symptomatic relief; therefore, the major goal in treating a patient with a viral URI is relieving irritating symptoms, specifically nasal congestion.

Rational Drug Selection

Drug Therapy

Although viral URI (the common cold) is a self-limited disease that requires no treatment, a huge industry touts nonprescription medications for treatment of colds. First, note that **antibiotics** have no place in the treatment of the common cold. Using **antibiotics** for a viral infection increases the likelihood of antimicrobial resistance to secondary bacterial infections that may occur in the upper respiratory tract. **Antihistamines** have not been proved to alter the course of a common cold, yet many over-the-counter (OTC) cold preparations contain some form of **antihistamine**, probably for their "drying" effect.

The mainstay of pharmacological management for a cold is the **decongestant**, either systemic or topical. **Decongestants** cause vasoconstriction of the capillaries in the nasal mucous membranes. This results in shrinkage of the mucous membrane, which promotes drainage and decreases the nasal stuffiness that accompanies a URI. Dosing of common **decongestants** can be found in Table 44–1. **Analgesics** such as **acetaminophen (Tylenol)**, **aspirin**, and **ibuprofen (Motrin)** can be given for malaise.

Nonpharmacological Therapy

Nonpharmacological therapy or lifestyle management includes increasing fluid intake, using **nasal saline spray** or **drops** to decrease the viscosity of nasal secretions, and obtaining rest. Patients and parents or other family members need to be reminded that anorexia is often associated with the common cold and that fluids often need to be forced on the ill person to maintain adequate hydration. Infants who are congested often cannot breathe and drink liquids from the bottle or breast at the same time; therefore, their fluid intake may be inadequate. Parents need to be encouraged to suction the infant's nose with a nasal bulb syringe to clear secretions before the infant eats or drinks. **Nasal saline spray** is also beneficial in thinning secretions at all ages to make blowing or bulbing secretions more effective. Patients can make their own **saline solution** by adding 1/4 tsp salt to 8 oz warm water. If a dropper is not available, patients can use a cotton ball saturated with **saline solution** to squeeze three or four drops into each nasal passage. Many patients are overcommitted and overworked and must be reminded of the restorative powers of rest. Encouraging patients to take a day or two off work is much more effective than prescribing an unnecessary **antibiotic.**

Monitoring

The patient with a viral URI should be monitored for signs of secondary bacterial infection. Monitor **decongestants** in cardiac patients, who may have increased hypertension from the added vasoconstriction caused by oral **decongestants**. Older adults are more likely to have adverse reactions from **decongestants.**

Outcome Evaluation

Secondary bacterial infections may complicate the common cold. The most common complication in adults is

Table 44–1. Drugs Commonly Used: Viral Upper Respiratory Infections

Drug	Adult Dose	Pediatric Dose	Strengths Available	Notes
Oral Decongestants				
Pseudoephedrine HCl (Sudafed, Genafed, Pseudotabs, Pediacare)	60 mg q4–6h Extended release: 120 mg q12h	*6–12 y:* 30 mg q4–6h *2–5 y:* 15 mg q4–6h *Infants–2 y:* 1 mg/kg or 0.1 mL/kg of 7.5 mg/0.8 mL drops	Tablets: 30 mg, 60 mg Capsules: 60 mg Extended release: 120 mg Liquid: 15 mg/5 mL, 30 mg/5 mL Drops: 7.5 mg/0.8 mL	*Adults:* do not exceed 120 mg in 24 h *Children:* do not exceed 4 doses/d
Pseudoephedrine sulfate (Afrin, Drixoral Non-Drowsy)	120 mg q12h	Not for use in children under age 12	Extended release: 120 mg	Do not crush or chew
Topical Decongestants				
Phenylephrine HCl (Neo-Synephrine, Nostril, Sinex, Alconefrin, Rhinall)	2–3 sprays each nostril; repeat q3–4h	*6–12 y:* 2 sprays each nostril q4h *>6 mo:* 1 to 2 drops each nostril q3h	Spray: 0.125%, 0.16%, 0.25%, 0.5%, 1% Drops: 0.25%, 0.5%, 1%	Do not use for longer than 3 days because of rebound congestion; rarely used in young children
Oxymetazoline HCl (Afrin, 12 Hour Nasal, Dristan Long Lasting, Allerest 12 Hour, Afrin Children's Nose Drops)	2 or 3 sprays or drops of 0.05% solution in each nostril bid or q10–12h	2 or 3 drops of 0.025% solution in each nostril bid, morning and evening	Solution: 0.05%, 0.025%	

Clinical Pearl

NUTRITIONAL OR HERBAL THERAPY

Nutritional or herbal therapy is often thought to decrease symptoms of the common cold. In the 1970s, Linus Pauling first brought forward the idea that **vitamin C** prevents and alleviates episodes of the common cold. Although this has still not been scientifically proved, many patients continue to take **vitamin C** at the first sign of a cold. **Zinc** lozenges have also been brought forth as a treatment for the common cold. Although one study did indicate that **zinc** lozenges decreased the duration and severity of cold symptoms, other studies have not been able to replicate the results. In a meta-analysis of eight published randomized clinical trials on the use of **zinc salts** lozenges in colds, Jackson and colleagues (1997) found evidence to be lacking for the effectiveness of **zinc salts** lozenges in reducing the duration of the common cold.

Another common herbal therapy patients may be using for their cold symptoms is **echinacea. Echinacea** is widely used in Europe for the prevention and treatment of colds and flu. Its use is increasing in the United States. A number of European studies have demonstrated the immune-enhancing properties of **echinacea**, specifically increasing T-cell activity and interferon (Brown, 1996). Among European providers, **echinacea** is the leading herbal recommendation for the prevention of colds and flu. **Echinacea** is available in tablet, liquid, and tea bags. The correct dosage is 900 mg daily divided into two or three doses or 40 drops of the juice three times a day. Length of therapy should not exceed 8 weeks. There are no reported side effects at the recommended dosages. It appears to be safe during pregnancy and lactation. The only true contraindication is having a progressive systemic disease such as tuberculosis or multiple sclerosis or an autoimmune illness. **Echinacea** is a relative of the daisy, and therefore patients who are allergic to daisies should also avoid any form of echinacea (Brown, 1996).

sinusitis, which occurs in approximately 1 percent of colds. In children, sinusitis is a common secondary infection (5% of colds), as is otitis media, which occurs in about 5 to 10 percent of children with colds. Some children appear more apt to get otitis media as a secondary infection, possibly because differences in middle ear and eustachian tube anatomy predispose them to ear infections. This chapter discusses both of these complications of URI. Another complication of viral URIs is exacerbation of asthma symptoms, occurring in 30 to 50 percent of the colds acquired by people with asthma. See Chapter 28 for asthma management.

Patient Education

Patient education for a viral URI is centered on symptomatic treatment and proper dosing of **decongestants**. Patients need to be assured that most URIs resolve in 7 days and that very little can be done to shorten the course of the disease. **Antibiotics** are not necessary for viral infections, and education regarding the signs and symptoms of a secondary bacterial infection needs to be provided.

Sinusitis

Diagnosis of sinusitis is based on clinical symptoms and the course of the illness. Any URI lasting longer than 10 days is, by definition, sinusitis. In adults, there is often pain or tenderness over the maxillary or frontal sinus area. They may have a headache that worsens when they bend over, and they may have a cough. Children have subtler symptoms. Because their frontal sinuses are not completely developed until they are 10 years old, children often do not have the classic frontal headache of sinusitis. Children often have colds more frequently than adults. Therefore, a careful history of whether the symptoms have actually been prolonged or whether the patient has a new viral URI is essential. Children and adults alike may have puffy eyes and a cough that worsens when they lie down. Radiologic studies are of questionable validity because sinus films look the same for a viral URI and a sinus infection. The length of the illness and the severity of symptoms often distinguish the two. Sinus infections can be either acute or chronic (lasting longer than 30 days).

Pathophysiology

The most common bacterial organisms found in acute sinusitis are *Streptococcus pneumoniae, Haemophilus influenzae, Moraxella catarrhalis*, and, more rarely, *Staphylococcus. Staphylococcus* and anaerobic bacteria are more common in chronic sinusitis. Rarely, the causative organism in chronic sinusitis is fungal, with *Aspergillus* the most common fungus found. Patients who are immunocompromised develop severe infection, even invasive infections with eye, mouth, and brain extensions. Culture of the nasal mucosa is not helpful in determining the causative agent in sinusitis. If the patient is not responding to therapy, sinus aspiration is the only accurate way to determine the organism involved.

Goals of Treatment

The overall goal for the treatment of sinusitis is absence of infection, demonstrated by the patient's freedom from all symptoms of a sinus infection.

Rational Drug Selection

Given the most likely organisms to be found in both children and adults, the first choice for **antibiotic therapy** in acute sinusitis is **amoxicillin** (Table 44–2). For adults, the dose is 500 mg given three times a day, and in children the daily dose is 50 to 90 mg/kg per day, divided in three doses. The usual length of treatment is 10 to 14 days; if the patient is responding slowly, treat until the patient is symptom-free and then an additional 7 days (Goodman & Brady, 1996). The course of treatment may be up to 21 days in acute sinusitis. If the patient is allergic to **penicillin, trimethoprim-sulfamethoxazole (Septra)** and **erythromycin** are also acceptable. Acute sinusitis may also be treated with many of the **cephalosporins**, but their cost keeps them from being considered first-line drugs. If the patient is not improving in 3 to 4 days, bacterial resistance needs to be considered, and then the drugs of choice are **amoxicillin-clavulanate (Augmentin), azithromycin (Zithromax)**, or a **beta-lactamase–stable cephalosporin antibiotic. Amoxicillin-clavulanate** is the drug of choice in chronic sinusitis. Patients who fail to respond to **antibiotics** may need referral to an otolaryngologist for sinus aspiration and possible endoscopic sinuscopy to facilitate sinus drainage. Figure 44–1 provides an algorithm for the treatment of sinusitis.

Monitoring

Patients who are being treated with **antibiotics** for sinusitis need to be monitored for adverse reactions to the **antibiotics** and for their response to treatment. They should begin to respond in 3 to 4 days. If there is no improvement in clinical symptoms, then bacterial resistance must be considered.

Table 44–2. Drugs Commonly Used: Sinusitis and Otitis Media

Drug	Dose	Length of Treatment	Strengths Available	Notes
Amoxicillin (Amoxil, Trimox)	*Adults and children >20 kg:* 250–500 mg q8h *Children:* 40–50 mg/kg/d divided in three doses	*Sinusitis:* 10–14 d or until 7 d after symptom-free (may need 21 d of treatment) *Otitis media:* 7–10 d	Capsules: 250 mg, 500 mg Chewable tablets: 125 mg, 200 mg, 250 mg, 400 mg Powder for suspension: 50 mg/mL, 125 mg/5 mL, 200 mg/5mL, 250 mg/5 mL, 400 mg/5mL	First choice for non-penicillin-allergic patients. Higher doses may be used for children who have recently been on antibiotics, up to 75 mg/kg/d.
Amoxicillin and clavulanate (Augmentin)	*Adults:* 500 mg q12h *or* 250 mg q8h *Children <3 mo:* 30 mg/kg/d of amoxicillin divided q12h *Children >3 mo:* 45 mg/kg/d of amoxicillin divided q12h (use 200 mg/5 mL or 400 mg/5 mL suspension) *or* 30–40 mg/kg/d of amoxicillin if using 125 mg/5 mL or 250/5 mL suspension (In children, may need to combine Augmentin with amoxicillin to dose amoxicillin at 80 mg/kg/d)	10–14 d for all patients	Tablets: 250 mg amoxicillin & 125 mg clavulanate; 500 mg amoxicillin & 125 mg clavulanate Chewable tablets: 125 mg amoxicillin & 31.25 mg clavulanate; 200 mg amoxicillin & 28.5 mg clavulanate; 250 mg amoxicillin & 62.5 mg clavulanate; 400 mg amoxicillin & 57 mg clavulanate Suspension: 125 mg amoxicillin & 31.25 mg clavulanate/5 mL; 200 mg amoxicillin & 28.5 mg clavulanate/5 mL; 250 mg amoxicillin & 62.5 mg clavulanate/5 mL; 400 mg amoxicillin & 57 mg clavulanate/5 mL; 400 mg amoxicillin & 57 mg clavulanate	Children's dose is based on amoxicillin content. Because of the clavulanate content, two 250-mg tablets are *not* the same as one 500-mg tablet. Because of the different clavulanate levels in the suspensions, it is not appropriate to dose the 125-mg/5 mL or the 250-mg/5 mL suspensions bid. Children should not be given the 250-mg tablet until they are >40 kg.
Azithromycin (Zithromax)	*Adults:* 500 mg single dose the first day, followed by 250 mg daily for days 2 through 5 *Children:* 10 mg/kg as one single dose on the first day, then 5 mg/kg/d on days 2 through 5; do not exceed adult dose	5 d	Capsules: 250 mg Z-pak (six 250-mg tablets with instructions for daily dosing) Suspension: 100 mg/5 mL, 200 mg/5mL	Broad spectrum. Use as second-line drug for otitis media. Convenient dosing. 5-d course of treatment.
Cefixime (Suprax)	*Adults and children >50 kg or >12 y:* 400 mg/d as a single 400 mg dose *or* 200 mg q12h *Children:* 8 mg/kg/d as one dose *or* divided into two doses 12 h apart	10–14 d	Tablets: 200 mg, 400 mg Suspension: 100 mg/5 mL	Expensive.

Continued on next page

Table 44–2. Drugs Commonly Used: Sinusitis and Otitis Media *(continued)*

Drug	Dose	Length of Treatment	Strengths Available	Notes
Cefpodoxime (Vantin)	*Adults:* 400 mg q12h *Children:* 10 mg/kg/d either as one dose or divided q12h (max dose 400 mg)	5–10 d	Tablets: 100 mg, 200 mg Suspension: 50 mg/5 mL, 100 mg/5 mL	Broad spectrum. Very expensive.
Cefprozil (Cefzil)	*Adults and children >12 y:* 500 mg q12h *Children:* 30 mg/kg/d divided into two doses 12 h apart	10–14 d	Tablets: 250 mg, 500 mg Suspension: 125 mg/5 mL, 250 mg/5 mL	Broad-spectrum coverage. Expensive.
Ceftibuten (Cedax)	*Adults:* 400 mg once daily *Children:* 9 mg/kg/d in one daily dose	10 d	Tablets: 400 mg Suspension: 90 mg/5 mL, 180 mg/5 mL	Must be given on an empty stomach.
Ceftriaxone (Rocephin)	*Children:* 50 mg/kg given as one IM dose (maximum of 1 g/dose)	One dose only	Powder for injection: 250 mg, 500 mg, 1 g	May be used as one-time dose for otitis media in children. Very expensive compared with amoxicillin. Broad spectrum.
Cefuroxime (Ceftin)	*Adults and children >12 y:* 250 mg or 500 mg q12h *Children:* 30 mg/kg/d given q12h up to 1000 mg/d	10 d	Tablets: 125 mg, 250 mg, 500 mg Suspension: 125 mg/5 mL Note: Tablets and suspension are *not* bioequivalent and are *not* substitutable on a mg-for-mg basis	Prolonged half-life in patients with renal failure. Suspension must be given with food. Broad spectrum. Expensive.
Erythromycin-sulfisoxazole (Pediazole)	*Children:* Dose by erythromycin content: 40/mg/kg/d in three divided doses	10–14 d	Suspension: 200 mg erythromycin with 600 mg sulfisoxazole/5 mL	Broad-spectrum activity. Used for treatment of otitis media in children.
Loracarbef (Lorabid)	*Adults and children >12 y:* 400 mg q12h *Children:* 30 mg/kg/d in divided doses given q12h	10 d	Capsules: 200 mg Suspension: 100 mg/5 mL	Broad spectrum, expensive.
Trimethoprim (TMP)-sulfamethoxazole (SMZ) (Bactrim, Septra, Cotrim)	*Adult:* 160 mg TMP & 800 mg SMZ q12h *Children >2 mo:* 8 mg/kg TMP & 40 mg/kg SMZ q12h	10–14 d for all patients	Tablets: 80 mg TMP & 400 mg SMZ Double-strength tablets: 160 mg TMP & 800 mg SMZ Oral suspension: 40 mg TMP & 200 mg SMZ/5 mL	Do not prescribe in children < 2 mo. *Dosing tip:* Dose of suspension is 1 mL/kg/d divided in two doses.

Outcome Evaluation

Sinusitis symptoms should resolve after 3 to 5 days of treatment. Chronic or recurrent sinusitis requires a referral to an otolaryngologist. Often surgical intervention is needed to provide adequate drainage from the sinuses.

Untreated sinusitis can lead to invasive disease such as orbital cellulitis or brain involvement. These are both medical emergencies and fortunately rare, usually seen only in immunocompromised patients. Like viral URIs, acute or chronic sinusitis may exacerbate asthma.

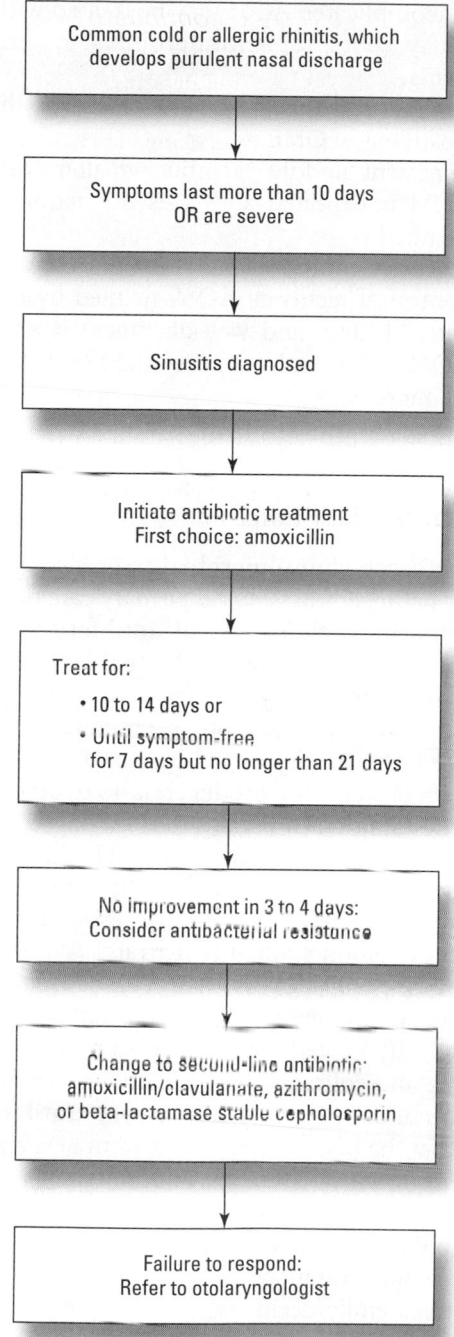

Figure 44–1. Algorithm for treatment of sinusitis.

The flowchart boxes contain:

- Common cold or allergic rhinitis, which develops purulent nasal discharge
- Symptoms last more than 10 days OR are severe
- Sinusitis diagnosed
- Initiate antibiotic treatment First choice: amoxicillin
- Treat for:
  - 10 to 14 days or
  - Until symptom-free for 7 days but no longer than 21 days
- No improvement in 3 to 4 days: Consider antibacterial resistance
- Change to second-line antibiotic: amoxicillin/clavulanate, azithromycin, or beta-lactamase stable cephalosporin
- Failure to respond: Refer to otolaryngologist

Patient Education

Nonpharmacological management includes **decongestants,** either topical or systemic, to improve nasal obstruction. Patients should be warned against long-term use of **topical decongestants,** but they can be very helpful in providing symptomatic relief during the few days it takes to respond to **antibiotics.** Adequate hydration is essential in liquefying secretions, as is the use of **saline nasal irrigation** to remove secretions. The facial pain and headache associated with sinusitis can be severe, and the patient should be encouraged to take **acetaminophen** or **ibuprofen** for pain. A warm pack to frontal and maxillary sinuses often provides pain relief. Running a humidifier at night can alleviate the dry mouth caused by mouth breathing during sleep. Breathing in hot steam often helps clear nasal passages, but caution patients about burns.

Sinusitis causes the air passages in the sinuses to become swollen and blocked and to trap air. Therefore, sinusitis poses a hazard to patients who dive because of the changing air pressures in the sinuses, and diving is contraindicated. Patients who are planning to fly or to drive over mountain ranges can use topical **decongestants** prior to the trip to prevent the pain associated with the changing air pressures in the air trapped in the sinuses.

Otitis Media

Treatment for otitis media (OM) is the most common reason for administering **antibiotics** to U.S. children; half of the office visits by ill children are for acute otitis media (AOM). OM may occur at any age, but the most common presentation is in children under age 10 years. The estimated annual cost of OM treatment is more than $3 billion. Every practitioner encounters OM, and those who work with children see OM daily. Defining AOM and otitis media with effusion (OME) would seem to be a simple task, yet there is great diversity in the criteria for diagnosis and management among primary care providers (Altemeier, 1998). Criteria for the diagnosis of AOM and OME, as well as their management, are discussed in this section of the chapter.

The hallmark symptom of otitis media is ear pain, often unilateral. Patients may also complain of hearing loss in the affected ear. Preverbal children may tug at the affected ear, be irritable, and sleep poorly. Fever often accompanies AOM. Patients may also report tinnitus, dizziness, an unsteady gait, or balance problems. In children, vomiting and diarrhea may be associated with OM.

Diagnosis of AOM is made from the combination of fluid in the middle ear and signs or symptoms of acute illness (Altemeier, 1998). OME is fluid in the middle ear without any signs or symptoms of acute illness. Erythema is nonspecific, and AOM should never be diagnosed on the basis of tympanic membrane (TM) color alone, as the TM can redden from crying or a fever. Fluid in the middle ear is assessed by observing white or yellow fluid, seeing air/fluid level, observing air bubbles, or noting decreased TM movement via pneumatic otoscopy. A thin-walled bulla is seen with bullous myringitis, a very painful form of AOM.

Pathophysiology

Acute otitis media occurs when there is a combination of eustachian tube dysfunction, which blocks the flow of secretions from the middle ear to the pharynx, and negative pressure developing in the middle ear, which causes reflux of bacteria into the middle ear space. This combination results in a middle ear effusion that becomes infected with nasopharyngeal bacteria. A predisposing factor in young children (under age 5 years) is that they have shorter, more horizontal, and more flaccid eustachian tubes, and bacteria are more easily drawn into the middle ear space. Certain risk factors predispose children to AOM: upper respiratory infections, Down syndrome, cleft palate, HIV infection, and Eskimo or Native American heritage. Children who are bottle-fed formula have a higher incidence of AOM than breast-fed infants. Children who live with one or more tobacco smokers have an increased risk of OM (Adair-Bischoff & Sauve, 1998). Immunocompromised patients and patients with indwelling nasogastric tubes have an increased incidence of OM, regardless of age.

S. pneumoniae and *H. influenzae* are the most common pathogens found in AOM. *S. pneumoniae* accounts for 25 to 50 percent of AOM, *H. influenzae* for 15 to 30 percent, and *M. catarrhalis* for 3 to 20 percent of pathogens found upon culture of middle ear aspirates (Adderson, 1998). Viruses alone or as a copathogen are found in 20 percent of AOM cases.

Goals of Treatment

The goal for the treatment of AOM is to clear infection from the middle ear fluid with the use of **antibiotics**. If the **antibiotic** chosen is effective against the pathogen, then the infection clears. Because the treatment of AOM is often based on the most commonly found pathogens, at times a change of **antibiotic** is necessary to treat the infection. The goal remains the same, clearing infection from the middle ear fluid.

Rational Drug Selection

Guidelines

There is much controversy regarding the treatment of OM. The different philosophies range from not using any **antibiotics** to using long-term prophylactic **antibiotics**. Dowell and colleagues (1998A) have proposed a set of principles for the judicious use of **antimicrobial agents** in the treatment of OM:

1. Episodes of OM should be classified as AOM or OME:
2. **Antimicrobials** are indicated for the treatment of AOM.

3. Uncomplicated AOM may be treated with a 5- to 7-day course of **antimicrobials** in certain patients.
4. **Antimicrobials** are not indicated for the initial treatment of OME.
5. Persistent middle ear effusion after therapy for AOM is expected and does not require retreatment.
6. **Antibiotic** prophylaxis should be reserved for control of recurrent AOM, defined by more than three distinct and well-documented episodes of AOM in 6 months or more than four episodes in 12 months.

Figure 44–2 provides an algorithm for treating OM.

Antimicrobial Resistance

The emergence of **antimicrobial** resistance among respiratory pathogens has caused primary care providers to reevaluate their routine use of **antibiotics** for all illnesses, especially otitis media. More than 95 percent of *M. catarrhalis* produces beta-lactamase, which can be resistant to **amoxicillin** and other **penicillins** (Chartrand & Pong, 1998; Hickey & Nelson, 1997). *H. influenzae*, another beta-lactamase producer, is 40 to 50 percent resistant to **amoxicillin** (Chartrand & Pong, 1998). Also of concern has been the emergence of highly resistant *S. pneumoniae*, which is currently in the range of less than 20 percent resistant to 83 percent resistant, depending on the population studied (Chartrand & Pong, 1998). Resistant *S. pneumoniae* is more common among children who are in daycare, have recurrent AOM, or have been recently treated with **beta-lactamase antibiotics**. Leibovitz and colleagues (1998) studied resistance patterns in children recently treated with **antibiotics** and found that the pneumococci isolated in new episodes of AOM are more likely to be intermittently resistant to **penicillin** (76% of patients) and highly resistant to **cefaclor** (63% of patients). In light of this increasing resistance among common OM pathogens, the provider needs to carefully decide whether an **antibiotic** is necessary and, in the case of treatment failure, consider the possibility of resistant bacterial strains. The common **antibiotics** used for OM and their dosages are listed in Table 44–2.

Dosing Regimen

Amoxicillin remains the first-line drug of choice for AOM in spite of resistance. Patients who have not recently been on **antibiotics**, are not in daycare, and are not currently on **amoxicillin** for OM prophylaxis should respond to **amoxicillin**. Conversely, patients who have had repeated episodes of AOM or have been on **antibiotics** recently should probably be treated with a second-

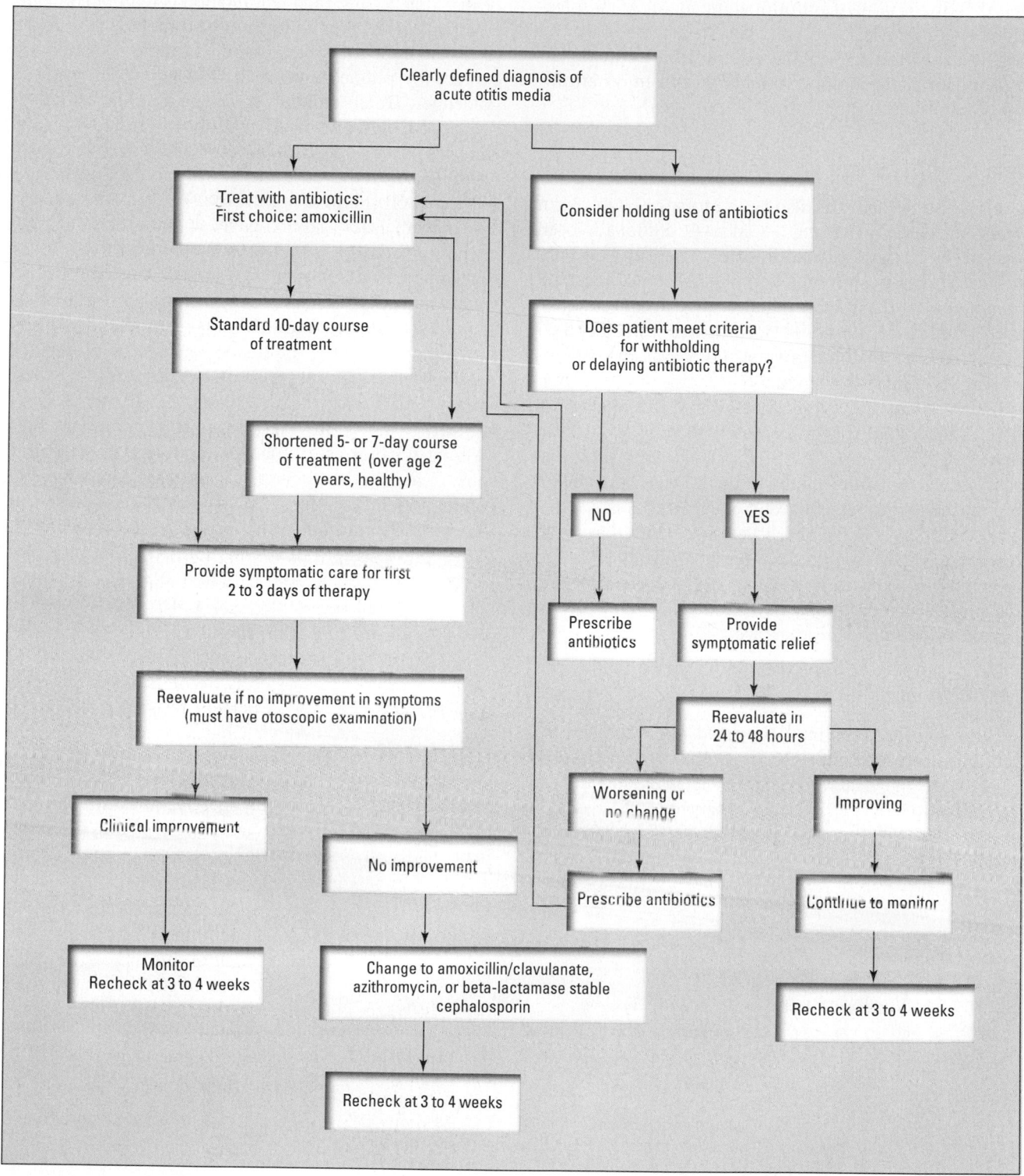

Figure 44–2. Algorithm for treatment of acute otitis media.

line drug that is beta-lactamase–stable (**amoxicillin-clavulanate, azithromycin,** or **beta-lactamase–stable cephalosporin**). Another option for patients who have been on **antibiotics** in the past month is to initially use high-dose **amoxicillin** (75 to 90 mg/kg daily).

Canafax and colleagues (1998) studied middle ear fluid penetration of **amoxicillin** at standard 40 to 50 mg/kg daily dosages and found that **amoxicillin** at that dose is inadequate to effectively eradicate resistant *S. pneumoniae*, particularly during viral coinfection. The authors felt that about 90 percent of pneumococcal AOM infections could be effectively treated with a higher dose, 75 mg/kg daily. Table 44–3 discusses **antibiotic** treatment options for AOM in patients who have been on **antibiotics** recently.

Length of Treatment

Length of treatment has also been investigated in recent years. In the United States, AOM has traditionally been treated for 10 days with **antibiotics.** There are few controlled studies to support the practice. Compliance and completion of the 10-day regimen have also been an issue. A number of studies have compared outcomes after 5 or 7 days of **antibiotics** versus 10 days. For patients over age 5 years, a shortened 5-day course of treatment is probably adequate (Paradise, 1997). In an analysis of nine studies comparing shortened therapy with traditional 10-day therapy, Paradise (1997) concluded that short-course **antimicrobial** treatment for AOM is probably not adequate for children under age 5 years, especially children age 2 years or younger. Dowell and colleagues (1998A) put forth a set of principles for the judicious use of **antimicrobial agents** in the treatment of OM, one of which is that uncomplicated AOM may be treated in patients older than age 2 for 5 to 7 days.

No Antibiotics

A number of authors have proposed not routinely prescribing **antibiotics** for AOM. Culpepper and Froom (1997) cite the Dutch College of General Practitioners' guidelines for children over age 2 years for AOM, in which symptomatic treatment is given for the first 3 days. If symptoms (pain or fever thought to be caused by AOM)

persist after 3 days, then reevaluation is required and **antibiotics** started. For children aged 6 months to 2 years, management is the same, except that there is mandatory contact (by phone or visit) after 24 hours. Using these guidelines, Dutch children have outcomes at 2 months similar to children from other countries treated with **antibiotics.** A previous study by van Buchem and colleagues (1985) studied the outcome of symptomatic treatment only on 4860 children, only 126 (2.7 %) of whom developed severe cases, defined as fever, pain, or discharge, after 3 to 4 days. Conrad (1998) reviewed five studies that compared the results of treating AOM with placebo versus **antimicrobials.** Although short-term outcomes were better in the **antimicrobial** groups (decreased pain), there was little difference between the groups in the long-term outcomes (persistence of middle ear fluid or recurrent AOM). Clearly, this topic needs to be studied further. For a provider who is considering not prescribing **antibiotics,** the patient and family need to meet some clear criteria to ensure a satisfactory outcome: (1) patient older than age 2 years, (2) normal host (no anatomic or immunologic abnormalities), (3) intact TM, (4) last previous episode of OM more than 3 months ago, (5) receptive parents, and (6) close follow-up ensured. Close follow-up is essential, and a plan of action has to be discussed with parents if the decision is made to not treat with **antibiotics.**

Pain Relief

Regardless of whether the patient receives **antibiotics,** all children require pain relief for the first 24 to 72 hours of treatment. Adequate dosing of **acetaminophen** (15 mg/kg per dose) or **ibuprofen** (5 to 10 mg/kg per dose) is necessary. It is the provider's responsibility to deter-

Table 44–3. Treatment Options for Otitis Media

Antibiotics in Prior Month	Initial Treatment	Treatment Failure (Days 3 to 5)	Treatment Failure (Days 10 to 28)
No	High-dose amoxicillin (75–90 mg/kg/d) *or* Usual dose amoxicillin (40–50 mg/kg/d)	*Amoxicillin & clavulanate Cefuroxime Cefpodoxime Azithromycin Ceftriaxone (IM) Cefixime	Same as day 3
Yes	High-dose amoxicillin (80–90 mg/kg/d) *or* *High-dose amoxicillin-clavulanate	IM ceftriaxone *or* Tympanocentesis	*High-dose amoxicillin-clavulanate *or* Cefuroxime *or* IM ceftriaxone *or* Tympanocentesis

*High-dose amoxicillin and clavulanate = 80–90 mg/kg/d of the amoxicillin component, with 6.4 mg/kg/d of clavulanate.

mine the dose of **analgesic** that ensures adequate pain relief. **Topical analgesia (Auralgan otic solution**, a combination of antipyrine, benzocaine, and glycerin) can be applied. In a study of children age 5 years or older who were being adequately dosed with **acetaminophen** (15 mg/kg), the study patients who received **Auralgan** reported lower ear pain scores than the control group who received the placebo (olive oil). A number of the study patients reported dramatic and immediate reductions in pain (Hoberman, Paradise, Reynolds, & Urkin, 1997). Some providers stock **Auralgan** in the clinic to provide immediate pain relief for their OM patients. **Auralgan** should never be used before the provider observes an intact TM.

Monitoring

Monitoring the effectiveness of the treatment chosen, either to prescribe **antibiotics** or to provide symptomatic care for the first 2 to 3 days, is essential to the optimal outcome for the patient. Although clinical symptoms may give some indication of whether the treatment is effective, pneumatic otoscopy is the only true measure of whether improvement is occurring. Patients may still experience pain with OME, even if the appearance of the TM improves. As mentioned previously, if no **antibiotics** are prescribed, a follow-up examination is essential in 2 to 3 days. All patients should be reexamined in 3 to 4 weeks after beginning **antibiotics,** with the understanding that at 4 weeks there is a 40 percent chance that fluid is still present in the middle ear and that effusions can last up to 3 months (Macon, 1996; Dowell et al., 1998A). **Antibiotics** are not appropriate for the initial treatment of OME, and there is controversy regarding their use at all for this indication, even after 3 months of persistent effusion.

Outcome Evaluation

The patient should be evaluated 3 to 4 weeks from the beginning of treatment to determine if the infection is completely resolved. The provider may choose to evaluate the patient sooner, with the understanding that some middle ear effusion may remain.

Patient Education

Two areas have to be covered in educating patients and families about OM: the proper use of the prescribed **antibiotic** and the predicted course of the infection once **antibiotics** are started. The instructions regarding the **antibiotic** dosage and timing of doses must be clear, and any questions regarding the medication answered. Expected adverse reactions, such as the mild diarrhea that may accompany many of the **antibiotics,** must be discussed. Patients and family members should be aware that the expected course of the ear infection, once **antibiotics** are started, is some symptomatic relief in 24 to 48 hours. Use of **acetaminophen** or **ibuprofen** for pain relief is necessary during this initial period to provide comfort. Parents should be encouraged to give their children a dose of **ibuprofen** or **acetaminophen** just before bedtime because children seem to complain of greater ear pain at night during the healing stages. Patients who are still having significant pain after 48 hours should be reexamined for the possibility of a resistant organism. Bacterial resistance ought to be mentioned, and the patient encouraged to complete the course of medication to prevent the development of antibacterial resistance to a partially treated organism.

Otitis Externa

Otitis externa (external otitis media) is an acute infection that causes an inflammatory reaction in the external auditory canal. It is also known as swimmer's ear.

The patient generally presents with severe ear pain, which may have begun as itching and irritation. The pain is generally unilateral and localized to the ear. Manipulation of the pinna or tragus causes moderate to severe pain, a finding that is usually absent in OM. The TM is normal in external otitis, but the external auditory canal may be swollen such that the TM is difficult to visualize. Malignant otitis externa is found in patients with diabetes and presents as severe cellulitis due to *Pseudomonas aeruginosa.*

Pathophysiology

Trauma or prolonged exposure to moisture predisposes to infection. The chlorine in swimming pools kills the normal flora in the external ear canal, which allows growth of pathogens. The most common organism found is *P. aeruginosa,* followed by *Staphylococcus aureus.*

Goals of Treatment

The goal of treatment of otitis externa is resolution of the infection and prevention of recurrence.

Rational Drug Selection

Treatment consists of irrigation and **antibiotic** eardrops. The medication of choice is **antibiotic-steroid** eardrops, which combine **hydrocortisone, neomycin sulfate,** and **polymyxin B (Cortisporin Otic, Pediotic).** The routine

Acute Maxillary Sinusitis

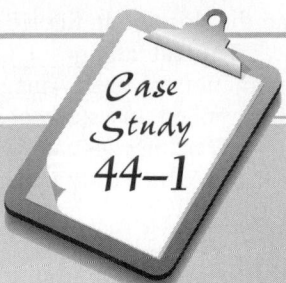

Case Study 44–1

Complaint

"I've got a cold."

History

George, a 45-year-old white man, presents with a 2-week history of green nasal discharge and cough. He states that for the past 48 hours he has had a headache that worsens when he bends over. He reports that his kids all have "colds" and that his symptoms are lasting longer than theirs.

George's history is notable for a 25-year history of smoking one pack per day of cigarettes, which he recently has been able to decrease to half a pack per day. He has no known drug allergies. He states he did have a sinus infection 4 or 5 years ago that cleared with antibiotics. He is generally healthy.

Asssessment

His vital signs are all within normal limits, except for an oral temperature of 100.6°F. His physical examination reveals the following:

1. Tympanic membranes are translucent gray, nasal turbinates are beefy red and swollen, and throat is clear with some green postnasal drip noted.
2. Patient complains of tenderness over his maxillary sinus area bilaterally.
3. Lymph glands show no adenopathy.
4. Heart has regular rhythm and rate, with no murmur.
5. Lungs show clear breath sounds in all fields.

Initial Management Plan

George is diagnosed with acute maxillary sinusitis. His management plan is as follows:

1. Amoxicillin 500 mg PO tid for 10 days.
2. Topical decongestants for the first 2 to 3 days of treatment.
3. Encourage adequate hydration.
4. Acetaminophen or ibuprofen for pain and fever.
5. He is to return to the clinic if there is no improvement in 3 to 4 days.
6. Decrease smoking, if possible.

Follow-up Visit

At his follow-up visit, George reported that he became symptom-free after 3 days of amoxicillin. He took the full 10 days of antibiotic therapy without incident.

Modifications to Management Plan

None needed.

Continuing Care

Patient education for prevention.

---

dosing is 3 to 4 drops administered four times a day. Suspension formulations are less ototoxic than solution preparations of eardrops. A cotton wick may be necessary if the ear canal is extremely swollen. For severe cellulitis, parenteral antistaphylococcal and antipseudomonas **antibiotics** are necessary.

Monitoring

The patient should begin to experience relief from pain in 3 or 4 days. Reevaluation in 1 week determines if the patient is clinically improving. Referral to a dermatologist or otolaryngologist may be necessary if there is no improvement.

Outcome Evaluation

To evaluate the effectiveness of otitis externa treatment, the provider determines if the infection is resolved after treatment with **antibiotic-steroid** eardrops.

Patient Education

Educate the patient to prevent external otitis media by avoiding pooling of water in the ears and by using a mildly acidic solution after swimming. Patients can instill 3 to 4 drops of a 1:1 solution of water and white vinegar or 70 percent **ethyl alcohol.** Commercially available products (**EarSol, Swim-Ear**) can also be used.

Explain proper irrigation of debris prior to instillation of eardrops to ensure that the medication contacts the affected area. Monitoring for increasing severity is essential to detect cellulitis early in the diabetic patient. The patient may take **ibuprofen** or another **analgesic** for the first 24 to 48 hours of treatment to provide pain relief.

REFERENCES

Adair-Bischoff, C. E., & Sauve, R. S. (1998). Environmental tobacco smoke and middle ear disease in preschool age children. *Archives of Pediatric and Adolescent Medicine, 152,* 127–133.

Adderson, E. E. (1998). Preventing otitis media: Medical approaches. *Pediatric Annals, 27,* 101.

Altemeier, W. A. (1998). A pediatrician's view: Earaches. *Pediatric Annals, 27,* 62–64.

Brown, D. J. (1996). *Phytotherapy: Herbal medicine meets clinical science.* Bothell, WA: Bastyr University.

Canafax, D. M., Yuan, Z., Chonmaitree, T., Deka, K., Russlie, H. Q., & Giebink, G. S. (1998). Amoxicillin middle ear fluid penetration and pharmacokinetics in children with acute otitis media. *Pediatric Infectious Disease Journal, 17*(2),149–155.

Chartrand, S. A., & Pong, A. (1998). Acute otitis media in the 1990s: The impact of antibiotic resistance. *Pediatric Annals, 27,* 86.

Conrad, D. A. (1998). Should acute otitis media ever be treated with antibiotics? *Pediatric Annals, 27,* 66.

Culpepper, L., & Froom, J. (1997). Routine antimicrobial treatment of acute otitis media: Is it necessary? *Journal of the American Medical Association, 278,* 1643.

Dowell, S. F., Butler, J. C., Giebink, G. S., Jacobs, M. R., Jernigan, D., Musher, D. M., Rakowsky, A., & Schwartz, B. (1999). Acute otitis media. Management and surveillance in an era of pneumococcal resistance: A report from the drug-resistant *Streptococcus pneumoniae* therapeutic working group (DRSPTWG). *Pediatric Infectious Disease Journal, 18*(1), 1–9.

Dowell, S. F., Mary, S. M., Phillips, W. R., Gerber, M. A., & Schwartz, B. (1998A). Otitis media: Principles of judicious use of antimicrobial agents. *Pediatrics, 101*(1, Suppl.), 165–169.

Dowell, S. F., Mary, S. M., Phillips, W. R., Gerber, M. A., & Schwartz, B. (1998B). Principles of judicious use of antimicrobial agents for pediatric upper respiratory tract infections. *Pediatrics, 101*(1, Suppl.) 163–165.

Goodman, M., & Brady, M. (1996). Respiratory disorders. In C. E. Burns, N. Barber, M. A. Brady & A. M. Dunn (Eds.), *Pediatric primary care: A handbook for nurse practitioners* (p. 643). Philadelphia: Saunders

Hendley, J. O. (1996). The common cold. In J. C. Bennett & F. Plum (Eds.), *Cecil textbook of medicine* (29th ed., p. 1747). Philadelphia: Saunders.

Hickey, S.M., & Nelson, J.D. (1997). Mechanisms of antibacterial resistance. *Advances in Pediatrics, 44,* 1.

Hoberman, A., Paradise, J. L., Reynolds, E. A., & Urkin, J. (1997). Efficacy of Auralgan for treating ear pain in children with acute otitis media. *Archives of Pediatric and Adolescent Medicine, 151,* 675.

Jackson J., Peterson, C., & Lesho, E. (1997). A meta-analysis of zinc salts lozenges and the common cold. *Archives of Internal Medicine, 157*(20), 2373–2376.

Liebovitz, E., Raiz, S., Piglanski, L., Greenberg, D., Yagupsky, P., Fliss, D. M., Lieberman, A., & Dagan, R. (1998). Resistance pattern of middle ear fluid isolates in acute otitis media recently treated with antibiotics. *Pediatric Infectious Disease Journal, 17,* 463.

Mason, W. H. (1996). The management of common infections in ambulatory children. *Pediatric Annals, 25,* 620.

O'Brien, K. L., Dowell, S. F., Schwartz, B., Marcy, S. M., Phillips, W. R., & Gerber, M. D. (1998). Acute sinusitis: Principles of judicious use of antimicrobial agents. *Pediatrics, 101*(Suppl.), 174.

Paradise, J. L. (1997). Short-course antimicrobial treatment for acute otitis media: Not best for infants and young children. *Journal of the American Medical Association, 278,* 1640.

Peterson-Smith, A. M. (1996). Ear disorders. In C. E. Burns, N Barber, M. A. Brady & A. M. Dunn (Eds.), *Pediatric primary care: A handbook for nurse practitioners* (p. 593). Philadelphia: Saunders.

Prince, A. (1998). Infectious diseases. In R. E. Behrman & R. M. Kliegman (Eds.), *Nelson essentials of pediatrics* (3rd ed., p. 341). Philadelphia: Saunders.

Simon, R. P. (1998). Parameningeal infections. In R. E. Behrman & R. M. Kliegman (Eds.), *Nelson essentials of pediatrics* (3rd ed., p. 2080). Philadelphia: Saunders.

Strohl, K. P. (1996). Upper airway diseases. In J. C. Bennett & F. Plum (Eds.), *Cecil textbook of medicine* (29th ed., p. 449). Philadelphia: Saunders.

Van Buchem, F., Peeters, M., & van't Hof, M. (1985). Acute otitis media: A new treatment strategy. *British Medical Journal* (Clinical Research Edition), 290(6474), 1033–1037.

CHAPTER 45

......

Urinary Tract Infections

CHAPTER OUTLINE

U rinary tract infections (UTIs) are responsible for more than 7 million office visits per year (Murdock & Munroe, 1999). UTIs are more common in women because the short female urethra provides easy access to the bladder for bacteria. Up to 50 percent of women experience a UTI at some time. Up to 40 percent experience at least one additional episode (Murdock & Munroe, 1999), and approximately 3 percent of adult women experience one episode or more annually. Some women have as many as seven UTIs a year (Leiner, 1995). UTIs also occur in men, most commonly related to urinary tract obstructions such as benign prostatic hyper-

trophy. Also one of the most common bacterial diseases in children, UTIs in male children under age 5 years are usually related to congenital abnormalities. In female children, the cause is usually the same as in adult women.

Most patients with UTIs do not experience long-term complications from these disorders. Those who do usually have a comorbid condition such as vesicoureteral reflux, renal stones, neurogenic bladder, diabetes, or obstruction. This chapter discusses the management of UTIs in otherwise healthy patients who do not have these comorbid conditions and who do not have retention catheters inserted.

Pathophysiology

A complex interaction between host and microbial factors leads to UTIs.

Host Factors

The Anatomy and Physiology of the Genitourinary Tract

The bladder has unique intrinsic defenses against infection. Periodic washout of the bacteria that perpetually colonize the urethra by voiding is one of the most important mechanisms. The bladder also deters microbial adherence to the mucosa through the antibacterial properties of the urinary bladder epithelium. Patients who have repeated UTIs appear to have altered bladder epithelial cells that facilitate adherence of bacteria to the mucosa rather than deter it (Leiner, 1995). The pH of the urine, urine osmolality, and a competent urethral valve that prevents backflow also decrease UTIs. These defense mechanisms are severely limited if residual urine is regularly present after voiding. Pregnancy increases the risk for UTIs because of pressure on the bladder from the enlarging fetus, increased incidence of residual urine, and changes in estrogen levels. Estrogen deficiency and concomitant decreased acidification of the vagina, with increased vaginal colonization by Enterobacteriaceae, also contribute to increased risk in postmenopausal women (Goroll, May, & Mulley, 1995; Leiner, 1995).

Behavioral Factors

Frequency of sexual intercourse, diaphragm or **spermicide** use, and failure to void within 10 to 15 minutes of coitus have all been associated with a higher risk for UTIs (Barker, Burton, & Zieve, 1995; Goroll et al., 1995; Leiner, 1995). Reasons for the increased risk may be urethral trauma, decreased urge to void, and residual urine. Diaphragm or **spermicide** use appears to compromise host defense mechanisms to the extent necessary for virulent strains of bacteria to become capable of causing an infection.

Other behavioral factors have been inconsistently associated with UTI and are subject to some controversy. Purposely resisting the urge to void has been associated with UTI in some studies and not in others. Increased fluid intake has also had an inconsistent association, although it is difficult to find a reason not to suggest adequate fluid intake for a variety of reasons, including increasing bacterial washout through more frequent voiding. Cranberry juice has an "on again, off again" history of association with prevention of UTI. A well-conducted, randomized, double-blind, placebo-controlled trial performed in Boston and published in the *Journal of the American Medical Association* (Avorn, Monane, Gurwitz, Glynn, Choodnovsky, & Lipitz, 1994) supports the ability of cranberry juice to reduce the incidence of UTI. There is little evidence to indicate that the direction of wiping after bowel movements, the use of **oral contraceptives** or tampons, or the habit of taking bubble baths or douching contributes to UTIs.

Microbial Factors

The Ability of the Bacteria to Adhere to Epithelial Cells

Escherichia coli, the organism responsible for 80 percent or more of UTIs in women and more than 50 percent of those in men, contain fimbriae that allow attachment to host cell receptor sites on the bladder mucosa.

The Virulence of the Organism

Coliforms cultured from women with recurrent UTIs were more virulent than those cultured from patients with first-time infections or from the fecal flora of patients who had no history of UTIs (Leiner, 1995).

The Ability of the Organism to Survive the Urinary Tract Environment

Some bacteria are more tolerant of the low pH of urine. Table 45–1 lists the factors shown by research to be associated with the occurrence of UTIs. It also lists those factors that have been inconsistently related to UTIs or not demonstrated by research to be associated with UTIs.

Diagnosis of UTI is based on symptoms and laboratory data. Presenting symptoms of UTI vary with age. Table 45–2 shows the various symptoms by age. Symptom presentation is similar for both men and women. All ages often exhibit dark, cloudy, and malodorous urine. Urethral discharge in men is more commonly associated with sexually transmitted diseases (STDs) than with UTIs. STDs are discussed in Chapter 42.

Laboratory data for diagnosis include urinalysis and urine culture and sensitivity. The most common findings from a clean-catch urine specimen are a positive leukocytes esterase or pyuria (usually more than 5 white blood cells [WBCs] per high-power field), the presence of bacteria, and a positive dipstick for nitrates. The presence of casts or hematuria suggests an upper UTI. Quantitative urine cultures are the most reliable method for diagnosing UTIs; however, they require trained personnel, are more expensive, and take time to complete, which might lead to postponing treatment of symptomatic patients. Cultures are usually reserved for children and men and for recurrent UTIs in women.

Pharmacodynamics

A wide range of **antimicrobial agents** are available for treatment of UTIs. They include **trimethoprim-**

Table 45–1. Factors Associated with Urinary Tract Infections

Host Factors	Microbial Factors	Inconsistent or Not Associated Factors
Anatomic and Physiological • Periodic washout with voiding* • Bladder epithelial cells that prevent adherence of bacteria* • Acid pH of urine* • Osmolality of urine* • Competent urethral valves to prevent backflow of urine* • Pregnancy • Estrogen deficiency • Residual urine	• Ability of the organism to adhere to epithelial cells • Virulence of the organism • Ability of the organism to survive the urinary tract environment	• Ingestion of cranberry juice* • Purposely resisting the urge to void • Increased fluid intake* • Wiping from front to back after defecation* • Oral contraceptive use • Tampon use • Bubble baths • Douching
Behavioral • Frequent sexual intercourse • Diaphragm use • Spermicide use • Failure to void 10–15 minutes after coitus		

*These factors are negatively associated with UTIs and may prevent them.

sulfamethoxazole (Bactrim, Septra), nitrofurantoin (Furadantin, Macrodantin), fluoroquinolones (ciprofloxacin [Cipro], ofloxacin [Floxin]), cephalosporins (cephalexin [Keflex], cefixime [Suprax]), and penicillins (amoxicillin [Amoxil], amoxicillin-clavulanate [Augmentin]). The spectrum of antimicrobial activity varies among these agents. Each of these agents is discussed in Chapter 22.

Another product, Azo-Cranberry, contains 450 mg of natural cranberry concentrate powder. Studies indicate that a substrate in cranberries may exert a bacteriostatic effect by inhibiting the adherence of organisms to the mucosal surface of the bladder. This product is marketed as an adjunct to **antimicrobial** regimens or as prophylactic therapy. It is not Food and Drug Administration (FDA)–approved for the treatment of UTI because it is officially a nutritional supplement, and the FDA does not evaluate the therapeutic claims of such supplements.

Symptomatic relief is often provided by urinary **anal-** gesics. The primary ingredient in these products is **phenazopyridine**, an azo dye taken orally that exerts a **topical analgesic** effect on the urinary tract mucosa when it is excreted into the urine. This dye is available in several different brands. **Azo-Standard, Prodium, Pyridium,** and **Urogesic** all contain **phenazopyridine** 95 mg.

Goals of Treatment

Eradication of the causative organism is the primary goal of therapy. Relief of symptoms and prevention of recurrent infections are also therapeutic goals.

Rational Drug Selection

Recommended treatments for UTIs include herbal remedies, cranberry juice, lifestyle modifications related to

Table 45–2. Urinary Tract Infection Symptoms by Age

Neonate	Failure to thrive, irritability, fever, hypothermia, sepsis, jaundice, vomiting, acidosis
Infant	Failure to thrive, irritability, fever, hypothermia, sepsis, jaundice, vomiting, acidosis, hematuria, urinary frequency, dysuria
Preschool child	Abdominal or suprapubic pain, dysuria, frequency, urgency, enuresis
Adult	• Dysuria, frequency, urgency, burning on urination, incontinence, urethral pain, suprapubic pain, low back pain, hematuria. • Significant fever is unusual in bladder infections but may occur, along with severe flank pain and costovertebral tenderness, in upper UTIs • Patients with upper UTIs may also demonstrate headache, malaise, nausea, and vomiting • Symptoms are similar for women and men

voiding and sexual intercourse, and drug therapies sometimes based on unsubstantiated opinions that health care providers have taken for granted. Herbal remedies are discussed in Chapter 9. Cranberry juice, which has been documented by research to be beneficial (Avorn et al., 1994), is discussed in the Patient Education section. Some lifestyle modifications have research support or make empiric sense and are discussed briefly here. The main focus of this section is appropriate selection and use of drugs to treat both upper and lower UTIs.

Algorithm

This chapter does not discuss the testing involved in the diagnosis of UTIs beyond that needed for treatment decisions. The treatment protocol here assumes accurate diagnosis of the UTI by means of the appropriate diagnostic tools, including laboratory data. Once the diagnosis has been made, treatment regimens are determined.

Treatment of UTIs is directed at the three goals cited previously. The infecting organism is eradicated with **antimicrobial therapy.** Treatment for symptom relief often includes urinary **analgesics.** Prevention of recurrence may involve prophylactic drug therapy but involves lifestyle management as well.

Lifestyle Management

Prevention is the key to management of UTIs. Although Leiner (1995) believes "there are no easily enacted measures that offer promise as effective UTI prevention," studies confirm several practices that may help to prevent UTIs, especially in women. The following lifestyle modifications and behavioral strategies have research support for their role in prevention:

1. Ingestion of cranberry juice or cranberry extract. Cranberry substrates exert a bacteriostatic effect. Most studies have been done in elderly women, but the same mechanism may prove effective in younger women and in men.
2. Avoidance of **spermicide** and diaphragms. Use of these products may cause a change in vaginal pH and flora that increases the potential for vaginal colonization with organisms likely to produce UTIs. **Nonoxynol-9 spermicides** are especially associated with increased incidence of bacteriuria. The essential first step to UTIs in women is thought to be frequently the colonization of the vaginal introitus.
3. Voiding 10 to 15 minutes after sexual intercourse. Urination washes out the bacteria from the urethra that may have entered the bladder during intercourse.

Additional measures that have inconsistent support but would not be harmful and are likely to be helpful include the following:

1. Maintaining fluid intake of at least 2000 cc per day of noncaffeinated fluids. Sufficient fluid is necessary to ensure regular voiding throughout the day. Caffeinated fluids have a mild diuretic effect but are less likely to maintain fluid volume balance.
2. Not resisting the urge to void. "Holding" urine may stretch the bladder and cause small breaks in the bladder mucosal layer that provide entrance for bacteria. It also increases the risk for growth of bacteria in residual urine.
3. Avoidance of douche products that change the vaginal pH and flora. This practice may decrease the likelihood of vaginal canal colonization (Murdock & Munroe, 1999).

Drug Therapy

Drug therapy is aimed at eradication of the infecting organism. Appropriate **antimicrobial** selection is based on drug variables (spectrum of activity of the drug, potential adverse drug reactions, patterns of resistance to the **antimicrobial,** and cost) and patient variables (age, gender, pregnancy, and the underlying cause of the UTI).

Drug Variables

Spectrum of Activity

Lower tract UTIs are most commonly caused by gram-negative bacteria (95% of UTIs), with *E. coli* the most prevalent organism (80% or more of all lower UTIs are caused by *E. coli*). Among community-acquired infections, *Staphylococcus saprophyticus* and gram-negative enteric bacilli cause almost all the UTIs not caused by *E. coli* (Preston, Abdel-Rahman, & Nahata, 1998). For children, additional organisms include *Klebsiella* in neonates and *Proteus* in boys. All of the **antimicrobial agents** mentioned have a spectrum of activity that covers these organisms. **Trimethoprim-sulfamethoxazole** is the most effective drug; the recommended dose is one double-strength tablet bid for 3 days (Barker et al., 1995; Gilbert, Moellering, & Sande, 1998; Goroll et al., 1995). **Nitrofurantoin** and the **fluoroquinolones** are also effective. The dose for **nitrofurantoin** is 50 to 100 mg bid for 3 days. During pregnancy, the dose must be given for 7 days. **Ciprofloxacin** is the **fluoroquinolone** of choice as second-line therapy (Gilbert et al., 1998). The dose is 250 mg bid for 3 days. Other **fluoroquinolones** may also be used, but studies show them to be no more effective than **trimethoprim-sulfamethoxazole** or any of the second-line drugs (Onrust, Lamb, & Barman Balfour, 1998). The **beta-lactams** (**amoxicillin** and the **cephalosporins**) are less effective and are usually reserved for children and pregnant women.

Any of these treatments generally sterilizes the urine and produces symptom relief in 24 hours or less. Patients who are very symptomatic or have severe burning on urination can have **phenazopyridine** 200 mg tid added to their treatment regimen for 2 to 3 days as a urinary **analgesic.**

All of these drugs may also be used for prophylaxis. The drug of choice for adults for prophylaxis or for recurrent infections (more than three infections in 1 year) is **trimethoprim-sulfamethoxazole** 1 single-strength tablet daily at bedtime for a minimum of 6 months or a self-administered single dose of two double-strength tablets at symptom onset (Gilbert et al., 1998). For children, the recommended dose of **trimethoprim-sulfamethoxazole** is 0.5 to 1 mg/kg daily. The **nitrofurantoin** dose for adults is 50 mg daily at bedtime. For children, the dose is 1 mg/kg daily (Mowry, 1997).

Patients with risk factors for STD, a positive dipstick for leukocyte esterase or hemoglobin, and a negative Gram's stain are likely to have a UTI complicated by *Chlamydia trachomatis*. The recommended drug for these patients is **doxycycline (Doxy-Caps, Vibramycin)** 100 mg bid for 7 days. The alternative drug is **azithromycin (Zithromax)** 1 g in a single dose. **Azithromycin** is the preferred drug if the patient's adherence to the 7-day regimen is questionable.

Upper UTIs (e.g., pyelonephritis) involve the same likely organisms because they are most often ascended from a bladder infection. The same drugs may be used to treat these infections by increasing the dose and extending the treatment period to 14 days. However, Gilbert and colleagues (1998) recommend **ciprofloxacin** 500 mg bid for 14 days as the first-line drug. Other **fluoroquinolones** may also be used at increased doses. The alternative drugs recommended are **amoxicillin-clavulanate** or an oral **cephalosporin** with the treatment extending for 14 days. Graber and Martinez-Bianchi (1999) suggest that failure of a short course of **antimicrobials** generally indicates an upper UTI. They recommend **trimethoprim-sulfamethoxazole** (double-strength 1 tablet bid) as first line, with **ciprofloxacin** 250 to 500 mg bid or **ofloxacin** 200 mg bid as second-line therapy. All of these drugs are to be given for 14 days. Patients with acute pyelonephritis who are not acutely ill may also benefit from 1 to 2 g **ceftriaxone** intramuscularly (IM) at the time of diagnosis. Acutely ill and pregnant patients require referral for hospitalization.

Potential Adverse Drug Reactions

A significant number of patients have allergies to **sulfonamides** and **penicillins.** Approximately 30 percent of patients allergic to **penicillin** are also allergic to the other class of **beta-lactam** drugs, **cephalosporins.** It is important to ask about allergies and to be aware that patients with allergies to other substances such as pet dander and pollens are at higher risk for drug allergies. Patients allergic to these drugs can be treated with **nitrofurantoin** 50 to 100 mg bid (Barker et al., 1995).

Amoxicillin and **cephalosporins** have a negative effect on bowel flora and often result in diarrhea. This adverse reaction is much less common with **trimethoprim,** and **nitrofurantoin** does not affect bowel flora. Patients with bowel disease should be given either of the latter two drugs.

Long-term therapy with **nitrofurantoin** has been associated with pulmonary fibrosis and peripheral neuropathy (Leiner, 1995). Short-term therapy has not been associated with this problem. If this drug is chosen for prophylaxis, it should be used for no more than 3 months.

Resistance Patterns

Drug resistance to **antimicrobial therapy** is a major factor in drug selection. In the United States, the resistance of *E. coli* to **trimethoprim-sulfamethoxazole** is approximately 11 percent (Gilbert et al., 1998), to **amoxicillin** is 33 percent (Preston et al., 1998), and to **fluoroquinolones** is 2 to 12 percent. There is increasing resistance to **fluoroquinolones** among *E. coli* isolates, however (Onrust et al., 1998), and they should be reserved for second-line therapy except in upper UTIs. Resistance patterns vary in other countries. Preston and colleagues (1998) present research data from Israel, the United Kingdom, the Netherlands, and South Africa that show a clear difference in resistance patterns. In all of these countries, however, resistance to **trimethoprim-sulfamethoxazole** is lower than to any other drugs. **Nitrofurantoin** resistance was less than 10 percent in all countries studied and only 2 percent in the United States.

Clearly, **amoxicillin** can no longer be recommended for empiric therapy in the United States in that one-third of the UTI organisms are resistant. **Trimethoprim-sulfamethoxazole** double-strength 1 tablet bid for 3 to 7 days remains an appropriate drug and dose for empiric therapy (Preston et al., 1998). A **fluoroquinolone** or **nitrofurantoin** is a reasonable alternative for patients who are allergic to **sulfonamides.**

Cost

Trimethoprim-sulfamethoxazole is the least expensive of the **antimicrobials,** especially when it can be given for 1 to 3 days. **Nitrofurantoin** is also relatively inexpensive. Cost comparisons for the **antimicrobials** are presented in Chapter 22.

Table 45–3 summarizes **antimicrobial** recommendations for upper and lower UTIs. Recommendations are included for adults and children. Figure 45–1 depicts the treatment protocol for management of UTI in adult women.

Table 45–3. Drugs Commonly Used: Upper and Lower Urinary Tract Infections

Indication	Primary Choices	Alternative Choices
Upper UTIs Simple, uncomplicated upper UTI Mild to moderately ill	• Ciprofloxacin 500 mg bid for 14 d • Trimethoprim-sulfamethoxazole double-strength 1 tablet bid for 14 d *or* • Ofloxacin 400 mg bid for 14 d	• Amoxicillin-clavulanate 500 mg bid for 14 d • Cefixime 200 mg bid for 14 d
Lower UTIs Simple, uncomplicated lower UTI in adults Symptomatic or asymptomatic and reinfection (single event)	• Trimethoprim-sulfamethoxazole double-strength 1 tablet bid for 3 d *or* • Ciprofloxacin 250 mg bid for 3 d • Ofloxacin 200 mg bid for 3 d	• Nitrofurantoin 50–100 mg bid for 3 d
Simple, uncomplicated lower UTI Serial reinfections (more than 3/y)	• Trimethoprim-sulfamethoxazole double-strength 1 tablet bid for 3 d with onset of symptoms	• Ciprofloxacin 250 mg bid for 3 d with onset of symptoms
Simple, uncomplicated lower UTI associated with intercourse: prophylaxis	• Trimethoprim-sulfamethoxazole double-strength 1 tablet single dose after intercourse	• Ciprofloxacin 250-mg single dose after intercourse
Simple, uncomplicated lower UTI recurrence: prophylaxis	• Trimethoprim-sulfamethoxazole double-strength 1 tablet daily at bedtime for at least 6 mo	• Nitrofurantoin 50 mg daily at bedtime for no more than 3 mo
Complicated lower UTI or symptomatic after 3 d of therapy	• Trimethoprim-sulfamethoxazole double-strength 1 tablet bid for 7–14 d • Ciprofloxacin 250 mg bid for 7–14 d • Ofloxacin 200 mg bid for 7–14 d	• Nitrofurantoin 100 mg bid for 7–14 d
Special Considerations Risk factors for STD	• Doxycycline 100 mg bid for 7 d	• Azithromycin 1-g single dose
Pregnancy	• Nitrofurantoin 100 mg bid for 7 d	• Amoxicillin 500 mg tid for 7 d • Cefixime 200 mg bid for 7 d
Children: over age 5 y	• Trimethoprim-sulfamethoxazole 0.5–1 mg/kg/d given in 2 divided doses	• Nitrofurantoin 1 mg/kg/d in 2 divided doses • Amoxicillin 20–40 mg/kg/d in 3 divided doses • Cefixime 8 mg/kg/d once daily
Estrogen deficiency/ postmenopausal female	• Vaginal estrogen cream 0.5–2 g intravaginally daily	
Advanced age	• No treatment if asymptomatic	

Patient Variables

Age

Children under age 5 years require referral to a pediatric urologist for workup. Any girl age 5 years or under, all boys regardless of age, children with evidence of pyelonephritis, and any girl over age 5 years with recurrent UTIs should be referred for anatomic abnormality studies (Mowry, 1997; Burns, Barber, Brady, & Dunn, 1996).

Adolescents with pyelonephritis or a second UTI with documented positive urine cultures and no history of recent sexual activity require at least consultation (Burns et al., 1996).

Older children can be treated with the same drugs as adults, whether they are asymptomatic or symptomatic, but the extent of treatment may need to be 7 to 10 days. Consideration should be given to the effect of the agent chosen on bowel flora, which is highly correlated with diarrhea. Younger children are more likely

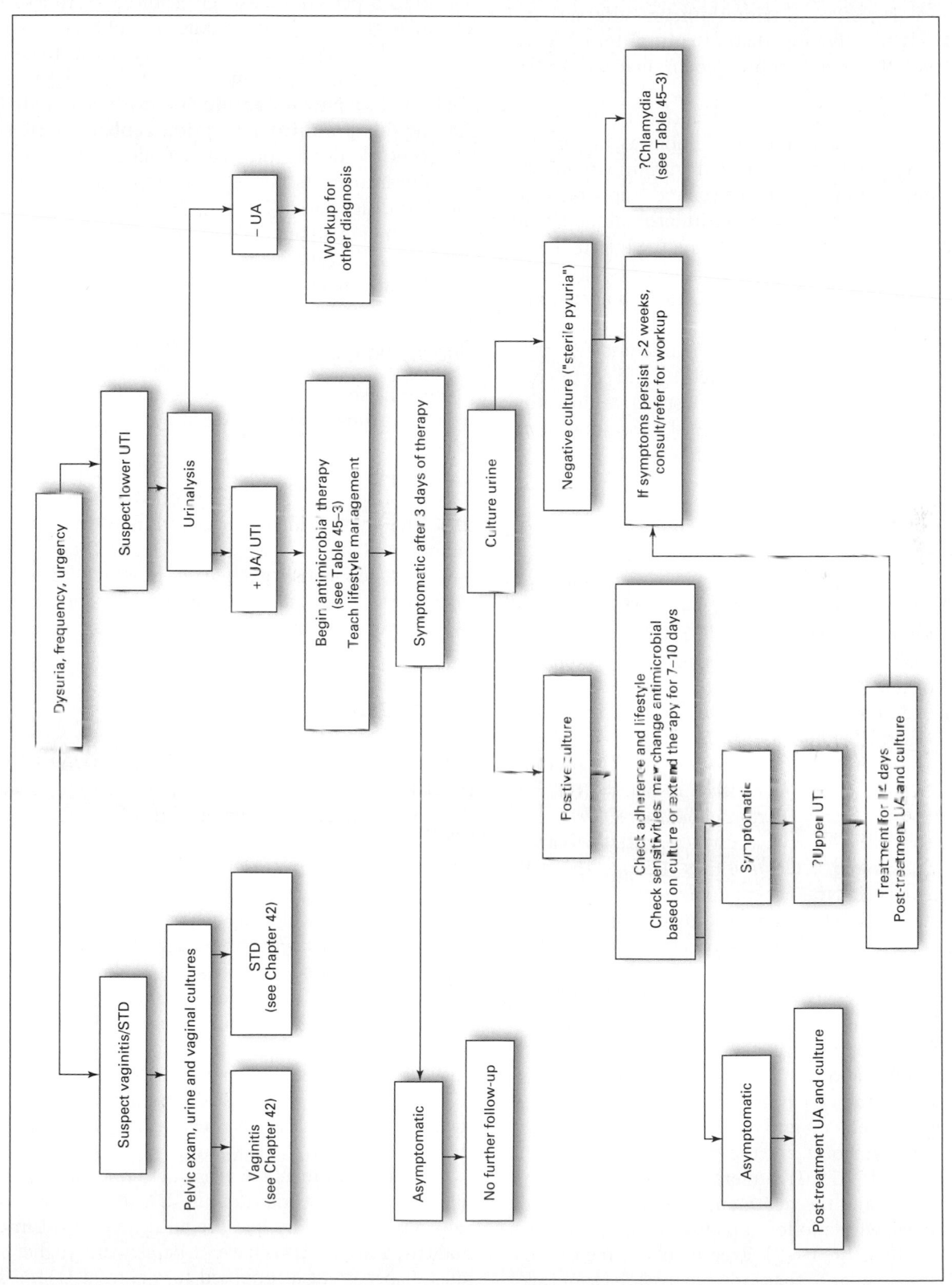

Figure 45–1. Treatment protocol: Urinary tract infections in women.

to experience fluid volume deficits secondary to diarrhea. Among the available drugs, **nitrofurantoin** has the least effect on bowel flora and **amoxicillin** has the most effect. The effect of **trimethoprim-sulfamethoxazole** is only slightly more than **nitrofurantoin**. Figure 45–2 depicts the treatment protocol for management of UTI in children.

After age 80, 22 percent of men and up to 50 percent of women have bacteriuria. In addition, asymptomatic bacteriuria is commonly associated with urinary incontinence, multiple medical illnesses, and impairment of mental status. Treatment with **antimicrobial** therapy is frequently unsuccessful in eradicating the infection and may be associated with the development of more resistant bacteria (Barker et al., 1995). Choice of **antimicrobial** should be based on culture and sensitivity tests rather than done empirically. No treatment is indicated in asymptomatic adults of advanced age unless in conjunction with surgery to correct obstructive uropathy (Gilbert et al., 1998) or after removal of an indwelling catheter (Graber & Martinez-Bianchi, 1999).

Male Gender

Signs and symptoms of UTI are similar in males and females. Urethral discharge in men is more commonly associated with STD than with a UTI.

In children and young men, UTIs are more commonly associated with congenital obstructive disorders. The risk of infection with *E. coli* is increased in homosexual men and heterosexual men with a colonized partner. The rate of UTI increases in men age 50 to 65 and parallels the increase in hyperplasia of the prostate gland. Glandular enlargement leads to bladder outflow obstruction and increased residual urine. Older adult men (age 65 and older) have further prostate enlargement and increased urine residuals. Despite the high prevalence of UTI in this age group, most remain asymptomatic and seem to be at low risk for serious complications. However, gram-negative sepsis from a UTI can occur and may be life-threatening.

Culture and sensitivity studies should be done in men with a history of UTI. In men, the organisms responsible for infection are slightly different. *E. coli* accounts for only about 25 percent of their infections. Gram-negative rods such as *Proteus* and *Pseudomonas* account for 50 percent, and enterococci and coagulase-negative staphylococci are the remaining 25 percent (Goroll et al., 1995). Treatment should be based on culture results, and the treatment period should be for 10 to 14 days, with a follow-up culture drawn (Graber & Martinez-Bianchi, 1999). Treatment for men of advanced age is similar to that for women of the same age. Figure 45–3 presents the treatment protocol for males with UTI.

Pregnancy

Asymptomatic bacteriuria is relatively common, affecting up to 6 percent of women in the first trimester. It should be treated because eradication of bacteriuria reduces the high incidence of symptomatic UTI that commonly occurs later; treatment may reduce the risk for preterm birth. **Nitrofurantoin** 100 mg bid, **amoxicillin** 500 mg tid, and **third-generation cephalosporins** are all acceptable during pregnancy (Gilbert et al., 1998). **Nitrofurantoin** has the best adverse reactions profile. All these drugs have a 7-day length of treatment for this indication. If treatment fails on the 7-day course, culture the urine and treat for 2 weeks with the appropriate antimicrobial (Gilbert et al., 1998).

Underlying Cause

If the UTI should develop in relation to intercourse, **trimethoprim-sulfamethoxazole** (double-strength, 1 tablet after coitus) may prevent the UTI. It is effective and inexpensive. A single dose of a **fluoroquinolone** is a second-line choice. It is also effective but more expensive. Patients should also void within 10 minutes after intercourse (Graber & Martinez-Bianchi, 1999).

In postmenopausal women, UTIs associated with estrogen deficiency can be reduced by daily application of **vaginal estrogen cream** 0.5 to 2 g intravaginally.

Monitoring

For lower UTIs, a standard urinalysis (UA) is cost-effective in diagnosing the disorder. Symptom resolution within 48 hours is considered sufficient monitoring of outcome. If symptoms persist, a urine culture is obtained, and any necessary changes in **antimicrobial** therapy are instituted. For these patients, a follow-up office visit in 10 to 14 days should be scheduled. For patients with recurrent infections, obtaining and documenting one urine culture is worthwhile, although it is generally unnecessary for women with acute UTI. As few as 10,000/mL colony count of gram-negative rods is diagnostic. If the culture is negative despite a positive UA, investigation is needed for organisms that do not grow on standard laboratory media, such as those that cause gonorrhea, chlamydia, and renal tuberculosis.

One post-treatment UA is useful to rule out persistent infection or hematuria. Routine UA to test for cure is generally unnecessary because all the main **antimicrobials** used to treat UTIs have 91 percent and higher cure rates. If persistent as opposed to recurrent UTI is suspected, a follow-up UA may be helpful in making this diagnosis.

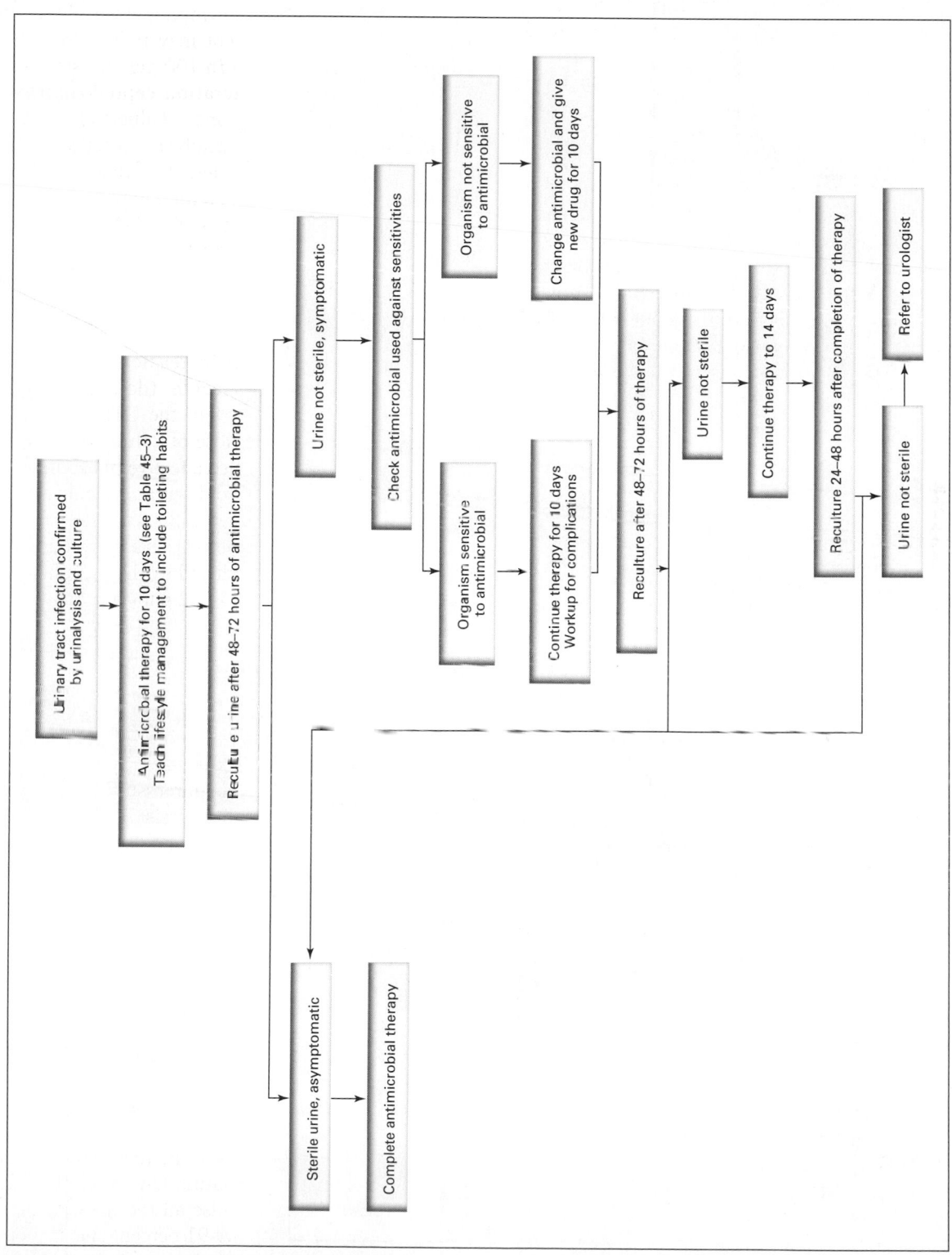

Figure 45–2. Treatment protocol: Urinary tract infections in children.

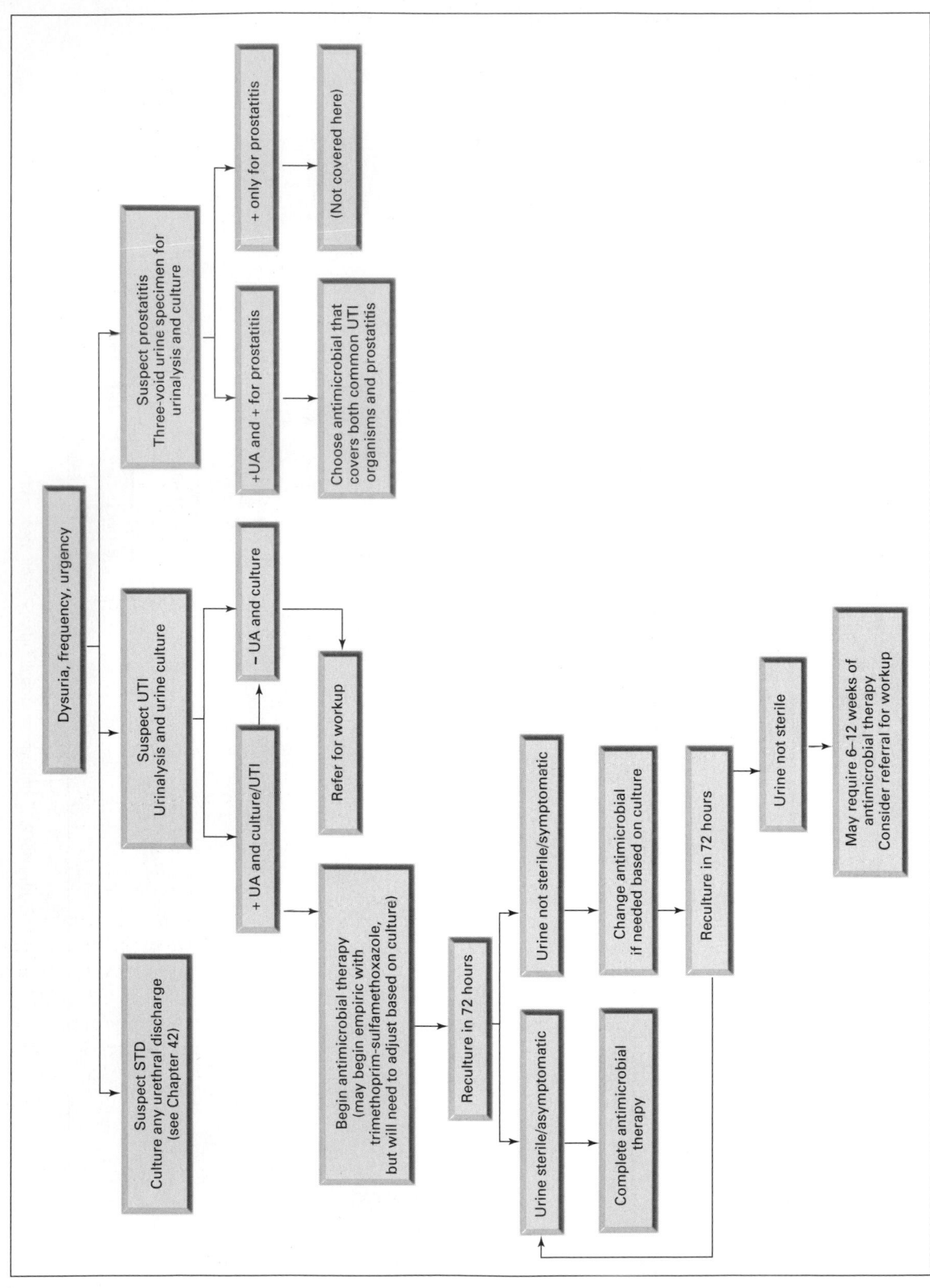

Figure 45–3. Treatment protocol: Urinary tract infections in men.

PATIENT EDUCATION

Urinary Tract Infections

Related to the Overall Treatment Plan or Disease Process

☐ Understanding the causes of UTIs and their prognoses
☐ Role of lifestyle modifications in preventing UTIs, especially ingestion of cranberry juice or cranberry extract; avoidance of diaphragms and spermicides, especially those containing nonoxynol-9; voiding 10 to 15 minutes after sexual intercourse to wash out the bacteria from the urethra that may have entered the bladder during intercourse; maintaining fluid intake of at least 2000 mL per day of noncaffeinated fluids; and not resisting the urge to void
☐ Importance of adherence to the treatment regimen
☐ Indications of relapse or complications that need to be reported
☐ Need for a follow-up visit only if patient remains symptomatic

Specific to the Drug Therapy

☐ Discussion of the reasons for taking the drug(s) and the anticipated action of the drug(s) on the disease process. The patient should be asymptomatic within 48 hours for simple, uncomplicated lower UTIs and within 7 days for upper UTIs. Urinary analgesics should relieve symptoms within 24 hours.
☐ Doses and schedules for taking the drug and the length of time the drug will need to be taken.
☐ Possible adverse reactions and what to do when they occur. For patients given phenazopyridine, warn them that the drug turns the urine bright orange and that this is not an indication of hematuria.

Additional patient education specific to antimicrobials is provided in Chapter 22.

All children age 5 years and under need referral to a pediatric urologist for workup. Older children with simple, uncomplicated UTI require urine culture for diagnosis of the offending organism, repeat cultures throughout their therapy, and a culture after completion of therapy. Failure to produce sterile urine after 14 days of therapy suggests referral.

Pregnant patients with a positive urine culture should have a follow-up urine culture every 2 weeks until delivery and at their postpartum evaluation to validate sterile urine. Reinfections require prophylactic **antimicrobial** therapy. For upper UTIs, an initial telephone assessment of the patient's symptoms and response to therapy is important within 24 hours. A second assessment with an office visit should occur in 2 to 3 days. If symptoms do not resolve or if they worsen, hospitalization may be required. A urine culture should be done 1 to 2 weeks after therapy in pregnant patients, children, patients who remain symptomatic, and those for whom suppression therapy is being considered. Follow-up cultures are optional for all other patients (Leiner, 1995).

Outcome Evaluation

Neonates, infants, and children under age 5 years who present with clinical and laboratory evidence of UTI should be referred to a pediatric urologist. The cause is likely to be an anatomic obstructive problem, especially in boys. Although adults often do not have long-term complications from UTIs, 10 percent of children with reflux nephropathy go on to develop hypertension with bilateral scarring of the kidney within 10 years. Risk for development of end-stage renal disease after UTI is rare in adults but is 1:500 for children who later develop hypertension. Recurrent UTI in girls leads to increased risk for new infection in pregnancy (Mowry, 1997).

Certain criteria in adults also suggest the need for an aggressive workup that requires referral to a urologist. Gross hematuria, persistent microscopic hematuria between episodes of infection, symptoms of obstruction, a clinical impression of persistent rather than recurrent UTI, or infection with urea-splitting bacteria, such as *Proteus mirabilis,* which are associated with staghorn calculi, suggests referral (Leiner, 1995). Graber and Martinez-Bianchi

Urinary Tract Infections

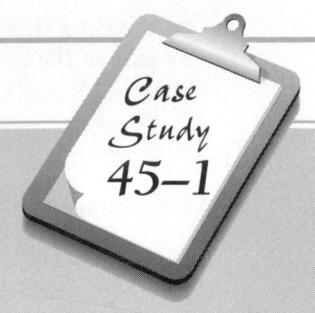

Complaint

"It hurts when I urinate."

History

Janice is a 26-year-old married woman who presents at the clinic with symptoms of dysuria, frequency, and urgency. Further history yields 2 days of these symptoms but no fever, chills, or flank pain. She describes a burning discomfort during and immediately following urination and feeling the need to void every half-hour. There is no vaginal discharge, itching, or odor. Janice uses a diaphragm and spermicide for birth control. She requests "a urine culture and some sulfa pills." When asked to explain, she says she has had many "bladder infections" over the last 3 years and "sulfa pills usually work." She was evaluated approximately 5 years ago with an intravenous pyelography and cystogram, and "nothing was wrong."

Assessment

A midstream urine specimen is collected for urinalysis and culture. A urine dipstick reveals 2+ pyuria, 1+ hematuria, and trace nitrates. Her pregnancy test is negative. She exhibits no costovertebral angle or abdominal tenderness. Her vital signs are within normal limits.

Janice looks essentially well. There are no symptoms suggestive of pyelonephritis or vaginal disorders.

Initial Management Plan

Janice is diagnosed with simple, uncomplicated lower UTI. Her initial management plan is as follows:

1. Trimethoprim-sulfamethoxazole double-strength 1 tablet bid for 3 days. The most likely cause of UTI in females is *Escherichia coli*, and it is susceptible to this drug with an incidence of resistance of only 11 percent. She is not pregnant so this is a safe drug.
2. To correct her discomfort and burning with urination, phenazopyridine 200 mg bid is also prescribed.
3. Urine culture is ordered. Although urine cultures are not usually required for females with acute UTI, she states that she has had "many" infections over the last 3 years so further evaluation may be needed.
4. Lifestyle management is discussed. She has been

married for only 4 years and noted that the frequent UTIs began since her marriage. Consideration will be given to postcoital suppression therapy if she continues to have these infections.

Two days later, Janice is completely asymptomatic. Her urine culture has grown 50,000 *E.coli* susceptible to trimethoprim-sulfamethoxazole. A post-treatment urinalysis is sterile.

Follow-up Visit

Six weeks later, Janice returns to the clinic with similar symptoms and is again diagnosed with acute UTI. She is again treated with trimethoprim-sulfamethoxazole, and her symptoms resolve within 24 hours, but she is not happy about the number of infections she is experiencing. She has been adherent to the suggestions about voiding after intercourse and has changed her birth control method to oral contraceptives. Her fluid intake is at least 2 quarts per day of noncaffeinated fluids, and these fluids include 4 oz cranberry juice.

Modifications to Management Plan

Suppression therapy is decided upon:

1. Because it is effective in curing her UTIs, trimethoprim-sulfamethoxazole 1 single-strength tablet at bedtime is prescribed. An alternative dosing schedule might be 1 double-strength tablet after intercourse, but she is afraid she might forget and chooses the once-daily dosing instead.
2. Continue the lifestyle management.

Continuing Care

For the next 6 months, Janice remains symptom-free. A urinalysis reveals sterile urine. The prophylactic antimicrobial is discontinued. Many women with recurrent UTI associated with intercourse require prophylactic drug therapy intermittently. To keep costs down and reduce the risk for the development of resistance, this regimen was chosen for Janice. She has not had a UTI for a full year since the prophylactic antimicrobial was discontinued.

(1999) add to these criteria any symptomatic pregnant patients and patients who have a high fever or appear dehydrated or septic. These patients may require hospitalization for intravenous (IV) therapy.

If patients remain symptomatic after 3 days of therapy for a simple, uncomplicated lower UTI or after completion of 10 to 14 days of therapy for an upper UTI, a culture should be done to determine the causative organism, and a different **antimicrobial** may be needed.

Patient Education

Patient education should include a discussion of information related to the overall treatment plan as well as

that specific to the drug therapy, reasons for taking the drug, drugs as part of the total treatment regimen, and adherence issues.

REFERENCES

Avorn, J., Monane, M., Gurwitz, J., Glynn, R., Choodnovsky, I., & Lipitz, L. (1994). Reduction of bacteriuria and pyuria after ingestion of cranberry juice. *Journal of the American Medical Association, 271,* 751–754.

Barker, L. R., Burton, J., & Zieve, P. (1995). *Principles of ambulatory medicine* (4th ed.). Baltimore: Williams & Wilkins.

Burns, C., Barber, N., Brady, M., & Dunn, A. (1996). *Pediatric primary care: A handbook for nurse practitioners.* Philadelphia: Saunders.

Gilbert, D., Moellering, R., & Sande, M. (1998). *The Sanford guide to antimicrobial therapy* (28th ed.). Vienna, VA: Antimicrobial Therapy, Inc.

Goroll, A., May, L., & Mulley, A. (1995). *Primary care medicine* (3rd ed.). Philadelphia: Lippincott.

Graber, M., & Martinez-Bianchi, V. (1999). Genitourinary and renal disease: Urinary tract infections. In *University of Iowa family practice handbook* (3rd ed.). Website: *http://www.vh.org/providers/clinref/fphandbook/chapter11/03-11.html.*

Hickey, S., & Nelson, J. (1997). Mechanisms of antibacterial resistance. *Advances in Pediatrics, 44,* 1–41.

Leiner, S. (1995). Recurrent urinary tract infections in otherwise healthy adult women. *Nurse Practitioner, 20*(2), 48–56.

Mowry, J. (1997). Urinary tract infections. Presentation at the 20th annual educational conference, Nurse Practitioner Oregon—Oregon Nurses Association, Bend, OR.

Murdock, A., & Munroe, W. (1999). Prevention and OTC options for urinary tract infections. *Drug facts and comparisons news,* April 1999, 26–29.

Onrust, S., Lamb, H., & Barman Balfour, J. (1998). Ofloxacin: A reappraisal of its use in the management of genitourinary tract infections. *Drugs, 56*(5), 895–928.

Preston, S., Abdel-Rahman, S., & Nahata, M. (1998). Empiric treatment of uncomplicated urinary tract infections. *Annals of Pharmacotherapy, 32,* 1231–1233.

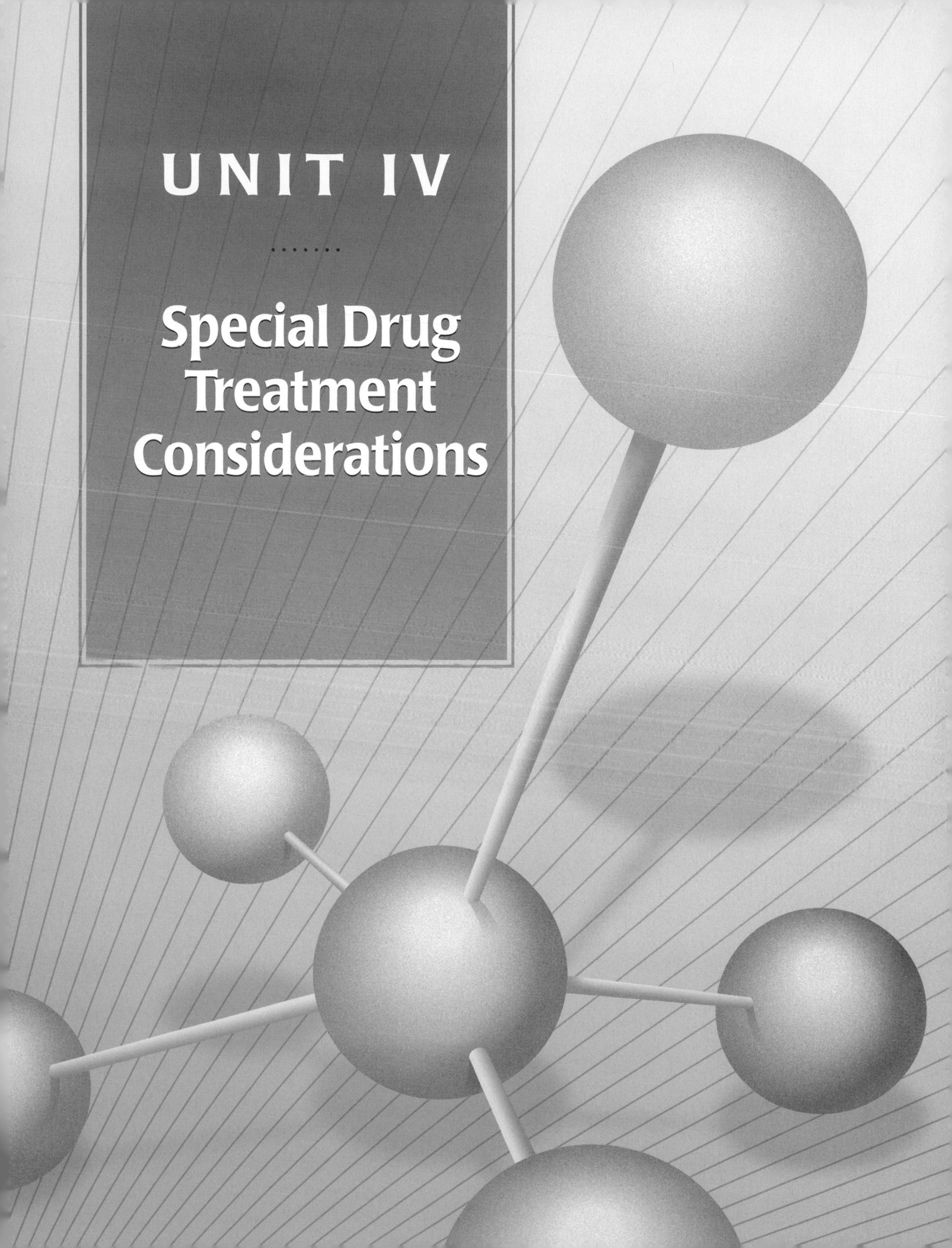

UNIT IV

·······

Special Drug Treatment Considerations

CHAPTER 46

......

Women as Patients

CHAPTER OUTLINE

omen as adult patients have different needs from male patients, besides the obvious differences in physiology and anatomy. Both male and female patients experience growth and development similarly until puberty, when estrogen and progesterone prepare women for fertility and reproduction. Roughly 2 years later, men come under the influence of androgens, triggering a cascade of changes such as increased height, weight, and muscle mass and the genital changes that signal the ability to reproduce. Women are born with all their gamete cells vulnerable to endogenous and environmental factors from birth. Men produce sperm throughout their adult lives until levels of testosterone start to wane, usually in their sixth or seventh decade.

Prescribing for women in their childbearing years requires knowledge of the possibility of pregnancy in order to avoid exposing the developing fetus to potential teratogens. Even women who use birth control can contract lifelong viral infections or silent bacterial infections that scar delicate fallopian tubes, rendering them infertile. Early sexual activity may expose them to infections and pregnancy when their bodies and emotions are not yet mature. Teenage pregnancy is associated with inconsistent prenatal care, smaller babies, and preterm labor.

These babies are then at high risk for development disorders and other medical conditions associated with low birth weight.

Breastfeeding is another time when prescribing for women requires special care and knowledge. (For information on pharmacokinetics about breastfeeding to assist the practitioner in making safe decisions about prescribing, see Chapter 49. Areas discussed there include maternal pharmacokinetics, infant suckling pattern, infant pharmacokinetics, variable infant susceptibility to drugs, and milk-to-plasma ratios.)

Caring for women from different cultures requires knowledge of their beliefs about health care and the treatments they will accept. Translation alone may not be the issue. They may not understand explanations if they lack basic education in their own country.

During the 1980s abuse of children and women was recognized as a significant public health problem. Prior to that time, it was handled in whispers and behind closed doors with therapists. Public outrage has brought this subject to television, movies, and literature. Generations of abuse proliferated until the abused learned that they could stop the behavior in their generation. Although boys have also been abused, most abuse has been against girls and women. Domestic violence often begins during the first pregnancy. Elder abuse can happen to men as well, but women have longer life expectancies and therefore more older women are abused and neglected. Nurse practitioners need nonpharmacological skills to identify and deal with potential problems. Many women have been helped by the newer **antidepressants.** A large percentage of abused and formerly abused women struggle with depression and chemical dependency. "Escape from reality" and "numb the pain" are comments that come out during group therapy in drug treatment programs.

Women of the 1990s are much more fortunate than their predecessors in that studies are currently being done with women as research subjects. Early on, reasons postulated for "male-only" trials related to fear of giving drugs to subjects who may become pregnant and the possibility of teratogenic effects. Later, these practices were attributed to the complexity of hormonal and menstrual cycles. More recently, the effects of hysterectomy, with or without oophorectomy, menopause, use of **hormone replacement therapy (HRT),** and **oral contraceptives** were thought to be confounding variables (Rosenfeld, 1997). Women are still prescribed many **antihypertensive** and **cardiovascular drugs** that had safety and efficacy trials performed with only men.

Pharmacokinetics and Pharmacodynamics in Women

There are gender differences in the pharmacokinetics between men and women besides the obvious ones of size and percentage of body fat. Women have longer gastric emptying times and secrete less total gastric acid, and both factors influence the absorption and bioavailability of some drugs (Rosenfeld, 1997). The volume of distribution of drugs is dramatically altered by body composition. **Tricyclic antidepressants** take longer to reach a steady state in women because of the drug's lipophilic distribution. As a result, women experience more adverse reactions after the drug saturates all the sites in adipose tissues and more active drug remains in the bloodstream.

Metabolism and excretion of drugs by the liver and kidney depend on weight, body surface area, age, and gender. Renal function in men is greater than in women. In addition, the liver enzyme system and cytochrome P-450 affect and are affected by drugs women take. **Oral contraceptives** and **HRT** increase hepatic glucuronidation. If the second drug prescribed has active metabolites, like **fluoxetine,** the reaction increases the levels instead of clearing the drug, with the potential for toxicity. Women also metabolize **alcohol** more slowly than men of the same size. The ethanol is absorbed into the bloodstream without being partially metabolized by the gastric tissue. Women's liver tissues are also more susceptible to cirrhosis than men's.

The effects of **cardiac** and **antihypertensive** drugs on women are different from their effects on men. Women between 15 and 50 have longer QT intervals, making them more vulnerable to cardiac arrhythmias. **Macrolide antibiotics** cause a woman's heart to repolarize more slowly. The incidence of life-threatening ventricular arrhythmias is twice as common in women who are taking **erythromycin** (Drici et al., 1998). Another example is **lithium** and its increased bioavailability because of renal excretion. The dosing literature does not indicate that levels of this drug could be less than 63 percent as high in women as a result of reduced clearance. Drug levels early in therapy must prevent toxicity in medications with narrow margins of safety, such as **lithium, digoxin, and theophylline.**

Factors That Influence Medication Administration

Women receive more prescriptive drugs than men the same age. Women are more apt to take medications for their skin, muscles, urinary tract, ophthalmologic and otologic problems, fatigue, extremity pain, weight, hypertension, and emotional complaints. Depression and connective tissue diseases are much more common in women. Because most of the research has been performed on male subjects, the clinician needs to anticipate a higher potential for toxicity and adverse reaction in women. Monitoring drug levels in medications that have a narrow margin of safety is recommended (Rosenfeld, 1997).

Differences between men and women start early in their lives. A slower intestinal absorption in women, independent of hormones and menstrual cycle, can be demonstrated by higher rates of iron absorption in prepubertal women than in prepubertal men (Fletcher, Acosta, & Strykowski, 1994). Because of the anatomic differences of a short urethra in girls, contamination with coliform bacteria is easier, resulting in more frequent urinary tract infections. (See Chapter 49 for a discussion of differences in children in relation to pharmacokinetics and their age-related development.)

Puberty

Puberty heralds great physiological change in both girls and boys. Female athletes, as demonstrated with ballet dancers, can prevent menarche by the training effect of reduced body fat. Other factors can cause delayed menarche such as genetic predisposition, dieting behavior, quantity and quality of diet, stress, and the amount of the athletic training that preceded menarche. Dancers who experienced menarche between ages 12 and 14 developed normal bone densities and reduced incidence of stress fractures and scoliosis (Graber, Brooks-Gunn, & Warren, 1999). Calcium intake can help to build bone mass and ease some of the luteal-phase premenstrual symptoms such as mood swings, depression, irritability, crying spells, headaches, and food cravings. Athletes, as well as teens with eating disorders such as anorexia nervosa, can become amenorrheic, resulting in the loss of bone mass. If this process is not quickly corrected, osteoporosis is possible. Hormonal therapy is not successful with this type of secondary hypogonadism. In a similar way, the wasting phase of human immunodeficiency virus (HIV) disease causes hypogonadism. Women lose more body fat than men with the same level of immune compromise in HIV disease (Kotler et al., 1999).

Iron-deficiency anemia is common in teenage girls and younger women, who may have quite heavy menstruation. Girls going through puberty may also be avoiding red meat, the best source of iron, in favor of lower-calorie salads and vegetables. Although green, leafy vegetables contain iron, the plant sources are not as fully absorbed. Some teenage girls and young women need to take an iron supplement at least 1 week each month to replenish iron loss during menstruation.

Pregnancy

Women change anatomically and physiologically with each week of gestation. Drug absorption through the lungs, skin, and mucous membranes is increased because of the 40 percent increase in cardiac output. Plasma volume is 50 percent higher by the third trimester; most of the volume is in the products of conception. **Anticonvulsants** are potentially teratogenic, but the risk of seizure is much more dangerous to the mother and the fetus. Phenytoin clearance is increased during the second and third trimesters, whereas theophylline levels are raised because of decreased clearance (Schoonover & Litell, 1998).

Iron-deficiency anemia is common (30 to 50 percent) because of the increased demands of a larger blood supply and the developing fetus. This physiological anemia is commonly treated with **ferrous sulfate.** This preparation is best given with **vitamin C** for increased absorption. There is less gastrointestinal irritation when it is given after meals. Most prenatal vitamins contain the required 60 to 120 mg of **iron.** Because not all women need large quantities of iron, monitoring hemoglobin and hematocrit is necessary.

Pregnancy may be a productive time to intervene in modifying a risky lifestyle. For example, illicit drug use may be corrected or reduced when the patient is motivated by anticipation of the birth of her child. Although legal, **caffeine, nicotine,** and **alcohol** are also harmful to the developing fetus. **Caffeine** is in coffee, teas, colas and some other sodas, chocolate, and some over-the-counter (OTC) pain relievers. **Caffeine** can cause mood swings and fetal or newborn cardiac arrhythmias. **Nicotine** causes vasoconstriction and has been associated with decreased uteroplacental blood flow, decreased birth weight, prematurity, abortion, and abruptio placentae. **Alcohol** causes decreased folic acid and thiamine absorption. The fetus is lower in birth weight and may have the mental retardation associated with the fetal alcohol syndrome (Kastrup, 1998).

Alternative therapies, such as the use of medicinal herbs, are currently being evaluated with randomized methodologies to evaluate their efficacy, but pregnant women should be cautioned about use of herbs that may be harmful to the fetus. Table 46–1 presents a listing of selected herbs that are contraindicated during pregnancy.

Menopause

The emphasis at this time of a woman's life is prevention of the diseases of older age. Although genetics play an important role in the diseases that afflict us at midlife, many preventive measures can be taught as well as prescribed. Primary prevention studies demonstrate that diets high in complex carbohydrates, high in fiber and protein, and low in animal fat are best. The "pyramid" type of diet recommended by national nutrition guidelines can lead to a lower body mass index (BMI). The recommended level of body mass is 26 percent or less. Those greater than 30 percent are associated with morbidity and shortened life expectancy. Exercise is another nonpharmacological prevention. Longitudinal studies demonstrate that 3 hours of exercise each week is associated with improved health.

Table 46–1. Herbs Contraindicated during Pregnancy

Strictly contraindicated	capsella bursa-pastoris, gossypium herbaceum
Contraindicated (but have been used during the last trimester in preparation for delivery)	aletris farinosa, caulopyllum thalictrodies, cimicifuga racemosa, mentha pulegium, sassafras albidum
Contraindicated	achillea millefolium, acorus calamus, agave americana, allium sativa, allium cepa, aloe barbadensis, anemone pulsatilla, angelica archangelica, angelica sylvestris, anthemis nobilis, apium graveolens, arctium lappa, areca catechu, arnica montana, artemesia absinthinium, artemesia vulgaris, berberis vulgaris, beta vulgaris, brayera anthelmintica, caffea arabica, calendula officinalis, capsicum frutescens, carica papaya, cephalis ipechacuanha, chelidonium majus, chenopodium ambrosodies, cichorum intybus, cinchona legederiana, cinnamomum camphora, cinnamomum cassia, cinnamomum zeylancium, citrullus colocynthis, citrus sp., claviceps purpurea, colchicim autumnale, commiphora myrrha, crocus sativa, croton tiglium, cytisus scoparius, daucus carota, dryopteris filix-mas, ephedra vulgaris, erythroxylon coca, ferula asafoetida, foeniculum vulgaris, gelsemium sempervirens, glycyrrhiza glabra, hedoma pulegioides, helleborous niger, hibiscus rosa-sinensis, hydrastis canadensis, hydrocotyle asiatica, hypericum perforatum, hyssopus officinalis, jateorhiza palmata, juniperis communis, lavandula officinalis, ledum palustre, leonurus cardciaca, linum usitatissimum, marrubium vulgare, matricaria chamomile, medicago sativa, mentha piperita, myristica fragrans, nasturtium officinale, nepeta cataria, nicotiana tobacum, origanum vulgare, oxalis acetosella, paeonia officinalis, papaver somniferum, passilora incarnata, petroselinum sativa, phytolacca americana, pilocarpus jaborandi, pinus palustris, piper nigrum, plantago sp., podophyllum peltatum, polygala senega, polygonum aviculare, prunus persica, prunus virginiana, prunus serotina, punica granatum, ranunculus sp., rauwolfia serpentina, rheum sp., ricinis communis, rosmarinus officinalis, ruta graveolens, salvia officinalis, sanguinaria canadensis, santalum album, senecio vulgaris, silybim marianum, strophanthus sp., strychonos nux-vomica, tanacetum parthenium, tanacetum vulgare, thuja occidentalis, thymus serpyllum, toxicodendron radicans, trigonella foenumgraecum, turnera sp., tussilago farfara, urtica dioica, veratrum sp., veronicastrum virginicum, vinca rosea, viscum album, zingiber officinale

Adapted from Brinker, B. F. (1996). *The Toxicology of Botanical Medicines.* Sandy, OR: Eclectic Medical Publishing.

The exercise does not have to be aerobic, just consistent. Walking, yard work, bicycling, and swimming are all good forms of exercise. Brisk walking has been the recommended activity by most health care providers.

Immunizations for diphtheria-tetanus need to be updated every 10 years.

Calcium supplementation is necessary during peak growth periods, pregnancy, lactation, and postmenopause. The requirements are 1500 mg per day and must be given with adequate **vitamin D,** 400 IU.

After menopause, the lipid profile of women changes, and they are no longer protected from heart disease. Women "catch up" to men and may soon experience "silent" coronary artery disease, which becomes their greatest risk factor for dying early. Fewer women than men survive their first heart attack. By age 55, 233,000 women have died from heart disease, 65,000 from complications related to hip fracture, and 45,000 from breast cancer.

Changes that we see in women at menopause are the results of aging that men also share. These changes include thinning and graying of the hair, weight gain, drying skin, vision changes associated with presbyopia, and increased healing time for musculoskeletal injuries.

Other changes, including atrophy of the genitourinary tract affecting the vagina and urinary system, are the result of the cessation of ovarian function. Loss of the ureterovesicular angle promotes urine leakage and increased residual volumes. Breast tissue loses the denser glandular tissue to fatty replacement.

Older Age

Women are living as long after menopause as before. If a woman reaches age 50 and is healthy, she has a good chance to live to age 100. Cardiovascular disease, including stroke, causes the greatest morbidity and mortality for the aging woman (Begley, 1999). Aging women experience more frequent autoimmune disease, which manifests itself in joint and soft tissue pain and deformity. Hip fractures cause the next greatest mortality, and yet more women worry more that the therapies cause breast cancer. Lung and colon cancers in women have increased in this century, and both men and women need to start screening procedures such as sigmoidoscopy and barium enema at age 50. Smoking by women has also increased during the post–World War II years, which is hypothesized as the reason for their increased lung cancer rates.

Aspirin has been shown to prevent myocardial infarction in both men and women, but after age 65, women have more risk of intracranial bleeding, reflecting higher blood levels of this **anticoagulant**. A primary prevention study of **aspirin** and **vitamin E** is currently in process from the Brigham and Women's Study in Boston. This randomized, double-blind study, including more than 160,000 middle-aged health professionals, has been extended to the year 2002. Some of the questions being asked are: What is the impact of **aspirin** and **vitamin E** on the prevention of cancer, heart disease, and Alzheimer's disease? Can we prevent some of these diseases with changes in lifestyle? When do we need to start exercise? How much exercise is helpful for strong bones, and how much is too much? It is already known that cigarette smoking, obesity, and a sedentary lifestyle are modifiable behaviors that are associated with shortened life expectancy.

Factors That Influence Positive Outcomes

Duration of Medication Therapy

Most patients can remember to take medications for a few days, especially if they are feeling ill, but drugs that must be taken daily and for many years are subject to poor compliance. Women may find themselves responsible for taking **birth control pills (BCPs)** for 10 to 40 years. Compliance with contraception use (as measured by annual continuation rates) are **spermicides**, 40 percent; diaphragm, 56 percent; **oral contraceptive**, 71 percent; **Depo-Provera**, 70 percent; and **Norplant** implants, 88 percent (Hatcher et al., 1998).

Remembering to take medications with other routine activities of daily living once or twice a day helps with compliance. Women are frequently the primary caregivers of children; that fact, plus remembering their own medications, can complicate medication administration and decrease compliance.

Number of Medications

The complexity of the regimen is inversely proportional to compliance. If several medications are necessary, plan a once-daily dosing schedule. Many prescription drugs can be administered once daily, before or after breakfast, and this simplicity increases the likelihood of compliance.

Fear That Medications Cause Disease

Women hear about medications such as hormones causing cancer or other disease from the media (e.g., television, newspapers) and from friends and relatives. Often the source is not specific enough to determine if the hormone is from BCPs or from postmenopausal **hormone** or **estrogen replacement therapy.** Many of the cancer studies reported are based on data from the 1960s, when much higher levels of potent **estrogen** were used in **BCP** formulations. Risk of breast cancer is very prevalent in our country. One in nine women will be diagnosed in her lifetime if she lives to be age 85. Woman have a hard time deciding to use **hormonal therapies** because they cannot calculate their own absolute risk. What they hear in the media are relative risks, which refer to populations of women in certain age brackets.

Safety of Medications While Breastfeeding

The benefits to infants, especially in the first year of life, conferred by breastfeeding are well described in the literature. Points to be considered are the acidity of breast milk in relation to the pH of plasma, the protein-binding effects of the drug prescribed, the liposolubility of the drug prescribed, and the molecular weight of the drug prescribed. Just think of the lactating woman as you would the pregnant woman. (See Chapter 47 for more information.)

Cost

The cost of the prescription always needs to be considered in the treatment plan. Even women who have prescription benefits through their health insurance may have high copay for nongeneric drugs. Many companies still do not pay for contraception. Samples can defray medication expenses. Many drug companies have a program of helping with 1 or 2 months of therapy for

Clinical Pearl

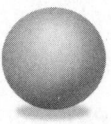

··

PRESCRIBING DURING BREASTFEEDING

When prescribing for a breastfeeding woman, ask yourself: IS this drug safe for infants?

··

Clinical Pearl

MOTHERS AND SMOKING

Mothers who smoke should be told that babies of mothers who smoked in the home had the same level of drug (**nicotine**) excreted in their urine as those babies with mothers who always smoked outside.

patients in need, especially for chronic diseases such as hypertension, diabetes, and asthma.

Family Preferences

Once women become adults or parents, the provider may assume that medications will be used as directed. However, many women talk with relatives, friends, and others about their problems and the drugs prescribed. It is important to ask your patient what her spouse or significant other thinks about the therapy for her problem. Frequently, the spouse accompanies the patient to the office visit, and then a discussion about the drug, adverse reactions, expected outcomes, and cost may ensue. Parents must be involved in prescribing medications for minors and need to know specific instructions for the drug's use and follow-up.

Ethnic, Cultural, and Religious Differences

Women from other cultures commonly seek health care more often than men in their culture; however, many other cultures are patriarchies. For example, the man makes the decisions about birth control, whether the woman works outside the home, and how much money she gets to run the household. The woman may not have a choice if she does not want to have sexual relations. These patients can present with multiple visits filled with somatic complaints and genital pain.

Religion can also bring conflict to the prescribing of medications. If the belief system does not support the practice the provider is prescribing, then compliance may be a problem. For example, if the woman is Roman Catholic and the provider suggests **BCPs** for treatment of acne, there may be difficulties.

Common Problems That Require Medications

Common problems in women that require medications include urinary tract infection and urinary incontinence, sexually transmitted diseases and vaginitis, birth control, menopause, osteoporosis, depression, and hypothyroidism. Each of these problems is discussed in the appropriate chapter; however, concerns and considerations specific to women are presented here.

Some diseases are gender-specific, for example, those diseases related to women's reproductive organs. Men develop urinary problems when their prostate gland becomes hypertrophied, but women experience urinary tract difficulties across their lifespan. The shorter urethra and the changes in pelvic support after vaginal childbirth contribute to urinary disease. Although men have used the latex condom for birth control and disease prevention, most **contraceptive** medications have been prescribed for women. Men may develop osteoporosis late in their seventh and eighth decades as their hormone levels wane, but women experience it dramatically within 2 to 5 years after menopause. Women live 20 to 40 years at risk from osteoporosis, and they start out with less dense bones in childhood. Women experience autoimmune diseases, such as rheumatoid arthritis, multiple sclerosis, and systemic lupus erythematosus, with greater frequency than men. Depression is another common disorder that affects women disproportionately. Whether the cause is hormonally driven, culturally nurtured, or genetically induced, mood changes account for many days of work loss and many dollars in health care cost for therapy and drug management. Hypothyroidism is another disease that develops more commonly in women. Whenever menstrual dysfunction occurs, this disease is at the top of the differential diagnosis list.

Clinical Pearl

PRESCRIBING FOR ADOLESCENTS

Become knowledgeable about the laws in your state regarding treatment of sexually transmitted diseases, contraception, and medical record confidentiality in minor patients.

Clinical Pearl

PRESCRIBING IN A DIVERSE CULTURE

Be aware of the common ethnic groups in your patient population. Get to know the cultures. Frequently, community programs that teach cultural awareness and some simple ethnic phrases are available for health care personnel. Bookstores carry pocket-sized books to facilitate a simple medical interview in many different languages.

Urinary Tract Infection and Urinary Incontinence

Lower urinary tract infection is caused by contamination by the perineal bacteria. Sometimes the trauma of sexual relations can infect the distal urethra. Another method of infection is instrumentation of the urinary tract by catheterization or endoscopy. The commonest urinary pathogens are *Escherichia coli, Staphylococcus aureus,* and group B streptococci. The usual treatment is **trimethoprim-sulfamethoxazole (Septra)** twice a day for 3 to 10 days. This drug is not safe during the first or last trimester of pregnancy. **Nitrofurantoin** (e.g., **Macrobid**) twice a day for 3 to 10 days, a **cephalosporin** (safe for pregnancy), and the **fluoroquinolones** (e.g., **Cipro**) 250 mg to 750 mg twice a day for 3 to 10 days (not to be used in pregnancy or in patients under age 18) may also be used.

Upper urinary tract infections may ascend from the untreated urinary bladder. They can also be caused by anatomic deformities of the ureters. Sometimes a kidney stone is a nidus of infection. The pathogens are similar, but the treatment may require hospitalization if the patient is toxic. When patients complain about pain with urination, diagnostic tests need to rule out sexually transmitted disease. Frequently, the patient is treated without cultures unless the problem becomes chronic (more than three episodes in 1 year). Patient education includes emphasis on hygiene, drinking enough water to produce dilute urine, and clothing that allows circulation of air. Some women need prophylactic treatment with a bolus of a **sulfa** preparation after intercourse. Chronic maintenance with **antibiotics** is not recommended because of the increasingly serious problem of drug-resistant microorganisms.

Both the loss of ovarian hormones and the anatomic changes due to aging and loss of muscular support affect the urinary system. Successful treatment of urinary incontinence often requires surgical as well as drug therapy.

Sexually Transmitted Disease and Vaginitis

Most sexually transmitted diseases are passed during genital contact with an infected partner. Some infections such as HIV infection have 6-week to 10-year latency so that the infecting partner may be hard to identify. The treatment guidelines from the Centers for Disease Control and Prevention (CDC) are presented in Chapter 42.

Vaginitis is a condition that crosses the lifespan of women. In the young girl, coliform bacteria from the intestinal tract can inflame the immature vaginal tissues. Cultures are necessary to rule out sexual abuse. The teenage girl may notice the leukorrhea characteristic of the cyclic hormonal changes of puberty. If sexually active, the girl needs to be screened for all pathogens, as well as have a Pap smear performed. The pregnant woman has vulnerability to all pathogens, several of which may lead to preterm labor. Those infections are bacterial vaginosis, chlamydia, gonorrhea, and syphilis. The latter two infections can cause congenital infections in the fetus. The menopausal woman returns to a vulnerable state because thinner vaginal epithelium and higher-pH secretions make her susceptible to infections. Atrophic vaginitis can lead to painful syndromes that make sexual relations intolerable. Inflammatory conditions of the vulva are more common in middle-aged and older women. Treatment is detailed in Chapter 12.

Birth Control (Contraception)

The **oral contraceptive (BCP)** brought a new freedom to women. Along with this freedom came the need for protection from pelvic infections. The "pill" has been available since the mid-1960s. Since then, the potency has been altered to provide the safest, most effective birth control product for women of all ages. **Oral contraceptives** have also been used as therapy for amenorrhea, menometrorrhagia, dysmenorrhea, polycystic ovary syndrome, and acne. It is safest in women of any age who do not smoke and in women who do not have thromboembolic tendencies or liver disease.

Menopause

Menopause is a physiological change in women that occurs between ages 42 to 56, with the mean being age

Table 46–2. Alternative Therapies for Symptoms of Menopause

Symptom	Alternative Therapy and Its Effects
Hot flashes	• **Vitamin E 400 bid:** affects blood vessel walls; some women have blood pressure changes; monitor patients with hypertension • **Soy 2 oz:** contains 45 mg phytoestrogens (genistein); may protect from cancer • **Evening primrose 3 oz:** eliminates breast tenderness; stabilizes hormone fluctuations • **Remifemin (black cohost) 1 tab bid:** suppresses LH but not FSH; progesterone precursor; reduces hot flashes; used in Germany • **Dong quai:** estrogen precursor
Lack of (or reduced) sex drive	• **Talking with the patient, therapy:** ensure that spousal issues are not a hidden factor; if the intimate relationship is not good, menopause may not be the primary problem • **Use of alternative therapies listed for weight fluctuation:** weight gain may hinder self-image; increases energy after loss of even 5–10 lb • **Use of alternative therapies listed for vaginal dryness or soreness:** reduces vaginal dryness and pain; allows for anticipation of positive sensations
Mood changes (irritability, depression)	• **Vitamin B$_6$ (pyridoxine) 1.3 mg daily:** turns amino acids into serotonin, which affects mood • **Meditation, yoga, prayer:** stimulates immunity; enhances personal control
Sleep disturbances	• **Valerian root, chamomile:** aids relaxation • **Exercise:** stimulates serotonin after 40 minutes; affects mood • **Decreased intake or avoidance of stimulants (caffeine, nicotine, large protein-rich meals):** allows relaxation of nervous system
Stress incontinence (urinary)	• **Decreased intake of caffeine beverages and diuretics:** reduces irritated detrusor muscle; results in less urgency • **Kegel exercises:** strengthens pelvic floor muscles • **Treat/reduce constipation:** relieves pressure on urethra and bladder
Vaginal dryness or soreness	• **Reduce or avoid use of medications such as antihistamines, decongestants, anticholinergics, and diuretics:** improves tissue moisture • **Use of alternative therapies listed for hot flashes:** increases epithelial lining of vaginal tissues • **Use of water-soluble lubricants daily (e.g., Replens, Astroglide, Lubrin):** facilitates penetration; enhances foreplay (ensure that the patient knows areas to apply for maximum stimulation)
Weight fluctuations	• **Exercise 20–40 min, 3–4 times weekly:** reduces weight gain; stabilizes mood; strengthens muscles; improves balance; stimulates good bone metabolism

50. Several years of gradual decline or erratic levels of estrogen precede cessation of ovarian function. Some women barely notice vasomotor instability, whereas hot flashes and insomnia incapacitate others. Estrogen and progesterone may interact at more than 200 receptor sites, so exogenous treatment may affect women in many different ways. All women experience changes in their secondary sexual characteristics. Alternative therapies for symptoms of menopause are presented in Table 46–2. When women are postmenopausal and choose to use drug therapy, then absolute risks versus benefits for the individual should be assessed and discussed.

Osteoporosis

Osteoporosis is a generalized metabolic disease characterized by decreased bone mass as a result of an imbalance in the bone-remodeling process. Weakening of the bony matrix increases the risk of fractures, most commonly in the hip, spine, and wrist. Good nutrition with calcium and vitamin D and exercise are preventive measures. Avoidance of cigarette smoking and excessive **alcohol** and **caffeine** consumption are other lifestyle choices women can make. **Estrogen** therapy is the most effective prevention and treatment modality. Some women cannot or will not take **estrogen,** so they may be offered **raloxifene, alen-**

dronate, and **calcitonin.** Chapter 36 has further discussion of these therapies.

Depression

Depression is a mood disorder characterized by irritability, lethargy, appetite changes, decreased libido, sleep disturbances, and feeling of hopelessness. Severe depression can drive patients to suicide. The very young (teenagers) patient and the older patient (age 65 or older) are at the highest risk to commit suicide. Women experience hormone changes from puberty to menopause, but the most dramatic fluctuations are at puberty, postpartum, and the perimenopause period, which are also the most common times for depression. Genetics also plays a role in a woman's vulnerability to depression. Her past medical history may reflect a previous depressive episode. Life experiences at the time of menopause may also be an emotional trigger. Treatment usually includes a combination of pharmacological and nonpharmacological measures. Within the last 10 years, new classes of **antidepressants** have been developed that are safer for women of all ages with relatively low incidence of adverse reactions. See Chapter 27 for more information.

Hypothyroidism

Primary hypothyroidism is characterized by atrophy or destruction of the thyroid tissue due to an immune response. Primary disease occurs in 90 percent of hypothyroid patients. Transient hypothyroidism can follow pregnancy or significant illness. It usually lasts 6 months or less and requires only monitoring. Older women often are affected, but their symptoms tend to be subtle and may be missed. The patient may complain of fatigue, depression, dry skin, constipation, and shortness of breath. Younger women may present with abnormal menstrual patterns or infertility. Hypothyroidism is treated with T_4, which is synthesized as **levothyroxine.** See Chapter 39 for a more detailed discussion of all thyroid disorders.

REFERENCES

Allen-Barash, N., Wu, R., LaCroix, K., & Foster, V. (1997). Barriers to breast cancer screening in Washington State. Paper presented at the 1997 meeting of the Centers for Disease Control and Prevention, Atlanta.

August, P. (1998). Sex, hormones, and hypertension: What is and is not known. *Women's Health in Primary Care, 1*(10), 21–28.

Begley, S. (1999). Understanding perimenopause. *Newsweek* (Spring-Summer Special Edition), 31–34.

Cauley, J., Lucas, F., Kuller, L., Stone, K., Browner, W., & Cummings, S. (1999). Elevated serum estradiol and testosterone concentrations are associated with a high risk for breast cancer. *Annals of Internal Medicine, 130*(4), 270–277.

Charney, P., Walsh, J., & Nattinger, A. (1998). Update in women's health. *Annals of Internal Medicine, 129*(7), 551–558.

Drici, M., Knollmann, B., Wang, W., & Woosley, R. (1998). Cardiac actions of erythromycin: Influence of female sex. *Journal of the American Medical Association, 280*(20), 1774–1776.

Einarson, A., Phillips, E., Mawji, F., DíAlimonte, D., Schick, B., Addis, A., Mastroiacova, P., Massone, T., Matsui, D., & Koren, G. (1998). A prospective controlled multicentre study of clarithromycin in pregnancy. *American Journal of Perinatology, 15*(9), 523–525.

Eisen, A., & Weber, B. (1999). Prophylactic mastectomy: The price of fear. *New England Journal of Medicine, 340*(2), 137–138.

Fletcher, C. V., Acosta, E. P., & Strykowski, J. M. (1994). Gender differences in human pharmacokinetics and pharmacodynamics, *Journal of Adolescent Health, 15*(8), 619–622.

Graber, J., Brooks-Gunn, J., & Warren, M. (1999). The vulnerable transition: Puberty and the development of eating pathology and negative mood. *Women's Health Issues, 9*(2), 107–114.

Hatcher, R., Trussell, J., Stewart, F., Cates, W., Stewart, G., Guest, F., & Kowal, D. (1998). *Contraceptive technology* (17th ed.). New York: Ardent Media.

Hwang, J., & Morrell, M. (1998). Coping with epilepsy in women. *Women's Health in Primary Care, 1*(6), 520–527.

Kastrup, E. (Ed.). (1998). *Drug facts and comparisons.* St. Louis: Facts and Comparisons.

Kotler, D., Thea, D., Heo, M., Allison, D., Engelson, E., Wang, J., Pierson, R., Jr, St. Louis, M., & Keusch, G. (1999). Relative influences of sex, race, environment, and HIV infection on body composition in adults. *American Journal of Clinical Nutrition, 69*(9), 432–439.

Letourneau, E., Holmes, M., & Chasedunn-Roark, J. (1999). Gynecologic health consequences to victims of interpersonal violence. *Women's Health Issues, 9*(2), 115–120.

Letter to the Editor. (1998). Alcohol consumption and breast cancer. *Journal of the American Medical Association, 280*(13), 1138–1139.

Levine, S. (1998). The sexual consequences of perimenopause and menopause. *Women's Health in Primary Care, 1*(10), 509–514.

Marchiondo, K. (1998). A new look at urinary tract infection. *American Journal of Nursing, 98*(3), 34–39.

Morgenstern, I. (1998). Slower care for female stroke patients. *Neurology, 51*, 427–432.

Mosca, L., Manson, J., Sutherland, S., et al. for the American Heart Association Writing Group. (1997). Cardiovascular disease in women: A statement for healthcare professionals from the American Heart Association. *Circulation, 96*, 2468–2482.

Oss, M., Yennie, H., & Birch, S. (1998). Managed care approaches and models for treatment and management of depression: Specific issues for women. *Women's Health Issues, 8*(5), 283–292.

Paganini-Hill, A. (1998). Alzheimer's disease in women: Can estrogen play a preventive role? *Female Patient, 23*(3), 12–18.

Page, D., & Dupont, W. (1998). Benign breast diseases and premalignant breast disease. *Archives of Pathology and Laboratory Medicine, 122*(12), 1048–1050.

Pan, C., & Boal, J. (1999). Letter to the Editor: Hormone replacement therapy for secondary prevention of coronary heart disease. *Journal of the American Medical Association, 281*(9), 794–797.

Rajaram, S., & Rashidi, A. (1998). Minority women and breast cancer screening: The role of cultural explanatory models. *Preventive Medicine, 27*, 757–764.

Rosenfeld, J. (1997). Pharmacokinetics: The female factor. *Female Patient, 22*(5), 37–38, 40–41, 45–47.

Sarto, G. (1998). How race, ethnicity, and culture influence women's health. *Women's Health in Primary Care, 1*(10), 7–14.

Schoonover, L., & Litell, C. (1998). How pregnancy affects pharmacokinetics. *Female Patient, 23*(6), 11–15, 19–20.

Stowe, Z., & Newport, J. (1998). Depression in women: Recognition and treatment. *Women's Health in Primary Care, 1*(10), 29–39.

Teegarden, D., Lyle, R., McCabe, G., McCabe, L., Proulx, W., Michon, K., Knight, A., Johnston, C., & Weaver, C. (1998). Dietary calcium, protein, and phosphorus are related to bone mineral density and content in young women. *American Journal of Clinical Nutrition, 68,* 749–754.

Thys-Jacob, S., Starkey, P., Bernstein, D., & Tian, J. (1998). Calcium carbonate and the premenstrual syndrome: Effects on premenstrual and menstrual symptoms. *American Journal of Obstetrics and Gynecology, 179,* 444–452.

Woosley, R. (1998). Why women are at greater risk for torsades de pointes drug toxicity. *Women's Health in Primary Care, 1*(10), 15–20.

CHAPTER 47

·······

Pediatric Patients

CHAPTER OUTLINE

*P*ediatric patients present a special challenge to the primary care practitioner; they are constantly changing, both physiologically and developmentally. The practitioner who is making a treatment decision must consider the parent and the family situation, as well as the patient, in determining if the treatment will be appropriate. In addition, information on use of medications in children is limited. Only 20 percent of prescription drugs on the market have dosing recommendations for pediatric patients (Gilman & Gal, 1992). This chapter discusses these issues.

Pharmacokinetic and Pharmaco-dynamic Differences in Children

Pharmacokinetics

Drug absorption, metabolism, and excretion can vary throughout infancy and early childhood. Even at puberty, there are differences in drug clearance between girls and boys as drug clearance rates reach adult levels. As more is learned about the metabolic pathways in the adult liver, more knowledge will be gained about how to study the differences in children. Past disasters caused by lack of understanding about the physiology of newborn metabolism have led to caution regarding the use of medications in infants. Gray baby syndrome caused by inadequate glucuronidation of **chloramphenicol**, which led to dangerous drug accumulation, and **sulfonamide**-induced kernicterus (caused by displacement of bilirubin from plasma proteins by **sulfonamides**) are two such disasters that have been hard lessons in the use of medication in newborns. Careful pharmacokinetic studies in the newborn and careful therapeutic drug monitoring have improved our knowledge of neonatal pharmacology, yet care is essential when any new therapy is tried. (Gupta & Waldhauer, 1997).

Drug Absorption

Drug absorption can be affected in children more than in adults by two factors: (1) the blood flow at the site of administration (intramuscular [IM] or subcutaneous [SC] administration) and (2) gastrointestinal (GI) function. Neonates have more variability in the blood flow to the muscles, especially ill newborns, and poor blood flow can lead to delayed or variable absorption of medications. If perfusion suddenly improves, there can be a rapid absorption of the medication from the muscle, leading to possible toxic levels. Care should be taken when administering potentially toxic drugs such as **cardiac glycosides, aminoglycoside antibiotics,** and **anticonvulsants** IM to ill infants. GI function is variable in neonates. Gastric acid function begins soon after birth and gradually increases over several hours. In premature infants, gastric acid secretion occurs more slowly and takes up to 4 days to reach normal levels. Gastric emptying time is prolonged in the first day of life, and medications absorbed from the stomach may therefore have increased absorption. The neonate also has slow and irregular peristalsis, and medications absorbed primarily from the small intestine should be monitored for potential toxic levels. It is known that the neonate has decreased oral absorption of **acetaminophen, phenobarbital,** and **phenytoin,** whereas **ampicillin** and **penicillin G** have increased bioavailability when taken orally. Diarrhea, a common ailment in young children, lessens the extent of absorption from the intestine, causing decreased drug levels.

Metabolism

The pathways of drug clearance develop variably over the first year of life and may be influenced by medications that induce drug-metabolizing enzymes (such as **phenobarbital**). In adults, much has been learned about the cytochrome P-450 enzymes, and much is still unknown. The exact developmental pattern is not known for most of the P-450 isoenzymes. Recent studies recognize that the small intestine is a major site of drug metabolism because it contains enterocytes in the bowel mucosa, which have P-450 drug metabolism enzymes. This new information enhances our knowledge of drug metabolism, but there may be large interindividual variation in the capacity of the small bowel to metabolize drugs. Studies of CYP-450 1A2 using **caffeine** as the test substrate demonstrate limited metabolic clearance in the newborn, with significant maturation in the first year of life to levels greater than weight-adjusted adult levels. At puberty, clearance begins to decline to adult levels, in girls sooner than in boys. This pattern is found in other medications such as **theophylline** and **anticonvulsants,** with much intersubject and metabolic pathway variability. **One essential consideration is that, during times of great physiological change (the premature, the neonate, puberty), there are likely to be major changes in pharmacokinetics.** More variability among individuals and within the individual is likely during these periods. Careful monitoring of therapeutic drug levels is critical to safe outcomes. In the neonatal period, frequent adjustments may be necessary because of the rapid changes the neonate is undergoing. A drug dosage that is at a therapeutic level in a 9-year-old girl has to be carefully monitored as she evolves through puberty to ensure that she will not develop toxic levels as her drug clearance reaches adult levels.

Excretion

Drug excretion rates are affected by the lower glomerular filtration rate in newborns, which is only 30 to 40 percent of adult values. By age 6 to 12 months, the glomerular filtration rate reaches adult values (per unit surface area). Drugs that depend on renal excretion are cleared more slowly in neonates. Drug dosages and dosing intervals in newborns are adjusted accordingly for medications such as **ampicillin, aminoglycoside antibiotics,** and **digoxin.** Renal blood flow is also reduced in neonates and reaches adult levels at approximately age 9 months.

Pharmacodynamics

There are pharmacodynamic differences between children and adults that need to be taken into consideration in prescribing for children. Like much medical knowledge, information on the differences between children and adults has been gained from an unexpected outcome in children in response to a medication that is safe for adults. The classic examples are **antihistamines** and **barbiturates,** which cause hyperactivity rather than sedation when given to children. Another classic example is **tetracycline,** which deposits in developing teeth and causes permanent stains. **Corticosteroids** stunt linear growth if taken for long periods, as well as producing all of the same adverse reactions found in adults. Some medications are less toxic in children, such as **isoniazid.**

Another concern in children is the vehicle in which the medication is administered or the formulation. Children have sometimes had toxic or unexpected results, not from the medication, but from the additives or preservatives used. As recently as the 1980s, **benzyl alcohol,** a preservative used in drugs, was discovered to cause "gasping syndrome" when medications containing it were administered to newborns.

Topical ointments and creams are routinely prescribed to adults and children, yet there is a major difference between adults and children in the absorption rates from the skin. Infants and children have a thinner stratum corneum that allows medications to be more readily absorbed. Compared with older children and adults, infants have a larger skin surface area that is capable of greater weight-adjusted absorption of hydrophilic drugs (Niederhauser, 1997). Occlusive dressings can increase the absorption of medications, which is of particular concern regarding **corticosteroids** in the diaper area. The plastic coating on the diaper can cause occlusion, thereby increasing absorption and producing systemic steroid effects.

Developmental Aspects of Pediatric Medication Administration

With adults, the provider can assume that, if reasonably clear instructions are given, the patient will take the medication as prescribed. With children, many added variables affect administration of the medication and compliance with the medication regimen. The first consideration is the developmental level of the child and the amount of parental control at each developmental level. This section addresses these differences and suggests strategies for improving compliance at each age level.

Breast-Fed Infants

Breastfeeding an infant the first year of life is beneficial both physically and emotionally to the infant. Therefore, when prescribing medications to a lactating woman, the practitioner needs to be aware of which medications can be used safely and which are contraindicated (Table 47–1).

Drug Excretion in Breast Milk

The mammary gland can be viewed as an elimination organ in relation to maternal medication ingestion. Like other elimination organs, the properties of the medication determine how much of the medication will be in the breast milk (Bailey & Ito, 1997). Because breast milk is more acidic than plasma, basic compounds may be slightly more concentrated in the milk, and the concentration of acidic compounds in the milk will be lower than plasma levels (Benet, Kroetz, & Sheiner, 1996). Protein binding also affects the transfer of medications into breast milk. Highly plasma protein–bound drugs have a lower amount of drug available to transfer into milk because only the free drug is available for transfer (Bailey & Ito, 1997). Liposolubility also affects the ability of drugs to cross the alveolar cells by diffusion and enter the milk. Another factor is the molecular weight of the drug: Drugs with high molecular weight are transferred less easily into milk than drugs with lower molecular weight.

Factors That Influence an Infant's Exposure to Drugs in Breast Milk

A number of factors must be accounted for in determining the infant's exposure to a drug (Table 47–2). The following variables encompass physiological processes in both the infant and the mother that influence the effects of a drug on the infant:

1. Maternal pharmacokinetics has a great impact on the level of drug found in breast milk. The higher the drug concentration in the maternal plasma, the higher the concentration in the milk. Pregnant women have altered pharmacokinetics in the last trimester of gestation. Failure to monitor doses and decrease medication dosages appropriately after delivery may lead to toxic effects in both the mother and the breast-fed infant. Higher maternal drug dose or decreased clearance leads to increased drug in breast milk.

2. The infant suckling pattern can determine the level of drug found in breast milk. The time of the feeding in relation to the maternal dosing determines how much of the drug is in the breast milk. A drug with a short half-life, given to the mother right after feeding, decreases the amount of drug the infant is exposed to. Likewise, drugs with a long half-life increase the infant's exposure to the drug. Infant suckling time and the number of feedings also have an impact on drug exposure. Some infants nurse for long periods or very

Table 47–1. Prescribing for Lactating Women

Prescribing medications for lactating women should be undertaken with the same caution as prescribing for a pregnant woman. Assume that any drug prescribed will, in some amount, be found in the breast milk. Therefore, knowledge regarding safety of medications for lactating women is essential for all primary care practitioners. When prescribing, take the following steps (Bailey & Ito, 1997):

1 Review the safety of the drug during lactation.
2 If the drug is relatively safe, discuss the risks with the mother and explain the symptoms of drug toxicity.
3 Explain that the drug should be taken just after nursing or before infant's sleep.
4 Measure drug concentrations in milk or infant's serum when toxicity is likely.
5 Monitor the infant for signs of pharmacological action or drug toxicity.
6 Report any symptoms or signs of drug toxicity to the American Academy of Pediatrics, Committee on Drugs.

A few medications are absolutely contraindicated in lactating women (Table 47–2). Contraindications include **antineoplastic drugs** because of immediate or delayed toxicity in the infant. Weekly use of **methotrexate** for rheumatic disease is acceptable during lactation, but the infant needs to be monitored closely, with routine laboratory analysis of complete blood count with differential, liver enzymes, and renal function essential to infant safety (Bailey & Ito, 1997; Kastrup, 1999). Another contraindication to breastfeeding is **iodine-containing radioactive medications** used in nuclear medicine studies. In this case, temporary cessation of breastfeeding ("pump and dump") is indicated. The length of time before resumption of breastfeeding is determined by the half-life of the **radiopharmaceutical** agent.

Drugs that should be avoided include **lithium** and **oral contraceptives,** yet both have been used in lactating women. **Lithium** is excreted in breast milk at about 40 percent of the concentration of maternal serum, and milk and infant serum levels are approximately equal (Kastrup, 1999). If, for maternal health reasons, **lithium** needs to be prescribed, the infant's serum **lithium** level needs to be monitored closely. The main contraindication to **oral contraceptives** containing **estrogen** is that they may decrease milk supply. An **oral contraceptive** with low **estrogen** levels can be prescribed once the milk supply is well established (more than 6 weeks postpartum), but the first choice should be a **progestin-only oral contraceptive**. Decreased milk supply should be discussed with the mother as an adverse effect of **estrogen-containing oral contraceptives** prior to prescribing.

All illicit drugs are contraindicated in lactating women, specifically **cocaine, heroin,** and **methamphetamine.** Infants exposed to **cocaine** via breast milk may show signs of toxicity (irritability, tremors, increased startle response). **Cocaine** metabolites can be found in breast milk for up to 36 hours after the mother's last dose (Kastrup, 1999). **Heroin** enters breast milk and can cause neonatal depression. **Amphetamines** are excreted in breast milk and cause excitation in the infant. **Methamphetamine** poses an additional concern because some of the chemicals used to manufacture the illicit drug are toxic to both mother and infant, specifically lead, which is quite harmful to the infant. **Any drug use during lactation should be explored and the mother encouraged to discontinue breastfeeding if illicit drug use is a concern.**

Alcohol and **tobacco** are two commonly used legal drugs that can affect the breast-fed infant. **Alcohol** passes freely into breast milk and reaches levels close to maternal serum levels (Kastrup, 1999). High levels of **alcohol** in the breast milk put the infant at risk for sedation and cause a reduction in the maternal milk-ejecting response. There is controversy regarding maternal **alcohol** use during lactation. It is probably safe for the mother to ingest small amounts of **alcohol** timed just after a feeding, when levels in the milk are the lowest possible. **Tobacco** is a concern because of both secondhand smoke exposure and the **nicotine** that passes into breast milk. **Nicotine** passes freely into breast milk, and therefore the breast-fed infant is exposed to this toxin. If a **nicotine replacement patch** is used for maternal smoking cessation, the **nicotine** blood levels and therefore breast milk levels are lower than with smoked **tobacco.**

Because drugs are almost never tested for use in lactating women prior to their release onto the market, there is always a question regarding their safety during breastfeeding. Understanding some basic principles regarding the transfer of drugs into breast milk and their pharmacokinetic actions helps the practitioner make decisions about safe prescribing. It is essential for the practitioner to have ready reference to the most current information available about drugs during lactation, including "Transfer of Drugs and Other Chemicals in Breast Milk" by the Committee on Drugs of the American Academy of Pediatrics, published in *Pediatrics; Drug Facts and Comparisons; Drugs in Pregnancy and Lactation* by Biggs, Freeman, and Yaffe; and *Teratogen Information Services,* available from your local Poison Control Center.

frequently, which will increase the amount of drug the infant ingests.

3. Infant pharmacokinetics also plays an important role in how maternal medication use affects the breast-fed infant. As mentioned at the beginning of this chapter, gastric acid production and gastric emptying time are decreased and variable in neonates. The volume of distribution in infants is greater because of their greater total body water and their lower body fat. Infants also have significant differences in drug metabolism by the liver, as previously mentioned. Renal excretion, too, is al-

tered in younger infants, which can affect their overall clearance rate of drugs. All of these factors need to be considered in prescribing to a lactating woman, especially if the breast-fed infant is very young (less than 1 month old).

4. Susceptibility to a drug's effects can vary among infants. There is some dose-related predictability to a drug's effects that are related to the pharmacological properties of the drug. In some infants, however, there are unique effects that are not dose related and instead are idiosyncratic and therefore unpredictable. This reaction is fortunately uncommon,

Table 47–2. Effects of Commonly Prescribed Medications
on Infants during Lactation

Drug	Effect on Infant	Comment
Amoxicillin (all penicillins)	Minimal	Excreted in breast milk in low concentrations. May cause mild diarrhea in infant.
Amoxicillin-clavulanate (Augmentin)	Minimal	Excreted in breast milk. Infant may have diarrhea.
Acetaminophen	Minimal	Found in breast milk. No adverse reactions reported. Safer than aspirin when lactating.
Aspirin	Minimal, rare complication of bleeding	Occasional doses probably safe.
Atenolol	Moderate to significant	Excreted in breast milk in a milk to plasma (M:P) ratio of 1.5–6.8 (one patient had an estimated dose of 0.13 mg atenolol per feeding with a maternal dose of 100 mg/d). Cyanosis and bradycardia have been reported in breast-fed infants with maternal intake of 100 mg/d. Use with caution.
Caffeine	Minimal	Excreted in breast milk. If mother has 1 cup of coffee, the infant probably ingests 1.5–3.1 mg of caffeine. Caffeine has a long half-life in young infants (82 h in term newborn, 14.4 h in 3- to 4 1/2-mo-old infants, and 2.6 h in 6-mo-old infants). Probably safe in small amounts, with variable reaction based on individual infant.
Bromocriptine	Minimal	Used to suppress lactation.
Carbamazepine	Unknown	Milk concentration approximately 60% of maternal plasma concentrations. Potential adverse reactions in infant. Avoid while breastfeeding.
Chloramphenicol	Significant	Avoid while lactating. Possible bone marrow suppression.
Cascara	Moderate	Excreted in breast milk. Causes colic and diarrhea in the infant. Avoid.
Cephalosporin antibiotics	Minimal	Excreted in small amounts in milk. Probably safe.
Chlorpromazine	Probably minimal	Excreted in breast milk. Safety not established.
Codeine	Minimal; infant may experience lethargy	Probably safe.
Diazepam (all benzo-diazepines)	Significant; infant may experience lethargy; apnea reported	Infants metabolize benzodiazepines more slowly than adults; accumulation of toxic levels of drug is possible. Avoid in nursing mothers.
Dicumarol	Minimal	Excreted in breast milk in **inactive** form. May want to monitor infant's prothrombin time.
Digoxin	Minimal	Small amounts excreted in breast milk. Probably safe.
Ergot	Significant; infant may experience vomiting, diarrhea, peripheral vasoconstriction	**Contraindicated** in lactation. May suppress lactation.
Fluoroquinolones	Unknown	Little is known about these antibiotics and breastfeeding. Because they have an adverse effect on children, they should probably be avoided during lactation.

Continued on next page

Table 47–2. Effects of Commonly Prescribed Medications
on Infants during Lactation *(continued)*

Drug	Effect on Infant	Comment
Fluconazole	Minimal or unknown	Fluconazole is excreted in breast milk at concentrations similar to plasma.
Furosemide	Minimal or unknown	Excreted in breast milk. Use with close monitoring of the infant.
Gold salts	Significant hepatonephro-toxicity	**Contraindicated** in lactation. May be excreted in milk after therapy is discontinued.
Iodine (radioactive)	Significant; may cause thyroid suppression in the infant	**Contraindicated.** Maternal testing requiring radioactive iodine requires breast milk to be discarded according to the half-life of the drug.
Isoniazid (INH)	Minimal; possibility of pyridoxine deficiency developing in the infant	Milk levels same as maternal plasma levels. Observe infant for adverse effects. Probably safe.
Lithium	Significant; infant may develop toxic lithium levels	Avoid breastfeeding if possible. If no other choice, lithium may be prescribed to the mother, but routine lithium levels need to be drawn on the infant and the infant observed for toxicity.
Macrolide antibiotics	Minimal	There is the most information available about the safety of erythromycin, and it is considered safe. Other macrolides are also probably safe.
Methadone	Significant	May be used under close medical supervision. Infant may exhibit signs of withdrawal if methadone is discontinued abruptly or if breastfeeding is discontinued abruptly.
Metoprolol	Minimal	Excreted in very small amounts in breast milk. Infant consuming 1 L breast milk will get <1 mg metoprolol.
Metronidazole	Unknown	Milk levels similar to maternal plasma levels. Half-life in breast milk 8–10 h. **Contraindicated:** Nursing mothers should express and discard milk during and for 24–48 h after stopping drug therapy.
Oral contraceptives	Minimal to moderate	Hormones are released into breast milk. May cause jaundice and breast enlargement in the infant. Estrogen compounds suppress lactation, decreasing the quantity and quality of breast milk. Use progestin-only preparations ("minipill") or wait until milk supply is well established (>6 wk postpartum) to use combined forms.
Phenobarbital	Moderate; lethargy in the infant	Excreted in breast milk. Monitor infant for lethargy and feeding problems.
Phenytoin	Moderate	Enters breast milk in amounts large enough to cause adverse effects in the infant. **Use with caution;** suggest alternative therapy or not breastfeeding.
Prednisone	Moderate	Excreted in breast milk and may suppress growth and interfere with exogenous steroid production in the infant. Low maternal doses (<20 mg/d) probably safe. Larger doses for a short time may not harm the infant. It is best to time the medication dose just after a feeding and wait 3–4 h for next feeding.
Propranolol	Minimal	Excreted in breast milk in amounts too small to have any effect.

Continued on next page

Table 47–2. Effects of Commonly Prescribed Medications
on Infants during Lactation *(continued)*

Drug	Effect on Infant	Comment
Propoxyphene	Minimal; possible lethargy	Excreted in small amounts in breast milk.
Propylthiouracil	Significant; can suppress thyroid function in the infant	**Use with caution.** Avoid if possible.
Radioactive material	Significant; carcinogenic	**Contraindicated.**
Spironolactone	Minimal	Very small amounts (0.2%) of metabolite of mother's daily dose is excreted in breast milk. Safe for use with breastfeeding.
Tetracycline	Moderate; discolored teeth	Excreted in breast milk, M:P ratio of 0.6 to 0.8. **Avoid when lactating.** Use safer antibiotics.
Theophylline	Moderate	Excreted in breast milk. May cause irritability in the infant. Monitor for signs of toxicity.
Warfarin	Minimal	Excreted in breast milk in inactive form. Safe during breastfeeding.

but must be considered if an infant is demonstrating some effects of maternal drug use.

5. The milk to plasma (M:P) drug ratio affects the infant's exposure to a medication because the infant's clearance of the drug affects the overall exposure. Even drugs with a low M:P ratio may produce a toxic level if the infant is unable to effectively clear the drug.

Infants

Infants are totally dependent on their parents to administer their medication. Although the infant may balk at the taste of a medication, the parent is still in control of administering the medication. Intervention at this age is aimed at teaching parents how to properly administer the medication. Parents need to be edified and encouraged as they take on the role of administering and monitoring a child's medication. Many parents are nervous the first time they give their child medication. Thorough education ensures better medication compliance. Discussing the reason for the medication, the dose, the length of treatment, medication administration tips, and expected and unexpected adverse effects (e.g., the mild diarrhea that is expected with some **antibiotics**) should increase a parent's comfort with administering medications. Written instructions are essential at all ages but especially for the infant because the parent is more likely to be fatigued and less likely to retain instructions given. Dosing medications for parental convenience increases compliance. Ask parents if they are working outside their home and who else

may be administering the medication. A medication with fewer daily doses may be indicated if the child is in a day-care setting or has multiple caregivers.

Toddlers and Preschoolers

Toddlers and preschoolers are beginning to exert their independence, and administering medications to this age group can be a challenge, even a battlefield. Even the most experienced parent can have difficulty administering oral medications to a toddler. The key to success with this age group is to discuss medication administration with the parent prior to prescribing and, if possible, choose a medication that poses the fewest problems with administration. Doses per day, palatability, and dosage forms should be taken into consideration. If the toddler is resistant to taking medication, prescribe a once- or twice-daily medication if possible. Using chewable formulations, if the child has molars, can increase compliance because the child can self-administer the medication. Using higher concentrations of medication, if possible, to decrease the volume administered can be helpful. By age 2 or 3, children can often begin to self-administer oral medication by using a vertical medication spoon or medicine cup. Parents can help a child practice this skill with juice or another liquid before taking the medication. Discussing administration of the prescribed medication while the family is still in the clinic is essential. Ask the parent what has worked in the past to ease medication administration and what has not worked. Listen to parents, who know their child and can anticipate what will ease the medication administration.

Clinical Pearl

INFANTS

- Parents are often unsure how to administer medication to an infant. While the parents are in the clinic with the child, the practitioner should address this issue and *demonstrate* how to administer medication to an infant. For ease of administration, use a medication syringe and insert the syringe into the mouth along the inner cheek. To decrease choking, advise parents to squirt small amounts (1 cc) of medication at a time into the inner buccal space. Wait until the infant swallows, and then administer another small amount until all the medication is administered. Direct parents *not* to administer the medication directly over the tongue, which increases choking and allows the infant to more easily spit out the medication.
- Advise parents to check with the pharmacist before mixing any medication with formula or breast milk; some medications are bound with the calcium or other ingredients in the formula, causing them to be less effective.
- Breast-fed infants often choke and sputter when medications are first administered because these infants are used to only the feel of the breast in their mouths. Warning parents of this response and teaching them proper technique will help them gain confidence in medication administration.
- Giving **acetaminophen** in suppository form is an option if administering oral medications to the infant is difficult. The practitioner can demonstrate this procedure, which works well in breast-fed infants especially.

School-Age Children

Giving medication to school-age children is often easier than other age groups. Developmentally, they are industrious and eager to learn. It is essential to include the child in the decision-making process, if possible. Let the child choose the formulation. Does he or she want liquid, chewable tablets, or pills to swallow? Some liquid medications get to be large volumes as the child gets to school age (e.g., **trimethoprim-sulfamethoxazole** and **prednisone**), so advise parents and the child who chooses a liquid formulation of this fact. Be sure the child can swallow pills before prescribing them. Some medications can be crushed and mixed with highly viscous fluid (e.g., chocolate syrup). Check with the pharmacist prior to suggesting this if you are not fa-

miliar with a medication. Teaching with this age group should be aimed at both the parent and the child. Children need to know the rationale for prescribing a particular medication. They are being taught in school to avoid "drugs," and they need clarification about helpful medication and illicit drugs. Schools have varying regulations regarding administration of medication at school. If possible, avoid school-hour dosing to simplify the medication regimen.

Adolescents

Adolescent patients often administer their own medications. The compliance rates with this age group vary. Some teenagers are excellent at medication self-admin-

Clinical Pearl

TODDLERS AND PRESCHOOLERS

- Using higher-concentration liquid formulations will often increase compliance at any age. It is easier to administer half a teaspoon than a full teaspoon of any medication.
- Have parents teach preschoolers to self-administer medication by practicing with a medicine spoon or cup filled with juice or other flavored liquid. This practice often increases compliance because the child has control over this aspect of medication taking.

Clinical Pearl

SCHOOL-AGE CHILDREN

- **Prednisone** is bitter in liquid form and has a disagreeable aftertaste. Crushing the tablet form and mixing it with chocolate syrup often increases compliance. Parents can also administer something sweet after **prednisone** syrup, which decreases the aftertaste.

istration, and others are poorly compliant. The adolescent is developmentally entering the period of formal operational thinking, characterized by propositional thinking and abstract reasoning. Younger adolescents may still be in the concrete thinking stage, and their interactions with the health care provider may reflect this stage, rather than the abstract thought process of older teenagers. Although adolescents may be able to self-administer medication and appear to be capable of the task, they may vary in their sophistication regarding medication use. The practitioner needs to make an alliance with teenagers and ask their perspective regarding their medications. Do they have an opinion regarding the medication? What schedule will work best with their lifestyle? Teenagers appreciate having their opinions taken into consideration as treatment is planned. When a medication history is taken with the parent present, the teenager may not be completely truthful. Practitioners need to be aware of the laws of the state in which they practice and, when treating teenagers, maintain confidentiality if necessary. Teenagers, too, must understand the confidentiality laws of their state and at what age they are able to receive confidential treatment. Parents often struggle with letting teenagers self-administer medications. The practitioner needs to be skilled at assisting family members as they move from parent-controlled to child- or teen-controlled medication administration. This transition varies by family.

Factors That Influence Positive Outcomes

Compliance with the medication regimen is an issue for all patients. Pediatric patients pose a unique dilemma because the practitioner has to address both the child's compliance and the parent's, plus possibly that of other caregivers. The many factors that influence compliance include length of medication regimen, number of medications prescribed, medication interval, palatability, cost, and family issues. The practitioner needs to consider all of these issues when prescribing to ensure successful treatment.

There is little agreement in the definitions of *compliance* and *noncompliance*. Is anything less than full compliance considered noncompliance? If the therapeutic outcome is adequate, is less than full compliance with the treatment regimen acceptable? Often, compliance of a certain set percentage (e.g., 70 percent or more) is considered to be compliant with the regimen (Matsui, 1997). Dose omission and delay are the most common dosing errors, yet other forms of noncompliance may occur, including failure to fill the prescription, incorrect dosing or dosing intervals, and discontinuation of the medication prior to the recommended time. Compliance rates vary from 7 to 89 percent for short-term medications and from 11 to 83 percent for long-term medications when rates are studied in pediatric patients (Matsui, 1997). There are few recent studies of medication compliance, but older studies indicate that of patients treated for otitis media only 7.3 percent had complete compliance with the prescribed **antibiotics** and 53 percent took less than half of the prescribed medicine (Matter et al., 1975). A study of sexually active female teenagers found that only 44.6 percent were compliant with taking their **oral contraceptives** (Litt, Cuskey, & Rudd, 1980). Even patients with life-threatening illnesses such as organ transplant or cancer report compliance rates as low as 52 to 60 percent (Matsui, 1997).

Monitoring compliance can be a challenge in children. Direct methods of measuring compliance with the medication regimen, such as serum drug levels, are invasive and costly. Less invasive methods are being explored, such as urinalysis for drug metabolites, saliva analysis (for **theophylline, phenytoin, phenobarbital, and carbamazepine** levels), and hair analysis (used currently for **cocaine** and **nicotine** exposure in utero, can be expanded to other medications) (Bailey, Klein, & Koren, 1997). Indirect methods, such as patient and parental reports, are the most widely used and the most practical method of measuring medication compliance, but it is limited by the reliability of the person who is reporting. Pill counts and other methods of determining compliance have also been found to be unreliable (Matsui, 1997). A diary of medication doses taken may give a clearer picture of what doses the child has received, although this is also only as accurate as the recorder.

Specific Factors That Influence Compliance

Long-Term versus Short-Term Medication Regimens

It is clear that compliance is poorer for long-term medications than for short-term medication regimens (Fotheringham & Sawyer, 1995). Compliance also decreases as soon as symptoms improve. For example, compliance with **antibiotics** is poor because the medication may be discontinued as soon as symptoms are relieved. Compliance in **penicillin** prescribed for streptococcal pharyngitis decreases sharply after symptoms improve. In a summary of eight randomized clinical trails, Paradise (1997) determined that a shortened course of **antibiotics** (5 days versus 10 days) for mild otitis media is often adequate treatment for children over age 6 years. This same analysis determined that in children younger than age 6 years—in particular, children younger than age 2 years—a shortened course of treatment is not adequate and that these younger children should be treated for 10 full days. Note that **azithromycin (Zithromax)**, which has a standard 5-day dosing schedule, was not included in this analysis. More studies are needed regarding a shortened length of treatment for other common childhood illnesses because briefer treatments could lead to increased compliance.

Chronic illness presents a number of problems for the family, often including a daily medication regimen. Compliance rates vary significantly for children with chronic illness (Matsui, 1997). Even patients for whom noncompliance can be life-threatening are not taking their medications as prescribed. Self-reported compliance among children and adolescents with cancer was 60.5 percent in one study (Tebbi, Cummings, & Zevon, 1986).

Number of Medications Prescribed

The number of medications prescribed can have an impact on compliance with the regimen. The more medications prescribed, the lower the compliance. Keeping medication schedules simple increases the likelihood of success for the treatment.

Medication Interval

Medication interval has a significant impact on the success of the treatment, especially given the number of families with both parents working and more children in daycare. In a review of the literature (Greenberg, 1984), once-a-day and twice-a-day regimens were associated with significantly better compliance (73 percent and 70 percent, respectively). Three-times-a-day regimens had 52 percent compliance, and four-times-a-day medications were likely to be given as directed only 42 percent of the time. Children who are in school or have parents who are both working are probably not receiving their medications as often as recommended if they are taking any medication that needs to be administered more than twice a day.

Palatability

Palatability is often overlooked as a reason for noncompliance, yet in children it is a critical factor in medication compliance. Two studies comparing the taste of a variety of **antibiotics** (Matsui, Barron, & Rieder, 1996; Ruff et al., 1991) determined that some **antibiotics** were ranked better tasting than others, with the **cephalosporins (cefixime,** cephalexin, and **cefaclor)** ranked as the best tasting overall. **Dicloxacillin** ranked the worst for taste in both studies. Although no published reports studied taste differences between name-brand and generic preparations, anecdotal reports from parents and patients suggest that name-brand preparations taste better. Of medications with the same efficacy profile, the best tasting is the easiest to administer to young children.

Cost

The cost of the medication needs to be addressed for patients who are not adequately insured for prescriptions. The cost of common **antibiotics** prescribed for otitis me-

Clinical Pearl

ELECTROLYTE SOLUTIONS

- Pediatric **electrolyte solutions** are often not well accepted by children. One trick is to use **electrolyte Popsicles (Pedialyte)** or freeze the bottled solution into homemade Popsicles. The cold taste seems to be better accepted.
- Sugar-free Kool-Aid or another drink mix sweetened with Nutrasweet can be added to unflavored **electrolyte solutions** to make the taste of the **electrolyte solution** more acceptable to children.

dia range from $6.10 to $53.95 to treat a 15-kg child for 10 days (Niederhauser, 1997). Prescribing an expensive **antibiotic** for a family who cannot afford to fill the prescription places the family in an uncomfortable position. Simply asking the family if they have insurance to cover the medication and then problem solving with them if they do not will increase the likelihood that the family will fill the prescription. If possible, give the family a few days of medication samples to defray the cost of the treatment if a less expensive medication is not available. Knowing which pharmacies in the local area are the least expensive or calling ahead for a price check before sending the family to the pharmacy is helpful. A family who knows the approximate amount that the medication will cost will not be surprised when the prescription is filled.

Family Issues

Family issues affect the family's ability to comply with the prescribed treatment regimen. Families in which both parents are working and therefore have limited time with their children have more problems with complex treatment regimens. Lack of social support can leave a parent isolated and make parenting more stressful. Parental fatigue is often overlooked as a factor in treatment outcomes. Parents who are fatigued can easily miss medication doses; even those who are usually well organized can miss medication doses when they are tired. Disruptive and dysfunctional families may have difficulty in following the plan of treatment because of the chaos present in the home. Another family situation that needs to be addressed when clinical improvement is less than satisfactory is parental use of the child's medications. For example, a child may be prescribed stimulants for attention deficit disorder, and a parent or other family member may be abusing the child's medication. This is a situation no practitioner wants to encounter, yet there should always be some index of suspicion when the family history

is not clear. All of these issues need to be accounted for when the practitioner is prescribing a medication and during follow-up on the patient's progress. They often present in an unclear fashion, and ferreting out the reason for noncompliance with the treatment regimen may take some time.

Improving Compliance in the Pediatric Patient

When poor compliance is identified, it is essential to address this issue and determine strategies with the patient and parent to improve the success of the treatment regimen. There are a variety of methods to improve the success of the treatment regimen, but first it is necessary to make sure that the diagnosis is accurate and that the drug therapy is beneficial.

Medication Concentration

Medication concentration can be adjusted in some of the liquid preparations. The practitioner can choose to prescribe a more concentrated form when a parent has difficulty administering medications to a patient. Many of the **antibiotics** come in different strengths, and giving half a teaspoon is easier than administering a full teaspoon. **Prednisone** comes in two different strengths, as well as in tablets that can be crushed. By involving the parents in the decision to use a more concentrated form of a medication, you are allowing them some control over the treatment regimen, and they may therefore be more likely to administer the medication that is prescribed (Table 47–3).

Written versus Oral Instructions

Most practitioners should address the issue of written versus oral instructions in their own practice. Studies

Table 47–3. Prescribing Over-the-Counter Pain Medications for Pediatric Patients

Pain in children can come from many areas, from teething pain to pain associated with otitis media. Parents often ask the practitioner about using **acetaminophen** or **ibuprofen** for the treatment of pain in children. It is essential for both the safety of the child and the efficacy of the medication that parents be taught how to properly administer over-the-counter (OTC) pain medication to their children.

The two most commonly used **analgesics** in pediatric patients are **acetaminophen** and **ibuprofen**. **Aspirin** should never be given to children for acute pain management, and the practitioner should teach parents this rule. **Acetaminophen** can be administered orally or rectally (suppository), and it peaks in 30 to 60 min. Dosage for children is 10 to 15 mg/kg/dose q4–6h. **Ibuprofen** is effective for pain control and has an additive anti-inflammatory effect, which appears to provide better pain control in acute otitis media than **acetaminophen**. The correct dosage is 5 to 10 mg/kg/dose q6–8h. Although both provide good pain relief for mild to moderate pain and both have antipyretic effects, **ibuprofen** may be the drug of choice for night pain associated with otitis media because of its longer duration. Both drugs are equally easy to administer, although **ibuprofen** is not available in suppository form.

Give parents a dosing chart with their child's dose based on weight. The different strengths of **acetaminophen** must be dosed correctly. New parents may not be aware that drops and liquid or suspension are different strengths, which can lead to dosing errors. There are also different strengths of chewable tablets available.

Clinical Pearl

ORAL MEDICATIONS

- Often, administering oral medications to breast-fed infants is hard. A more concentrated formula decreases the volume administered, which often makes it easier to give the medication.

Clinical Pearl

EDUCATIONAL HANDOUTS

- Having available in the examination room printed handouts for common acute illnesses that require prescriptions can streamline the education process. Briefly discuss on each handout a disease process such as otitis media, streptococcol pharyngitis, or pneumonia, and leave a blank space for the **antibiotic** to be filled in. Educating families about the prescription is then much easier.

show that only 50 percent of instructions given by physicians are recalled immediately after the visit (Liptak, 1996). Therefore, giving written instructions along with the oral directions will improve compliance.

Self-Monitoring Calendars

Self-monitoring calendars should be a standard in the treatment of preschool and school-age children. Children can apply a sticker or color in a box as each dose is taken. Parents should be involved in the process and set a reward for completion of the medication regimen. In acute illness such as otitis media, in which the patient will be returning to the clinic, the practitioner may offer a reward for a full calendar. Children with chronic illness, who are often on long-term medication, need to have a set reward for a certain number of days of successfully taking their medication. Parents need to take an active role in medication calendar usage, and they, too, should be praised for their participation in the medication regimen.

Telephone Reminders

Telephone reminders are helpful in increasing compliance, especially if the parent is leaving the clinic with multiple prescriptions. A quick telephone call allows the parent to clarify the treatment regimen and reinforces teaching that took place in the clinic.

Contracts and Reinforcement Programs

Contracts or reinforcement programs may be necessary if compliance continues to be a problem. The practitioner, the patient, and the family need to be in agreement about the goals of the treatment contract and the consequences of noncompliance. A case conference may be necessary to involve other disciplines in the treatment. A home visit may provide information that leads to an altered treatment program that will be better tolerated by the family. The role of the practitioner is to attempt to simplify the medication treatment and still have an adequate therapeutic outcome. This goal should be shared with the patient and family.

Clinical Pearl

MOTIVATIONAL CALENDARS

- Pharmaceutical companies often have motivational calendars available for specific name-brand medications.

Clinical Pearls

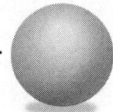

IMPROVING COMPLIANCE WITH OPHTHALMIC PREPARATIONS

- Administration of ophthalmic preparations to toddlers and preschoolers is often difficult, and the incidence of noncompliance increases with each dose that is a battle to administer. Parents can safely restrain the child to administer eye medications as follows: (1) Sit on the floor with the child sitting on the floor between the parent's legs. (2) The child's feet should be near the parent's feet, and the child's head between the parent's thighs. (3) Slip the child's arms under the parent's thighs and, with the legs, hold the child's head and arms still. (4) The parent then has both hands free to administer the eye medication. Although this procedure may sound drastic, it is a quick way for a parent to administer the medication when there is no other adult around to assist with a squirming, resistant child.
- Older preschoolers and school-age children often cooperate with administration of eyedrops if they are told to lie back and *close their eyes*. Eyedrops can then be applied to the inner corner of the eyes (while the eyes are closed). Next, children are told to open their eyes, without any head movement. The medication rolls into the eye when the eye is opened. This is much easier than the bull's-eye approach of trying to get children to keep their eyes open for drops to be squeezed in.

REFERENCES

American Academy of Pediatrics, Committee on Drugs. (1994). Transfer of drugs and other chemicals into human milk. *Pediatrics, 93,* 137.

Bailey, B., & Ito, S. (1997). Breast-feeding and maternal drug use. *Pediatric Clinics of North America, 44*(1), 41–54.

Bailey, B., Klein, J., & Koren, G. (1997). Noninvasive methods for drug measurement in pediatrics. *Pediatric Clinics of North America, 44*(1), 15–25.

Barber, N. (1996). Genitourinary disorders. In C. E. Burns & A. Dunn (Eds.), *Pediatric primary care: A handbook for nurse practitioners.* Philadelphia: Saunders.

Benet, L., Kroetz, D., & Sheiner, L. (1996). Pharmacokinetics: The dynamics of drug absorption, distribution, and elimination. In J. G. Hardman, & L. E. Limbird (Eds. in Chief), *Goodman & Gillman's the pharmacological basis of therapeutics* (9 ed., pp. 16–17). New York: McGraw Hill.

Berlin, C. M. (1997). Advances in pediatric pharmacology and toxicology. *Advances in Pediatrics, 44,* 545.

Biggs, G. G., Freeman, R. K., & Yaffe, S. J. (1994). *Drugs in Pregnancy and Lactation.* Williams & Wilkins, Baltimore.

Bolinger, A. M., & Chan, C. Y. J. (1996). Pediatric considerations. In L. Y. Young & M.A. Koda-Kimble (Eds.), *Applied therapeutics.* Vancouver, WA.

Brady, M. A. (1996). Atopic disorders and rheumatic diseases. In C. E. Burns, N. Barber, M. A. Brady and A. M. Dunn (Eds.), *Pediatric primary care: A handbook for nurse practitioners.* Philadelphia: Saunders.

Fotheringham, M. J., & Sawyer, M. G. (1995). Adherence to recommended medical regimens in childhood and adolescence. *Journal of Pediatrics and Child Health, 31,* 72.

Friedman, A. L. (1998). Nephrology: Fluids and electrolytes. In R. E. Behrman & R. M. Kliegman (Eds.), *Nelson essentials of pediatrics* (3rd ed., p. 609). Philadelphia: Saunders.

Goodman, J., & Gal, P. (1992). Pharmacokinetic and pharmacodynamic data collection in children and neonates. *Clinical Pharmacokinetics, 23*(1), 1–9.

Greenberg, R. N. (1984). Overview of patient compliance with medication dosing: A literature review. *Clinical Therapeutics, 6,* 592.

Gupta, A. & Waldhauer, L. K. (1997). Adverse drug reactions from birth to early childhood. *Pediatric Clinics of North America, 44*(1), 79–92.

Kastrup, E. (Founding Ed.). (1999). *Drug facts & comparisons.* St. Louis: Facts & Comparisons.

Liptak, G. S. (1996). Enhancing patient compliance in pediatrics. *Pediatrics in Review, 17,* 128.

Litt, I. F., Cuskey, W. R., & Rudd, S. (1980). Identifying adolescents at risk for noncompliance with contraceptive therapy. *Journal of Pediatrics, 96,* 742.

MacDonald, M. (1996). Eye problems. In C. E. Burns & A. Dunn. (Eds.). *Pediatric primary care: A handbook for nurse practitioners.* Philadelphia: Saunders.

Mason, W. H. (1996). The management of common infections in ambulatory children. *Pediatric Annals, 25,* 621.

Matsui, D. M. (1997). Drug compliance in pediatrics. *Pediatric Clinics of North America, 44*(1), 1–13.

Matsui, D. M., Barron, A., & Rieder, M. J. (1996). Assessment of the palatability of antistaphylococcal antibiotics in pediatric volunteers. *Annals of Pharmacotherapy, 30,* 586–588.

Matter, M. E., Markello, J., Yaffe, S. J. (1975). Inadequacies in the pharmacological management of ambulatory children. *Journal of Pediatrics, 87,* 137.

Niederhauser, V. P. (1997). Prescribing for children: Issues in pediatric pharmacology. *Nurse Practitioner, 22*(3), 16–30.

Nies, A. S., & Spielberg, S. P. (1996). Principles of therapeutics. In *Goodman & Gilman's the pharmacological basis of therapeutics* (9th ed.). New York: McGraw-Hill.

O'Brien, K. L., Dowell, S. F., Schwartz, B., Marcy, S. M., Phillips, W. R., & Gerber, M. A. (1998). Acute sinusitis: Principles of judicious use of antimicrobial agents. *Pediatrics, 101*(Suppl.), 174.

Paradise, J. L. (1997). Short-course antimicrobial treatment for acute otitis media: Not best for infants and young children. *Journal of the American Medical Association, 278,* 1640.

Peterson-Smith, A. M. (1996). Gastrointestinal disorders. In C. E.

Burns & A. Dunn. (Eds.), *Pediatric primary care: A handbook for nurse practitioners.* Philadelphia: Saunders.

Prince, A. (1998). Infectious disease. In R. E. Behrman & R. M. Kliegman (Eds.), *Nelson essentials of pediatrics* (3rd ed., p. 315). Philadelphia: Saunders.

Ruff, M. E., Schotic, D. A., Bass, J. W., & Vincent, J. M. (1991). Antimicrobial drug suspensions: A blind comparison of taste of fourteen common pediatric drugs. *Pediatric Infectious Disease Journal, 10,* 30.

Schwartz, B., Marcy, S. M., Phillips, W. R., Gerber, M. A., & Dowell, S. F. (1998). Pharyngitis: Principles of judicious use of antimicrobial agents. *Pediatrics, 101*(Suppl.), 171.

Tebbi, C. K., Cummings, M., & Zevon, M. A. (1986). Compliance of pediatric and adolescent cancer patients. *Cancer, 58,* 1179.

Tershakovec, A. M., & Stallings, V. A. (1998). Pediatric nutrition and nutritional disorders. In R. E. Behrman & R. M. Kliegman (Eds.), *Nelson essentials of pediatrics* (3rd ed., p. 56). Philadelphia: Saunders.

Umetsu, D. T. (1998). Immunology and allergy. In R. E. Behrman & R. M. Kliegman (Eds.), *Nelson essentials of pediatrics* (3rd ed., p. 263). Philadelphia: Saunders.

CHAPTER 48

·······

Geriatric Patients

CHAPTER OUTLINE

W orking with older adults is exciting and challenging. They are about 12.6 percent of the population, but it is estimated that this group consumes about 30 percent of prescription drugs and about 40 percent of over-the-counter (OTC) medications (Graitzer, 1998; Mahoney, Zhan, & Eckler, 1999; Ross, 1997). With the high cost of prescribed medications (rarely covered by insurance programs), complex medication schedules, inadequate teaching, poor vision, and loss of dexterity, it is not unusual for older adults to have unintended noncompliance with their medication regimens (Conn, Taylor, & Miller, 1994; Graitzer, 1998; Mahoney, Zhan, & Eckler, 1999).

Pharmacokinetics and Pharmacodynamic Changes

The nurse practitioner must be aware of all the compounding factors that make pharmacotherapeutics especially difficult with the geriatric population. Older adults are like sleeping giants. They may not report their symptoms because they fear the diagnosis or fear loss of acceptance by peers if they have a stigmatized diagnosis (e.g., Alzheimer's disease, cancer, psychiatric disorder). Older adults have the possibility of complex medical, emotional, and social aspects that predispose them to adverse drug reactions (Graitzer, 1998). Caution, wisdom, and creativity are the guidelines for interaction.

General absorption of medications is not dramatically different in the older adult versus the younger population for the vast majority of prescribed and OTC medications. But general metabolism does appear to be affected by the general aging process. When evaluating adverse drug reactions, compounded by increased age and several disease processes, the practitioner must be careful and cautious.

The well older adult does not have an increase in possible drug reactions because of the drug. What happens is that the normal physiological changes that occur with aging (e.g., decreased metabolism) increase the risk of adverse drug reactions. As an example, renal function declines by about a third with normal aging; therefore, normal renal function tests may not mean normal renal function. It takes adequate protein ingestion to produce an accurate blood urea nitrogen level and adequate muscle mass to have an accurate serum creatinine level. If the patient has poor nutrition, renal function tests are affected. Many drugs are highly protein-bound. With decreased clearing ability, more free drug is available, necessitating lower drug doses to prevent adverse drug interactions.

Table 48–1 presents common pharmacokinetic and pharmacodynamic age-related changes and the drug implications.

As a person ages, body fat stores change from 14 to 30 percent, with a decrease in lean body mass. Lipid-soluble drugs, such as **benzodiazepines,** have a greater volume of distribution with a prolonged or erratic effect in the older adult. Along with the fat and lean body mass changes, total body water also decreases. Water-soluble drugs, such as **lithium** and **digoxin,** can have a smaller volume of distribution, resulting in higher peak plasma concentration at normal dosages.

The older adult may exhibit increased sensitivity to drug effects. **Anticholinergic agents** may cause urinary retention because the detrusor muscle tone of the bladder is decreased. **Tricyclic antidepressants** may cause confusion in the depressed patient, secondary to the anticholinergic adverse reactions. **Narcotic** and **psychoactive drugs** can cause oversedation, confusion, and respiratory depression and distort the patient's sense of

Table 48–1. Common Pharmacokinetic and Pharmacodynamic Changes in the Geriatric Patient

Pharmacokinetics and Pharmacodynamics	Changes in the Geriatric Patient	Implications
Absorption	• None, or if there is a change, the change is due to age-related delay in gastric emptying and reduced blood flow to the gastrointestinal (GI) tract	• May decrease the rate of absorption for some OTC drugs (e.g., antacids, laxatives)
Distribution	• Increase in fat stores • Decrease in lean body mass • Decrease in total body water • Decrease in serum albumin concentration	• Increases the effect of lipid-soluble drugs • Increases drug effects due to higher plasma concentration • Changes the onset and duration of action of highly tissue-bound, water-bound, and protein-bound drugs
Metabolism	• Change in the capacity of the liver to metabolize certain drugs because of decreased liver mass and blood flow • Decrease in the breakdown of enzymes	• Inhibits oxidative reaction, prolonging the effects of some drugs • Increases the plasma concentration of some drugs
Excretion	• Reduction in the efficiency of renal elimination of drugs because of reduced renal mass, decreased glomerular filtration rate, and reduced tubular secretion	• Decreases renal clearance of drugs

Adapted from Mahoney, D., Zhan, L. M., & Eckler, M. (1999). Preventing drug-drug interactions among older adults: Guidelines and clinical application. *American Journal for Nurse Practitioners, 3*(1), 7–20.

Clinical Pearl

....

The Golden Rule of geriatrics: Go low, go slow, but go! Treat the problem, starting at lower dosages and titrate up slowly, over a longer period of time than for a younger person. You will be able to evaluate for adverse reactions before they become serious and costly.

....

balance. Some OTC cold remedies with anticholinergic adverse reactions may cause the patient with glaucoma to experience vision loss secondary to the increase of intraoptic pressure or urinary retention in the patient with benign prostatic hypertrophy.

As a contrast, some older adults are less sensitive to certain other drugs, such as **beta blockers** and **beta agonists** (Mahoney, Zhan, & Eckler, 1999). The older adult may have a decreased response to a **beta blocker** (e.g., **propranolol**), resulting in less of a slowed heart rate than a younger person or only a mild increase in response to a **beta agonist** (e.g., **epinephrine**).

The best advice for evaluating pharmacological intervention is to assess for drug-disease interactions, drug-drug interactions, and drug-metabolism interactions. The older adult reacts to medications like individuals of all other ages, but the practitioner has to be aware of all compounding factors. Drugs may cause an adverse reaction, but this reaction occurs later than with a younger person, the half life of the drug takes longer to clear the older adult's system because of slower metabolism.

Assessing Pharmacological Problems and Concerns of Geriatric Patients

Older adults are at higher risk for drug interactions, not only because of physiological changes but also because of the medication practices of both health care provider and patients. Nonadherence with drug therapy, either intentional or unintentional, is reported in about 40 to 45 percent of older adults (Thwaites, 1999).

Physicians and nurse practitioners practice in similar ways; in many clinical situations, however, nurse practitioners are more likely than physicians to explore a patient's lifestyle practices and less likely to write a prescription when an appropriate nondrug alternative is available (Mahoney, 1994). These practice differences not only differentiate the nurse practitioner prescriber from the physician prescriber but also help to reduce the risk of pharmacological interactions in the older adult.

The nurse practitioner must be aware of all the compounding factors that make pharmacotherapeutics especially difficult with the older adult population. Using a thorough and quick checklist at each clinic visit with the older adult provides an accurate evaluation of the patient's understanding of the medications and ability to manage the regimen. Table 48–2 is a questionnaire that may be used for this purpose.

Common Pharmacological Concerns of Geriatric Patients

Polypharmacy

Drug-Drug Interactions

Actual data about drug-drug interactions in community-living geriatric patients are very likely underestimated.

Table 48–2. Questionnaire for Assessing Medication Management

- Did you bring all of your medications with you?
- List your medications, and tell me how you take them.
- Do you have any new eyedrops, either over the counter or from your eye doctor?
- What over-the-counter medications are you taking, such as food supplements, vitamins, laxatives, pain relievers, and herbal or natural products?
- Do you have any problems opening the bottles?
- Do you sometimes skip some of the medicine? Why?
- What do you do when you run out of your pills?
- At what time of the day do you take your pills, and do you do this the same every day?
- How do you remember to take your pills?
- How do you tell the difference between your medications (size, color)?
- What questions do you have about your medications?

Pharmacological interventions contribute significantly to the treatment of diseases; however, adverse drug reactions also occur more commonly. Adverse drug reactions are implicated in about 10 to 20 percent of acute geriatric admissions (Atkin et al., 1999). An older adult with chronic illnesses may not recognize a new symptom as drug related but as a manifestation of the ongoing disease process and therefore may not report the new symptom to the health care provider. Drug-induced confusion, incontinence, depression, or fatigue may be, in error, attributed to the aging process.

Self-Medication Practices

The older adult can be a very independent thinker, resulting in self-medication practices. Self-medication is often the first or primary response to symptoms of illness but can also be a complicating factor. **Aspirin (acetylsalicylic acid), nonsteroidal anti-inflammatory drugs (NSAIDs), cardiovascular agents** (e.g., **diuretics, digoxin**), and **psychotropic agents** (e.g., **benzodiazepines, antidepressants, antipsychotics**) are most frequently implicated in adverse drug reactions (Atkin et al., 1999). However, it is not the drug classes themselves but the absolute numbers of how many classes of drugs are used that are the important predictors for risk of adverse drug reactions (Atkin et al., 1999).

Someone Else's Medication

A second area of concern is the older adult's practice of using someone else's prescribed medication. The symptoms may sound the same, and to save cost, the kindly neighbor or family member offers to help out by sharing a medication. Then, out of embarrassment or concern for the "helpful" friend, the patient may not tell the health care provider about using someone else's medication. This results in poor medication practices for both the uninformed provider and the patient. Table 48–3 presents poor medication practices commonly seen with geriatric patients and their health care providers.

Alternative Medicines

Utilization of alternative medicines is well worth investigating, and knowledge about this area is valuable. Diverse

Table 48–3. Poor Medication Practices Commonly Seen with Geriatric Patients and the Health Care Provider

Patients
- Using neighbors' or friends' medications or remedies
- Changing the prescribed medication regimen without informing the provider
- Utilizing self-care practices based on no or poor information
- Neglecting to inform the health care provider about all therapies being utilized

Providers
- Failure to thoroughly question about current medication use, including OTCs, herbal, or alternative medicines
- Failure to provide thorough individualized patient education about medication regimen
- Poor follow-up monitoring of therapeutic treatments
- Prescribing medication in a clinically inappropriate manner.
- Using medications as the first line of treatment without first considering alternatives
- Treating drug-induced symptoms as "normal aging"

cultures, fads, and advertising have combined to make alternative medicines more prevalent now in the American culture, and problems have developed. Regarding herbal medications, for example, **St. John's wort** is advertised as a safe natural **antidepressant.** If it is combined with **monoamine oxidase inhibitors (MAOIs),** however, both adverse reactions and drug interactions may occur. Many practitioners utilize herbal medications, but the practice is very diverse and complicated. If the practitioner has only a limited knowledge of herbal medications or cultural practices, opening the dialogue with the older adult to understand the patient's practices will help in avoiding the adverse reactions of polypharmacy. Contact with a local person who is knowledgeable on these topics will help the practitioner prescribe and recommend appropriate treatment.

The Patient's "Peace of Mind"

Knowing the patient is important. Some patients feel as if they are being slighted and discounted if they are not given a prescription. Provide education and a rationale if a prescription drug is not indicated. Work as a team, of-

Clinical Pearl

The first step in avoiding adverse drug reactions is to establish risk predictions. Polypharmacy is only part of the picture. Take into account age, gender, multiple comorbidities, body weight, renal and hepatic failure, and previous drug reactions.

Table 48–4. Factors Influencing Therapeutic Outcomes

Factor	Pharmaceutical Effects	Therapeutic Outcome
Physiological decline	Altered pharmacokinetics	Increased potential for adverse reactions
Increase in disease process or severity of disease	Increased total number of medications	Increased potential for drug interactions
Decreased mental abilities Decreased income	Decreased reporting of drug compliance	Increased potential for decreased therapeutic effects

fering negotiations and, if indicated, a contract in providing care to the patient. If it is necessary for the patient's peace of mind and compliance, write a prescription to be filled by a pharmacist. The prescription may be for an OTC medication, but it can prevent a patient from feeling discounted and instead create a satisfied "customer."

Factors Influencing Positive Outcomes or Compliance

Polypharmacy is only one of the possible influences that affects the outcome in the management of medications with the geriatric patient. Several other factors such as income, mobility, complicated dosages, and the patient's functional ability can also influence the older adult's ability to be compliant with a medication regimen. Table 48–4 presents factors associated with geriatric patients, pharmaceutical effects, and therapeutic outcomes.

Assessing functional ability may be one of the most important steps in evaluating appropriate pharmaceutical interventions (von Welsheim, 1998). Older adults' abilities to manage their activities of daily life and their cognitive and social status are strong indicators in their ability to manage pharmaceutical interventions (Crigger & Forbes, 1997; von Welsheim, 1998).

Several functional assessment tools (e.g., Folstein Mini Mental, Geriatric Depression Scale) are short, quick, and accurate. In addition, assessing the geriatric patient's sensory functions (sight, hearing, taste, touch) is important because of the possible impairments that occur with aging that may affect the patient's ability to know what is expected in managing a medication regimen. An accurate functional assessment helps the nurse practitioner assess risk behaviors, prevent catastrophic events triggered by adverse drug reactions or inadvertent misuse of medications, and improve a patient's quality of life.

Physical Changes Associated with Aging

Mental Changes

Mental changes in the healthy older adult are minimal. Although white brain matter does begin to deteriorate at about age 60, an inability of the older adult to function independently is not a normal part of the aging process. Disease processes are the culprits that rob the geriatric patient of the ability to think clearly and maintain independence. Several diseases, such as Alzheimer's disease and cerebrovascular accidents, may impair the patient's mental status. In addition, evaluation of the patient's pharmaceutical practices may provide insight into the actual causes of a "dementia."

Dementia may present as mild confusion or as inability to perform even the simplest of tasks. Abrupt changes in an older adult's abilities are usually readily recognizable and often attributed to disease processes, whereas insidious, slow changes are attributed to "aging." However, both abrupt and slow changes could be the result of adverse medication reactions, a situation the practitioner should investigate. For example, "simple" cystitis, which may also bring complaints of dizziness or ataxia, could be a result of a disease process, changes associated with aging, or an adverse medication reaction.

Clinical Pearl

When ordering laboratory tests, always order at least a urine dip. A "simple" cystitis can cause dizziness, delirium, or ataxia, which may not be recognized as cystitis because the normal complaints of urinary burning, urgency, or frequency may not be present. Simple cystitis is much easier to manage pharmaceutically than the complications of ataxia.

Sensory Changes

Sight

The eye undergoes several changes (e.g., shape) with natural aging. Conditions associated with aging, such as cataracts, glaucoma, and macular degeneration, can present challenges to the practitioner who is prescribing and managing the patient's medication regimen. Fortunately, most of these changes can be either corrected or easily managed if identified, and most geriatric patients have insurance coverage, such as Medicare, that allows for at least one examination every 2 years for general eye health.

If the patient's vision is affected, it is important to adjust the medication regimen to accommodate these changes. For example, simplifying the medication regimen to once or twice a day, if possible, enables greater compliance; reducing the total number of medications prescribed, if possible, also helps. For some patients with vision loss, having more than three medications can create inadvertent devastating medication errors. Medisets or pill containers that can be set up for the week also greatly reduce the possibility of inadvertent medication mismanagement.

Hearing

The practitioner who is providing directions for pharmaceutical interventions must assess the patient's hearing accurately. Inability to distinguish high-pitched sounds and muffling of the spoken word are two common occurrences of the aging process. Also, the cerumen may become hardened near the tympanic membrane and form a plug that becomes almost impossible to hear through. Removal of this plug is simple and creates a remarkable hearing improvement.

Geriatric patients may have lost their hearing gradually and not be aware that they are not fully hearing what is spoken. Missing one or two words in the instructions for a prescribed medication could have devastating consequences.

Smell and Taste

The senses of smell and taste are usually lost only through a disease process or in the very old (above age 90). Aging may reduce the perceived intensity of taste sensations, but the changes are usually small. This problem therefore very rarely causes any kind of medication mismanagement, but it may create a situation of poorer nutrition secondary to the lack of stimulus in eating. Lack of dietary iron or the B vitamins can lead to atrophic changes of the oral mucosa, resulting in dry mouth and a change in taste.

Some older adults may complain of a burning mouth and tongue. Local trauma, poor nutrition, diabetes, or anemia can cause these symptoms. Thorough investigation and treatment of the cause, if possible, are the easy parts of managing this irritating problem. Reassurance and empathy are the tools of management if no medical cause can be found.

Musculoskeletal Changes

Musculoskeletal changes associated with aging range from impaired manual dexterity, which can prevent a patient from opening medication containers, to mobility problems, which can keep a patient from getting to the drugstore. These musculoskeletal changes can cause geriatric patients to experience difficulty with medication administration and compliance.

Mobility problems, including disorders affecting gait, limb function, manual dexterity, and driving, can threaten the independence and functioning of older adults, specifically their adherence to pharmaceutical interventions. Nonadherence to drug therapy occurs in 40 to 45 percent of older adults (Thwaites, 1999), and impaired mobility plays an important role in their inability to comply with pharmaceutical interventions.

Neurological diseases, such as cerebrovascular disease, Parkinson's disease, and motor neuron disease, can lead to increased difficulties in the practical application of drug treatments. Such problems may range from the inability to visit the health care provider's office to the inability to open the childproof containers that contain the medications designed to help the patient.

Immobility from joint deformity, pain, and impaired manual dexterity may make activating inhalers or nebulizers or applying eyedrops impossible to perform. Some medications may dramatically improve patients' mobility (e.g., medications to treat Parkinson's disease), but others may dramatically exacerbate mobility problems (e.g., **antihypertensives, tricyclic antidepressants**).

Clinical Pearl

Have the older adult repeat back the directions you have given them orally. Write the directions out clearly, concisely, and in lay language. Find an interpreter if indicated.

So how does a nurse practitioner manage the multi-faceted problems associated with impaired mobility in the older adult? Following are some practical guidelines that can be applied in most settings:

1. While writing a prescription, assess potential problems that may create unintentional medication noncompliance. Can the patient open and remove the tablets from the childproof bottle or the prepackaged blister packs? Can the patient being asked to take half a tablet see the tablet well enough and have the manual dexterity to break or cut the tablet in half?

2. If an inhaler has been prescribed, does the older adult have the manual dexterity and strength to activate the inhaler? If a metered-dose inhaler (MDI) is more applicable to the situation, can the older adult actually utilize this device, which is difficult for about 40 percent of patients (Thwaites, 1999)? Breath-activated inhalers (BAIs) have been developed to assist the patient with manual dexterity problems. The effectiveness and compliance in appropriate use of BAIs over MDIs have been demonstrated in studies justifying the use of BAIs by such patients (Connolly, 1995; Gray et al., 1996).

3. Home pharmacy assessments of frail, older adults have revealed multiple drug administration problems, including incorrect dosages, incorrect frequency, expired medication use, and medication omission (Hsia Der, Rubenstein, & Choy, 1997). This particular study suggests that home visits could lead to improved pharmaceutical interventions and compliance. Nurse practitioners are perfect for this type of assessment. With the recent changes in Medicare reimbursement, the nurse practitioner can be reimbursed for such a home visit.

4. Another study showed that, of patients who were asked whether they could manage application of medications, 72 percent stated that this was the first time they had been asked and 69 percent said they would not tell their doctor about the problem even if asked (Thwaites, 1999). This area is obviously a concern for the practitioner and the patient. Ask patients not only how they are feeling but also if they have the mobility and manual dexterity to manage their medications.

5. Utilize the local pharmacist, who certainly has a wealth of information that can help the practitioner and the patient create a manageable, easy-to-follow pharmaceutical regimen.

Common Problems and Concerns of Geriatric Patients

Nutrition

The economic position of the majority of geriatric patients has improved greatly over the last 15 years. However, the reality is that many of these patients are still poor, with 22.4 percent of older adults living in poverty or near poverty (Lawton, 1995). Although many geriatric patients are eligible for social welfare programs, many do not receive them. Explanations for this phenomenon include: (1) older adults are unable to initiate and follow through the bureaucratic requirements to establish their eligibility, (2) older adults are unaware of the various benefits they are entitled to, and (3) many older adults have an ethical rejection of accepting "charity."

So what does this have to do with nutrition and pharmaceutical interventions? Malnutrition by itself is a major common health problem for older adults. Medication compliance is a strong component of malnutrition in that the older adult may forgo buying food in order to pay for medication. The older adult tends to have a gradual weight loss and a reduction in energy requirements as activity declines and body composition changes. It would be very easy to neglect gradually developing malnutrition and instead attribute the weight loss to a secondary effect of the aging process. Malnutrition can be the cause of many other disease problems and may have a role in the decline of the body's immune system. Alterations in the older person's ability to chew, taste, or smell decrease interest in food. Poor health and limited functional ability lower the nutritional well-being of the older adult (Miller, 1995).

In the control of diabetes, nutrition plays a major role in the start or adjustment of pharmaceutical interventions. Control of blood glucose is the most important factor in preventing or delaying the chronic complications of diabetes (Reynolds, 1998; Sinsel-Phillips, 1996).

Clinical Pearl

Remember that drugs present a double-edged sword of either a positive or negative effect on mobility. If the patient has an increase in difficulty with dexterity or an increase in falls, closely scrutinize the medication regimen.

Polypharmacy may contribute to decreased appetite or to gastric discomfort and thus contribute to a changed nutritional intake.

The majority of older adults have limited income and do not eat the recommended amounts of nutritional intake daily. Utilize the DETERMINE chart developed by the Nutrition Screening Initiative Agency for Health Care Policy and Research, (1992):

D: disease
E: eating poorly
T: toothless or mouth pain
E: economic hardship
R: reduced social contact
M: multiple medications
I: involuntary weight loss or gain
N: needs assistance in self-care
E: elder years above age 80

By assessing each of these components, the nurse practitioner is better able to assess the geriatric patient's nutritional status and determine if nutrition is playing a part in poor health. Consultation with a nutritionist or dietitian is also usually indicated.

Sleep Problems

Sleep problems are common complaints of about half of older adults (Dexter, 1999). Sleep-wake disturbances may be a result of physiological changes that appear to be part of the normal aging process, a primary sleep disorder, or a secondary sleep disorder resulting from numerous causes. Patients may complain, "I sleep all night, but I wake up so tired," indicating that they are not obtaining high-quality sleep.

Studies reveal that older adults have decreased rapid eye movement (REM) sleep and increased nighttime wakefulness as part of normal aging. As a result, the older adult often naps during the daytime. When sleep disorder becomes a problem for the patient, such as missing meals or appointments or contributing to limited energy, the practitioner must figure out the problem and treat accordingly. Table 48–5 lists common age-related factors that influence sleep problems.

Sleep problems affect more than half of older adults residing at home and about two-thirds of those residing in long-term care facilities (Beck-Little & Weinrich, 1998). Clearly, sleep affects the mental and physical health of all adults, but older adults have particular difficulties with two classifications of sleep problems: (1) age-related sleep disturbances and (2) sleep disorders.

Age-Related Sleep Disturbances

Age-related sleep disturbances are reported as spending more time in bed but having less sleep time, having difficulty in falling asleep, waking frequently at night, and ex-

Table 48–5. Age-Related Factors Influencing Sleep Problems

Biological Factors
- Increased micturition
- Apnea
- Restless legs
- Muscle cramps
- Arthritic pain
- Vascular changes
- Depression
- Dementia

Social/Psychological Factors
- Death of loved loves
- Loneliness
- Financial hardships
- Institutionalization

periencing early morning awakenings (Asplund, 1999; Beck-Little & Weinrich, 1998; Dexter, 1999). These sleep problems can usually be managed with environmental changes, sleep hygiene, or occasionally medications.

Sleep Disorders

Sleep disorders are considered to be more severe than age-related sleep disturbances because of their relation to increased morbidity and mortality (Asplund, 1999; Beck-Little & Weinrich, 1998). According to the 1990 International Classification Sleep Disorders Diagnostic and Coding Manual (ICSD), sleep disorders are classified into three major categories: (1) dyssomnias, (2) parasomnias, and (3) medical-psychiatric disorders. The more prevalent disorders in the older adult are dyssomnias (produce insomnia or excessive sleepiness) and medical-psychiatric disorders (medical, psychiatric, and neurological disorders).

DYSSOMNIAS. Dyssomnias that affect older adults include obstructive sleep apnea, periodic limb movement, and restless legs syndrome. Pharmaceutical interventions are at times used alone or in conjunction with environmental or surgical interventions. Surgery, weight loss, and use of continuous positive airway pressure may assist the patient with obstructive sleep apnea. The patient who has periodic limb movement disease, resulting in frequent waking, nocturnal restlessness, and daytime fatigue, may benefit from **clonazepam, trazodone,** or **benzodiazepines.** The parkinsonian symptoms of muscle ache, stiffness, and pain respond better to controlled-release **levodopa.** Patients with restless legs syndrome may respond to standard **levodopa** or to high doses of vitamin E. Recent literature has reviewed using **gabapentin** (**Neurontin**) in small doses for managing restless legs syndrome.

MEDICAL-PSYCHIATRIC DISORDERS. Medical disorders that contribute to sleep problems in the older adult include cardiovascular disease, diabetes, gastrointestinal reflux, and arthritis. Psychiatric disorders that affect sleep include anxiety disorder, depression, and cognitive deficits. Cardiovascular problems may cause nocturnal awakenings because of the increased heart rate that occurs during REM sleep (Asplund, 1999). Sustained-release **cardiac vasodilator agents** may resolve this problem. **Diuretics** and fluids should be avoided in late afternoon to prevent nocturnal enuresis. Hypoglycemia related to diabetes that occurs at night could be relieved by a bedtime snack. Evaluation of **insulin** doses or **oral hypoglycemics** may resolve this particular problem. Gastrointestinal reflux, which may result in prolonged sleep latency or awakenings, may be relieved by restricting intake after dinner, administering **antacids,** and elevating the head of the bed. The pain and muscle stiffness of arthritis often results in early morning awakenings. Prescribing a sustained-release **analgesic** to be taken at bedtime may help. Providing supportive care and **antianxiety medications** such as **anxiolytics** may assist the patient with an anxiety disorder. Depression may result in early morning awakenings with a decreased energy level. Providing counseling, encouraging socialization, and prescribing low-dose **tricyclic antidepressants** may help the patient overcome this sleep problem. Agitation at bedtime or nocturnal wandering, resulting in reduced sleep, may be a result of cognitive deficits. Providing a structured environment and prescribing **antipsychotic medications** may be indicated.

Melatonin has been used with limited success to treat sleep disorders. It appears to have a greater effect in "resetting" the circadian rhythm than in treating insomnia. Resetting the circadian rhythm enables the patient to sleep at "normal" times of the night. This treatment is certainly more relevant for patients with age-related sleep problems than for those with sleep disorders.

Management of sleep disorders is second to incontinence in the diagnosis of admissions to long-term care facilities for the older adult. With improved sleep, the older adult has the potential for greater alertness and more social interaction. Recognition and proper treatment of sleep disorders improve quality of life.

Urinary Incontinence

Urinary incontinence affects approximately 12 to 13 million people in the United States, with an annual treatment cost about $16 billion (Agency for Health Care Policy and Research, 1996). It is estimated that 50 to 74 percent of women in long-term care facilities and 20 percent of women age 40 to 60 have some degree of incontinence (Maloney, 1998). About 1.5 to 2.5 percent of men age 15 to 64 are affected by incontinence, with this percentage growing to 15 to 25 percent after age 60 (Maloney, 1998).

Urinary incontinence is not a disease in itself but a symptom of an underlying disorder. Urinary incontinence is important to mention because of its social and fiscal impact. Many patients are embarrassed to mention their incontinence or simply accept it as a part of the "normal" aging process. The person with urinary incontinence may stop attending social events because of the fear of "being wet." This fear of incontinence may also interfere with normal sexual relations, putting strain on both partners. The cost of incontinence products can create a financial burden. The nurse practitioner can identify this problem and help their patients find a solution.

There are several types of chronic urinary incontinence, each with a different etiology: stress incontinence, urge incontinence, overflow incontinence, and functional urinary incontinence. Stress and urge urinary incontinence usually occur because of a weakened pelvic floor, whereas overflow and functional urinary incontinence stem from a neurological impairment.

Medications play a dominant role in the causes and cures of urinary incontinence. Nonneurological causes of urinary incontinence are predominantly related to medications that directly affect smooth muscle (Gallo, Fallon, & Staskin, 1997). Commonly prescribed medications for psychiatric, cardiac, and gastrointestinal disorders, as well as those prescribed for the treatment of colds and pain, have an anticholinergic effect that directly affects the smooth muscle of the bladder by relaxing the sphincter. This information again makes it important for the practitioner to obtain an accurate and complete list of the medications that the patient is taking. Medications also play an important part in "curing" stress and urge urinary incontinence by strengthening tissue.

Stress incontinence can usually be diagnosed through a basic health examination, including a history of duration and the situations of occurrence, a urinalysis, and a pelvic, rectal, and neurological examination (Gallo, Fallon, & Staskin, 1997; Maloney, 1998; Peters, 1997). Treatments for stress incontinence include behavioral interventions, medications, and surgical repair.

Medications prescribed for stress urinary incontinence include the **alpha-adrenergic agonists (pseudoephedrine, phenylpropanolamine),** which increase the bladder outlet resistance. However, in the older adult these medications may be poorly tolerated. The **alpha-adrenergic agonists** also may increase blood pressure, create a dry mouth, and induce tachycardia, headache, or palpitations (Maloney, 1998). Use this type of drug with caution in the older adult.

The older female patient with stress incontinence may benefit from the addition of **estrogen,** which may relieve many of the symptoms. However, some women are unwilling to tolerate symptoms of vaginal bleeding and breast tenderness secondary to the **hormone replacement.** Use of the lowest amount of **estrogen** appears to improve the urethral closure without causing the adverse reactions seen in many women. More recently, use of **estrogen** creams vaginally appears to be effective in treating this type of incontinence (Maloney, 1998). Recommended effective dosage is application every night for 2 weeks, then 2 nights a week. **Vaginal estrogens** spare the patient the adverse reactions of the oral products. Inform the patient that it may take about 4 to 6 weeks before the beneficial effect is apparent.

Urge incontinence may have a functional or medication-related cause. **Diuretics** may cause urgency and frequency, which may create such emotional stress that patients may either not leave their room or not take the medication. If a patient has urge incontinence and must take diuretics, work with the patient about timing the medication so it does not interfere with his or her social life.

Functional urge incontinence can be caused by problems of the nervous system, bladder infection, thinning of the urethral tissue, fecal impaction, or enlarged prostate (Peters, 1997). Pharmacological interventions are **vaginal estrogen** as mentioned previously, **anticholinergics (oxybutynin, propantheline),** or **tricyclic antidepressants (imipramine).** The **anticholinergics** and **antidepressants** both have their particular adverse reactions, but the emotional relief of controlling the urine problem may outweigh them.

The Agency for Health Care Policy and Research has established basic criteria for a primary care provider for referral to a specialist for the incontinent patient. This guideline is helpful in following treatment plans and well worth the practitioner's time to have the resource available.

Many practitioners use behavioral interventions first in treating urge and stress incontinence with relatively frequent success. Pharmacological interventions may become necessary, but keep in mind the possible adverse reactions.

Constipation

Of the possible gastroenteritis problems, constipation is the most frequently encountered in the older adult population. There are several pathogenic reasons. Ignoring the urge to defecate; inadequate ingestion of food, fluid, and fiber; diuretic therapy; sedentary lifestyle; and the early, lifelong attitude that one must defecate every day (chronic laxative use) are common behaviors that are hard to treat. The various medication interactions, metabolic disorders, neurological diseases, and colonic disorders are more readily recognizable.

The complaint of constipation accounts for about 2.5 million health care visits every year (Uphold & Graham, 1994). Despite this high number of health care visits, rarely does a significant abnormality exist. The abuse of OTC laxatives may contribute to the problem. Careful history taking and continued education are the keys to helping the older adult stop fearing constipation.

Constipation is a real problem with real consequences. Some patients have been told that no one has ever died from constipation. This attitude discredits patients' complaints and may cause them to use alternative therapies that are less than desirable. Some older adults have been taught that they should be "cleansed" at least weekly or daily, which means an enema. Others believe that they must have a daily bowel movement. To the younger population, many of these ideas are not consistent with their beliefs, and bias may create a barrier to open communication.

So how does a practitioner treat constipation in the older adult? Use patience and understanding at each encounter. Consider the patient's living situation. Is the recommendation of increased dietary fiber a reality? Does the patient have the ability to add this to the diet, or does he or she eat only once a day, when a Meal on Wheels is delivered? The practitioner must suggest acceptable ways to add the fiber, such as buying whole wheat and bran breads and cereals.

Encourage the intake of up to 3000 cc of "free" water every day, if there is no contradictory disease process (e.g., congestive heart failure). Have the older adult fill a 2-quart (2000 cc) container with water in the morning and drink it throughout the day until it is gone. The other 1000 cc can be obtained by various other sources (e.g., juice, herbal teas). For better compliance, encourage the patient to drink the water before 6 P.M., so the patient is not getting up more frequently at night to urinate.

Encourage exercise. If the older adult has the mobility, encourage abdominal and pelvic exercises in the morning. Walking is a terrific overall exercise but can be problematic if the older adult has physical limitations. Many who cannot tolerate the joint impact of walking can ride a stationary bike. Swimming is another overall exercise that can maintain the level of muscle activity needed without causing undue stress on joints. Exercise is good for the overall conditioning of the older adult's psychosocial well-being, but many will not see the necessity. Exercise must be tailored to the individual and may not be an option in reducing the constipation complaint.

Laxatives may be the only choice available to the practitioner if the constipation is not relieved through the preceding methods. The practitioner has the choice of **stool softeners, stimulant** or **saline laxatives,** and **bulk laxatives. Stool softeners** are used when the complaint is consistent with hard, dry stools. **Mineral oil** is a poorly tolerated **laxative** because of its interference with the absorption of the fat-soluble vitamins, calcium, phosphate, and other nutrients. Aspiration of **mineral oil** can cause lipid pneumonia and pulmonary fibrosis.

Bulk-forming laxatives include bran, methylcellulose, and psyllium. They act like **laxatives** because of their ability to hold water, which in turn softens the stool and promotes peristalsis. Do not recommend **bulk laxatives**

to patients with bowel strictures, diabetics, and those on **salicylate** and **digoxin** therapy.

For appropriate patients, a very simple recipe can create a satisfied patient. Two cups all-bran cereal, 2 cups applesauce, and 1 cup prune juice, mixed together and refrigerated, make an easy, inexpensive **laxative** (Brown & Everett, 1990). Alternative recipes include ground figs, raisins, and a different fruit juice. The prescribed amount for ingestion is variable, from 1 to 5 tablespoons per day. This mixture can be simply eaten, spread on toast or crackers, and is extremely palatable.

Stimulant laxatives should be used only short term and only under specific conditions. They can be habit forming, in that the colon becomes dependent on the outside stimulation for peristalsis. There are appropriate times for this type of **laxative,** but proceed with caution in prescribing them. The **stimulant laxative** is normally utilized as the last choice when other **laxatives** have failed.

Complaints of constipation can drive both practitioner and patient crazy. Patience, education, and encouraging small lifestyle changes can maintain the equanimity of both.

REFERENCES

Agency for Health Care Policy and Research. (1992). *Nutrition screening initiative.* Rockville, MD: U.S. Department of Health and Human Services.

Agency for Health Care Policy and Research. (1996). Management of urinary incontinence (AHCPR publication No 96–0682). Rockville, MD: U.S. Department of Health and Human Services.

Asplund, R. (1999). Sleep disorders in the elderly. *Drugs and Aging, 11(2), 91 104.*

Atkin, P. A., Veitch, P. C., Veitch, E. M., & Ogle, S. J. (1999). The epidemiology of serious adverse drug reactions among the elderly. *Drugs and Aging, 14(2), 141–152.*

Beck-Little, R., & Weinrich, S. P. (1998). Assessment and management of sleep disorders in the elderly. *Journal of Gerontological Nursing, 24(4), 21–29.*

Brown, M. K., & Everett, I. (1990). Gentler bowel fitness with fiber. *Geriatric Nursing, 2, 26–27.*

Conn, V., Taylor, S., & Miller, R. (1994). Cognitive impairment and medication adherence. *Journal of Gerontological Nursing, 7, 41–47.*

Connolly, M. J. (1995). Inhaler technique of elderly patients: Comparison of metered-dose inhalers and large volume spacer devices. *Age and Ageing, 17, 190–192.*

Crigger, N., & Forbes, W. (1997). Assessing neurologic function in older patients. *American Journal of Nursing, 3(97), 37–40.*

Dexter, D. (1999). Sleep disorders in the elderly. *Annals of long-term care, 7, 33–36.*

Gallo, M., Fallon, P. J., & Staskin, D. R. (1997). Urinary incontinence: Steps to evaluation, diagnosis and treatment. *Nurse Practitioner, 22(2), 21–44.*

Graitzer, H. M. (1998). *Therapeutic considerations in the elderly.* Lecture presented at meeting for the Oregon Pharmacists Association, Portland.

Gray, S. L., Williams, D. M., & Pulliam, C. C., (1996). Characteristics predicting incorrect metered-dose inhaler technique in older subjects. *Archives of Internal Medicine, 156, 984–988.*

Hsia Der, E., Rubenstein, L., & Choy, G. (1997). The benefits of in-home pharmacy evaluation for older persons. *Journal of the American Geriatric Society, 45, 211–214.*

Lawton, M. P. (Ed.). (1995). *Annual review of gerontology and geriatrics: Focus on nutrition.* New York: Springer.

Levy, M. L. (1998). Cholinergic therapy for Alzheimer's disease. *Annals of Long-Term Care, 6(3), 92–96.*

Mahoney, D. (1994). The appropriateness of geriatric prescribing decisions made by nurse practitioners and physicians. *Image: Journal of Nursing Scholarship, 26(1), 41–46.*

Mahoney, D., Zhan, L., & Eckler, M. (1999). Preventing drug-drug interactions among older adults: Guidelines and clinical application. *The American Journal for Nurse Practitioners, 3(1), 7–20.*

Maloney, C. (1998). Urinary incontinence: A guide to the diagnosis of chronic and reversible causes in a primary care setting. *American Journal for Nurse Practitioners, 2(3), 8–13.*

Meiner, S. (1997). Polypharmacy in the elderly: Early intervention can prevent complications. *Advance for Nurse Practitioners, 5(7), 29–35.*

Miller, C. A. (1995). *Nursing care of the older adult: Theory and practice* (2nd ed.). Philadelphia: Lippincott.

Peters, S. (1997). Don't ask, don't tell: Breaking the silence surrounding female urinary incontinence. *Advance for Nurse Practitioners, 5(5), 41–45.*

Reynolds, H. R. (1998). Recipe for success: Medical nutrition therapy in diabetes care. *Advance for Nurse Practitioners, 6(7), 46–49.*

Ross, C. (1997). A comparison of osteoarthritis and rheumatoid arthritis: Diagnosis and treatment. *Nurse Practitioner, 22(9), 20–41.*

Sinsel-Phillips, P. (1996). Syndrome X: Primary care provider's role in health promotion and disease prevention. *Nurse Practitioner 21(6), 66–70.*

Thwaites, J. H. (1999). Practical aspects of drug treatment in elderly patients with mobility problems. *Drugs and Aging, 2, 105–114.*

Uphold, C. R., & Graham, M. V. (1994). *Clinical guidelines in adult health.* Gainesville, FL: Barmarrae.

Von Welsheim, L. (1998). *Functional assessment of older patients.* Lecture presented at Nurse Practitioner Organization conference, Eugene, OR.

CHAPTER 49

······

Chronically Ill and Long-Term Care

CHAPTER OUTLINE

aring for patients with chronic diseases can challenge the most experienced health care provider. Chronic diseases create emotional, physical, social, and economic challenges for the patient, the health care provider, and the health care system. For example, the annual cost of caring for patients with osteoporosis, only one of the multiple chronic disease processes in the United States, is estimated at $10 billion. The psychosocial and medical costs to the patient and health care provider for all chronic diseases are unfathomable. This chapter discusses pharmocotherapeutic interventions to reduce some of these challenges to the patient and health care provider.

Assessing the Pharmacological Problems and Concerns of the Chronically Ill Patient

Assessing a patient's pharmacological responses to prescribed medications has multiple layers. Each disease process has its own guidelines in treatment, but a repetitive theme runs throughout most thoroughly researched articles. Does the patient have the ability to comply with the prescribed therapy, and how does the provider assess the compliance?

Take, for example, chronic lung diseases (e.g., asthma, chronic obstructive pulmonary disease), which are usually lifelong. The goal in treating asthma in children is to establish quick control and maintain it with the least medication and minimal risk of adverse effects (Autio & Rosenow, 1999). The major goal in treating chronic obstructive pulmonary lung disease in the older adult is to alleviate symptoms and improve exercise tolerance with the fewest medications and adverse reactions (Witta, 1997). Obviously, the theme of treatment is the same whether the patient is 5 years old or 70. How can the provider assess that therapy is being followed?

First, never assume that because the patient has been provided with information about the treatment regimen that the outlined treatment or regimen will be followed correctly. Is the pharmaceutical intervention not relieving the symptoms because it is not the right medication or because adherence to the pharmaceutical intervention was impossible for the patient to follow?

A child or adult with a chronic condition can cause major life changes within the family. Coping patterns can alter the family unit's original goals (Bowden, Dickey, & Greenberg, 1998). If the family unit was unstable prior to the chronic disease process, the added stress may alter the family unit, creating several possible scenarios.

It is not uncommon for the person or family with the chronic disease processes to deny the disease process. Denial is a very strong protective emotion. By utilizing this concept, the patient and family can, in their minds, change the pharmaceutical interventions to suit their particular needs at the time.

Correct assessment utilizes all the biopsychosocial training that the health care provider has learned through education, formal and informal: review of medications and how they are utilized; review of any unprescribed medications, over-the-counter or herbal; and review of the system in place in the home to remember how and when to take medications. The provider's open, accepting, nonjudgmental approach can create an atmosphere in which the patient or family is more willing to share any changes they have made at home in the medication regimen.

Lack of adherence to the regimen on the part of the child or adult with a chronic disease can stem from any number of causes: medication administration, misuse, financial inability to afford the medication, or any number of other problems. Table 49–1 presents questions to assess nonadherence to a medication regimen. The next section presents tips to overcome the myriad of problems faced by the patient, family, and provider.

Methods to Overcome Nonadherence in Patients with Chronic Diseases

Patient education is the mainstay of an effective pharmacological treatment program. Education improves patient adherence to medication regimens, improves self-management skills, and reduces hospital stays (Voelker, 1997). So how does a health care provider in a managed care clinic setting provide this kind of treatment?

From the patient's point of view, there is concern expressed whether primary health care providers will be willing and able to provide long-term chronic care. These concerns are justified, considering that few primary care protocols have been adjusted for the needs of the chronic illness. Too often basic education programs do not allocate significant content or clinical practice to prepare providers to work with the patient who has chronic medical needs.

This is a huge concern for health care. Evidence suggests that patients take only a small percentage of prescribed medications (Haynes, McKibbon, & Kanani, 1996; Williams et al., 1998). One study showed that fewer than half of the patients who are on a 2-week course of medication take less than the amount necessary for effective pharmaceutical results (Dwyer, Levy, & Menander, 1986). Unfortunately, very little research has been done to determine accurate interventions for greater compliance with the chronic medication regimens.

Two different approaches that can be combined have shown greater success. One approach is utilizing multidisciplinary teams. The second approach, by the primary care provider, utilizes the self-determination theory.

Utilizing Multidisciplinary Teams

Multidisciplinary intervention is a continual process that provides the primary health care provider with much-needed information regarding the ability of the patient with chronic disease processes to adhere to pharmacological interventions.

Social workers, nurses, specialists, and psychologists, to name a few, can all be part of the multidisciplinary team. The primary care provider must be identified clearly, both to the rest of the team and to the patient and family. The primary care provider then acts as the team leader in coordinating the health care and interventions. This process saves repeated use or misuse of the team and creates the atmosphere for the patient that just one health care provider is in control of the patient's disease process.

Utilizing the Self-Determination Theory

Utilizing the self-determination theory (or goal-oriented theory) works well in increasing the potential of correct pharmaceutical interventions. By using the self-determination theory, the patient and family experience a sense of volition, choice, and action because the intervention is of personal importance (Williams et al., 1998). The feeling of pressure to comply with a regimen, either external or intrapsychic, is removed. This then improves the pharmaceutical interventions that the health care provider encourages.

Table 49–1. Assessment of Nonadherence to a Medication Regimen

- Does the medicine taste bad or leave a bad taste in the mouth?
- How often is the medication supposed to be taken? The more often within a day that the medication should be taken, the more likely it is that the medication will not be taken.
- What is the total number of medications being taken? The more medications that are taken, the greater the chance that the wrong drug will be taken or a dose will be missed.
- Does the patient have to be wakened at night to take the medication? This creates a very difficult problem, which increases the chance of missed doses.

Clinical Pearl

Self-motivation and multidisciplinary support improve the likelihood of correct pharmaceutical interventions.

Administration Problems

Several chronic pulmonary diseases require inhaled medications for treatment. However, several studies have revealed that only about half the patients are able to correctly use the inhalers (Autio & Rosenow, 1999; Gaine & Terry, 1997). The adverse reactions of tremors and nervousness lead to decreased compliance. Correct use of the inhaler is a second problem that leads to unintentional noncompliance. Having the patient or caregiver demonstrate use of equipment to deliver medications, with a return demonstration later, helps to decrease the chances of inadvertent noncompliance. Education and reassurance are other components of successful pharmacological interventions.

Depression as a secondary problem in chronic illness is estimated to occur in more than 49 percent of patients (Barlow-Pieterick & Coehlo, 1999). Some estimates indicate that between 6 and 25 percent of the patients have a major depressive order; others suggest that 30 to 50 percent of patients have depressive symptoms. The biopsychosocial components are intermeshed and difficult to separate. True depression is pervasive, persistent, and intense and interferes with functioning, including the patient's ability to adhere to an outlined, chronic medication regimen. Careful evaluation of whether the depression is a reaction to a combination of medications, a psychological reaction to the illness, or a sense of loss of oneself is done by either the primary care provider or in conjunction with other disciplines.

Recognizing the cultural beliefs and values of the patient plays an active role in appropriate diagnosis for the patient. Depression and grieving for loss of health occur in the patient and family coping with chronic illness. Again, the multidisciplinary team can play a role in defining the care needs of the chronically ill person, and this also helps to enable the patient to adhere to the medication program.

Socioeconomic Concerns

Many patients with chronic health care needs are on some kind of government support, secondary to economic hardships (Hoeman, 1997) created by the chronic medical condition. Health care providers in managed care environments are struggling with ways to locate and use the array of services and resources required for persons with chronic, disabling conditions, as well as ways to collaborate with case managers.

Nurse practitioners have had the opportunity through their educational process to learn about the multidisciplinary process; however, in primary practice they may struggle to develop this process fully (Burns et al., 1996; Hoeman, 1997) Time management becomes a stressful element in further developing a cohort of resource people that the practitioner trusts to follow a regimen outlined by the practitioner. Utilization of a multidisciplinary team does, however, work in treating patients and families who are coping with chronic diseases. Contact your local state or county services and build a cohort of contacts who will cooperate with providing appropriate care. One practitioner alone cannot provide all of the care needed in creating a successful environment for the patient and family who are dealing with a chronic disease.

Education for the patient and family remains the key component in medication adherence. Table 49–2 presents

Table 49–2. Improving Compliance to Medication Therapy

Questions to Answer
- What is the purpose of the medication?
- Why and how does the medication affect the body and disease process?
- What are the signs and symptoms of the medication's effects, both good and bad?
- What drug interactions are possible?
- Will any over-the-counter medications create serious interactions?

Components to Include
- Encourage return demonstrations with medicinal delivery adjuncts.
- Monitor the parameters for safe efficacy of the pharmaceutical interventions carefully.
- If pregnancy is suspected or possible (women of childbearing age), perform pregnancy screens for specific medications that will cause adverse interactions in a fetus.

questions to help develop an individualized educational plan for improving compliance to medication therapy. This education can and should be delivered by the whole team. The primary care provider needs to coordinate the team so the same information is delivered in a multitude of fashions. The team is then responsible to keep the primary provider informed of changes or problems. This process can be very time-consuming.

Because the main issue for the patient and family who are coping with chronic illnesses is adherence, the practitioner must be equally compliant in providing the correct care and the best pharmaceutical interventions. Table 49–3 presents guidelines for improving adherence.

Special Considerations When Prescribing for Patients in Long-Term Care Facilities

Long-term care (LTC) facilities are varied in the type of care provided. Traditional nursing homes are only one of the possibilities. The current trend of creating a more homelike institution has provided the ailing elder a multitude of choices. Assisted living, residential care, and adult foster homes are some of the alternatives now available for the older adult who needs supportive or LTC.

These alternative living situations provide the health care provider with different challenges in prescribing medication. Most, but not all, of the residents have medications either administered or supervised by a caregiver. That caregiver may be licensed staff, a medication aide, or an individual with delegated authority. The ability of residents to manage their own medication regimen may be evaluated by the practitioner or the licensed staff. Knowledge of the specific living situation is a must for appropriate evaluation by the practitioner.

Intermediate-care and LTC facilities are highly regulated by the state and federal governments. This provides many safeguards for the patient. The practitioner can assume some givens in these situations. First, medications are given at a designated time, which can be of utmost importance for some medications. Compliance with timed delivery is less of a problem because a patient's

memory or sensory disabilities are not an issue. A complicated polypharmacy regimen is more likely to be correct because staff monitors it. Many facilities utilize a bubblepack system, which lessens the risk of error in medication setup. It also reduces the chance of running out of medications or skipping doses. A route of administration other than oral is less of an issue because of the availability of licensed staff.

Any licensed LTC facility is mandated to have a consulting pharmacy, which reviews a patient's medication regimen at least quarterly. The pharmacist can help identify potential drug interactions; suggest changes; and recommend limitations, laboratory monitoring, or discontinuing the medication. Laboratory monitoring is usually more easily obtained, which makes interventions for abnormal results quicker.

Therapeutic effects of medications are also closely monitored (e.g., **analgesics, laxatives**), and titration of the medications can be done more promptly. There is much better control over the addition of unknown medications or over-the-counter or natural products. Potential drug abuse is less likely because of adherence to prn dosing instructions. As a side note, prescription orders are required for all medications, including over-the-counter medications, topical or oral medications, and **oxygen.** Some practitioners become irritated with LTC nurses' requests, but practitioners need to remember that the LTC facility has specific rules and regulations the nurses must comply with or the facility will lose its license.

A special consideration with LTC is adult foster care homes. The caregivers may have limited pharmacology knowledge and training. Errors of duplication related to generic versus brand names may occur. The wrong medication to the wrong patient is more possible than in the licensed facilities. Topical medications may receive less focus than oral delivery because the topicals are viewed as less important. The primary care provider may have less knowledge of what medications are being delivered. Caregivers may call other providers, which may add or delete medications per request of family or caregiver, resulting in a medication list that may or may not be up to date with the primary provider's current list. Caregivers can put tremendous pressure on the provider to prescribe specific products or to change the current medication dosing because of behavior problem manage-

Table 49–3. Guidelines for the Provider for Improving Adherence

- Utilize the five rights (the right patient, dose, medication, route, and time) when informing the patient of the new medication.
- Compare cost. Is an alternative less expensive, but as therapeutic?
- Review the patient's medication list. Can some of the medication be discontinued? Do you know what over-the-counter medications and herbals are being used?
- Request that the patient fill the prescriptions through one pharmacy. The pharmacist can then help to avoid interactions.
- Utilize a multidisciplinary team.
- Ask the patient and family questions regarding biopsychosocial events.

Clinical Pearl

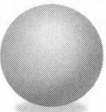

Long-term care facilities utilize multidisciplinary teams. The nurse practitioner can benefit patients with chronic illness by forming a base knowledge of who and what are available.

ment of the patient. Because of closer patient observation, the provider may receive more requests for **antibiotics, hypnotics, antidepressants,** or **antipsychotics.**

A huge opportunity exists for education to the caregiver staff, patient, and family. Use these opportunities to provide the rationale for therapy, desired outcomes, and specific assessments for evaluating the effectiveness of the pharmacotherapeutics. The caregivers and family are eager to provide appropriate care.

Caregivers in LTC facilities, whether they are licensed personnel or laypeople, are the eyes and ears for the provider. Over-the-phone consultation is very common because of the decreased mobility of the patient. This results in indirect assessment by the provider. The provider must be a skilled interviewer of staff to elicit complete and accurate patient assessment data from the caregiver. It is extremely important that the "reporter" has actually looked at the patient and is not reporting secondhand information. Ask specifically whether the patient has had any new medications added or has had a change in dosage since you were last consulted. Ask for specific symptoms that are different, not just a change in behavior. This type of assessment can easily result in mismanagement of medications, and caution is a must.

A philosophical discussion of pharmacotherapeutics may occur more often in an LTC facility. Often the patient is facing the end of life. Does a point exist where selected medications for chronic illnesses should be discontinued? Discussion with the patient, family, significant others, and caregivers early in the institutionalization may avoid crisis intervention at a later date. Determination of resuscitation status is only the beginning of the decision tree. Reviewing and documenting the patient's and family's wishes regarding intravenous therapy, parenteral tube feeding for hydration and nutrition, **antibiotic** use in potentially reversible conditions, and the aggressiveness in implementation of preventive measures the provider should take are important steps to review prior to a crisis. LTC facilities

often have a social worker to help with these difficult decisions. It is the primary care provider's responsibility to qualify the patient's, family's, or significant other's understanding of these types of interventions prior to implementation.

Placement in LTC facilities is often appropriate for a great number of older adults. There are rewards and problems. The provider has to be aware of the situation so as to provide appropriate interventions. Ignorance of the living situation is a source of great detriment and frustration. The nurse practitioner has great potential to appropriately care for the older adult. Satisfaction in knowing the best care and interventions are being carried out is a wonderful personal reward.

REFERENCES

Autio, L., & Rosenow, D. (1999). Effectively managing asthma in young and middle adulthood. *Nurse Practitioner, 24*(1), 100–111.

Barlow-Pieterick, M., & Coehlo, D. P. (1999). Keynote speech at Oregon Geriatric Education Conference, Corvalis.

Bowden, V. R., Dickey, S. B., & Greenberg, C. S. (1998). *Children and their families: A continuum of care.* Philadelphia: Saunders.

Burns, C., Barber, N., Brady, M. A., & Dunn, A. M. (1996). *Pediatric primary care: A handbook for nurse practitioners.* Philadelphia: Saunders.

Dwyer, M. S., Levy, R. A., & Menander K. B. (1986). Improving medication compliance through the use of modern dosage forms. *Journal of Pharmacology Technology, 2*(7), 166–170.

Gaine, S. P., & Terry, P. (1997). Treatment modalities for COPD in the institutionalized elderly. *Nursing Home Medicine, 5*(11), 390–397.

Haynes, R. B., McKibbon, K. A., & Kanani, R. (1996). Systematic review of randomized trials of interventions to assist patients to follow prescriptions for medications. *Lancet, 348,* 383–386.

Hoeman, S. P. (1997). Primary care for children with spina bifida. *Nurse Practitioner, 22*(9), 60–72.

Voelker, R. (1997). Taking asthma seriously. *Journal of American Medical Association, 278*(1), 11.

Williams, G. C., Ryan, R. M., Rodin, G. C., Grolinick, W. S., & Deci, E. L. (1998). Autonomous regulation and long-term medication adherence in adult outpatients. *Health Psychology, 17*(3), 269–276.

Witta, K. M. (1997). COPD in the elderly: Controlling symptoms and improving quality of life. *Advance for Nurse Practitioners, 5*(97), 18–27.

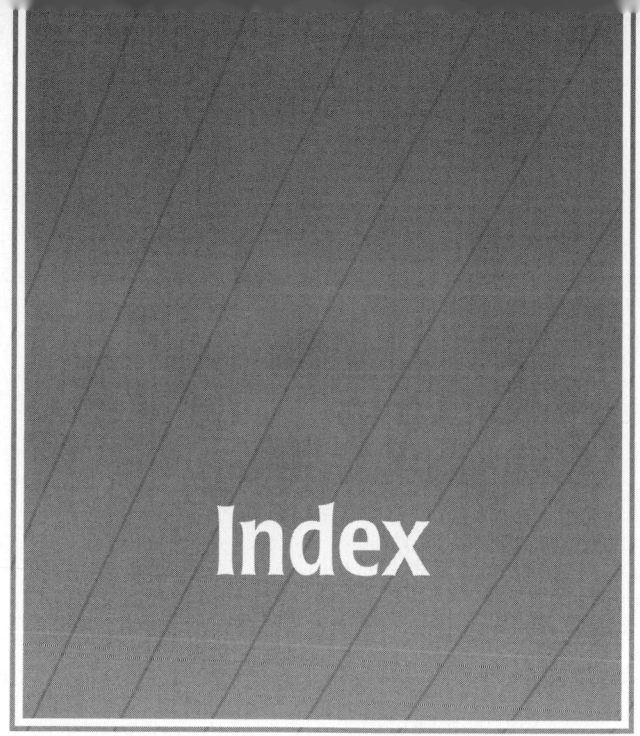

Index

Page numbers followed by "f" indicate figures; page numbers followed by "t" indicate tables.

AAP-0683

For Reference

Not to be taken from this room

AAP-0683